Psychiatric Nursing

Contemporary Practice

EIGHTH EDITION

Mary Ann Boyd, PhD, DNS, RN, PMHCNS-BC
Professor Emerita
Southern Illinois University Edwardsville
Edwardsville, Illinois

Rebecca Luebbert, PhD, RN, PMHCNS-BC
Professor
Associate Dean
Southern Illinois University Edwardsville
Edwardsville, Illinois

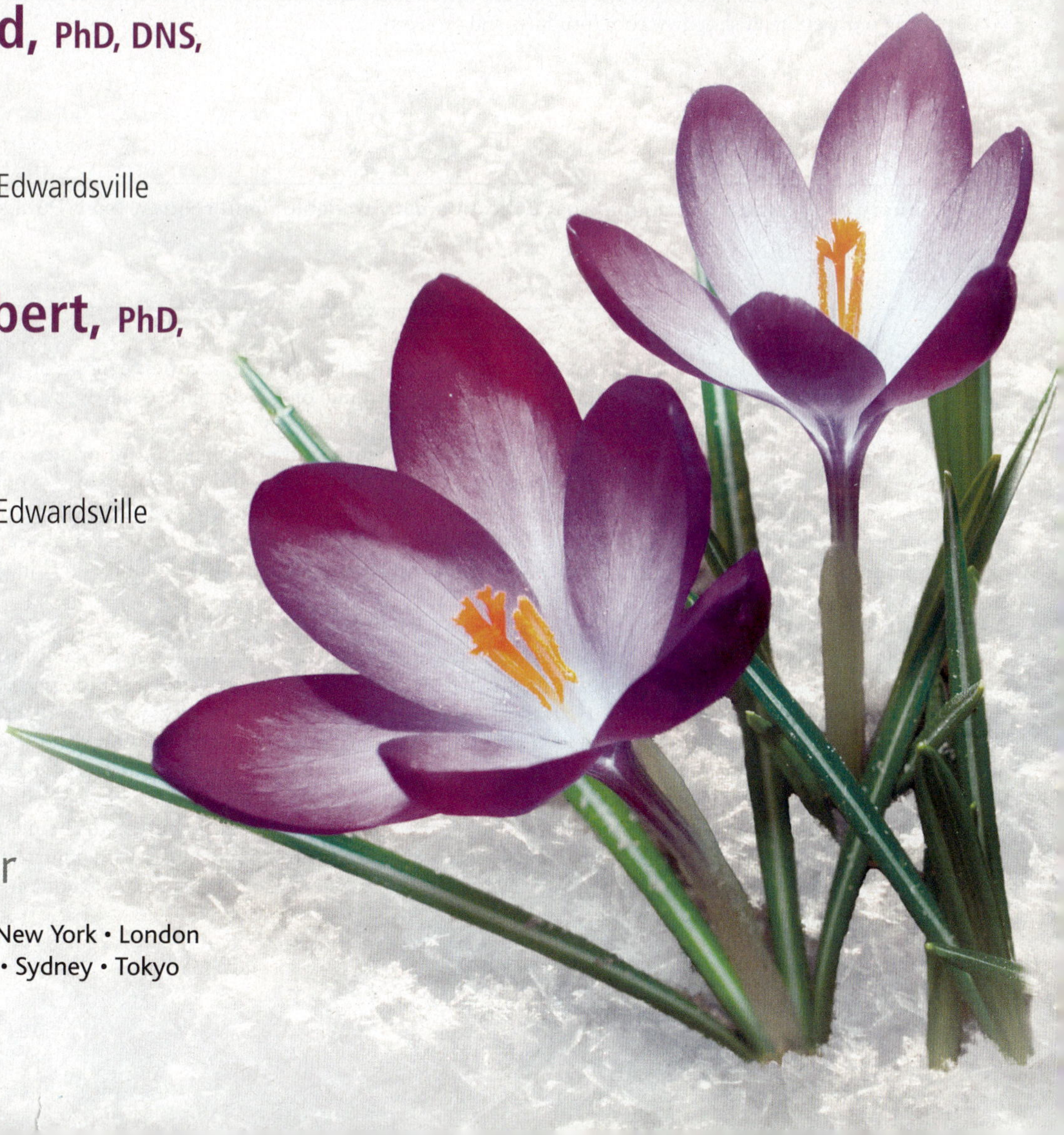

Wolters Kluwer

Philadelphia • Baltimore • New York • London
Buenos Aires • Hong Kong • Sydney • Tokyo

Vice President, Nursing Segment: Julie Stegman
Director, Nursing Education and Practice Content: Jamie Blum
Acquisitions Editor: Jodi Rhomberg
Development Editor: Meredith Brittain/Devika Kishore
Freelance Development Editor: Rose Foltz
Editorial Coordinator: Ann Francis
Editorial Assistant: Sara Thul
Marketing Manager: Wendy Mears
Production Project Manager: Matthew West
Design Coordinator: Stephen Druding
Art Director: Jennifer Clements
Manufacturing Coordinator: Margie Orzech
Prepress Vendor: Aptara, Inc.

Eighth Edition

9 8 7 6 5 4 3 2 1

Printed in Mexico

Library of Congress Cataloging-in-Publication data available upon request from Publisher.

U.S. Edition ISBN-13: 978-1-9752-3904-6
International Edition ISBN: 978-1-9752-3905-3

shop.LWW.com

QUADM0925

In loving memory of my parents Edward and Emma Long, who provided the opportunity to begin my nursing journey.

MAB

To Adam, for your love, support, and encouragement through every step of this journey. And to the countless students who remind me why this work matters—may this text serve you well as you serve others.

RL

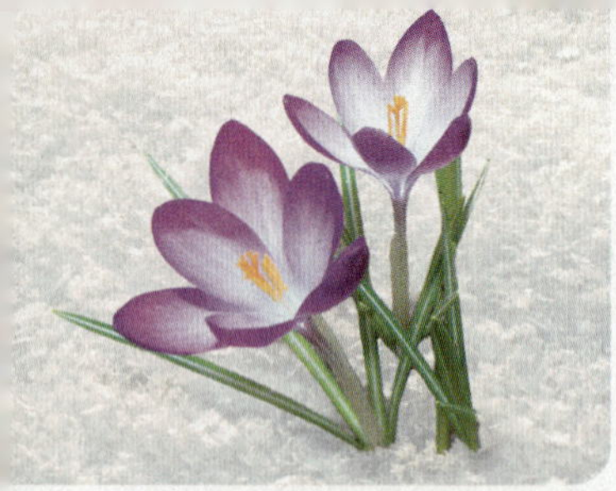

Contributors

Beverly Baliko, PhD, APRN, PMHNP-BC
Associate Professor
College of Nursing
University of South Carolina
Columbia, South Carolina
Chapter 23: Mental Health Care for People Who Have Experienced Violence

Rachel S. Bush, DNP, PMHNP-BC, LPC
Assistant Professor
Department of Nursing
University of South Carolina
Columbia, South Carolina
Chapter 23: Mental Health Care for People Who Have Experienced Violence

Andrea C. Bostrom, PhD, PMHCNS-BC
Professor Emeritus
Kirkhof College of Nursing
Grand Valley State University
Allendale, Michigan
Chapter 24: Schizophrenia and Related Disorders

Mary Ann Boyd, PhD, DNS, RN, PMHCNS-BC
Professor Emerita
Southern Illinois University Edwardsville
Edwardsville, Illinois

Jennifer Caires-Kennel, MSN, RN
Instructor
Southern Illinois University Edwardsville
Edwardsville, Illinois
Chapter 32: Eating Disorders

Sheri Compton-McBride, DNP, RN
Assistant Professor
Department Chair
Director of RN/BS Nursing Program and Contract Management
Southern Illinois University Edwardsville—School of Nursing
Edwardsville, Illinois
Chapter 34: Sleep–Wake Disorders

Dorothy M. Corrigan, DMin, APNP, CNP, GNP-BC, CARN-AP
CEO-The Knock Institute LLC
La Crosse Wisconsin
Chapter 43: Care of People Who Are Medically Compromised

Susan Dawson, EdD, PMHNP-BC
Adult Psychiatric Nurse Practitioner
Compassionate Healthcare
St. Louis, Missouri
Chapter 31: Substance-Related Disorders

Catherine Deering, PhD, ABPP
Professor of Psychology, Clayton State University
Adjunct Professor of Psychiatry & Behavioral Sciences
Emory University School of Medicine
Chapter 16: Mental Health Promotion for Childhood and Adolescence

Cheryl Forchuk, RN, PhD, O Ont, FCAHS, FRSC, FCAN
Distinguished University Professor
Nursing and Psychiatry
Western University
Scientist, Lawson Health Research Institute
St. Joseph's Health Care Centre
London, Ontario, Canada
Chapter 10: Clinical Judgment Nursing Care Planning in Psychiatric–Mental Health

Patricia E. Freed, MSN, EdD
Associate Professor
Trudy Bush Valentine School of Nursing
Saint Louis University
St. Louis, Missouri
Chapter 1: Psychiatric–Mental Health Nursing and Evidence-Based Practice
Chapter 28: Obsessive-Compulsive and Related Disorders
Chapter 31: Substance-Related Disorders
Chapter 33: Somatic Symptoms and Related Disorders

Valerie Griffin, DNP, PPCNP-BC, FNP-BC, PMHS, FAANP
Associate Professor and Director of Nurse Practitioner Specializations
Southern Illinois University Edwardsville
School of Nursing
Edwardsville, Illinois
Chapter 36: Mental Health Assessment of Children and Adolescents
Chapter 37: Mental Disorders of Childhood and Adolescence

Rebecca Luebbert, PhD, RN, PMHCNS-BC
Professor
Associate Dean
Southern Illinois University Edwardsville
Edwardsville, Illinois

Kelley McGuire, PhD, RN, CNE
Assistant Professor, Nursing
University of Wisconsin—Green Bay
Green Bay, Wisconsin
Chapter 19: Stress and Mental Health

Rita Tadych, PhD, MSN, MS, BSN, RN, APRN-BC, & Licensed Psychologist/Health Service Provider
Adjunct Assistant Professor
Trudy Busch Valentine School of Nursing
Saint Louis University
St. Louis, Missouri
Chapter 14: Group Interventions
Chapter 15: Family Assessment and Interventions

Sandra P. Thomas, PhD, RN, FAAN
Editor, "Issues in Mental Health Nursing"
Professor and PhD Program Chair
University of Tennessee, Knoxville
College of Nursing
Knoxville, Tennessee
Chapter 20: Safety and De-Escalation Practices

Barbara Jones Warren, PhD, RN, PMH APRN-CNS, FNAP, FAAN
Emeritus Professor
The Ohio State University
Columbus, Ohio
Adult & Adolescent Psychiatric Clinical Nurse Specialist
NIMH ANA Racial/Ethnic Minority Fellow
Orleans Psychological Services
Powell, Ohio
Chapter 25: Depression

Crystal Jordan, MSN, RN
Southwest Mississippi Community College
Summit, Mississippi
PrepU Writer

Jessica Clairmont, MSN, BSN, RN
Assistant Professor of Nursing, Minnesota State University-Moorhead
Moorhead, Minnesota
PrepU Reviewer

Maryann Foley, BSN, RN
Clinical Consultant
Horsham, Pennsylvania
Test Bank Writer

Linda Turchin, MSN, RN, CNE
Associate Professor Emeritus of Nursing, Fairmont State University
Fairmont, West Virginia
Test Bank Reviewer

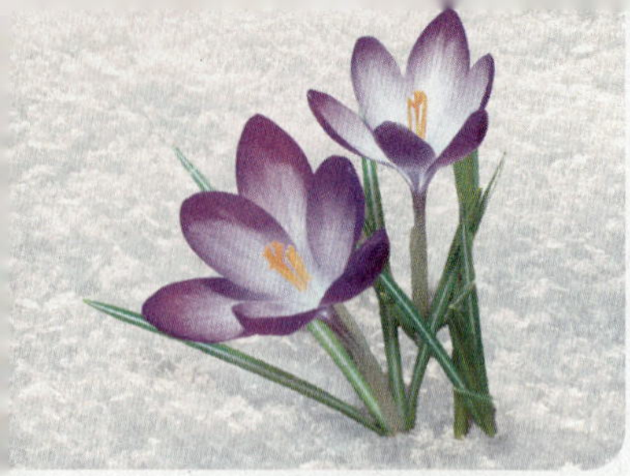

Reviewers

Jessica Bower, DNP, RN
Commonwealth University, Bloomsburg
Bloomsburg, Pennsylvania

Renee L. Fox, MSN, MA, RN, CMSRN, CRC
GateWay Community College
Phoenix, Arizona

Karmie Johnson, DNP, RN, PMHNP-BC, CNE
University of Alabama at Birmingham
Columbus, Indiana

Lisa Johnson, PhD, RN, CPN
Community College of Philadelphia
Philadelphia, Pennsylvania

Moniaree Parker Jones, EdD, MSN, RN, COI
Samford University
Birmingham, Alabama

Kim Link, DNP, APRN, PMHNP-BC
Western Kentucky University
Bowling Green, Kentucky

Elizabeth Lucas, MSN, RN, NP, PMHNP-BC
Macomb Community College
Clinton Township, Michigan

Stacy Mikel, DNP, MSN, RN
Jacksonville State University
Jacksonville, Alabama

Christa Moore, MSN, RN, CNE, COI
Samford University
Birmingham, Alabama

Crystal Schauerte, MScN, BScN
Algonquin College
Ottawa, Ontario

Laura Sooby, MSN, RN
Wichita State University
Wichita, Kansas

Susan Tschirhart, MSN, RN
Macomb Community College
Clinton Township, Michigan

Margaret Touw, DNP, RN, CNE
UTMB School of Nursing
Galveston, Texas

Susan K. Tucker, DNP, RN, CNE
Gadsden State Community College
Gadsden, Alabama

David Vander Ark, DNP, MSN, RN, PMH-BC
Grand Valley State University
Grand Rapids, Michigan

Kennetha Williams, DNP, MS, APRN, PMHNP-BC
University of Louisville
Louisville, Kentucky

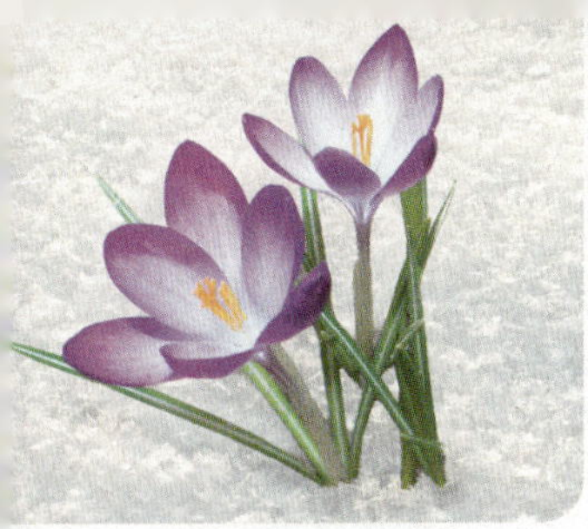

Preface

Psychiatric–mental health nurses are the forefront of health care delivery. At no other time in the history of the United States have the nursing skills of a psychiatric–mental health nurse been more essential. Mental disorders continue to be recognized as a major societal burden, contributing to high rates of morbidity and mortality, as well as lost economic productivity. One in five people will experience a mental disorder in their lifetime.

The landscape of mental health care is constantly evolving, moving from specialized psychiatric settings to primary care. Our understanding of how emotional and mental health influence overall well-being continues to deepen. While only a small number of nurses may choose a mental health practice setting, all nurses will be challenged to care for patients with psychiatric needs in their day-to-day practice. This dynamic evolution requires nursing students to have a strong background in understanding mental disorders, the knowledge of underlying principles, and the skills to implement evidence-based psychiatric–mental health care.

In the eighth edition of *Psychiatric Nursing: Contemporary Practice*, we introduce the Clinical Judgment Measurement Model, which is used throughout the text. This model challenges students to enhance their clinical judgment by identifying assessment cues, establishing priority hypotheses, and taking action. The purpose of this text is to prepare nurses to care for all people with mental health issues across all clinical settings. We address the mental health needs of underrepresented groups and those groups traditionally excluded from mainstream health care delivery. Many people with mental health needs face inequities in access and health care delivery, compounding physical and mental health needs. Factors such as ethnicity, race, and gender contribute to inequities and exclusion in accessing health care. This edition includes evidence-based discussions on these inequities and their impact on care delivery. Gender-neutral, bias-free language is used throughout the text.

A key enhancement in this edition is the increased emphasis on the holistic care of people with mental health disorders. The biopsychosocial organizing framework is expanded to include the Biopsychosocial-Spiritual Model instead of the traditional biopsychosocial approach. We emphasize spiritual assessment to support a more holistic approach to nursing care. Spiritual interventions are threaded throughout the text. In addition, we explore complementary therapies—including nutrition, dietary and herbal supplements, and essential vitamins and minerals—in a dedicated chapter and throughout the text, ensuring a well-rounded and inclusive approach to mental health care.

TEXT ORGANIZATION

The first three units of *Psychiatric Nursing: Contemporary Practice, Eighth Edition* present the conceptual underpinnings and principles of psychiatric–mental health nursing. In Unit I, students are introduced to mental health nursing care in contemporary society as an evidenced-based practice. Students are introduced to stigma and recovery in Chapter 2, which sets the stage for a more detailed discussion of recovery in Chapter 9. Chapter 3 prepares students for later discussions of cultural, spiritual, and gender-based considerations.

Unit II provides the theoretical foundations of psychiatric nursing including several nursing and recovery frameworks as well as biological and psychosocial theoretical underpinnings. Unit III is the essence of psychiatric–mental health nursing with a detailed discussion of psychiatric–mental health clinical judgment planning including explanations of evidence-based and spiritual interventions. Therapeutic communication skills, psychopharmacology, cognitive interventions, group interventions, complementary therapies, and family assessment and interventions are presented in a clear and understandable language. A new chapter, Complementary Therapies and Integrative Health, is introduced in this unit. This unit prepares the student for making clinical judgments and sound decisions in caring for patients.

Units IV and V present mental health promotion and prevention content, including comprehensive chapters on stress and mental health, crises, safety and de-escalation, and suicide prevention. Unit VI discusses the care of people with mental disorders within a recovery-oriented, evidence-based practice. For each disorder, students will find discussions on spirituality, considerations of inequities in mental health care, complementary therapies, SBAR examples for clinical decision-making, trauma-informed approaches, and clinical vignettes.

Units VII and VIII focus on the assessment and care of children and older adults with mental disorders characteristic of each age group. Unit IX includes chapters related to the mental health needs of veterans, care of people experiencing housing instability, and those with co-occurring mental disorders. Chapter 43 addresses the care of people with selected medical disorders that are typically found in people with mental disorders.

The text presents complex concepts in easy-to-understand language with multiple examples and explanations. Students find the text easy to comprehend, filled with meaningful information, and applicable to all areas of nursing practice.

PEDAGOGICAL FEATURES

The eighth edition of *Psychiatric Nursing: Contemporary Practice* incorporates a multitude of pedagogical features to focus and direct student learning, including the following:

By including evidence-based content from which students can draw valid inferences, students can develop clinical judgment and decision-making skills.

- **Expanded Table of Contents** allows readers to find and refer to concepts from one location.
- **Learning Objectives**, **Key Terms**, and **Key Concepts** in the chapter openers cue readers on what will be encountered and what is important to understand in each chapter.
- **Summary of Key Points** listed at the end of each chapter provides quick access to important chapter content to facilitate study and review.
- **Developing Clinical Judgment** includes competency-based statements and asks questions that require students to think critically about chapter content and the important actions to include in their nursing practice.
- **Movie, TV, or Streaming Viewing Guides** list current examples of movies that depict various mental health disorders and that are widely available. Viewing points are provided to serve as a basis for discussion in class and among students.

SPECIAL FEATURES

- **Case Studies** threaded in the disorder chapters are related to the Nursing Care Plan and Therapeutic Dialogue features, giving students the opportunity to apply content. Cases will come from the Patient Experience Videos, to help tie content from the book to the videos. For chapters without a corresponding video, a new case study has been created. Exposure to patients builds student confidence and provides a seamless transition to the practice world.
- **Wellness Challenges** threaded in disorder chapters focus on keeping patients healthy and utilize case study "patient" information to apply the content.
- **Integration with Primary Care,** also threaded in disorder chapters and utilizing case study content, addresses integration of psychiatric disorders with basic health needs blended.
- **NCLEX Notes** help students focus on important application areas to prepare for the NCLEX.
- **Emergency Care Alerts** highlight important situations in psychiatric nursing care that the nurse should recognize as emergencies.
- **Research for Best Practice** boxes highlight today's focus on evidence-based practice for best practice, presenting findings and implications of studies that are applicable to psychiatric nursing practice.
- **Mental Health Inequities** boxes present evidence-based information demonstrating the impact of social determinants, discrimination, and structural barriers that result in vulnerabilities to mental health issues, care, and access to treatment.
- **Trauma-Informed Approach** boxes illustrate the impact of trauma on mental health as well as principles of trauma informed care for nursing students to include in their mental health nursing practice.
- **Reflection of a Nurse** boxes present a scenario that was not effective followed by a reflection of the intervention. Students are provided with reflection questions relevant to the scenario.
- **Building Clinical Judgment with SBAR** boxes consist of an SBAR communication followed by brief questions for the student to provide rationale for the recommendation.
- **Therapeutic Dialogue** boxes compare and contrast therapeutic and nontherapeutic conversations to encourage students by example to develop effective communication skills.
- **Psychoeducation Checklists** identify content areas for patient and family education related to specific disorders and their treatment. These checklists support critical thinking by encouraging students to develop patient-specific teaching plans based on chapter content.
- **Clinical Judgment Vignette** boxes are twofold and present reality-based clinical portraits of patients who exhibit the symptoms described in the text, followed by short-answer clinical judgment questions for the student to identify relevant cues, analyze cues, prioritize hypotheses, and generate solutions.
- **Medication Profile** boxes present a thorough picture of commonly prescribed medications for patients with mental health problems. The profiles complement the text discussions of biologic processes known to be associated with various mental health disorders.
- **Key Diagnostic Characteristics** summaries describe diagnostic criteria, target symptoms, and target associated

findings for select disorders, adapted from the *DSM-5* by the American Psychiatric Associations.

- **Concept Mastery Alerts** clarify common misconceptions as identified by Lippincott's Adaptive Learning Powered by PrepU.
- **Evidence-Based Nursing Practice of People with Selected Mental Health Disorders** sections provide an in-depth study of the more commonly occurring major psychiatric disorders.

TEACHING/LEARNING PACKAGE

To facilitate mastery of this text's content, a comprehensive teaching and learning package has been developed to assist faculty and students.

Instructor Resources

Tools to assist you with teaching your course are available upon adoption of this text at http://thePoint.lww.com/Boyd8e.

- **A Test Bank** lets you put together exclusive new tests from a bank containing hundreds of questions to help you in assessing your students' understanding of the material. Test questions link to chapter learning objectives.
- **PowerPoint Presentations** provide an easy way for you to integrate the textbook with your students' classroom experience, either via slide shows or handouts. Multiple choice and true/false questions are integrated into the presentations to promote class participation and allow you to use i-clicker technology.
- **An Image Bank** lets you use the photographs and illustrations from this textbook in your PowerPoint slides or as you see fit in your course.
- **Guided Lecture Notes** walk you through the chapters, objective by objective.
- **Watch & Learn Videos,** *Lippincott Theory to Practice Video Series: Psychiatric–Mental Health Nursing*, includes videos of true-to-life patients displaying mental health disorders, allowing students to gain experience and a deeper understanding of mental health patients. This edition includes five new Watch and Learn videos.
- **Movies, TV, or Streaming Viewing Guides** list current examples of movies that depict various mental health disorders and that are widely available. Viewing points are provided to serve as a basis for discussion in class and among students.
- Also available are the **AACN Competency Map, Syllabi,** and **Journal Articles**.

A FULLY INTEGRATED COURSE EXPERIENCE

We are pleased to offer an expanded suite of digital solutions and ancillaries to support instructors and students using *Psychiatric Nursing: Contemporary Practice*, Eighth Edition. To learn more about any solution, please contact your local Wolters Kluwer representative.

The same trusted solution, innovation and unmatched support that you have come to expect from *Lippincott CoursePoint+* is now enhanced with more engaging learning tools and deeper analytics to help prepare students for practice. This powerfully integrated, digital learning solution combines learning tools, case studies, virtual simulation, real-time data, and the most trusted nursing education content on the market to make curriculum-wide learning more efficient and to meet students where they're at in their learning. And now, it's easier than ever for instructors and students to use, giving them everything they need for course and curriculum success!

Lippincott CoursePoint+ includes the following:

- Engaging course content provides a variety of learning tools to engage students of all learning styles.
- A more personalized learning approach, including adaptive learning powered by PrepU, gives students the content and tools they need at the moment they need it, giving them data for more focused remediation and helping to boost their confidence.
- Varying levels of case studies, virtual simulation, and access to Lippincott Advisor help students learn the critical thinking and clinical judgment skills to help them become practice-ready nurses.
- Unparalleled reporting provides in-depth dashboards with several data points to track student progress and help identify strengths and weaknesses.
- Unmatched support includes training coaches, product trainers, and nursing education consultants to help educators and students implement CoursePoint with ease.

vSim for Nursing

vSim for Nursing, jointly developed by Laerdal Medical and Wolters Kluwer Health, offers innovative scenario-based learning modules consisting of web-based virtual simulations, course learning materials, and curriculum tools designed to develop critical thinking skills and promote clinical confidence and competence. vSim for Nursing | Mental Health includes 10 mental health scenarios authored by the National League for Nursing. Students can progress through suggested readings, pre- and postsimulation assessments, documentation assignments, and guided reflection questions, and will receive an individualized feedback log immediately upon completion of the simulation. Throughout the student learning experience, the product offers remediation back to trusted Lippincott resources, including Lippincott Nursing Advisor and Lippincott Nursing Procedures—two online, evidence-based, clinical information solutions used in health care facilities throughout the United States. This innovative product provides a comprehensive patient-focused solution for learning and integrating simulation into the classroom.

Contact your Wolters Kluwer sales representative or visit http://thepoint.lww.com/vsim for options to enhance your mental health nursing course with vSim for Nursing.

Lippincott DocuCare

Lippincott DocuCare combines web-based academic electronic health record (EHR) simulation software with clinical case scenarios, allowing students to learn how to use an EHR in a safe, true-to-life setting, while enabling instructors to measure their progress. Lippincott DocuCare's nonlinear solution works well in the classroom, simulation lab, and clinical practice.

Contact your Wolters Kluwer sales representative or visit http://thepoint.lww.com/DocuCare for options to enhance your mental health nursing course with DocuCare.

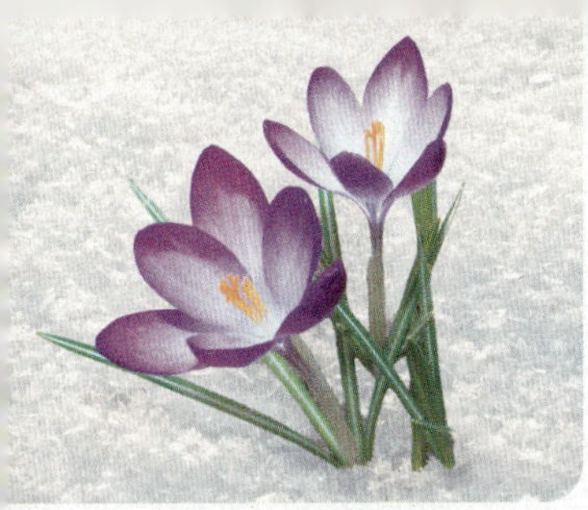

Acknowledgments

This text is a result of many long hours of diligent work by the contributors, editors, and assistants. Psychiatric nurses are constantly writing about and discussing new strategies for caring for people with mental disorders. Consumers of mental health services provided directions for nursing care and validated the importance of nursing interventions. I wish to acknowledge and thank these individuals.

Meredith Brittain and Jodi Rhomberg were instrumental to the development and publication of this edition. I especially want to acknowledge their attention to detail and their commitment to excellence. They provided direction, support, and valuable input throughout this project. They were extraordinary partners during revision of this update. They brought a broad knowledge base and extreme patience during the whole update process. I want to thank Ann Francis for the organizational skills that kept the project on target. This text would not be possible without Parul Mehta and the highly committed team of Aptara.

A NOTE ABOUT THE LANGUAGE USED IN THIS BOOK

Wolters Kluwer recognizes that people have a diverse range of identities, and we are committed to using inclusive and nonbiased language in our content. In line with the principles of nursing, we strive not to define people by their diagnoses, but to recognize their personhood first and foremost, using as much as possible the language diverse groups use to define themselves, and including only information that is relevant to nursing care.

We strive to better address the unique perspectives, complex challenges, and lived experiences of diverse populations traditionally underrepresented in health literature. When describing or referencing populations discussed in research studies, we will adhere to the identities presented in those studies to maintain fidelity to the evidence presented by the study investigators. We follow best practices of language set forth by the Publication Manual of the American Psychological Association, 7th edition, but acknowledge that language evolves rapidly, and we will update the language used in future editions of this book as necessary.

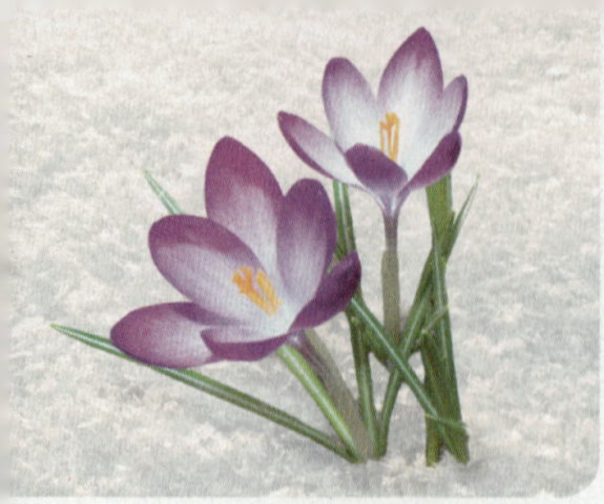

Contents

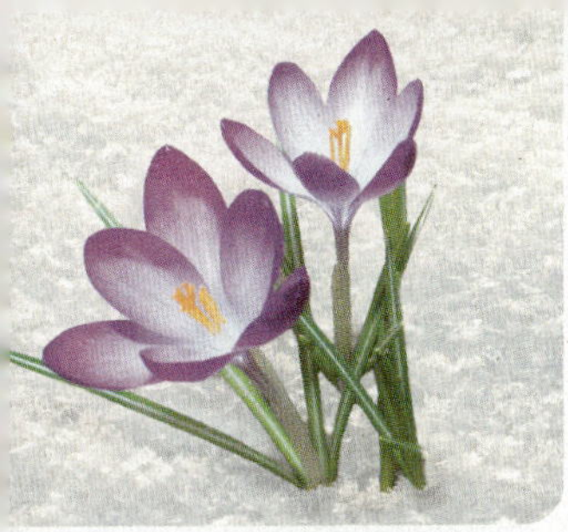

Case Studies in This Book

CASES THAT UNFOLD ACROSS UNITS

CASES THAT UNFOLD WITHIN CHAPTERS

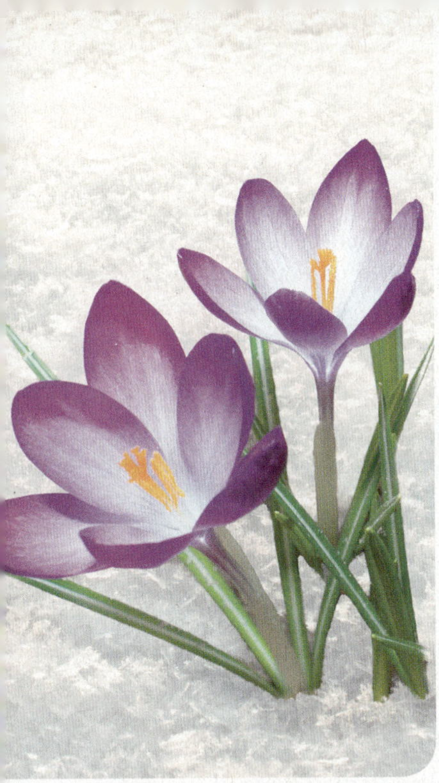

UNIT I
Mental Health Care in Contemporary Society

1 Psychiatric–Mental Health Nursing and Evidence-Based Practice

Patricia E. Freed

KEYCONCEPTS

- evidence-based practice
- psychiatric–mental health (PMH) nursing

LEARNING OBJECTIVES

After studying this chapter, you will be able to:

1. Identify the dynamic scope of psychiatric–mental health nursing practice.
2. Relate the history of psychiatric–mental health nursing to contemporary nursing practice.
3. Discuss the importance of evidence-based psychiatric–mental health nursing practice in all health care settings.
4. Describe populations that have specialized mental health needs.
5. Outline the evolution of recovery in mental health care.
6. Discuss the impact of recent legislative and policy changes in the delivery of mental health evidence.

KEY TERMS

• asylum • deinstitutionalization • institutionalization • moral treatment • neurosis • psychoanalysis • psychosis

INTRODUCTION

Everyone experiences emotional and mental health issues at some time in their lives. During periods of illness and stress, mental health issues often become overwhelming to individuals and their families. Every nurse provides mental health interventions, no matter the practice site or patient population served. Nurses in acute care settings are likely to care for people in mental health crises because medical issues are treated before any mental health issues (e.g., physical injuries from a suicide attempt are treated before the underlying depression). Like people with physical ailments, people with psychiatric disorders seek health care for their medical illnesses. The stress of the medical illness can also exacerbate psychiatric symptoms.

Psychiatric nurses care for patients with a wide range of emotional issues and mental disorders These nurses, specializing in mental health nursing, are experts in caring not only for people with a primary diagnosis of a mental disorder but also for those with self-concept and body image issues, developmental crises, co-occurring disorders, end-of-life changes, and emotional stress related to illness, disability, or loss. Psychiatric nurses are called when violence, suicide, or a disaster erupts. In this text, the terms *psychiatric nursing* and *psychiatric–mental health nursing* are used interchangeably.

> **KEYCONCEPT** Grounded in nursing theories, **psychiatric–mental health (PMH) nursing** "is a science and an art, based on evidence and the purposeful use of self and the therapeutic relationship. PMH nurses provide care at the individual, family/relationship, community, and societal levels to promote well-being and quality of life, as well as to sustain positive health outcomes" (American Nurses Association, American Psychiatric Nurses Association, & International Society of Psychiatric-Mental Health Nurses, 2022).

THE PAST AND PRESENT

The history of psychiatric nursing can be traced back to the early days of nursing practice. Today, the specialty has developed into one of the core mental health professions, with an emphasis on evidence-based practice.

Early Founders

The roots of contemporary PMH nursing can be traced to Florence Nightingale's holistic view of a patient who lives within a family and community. She was especially sensitive to human emotions and recommended interactions that today would be classified as therapeutic communication (see Chapter 9). For example, this early nursing leader's intervention for reducing anxiety about an illness was to encourage independence and self-care (Nightingale, 1859).

Linda Richards, the first trained nurse in the United States, opened the Boston City Hospital Training School for Nurses in 1882 at McLean Hospital, a mental health facility (Box 1.1) (Cowles, 1887). Employees of McLean were recruited into the nursing program to learn to provide physical care for patients with mental disorders who developed medical illnesses. In 1913, Effie Taylor integrated psychiatric nursing content into the curriculum at Johns Hopkins' Phipps Clinic. Taylor, like Nightingale before her, encouraged nurses to avoid the dichotomy of mind and body (Church, 1987). The first psychiatric nursing textbook, *Nursing Mental Disease*, was written by Harriet Bailey in 1920 (Bailey, 1920). Gradually, nursing education programs in psychiatric hospitals were phased into mainstream nursing education programs.

BOX 1.1

History of PMH Nursing

1882 First training school for psychiatric nursing at McLean Asylum by E. Cowles; first nursing program to admit men.

1913 First nurse-organized program of study for psychiatric training by Euphemia (Effie) Jane Taylor at Johns Hopkins Phipps Clinic.

1914 Mary Adelaide Nutting emphasized nursing role development.

1920 First psychiatric nursing text published, *Nursing Mental Disease,* by Harriet Bailey.

1950 Accredited schools required to offer a psychiatric nursing experience.

1952 Publication of Hildegard E. Peplau's *Interpersonal Relations in Nursing.*

1954 First graduate program in psychiatric nursing established at Rutgers University by Hildegard E. Peplau.

1963 *Perspectives in Psychiatric Care and Journal of Psychiatric Nursing* published.

1967 *Standards of Psychiatric–Mental Health Nursing Practice* published; American Nurses Association (ANA) initiated the certification of generalists in PMH nursing.

1979 *Issues in Mental Health Nursing* published; ANA initiated the certification of specialists in PMH nursing.

1980 *Nursing: A Social Policy Statement* published by the ANA.

1982 *Revised Standards of Psychiatric and Mental Health Nursing Practice* issued by the ANA.

1985 *Standards of Child and Adolescent Psychiatric and Mental Health Nursing Practice* published by the ANA.

1987 *Archives of Psychiatric Nursing and Journal of Child and Adolescent Psychiatric and Mental Health Nursing* published.

1994 *Statement on Psychiatric–Mental Health Clinical Nursing Practice and Standards of Psychiatric–Mental Health Clinical Nursing Practice* published.

1996 Guidelines specifying course content and competencies published by the Society for Education and Research in Psychiatric–Mental Health Nursing.

2000 *Scope and Standards of Psychiatric–Mental Health Nursing Practice* published.

2003 A second advanced practice role, Psychiatric–Mental Health Nurse Practitioner, was delineated.

2014 *Psychiatric–Mental Health Nursing: Scope and Standards of Practice* was revised to reflect the expanding role of PMH nurses practicing in a recovery-oriented environment.

2016 *Issues in Mental Health Nursing* concluded its first year of collaboration with the Cochrane Nursing Care Field, allowing readers easier access to patient care research.

2018 As deaths by suicide in the United States were recognized as a major public health issue, the *American Psychiatric Nursing Association* began safety training for acute care nurses.

2020 The Keynote presentation at the *American Psychiatric Nursing Association* (APNA) featured an address on how racism, socioeconomic status, and stress affect mental health and what nurses can do about it.

2022 *The Mental Health Wellness Resource Center* focused on supporting mental health and well-being in nurses, as nurses rated their current health declining 26% from pre-COVID-19 levels.

2022 *Psychiatric–Mental Health Nursing: Scope and Standards of Practice* (3rd edition) was updated and revised to reflect contemporary practice and the evolution of mental health care.

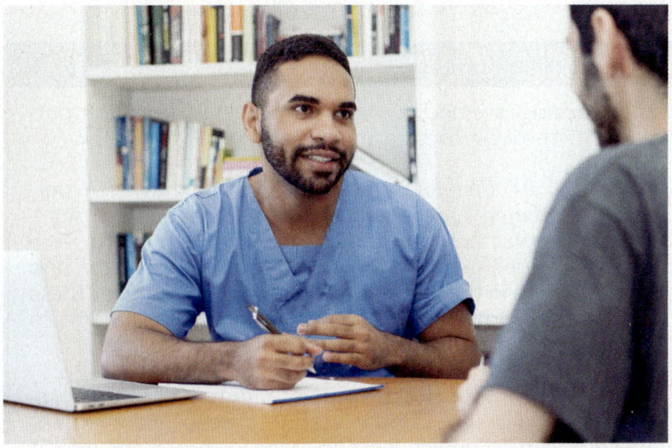
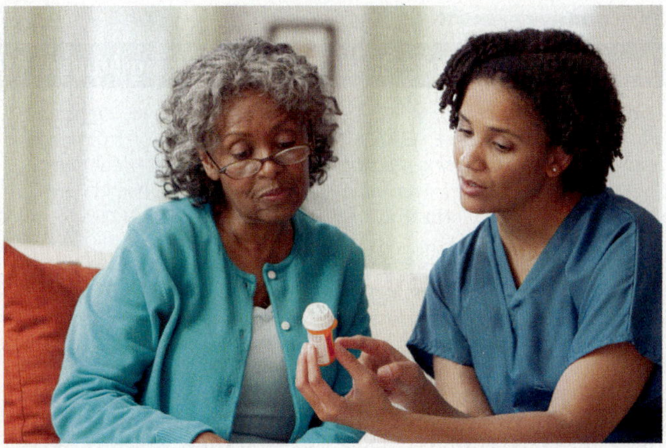

FIGURE 1.1 Contemporary PMH nursing is a versatile and rewarding field of practice. (First photo: Shutterstock/Daniel M Ernst.)

Emergence of Modern Nursing Perspectives

As PMH nursing developed as a profession in the 20th century, modern perspectives of mental illness emerged, and these new theories profoundly shaped mental health care (see Units II and III). In 1952, Hildegard E. Peplau published the landmark work *Interpersonal Relations in Nursing* (Peplau, 1952). This publication introduced PMH nursing practice to the concepts of interpersonal and therapeutic relationships. Peplau conceptualized nursing practice as independent of physicians. The use of self as a nursing tool was outside the domains of both hospital administrators and physicians.

Peplau also contributed to educational programs for psychiatric nursing, developing a specialty training program in psychiatric nursing—the first graduate nursing program—in 1954 at Rutgers University. Subspecialties began to emerge, focusing on children, adolescents, and older adults.

In 1967, the Division of Psychiatric and Mental Health Nursing Practice of the ANA published the first *Statement on Psychiatric Nursing Practice*. This publication was the first official sanction of a holistic approach of PMH nurses practicing in a variety of settings with a diverse clientele, emphasizing health promotion as well as health restoration. Since 1967, there have been several updates of the official practice statement that reflect the expansion of the role of psychiatric nurses with a delineation of functions.

Over the past century, psychiatric nursing practice expanded from the hospital to the community. Today in the United States, many nursing graduate degree programs offer specializations in PMH. Subspecialities in substance use disorders, forensic psychiatric nursing, military mental health, child and adolescent psychiatric nursing, geriatric psychiatric nursing, and psychosomatic consultation-liaison psychiatric nursing are flourishing. Micro-credentials, also known as badges, are available on a range of timely topics. These are increasingly available from universities and other reputable sources. Unlike certifications, which are standardized and accredited, microcredentials demonstrate alignment with various job descriptions, and highlight particular skills. Although these are trending and gaining popularity, rules around them and their actual market benefit is still being investigated (American Nurse, 2021).

Psychiatric nurses sit on corporate boards; serve in the armed forces; lead major health care initiatives; teach in major universities; and care for young and old people, families, and communities. Psychiatric nursing is truly a versatile and rewarding field of nursing practice (Fig. 1.1).

Evidence-Based Practice and Current Psychiatric Nursing

Evidence-based practice is the standard of care in psychiatric nursing and mental health care. Clinical decisions that lead to high-quality patient outcomes are based on research and evidence-based theories, clinical expertise, and patient preferences and values. By combining data from various sources such as expert opinion, patient data, and clinical experiences, the nurse can be objective, yet open to innovative ideas. For example, using epidemiologic data alerts nurses to the increase in suicide rates among young men, that experts were predicting, but whether the trend continues or the factors behind it remains unknown.

> **KEYCONCEPT Evidence-based practice** is a lifelong problem-solving approach to clinical practice that integrates "the best evidence from a body of research with the patient/family's preferences and values to achieve the quadruple aims of healthcare, which are: enhancing the patient experience to provide better healthcare quality and safety, improving patient outcomes, reducing costs and empowering clinicians while improving their work life experiences" (Melnyk & Fineout-Overholt, 2023, p. 1).

In an evidence-based approach, clinical questions are defined, evidence is discovered and analyzed, the research

BOX 1.2

Research for Evidence-Based Practice: Nursing Student Mentorship

Lillekroken, D., Kvalvaag, H. M., Lindeflaten, K., Fløl o, T. N., Krogstad, K., & Hessevaagbakke, E. (2024). Educating the nurses of tomorrow: exploring first-year nursing students' reflections on a one-week senior peer-mentor supervised inspiration practice in nursing homes. BMC Nursing, *23(1), 1–15. https://doi.org/10.1186/s12912-024-01768-5*

THE QUESTION: What are the perceptions and experiences of first-year nursing students with peer mentoring during their clinical experiences at long-term care nursing facilities?

METHODS: Using a qualitative exploratory descriptive design, 53 first-year nursing students were assigned third-year mentors during 1 week of inspiration practice at a nursing home by employing peer mentoring as a teaching and learning method. Data were collected from the participants through focus groups.

FINDINGS: All first-year students reported that their perception of being supervised by third-year students at nursing homes was being inspired and moving forward. Two categories emerged: (1) feeling close to the mentor and (2) confidence in the mentors' professional knowledge. These findings were interpreted as enabling first-year students to learn more about the nurses' roles and responsibilities.

IMPLICATIONS FOR NURSING: Peer mentoring can be useful in clinical practice by facilitating practice from experienced nurses to novice learners. Mentorship is possible at all levels of nursing education and practice.

findings are applied in a practical manner and in collaboration with the patient/family, and outcomes are evaluated. One of the first steps is seeking out a mentor who can help through the evidence-based process because this approach requires using literature search skills, followed by careful reading and critiquing of the current studies and seeking the advice of experts in the field. A nurse might start with a clinical question, such as "Do social and environmental adversities effects recovery among people with serious mental illness being treated in community mental health centers?"

The nurse and mentor will narrow the question and begin a critique of the literature. Even though the process results in directions for practice, the nurse will face many challenges. See Box 1.2.

EVOLUTION OF MENTAL HEALTH RECOVERY

Throughout history, popular beliefs of the time served as the basis for understanding and treating people with mental illnesses. Prehistoric healers practiced an ancient surgical technique of removing a disk of bone from the skull to let out the so-called evil spirits, which healers believed were the cause of mental disorders. In the early Christian period (1–100 CE), when alleged sin or supposed demonic possession were thought to cause mental disorders, clergymen treated patients, often through prescribed exorcisms. When such measures would inevitably fail, patients were excluded from the community and sometimes even put to death. Later in the medieval era (1000–1300 CE), contaminated environments were believed to cause *mental illness*. Consequently, individuals were removed from their "sick" environments and placed in protected asylums. Table 1.1 provides a summary of historical events and correlating perspectives on mental health during the premoral treatment era (from ancient times to the colonial period).

Moral Treatment and Asylums

As evidence mounted that a mental disorder was an illness and recovery was possible, existing primitive physical treatments, such as venesections (bloodletting) and gyrations (strapping patients to a rotating board), began to be viewed as either painful or barbaric (Fig. 1.2). With science not advanced enough to offer reasonable treatment approaches, a safe haven, or **asylum**, was considered the best option for treatment. In the moral treatment period (1790–1900), **moral treatment**, that is, the use of kindness, compassion, and a pleasant environment, was adopted. Individuals with mental disorders were routinely removed from their communities and placed in asylums, which were thought to be best for their safety and comfort (Fig. 1.3).

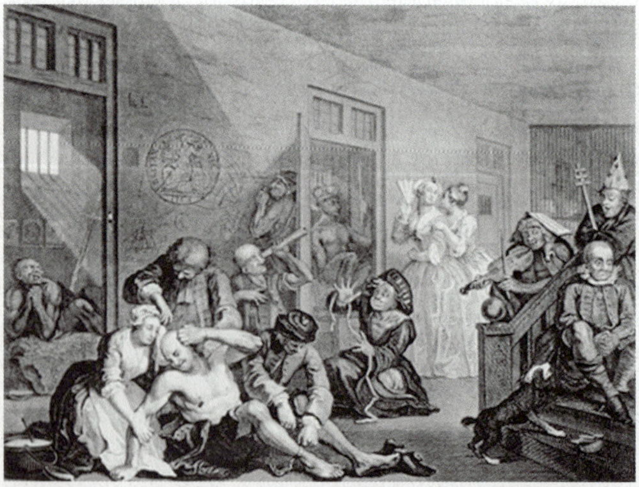

FIGURE 1.2 Interior of Bethlehem Asylum, London. (William Hogarth, 1697–1765. The Rake's Progress: Scene in Bedlam.) (Reprinted from U.S. National Library of Medicine. Images from the history of medicine. Washington, DC: National Institutes of Health, Department of Health and Human Services. http://resource.nlm.nih.gov/101394076)

TABLE 1.1 PREMORAL TREATMENT ERA

Period	Beliefs About Mental Illness	Mental Health Care
Ancient times to 800 BCE	Sickness was viewed as an indication of the displeasure of deities for sins; viewed as supernatural.	People with psychiatric symptoms were driven from homes and ostracized by relatives. When behavioral manifestations were viewed as supernatural powers, the people who exhibited them were revered.
Periods of inquiry: 800 BCE to 1 CE	Egypt and Greek periods of inquiry. Physical and mental health were viewed as interrelated. Hippocrates argued atypical behaviors were due to brain disturbances. Aristotle related mental disorders to physical disorders.	Counseling, work, and music were provided in temples by priests to relieve the distress of those with mental disorders. Observation and documentation were a part of the care. The mental disorders were treated as diseases. The aim of treatment was to correct imbalances.
Early Christian and early medieval: 1–1000 CE	Power of Christian church grew. St. Augustine pronounced all diseases were ascribed to demons.	People with psychiatric symptoms were incarcerated in dungeons, beaten, and starved.
Later medieval: 1000–1300	In Western Europe, spirit of inquiry was dead. Healing was taken over by theologians and witch doctors. People with psychiatric symptoms were incarcerated in dungeons, beaten, and starved. In the Middle East, Avicenna said mental disorders are illnesses.	First asylums were built by Muslims. People with psychiatric symptoms were treated as being sick.
Renaissance: 1300–1600	In England, people with mental illness were differentiated from those considered criminals. In colonies, mental illnesses were believed to be caused by demonic possession. Witch hunts were common.	People with psychiatric symptoms who presented a threat to society were apprehended and locked up. There were no public provisions for people with mental disorders except jail. Private hospitalization for the wealthy who could pay. Bethlehem Asylum was used as a private institution.
Colonial: 1700–1790	1751: Benjamin Franklin established Pennsylvania Hospital (in Philadelphia)—the first institution in United States to receive those with mental disorders for treatment and cure. 1773: First public, freestanding asylum at Williamsburg, Virginia. 1783: Benjamin Rush categorized mental illnesses and began to treat mental disorders with medical interventions, such as bloodletting, mechanical devices.	The beginnings of mental diseases were viewed as illness to be treated.

Despite the good intentions that may have been at the root of the moral treatment movement, within the asylums, patients were often treated inhumanely. A turning point occurred at Bicêtre, a men's hospital in France that had the distinction of being the worst asylum in the world, when physician Philippe Pinel (1745–1826) ordered the removal of the chains, stopped the drugging and bloodletting, and placed the patients under the care of physicians. Three years later, the same standards were extended to Salpêtrière, the asylum for female patients. At about the same time in England, William Tuke (1732–1822), a member of the Society of Friends, raised funds for a retreat for members who had mental disorders. The York Retreat was opened in 1796; restraints were abandoned, and sympathetic care in quiet, pleasant surroundings with some form of industrial occupation, such as weaving or farming, was provided (Fig. 1.4).

In the United States, the Quakers were instrumental in stopping the practice of bloodletting; they also placed great emphasis on providing a proper religious atmosphere (Deutsch, 1949). The Quaker Friends Asylum was proposed in 1811 and opened 6 years later in Frankford, Pennsylvania (now Philadelphia), to become the second asylum in the United States. The humane and supportive rehabilitative attitude of the Quakers was seen as an extremely important influence in changing the techniques of caring for those with mental disorders. As

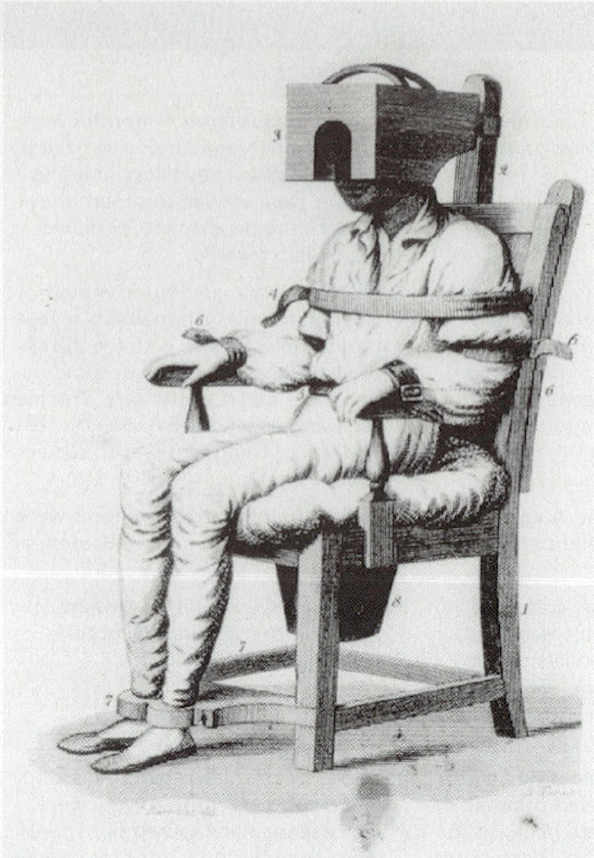

FIGURE 1.3 The Tranquilizer Chair of Benjamin Rush. A patient is sitting in a chair, his body immobilized, a bucket attached beneath the seat. (Benjamin Rush, 1746–1813. [1811].) (Reprinted from U.S. National Library of Medicine. Images from the history of medicine. Washington, DC: National Institutes of Health, Department of Health and Human Services. http://resource.nlm.nih.gov/101436673)

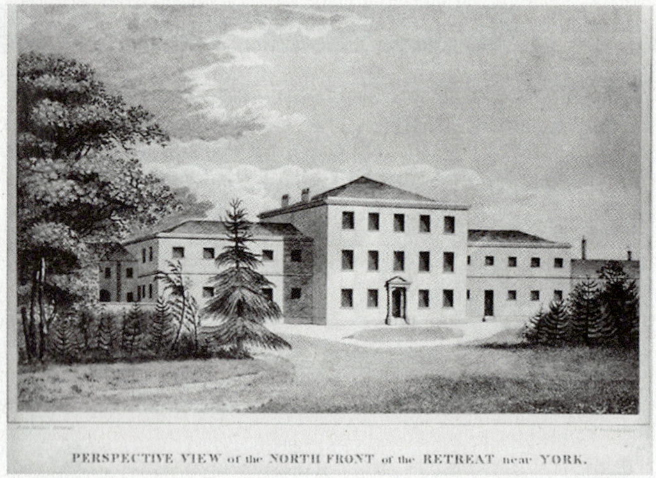

FIGURE 1.4 The perspective view of the north front of the retreat near York Samuel Tuke, 1784–1857 (1813). (Reprinted from U.S. National Library of Medicine. Images from the history of medicine. National Institutes of Health, Department of Health and Human Services. http://resource.nlm.nih.gov/101436033)

states were founded, new hospitals were opened that were dedicated to the care of patients with mental disorders.

Even with these hospitals, only a fraction of people with mental disorders received treatment. Those who were judged dangerous were hospitalized; those deemed harmless or with mild illness were treated the same as people who were indigent—that is, they were given no public support. In farm communities during the first half of the 19th century, individuals who were poor or who had a mental illness were often auctioned and bought by landowners seeking inexpensive labor. Some states used almshouses (poorhouses) for housing individuals with mental illness.

Public Funding, Dorothea Dix, and State Hospitals

Hospitals for individuals with mental illness were few because of financing; there were no funding mechanisms to support these large institutions. The first step in resolving the funding problem was defining responsibility—that is, which agency would be responsible for paying for care. In 1828, Horace Mann, a representative in the Massachusetts state legislature, saw his plea that the "insane are wards of the state" become a reality. State governments were mandated to assume fiscal responsibility for the care of people with mental illnesses (Beers, 1908).

After states were designated as being financially responsible for the treatment of their residents with mental illnesses, the next step was ensuring that each state appropriated funds. Dorothea Lynde Dix (1802 to 1887), a vigorous crusader for the humane treatment of patients with mental illness, was responsible for much of the reform of the mental health care system in the 19th century. Her solution was state hospitals. She first influenced the Massachusetts legislature to expand the Massachusetts State Hospital. Then, through public awareness campaigns and lobbying efforts, she managed to convince state after state to build hospitals. At the end of Dix's lengthy career, 20 states had responded directly to her appeals by establishing or enlarging state hospitals (Box 1.3).

Institutionalization and Its Outcomes

In state hospitals, **institutionalization**, the forced confinement of individuals for extended periods of time in large facilities, became the primary treatment for more than 50 years (1900–1955). Institutions had little more to offer than food, clothing, pleasant surroundings, and some means of employment and exercise. Outcomes of institutionalization were consistently negative. Thousands of people were warehoused within the walls of institutions for months and years with little hope of reentering society. Patients were socially isolated from their families and community life. The medical superintendent's major concern was the day-to-day operation of the large, aging

BOX 1.3

Dorothea Lynde Dix

At nearly 40 years of age, Dorothea Dix, a retired school teacher living in Massachusetts, was solicited by a young theology student to help in preparing a Sunday school class for women inmates at the East Cambridge Jail. Dix led the class herself and was shocked by the filth and dirt in the jail. She was particularly struck by the treatment of inmates with mental disorders. It was the dead of winter, and no heat was provided. When she questioned the jailer about the lack of heat, his answer was that "the insane need no heat." The prevailing myth was that people with mental illnesses were insensible to extremes of temperature. Dix's outrage initiated a long struggle in the reform of care.

An early feminist, Dix disregarded the New England role of a Puritan woman and diligently investigated the conditions of jails and the plight of those with mental illness. During the Civil War, she was appointed to the post of Superintendent of Women Nurses, the highest position held by a woman during the war.

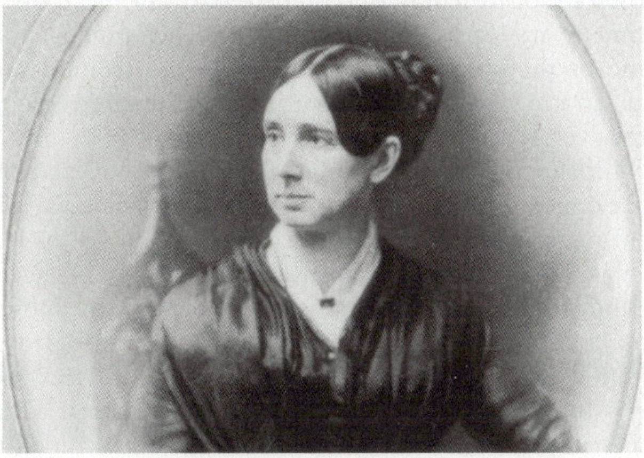

Dorothea Lynde Dix.

Image reprinted from U.S. National Library of Medicine. Image from the history of medicine. National Institutes of Health, Department of Health and Human Services. http://resource.nlm.nih.gov/101413738.

physical structures. Untrained attendants who had little understanding of mental illnesses were responsible for the care, which was often cruel and inhumane. There were few educated nurses. Patients suffered adverse physical and psychological effects. There were few trained mental health providers. Early institutions eventually evolved into self-contained communities that produced their own food and made their own clothing. Institutionalization was a dismal failure.

Women had a particularly difficult time and often were institutionalized at the convenience of their fathers or husbands. Because American society in the late 1800s expected a woman to function as a domestic extension of her husband, any behaviors or beliefs that did not conform to male expectations could be used to justify the claim of insanity. Some women were held prisoner for years. In the asylums, women were psychologically degraded, used as servants, and physically tortured by male physicians and female attendants (Bly, 1887).

Primitive and often misguided biologic treatments were unsuccessful. For example, the use of hydrotherapy, or baths, was an established procedure in mental institutions. Warm baths and, in some instances, ice cold baths produced calming effects for patients with mental disorders. However, this treatment's success at that time was attributed to the restraint of patients during the bath rather than the physiologic responses that hydrotherapy produced. Baths were then applied indiscriminately and used as a form of restraint rather than a therapeutic practice.

Clifford Beers (1876–1943) recovered from a mental disorder, became an advocate of humane treatment, and published an autobiography, *A Mind That Found Itself* (1908), depicting his 3-year hospitalization experience in the 18th century. He was beaten; choked; imprisoned for extended periods in dark, dank, padded cells; and confined for many days in a straitjacket. By 1909, Beers formed the National Committee for Mental Hygiene. Through the committee's advocacy efforts, other mental health services were initiated, such as child guidance clinics, prison clinics, and industrial mental health care.

Freud's Contribution

While the institutionalization movement was gaining strength, Sigmund Freud (1856–1939) and the psychoanalytic movement of the early 1900s exerted influence on the mental health community. Trained as a neuropathologist, Freud developed a personality theory based on unconscious motivations for behavior or drives. According to the Freudian model, development occurred in stages, with the first three—oral, anal, and genital—being the most important. Infants progressed through the oral stage, experiencing the world through symbolic oral ingestion; through the anal stage, in which toddlers develop a sense of autonomy through withholding; and on to the genital stage, in which a beginning sense of sexuality emerges within the framework of the oedipal relationship. If there was any interference in development, such as psychological trauma, psychosis or neurosis would develop (Freud, 1905).

Freud and his followers believed the primary causes of mental illnesses were psychological and a result of disturbed personality development and faulty parenting (Freud, 1927). Mental illnesses were categorized either as a **psychosis** (severe) or as a neurosis (less severe). A psychosis impaired daily functioning because of breaks in contact with reality. A neurosis was less severe, but individuals were often distressed about their issues. Soon, Freud's ideas represented the forefront of psychiatric thought and began to shape society's view of mental health care. Freudian ideology dominated psychiatric thought well into the 1970s.

Intensive **psychoanalysis**, therapy that focused on repairing the trauma of the original psychological injury, was the Freudian treatment of choice. However, psychoanalysis was costly, time-consuming, and required lengthy training. Few could perform it. Thousands of patients in state institutions with severe mental illnesses were ignored.

Freud's view of mental illness as a psychological disorder gained credibility. He was a prolific writer who reported that his patients improved through psychoanalysis and interpretation of dreams (Freud, 1900). His outcomes were not judged by contemporary standards or subjected to meta-analysis processes. Today, psychoanalysis remains as a treatment option for a select group of patients who have the cognitive abilities to discuss and to understand complex psychological concepts. In addition, the use of time-limited, briefer psychoanalytic therapy is being explored, and a recent research article featured a promising role for psychoanalysis in post trauma brain rehabilitation (Bruguiere et al., 2023).

National Action

During World War II (1939–1945), mental illness was beginning to be seen as an issue that could happen to anyone. Many people who volunteered for the armed services were disqualified on the grounds that they were psychologically unfit to serve. Others who had already served tours of duty developed psychiatric and emotional issues related to their wartime experiences. Today, these issues are recognized as a distinct disorder: posttraumatic stress disorder (see Chapter 29).

In 1946, the National Mental Health Act created a six-member National Mental Health Advisory Council that established the National Institute of Mental Health, which was responsible for overseeing and coordinating research and training. Under the Act's provisions, the federal government also provided grants to states to support existing outpatient facilities and programs to establish new ones. Before 1948, more than half of all states had no clinics; by 1949, all but five had one or more. Six years later, there were 1,234 outpatient clinics. Also passed in 1946, the Hill–Burton Act provided substantial federal support for hospital construction, which expanded the number of psychiatric units in general hospitals.

Impact of Psychopharmacology

Psychopharmacology revolutionized the treatment of people with mental illness. Initially, barbiturates, particularly amobarbital sodium (Amytal sodium), were tried for treating mental diseases in the 1930s (Malamud, 1944). When chlorpromazine was introduced in the 1950s, the mental health community was hopeful that a medication had been discovered to cure severe mental illness. The phenothiazines were the first of many antipsychotics to be developed (see Chapter 11). The medications calmed the patients and reduced some of the symptoms.

A New National Objective: Community Treatment

In 1961, *Action for Mental Health*, a report of the Joint Commission on Mental Illness and Health Commission, called for larger investments in basic research; national personnel recruitment and training programs; one full-time clinic for every 50,000 individuals supplemented by general hospital units and state-run regional intensive psychiatric treatment centers; and access to emergency care and treatment in general, both in mental hospitals and in community clinics. The funding for the construction and operation of the community mental health system would be shared by federal, state, and local governments. The ideas expressed in the report clearly shifted authority for mental health programming to the federal government and were the basis of the federal legislation, the Mental Retardation Facilities and Community Mental Health Centers Construction Act, signed into law by John F. Kennedy in 1963. Unfortunately, this act funded only some of the approaches proposed by the Commission and did not support the operation of state-run regional intensive psychiatric centers.

The supporters of this 1963 legislation believed the exact opposite of what Dorothea Dix believed during the previous century. That is, instead of viewing an institution as a peaceful asylum, institutionalization was viewed as contributing to the illness. If patients were moved from an asylum into a community-living setting, it was believed that the symptoms of mental disorders could easily be treated and eventually would disappear. Thus, **deinstitutionalization**, the release of those confined to mental institutions for extended periods of time into the community for treatment, support, and rehabilitation, became a national movement.

The inpatient state hospital population fell by about 15% between 1955 and 1965 and by about 59% during the succeeding decade. The 2,000 projected community mental health centers (CMHCs) that should have been in place by 1980 were never established. By 1990, only about 1,300 programs provided several types of psychosocial rehabilitation services, such as vocational, educational, or social–recreational services (International Association of Psychosocial Rehabilitation, 1990).

Deinstitutionalization: A Failed Approach

There is no evidence that most people discharged from state hospitals benefited from CMHC services. The CMHCs ignored the legions of people with serious mental illnesses and instead focused on the treatment of alcohol and substance use disorders. Individual psychotherapy, the primary treatment offered in most centers, was insufficient for those who needed other types of treatment, housing, and vocational opportunities. By the 1990s, deinstitutionalization was considered a failure.

MENTAL HEALTH LEGISLATIVE ACTIONS

Millions of adults and children are disabled by mental illness every year. Compared with all other diseases, major depressive disorder, anxiety disorder, and opioid use disorders ranked in the top eight conditions responsible for chronic disability in the United States from 1990 to 2019 (GBD 2019 Mental Disorders Collaborators, 2022). Government initiatives are attempting to increase the public's understanding of mental disorders and related issues.

In 1999, *Mental Health: A Report of the Surgeon General* summarized evidence for the treatment of mental illness. As the first report addressing mental health by the Office of the Surgeon General, two main findings were presented (U.S. Department of Health and Human Services [USDHHS], 1999):

- The efficacy of mental health treatments is well documented.
- A range of treatments exist for most mental disorders.

The following year, another landmark report, *Report of the Surgeon General's Conference on Children's Mental Health: A National Action Agenda*, was published. This report highlights consensus recommendations for identifying, recognizing, and referring children to services; increasing access to services for families; and using evidence for evaluating treatment services, systems of care, and financing (U.S. Public Health Service, 2000).

In 2003, the *President's New Freedom Commission on Mental Health* recommended that the mental health system be transformed. The report identified six goals as the foundation for transforming mental health care in the United States into a consumer-centered, family-centered, and recovery-oriented system (Box 1.4) (New Freedom Commission on Mental Health, 2003).

The Mental Health Parity and Addiction Equity Act was enacted in 2008 to ensure that health plans cover mental health and/or substance use disorder benefits equally to medical/surgical benefits. Under this law, insurance companies are prevented from imposing less favorable benefits on mental health or substance use disorders than on medical disorders. The final rules, effective July 1, 2014, were implemented in 2015.

Passage of the Patient Protection and Affordable Care Act in 2010 provided more people with access to affordable, effective treatments for their mental health needs. This law also prevents insurance companies from excluding people because of preexisting conditions. The intent of this legislation was to ensure the consumers of mental health care were in charge of their own care. Access through Medicaid coverage and establishing state marketplaces improved access to care for millions of Americans, who, unlike those who remained uninsured, were less likely to experience delays or be unable to get care due to costs (Lieff et al., 2024). A variety of provisions under the Affordable Care Act brought the biggest expansion of services for those with substance use disorders in a generation (Jayawardhana, 2023). The future of mental health care in the United States looked promising, as legislation was propelling mental health care forward.

But then the COVID-19 pandemic hit hard, bringing a heavy death toll and disrupting the lives of millions of Americans. Health care workers themselves were not immune, and many front-line nurses fell ill with COVID-19 and/or developed trauma and stress-related symptoms (Ayotte et al., 2022; Wild et al., 2023). In 2020, the CARES ACT (Coronavirus Aid, Relief, and Economic Security) was passed to provide fast, direct economic aid and relief to Americans suffering through the pandemic. Funding included $425 million to the Substance Abuse and Mental Health Services Administration (SAMHSA) to address mental health and substance use disorders, $250 million for Certified Community Behavioral Health Clinics to increase access to mental health care services, and $50 million for suicide prevention (USDHHS, 2021).

When the pandemic quarantine was finally lifted, notable increases in the rates of mental illness, as well as exacerbations and relapses in preexisting conditions, became apparent (Devoe et al., 2023; KFF, 2023; MHA, 2023a). High rates of mental health issues were reported in children and adolescents during the pandemic (Theberath et al., 2022), and these rates have remained high (KFF, 2023). A culture of increasing violence and mass school shootings has only exacerbated the situation, and addressing the mental health needs of American youth and families is a national concern (Rapa et al., 2024).

An urgent call to engage psychiatric nurses in promoting pediatric mental health has already been raised (Kumar et al., 2020), and several innovative models proposing a national response to prioritize the well-being of youth via a collective and coordinated effort are available for consideration (see Hoagwood et al., 2021). Conscientious

BOX 1.4

U.S. Goals in a Transformed Mental Health System

Goal 1 Americans understand that mental health is essential to overall health.

Goal 2 Mental health care is consumer and family driven.

Goal 3 Disparities in mental health services are eliminated.

Goal 4 Early mental health screening, assessment, and referral to services are common practices.

Goal 5 Excellent mental health care is delivered, and research is accelerated.

Goal 6 Technology is used to access mental health care and information.

Reprinted from New Freedom Commission on Mental Health. (2003). Achieving the promise: Transforming mental healthcare in America (p. 8). DHHS Publication No. SMA-03–3831. U.S. Department of Health and Human Services.

assessment for trauma-stress symptoms and disorders must remain a priority for many years to come, and the lasting effects of long COVID (post-COVID) conditions, now recognized as severe and potentially disabling, are still under investigation (CDC, 2025; Davis, 2023).

Today, 90% of adults in the United States believe that the country is facing a mental health crisis (Panchai et al., 2023). The future of America's mental health services depends on what advocates, consumers, and voters can accomplish by supporting government policies that fund mental health services. Psychiatric nurses need to be ever vigilant of the gains previously made and to stand with the populations we serve.

POPULATIONS WITH SPECIAL MENTAL HEALTH NEEDS

Mental disorders affect populations differently, including variations in rates, symptom expression, treatment and management needs, influencing factors, resource needs, and even cultural and public attitudes. Within the United States, several population groups have unique mental health needs when compared to the general population. These groups include people assigned female at birth, LGBTQ+ (lesbian, gay, bisexual, transgender, queer) individuals, and individuals who are members of underrepresented racial and ethnic groups. Unique mental health needs exist for these populations because they are often discriminated against.

Mental Health Needs of People Assigned Female at Birth

People assigned female at birth (referred to as "female" in the remainder of this section) with mental illnesses are vulnerable to discrimination and power inequities in mental health care systems. In one survey, over half of young females and females with low incomes reported the need for mental health care. Females experience more challenges in accessing and receiving mental health care when compared to the general population and when compared to men with mental illnesses (KFF, 2022). Mental health challenges of females are well documented and include gender differences in mental and medical health outcomes, treatment bias, barriers to care, and service utilization. Females report that providers doubt and question the legitimacy of their symptoms and concerns, and they report instances of sexual exploitation by their providers (Mizock & Brubaker, 2021) and either long waiting times at appointments or inability to attain mental health appointments. Two in 10 females reported that their insurance was refused, and many others do not seek mental health treatment (KFF, 2023).

Reproductive health care is linked to mental health care. The June 24, 2022, U.S. Supreme Court decision in the case of Dobbs v. Jackson Women's Health Organization has led to the proliferation of legislative restrictions on reproductive care. These restrictions have led to increasing emotional distress, traumatization, and victimization of underrepresented populations (Stotland, 2023). Because of restrictions on female reproductive rights, increased infant mortality rates, maternal health complications and mortality, and greater family poverty are expected to occur (Arey et al., 2022; Foster et al., 2022; Pabayo et al., 2020). It is predicted that racially underrepresented groups will be disproportionately affected by the new restrictions on reproductive care (Hill et al., 2024).

During the pandemic, nurses mobilized and reached out to those in quarantine via telehealth and online therapy. The USDHHS increased the flexibility of providing and obtaining telehealth services; some of these changes were temporary, and others were permanent (USDHHS, 2023). Use of these digital modalities took some adjustment on the part of providers, but they have been effective (Janka-Beltane et al., 2023). Digital modes of delivery continue to be popular or legitimized post-COVID, especially in youth-centered mental health care services (Ding et al., 2023).

Mental Health Needs of Sexual and Gender Underrepresented Groups

Disparities in care for sexual and gender underrepresented groups are supported by a large body of research (Gonzales & Ehrenfeld, 2018; Hoy-Ellis, 2023; Stacey & Wislar, 2023.) Research is needed to help guide the nursing care of these populations (Hughes et al., 2022).

When compared to non-LGBTQ+ people, LBGTQ+ individuals are more than twice as likely to have a mental health disorder in their lifetime and to experience depression, anxiety, and substance misuse (Orlov & Calixte, 2024). Research also suggests that LGBTQ+ individuals, of whom over 50% identify as female, face disparities linked to social stigma, discrimination, and denial of their civil and human rights (MHA, 2023b). However, despite the promises inherent in the Affordable Care Act, funding via the CARES Act, and prohibition of discrimination by the U.S. Constitution, mental health and substance use services have not improved among sexual underrepresented groups (Kim et al., 2023; Newman et al., 2022).

Mental Health Needs of Racial and Ethnic Underrepresented Groups

Racial and ethnic disparities exist in the United States in mental health care. There is a gap in the use of mental health services among members of Hispanic and Black communities, who access fewer services than White individuals. One explanation may be financial, but there may be nonfinancial reasons as well, including language barriers, mistrust of the medical profession, and systemic barriers such as limited availability of mental health services (Kim et al., 2023). See Chapters 2 and 3.

RECOVERY AND THE CONSUMER MOVEMENT

Recovery from mental illness is realistic and is now a worldwide goal. Consumers are demanding that mental health services receive the same support and attention as other health services. The traditional medical model, which is viewed as autocratic and paternalistic, is being replaced by a collaborative model whereby mental health professionals work in partnership with consumers to help rebuild their lives. Consumer advocacy efforts have led to the implementation of recovery philosophy and practices (see Chapters 2 and 8). In this text, the terms *consumers* and *patients* are used interchangeably. The basic nature of advocacy emphasizes standing up for what you believe and, by forming relationships and educating others, to stand with them in making a difference (Basloe, 2022).

National Mental Health Objectives

The vision of Healthy People 2030 is to build a healthier future for all. The overarching mental health goals are to improve mental health, eliminate health disparities, and achieve equity through prevention and by ensuring access to appropriate, high-quality mental health services. Healthy People Objectives for 2030 were written to focus on mental health and mental disorders to provide guidance for all health care professionals (Box 1.5). But new mental health issues have emerged in the past decade that are not yet reflected in the Healthy People Objectives: sexual and mental trauma experienced by military members and veterans, large-scale psychological trauma in communities caused by violence and natural disasters, devastating and continuing effects of COVID-19 on mental and physical health, increased emotional needs of employees and students, complex caregiving issues for families around trauma and social media use, health consequences of restrictions on reproductive care of people assigned female at birth and medical care for sexual underrepresented groups, and ongoing issues with substance misuse and overdose, to name a few.

The challenge for psychiatric nursing is to work toward these goals through direct practice, advocating for people with emotional and mental disorders, and improving the social and physical environments of care.

BOX 1.5

Mental Health and Mental Disorders Objectives for the Year 2030

MENTAL HEALTH STATUS IMPROVEMENT

- Reduce the suicide rate.
- Reduce suicide attempts by adolescents.
- Reduce the proportion of adolescents who engage in disordered eating behaviors in an attempt to control their weight.
- Reduce the proportion of people who experience major depressive episodes.

TREATMENT EXPANSION

- Increase the proportion of primary care facilities that provide mental health treatment onsite or by paid referral.
- Increase the proportion of children with mental health issues who receive treatment.
- Increase the proportion of juvenile residential facilities that screen admissions for mental health issues.
- Increase the proportion of people with serious mental illness who are employed.
- Increase the proportion of adults with mental health disorders who receive treatment.
- Increase the proportion of people with co-occurring substance use and mental disorders who receive treatment for both disorders.
- Increase depression screening by primary care providers.
- Increase the proportion of primary care provider office visits that screen youth ages 12 to 18 years for depression.
- Increase the proportion of adults with mental health issues who are homeless who receive mental health services.

Adapted from Office of Disease Prevention and Health Promotion. 2021. *Healthy People 2030*. U.S. Department of Health and Human Services. Mental Health and Mental Disorders; Healthy People 2030. health.gov

SUMMARY OF KEY POINTS

- Every practicing nurse cares for people with an emotional or mental disorder. Every nurse needs basic psychiatric nursing knowledge and skills.
- PMH nursing is a specialized area of nursing that promotes mental health through applying the nursing process. Psychiatric nurses care for people with a wide range of emotional issues and mental disorders.
- The need for PMH nursing was recognized near the end of the 19th century when Linda Richards opened the Boston City Hospital Training School for Nurses in 1882. Today, psychiatric nursing is recognized as one of the core mental health professions.
- Evidence-based practice is the standard of care in psychiatric nursing and in the mental health field. Historically, popular beliefs about the source of mental illnesses and treatment served as evidence.
- Over time, most treatment approaches, including institutionalization and deinstitutionalization, did not result in positive outcomes.
- Freud contributed to the psychoanalytic understanding of personality development and showed the strength of psychoanalysis. However, the psychoanalytic model was not effective in the treatment of people with severe mental illnesses.

- The U.S. Surgeon General's reports, the President's New Freedom Commission on Mental Health, and the goals of Healthy People 2030 continue to highlight the need for resources for the care of people with mental illness.
- The Patient Protection and Affordable Care Act prevents third-party payers from excluding people from insurance coverage for preexisting disorders.
- In the United States, people assigned female at birth, LGBTQ+ individuals, and individuals who are members of underrepresented racial and ethnic groups have special mental health needs.
- Today, consumers of mental health services insist on building partnerships with providers to recover from mental illness. The traditional medical model is being replaced by a collaborative approach in which consumers and mental health care providers develop a partnership in recovery-oriented care.

DEVELOPING CLINICAL JUDGMENT

1. Discuss whether you would expect the patients described below to have mental health needs:
   a. A 32-year-old recently divorced individual with obesity and diabetes, who recently lost their job and can no longer pay for medications.
   b. A 25-year-old veteran whose war injuries have left him paralyzed from the waist down.
   c. An 86-year-old whose husband recently died now must move to a nursing home.
2. Give three examples of changes in nursing practice based on new evidence.
3. Discuss the rationale for the moral treatment of people with mental disorders. Was moral treatment effective?
4. Identify common themes in the 1999 *Mental Health: A Report of the Surgeon General*, the *President's New Freedom Commission of Mental Health Report*, and *Healthy People 2030: National Health Promotion and Disease Prevention Objectives*.
5. Research and discuss a federal law (pending or enacted) or U.S. Supreme Court ruling that affects (or will affect) the health of vulnerable people and sexual underrepresented groups.

MOVIE, TV, OR STREAMING PROGRAMS

***Mysteries of Mental Illness: Episode 1: Evil or Illness* (2021).** The first episode of this excellent contemporary PBS documentary documents the impact of mental illness on the lives of individuals with psychiatric disorders. The evolution in the understanding of mental illness is traced from the beginning of recorded history to modern times. Originally viewed as a curse of the Gods, mental illness was eventually viewed by early philosophers as a mind-body illness. As physicians tried to make sense of unusual thoughts and behaviors, the explanations were often determined by the cultural beliefs and stigma of the time. Women were often targeted as having mental illness because of socially unacceptable thoughts and behaviors, such as wanting to live independently or own property. Mental illness is shown to be highly stigmatized, which reinforced hopelessness, low self-esteem, and suicidal thoughts.

Viewing Points:

1. How did Jenny manage to compete in the Olympics and yet have a serious mental illness? Why did she not disclose her disorder until she had roommates? How would Jenny have been treated if she had lived in the 18th century?
2. Is Cecelia's illness incompatible with being a student of astrophysics? How do contemporary cultural norms influence the care that Cecelia is receiving?
3. What beliefs underlie the use of machinery such as the tranquilizer chair?

REFERENCES

American Nurse (ANA). (2021). *Micro-credentials and badges in healthcare*. https://www.myamericannurse.com/micro-credentials-and-badges-in-healthcare/

American Nurses Association, American Psychiatric Nurses Association, & International Society of Psychiatric-Mental Health Nurses. (2022). *Psychiatric-mental health nursing: Scope and standards of practice* (3rd ed.). ANA.

Arey, W., Lerma, K., Beasley, A., Harper, L., Moayedi, G., & White, K. (2022). A preview of the dangerous future of abortion bans—Texas Senate Bill 8. *New England Journal of Medicine*, *387*, 388–390. https://doi.org/10.1056/NEJMp2207423

Ayotte, B. J., Schierberl Scherr, A. E., & Kellogg, M. B. (2022) PTSD symptoms and functional impairment among nurses treating COVID-19 patients. *SAGE Open Nursing*, *8*, 23779608221074651.

Bailey, H. (1920). *Nursing mental diseases*. Macmillan.

Basloe, M. (2022). *Advocacy matters: Standing up for what you believe in makes a difference*. Child Care Services Association, https://www.childcareservices.org/2022/06/24/advocacy-matters-standing-up-for-what-you-believe-in-makes-a-difference/#:~:text=However%2C%20the%20basic%20nature%20of,understand%20the%20issues%20at%20hand/

Beers, C. W. (1908). *A mind that found itself*. Longmans, Green, & Co.

Bly, N. (1887). *Ten days in a mad-house*. Ian L. Munro.

Bruguiere, P., Morin, C., Maddux, B., & Pradat-Diehl, P. (2023). Contribution of psychoanalytic psychotherapy to the rehabilitation setting for a patient with acquired brain injury. *Journal of Psychosocial Rehabilitation and Mental Health*, *10*(1), 107–117.

Centers for Disease Control and Prevention (CDC). (2025). *Long COVID Basics*. https://www.cdc.gov/covid/long-term-effects/index.html

Church, O. M. (1987). From custody to community in psychiatric nursing. *Nursing Research*, *36*(10), 48–55.

Cowles, E. (1887). Nursing reform for the insane. *American Journal of Psychiatry*, *44*(176), 176–191.

Davis, H. E., McCorkell, L., Vogel, J. M., & Topol, E. J. (2023). Long COVID: Major findings, mechanisms and recommendations. *Nature Reviews Microbiology*, *21*, 133–146.

Devoe, D., Han, A., Anderson, A., Katzman, D. K., Patten, S. B., Soumbasis, A., Flanagan, J., Paslakis, G., Vyver, E., Marcoux, G., & Dimitropoulos, G. (2023). The impact of the COVID-19 pandemic on eating disorders: A systematic review. *International Journal of Eating Disorders*, *56*(1), 5–25.

Deutsch, S. (1949). *The mentally ill in America*. Oxford University Press.

Ding, X., Wuerth, K., Sakakibara, B., Schmidt, J., Parde, N., Holsti, L., & Barbic, S. (2023). Understanding mobile health and youth mental health:

Scoping review. *JMIR mHealth and uHealth*, *11*, e44951. https://doi.org/10.2196/44951

Freud, S. (1900). Interpretation of dreams. In J. Strachey, A. Freud, A. Strachey, & A. Tyson (Eds.). (1953). *The standard edition of the complete psychological works of Sigmund Freud* (Vol. 4). Hogarth Press.

Freud, S. (1905). Three essays on the theory of sexuality. In J. Strachey, A. Freud, A. Strachey, & A. Tyson (Eds.). (1953). *The standard edition of the complete psychological works of Sigmund Freud* (pp. 135–248). Hogarth Press.

Freud, S. (1927). The ego and the id. In E. Jones (Ed.). (1957). *The international psycho-analytical library*, *N. 12*. Hogarth Press.

Foster, D. G., Biggs, M. A., Ralph, L., Gerdts, C., Roberts, S., & Glymour, M. M. (2022). Socioeconomic outcomes of women who receive and women who are denied wanted abortions in the United States", *American Journal of Public Health*, *112*(9), 1290–1296. https://doi.org/10.2105/AJPH.2017.304247

GBD 2019 Mental Disorders Collaborators. (2022). Global, regional, and national burden of 12 mental disorders in 204 countries and territories, 1990–2019: a systematic analysis for the Global Burden of Disease Study 2019. *The Lancet. Psychiatry*, *9*(2), 137–150. https://doi.org/10.1016/S2215-0366(21)00395-3

Gonzales, G., & Ehrenfeld, J. M. (2018). The association between state policy environments and self-rated health disparities for sexual minorities in the United States. *International Journal of Environmental Research Public Health*, *15*(5), 1136.

Hill, L., Artiga, S., Ranji, U., Gomez, I., and Ndugga, N. (2024). What are the implications of the Dobbs ruling for racial disparities. https://www.kff.org/racialequity-and-health-policy/issue-brief/what-are-the-implications-of-theoverturning-of-roe-v-wade-for-racial-disparities/"https://www.kff.org/racial-equity-and-health-policy/issue-brief/what-are-the-implicationsof-the-overturning-of-roe-v-wade-for-racial-disparities/

Hoagwood, K. E., Gardner, W., & Kelleher, K. J. (2021). Promoting children's mental, emotional, and behavioral (MEB) health in all public systems, Post-COVID-19. *Administration and Policy in Mental Health*, *48*, 379–387.

Hughes, T. L., Jackman, K., Dorsen, C., Arslanian-Engoren, C., Ghazal, L., Christenberry-Deceased, T., Lance Coleman, C., Mackin, M., Moore, S. E., Mukerjee, R., Sherman, A., Smith, S., & Walker, R. (2022). How can the nursing profession help reduce sexual and gender minority related health disparities. Recommendations from the national nursing LGBTQ health summit. *Nursing Outlook*, *70*(3), 513–524.

Hoy-Ellis, C. P. (2023). Minority stress and mental health: A review of the literature. *Journal of Homosexuality*, *70*(5), 806–830. https://doi.org/10.1080/00918369.2021.2004794

International Association of Psychosocial Rehabilitation. (1990). *A national directory: Organizations providing psychosocial rehabilitation and related community support services in the United States*. Center for Psychiatric Rehabilitation.

Jayawardhana, J. (2023). The impact of Medicaid expansion on mental health and substance use related inpatient visits. *The International Journal on Drug Policy*, *119*, 104140. https://doi.org/10.1016/j.drugpo.2023.104140

KFF. (2022). *Access and coverage for mental health care: Findings from the 2022 Kff Women's Health Survey*. https://www.kff.org/womens-health-policy/issue-brief/access-and-coverage-for-mental-health-care-findings-from-the-2022-kff-womens-health-survey/

KFF. (2023). *The implications of COVID-19 for mental health and substance use*. https://www.kff.org/coronavirus-covid-19/issue-brief/the-implications-of-covid-19-for-mental-health-and-substance-use/

Kim, L. H., Hodgkin, D., Larson, M. J., & Doonan, M. (2023). Changes in racial and ethnic disparities in use of mental health services under the Affordable Care Act: Evidence from California. *Journal of Mental Health Policy and Economics*, *26*(1), 19–32.

Kumar, A., Kearney, A., Hoskins, K., & Iyengar, A. (2020). The role of psychiatric mental health nurse practitioners in improving mental and behavioral health care delivery for children and adolescents in multiple settings. *Archives of Psychiatric Nursing*, *34*(5), 275–280.

Lieff, S. A., Mijanovich, T., Yang, L., & Silver, D. (2024). Impacts of the Affordable Care Act Medicaid expansion on mental health treatment among low-income adults across racial/ethnic subgroups, 2010–2017. *The Journal of Behavioral Health Services & Research*, *51*(1), 57–73. https://doi.org/10.1007/s11414-023-09861-4

Malamud, W. (1944). The history of psychiatric therapies. In J. K. Hall, G. Zilboorg, & H. Bunker (Eds.). *One hundred years of American psychiatry* (pp. 273–323). Columbia University Press.

Merle Janka, B. M., Allen, V., Blackley, G., Hare, D. J., Frank, R., & Brown, K. (2023). "I am surprised that it works so well": Clinicians' views on delivering psychological assessments and therapy to young people in a fully-digital mental health service. *The Journal of Mental Health Training, Education, and Practice*, *18*(3), 228–247. doi:https://doi.org/10.1108/JMHTEP-04-2022-0020

Mental Health American (MHA). (2023a). *The state of mental health in America*. https://mhanational.org/issues/state-mental-health-america

Mental Health America (MHA). (2023b). *LGBTQ+ Communities and Mental Health*. https://mhanational.org/issues/lgbtq-communities-and-mental-health

Melnyk, B. M., & Fineout-Overholt, E. (2023). *Evidence-based practice in nursing & healthcare: A guide to best practice* (4th ed.). Wolters Kluwer.

Mizock, L., & Brubaker, M. (2021). Treatment experiences with gender and discrimination among women with serious mental illness. *Psychological Services*, *18*(1), 64–72. https://doi.org/10.1037/ser0000346

New Freedom Commission on Mental Health. (2003). *Achieving the promise: Transforming mental health care in America (Publication No. SMA-03-3831)*. Department of Health and Human Services.

Newman, M. W., Hawrilenko, M., Jakupcak, M., Chen, S., & Fortney, J. C. (2022). Access and attitudinal barriers to engagement in integrated primary care mental health treatment for rural populations. *Journal of Rural Health*, *38*(4), 721–727.

Nightingale, F. (1859). *Notes on nursing: What it is and what it is not*. Harrison & Son.

Orlov, D., & Calixte, R. (2024). The association of sexual minority status with the prevalence, diagnosis, and treatment of depression among NYC adults. *Journal of Community Health*, *49*(6), 954–958. Advance online publication. https://doi.org/10.1007/s10900-024-01336-7

Pabayo, R., Ehntholt, A., Cook, D. M., Reynolds, M., Muennig, P., & Liu, S. Y. (2020). Laws restricting access to abortion services and infant mortality risk in the United States. *International Journal of Environmental Research and Public Health*, *17*(11), 3773. https://doi.org/10.3390/ijerph17113773

Panchai, N., Suaders, H., Rudowitz, R., & Cox, C. (2023). *The implications of COVID-19 for mental health and substance use. KFF The Independent Source for Health Policy research*, Poling and News. https://www.kff.org/coronavirus-covid-19/issue-brief/the-implications-of-covid-19-for-mental-health-and-substance-use/

Peplau, H. (1952). *Interpersonal relations in nursing*. Putnam.

Rapa, L. J., Katsiyannis, A., Scott, S. N., & Durham, O. (2024). School shootings in the United States: 1997–2022. *Pediatrics*, *153*(4), e2023064311. https://doi.org/10.1542/peds.2023-064311

Stacey, L., & Wislar, W. (2023). Physical and mental health disparities at the intersection of sexual and gender minority statuses: Evidence from population-level data. *Demography*, *60*(3), 731–760. https://doi.org/10.1215/00703370-10708592

Stotland, N. L. (2023). Reproductive rights and women's mental health. *The Psychiatric Clinics of North America*, *46*(3), 607–619. https://doi.org/10.1016/j.psc.2023.04.014

Theberath, M., Bauer, D., Chen, W., Salinas, M., Mohabbate, A. B., Yang, J., Chon, T. Y., Bauer, B. A., & Wahner-Roedler, D. L. (2022). Effects of COVID-19 pandemic on mental health of children and adolescents A systematic review of survey studies. *SAGE Open Medicine*, *10*, 20503121221086712.

U.S. Department of Health and Human Services (USDHHS). (1999). *Mental health: A report of the surgeon general*. U.S. Department of Health and Human Services, Substance Abuse and Mental Health Services Administration, Center for Mental Health Services, National Institutes of Health, National Institute of Mental Health.

U.S. Department of Health and Human Services (USDHHS). (2021). *SAMHSA awards $250 million to 100 certified community behavior health centers to improve community substance use disorder and mental health treatment plan*. https://www.aha.org/news/headline/2021-07-30-samhsa-awards-grants-expand-certified-community-behavioral-health-clinics

U.S. Department of Health and Human Services (USDHHS). (2023). Telehealth policy changes after the COVID-19 public health emergency. https://www.myamericannurse.com/micro-credentials-and-badges-in-healthcare/

U.S. Public Health Service. (2000). *Report of the Surgeon General's Conference on Children's Mental Health: A national action agenda*. Department of Health and Human Services.

Wild, J., McKinnon, A., Wilkins, A., & Browne, H. (2021). Post-traumatic stress disorder and major depression among frontline healthcare staff working during the COVID-19 pandemic. *British Journal of Clinical Psychology*, *61*(3), 859–866.

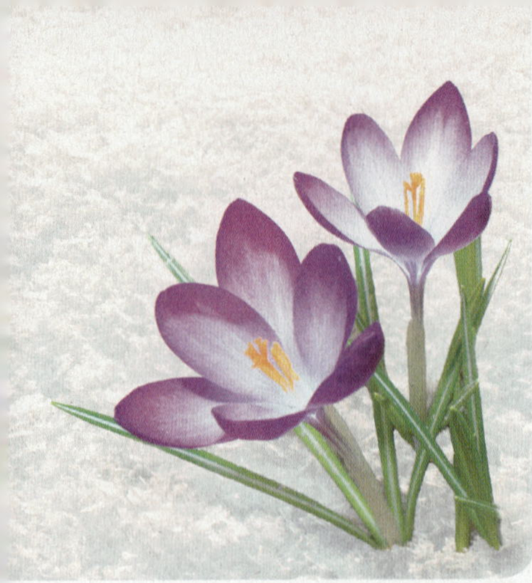

2 Mental Health and Mental Disorders

Fighting Stigma and Promoting Recovery

Rebecca Luebbert and Mary Ann Boyd

KEYCONCEPTS

- mental disorder
- mental health
- recovery
- resilience
- social determinants of health
- stigma
- trauma
- wellness

LEARNING OBJECTIVES

After studying this chapter, you will be able to:

1. Relate the concept of mental health to wellness.
2. Identify the rationale for promoting wellness for people with mental health challenges.
3. Differentiate the concepts of mental health and mental illness.
4. Discuss the factors contributing to behavioral health inequity.
5. Identify social determinants of health influencing mental health and mental illness.
6. Discuss the significance of epidemiologic evidence in studying the occurrence of mental disorders.
7. Describe the consequences of the stigma of mental illness on individuals and families.
8. Describe the impact of resiliency in recovery.
9. Identify recovery components and their role in the treatment of mental illness.
10. Discuss the impact of adverse childhood experiences on mental health.
11. Discuss the role of trauma-informed approaches in recovery-oriented nursing practice.

KEY TERMS

• adverse childhood experiences • behavioral health equity • *DSM-5-TR* • epidemiology • incidence • label avoidance • othering • point prevalence • prevalence • public stigma • racial trauma • rate • recovery-oriented care • resilience • self-stigma • trauma-informed approach

INTRODUCTION

To understand health and illness in any practice area, nurses need a basic understanding of mental health and its relationship with wellness. This chapter discusses concepts of mental health and wellness, the diagnosis of mental disorders, inequities, and disparities among historically minoritized groups, how the stigma of mental illness can be a barrier to treatment, and the importance of focusing on recovery from mental illness.

MENTAL HEALTH AND WELLNESS

Mental health is defined as a state of well-being in which the individual realizes their own abilities, can cope with life's usual stresses, can work productively and fruitfully, and can contribute to society. Mental health is essential to personal well-being, interpersonal relationships, and contributing to the community. An individual cannot be healthy without being *mentally* healthy, but it is possible to be mentally healthy and have a mental or physical disorder (World Health Organization [WHO], 2022). With mental health treatment, including therapy, medication, and self-care, recovery is a reality for most people experiencing mental illness (NAMI, 2023).

> **KEYCONCEPT Mental health** includes our emotional, psychological, and social well-being. It affects how we think, feel, and act. It also helps determine how we handle stress, relate to others, and make choices. Mental health is important at every stage of life, from childhood and adolescence through adulthood (U.S. DHHS, SAMHSA, 2022, 2023a).

Mental health is an essential piece of total wellness. The concept of wellness encompasses both physical and mental health. Issues in one area impact the other area. Wellness is not the absence of disease or stress; it involves having a purpose in life, being actively involved in satisfying work and play, having joyful relationships, having a healthy body and living environment, and being happy. It includes the mental, emotional, physical, occupational, intellectual, and spiritual aspects of an individual's life (U.S. Department of Health and Human Services, Substance Abuse and Mental Health Services Administration [U.S. DHHS, SAMHSA], 2016) (see Fig. 2.1).

> **KEYCONCEPT Wellness** is being in good physical and mental health. Improving physical health can benefit mental health, and vice versa. Wellness is not the absence of disease. There are eight dimensions of wellness: emotional, financial, social, spiritual, occupational, physical, intellectual, and environmental (U.S. DHHS, SAMHSA, 2016). See Figure 2.1.

Mental health issues significantly impact the process of wellness, as mental illness can impact physical health

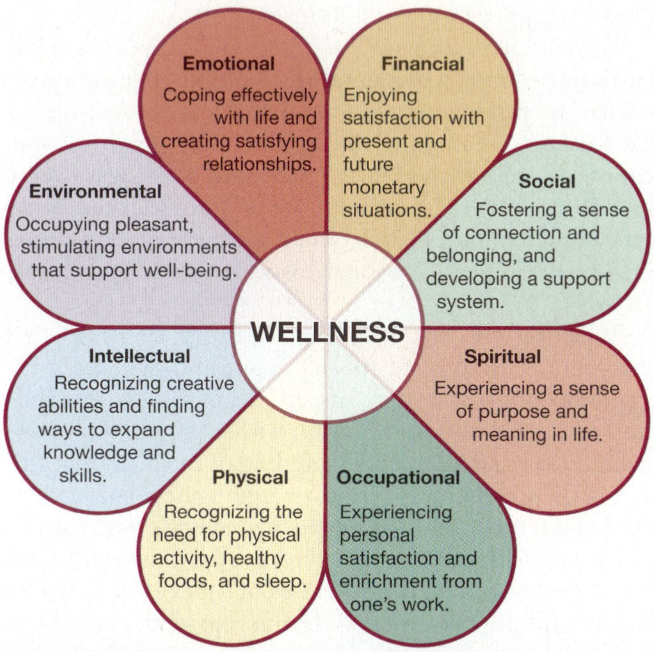

FIGURE 2.1 Eight dimensions of wellness. (Adapted from U.S. DHHS, SAMHSA. [2016]. *Learn the eight dimensions of wellness.* SMA16-4958. https://store.samhsa.gov/sites/default/files/d7/priv/sma16-4958.pdf)

as well. For example, research has found that individuals with depression have a 40% higher risk of developing cardiovascular and metabolic diseases than the general population. A third of adults with mental illness also experience a substance use disorder (NAMI, 2023). Although many evidence-based treatments exist for mental illnesses, there is a significant gap in mental health services. A shortage of mental health providers, a fragmented behavioral health system, and persistent stigma contribute to barriers in treatment (McGinty, 2023).

In recent years, stressors associated with the COVID-19 pandemic have increased psychological distress, anxiety, and depression worldwide. Socially or economically marginalized groups, including racial and ethnic minorities, women and LGBTQ+ communities, individuals in poverty, immigrants and migrants, children and individuals with a history of childhood adversity, and people in social isolation were disproportionally affected by COVID-19, experiencing greater mental health challenges (Parenteau et al., 2023). Throughout the pandemic, disparities in socioeconomic disparities between racial groups worsened (Lopez et al., 2021). Consistent with previous public health crises, Black Americans were disproportionally affected by COVID-19, experiencing higher hospitalization and mortality rates. People of color have been more severely affected by rises in overdose and suicide deaths (Pachal et al., 2024).

Behavioral Health Equity

People with serious mental health issues often face social, economic, and/or environmental disadvantages that result in lack of access to health care, lack of information, and lack of culturally and linguistically competent care and programs (Gnanapragasam et al., 2023). Racial and ethnic inequalities in mental health treatment also exist, with underrepresented ethnic groups having higher unmet mental health needs than White Americans (Thomeer et al., 2023). People of color are less likely to receive mental health services. Barriers to accessing services include cost, uncertainty of where to obtain care, and limited provider options. People of color face additional barriers, including lack of diversity of care providers, insufficient culturally informed treatment options, stereotypes, and discrimination associated with mental illness (Pachal et al., 2024; Rice & Harris, 2021). Structural and cultural racism contribute to the worsening of these inequalities. Mental health is a basic human right. **Behavioral health equity** is the right of all individuals, regardless of race, age, ethnicity, gender, disability, socioeconomic status, sexual orientation, or geographical location, to access high-quality and affordable health care and support (Substance Abuse and Mental Health Services Administration [SAMHSA], 2023b). Eliminating the persistent disparities in health require expanded access to health care, establishing equitable care models, and addressing the social determinants of health (Lopez et al., 2021).

Social Determinants of Health

Advancing behavioral health equity requires addressing the social determinants of health, racial/ethnic disparities, service access barriers, and language access barriers, as all of these have an impact on mental health outcomes (SAMHSA, 2023b). The presence of mental health inequities will be illustrated in future chapters throughout this textbook.

> **KEYCONCEPT Social determinants of health (SDOH)** are conditions in the places where people live, learn, work, and play that affect a wide range of health risks and outcomes (Office of Disease Prevention and Health Promotion, U.S. DHHS, 2023; Centers for Disease Control and Prevention [CDC], 2021).

The U.S. Department of Health and Human Services, Office of Disease Prevention and Health Promotion outlines five key areas of SDOH: health care access and quality, education access and quality, social and community context, economic stability, and neighborhood and built environment (2023). See Figure 2.2. SDOH contribute to health disparities and inequities, and have been shown to have a greater impact on health outcomes than either genetic factors or access to health services (CDC, 2022).

The COVID-19 pandemic, which was declared by the Centers for Disease Control and Prevention in March 2020, made the issues of health disparities even more evident. Social and cultural factors not only contribute to illness, but also impact how an individual experiencing illness responds and seeks help (Gnanapragasam et al., 2023). Studies show that racial and ethnic underrepresented groups have less access to mental health services and are more likely to receive inadequate care (Gnanapragasam et al., 2023; Thomeer et al., 2023). Healthy People 2030 prioritizes the need to "create social, physical, and economic environments that promote attaining the full potential for health and well-being for all" (Office of Disease Prevention and Health Promotion, U.S. DHHS, 2023).

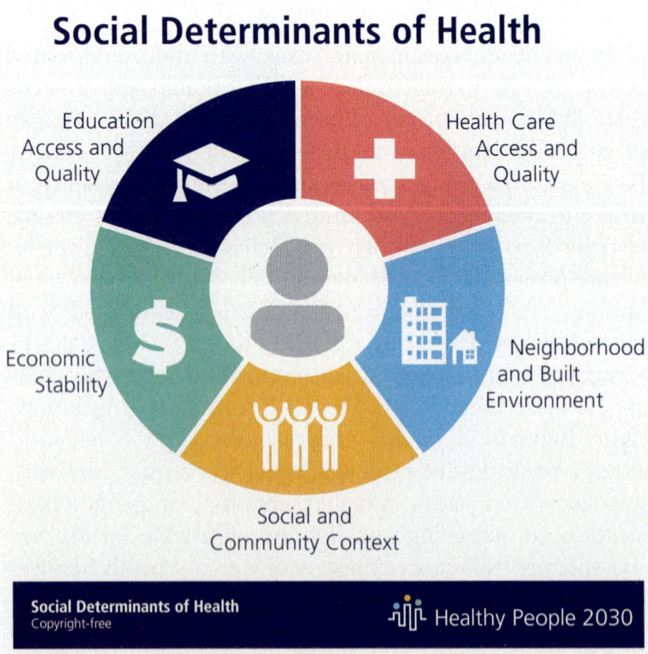

FIGURE 2.2 Social determinants of health. (Office of Disease Prevention and Health Promotion, U.S. DHHS, 2023.)

OVERVIEW OF MENTAL HEALTH DISORDERS

Mental disorders can disrupt mental health and result in one of the most common causes of disability. In this text, the terms *mental disorder*, *mental health disorder*, and *mental illness* will be used interchangeably.

> **KEYCONCEPT** A **mental disorder** is a syndrome characterized by clinically significant disturbance in an individual's cognition, emotion regulation, or behavior that reflects a dysfunction in the psychological, biologic, or developmental processes underlying mental functioning. Mental disorders are usually associated with significant distress or disability in social, occupational, or other important activities (American Psychiatric Association [APA], 2022).

A mental illness or mental disorder is a syndrome, a set of symptoms that cluster together that may have multiple causes and may represent several different disease states that have not yet been defined. Unlike many medical diseases, mental disorders are defined by clusters of behaviors, thoughts, and feelings, not by underlying biologic pathology. In general, laboratory tests are not used in diagnosing mental disorders.

The landmark study *Global Burden of Disease 2010* found an alarming impact of mental and behavioral disorders on health and productivity in the world. Depression is one of the leading disease burdens in middle- and high-income countries such as the United States. In 2021, just over 1 in 5 US adults (57.8 million people) experienced some type of mental illness, and 1 in 20 adults experienced serious mental illness (National Institute of Mental Health [NIMH], 2023).

Evidence for this very high occurrence of mental disorders is established through epidemiologic research. **Epidemiology**, the study of patterns of disease distribution and determinants of health within populations, contributes to the overall understanding of the mental health status of population groups, or aggregates, and associated factors. Epidemiologic studies examine associations among possible factors related to an area of investigation, but they do not determine causes of illnesses. The CDC tracks and reports mental health epidemiologic data. Throughout this book, epidemiologic data, including inequities in mental health care, are included in discussions of mental health issues and mental disorders. See Box 2.1 for an explanation of terms.

BOX 2.1

Epidemiologic Terms

In epidemiology, certain terms have specific meanings relative to what they measure. When expressing the number of cases of a disorder, population rates, rather than raw numbers, are used.

Rate is the proportion of the cases in the population when compared with the total population. It is expressed as a fraction, in which the numerator is the number of cases, and the denominator is the total number in the population, including the cases and noncases. The term average rate is used for measures that involve rates over specified time periods:

$$\text{Rate} = \frac{\text{Case in population}}{\text{Total population (cases and non-cases)}}$$

Prevalence refers to the total number of people who have the disorder within a given population at a specified time regardless of how long ago the disorder started.

Point prevalence is a basic measure that refers to the proportion of individuals in the population who have the disorder at a specified point in time (t). This point can be a day on the calendar, such as April 1, 2027, or a point defined in relation to the study assessment, such as the day of the interview. This is also expressed as a fraction:

$$\text{Point prevalence rate} = \frac{\text{Cases at } t}{\text{Population at } t}$$

Incidence refers to a rate that includes only new cases that have occurred within a clearly defined time. The most common time evaluated is 1 year. A study of incidence cases is more difficult than a study of prevalent cases because a study of incidence cases requires at least two measurements to be taken: one at the start of the prescribed time and another at the end of it.

Diagnosis of Mental Health Conditions

Mental disorders are organized and diagnosed according to the criteria published in the *Diagnostic and Statistical Manual of Mental Disorders, Fifth Edition, Text Revision (DSM-5-TR;* APA, 2022*)*. The current ***DSM-5-TR*** system contains subtypes and other specifiers that further classify disorders. Although the *DSM-5-TR* specifies criteria for diagnosing mental disorders, there are no absolute boundaries separating one disorder from another, and disorders often have different manifestations at different points in time.

In a mental disorder, alterations in behaviors, thoughts, and feelings are unexpected and are outside usual culturally defined limits. If a behavior is considered typical within a specific culture, it is not viewed as a psychiatric symptom. For example, members of some religious groups "speak in tongues." To an observer, it appears that the individuals are hallucinating (see Chapter 24), but this behavior is typical for this group within a particular setting.

The amount of disability or impairment in functioning is an important consideration when assessing an individual with a mental disorder. The ability to understand, communicate, and get along with others is important in the recovery process. If symptoms impair an individual's ability to independently perform self-care and daily activities, recovery will be more difficult. The WHO's Disability Assessment Schedule 2.0 is an instrument that can be used for measuring the amount of impairment that the individual experiences.

STIGMA

Stigma is a persistent major barrier to treatment, recovery, and social integration for individuals with mental health issues. Social stereotypes, culture, prejudices, and lack of knowledge and understanding surrounding mental illness contribute to the discrimination and human rights violations experienced by people living with mental illness. Stigma impacts the importance given to an individual's complaints related to mental health, access to adequate mental health care, and the likelihood that treatment for their mental health concerns will be pursued (Mahdanian et al., 2023; Torales et al., 2023). Individuals may be less likely to pursue treatment because of perceived stigma or a history of negative experiences, even with their health care providers. Examples of stigma by a health care provider include making assumptions about the person, suggesting blame for a health issue, not being responsive to requests, or withholding needed medication (Pachal et al., 2024). Public stigma, self-stigma, and label avoidance are three types of stigma people with mental illnesses experience.

> **KEYCONCEPT Stigma** is a dynamic social/interactional process in which the individual who is stigmatized is labeled as different and linked to negative stereotypes. People with stigmatizing beliefs socially distance themselves from the individual who is stigmatized.

Public Stigma

Public stigma occurs after individuals are publicly "marked" as having a mental illness. When they act or say things that are odd or unusual or tell others that they have a mental illness, these individuals are at risk of being subjected to prejudice and discrimination. Stigma and discrimination is particularly severe for individuals with serious mental illness, such as schizophrenia. Common stereotypes include being incompetent, incurable, violent, and dangerous. These stereotypes are neither justified nor based on evidence and inevitably lead to discrimination and coercive practices, such as involuntary hospitalization, overmedicating, and arbitrary legal incapacitation. Ultimately, this deep-rooted stigma leads to a reduction in an individual's access to meaningful social relationships, independent living, job opportunities, and overall autonomy (Mahdanian et al., 2023; Torales et al., 2023).

When people with mental illnesses or emotional issues are stigmatized by society, they are often ostracized by the society in which they live. The stigma associated with all forms of mental illness is strong but generally increases the more an individual's behavior differs from the cultural norm. Reducing stigma has been identified as a public health priority.

Media perpetuates the stigma of mental disorders and treatment. News coverage often associates mental illness with violence, fear, and madness (Pavlova & Berkers, 2022). Few media sources describe successful treatment or recovery. In films, psychiatric hospitals are often portrayed as dangerous and unwelcoming places, as in *The Snake Pit* (1948), *One Flew Over the Cuckoo's Nest* (1975), *Instinct* (1999), *Twelve Monkeys* (1995), *Sling Blade* (1996), *Girl, Interrupted* (1999), *Don Juan Demarco* (1994), *A Beautiful Mind* (2001), and *Analyze That* (2002). Nurses are dressed in white in contrast to the dark, gloomy surroundings, and patients seemingly have little to do other than to walk the halls of the institution, acting odd.

One of the best ways to counteract the negative effects of stigma is to have contact with the group that is stigmatized (Diouf et al., 2022). Another way is to use nonstigmatizing language. Just as a person with diabetes mellitus should not be referred to as "a diabetic" but rather as "an individual with diabetes," a person with a mental disorder should never be referred to as "a schizophrenic" or "bipolar" but rather as "an individual with schizophrenia" or "an individual with bipolar disorder." Jokes that depict people with mental illness as stupid, dangerous, or incompetent perpetuate negative myths. Strategies for therapeutic communication and building trust are discussed in Chapter 9.

Self-Stigma

Self-stigma occurs when negative stereotypes are internalized by people with mental illness. **Othering** can occur when people with mental illness perceive themselves as different and inferior from those without illness. Othering contributes to stigma and discrimination. Patients are aware of the public's negative view of mental illness and agree with the public's perceptions. As they become aware of the negative stereotypes, they begin agreeing with the stereotype. Then they may begin applying the stigma to themselves: "I have a mental illness, so I must be incompetent." As a result of the application of the negative stereotype to self, the patient develops low self-esteem. Othering can worsen psychological distress and can negatively impact relationships, help-seeking behaviors, therapeutic outcomes, and overall well-being (Allchin & Isobel, 2024; Bhugra et al., 2023).

Label Avoidance

Label avoidance, which is avoiding treatment or care in order not to be labeled as being mentally ill, is another type of stigma and one of the reasons that so few people with mental health issues receive help. By avoiding treatment, they avoid the stigma of mental illness. Talking about mental health is often considered a "taboo." Consequently, individuals may ignore their symptoms or refuse to seek treatment because of the stigma associated with being mentally ill (Ventriglio et al., 2022).

RECOVERY FROM MENTAL ILLNESS

Recovery is the single most important goal for individuals with mental disorders. The following definition of recovery was released following a lengthy consensus-seeking process that began in 2010 and involved government agency officials, experts, consumers, family members, advocates, researchers, managed care representatives, and others.

> **KEYCONCEPT Recovery** from mental disorders and/or substance use disorders is a process of change through which individuals improve their health and wellness, live a self-directed life, and strive to reach their full potential (U.S. DHHS, SAMHSA, 2020, 2023c).

Recovery-oriented treatment is based on the belief that mental illnesses and challenges are treatable, and that recovery is an expectation. There are four dimensions that support recovery: *health* (managing disease and living in a physically and emotionally healthy way), *home* (a safe and stable place to live), *purpose* (meaningful daily activities and independence, resources, and income), and *community* (relationships and social networks) (U.S. DHHS, SAMHSA, 2023c). Consumers and families have real and meaningful choices about treatment options and providers. In **recovery-oriented care,** people with mental health issues develop a partnership with a clinician to manage the illness, strengthen coping abilities, and build **resilience** for life's challenges (Box 2.2). Resilience refers to the ability to cope with change and adversity. Resilience is dynamic, developing over time. It varies from individual to individual and is impacted by both environmental and personal factors (SAMHSA, 2023d). Resilience can act as a protective factor and temper the effects of stressful life effects. People with higher resilience tend to report fewer mental health symptoms (Watters et al., 2023).

Mental health recovery benefits not only the individual and family but also society by ultimately reducing the global burden of mental health issues. Recovery is guided by 10 fundamental principles (Box 2.3). See Chapter 8 for further discussion of recovery.

Recovery-Oriented Care and Trauma-Informed Approaches

Mental health professionals increasingly focus on the harmful effects of trauma on both physical and mental

BOX 2.2

Research for Best Practice: Association Between Adverse Childhood Experiences and Mental Disorders

Sahle, B. W., Reavley, N. J., Li, W., Morgan, A. J., Yap, M. B. H., Reupert, A., & Jorm, A. F. (2022). The association between adverse childhood experiences and common mental disorders and suicidality: An umbrella review of systematic reviews and meta-analysis. European Child & Adolescent Psychiatry, 31, *1489–1499.*

THE QUESTION: What are the key adverse childhood experiences (ACEs) that are consistently associated with increased risk of mental disorders and suicidality?

METHODS: An umbrella review of systematic reviews and meta-analyses on the association between ACEs and common mental disorders or suicidality was completed using PsycINFO, PubMed, and Google Scholar. Sixty-eight articles published between January 2009 and July 2019 were included. The methodologic quality of reviews was evaluated using the AMSTAR2 checklist.

FINDINGS: Twenty-four ACEs were significantly associated with increased risk of anxiety disorders, internalizing disorders, depression, or suicidality. The most frequently occurring ACEs included childhood maltreatment (including physical abuse, sexual abuse, and maladaptive parenting), bullying, parental mental illness, and inter-parental conflict. Low socioeconomic status, discrimination, exposure to violence, and parental incarceration were also associated with one of the four outcomes.

IMPLICATIONS FOR NURSING: Identification of risk factors for ACEs is important. Preventative interventions may reduce the substantial burden of mental disorders and suicidality. Interventions may include promoting healthy caregiving, strengthening economic support to families, providing quality care and education in early life, mental health treatment, and social service referrals.

health. Individuals who experience trauma, particularly in childhood, have a higher incidence of mental disorders (see Box 2.2). **Adverse childhood experiences** (ACEs) are defined as potentially traumatic events occurring in childhood (0 to 17 years). Examples of ACEs include a child witnessing or experiencing violence, abuse, or neglect, or having a family member attempt or die by suicide. Growing up with family members who have substance use or mental health issues, or living in an unstable household due to caregiver separation or incarceration, may also contribute to ACEs. ACEs are common, with 64% of US adults reporting having experienced at least one type of ACE, and one in six reporting having experienced four or more types of ACEs (CDC, 2023). ACEs are preventable. Prevention requires addressing SDOH. Identifying families at high risk for ACEs is critical and includes assessment of individual, family, and community risk factors (Kameg, 2023).

Another common form of trauma found in the United States, Canada, and most Western nations is **racial trauma**, the development of mental disorder after a traumatic or stressful event due to perceived race or ethnicity. There is a documented link between racism and posttraumatic stress disorder. Racial trauma has also been linked

BOX 2.3

Guiding Principles of Recovery

Recovery emerges from hope: The belief that recovery is real provides the essential and motivating message of a better future—that people can and do overcome the internal and external challenges, barriers, and obstacles that confront them.

Recovery is person driven: Self-determination and self-direction are the foundations for recovery, as individuals define their own life goals and design their unique path(s).

Recovery occurs via many pathways: Individuals are unique with distinct needs, strengths, preferences, goals, culture, and backgrounds, including trauma experiences that affect and determine their pathway(s) to recovery. Abstinence is the safest approach for those with substance use disorders.

Recovery is holistic: Recovery encompasses an individual's whole life, including mind, body, spirit, and community. The array of services and supports available should be integrated and coordinated.

Recovery is supported by peers and allies: Mutual support and mutual aid groups, including the sharing of experiential knowledge and skills, as well as social learning, play an invaluable role in recovery.

Recovery is supported through relationship and social networks: An important factor in the recovery process is the presence and involvement of people who believe in the person's ability to recover; who offer hope, support, and encouragement; and who also suggest strategies and resources for change.

Recovery is culturally based and influenced: Culture and cultural background in all of its diverse representations including values, traditions, and beliefs are key in determining a person's journey and unique pathway to recovery.

Recovery is supported by addressing trauma: Services and supports should be trauma informed to foster safety (physical and emotional) and trust as well as to promote choice, empowerment, and collaboration.

Recovery involves individual, family, and community strengths and responsibility: Individuals, families, and communities have strengths and resources that serve as a foundation for recovery.

Recovery is based on respect: Community, systems, and societal acceptance and appreciation for people affected by mental health and substance use issues—including protecting their rights and eliminating discrimination—are crucial in achieving recovery.

Adapted from U.S. DHHS, SAMHSA. (2023c). *Recovery and recovery support.*

to depressive disorder, social anxiety disorder, substances use disorders, and psychosis (Holmes et al., 2024).

> **KEYCONCEPT Trauma** results from an event, a series of events, or a set of circumstances experienced by an individual as physically or emotionally harmful or life threatening and that has lasting adverse effects on the individual's functioning and mental, physical, social, emotional, or spiritual well-being (U.S. DHHS, SAMHSA, 2023d).

A **trauma-informed approach** is integral to recovery-oriented nursing care for people with emotional issues and mental disorders. Adopting a trauma-informed approach requires shifting the focus from "what is wrong with you?" to "what has happened to you?" (Center for Health Care Strategies, 2021). Trauma-informed approaches seek to:

- Realize the widespread impact of trauma and understand paths for recovery.
- Recognize signs and symptoms of trauma in patients, families, and those involved in their care.
- Integrate knowledge about trauma into policies, procedures, and practices.
- Actively resist re-traumatization.

Six principles of a trauma-informed approach include: safety, trustworthiness and transparency, peer support, collaboration and mutuality, empowerment, and cultural, historical, and gender issues (SAMHSA, 2023d). See Table 2.1. Trauma-informed practices should consider the impact of the individual's resilience in being able to successfully adapt from traumatic experiences (Watters et al., 2023).

TABLE 2.1 SIX PRINCIPLES OF A TRAUMA-INFORMED APPROACH

Safety	Safety in physical settings and interpersonal interactions
Trustworthiness and Transparency	Operations are conducted and decisions are made with transparency, consistency, respect, and fairness so as to build and maintain trust.
Peer Support	Support from those with lived experiences of trauma or, in case of children with history of trauma, their family members.
Collaboration and Mutuality	Partnering, leveling of power differences between and among staff and patients
Empowerment	Individuals' strengths and experiences are recognized and built upon
Cultural, Historical, and Gender Issues	Organization moves beyond the cultural stereotypes and biases

Source: U.S. Department of Health and Human Services, Substance Abuse and Mental Health Services Administration (U.S. DHHS, SAMHSA). (2023d). *Practical guide for implementing a trauma-informed approach.* p. 18. SAMHSA Publication No. PEP23-06-05-005. National Mental Health and Substance Use Policy Laboratory.

Individuals with mental illnesses can regain mental health with the support of families, mental health providers, and society. The contributions of these individuals strengthen communities and support the overall health of a nation.

SUMMARY OF KEY POINTS

- Mental health is the emotional and psychological well-being of an individual. To be mentally healthy means that one can interact with others, deal with daily stress, and perceive the world realistically. Mental disorders are health conditions characterized by alterations in thinking, mood, or behavior and are associated with distress or impaired functioning.
- Good physical and mental health characterize wellness. Individuals can have a mental disorder and experience wellness.
- Epidemiology is important to understanding the distribution of mental illness and determinants of health within a given population. The rate of occurrence refers to the proportion of the population that has the disorder. Incidence is the rate of new cases within a specified time. Prevalence is the rate of occurrence of all cases at a particular point in time.
- SDOH and provider bias contribute to health disparities and inequities and must be addressed in order to advance behavioral health equity.
- Stigma toward mental illness can be viewed in three ways. Public stigma marks a person as having a mental illness. When an individual with a mental illness shares the public's negative view of mental illness, self-stigma occurs. If the individual with a mental illness does not seek treatment because of fear of being labeled "mentally ill," label avoidance occurs.
- The *DSM-5-TR* organizes psychiatric diagnoses according to behaviors and symptom patterns.
- Mental health recovery is the single most important goal for the mental health delivery system. Recovery is viewed as a process of changes through which individuals improve their health and wellness, live a self-directed life, and strive to reach their full potential.
- ACEs are common, yet preventable. Identifying families at higher risk for ACEs requires addressing the SDOH is critical in mitigating negative outcomes.
- Trauma is experienced by many individuals as physically or emotionally harmful or life threatening and has lasting adverse effects on the individual. Trauma-informed approaches are integral to recovery-oriented care.

DEVELOPING CLINICAL JUDGMENT

1. An individual who is seeking help for a mental disorder asks why physical health is important to the nurse.
2. How do the SDOH contribute to behavioral health inequity? What might the nurse do to address these inequities?
3. How does resilience impact recovery?
4. Examine how family and friends describe people with mental illness. Do you think their description of mental illness is based on fact or myth? Explain.
5. Discuss the negative impact of labeling someone with a psychiatric diagnosis.
6. Using the components of mental health recovery as a framework, compare the goals for an individual with schizophrenia with the goals for an individual with a medical disease such as diabetes.
7. Discuss the application of trauma-informed approaches with a patient who has experienced multiple ACEs.

MOVIES, TV, OR STREAMING PROGRAMS

***Mysteries of Mental Illness:* Episode 2; Who's Normal? (2021).** This episode is the second of four in the PBS documentary series. (Episode 1 is featured in Chapter 1.) In Episode 2, the filmmakers describe the evolution of diagnosing mental disorders and the introduction of the *Diagnostic and Statistical Manual of Mental Disorders (DSM)*. The viewer will see how deeply entwined science and societal factors have been in defining and diagnosing mental illness over the years. Although diagnostic reliability increased when the DSM-III provided standardized definitions and criteria for diagnoses, because there are no biologic tests to diagnose mental illness, there remains a level of interpretation and subjectivity when determining a diagnosis. The boundary between "normal" and "illness" is very fluid.

Viewing Points:

1. The *DSM-5-TR* provides diagnoses by symptoms, not biology. What are the implications of this system?
2. Are psychiatric labels helpful or harmful?
3. How might a psychiatric diagnosis contribute to stigma?

Unfolding Patient Stories: Sandra Littlefield • Part 1

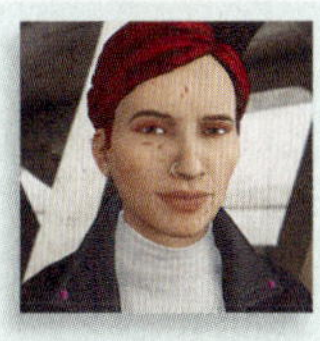

Sandra Littlefield is a 36-year-old diagnosed with borderline personality disorder. Her history includes several divorces, substance use disorder, poor impulse control, anxiety, cutting, suicide attempts, prostitution, and incarceration. How could her diagnosis of borderline personality disorder create a stereotype and bias even before the health care team meets her? How might the stigma of mental illness affect her as an inmate, in the community, and with recovery. How might Sandra's behavior be influenced by internalizing how others may perceive her? (Sandra Littlefield's story continues in Chapter 23.)

Care for Sandra Littlefield and other patients in a realistic virtual environment: ***vSim** for Nursing* (thepoint.lww.com/vSimMentalHealth). Practice documenting these patients' care in DocuCare (thepoint.lww.com/DocuCareEHR).

REFERENCES

Allchin, B., & Isobel, S. (2024). Re-imagining the vulnerability and risk framing of parents with mental illness and their children. *Frontiers in Public Health, 12*, 1373603.

American Psychiatric Association (APA). (2022). *Diagnostic and statistical manual of mental disorders* (5th ed., text rev.). Author.

Bhugra, D., Smith, A., Liebrenz, M., Ventriglio, A., Gnanapragasam, S. N., Buadze, A., Pemberton, M., & Poulter, D. (2023). "Otherness," otherism, discrimination, and health inequalities: Entrenched challenges for modern psychiatric disciplines. *International Review of Psychiatry, 35*(3–4), 234–241.

Centers for Disease Control and Prevention. (2022). Why is addressing social determinants of health important for CDC and public health? Retrieved August 12, 2023, from https://www.cdc.gov/about/sdoh/addressing-sdoh.html#:~:text=SDOH%20have%20been%20shown%20to%20have%20a%20greater,drivers%20of%20health%20inequities%20within%20communities%20of%20color

Centers for Disease Control and Prevention. (2023). Fast facts: Preventing adverse childhood experiences. Retrieved August 22, 2023, from https://www.cdc.gov/violenceprevention/aces/fastfact.html

Center for Health Care Strategies. (2021). What is trauma informed care? Retrieved August 22, 2023, from https://www.traumainformedcare.chcs.org/what-is-trauma-informed-care/

Diouf, F., Lemley, B., Barth, C., Goldbarg, J., Helgenberger, S., Grimm, B., Wartella, E., Smyser, J., & Bonnevie, E. (2022). Mental health stigma reduction in the midwestern United States: Evidence from a digital campaign using a collective impact model. *Journal of Community Health, 47*(6), 924–931.

Gnanapragasam, S. N., Wright, L. A., Pemberton, M., & Bhugra, D. (2023). Outside/inside: Social determinants of mental health. *Irish Journal of Psychological Medicine, 40*, 63–73.

Holmes, S. C., Zare, M., Haeny, A. M., & Williams, M. T. (2024). Racial stress, racial trauma, and evidence-based strategies for coping and empowerment. *Annual Review of Clinical Psychology, 20*(1), 77–95. https://doi.org/10.1146/annurev-clinpsy-081122-020235

Kameg, B. (2023). Adverse childhood experiences: An update on preventative and treatment interventions. *The Journal for Nurse Practitioners, 19*, 104482.

Lopez, L., Hart, L. H., & Katz, M. H. (2021). Racial and ethnic health disparities related to COVID-19. *Journal of the American Medical Association, 325*(8), 719–720.

Mahdanian, A. A., Laporta, M., Bold, N. D., Funk, M., & Puras, D. (2023). Human rights in mental healthcare: A review of current global situation. *International Review of Psychiatry, 35*(2), 150–162.

McGinty, B. (2023). The future of public mental health: Challenges and opportunities. *Milbank Quarterly, 101*(S1), 532–551.

National Alliance on Mental Illness. (2023). Mental health by the numbers. Retrieved August 12, 2023, from https://nami.org/mhstats

National Institute of Mental Health (NIMH). (2023). *Mental health by the numbers*. Retrieved August 12, 2023, from https://nami.org/mhstats

Office of Disease Prevention and Health Promotion, U.S. Department of Health and Human Services (U.S. DHHS). (2023). *Social determinants of health. Healthy People 2030*. Retrieved August 12, 2023, from https://health.gov/healthypeople/priority-areas/social-determinants-health

Pachal, N., Hill, L., Artiga, S., & Hamel, L. (2024). Racial and ethnic disparities in mental health care: Findings from the KFF survey of racism, discrimination, and health. https://www.kff.org/racial-equity-and-health-policy/issue-brief/racial-and-ethnic-disparities-in-mental-health-care-findings-from-the-kff-survey-of-racism-discrimination-and-health/

Parenteau, A. M., Boyer, C. J., Campos, L. J., Carranza, A. F., Deer, L. K., Hartman, D. T., Bidwell, J. T., & Hostinar, C. E. (2023). A review of mental health disparities during COVID-19: Evidence, mechanisms, and policy recommendations for promoting societal resilience. *Development and Psychopathology*, *35*(4), 1821–1842.

Pavlova, A., & Berkers, P. (2022). "Mental health" as defined by Twitter: Frames, emotions, stigma. *Health Communication*, 37(5), 637–647.

Rice, A. N., & Harris, S. C. (2021). Issues of cultural competence in mental health care. *Journal of the American Pharmacists Association*, *61*(1), e65–e68.

Thomeer, M. B., Moody, M. D., & Yahirun, J. (2023). Racial and ethnic disparities in mental health and mental health care during the COVID-19 pandemic. *Journal of Racial and Ethnic Health Disparities, 10*, 961–976.

Torales, J., Aveiro-Robalo, T. R., Rios-Gonzalez, C., Barrios, I., Almiron-Santacruz, J., Gonzalez-Urbieta, I., Caycho-Rodriguez, T., Castaldelli-Maia, J. M., & Ventriglio, A. (2023). Discrimination, stigma and mental health: What's next? *International Review of Psychiatry*, *35*(3–4), 242–250.

U.S. Department of Health and Human Services, Substance Abuse and Mental Health Services Administration (U.S. DHHS, SAMHSA). (2016). *Learn the eight dimensions of wellness.* SMA 16–4958. https://store.samhsa.gov/sites/default/files/d7/images/sma16-4958.jpg

U.S. Department of Health and Human Services, Substance Abuse and Mental Health Services Administration (U.S. DHHS, SAMHSA). (2023a). *What is mental health?* Retrieved August 12, 2023, from https://www.samhsa.gov/mental-health

U.S. Department of Health and Human Services, Substance Abuse and Mental Health Services Administration (U.S. DHHS, SAMHSA). (2023b). *Behavioral health equity.* Retrieved August 7, 2023, from https://www.samhsa.gov/behavioral-health-equity

U.S. Department of Health and Human Services, Substance Abuse and Mental Health Services Administration (U.S. DHHS, SAMHSA). (2023c). *Recovery and recovery support.* Retrieved August 13, 2023, from https://www.samhsa.gov/find-help/recovery

U.S. Department of Health and Human Services, Substance Abuse and Mental Health Services Administration (U.S. DHHS, SAMHSA). (2023d). *Practical guide for implementing a trauma-informed approach.* SAMHSA Publication No. PEP23-06-05-005. National Mental Health and Substance Use Policy Laboratory.

Ventriglio, A., Castaldelli-Maia, J. M., Torales, J., Chumakov, E., De Berardis, D., & Bhugra, D. (2022). New approaches for mental health of social minorities. *International Review of Psychiatry*, *34*(7–8), 760–769.

Watters, E. R., Aloe, A. M., & Wojciak, A. S. (2023). Examining the associations between childhood trauma, resilience, and depression: A multivariate meta-analysis. *Trauma, Violence, and Abuse*, *24*(1), 231–244.

World Health Organization (WHO). (2022). *Mental health.* Retrieved August 12, 2023, from https://www.who.int/news-room/fact-sheets/detail/mental-health-strengthening-our-response

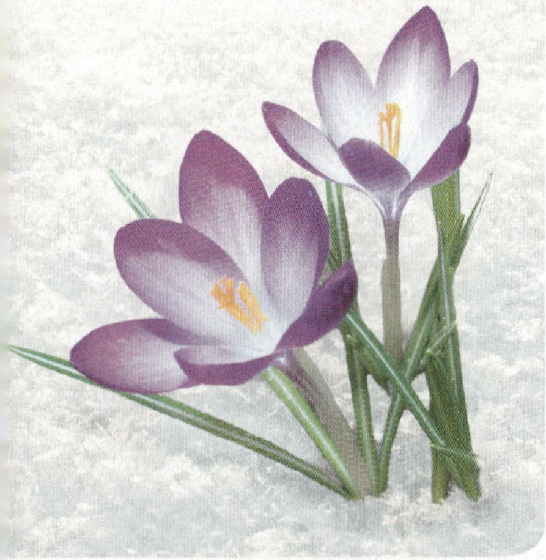

3 Cultural, Gender, Sexual, Social, and Spiritual/Religious Considerations

Sheri Compton-McBride

KEYCONCEPTS

- Cultural competence
- Cultural humility
- Cultural identity
- Culture
- Gender
- Gender identity
- Health literacy
- Intersectionality
- Sexuality
- Sexual orientation
- Spirituality

LEARNING OBJECTIVES

After studying this chapter, you will be able to:

1. Discuss the ways that cultural competence and cultural humility are demonstrated in psychiatric–mental health nursing.
2. Describe the beliefs about mental health and illness in different cultural and cross-cultural groups.
3. Explore the impact of gender diversity on mental health.
4. Identify opportunities to integrate diverse perspectives and social determinants of health into psychiatric–mental health nursing practices.
5. Differentiate concepts of religiousness and spirituality and their implications for mental health.
6. Explore inclusive practices to increase educational awareness of the importance of cultural and social mores of various groups.

KEY TERMS

• 2SLGBTQIA+ • acculturation • assimilation • bisexual • cisgender • cultural idiom of distress • culture • ethnicity • gay • Hispanic • Latinx • lesbian • LGBTQ+ • linguistic competence • nonbinary • queer • religiousness • social determinants of health • spirituality • transgender • two-spirit • underrepresented population groups

INTRODUCTION

All societal groups have sets of values, beliefs, and patterns of accepted behavior, and it is often difficult for those of one group to understand those of another. This is especially true regarding mental illness, where a wide range of beliefs and practices exist among different groups of people. Approaches to care and treatment also vary; some groups have historically practiced punishment, ostracization, or institutionalization of individuals with mental health conditions, whereas others emphasize the importance of family and community involvement in care. Nurses and patients often have different religious backgrounds, cultural heritages, and identities from each other, so it is important for nurses to clearly understand the thinking and perspectives of those they serve.

This chapter examines cultural and social mores of various groups. Understanding cultural, sexual, social, and spiritual considerations is crucial when caring for people with mental health issues. These beliefs and practices can define and shape the experience of being mentally ill and influence the willingness to seek care. Treating mental disorders is intertwined with people's attitudes about themselves and their beliefs, values, and ways.

UNDERSTANDING CULTURE

KEYCONCEPT Culture is not only a way of life for people who identify or associate with one another based on some common purpose, need, or similarity of background but also the totality of learned, socially transmitted beliefs, values, and behaviors that emerge from its members' interpersonal transactions that can be used to define them as a collective. Culture is a term that goes beyond just race or ethnicity. It can also refer to such characteristics as age, gender, sexual orientation, disability, religion, class, education, geographical location, or profession.

Cultures are dynamic and continually changing. **Acculturation** is the term used to describe the socialization process by which one (usually smaller) group learns and adopts selective aspects of another (usually dominant) culture while still retaining cultural markers such as food and language. Cultures change when influenced by a new environment. Eventually, a new, smaller culture evolves, transformed by the new residents, that is different from the native culture and different from the dominant culture. When **assimilation** occurs, both cultures change, and a new culture emerges.

Cultural Identity

KEYCONCEPT Cultural identity is an enduring, fundamental aspect of self that includes membership to a cultural group with a set of attitudes, beliefs, feelings, and behaviors associated with that group.

Even though cultural beliefs and knowledge are passed down through generations, the individual receives and interprets the information to create a personal meaning according to their social situation. People can have multiple cultural identities that often conflict with each other because of opposing beliefs and values. For example, cultural behavior expectations may be in direct conflict with an individual's gender identity (see the "Understanding Gender and Sexual Diversity" section later in this chapter). Having conflicting identities can lead to distress that impacts an individual's health and well-being (Chen & Tung, 2023).

Often, the nurse is challenged to provide culturally appropriate care for individuals from cultures other than the nurse's culture. Uncertainty about cultural beliefs and practices can result in feelings of anxiety and vulnerability when interacting with patients from other cultures. Patients may interpret the nurse's anxiety as a lack of caring or competence.

Cultural Competence and Humility

Cultural competence can reinforce an individual's engagement in treatment, therapeutic relations, and treatment outcomes. Although being culturally competent is important, it also has the potential of stereotyping, ignoring the power differences in relationships (nurse vs. patient), and exacerbating the notion that some individuals and groups do not fit in with the norms of a social group. Despite the best intentions, in the United States being culturally competent may not be enough to change the dominant White, middle-class standards of behavior that can contribute to a lack of understanding between patient and nurse. An approach that expands cultural competency and focuses on and fosters an appreciation of human diversity is cultural humility.

Although definitions of cultural humility can vary, there is a consensus that it involves an adjustment or recognition of one's own culture to understand the culture of another individual. Cultural humility and the related concept of linguistic competence are especially important for psychiatric–mental health nurses because of the significance of therapeutic communication.

KEYCONCEPT Cultural competence, the ability to interact effectively with people of different cultures, involves a set of academic and interpersonal skills that are respectful of and responsive to the health beliefs, health care practices, and cultural and linguistic needs of diverse patients to bring about positive health care outcomes (Centers for Disease Control and Prevention [CDC], 2023). The ideal of cultural competence can be challenging because it implies a finite set of knowledge or skills that one can master, which may overlook the complexity and fluidity of cultural identities and experiences. Cultural humility emphasizes ongoing self-reflection, openness, and a willingness to learn from individuals' unique cultural perspectives, recognizing that cultural understanding is an evolving process rather than a fixed goal.

Cultural humility is a way of being and an evolution in perspective. This approach implies that the patients are the experts of their experiences, and nurses engage in ongoing self-reflection and education to gain an awareness of their own assumptions and biases that contribute to health disparities (Tham & Solomon, 2023). The culturally humble nurse expresses openness, is egoless, and has supportive interactions, respecting the patient's culture. The nurse does not assume competence simply based on prior experience with or knowledge of people from a similar background (Tschannen et al., 2024).

KEYCONCEPT Cultural humility is active engagement in an ongoing process to self-reflect on oneself as a cultural being and to be open to hearing about, respecting, and striving to understand the cultural background and identity of others (Foronda, 2020).

Linguistic Competence

There are linguistic variations within cultural groups as well as cultural variations within language groups. Speaking the same language does not guarantee shared meaning and understanding. In the United States, communication may be adversely affected when patients are unable to fully express themselves in English. Understanding the impact of literacy is integral to providing culturally competent care. Demonstrating an understanding that literacy contributes to the interpretation of personal, psychological experiences is critical.

Linguistic competence, the capacity to provide readily available, culturally appropriate oral and written language, is an important part of cultural awareness in care delivery (Agency for Healthcare Research and Quality [AHRQ], 2024). Linguistic competence not only refers to the appropriate use of words, grammar, and syntax, but also to the practical aspects such as choice of discussion topics, taking turns, use of metaphors, and the "hidden rules" of interactions. The following is an example of a hidden rule: For one patient, it is a cultural expectation for a nurse to sit down and "chit chat" before providing care; for another patient, limited eye contact is best. A culturally aware and responsive nurse values diversity; understands and appreciates differences and similarities in health care practices within, among, and between individuals and groups; and strives to create space where diversity, equity, and inclusion are integrated.

Cultural beliefs and practices influence how patients communicate and manifest their symptoms, cope with their illnesses, and receive family and community support. The *DSM-5-TR* discusses the **cultural idiom of distress**, a commonly used term or phrase that describes the suffering within a cultural group, from cultural explanations, which are perceived causes for symptoms (American Psychiatric Association [APA], 2022). While cultural idioms of distress may offer insights into how mental illness is framed within different cultural contexts, it can also reinforce stereotypes by oversimplifying complex, individualized experiences.

Health Literacy

Most people face challenges in understanding and using health information (Brach, 2024). Mental health information can be even more complicated because of the unfamiliar terms, multiple treatment approaches, and various disciplines involved in care. A key role of the mental health nurse is to synthesize the information and help the patient understand symptoms and treatment options.

KEYCONCEPT Health literacy is the ability to use reading, writing, verbal, and numerical skills in the context of health. It is the "ability to find, understand, and use information and services to inform health-related decisions and actions for themselves and others" (AHRQ, 2024).

Healthy People 2030 has six objectives related to health literacy specifically toward the goal to "Eliminate health disparities, achieve health equity, and attain health literacy to improve the health and well-being of all" (Office of Disease Prevention and Health Promotion, n.d.). If an individual has limited health literacy and cannot process and understand basic health information and services, it is unlikely the individual will be able to follow discharge instructions, take prescribed medication, and adhere to a treatment plan (Pappadis et al., 2023; see Boxes 3.1 and 3.2).

Barriers to health literacy are closely linked to the social determinants of health (SDOH), such as education, income, housing, and access to health care. It is important to approach individuals with sensitivity, recognizing

BOX 3.1

Health Literacy Healthy People 2030 Objectives

- Increase the proportion of adults whose health care provider checked their understanding.
- Decrease the proportion of adults who report poor communication with their health care provider.
- Increase the proportion of adults whose health care providers involved them in decisions as much as they wanted.
- Increase the proportion of people who say their online medical record is easy to understand.
- Increase the proportion of adults with limited English proficiency who say their providers explain things clearly.
- Increase the health literacy of the population.

Source: Office of Disease Prevention and Health Promotion. (n.d.). Health literacy. *Healthy People 2030*. U.S. Department of Health and Human Services. https://health.gov/healthypeople/priority-areas/health-literacy-healthy-people-2030

BOX 3.2

Health Literacy Universal Precautions

- Health professionals should assume that all patients and caregivers may have difficulty comprehending health information.
- Health professionals should communicate in ways that anyone can understand.
- Health literacy universal precautions are aimed at the following:
  - Simplifying communication with and confirming comprehension for all patients, so that the risk of miscommunication is minimized.
  - Making the office environment and health care system easier to navigate.
  - Supporting patient's efforts to improve their health.
- Important key areas for promoting health literacy include:
  - Practice change
  - Spoken communication
  - Written communication
  - Self-management and empowerment
  - Supportive systems

Adapted from Agency for Healthcare Research & Quality (AHRQ). (2020). *Health literacy universal precautions toolkit* (2nd ed.). Agency for Healthcare Research and Quality. https://www.ahrq.gov/health-literacy/quality-resources/tools/literacy-toolkit/healthlittoolkit2-intro.html

that everyone has unique needs and experiences that shape their health literacy, rather than making assumptions based on socioeconomic status (SES) or cultural background.

UNDERSTANDING GENDER AND SEXUAL DIVERSITY

While some cultures teach that gender can be neatly divided into male and female and sexuality into straight and gay, many others have long taught that both gender and sexuality are far more complex. Modern scientific, medical, and psychological perspectives are increasingly upholding the truth that variances in gender and sexuality are not pathologies, but naturally occurring dimensions of human diversity. For example, nonheterosexual sexual orientations and noncisgender gender identities were once treated as mental health disorders under the DSM in its earlier editions, but the APA now recognizes both to be variations of the human experience.

The concepts of gender identity and sexual orientation are not the same. The following section differentiates these complex concepts. Although the discussion in this section offers a glimpse into concepts related to gender and human sexuality, it is essential to note that a comprehensive discussion is beyond the scope of this chapter. Because these concepts are core aspects of the human experience, it is important that nurses acknowledge and embrace these biopsychosocial concepts for patient-centered nursing care.

Gender and Identity: Beyond Binary

KEYCONCEPT Gender is a complex term that refers to the social, relational, cultural, psychological, and emotional traits that are associated with being male, female, both, or neither. Individuals are assigned a legal sex at birth based on biologic characteristics, but a person's innermost concept of self can be different from their physical state. Gender-related traits are often influenced by societal expectations and norms.

KEYCONCEPT Gender identity is an individual's psychological sense of their gender—male, female, neither, or both. Gender identity is not visible to others. According to the American Psychological Association (APA, 2023), individuals typically develop a sense of their gender identity between the ages of 2 and 5.

It is important to recognize and respect the diversity of human gender identities. **Cisgender** is a term used to describe a gender identity that aligns with the sex that was assigned at birth. **Transgender** is an umbrella term for individuals whose gender identity is different from the sex they were assigned at birth, such as transgender men, transgender women, and nonbinary people. Some gender identities go beyond the **binary** understanding of male or female. **Nonbinary** people have gender identities that fall outside the male–female binary, encompassing a range of identities such as genderqueer, agender, Two-Spirit, genderfluid, and more, with some individuals who identify as transgender also embracing nonbinary identities (Bindman et al., 2022).

Being subjected to transphobic biases, including misgendering, discrimination, and a lack of recognition, can result in diminished feelings of belongingness and lower self-esteem among transgender people. Experiencing such treatment, whether in everyday interactions or within health care settings, reinforces a sense of invisibility or invalidation. Nonbinary people in particular often face significant challenges in expressing their authentic selves, largely due to societal and interpersonal biases against individuals identifying outside the male–female binary. Such ignorance, rooted in rigid gender norms and prejudice, creates barriers to mental and emotional well-being and contributes to health disparities within the transgender population. Transgender individuals are more likely to experience higher rates of mental health conditions, and their experiences of marginalization can limit access to appropriate health care. The compounded effects of bias, and inadequate care contribute to poor health outcomes and diminished well-being for transgender individuals (Wickham et al., 2023).

Gender Dysphoria

Gender dysphoria is the term used to describe an individual's discomfort or distress regarding the gender that is assigned by society. These symptoms occur because of the way society labels and responds to gender-diverse people. If society were more open to a spectrum of gender expression, these symptoms might not be present (Garg et al., 2023). One of the biggest issues faced by the transgender community is lack of access to competent gender-affirming care.

Recovery-Oriented Care for People With Gender Dysphoria

Teamwork and Collaboration: Working Toward Recovery. Individuals with gender dysphoria deserve support and care from gender-affirming clinicians. Some individuals may decide to align their physical state to their true gender identity. Hormones may be used to feminize (estrogen) or masculinize (testosterone) the body. For those who want to feminize their bodies, a testosterone blocker is usually given along with estrogen. The changes that occur take months to years. Others may decide on surgical procedures that are increasingly possible as third-party payers are starting to cover the cost. There is much to learn about gender and its expression (Garg et al., 2023).

Sexuality

Humans are sexual beings. Sexuality is a part of who we are, not what we do—the sum total of all our biologic and experiential influences.

> **KEYCONCEPT Sexuality** is the way people experience and express themselves sexually. This involves biologic, psychological, physical, erotic, emotional, social, or spiritual feelings and behaviors.

Various psychiatric disorders encompass a spectrum of symptoms impacting sexual life, including impaired arousal, desire, and/or satisfaction. Depression, bipolar disorder, anxiety, and even psychosis may impact an individual's sexual well-being. Recognizing, understanding, and addressing symptoms are paramount to providing comprehensive mental health care. Individuals who do not engage in an active sex life still have unique sexual needs and concerns, underscoring sexuality's connection and impact on mental health and well-being.

Sexual Orientation

> **KEYCONCEPT Sexual orientation** describes an enduring pattern of emotional, romantic, or sexual attraction to other people. Some people are attracted to a single gender and some are attracted to more than one gender. Some people experience strong sexual attractions and some experience little or no sexual attraction. Sexual orientation is independent of gender identity.

Sexual orientation profoundly influences people's daily experiences, including sexual and romantic relationships. Research shows that sexual orientation has a genetic, hormonal, and immunologic basis in brain development that is well established before birth. The precise mechanisms are not clearly understood (VanderLaan et al., 2023).

FACTORS RELATED TO MENTAL ILLNESS

Social factors contribute to the development of mental disorders. Children, Indigenous populations, people of color, people who do not speak English, individuals from low- or no-income backgrounds, and LGBTQ+ (lesbian, gay, bisexual, transgender, queer) people encounter heightened vulnerability to risk factors and encounter reduced access to health care services (Edyburn et al., 2022).

Underrepresented population groups in the United States live in a social environment of inequality that increases their exposure to racism, discrimination, violence, and poverty, which contribute to the experience of their illnesses (Funer, 2023). Slavery, segregation, and discriminatory practices in areas such as housing, education, and employment have led to generations of marginalized communities facing limited access to resources and opportunities. This history has also resulted in significant disparities in the quality of health care available to marginalized communities (Smallwood et al., 2021). Underrepresented racial–ethnic groups are less likely to receive mental health services and more likely to receive substandard quality care.

Poverty stigma is deemed a key determinant of mental health and is found in all cultural groups (Inglis et al., 2023). In the United States in 2022, 11.5% of residents were living in poverty (United States Census Bureau, 2023). Of those living below the poverty line, 25.6% were single mothers and their children, 19.5% were Black, 17.0% were Hispanic, and 10.1% were White (Shrider et al., 2021). Currently in the United States, the poverty guidelines for a family of four is a yearly income of $31,200 or less in the 48 mainland states; $39,000 or less in Alaska; and $35,880 or less in Hawaii (U.S. DHHS, 2024). Bias impacts care delivery and perpetuates systemic inequalities. Increased awareness of provider biases can reduce errors, improve patient safety, and translate to improved care for marginalized communities who experience the poorest health care outcomes (Gopal et al., 2021).

Families living in poverty are under tremendous financial and emotional stress, which may trigger or exacerbate mental issues. Along with the daily stressors of trying to provide food and shelter for themselves and their families, their lack of time, energy, and money prevents them from attending to their psychological needs. Often, these families become trapped in a downward economic spiral as tension and stress mount. The inability to gain employment and the lack of financial independence only add to the feelings of powerlessness and low self-esteem. Being self-supporting gives one a feeling of control over life and bolsters self-esteem. Alcohol use disorder, depression, and child and partner abuse may become a means of coping with such hopelessness and despair.

The population that is unhoused is the group most at risk of being unable to escape this spiral of poverty. Individuals who are unhoused encounter significant challenges accessing support and resources. Traditional approaches in health systems can unintentionally retraumatize individuals. Nurses should avoid exclusionary behaviors, dismissing their experiences, or making assumptions about their needs, as these actions can perpetuate stigma and harm. Considering the rates of trauma in people experiencing housing insecurity, nurses should view each interaction as an opportunity to establish trust and implement trauma-informed approaches (Albert et al., 2023).

Social determinants of health (SDOH) consist of five domains addressing environments where individuals are born and live, economic resources and opportunities, social and community support as well as access to quality education and health care services (Office of Disease Prevention and Health Promotion, n.d.). SDOH impacts mental health and well-being. See Chapter 2.

Underrepresented Population Groups

Underrepresented population groups are people from various ethnic and nondominant groups that have disproportionately low representation (in health care, research, and education) relative to their numbers in the general population. Whereas the term ethnic group or **ethnicity** refers to common geographic origin and ancestry or cultural traditions, the term *race* is a social construct that has been conceptualized as a biologic variable, supported by a false historical narrative that there are inherent biologic differences between groups. The use of the concept of race as a biologic determinant in research has contributed to perpetuating negative stereotypes and further stigmatizing underrepresented nondominant and ethnic groups (Bryant et al., 2022; Braveman & Parker Dominguez, 2021). The concept of race continues to be used inaccurately to differentiate human groups. It is important that nurses recognize that the concept of race is not genetically discrete, is not a reliable measure, and may not be biologically relevant.

Race and Ethnicity

The U.S. Census Bureau collects population data every 10 years; this occurred most recently in the 2020 Census, which asked respondents to self-identify both race and ethnicity by choosing one of the following general categories: (1) White non-Hispanic, (2) White Hispanic or Latino, (3) Black or African American, (4) American Indian and Alaska Native (AI/AN), (5) Asian, (6) native Hawaiian and other Pacific Islander, and (7) some other (multiracial and multiethnic). The 2020 Census found that the most prevalent racial or ethnic group in the United States was the White, non-Hispanic population at 57.8%, a decrease from 63.7% from the 2010 census (U.S. Census Bureau, 2021a). The categories are for the purposes of data collection often detailed by government agencies and forms. It is vital to remember that race and ethnicity are social constructs. The way we categorize people can unintentionally reinforce stereotypes and limit our understanding of individuals, making it essential to recognize the complexity and fluidity of identity beyond these prescribed population categories.

Hispanic and Latinx

The number of Hispanic or Latinx Americans living in the United States has been gradually increasing, and this group is now the second largest racial or ethnic group in the United States, constituting 41.1 million (18.7% of the total population) in 2020 (U.S. Census Bureau, 2021b). **Hispanic** groups are Spanish speaking or have a background in a Spanish-speaking country such as Mexico. **Latinx** is a gender-neutral term that refers to those who are from or have a background in a Latin American country. The nurse should remember that these terms, though widely used and sometimes useful for statistical analysis, are still ways of categorizing people that can result in stereotyping individuals and groups leading to discriminatory practices. In the United States, the largest Hispanic population groups are from Mexico (35.9 million), followed by Puerto Rico (5.6 million), and El Salvador (2.3 million) (U.S. Census Bureau, 2023).

Studies indicate that Hispanic and Latinx Americans tend to use available resources before seeking help from mental health professionals. They are more likely to seek help at nonprofit hospitals or community health centers that also offer mental health services. Reasons for this are unclear, but possible barriers to treatment include beliefs that mental health facilities do not accommodate their cultural needs (e.g., language, beliefs, values), cost of care, availability of services, accessibility of services, and concerns regarding immigration status (Mallonee et al., 2023; Swetlitz et al., 2024). Consequences of the COVID-19 pandemic—including exposure to illness, financial and social burdens, and social isolation—have exacerbated mental health issues in Latinx communities (Saltzman et al., 2021). The National Alliance on Mental Illness (NAMI) notes that language and linguistically competent care barriers, limited or lack of health coverage, SES, stigma, and acculturation are all factors that contribute to disparities in communities of color (National Alliance on Mental Illness, n.d.).

Black or African American

In 2020, the estimated population of Black or African American people living in the United States was 41.1 million (12.4% of the total population) (U.S. Census Bureau, 2021b). The U.S. Census Bureau does not differentiate people who self-identify as Black (racial identification) from those who self-identify as African American (ethnicity with ancestry from the African continent).

Black or African American individuals living with or diagnosed with mental illness or a mental health disorder suffer from the stresses of double stigma—not only from the stigma of mental illness but also from long-time racism, discrimination, and inequity. Discrimination, in turn, contributes to poor health outcomes (Box 3.3).

Research shows that diagnoses and treatment for African Americans often are racially biased. African Americans are disproportionately diagnosed as having schizophrenia compared to other groups. The racial gap observed in schizophrenia-spectrum disorder diagnoses has become a focal point in understanding mental health disparities. This gap does not appear to be rooted in genetic differences but rather emerges from societal factors (Faber et al., 2023). This disparity in the diagnosis of schizophrenia has been stable over the past three decades. Using subjective assessment methods may account for this. Misunderstandings about culture can further complicate diagnostic and treatment approaches for Black

BOX 3.3

Research for Evidence-Based Practice: Discrimination and Health Outcomes

Hudson, D., Collins-Anderson, A., & Hutson, W. (2023). Understanding the impact of contemporary racism on the mental health of middle-class Black Americans. International Journal of Environmental Research and Public Health, 20*(3), 1660. https://doi.org/10.3390/ijerph20031660*

THE QUESTION: Mental health inequities do not disappear even when socioeconomic status (SES) of Black and White Americans is similar. How do perceptions of unfair treatment affect the mental health of middle-class Black Americans?

METHODS: A sample of 526 college-educated, self-identified Black Americans answered a Qualtrics survey consisting of gender, age, participant race/ethnicity, marital status, and extensive SES information. The Patient Health Questionnaire 9-item (PHQ-9) was used to measure depression, and a major discrimination scale was used to determine everyday discrimination.

FINDINGS: Significant associations were found among depression and major discrimination. The participants' SES had no affect; that is, SES did not diminish the effect of discrimination. This study provided additional evidence that discrimination is prevalent among middle-class Black Americans.

IMPLICATIONS FOR NURSING: The nurse should recognize that discrimination is a common experience among Black Americans, which contributes to poorer health outcomes.

and African American individuals and contribute to disparity (Merritt et al., 2023).

Asian American and Pacific Islander (AAPI)

More than 20.6 million Asian American individuals and Pacific Islanders, encompassing over 40 distinct ethnicities, live in the United States (more than 6.2% of the U.S. population). This group represents one of the fastest-growing underrepresented groups (Schlossberg, 2023). This large multicultural group includes Chinese, Filipino, Japanese, Asian Indian, Korean, Vietnamese, Laotian, Cambodian, Hawaiian, Samoan, and Guamanian people. Most Chinese, Japanese, Korean, Asian Indian, and Filipino immigrants have migrated to urban areas, whereas Vietnamese individuals have settled throughout the United States (U.S. Census Bureau, 2022a).

Some Asian cultures have a tradition of denying or disguising the existence of mental illnesses. In some Asian cultures, people may view having a family member treated for mental illness as a weakness and an embarrassment. This cultural bias may explain the extremely low utilization of mental health services by Asian Americans (Chu et al., 2021; Schlossberg, 2023).

American Indian and Alaska Native

In 2021, the population of AI/AN individuals comprised 9.7 million people (U.S. Census Bureau, 2022b). Indigenous peoples, specifically AI/AN communities, grapple with substantial disparities, consistently ranking at or near the bottom across various social, health, and economic indicators. Colonization, intergenerational trauma, and discrimination contribute to the social and economic disparities of the AI/AN communities. Additionally, mental health providers and Western-based medicine were often complicit in removing Native people from their home and placing them into boarding schools and asylums (Oldani & Prosen, 2021). These challenges manifest in lower life expectancy and a disproportionate burden of diseases, stemming from interconnected issues such as inadequate education, disproportionate poverty, food insecurity, discrimination in health service delivery, and cultural differences. Various data suggest that rates of suicide among AI/AN adolescents are higher than those of other adolescents in the United States (Ross et al., 2023).

Arab American

Although the number of Arab Americans is not captured by the US census, this population is discussed in this text because there is evidence that Arab American individuals are at high risk for adverse mental health issues (Alsaidi et al., 2023). The Arab American community includes immigrants and their descendants from several Arab world countries including Syria, Lebanon, Egypt, Palestine, Iraq, Jordan, and Yemen. There are an estimated 3.7 million Arab Americans in the United States, with two thirds living in 10 states (California, Michigan, New York, Florida, Texas, New Jersey, Illinois, Ohio, Pennsylvania, and Virginia). More than one third live in Los Angeles, Detroit, and New York, and more than 82% are U.S. citizens. The first wave of Arab immigrants that came to the United States during the 19th and 20th centuries was primarily Christian. In the 1960s, Muslim Arabs began immigrating in greater numbers to the United States. Most Arab Americans in the United States practice Christianity (Arab American Institute Foundation, 2021).

Although there is little research about the views of Arab Americans, there is emerging evidence that stigma toward mental health treatment may prevent individuals from accessing treatment. They are more likely to visit a primary care provider than a mental health provider (Ali et al., 2022; Shaimaa & Bialous, 2024).

There is research evidence that Arab Americans are at an increased risk of adverse mental health, specifically with discrimination at the intersection of racial, ethnic, and religious identities (Alsaidi et al., 2023).

Depression in Arab American people is associated with being an individual who is assigned female at birth, unmarried, unemployed, and having experienced abuse as a child (Abuelezam & El-Sayed, 2021). Frequent contact with family and community is linked to well-being within those identifying as Arab American, resulting in increased rates of depression during imposed social distancing during the COVID-19 pandemic (Sayad et al., 2023).

Women of Underrepresented Groups

Women within many immigrant racial or ethnic groups may experience more conflicting feelings and psychological stressors than do men in trying to adjust to both their defined role in their new culture and a different role in the larger predominant society. Stress from acculturation, stigma toward mental illness, and lack of social support contribute to depression among immigrant women (Salameh et al., 2023).

The disparities in mental health outcomes among racial and ethnic underrepresented women highlight a concerning trend where diagnosis rates are high, yet access to treatment remains disproportionately low. Stigma, cultural influence, racism, and family influence of past experiences contribute to the lack of treatment (Ballone & Richards, 2023). Fear that health care providers may be biased toward members of underrepresented groups may also contribute to reluctance to access mental health care (LeBlanc et al., 2024). The heart of effective interventions lies in adopting a multidisciplinary approach and prioritizing culturally sensitive components of care (Ballone & Richards, 2023).

Rural Cultures

According to the U.S. Census Bureau, 20% of the U.S. population resides in a rural area. Rural areas are diverse in both geography and culture. For example, access to mental health services for those in the rural deep South differs from access for those in the rural Northwest, and treatment approaches may be accepted in one part of the country but not in another.

When compared to urban counterparts, individuals who reside in rural communities experience high rates of poverty and less access to health care (CDC, 2023). Most mental health services are in urban areas because most people live near cities. Because rural occupants have less access to mental health resources and health care providers with specialized mental health training, individuals are less likely to be diagnosed with a mental health issue (Edwards et al., 2023). Even though rural residents are less likely than urban residents to have mental health diagnoses or receive mental health care, the suicide rate is higher in rural areas, where firearms are most used. Rural cultures had additional mental health service challenges, such as social isolation and access to firearms (Monteith et al., 2021). The highest rates of suicide in rural areas occur in non-Hispanic AI/AN people (CDC, 2023).

LGBTQ+ Community

Delivery of culturally competent care within the context of cultural humility is important in mental health care for the LGBTQ+ community. In this text, the acronym **LGBTQ+** refers to **lesbian, gay, bisexual, transgender, and queer** individuals, as well as others with nondominant gender identities and/or sexual orientations. For example, an expanded acronym **2SLGBTQIA+** means two-spirit, lesbian, gay, bisexual, transgender, questioning/queer, intersex, and asexual. **Two-spirit** is a term that should be used only when discussing Canadian and U.S. Indigenous communities and refers to individuals as having masculine and feminine spiritual or religious energies and who express their gender differently than assigned at birth.

Fear of discrimination is a barrier to many LGBTQ+ individuals seeking health care, and nurses often lack knowledge about the health care needs of LGBTQ+ individuals. Developing gender-neutral, affirming, and respectful terminology and staying up to date on LGBTQ+ health issues and disparities are important in reducing stigma and discrimination (Cooper et al., 2023).

The estimate of the percent of U.S. adults who identify as LGBTQ+ was 7% in 2022; this includes 17% of those age 30 or younger compared with 8% of those ages 30 to 49 (Brown, 2023). LGBTQ+ individuals are at elevated risks for violent victimization and experience increased health disparities compared to their heterosexual and cisgender counterparts (Medina-Martinez et al., 2021; Beaudry et al., 2024). Polyvictimization (multiple traumas) is associated with poor health, anxiety, depression, drug misuse, and suicidality (Kassing et al., 2021).

Intersectionality

Identifying the compounding effects of occupying two or more social identities can be a useful framework for understanding the lived experience of people with mental health issues.

> **KEYCONCEPT Intersectionality** is the impact of interconnected, overlapping social categories (race, ethnicity, gender, etc.) within an individual or group that are social systems of discrimination or disadvantage.

Intersectionality theory, introduced by legal scholar Kimberlé Crenshaw, initially focused on discrimination against Black women. According to the theory, Black women should be understood by the effects of the interactions between being "Black" and "female"—that is, racism and sexism—which frequently compound each other and create a unique experience of oppression that cannot be addressed simply by addressing racism and sexism independently. Crenshaw examined how overlapping social identities related to systems and structures of oppression, dominance, or discrimination (Crenshaw, 1989).

Although an in-depth discussion of intersectionality is beyond the scope of this text, nurses should appreciate the complexity of overlapping social identities and consider their effects on physical health and mental health. The National Institutes of Health is supporting research that moves beyond the biomedical model and individual-level determinants of health to the health effects from the intersection of structural power dynamics, such as racism and sexism (Alvidrez et al., 2021).

SPIRITUALITY, RELIGION, AND MENTAL ILLNESS

Both spirituality and religion are factors that may influence beliefs about mental illness and impact treatment and recovery. There is no one widely accepted definition of spirituality (Pew Research Center, 2023). In Geneva, Switzerland, in 2013, the International Consensus Conference on Improving the Spiritual Dimension of Whole Person Care defined spirituality. The following definition continues to be used today and will be used throughout this text (Balboni et al., 2022; Long et al., 2024).

> **KEYCONCEPT** "**Spirituality** is a dynamic and intrinsic aspect of humanity through which persons seek ultimate meaning, purpose, and transcendence and experience relationship to self, family, others, community, society, nature, and the significant or sacred. Spirituality is expressed through beliefs, values, traditions, and practices" (Puchalski et al., 2014).

Related to but different from spirituality, **religiousness** is the participation in a community of people who gather around common ways of worshiping. Spirituality can be expressed through adhering to a set of religious beliefs. Religious beliefs often define an individual's relationship within a family and community. Many religions are practiced throughout the world. Judeo-Christian thinking tends to dominate Western societies. Other religions, such as Islam, Hinduism, and Buddhism, dominate Eastern and Middle Eastern cultures. Because religious beliefs often influence approaches to mental health, it is important to understand the basis of various religions in the United States. Both religion and spirituality can provide support and strength in dealing with mental illnesses and emotional issues.

People with a diagnosis of, or who are living with, mental illness benefit from spiritual assessment and interventions (see Chapter 10). Perception of well-being and health in people with severe mental illness has been positively associated with spirituality and religiousness. To carry out spiritual interventions, the nurse enters a therapeutic relationship with the patient and uses the self as a therapeutic tool. Examples of spiritual interventions to connect with inner sources of solace and hope include meditation, guided imagery, and prayer (if participation is requested by the patient and prayer is practiced within the facility). If a nurse is uncomfortable or unfamiliar with prayer, a chaplain referral can be made.

SUMMARY OF KEY POINTS

- The term *culture* is defined as a way of life that manifests the learned beliefs, values, and accepted behaviors that are transmitted socially within a specific group. Mental illnesses are stigmatized in many cultural groups. A variety of cultural and religious beliefs underlie this stigma.
- Cultural identity is a fundamental aspect of self and helps to define expected behavior.
- Cultural competence and cultural humility are goals for nurses to achieve to understand patients from different cultures. Cultural competence is demonstrated by valuing cultural beliefs, bridging any language gap, and considering the patient's literacy level when planning and implementing care.
- Cultural humility is being open and willing to reflect on oneself as a cultural being, focusing on civility, kindness, and respect. It is being open and willing to learn about the cultural background and identity of another.
- Linguistic competence is based on a set of skills that allows individuals to increase their understanding and appreciation of cultural differences and similarities within, among, and between groups.
- Sexuality is an enduring pattern of emotional, romantic, or sexual attraction to other people.
- Gender identity is an individual's psychological sense of their gender—male, female, neither, or both. Gender identity is not visible to others. Most people develop a gender identity between the ages 2 and 5 years old.
- Gender dysphoria occurs when the individual is distressed with assigned sex or gender role.
- Social factors contribute to the development of mental disorders. Intersectionality occurs when an individual or group has multiple social identities that are subject to systemic discrimination.
- Members of underrepresented groups (various nondominant groups with disproportionately low representation in health care, research, and education) experience racism, discrimination, violence, and poverty, which contribute to their experience of mental disorders.
- Access to mental health treatment is particularly limited for underrepresented ethnic and cultural groups.

- Spirituality can be a source of strength and support for both the patient with mental illness and the nurse providing the care.
- Religious beliefs are closely intertwined with beliefs about health and mental illness.

DEVELOPING CLINICAL JUDGMENT

1. Differentiate the concepts of cultural competence and cultural humility.
2. A nurse is discharging a patient who does not use English for medical conversations. What considerations should the nurse have as discharge instructions are being given?
3. During an initial consult with a new patient, the nurse realizes that the patient has left the "gender" field on the intake paperwork blank. When asked about it, the patient explains that neither "male" nor "female" fully represents them. What gender identity might they be describing?
4. During a nursing assessment, a young individual reveals that she identifies as a lesbian and that she is currently living with her partner. She has not yet told her parents about her sexual orientation and is experiencing some anxiety about sharing this part of her life with her family. Her partner is supportive and encourages the young person to take her time in telling her family members. Is this patient experiencing symptoms of a gender dysphoria? Explain.
5. Discuss the differences between spirituality and religiousness. Is it possible that someone can be spiritual and not religious?
6. Reflect on how bias may impact interactions with individuals who are affected by social factors.

Unfolding Patient Stories: Li Na Chen • Part 1

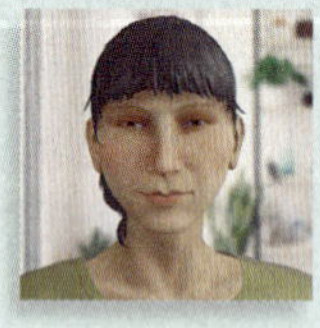

Li Na Chen is a 40-year-old Chinese female diagnosed with major depressive disorder who attempted suicide by drug overdose. She is married with two children, ages 12 and 14. Why is it important for the nurse to conduct a cultural assessment of the client and her family? Describe methods the nurse can use to demonstrate cultural competence and avoid inaccurate assumptions about the Chinese culture. What questions can the nurse ask to assess cultural beliefs, practices, and influences on Li Na's mental illness and family functioning? (Li Na Chen's story continues in Chapter 25.)

Care for Li Na and other patients in a realistic virtual environment: ***vSim** for Nursing* for Nursing (thepoint.lww.com/vSimMentalHealth). Practice documenting these patients' care in DocuCare (thepoint.lww.com/DocuCareEHR).

REFERENCES

Abuelezam, N. N., & El-Sayed, A. M. (2021). Objective and subjective poor mental health indicators among Arab Americans in Michigan: A population-based study. *Ethnicity & Health*, *26*(2), 225–234. https://doi.org/10.1080/13557858.2018.1494822

Agency for Healthcare Research and Quality (AHRQ). (2024). *About health literacy*. Retrieved September 20, 2024, from https://www.ahrq.gov/health-literacy/about/index.html

Albert, R., Baillie, D., & Neal, H. (2023). Unmet needs in street homeless people: A commentary on multiple interconnected needs in a vulnerable group. *Future Healthcare Journal*, *10*(2), 103–106.

Ali, S., Elsayed, D., Elahi, S., Zia, B., & Awaad, R. (2022). Predicting rejection attitudes toward utilizing formal mental health services in Muslim women in the US: Results from the Muslims' perceptions and attitudes to mental health study. *The International Journal of Social Psychiatry*, *68*(3), 662–669. https://doi.org/10.1177/00207640211001084

Alsaidi, S., Velez, B. L., Smith, L., Jacob, A., & Salem, N. (2023). "Arab, brown, and other": Voices of Muslim Arab American women on identity, discrimination, and well-being. *Cultural Diversity and Ethnic Minority Psychology*, *29*(2), 163–171. https://doi.org/10.1037/cdp0000440

Alvidrez, J., Greenwood, G. L., Johnson, T. L., & Parker, K. L. (2021). Intersectionality in public health research: A view from the National Institutes of Health. *American Journal of Public Health*, *111*(1), 95–97. https://doi.org/10.2105/AJPH.2020.305986

American Psychiatric Association (APA). (2022). *Diagnostic and statistical manual of mental disorders* (5th ed., text rev.). Author.

American Psychological Association. (2023). *Understanding transgender people, gender identity and gender expression*. Retrieved September 4, 2023, from https://www.apa.org/topics/lgbtq/transgender-people-gender-identity-gender-expression

Arab American Institute Foundation. (2021). *Who are Arab Americans*? https://www.aaiusa.org/demographics

Balboni, T. A., VanderWeele, T. J., Doan-Soares, S. D., Long, K. N. G., Ferrell, B. R., Fitchett, G., Koenig, H. G., Bain, P. A., Puchalski, C., Steinhauser, K. E., Sulmasy, D. P., & Koh, H. K. (2022). Spirituality in serious illness and health. *JAMA*, *328*(2), 184–197. https://doi.org/10.1001/jama.2022.11086

Ballone, N., & Richards, E. (2023). Racial/ethnic disparities and women's mental health. *Psychiatric Clinics of North America*, *45*(3), 571–582. https://doi.org/10.1016/j.psc.2023.04.011

Beaudry, S., Duff, E., & Ziegler, E. (2024). 2-Spirit indigenous health care and cultural humility. *The Journal for Nurse Practitioners*, *20*(2), 104892.

Bindman, J., Ngo, A., Zamudio-Haas, S., & Sevelius, J. (2022). Health care experiences of patients with nonbinary gender identities. *Transgender Health*, *7*(5), 423–429.

Brach, C. (Ed.). (2024). *AHRQ health literacy universal precautions toolkit* (3rd ed.). Agency for Healthcare Research and Quality. AHRQ Publication No. 23-0075.

Braveman, P., & Parker Dominguez, T. (2021). Abandon "race." Focus on racism. *Frontiers in Public Health*, *9*, 689462. https://doi.org/10.3389/fpubh.2021.689462

Brown, A. (2023). *5 key findings about LGBTQ+ Americans*. Pew Research Center. Retrieved January 13, 2024, from https://www.pewresearch.org/short-reads/2023/06/23/5-key-findings-about-lgbtq-americans/

Bryant, B. E., Jordan, A., & Clark, U. S. (2022). Race as a social construct in psychiatry research and practice. *JAMA Psychiatry*, *79*(2), 93–94. https://doi.org/10.1001/jamapsychiatry.2021.2877

Centers for Disease Control and Prevention (CDC). (2023). *Rural health*. Retrieved November 30, 2023, from https://www.cdc.gov/ruralhealth/about.html

Centers for Disease Control and Prevention (CDC). (2023). *Cultural understanding and awareness*. Retrieved May 31, 2025, from https://www.cdc.gov/std-ips/php/about/cultural-understanding-and-awareness.html#:~:text=Cultural%20competence%20is%20the%20ability%20to%20%22deliver,diverse%20patients%22%20(NIH%2C%20Clear%20Communication.%20Retrieved%2011/1/2019)

Chen, E. Y., & Tung, E. Y. (2023). Similarities and differences in the longitudinal trajectories of depressive symptoms from mid-adolescence to young adulthood: The intersectionality of gender, race/ethnicity, and levels of depressive symptoms. *Journal of Racial and Ethnic Health Disparities*. https://doi.org/10.1007/s40615-023-01630-5

Chu, K. M., Garcia, S., Koka, H., Wynn, G. H., & Kao, T. C. (2021). Mental health care utilization and stigma in the military: Comparison of Asian Americans to other racial groups. *Ethnicity and Health*, *26*(2), 235–250. https://doi.org/10.1080/13557858.2018.1494823

Cooper, R. L., Ramesh, A., Radix, A. E., Reuben, J. S., Juarez, P. D., Holder, C. L., Belton, A. S., Brown, K. Y., Mena, L. A., & Matthews-Juarez, P. (2023). Affirming and inclusive care training for medical students and residents to reduce health disparities experienced by sexual and gender minorities: A systematic review. *Transgender Health*, *8*(4), 307–327.

Crenshaw, K. (1989). *Demarginalizing the intersection of race and sex: A black feminist critique of antidiscrimination doctrine, feminist theory and antiracist politics*. University of Chicago Legal Forum: Vol. 1989: Issue 1, Article 8. http://chicagounbound.uchicago.edu/uclf/vol1989/iss1/8

Edwards, A., Hung, R., Levin, J. B., Forthun, L., Sajatovic, M., & McVoy, M. (2023). Health disparities among rural individuals with mental health conditions: A systematic literature review. *Rural Mental Health*, *47*(3), 163–178. https://doi.org/10.1037/rmh0000228

Edyburn, K. L., Bertone, A., Raines, T. C., Hinton, T., Twyford, J., & Dowdy, E. (2023). Integrating intersectionality, social determinants of health, and healing: A new training framework for school-based mental health. *School Psychology Review*, *52*(5), 563–585.

Faber, S. C., Khanna Roy, A., Michaels, T. I., & Williams, M. T. (2023). The weaponization of medicine: Early psychosis in the Black community and the need for racially informed mental healthcare. *Frontiers in Psychiatry*, *14*, 1098292. https://doi.org/10.3389/fpsyt.2023.1098292

Foronda, C. (2020). A theory of cultural humility. *Journal of Transcultural Nursing*, *31*(1), 7–12. https://doi.org/10.1177/1043659619875184

Funer, F. (2023). Admitting the heterogeneity of social inequalities: Intersectionality as a (self-)critical framework and tool within mental health care. *Philosophy, Ethics, and Humanities in Medicine*, *18*(1), 21. https://doi.org/10.1186/s13010-023-00144-6

Garg, G., Elshimy, G., & Marwaha, R. (2023). Gender dysphoria. In *StatPearls*. StatPearls Publishing. https://www.ncbi.nlm.nih.gov/books/NBK532313/

Gopal, D. P., Chetty, U., O'Donnell, P., Gajria, C., & Blackadder-Weinstein, J. (2021). Implicit bias in healthcare: Clinical practice, research and decision making. *Future Healthcare Journal*, *8*(1), 40–48.

Human Rights Campaign. (2023). *Resources: Glossary of terms*. Retrieved January 11, 2024, from https://www.hrc.org/resources/glossary-of-terms

Inglis, G., Jenkins, P., McHardy, F., Sosu, E., & Wilson, C. (2023). Poverty stigma, mental health, and well-being: A rapid review and synthesis of quantitative and qualitative research. *Journal of Community & Applied Social Psychology*, *33*(4), 783–806.

Kassing, F., Casanova, T., Griffin, J. A., Wood, E., & Stepleman, L. M. (2021). The Effects of polyvictimization on mental and physical health outcomes in an LGBTQ sample. *Journal of Traumatic Stress*, *34*(1), 161–171. https://doi.org/10.1002/jts.22579

LeBlanc, M. E., Trinh, M. H., Zubizarreta, D., & Reisner, S. L. (2024). Healthcare stereotype threat, healthcare access, and health outcomes in a probability sample of U.S. transgender and gender diverse adults. *Preventive Medicine Reports*, *42*, 102734. https://doi.org/10.1016/j.pmedr.2024.102734

Long, K. N. G., Symons, X., VanderWeele, T. J., Balboni, T. A., Rosmarin, D. H., Puchalski, C., Cutts, T., Gunderson, G. R., Idler, E., Oman, D., Balboni, M. J., Tuach, L. S., & Koh, H. K. (2024). Spirituality as a determinant of health: Emerging policies, practices, and systems. *Health Affairs (Project Hope)*, *43*(6), 783–790. https://doi.org/10.1377/hlthaff.2023.01643.

Mallonee, J., Escalante, R., Robles, E. H., & Tucker, C. (2023). "Something very taboo": a qualitative exploration of beliefs, barriers, and recommendations for improving mental health care and access for Hispanic adults in the Paso del Norte U.S.-Mexico border region. *Frontiers in Public Health*, *11*, 1134076. https://doi.org/10.3389/fpubh.2023.1134076

Medina-Martínez, J., Saus-Ortega, C., Sánchez-Lorente, M. M., Sosa-Palanca, E. M., García-Martínez, P., & Mármol-López, M. I. (2021). Health inequities in LGBT people and nursing interventions to reduce them: A systematic review. *International Journal of Environmental Research and Public Health*, *18*(22), 11801.

Merritt, C. C., Halverson, T. F., Elliott, T., Jarskog, L. F., Pedersen, C. A., & Penn, D. L. (2023). Racial disparities and predictors of functioning in schizophrenia. *The American Journal of Orthopsychiatry*, *93*(3), 177–187. https://doi.org/10.1037/ort0000661

Monteith, L. L., Holliday, R., Brown, T. L., Brenner, L. A., & Mohatt, N. V. (2021). Preventing suicide in rural communities during the COVID-19 pandemic. *The Journal of Rural Health*, *37*(1), 179–184. https://doi.org/10.1111/jrh.12448

National Alliance on Mental Illness (NAMI). (n.d.). *Mental health inequities: Racism and racial discrimination*. Retrieved September 21, 2024, from https://www.nami.org/advocacy/policy-priorities/supporting-community-inclusion-and-non-discrimination/mental-health-inequities-racism-and-racial-discrimination/

National Council on Aging. (2023). *American Indians and Alaska Natives: Key demographics and characteristics*. Retrieved January 13, 2024, from https://www.ncoa.org/article/american-indians-and-alaska-natives-key-demographics-and-characteristics

Oldani, M. J., & Prosen, D. (2021). Trauma-informed caring for Native American patients and communities prioritizes healing, not management. *AMA Journal of Ethics*, *23*(6), E446–E455. https://doi.org/10.1001/amajethics.2021.446

Pappadis, M. R., Sander, A. M., Juengst, S. B., Leon-Novelo, L., Ngan, E., Bell, K. R., Corrigan, J. D., Driver, S., Dreer, L. E., & Lequerica, A. H. (2023). The relationship of health literacy to health outcomes among individuals with traumatic brain injury: A traumatic brain injury model systems study. *The Journal of Head Trauma Rehabilitation*. https://doi.org/10.1097/HTR.0000000000000912

Pew Research Center. (2023). *Spirituality among Americans*. Retrieved September 25, 2024, from https://www.pewresearch.org/religion/2023/12/07/spirituality-among-americans/

Puchalski, C. M., Vitillo, R., Hull, S. K., & Reller, N. (2014). Improving the spiritual dimension of whole person care: Reaching national and international consensus. *Journal of Palliative Medicine*, *17*(6), 642–656. https://doi.org/10.1089/jpm.2014.9427

Ross, K., Schell, L., & Hubicki, L. (2023). American Indian/Alaskan Native child and adolescent mortality. *Journal of Racial and Ethnic Health Disparities*. https://doi.org/10.1007/s40615-023-01641-2

Salameh, T. N., Nyakeriga, D. B., & Hall, L. A. (2023). Telehealth care for perinatal depression in immigrant and refugee women: A scoping review. *Issues in Mental Health Nursing*, *44*(12), 1216–1225. https://doi.org/10.1080/01612840.2023.2258222

Saltzman, L. Y., Lesen, A. E., Henry, V., Hansel, T. C., & Bordnick, P. S. (2021). COVID-19 mental health disparities. *Health Security*, *19*(S1), S5–S13. https://doi.org/10.1089/hs.2021.0017

Sayed, L., Alanazi, M., & Ajrouch, K. J. (2023). Self-reported cognitive aging and well-being among older Middle Eastern/Arab American immigrants during the COVID-19 pandemic. *International Journal of Environmental Research and Public Health*, *20*(11), 5918.

Schlossberg, J. (2023). *Confronting mental health barriers in the Asian American and Pacific Islander community*. UCLA Health. https://www.uclahealth.org/news/confronting-mental-health-barriers-asian-american-and-2

Shaimaa, E., & Bialous, S. (2024). Mental health care access among Arab Immigrants in the United States: Application of Public Arena Model. *Community Mental Health Journal*, *60*(2), 376–384. https://doi.org/10.1007/s10597-023-01182-2

Shrider, E. A., Kollar, M., Chen, F., & Semega, J. (2021). Current population reports. *Income and Poverty in the United States: 2020*. pp. 60–273. U.S. Census Bureau.

Smallwood, R., Woods, C., Power, T., & Usher, K. (2021). Understanding the impact of historical trauma due to colonization on the health and well-being of indigenous young peoples: A systematic scoping review. *Journal of Transcultural Nursing*, *32*(1), 59–68.

Swetlitz, N., Hinton, L., Rivera, M., Liu, M., Fernandez, A. C., & Garcia, M. E. (2024). Barriers and facilitators to depression care among Latino men in a primary care setting: A qualitative study. *BMC Primary Care*, *25*(1), 30. https://doi.org/10.1186/s12875-024-02275-x

Tham, S. S., & Solomon, P. (2023). Practicing cultural humility will achieve recovery-oriented mental health practice and service delivery. *Administration and Policy in Mental Health*. https://doi.org/10.1007/s10488-023-01307-5.

Tschannen, D., Tillman-Meakins, P., Keiser, M., Bathish, M., & Turkelson, C. (2024). Development of the "through the eyes of …" program for improving cultural awareness. *The Journal of Nursing Education*, 1–5. https://doi.org/10.3928/01484834-20240422-04

U.S. Census Bureau. (2021a). *2020 U.S. population more racially and ethnically diverse than measured in 2010*. America counts: Stories behind the numbers. Retrieved August 22, 2021, from https://www.census.gov/library/stories/2021/08/2020-united-states-population-more-racially-ethnically-diverse-than-2010.html

U.S. Census Bureau. (2021b). *2020 Census illuminations racial and ethnic composition of the country*. America counts: Stories behind the numbers. Retrieved October 29, 2024, from https://www.census.gov/library/stories/2021/08/improved-race-ethnicity-measures-reveal-united-states-population-much-more-multiracial.html

U.S. Census Bureau. (2022a). *20.6 Million people in the U.S. identify as Asian, Native Hawaiian or Pacific Islander*. Broad diversity of Asian, native Hawaiian, Pacific Islander Population. Retrieved January 12, 2023, from https://www.census.gov/library/stories/2022/05/aanhpi-population-diverse-geographically-dispersed.html

U.S. Census Bureau. (2022b). *Facts for features: American Indian and Alaska Native Heritage Month*. Retrieved May 31, 2025, from November 2022. https://www.census.gov/newsroom/facts-for-features/2022/aian-month.html

U.S. Census Bureau. (2023). *Census bureau releases 202 census data for nearly 1,500 detailed race and ethnicity groups, tribes and villages*. https://www.census.gov/newsroom/press-releases/2023/2020-census-detailed-dhc-file-a.html

U.S. Department of Health and Human Services. (2024). HHS poverty guidelines for 2024. Retrieved January 12, 2024, from https://aspe.hhs.gov/topics/poverty-economic-mobility/poverty-guidelines

VanderLaan, D. P., Skorska, M. N., Peragine, D. E., & Coome, L. A. (2023). Carving the biodevelopment of same-sex sexual orientation at its joints. *Archives of Sexual Behavior, 52*(7), 2939–2962. https://doi.org/10.1007/s10508-022-02360-1

Wickham, M. I., van Nunspeet, F., & Ellemers, N. (2023). Gender identification beyond the binary and its consequences for social well-being. *Archives of Sexual Behavior*, *52*(3), 1073–1093.

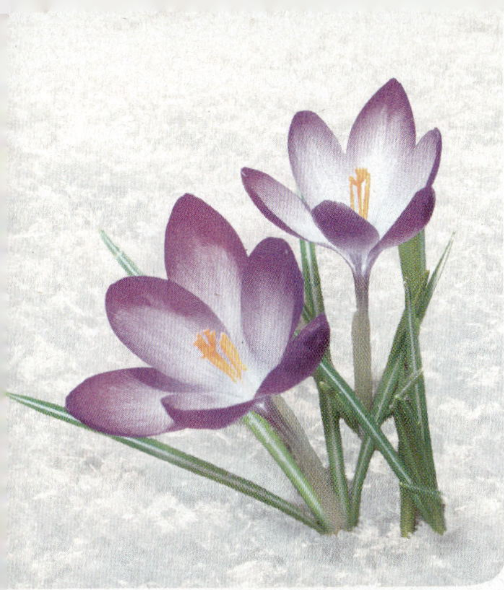

4 Nursing Ethics, Patient Rights, and Legal Issues

Rebecca Luebbert

KEYCONCEPT

- self-determinism

LEARNING OBJECTIVES

After studying this chapter, you will be able to:

1. Describe the importance of the ethical principles of respect for autonomy, beneficence, justice, nonmaleficence, veracity, and fidelity for considering ethical situations in psychiatric–mental health (PMH) nursing practice.
2. Define self-determinism and its implications in mental health care.
3. Discuss the legal protection of the rights of people with mental illness.
4. Distinguish decisional capacity and competency.
5. Discuss the significance of treatment in the least restrictive environment.
6. Describe the implications of seclusion and restraint use.
7. Identify the impact of trauma-informed approaches.
8. Delineate the differences between voluntary and involuntary treatment.
9. Discuss the difference between privacy and confidentiality.
10. Discuss Health Insurance Portability and Accountability Act and mandates to inform and their implications in PMH care.
11. Examine the presence and impact of mental illness in forensic settings.
12. Discuss the stigma of mental illness and criminality.
13. Describe legal outcomes for people with mental illness in forensic settings.
14. Identify the importance of accurate, quality documentation in electronic and nonelectronic patient records.

KEY TERMS

• accreditation • advance care directives • assault • autonomy • beneficence • breach of confidentiality • chemical restraint • competence • confidentiality • durable power of attorney • external advocacy system • fidelity • incompetent • informed consent • internal rights protection system • involuntary commitment • justice • least restrictive environment • living will • medical battery • negligence • nonmaleficence • paternalism • power of attorney • privacy • restraint • seclusion • trauma-informed approach • veracity • voluntary admission • voluntary commitment

INTRODUCTION

Because individuals with mental disorders are often vulnerable to mistreatment and abuse, their legal rights and the ethical health care practices of mental health providers are ongoing concerns for PMH nurses. For example, can an individual be forced into a hospital if their behavior is bizarre but harmless? What human rights can be denied to an individual who has a mental disorder and under what circumstances? These questions are not easily answered. This chapter summarizes some of the key patient rights and legal issues that underlie PMH nursing practice across the continuum of care.

ETHICS OF PSYCHIATRIC–MENTAL HEALTH NURSING

PMH nursing practice is guided by the *Code of Ethics for Nurses with Interpretive Statements*. The *Code* communicates nursing's ethical values, obligations, duties, and professional ideals; establishes ethical standards; and confirms the profession's commitment to society (American Nurses Association [ANA], 2015).

Four primary health care ethical principles—respect for autonomy, beneficence, nonmaleficence, and justice—guide nurses' consideration of ethical concerns. In health care decisions and conduct, these principles highlight the ethical aspects of the patient situations, decision dilemmas, and relationships. Each of the four primary principles prompts nurses to focus on different aspects of an ethical decision or relationship. Sometimes, the value(s) inherent in one principle may be in tension with one or more of the other principles. For example, a patient may decide to stop taking a medication (respect for autonomy), but the nurse believes that harm could likely come to the patient or others without medication use. In ethical dilemmas, all of the principles are important and relevant. In a situation of ethical conflict, the PMH nurse weighs the values protected in each principle and helps others to see the different sides of an ethical question.

Autonomy

The principle of **autonomy** is based on the understanding that each individual has the fundamental right to make voluntary decisions about their health care and life decisions. People are to be regarded as self-determining. The principle of respect for autonomy gives rise to expectations for ethical conduct, namely, the use of informed consent in health care practices. To give consent to a treatment or procedure, an individual must have the needed relevant information, be able to rationally deliberate, and not be forced into a decision. The PMH nurse protects patient autonomy by assessing an individual's decisional capacity and ability to act in their own best interests. Nurses are also obligated by the principle of respect for autonomy to protect individuals' privacy. People lose the ability to be self-determining when information about their health conditions is shared without their permission. Privacy can be important especially in mental health practice because of mental health stigmatization and the patient's potential vulnerability.

Beneficence

The principle of **beneficence** (goodness) rests on the assumption that professionals have a duty to act in ways that benefit a patient or community, and they take the steps necessary to minimize harm. The scope and standards of nursing practice (discussed later in this chapter) describe how PMH nurses act in a beneficent way toward those in their care.

Nonmaleficence

Nonmaleficence is the duty one has to never intentionally harm another. Often in health care decisions, negative outcomes may occur as a result of any choice that is made. The professional is obligated to minimize the harm and risks as much as possible for both the individual and others who may be involved.

Justice

The principle of **justice** encourages providers to consider how the goods of a society, including health care, are distributed. As noted in the first provision of the *Code of Ethics for Nurses*, providers have an ethical duty to treat all people with dignity, respect, and fairness. Those "goods" of health care, including access to care, should be distributed equally. Justice also requires that we consider how to distribute resources so that those with greater needs get what is essential for their health and survival, even if they should get more than others. The principle of justice is violated when mental health services are not readily available to those most in need.

NCLEXNOTES Be prepared to consider the ways in which ethical principles may be in tension with one another in situations of ethical conflict in PMH nursing.

Veracity and Fidelity

Two secondary ethical principles, veracity and fidelity, provide additional guidance for mental health care practice. **Veracity** highlights one's duty to tell the truth. Being honest with others provides a foundation for the development of trust in a helping, healing relationship. Often, "telling the truth" requires judgment and sensitivity. For example, giving others more information than is necessary, even if that information is true, could cause fear, anxiety, and harm. Or, there may be times when the nurse cannot truthfully respond to a patient's question. A nurse cannot promise, for example, that a medication will eliminate all mental health symptoms, even if that is what the patient wants to hear.

Fidelity implies that nurses should be faithful to their obligations and duties toward others, society, and the nursing profession. Fidelity is also essential for the maintenance of trusting relationships because it is centered on doing what one says will be done (keeping promises).

Paternalism

At times, health care professionals use the principle of **paternalism** to guide their actions and decisions. A paternalistic approach assumes that because professionals have specialized knowledge and education, they are best equipped to make decisions for others. Indeed, often professionals' expert knowledge of the medical aspects of a situation makes their judgment extremely valuable. Professionals may not know, however, the details of an individual's life and values. Nurses protect against unwarranted use of paternalism by encouraging patient, family, and community involvement in decisions. Paternalism may be justified in some mental health conditions in which an individual is temporarily unable to deliberate in the best interests of self or others. Some health care decisions—such as the legally mandated use of seat belts, face masks, or motorcycle helmets—are made to protect others. Paternalism can be in direct conflict with the mental health recovery belief of self-determination (see Chapters 1 and 8).

NCLEXNOTES Be able to identify ethical situations encountered by PMH nurses in inpatient and outpatient settings.

Overcoming Stigma

All nurses, based on their knowledge and adherence to the professional code of ethics, play an important role in dispelling myths and stigma often associated with mental illness. Stigma often prevents individuals from seeking help for mental health problems and is a form of injustice (see Chapter 2). PMH nurses have a unique insight into the harm caused by stigmatization. The principle of beneficence underlies the nurse's responsibility to reduce the burden of mental illness by addressing stigma, improving access to care, and educating patients, family members, communities, and society about the etiology, symptoms, and treatment of mental illnesses.

SELF-DETERMINISM: A FUNDAMENTAL RIGHT AND NEED

At the foundation of many questions related to the rights of patients with mental disorders is the issue of self-determinism and preservation of this right.

A self-determined individual is internally motivated to make choices based on personal goals, not to please others or to be rewarded. That is, an individual engages in activities that are interesting, challenging, pleasing, exciting, or fun, requiring no rewards other than the positive feelings that accompany them because of inner goals, needs, drives, or preferences. Personal autonomy and avoidance of dependence on others are key values of self-determinism, which is integral to the recovery process.

In mental health care, self-determinism is the right to choose one's own health-related behaviors, which at times differ from those recommended by health professionals. A patient's right to refuse treatment, to choose an alternative treatment, and to seek a second opinion are all self-deterministic acts. In mental health care, adhering to treatment regimens may be at odds with the self-deterministic views of an individual. Patients may decline taking medication for many reasons, including denial or lack of awareness or understanding about their illness and medication, concerns about potential side effects or cost of medications, and perceived stigma associated with taking a psychotropic medication (Alvear Velasquez et al., 2024). Supporting an individual's ability to choose treatment becomes complex because of related issues of competency, informed consent, voluntary and involuntary commitment, and public safety; these issues are discussed later in this chapter.

KEYCONCEPT Self-determinism is based on an individual's fundamental right to autonomy. Exercising this right, patients may choose to "accept, refuse, or terminate treatment without deceit, undue influence, duress, coercion, or prejudice" (American Nurses Association, 2015, p. 2).

PROTECTION OF PATIENT RIGHTS

Because people with psychiatric problems are vulnerable to mistreatment, coercion, and abuse, laws exist that guarantee them legal protection. These laws offer protection of self-determinism, protection against discrimination in employment, and protection against mistreatment in health care settings.

Self-Determination Act

The Patient Self-Determination Act (PDSA) is a federal law that became effective in 1991, as a part of the Omnibus Budget Reconciliation Act of 1990. The PDSA requires hospitals, health maintenance organizations, skilled nursing facilities, home health agencies, and hospice organizations receiving Medicare and Medicaid reimbursement to inform patients at the time of admission of their right to be a central part of any and all health care decisions made about them or for them. Patients have the following rights:

- Be provided with information regarding advance care directives
- Be asked at admission or enrollment whether they have an advance care document and that this fact be recorded in the medical record
- Be provided with information on their rights to complete advance care documents and refuse medical care (Omnibus Budget Reconciliation Act, 1990)

The Act also requires health care institutions receiving Medicare and Medicaid reimbursement to educate health care personnel and the local community about advance care planning.

Advance Care Directives in Mental Health

At different times during the course of an illness, people with mental disorders may be unable to make sound decisions regarding their treatment and care. Fortunately, advance care directives legally protect them from their periodic poor decision-making abilities. A competent individual can make a decision about a treatment—a decision that can be honored even if the individual is no longer able to make decisions. (See later discussion for how competency is determined.)

Advance care directives are written instructions for health care when individuals are incapacitated. Living wills and appointment directives, often referred to as **power of attorney** or health proxies, are recognized under state laws and their courts. **A living will** specifies what treatment should be omitted or refused in the event that an individual is unable to make those decisions. A **durable power of attorney** for health care appoints a proxy, usually a relative or trusted friend, to make health care decisions on an individual's behalf if that individual is incapacitated.

An advance directive does not need to be written, reviewed, or signed by an attorney. It must be witnessed by two people and notarized and applies only if the individual is unable to make their own decisions as a result of being incapacitated or if, in the opinion of two providers, the individual is otherwise unable to make decisions for themselves.

Psychiatric advance directives (PADs) allow patients, while competent, to document their choices of treatment and care. This declaration must be made in advance and signed by the patient and two witnesses. Through the use of a PAD, individuals are empowered to direct their treatment such as choice of medication and hospitalization. Although a physician can override this declaration during times when the patient's decision-making capacity is clearly distorted because of mental illness, the patient must be informed first and the order made by the court. During periods of competency, the PAD can be revoked.

Bill of Rights for Patients With Mental Disorders

Rights of people with mental disorders receive additional protection beyond that afforded to patients in other health care areas (Box 4.1). The Mental Health Systems Act [42 U.S.C. 9501 et seq.] of 1980 requires that each state review and revise, if necessary, its laws to ensure that patients with mental disorders receive these human rights protections and services that they require.

Americans With Disabilities Act and Job Discrimination

The Americans with Disabilities Act of 1990 ensures that people with disabilities, including those with mental impairment, have legal protection against discrimination in the workplace, housing, public programs, transportation, and telecommunications. An employer is free to select the most qualified applicant available, but if the most qualified individual has a physical or mental impairment, this law mandates that reasonable accommodations are made for that individual to be able to perform the

BOX 4.1

Bill of Rights for People Receiving Mental Health Services

- The right to appropriate treatment and related services under conditions that support the person's personal liberty and restrict such liberty only as necessary to comply with treatment needs, laws, and judicial orders.
- The right to an individualized, written treatment or service plan (to be developed promptly after admission), treatment based on the plan, periodic review and reassessment of needs, and appropriate revisions of the plan, including a description of services that may be needed after discharge.
- The right to ongoing participation in the planning of services to be provided and in the development and periodic revision of the treatment plan, and the right to be provided with a reasonable explanation of all aspects of one's own condition and treatment.
- The right to refuse treatment, except during an emergency situation or as permitted under law in the case of an individual committed by a court for treatment.
- The right not to participate in experimentation in the absence of the patient's informed, voluntary, written consent; the right to appropriate protections associated with such participation; and the right to an opportunity to revoke such consent.
- The right to freedom from restraints or seclusion, other than during an emergency situation.
- The right to a humane treatment environment that affords reasonable protection from harm and appropriate privacy.
- The right to confidentiality of records.
- The right to access, upon request, one's own mental health care records.
- The right (in residential or inpatient care) to converse with others privately and to have access to the telephone and mails unless denial of access is documented as necessary for treatment.
- The right to be informed promptly, in appropriate language and terms, of the rights described in this section.
- The right to assert grievances with respect to infringement of the Bill of Rights, including the right to have such grievances considered in a fair, timely, and impartial procedure.
- The right of access to protection, service, and a qualified advocate in order to understand, exercise, and protect one's rights.
- The right to exercise the rights described in this section without reprisal, including reprisal in the form of denial of any appropriate, available treatment.
- The right to referral as appropriate to other providers of mental health services upon discharge.

Adapted from 42 (U.S. Code § 10841)—Restatement of bill of rights. Title V of the Mental Health Systems Act [42 U.S.C. 9501 et seq.].

essential functions of the job. Accommodations include any adjustments to a job or work environment, such as restructuring a job, modifying work schedules, and providing or modifying equipment (U.S. Equal Employment Opportunity Commission, Office of the Americans with Disabilities Act, 2023).

Access to Mental Health Services

Mental health and substance use disorder services are one of the 10 designated Essential Health Benefits requiring coverage through plans established by the Patient Protection and Affordable Care Act. Services required include behavioral health treatment, counseling, and psychotherapy. The Mental Health Parity and Addiction Equity Act requires insurance plans to offer benefits and coverage for mental health and substance use disorders that are comparable to coverage for other medical conditions. Treatment fees and limitations for mental health services or substance use disorders cannot be any more restrictive than those designated for medical care (Substance Abuse and Mental Health Services Administration [SAMHSA], 2022a).

Internal Rights Protection Systems

Mental health care systems have **internal rights protection systems** or mechanisms to combat any violation of their patients' rights. Public Law 99–319, the Protection and Advocacy for Mentally Ill Individuals Act of 1986, requires each state mental health provider to establish and operate a system that protects and advocates for the rights of individuals with mental illnesses and investigates any incidents of abuse, neglect, and rights violations.

External Advocacy Systems

Health organizations such as the American Hospital Association, American Healthcare Association, and the American Public Health Association serve as advocates for the rights and treatment of patients with mental disorders and are a part of an **external advocacy system**. They are financially and administratively independent from the mental health agencies. These groups advocate through negotiation and recommendations but have no legal authority. They can resort to litigation that leads to lawsuits and consent decrees (legal mandates that are monitored by the U.S. Department of Justice) or, in some instances, a denial of accreditation to the health care institution by their certifying body.

Accreditation of Mental Health Care Delivery Systems

Patient rights are also assured of protection by an agency's **accreditation**, the recognition or approval of an institution according to the accrediting body's criteria. Accrediting bodies such as The Joint Commission require patient rights standards. The Centers for Medicare & Medicaid Services (CMS) sets patient rights standards for institutions seeking Medicare and Medicaid funding. Community mental health centers are not accredited by either The Joint Commission or CMS but by another agency, the Commission on Accreditation of Rehabilitation Facilities.

TREATMENT AND PATIENT RIGHTS

When patients are involved in decision making, they are more likely to be adherent to their treatment regimen (Calcedo-Barba et al., 2020). In caring for patients receiving mental health services or treatment, it is important for nurses to understand several issues related to the patient's rights to determine choices about their own treatment. These issues are related to competency, informed consent, least restrictive environment, and voluntary and involuntary treatment.

Competency

One of the most important concepts underlying the legal rights of individuals is the competency to consent to or to refuse treatment. Although competency is a legal determination, it is not clearly defined across the states. It is generally agreed that **competence**, or the degree to which the patient can understand and appreciate the information given during the consent process, refers to a patient's cognitive ability to process information at a specific time. A patient may be competent to make a treatment decision at one time and not be competent at another time. Similarly, competence is also decision specific—a patient may be competent to decide on a simple treatment with a relatively clear consequence but may not be competent to decide about a treatment with a complex set of outcomes. A competent patient can refuse any aspect of the treatment plan (Marshall et al., 2024; Steinert & Henking, 2022).

Competency is different from rationality, which is a characteristic of a patient's decision, not of the patient's ability to make a decision. An irrational decision is one that involves hurting oneself pointlessly, such as stopping recommended treatment even though symptoms return. An individual who is competent may make what appears to be an irrational decision, and it cannot be overruled by health care providers; however, if an individual is judged **incompetent** (i.e., unable to understand and appreciate the information given during the consent process), it is possible to force treatment on the individual. Strong arguments are, however, made against forced treatment under these circumstances. Forced treatment denigrates individuals, and according to self-determinism theory

BOX 4.2

Research for Evidence-Based Practice: Assessing Decisional Capacity of Patients With Severe Mental Disorders

Calcedo-Barba, A., Fructuoso, A., Martinez-Raga, J., Paz, S., Sanchez de Carmona, M., & Vicens, E. (2020). A meta-review of literature reviews assessing the capacity of patients with severe mental disorders to make decisions about their healthcare. BMC Psychiatry, 20*(1), 339.*

THE QUESTION: Do psychiatric patients have the mental capacity to make health care–related decisions?

METHODS: A systematic review of studies on the capacity of patients with serious mental illnesses to make health care and treatment-related decisions was conducted. Literature reviews, meta-analyses, and summarizing studies were included. In total, eleven publications were reviewed.

FINDINGS: Up to three quarters of psychiatric patients, including those with serious illnesses such as schizophrenia or bipolar disorder may have decisional capacity to make their own medical decisions. The capacity of patients with stable psychiatric disorders to make decisions related to their own health care may be similar to that of non-psychiatric patients. Patients with mental illness are able to judge risk-reward situations and make a decision about their treatment outcomes. There are some symptoms that might impair different domains of the decisional capacity of psychotic patients. These impairments are temporal and efforts should be made to simplify information, provide education, and encourage shared decision making.

IMPLICATIONS FOR NURSING: Although some patients with severe mental disorders may lack decisional capacity, most individuals are able to make rational decisions about their own health care. Nurses should advocate for patient's rights to determine their own treatment.

and recovery concepts, individuals are not as likely to experience treatment success if it is externally imposed.

Although some individuals with mental illness have limited decisional capacity, most patients with a mental disorder are deemed competent to make rational decisions about their health care plan (Box 4.2). How is it determined that a patient is competent? Mental health legal experts generally agree that four areas should be directly assessed (Appelbaum, 2007). Table 4.1 outlines these assessment areas. A patient who is competent to give **informed consent** should be able to achieve the following:

- Communicate choices
- Understand relevant information
- Appreciate the situation and its consequences
- Use a logical thought process to compare the risks and benefits of treatment options

Informed Consent

Individuals seeking mental health care must provide informed consent, a legal procedure to ensure that they know the benefits and costs of treatment. Informed consent is not an option but is mandated by state laws. Merely signing a consent document does not imply an informed consent. To provide informed consent for care, the patient must be given adequate information upon which to base decisions and actively participate in the decision-making process. A mental health provider must provide information about the risks and benefits of treatment in such a way that an average reasonable person would be able to make an educated decision about the interventions. Providing insufficient information and education to the patient may limit their ability to provide an autonomous decision about their plan of care, which in turn may lead to nonadherence (Steinert & Henking, 2022).

TABLE 4.1 DETERMINATION OF COMPETENCY

Assessment Area	Definition	Patient Attributes
Communicate choices	Ability to express choices	Patient should be able to clearly indicate their treatment choice
Understand relevant information	Capacity to comprehend the meaning of the information given about treatment	Patient should be able to paraphrase understanding of treatment
Appreciate the situation and its consequences	Capacity to grasp what the information means specifically to the patient	Patient should be able to discuss the disorder, the need for treatment, the likely outcomes, and the reason the treatment is being suggested
Use a logical thought process to compare the risks and benefits of treatment options	Capacity to reach a logical conclusion consistent with the starting premise	Patient should be able to discuss logical reasons for the choice of treatment

Adapted from Appelbaum, P. S. (2007). Clinical practice. Assessment of patients' competence to consent to treatment. *New England Journal of Medicine, 357*(18), 1834–1840.

Informed consent is complicated in mental health treatment. A patient must be competent to give consent, but the individual's decision-making ability may be compromised by their mental illness. This dilemma might be illustrated by a situation in which an individual who is informed of medication side effects refuses treatment, not because of the potential negative impact of the medication but because they deny the illness outright. The health care provider knows that when the individual begins taking the medication, the symptoms of the illness may subside, and the decision-making ability will return.

Most institutions have policies that outline the nursing responsibilities within the informed consent process. The nurse has a key role in the process of informed consent, from structuring the written informed consent document to educating the patient about a particular treatment. The nurse makes sure that consent has been obtained before any treatment is given. Informed consent is especially important in research projects involving experimental drugs or therapies.

Least Restrictive Environment

The right to refuse treatment is related to a larger concept—the right to be treated in the **least restrictive environment**, which means that an individual cannot be restricted to an institution when they can be successfully treated in the community. In 1975, the courts ruled that an individual committed to psychiatric treatment had a right to be treated in the least restrictive environment (Dixon v. Weinberger, 1975). Medication cannot be given unnecessarily. An individual cannot be secluded in a room or restrained unless all other *less restrictive* interventions are tried first.

Seclusion and Restraint

Seclusion is the involuntary confinement of an individual alone in a room or an area where the person is physically prevented from leaving. A patient is placed in seclusion for purposes of safety or behavioral management. The seclusion room has no furniture except a mattress and a blanket. The walls are usually padded. The room is environmentally safe, with no hanging devices, electrical outlets, or windows from which the patient could jump. When a patient is placed in seclusion, they are observed at all times.

There are several types of seclusion arrangements. Some facilities place seclusion rooms next to the nurses' stations. These seclusion rooms have an observation window. Other facilities use a modified patient room and assign a staff member to view the patient at all times.

The most restrictive safety intervention is the use of **restraint,** any manual method, physical or mechanical, that immobilizes or reduces the ability of the patient to move freely. The nurse must choose the least restrictive type of restraint to keep a patient safe. Wrist restraints restrict arm movement. Walking restraints or ankle restraints are used if a patient cannot risk the impulse to run from a facility but is safe to go outside and to activities. Three- and four-point restraints are applied to the wrist and ankles in bed. When five-point restraints are used, all extremities are secured, and another restraint is placed across the chest. **Chemical restraint** is the use of medications for restricting patients' behavior or their freedom of movement. These chemical restraints include medications that are not a part of their standard psychiatric treatment or that are at a higher dosage than their standard medication.

Seclusion and restraint should never be used as a means of coercion or punishment or for the convenience of staff. Use of restraints is the most intrusive intervention against patient autonomy and therefore should only be used when less restrictive measures have been proven ineffective and the behavioral emergency poses serious and imminent danger to the person, self, or others. If it is determined that seclusion or restraint is needed, it must be used for the minimal amount of time necessary to ensure the safety of the patient or others. When mechanical restraint is necessary, only the least restrictive and least number of restraint points should be used (APNA, 2022; Steinert & Henking, 2022).

The use of seclusion or restraint requires an order from a physician or licensed practitioner who is responsible for the care and treatment of the patient. Within an hour of initiation of seclusion or restraint, a face-to-face evaluation by a physician, licensed provider, or trained and competent registered nurse is necessary to evaluate the patient's response and determine whether seclusion/restraint is to continue. While in seclusion/restraint, the patient must be under continuous observation in accordance with federal, state, and regulatory agency guidelines. Continuous monitoring is critical to ensure the safety of the patient and to ensure that they are released from seclusion or restraint as soon as it is determined safe to do so. As soon as possible following the discontinuation of seclusion or restraint, the nurse, the patient, and others as appropriate should participate in a debriefing (APNA, 2022). Documentation in the clinical record is required and should include:

- The events and behavior resulting in seclusion/restraint.
- A description of the least restrictive interventions that were attempted and the patient's response.
- All necessary notifications of attending physicians/providers, parent/guardian, or others requiring notification.
- A timeline of the episode and events, including time of initiation and the patient's response to the intervention.
- Assessment of the patient to include position, circulation, range of motion, etc.

BOX 4.3

Research for Evidence-Based Practice: Patient Experience of Physical Restraint

Douglas, L, Donohue, G., & Morrissey, J. (2022). Patient experience of physical restraint in the acute setting: A systematic review of the qualitative research evidence. Issues in Mental Health Nursing, *43(5), 473–481.*

THE QUESTIONS: (1) What are the experiences of physical restraint for adult inpatients receiving mental health services? (2) What are the implications of physical restraint use on the therapeutic relationship in inpatient mental health services?

METHODS: The literature was systematically searched using keywords "physical restraint" and "patient experience" and "acute setting." The search yielded 482 papers. Of these, nine were considered suitable for the review.

FINDINGS: Following analysis, three themes were identified: the bio-psychosocial impact of restraint on patients, the impact of restraint on the therapeutic relationship, and patient needs concerning the use of restraint.

IMPLICATIONS FOR NURSING: Overall, the use of restraint is experienced by those receiving it as negative, contributing to traumatic feelings of fear and distress. Patients with a history of abuse or trauma are predisposed to being retraumatized by the restraint process. Alternatives to restraint that promote patient autonomy and safety are important.

- Interventions provided to promote comfort and safety as well as those to expedite release of seclusion/restraint.
- Criteria for release, including the patients understanding of the criteria.
- Time of release from seclusion/restraint.
- Debriefing with the person involved, staff, and caregivers as indicated (APNA, 2022).

Definite risks are associated with the use of seclusion and restraint. Patient outcomes may actually be worsened (Box 4.3). As a result, many facilities have completely abandoned its practice. The use of seclusion and restraint can result in psychological harm and physical injury to both the patient and staff members involved in its use. Injury rates to staff in settings involving the use of seclusion and restraint are found to be higher than in other high-risk industries. Additionally, studies have shown that patients who have been secluded or restrained prolong their treatment time and are more likely to be readmitted for further treatment (SAMHSA, 2022b).

In recovery-oriented practice, the nurse is particularly sensitive to recognizing the relationship between earlier trauma and retraumatizing an individual by using restraint. Using a **trauma-informed approach** is important in recovery-oriented practice and includes understanding the widespread impact of trauma, recognizing the symptoms of trauma, avoiding retraumatization, and supporting paths to recovery (SAMHSA, 2023). In order to use a trauma-informed approach, the patient needs to feel connected, valued, informed, and hopeful of recovery. Nursing interventions should be perceived by the patient as safe, responsive, empowering, and collaborative. A trusting relationship between the patient and the nurse is critical (Nizum et al., 2020).

Voluntary and Involuntary Treatment

Accessing the mental health delivery system is similar to seeking any other type of health care. Whether in a public or private system, the treatment setting is usually for outpatient. Treatment strategies (e.g., medication, psychotherapy) are recommended and agreed on by both the provider and the individual. Arrangements for treatment and follow-up are then made. The patient leaves the outpatient setting and is responsible for following the plan.

Inpatient treatment is generally reserved for patients who are acutely ill or have a forensic commitment. If hospitalization is required, the individual enters the treatment facility, participates in the treatment planning process, and follows through with the treatment. The individual maintains all civil rights and is free to leave at any time even if it is against medical advice. In most settings, this type of admission is called a **voluntary admission**. If an individual is admitted to a public facility, the state statute may refer to the process as **voluntary commitment** rather than admission; however, in both instances, full legal rights are retained.

Involuntary commitment is the mandated treatment without the individual's consent but with a court order. There are also legal provisions for people to be involuntarily committed to outpatient mental health facilities through state civil laws. Because involuntary commitment is a prerogative of the state agency, each state and the District of Columbia have separate commitment statutes; however, three common elements are found in most of these statutes. There should be evidence that the individual is (1) mentally ill to the degree that their thought or mood grossly impairs judgment, behavior, or ability to negotiate demands of life, (2) dangerous to self or others, or (3) unable to provide for basic needs (i.e., *gravely disabled*) (SAMHSA, 2019).

Patients who are involuntarily committed have the right to receive treatment, but they also may have the right to refuse it. Arguments over the rights of patients who are civilly committed to refuse treatment first surfaced in 1975 when a federal district court judge issued a temporary restraining order prohibiting the use of psychotropic medication against the patient's will at a state hospital in Boston. Laws about commitment and refusal of medication vary from state to state. A separate judicial

BOX 4.4

Mental Health Inequities: Inequities in Inpatient Psychiatric Commitment

The legal status of admission of all patients admitted to an inpatient psychiatric unit over a 6-year period was recorded. Of the 4,393 patients admitted, 28% were involuntarily admitted, and court commitment petitions were filed for 7%. Patients of color were more likely than White patients to be involuntarily admitted, and Black and Asian patients were more likely to have court commitment petitions filed. Proposed causes of ethnoracial inequities in commitment found in prior studies include interpersonal racism, implicit bias, and differences between racial groups in terms of illness severity, access to treatment, and social determinants of health (SDOH).

Shea, T., Dotson, S., Tyree, G., Obgu-Nwodbodo, L., Beck, S., & Shtasel, D. (2022). Racial and ethnic inequities in inpatient psychiatric civil commitment. *Psychiatric Services, 73*(12), 1322–1329.

process may be necessary if an individual is determined to be incompetent to refuse medication. Forcing a patient to take medication against their will without a legal provision to do so may expose the nurse to liability.

Commitment procedures vary considerably among the states. Most have provisions for an emergency short-term hospitalization of 48 to 92 hours authorized by a certified mental health provider without court approval. These emergency hospitalizations are often initiated by a concerned family member or friend. At the end of this time-limited period, either the individual agrees to voluntary treatment or extended commitment procedures are begun. The judge must order the commitment, and the individual is afforded several legal rights, including notice of the proceedings, a full hearing (jury trial if requested) in which the government must prove the grounds for commitment, and the right to legal counsel at state expense (see Box 4.4).

NCLEXNOTES Patients who are unable to care for their basic needs or who pose an immediate danger to themselves or others are candidates for involuntary commitment.

PRIVACY AND CONFIDENTIALITY

In addition to issues related to self-determinism, privacy and confidentiality are rights requiring protection for patients with mental disorders. **Privacy** refers to the part of an individual's personal life that is not governed by society's laws and government intrusion. Protecting an individual from intrusion is a responsibility of health care providers. **Confidentiality** pertains to an ethical duty of nondisclosure. Patients often share intimate details of their lives during the course of treatment, including personal thoughts, experiences, and behaviors. Providers who receive confidential information within their nurse–patient relationship must protect that information from being accessed by others and resist disclosing it. Confidentiality involves two people: the individual who discloses and the person with whom the information is shared. If confidentiality is broken, an individual's privacy is also violated; however, an individual's privacy can be violated but confidentiality maintained. For example, if a nurse observes an adult patient reading pornography alone in their room, the patient's privacy has been violated. If the patient asks the nurse not to tell anyone and the request is honored, confidentiality is maintained.

A **breach of confidentiality** occurs when a nurse divulges a patient's personal information without the patient's consent. Examples of a breach in confidentiality include discussing a patient's problem with one of their relatives without the patient's consent and sharing patient information with another professional who is not involved in the patient's care when the individual has not given permission for the information to be shared. Maintaining confidentiality is not as easy as it first appears. For example, family members are legally excluded from receiving any information about an adult member without consent even if that member is receiving care from the family. Ideally, a patient gives consent for information to be shared with the family or has psychiatric advance care directive. Ultimately, it is the nurse's duty to safeguard both personal and clinical information in the work setting as well as off duty in all venues, including social media (American Nurses Association, 2015).

Concept Mastery Alert

Privacy is the part of the person's life that is not governed by laws. *Confidentiality* is the responsibility of the health care worker to limit sharing of patient information with only those mandated to know. Confidentiality affords the patient privacy.

Health Insurance Portability and Accountability Act, and Protection of Health Information

The Health Insurance Portability and Accountability Act of 1996 (HIPAA) provides legal protection in several areas of health care, including privacy and confidentiality. This act protects working Americans from losing existing health care coverage when changing jobs and increases opportunities for purchasing health care. It regulates the use and release of patient information, especially electronic transfer of health information. Effective April 2003, HIPAA regulations require patient authorization for the release of information with the exception of that required for treatment, payment, and health care administrative operations. The release of information related to psychotherapy requires patient permission.

The underlying intent is to prevent the release of information to agencies not related to health care, such as employers, without the patient's consent. When information is released, the patient must agree to the exact information that is being disclosed, the purpose of disclosure, the recipient of the information, and an expiration date for the disclosure of information (U.S. Department of Health and Human Services, 2002).

The American Recovery and Reinvestment Act of 2009 includes several provisions affecting the management of health information. For the most part, this law focuses on maintaining the privacy of electronic transfer and storage of health information and communication. In the clinical area, one way of maintaining privacy is by restricting access to records by staff members unless there is a specific reason such as caring for a patient.

Mandates to Inform

At certain times, health care professionals are legally obligated to breach confidentiality. When there is a judgment that the patient has harmed any person or is about to injure someone, professionals are mandated by law to report it to authorities. The legal *duty to warn* was a result of the 1976 decision of Tarasoff v. Regents of the University of California (1976). In this case, a 26-year-old graduate student told university psychologists about his obsession with another student, Tatiana Tarasoff, whom he subsequently killed. Tatiana Tarasoff's parents initiated a separate civil action and brought a lawsuit against the therapists, the university, and the campus police, claiming that Tatiana's death was a result of negligence on the part of the defendants.

The plaintiffs claimed that the therapists should have warned Ms. Tarasoff that the graduate student presented a danger to her and that he should have been confined to a hospital. Both claims were originally dismissed in the lower courts, but in 1974, the California Supreme Court reversed the lower courts' decisions and said that Ms. Tarasoff should have been warned. The high court said that psychotherapists have a duty to warn the foreseeable victims of their patients' violent actions. Because of the outcry from professional mental health organizations, the court agreed to review the case, and in 1976, the original decision was revised by the ruling that psychotherapists have a duty to exercise reasonable care in protecting the foreseeable victims of their patients' violent actions. The results of this case have had far-reaching consequences and have influenced many decisions in the United States. Although many lawsuits have been based on the *Tarasoff* case, most have failed. Usually, if there are clear threats of violence toward others, the therapist is mandated to warn potential victims.

NCLEXNOTES If a patient tells the nurse that they intend to hurt a family member, the nurse is legally obligated to breach confidentiality and report the threat.

CRIMINAL JUDICIAL PROCESSES

In mental health, the term *forensic* pertains to legal proceedings and mandated treatment of people with mental illness. Individuals with mental illnesses are at higher risk for arrest than the general population and are more likely to have encounters with the criminal justice system and be convicted of a crime than those without a mental illness. Approximately 2 million individuals with mental illness are incarcerated in prisons and jails in the United States each year, with nearly 40% of those incarcerated having a history of mental illness (National Alliance on Mental Illness [NAMI], 2023). Overall, more individuals with serious mental illness reside in jails and prisons than in psychiatric facilities (Thordarson & Rector, 2020; Treatment Advocacy Center, 2023). High rates of substance use and substance use disorders are found in incarcerated adults and youth of all genders. The prevalence of post-traumatic stress disorder and mood and anxiety disorders is also higher in incarcerated individuals than in the general population (Baranyi et al., 2022). Individuals with schizophrenia or bipolar disorder are 10 times more likely to be in a prison or jail than in a psychiatric treatment facility (Treatment Advocacy Center, 2023). Despite the large number of people with mental illnesses that commit crimes, the majority of the encounters with the justice system occur when individuals with mental illness are victims of crime.

As the number of state hospitals was dramatically reduced beginning in the 1960s, the number of people with mental illness incarcerated in jails and prisons increased. Individuals in crisis are now more likely to encounter the police versus the mental health care system. Many factors contribute to the criminalization of individuals with mental illness, including "zero tolerance" policing and mandatory sentences for drug offenses, an inadequate mental health crisis response infrastructure, and the assumption that people with mental illness are violent (NAMI, 2023). Individuals with mental illnesses are treated in a variety of forensic settings, including county jails, correctional facilities, psychiatric hospitals, and the community. Forensic patients often do not receive sufficient treatment for their illness while they are incarcerated, however, and as a result are at risk for further deterioration and revictimization (Flores et al., 2023; NAMI, 2023). Further, people of color who are incarcerated are less likely to be recognized as having a mental health problem and, consequently, are less likely to receive access to treatment for their mental illness (Edwards et al., 2024).

Stigma of Criminality

Patients who are incarcerated suffer the combined effects of the stigma of mental illness and criminality. Although stigma is an issue for all people with a mental illness, it is magnified for those who have committed a crime. There is often reluctance on the part of mental health professionals to treat these patients, especially if murder and childhood sexual abuse are involved. Even if the worry is unfounded, clinicians express safety concerns for themselves and other patients and may refuse to care for these patients. However, patients with serious mental illness are far more likely than the general population to be *victims* of trauma or violence than perpetrators (Gupta et al., 2023; Ponte, 2021).

When nonforensic patients receive the maximum benefit from hospitalization, they are usually discharged back into the community. For forensic patients, the community often wants a more stringent discharge threshold and unrealistically expects the hospital to guarantee adherence to community rules and structure. Treatment and the criminal justice systems are often in conflict with each other. The promotion and utilization of community resources helps to reduce the risk of an individual with serious mental illness from entering or reentering the criminal justice system. Those eligible for access to government benefits such as Supplemental Security Income (SSI), Social Security Disability Insurance (SSDI), Medicaid, Medicare, Veterans Affairs' benefits, food stamps, and public housing programs may need assistance in securing these benefits. Ensuring adequate access to mental health care, medical care, and substance use treatment is critical. Successful employment and educational opportunities also lead to a lower risk of criminal justice involvement (Buck et al., 2022; Ponte, 2021).

Fitness to Stand Trial

Once a mental illness is diagnosed in an individual who has committed a crime, the individual's **fitness to stand trial** is determined. Fitness means that an individual is able to consult with a lawyer with a reasonable degree of rational understanding of the facts of the alleged crime and of the legal proceedings as spelled out in the court case of *Dusky v. United States* of 1960 (Beran & Toomey, 1979, p. 12). An individual is found **unfit to stand trial** if, because of mental or physical condition, they are unable to understand the nature and purpose of the proceedings or to assist in the defense (West, 2021).

In most states, when an individual with a mental illness is found unfit to stand trial, hospitalization in a forensic mental health facility follows. The goal of this hospitalization is to help the person become *fit* to stand trial, not to treat the mental illness. Sometimes, the patient's mental illness has to be treated to attain fitness. Simply stated, to be fit to stand trial, the person must be able to communicate with counsel and assist in the defense; be able to appreciate their presence in relation to time, place, and things; be able to understand that they are in a court of justice charged with a criminal offense; show an understanding of the charges and their consequences, as well as court procedures and the roles of the judge, jury, prosecutor, and defense attorney; and have sufficient memory to relate the circumstances surrounding the alleged criminal offense.

An individual cannot be *unfit* forever. If fitness cannot be attained usually within 1 year, a hearing is held, during which the facts of the alleged crime are presented to a judge who rules on the case. If the charges are dismissed, the judge could order a civil commitment. If there is sufficient evidence to convict, the individual could be sent back to the hospital for further treatment to attain fitness. The maximum length of this additional treatment is based on the severity of the charge. For those accused of sexual-related offenses (because of a mental disorder), states usually have special statutes for hospitalization and discharge (e.g., registration and community notification).

Not Guilty by Reason of Insanity

Once fitness to stand trial is established, the trial or hearing can proceed. One possible outcome is **not guilty by reason of insanity (NGRI)**. The accused is judged unable to distinguish right from wrong or to be unable to control their actions at the time of the crime. The rationale underlying this ruling is one of fairness. It is unfair to hold an individual responsible if that individual does not know that the action is wrong or does not have control over their behavior.

Nearly all individuals found NGRI are also subject to involuntary commitment in a *secure* setting. The patient cannot leave the hospital grounds without court approval. An individual sentenced to NGRI is given a date that is equal to the time or sentence to be served if they had been guilty of the crime.

Guilty but Mentally Ill

Different from NGRI, in which individuals judged *not guilty* are committed to the mental health system, **guilty but mentally ill (GBMI)** is a criminal conviction, and the person is sent to the correctional system. Mental illness is considered a factor in the crime but not to the extent that the individual is incapable of knowing right from wrong or controlling their actions. The sentence for the GBMI is the same type of determinate sentence any inmate receives. Before release, every effort is made to ensure that patients will receive proper follow-up care in the community and close monitoring by parole staff. Individuals with either an NGRI or a GBMI are treated for their mental disorders, but one is treated in jail and the other in a hospital. The conditions of release are different. Whereas individuals with a GBMI are subject to the correctional system's parole decisions, those with an NGRI are discharged from the hospital through the courts upon recommendations of the forensic mental health professionals.

Probation

Probation is a sentence of conditional or revocable release under the supervision of a probation officer for a specified time. For individuals with a mental illness who have committed minor offenses, probation is sometimes used instead of jail as long as care in a treatment facility can be arranged. If treatment and rehabilitation are successful, criminal charges may be dropped and a prison record avoided. Probation is also used when a criminal has served time and continued monitoring is needed after being released from the correctional facility.

Misconceptions Regarding Insanity Pleas

There are many misconceptions about the insanity plea. One is that the insanity defense provides a loophole through which criminals can escape punishment for illegal acts. In reality, the insanity defense is extremely difficult to use even in the cases of individuals who are severely ill. As a result, despite popular belief, the insanity defense is used in fewer than 1% of criminal cases (Box 4.5).

Countless newspaper articles, talk shows, and news commentaries concerning the insanity defense have bombarded the public. Some of the cases have been highly publicized. One such case was that of John Hinckley, who attempted to assassinate President Ronald Reagan in 1981 and who was found NGRI. On psychiatric examination, Hinckley was found to be living in a "fantasy world with magical and grandiose expectations of impressing and winning over" the famous person he was obsessed with, actress Jodie Foster (Goldstein, 1995, p. 309). Hinckley attempted to commit a historic deed that would make him famous and would unite him with the love object of his delusions. His acquittal stimulated public cries for reform of the insanity defense. Within 2.5 years of John Hinckley's acquittal, 34 states changed their insanity defense statutes to limit its use or to prevent the premature release of dangerous people. After 41 years of imprisonment, Hinckley was unconditionally released in 2022.

BOX 4.5

The Case of Andrea Yates

In March 2002, Andrea Yates, age 37 years, was convicted of murder for drowning her five children. She was sentenced to life in prison despite past treatment for postpartum depression and psychosis, four hospitalizations, and two suicide attempts. Andrea Yates was found guilty because in her testimony to the police, she stated that she knew the criminal justice system would punish her for her actions, implying that she knew the acts were wrong in the eyes of the law. Texas law does not recognize that for someone as ill as Andrea Yates, mental illnesses can create more powerful hierarchies of right and wrong than societal law. In July 2006, Andrea was granted a retrial because the previous verdict was overturned on appeal because of erroneous testimony. At the second trial, Andrea was found not guilty by reason of insanity. She was committed to a state mental hospital with periodic hearings before a judge to determine whether she should be released (Biography.com, 2021).

Gun Laws and Mental Illness

The Brady Handgun Violence Prevention Act of 1993, commonly referred to as the Brady Act or Brady Bill, was originally proposed in response to Hinckley's assassination attempt on President Reagan. The Brady Act requires a background check on individuals seeking ownership of a firearm. Under this Act, individuals considered mentally incompetent, having severe mental illness, or those having been committed to a mental institution are prohibited from gun ownership. There is much controversy surrounding gun control for people with mental illness. Although the laws are intended to restrict firearms in those determined to be of significant danger to others, the reality is that only a very small percentage of all violent crimes are perpetrated by individuals diagnosed with mental illness. In fact, evidence shows that individuals with serious mental illness are more likely to be victims—not perpetrators—of gun violence. Therefore, insisting that gun violence is strictly a mental health problem unfairly stigmatizes those with mental illness (O'Brien, 2023).

ACCOUNTABILITY FOR NURSES AND OTHER MENTAL HEALTH CARE PROFESSIONALS

Nurses and other health care professionals are accountable for the care they provide in mental health as well as any other practice area.

Legal Liability in Psychiatric Nursing Practice

Malpractice is based on a set of torts (a civil wrong not based on contract committed by one person that causes injury to another). An **assault** is the threat of unlawful force to inflict bodily injury upon another. An assault must be imminent and cause reasonable apprehension in the individual. Battery is the intentional and unpermitted contact with another. **Medical battery**, intentional and unauthorized harmful or offensive contact, occurs when a patient is treated without informed consent. For example, a clinician who fails to obtain consent before performing a procedure is subject to being accused of medical battery. Also, failure to respect a patient's advance directives is considered medical battery. False imprisonment is the detention or imprisonment contrary to provision of the law. Facilities that do not discharge patients who were voluntarily committed upon request can be subject to this type of litigation.

Negligence is a breach of duty of reasonable care for a patient for whom a nurse is responsible that results in personal injuries. A clinician who does get consent but does not disclose the nature of the procedure and the risks involved is subject to a negligence claim. Five elements are required to prove negligence: duty (accepting assignment to care for patient), breach of duty (failure to practice according to acceptable standards of care), cause in fact (the injury would not have happened if the standards had been followed), cause in proximity (harm actually occurred within the scope of foreseeable consequence), and damages (physical or emotional injury caused by breach of standard of care). Simple mistakes are not negligent acts.

Lawsuits in Psychiatric–Mental Health Care

Few lawsuits are filed against mental health clinicians and facilities compared with other health care areas. If psychiatric nurses are included in lawsuits, they are usually included in the lawsuit filed against the agency. Common areas of litigation surround the nursing care of patients who are suicidal or violent. Maintaining and documenting an appropriate standard of care can protect nurses from complicated legal proceedings. The following can help prevent negative outcomes of malpractice litigations:

- Evaluate risks, especially when privileges broaden or care is transferred.
- Document decisional processes and reasons for choices among alternatives.
- Involve family in important decisions.
- Make decisions within team model and document this shared responsibility.
- Adhere to agency's policy and procedures.
- Seek consultation and record input.

Nursing Documentation

Careful documentation is important both to help ensure protection of patient rights and for nurse accountability. Documentation can be handwritten or electronic. It is very common in psychiatric facilities that all disciplines record one progress note. Nursing documentation is based on nursing standards and the policies of the particular facility. Many documentation styles are problem focused. That is, documentation is structured to address specific problems that are identified on the nursing care plan or interdisciplinary treatment plan. No matter the setting or structure of the documentation, nurses are responsible for documenting the following:

- Observations of the patient's subjective and objective physical, psychological, and social responses to mental disorders and emotional problems
- Interventions implemented and the patient's response
- Observations of therapeutic effects and side effects of medications
- Evaluation of outcomes of interventions

Particular attention should be paid to the reason the patient is admitted for care. If the person's initial problem was suicide or homicidal ideation, the patient should routinely be assessed for suicidal and homicidal thoughts even if the treatment plan does not specifically identify suicide and homicide as potential problems. Careful documentation is always needed for patients who are suicidal, homicidal, aggressive, or restrained in any way. It is important to document both symptoms that are present as well as symptoms that are absent. Medications prescribed as needed (pro re nata) also require a separate entry, including reason for administration, dosage, route, and response to the medication.

A patient record is the primary documentation of a patient's problems, verifies the behavior of the patient at the point of care, and describes the care provided. The patient record is considered a legal document. Courts consider acts not recorded as acts not done. Patients also have legal access to their records. For handwritten documentation, the entries should always be written in pen with no erasures. If an entry is corrected, it should be initialed by the person making the correction. All entries should be clear, well written, and void of jargon. Judgmental statements, such as *patient is manipulating staff*, have no place in patients' records. Only meaningful, accurate, objective descriptions of behavior should be used. General, stereotypic statements, such as *had a good night* or *no complaints*, are meaningless and should be avoided.

With the universal use of electronic records, meaningful documentation is sometimes more difficult. Many institutions require health care workers to enter observations, assessment data, and interventions into a template that requires a *click* in a box on the monitor screen. Additional narrative entries are usually required to provide quality, individualized care. Nurses should adhere to the same standards of practice and documentation when entering electronic data as when entering data in a nonelectronic record.

SUMMARY OF KEY POINTS

- The ANA's Code of Ethics establishes the ethical standards used by all nurses and communicates those standards to others.
- Several primary and secondary ethical principles provide guidance to nurses for making ethical decisions

and forming trusting relationships with patients. These include autonomy, beneficence, nonmaleficence, justice, veracity, and fidelity.

- The right of self-determinism entitles all patients to refuse treatment, to obtain other opinions, and to choose other forms of treatment. It is one of the basic patients' rights established by Title II, Public Law 99–139, outlining the Universal Bill of Rights for Mental Health Patients.
- Laws and systems are established to protect the rights of people with mental health issues. Some of these include the Self-Determination Act, advance directives, a patient Bill of Rights, the Americans with Disabilities Act, internal rights protection systems, external advocacy systems, and accreditation of mental health care delivery systems.
- Informed consent is another protective right that helps patients decide what can be done to their bodies and minds. It must be obtained from a competent individual before any treatment is begun to ensure that the information is not only received but also understood.
- A competent person can refuse any treatment. Incompetence is determined by the court when the patient cannot understand the information or appreciate its relevance to their own situation.
- The right to the least restrictive environment entitles patients to be treated in the least restrictive setting and by the least restrictive means and protects patients from unnecessary confinement and medication.
- Seclusion or restraint should be used as a last resort and only when there is a serious and imminent risk of harm to the patient or someone else. Its use can contribute to physical and psychological harm. Patients secluded or restrained must be under continuous observation by staff.
- Involuntary commitment procedures are specified at the state level. Patients who are involuntarily committed have the right to refuse treatment and medication.
- Patient privacy is protected through Health Insurance Portability and Accountability Act (HIPAA) regulations related to the transfer and storage of information. A breach in confidentiality is legally mandated when there is a threat of violence toward others.
- Nursing documentation is guided by practice standards and policies of the agency. Nurses are responsible for individualized documentation in both electronic and nonelectronic health records.

DEVELOPING CLINICAL JUDGMENT

1. Consider the relationship of self-determinism to competence by differentiating patients who are competent to give consent and those who are incompetent. Discuss the steps in determining whether a patient is competent to provide informed consent for a treatment.
2. A patient is involuntarily admitted to a psychiatric unit and refuses all medication. After being unable to persuade the patient to take prescribed medication, the nurse documents the patient's refusal and notifies the prescriber. Should the nurse attempt to give the medication without patient's consent? Support your answer.
3. A patient with a history of trauma is placed in seclusion and physical restraint after posing a serious and imminent danger to others. What implications should the nurse consider, and what responsibilities does the registered nurse have when caring for the patient?
4. Identify the legal and ethical issues underlying the Tarasoff case and mandates to inform.

MOVIES, TV, OR STREAMING PROGRAMS

***Mysteries of Mental Illness: Episode 3; The Rise and Fall of the Asylum:* 2021.** In the third episode of the PBS documentary series *Mysteries of Mental Illness*, the filmmakers illustrate the origin and downfall of mental asylums in the United States. People with mental illness were confined in institutions far exceeding the intended capacity, and without sufficient resources to provide adequate care. They were kept apart from their communities, out of sight and out of mind. Though well-intentioned, desperate physicians implemented therapies and extreme treatments based on speculation that were often proven wrong. Because patients were seen as degenerate, treatments were provided without patient consent and, often times, even without their knowledge.

Viewing Points:

1. Eugenics programs, discriminatory and destructive acts, were used as a means of controlling the so-called "undesirable" populations, with a stated purpose to protect society from the offspring of people considered to be inferior or dangerous. How was this practice applied to people with mental illness?
2. In the 1950s, when mental asylums were at their peak, approval of the first antipsychotic medications empowered these facilities to discharge patients home. What were the implications of this?
3. Today, America's largest mental health facilities are not hospitals; rather, they are prisons and jails. What factors contribute to prisons and jails becoming front-line treatment facilities for those with mental illness?

REFERENCES

Alvear Velásquez, M. J., & Sandoval Carrión, I. P. (2024). Adherence to psychopharmacological treatment in patients with severe and persistent mental disorders: A systematic review. *Revista Colombiana de Psiquiatria (English Ed.)*, *53*(2), 192–205. https://doi.org/10.1016/j.rcpeng.2022.01.004

American Nurses Association. (2015). *Code of ethics for nurses with interpretive statements*. American Nurses Association.

American Psychiatric Nurses Association. (2022). *APNA position statement on the use of seclusion and restraint*. https://www.apna.org/publications/position-papers/

Appelbaum, P. S. (2007). Clinical practice. Assessment of patients' competence to consent to treatment. *New England Journal of Medicine*, *357*(18), 1834–1840.

Baranyi, G., Fazel, S., Langerfeldt, S. D., & Mundt, A. P. (2022). The prevalence of comorbid serious mental illnesses and substance use disorders in prison populations: A systematic review and meta-analysis. *The Lancet Public Health*, 7(6), e557–e568.

Beran, N. J., & Toomey, B. G. (1979). *Mentally ill offenders and the criminal justice system: Issues in forensic services* (pp. 1–23). Praeger Special Studios.

Biography.com (Editors). (2021). Andrea Yates biography. https://www.biography.com/crime/andrea-yates

Brady Handgun Violence Prevention Act of 1993. 18 U.S. Code §921–922 (Public Law 103–159, 107 Stat. 1536, November 30, 1993).

Buck, K., Cochran, A., Young, H., Gordon, M. J., Yuen, H. K., & Tucker, S. C. (2022). The facilitators and barriers faced when transitioning back into the community following a prison sentence. *International Journal of Offender Therapy and Comparative Criminology*, *66*(10–11), 1156–1174.

Calcedo-Barba, A., Fructuoso, A., Martinez-Raga, J., Paz, S., Sanchez de Carmona, M., & Vicens, E. (2020). A meta-review of literature reviews assessing the capacity of patients with severe mental disorders to make decisions about their healthcare. *BMC Psychiatry*, *20*(1), 339.

Dixon v. Weinberger, 405 F. Supp. 974 (D.D.C. 1975).

Douglas, L, Donohue, G., & Morrissey, J. (2022). Patient experience of physical restraint in the acute setting: A systematic review of the qualitative research evidence. *Issues in Mental Health Nursing*, *43*(5), 473–481.

Edwards, E. R., Epshteyn, G., Diehl, C. K., Ruiz, D., Coolidge, B., Weiss, N. H., & Stein, L. (2024). Prison or treatment? Gender, racial, and ethnic inequities in mental health care utilization and criminal justice history among incarcerated persons with borderline and antisocial personality disorders. *Law and Human Behavior*, *48*(2), 104–116. https://doi.org/10.1037/lhb0000557

Flores, M. W., Sharp, A., Moyer, M., Fung, V., Rotter, M. R., & Le Cook, B. (2023). Criminal legal involvement among U.S. adults with serious psychological distress and differences by race-ethnicity. *Psychiatric Services*, *74*(7), 702–708.

Goldstein, R. L. (1995). Paranoids in the legal system: The litigious paranoid and the paranoid criminal. *Psychiatric Clinics of North America*, *18*(2), 303–315.

Gupta, G., Sachdeva, A., Kumar, M., & Singh, M. (2023). Spectrum of intimate partner violence in patients with psychiatric illness–From victimization to perpetration. *International Journal of Psychiatry in Medicine*, *58*(1), 20–36. https://doi.org/10.1177/00912174211053726

Marshall, K. D., Derse, A. R., Weiner, S. G., & Joseph, J. W. (2024). Revive and refuse: Capacity, autonomy, and refusal of care after opioid overdose. *American Journal of Bioethics*, *24*(5), 11–24. https://doi.org/10.1080/15265161.2023.2209534

National Alliance on Mental Illness (NAMI). (2023). *Criminalization of people with mental illness*. Retrieved July 22, 2023, from https://nami.org/Advocacy/Policy-Priorities/Stopping-Harmful-Practices/Criminalization-of-People-with-Mental-Illness

Nizum, N., Yoon, R., Ferreira-Legere, L., Poole, N., & Lular, Z. (2020). Nursing interventions for adults following a mental health crisis: A systematic review guided by trauma-informed principles. *International Journal of Mental Health Nursing*, *29*(3), 348–363.

O'Brien, E. (2023). Changing the narrative: Mental illness and gun violence. *Psychiatric Times*, *40*(4), 1–10.

Omnibus Budget Reconciliation Act of 1990. Public Law No. 101–158, Paragraph 4206, 4751.

Ponte, K. (2021). *Criminal justice involvement of people with serious mental illness*. Retrieved October 15, 2021, from https://www.nami.org/Blogs/NAMI-Blog/March-2021/Criminal-Justice-Involvement-of-People-with-Serious-Mental-Illness

Steinert, T., & Henking, T. (2022). Laws and psychiatry-current and future perspectives. *Frontiers in Public Health*, *10*, 968168.

Substance Abuse and Mental Health Services Administration (SAMHSA). (2019). *Civil commitment and the mental health care continuum: Historical trends and principles for law and practice*. Retrieved August 17, 2024, from https://www.samhsa.gov/sites/default/files/civil-commitment-continuum-of-care.pdf

Substance Abuse and Mental Health Services Administration (SAMHSA). (2022a). *Alternatives to seclusion and restraint*. Retrieved July 22, 2023, from https://www.samhsa.gov/trauma-violence

Substance Abuse and Mental Health Services Administration (SAMHSA). (2022b). *Laws, regulations, and guidelines*. Retrieved July 22, 2023, from https://www.samhsa.gov/about-us/who-we-are/laws-regulations

Substance Abuse and Mental Health Services Administration (SAMHSA). (2023). *Practical guide for implementing a trauma-informed approach*. SAMHSA Publication No. PEP23-06-05-005. National Mental Health and Substance Use Policy Laboratory.

Tarasoff v. Regents of the University of California. 551 P.2d 334 (Cal. 1976).

Thordarson, H., & Rector, T. (2020). From trauma-blind to trauma-informed: re-thinking criminalization and the role of trauma in persons with serious mental illness. *CNS Spectrums: The International Journal of Neuropsychiatric Medicine*, *25*(5), 577–583.

Treatment Advocacy Center. (2023). *Criminalization of mental illness*. Retrieved July 22, 2023, from https://www.treatmentadvocacycenter.org/key-issues/criminalization-of-mental-illness

U.S. Department of Health and Human Services. (2002). Standards for privacy of individually identifiable health information; final rule. *Federal Register*, *65*, 53182–53273.

U.S. Equal Employment Opportunity Commission, Office of the Americans with Disabilities Act. (2023). *Your employment rights as an individual with a disability*. Retrieved July 22, 2023, from https://www.eeoc.gov/laws/guidance/your-employment-rights-individual-disability

West, T. (Ed.). (2021). *West's Illinois criminal law and procedure*. Thompson Reuters.

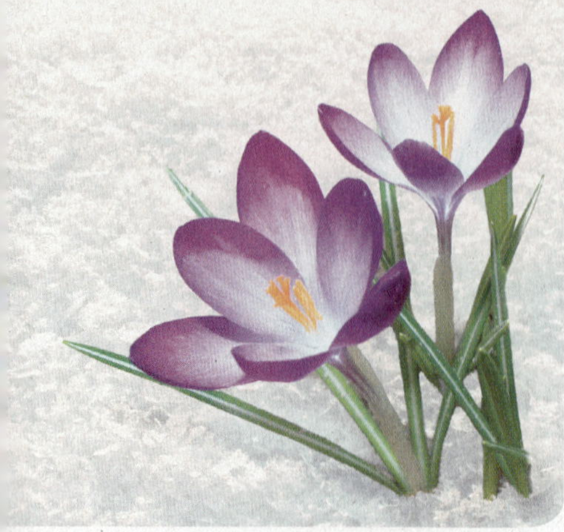

5 Mental Health Care in the Community

Mary Ann Boyd

KEYCONCEPTS

- case management
- continuum of care

LEARNING OBJECTIVES

After studying this chapter, you will be able to:

1. Define and explain the continuum of care for mental health services.
2. Explain how the concept of the least restrictive environment influences the choice of treatment settings.
3. Identify various mental health treatment settings and associated programs along the continuum of care.
4. Discuss the role of the nurse at different points along the continuum of mental health care.
5. Describe the integration of psychiatric and medical care in community settings.

KEY TERMS

• 23-hour observation • assertive community treatment • board-and-care homes • case management • coordination of care • crisis intervention • crisis intervention teams • digital applications • in-home mental health care • integrated care • intensive case management • intensive outpatient program • intensive residential services • medical home • outpatient detoxification • partial hospitalization • peer support services • psychiatric rehabilitation programs • recovery centers • reintegration • relapse • residential services • telehealth • therapeutic foster care • transfer • transitional care

INTRODUCTION

The evolution of a behavioral health care system is affected by scientific advances and social factors. Recovery from mental illness is a goal at all stages of treatment. Mental health care now features integrated community-based services where culturally competent, high-quality nursing care is needed to meet the mental health care needs of patients and communities. The long-term nature of mental disorders requires varying levels of care at different stages of the disorders as well as family and community support. Treatment costs are shared among public and private sectors. A demand exists for a comprehensive, holistic approach to care that encompasses all levels of need. Consumers, families, providers, advocacy groups, and third-party payers of mental health care no longer accept long-term institutionalization, once the hallmark of psychiatric care. Instead, they advocate for short-term treatment in an environment that promotes dignity and well-being while meeting the patient's biologic, psychological, social, and spiritual needs.

Reimbursement issues influence health care delivery. In the United States, health maintenance organizations, preferred provider organizations, Medicaid, and Medicare have set limits on the types and lengths of treatment for which they provide reimbursement coverage, which in turn influences the kind of care the patient receives. In other countries, other regulatory bodies influence access and treatment options. Fragmentation of services is a constant threat. Today, psychiatric–mental health nurses face the challenge of providing mental health care within a complex system that is affected by financial constraints and narrowed treatment requirements.

DEFINING THE CONTINUUM OF CARE

A continuum of care that supports recovery can be viewed from various perspectives and ranges from intensive treatment (hospitalization) to supportive interventions (outpatient therapy). An individual's needs for ongoing clinical treatment and care are matched with the intensity of professional health services.

In a continuum, continuity of care is provided over an extended time. The appropriate medical, nursing, psychological, or social services may be delivered within one organization or across multiple organizations. The continuum facilitates the stability, continuity, and comprehensiveness of service to an individual and maximizes the coordination of care and services.

> **KEYCONCEPT** A **continuum of care** consists of an integrated system of settings, services, health care clinicians, and care levels, spanning illness-to-wellness states.

Least Restrictive Environment

The primary goal of the continuum of care is to provide treatment that supports recovery in the least restrictive environment (see Chapter 4). In 1999, the U.S. Supreme Court reinforced the principle of least restrictive environment with the Olmstead decision, which states that it is a violation of the Americans with Disabilities Act to institutionalize people with severe mental illnesses when services in the community are equally effective (Olmstead v. L.C., 1999). Therefore, treatment is usually delivered in the community (as opposed to a hospital or institution) and, ideally, in an outpatient setting.

Coordination of Care

Coordination of care is the integration of appropriate services so that individualized care is provided. Appropriate services are those that are tailored to address a client's strengths and weaknesses, cultural context, service preferences, and recovery goals, including referral to community resources and liaisons with others (e.g., providers, health care organizations, and community services). Several agencies could be involved, but when care is coordinated, an individual's needs are met without duplication of services. Coordination of care requires collaborative and cooperative relationships among many services, including primary care, public health, mental health, social services, housing, education, and criminal justice, to name a few.

In some instances, a whole array of integrated services is needed. For example, children can benefit from treatment and specialized support at home and school. These wraparound services represent a unique set of community services and natural supports individualized for the child or adult and family to achieve a positive set of outcomes.

Case Management

Coordinated care is often accomplished through a **case management** service model in which a case manager locates services, links the patient with these services, and then monitors the patient's receipt of these services. This type of case management is referred to as the broker model. Case management can be provided by an individual or a team; it may include both face-to-face and telephone contact with the patient as well as contact with other service providers. **Intensive case management** is targeted for adults with serious mental illnesses and children with serious emotional disturbances. Managers of such cases have fewer caseloads and higher levels of professional training than traditional case managers.

> **KEYCONCEPT Case management** is a process that assesses, plans, implements, coordinates, monitors, and evaluates the options and services required to meet an individual's health needs (Commission for Case Manager Certification [CCMC], 2024).

Case management services are built on a strong working alliance between the patient and the case manager. Quality is assessed by measuring patient outcomes that result from the services, such as symptom reduction, improved functioning and community integration, and patient satisfaction with the services provided. In addition, case managers can optimize a patient's use of resources by developing a treatment plan that closely matches the individual needs of the patient and by matching the most appropriate treatment to the patient's phase of illness.

The Nurse as Case Manager

Case managers practice in a variety of settings, including clinics, long-term care facilities, insurance companies, hospitals, workers' compensation programs, and independent organizations. Psychiatric nurse case managers serve in various pivotal functions across the continuum of care. These functions can involve both direct care and coordination of the care delivered by others. The repertoire of required skills includes collaboration with members of a multidisciplinary team, teaching, management, leadership, group, and research skills. The case manager assesses the patient including the patient's level of health literacy, as well as that of the patient's caregiver and family. A plan of care is developed with the patient, and the case manager arranges and ensures that care is delivered, usually in multiple settings (American Case Management Association, 2023). The nurse case manager must have firm knowledge of psychiatric nursing and be able to function independently. This role is probably the most diverse role within the continuum of care.

Virtual Health Care

Telehealth, the delivery of health-related services and information via digital communication technologies, is rapidly appearing as a primary strategy in the delivery of health care, particularly mental health throughout the continuum of care. Telehealth had its beginning in the early 1900s, and as technology advanced, the impact of digital communication has assumed increasing importance (see Table 5.1). The technology was initially used as a method of storing and forwarding medical information, but its use quickly expanded to remote medical monitoring. The coronavirus disease (COVID-19) pandemic drove dramatic acceleration in the use and acceptance of digital health care as a credible option to in-person visits. Today, it is widely used for real-time interactive services. **Digital applications** or apps are used for all three—storing and forwarding, remote medical monitoring, and interactive services (Tong et al., 2022). Now, telehealth is preferred by many clinicians and patients in certain situations (Crouch et al., 2023).

TABLE 5.1 HISTORY OF TELEHEALTH IN U.S. HEALTH CARE

Date	Events
Early 1900s	Patient interview is conducted over telephone.
1950s	Psychiatrist–patient interaction occurs over closed-circuit television.
1960s	U.S. space program introduces remote medical monitoring.
1990s	With introduction of the internet, health professionals begin sharing information electronically.
1996	Publication of Institute of Medicine report—Telemedicine: A Guide to Assessing Telecommunication for Healthcare.
2010	Affordable Care Act results in improvement in broadband support, medical networks, and electronic health records.
2020	Coronavirus pandemic causes a need for remote health care delivery, leading to reduction in barriers and widespread use of telehealth.
2025 and beyond	The demand for telehealth modalities increases. Clinicians are challenged to decrease digital health inequities and to provide coordinated care.

In mental health care, telehealth was initially viewed as a way of providing access to mental health services in rural communities because of clinician shortages, lack of public transportation, and poverty. Telehealth contact with patients after discharge from the hospital allowed nurses to assess psychiatric symptoms, check on medication adherence, discuss approaches to solving problems associated with community living, and provide emotional support. As technology advanced, more telehealth applications became available to those in rural areas.

Even though the technology supported virtual interaction, there were several barriers that prevented utilization of the service. Internet connectivity was not always available. Clinicians were often reluctant to use technology for fear of missing indications of suicide or other safety issues. Third-party insurers were unwilling to pay for telehealth visits. An in-person visit was required before controlled substances could be prescribed, and the Health Insurance Portability and Accountability Act and Privacy Standards required strict secure two-way communication preventing the use of Zoom, Skype, or FaceTime.

These barriers were relaxed or removed during the COVID-19 pandemic. Medicare began paying for office, hospital, and other visits furnished via telehealth across the country in 2020. The Health Insurance Portability and Accountability Act and Privacy Standards were relaxed; visits were no longer limited to rural settings. Prescribers were able to issue prescriptions for controlled substances to patients using telemedicine without a prior in-person patient medical evaluation.

Telehealth interventions for the treatment, prevention, diagnosis, and management of depression, serious mental illness, and substance use are now used in most urban and rural settings (Box 5.1). Videoconferencing, e-mail, mobile apps, and texting are being used (Watanabe et al., 2023).

MENTAL HEALTH SERVICES IN A CONTINUUM OF CARE

Crisis Care

An organized approach is required to treat individuals in crisis, including a mechanism for rapid access to care (within 24 hours), a referral for hospitalization, or access to outpatient services.

Crisis Intervention

Crisis intervention—a specialized short-term, goal-directed therapy for those in acute distress—is brief, usually lasting fewer than 6 hours (see Chapter 21). This type of short-term care focuses on stabilization, symptom

BOX 5.1

Evidence-Based Research for Evidence-Based Practice: Telehealth Use Among Hispanic Veterans

Guajardo, E., Amspoker, A. B., Stanley, M. A., Hogan, J., Ecker, A. H., & Lindsay, J. A. (2023). Patterns of telehealth use for mental health treatment among Hispanic veterans. Telemedicine Journal and E-Health, *29(5), 788–792. https://doi.org/10.1089/tmj.2022.0300*

THE QUESTION: Does video-to-home (VTH) telehealth reduce barriers in accessing mental health care while maintaining clinical effectiveness?

METHODS: Use of VTH for at least one mental health visit from October 2019 to September 2020 by Hispanic/Latino veterans (155,492) was compared to use of VTH by non-Hispanic/Latino veterans (1,544,988) through a retrospective cohort investigation. The VA Video Connect (VVC) system involved face-to-face synchronous video-based teleconference between patients and providers. Patients were at home or at a private location. The main measures were the percentage of mental health encounters delivered through VCC.

RESULTS: Hispanic veterans accessed VTH at a higher rate than their non-Hispanic counterparts. Compared to non-Hispanic/non-Latino veterans, Hispanic veterans had a 3.28% greater percentage of VVC mental health encounters. There was also a 2.65% increase per month in percentage of VVC mental health encounters by Hispanic veterans.

IMPLICATIONS FOR NURSING: Nurses should embrace the use of telehealth when the opportunity is available. These findings challenge the conventional narrative that Hispanic veterans access telehealth services less than non-Hispanic veterans. More research is needed to determine whether these findings are applicable to the general Hispanic population who are not veterans.

reduction, and prevention of relapse requiring inpatient services. Crisis intervention services can be viewed on a continuum including crisis hotline, mobile teams, observations, crisis residential programs, and peer wraparound services.

Crisis intervention units can be found in the emergency departments of general and psychiatric hospitals and in crisis centers within community mental health centers. Patients in crisis demonstrate severe symptoms of acute mental illness, including labile mood swings, suicidal ideation, or self-injurious behaviors. Therefore, this treatment option commands a high degree of nursing expertise. Patients in crisis usually require medications such as anxiolytics or benzodiazepines for symptom management. Key nursing roles include assessment, short-term therapeutic interventions, and medication administration. Nurses also facilitate referrals for admission to the hospital or for outpatient services.

Crisis intervention teams (CIT)—interdisciplinary mental health specialists and first responders—provide protection to individuals with mental illness symptoms who are a threat to self or others. Law enforcement personnel, such as police officers, are often the first responders when crises occur in the community. Police officers need to accurately assess and intervene in crisis situations and determine whether the people involved in the crisis are experiencing behavioral problems due to symptoms of mental illness. CIT have been developed to train police officers to recognize and intervene in crisis situations in the community and determine whether emergency psychiatric services are needed. Crisis intervention by CIT-trained police officers can avoid inappropriate involvement of the patient in the criminal justice system and ensure that patients with behavioral problems due to mental illnesses receive appropriate psychiatric treatment (Balfour & Zeller, 2023).

23-Hour Observation

The use of **23-hour observation** is a short-term treatment that serves the patient in immediate but short-term crisis. This type of care admits individuals to an inpatient setting for as long as 23 hours, during which time services are provided at a less-than-acute care level. The clinical problem usually is a transient disruption of baseline function, which will resolve quickly. Usually, the individual is experiencing suicidal or homicidal ideation, which presents a threat to themselves or others. The nurse's role in this treatment modality is assessment and monitoring. Medications are also usually administered. This treatment is used for acute trauma such as rape, for alcohol and narcotic detoxification, and for individuals with personality disorders who present with self-injurious behaviors.

Crisis Stabilization

When the immediate crisis does not resolve quickly, crisis stabilization is the next step. This type of care usually lasts fewer than 7 days and has a symptom-based indication for hospital admission. The primary purpose of stabilization is control of precipitating symptoms through medications, behavioral interventions, and coordination with other agencies for appropriate aftercare. The major focus of nursing care in a short-term inpatient setting is symptom management. Ongoing assessment; short-term, focused interventions; and medication administration and monitoring of efficacy and side effects are major components of nursing care during stabilization. Nurses may also provide focused group psychotherapy designed to develop and strengthen the personal management strategies of patients. When treating patients who act aggressively or violently, the nurse implements the appropriate use of seclusion and restraints according to facility policy.

Acute Inpatient Care

Acute inpatient hospitalization is the most intensive treatment and occurs in the most restrictive setting in the continuum. Inpatient treatment is reserved for patients who are acutely ill and who, because of a mental illness, meet one or more of three criteria: high risk for harming themselves, high risk for harming others, or unable to care for their basic needs. Delivery of inpatient care can occur in a psychiatric hospital, psychiatric unit within a general hospital or public-operated facility. Nursing care is critical in the acute care setting and is provided around the clock.

Admission to inpatient environments can be voluntary or involuntary (see Chapter 4). The average length of stay for an involuntary admission ranges between 24 hours and several days, depending on the state or province laws; the length of stay for a voluntary admission depends on the acuity of symptoms and the patient's ability to pay the costs of treatment. It is unconstitutional in the United States to confine people with mental illness who are not a danger to self or others if they can survive independently with the help of willing and responsible family or friends. Nevertheless, the interdisciplinary treatment team determines that the patient is no longer at risk to themselves or others before discharge can occur. Court orders can mandate hospitalization.

Both the number of available beds in psychiatric hospitals in the United States and length of inpatient stay have continually decreased since the 1980s, a trend attributed to managed care and expansion of multidisciplinary, intensive community-based services, such as **assertive community treatment (ACT)**. Additional contributors to decreased length of stay include strict admission criteria and regulations that determine the need for continued hospitalization. Currently, admission to a hospital is determined based on medical necessity, such as dangerousness or the need for crisis stabilization. Discharge is a complex process that varies from setting to setting often depending on the resources of individual, hospital, and community systems.

Partial Hospitalization

Partial hospitalization programs (PHPs), also referred to as day treatment programs, were developed to complement inpatient mental health care and outpatient services and provide treatment to patients with acute psychiatric symptoms who are experiencing a decline in social or occupational functioning, who cannot function autonomously daily, or who do not pose imminent danger to themselves or others. It is a time-limited, ambulatory, active treatment program that offers therapeutically intensive, coordinated, and structured clinical services within a stable milieu. The aim of PHPs is patient stabilization without hospitalization or reduced length of inpatient care. An alternative to inpatient treatment, PHP usually provides the resources to support therapeutic activities both for full-day and half-day programs. This level of care does not include overnight hospital care; however, the patient can be admitted for inpatient care within 24 hours.

In **partial hospitalization,** the interdisciplinary treatment team partners with the patient and devises and executes a comprehensive plan of care encompassing behavioral therapy, social skills training, basic living skills training, education regarding illness and symptom identification and relapse prevention, community survival skills training, relaxation training, nutrition and exercise counseling, and other forms of expressive therapy. Group-based services such as wellness education and counseling for comorbid serious mental illnesses and substance use are also provided (Gautam et al., 2023). Compared with other outpatient programs, PHPs offer more intensive nursing care.

Residential Services

Residential services provide a place for people to reside during a 24-hour period or any portion of the day on an ongoing basis. A residential facility can be publicly or privately owned. **Intensive residential services** are intensively staffed for patient treatment. These services may include medical, nursing, psychosocial, vocational, recreational, or other support services. Combining residential care and mental health services, this treatment form offers rehabilitation and therapy to people with serious and persistent mental illnesses, including chronic schizophrenia, bipolar disorder, and unrelenting depression. These services may provide short-term treatment for stays from 24 hours to 3 or 6 months or long-term treatment for several months to years.

As a result of deinstitutionalization, many patients who were unable to live independently were discharged from state hospitals to intermediate- or skilled-care nursing facilities. The use of nursing homes for residential care is controversial because many of these facilities lack mental health services. Residential care in nursing homes varies from state to state. If a facility serves a primarily older adult population, placement of younger people there can be problematic. If a facility with more than 16 beds is engaged primarily in providing diagnosis, treatment, or care of people with mental disorders (including medical attention, nursing care, and related services), it is designated by the federal government as an institution for mental disease (IMD). A Medicare-certified facility having more than 16 beds and at least 50% of residents with a mental disorder is also considered an IMD. An IMD may not qualify for matching federal Medicaid dollars, which means that the state has principal responsibility for funding inpatient psychiatric services (Medicaid and CHIP Payment and Access Commission, 2023).

Nursing plays an important role in the care of people who have severe and persistent mental illnesses and who require partial hospitalization or long-term stays at residential treatment facilities. Nurses provide recovery-oriented psychiatric nursing care with a focus on psychoeducation, basic social skills training, aggression management, activities of daily living training, and group living. Education on symptom management, understanding mental illnesses, and medication is essential for recovery. *The Psychiatric–Mental Health Nursing: Scope and Standards of Practice* and *Addiction Nursing Scope and Standards of Practice* guide nurses in delivering patient care (American Nurses Association, American Psychiatric Nurses Association, & International Society of Psychiatric-Mental Health Nurses, 2022; Fornili & Fogger, 2022) (see Chapter 10).

Respite Residential Care

Sometimes, the family of an individual with mental illness who lives at home may be unable to provide care continuously. In such cases, respite residential care can provide short-term necessary housing for the patient and periodic relief for the caregivers.

Transitional Care

Health service systems have established a goal of reducing readmission following discharge from the hospital. People with serious mental illnesses need support and access to community resources when they are discharged from inpatient hospitalization but are often unable to access resources due to cognitive impairments, poor problem-solving skills, social isolation, unstable housing, and poverty. Access to these resources is critically important to promote medication adherence and attendance at the first follow-up appointment following discharge from the hospital.

Transitional care interventions have been used in the community to ensure that people with mental illnesses stay engaged in treatment between discharge from the hospital and the first follow-up appointment. Some programs provide intensive interventions immediately after discharge with reducing the intensity when the individual returns for a follow-up appointment; some use peer support specialists over a long length of time (Mullen et al., 2023).

In-Home Mental Health Care

If possible, people with mental illnesses live at home, not in a residential treatment setting. The goals are choices, not placement; physical and social integration, not segregated and congregate grouping by disability; and individualized flexible services and support, not standardized levels of service. When an individual can live at home, but outpatient care does not meet the treatment needs, **in-home mental health care** may be provided. Home care emphasizes the personal autonomy of the patient and the need for a trusting, collaborative relationship between the nurse and the patient (Han et al., 2023). In this setting, direct patient care and case management skills are used to decrease hospital stays and increase the functionality of the patient within the home. Individuals who most benefit from in-home mental health care include patients with chronic, persistent mental illness or patients with mental illness and comorbid medical conditions that require ongoing monitoring.

In-home mental health care services rely on the skills of the mental health nurse in providing ongoing assessment and implementing a comprehensive, individualized treatment plan of care. Components of the care plan and the ongoing assessment include data on mental health status, the environment, medication adherence, family dynamics and home safety, supportive psychotherapy, psychoeducation, coordination of services delivered by other home care staff, and communication of clinical issues to the patient's psychiatrist. In addition, the plan should address care related to collecting laboratory specimens (blood tests) and crisis intervention to reduce rehospitalization.

Outpatient Care

Outpatient care is a level of care that occurs outside of a hospital or institution. Outpatient services usually are less intensive and are provided to patients who do not require inpatient, residential, or home care environments. Many patients enroll in outpatient services immediately upon discharge from an inpatient setting. Outpatient treatment can include ongoing medication management, skills training, supportive group therapy, substance use disorder counseling, social support services, and case management. People with severe mental illnesses have high rates of comorbid medical illnesses, and many outpatient mental health clinics have developed integrated mental health–primary care treatment models to address the physical health needs of those with mental illnesses. These varying services promote community **reintegration** (return and acceptance of an individual as a fully participating member of a community), symptom management, and a healthy lifestyle (Edwards et al., 2023).

Intensive Outpatient Programs

The primary focus of **intensive outpatient programs** is on stabilization and relapse prevention for highly vulnerable individuals who function autonomously daily. People who meet these criteria have returned to their previous lifestyles (e.g., interacting with family, resuming work, and returning to school). Attendance in this type of program benefits individuals who still require frequent monitoring and support within a therapeutic milieu that enables them to remain connected to the community. The duration of treatment and level of services rendered are based on the patient's immediate needs. The treatment duration usually is time limited, with sessions offered 3 to 4 hours per day and 2 to 3 days per week. The treatment activities of the intensive outpatient program are like those offered in PHPs; whereas PHPs emphasize social skills training, intensive outpatient programs teach patients about stress management, illness, medication, and relapse prevention.

Other Services Integrated into a Continuum of Care

Within the continuum of care, other outpatient services may be received separately or simultaneously within various settings. They involve discrete services and patient variables.

Peer Support Services

Peer support services are provided by mental health consumers who have experienced symptom remission and are actively involved in their own recovery from mental illness. Peer support specialists are part of the behavioral health workforce, with their services offered in substance use and mental health programs. More peer support specialists are found in substance use programs than in mental health. They typically work in outpatient settings, such as community mental health centers, therapeutic rehabilitation centers, and **recovery centers**. The peer support specialist works with other mental health consumers who are in the process of moving toward recovery goals (Høgh Egmose et al., 2023). The relationship between peer specialists and mental health consumers offers an opportunity for mutual support for coping with mental illness and reciprocal sharing of personal experiences in the process of recovery. Peer support specialists assist consumers with self-determination and personal responsibility for recovery. They can also teach mental health consumers effective self-management skills and self-advocacy and encourage participation in wellness and recovery activities (Videka et al., 2023).

Outpatient Detoxification

There is an increasing shift toward providing alcohol and drug detoxification in an outpatient setting. The decision to use outpatient detoxification depends on symptom severity and the types of drugs the patient uses. Patients with alcohol use disorder who show signs of tolerance and withdrawal can undergo detoxification in an outpatient setting. However, patients who undergo ambulatory detoxification must have reliable family members who are available to provide monitoring. Outpatient detoxification is not suitable for situations involving severe or complicated withdrawal, especially with delirium. In addition, patients who are pregnant or have a history of a seizure disorder are hospitalized for detoxification.

Outpatient detoxification is a specialized form of partial hospitalization for patients requiring medical supervision. During the initial withdrawal phase, use of a 23-hour bed may be a treatment option, depending on the stage of withdrawal and the type of substance used. Or the patient may be required to attend a detoxification program 4 to 5 days per week until symptoms resolve. The length of participation depends on the severity of substance use disorder.

Outpatient detoxification includes a 12-step recovery model, such as Alcoholics Anonymous (AA) and Narcotics Anonymous (NA), which provides outpatient involvement with professionals experienced in substance use disorder counseling. It encourages abstinence and provides training in stress management and relapse prevention. Al-Anon and Alateen rely on 12-step support for families, who are usually included in the treatment program.

In-Home Detoxification

Detoxification from alcohol may be done in the home. For home detoxification to be safe and effective, symptoms of withdrawal must be mild, and a family member must be always present. The nurse is required to visit the patient daily for medication monitoring during the patient's first week of sobriety. Daily visits are necessary until the patient is in a medically stable condition. Referrals may come from primary care providers, court mandates, or employee assistance programs.

Assertive Community Treatment

The ACT model is a multidisciplinary clinical team approach providing 24-hour, intensive community-based services. ACT typically includes low staff-to-patient ratios, but this may not be possible in rural areas with shortages of qualified mental health professionals and few services. The ACT model helps individuals with serious mental illness live in the community by providing a comprehensive range of treatments, rehabilitation, and supportive services to help patients meet the requirements of community living. Concentration of services for high-risk patients within a single multiservice team enhances continuity and coordination of care, which improves the quality of care. ACT can reduce length of hospitalization and emergency department services, which reduces the cost of mental health treatment for patients with serious mental illnesses (Abufarsakh et al., 2023).

DISPARITIES IN MENTAL HEALTH SERVICE THROUGHOUT THE CONTINUUM OF CARE

A discussion of the mental health continuum of care would be incomplete without recognition of the inequities that exist for underserved and discriminated populations. Factors such as age, gender identity, and race/ethnicity influence the complexity of mental health needs associated with the lack of available services and access to care (see Box 5.2). Groups with complex mental health needs may not receive the same level of care as others. For example, during the COVID-19 pandemic, individuals who were Black or American Indian were more likely to have a higher number of needs that interfered with functioning than their White peers (Hong et al., 2023).

Access to the continuum of mental health services is dependent upon resources. For many individuals, resources are minimal or nonexistent. Without health insurance or government support, access to mental health services is not available. People without health insurance often have complex health and mental health needs. For example, individuals who are unhoused often have a mental disorder, substance use disorder, and poor health. Many states are not prepared to support the needed services for these individuals (Subica et al., 2023).

Screening for mental health issues can easily be influenced by social bias (Kiperman et al., 2024). People who identify as LGBTQ+ often have elevated rates of depression, anxiety, substance use disorders, and suicidality. When visiting a mental health provider, these individuals report experiencing stigma and microaggressions (insults, slights, offensive behavior) during the screening process (Williams et al., 2022). This discriminatory behavior is often unconscious and unintentional.

Nurses should reflect upon their explicit (known) personal prejudice and attitudes toward certain groups and implicit (unconscious) attitudes that precipitate unintentional discriminatory behavior. Unconscious negative bias toward a particular group can be reduced by recognizing them and having positive contacts with that group. See Chapter 10.

BOX 5.2

Mental Health Inequities: Gaps in Outpatient Mental Health Care in the United States

Outpatient mental health care services used by non-Hispanic White (*N* = 29,126), non-Hispanic Black (*N* = 7,965) and Hispanic (*N* = 12,640) individuals from 2018 to 2019 were analyzed for use of psychotropic medications, psychotherapy, or both and on receipt of minimally adequate mental health care. The annual rate per 100 people was twice as high for White individuals (25.3) as for Black (12.2) or Hispanic (11.4) individuals. Large racial-ethnic gaps in mental health services require dedicated efforts to promote greater mental health access for Black and Hispanic individuals in need.

Olfson, M., Zuvekas, S. H., McClellan, C., Wall, M. M., Hankerson, S. H., & Blanco, C. (2023). Racial-ethnic disparities in outpatient mental health care in the United States. *Psychiatric Services, 74*(7), 674–683. https://doi.org/10.1176/appi.ps.20220365

RECOVERY-ORIENTED REHABILITATION SETTINGS

Psychiatric rehabilitation programs, also termed psychosocial rehabilitation, focus on the reintegration of people with psychiatric disabilities into the community through work, education, and social avenues while addressing their medical and residential needs. The goal is to empower patients to achieve the highest level of functioning possible. Therapeutic activities or interventions are provided individually or in groups. They may include development and maintenance of daily and community living skills, such as communication (basic language), vocational, self-care (grooming, bodily care, feeding), and social skills that help patients function in the community. These programs promote increased functioning with the least necessary ongoing professional intervention. Psychiatric rehabilitation provides a highly structured environment, like a PHP, in a variety of settings, such as office buildings, hospital outpatient units, and freestanding structures.

The mental health nurse's role continues to focus on the consumer's recovery goals in all treatment settings. As behavioral health care delivery occurs more in outpatient settings, so does the work of nurses. Most rehabilitation programs have a full-time nurse who functions as part of the multidisciplinary team.

Psychiatric rehabilitation nurses are concerned with the recovery-oriented, holistic evaluation of the individual and with assessing and educating the patient on adherence issues, necessary laboratory work, and environmental and lifestyle issues. This evaluation assesses the five dimensions of an individual—physical, emotional, intellectual, social, and spiritual—and emphasizes recovery. Issues of psychotropic medication—evaluation of response, monitoring of side effects, and connection with pharmacy services—also fall to the nurse.

Self-Help Groups

Self-help groups are available in the community. These include AA, NA, and related 12-step programs. AA and NA use peer support as a strategy for helping people who are attempting to abstain from alcohol or drug use.

Counseling, mentoring, and support are provided by individuals with alcohol or substance use disorders who successfully abstain from substance use. In many cases, people with comorbid substance use and psychiatric diagnoses, such as schizophrenia and bipolar disorder, are unable to benefit from traditional AA self-help groups because of their psychiatric symptoms. For this reason, AA groups are available to meet the needs of individuals with comorbid psychiatric and substance use issues. Nurses may be asked to serve as consultants to these groups.

Relapse Prevention Aftercare Programs

Relapse of mental illness symptoms and substance use is the major reason for rehospitalization in the United States. **Relapse** is the recurrence or marked increase in severity of the symptoms of a disease, especially after a period of apparent improvement or stability. Many issues affect an individual's well-being. First and foremost, patients must believe that their lives are meaningful and worthwhile. Homelessness and unemployment create tremendous threats to an individual's identity and feelings of wellness.

Much work has gone into relapse prevention programs for the major mental illnesses and substance use disorders. Relapse prevention programs involve both patients and families and seek to (1) educate them about the illness, (2) enable them to cope with the chronic nature of the illness, (3) teach them to recognize early warning signs of relapse, (4) educate them about prescribed medications and the need for adherence, and (5) inform them about other disease management strategies (i.e., stress management, exercise) in preventing relapse.

Nurses become involved in relapse prevention programs in several different ways. They can act as referral sources for the programs, trainers or leaders of the programs, or aftercare sources for patients when the programs are completed. In addition, mental health nurses can help patients and family members by promoting optimism, sticking to goals and aspirations, and focusing on individual strengths.

Supported Employment

The ability to work in a competitive job is important in recovery from severe mental illness. Supported employment services assist individuals to find work; assess individuals' skills, attitudes, behaviors, and interest relevant to work; offer vocational rehabilitation or other training; and provide work opportunities. Consumers receive onsite support and job-coaching services on a one-to-one basis. They occur in real work settings and are used for patients with severe mental illnesses. The primary focus is to maintain attachment between the individual with a mental illness and the workforce.

ALTERNATIVE HOUSING ARRANGEMENTS

Housing is an important factor in successful community transition. Patients with psychiatric disabilities who are homeless are a vulnerable population. One of the largest hurdles to overcome in treating people with mental illness is finding appropriate housing that will meet the individual's immediate social, financial, and safety needs. Caring for people with severe mental illnesses in the home can be very stressful for family members because of the individual's symptom severity and unpredictable behaviors. Many individuals with a mental illness live in some form of supervised or supported community living situation, which ranges from highly supervised congregate settings to independent apartments. The following discussion focuses on four models of alternative housing and the role of the nurse. These are personal care homes, board-and-care homes, therapeutic foster care, and supervised apartments.

Personal Care Homes

Personal care homes operate within houses in the community. Usually, 6 to 10 people live in one house with a health care attendant providing 24-hour supervision to assist with medication monitoring or other minor activities, including transportation to appointments, meals, and self-care skills. The clientele generally is heterogeneous and includes older adults, people with mild intellectual disability, and patients with chronic and subacute mental illness. Most states require these homes to be licensed.

Board-and-Care Homes

Board-and-care homes provide 24-hour supervision and assistance with medications, meals, and some self-care skills. Individualized attention to self-care skills and other activities of daily living generally is not available. These homes are licensed to house 50 to 150 people in one location. Rooms are shared, with two to four occupants per bedroom.

Therapeutic Foster Care

Therapeutic foster care is indicated for patients in need of a family-like environment and a high level of support. Therapeutic foster care is available for child, adolescent, and adult populations. This level of care places patients in residences of families specially trained to handle individuals with mental illnesses. The training usually consists of crisis management, medication education, and illness education. The family provides supervision, structure, and support for the individual living with them. The person who receives these services shares the responsibility of completing household chores and may be required to attend an outpatient program during the day.

Supervised Apartments

In a supervised apartment setting, individuals live in their own apartments, usually alone or with one roommate, and are responsible for all household chores and self-care. A staff member or *supervisor* stops by each apartment routinely to evaluate how well the patients are doing, make sure they are taking their medications, and ensure that the household is being maintained. The supervisor may also be required to mediate disagreements between roommates.

Role of Nurses in Alternative Housing

Professional registered nurses typically are not employed in alternative housing settings. However, nurses play a pivotal role in the successful reintegration of patients from more restrictive inpatient settings into society. Nurses are employed in PHPs and inpatient units and as case managers. Therefore, nurses act as liaisons for the residential placement of patients. Nurses are employed directly as consultants or provide consultation to treatment teams during discharge planning in determining appropriate outpatient settings, evaluating medication follow-up needs, and making recommendations for necessary medical care for existing physical conditions. Feedback from the residential care providers and follow-up by the treatment team regarding the patient's response to treatment interventions are essential. Rehospitalization can be curtailed if the residential care operators identify and forward specific problems to the treatment teams. Patient interventions can be modified in an outpatient setting.

INTEGRATED CARE

People diagnosed with psychiatric disorders frequently have complex comorbid medical illnesses, such as hypertension, cardiac disease, metabolic syndrome, and diabetes, that require regular and ongoing treatment and engagement in self-management. However, access to care for complex health problems is often very limited in this population. Collaboration between medical and psychiatric providers is important to ensure that patients receive holistic care that addresses all illnesses. **Integrated care** is a health systems delivery model that ensures people receive a continuum of health promotion, disease management, rehabilitation, and palliative care services at different levels and settings according to their needs throughout life (Ganesh et al., 2023).

Medical Home

Integrated care can also be delivered in a **medical home**, a treatment setting that uses a team approach to deliver comprehensive patient-centered care that addresses all aspects of patients' health-related needs. There are five key functions of the medical home:

- Comprehensive care that meets most the individual's physical and mental health care needs through a team-based approach.
- Patient-centered care that delivers primary care that is oriented toward the whole person.
- Coordinated care across all elements of the health care system.
- Accessible services through minimizing wait times, enhanced office hours, and after-hours access to providers through alternative methods such as telephone or mail.
- Quality and safety through providing safe, high-quality care through clinical judgment, decision support tools, evidence-based care, shared decision making, performance measurement, improvement activities (Agency for Healthcare Quality and Research, 2022).

Health and Illness Management in the Community

High rates of medical illnesses among people with serious mental illnesses are often attributed to side effects of medication and lifestyle factors. Rates of smoking and obesity are very high among people diagnosed with posttraumatic stress disorder. They often do not engage in wellness and health promotion activities because of psychiatric symptoms, of lack of understanding of what they need to do to promote health, and their residing in unsafe communities (Søegaard et al., 2022).

Community mental health centers and therapeutic rehabilitation centers are convenient and safe settings to provide services that promote wellness in this population. These community centers can provide health education, self-management programs, healthy eating and cooking classes, group exercise or walking programs, weight loss groups, smoking cessation counseling, and screening for medical comorbidities.

MANAGED CARE

The concept of managed care emerged in efforts to coordinate patient care efficiently and cost-effectively. Managed care organizations provide services through health maintenance organizations or preferred provider organizations. Purchasers of health care, such as employers and government health agencies, contract with managed care organizations to provide mental health services. Traditionally, these services were separated from general medical care packages and reimbursed differently than other health care services. With the passage of the Affordable Care Act (see Chapter 1), the mental health services are supposed to be reimbursed at the same level as other health care problems. The recent trend is integration of many mental health services within a primary care setting. The goals of this approach to care are to increase access to care and to provide the most appropriate level of services in the least restrictive setting. Efforts focus on providing more outpatient and alternative treatment programs and avoiding costly inpatient hospitalizations. When properly conducted and administered, an integrated primary care allows patients better access to quality services while using health care dollars wisely.

Today, managed behavioral health care has succeeded in standardizing admissions criteria, reducing length of patient stay, and directing patients to the proper level of care—inpatient and outpatient—all while attempting to control the costs. Across the continuum of care nurses encounter integrated or collaborative organizations, and they must be familiar with the policies, procedures, and clinical judgment criteria established by managed care organizations. As the delivery of mental health care services becomes more integrated into primary care and growing numbers of patients with mental illnesses reach older age, increasing demands are placed on the health and mental health care systems to accommodate the needs of this population. Rates of comorbid medical illnesses are high in older adults with severe mental illnesses, and the need is great for services that provide adequate psychiatric and medical care for this population, ideally in the same treatment setting (Lovett et al., 2023).

The Nurse's Role in Negotiating the Mental Health Delivery Systems

Because of shorter inpatient stays, nurses maximize the short time they have by educating patients about their illness, available community resources, and medications to minimize the potential for relapse. These nurses focus on teaching social skills and self-reliance and creating empowering environments that in turn build self-confidence and help the patient move toward recovery.

The interface of psychiatric–mental health nurses with other nurses in managed care organizations and integrated primary care systems is primarily in the form of communicating the progress of individual patients to the nurses (mental health and nonmental health) and other health care workers who maintain a long-term relationship with the patient and family.

Public and Private Collaboration

Today, there are many public–private sector collaborations. The need for public–private collaboration prompted the National Association of State Mental Health Program Directors, an organization representing the 55 state and territorial public mental health systems, and the American Managed Behavioral Healthcare Association, an organization representing private managed behavioral health care firms, to work together. Nurses can expect to see more strategic alliances and joint ventures between the public and private sectors.

NURSING PRACTICE IN THE CONTINUUM OF CARE

Throughout this chapter, nurses' roles in different settings have been explained. Regardless of the situation or setting, nurses conduct assessments at the point of first patient contact. The individual's needs are then matched with the most appropriate setting, service, or program that will meet those needs. If a patient is admitted for services, the nurse also begins discharge planning upon first admission.

Assessment and Identification of Services

Choosing the level of care begins with an initial assessment to determine the need for care, the type of care to be provided, and the need for additional assessment. The nurse must discuss with the patient suicidal and homicidal thoughts. Nurses also need to consider financial issues because funding considerations may play a part in placement options. Other factors affecting the selection of care include the type of treatment the individual seeks, their current physical condition and ability to consent to treatment, and the organization's ability to provide direct care or to deflect care to another service provider.

Based on the results of the initial assessment, the nurse may admit the patient into services provided at that agency or initiate a referral or transfer to provide the intensity and scope of treatment required by the individual at that point in time (Fig. 5.1). Referral involves sending an individual from one clinician to another or from one service setting to another for care or consultation. Transfer involves formally shifting responsibility for the care of an individual from one clinician to another or from one care unit to another. The processes of referral and transfer to other levels of care are integral for effective use of services along the continuum. These processes are based on the individual's assessed needs and the organization's capability to provide the care. Figure 5.1 depicts the process of assessment, treatment, transfer, and referral when considering appropriate levels of care.

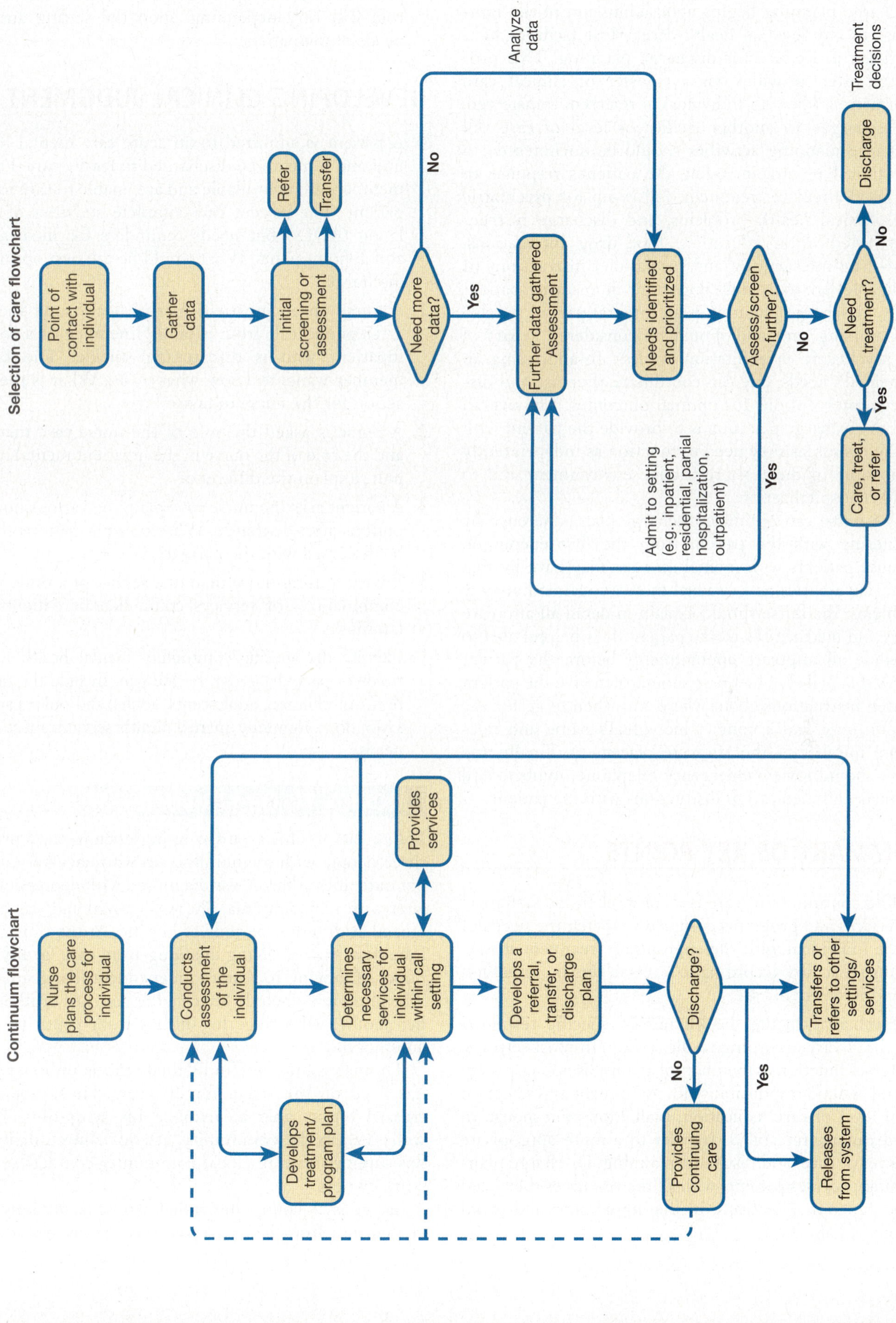

FIGURE 5.1 Flowcharts illustrating nursing care in the mental health care continuum and selection of care.

Discharge Planning

Discharge planning begins upon admission of the individual to any level of health care. Most facilities have a written procedure for discharge planning. This procedure often provides for a transfer of clinical care information when an individual is referred, transferred, or discharged to another facility or level of care. All discharge planning activities should be documented in the clinical record, including the patient's response to proposed aftercare treatment, follow-up for psychiatric and physical health problems, and discharge instructions. Medication education, food–drug interactions, drug–drug interactions, and special diet instructions (if applicable) are extremely important in ensuring patient safety. Discharge planning is an integral part of psychiatric nursing care and should be considered a part of the psychiatric rehabilitation process. In addressing an individual's needs, one can coordinate aftercare and discharge interventions for optimal outcomes. The overall goal of discharge planning is to provide the patient with all the resources they need to function as independently as possible in the least restrictive environment and to avoid rehospitalization.

The nurse can optimize discharge plan adherence by partnering with the patient from the first encounter. Because patients with mental illnesses may have limited cognitive abilities and residual motivational and anxiety problems, the nurse should explain in detail all aftercare plans and instructions to the patient. It is helpful also to schedule all aftercare appointments before the patient leaves the facility. The nurse should then give the patient written instructions about where and when to go for the appointment and a contact individual's name and telephone number at the aftercare placement. Finally, the nurse should review emergency telephone numbers and contacts and medication instructions with the patient.

SUMMARY OF KEY POINTS

- The continuum of care is a comprehensive system of services and programs designed to match the needs of the individual with the appropriate treatment in settings that vary according to levels of service, structure, and intensity of care.
- Psychiatric–mental health nurses' specific responsibilities vary according to the setting. In most settings, nurses function as members of a multidisciplinary team and assume responsibility for assessment and selection of level of care, education, evaluation of response to treatment, referral or transfer to a more appropriate level of care, and discharge planning. Discharge planning provides patients with all the resources they need to function effectively in the community and avoid rehospitalization.
- Mental health care can be given within an integrated primary care setting or a separate system. The nurse's role will vary depending upon the setting and the needs of the patient.

DEVELOPING CLINICAL JUDGMENT

1. A patient is admitted to an acute care mental health unit and wants to be discharged to family care. Family members are unavailable and are unable to care for the patient. The patient can complete activities of daily living (ADLs) but needs reminders for medications and appointments. What would be the best option for discharge?
2. A nurse on an inpatient mental health unit receives a telephone call from a family member of a former inpatient who is threatening suicide. The family member wants to know what to do. What is the best action for the nurse to take?
3. A nurse is asked the role of the nurse case manager and the role of the nurse in the inpatient mental health unit. Explain the difference.
4. A patient asks the nurse to explain the various housing options after discharge. What housing options should be discussed with the patient?
5. Envision using more than one service at a time. What combinations of services could benefit patients and families?
6. Identify the specific community mental health service needs of patients across the lifespan. Include the unique needs of children, adolescents, adults, and older patients. How do community mental health services meet these needs?

MOVIES, TV, OR STREAMING PROGRAMS

Voices: 2015. This award-winning documentary profiles three people with mental illnesses who have very different outcomes. Sharon was diagnosed with depression and later with schizophrenia. She was treated and was hospitalized at different periods of her life. At the time of the interview, she was living in a long-term care facility with hopes of moving to a more independent living situation. The interviews include Sharon, her son, her brother, and her mother who trace her illness from youth to older adulthood.

Thomas is an older individual who is unhoused and has lived on the street for 20 years. He is not being treated but is able to manage his symptoms. He is well-liked in the community, attends church daily, and has support from his local community contacts such as store owners.

Aaron is a young individual whose symptoms prevented him from being treated. His family reached out for help from the mental health center, but the family could not intervene because Aaron was an adult. By the time the legal system could intervene, it was too late.

Viewing Points:

1. Sharon, Thomas, and Aaron had similar psychotic symptoms but different outcomes. What role did their families play in helping them cope with their mental illness?
2. What type of services will Thomas need? Is housing a priority?

REFERENCES

Abufarsakh, B., Kappi, A., Pemberton, K. M., Williams, L. B., & Okoli, C. T. C. (2022). Substance use outcomes among individuals with severe mental illnesses receiving assertive community treatment: A systematic review. *International Journal of Mental Health Nursing*, *32*(3), 704–726. https://doi.org/10.1111/inm.13103

Agency for Healthcare Quality and Research. (2022). *5 key functions of the medical home*. Department of Health and Human Services. https://www.ahrq.gov/ncepcr/research/care-coordination/pcmh/define.html

American Case Management Association. (2023). *Case management: Standards of practice and scope of services*. https://www.acmaweb.org/forms/Standards_of%20Practice_Scope_of%20Services_Brochure.pdf

American Nurses Association, American Psychiatric Nurses Association, & International Society of Psychiatric-Mental Health Nurses. (2022). *Psychiatric-mental health nursing: Scope and standards of practice* (3rd ed.). American Nurses Association.

Balfour, M. E., & Zeller, S. L. (2023). Community-based crisis services, specialized crisis facilities, and partnerships with law enforcement. *Focus*, *21*(1), 18–27. https://doi.org/10.1176/appi.focus.20220074

Commission for Case Manager Certification. (2024). *Definition of case management. Case management body of knowledge*. Retrieved July 23, 2024, from https://cmbodyofknowledge.com/content/introduction-case-management-body-knowledge

Crouch, J., Winters, K., Zhang, L., & Stewart, M. W. (2023). Telehealth during the pandemic: Patient perceptions and policy implications. *Journal of Nursing Scholarship*, *55*(1), 141–148. https://doi.org/10.1111/jnu.12832

Edwards, J., Wang, L., Fuller, A. E., Anderson, K. K., & Georgiades, K. (2023). Comparing youth with vs without outpatient mental health services on subsequent acute mental health care visits. *Social Psychiatry and Psychiatric Epidemiology*, *58*(3), 501–504. https://doi.org/10.1007/s00127-022-02418-4

Fornili, K., & Fogger, S. (2022). *Addictions nursing: Scope and standards of practice.* (3rd. ed.). American Nurses Association & International Nurses Society on Addictions.

Ganesh, N., Sun, S., Feder, A., Galfalvy, H., Yehuda, R., Byma, L., & Haghighi, F. (2023). Delivery of telehealth complementary and integrated health interventions improves mental health and overall wellness to broaden veterans' access to care. *Journal of Integrative & Complementary Medicine*, *29*(2), 127–130. https://doi.org/10.1089/jicm.2022.0614

Gautam, R., Healey, D. N., & Batwara, S. (2023). Editorial: The untapped potential of partial hospitalization programs. *Journal of the American Academy of Child and Adolescent Psychiatry*, *63*(2), 111–113. https://doi.org/10.1016/j.jaac.2023.06.003

Han, J. H., Koch, E., Jeffery, A. D., Reese, T. J., Dorn, C., Pugh, S., Rubenstein, M., Wilson, J. E., Campbell, C., & Ward, M. J. (2023). The effect of telemental versus in-person mental health consults in the emergency department on 30-day utilization and processes of care. *Academic Emergency Medicine*, *30*(4), 262–269. https://doi.org/10.1111/acem.14688

Høgh Egmose, C., Heinsvig Poulsen, C., Hjorthøj, C., Skriver Mundy, S., Hellström, L., Nørgaard Nielsen, M., Korsbek, L., Serup Rasmussen, K., & Falgaard Eplov, L. (2023). The effectiveness of peer support in personal and clinical recovery-systematic review and meta-analysis. *Psychiatric Services*, *74*(8), 847–858. https://doi.org/10.1176/appi.ps.202100138

Hong, S., Walton, B., Kim, H. W., Kaboi, M., Moynihan, S., & Rhee, T. G. (2023). Exploring disparities in behavioral health service use in the early stages of the COVID-19 pandemic. *International Journal of Behavioral Medicine*, *31*(4), 549–562. https://doi.org/10.1007/s12529-023-10192-z

Kiperman, S., Clark, K., Renshaw, T. L., Anderson, J. R., Bernstein, E., & Willenbrink, J. B. (2024). Guidelines toward more socially just mental health screening in schools. *School Psychology*, *39*(2), 151–166. https://doi.org/10.1037/spq0000558

Lovett, R. M., Benavente, J. Y., Opsasnick, L. A., Weiner-Light, S., Curtis, L. M., & Wolf, M. S. (2023). Associations between cognitive impairment severity and barriers to healthcare engagement among older adults. *Journal of Applied Gerontology*. *42*(7), 1387–1396. https://doi.org/10.1177/07334648231166289

Medicaid and CHIP Payment and Access Commission. (2023). *Payment for services in institutions for mental diseases*. Retrieved July 18, 2023, from https://www.macpac.gov/subtopic/payment-for-services-in-institutions-for-mental-diseases-imds

Mullen, J. N., Levitt, A., & Markoulakis, R. (2023). Supporting individuals with mental health and/or addictions issues through patient navigation: A scoping review. *Community Mental Health Journal*, *59*(1), 35–56. https://doi.org/10.1007/s10597-022-00982-2

Olmstead v. L.C. (1999). 527 U.S. 581; 119 S.Ct. 2176. Brief Filed: 3/99 Court: Supreme Court of the United States.

Søegaard, E. G. I., Kan, Z., Aass, H. C. D., Koirala, R., Hauff, E., & Thapa, S. B. (2022). Abnormal cytokines in trauma patients explained by obesity, musculoskeletal disease, smoking, and lung disease. *Neuropsychobiology*, *81*(6), 516–530. https://doi.org/10.1159/000526806

Subica, A. M., Sampaga, D. S., Ortiz-Misiaszek, J., Martin, T. K. K., & Okamoto, S. K. (2023). The mental health, substance use, physical health, and mental health treatment need of community individuals experiencing homelessness in Hawai'i. *Community Mental Health Journal*, *59*(5), 1021–1026. https://doi.org/10.1007/s10597-022-01076-9

Tong, F., Lederman, R., D'Alfonso, S., Berry, K., & Bucci, S. (2022). Digital therapeutic alliance with fully automated mental health smartphone apps: A narrative review. *Frontiers in Psychiatry*, *13*, 819623. https://doi.org/10.3389/fpsyt.2022.819623

Videka, L., Page, C., Buche, J., Neale, J., Evans, E., Beck, A. J., Grazier, K. L., Railey, J. A., & Gaiser, M. (2023). Peer support services in behavioral health facilities: Secondary analysis from two national surveys. *Psychiatric Services*, *74*(12), 1247–1255. https://doi.org/10.1176/appi.ps.20220366

Watanabe, J., Teraura, H., Nakamura, A., & Kotani, K. (2023). Telemental health in rural areas: A systematic review. *Journal of Rural Medicine*, *18*(2), 50–54. https://doi.org/10.2185/jrm.2022-059

Williams, N. D., Turpin, R. E., Akré, E. L., Boekeloo, B. O., & Fish, J. N. (2022). Disparities in mental health care access among persons differing in sexual identity: Nationally representative findings. *Psychiatric Services (Washington, D.C.)*, *73*(4), 456–459. https://doi.org/10.1176/appi.ps.202100045

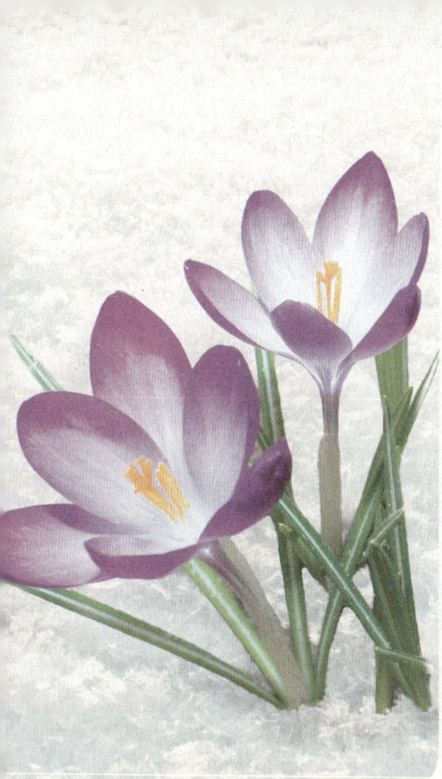

UNIT II
Foundations of Psychiatric Nursing

6 Psychosocial–Spiritual Basis of Psychiatric Nursing

Mary Ann Boyd

KEYCONCEPTS

- anxiety
- cognition
- empathic linkage

LEARNING OBJECTIVES

After studying this chapter, you will be able to:

1. Discuss psychosocial theories and spiritual concepts that support psychiatric nursing practice.
2. Identify the underlying theories and concepts that contribute to the understanding of human beings and behavior.
3. Compare the key elements of each theory that provides a basis for psychiatric–mental health (PMH) nursing practice.
4. Identify common nursing theoretic models used in PMH nursing.

KEY TERMS

• behaviorism • classical conditioning • cognitive interventions • cognitive theory • collective efficacy • countertransference • defense mechanisms • empathy • family dynamics • formal support systems • informal support systems • interpersonal relations • libido • modeling • object relations • operant behavior • principle of frequency • principle of recency • psychoanalysis • religion • self-efficacy • self-system • social distance • spiritual interventions • spirituality • transaction • transference • unconditional positive regard

INTRODUCTION

This chapter presents an overview of selected psychodynamic, cognitive-behavioral, developmental, social, and nursing theories that serve as the knowledge base for PMH nursing practice. Many of these theories are covered in more depth in other chapters. Biologic theories are discussed in Chapters 7 and 11.

PSYCHODYNAMIC THEORIES

Psychodynamic theories explain the development of mental or emotional processes and their effects on behavior and relationships. Many of the psychodynamic concepts and models that are important in psychiatric nursing began with the Austrian physician Sigmund Freud (1856–1939). Since his time, Freud's theories have been enhanced by interpersonal and humanist models. These theories proved to be especially important in the development of therapeutic relationships, techniques, and interventions (Table 6.1).

Psychoanalytic Theory

In Freud's psychoanalytic model, the human mind is conceptualized in terms of conscious mental processes (an awareness of events, thoughts, and feelings with the ability to recall them) and unconscious mental processes (thoughts and feelings that are outside awareness and are not remembered).

Study of the Unconscious

Freud believed that the unconscious part of the human mind is only rarely recognized by the conscious, as in remembered dreams. The term *preconscious* is used to describe unconscious material that can enter consciousness.

TABLE 6.1 PSYCHODYNAMIC MODELS

Theorist	Overview	Major Concepts	Applicability
Psychoanalytic Models			
Sigmund Freud (1856–1939)	Founder of psychoanalysis Believed that the unconscious could be accessed through dreams and free association Developed a personality theory and theory of infantile sexuality	Id, ego, superego Consciousness Unconscious mental processes Libido Object relations Anxiety and defense mechanisms Free associations, transference, and countertransference	Individual therapy approach used for enhancement of personal maturity and personal growth
Anna Freud (1895–1982)	Application of ego psychology to psychoanalytic treatment and child analysis with emphasis on the adaptive function of defense mechanisms	Refinement of concepts of anxiety, defense mechanisms	Individual therapy, childhood psychoanalysis
Neo-Freudian Models			
Alfred Adler (1870 1937)	First defected from Freud Founded the school of individual psychology	Inferiority	Added to the understanding of human motivation
Carl Gustav Jung (1875–1961)	After separating from Freud, founded the school of psychoanalytic psychology Developed new therapeutic approaches	Redefined libido Introversion Extroversion Persona	Personalities are often assessed on the intro-version and extroversion dimensions
Otto Rank (1884–1939)	Introduced the idea of primary trauma of birth Active technique of therapy, including more nurturing than Freud Emphasized feeling aspect of analytic process	Birth trauma Will	Recognized the importance of feelings within psychoanalysis
Erich Fromm (1900–1980)	Emphasized the relationship of the individual to society	Society and individual are not separate	Individual desires are formed by society
Melanie Klein (1882–1960)	Devised play therapy techniques Believed that complex unconscious fantasies existed in children younger than 6 months of age Principal source of anxiety arose from the threat to existence posed by the death instinct	Pioneer in object relations Identification	Developed separate ways of applying psychoanalysis to children; influenced present-day English and American schools of child psychiatry
Karen Horney (1885–1952)	Opposed Freud's theory of castration complex in women and his emphasis on the oedipal complex Argued that neurosis was influenced by the society in which one lived	Situational neurosis Character	Beginning of feminist analysis of psychoanalytic thought

TABLE 6.1 PSYCHODYNAMIC MODELS (*Continued*)

Theorist	Overview	Major Concepts	Applicability
Interpersonal Relations			
Harry Stack Sullivan (1892–1949)	Impulses and striving need to be understood in terms of interpersonal situations	Participant observer Parataxic distortion Consensual validation	Provided the framework for the introduction of the interpersonal theories in nursing
Humanist Theories			
Abraham Maslow (1908–1970)	Concerned himself with healthy rather than sick people Approached individuals from a holistic-dynamic viewpoint	Needs Motivation	Used as a model to understand how people are motivated and needs that should be met
Frederick S. Perls (1893–1970)	Awareness of emotion, physical state, and repressed needs would enhance the ability to deal with emotional problems	Reality Here and now	Used as a therapeutic approach to resolve current life problems that are influenced by old, unresolved emotional problems
Carl Rogers (1902–1987)	Based theory on the view of human potential for goodness Used the term *client* rather than *patient* Stressed the relationship between therapist and client	Empathy Positive regard	Individual therapy approach that involves never giving advice and always clarifying client's feelings

Personality and Its Development

Freud's personality structure consists of three parts: the id, ego, and superego (Freud, 1927). The *id* is formed by unconscious desires, primitive instincts, and unstructured drives, including sexual and aggressive tendencies that arise from the body. The *ego* consists of the sum of certain mental mechanisms, such as perception, memory, and motor control, as well as specific defense mechanisms (discussed below). The ego controls movement, perception, and contact with reality. The capacity to form mutually satisfying relationships is a fundamental function of the ego, which is not present at birth but is formed throughout the child's development. The *superego* is that part of the personality structure associated with ethics, standards, and self-criticism. A child's identification with important and esteemed people in early life, particularly parents, helps form the superego.

Object Relations and Identification

Freud introduced the concept of **object relations**, the psychological attachment to another person or object. He believed that the choice of a sexual partner in adulthood and the nature of that relationship depended on the quality of the child's object relationships during the early formative years.

The child's first love object is the parent who gives birth to the child, who is the source of nourishment and the provider of pleasure. Gradually, as the child separates from this parent, the nature of this initial attachment influences future relationships. The development of the child's capacity for relationships with others progresses from a state of narcissism to social relationships, first within the family and then within the larger community. Although the concept of object relations is abstract, it can be understood in terms of a child who imitates the parent who gave birth to them and then becomes like them in adulthood. This process—incorporating that parent as a love object, identifying with them, and growing up to become like them—is especially important in understanding an abused child who, under certain circumstances, becomes an adult who abuses children.

Anxiety and Defense Mechanisms

For Freud, anxiety is the reaction to danger and is experienced as a specific state of physical unpleasantness. **Defense mechanisms** are coping styles that protect people from unwanted anxiety. Although they are defined differently than in Freud's day, defense mechanisms still play an explanatory role in contemporary PMH practice. Defense mechanisms are discussed in Chapter 9.

Sexuality

The energy or psychic drive associated with the sexual instinct, or **libido**, literally translated from Latin to mean "pleasure" or "lust," resides in the id. When sexual desire is controlled and not expressed, tension results and is transformed into anxiety (Freud, 1905). Freud believed that adult sexuality is a product of a complex process of development that begins in early childhood and involves a variety of body functions or areas (oral, anal, and genital zones) that correspond to stages of relationships, especially with parents.

Psychoanalysis

Freud developed **psychoanalysis**, a therapeutic process of accessing the unconscious conflicts that originate in childhood and then resolving the issues with a mature adult mind. As a system of psychotherapy, psychoanalysis attempts to reconstruct the personality by examining free associations (spontaneous, uncensored verbalizations of whatever comes to mind) and the interpretation of dreams. Therapeutic relationships had their beginnings within the psychoanalytic framework (Sharma & Spiro, 2023).

Transference and Countertransference

Transference is the displacement of thoughts, feelings, and behaviors originally associated with significant others onto a person in a current therapeutic relationship. For example, an adult's feelings toward their parents as a child may be directed toward their therapist. If a person was unconsciously angry with their parents, they may feel unexplainable anger and hostility toward their therapist. In **psychoanalysis**, the therapist uses transference as a therapeutic tool to help the patient understand emotional problems and their origin.

Countertransference, on the other hand, is defined as the direction of all the health professional's feelings and attitudes toward the patient. Countertransference becomes a problem when these feelings and perceptions are based on other interpersonal experiences. For example, a patient may remind a nurse of a beloved relative. Instead of therapeutically interacting with the patient from an objective perspective, the nurse feels an unexplained attachment to the patient, treating them as if they were the nurse's relative. Because of this approach, the nurse misses important assessment and intervention data.

Neo-Freudian Models

Many of Freud's followers ultimately broke away, establishing their own forms of psychoanalysis. Freud did not receive criticism well. The rejection of some of his basic tenets often cost his friendship as well. Various psychoanalytic schools have adopted other names because their doctrines deviated from Freudian theory.

Adler's Foundation for Individual Psychology

Alfred Adler (1870–1937), a Viennese psychiatrist and founder of the school of individual psychology, was a student of Freud, who believed that the motivating force in human life is an intolerable sense of inferiority. Some people try to avoid these feelings by developing an unreasonable desire for power and dominance. This compensatory mechanism can get out of hand, and these individuals become self-centered and neurotic, overcompensate, and retreat from the real world and its problems.

Today, Adler's theories and principles are adapted and applied to both psychotherapy and education. Adlerian theory is based on principles of mutual respect, choice, responsibility, consequences, and belonging.

Jung's Analytical Psychology

One of Freud's earliest students, Carl Gustav Jung (1875–1961), a Swiss psychoanalyst, created a model called analytical psychology. Jung believed in the existence of two basically different types of personalities: extroverted and introverted. Whereas extroverted people tend to be generally interested in other people and objects of the external world, introverted people are more interested in themselves and their internal environment. According to Jung, both extroverted and introverted tendencies exist in everyone, but the libido usually channels itself mainly in one direction or the other. He also developed the concept of *persona*—what a person appears to be to others in contrast to who they really are (Jung, 1966).

Horney's Feminine Psychology

Karen Horney (1885–1952), a German American psychiatrist, challenged many of Freud's basic concepts and introduced principles of feminine psychology. Freud believed that people assigned female at birth felt inferior to those assigned male at birth because their bodies were less completely equipped, a theory he described as "penis envy." Recognizing a male bias in psychoanalysis, Horney rejected this concept, as well as the oedipal complex, arguing that such individuals were at a disadvantage because of the paternalistic culture in which they lived, which is the reason they strived to obtain qualities or privileges that were defined by society as being masculine, such as a university education, the right to vote, or economic independence (Horney, 1939).

Other Neo-Freudian Theories

Otto Rank: Birth Trauma

Otto Rank (1884–1939), an Austrian psychologist and psychotherapist, was also one of Freud's students. He attributed all neurotic disturbances to the primary trauma of birth. For Rank, human development is a progression from complete dependence on the person who gives birth to the child, as well as the family; to physical independence coupled with intellectual dependence on society; and finally to complete intellectual and psychological emancipation. A person's will guides and organizes the integration of self.

Erich Fromm: Societal Needs

Erich Fromm (1900–1980), an American psychoanalyst, focused on the relationship of society and the individual. He argued that individual and societal needs are not separate and opposing forces; their relationship is determined by the historic background of the culture. Fromm also believed that the needs and desires of individuals are largely formed by their society. For Fromm, the fundamental purpose of psychoanalysis and psychology is to bring harmony and understanding between the individual and society (Fromm-Reichmann, 1950).

Melanie Klein: Play Therapy

Melanie Klein (1882–1960), an Austrian psychoanalyst, devised play therapy techniques to demonstrate how a child's interaction with toys reveals earlier infantile fantasies and anxieties. She believed that complex, unconscious fantasies exist in children younger than 6 months of age. She is generally acknowledged as a pioneer in presenting an object relations viewpoint to the psychodynamic field, introducing the idea of early identification, a defense mechanism by which one patterns oneself after another person, such as a parent (Klein, 1963).

Harry Stack Sullivan: Interpersonal Forces

Interpersonal theories stress the importance of human relationships; instincts and drives are less important. Harry Stack Sullivan (1892–1949), an American psychiatrist, viewed **interpersonal relations** as a basis of human development and behavior. He believed that the health or sickness of one's personality is determined by the characteristic patterns in which one deals with other people. For example, a person is passive aggressive to everyone who contradicts them. This maladaptive behavior began when they were unable to express their disagreement to their parents. Health depends on managing the constantly changing physical, social, and interpersonal environment as well as past and current life experiences (Sullivan, 1953).

Humanistic Theories

Humanistic theories are based on the belief that all human beings have the potential for goodness. Humanist therapists focus on patients' ability to learn about and accept themselves. They do not investigate repressed memories. Through therapy, patients explore personal capabilities to develop self-worth. They learn to experience the world in a different way.

Rogers' Client-Centered Therapy

Carl Rogers (1902–1987), an American psychologist, introduced client-centered therapy. **Empathy**, the capacity to assume the internal reference of the client to perceive the world in the same way as the client, is used in the therapeutic process (Rogers, 1980). The counselor is genuine but nondirect and uses **unconditional positive regard**, a nonjudgmental caring for the client. In this therapy, the counselor's attitude and nonverbal communication are crucial. The therapist's emotional investment (i.e., true caring) in the client is essential in the therapeutic process (Rogers, 1980).

Abraham Maslow's Hierarchy of Needs

Abraham Maslow's (1921–1970) hierarchy of needs is a fixture in social science and nursing (see Fig. 6.1) (Maslow, 1970). In nursing, Maslow's model is used to prioritize care. Basic needs (food, shelter) should be met before higher-level needs (self-esteem) can be met. This model serves as a framework in understanding the needs of people who are without housing. Basic needs such as food, clothing, shelter, and funds are the strongest needs followed by health and social services and safety (Fleury et al., 2021).

Applicability of Psychodynamic Theories to Psychiatric–Mental Health Nursing

Several psychodynamic concepts are important in the practice of PMH nursing, such as interpersonal relationships, defense mechanisms, transference, countertransference,

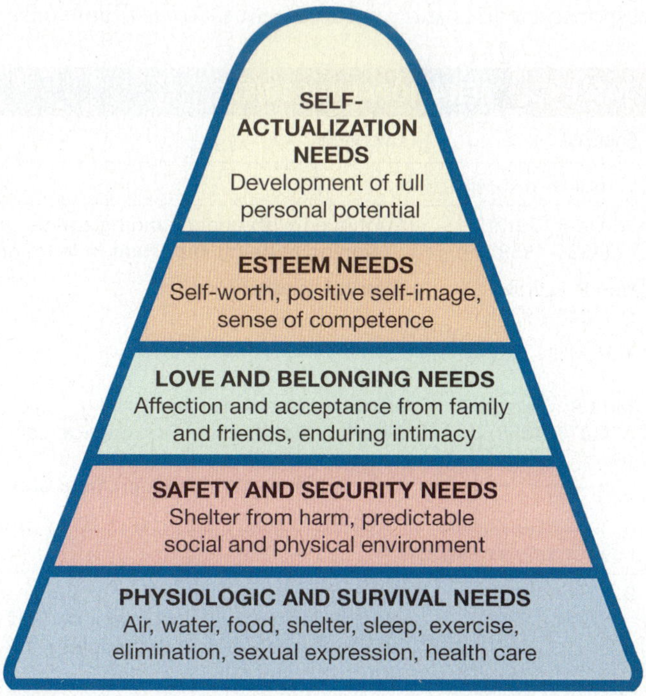

FIGURE 6.1 Maslow's hierarchy of needs. (Adapted from Maslow, A. H. [1954]. *Motivation and personality*. Harper & Row.)

and internal objects. A therapeutic interpersonal relationship is a core of PMH nursing intervention (see Chapter 10 for nursing interventions). Even though there is consensus that most of these theories are useful, the nurse should continue to critically analyze them for utility and relevance. For example, Maslow's theory may be useful when a person with mental illness is homeless and wants food and shelter. But another person in a similar situation may reject food and shelter because self-esteem is associated with being free to reject the confines of an institution. In this case, self-esteem need is more important than food or shelter.

There is renewed interest in psychodynamic treatment for depression. Psychodynamic therapists have a strong emphasis on affect and emotional expression, examination of topics that the patient avoids, recurring patterns of behaviors, feelings, experiences, and relationships, the past and its influence on the present, interpersonal relationships, and exploration of wishes, dreams, and fantasies (Wienicke et al., 2023).

COGNITIVE-BEHAVIORAL THEORIES

Behavioral Theories

Behavioral theories attempt to explain how people learn and act. Behavioral theories never attempt to explain the cause of mental disorders; instead, they focus on typical human behavior. Research results are then applied to the clinical situation. Two areas of behavioral theories relevant to psychiatric–nursing practice are stimulus–response theories and reinforcement theories (Table 6.2).

Early Stimulus–Response Theories

Pavlovian Theory

One of the earliest behavioral theorists was Ivan P. Pavlov (1849–1936), who noticed that stomach secretions of dogs were stimulated by triggers other than food reaching the stomach. He found that the sight and smell of food triggered stomach secretions, and he became interested in this anticipatory secretion. Through his experiments, he was able to stimulate secretions with a variety of other laboratory nonphysiologic stimuli. Thus, a clear connection was made between thought processes and physiologic responses.

In Pavlov's model, there is an unconditioned stimulus (not dependent on previous training) that elicits an unconditioned (i.e., specific) response. In his experiments, meat is the unconditioned stimulus, and salivation is the unconditioned response. Pavlov taught the dog to associate a bell (conditioned stimulus) with the meat (unconditioned stimulus) by repeatedly ringing the bell before presenting the meat. Eventually, the dog salivated when hearing the bell. This phenomenon is called **classical conditioning** (or Pavlovian conditioning) (Pavlov, 1927/1960).

John B. Watson and the Behaviorist Revolution

At about the same time Pavlov was working in Russia, **behaviorism**, a learning theory that only focuses on objectively observable behaviors and discounts any independent activities of the mind, was introduced in the United States by John B. Watson (1878–1958). He

TABLE 6.2 BEHAVIORAL THEORISTS

Theorist	Overview	Major Concepts	Applicability
Stimulus–Response			
Edwin R. Guthrie (1886–1959)	Continued with understanding conditioning as being important in learning	Recurrence of responses tends to follow a specific stimulus	Important in analyzing habitual behavior
Ivan P. Pavlov (1849–1936)	Classical conditioning	Unconditioned stimuli Unconditioned response Conditioned stimuli	Important in understanding learning of automatic responses such as habitual behaviors
John B. Watson (1878–1958)	Introduced behaviorism Believed that learning was classical conditioning called *reflexes* Rejected distinction between mind and body	Principle of frequency Principle of recency	Focuses on the relationship between the mind and body
Reinforcement Theories			
B. F. Skinner (1904–1990)	Developed an understanding of the importance of reinforcement and differentiated types and schedules	Operant behavior Respondent behavior Continuous reinforcement Intermittent reinforcement	Important in behavior modification
Edward L. Thorndike (1874–1949)	Believed in the importance of effects that followed behavior	Reinforcement	Important in behavior modification programs

rejected the distinction between body and mind and emphasized the study of objective behavior (Watson & Rayner, 2000). He developed two principles: frequency and recency. The ***principle of frequency*** states that the more often a response is made to a stimulus, the more likely the response to that stimulus will be repeated. The ***principle of recency*** states that the closer in time a response is to a particular stimulus, the more likely the response will be repeated.

Reinforcement Theories

Edward L. Thorndike

A pioneer in experimental animal psychology, Edwin L. Thorndike (1874–1949), studied the problem-solving behavior of cats to determine whether animals solved problems by reasoning or instinct. He found that neither choice was completely correct; animals gradually learn the correct response by "stamping in" the stimulus–response connection. The major difference between Thorndike and behaviorists such as Watson was that Thorndike believed that reinforcement of positive behavior was important in learning. He was the first reinforcement theorist, and his view of learning became the dominant view in American learning theory (Thorndike, 1906).

B. F. Skinner

One of the most influential behaviorists, B. F. Skinner (1904–1990), studied **operant behavior** or conditioning. In this type of learning, the focus is on the consequence of the behavioral response, not on a specific stimulus. If a behavior is reinforced or rewarded with success, praise, money, and so on, the behavior will probably be repeated. For example, if a child climbs on a chair, reaches the faucet, and can get a drink of water successfully, it is more likely that the child will repeat the behavior (Skinner, 1935). If a behavior does not have a positive outcome, it is less likely that the behavior will be repeated. Nurses use this knowledge to create behavior management plans to reinforce healthy, positive behaviors.

Cognitive Theories

The initial behavioral studies focused on human actions without much attention to the internal thinking process. When complex behaviors could not be accounted for by strict behavioral explanations, thought processes became new subjects for study. **Cognitive theory**, an outgrowth of different theoretic perspectives, including the behavioral and the psychodynamic, attempted to link internal thought processes with human behavior (Table 6.3).

KEYCONCEPT Cognition can be defined as an internal process of perception, memory, and judgment through which an understanding of self and the world is developed.

Cognitive interventions aim to change or reframe an individual's automatic thought patterns that have developed over time and that interfere with the individual's ability to function optimally. The skills and techniques that were developed based on **cognitive theory** result in a new view of self and the environment. Cognitive therapies incorporate additional therapeutic modalities such as mindfulness and targeting for people with anxiety and depressive disorders (Maas Genannt Bermpohl et al., 2023).

Albert Bandura's Social Cognitive Theory

Learning by watching others is the basis of Albert Bandura's (1925–2021) social cognitive theory. He developed his ideas after being concerned about television violence contributing to aggression in children. He showed learning occurs by internalizing the behaviors of others through a process of **modeling** called pervasive imitation, or one person trying to be like another. The model does not have to be a real person who is currently alive but could be a character in history or generalized to an ideal person (Bandura, 1977, 1986; Ozer, 2022).

Self-efficacy, an important concept in his theory, is a person's sense of their ability to deal effectively with the environment (Bandura, 1993). Efficacy beliefs influence how people feel, think, motivate themselves, and behave.

TABLE 6.3 COGNITIVE THEORISTS

Theorist	Overview	Major Concepts	Applicability
Aaron Beck (b. 1921)	Conceptualized distorted cognitions as a basis for depression	Cognitions Beliefs	Important in cognitive therapy
Kurt Lewin (1890–1947)	Developed field theory, a system for understanding learning, motivation, personality, and social behavior	Life space Positive valences	Important in understanding motivation for changing behavior
Edward Chace Tolman (1886–1959)	Introduced the concept of cognitions: believed that human beings act on beliefs and attitudes and strive toward goals	Negative valences Cognition	Important in identifying person's beliefs

The stronger the self-efficacy, the higher the goals people set for themselves and the firmer their commitment to them (Kuchenbaur & Peter, 2021).

Collective efficacy, an expansion of self-efficacy, is a family or neighborhood's shared beliefs about how well the family works together to achieve desired outcomes. The positive **collective efficacy** can protect against risky health behaviors (violence, substance use, sexual behavior, unhealthy diet, and physical inactivity) despite adolescent depressive symptoms (Rivera & Doom, 2023).

One of Bandura's contributions is showing that intentions and self-motivation play roles in determining behavior, significantly expanding the reinforcement model. He believed that the human mind is not only reactive to a stimulus but is also creative, proactive, and reflective (Bandura, 2001). Recent research supports Bandura's ideas in explaining goal achievement in entrepreneurship (Egana-delSol et al., 2023).

Aaron Beck: Thinking and Feeling

American psychiatrist Aaron T. Beck (1921–2021) of the University of Pennsylvania devoted his career to understanding the relationship between cognition and mental health. For Beck, cognitions are verbal or pictorial events in the stream of consciousness. He realized the importance of cognition when treating people with depression. He found that depression improved when patients began viewing themselves and situations in a positive light.

He believed that people with depression have faulty information-processing systems that lead to biased cognitions. These faulty beliefs cause errors in judgment that become habitual errors in thinking. These individuals incorrectly interpret life situations, judge themselves too harshly, and jump to inaccurate negative conclusions. A person may truly believe that they have no friends, and therefore no one cares. On examination, the evidence for the beliefs is since there has been no contact with anyone because of moving from one city to another. Thus, a distorted belief is the basis of the cognition. Beliefs are important because they are related to a person's mood. For example, negative beliefs of caregivers of family members with Alzheimer disorder are related to depression. Judith Beck and colleagues continue to develop cognitive therapy, a successful approach for the treatment of depression (Beck, 2021).

Applicability of Cognitive-Behavioral Theories to Psychiatric–Mental Health Nursing

Basing interventions on behavioral theories is widespread in psychiatric nursing. For example, patient education interventions are usually derived from the behavioral theories. Teaching patients new coping skills for their symptoms of mental illnesses is another example. Changing an entrenched habit involves helping patients identify what motivates them and how these new lifestyle habits can become permanent. In psychiatric units, behavioral interventions include the privilege systems and token economies. Cognitive-behavioral approaches are discussed throughout this text.

DEVELOPMENTAL THEORIES

Developmental theories explain typical human growth and development over time. Many developmental theories are presented in terms of stages based on the assumption that typical development proceeds longitudinally from the beginning to the ending stage.

Erik Erikson: Psychosocial Development

Freud and Sullivan both published treatises on stages of human development, but Erik Erikson (1902–1994) outlined the psychosocial developmental model most often used in nursing. Erikson's model is an expansion of Freud's psychosexual development theory. Whereas Freud's model emphasizes intrapsychic experiences, Erikson's model recognizes the role of the psychosocial environment. For example, parental divorce disrupts the family interaction pattern, and the financial and housing environment impacts the development of the children.

Each of Erikson's eight stages is organized by age and developmental conflicts: basic trust versus mistrust, autonomy versus shame and doubt, initiative versus guilt, industry versus inferiority, identity versus role diffusion, intimacy versus isolation, generativity versus stagnation, and ego integrity versus despair. Successful resolution of a conflict or crisis leads to essential strength and virtues (Table 6.4). For example, a positive outcome of the trust versus mistrust crisis is the development of a basic sense of trust. If the crisis is unsuccessfully resolved, the infant moves into the next stage without a sense of trust. According to this model, a child who is mistrustful will have difficulty completing the next crisis successfully and, instead of developing a sense of autonomy, will more likely be full of shame and doubt (Erikson, 1963).

Identity and Adolescence

One of Erikson's major contributions is the recognition of the turbulence of adolescence and identity formation. When adolescence begins, childhood ways are given up, and bodily changes occur. An identity is formed. Trying to reconcile a personal view of self with society's perception can be overwhelming and lead to role confusion and alienation (Erikson, 1968).

TABLE 6.4 ERIKSON'S EIGHT AGES OF DEVELOPMENT

Approximate Chronologic Age	Developmental Conflict[a]	Long-Term Outcome of Successful Resolution
Infant	Basic trust vs. mistrust	Drive and hope
Toddler	Autonomy vs. shame and doubt	Self-control and willpower
Preschool-aged child	Initiative vs. guilt	Direction and purpose
School-aged child	Industry vs. inferiority	Method and competence
Adolescence	Identity vs. role diffusion	Devotion and fidelity
Young adult	Intimacy vs. isolation	Affiliation and love
Adulthood	Generativity vs. stagnation	Production and care
Maturity	Ego integrity vs. despair	Renunciation and wisdom

[a]Successful outcome is evidenced by the development of the characteristic listed first.
Adapted from Erikson, E. (1963). *Childhood and society* (2nd ed., pp. 273–274). W. W. Norton & Company.

Research Evidence for Erikson's Models

Evidence is mixed that every person follows the eight stages of development as outlined by Erikson. In early studies, male college students who measured low on identity also scored low on intimacy ratings (Orlofsky et al., 1973). These results lend support to the idea that identity precedes intimacy. In another study, intimacy was found to begin developing early in adolescence before the development of identity (Ochse & Plug, 1986). Studying fathers with young children, Christiansen and Palkovitz (1998) found that *generativity* (defined as the need or drive to produce, create, or effect a change) was associated with a paternal identity, psychosocial identity, and psychosocial intimacy. In addition, fathers who had a religious identification also had higher generativity scores than others.

A study of autobiographical memories of 112 older adults (61 to 92 years) rated memories according to themes of Erikson's theory of psychosocial development—trust/mistrust, identity/confusion, intimacy/isolation, and generativity/stagnation. Results supported Erikson's theory and showed that childhood memories were associated with trust, memories from youth were related to identity and intimacy, and adulthood memories were associated with intimacy and generativity (Nusser et al., 2023). The study reported by Chen et al. (2021) also supports the relationship of the eight stages to each other and the importance of the first seven stages to a successful eighth stage of generativity. The model is also used as a framework for psychodynamic psychotherapy (Corradi, 2024).

Studies show that generativity is significantly associated with successful relationships, work achievements, close friendships, altruistic behaviors, and overall mental health. Generativity is also associated with optimism and forgiveness in dealing with grandparenting problems within the family (Paul, 2023). Generativity is emerging as a useful concept in understanding attitudes toward death (Tomoi, 2024).

Jean Piaget: Learning in Children

One of the most influential people in child psychology is Jean Piaget (1896–1980), who contributed more than 40 books and 100 articles on child psychology alone. Piaget's theory views intelligence as an adaptation to the environment. He proposes that cognitive growth is like embryologic growth: an organized structure becomes more and more differentiated over time. Piaget's system explains how knowledge develops and changes (Table 6.5).

Each stage of cognitive development represents a particular structure with major characteristics. Piaget's theory was developed through observation of his own children and therefore never received formal testing.

The major strength of his model is its recognition of the central role of cognition in development and the discovery of surprising features of young children's thinking. For example, children in middle childhood become capable of considering more than one aspect of an object or situation at a time. Their thinking becomes more complex. They can understand that the area of a rectangle is determined by the length *and* width. For PMH nurses, Piaget's model provides a framework to recognize different levels of thinking in the assessment and intervention processes. For example, the assessment of concrete thinking is typical of some people with schizophrenia who are unable to perform abstract thinking.

One of the criticisms of this theory from a moral perspective is that it does not account for inequality—that is, children preferentially allocate resources to the rich rather than the poor. Piaget explained that children acquired behavioral routines in which they match items to already preexisting distributions. This should be particularly true for very young children who have not yet developed rule consciousness or whose appreciation of rules does not allow them to solve the problem. In addition, children could accept and even perpetuate a

TABLE 6.5 PIAGET'S PERIODS OF INTELLECTUAL DEVELOPMENT

Age (years)	Period	Cognitive Developmental Characteristics	Description
Birth to 2	Sensorimotor	Divided into six stages, characterized by (1) inborn motor and sensory reflexes, (2) primary circular reaction and first habit, (3) secondary circular reaction, (4) use of familiar means to obtain ends, (5) tertiary circular reaction and discovery through active experimentation, and (6) insight and object permanence	The infant understands the world in terms of overt, physical action on that world. The infant moves from simple reflexes through several steps to an organized set of schemes. Significant concepts are developed, including space, time, and causality. Above all, during this period, the child develops the scheme of the permanent object.
2–7	Preoperational	Deferred imitation; symbolic play, graphic imagery (drawing); mental imagery; and language Egocentrism, rigidity of thought, semi-logical reasoning, and limited social cognition	Child no longer only makes perceptual and motor adjustment to objects and events. Child can now use symbols (mental images, words, gestures) to represent these objects and events; uses these symbols in an increasingly organized and logical fashion.
7–11	Concrete operations	Conservation of quantity, weight, volume, length, and time based on reversibility by inversion or reciprocity; operations: class inclusion and seriation	Conservation is the understanding of what values remain the same. For example, if liquid is poured from a short, wide glass into a tall, narrow one, the preoperational child thinks that the quantity has changed. For the concrete operation child, the amount stays the same.
11 through the end of adolescence	Formal operations	Combination system whereby variables are isolated and all combinations are examined; hypothetical–deductive thinking	Mental operations are applied to objects and events. The child classifies, orders, and reverses them. Hypotheses can be generated from these concrete operations.

preexisting inequality insofar as it is endorsed by adult authority (Orsholits et al., 2022; Paulus & Essler, 2020).

Carol Gilligan: Gender Differentiation in Moral Development

Carol Gilligan (b. 1936) argued that most development models are male centered and therefore inappropriate for girls and women. (Please note that Gilligan was doing research at a time when gender was considered binary instead of a continuum, as it is today.) She challenged Erik Erikson's (psychosocial development) and Kohlberg's (moral) theories as being biased against women because they are based on primarily privileged White men and boys. For Gilligan, attachment within relationships was the important factor for successful development. In developing identity, she said that whereas boys separate from the person who gave birth to them, girls attach, most likely learning to value relationships and becoming interdependent at an earlier age (Gilligan, 2004). She said girls learn to value the ideal of care, begin to respond to human needs, and want to take care of the world by sustaining attachments. Her model of moral development, *Ethic of Care*, is divided into three stages beginning with *preconventional* or selfishness (what is best for me) to *conventional* or responsibility to others (self-sacrifice is goodness) to *postconventional* or do not hurt others or self (she is a person too) (Gilligan, 2011).

Traditional models that advocate separation as the primary goal of human development immediately place women at a disadvantage. According to Gilligan (1982), negating the value and importance of attachments within relationships impairs the natural development of women. If Erikson's model is applied to women, their failure to separate then becomes defined as a developmental failure (Gilligan, 1982). She continues to challenge the traditions and conventional power relationships that exist in today's patriarchal society (Gilligan, 2020).

Applicability of Developmental Theories to Psychiatric–Mental Health Nursing

Developmental theories are one tool that can be used to help understand child and adolescent experiences and mood, and their manifestations as adult problems; however, their application is limited. Most of the models are based on the assumptions of the linear progression of stages, have not been adequately tested, and do not account for gender differences and diversity in lifestyles and cultures. Emerging research points to the importance of considering social inequities and their impact on health care access and delivery.

SOCIAL THEORIES

Numerous social theories underlie PMH nursing practice. Chapter 3 presents some of the sociocultural issues and discusses various social groups. This section represents a sampling of important social theories that a nurse uses. This discussion is not exhaustive and should be viewed by the student as including a few of the important social theoretic perspectives.

Family Dynamics

Family dynamics are the patterned interpersonal and social interactions that occur within the family structure over the life of a family. Family dynamics models are based on systems theory in which the change of one part affects the total functioning of the system. The family is viewed organizationally as an open system in which one member's actions influence the functioning of the total system. Family theories are especially useful to nurses who are assessing family dynamics and planning interventions. Family systems models are used to help nurses form collaborative relationships with patients and families dealing with health issue s. Generalist PMH nurses will not be engaged in family therapy. However, they will be caring for individuals and families. Understanding family dynamics is important in every nurse's practice.

Formal and Informal Social Support

Assisting patients in the recovery process means helping patients identify supportive family and community systems. **Formal support systems** are large organizations, such as hospitals and nursing homes that provide care to individuals. **Informal support systems** are family, friends, and neighbors. Individuals with strong informal support networks live longer than those without this type of support. Adolescents who are sexually assaulted are more likely to seek support from informal support systems than formal supports (Klein et al., 2024). Studies show that those without informal support who are socially isolated have significantly higher mortality rates (Wang et al., 2023).

An important concept is **social distance,** the degree to which the values of the formal organization and primary group members differ. In the United States, the most closely located, accessible, and available family member is expected to provide the care to a family member. Spouses are the first choice, then children, other family members, friends, and finally formal support. On the other hand, care-related stress can result in the informal caregiver changing the balance by placing a family member in an institution (Friedemann et al., 2014).

Formal and informal support systems are balanced when they are at a midpoint of social distance, that is, close enough to communicate but not so close to destroy each other—neither enmeshment nor isolation (Litwak et al., 1990; Messeri et al., 1993). Conflicts arise when the relationship becomes unbalanced. For example, if the primary group and the formal care system begin performing similar caregiving services, there may be disagreements. Balance is reestablished when the formal system increases the social distance by developing relationships and providing support to the caregiver and reducing contact with the patient. Thus, a balance is maintained between the two systems. In another instance, when a patient relies only on the health care provider for care and support (e.g., calls the nurse every day, visits the provider weekly, refuses any help from family), balance can be reestablished by linking the patient to an informal support system for help with some of the caregiving tasks.

By applying frameworks of formal and informal support systems to their patients, psychiatric nurses can understand the complex social forces that patients with mental disorders and their caregivers experience. This framework is useful in looking at domestic violence and sources of support (Gauthier et al., 2021). Nurses can help adjust the social distance between the formal and informal systems by identifying communication barriers and helping the two groups work together. For example, a patient misses an appointment because of a lack of transportation. The case manager helps the patient communicate the problem to the system to obtain another appointment. Informal caregivers are valued by the case manager, who recognizes the important services performed by family and friends. Thus, linkages between mental health providers (formal support) and the consumer network (informal support) are reinforced.

Role Theories

A role is a person's social position and function within an environment. Anthropologic theories explain members' roles that relate to a specific society. For example, the universal roles of healers may be assumed by a nurse in one culture and a spiritual leader in another. Societal expectations, social status, and rights are attached to these roles. Psychological theories, which are concerned about roles from a different perspective, focus on the relationship of an individual's role: the self. The responsibilities of a parent are often in conflict with the personal needs for time alone. All the neo-Freudian and humanist models that have been discussed focus on reciprocal social relationships or interactions that determine how the mind develops.

Role theories emphasize the importance of social interaction in either the individual's choice of a particular role or society's recognition of it. PMH nursing uses role concepts in understanding group interaction and the role of the patient in the family and community. In addition, milieu therapy approaches discussed in later chapters are based on the patient's assumption of a role within the psychiatric environment.

Sociocultural Perspectives

Margaret Mead: Culture and Gender

American anthropologist Margaret Mead (1901–1978) is widely known for her studies of primitive societies and her contributions to social anthropology. She conducted studies in New Guinea, Samoa, and Bali and devoted much of her studies to the patterns of child-rearing in various cultures. She was particularly interested in the cultural influences determining gender-related behavior (Mead, 1970). Influenced by Carl Jung and Erik Erikson, she had a vision of unity and diversity in the psychosocial development of a single human species (Sullivan, 2004). Although her research is often criticized as not having scientific rigor and containing misinterpretations, it is accepted as a classic in the field of anthropology (Sullivan, 2004). She established the importance of culture in determining human behavior.

Madeleine Leininger: Transcultural Health Care

Concern about the impact of culture on the treatment of children with psychiatric and emotional problems led Madeleine Leininger (1924–2012) to develop a new field, transcultural nursing, directed toward holistic, congruent, and beneficent care. Leininger developed the *Theory of Culture Care Diversity and Universality*, which explains diverse and universal dimensions of human caring (Fig. 6.2). Nursing care in different cultures varies because health, illness, and care are culturally defined

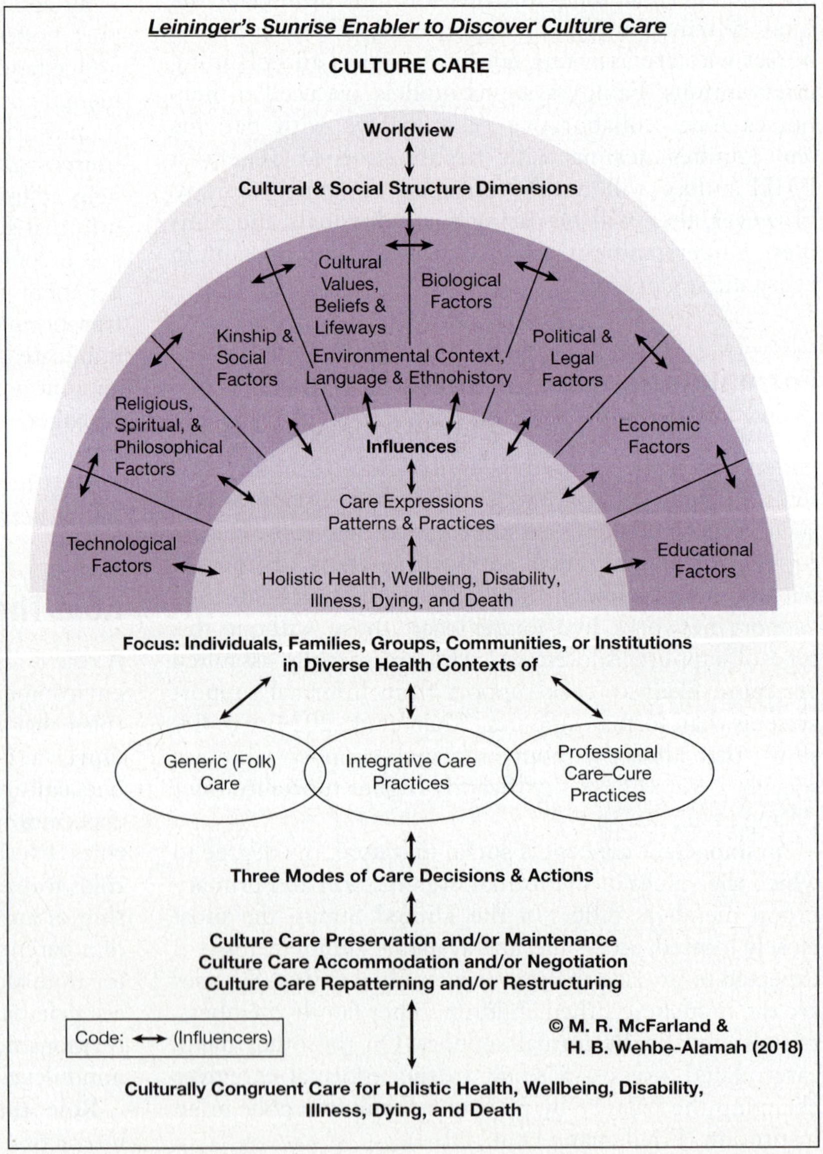

FIGURE 6.2 Leininger sunrise model to depict theory of cultural care diversity and universality. (Reprinted with permission from McFarland, M. R., & Wehbe-Alamah, H. B. (2018). *Transcultural nursing concepts, theories, research, & practice*. (4th ed.). McGraw-Hill Education.)

BOX 6.1

Research for Evidence-Based Practice: Cultural Perceptions of Healthy Eating in Mexican American Children

Ribar, A. K., Kilanowski, J. F., & Zoucha, R. (2021). The cultural perceptions of healthy eating in Mexican American children: A focused ethnography. Journal of Transcultural Nursing, *32(3), 221–229.*

THE QUESTION: What are the meanings and experiences associated with healthy eating from the perspective of Mexican American children?

METHODS: Using a focused ethnography, 21 midwestern children aged 11 to 13 years were interviewed in home and school settings. Leininger's four phases of qualitative data analysis were used.

FINDINGS: Two themes emerged. Mexican American children connect healthy eating with familiar foods in the context of their ethnic culture. Foods that provide feelings of happiness and well-being are associated with healthy eating.

IMPLICATIONS FOR NURSING: This study provides an understanding of the meaning and perceptions of healthy eating for Mexican American children.

(Leininger & McFarland, 2006). Leininger theory was developed with the goal of understanding these variations (Leininger, 2007). Leininger's model continues to be used today as a research framework. For example, the model was used to understand obesity in African American women (Omondi & Freysteinson, 2024), and the influence of culture on health beliefs and health behaviors of older adults (Nguyen et al., 2024), cultural care needs of Spanish-speaking parents (Stephen et al., 2023), and healthy eating in Mexican American children. See Box 6.1.

Applicability of Social Theories to Psychiatric–Mental Health Nursing

The use of social and sociocultural theories is especially important for PMH nurses. In any individual or family assessment, the sociocultural aspect is integral to mental health. It would be impossible to complete an adequate assessment without considering the role of the individual within the family and society. Interventions are based on the understanding and significance of family and cultural norms. It would be impossible to interact with the family in a meaningful way without an understanding of the family's cultural values. In the inpatient setting, the nurse is responsible for designing the social environment of the unit as well as ensuring that the patient is safe from harm. To accomplish this complex task, an understanding of the unit as a small social community helps the nurse use the environment in patient treatment (see Chapter 10). In addition, many group interventions are based on sociocultural theories.

SPIRITUAL CONCEPTS

The inclusion of spiritual concepts in the biopsychosocial approach is gaining support in mental health care (Van Denend et al., 2022). Patients want nurses to be sensitive to their spiritual or religious needs, which is a fundamental aspect of holistic nursing. Although the terms religion and spirituality are sometimes used interchangeably, in this text the terms are viewed as separate concepts. **Religion** denotes an organized set of beliefs, practices, ceremonies, and rituals associated with a specific community or group, whereas **spirituality** is "a dynamic and intrinsic aspect of humanity through which persons seek ultimate meaning, purpose, and transcendence and experience relationship to self, family, others, community, society, nature, and the significant or sacred. Spirituality is expressed through beliefs, values, traditions, and practices" (Puchalski et al., 2014). For more on spirituality, see Chapter 3.

Spiritual Interventions

Spiritual interventions help the patient find meaning, provide a nursing presence, and offer support. These interventions are important during periods of suffering, pain, and negative emotional experiences. Spiritual interventions can help alleviate suffering, improve hope, decrease depressive symptoms, and improve quality of life (de Diego-Cordero et al., 2022). The focus of spiritual interventions is on the patient's spiritual needs and creating a sense of well-being. It may mean referring a patient to a chaplain for in-depth religious and spiritual care. See Box 6.2.

Jean Watson: Theory of Transpersonal Caring

The theory of transpersonal caring was initiated by Jean Watson (b. 1940). Watson believes that caring is the foundation of nursing and recommends that specific theories of caring be developed in relation to specific human conditions and health and illness experiences (Watson, 2005, 2022). Her conceptualizations transcend conventional views of illness and focus on the meaning of health and quality of life (Watson, 2007). There are three foundational concepts of her theory:

BOX 6.2

Research for Evidence-Based Practice: Appalachian Older Adults' Health and Spiritual Engagement

Strange, K. E., Troutman-Jordan, M., & Mixer, S. J. (2023). Influence of spiritual engagement on Appalachian older adults' health: A systematic review. Journal of Psychosocial Nursing & Mental Health Services, 61*(5), 45–52. https://doi.org/10.3928/02793695-20221026-02*

THE QUESTION: Do many older adults in Appalachian culture use spiritual engagement to cope with health challenges?

METHODS: In this systematic review, 11 qualitative and 3 mixed-methods studies were analyzed using thematic synthesis (a technique that analyzes findings from multiple studies, typically by the coding of text line-by-line, then developing descriptive themes and generating analytical themes).

FINDINGS: Spiritual engagement positively impacts holistic health through adaptive coping, guided partnerships with God, decreased loneliness, and enhanced sense of purpose.

IMPLICATIONS FOR NURSING: Understanding the impact of spiritual engagement on older adults in Appalachia could help nurses reduce disparities and improve health outcomes; nurses could encourage spiritual engagement in patients, which in turn could help them cope with health issues, decrease loneliness, and develop a sense of purpose.

- Transpersonal Caring–Healing Relations: a relational process related to philosophic, moral, and spiritual foundation.
- 10 Caritas Processes: the original 10 Carative Factors have evolved into the 10 Caritas Processes (Box 6.3).
- Caritas Field: a field of consciousness created when the nurse focuses on love and caring as their way of being and consciously manifests a healing presence with others.

Watson's theory is especially applicable to the care of those who seek help for mental illness. This model emphasizes the importance of sensitivity to self and others; the development of helping and trusting relations; the promotion of interpersonal teaching and learning; and provision for a supportive, protective, and corrective mental, physical, sociocultural, and spiritual environment. Watson's caring science–based interventions have been shown to decrease patients' emotional strains; increase patients' self-management, confidence, and emotional well-being; increase nurses' job satisfaction and engagement; and improve nursing students' confidence in the conical performance and the awareness of caring behaviors (Holly et al., 2019). Watson's model was recently used as a beginning theoretical frame for understanding ICU nurses' experience of seeking increased spiritual development (Leone-Sheehan et al., 2024).

NURSING THEORIES

Nursing theories are useful to PMH nursing in conceptualizing the individual, family, or community and in planning nursing interventions (see Chapter 10). The use of a specific theory depends on the patient's situation. For example, in people with schizophrenia who have problems related to maintaining self-care, Dorothea Orem's theory of self-care is useful. By contrast, Hildegarde Peplau's theories are appropriate when a nurse is developing a relationship with a patient. Because of the wide range of possible problems requiring different approaches, familiarity with several nursing theories is essential.

Interpersonal Relations Models

Hildegarde Peplau: The Power of Empathy

Hildegarde Peplau (1909–1999) introduced the first systematic theoretic framework for psychiatric nursing and focused on the nurse–patient relationship in her 1952 book *Interpersonal Relations in Nursing* (Peplau, 1952). She led PMH nursing out of the confinement of custodial care into a theory-driven professional practice. One of her major contributions was the introduction of the nurse–patient relationship (see Chapter 9). See Box 6.4.

Peplau believed in the importance of the environment, defined as external factors considered essential to human development (Peplau, 1992): cultural forces, presence of adults, secure economic status of the family, and a healthy prenatal environment. Peplau emphasized the importance of empathic linkage.

KEYCONCEPT Empathic linkage is the ability to feel in oneself the feelings experienced by another person.

The interpersonal transmission of anxiety or panic is the most common empathic linkage. According to Peplau, other feelings, such as anger, disgust, and envy, can also be communicated nonverbally by way of empathic transmission to others. She believes that although the process is not yet understood, empathic communication occurs—that is, if nurses pay attention to what they feel during a relationship with a patient, they can gain invaluable observations of feelings a patient is experiencing and has not yet noticed or talked about.

BOX 6.3

Nursing: Human Science and Human Care Assumptions, and Factors in Care

ASSUMPTIONS

1. Caring can be effectively demonstrated and practiced only interpersonally.
2. Caring consists of factors that result in the satisfaction of certain human needs.
3. Effective caring promotes health and individual or family growth.
4. Caring responses accept a person not only as they are now but also as what they may become.
5. A caring environment offers the development of potential while allowing the person to choose the best action for themselves at a given point in time.
6. Caring is more "healthogenic" than is curing. It integrates biophysical knowledge with knowledge of human behavior to generate or promote health and provide ministrations to those who are ill. The science of caring is complementary to the science of curing.
7. The practice of caring is central to nursing.

10 CARITAS PROCESSES®

1. Embrace (*Loving-Kindness*)
   Sustaining humanistic-altruistic values by practice of loving-kindness, compassion, and equanimity with self/others.
2. Inspire (*Faith-Hope*)
   Being authentically present, enabling faith/hope/belief system; honoring subjective inner, life-world of self/others.
3. Trust (*Transpersonal*)
   Being sensitive to self and others by cultivating own spiritual practices; beyond ego-self to transpersonal presence.
4. Nurture (*Relationship*)
   Developing and sustaining loving, trusting-caring relationships.
5. Forgive (*All*)
   Allowing for expression of positive and negative feelings—authentically listening to another person's story.
6. Deepen (*Creative Self*)
   Creatively problem-solving-'solution-seeking' through caring process; full use of self and artistry of caring-healing practices via use of all ways of knowing/being/doing/becoming.
7. Balance (*Learning*)
   Engaging in transpersonal teaching and learning within context of caring relationship; staying within other's frame of reference-shift toward coaching model for expanded health/wellness.
8. Co-create (*Caritas Field*)
   Creating a healing environment at all levels; subtle environment for energetic authentic caring presence.
9. Minister (*Humanity*)
   Reverentially assisting with basic needs as sacred acts, touching mindbodyspirit of spirit of other; sustaining human dignity.
10. Open (*Infinity*)
   Opening to spiritual, mystery, unknowns—allowing for miracles.

---

10 Caritas Processes reprinted with permission from Jean Watson and Watson Caring Science Institute, International Caritas Consortium. (2021). *Dr. Jean Watson's human caring theory: 10 Caritas Processes®*. https://www.watsoncaring-science.org/jean-bio/caring-science-theory/10-caritas-processes/

Anxiety is a key concept for Peplau, who contends that professional practice is unsafe if this concept is not understood.

KEYCONCEPT Anxiety, according to Peplau, is an energy that arises when expectations that are present are not met.

If anxiety is not recognized, it continues to rise and escalates toward panic. There are various levels of anxiety, each having its observable behavioral cues (Box 6.5). These cues are sometimes called *defensive*, but Peplau argues that they are often "relief behaviors." For example, some people may relieve their anxiety by yelling and swearing; others seek relief by withdrawing. In both instances, anxiety was generated by an unmet security need.

NCLEXNOTE Peplau's model of anxiety continues to be an important concept in psychiatric nursing. Severe anxiety interferes with learning. Mild anxiety is useful for learning.

The **self-system** is another important concept in Peplau's model. Drawing from Sullivan, Peplau defined the self as an "anti-anxiety system" and a product of socialization. The self proceeds through personal development that is always open to revision but tends toward stability. For example, in parent–child relationships, patterns of parental approval, disapproval, and indifference are used by children to define themselves. If the verbal and nonverbal messages have been derogatory, children incorporate these messages and view themselves negatively.

The concept of need is important to Peplau's model. Needs are primarily of biologic origin but need to be met within a sociocultural environment. When a biologic need is present, it gives rise to tension that is reduced and relieved by behaviors meeting that need. According to Peplau, nurses should recognize and support the patients' patterns and style of meeting their health care needs.

Ida Jean Orlando: Theory of Effective Nursing Practice

In 1954, Ida Jean Orlando (1926–2007) studied the factors that enhanced or impeded the integration of mental health principles in the basic nursing curriculum. From this study, she published *The Dynamic Nurse–Patient Relationship* to offer nursing students a theory of effective nursing practice. She studied nursing care of patients on medical–surgical units, not people with psychiatric issues in mental hospitals. Orlando identified three areas of nursing concern: the nurse–patient relationship, the nurse's professional role, and the identity and development of knowledge that is distinctly nursing (Orlando, 1961). A nursing situation involves the behavior of the patient, the reaction of the nurse, and anything that does not relieve the distress of the patient. Patient distress is related to the inability of the individual to meet or communicate their own needs (Orlando, 1961, 1972).

BOX 6.4

Research for Evidence-Based Practice: Patient Outcomes of the Nurse–Patient Relationship

Desmet, K., Bracke, P., Deproost, E., Goossens, P. J. J., Vandewalle, J., Vercruysse, L., Beeckman, D., Van, H. A., Kinnaer, L., & Verhaeghe, S. (2023). Patient-reported outcomes of the nurse–patient relationship in psychiatric inpatient hospitals: A multicentred descriptive cross-sectional study. Journal of Psychiatric & Mental Health Nursing, 30*(3), 568–579. https://doi.org/10.1111/jpm.12895*

THE QUESTION: Are there measurable patient outcomes related to the implementation of the nurse–patient relationship?

METHODS: In a multicenter cross-sectional study, patients (*N* = 296) admitted to one of 30 psychiatric units in five participating hospitals for at least 2 weeks were asked to complete questions about their most "meaningful" nurse–patient relationship, and an instrument (Mental Health Nurse-Sensitive Patient Outcome-Scale [MH-NURSE-POS], a six-point Likert scale) measured changes that the patient perceived occurred because of the nurse–patient interaction. The MH-NURSE-POS measured four domains: *growth* (sense of self), *expression* (attunement, mentalization, and coping with personal emotions and/or problems), *control* (self-control in risk-taking, building and establishing safe and meaningful contacts), and *motivation* (personal motivation to change). A primary care nursing model was usually used, with one primary nurse assigned to a patient. The primary nurse was responsible for shared decision-making, assessing, planning, organizing and evaluating care, and delegating planned care to unit nurses. Patients interacted with primary and unit nurses.

FINDINGS: Of the 296 participants, 241 had a primary nurse. Of those with a primary nurse, 83% (*N* = 200), defined their relationship with the primary nurse as the most meaningful nurse–patient relationship during hospitalization. Survey results indicated positive changes occurred in all four domains, with the most changes occurring in motivation to stay committed to treatment (4.97 SD = 1.22) and the least changes occurring in control in risk taking (3.71, SD = 1.49).

IMPLICATIONS FOR NURSING: These findings support the importance of the nurse–patient relationship because it promotes positive, measurable changes in patients.

Orlando helped nurses focus on the whole patient rather than on the disease or institutional demands. Her ideas continue to be useful today and guide nursing care. She was an early advocate of the use of the nursing process, with an emphasis on critical thinking and evidence-based practice (Toney-Butler & Thayer, 2023). Orlando's model has been used in many settings, including intensive care units (Fahmi et al., 2022). Orlando's theory is also proposed as a model for reinforcing the use of the nursing process in the practice setting (Areri et al., 2024).

Existential and Humanistic Theoretical Perspectives

Rosemarie Rizzo Parse: Humanbecoming Theory

The ***Humanbecoming Theory*** views humans as indivisible, unpredictable, ever-changing coauthors and experts about their lives (Parse, 1998, 2007). Three major themes underlie this theory: meaning (personal meaning to the situation), rhythmicity (the paradoxical patterning of the human–universe mutual processes—the ups and downs of life), and transcendence (power and originating of transforming) (Parse, 1996, 1998, 2008). The postulates involved in living a human life are ***illuminating*** (unbound knowing extended to infinity), ***paradox*** (intricate rhythm expressed as a pattern preference), ***freedom*** (liberation), and ***mystery*** (unexplainable) (Parse, 2007).

The theory was expanded to address the ethos of humanbecoming with the core knowings of living quality. The four tenets of humanbecoming are *reverence* (solemn regard for humanuniverse presence), *awe* (beholding the unexplainable of humanuniverse existence), *betrayal* (the violation of humanuniverse trust), and *shame* (humiliation with dishonoring humanuniverse worth) (Parse, 2018).

As one of the more abstract nursing theories, *humanbecoming* can be used in understanding patients' life experiences and connecting psychologically with a patient. This theory has been widely studied in nursing and adds qualitative dimension to understanding the patient's human experience. For example, one of the studies explores freedom from a humanbecoming perspective (Bunkers, 2020). Parse's theory is recommended as an alternative to the medical approach for a grieving family who has experienced a pregnancy loss, still birth, or neonatal death. The theory of humanbecoming focuses on quality of life as experienced and the meaning of the experience as perceived by the parents (Wilson, 2016) and community (Ortiz, 2021).

BOX 6.5

Levels of Anxiety

Mild: awareness heightens
Moderate: awareness narrows
Severe: focused, narrow awareness
Panic: unable to function

Systems Models

Imogene M. King: Theory of Goal Attainment

The theory of goal attainment developed by Imogene King (1923–2007) is based on a systems model that includes three interacting systems: personal, interpersonal, and social. In this model, human beings interact with the environment, and the individual's perceptions influence reactions and interactions. Nursing involves caring for the human being, with the goal of health defined as adjusting to the stressors in both internal and external environments (King, 2007). She defines nursing as a "process of human interactions between nurse and patient whereby each perceives the other and the situation; and through communication, they set goals, explore means, and agree on means to achieve goals" (King, 1981, p. 144). This model focuses on the process that occurs between a nurse and a patient. The process is initiated to help the patient cope with a health issue that compromises their ability to maintain social roles, functions, and activities of daily living (King, 1992).

In this model, the person is goal oriented and purposeful, reacting to stressors, and is viewed as an open system interacting with the environment. The variables in nursing situations are as follows:

- Geographic place of the transacting system, such as the hospital
- Perceptions of the nurse and patient
- Communications of the nurse and patient
- Expectations of the nurse and patient
- Mutual goals of the nurse and patient
- The nurse and patient as a system of interdependent roles in a nursing situation (King, 1981, p. 88)

The quality of nurse–patient interactions may have positive or negative influences on the promotion of health in any nursing situation. It is within this interpersonal system of nurse and patient that the healing process is performed. Interaction is depicted in which the outcome is a **transaction**, defined as the transfer of value between two or more people. This behavior is unique, based on experience, and is goal directed.

King's work reflects her understanding of the systematic process of theory development. Her model continues to be used in exploring inherent systematic health care inequities affecting Black communities (Flynn & Graham-O'Gilvie, 2022).

Betty Neuman: Systems Approach

Betty Neuman (1924–2022) used a systems approach as a model of nursing care. Neuman wanted to extend care beyond an illness model, incorporating concepts of problem finding and prevention and behavioral science concepts, and environmental approaches to wellness. Neuman developed her framework in the late 1960s as chairwoman of the University of California at Los Angeles graduate nursing program. The key components of the model are a client system (physiologic, psychological, sociocultural, developmental, spiritual) interacting with the environment. The wholistic model can be applied to prevention and treatment.

Neuman was one of the first psychiatric nurses to include the concept of stressors in understanding nursing care. The Neuman systems model is applied to practice and educational settings, including community health, care of patients with cancer, children with medically complex illnesses, stroke patients, palliative care, and mental health nursing of older adults (Böger et al., 2022; Choi & Kim, 2022; Domingues Sousa et al., 2022; Van Orne, 2024).

Dorothea Orem: Focus on Self-Care

Self-care is the focus of the general theory of nursing initiated by Dorothea Orem (1914–2007) in the early 1960s. The Self-Care Deficit Nursing Theory consists of three separate parts: a theory of self-care, theory of self-care deficit, and theory of nursing systems (Biggs, 2008; Orem, 2001; Orem & Taylor, 2011). The theory of self-care defines the term as activities performed independently by an individual to promote and maintain personal well-being throughout life. The central focus of Orem's theory is the self-care deficit theory, which describes how people can be helped by nursing. Nurses can help meet self-care requisites through five approaches: acting or doing for, guiding, teaching, supporting, and providing an environment to promote the patient's ability to meet current or future demands. The nursing systems theory refers to a series of actions a nurse takes to meet the patient's self-care requisites. This system varies from the patient being totally dependent on the nurse for care to needing only some education and support.

Orem's model is used in nursing because of its emphasis on promoting independence of the individual and on self-care activities (Kennel et al., 2024; Khoramabad & Khoramabad, 2022). Although many psychiatric disorders have an underlying problem, such as motivation, these problems are generally manifested as difficulties conducting ordinary self-care activities (e.g., personal hygiene) or developing independent thinking skills.

Other Nursing Theories

Other nursing models that are applied in psychiatric settings include Martha Rogers' model of unitary human beings and Calista Roy's adaptation model. Discussion of these models is beyond the scope of this textbook.

SUMMARY OF KEY POINTS

- The traditional psychodynamic framework helped form the basis of early nursing interpersonal interventions, including the development of therapeutic relationships and the use of such concepts as transference, countertransference, empathy, and object relations.

- The behavioral theories are often used in strategies that help patients change behavior and thinking.
- Sociocultural theories remain important in understanding and interacting with patients as members of families and cultures.
- Nursing theories form the conceptual basis for nursing practice and are useful in a variety of PMH settings.

DEVELOPING CLINICAL JUDGMENT

1. Identify the similarities and differences among Freud's ideas and those of the neo-Freudians, including Jung, Adler, Horney, and Sullivan.
2. Hypothesize how the basic ideas of psychodynamic and behavioral theories have influenced mental health nursing.
3. What is the difference between classical conditioning from operant conditioning? How are they applied in nursing?
4. Hypothesize how Erikson and Piaget influence nursing. Are their models evidence based?
5. Define formal and informal support systems. How does the concept of social distance relate to these two systems?
6. Using Watson's theory of transpersonal caring, give an example of a patient who would benefit from this approach.
7. A patient admitted to the emergency room is hearing voices that others do not hear. They do not have a place to stay and have not eaten for a day. What psychosocial–spiritual theory is best applied to this situation?
8. A patient is experiencing depression with sadness, frequent crying, and expressing hopelessness about their current marital situation. Using a cognitive-behavioral approach, develop a brief intervention plan with the patient.

MOVIES, TV, OR STREAMING PROGRAMS

***An Angel at My Table:* 1990.** This three-part television mini-series tells the story of Janet Frame, New Zealand's premiere novelist and poet. Based on her autobiography, the film portrays Frame as a shy, awkward child who experiences a family tragedy that alienates her socially. She studies in England to be a teacher, but her shyness and social ineptness cause extreme anxiety. Seeking mental health care, she receives a misdiagnosis of schizophrenia and spends 8 years in a mental institution. This movie shows the inhumane treatment of patients in a mental asylum. She barely escapes a lobotomy when she is notified of a literary award. She then begins to develop friendships and a new life.

Viewing Points:

1. What are the significant events of Janet Frame's childhood that would impact her development and her adult life?
2. Does Janet "fit" any of the models that are discussed in this chapter?
3. Consider Janet's life in light of Gilligan's theory that it is important for women to have a sense of connection.
4. How did the hospitalization negatively affect Janet's mental health?

Unfolding Patient Stories: Randy Adams • Part 1

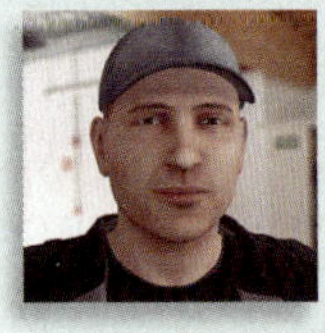

Randy Adams, a 28-year-old veteran exposed to bomb blasts during combat in the Middle East, has symptoms of posttraumatic stress disorder (PTSD) and neurocognitive symptoms. How could cognitive-behavioral and social theories be applied to his condition? How could an understanding of psychosocial theories assist the nurse in selecting suitable interventions to promote psychological and social functioning? (Randy Adams' story continues in Chapter 14.)

Care for Randy Adams and other patients in a realistic virtual environment: ***vSim** for Nursing* (thepoint.lww.com/vSimMentalHealth). Practice documenting these patients' care in DocuCare (thepoint.lww.com/DocuCareEHR).

Unfolding Patient Stories: Linda Waterfall • Part 1

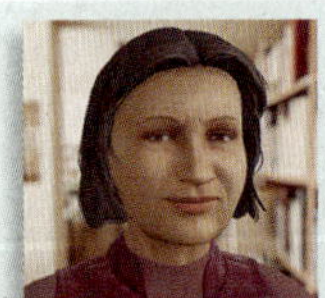

Linda Waterfall, age 48, was recently diagnosed with an aggressive form of breast cancer and is in the hospital for a mastectomy. She is Native American, and she initially refused her family's request for her to meet with tribal healers about the surgery. Her anxiety escalates, and when she realizes she forgot her medicine bundle at home, she is now reconsidering meeting with tribal healers. She is refusing the preoperative medication, lorazepam. What ethical principles will help to guide the nurse in the care of Linda in this situation? What values and beliefs of a nurse might conflict with Linda's? How might the nurse reconcile the conflicts in these values and beliefs? How does understanding the patient's values influence the nurse's response to Linda's beliefs and inform ethical decision-making? (Linda Waterfall's story continues in Chapter 27.)

Care for Linda Waterfall and other patients in a realistic virtual environment: ***vSim** for Nursing* (thepoint.lww.com/vSimMentalHealth). Practice documenting these patients' care in DocuCare (thepoint.lww.com/DocuCareEHR).

REFERENCES

Areri, H. A., Getie, H., Guta, A., & Simegn, B. (2024). Exploring the experience of nurses on nursing process implementation in northwest Ethiopia: a qualitative study. *Nursing: Research & Reviews*, *14*, 81–89. https://doi.org/10.2147/NRR.S449968

Bandura, A. (1977). *Social learning theory*. Prentice-Hall.

Bandura, A. (1986). *Social foundations of thought and action: A social-cognitive theory*. Prentice Hall.

Bandura, A. (1993). Perceived self-efficacy in cognitive development and function. *Educational Psychologist*, *28*(2), 117–148.

Bandura, A. (2001). Social cognitive theory: an agentic perspective. *Annual Review of Psychology*, *52*, 1–26.

Beck, J. S. (2021). *Cognitive behavior therapy: Basics and beyond* (3rd ed.). Guilford Press.

Biggs, A. (2008). Orem's self-care deficit nursing theory: update on the state of the art and science. *Nursing Science Quarterly*, *21*(3), 200–206.

Böger, R., dos Reis Bellaguarda, M. L., da Silva Knihs, N., Manfrini, G. C., Martins da Rosa, L., dos Santos, M. J., & Alonso Caravaca-Morera, J. (2022). Palliative professionals: stressors imposed on the team in the death and dying process. *Texto & Contexto Enfermagem*, *31*, 1–15. https://doi.org/10.1590/1980-265X-TCE-2021-0401en

Bunkers, S. S. (2020). Freedom and humanbecoming. *Nursing Science Quarterly*, *33*(1), 7–11.

Chen, P. Y., Ho, W. C., Lo, C., & Yeh, T. P. (2021). Predicting ego integrity using prior ego development stages for older adults in the community. *International Journal of Environmental Research and Public Health*, *18*(18), 9490. https://doi.org/10.3390/ijerph18189490

Choi, E. J., & Kim, H. Y. (2022). Relationship between multidimensional stressors and quality of life in people with stroke. *Nursing & Health Sciences*, *24*(3), 764–773. https://doi.org/10.1111/nhs.12976

Christiansen, S. L., & Palkovitz, R. (1998). Exploring Erikson's psychosocial theory and development: generativity and its relationship to paternal identity, intimacy, and involvement in childcare. *The Journal of Men's Studies*, 7(1), 133–156.

Corradi, R. B. (2024). Psychoanalytic contributions to psychodynamic psychiatry and psychotherapy: Erik Erikson's psychosocial developmental theory. *Psychodynamic Psychiatry*, *52*(1), 18–24. https://doi.org/10.1521/pdps.2024.52.1.18

de Diego-Cordero, R., Suárez-Reina, P., Badanta, B., Lucchetti, G., & Vega-Escaño, J. (2022). The efficacy of religious and spiritual interventions in nursing care to promote mental, physical and spiritual health: a systematic review and meta-analysis. *Applied Nursing Research*, *67*, 151618. https://doi.org/10.1016/j.apnr.2022.151618

Domingues Sousa, A. F., Simões Marques Santos, D. G., Baptista Costeira, C. R., da Silva Reis dos Santos Ferreira, M. M., & Lopes de Freitas Lomba, M. de L. (2022). Experiencing parental cancer: a case study with application of Neuman's Model. *Texto & Contexto Enfermagem*, *31*, 1–12. https://doi.org/10.1590/1980-265X-TCE-2022-0201en

Egana-delSol, P., Sun, X., & Sajda, P. (2023). Neurophysiological markers of emotion regulation predict efficacy of entrepreneurship education. *Scientific Reports*, *13*(1), 7206. https://doi.org/10.1038/s41598-023-34148-1

Erikson, E. (1963). *Childhood and society* (2nd ed.). W. W. Norton & Company.

Erikson, E. (1968). *Identity: Youth and crisis*. W. W. Norton & Company.

Fahmi, I., Nurachmah, E., Dianingtyas, H. E., Kamal, M., & Ganefianty, A. (2022). Application of breathing exercises using Ida Jean Orlando's dynamic nurse-patient relationship model in overcoming postoperative hypoxia (POH) after coronary artery bypass grafting: a case-series. *Nurse Media Journal of Nursing*, *12*(2), 249–257. https://doi.org/10.14710/nmjn.v12i2.45394

Fleury, M. J., Grenier, G., Sabetti, J., Bertrand, K., Clément, M., & Brochu, S. (2021). Met and unmet needs of homeless individuals at different stages of housing reintegration: a mixed-method investigation. *PLoS One*, *16*(1), e0245088. https://doi.org/10.1371/journal.pone.0245088

Flynn, C., & Graham-O'Gilvie, A. (2022). Breastfeeding disparities among communities lacking access to lactation consultants during the COVID-19 pandemic: a theory-guided paper. *Journal of the New York State Nurses Association*, *49*(1), 5–10.

Freud, S. (1905). Three essays on the theory of sexuality. In J. Strachey, A. Freud, A. Strachey & A. Tyson (Eds.), *The standard edition of the complete psychological works of Sigmund Freud* (pp. 135–248). Hogarth Press.

Freud, S. (1927). The ego and the id. In E. Jones (Ed.), *The international psychoanalytical library* (No. 12). Hogarth Press.

Friedemann, M. L., Newman, F. L., Buckwalter, K. C., & Montgomery, R. J. V. (2014). Resource need and use of multiethnic caregivers of elders in their homes. *Journal of Advanced Nursing*, *70*(3), 662–673.

Fromm-Reichmann, F. (1950). *Principles of intensive psychotherapy*. University of Chicago Press.

Gauthier, G. R., Francisco, S. C., Khan, B., & Dombrowski, K. (2021). Social integration and domestic violence support in an indigenous community: women's recommendations of formal versus informal sources of support. *Journal of Interpersonal Violence*, *36*(7–8), 3117–3141.

Gilligan, C. (1982). *In a different voice*. Harvard University Press.

Gilligan, C. (2004). Recovering psyche: reflections on life-history and history. *Annual of Psychoanalysis*, *32*, 131–147.

Gilligan, C. (2011). *Joining the resistance*. Polity Press.

Gilligan, C. (2020). Disrupting the story: enter Eve. *Journal of the American Psychoanalytic Association*, *68*(4), 675–693.

Holly, W., Fazzone, P. A., Sitzman, K., & Hardin, S. R. (2019). The current intervention studies based on Watson's Theory of Human Caring: a systematic review. *International Journal for Human Caring*, *23*(1), 4–22.

Horney, K. (1939). *New ways in psychoanalysis*. W. W. Norton & Company.

Jung, C. (1966). On the psychology of the unconscious. The personal and the collective unconscious. In C. Jung (Ed.), *Collected works of C. G. Jung* (2nd ed., Vol. 7, pp. 64–79). Princeton University Press.

Kennel, K. D., Barrett, T., Brown, S. J., & Tucker, J. (2024). Self-care in nursing education. *Journal of Nursing Education*, *63*(6), 394–398. https://doi.org/10.3928/01484834-20240404-08

Khoramabad, N. N. (2022). Implementation of Orem's self-care model in early stages of breast cancer. *Indian Journal of Cancer*, *59*(1), 142–143. https://doi.org/10.4103/ijc.IJC_1115_20

King, I. M. (1981). *A theory for nursing: Systems, concepts, process*. Wiley.

King, I. M. (1992). King's theory of goal attainment. *Nursing Science Quarterly*, *5*(1), 19–26.

King, I. M. (2007). King's conceptual system, theory of goal attainment, and transaction process in the 21st century. *Nursing Science Quarterly*, *20*(2), 109–111.

Klein, M. (1963). *Our adult world and other essays*. Heinemann Medical Books.

Klein, L. B., Melnik, J., Curran, K., Luebke, J., Moore, K. M., Ruiz, A. M., Brown, C., Parker, D., Hernandez-White, I., & Walsh, K. (2024). Trauma- and violence-informed empowering care for sexual assault survivors. *Journal of Forensic Nursing*, *20*(3):166–173. https://doi.org/10.1097/JFN.0000000000000483

Kuchenbaur, M., & Peter, R. (2021). Assessing the role of collective efficacy beliefs during participative occupational health interventions. *Frontiers in Public Health*, *9*, 797838. https://doi.org/10.3389/fpubh.2021.797838

Leininger, M. (2007). Theoretical questions and concerns: Response from the theory of culture care diversity and universality perspective. *Nursing Science Quarterly*, *20*(1), 9–13.

Leininger, M., & McFarland, M. (2006). *Cultural care diversity and universality theory. A theory of nursing* (2nd ed.). Jones & Bartlett Publishers.

Leone-Sheehan, D., Flanagan, J., & Willis, D. (2024). Intensive care unit nurses' experience of Watson's Theory of Human Caring Caritas Process III: developing spiritual self to provide spiritual nursing care. *Advances in Nursing Science*, *47*(1):59–72. https://doi.org/10.1097/ANS.0000000000000489

Litwak, E., Messeri, P., & Silverstein, M. (1990). The role of formal and informal groups in providing help to older people. *Marriage and Family Review*, *15*(1–2), 171–193.

Maas Genannt Bermpohl, F., Hülsmann, L., & Martin, A. (2023). Efficacy of mindfulness- and acceptance-based cognitive-behavioral therapies for bodily distress in adults: a meta-analysis. *Frontiers in Psychiatry*, *14*, 1160908. https://doi.org/10.3389/fpsyt.2023.1160908

Maslow, A. (1970). *Motivation and personality* (rev. ed.). Harper & Brothers.

Mead, M. (1970). *Culture and commitment: A study of the generation gap*. Natural History Press/Doubleday & Co.

Messeri, P., Silverstein, M., & Litwak, E. (1993). Choosing optimal support groups: a review and reformulation. *Journal of Health and Social Behavior*, *34*(2), 122–137.

Nguyen, T. N. M., Saunders, R., Dermody, G., & Whitehead, L. (2024). The influence of culture on the health beliefs and health behaviours of older Vietnam-born Australians living with chronic disease. *Journal of Advanced Nursing*, *80*(9), 3781–3796. https://doi.org/10.1111/jan.16283

Nusser, L., Zimprich, D., & Wolf, T. (2023). Themes of trust, identity, intimacy, and generativity in important autobiographical memories: associations with life periods and life satisfaction. *Journal of Personality*, *91*(5), 1110–1122. https://doi.org/10.1111/jopy.12786

Ochse, R., & Plug, C. (1986). Cross-cultural investigation of the validity of Erikson's theory of personality development. *Journal of Personality and Social Psychology*, *50*(6), 1240–1252.

Omondi, H., & Freysteinson, W. (2024). Understanding obesity in African American women using Leininger's theory. *Nursing Science Quarterly*, *37*(1), 71–75. https://doi.org/10.1177/08943184231207383

Orem, D. (2001). *Nursing concepts of practice* (6th ed.). Mosby.

Orem, D. E., & Taylor, S. G. (2011). Reflections on nursing practice science: the nature, the structure, and the foundation of nursing sciences. *Nursing Science Quarterly*, *24*(1), 35–41.

Orlando, I. J. (1961). *The dynamic nurse–patient relationship*. G. P. Putnam's Sons.

Orlando, I. J. (1972). *The discipline and teaching of nursing process*. G. P. Putnam's Sons.

Orlofsky, J. L., Marcia, J. E., & Lesser, I. M. (1973). Ego identity status and the intimacy versus isolation crisis of young adulthood. *Journal of Personality and Social Psychology*, *27*(2), 211–219.

Orsholits, D., Cullati, S., Cheval, B., Ghisletta, P., Oris, M., Maurer, J., Studer, M., Marques, A., Marconcin, P., Gouveia, É. R., Kliegel, M., & Ihle, A. (2022). Residential trajectories across the life course and their association with cognitive functioning in later life. *Scientific Reports*, *12*(1), 17004. https://doi.org/10.1038/s41598-022-18501-41–76

Ortiz, M. R. (2021). Community change concepts and health policy implications. *Nursing Science Quarterly*, *34*(1), 88–92.

Ozer E. M. (2022). Albert Bandura (1925-2021). *The American Psychologist*, 77(3), 483–484. https://doi.org/10.1037/amp0000981.

Parse, R. R. (1996). Reality: a seamless symphony of becoming. *Nursing Science Quarterly*, *9*(4), 181–184. https://doi.org/10.1177/089431849600900411

Parse, R. R. (1998). *The humanbecoming school of thoughts: A perspective for nurses and other health professionals*. Sage.

Parse, R. R. (2007). The humanbecoming school of thought in 2050. *Nursing Science Quarterly*, *20*(4), 308–311.

Parse, R. R. (2008). The humanbecoming leading-following model. *Nursing Science Quarterly*, *21*(4), 369–375.

Parse, R. R. (2018). Dignity: the ethos of humanbecoming. *Nursing Science Quarterly*, *31*(3), 259–262.

Paul R. A. (2023). Identity and community: Erikson reconsidered. *The Psychoanalytic Quarterly*, *92*(3), 377–405. https://doi.org/10.1080/00332828.2023.2267527

Paulus, M., & Essler, S. (2020). Why do preschoolers perpetuate inequalities? Theoretical perspectives on inequity preferences in the face of emerging concerns for equality. *Developmental Review*, *58*, 100933. https://doi.org/10.1016/j.dr.2020.100933

Pavlov, I. P. (1927/1960). *Conditioned reflexes: An investigation of the physiological activity of the cerebral cortex*. Dover Publications.

Peplau, H. (1952). *Interpersonal relations in nursing: Conceptual frame of reference for psychodynamic nursing*. G. Putnam & Sons.

Peplau, H. E. (1992). Interpersonal relations: a theoretical framework for application in nursing practice. *Nursing Science Quarterly*, *5*(1), 13–18.

Puchalski, C. M., Vitillo, R., Hull, S. K., & Reller, N. (2014). Improving the spiritual dimension of whole person care: reaching national and international consensus. *Journal of Palliative Medicine*, *17*(6), 642–656. https://doi.org/10.1089/jpm.2014.9427

Rivera, K. M., & Doom, J. R. (2023). The role of neighborhood collective efficacy in moderating associations between adversity and internalizing and externalizing problems in adolescents. *Journal of Community Psychology*, *51*(4), 1736–1755. https://doi.org/10.1002/jcop.22956

Rogers, C. (1980). *A way of being*. Houghton Mifflin.

Sharma, N. P., & Spiro, P. M. (2023). Psychoanalytic Therapy. In *StatPearls*. StatPearls Publishing. NCBI Bookshelf. https://www.ncbi.nlm.nih.gov/books/NBK592398/

Skinner, B. F. (1935). The generic nature of the concepts of stimulus and response. *Journal of General Psychology*, *12*, 40–65.

Stephen, J. M., Zoucha, R., Cazzell, M., & Devido, J. (2023). Cultural care needs of Spanish speaking parents with limited English proficiency whose children are hospitalized: an ethnonursing study. *Journal of Pediatric Nursing*, *69*, 62–70. https://doi.org/10.1016/j.pedn.2022.12.019

Sullivan, H. (1953). *The interpersonal theory of psychiatry*. W. W. Norton & Company.

Sullivan, G. (2004). A four-fold humanity: Margaret Mead and psychological types. *Journal of the History of the Behavioral Sciences*, *40*(2), 183–206.

Thorndike, E. L. (1906). *The principles of teaching, based on psychology*. A.G. Seiler.

Tomoi, K. (2024). Death attitudes among middle-aged and older adults in Japan: a qualitative study based on Erikson's theory of generativity. *Omega (Westport)*, *90*(2), 536–553. https://doi.org/10.1177/00302228221108296

Toney-Butler, T. J., & Thayer, J. M. (2023). Nursing process. In *StatPearls*. StatPearls Publishing. Nursing Process. https://www.ncbi.nlm.nih.gov/books/NBK499937/

Van Denend, J., Ford, K., Berg, P., Edens, E. L., & Cooke, J. (2022). The body, the mind, and the spirit: Including the spiritual area in mental health care. *Journal of Religion & Health*, *61*(5), 3571–3588. https://doi.org.libproxy.siue.edu/10.1007/s10943-022-01609-2

Van Orne, J. A. (2024). Improving transitions in care for the child with medical complexity using Betty Neuman's Systems Model. *Nursing Science Quarterly*, *37*(2), 142–147. https://doi.org/10.1177/08943184231224471

Wang, F., Gao, Y., Han, Z., Yu, Y., Long, Z., Jiang, X., Wu, Y., Pei, B., Cao, Y., Ye, J., Wang, M., & Zhao, Y. (2023). A systematic review and meta-analysis of 90 cohort studies of social isolation, loneliness and mortality. *Nature Human Behaviour*, 7(8), 1307–1319. https://doi.org/10.1038/s41562-023-01617-6

Watson, J. (2005). *Caring science as sacred science*. F. A. Davis.

Watson, J. (2007). Theoretical questions and concerns: Response from a caring science framework. *Nursing Science Quarterly*, *20*(1), 13–15.

Watson, J. (2022). Revisiting *'Discipline'* in relation to caring science as sacred science: revisiting *Discipline* of nursing. *Journal of Holistic Nursing*, *40*(1), 58–63. https://doi.org/10.1177/08980101211041187

Watson, J. B., & Rayner, R. (2000). Conditioned emotional reactions. 1920. *American Psychologist*, *55*(3), 313–317.

Wienicke, F. J., Beutel, M. E., Zwerenz, R., Brähler, E., Fonagy, P., Luyten, P., Constantinou, M., Barber, J. P., McCarthy, K. S., Solomonov, N., Cooper, P. J., De Pascalis, L., Johansson, R., Andersson, G., Lemma, A., Town, J. M., Abbass, A. A., Ajilchi, B., Connolly Gibbons, M. B., … Driessen, E. (2023). Efficacy and moderators of short-term psychodynamic psychotherapy for depression: A systematic review and meta-analysis of individual participant data. *Clinical Psychology Review*, *101*, 102269. https://doi.org/10.1016/j.cpr.2023.102269

Wilson, D. R. (2016). Parse's nursing theory and its application to families experiencing empty arms. *International Journal of Childbirth Education*, *31*(2), 29–33.

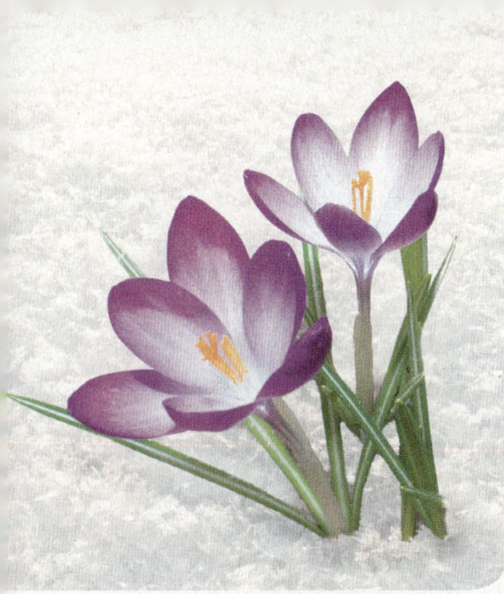

7 Biologic Foundations of Psychiatric Nursing

Mary Ann Boyd

KEYCONCEPTS

- neuroplasticity
- neurotransmitters

LEARNING OBJECTIVES

After studying this chapter, you will be able to:

1. Describe the association between biologic functioning and symptoms of psychiatric disorders.
2. Locate brain structures primarily involved in psychiatric disorders and describe the primary functions of these structures.
3. Describe basic mechanisms of neuronal transmission.
4. Identify the location and function of neurotransmitters significant to hypotheses regarding major mental disorders.
5. Discuss the role of genetics in the development of psychiatric disorders.
6. Discuss the basic utilization of new knowledge gained from fields of study, including psychoneuroimmunology and chronobiology.

KEY TERMS

• acetylcholine • amino acids • autonomic nervous system • basal ganglia • biogenic amines • biologic markers • brain stem • cerebellum • chronobiology • circadian cycle • cortex • dopamine • enteric nervous system • epigenetics • extrapyramidal motor system • frontal, parietal, temporal, and occipital lobes • functional imaging • GABA • genetic susceptibility • glutamate • gut–brain axis • gut microbiota • hippocampus • histamine • hypothalamus–pituitary–thyroid axis • limbic system • locus coeruleus • neurocircuitry • neurohormones • neuromodulators • neurons • neuropeptides • norepinephrine • phenotype • pineal body • population genetics • prefrontal cortex • proband • psychoneuroimmunology • receptors • serotonin • structural imaging • synaptic cleft • zeitgebers

INTRODUCTION

All behavior recognized as human results from actions that originate in the brain and its amazing interconnection of neural networks. Modern research has increased understanding of how the complex circuitry of the brain interacts with the external environment, memories, and experiences. Through the spinal column and peripheral nerves, along with other systems, such as the endocrine and immune systems, the brain constantly receives and processes information. As the brain shifts and sorts through the amazing amount of information it processes every hour, it decides on actions and initiates behaviors, allowing each person to act in entirely unique and very human ways.

Mental disorders cannot be traced to specific physiologic problems but rather are complex syndromes consisting of symptoms that more or less cluster together. Therefore, it is important for the nurse to understand basic nervous system functioning, as well as some of the research that is exploring the biologic basis of mental disorders.

This chapter reviews the basic information necessary for understanding the neuroscience that underlies the connection among (1) psychiatric symptoms, (2) the probable alterations in brain functioning linked to those symptoms, and (3) the rationale for treatment and care practices. It reviews basic central nervous system (CNS) structures and functions, the peripheral nervous system (PNS), general functions of the major neurotransmitters and receptors, basic principles of neurotransmission, genetic models, circadian rhythms, and biologic tests. It is not intended as a full presentation of neuroanatomy and physiology. The chapter assumes that the reader has a basic knowledge of human biology, anatomy, and pathophysiology.

NEUROANATOMY OF THE CENTRAL NERVOUS SYSTEM

Although this section discusses functioning areas of the brain separately, each area is intricately connected with the others, and each functions interactively. The CNS contains the brain, **brain stem**, and spinal cord, and the PNS consists of the **neurons** that connect the CNS to the muscles, organs, and other systems in the periphery of the body. Whatever affects the CNS may also affect the PNS and vice versa.

Cerebrum

The largest region of the human brain, the cerebrum, fills the entire upper portion of the cranium. The **cortex**, or the outermost surface of the cerebrum, makes up about 80% of the human brain. The cortex is four to six cellular layers thick, and each layer is composed of cell bodies mixed with capillary blood vessels. This mixture makes the cortex gray brown (thus the term *gray matter*). The cortex consists of numerous bumps and grooves in a fully developed adult brain, as shown in Figure 7.1. This "wrinkling" allows for a large amount of surface area to be confined in the limited space of the skull. The increased surface area allows for more potential connections among cells within the cortex. The grooves are called *fissures* if they extend deep into the brain and *sulci* if they are shallower. The bumps or convolutions are called *gyri*. Together they provide many of the landmarks for the subdivisions of the cortex. The longest and deepest groove, the longitudinal fissure, separates the cerebrum into left and right hemispheres. Although these two divisions are nearly symmetric, there is some variation in the location and size of the sulci and gyri in each hemisphere. Substantial variation in these convolutions is found in the cortex of different individuals.

Left and Right Hemispheres

The cerebrum can be roughly divided into two halves, or hemispheres. The left hemisphere is dominant in about 95% of people, but about 5% of individuals have mixed dominance. Each hemisphere controls functioning mainly on the opposite side of the body. Aside from controlling activities on the left side of the body, the right hemisphere also provides input into receptive nonverbal communication, spatial orientation and recognition, intonation of speech and aspects of music, facial recognition and facial expression of emotion, and nonverbal learning and memory. In general, the left hemisphere is more involved with verbal language function, including areas for both

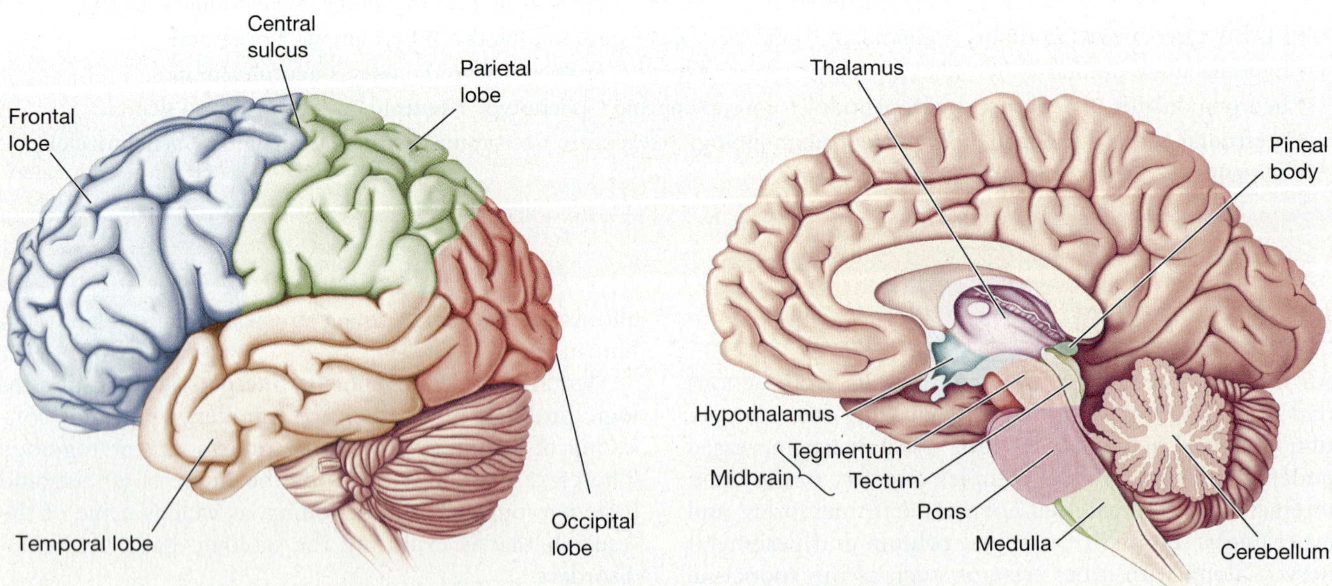

FIGURE 7.1 Lateral and medial surfaces of the brain. **Left:** The left lateral surface of the brain. **Right:** The medial surface of the right half of a sagittally hemisected brain. (Reprinted with permission from Bear, M. F., Conners, B. W., & Paradiso, M. A. [2016]. Neuroscience: Exploring the brain [4th ed.]. Wolters Kluwer.)

receptive and expressive speech control, and provides strong contributions to temporal order and sequencing, numeric symbols, and verbal learning and memory.

The two hemispheres are connected by the corpus callosum, a bundle of neuronal tissue that allows information to be exchanged quickly between the right and left hemispheres. An intact corpus callosum is required for the hemispheres to function in a smooth and coordinated manner.

Lobes of the Brain

The lateral surface of each hemisphere is further divided into four lobes: the **frontal, parietal, temporal, and occipital lobes** (Fig. 7.1). The lobes work in coordinated ways, but each is responsible for specific functions. An understanding of these unique functions clarifies how damage to these areas produces the symptoms of mental illness and how medications that affect the functioning of these lobes can produce certain effects.

Frontal Lobes

The right and left frontal lobes make up about one-fourth of the entire cerebral cortex and are proportionately larger in humans than in any other mammal. The frontal lobe has several functional areas. The **precentral gyrus**, the gyrus immediately anterior to the central sulcus, contains the primary motor area, or homunculi. Damage to this gyrus or to the anterior neighboring gyri causes spastic paralysis in the opposite side of the body. The frontal lobe also contains **Broca area**, which controls the motor function of speech. Damage to Broca area produces expressive aphasia or difficulty with the motor movements required for speech. The **prefrontal cortex** lies in the very front of the brain and is responsible for higher-level cognitive function including decision-making, problem solving, intelligence, and emotion regulation. It has also been associated with social skills and personality of human.

Insight, judgment, reasoning, concept formation, problem-solving skills, abstraction, and self-evaluation are all abilities that are modulated and affected by the actions of the frontal lobes. These skills are often referred to as *executive functions* because they modulate more primitive impulses through numerous connections to other areas of the cerebrum.

When frontal lobe functioning is altered, executive functioning is decreased, and modulation of impulses can be lost, leading to changes in mood and personality. The importance of the frontal lobe and its role in the development of symptoms common to psychiatric disorders are emphasized in later chapters that discuss disorders such as schizophrenia, attention-deficit hyperactivity disorder, and dementia. Box 7.1 describes how altered frontal lobe function can affect mood and personality.

BOX 7.1

Frontal Lobe Syndrome

In the 1860s, Phineas Gage became a famous example of frontal lobe dysfunction. Mr. Gage was a New England railroad worker who had a thick iron-tamping rod propelled through his frontal lobes by an explosion. He survived but suffered significant changes in his personality. Mr. Gage, who had previously been a capable and calm supervisor, began to show impatience, labile mood, disrespect for others, and frequent use of profanity after his injury (Harlow, 1869). Similar conditions are often called *frontal lobe syndrome*. Symptoms vary widely from individual to individual. In general, after damage to the dorsolateral (upper and outer) areas of the frontal lobes, the symptoms include a lack of drive and spontaneity. With damage to the most anterior aspects of the frontal lobes, the symptoms tend to involve more changes in mood and affect, such as impulsive and inappropriate behavior.

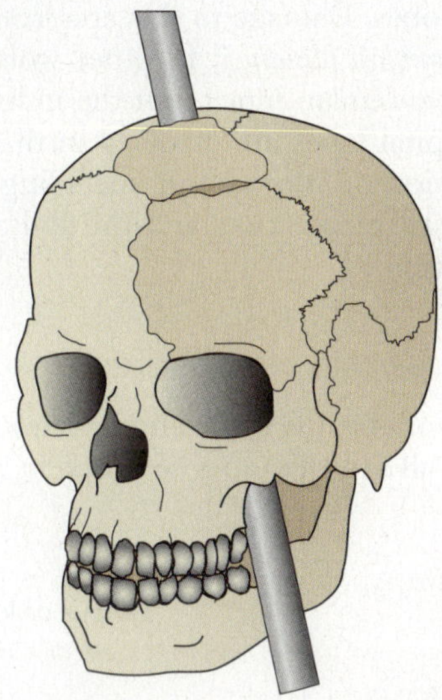

The skull of Phineas Gage, showing the route the tamping rod took through his skull. The angle of entry of the rod shot it behind the left eye and through the front part of the brain, sparing regions that are directly concerned with vital functions like breathing and heartbeat.

Parietal Lobes

The postcentral gyrus, immediately behind the central sulcus, contains the primary somatosensory area. Damage to this area and neighboring gyri results in deficits in discriminative sensory function but not in the ability to perceive sensory input. The posterior areas of the parietal lobe appear to coordinate visual and somatosensory information. Damage to this area produces complex sensory deficits, including neglect of contralateral sensory stimuli and spatial relationships. The parietal lobes contribute to the ability to recognize objects by touch, calculate, write, recognize fingers of the opposite hands, draw, and organize spatial directions (e.g., how to travel to familiar places).

Temporal Lobes

The temporal lobes contain the primary auditory and olfactory areas. Wernicke area, located at the posterior aspect of the superior temporal gyrus, is primarily responsible for receptive speech. The temporal lobes also integrate sensory and visual information involved in control of written and verbal language skills as well as visual recognition. The hippocampus, an important structure discussed later, lies in the internal aspects of each temporal lobe and contributes to memory. Other internal structures of this lobe are involved in the modulation of mood and emotion.

Occipital Lobes

The primary visual area is in the most posterior aspect of the occipital lobes. Damage to this area results in a condition called *cortical blindness*. In other words, the retina and optic nerve remain intact, but the individual cannot see. The occipital lobes are involved in many aspects of visual integration of information, including color vision, object and facial recognition, and the ability to perceive objects in motion.

Association Cortex

Although not a lobe, the association cortex is an important area that allows the lobes to work in an integrated manner. Areas of one lobe of the cortex often share functions with an area of the adjacent lobe. When these neighboring nerve fibers are related to the same sensory modality, they are often referred to as *association areas*. For example, an area in the inferior parietal, posterior temporal, and anterior occipital lobes integrates visual, somatosensory, and auditory information to provide the abilities required for basic academic skills. These areas, along with numerous connections beneath the cortex, are part of the mechanisms that allow the human brain to work as an integrated whole.

Subcortical Structures

Beneath the cortex are layers of tissue composed of the axons of cell bodies. The axonal tissue forms pathways that are surrounded by glia, a fatty or lipid substance, which has a white appearance and gives these layers of neuron axons their name—white matter. Structures inside the hemispheres, beneath the cortex, are considered subcortical. Many of these structures, essential in the regulation of emotions and behaviors, play important roles in our understanding of mental disorders. Figure 7.2 provides a coronal section view of the gray matter, white matter, and important subcortical structures.

The **basal ganglia** are subcortical gray matter areas in both the right and left hemispheres that contain many cell bodies or nuclei. The primary subdivisions

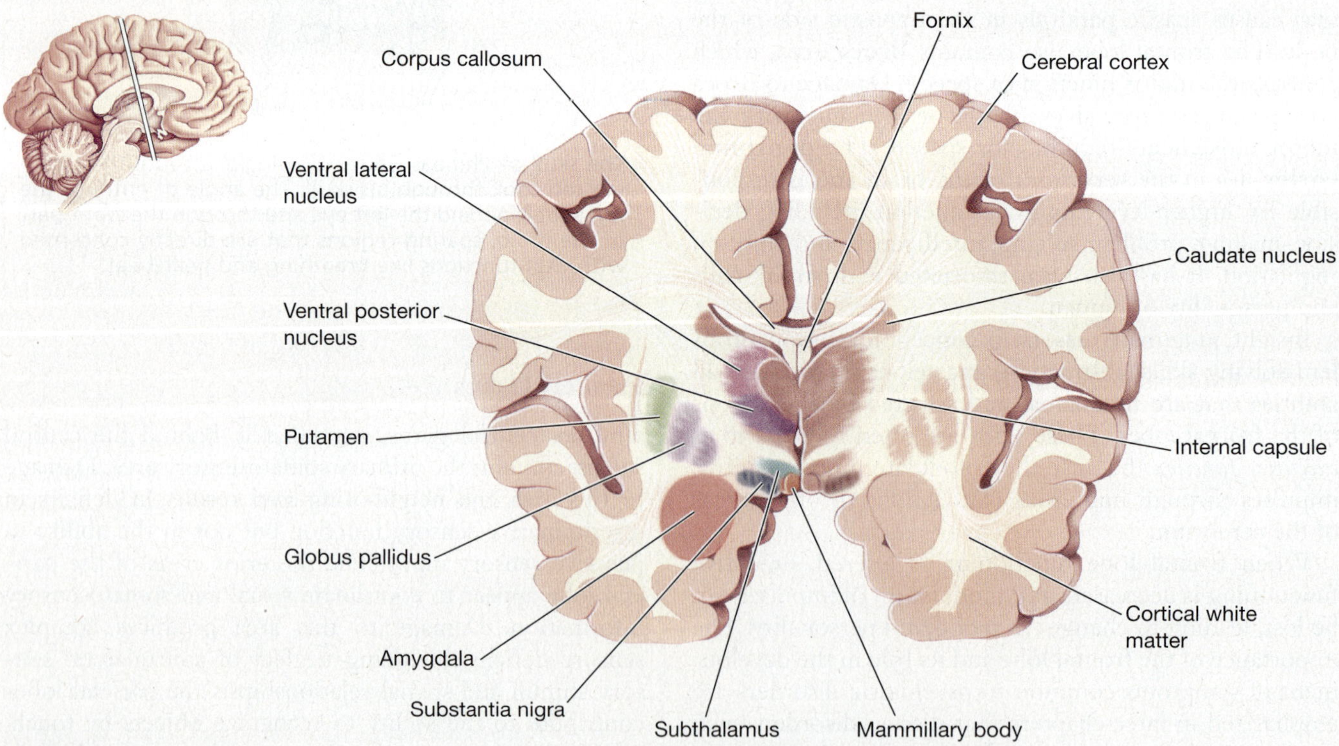

FIGURE 7.2 Coronal section of the brain, illustrating the corpus callosum, basal ganglia, and lateral ventricles. (Reprinted with permission from Bear, M. F., Conners, B. W., & Paradiso, M. A. [2016]. *Neuroscience: Exploring the brain* [4th ed.]. Wolters Kluwer.)

of the basal ganglia are the putamen, globus pallidus, and caudate. The basal ganglia are involved with motor functions and the learning and the programming of behavior or activities that are repetitive and, done over time, become automatic. The basal ganglia have many connections with the cerebral cortex, thalamus, midbrain structures, and spinal cord. Damage to portions of these nuclei may produce changes in posture or muscle tone. In addition, damage may produce atypical movements, such as twitches or tremors. The basal ganglia can be adversely affected by some of the medications used to treat psychiatric disorders, leading to side effects and other motor-related problems.

Limbic System

The **limbic system** is essential to understand the many hypotheses related to psychiatric disorders and emotional behavior in general. The limbic system is called a "system" because it comprises several small structures that work in a highly organized way. These structures include the hippocampus, thalamus, hypothalamus, amygdala, and limbic midbrain nuclei. See Figure 7.3 for identification and location of the structures within the limbic system and their relationships to other common CNS structures.

Basic emotions, needs, drives, and instincts begin and are modulated in the limbic system. Hate, love, anger, aggression, and caring are basic emotions that originate within the limbic system. Not only does the limbic system function as the seat of emotions, but because emotions are often generated based on our personal experiences, the limbic system is also involved with aspects of memory. Hypothesized changes in the limbic system play a significant role in many theories of major mental disorders, including schizophrenia, depression, and anxiety disorders (discussed in later chapters).

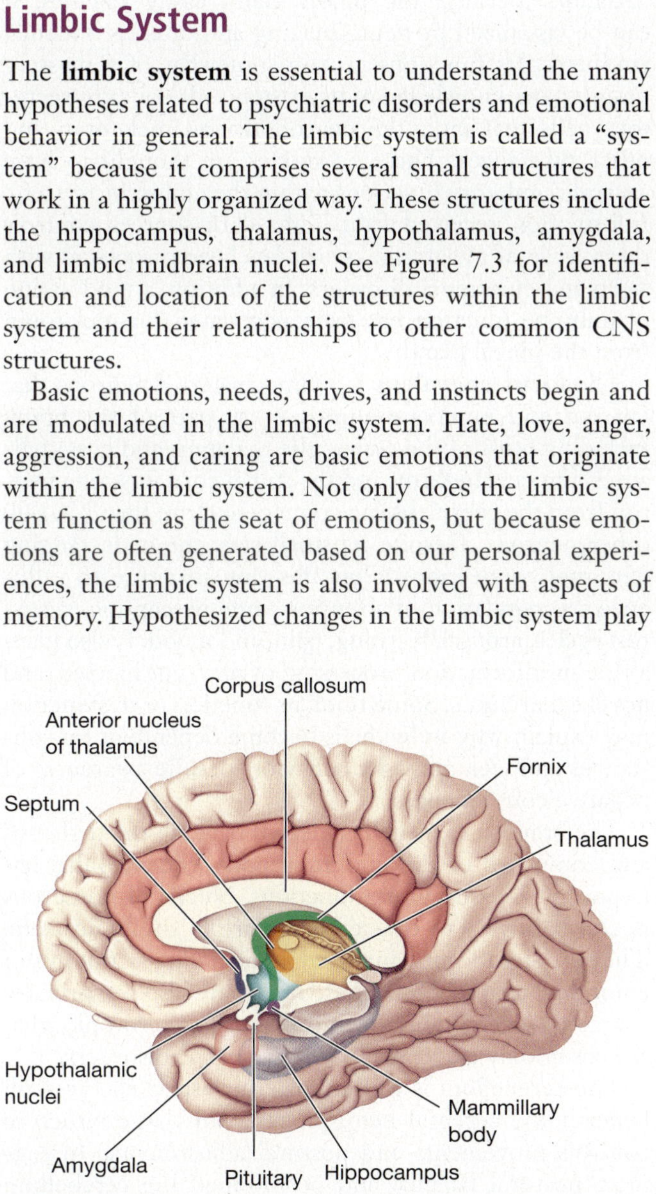

FIGURE 7.3 The structures of the limbic system are integrally involved in memory and emotional behavior. Theories link changes in the limbic system to many major mental disorders, including schizophrenia, depression, and anxiety disorders.

Hippocampus

The **hippocampus** is involved in storing information, especially the emotions attached to a memory. Our emotional responses to memories and our associations with other related memories are functions of how information is stored within the hippocampus. Although memory storage is not limited to one area of the brain, destruction of the left hippocampus impairs verbal memory and damage to the right hippocampus results in difficulty with recognition and recall of complex visual and auditory patterns. Deterioration of the nerves of the hippocampus and other related temporal lobe structures found in Alzheimer disease produces the disorder's hallmark symptoms of memory dysfunction.

Thalamus

Sometimes called the "relay-switching center of the brain," the thalamus functions as a regulatory structure to relay all sensory information, except smell, sent to the CNS from the PNS. From the thalamus, the sensory information is relayed mostly to the cerebral cortex. The thalamus relays and regulates by filtering incoming information and determining what to pass on or not pass on to the cortex. In this fashion, the thalamus prevents the cortex from becoming overloaded with sensory stimulus. The thalamus is thought to play a part in controlling electrical activity in the cortex. Because of its primary relay function, damage to a very small area of the thalamus may produce deficits in many cortical functions, thus causing behavioral anomalies.

Hypothalamus

Basic human activities, such as sleep–rest patterns, body temperature, and physical drives such as hunger and sex, are regulated by another part of the limbic system that rests deep within the brain and is called the hypothalamus. Dysfunction of this structure, whether from disorders or because of an adverse effect of drugs used to treat mental illness, produces common psychiatric symptoms, such as appetite and sleep problems.

Nerve cells within the hypothalamus secrete hormones, for example, antidiuretic hormone, which, when sent to the kidneys, accelerates the reabsorption of water; and oxytocin, which acts on smooth muscles to promote contractions, particularly within the walls of the uterus. Because cells within the nervous system produce these hormones, they are often referred to as **neurohormones** (hormones that are produced by cells within the nervous system) and form a communication mechanism through the bloodstream to control organs that are not directly connected to nervous system structures.

The pituitary gland, often called the *master gland*, is directly connected by thousands of neurons that attach it to the ventral aspects of the hypothalamus. Together with the pituitary gland, the hypothalamus functions as one of the primary regulators of many aspects of the endocrine system. Its functions are involved in control of visceral activities, such as body temperature, arterial blood pressure, hunger, thirst, fluid balance, gastric motility, and gastric secretions. Deregulation of the hypothalamus can be manifested in symptoms of certain psychiatric disorders. For example, in schizophrenia, patients often wear heavy coats during the hot summer months and do not appear hot. Before the role of the hypothalamus in schizophrenia was understood, psychological reasons were used to explain such symptoms. Now it is increasingly clear that such a symptom relates to deregulation of the hypothalamus' usual role in temperature regulation and is a biologically based symptom (Rogers et al., 2024).

Amygdala

The amygdala is directly connected to more primitive centers of the brain involving the sense of smell. It has numerous connections to the hypothalamus and lies adjacent to the hippocampus. The amygdala provides an emotional component to memory and is involved in modulating aggression and sexuality. Impulsive acts of aggression and violence have been linked to dysregulation of the amygdala, and erratic firing of the nerve cells in the amygdala is a focus of investigation in bipolar mood disorders (see Chapter 26).

Limbic Midbrain Nuclei

The limbic midbrain nuclei are a collection of neurons (including the ventral tegmental area and the locus coeruleus) that appear to play a role in the biologic basis of dependency. Sometimes referred to as the pleasure center or reward center of the brain, the limbic midbrain nuclei function to chemically reinforce certain behaviors, ensuring their repetition. Emotions such as feeling satisfied with good food, the pleasure of nurturing young, and the enjoyment of sexual activity originate in the limbic midbrain nuclei. The reinforcement of activities such as nutrition, procreation, and nurturing young are all primitive aspects of ensuring the survival of a species. When functioning in atypical ways, the limbic midbrain nuclei can begin to reinforce unhealthy or risky behaviors, such as drug misuse. Exploration of this area of the brain is in its infancy but offers potential insight into dependencies and their treatment.

Other Central Nervous System Structures

The **extrapyramidal motor system** is a bundle of nerve fibers connecting the thalamus to the basal ganglia and cerebral cortex. Muscle tone, common reflexes, and automatic voluntary motor functioning (e.g., walking) are controlled by this nerve track. Dysfunction of this motor track can produce hypertonicity in muscle groups. In Parkinson disease, the cells that compose the extrapyramidal motor system are severely affected, producing many involuntary motor movements. Several medications, which are discussed in Chapter 11, also affect this system.

The **pineal body** is located above and medial to the thalamus. Because the pineal gland easily calcifies, it can be visualized by neuroimaging and often is a medial landmark. Its functions remain somewhat of a mystery despite long knowledge of its existence. It contains secretory cells that emit the neurohormone melatonin and other substances. These hormones are thought to have several regulatory functions within the endocrine system. Information received from light–dark sources controls the release of melatonin, which has been associated with sleep and emotional disorders. In addition, a modulation of immune function has been postulated for melatonin from the pineal gland.

The **locus coeruleus** is a tiny cluster of neurons that fan out and innervate almost every part of the brain, including most of the cortex, the thalamus and hypothalamus, the **cerebellum**, and the spinal cord. Just one neuron from the coeruleus can connect to more than 250,000 other neurons. Despite its small size, the wide-ranging neuronal connections allow this tiny structure to influence the regulation of attention, time perception, sleep–rest cycles, arousal, learning, pain, and mood. It also plays a role in information processing of new, unexpected, and novel experiences. Some think its function or dysfunction may explain why individuals become dependent on substances and seek out risky behaviors despite awareness of negative consequences.

The brain stem, which is located beneath the thalamus and composed of the midbrain, pons, and medulla, has important life-sustaining functions. Nuclei of numerous neural pathways to the cerebrum are in the brain stem. They are significantly involved in mediating symptoms of emotional dysfunction. These nuclei are also the primary source of several neurochemicals, such as serotonin, that are commonly associated with psychiatric disorders.

The cerebellum is in the posterior aspect of the skull beneath the cerebral hemispheres. This large structure controls movements and postural adjustments. To regulate postural balance and positioning, the cerebellum receives information from all parts of the body, including the muscles, joints, skin, and visceral organs, as well as from many parts of the CNS.

Autonomic Nervous System

Closely associated with the spinal cord but not lying entirely within its column is the **autonomic nervous system (ANS)**, a subdivision of the PNS. It was originally given this name for being independent of conscious thought, that is, automatic. However, it does not necessarily function as autonomously as the name indicates. This system contains efferent (nerves moving away from the CNS), or motor system neurons, which affect target tissues such as cardiac muscle, smooth muscle, and the glands. It also contains afferent nerves, which are sensory and conduct information from these organs back to the CNS.

The autonomic nervous system is further divided into the sympathetic and parasympathetic nervous systems. These systems, although peripheral, are included here because they are involved in the emergency, or "fight-or-flight," response as well as the peripheral actions of many medications (see Chapter 11). Figure 7.4 illustrates the innervations of various target organs by the autonomic nervous system. Table 7.1 identifies the actions of the sympathetic and parasympathetic nervous systems on various target organs.

TABLE 7.1 PERIPHERAL ORGAN RESPONSE IN THE AUTONOMIC NERVOUS SYSTEM

Effector Organ	Sympathetic Response (Mostly Norepinephrine)	Parasympathetic Response (Acetylcholine)
Eye		
• Iris sphincter muscle	Dilation	Constriction
• Ciliary muscle	Relaxation	Accommodation for near vision
Heart		
• Sinoatrial node	Increased rate	Decrease in rate
• Atria	Increased contractility	Decrease in contractility
• Atrioventricular node	Increased contractility	Decrease in conduction velocity
Blood Vessels	Constriction	Dilation
Lungs		
• Bronchial muscles	Relaxation	Bronchoconstriction
• Bronchial glands		Secretion
Gastrointestinal Tract		
• Motility and tone	Relaxation	Increased
• Sphincters	Contraction	Relaxation
• Secretion		Stimulation
Urinary Bladder		
• Detrusor muscle	Relaxation	Contraction
• Trigone and sphincter	Contraction	Relaxation
Uterus	Contraction (pregnant) Relaxation (nonpregnant)	Variable
Skin		
• Pilomotor muscles	Contraction	No effect
• Sweat glands	Increased secretion	No effect
Glands		
• Salivary, lachrymal		Increased secretion
• Sweat		Increased secretion

NEUROPHYSIOLOGY OF THE CENTRAL NERVOUS SYSTEM

At their most basic level, the human brain and connecting nervous system are composed of billions of cells. Most are connective and supportive glial cells with ancillary functions in the nervous system.

> **KEYCONCEPT Neuroplasticity** is a continuous process of modulation of neuronal structure and function in response to the changing environment.

The changes in neural environment can come from internal sources, such as a change in electrolytes, or from external sources, such as a virus or toxin. Because of neuroplasticity, nerve signals may be rerouted, cells may learn new functions, the sensitivity or number of cells may increase or decrease, and some nerve tissue may undergo limited regeneration. Brains are mostly plastic during infancy and young childhood, when large adaptive learning tasks typically occur. With age, brains become less plastic, which explains why it is easier to learn a second language at the age of 5 years than 55 years. Neuroplasticity contributes to understanding how function may be restored over time after brain damage occurs, or how an individual may react over time to continuous pharmacotherapy regimens.

Neurons and Nerve Impulses

In the human body, approximately 10 billion nerve cells, or neurons, function to receive, organize, and transmit information (Fig. 7.5). Each neuron has a cell body, or soma, which holds the nucleus containing most of the cell's genetic information. The soma also includes other organelles, such as ribosomes and endoplasmic reticulum, which carry out protein synthesis; the Golgi apparatus, which contains enzymes to modify the proteins for specific functions; vesicles, which transport and store proteins; and lysosomes, which are responsible for

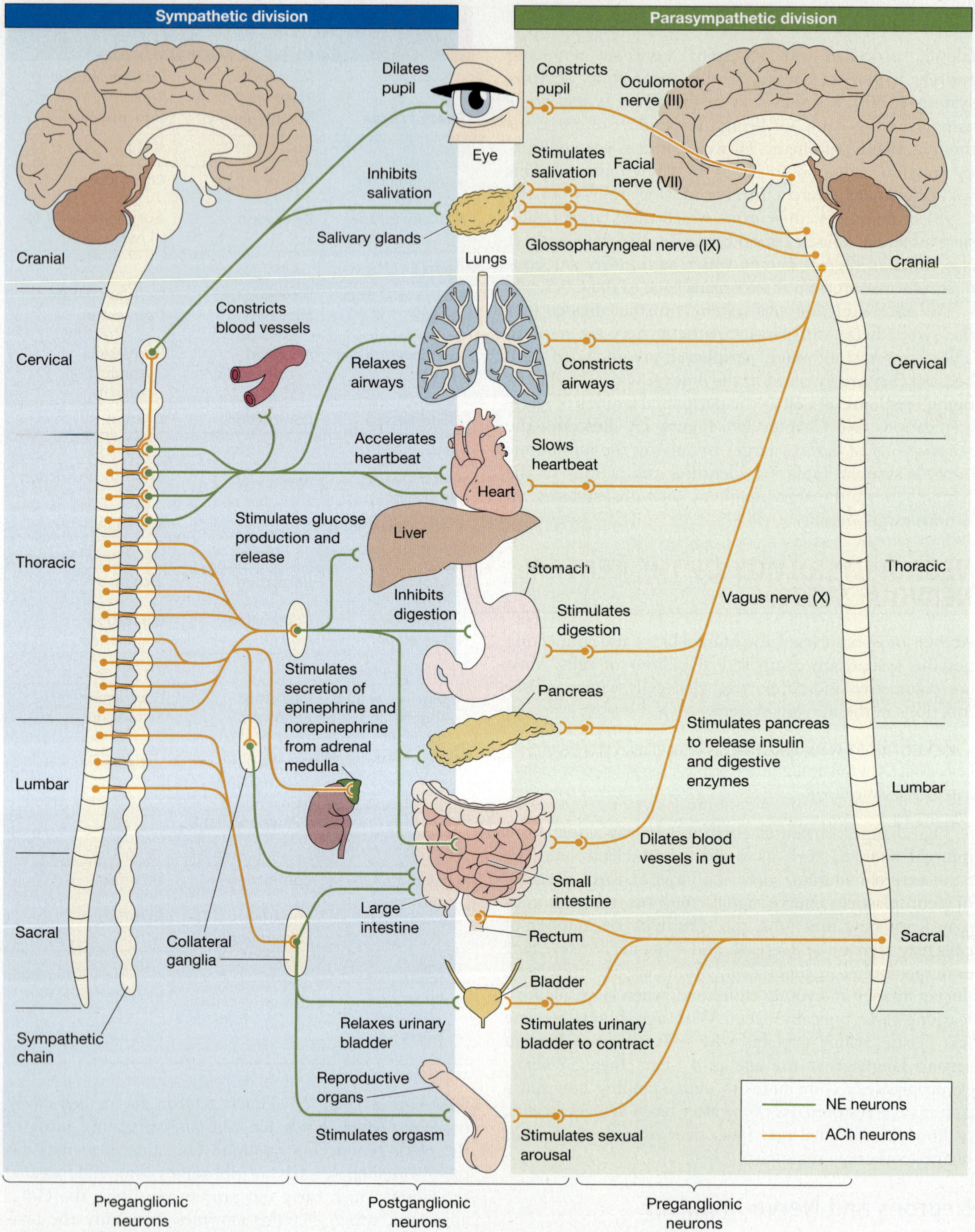

FIGURE 7.4 Diagram of the autonomic nervous system. Note that many organs are innervated by both sympathetic and parasympathetic nerves. ACh, acetylcholine; NE, norepinephrine. (Reprinted with permission from Bear, M. F., Conners, B. W., & Paradiso, M. A. [2016]. *Neuroscience: Exploring the brain* [4th ed.]. Wolters Kluwer.)

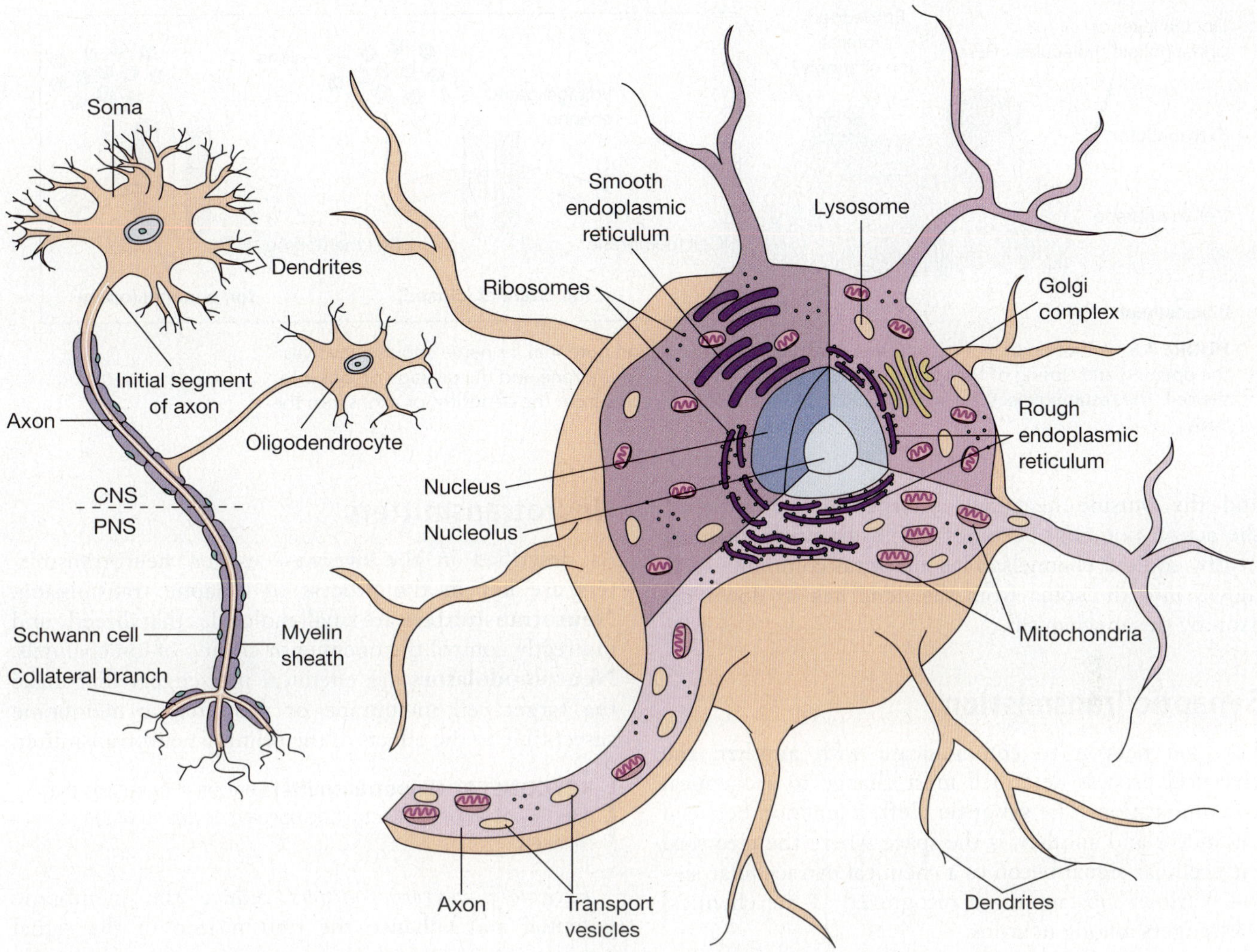

FIGURE 7.5 Cell body and organelles of neuron. CNS, central nervous system; PNS, peripheral nervous system.

degradation of these proteins. Located throughout the neurons, mitochondria, containing enzymes and often called the "powerhouse," are the sites of many energy-producing chemical reactions. These cell structures provide the basis for secreting numerous chemicals by which neurons communicate.

It is not just the vast number of neurons that accounts for the complexities of the brain but also the enormous number of neurochemical interconnections and interactions among neurons. A single motor neuron in the spinal cord may receive signals from more than 10,000 sources of interconnections with other nerves. Although most neurons have only one axon, which varies in length and conducts impulses away from the soma, each has numerous dendrites, receiving signals from other neurons. Because axons may branch as they terminate, they also have multiple contacts with other neurons.

Nerve signals are prompted to fire by a variety of chemical or physical stimuli. This firing produces an electrical impulse. The cell's membrane is a double layer of phospholipid molecules with embedded proteins. Some of these proteins provide water-filled channels through which inorganic ions may pass (Fig. 7.6). Each of the common ions—sodium, potassium, calcium, and chloride—has its own specific molecular channel. Many of these channels are voltage gated and thus open or close in response to changes in the electrical potential across the membrane. At rest, the cell membrane is polarized with a positive charge on the outside and about a 270 mV charge on the inside, owing to the resting distribution of sodium and potassium ions. As potassium passively diffuses across the membrane, the sodium pump uses energy to move sodium from the inside of the cell against a concentration gradient to maintain this distribution. An action potential, or *nerve impulse,* is generated as the membrane is depolarized and a threshold value is reached, which triggers the opening of the voltage-gated sodium channels, allowing sodium to surge into the cell. The inside of the cell briefly becomes positively charged

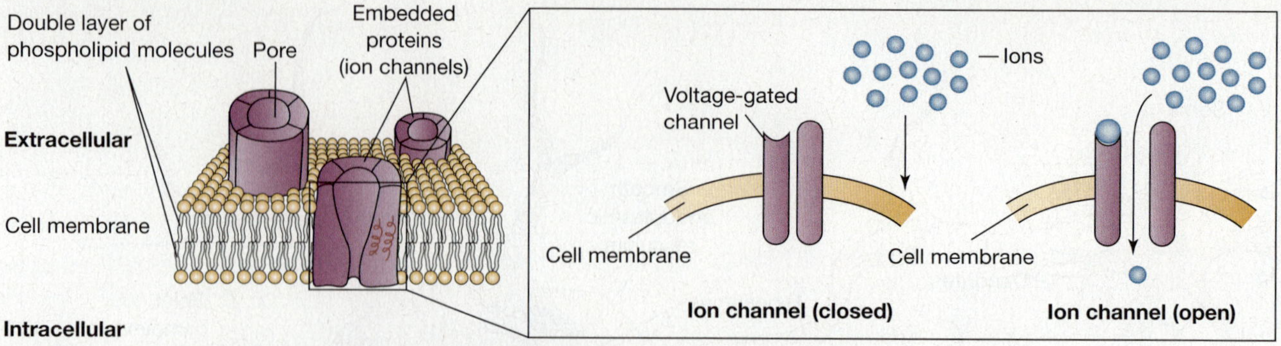

FIGURE 7.6 Initiation of a nerve impulse. The initiation of an action potential, or nerve impulse, involves the opening and closing of the voltage-gated channels on the cell membrane and the passage of ions into the cell. The resulting electrical activity sends communication impulses from the dendrites or axons into the body.

and the outside negatively charged. Once initiated, the action potential becomes self-propagating, opening nearby sodium channels. This electrical communication moves into the soma from the dendrites or down the axon by this mechanism.

Synaptic Transmission

For one neuron to communicate with another, the electrical process described must change to a chemical communication. The **synaptic cleft,** a junction between one nerve and another, is the space where the electrical intracellular signal becomes a chemical extracellular signal. Various substances are recognized as the chemical messengers among neurons.

As the electrical action potential reaches the ends of the axons, called *terminals,* calcium ion channels are opened, allowing an influx of Ca^{++} ions into the neuron. This increase in calcium stimulates the release of neurotransmitters into the synapse. Rapid signaling among neurons requires a ready supply of neurotransmitters. These neurotransmitters are stored in small vesicles grouped near the cell membrane at the end of the axon. When stimulated, the vesicles containing the neurotransmitter fuse with the cell membrane, and the neurotransmitter is released into the synapse (Fig. 7.7). The neurotransmitter then crosses the synaptic cleft to a receptor site on the postsynaptic neuron and stimulates adjacent neurons. This is the process of neuronal communication.

When the neurotransmitter has completed its interaction with the postsynaptic receptor and stimulated that cell, its work is done, and it needs to be removed. It can be removed by natural diffusion away from the area of high neurotransmitter concentration at the receptors by being broken down by enzymes in the synaptic cleft or through reuptake through highly specific mechanisms into the presynaptic terminal. The primary steps in synaptic transmission are summarized in Figure 7.7.

Neurotransmitters

As described in the overview earlier, neurotransmitters are key in the process of synaptic transmission. **Neurotransmitters** are small molecules that directly and indirectly control the opening or closing of ion channels. **Neuromodulators** are chemical messengers that make the target cell membrane or postsynaptic membrane susceptible to the effects of the primary neurotransmitter.

> **KEYCONCEPT Neurotransmitters** are small molecules that directly and indirectly control the opening or closing of ion channels.

Excitatory neurotransmitters reduce the membrane potential and enhance the transmission of the signal between neurons. *Inhibitory neurotransmitters* have the opposite effect and slow down nerve impulses. Although some are synthesized from dietary precursors, such as tyrosine or tryptophan, most synthesis occurs in the terminals or the neuron itself. Neurotransmitters are commonly classified as the following: cholinergic, biogenic amine (monoamines or bioamines), amino acid, and neuropeptides. Table 7.2 summarizes some of the key neurotransmitters and their proposed functions.

Acetylcholine

Acetylcholine (ACh) is the primary cholinergic neurotransmitter. Found in the greatest concentration in the PNS, ACh provides the basic synaptic communication for the parasympathetic neurons and part of the sympathetic neurons, which send information to the CNS.

ACh is an excitatory neurotransmitter that is found throughout the cerebral cortex and limbic system. It arises primarily from cell bodies in the basal forebrain constellation, which provides innervations to the cerebral cortex, amygdala, hippocampus, and thalamus as well as from the dorsolateral tegmentum of the pons that projects to the basal ganglia, thalamus, hypothalamus, medullary

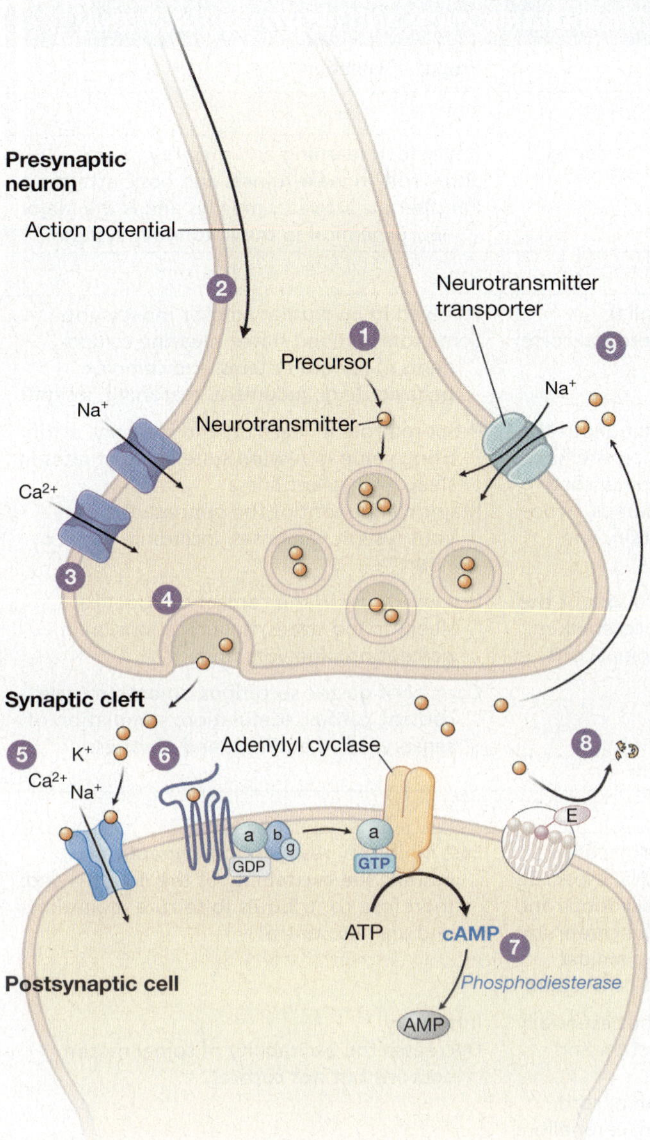

FIGURE 7.7 Synaptic transmission. The most significant events that occur during synaptic transmission are as follows: (*1*) the action potential reaches the presynaptic terminal; (*2*) membrane depolarization causes Ca^{++} terminals to open; (*3*) Ca^{++} mediates fusion of the vesicles with the presynaptic membrane; (*4*) transmitter molecules are released into the synaptic cleft by exocytosis; (*5*) transmitter molecules bind to postsynaptic receptors and activate ion channels; (*6*) conductance changes cause an excitatory or inhibitory postsynaptic potential, depending on the specific transmitter; (*7*) current flow spreads along the postsynaptic membrane; (*8*) transmitter remaining in the synaptic cleft returns to the presynaptic terminal by reuptake; and (*9*) the transmitter diffuses into the extracellular fluid. AMP, adenosine monophosphate; ATP, adenosine triphosphate; cAMP, cyclic adenosine monophosphate; GDP, guanosine diphosphate; GTP, guanosine triphosphate. (Reprinted with permission from Bear, M. F., Conners, B. W., & Paradiso, M. A. [2016]. *Neuroscience: Exploring the brain* [4th ed.]. Wolters Kluwer.)

reticular formation, and deep cerebellar nuclei (Fig. 7.8) (Sam & Bordoni, 2023). These connections suggest that ACh is involved in higher intellectual functioning and memory. Individuals who have Alzheimer disease or Down syndrome often exhibit patterns of cholinergic neuron loss in regions innervated by these pathways (e.g., the hippocampus), which may contribute to their memory difficulties and other cognitive deficits. Some cholinergic neurons are afferent to these areas bringing information from the limbic system, highlighting the role that ACh plays in communicating one's emotional state to the cerebral cortex.

Biogenic Amines

The **biogenic amines** (bioamines) consist of small molecules manufactured in the neuron that contain an amine group, thus the name. The catecholamines (amine attached to a catechol group) include dopamine, norepinephrine, and epinephrine, which are all synthesized from the amino acid tyrosine. Another monoamine, serotonin, is synthesized from tryptophan. Melatonin is derived from serotonin. All these neurotransmitters are critical in many mental disorders.

Dopamine

Dopamine is an excitatory neurotransmitter found in distinct regions of the CNS and is involved in learning, movement, motivation, and neuroendocrine functions. Dopamine is the neurotransmitter that stimulates the body's natural "feel good" reward pathways, producing a pleasant euphoric sensation under certain conditions. It is involved in the regulation of action, emotion, motivation, and attention. Dopamine levels are decreased in Parkinson disease, and unusually high activity of dopamine has been associated with schizophrenia (discussed in more detail in Chapter 24). Anomalies of dopamine activity within the reward system pathways are a critical aspect of the development of drugs and other dependencies. The dopamine pathways are distinct neuronal areas within the CNS in which the neurotransmitter dopamine predominates. Three major dopaminergic pathways have been identified.

The *mesocortical* and *mesolimbic pathways* originate in the ventral tegmental area and project into the medial aspects of the cortex (mesocortical) and the limbic system inside the temporal lobes, including the hippocampus and amygdala (mesolimbic). Sometimes, there is one pathway and at other times two separate pathways. The mesocortical pathway has major effects on cognition, including functions such as judgment, reasoning, insight, social conscience, motivation, the ability to generalize learning, and reward systems in the human brain. It contributes to some of the highest seats of cortical functioning. The

TABLE 7.2 CLASSIC AND PUTATIVE NEUROTRANSMITTERS: THEIR DISTRIBUTION AND PROPOSED FUNCTIONS

Neurotransmitter	Cell Bodies	Projections	Proposed Function
Acetylcholine			
Dietary precursor: choline	Basal forebrain Pons Other areas	Diffuse throughout the cortex, hippocampus PNS	Key role in learning and memory Some role in wakefulness and basic attention Peripherally activates muscles and is the major neurochemical in the autonomic system
Monoamines			
Dopamine (dietary precursor: tyrosine)	Substantia nigra Ventral tegmental area Arcuate nucleus Retina olfactory bulb	Striatum (basal ganglia) Limbic system and cerebral cortex Pituitary	Involved in involuntary motor movements Some role in mood states, pleasure components in reward systems, and complex behavior (e.g., judgment, reasoning, insight)
Norepinephrine (dietary precursor: tyrosine)	Locus coeruleus Lateral tegmental area and others throughout the pons and medulla	Very widespread throughout the cortex, thalamus, cerebellum, brain stem, and spinal cord Basal forebrain, thalamus, hypothalamus, brain stem, and spinal cord	Proposed role in learning and memory, attributing value in reward systems, fluctuates in sleep and wakefulness Major component of the sympathetic nervous system responses, including "fight or flight"
Serotonin (dietary precursor: tryptophan)	Raphe nuclei Others in the pons and medulla	Very widespread throughout the cortex, thalamus, cerebellum, brain stem, and spinal cord	Proposed role in the control of appetite, sleep, mood states, hallucinations, pain perception, and vomiting
Histamine (pre cursor: histidine)	Hypothalamus	Cerebral cortex Limbic system Hypothalamus Found in all mast cells	Control of gastric secretions, smooth muscle control, cardiac stimulation, stimulation of sensory nerve endings, and alertness
Amino Acids			
GABA	Derived from gluta mate without localized cell bodies	Found in cells and projections throughout the CNS, especially in intrinsic feedback loops and interneurons of the cerebrum; also in the extrapyramidal motor system and cerebellum	Fast inhibitory response postsynaptically inhibits the excitability of the neurons and therefore contributes to seizure, agitation, and anxiety control
Glycine	Primarily the spinal cord and brain stem	Limited projection, but especially in the auditory system and olfactory bulb Also found in the spinal cord, medulla, midbrain, cerebellum, and cortex	Inhibitory Decreases the excitability of spinal motor neurons but not cortical
Glutamate	Diffuse	Diffuse, but especially in the sensory organs	Excitatory Responsible for the bulk of information flow
Neuropeptides			
Endogenous opioids (i.e., endorphins, enkephalins)	A large family of neuropeptides that has three distinct subgroups, all of which are manufactured widely throughout the CNS	Widely distributed within and outside of the CNS	Suppress pain, modulate mood, and stress Likely involvement in reward systems and dependency Also may regulate pituitary hormone release Implicated in the pathophysiology of diseases of the basal ganglia
Melatonin (one of its precursors: serotonin)	Pineal body	Widely distributed within and outside of the CNS	Secreted in dark and suppressed in light, helps regulate the sleep–wake cycle as well as other biologic rhythms
Substance P	Widespread, significant in the raphe system, and spinal cord	Spinal cord, cortex, brain stem, and especially sensory neurons associated with pain perception	Involved in pain transmission, movement, and mood regulation
Cholecystokinin	Predominates in the ventral tegmental area of the midbrain	Frontal cortex, where it is often colocalized with dopamine Widely distributed within and outside of the CNS	Primary intestinal hormone involved in satiety; also has some involvement in the control of anxiety and panic

CNS, central nervous system; GABA, gamma-aminobutyric acid; PNS, peripheral nervous system.

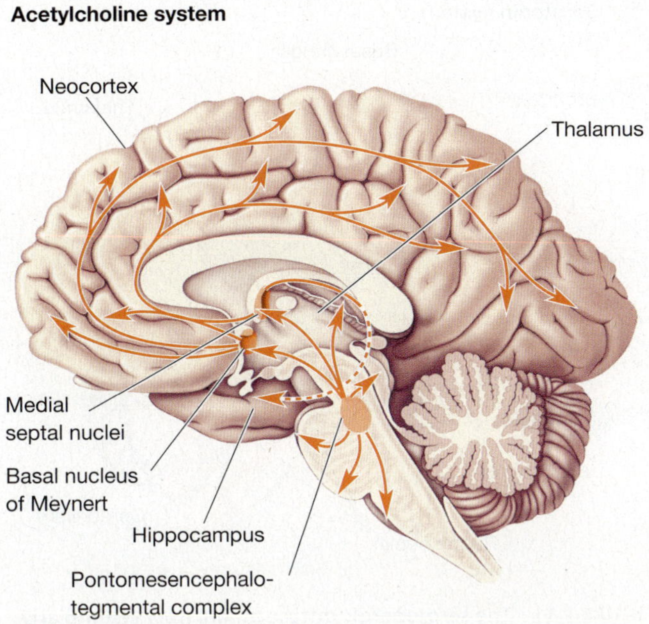

FIGURE 7.8 Cholinergic pathways. (Reprinted with permission from Bear, M. F., Conners, B. W., & Paradiso, M. A. [2016]. *Neuroscience: Exploring the brain* [4th ed.]. Wolters Kluwer.)

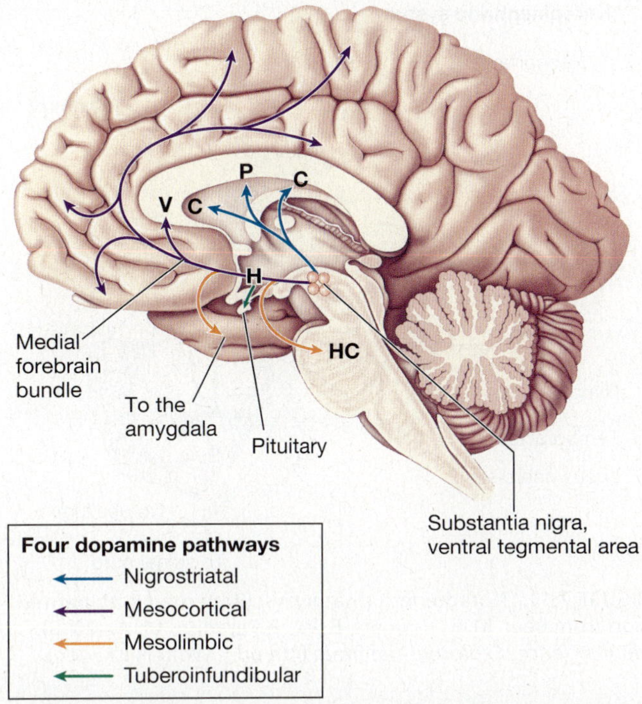

FIGURE 7.9 Dopaminergic pathways. The dopaminergic diffuse modulatory systems arising from the substantia nigra and the ventral tegmental area. The substantia nigra and ventral tegmental area lie close together in the midbrain. They project to the striatum (caudate nucleus and putamen) and limbic and frontal cortical regions, respectively. *C*, caudate nucleus; *H*, hypothalamus; *HC*, hippocampal formation; *P*, putamen; *V*, ventral striatum. (Reprinted with permission from Bear, M. F., Conners, B. W., & Paradiso, M. A. [2016]. *Neuroscience: Exploring the brain* [4th ed.]. Wolters Kluwer.)

mesolimbic pathway also strongly influences emotions and has projections that affect memory and auditory reception. Anomalies in these pathways have been associated with schizophrenia.

Another major dopaminergic pathway begins in the substantia nigra and projects into the basal ganglia, parts of which are known as the *striatum*. Therefore, this pathway is called the *nigrostriatal pathway*. This influences the extrapyramidal motor system, which serves the voluntary motor system and allows involuntary motor movements. This pathway is associated with not only the motor system, but also with reward-related and associative learning. Destruction of dopaminergic neurons in this pathway has been associated with Parkinson disease. See Figure 7.9.

There are at least three other dopamine pathways. The *tuberoinfundibular pathway* originates from projections of the mesolimbic pathway and continues into the hypothalamus, which then projects into the pituitary gland. This pathway regulates prolactin secretion and impacts other functions, such as metabolism, hunger, thirst, sexual function, circadian rhythms, digestion, and temperature control. The *hypothalamospinal* tract projects from the hypothalamus to the spinal cord and is associated with motor function. Restless leg syndrome is an associated disorder. The *incertohypothalamic* pathway projects from the subthalamus to the brain stem and amygdala and influences the hypothalamus and locomotor centers in the brain stem. This pathway is associated with visceral and sensorimotor activities and can result in tremors.

Norepinephrine

Norepinephrine is an excitatory neurochemical that plays a major role in generating and maintaining mood states. Because norepinephrine is so heavily concentrated in the terminal sites of sympathetic nerves, it can be released quickly to ready the individual for a fight-or-flight response to threats in the environment. Norepinephrine is associated with attention and reward systems and is thought to play a role in the physical symptoms of anxiety, substance use disorders, and eating disorders (Zhang et al., 2023).

Nerve tracts and pathways containing predominantly norepinephrine are called *noradrenergic* and are less clearly delineated than the dopamine pathways. In the CNS, noradrenergic neurons originate in the locus coeruleus, where more than half of the noradrenergic cell bodies are located. Because the locus coeruleus is one of the major timekeepers of the human body, norepinephrine is involved in sleep and wakefulness. From the locus coeruleus, noradrenergic pathways ascend into the neocortex, spread diffusely (Fig. 7.10), and enhance the ability of neurons to respond to whatever input they

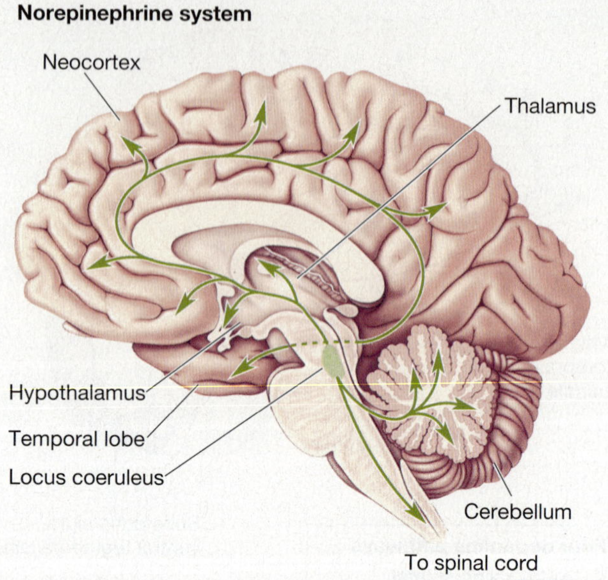

FIGURE 7.10 Noradrenergic pathways. (Reprinted with permission from Bear, M. F., Conners, B. W., & Paradiso, M. A. [2016]. *Neuroscience: Exploring the brain* [4th ed.]. Wolters Kluwer.)

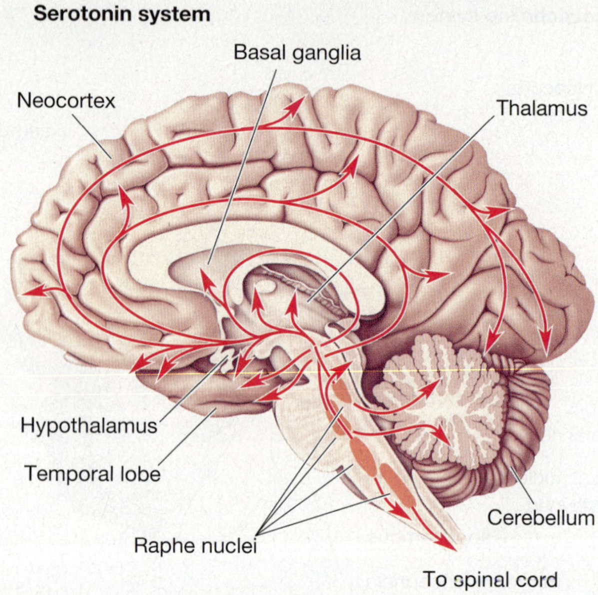

FIGURE 7.11 The serotonergic diffuse modulatory systems arising from the raphe nuclei. The raphe nuclei are clustered along the midline of the brain stem and project extensively to all levels of the central nervous system. (Reprinted with permission from Bear, M. F., Conners, B. W., & Paradiso, M. A. [2016]. *Neuroscience: Exploring the brain* [4th ed.]. Wolters Kluwer.)

may be receiving. In addition, norepinephrine appears to be involved in the process of reinforcement, which facilitates learning. Noradrenergic pathways innervate the hypothalamus and thus are involved to some degree in endocrine function. Anxiety disorders and depression are examples of psychiatric illnesses in which dysfunction of the noradrenergic neurons may be involved. (Refer to Table 7.1 for the effects of ACh on various organs in the parasympathetic system.)

Serotonin

Serotonin (also called 5-hydroxytryptamine or 5-HT) is primarily an excitatory neurotransmitter that is diffusely distributed within the cerebral cortex, limbic system, and basal ganglia of the CNS. Serotonergic neurons also project into the hypothalamus and cerebellum. Figure 7.11 illustrates serotonergic pathways. Serotonin plays a role in emotions, cognition, sensory perceptions, and essential biologic functions, such as sleep and appetite. During the rapid eye movement (REM) phase of sleep, or the dream state, serotonin concentrations decrease, and muscles subsequently relax. Serotonin is also involved in the control of food intake, hormone secretion, sexual behavior, thermoregulation, and cardiovascular regulation. Some serotonergic fibers reach the cranial blood vessels within the brain and the *pia mater* where they have a vasoconstrictive effect. The potency of some new medications for migraine headaches is related to their ability to block serotonin transmission in the cranial blood vessels. Descending serotonergic pathways are important in central pain control. Whereas depression and insomnia have been associated with decreased levels of 5-HT, mania has been associated with increased 5-HT. Some of the most well-known antidepressant medications, such as fluoxetine and sertraline, which are discussed in more depth in Chapter 11, function by raising serotonin levels within certain areas of the CNS. Melatonin, which is derived from serotonin, is produced by the pineal gland and plays a role in sleep, aging, and mood changes.

Amino Acids

Amino acids, the building blocks of proteins, have many roles in intraneuronal metabolism. In addition, amino acids can function as neurotransmitters in as many as 60% to 70% of the synaptic sites in the brain. Amino acids are the most prevalent neurotransmitters. Virtually all the neurons in the CNS are activated by excitatory amino acids, such as glutamate, and inhibited by inhibitory amino acids, such as **GABA** (gamma-aminobutyric acid) and glycine. Many of these amino acids coexist with other neurotransmitters.

Histamine

Histamine, derived from the amino acid histidine, has been identified as a neurotransmitter. Its cell bodies originate predominantly in the hypothalamus and project to all major structures in the cerebrum, brain stem, and spinal cord. Its functions are not well known, but it appears to have a role in autonomic and neuroendocrine regulation. Many psychiatric medications can block the effects of histamine postsynaptically and produce side effects such as sedation, weight gain, and hypotension.

Gamma-Aminobutyric Acid

GABA is the primary inhibitory neurotransmitter for the CNS. The pathways of GABA exist almost exclusively in the CNS, with the largest GABA concentrations in the hypothalamus, hippocampus, basal ganglia, spinal cord, and cerebellum. GABA functions in an inhibitory role in control of spinal reflexes and cerebellar reflexes. It has a major role in the control of neuronal excitability through the brain. In addition, GABA has an inhibitory influence on the activity of the dopaminergic nigrostriatal projections. GABA also has interconnections with other neurotransmitters. For example, dopamine inhibits cholinergic neurons, and GABA provides feedback and balance. Dysregulation of GABA and GABA receptors has been associated with anxiety disorders, and decreased GABA activity is involved in the development of seizure disorders.

Glutamate

Glutamate, the most widely distributed excitatory neurotransmitter, is the main transmitter in the associational areas of the cortex. Glutamate is the single most potent neurotransmitter in the entire brain and can be found in several pathways from the cortex to the thalamus, pons, striatum, and spinal cord. It plays a large role in learning, cognition, and mood. Glutamate pathways have several connections with the hippocampus. Some glutamate receptors may play a role in the long-lasting enhancement of synaptic activity. In turn, in the hippocampus, this enhancement may have a role in learning and memory. Too much glutamate is harmful to neurons, and considerable interest has emerged regarding its neurotoxic effects.

Conditions that produce an excess of endogenous glutamate can cause neurotoxicity by overexcitation of neuronal tissue. This process, called excitotoxicity, increases the sensitivity of glutamate receptors, produces overactivation of the receptors, and is increasingly being understood as a critical piece of the cascade of events involved in physical symptoms of alcohol withdrawal in dependent individuals. Excitotoxicity is also believed to be part of the pathology of conditions such as ischemia, hypoxia, hypoglycemia, and hepatic failure. Damage to the CNS from chronic malfunctioning of the glutamate system may be involved in the psychiatric symptoms seen in neurodegenerative diseases such as Huntington, Parkinson, and Alzheimer diseases; vascular dementia; amyotrophic lateral sclerosis; and AIDS-related dementia. Glutamate is implicated in the development of schizophrenia, substance use disorders, and major depression.

Neuropeptides

Neuropeptides, short chains of amino acids, exist in the CNS and have several important roles as neurotransmitters, neuromodulators, or neurohormones. Neuropeptides were first thought to be pituitary hormones, such as adrenocorticotropin, oxytocin, and vasopressin, or hypothalamic-releasing hormones (e.g., corticotropin-releasing hormone and thyrotropin-releasing hormone). However, when an endogenous morphine–like substance was discovered in the 1970s, the term *endorphin,* or endogenous morphine, was introduced. Although the amino acids and monoamine neurotransmitters can be produced directly from dietary precursors in any part of the neuron, neuropeptides are, almost without exception, synthesized from messenger ribonucleic acid in the cell body. Currently, two types of neuropeptides have been identified. Opioid neuropeptides, such as endorphins, enkephalins, and dynorphins, function in endocrine functioning and pain suppression. The nonopioid neuropeptides, such as substance P and somatostatin, play roles in pain transmission and endocrine functioning, respectively.

There are considerable variations in the distribution of individual neuropeptides, but some areas are especially rich in cell bodies containing neuropeptides. These areas include the amygdala, striatum, hypothalamus, raphe nuclei, brain stem, and spinal cord. Many of the interneurons of the cerebral cortex contain neuropeptides, but there are considerably fewer in the thalamus and almost none in the cerebellum.

Receptors

Embedded in the postsynaptic membrane are several proteins that act as **receptors** for the released neurotransmitters. Each neurotransmitter has a specific receptor, or protein, for which it and only it will fit.

Lock and Key

The "lock-and-key" analogy has often been used to describe the fit of a given neurotransmitter to its receptor site. The target cell, when stimulated by the neurotransmitter, will then respond by evoking its own action potential and either producing some action common to that cell or acting as a relay to keep the messages moving throughout the CNS. This pattern of the electrical signal from one neuron, converted to chemical signal at the synaptic cleft, picked up by an adjacent neuron, again converted to an electrical action potential, and then to a chemical signal, occurs billions of times a day in billions of different neurons. This electrical–chemical communication process allows the structures of the brain to function together in a coordinated and organized manner.

Receptor Sensitivity

Both pre- and postsynaptic receptors have the capacity to change, developing either a greater-than-usual response to the neurotransmitter, known as supersensitivity, or a less-than-usual response, called subsensitivity. These changes represent the concept of neuroplasticity of brain tissue discussed earlier in the chapter. The change in sensitivity of the receptor is most commonly caused by the effect of a drug on a receptor site or by disease that affects the usual functioning of a receptor site. Drugs can affect the sensitivity of the receptor by altering the strength of attraction or affinity of a receptor for the neurotransmitter, by changing the efficiency with which the receptor activity translates the message inside the receiving cell, or by decreasing over time the number of receptors.

These mechanisms may account for the long-term, sometimes severely adverse, effects of psychopharmacologic drugs, the loss of effectiveness of a given medication, or the loss of effectiveness of a medication after repeated use in treating recurring episodes of a psychiatric disorder. Disease may cause a change in the number or function of receptors, thereby altering their sensitivity. For example, depression is associated with a reduction in the usual number of certain receptors, leading to an anomaly in their sensitivity to neurotransmitters such as serotonin and norepinephrine (Bamalan et al., 2023). A decreased response to continued stimulation of these receptors is usually referred to as *desensitization* or *refractoriness*. This suspected subsensitivity is referred to as *downregulation* of the receptors.

Receptor Subtypes

The nervous system uses many different neurochemicals for communication, and each specific chemical messenger requires a specific receptor on which the chemical can act. More than 100 different chemical messengers have been identified, with new ones being uncovered. In addition to the sheer number of receptors needed to accommodate these chemicals, the neurotransmitters may produce different effects at different synaptic sites.

Each major neurotransmitter has several different subtypes of receptors, allowing the neurotransmitter to have different effects in different areas of the brain. The receptors usually have the same name as the neurotransmitter, but the classification of the subtypes varies. For example, dopamine receptors are named D1, D2, D3, and so on. Serotonin receptors are grouped in families such as 5-HT1A and 5-HT1B. The receptors for ACh have completely different names: muscarinic and nicotinic. Two specific subtype receptors have been identified for GABA: A and B (Table 7.3).

Brain structures such as the prefrontal cortex, striatum, hippocampus, and amygdala are linked through complex neural functional networks (Xia et al., 2022).

TABLE 7.3 SELECTED NEUROTRANSMITTERS AND RECEPTORS

Neurotransmitter	Receptor Subtypes
Acetylcholine (ACh)	Muscarinic receptors (M_1, M_2, M_3, M_4, M_5) Nicotinic receptor
Glutamate (Glu)	AMPA, NMDA, kainate receptors
Gamma-aminobutyric acid (GABA)	$GABA_A$, $GABA_B$
Serotonin (5-HT)	5-HT_{1A}, 5-HT_{1B}, 5-HT_{1D}, 5-HT_{1E}, 5-HT_{2A}, 5-HT_{2B}, 5-HT_C, 5-HT4, 5-HT_{5A}
Dopamine (DA)	D1, D2, D3, D4, D5
Norepinephrine (NE)	α_1, α_2, β_1, β_2

Reprinted with permission from Bear, M. F., Conners, B. W., & Paradiso, M. A. (2016). *Neuroscience: Exploring the brain* (4th ed.). Wolters Kluwer.

Recent research indicates that a dysfunctional **neurocircuitry** underlies most psychiatric disorders (Fig. 7.12). Various neurocircuits are the focus of study of different illnesses. For example, the cingulo–frontal–parietal network is associated with attention-deficit disorder, and the amygdalocortical circuitry is the focus in psychosis and schizophrenia.

STUDIES OF THE BIOLOGIC BASIS OF MENTAL DISORDERS

As described earlier, mental disorders are complex syndromes consisting of clusters of biopsychosocial

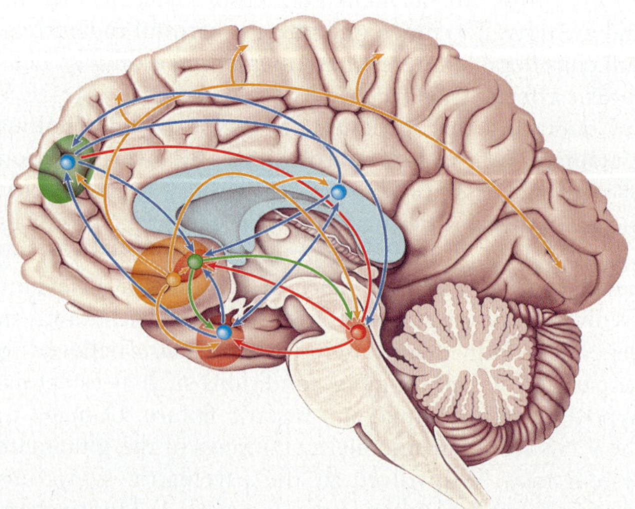

FIGURE 7.12 Complex neural functional networks involved in psychiatric disorders. *Arrows* illustrate projections. (Redrawn by permission from Nature, Haber, S. N., & Rauch, S. L. [2010]. Neurocircuitry: A window into the networks underlying neuropsychiatric disease. *Neuropsychopharmacology*, *35*[1], 1–3. https://doi.org/10.1038/npp.2009.146. Copyright © 2009 Springer Nature.)

symptoms. These syndromes are not specific physiologic disorders, and research efforts are focused on piecing the puzzle together. One important area of study is genetics; it is well established that genetic factors play an important role in the development of mental disorders. In addition, as the complexity of the nervous system and its interrelationship with other body systems and the environment have become more fully understood, new fields of study have emerged. One field worth noting is **psychoneuroimmunology (PNI).** Although it has long been observed that individuals under stress have compromised immune systems and are more likely to acquire common diseases, only recently have changes in the immune system been noted as widespread in some psychiatric illnesses. Another field, **chronobiology,** has provided new information suggesting that dysfunction of biologic rhythms may not only result from a psychiatric illness but also contribute to its development.

Genetics

The sequence of the human genome is the beginning of our understanding of complex genetic connections that leads to a **phenotype** or observable characteristics or expressions of a specific trait. The genome provides researchers with a road map of the exact sequence of the three billion nucleotide bases that make up human organisms. Many thought that after the human genome was mapped, it would be easy to determine the genes responsible for mental disorders. Unfortunately, it is not that simple. Knowing the location of the gene and its sequence is just a piece of the complex puzzle. The location of the genes does not tell us which genes are responsible for a mental illness or how mutations occur.

Population Genetics

Inheritance of mental disorders is studied by using epidemiologic methods that identify risks and patterns of illness or traits from generation to generation. Beginning with a **proband,** a person who has the disorder or trait, **population genetics** relies on the following principal epidemiologic methods:

- **Family studies** analyze the occurrence of a disorder in first-degree relatives (biologic parents, siblings, and children), second-degree relatives (biologic grandparents, uncles, aunts, nieces, nephews, and grandchildren), and so on.
- **Twin studies** analyze the presence or absence of the disorder in pairs of twins. The *concordance rate* is the measure of similarity of occurrence in individuals with a similar genetic makeup.
- **Adoption studies** compare the risk for the illness developing in offspring raised in different environments. The strongest inferences may be drawn from studies that involve children separated from their biologic parents at birth.

Mental disorders and their symptoms are not an expression of a single gene. The transmission pattern does not follow classic Mendelian genetics in which the dominant allele (variant) on only one chromosome or recessive alleles on both chromosomes are responsible for manifestation of a disorder. Monozygotic (identical) twins do not manifest the same mental disorder with 100% concordance rate, but they have a higher rate of a disorder than dizygotic (fraternal) twins, who share roughly the same proportion of genes that ordinary siblings do (50%). Internal and external environmental events influence the development of a disorder with a genetic contribution. This interaction between the environment and a genetic predisposition underlies several mental disorders such as schizophrenia, autism, and attention-deficit hyperactivity disorder.

Molecular Genetics

A gene comprises short segments of deoxyribonucleic acid (DNA) and is packed with the instructions for making proteins that have a specific function. When genes are absent or malfunction, protein production is altered, and bodily functions are disrupted. In this fashion, genes play a role in cancer, heart disease, diabetes, and many psychiatric disorders. Although no conclusive evidence exists for a complete genetic cause of most psychiatric disorders, significant evidence suggests that strong genetic contributions exist for most (Peedicayil, 2023).

Intracellular genes direct protein production responsible for genetic expression. Individual nerve cells outside of the cell respond to these changes, modifying proteins to adapt to the new environment. This dynamic nature of gene function highlights the way the body and the environment interact and how environmental factors influence gene expression.

The study of molecular genetics in psychiatric disorders is in its infancy. It is likely that psychiatric disorders are polygenic. This means that psychiatric disorders develop when genes interact with each other and with environmental factors such as stress, infections, poor nutrition, catastrophic loss, complications during pregnancy, and exposure to toxins. Thus, genetic makeup conveys vulnerability, or a risk for the illness, but the right set of environmental factors must be present for the disorder to develop in an at-risk individual (Peedicavil, 2023).

Genetic Susceptibility

The concept of **genetic susceptibility** suggests that an individual may be at increased risk for a psychiatric disorder. Specific risk factors for psychiatric disorders are just beginning to be understood, and environmental influences are examples of risk factors. In the absence of one specific gene for the major psychiatric disorders, risk factor assessment is a logical alternative for predicting who is more likely to experience psychiatric disorders or certain conditions, such as aggression or suicidality (Hill et al., 2024).

When considering information regarding risks for genetic transmission of psychiatric disorders, there are several key points to remember:

- Psychiatric disorders have been described and labeled quite differently across generations, and errors in diagnosis may occur.
- Similar psychiatric symptoms may have considerably different causes, just as symptoms such as chest pain may occur in relation to many different causes.
- Genes that are present may not always cause the appearance of the trait.
- Several genes work together in an individual to produce a given trait or disorder.
- A biologic cause is not necessarily solely genetic in origin. Environmental influences alter the body's functioning and often mediate or worsen genetic risk factors.

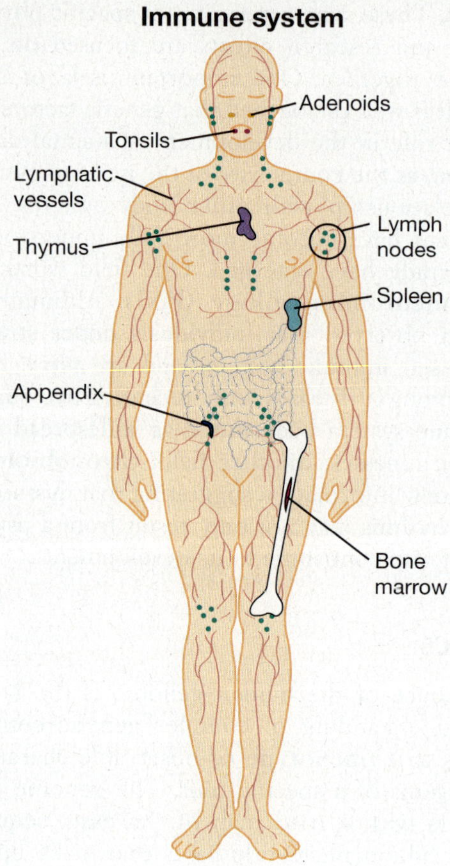

FIGURE 7.13 The immune system.

Epigenetics, Environmental Factors, and Mental Disorders

The environment cannot interact directly with the genome, but it can change the expression of the gene. **Epigenetics,** study of changes in organisms caused by modification of gene expression rather than alteration of the genetic code itself, has transformed the understanding of the impact of the environment on mental disorders. There is growing evidence that social determinants of health that result in early life adversity and stress lead to the development of mental disorders. Maternal prenatal stress, poverty, migration, urban dwelling, pregnancy and birth complications, alcohol use, microbiota, and pre- and postnatal infections are associated with mental disorders (Peedicavil, 2023).

Psychoneuroimmunology

PNI examines the relationships among the immune system, nervous system, and endocrine system and our behaviors, thoughts, and feelings. The immune system is composed of the thymus, spleen, lymph nodes, lymphatic vessels, tonsils, adenoids, and bone marrow, which manufacture all the cells that eventually develop into T cells, B cells, phagocytes, macrophages, and natural killer (NK) cells (Fig. 7.13). Many contemporary stress research studies are examining the role of the NK cells in the early recognition of foreign bodies. Lower NK cell function is related to increased disease susceptibility. NK cell function is affected by stress-induced physiologic arousal in humans. NK cell activity has been shown to vary in response to many emotional, cognitive, and physiologic stressors, including anxiety, depression, perceived lack of personal control, bereavement, pain, and surgery (Rahman & Bordoni, 2023; Rust et al., 2023).

Overactivity of the immune system can occur in autoimmune diseases such as systemic lupus erythematosus, allergies, and anaphylaxis. Evidence suggests that the nervous system regulates many aspects of immune function. Specific immune system dysfunctions may result from damage to the hypothalamus, hippocampus, or pituitary and may produce symptoms of psychiatric disorders. Figure 7.14 illustrates the interaction between stress and the immune system. This figure also demonstrates the true biopsychosocial nature of the complex interrelationship of the nervous system, the endocrine system, the immune system, and environmental or emotional stress.

Immune dysregulation may also be involved in the development of psychiatric disorders. This can occur by allowing neurotoxins to affect the brain, damaging neuroendocrine tissue, or damaging tissues in the brain at locations such as the receptor sites. Some antidepressants

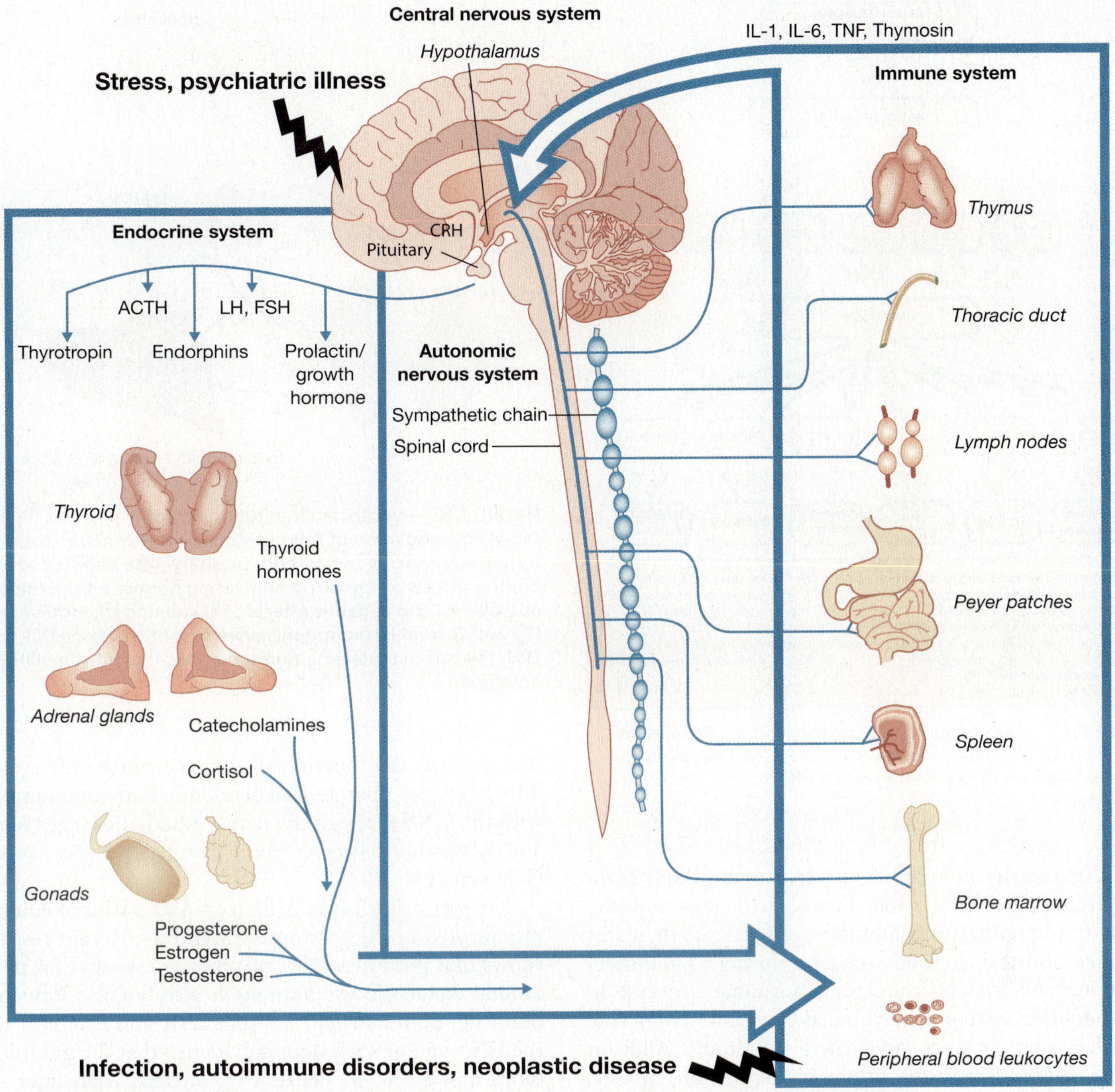

FIGURE 7.14 Examples of the interaction between stress or psychiatric illness and the immune system through the endocrine system. ACTH, adrenocorticotropic hormone; CRH, corticotropin-releasing hormone; FSH, follicle-stimulating hormone; IL, interleukin; LH, luteinizing hormone; TNF, tumor necrosis factor.

have been thought to have antiviral effects. Symptoms of diseases such as depression may occur after an occurrence of serious infection, and prenatal exposure to infectious organisms has been associated with the development of schizophrenia. Stress and conditioning have specific effects on the suppression of immune function (Cao et al., 2023; Chan et al., 2023).

Functioning of the endocrine system is often disturbed in people with psychiatric disorders. For example, thyroid functioning is often low in those with bipolar disorder, and people with schizophrenia have a higher incidence of diabetes (see Unit VI). The hypothalamus sends and receives information through the pituitary, which then communicates with structures in the peripheral aspects of the body. Figure 7.15 presents an example of the communication of the anterior pituitary with several organs and structures.

Axes, the structures within which the neurohormones are providing messages, are the most often studied aspect of the neuroendocrine system. These axes always involve a feedback mechanism. For example, the **hypothalamus–pituitary–thyroid axis (HPT)** regulates the release of thyroid hormone by the thyroid gland using thyrotropin-releasing hormone from the hypothalamus to the

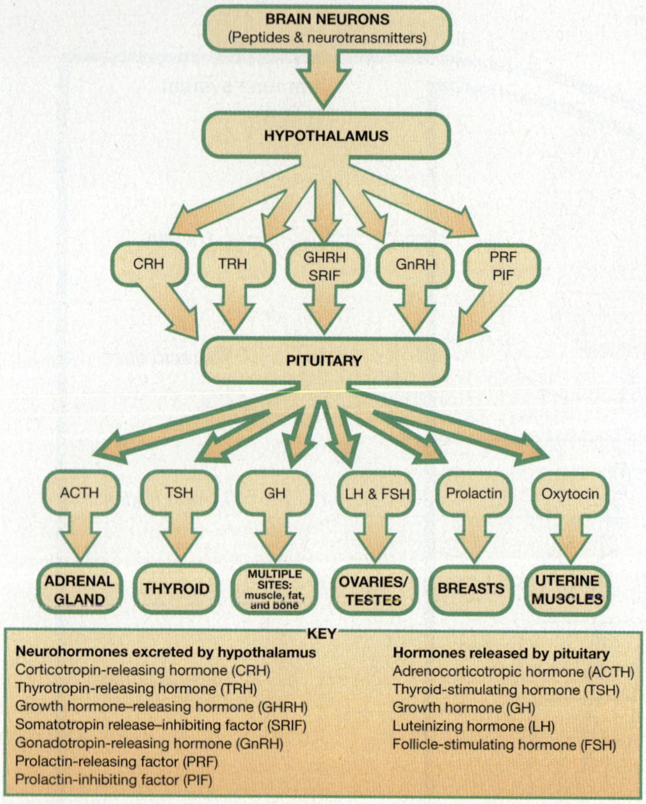

FIGURE 7.15 Hypothalamic and pituitary communication system. The neurohormonal communication system between the hypothalamus and the pituitary exerts effects on many organs and systems.

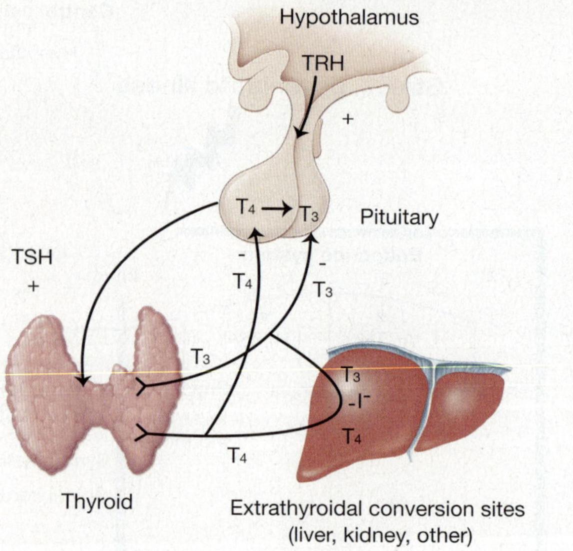

FIGURE 7.16 Hypothalamic–pituitary–thyroid axis. This figure shows the regulation of thyroid-stimulating hormone (or thyrotropin) secretion by the anterior pituitary. Also depicted are the positive effects of thyrotropin-releasing hormone from the hypothalamus and negative effects of circulating triiodothyronine (T_3) and T_3 from intrapituitary conversion of thyroxine (T_4). TRH, thyrotropin-releasing hormone; TSH, thyroid-stimulating hormone.

pituitary and thyroid-stimulating hormone (TSH) from the pituitary to the thyroid. Figure 7.16 illustrates the HPA. The hypothalamic–pituitary–gonadal axis regulates estrogen and testosterone secretion through luteinizing hormone and follicle-stimulating hormone. Interest in the endocrine system is heightened by various endocrine disorders that produce psychiatric symptoms. Addison disease (hypoadrenalism) produces depression, apathy, fatigue, and occasionally psychosis. Hypothyroidism produces depression and some anxiety. Administration of steroids can cause depression, hypomania, irritability, and in some cases, psychosis. Some psychiatric disorders have been associated with endocrine system dysfunction. For example, some individuals with mood disorders show evidence of dysregulation in adrenal, thyroid, and growth hormone axes (see Chapter 26).

Gut–Brain Axis

The **gut–brain axis** is the term used to define the relationship among the CNS, neuroendocrine, and neuroimmune systems including the HPA, sympathetic and autonomic nervous systems, the **enteric nervous system (ENS)**, the vagus nerve, and the gut microbiota. The ENS or "second brain" is a mesh-like system of neurons that governs the function of the gastrointestinal system. The ENS can operate independently and communicates with the CNS through the parasympathetic (vagus nerve) and sympathetic (prevertebral ganglia) nervous systems (Nguyen et al., 2023).

The **gut microbiota** is the complex bacterial community located in the gastrointestinal tract. Recent research shows that gut microbiota not only is essential for maintaining metabolic and immune health but also influences brain development and neurogenesis and interacts with the ENS and CNS. There is evidence that the gut microbiota has a role in depression, anxiety, Alzheimer disease, and autism spectrum disorder (Kumar et al., 2023; Nguyen et al., 2023; Yao et al., 2023). It appears that bacteria can respond to and produce neurotransmitters such as the dopamine, norepinephrine, serotonin, and GABA (Marano et al., 2023).

Chronobiology

Chronobiology involves the study and measuring of time structures or biologic rhythms. Some rhythms have a **circadian cycle,** or 24-hour cycle, but others, such as the menstrual cycle, operate in different periods. Rhythms exist in the human body to control endocrine secretions, sleep–wake, body temperature, neurotransmitter synthesis, and more. These cycles may become deregulated and may begin earlier than usual, known as a phase advance, or later than usual, known as a phase delay.

Zeitgebers are specific events that function as time givers or synchronizers and that set biologic rhythms. Light is the most common example of an external zeitgeber. The suprachiasmatic nucleus of the hypothalamus is an example of an internal zeitgeber. Some theorists think that psychiatric disorders may result from one or more biologic rhythm dysfunctions. For example, depression may be, in part, a phase advance disorder, including early morning awakening and decreased time of onset of REM sleep. Seasonal affective disorder may be the result of shortened exposure to light during the winter months. Exposure to specific artificial light often relieves symptoms of fatigue, overeating, hypersomnia, and depression (see Chapters 11, 26, and 34).

DIAGNOSTIC APPROACHES

Although no commonly used laboratory tests exist that directly confirm a mental disorder, they are still used as part of the diagnosis of these illnesses. **Biologic markers** are diagnostic test findings that occur only in the presence of the psychiatric disorder and include such findings as laboratory and other diagnostic test results and neuropathologic changes noticeable in assessment. These markers increase diagnostic certainty and reliability and may have predictive value, allowing for the possibility of preventive interventions to forestall or avoid the onset of illness. In addition, biologic markers could assist in developing evidence-based care practices. If markers are used reliably, it is much easier to identify the most effective treatments and to determine the expected prognoses for given conditions. The psychiatric–mental health (PMH) nurse should be aware of the most current information on biologic markers so that information, limitations, and results can be discussed knowledgeably with the patient.

Laboratory Tests

For many years, laboratory tests have attempted to measure levels of neurotransmitters and other CNS substances in the bloodstream. Many of the metabolites of neurotransmitters can be found in the urine and cerebrospinal fluid as well. However, these measures have had only limited utility in elucidating what is happening in the brain. Levels of neurotransmitters and metabolites in the bloodstream or urine do not necessarily equate with levels in the CNS. In addition, availability of the neurotransmitter or metabolite does not predict the availability of the neurotransmitter in the synapse, where it must act, or directly relate to the receptor sensitivity. Nonetheless, numerous research studies have focused on changes in neurotransmitters and metabolites in blood, urine, and cerebrospinal fluid. These studies have provided clues but remain without conclusive predictive value and therefore are not routinely used.

Another laboratory approach to the study of some of the psychiatric disorders is the challenge test. A challenge test has been most often used in the study of panic disorders. These tests are usually conducted by intravenously administering a chemical known to produce a specific set of psychiatric symptoms. For example, lactate or caffeine may be used to induce the symptoms of panic in people who have panic disorder. The biologic response of the individual is then monitored.

Beyond their role in helping to diagnose mental disorders, laboratory tests are also an active part of the care and assessment of patients with psychiatric disorders. Many physical conditions mimic the symptoms of mental illness, and many of the medications used to treat psychiatric illness can produce health issues. For these reasons, the routine care of patients with psychiatric disorders includes the use of laboratory tests such as complete blood counts, thyroid studies, electrolytes, hepatic enzymes, and other evaluative tests. PMH nurses need to be familiar with these procedures and assist patients in understanding the use and implications of such tests.

Neurophysiologic Procedures

Several neurophysiologic procedures are used in mental health for diagnostic purposes.

Electroencephalography

Electroencephalography (EEG) is a tried-and-true method for investigating what is happening inside the living brain. Developed in the 1920s, EEG measures electrical activity in the uppermost nerve layers of the cortex. Usually, 16 electrodes are placed on the patient's scalp. The EEG machine, equipped with graph paper and recording pens, is turned on, and the pens then trace the electrical impulses generated over each electrode. Until the use of computed tomography (CT) in the 1970s, EEG was the only method for identifying brain anomalies. It remains the simplest and most noninvasive method for identifying some disorders. It is increasingly being used to identify individual neuronal differences.

An EEG may be used in psychiatry to differentiate possible causes of the patient's symptoms. For example, some types of seizure disorders, such as temporal lobe epilepsy, head injuries, or tumors, may present predominantly with psychiatric symptoms. In addition, metabolic dysfunction, delirium, dementia, altered levels of consciousness, hallucinations, and dissociative states may require EEG evaluation.

Spikes and wave-pattern changes are indications of brain anomalies. Spikes may be the focal point from which a seizure occurs. However, atypical activity often is not discovered on a routine EEG while the individual is awake. For this reason, additional methods are sometimes used. Nasopharyngeal leads may be used to get physically closer to the limbic regions. The patient may be exposed to a flashing strobe light while the examiner looks for activity that is not in phase with the flashing light or the patient may be asked to hyperventilate for 3 minutes to induce atypical activity if it exists. Sleep deprivation may also be used. This involves keeping the patient awake throughout the night before the EEG evaluation. The patient may then be drowsy and fall asleep during the procedure. Anomalies are more likely to occur when the patient is asleep. Sleep may also be induced using medication; however, many medications change the wave patterns on an EEG. For example, the benzodiazepine class of drugs increases the rapid and fast beta activity. Many other prescribed and illicit drugs, such as lithium, which increases theta activity, can cause EEG alterations.

In addition to reassuring, preparing, and educating the patient for the examination, the nurse should carefully assess the history of substance use and report this information to the examiner. If a sleep deprivation EEG is to be done, caffeine or other stimulants that might assist the patient in staying awake should be withheld because they may change the EEG patterns.

Polysomnography

Polysomnography is a special procedure that involves recording the EEG throughout a night of sleep. This test is usually conducted in a sleep laboratory. Other tests are usually performed at the same time, including electrocardiography and electromyography. Blood oxygenation, body movement, body temperature, and other data may be collected as well, especially in research settings. This procedure is usually conducted for evaluating sleep disorders, such as sleep apnea, enuresis, or somnambulism. However, sleep pattern changes are frequently researched in mental disorders as well.

Researchers have found that sleep divisions and stages are affected by many factors, including drugs, alcohol, general medical conditions, and psychiatric disorders. For example, REM latency, the length of time it takes an individual to enter the first REM episode, is shortened in depression. Reduced delta sleep is also observed. These findings have been replicated so frequently that some researchers consider them biologic markers for depression.

Concept Mastery Alert

Polysomnography involves recording an EEG throughout a night of sleep. A sleep deprivation EEG involves keeping a client awake the night before the EEG evaluation.

Structural and Functional Imaging

Neuroimaging of the brain involves **structural imaging**, which visualizes the structure of brain and allows diagnosis of gross intracranial disease and injury, and **functional imaging**, which visualizes the processing of information. One of the most well-known examples of structural imaging is magnetic resonance imaging (MRI), which produces two- or three-dimensional images of brain structures without the use of x-rays or radioactive tracers. An MRI creates a magnetic field around the patient's head through which radio waves are sent. A functional MRI (fMRI) that creates functional images relies on the properties of oxygenated and deoxygenated hemoglobin to see images of changes in blood flow. The advantage of fMRI is that it is possible to see how the brain works when different stimuli are presented and issues that exist, such as a stroke. The fMRI has replaced most use of positron emission tomography (PET), which measures blood flow and oxygen and glucose metabolism. The emissions from the injected radioactive tracers are rapidly decayed and limit the monitoring of PET to short tasks.

Neuroimaging has limited clinical use in mental health, but its use is increasing in diagnosis and treatment of some disorders such as Alzheimer disease and traumatic brain injury (Casagrande et al., 2023). Neuroimaging has promising potential for unlocking the pathophysiology of several mental disorders. With the introduction of the fMRI, it is now possible to study the circuitry and pinpoint genetic-based predisposing factors. An MRI technique, diffusion tensor imaging, allows for viewing macroscopic changes that occur at the axon level (Jameei et al., 2023).

Other Neurophysiologic Methods

Evoked potentials (EPs), also called event-related potentials, use the same basic principles as an EEG. They measure changes in electrical activity of the brain in specific regions as a response to a given stimulus. Electrodes placed on the scalp measure a large waveform that stands out after the administration of repetitive stimuli, such as a click or flash of light. There are several different types of EPs to be measured, depending on the sensory area affected by the stimulus, the cognitive task required, or the region monitored, any of which can change the length of time until the wave occurrence. EPs are used extensively in psychiatric research. In clinical practice, EPs are used primarily in the assessment of demyelinating disorders, such as multiple sclerosis.

However, brain electrical activity mapping studies, which involve a 20-electrode EEG that generates computerized maps of the brain's electrical activity, have found a slowing of electrical activity in the frontal lobes of individuals who have schizophrenia.

SUMMARY OF KEY POINTS

- Neuroscientists now view behavior and cognitive function as a result of complex interactions within the CNS and its plasticity, or its ability to adapt and change in both structure and function.
- Each hemisphere of the brain is divided into four lobes: the frontal lobe, which controls motor, speech function, personality, and cognitive ability—often called executive functions that govern one's ability to plan and initiate action; the parietal lobe, which controls the sensory functions; the temporal lobe, which contains the primary auditory and olfactory areas; and the occipital lobe, which controls visual integration of information.
- The structures of the limbic system are integrally involved in memory and emotional behavior. Dysfunction of the limbic system has been linked with major mental disorders, including schizophrenia, depression, and anxiety disorders.
- Neurons communicate with each other through synaptic transmission. Neurotransmitters excite or inhibit a response at the receptor sites and have been linked to certain mental disorders. These neurotransmitters include ACh, dopamine, norepinephrine, serotonin, GABA, and glutamate.
- Although no one gene has been found to produce any psychiatric disorder, significant evidence indicates that most psychiatric disorders have a genetic predisposition or susceptibility. For individuals who have such genetic susceptibility, the identification of risk factors is crucial in helping to plan interventions to prevent the development of that disorder or to prevent certain behavior patterns, such as aggression or suicide.
- PNI examines the relationship among the immune system; the nervous system; the endocrine system; and thoughts, emotions, and behavior.
- The gut microbiota is not only essential for maintaining metabolic and immune health, but also has a role in depression, anxiety, and other mental disorders. It appears that the bacteria can respond to and produce neurotransmitters.
- Chronobiology focuses on the study and measure of time structures or biologic rhythms occurring in the body and associates dysregulation of these cycles as contributing factors to the development of psychiatric disorders.
- Biologic markers are physical indicators of disturbances within the CNS that differentiate one disease process from another, such as biochemical changes or neuropathologic changes. These biologic markers can be measured by several methods of testing, including challenge tests, EEG, polysomnography, EPs, CT scanning, MRI, PET, and single-photon emission CT; the psychiatric nurse must be familiar with all these methods.

DEVELOPING CLINICAL JUDGMENT

1. A patient has experienced a "ministroke" with brain damage. Cognitive function continues to improve months after the stroke. The patient questions whether a stroke occurred. How would you approach patient teaching and counseling to explain the cognitive improvement after the stroke?
2. Your patient has "impaired executive functioning." Consider what would be a reasonable follow-up schedule for this patient for counseling sessions. Would it be reasonable to schedule visits at 1 PM weekly? Is the patient able to keep to this schedule? Why or why not?
3. Your patient is unable to sleep after watching an upsetting documentary. Identify the neurotransmitter activity that may be interfering with sleep. (Hint: fight or flight.)
4. For each of the following brain areas, describe what behavioral symptoms or issues may be present in a patient with dysfunction of that brain area.
   a. Basal ganglia
   b. Hippocampus
   c. Limbic system
   d. Thalamus
   e. Hypothalamus
   f. Frontal lobe
5. Identify the major neurotransmitters of the sympathetic and parasympathetic nervous systems.
6. Examine how a receptor's usual response to a neurotransmitter might change.
7. Discuss the significance of the gut–brain relationship.
8. Discuss how the fields of psychoneuroimmunology (PNI) and chronobiology overlap. What is the clinical significance?

REFERENCES

Bamalan, O. A., Moore, M. J., & Al Khalili, Y. (2023). Physiology, serotonin. In *StatPearls*. StatPearls Publishing. www.ncbi.nlm.nih.gov/books/NBK545168

Cao, Y., Ji, S., Chen, Y., Zhang, X., Ding, G., & Tang, F. (2023). Association between autoimmune diseases of the nervous system and schizophrenia: a systematic review and meta-analysis of cohort studies. *Comprehensive Psychiatry*, *122*, 152370. https://doi.org/10.1016/j.comppsych.2023.152370.

Casagrande, C. C., Rempe, M. P., Springer, S. D., & Wilson, T. W. (2023). Comprehensive review of task-based neuroimaging studies of cognitive deficits in Alzheimer's disease using electrophysiological methods. *Ageing Research Reviews*, *88*, 101950. https://doi.org/10.1016/j.arr.2023.101950

Chan, V. K. Y., Luo, H., Chan, S. S. M., Lau, C. S., Yeung, W. W. Y., Peng, K., Tong, X., Lam, M. P. S., Wong, I. C. K., & Li, X. (2023). Treatment-resistant depression and risk of autoimmune diseases: evidence from a population-based cohort and nested case-control study. *Translational Psychiatry*, *13*(1), 76. https://doi.org/10.1038/s41398-023-02383-9

Harlow, J. M. (1869). *Passage of an iron bar through the head.* David Clapp & Son.

Hill, M. D., Gill, S. S., Le-Niculescu, H., MacKie, O., Bhagar, R., Roseberry, K., Murray, O. K., Dainton, H. D., Wolf, S. K., Shekhar, A., Kurian, S. M., & Niculescu, A. B. (2024). Precision medicine for psychotic disorders: objective assessment, risk prediction, and pharmacogenomics. *Molecular Psychiatry*, *29*(5), 1528–1549. https://doi.org/10.1038/s41380-024-02433-8

Jameei, H., Rakesh, D., Zalesky, A., Cairns, M. J., Reay, W. R., Wray, N. R., & Di Biase, M. A. (2023). Linking polygenic risk of schizophrenia to variation in magnetic resonance imaging brain measures: a comprehensive systematic review. *Schizophrenia Bulletin*, 50(1), 32–46. https://doi.org/10.1093/schbul/sbad087

Kumar, A., Pramanik, J., Goyal, N., Chauhan, D., Sivamaruthi, B. S., Prajapati, B. G., & Chaiyasut, C. (2023). Gut microbiota in anxiety and depression: unveiling the relationships and management options. *Pharmaceuticals*, *16*(4), 565. https://doi.org/10.3390/ph16040565

Marano, G., Mazza, M., Lisci, F. M., Ciliberto, M., Traversi, G., Kotzalidis, G. D., De Berardis, D., Laterza, L., Sani, G., Gasbarrini, A., & Gaetani, E. (2023). The microbiota-gut-brain axis: psychoneuroimmunological insights. *Nutrients*, *15*(6), 1496. https://doi.org/10.3390/nu15061496

Nguyen, N. M., Cho, J., & Lee, C. (2023). Gut microbiota and Alzheimer's Disease: how to study and apply their relationship. *International Journal of Molecular Sciences*, *24*(4), 4047. https://doi.org/10.3390/ijms24044047

Nguyen, T. T., Baumann, P., Tüscher, O., Schick, S., & Endres, K. (2023). The aging enteric nervous system. *International Journal of Molecular Sciences*, *24*(11), 9471. https://doi.org/10.3390/ijms24119471

Peedicayil J. (2023). Genome–environment interactions and psychiatric disorders. *Biomedicines*, *11*(4), 1209. https://doi.org/10.3390/biomedicines11041209.

Rahman, M., & Bordoni, B. (2023). Histology, Natural killer cells. In *StatPearls*. StatPearls Publishing. https://www.ncbi.nlm.nih.gov/books/NBK565844/

Rogers, J. F., Vandendoren, M., Prather, J. F., Landen, J. G., Bedford, N. L., & Nelson, A. C. (2024). Neural cell-types and circuits linking thermoregulation and social behavior. *Neuroscience and Biobehavioral Reviews*, *161*, 105667. https://doi.org/10.1016/j.neubiorev.2024.105667

Rust, C., Malan-Muller, S., van den Heuvel, L. L., Tonge, D., Seedat, S., Pretorius, E., & Hemmings, S. M. J. (2023). Platelets bridging the gap between gut dysbiosis and neuroinflammation in stress-linked disorders: a narrative review. *Journal of Neuroimmunology*, *382*, 578155. https://doi.org/10.1016/j.jneuroim.2023.578155

Sam, C., & Bordoni, B. (2023). Physiology, Acetylcholine. In *StatPearls*. StatPearls Publishing. https://www.ncbi.nlm.nih.gov/books/NBK557825/

Xia, H., He, Q., & Chen, A. (2022). Understanding cognitive control in aging: a brain network perspective. *Frontiers in Aging Neuroscience*, *14*, 1038756. https://doi.org/10.3389/fnagi.2022.1038756

Yao, H., Zhang, D., Yu, H., Shen, H., Liu, H., Meng, F., Wu, X., Zhang, G., & Wang, X. (2023). The microbiota-gut-brain axis in pathogenesis of depression: a narrative review. *Physiology & Behavior*, *260*, 114056. https://doi.org/10.1016/j.physbeh.2022.114056

Zhang, Y., Chen, Y., Xin, Y., Peng, B., & Liu, S. (2023). Norepinephrine system at the interface of attention and reward. *Progress in Neuro-Psychopharmacology and Biological Psychiatry*, *125*, 110751. https://doi.org/10.1016/j.pnpbp.2023.110751

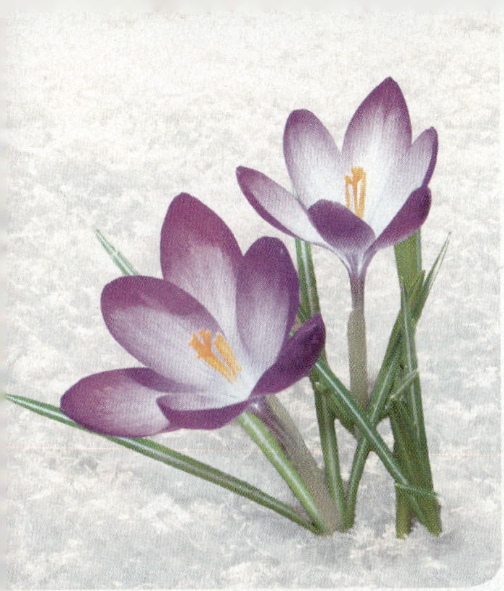

8 Recovery Framework for Psychiatric–Mental Health Nursing

Mary Ann Boyd

KEYCONCEPTS

- advocacy
- engagement
- hope
- peer support specialists
- person-centered care
- positive mental health
- psychoeducation
- recovery-oriented nursing care
- shared decision-making

LEARNING OBJECTIVES

After studying this chapter, you will be able to:

1. Identify major concepts underlying the recovery framework.
2. Delineate the phases of change according to the Transtheoretical Model.
3. Compare and contrast recovery-oriented interventions.
4. Identify the barriers to recovery from mental health issues.
5. Discuss the factors that contribute to a recovery-oriented environment.

KEY TERMS

• action • collaboration • contemplation • employment • empowerment • illness management and recovery program • informed choice model • insecure housing • instilling hope • integrated person-centered health service • maintenance • motivation • paternalistic model • poverty • precontemplation • preparation • relationship building • social inclusion • spiritual connections • stigma resilience • transtheoretical model • well-being

INTRODUCTION

The practice of psychiatric–mental health (PMH) nursing incorporates the whole person, not only active symptoms and treatment.

> **KEYCONCEPT Recovery-oriented nursing care** is a holistic approach characterized by collaborating with people with mental health issues and disorders to improve health and wellness, live a self-directed life, and strive to meet their full potential.

The overall goal of nursing care is to facilitate an individual's recovery. Chapter 2 discussed the concept of recovery and delineated the principles of recovery. This chapter explores recovery concepts, explains recovery interventions, identifies barriers, and covers approaches that promote societal support for recovery.

MENTAL HEALTH RECOVERY

Recovering from mental health disorders is not a new concept. In 1830, John Perceval, son of one of England's prime ministers, wrote of his personal recovery from schizophrenia despite the psychiatric treatment he received (Bateson, 1974). In the United States, the recovery model was initially applied only to the care of people with substance use issues. Recently, the recovery model application was expanded to all people with mental health issues. This change grew out of the consumer/survivor/ex-patient movement following the civil rights movement in the late 1960s (Vine, 2023). Today, recovery concepts and principles are embraced worldwide in the care and treatment of people with mental disorders.

Recovery involves achieving a balance between clinical and personal recovery. There are often differing views of mental health recovery between the individual with mental health issues and the clinician. The individual is often more focused on developing meaning in life and transforming an illness identity into a healthy one, whereas the clinician may want to focus on the reduction of symptoms, a return to preillness states, and a reduction or cessation of medication (Gyamfi et al., 2021). It is important that clinicians understand that the therapeutic relationship is collaborative and involves much more than symptom reduction. Building upon trust, the clinician acknowledges the negative impact of mental illness on self-esteem, builds a supportive relationship, listens to personal viewpoints, conveys the belief that recovery is possible, recognizes the individual's capacity for recovery, and promotes access to resources.

Positive Mental Health

Positive mental health is a useful concept when collaborating with a person in recovery.

> **KEYCONCEPT Positive mental health** is experiencing more desirable health-related quality-of-life events than undesirable ones (Velten et al., 2022).

Positive mental health can be viewed from different perspectives. A biologic perspective supports increasing serotonin and dopamine activity as an indicator of positive moods. A psychosocial–spiritual perspective supports spending less time in social isolation and more time in social activities, such as connecting with family or friends.

Positive mental health includes satisfying experiences with family, friends, and work. **Spiritual connections** to self, others, nature, and the transcendent (condition of moving beyond physical needs and realities) are associated with positive mental health (Michaelson et al., 2023). Feelings of well-being are important. **Well-being** comprises overall life satisfaction, as well as cognitive, emotional, social, spiritual, and moral growth and development. Self-acceptance, personal growth, purpose in life, autonomy, and positive relations with others contribute to positive mental health (Velten et al., 2022).

Person-Centered Care

One of the key concepts in recovery-oriented care is person-centered care. The individual is at the center of care—that is, the individual is actively involved in determining the best options for their health care circumstances and no longer passively receives a prescription for treatment of a disease. For people to participate in their care and make meaningful decisions, the individual must be educated about the disorder and treatment options and use collaboration skills to interact with the clinician.

> **KEYCONCEPT Person-centered care** is an approach to health care that is organized around health needs and expectations, rather than diseases (World Health Organization [WHO], 2022).

In person-centered care, the individual is actively engaged in planning interventions based upon personal strengths and needs. The plan, which reflects preferences and values, provides the structure in which the individual, in partnership with the clinician, can identify long- and short-term life goals and skills. The patient–clinician partnership plans and manages mental health and health care issues, provides an opportunity for collaborative and creative thinking, and serves as a tool for gauging progress toward goals. Research on this approach shows improved engagement in health care and medication adherence (Stanhope et al., 2021).

Person-centered care in nursing practice is built on a strong nurse–patient relationship. A solid therapeutic relationship can help reduce symptom severity and improve global function, community living skills, quality of life, and patient satisfaction with treatment (Wand et al., 2022). The therapeutic relationship and the care planning process are linked to each other, each influencing the other. A sense of connection based on caring, support, and continuity enables the individual to engage in behavior change needed to improve health and well-being (Cheng et al., 2021).

Health care systems oriented to the needs of people and communities are better prepared to respond to health crises.

An **integrated person-centered health service** provides equal access to quality health care for all people. This system of care empowers patients, fights health system fragmentation, and fosters greater coordination and collaboration with organizations. An integrated system is based on a continuum of care that provides health promotion, disease prevention, diagnosis, treatment, disease management, rehabilitation, and palliative care (WHO, 2022).

Empowerment

A related concept is **empowerment**, the process of supporting people and communities to take control of their own health needs with the goal of healthy behaviors, positive mental health, self-management of illnesses, and well-being (Peterson et al., 2021). Empowerment facilitates patient independence, self-management, and self-efficacy.

Empowerment can lead to better decision making and foster permanent changes in health. To feel empowered, the individual must have the knowledge and skill to manage a particular issue. By sharing health and mental health care information, patients can develop self-management skills. Empowerment and hope are enhanced through patient self-management. See Box 8.1.

BOX 8.1

Research for Evidence-Based Practice: Empowerment in Medication Adherence

Hsieh, W. L., Li, I. H., & Liu, W. I. (2023). Effects of empowerment-based illness management on the medication adherence and recovery of persons with schizophrenia: A systematic review and meta-analysis. International Journal of Mental Health Nursing, *32(4), 1008–1024. https://doi.org/10.1111/inm.13123*

THE QUESTION: What are the effects of specific intervention connotations of empowerment-based illness management on the medication adherence and recovery of people with schizophrenia?

METHODS: This study was a systematic review of empowerment interventions with people with schizophrenia according to the International Prospective Register of Systematic Reviews. Empowerment intervention was defined as having the elements of autonomy, competence, relationship, or motivation. Interventions focusing on only life management were excluded.

FINDINGS: From 1,006 articles, 8 randomized controlled trials (RCTs) with 859 participants were pooled for meta-analysis of medication adherence. Ten RCTs with 1,473 participants were pooled for meta-analysis of recovery. Empowerment-based illness management can improve medication adherence and recovery in people with schizophrenia with the overall effect being moderate. The empowerment interventions for medication adherence included inducing medication motivation, promoting self-medication management, and providing support resources. The empowerment interventions to promote recovery included using self-strength, connecting external forces, understanding personal needs, and overcoming self-stigma.

IMPLICATIONS FOR NURSING: Empowerment is important for medication adherence and recovery of people with schizophrenia. Nurses can operationalize empowerment strategies by focusing on increasing motivation to take medication, encouraging self-medication management, supporting individual strengths, encouraging connection with family and friends, and providing opportunities for patients to explore personal needs.

Engagement

Engaging an individual in mental health care is the first step in supporting recovery. The interaction between a clinician and an individual seeking help can set the tone and course of treatment. The first interaction can start the recovery journey, or it can leave the individual feeling hopeless and unwilling to return. Many people who seek mental health care drop out after their first or second visit. Engagement in treatment begins with trusting and respectful relationships with providers (National Alliance on Mental Illness [NAMI], 2016).

KEYCONCEPT Engagement is the strengths-based process through which individuals with mental health conditions form a healing connection with people that support their recovery and wellness within the context of family, culture, and community (NAMI, 2016).

Engagement is not adherence or compliance but a broader concept involving active participation from people who are seeking care and those who deliver care. Lack of effective engagement can result in serious consequences such as hospitalization, housing challenges, or even death.

Stigma and discrimination can prevent individuals from seeking help or engaging in a therapeutic relationship. Hospital policies and procedures requiring removal of personal items, locked doors, and sterile environments can magnify feelings of dehumanization and self-stigma. Preventing or treating self-stigma may be important in promoting active engagement (Chan & Tsui, 2023; Falgas-Bague et al., 2023).

Shared Decision-Making

Shared decision-making (SDM) is central in the recovery model; in this approach, the individual is an active participant, and decision making is shared. In SDM, clinician–patient communication and decision making differ from the following two types of models: a **paternalistic model**, in which the decisions are made by only the clinician and given to the patient, and the **informed choice model**, in which information is given to the patient and the patient makes the decision.

Because patients almost always view psychiatric hospitalization and treatment as unwanted, many people believe that having a mental disorder means a lifelong process of losing power and control over their lives, particularly if their treatment is not voluntary. In the paternalistic model, individuals can feel coerced into treatment and believe they have lost their ability to make decisions. However, empowering the patient to make the decision, as in the informed choice model, excludes clinician expertise and support, which may lead to poor choices.

KEYCONCEPT Shared decision-making is a "health communication process requiring at least two autonomous decision makers or advocates: a client, who draws on lived experience of mental health challenges and use of psychiatric services, and a provider, who is a knowledgeable and certified content expert for the decision at stake" (Zisman-Ilani et al., 2022).

SDM helps people make decisions about their care and treatment based on facts and recommendations provided by the clinician. It changes the power imbalance, where

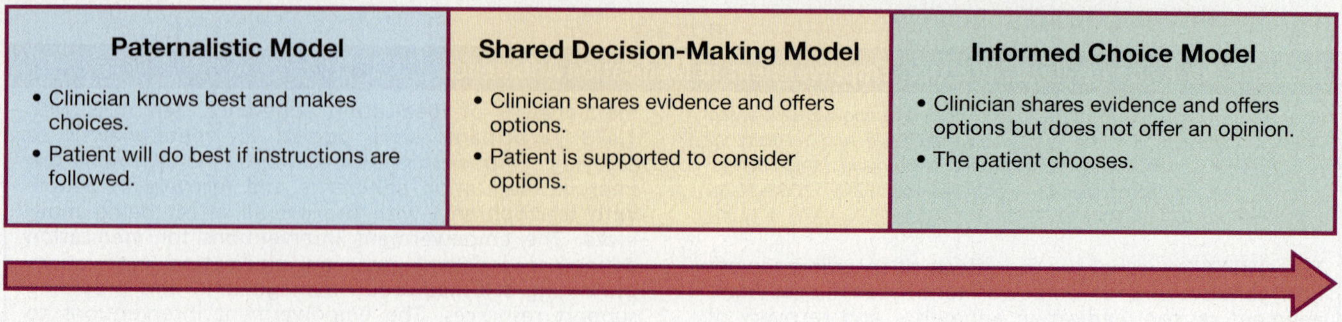

FIGURE 8.1 Continuum of decision making.

the clinician makes the decision, to shared decisions based on relevant information. SDM is *how* a decision is made, not *what* the final decision is (see Figure 8.1 for the continuum of decision making).

The advantages of SDM are reduced symptoms, improved self-esteem, increased service satisfaction, and improved treatment adherence. Other positive outcomes include improved patient knowledge, increased confidence in decision making, and more active patient involvement (Pearson et al., 2021).

STAGES OF CHANGE

Recovery is dependent on a change of thoughts, feelings, and behaviors. The **Transtheoretical Model** of health behavior change is often used as a guide in supporting people in their recovery. Developed in the 1980–1990s for smoking cessation (Prochaska & DiClemente, 1983), it was expanded to apply to other mental health issues, substance use disorders, and dysfunctional behaviors (Raihan & Cogburn, 2023). The model consists of a series of five steps toward change.

Precontemplation

The first stage of change is **precontemplation.** In this stage, there is limited or no awareness of the problem. The individual does not believe a problem exists. People often resist trying to change and are not motivated or are unwilling or unready to work toward change. Any benefits from changing is outweighed by negative consequences. For example, fear of losing friendships and social activities associated with unhealthy behaviors, such as using drugs, outweighs the benefits of changing to a healthier lifestyle. People may engage in treatment if pressured by family but will quickly return to former behaviors when the pressure is no longer present. People continue in the precontemplation stage until they can critically evaluate their behavior and gain insight into the significance of the issue.

Contemplation

The next stage of change is **contemplation.** In this stage, people begin to realize and acknowledge that there is a problem. There is no commitment to change, but they are amenable to receiving information and finding solutions to correct the problem.

Preparation

In the **preparation** stage, people easily acknowledge that there are problematic behaviors and can make a commitment to change. The advantages of changing behaviors outweigh the disadvantages of maintaining the behaviors. They will gather information from various sources and start to develop a plan. Gathering information is important for a successful plan. Once planning is completed, action usually occurs within 30 days.

Action

Change happens during the **action** phase. People gain confidence and they believe that they have the willpower to continue their journey. Overt behavior change occurs but relapse is a risk unless plans for potential triggers are established. Depending on the behavior change, this stage can last 6 months.

Maintenance

Continuing the behavior change is the focus of the **maintenance** stage. This stage may last from months to years. People become more confident in their ability to sustain the positive lifestyle changes and can resist temptations to return to previous behaviors. They can anticipate triggers and maintain their coping strategies.

If relapse occurs, it is not viewed as a failure. Instead, relapse is viewed as an opportunity to re-engage in the change process by re-evaluating triggers, reassessing motivation to change, and developing other contingency plans.

RECOVERY INTERVENTIONS

During the patient assessment, the astute nurse will listen for readiness to change. Based on the assessment, the nurse can tailor recovery interventions according to the patient's stage of readiness. For example, if the patient is in the precontemplation stage and is denying that drug use is a problem, focusing on relationship building and general discussion of the evidence about the drug use may be the best approach. If a patient is in the action phase, the nurse can help the patient evaluate the success of specific approaches.

The aim of every intervention is to support the journey of recovery. Effective interventions are based on the individual's needs, preparedness to engage, and stage of change. Along the way, specific interventions that focus on treating underlying illnesses place the individual in the best position to continue the recovery journey. Many of these interventions are discussed in later chapters. Successful outcomes of these interventions lead to engagement of other evidence-based strategies that support the journey (Sly et al., 2020; Solmi et al., 2023; Winsper et al., 2020).

Relationship Building

Recovery-oriented practice is based on **relationship building**, which is defined as building and maintaining therapeutic interpersonal relationships developed on trust, communication, and rapport. The relationship is framed through a recognition of the uniqueness of individuals and their families, and that well-being and positive mental health are ultimate goals. Focus on the mental illness and the patient's symptoms is only a part of recovery-oriented practice.

Specific relationship-building strategies include active listening to the patient and valuing the individual's perspective. It is important to convey the feeling of acceptance to the individual who may have values and beliefs different than the nurse. Through a nonjudgmental attitude, the nurse allows the patient to express feelings of vulnerability and hopelessness in a safe, interactive environment.

Instilling Hope

Hope, which is intrinsic to recovery, can be viewed as having energy for life and a sense of possibility (Murphy et al., 2023). Evidence shows that hope can decrease stress, anxiety, and depression. Hope is positively related to self-esteem, self-efficacy, spirituality, and well-being (Senger 2023).

> **KEYCONCEPT Hope** consists of goals or attainable targets, motivation or urge to pursue goals, and the ability to think of ways or pathways to pursue goals (Senger, 2023).

Instilling hope starts with the nurse projecting a hopeful, empathetic attitude. Verbally expressing confidence that the recovery is possible demonstrates belief in the patient. Instilling hope is shown in collaborating with the patient. **Collaboration** is identifying concrete, realistic goals that will foster a sense of control. Goals can be small steps to a larger goal. For example, a patient wants to get a job, but the first step is finishing high school. A smaller, realistic goal might be enquiring about the requirements for finishing high school.

Motivation improves the sense of hope for the future through increasing energy for life. A motivated individual has a sense of purpose. Motivation is developed collaboratively through encouragement and confidence that a goal is achievable. Defining several ways of achieving the goal improves the likelihood of success (Cheavens & Whitted, 2023).

Obstacles to developing a sense of hope include self-stigma and public stigma. In addition, perceived stigma from mental health clinicians can negatively impact personal recovery by reinforcing self-stigma and prompting disengagement from services (Chan & Tsui, 2023). Illness symptoms can also interfere with feeling hopeful. Strategies to counteract stigma and illness management approaches should be included among interventions used to instill hope. Group interventions are effective in instilling hope because of the interaction and social support received in this setting. Social support is important in counteracting the negative effects of stigma.

Illness Management and Recovery (IMR)

Illness Management and Recovery program is an evidence-based curriculum designed to provide people with mental illness the knowledge and skills to cope with their mental illness and achieve recovery goals. Mental health clinicians, including nurses, use psychoeducation (PE), behavioral techniques, relapse prevention training, and coping skills training to assist in symptom management and goal formulation. In this curriculum, people learn about mental illness and strategies for treatment, medication education, medication adherence, symptom management, relapse prevention, and social support network creation.

IMR toolkit consists of 10 booklets that leaders use in setting up an IMR mental health program. The toolkit includes instructions on setting up the IMR for administrators, training the frontline staff, and evaluating the program (SAMHSA, 2010). The program has shown to be effective for people with severe mental illness (Goh et al., 2023).

Psychoeducation

> **KEYCONCEPT Psychoeducation (PE)** is an individual, family, group, or community education intervention with systematic, structured, and didactic teaching–learning interaction that focuses on enhancing knowledge and skills related to a mental health and wellness through emotional support and motivation to enable individuals to recover from mental health issues and disorders and lead meaningful, productive lives.

PE is not a new idea in mental health care with its beginnings in the early 20th century and the deinstitutional movement of the 1950s and 1960s (see Chapter 1). As PE developed, it became recognized as a useful and effective approach in helping people with mental health issues actively participate in treatment. PE combines cognitive-behavioral, educational, and motivational approaches with the goal of providing the individual and family with knowledge about the disorder and treatment, and the skills to participate in treatment decisions.

PE is conducted by several mental health disciplines, including nurses, psychiatrists, social workers, psychologists, peer support specialists, and others. Not only does PE provide knowledge and competence about the disorder, but it also promotes insight into the disorders, promotes relapse prevention, and provides skills for crisis management and suicide prevention.

PE empowers the patient to collaborate in their treatment. The content should be understandable, and evidence based. Because giving information does not guarantee understanding, the leader should ask open-ended questions and continuously evaluate the learner's comprehension of the content. The PE sessions should be interactive with the leader using facilitation as well as other teaching skills. Most importantly, the sessions should be tailored to the individual needs of the learner (Magill et al., 2021).

Social Inclusion

Social inclusion, receiving social support, and participation in a family and community, is important in a successful recovery. Social inclusion is multidimensional with interrelated dimensions including employment or education, housing and neighborhood, and participation in social activities (Filia et al., 2022).

Employment and Education

Employment is one of the most important factors that impact mental health recovery. Employment gives individuals a sense of purpose and a reason to get up in the morning. Mental health issues, including functional impairment and psychosocial disability, frequently interfere with the ability to work, resulting in absences, interpersonal conflicts, and poor work performance. Symptoms of the illness, side effects of medications, stigma, poor social support, academic underachievement, and poor workplace environment are factors that contribute to difficulty in obtaining and maintaining employment. Individuals who quit work or are fired often find that it is difficult to regain employment.

Even when their symptoms are treated, they still may not be hired. Once employed, workers have the choice of disclosing their illness. Nondisclosure is widespread, but suppressing the information can affect productivity and eliminate access to employer-provided job accommodations. Research shows that disclosure is related to the probability of gainful employment. That is, employees evaluate the risks of disclosure based on their assessment of workplace culture and job security (Baldwin et al., 2023).

Lack of educational opportunities can lead to lack of skills or qualifications required for employment. Unrecognized learning disabilities can lead to mental health issues that culminate in dropping out of school prior to high school completion (Aro et al., 2024). Education and employment are important goals for people with mental illness. Employment improves mental health and reduces the overall cost of mental health care (Taubman & Parikh, 2023). Recovery-oriented care recognizes employment potential and provides social support for gaining meaningful employment. Factors that facilitate obtaining and maintaining employment include personal strengths, social support, accommodative work environment, disclosure, and support from mental health professionals and services (Noteboom et al., 2024).

Housing and Neighborhood

Housing is critical to recovery from mental and substance use disorders. Recovery-oriented care promotes safe, affordable, and permanent housing in the community, with access to benefits and services for individuals, families, and communities. In some instances, housing is sought after the mental disorder is treated and is in remission. In other instances, securing housing is a necessary first step to set the stage for strengthening coping skills and addressing the mental disorder.

Housing is more than a place to live. Housing within a safe neighborhood with low crime rates, grocery stores, and access to transportation is critical for a recovery. There should be opportunities to develop social relationships within the neighborhood environment.

Social Activities

The opportunity to engage in social activities results in several positive outcomes. When engaging in social activities, the individual is not alone in a room or apartment and can interact and connect with others. Social activities provide opportunities for the individual to grow and develop as a member of society. Within the context of social activities, social support from others can emerge (Filia et al., 2022).

Peer Support

Peer support is an integral component of the recovery model.

BOX 8.2

Core Competencies for Peer Workers in Behavioral Health Services

1. Engages peers in collaborative and caring relationships.
2. Provides support.
3. Shares lived experiences of recovery.
4. Personalizes peer support.
5. Supports recovery planning.
6. Links to resources, services, and supports.
7. Provides information about skills related to health, wellness, and recovery.
8. Helps peers to manage crises.
9. Values communication.
10. Supports collaboration and teamwork.
11. Promotes leadership and advocacy.
12. Promotes growth and development.

Reprinted from Substance Abuse and Mental Health Services Administration. (2015). Core competencies for peer workers in behavioral health services. https://www.samhsa.gov/sites/default/files/programs_campaigns/brss_tacs/core-competencies_508_12_13_18.pdf

KEYCONCEPT Peer support specialists (also called peer workers) are people who have been successful in their recovery who help others experiencing similar situations. These specialists are trained and certified to use their experiences to help others and work with the other mental health disciplines in recovery-oriented care. They have well-defined competencies (see Box 8.2).

Peer support specialists form voluntary relationships with patients based on mutual fit. Peer support specialists engage in a wide range of activities, including advocacy, linkage to resources, sharing of experiences, community and relationship building, group facilitation, skill-building mentoring, and goal setting. They also plan and develop groups, services, or activities, provide training, and administer programs. Because they can describe their mental health experiences and can explain their journey of recovery, they are especially well suited to educate the public and policymakers and can challenge negative stereotypes.

Research supports the effectiveness of peer support specialists in a variety of settings, including urban and rural areas (Wallis et al., 2023; Zeng & McNamara, 2021). For example, the Veterans Administration is using certified peer support specialists in remote, community-based clinics to support trauma-affected veterans in a group setting. The veterans can share their experiences involving service-related trauma and interpersonal violence in a supportive environment with other veterans and a peer specialist. In this setting, skills are taught to defuse violent thoughts and to prevent further violence (Chalker et al., 2024).

BARRIERS TO RECOVERY

Poverty

A major barrier in accessing recovery-oriented care is **poverty**. Individuals with schizophrenia are more likely than the general population to experience poverty and housing challenges. Poverty is associated with mental disorders such as depression (Rivera et al., 2023) and schizophrenia (Jester et al., 2023).

The lack of monetary resources is the primary definition of what it means to be poor (McAlpine & Alang, 2021). Without economic resources such as an income or savings, people are unable to fully participate in society. Individuals and families who meet a certain income threshold are eligible for government supplement, which is minimal and cannot meet basic needs. People with a disability such as a mental illness may qualify for additional support through Social Security Disability Insurance. Their ability to survive on this income will depend on the availability of other resources, such as support from family, friends, and neighbors, available social services, and cost of living (which varies depending on where people live).

Poverty can result in a lack of permanent housing, no transportation, and inability to pay for services. Access to health care in the United States is highly dependent on employment; many people with mental health issues are unemployed, resulting in lack of income and health insurance. People with mental illnesses are frequently reliant on public health care, but they may not be able to access services. Public mental health care often involves long wait times for appointments at inconvenient hours. Medications may not be affordable, and even if individuals are able to obtain them, they may have no place to store them. Interpersonal aspects of health care also play a role in people seeking mental health care. Individuals may perceive that they cannot talk to their provider or that their provider does not care about them (Torres Sanchez et al., 2022).

Housing Challenges

Insecure housing is a lack of a fixed, regular, and adequate nighttime residence, and it can be considered as either sheltered or unsheltered (see Chapter 41). Shelters provide temporary or transitional housing operated by public and private agencies for individuals and families who have no stable housing, including a hotel or motel paid for by government or charitable organization. People who are unsheltered live in places that are not ordinarily used for housing such as cars, parks, abandoned building, tents, and bus/train stations (National Alliance to End Homelessness, 2023).

Insecure housing is stressful and coping with it is challenging. Substance use can be an issue, and people who are unhoused are often victims of crime. The incidence of posttraumatic stress disorder among individuals who are unhoused may be higher than in the general population (Ayano et al., 2020). Among those who are unsheltered, women (both individuals and those in families) and people who identify as transgender, nonbinary, and questioning are especially in danger of being assaulted, abused, or raped. Individuals with mental illnesses who do not have a place to live fear being hospitalized or "locked up."

Stigma

Antistigma approaches have had a positive impact in reducing public stigma for people with mental illness (Corrigan & Nieweglowski, 2021) (see Chapter 2). Self-stigma is a barrier to recovery because individuals internalize the community's negative views of people with mental disorders. Self-stigma is associated with increased severity of symptoms of mental disorders. The challenge for nurses and other clinicians is to support **stigma resilience,** a personal trait that means the patient has the capacity to withstand or recover from significant challenges that threaten stability, viability, or development (Hofer et al., 2019; Mackali et al., 2023).

Lack of Services

Mental health services vary from state to state. Factors that contribute to whether people with mental health disorders can be treated include access to insurance, access to treatment, quality and cost of insurance, access to special education, and workforce availability. In the United States, 10.1% of adults with mental illness are uninsured, limiting access to services. The number of uninsured declined under the Affordable Care Act. The state prevalence of uninsured adults with mental illness ranges from 2.6% in Washington D.C. to 22.9% in Texas (Reinert et al., 2024).

More than 55% of adults with a mental health disorder receive no treatment in the United States (ranging from 40.6% in Montana to 69.1% in Hawaii [Reinert et al., 2022]). Twenty-eight percent of all adults with a mental illness report inability to receive needed services. There are several reasons for lack of treatment, including no insurance or limited coverage of services; shortage of psychiatrists, nurses, and other mental health professionals; and lack of treatment services such as inpatient treatment, individual therapy, and community services. In addition, there is a disconnect between primary care systems and mental health systems (Reinert et al., 2022).

Services for children and youth are even more sparse. Only 28% of youth with major depression receive some consistent treatment (7 to 25 visits per year). Most youth (57.3%) with severe depression do not receive any care. Prevalence of youth with depression who are untreated varies by state, with 77.1% in South Carolina and 32.6% in the District of Columbia untreated (Reinert et al., 2022).

Access to mental health care is very limited in rural areas. Health care providers are concentrated in urban areas, leaving rural counties without an adequate number of health care professionals. It is estimated that 1,600 counties in the United States do not have an accredited mental health provider. Farmers and their families need mental health support and treatment; stress among farm families is high, and they need to know how to manage the stress effectively (Newman et al., 2022). The use of telehealth has increased access to mental health service in rural areas (Watanabe et al., 2023).

SOCIETAL ROLE IN PROMOTING A RECOVERY-ORIENTED ENVIRONMENT

Advocacy

The World Health Organization recognized the need for mental health advocacy to promote the human rights of people with mental disorders and to reduce stigma and discrimination in a 2003 publication, *Advocacy for Mental Health* (WHO, 2003).

KEYCONCEPT Advocacy is various actions aimed at changing the major structural and attitudinal barriers to achieving positive mental health outcomes. It is an important means of raising awareness of mental health issues.

Mental health advocacy began when families of people with mental disorders made their voices heard and raised awareness of the needs and mistreatment of their loved ones. Individuals with the disorders joined their families to develop advocacy organizations to influence legislation and policy development. Today, many mental health workers and their organizations have joined the movement to advocate for the mental health needs, rights, and recovery of the general population.

The concept of advocacy includes several elements such as awareness raising; providing information, education, training, and counseling; and mutual help, mediating, defending, and denouncing. Through the advocacy movement, society's negative perception of people with mental disorders is being challenged and gradually replaced with more realistic, empathic perceptions.

Advocacy occurs at many levels. Individuals with mental disorders advocate for their own recovery. They are often motivated to contact advocacy groups in the hope that advocates will intervene on their behalf through effective communication with health care providers (Webster et al., 2021). They may contact the local advocacy service in their facility or a local community advocacy group such as *National Alliance on Mental Illness* or *Mental Health America*.

Advocacy groups and organizations play important roles in promoting national and international agendas. These groups develop databases with patient groups, families, and organizations. Establishing a regular flow of information with governmental decision-making groups and other organizations, they are instrumental in formulating and evaluating policy, plans, programs, legislation, and quality improvement standards. Other activities include establishing educational initiatives, conducting media activities, and organizing public events to raise awareness of mental health issues.

Removing Social, Economic, and Political Barriers

An important step in promoting a recovery-oriented environment is the reduction of stigma and stigmatizing messages. Education about mental health disorders and treatment is critical in reducing discrimination of people with mental disorders. National media organizations should use nonstigmatizing language in their publications.

Universal access to mental health services would help reduce the disparities between those who are insured and those who are not. More national mental health programs such as the National Suicide Hotline, a 24-hour crisis intervention hotline offering counseling and referral, would also be helpful.

Health care workers can play an important role in advocating for quality mental health care through participating in activities of patient and family groups. They can educate communities and support access to services.

RECOVERY-ORIENTED PSYCHIATRIC–MENTAL HEALTH NURSING PRACTICE

Recovery-oriented care is integral to the practice of PMH nursing and consistent with relationship-based care. PMH nurses develop collaborative partnerships with patients through therapeutic relationships. PMH nursing approaches are based on SDM. Interventions are determined by both the nurse and the patient.

As the care paradigm has shifted from nurse-directed care to recovery-oriented care with SDM, nurses can truly practice from a holistic perspective. Also, nurses are now able to engage peer support specialists in supporting patients through recovery.

SUMMARY OF KEY POINTS

- Mental health recovery is based on concepts of person-centered care, empowerment, SDM, employment, housing, and peer support.
- Positive mental health comprises overall life satisfaction and includes cognitive, emotional, social spiritual, and moral growth and development.
- Person-centered care places the individual in the center of the care process. The individual becomes a partner to the clinician and together they decide the best approach based on people circumstances. The care approach is individualized; one individual's care plan will look different from another.
- Empowering the patient to engage in the care process requires that the individual is educated on health and mental health issues and approaches. The individual must have the knowledge and skills to engage in a meaningful collaborative process.
- Engagement of an individual in mental health care is the first step toward recovery.
- In SDM, the patient is an active participant in the decision. The advantages of SDM include reduced symptoms, improved self-esteem, increased service satisfaction, and improved treatment adherence.
- The Transtheoretical Model of health behavior change guides the journey of recovery and includes precontemplation, contemplation, preparation, action, and maintenance phases. Clinician interaction is adapted to support the patient in each phase.
- Relationship building and instilling hope are key interventions in support recovery. Other intervention that may be used is the IMR.
- Employment is a goal of recovery. In some instances, supportive employment will be needed to accommodate disabilities.
- Housing is critical to recovery. There are several types of housing arrangements such as independent, transitional, and supportive.
- Peer support is an integral component of recovery. Peer support specialists are new members of the mental health team who are recovering from mental health issues. These individuals use their experiences to help others.
- Barriers to recovery include poverty, housing challenges, stigma, and lack of services. Advocacy plays an important role in promoting a recovery-oriented environment and seeks to remove social, economic, and political barriers.
- Recovery-oriented PMH nursing practice is based on developing collaborative partnerships with patients using the therapeutic relationship.

DEVELOPING CLINICAL JUDGMENT

1. Compare a traditional medical approach to care with recovery-oriented care.
2. You are asked by the provider to educate the patient about schizophrenia. The patient states, "I'm not interested in treatment. There is nothing wrong

with me." What phase of change does this statement demonstrate? How would you approach the patient?

3. A psychiatric nurse is teaching a patient about the benefits of exercise. The patient questions why a psychiatric nurse would be concerned with exercise. What should the nurse tell the patient?
4. A patient is feeling hopeless and expresses feelings of failure. What recovery-oriented interventions would be appropriate to use?
5. What factors might interfere with the ability of the individual who has a mental illness to participate in treatment?

MOVIES, TV, OR STREAMING PROGRAMS

Recovery Boys: **2018.** This documentary follows the recovery journey of four residents (Jeff, Rush, Adam, and Ryan) who had substance use issues and sought treatment at Jacob's Ladder at Brookside Farm in West Virginia, which is operated by psychiatrist Kevin Blankenship. This documentary shows the reality of substance use disorders and the hard work of recovery. While humanizing substance use disorder, the movie highlights the many challenges in sustaining recovery.

Viewing Points:

1. The documentary demonstrates the importance of approaching recovery from a holistic perspective. Identify the recovery interventions used that focused on health.
2. Describe instances of self-stigma and efforts directed toward developing stigma resilience.
3. What role did employment play in sustaining or destroying attempts at recovery?
4. What role did "instilling hope" play in their recovery journeys?

REFERENCES

Aro, T., Özbek, A. B., & Torppa, M. (2024). Predicting adult-age mental health with childhood reading and math disability: do resilience and coping styles matter? *Annals of dyslexia*, 74(1), 97–122. https://doi.org/10.1007/s11881-023-00290-8

Ayano, G., Solomon, M., Tsegay, L., Yohannes, K., & Abraha, M. (2020). A systematic review and meta-analysis of the prevalence of post-traumatic stress disorder among homeless people. *The Psychiatric Quarterly*, *91*(4), 949–963. https://doi.org/10.1007/s11126-020-09746-1

Baldwin, M. L., DeSerpa, A. C., & Marcus, S. C. (2023). Workplace disclosure of serious mental illness and gainful employment: Theory and evidence. *The Journal of Mental Health Policy and Economics*, *26*(1), 3–17.

Bateson, G. (Ed.) (1974). *Perceval's narrative: A patient's account of his psychosis* (pp. 1830–1832). William Morrow & Company.

Brown, C. E., Marshall, A. R., Snyder, C. R., Cueva, K. L., Pytel, C. C., Jackson, S. Y., Golden, S. H., Campelia, G. D., Horne, D. J., Doll, K. M., Curtis, J. R., & Young, B. A. (2023). Perspectives about racism and patient-clinician communication among black adults with serious illness. *Journal of the American Medical Association Network Open*, *6*(7), e2321746. https://doi.org/10.1001/jamanetworkopen.2023.21746.

Chalker, S. A., Serafez, J., Imai, Y., Stinchcomb, J., Mendez, E., Depp, C. A., Twamley, E. W., Fortuna, K. L., Goodman, M., & Chinman, M. (2024). Suicide prevention by peers offering recovery tactics (SUPPORT) for US veterans with serious mental illness: Community engagement approach. *Journal of Participatory Medicine*, *16*, e56204. https://doi.org/10.2196/56204

Chan, K. K. S., & Tsui, J. K. C. (2023). Perceived stigma from mental health service providers and its adverse impact on service engagement and recovery among people with mental illness. *The American Journal of Orthopsychiatry*, *93*(5), 365–374. https://doi.org/10.1037/ort0000680

Cheng, A. W., Nakash, O., Cruz-Gonzalez, M., Fillbrunn, M. K., & Alegría, M. (2021). The association between patient-provider racial/ethnic concordance, working alliance, and length of treatment in behavioral health settings. *Psychological Services*, *20*(Suppl 1), 145–156. https://doi.org/10.1037/ser0000582

Cheavens, J. S., & Whitted, W. M. (2023). Hope therapy. *Current Opinion in Psychology*, *49*, 101509. https://doi.org/10.1016/j.copsyc.2022.101509

Corrigan, P. W., & Nieweglowski, K. (2021). Difference as an indicator of the self-stigma of mental illness. *Journal of Mental Health*, *30*(4), 417–423. https://doi.org/10.1080/09638237.2019.1581351

Falgas-Bague, I., Zhen-Duan, J., Ferreira, C., Tahanasab, S. A., Cuervo-Torello, F., Fukuda, M., Markle, S. L., & Alegría, M. (2023). Uncovering barriers to engagement in substance use disorder care for Medicaid enrollees. *Psychiatric Services*, *74*(11), 1116–1122. https://doi.org/10.1176/appi.ps.20220193

Filia, K., Menssink, J., Gao, C. X., Rickwood, D., Hamilton, M., Hetrick, S. E., Parker, A. G., Herrman, H., Hickie, I., Sharmin, S., McGorry, P. D., & Cotton, S. M. (2022). Social inclusion, intersectionality, and profiles of vulnerable groups of young people seeking mental health support. *Social Psychiatry and Psychiatric Epidemiology*, *57*(2), 245–254. https://doi.org/10.1007/s00127-021-02123-8

Goh, Y. S. S., Ow Yong, J. Q. Y., & Li, A. Z. (2023). Effectiveness of Illness Management and Recovery program on people with severe mental illnesses: A systematic review and meta-analysis. *Frontiers in Psychiatry*, *14*, 1162288. https://doi.org/10.3389/fpsyt.2023.1162288

Gyamfi, N., Bhullar, N., Islam, M. S., & Usher, K. (2021). A systematic review of measures assessing mental health professionals' perspectives of recovery. *International Journal of Mental Health Nursing*, *30*(4), 847–874. https://doi.org/10.1111/inm.12895

Hofer, A., Post, F., Pardeller, S., Frajo-Apor, B., Hoertnagl, C. M., Kemmler, G., & Fleischhacker, W. W. (2019). Self-stigma versus stigma resistance in schizophrenia: associations with resilience, premorbid adjustment, and clinical symptoms. *Psychiatry Research*, *271*, 396–401.

Jester, D. J., Thomas, M. L., Sturm, E. T., Harvey, P. D., Keshavan, M., Davis, B. J., Saxena, S., Tampi, R., Leutwyler, H., Compton, M. T., Palmer, B. W., & Jeste, D. V. (2023). Review of major social determinants of health in schizophrenia-spectrum psychotic disorders: I. Clinical outcomes. *Schizophrenia Bulletin*, *49*(4), 837–850. https://doi.org/10.1093/schbul/sbad023

Mackali, Z., Çetinkaya, S., & Ay, N. (2023). The mediating role of self-compassion in the relationship between internalized stigma and psychological resilience in bipolar disorder. *Psychology and Psychotherapy*, *96*(4), 952–966. https://doi.org/10.1111/papt.12488

Magill, M., Martino, S., & Wampold, B. (2021). The principles and practices of psychoeducation with alcohol or other drug use disorders: A review and brief guide. *Journal of Substance Abuse Treatment*, *126*, 108442. https://doi.org/10.1016/j.jsat.2021.108442

McAlpine, D. D., & Alang, S. M. (2021). Employment and economic outcomes of persons with mental illness and disability: The impact of the Great Recession in the United States. *Psychiatric Rehabilitation Journal*, *44*(2), 132–141. https://doi.org/10.1037/prj0000458

Michaelson, V., Šmigelskas, K., King, N., Inchley, J., Malinowska-Cieślik, M., Pickett, W., & HBSC Spiritual Health Writing Group (2023). Domains of spirituality and their importance to the health of 75 533 adolescents in 12 countries. *Health Promotion International*, *38*(3), daab185. https://doi.org/10.1093/heapro/daab185

Murphy, J., Mulcahy, H., Mahony, J. O., & Bradley, S. (2023). Exploring individuals' experiences of hope in mental health recovery: An interpretative phenomenological analysis. *Journal of Psychiatric and Mental Health Nursing*, *30*(1), 101–109. https://doi.org/10.1111/jpm.12833

National Alliance on Mental Illness. (2016). Engagement: A new standard for mental health care. Retrieved July 16, 2024, from https://www.nami.org/Support-Education/Publications-Reports/Public-Policy-Reports/Engagement-A-New-Standard-for-Mental-Health-Care/NAMI_Engagement_Web#:~:text=Engagement%20is%20the%20strengths%2Dbased,of%20family%2C%20culture%20and%20community

National Alliance to End Homelessness. (2023). *State of homelessness: 2023 Edition*. Homelessness Research Institute. Retrieved September 11, 2023, from https://endhomelessness.org/homelessness-in-america/homelessness-statistics/state-of-homelessness/#key-facts

Newman, M. W., Hawrilenko, M., Jakupcak, M., Chen, S., & Fortney, J. C. (2022). Access and attitudinal barriers to engagement in integrated primary care mental health treatment for rural populations. *The Journal of Rural Health*, *38*(4), 721–727. https://doi.org/10.1111/jrh.12616

Noteboom, Y., van Nassau, F., Bosma, A. R., van der Hijden, E. J. E., Huysmans, M. A., & Anema, J. R. (2024). A roadmap for sustainable implementation of vocational rehabilitation for people with mental disorders and its outcomes: A qualitative evaluation. *International Journal of Mental Health Systems*, *18*(1), 7. https://doi.org/10.1186/s13033-023-00620-8

Pearson, M., Sibson, T., & Carter, T. (2021). A qualitative study of service users' experiences of mental health nurses' knowledge and skills in relation to medication. *Journal of Psychiatric and Mental Health Nursing*, *28*(4), 682–691. https://doi.org/10.1111/jpm.12718

Peterson, N. A., Lardier, D. T., Powell, K. G., Mankopf, E., Rashid, M., Morton, C. M., & Borys, S. (2021). Psychometric properties of a recovery empowerment scale: testing emotional, cognitive, behavioral, and relational domains. *Journal of Community Psychology*, *49*(7), 2874–2891. https://doi.org/10.1002/jcop.22592

Prochaska, J. O., & DiClemente, C. C. (1983). Stages and processes of self-change of smoking: Toward an integrative model of change. *Journal of Consulting and Clinical Psychology*, *51*(3), 390–395. https://doi.org/10.1037//0022-006x.51.3.390.

Raihan, N., & Cogburn, M. (2023). Stages of change theory. In *StatPearls*. StatPearls Publishing. NCBI Bookshelf (nih.gov).

Reinert, M. Fritze, D. & Nguyen, T. (2022). The state of mental health in American 2023. Mental Health America, Alexandria VA. https://mhanational.org/research/state-of-mental-health-in-america-2023/

Reinert, M, Fritze, D & Nguyen, T. (2024). The state of mental health in America 2024." Mental Health America, Alexandria VA. https://mhanational.org/wp-content/uploads/2024/12/2024-State-of-Mental-Health-in-America-Report.pdf

Rivera, R., Capers, T., Chandler, M., Matthews, E., Rzewinski, J., Rees, J., Israel, S., & Lushin, V. (2023). Socioeconomic stability buffers racial discrimination effect on depression in a marginalized community. *Journal of Racial and Ethnic Health Disparities*, *10*(1), 130–140. https://doi.org/10.1007/s40615-021-01203-4

Senger, A. R. (2023). Hope's relationship with resilience and mental health during the COVID-19 pandemic. *Current Opinion in Psychology*, *50*, 101559. https://doi.org/10.1016/j.copsyc.2023.101559

Sly, K. A., Lewin, T. J., Frost, B. G., Tirupati, S., Turrell, M., & Conrad, A. M. (2020). Care pathways, engagement and outcomes associated with a recovery-oriented intermediate stay mental health program. *Psychiatry Research*, *286*, 112889. https://doi.org/10.1016/j.psychres.2020.112889

Solmi, M., Cortese, S., Vita, G., De Prisco, M., Radua, J., Dragioti, E., Köhler-Forsberg, O., Madsen, N. M., Rohde, C., Eudave, L., Aymerich, C., Pedruzo, B., Rodriguez, V., Rosson, S., Sabé, M., Hojlund, M., Catalan, A., de Luca, B., Fornaro, M., … Correll, C. U. (2023). An umbrella review of candidate predictors of response, remission, recovery, and relapse across mental disorders. *Molecular psychiatry*, *28*(9), 3671–3687. https://doi.org/10.1038/s41380-023-02298-3

Stanhope, V., Choy-Brown, M., Williams, N., & Marcus, S. C. (2021). Implementing person-centered care planning: A randomized controlled trial. *Psychiatric Services*, 72(6), 641–646. https://doi.org/10.1176/appi.ps.202000361

Substance Abuse and Mental Health Services Administration (SAMHSA). (2010). *Illness management and recovery evidence-based practices (EBP) kit*. Retrieved July 16, 2024, from https://store.samhsa.gov/product/Illness-Management-and-Recovery-Evidence-Based-Practices-EBP-KIT/SMA09-4462

Substance Abuse and Mental Health Services Administration (SAMHSA). (2015). *Core competencies for peer workers in behavioral health services*. Retrieved July 16, 2024, from https://www.samhsa.gov/sites/default/files/programs_campaigns/brss_tacs/core-competencies_508_12_13_18.pdf

Taubman, D. S., & Parikh, S. V. (2023). Understanding and addressing mental health disorders: A workplace imperative. *Current Psychiatry Reports*, *25*(10), 455–463. https://doi.org/10.1007/s11920-023-01443-7

Torres Sanchez, A., Park, A. L., Chu, W., Letamendi, A., Stanick, C., Regan, J., Perez, G., Manners, D., Oh, G., & Chorpita, B. F. (2022). Supporting the mental health needs of underserved communities: A qualitative study of barriers to accessing community resources. *Journal of Community Psychology*, *50*(1), 541–552. https://doi.org/10.1002/jcop.22633

Velten, J., Brailovskaia, J., & Margraf, J. (2022). Positive Mental Health Scale: validation and measurement invariance across eight countries, genders, and age groups. *Psychological Assessment*, *34*(4), 332–340. https://doi.org/10.1037/pas0001094

Vine, P. (2023). *Fighting for recovery*. Beacon Press.

Wallis, R., Signorelli, M., Linn, H., Bias, T., Allen, L., & Davis, S. M. (2023). Lessons learned from employing Medicaid-funded peer recovery support specialists in residential substance use treatment settings: An exploratory analysis. *Journal of Substance Use and Addiction Treatment*, *154*, 209136. https://doi.org/10.1016/j.josat.2023.209136

Wand, T., Glover, S., & Paul, D. (2022). What should be the future focus of mental health nursing? Exploring the perspectives of mental health nurses, consumers, and allied health staff. *International Journal of Mental Health Nursing*, *31*(1), 179–188. https://doi.org/10.1111/inm.12947

Watanabe, J., Teraura, H., Nakamura, A., & Kotani, K. (2023). Telemental health in rural areas: A systematic review. *Journal of Rural Medicine*, *18*(2), 50–54. https://doi.org/10.2185/jrm.2022-059

Webster, D., Willey, A., & Seldomridge, L. A. (2021). Advocacy, collaboration, and conflict management: Teaching core skill sets in mental health nursing. *Journal of Psychosocial Nursing and Mental Health Services*, *59*(9), 26–29. https://doi.org/10.3928/02793695-20210427-01

Winsper, C., Crawford-Docherty, A., Weich, S., Fenton, S. J., & Singh, S. P. (2020). How do recovery-oriented interventions contribute to personal mental health recovery? A systematic review and logic model. *Clinical Psychology Review*, *76*, 101815. https://doi.org/10.1016/j.cpr.2020.101815

World Health Organization. (2003). *Advocacy for mental health*. World Health Organization (Mental Health Policy and Service Guidance Package). https://www.who.int/mental_health/policy/services/essentialpackage1v7/en/

World Health Organization. (2022). *Integrated people-centred care*. https://www.who.int/health-topics/integrated-people-centered-care#tab=tab_1

Zeng, G., & McNamara, B. (2021). Strategies used to support peer provision in mental health: A scoping review. *Administration and Policy in Mental Health*, *48*(6), 1034–1045. https://doi.org/10.1007/s10488-021-01118-6

Zisman-Ilani, Y., & Byrne, L. (2022). Shared decision making and peer support: New directions for research and practice. *Psychiatric Services*, 74(4), 427–428.

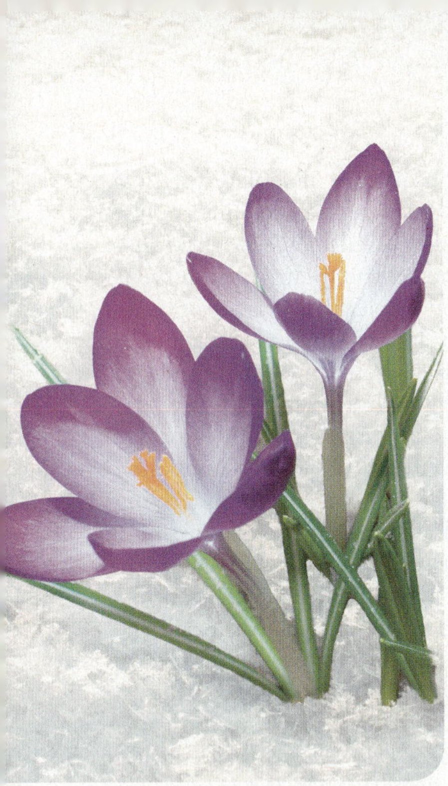

UNIT III

Contemporary Psychiatric Nursing Practice

9 Communication and the Therapeutic Relationship

Cheryl Forchuk and Rebecca Luebbert

KEYCONCEPTS

- nurse–patient relationship
- self-awareness
- therapeutic communication

LEARNING OBJECTIVES

After studying this chapter, you will be able to:

1. Identify the importance of self-awareness in nursing practice.
2. Demonstrate the appropriate use of verbal and nonverbal communication skills.
3. Distinguish between active and passive listening.
4. Incorporate therapeutic communication strategies when working with patients.
5. Identify common barriers to therapeutic communication.
6. Explain how the nurse can establish a therapeutic relationship with patients by using rapport and empathy.
7. Understand the physical, emotional, and social boundaries of the nurse–patient relationship.
8. Appreciate the significance of adaptive and maladaptive defense mechanisms.
9. Explain what occurs in each of the three phases of the nurse–patient relationship: orientation, working, and resolution.
10. Describe what characterizes a nontherapeutic or deteriorating nurse–patient relationship.

KEY TERMS

• active listening • boundaries • communication blocks • content themes • countertransference • defense mechanisms • deteriorating relationship • empathic linkages • empathy • introspective • motivational interviewing • nontherapeutic relationship • nonverbal communication • orientation phase • passive listening • process recording • rapport • resolution phase • self-disclosure • strength-based communication • symbolism • transference • verbal communication • working phase

INTRODUCTION

Patients with psychiatric disorders have special communication needs that require advanced therapeutic communication skills. In psychiatric nursing, the nurse–patient relationship is an important tool used to reach treatment goals. The purpose of this chapter is to help the nurse (1) develop self-awareness and communication techniques needed for a therapeutic nurse–patient relationship, (2) examine the specific stages or steps involved in establishing the relationship, (3) explore the specific factors that make a nurse–patient relationship successful and therapeutic, (4) differentiate therapeutic from nontherapeutic relationships, and (5) recognize the significance and impact of a patient's use of **defense mechanisms**.

SELF-AWARENESS

Self-awareness is the process of understanding one's own beliefs, thoughts, motivations, biases, and limitations and recognizing how they affect others. Without self-awareness, nurses will find it impossible to establish and maintain therapeutic relationships with patients. "Know thyself" is a basic tenet of psychiatric–mental health nursing (Box 9.1).

A well-developed sense of self-awareness can only come after nurses carry out self-examination. Self-awareness requires a willingness to be **introspective** and to examine one's own personal beliefs, attitudes, and motivations. Although this process may be uncomfortable and time consuming, this objective examination is an essential exercise for a professional nurse. Self-examination should be an ongoing process and involves reflecting on the personal meaning of the current situation. This reflection can relate to the nurse's past situations and issues related to their own personal values. Self-examination without the benefit of another's perspective might lead to a biased view of self. Therefore, conducting self-examinations with a trusted individual who can give objective, but realistic, feedback is best.

KEYCONCEPT Self-awareness is the process of understanding one's own beliefs, thoughts, motivations, biases, and limitations and recognizing how they affect others.

Know Thyself

Each nurse brings an identity, a *sense of self*, to their nursing practice that includes biologic, psychological, experiential, and social influences. The patient perceives the biologic dimension of the nurse in terms of physical characteristics such as age, gender, body weight, height, and ethnicity. Additionally, the nurse's response to a patient can be influenced by unobservable personal physical characteristics, such as an existing chronic illness. The nurse's psychological state also influences how they analyzes patient information and selects treatment interventions. An emotional state or behavior can inadvertently influence the therapeutic relationship. For example, a nurse who has just learned that their child is using illegal drugs and who has a patient with a history of drug use may inadvertently project a judgmental attitude toward the patient, which would interfere with therapeutic communication. The nurse needs to examine underlying emotions, motivations, and beliefs and determine how these factors shape behavior (Bhugra et al., 2023).

BOX 9.1

"Know Thyself"

- What physical issues or illnesses have you experienced?
- What significant traumatic life events (e.g., divorce, death of a significant person, abuse, disaster) have you experienced?
- What prejudiced or embarrassing beliefs and attitudes about groups different from yours can you identify from your family, significant others, and yourself?
- Which sociocultural factors in your background could contribute to your being rejected by members of other cultures?
- How would the above experiences affect your ability to care for patients?

The nurse's social biases can be particularly problematic for the nurse–patient relationship. Although the nurse may not verbalize these values to patients, some are readily evident in the nurse's behavior and appearance. A patient may perceive biases in the nurse because of how the nurse acts or appears at work. Other sociocultural values may not be immediately obvious to the patient; for example, the nurse's religious or spiritual beliefs or feelings about death, divorce, abortion, or sexual orientation. These beliefs and thoughts can influence how the nurse interacts with a patient who is dealing with such issues. Similarly, how one's cultural beliefs and patterns of communicating conform to or confront cultural norms may influence the emerging relationship.

Understanding Personal Feelings and Beliefs and Changing Behavior

Nurses must understand their own personal feelings and beliefs and try to avoid projecting them onto patients. Nurses who are not self-aware cannot recognize the effect their communication or behavior can have on others (Wright, 2021). The development of self-awareness will enhance the nurse's objectivity and foster a nonjudgmental attitude, which is so important for building and maintaining trust throughout the nurse–patient interaction. Soliciting feedback from colleagues and supervisors about how personal beliefs or thoughts are being projected onto others is a useful self-assessment technique. One of the reasons that ongoing clinical supervision is so important is that the supervisor really knows the nurse and can continually support positive interactions, observe for inappropriate communication, and question assumptions that the nurse may hold. Clinical supervision is different from administrative supervision in that the focus is on supporting the growth of the nurse and does not generally involve an administrative or reporting relationship.

After a nurse has identified and analyzed their personal beliefs and attitudes, behaviors that were driven by prejudicial ideas may change. The change process requires introspective analysis that may result in viewing the world differently. Through self-awareness and conscious effort, the nurse can change learned behaviors to engage effectively in therapeutic communication with patients. Nevertheless, sometimes a nurse realizes that some attitudes are too ingrained to support an effective interaction with a patient with different beliefs. In such cases, the nurse should refer the patient to someone with whom the patient is more likely to develop a successful therapeutic relationship.

EFFECTIVE COMMUNICATION

Effective communication, including verbal and nonverbal techniques, is a building block for all successful relationships. The nurse–patient relationship is built on therapeutic communication, the ongoing process of interaction through which meaning emerges (Box 9.2). **Verbal communication**, which is principally achieved by spoken words, includes the underlying emotion, context, and connotation of what is said. **Nonverbal communication** includes gestures, expressions, and body language. Both the patient and the nurse use verbal and nonverbal communication. To respond therapeutically in a nurse–patient relationship, the nurse is responsible for assessing and interpreting all forms of patient communication.

NCLEXNOTE In analyzing patient–nurse communication, nonverbal behaviors and gestures are communicated first. If a patient's verbal and nonverbal communications are contradictory, priority should be given to the nonverbal behavior and gestures.

Verbal Communication

The process of verbal communication involves a sender, a message, and a receiver. The patient is often the sender,

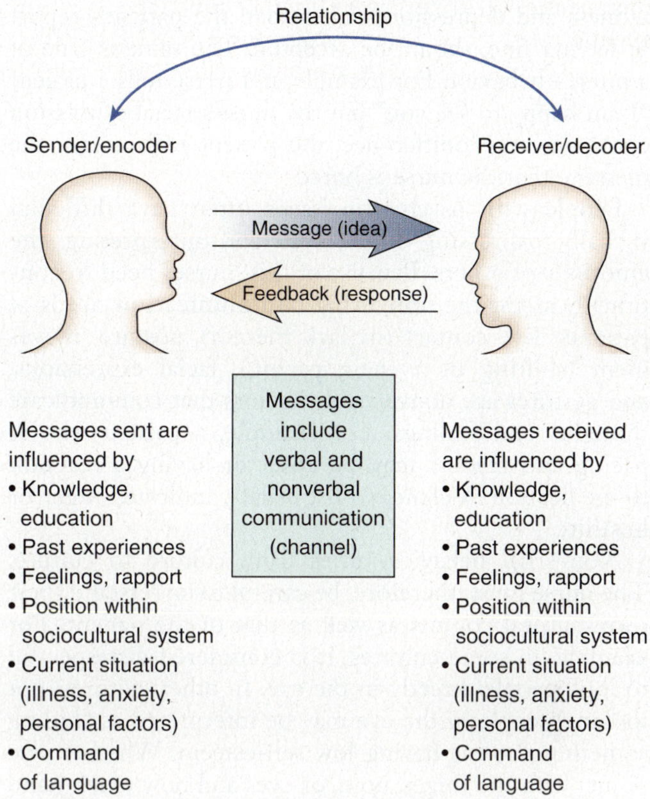

FIGURE 9.1 The communication process. (Reprinted with permission from Rosdahl, C. [2022]. *Rosdahl's textbook of basic nursing* [12th ed., Fig. 44-2]. Wolters Kluwer.)

and the nurse is often the receiver, but communication is always two ways (Fig. 9.1). The patient formulates an idea, encodes that message (puts ideas into words), and then transmits the message with emotion. The patient's words and their underlying emotional tone and connotation communicate the individual's needs and emotional issues. The nurse receives the message, decodes it (interprets the message, including its feelings, connotation, and context), and then responds to the patient.

On the surface, this interaction is deceptively simple; unseen complexities lie beneath. Is the message the nurse receives consistent with the patient's original idea? Did the nurse interpret the message as the patient intended? Is the verbal message consistent with the nonverbal flourishes that accompany it? Validation is essential to ensure that the nurse has received the information accurately.

BOX 9.2

Principles of Therapeutic Communication

- The patient should be the primary focus of the interaction.
- A professional attitude sets the tone of the therapeutic relationship.
- Use self-disclosure cautiously and only when the disclosure has a therapeutic purpose.
- Avoid social relationships with patients.
- Maintain patient confidentiality.
- Assess the patient's intellectual competence to determine the level of understanding.
- Implement interventions from a theoretic base.
- Maintain a nonjudgmental attitude. Avoid making judgments about the patient's behavior.
- Avoid giving advice. By the time the patient sees the nurse, they have had plenty of advice.
- Guide the patient to reinterpret their experiences rationally.
- Track the patient's verbal interaction by clarifying statements.
- Avoid changing the subject unless the content change is in the patient's best interest.

Nonverbal Communication

Gestures, facial expressions, and body language communicate more than verbal messages. Under the best circumstances, body language mirrors or enhances what is verbally communicated. However, if verbal and nonverbal messages conflict, the listener should rely on the nonverbal message. For example, if a patient says that they feel fine but has a sad facial expression and is slumped in a chair away from others, the message of sadness and depression, rather than the patient's report of feeling fine, should be accepted. The same is true of a nurse's behavior. For example, if a nurse tells a patient "I am happy to see you" but the nurse's facial expression communicates indifference, the patient will receive the message that the nurse is bored.

People with psychiatric issues often have difficulty verbally expressing themselves and interpreting the emotions of others. Because of this, nurses need to continually assess the **nonverbal communication** needs of patients. Eye contact (or lack thereof), posture, movement (shifting in a chair, pacing), facial expressions, and gestures are nonverbal behaviors that communicate thoughts and feelings. For example, a patient who is pacing and restless may be upset or having a reaction to medication. A clenched fist usually indicates anger or hostility.

Nonverbal behavior varies from culture to culture. The nurse must, therefore, be careful to understand their own cultural context as well as that of the patient. For example, in some cultures, it is considered disrespectful to look people directly in the eye. In other cultures, not looking people in the eye may be interpreted as "hiding something" or as having low self-esteem. Whether one points with the finger, nose, or eyes and how much hand gesturing is used are other examples of nonverbal communication that may vary considerably among cultures. The nurse needs to be aware of cultural differences in communication in the context of each relationship and may need to consult with a cultural interpreter or use other learning opportunities to ensure that their communication is culturally congruent.

Nurses should use positive body language, such as sitting at the same eye level as the patient with a relaxed posture that projects interest and attention. Leaning slightly forward helps engage the patient. Generally, the nurse should not cross their arms or legs during therapeutic communication because such postures pose a barrier to interaction. Uncrossed arms and legs project openness and a willingness to engage in conversation (Fig. 9.2). Any verbal message should be consistent with nonverbal messages.

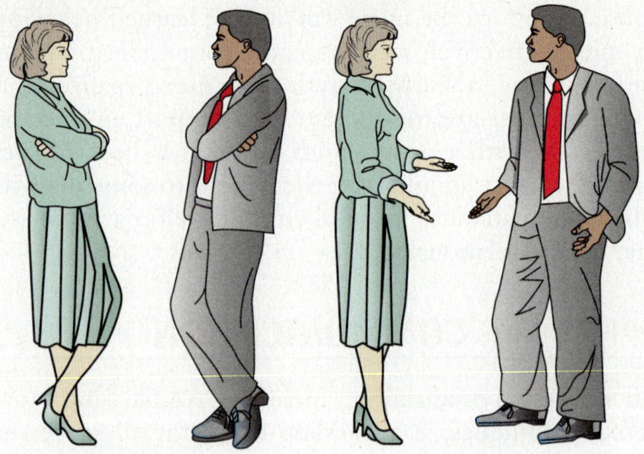

FIGURE 9.2 Open and closed body language.

Limiting Self-Disclosure

One of the most important principles of therapeutic communication for the nurse to follow is to focus the interaction on the patient's concerns. **Self-disclosure**, telling the patient personal information, generally is not a good idea. The conversation should focus on the patient, not the nurse. If a patient asks the nurse personal questions, the nurse should elicit the underlying reason for the request. The nurse can then determine how much personal information to disclose, if any. In revealing personal information, the nurse should be purposeful and have identified therapeutic outcomes. For example, a patient who was struggling with the implications of marriage and fidelity asked a nurse of the same gender if they had ever had an extramarital affair. The nurse interpreted the patient's statement as seeking role-modeling behavior and judged self-disclosure in this instance to be therapeutic. The nurse honestly responded that they did not engage in affairs and redirected the discussion back to the patient's concerns.

Nurses sometimes may feel uncomfortable avoiding patients' questions for fear of seeming rude. As a result, they might sometimes disclose too much personal information because they are trying to be "nice." However, being nice is not necessarily therapeutic. As appropriate, redirecting the patient, giving a neutral or vague answer, or saying "Let's talk about you" may be all that is necessary to limit self-disclosure. In some instances, nurses may need to tell the patient directly that the nurse will not share personal information (Table 9.1).

Active Listening

Listening is an ongoing activity by which the nurse attends to the patient's verbal and nonverbal communication. The art of listening is developed through careful attention to the content and meaning of the patient's speech. There are two types of listening: passive and active. **Passive listening** involves sitting quietly and letting the patient

THERAPEUTIC COMMUNICATION STRATEGIES AND TECHNIQUES

KEYCONCEPT Therapeutic communication is the ongoing process of interaction through which meaning emerges.

Therapeutic and social interactions are very different. In therapeutic communication, the nurse focuses on the patient and patient-related issues. Activities should have a definite purpose, and conversation should focus only on the patient. The nurse must not attempt to meet their own social or other needs during the activity.

TABLE 9.1 SELF-DISCLOSURE IN THERAPEUTIC VERSUS SOCIAL RELATIONSHIPS

Situation	Appropriate Therapeutic Response	Inappropriate Social Response with Rationale
A patient asks the nurse if they had fun over the weekend.	"The weekend was fine. How did you spend your weekend?"	"It was great. My partner and I went to dinner and a movie." *(This self-disclosure has no therapeutic purpose. The response focuses the conversation on the nurse, not the patient.)*
A patient asks a student nurse if they have ever been to a particular bar.	"Many people go there. I'm wondering if you have ever been there?"	"Oh yes—all the time. It's a lot of fun." *(Sharing information about outside activities is inappropriate.)*
A patient asks a nurse if mental illness is in the nurse's family.	"Mental illnesses do run in families. I've had a lot of experience caring for people with mental illnesses."	"My sister is being treated for depression." *(This self-disclosure has no purpose, and the nurse is missing the meaning of the question.)*
While shopping with a patient, the nurse sees a friend, who approaches them.	To the friend: "I know it looks like I'm not working, but I really am. I'll see you later."	"Hi, Bob. This is Jane Doe, a patient." *(Introducing the patient to the friend is very inappropriate and violates patient confidentiality.)*

talk. A passive listener allows the patient to ramble and does not focus or guide the thought process. This form of listening does not foster a therapeutic relationship. Body language during passive listening usually communicates boredom or indifference (Fig. 9.3).

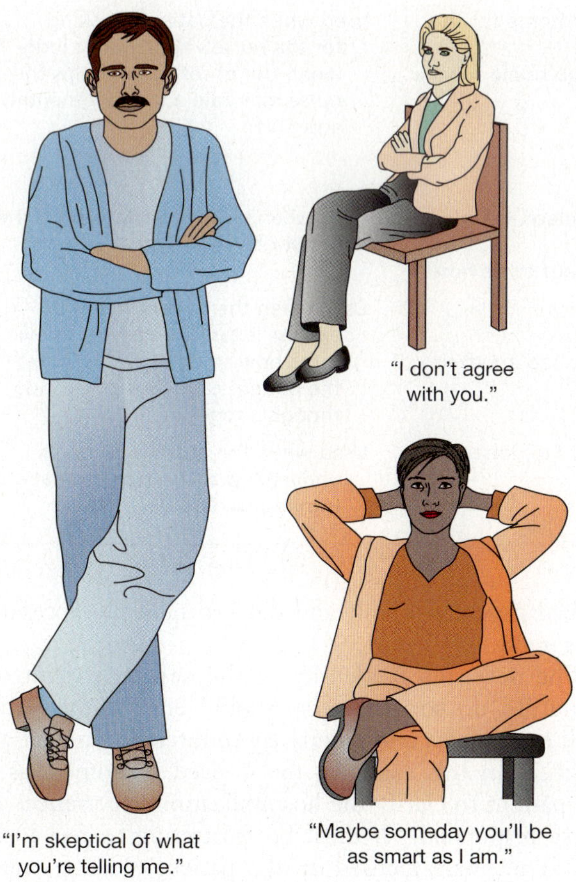

FIGURE 9.3 Negative body language.

Active listening is the most important strategy in developing a therapeutic relationship with a patient. Through **active listening**, the nurse focuses on what the patient is saying, interprets the underlying meaning, and responds to the message objectively. The nurse's verbal and nonverbal behaviors indicate active listening. The nurse usually responds indirectly using techniques such as open-ended statements, reflection (see Table 9.2), and questions that elicit additional responses from the patient. In active listening, the nurse should avoid changing the subject and instead follow the patient's lead. At times, however, it is necessary to direct a patient's focus on a specific topic or to clarify their thoughts or beliefs about that topic.

NCLEXNOTE Self-disclosure can be used in very specific situations but is not the first intervention to consider. In prioritizing interventions, active listening is one of the first to use.

Selection of Communication Techniques

Psychiatric nurses use many therapeutic techniques in establishing relationships and helping patients focus on their issues. Asking a question, restating, and reflecting are examples of such techniques. These techniques may at first seem artificial, but with practice, they can be useful. Table 9.2 lists useful therapeutic techniques along with examples. Choosing the best response begins with assessing and interpreting the meaning of the patient's communication—both verbal and nonverbal. For example, if a patient is angry and upset, the nurse might need to decide whether to invite the patient to sit down and discuss the issue, walk quietly with the patient, or simply observe the patient from a distance and not initiate conversation.

TABLE 9.2 VERBAL COMMUNICATION TECHNIQUES

Technique	Definition	Example	Use
Acceptance	Encouraging and receiving information in a nonjudgmental and interested manner	*Patient:* I have done something terrible. *Nurse:* I would like to hear about it. It's OK to discuss it with me.	Used in establishing trust and developing empathy
Confrontation	Presenting the patient with a different reality of the situation	*Patient:* My doctor won't talk to me. *Nurse:* I was in the room yesterday when you refused to speak with the doctor.	Used cautiously to immediately redefine the patient's reality. However, it can alienate the patient if used inappropriately. A nonjudgmental attitude is critical for confrontation to be effective.
Doubt	Expressing or voicing doubt when a patient relates a situation	*Patient:* My best friend hates me. They never call me. *Nurse:* From what you've told me, that doesn't sound like them. When did they call you last?	Used carefully and only when the nurse feels confident about the details. It is used when the nurse wants to guide the patient toward other explanations.
Interpretation	Putting into words what the patient is implying or feeling	*Patient:* I couldn't sleep because someone would come into my room and rape me. *Nurse:* It sounds like you were scared last night.	Used in helping the patient identify underlying thoughts or feelings
Observation	Stating to the patient what the nurse is observing	*Nurse:* You are trembling and perspiring. When did this start?	Used when a patient's behaviors (verbal or nonverbal) are obvious and unusual for that patient
Open-ended statements	Introducing an idea and letting the patient respond	*Nurse:* Trust means… *Patient:* That someone will keep you safe.	Used when helping the patient explore feelings or gain insight
Reflection	Redirecting the idea back to the patient for classification of important emotional overtones, feelings, and experiences; it gives patients permission to have feelings they may not realize they have	*Patient:* Should I go home for the weekend? *Nurse:* Should you go home for the weekend?	Used when the patient is asking for the nurse's approval or judgment; use of reflection helps the nurse maintain a nonjudgmental approach
Restatement	Repeating the main idea expressed lets the patient know what was heard	*Patient:* I hate this place. I don't belong here. *Nurse:* You don't want to be here.	Used when trying to clarify what the patient has said
Silence	Remaining quiet but nonverbally expressing interest during an interaction	*Patient:* I am angry! *Nurse:* (Silence) *Patient:* My partner had an affair.	Used when the patient needs to express ideas but may not know quite how to do it; with silence, the patient can focus on putting thoughts together
Validation	Clarifying the nurse's understanding of the situation	*Nurse:* Let me see if I understand.	Used when the nurse is trying to understand a situation the patient is trying to describe

Nurses should not necessarily take verbal messages literally, especially when a patient is upset or angry. For example, one nurse walked into the room of a newly admitted patient, who accused, "You locked me up and threw away the key." The nurse could have responded defensively that they had nothing to do with the patient being admitted; however, that response could have ended in an argument, and communication would have been blocked. Fortunately, the nurse recognized that the patient was communicating frustration at being in a locked psychiatric unit and did not take the accusation personally.

The next step is identifying the desired patient outcome. To do so, the nurse should engage the patient with eye contact and quietly try to interpret the patient's feelings. In this example, the desired outcome was for the patient to clarify the hospitalization experience. The nurse responded, "It must be frustrating to feel locked up." The nurse focused on the patient's feelings rather than on the accusations, which reflected an understanding of the patient's feelings. The patient knew that the nurse accepted these feelings, which led to further discussion. It may seem impossible to plan reactions for each situation, but with practice, the nurse will begin to respond automatically in a therapeutic way.

Silence

Silence consists of deliberate pauses to encourage the patient to reflect and eventually respond. One of the most difficult but often most effective communication techniques is the use of silence during verbal interactions. By maintaining silence, the nurse allows the patient to gather thoughts and to proceed at their own pace. It is important that the nurse not interrupt periods of silence because of their own anxiety or concern of "not doing anything" if sitting quietly with a patient.

Validation

Another important technique is validation, which means explicitly checking one's own thoughts or feelings with another person. To do so, the nurse must own their own thoughts or feelings by using "I" statements (Orlando, 1961). Validation generally refers to observations, thoughts, or feelings and seeks explicit feedback. For example, a nurse who sees a patient pacing the hallway before a planned family visit may conclude that the patient is anxious. Validation may occur with a statement such as, "I notice you pacing the hallway. I wonder if you are feeling anxious about the family visit." The patient may agree, "Yes. I keep worrying about what is going to happen!" or disagree, "No. I have been trying to get into the bathroom for the last 30 minutes, but my roommate is still in there!"

Strength-Based Communication

Strength-based communication should be supportive, focusing on the patient's strengths instead of potential deficits. Language that promotes acceptance and respect should be favored over language that distracts from acceptance of the person. For example, instead of stating that a patient is "manipulative," an alternate consideration is that the person is "resourceful; trying to get help." An "entitled" person might be viewed instead as someone who is "aware of their rights." Instead of noting that a patient is "resistant to treatment," it may be that the person is instead "choosing a different treatment." The nurse should incorporate language that promotes the strengths and unique characteristics of their patients (Kwame & Petrucka, 2021).

Avoiding Blocks to Communication

Some verbal techniques block interactions and inhibit therapeutic communication (Table 9.3). One of the biggest blocks to communication is giving advice, particularly when others have already given the same advice. Giving advice is different from supporting a patient through decision-making. The therapeutic dialogue presented in Box 9.3 differentiates between advice (telling the patient what to do or how to act) and therapeutic communication, through which the nurse and patient

TABLE 9.3 TECHNIQUES THAT INHIBIT COMMUNICATION

Technique	Definition	Example	Problem
Advice	Telling a patient what to do	*Patient:* I am struggling at work. *Nurse:* You should probably find a new job.	The nurse solves the patient's problem, which implies that the nurse knows best, and it may not be the appropriate solution; it also encourages dependency on the nurse.
Agreement	Agreeing with a particular viewpoint of a patient	*Patient:* Abortions are sinful. *Nurse:* I agree.	The patient is denied the opportunity to change their view now that the nurse agrees.
Challenges	Disputing the patient's beliefs with arguments, logical thinking, or direct order	*Patient:* I'm a cowpoke. *Nurse:* If you're a cowpoke, what are you doing in the hospital?	The nurse belittles the patient and decreases the patient's self-esteem. The patient will avoid relating to the nurse who challenges.
Reassurance	Telling a patient that everything will be OK	*Patient:* I don't think I will ever get better. *Nurse:* Hang in there. Everything will turn out just fine.	The nurse makes a statement that may not be true. The patient is blocked from exploring their feelings.
Disapproval	Judging the patient's situation and behavior	*Patient:* I'm so sorry. I did not mean to kill my mother. *Nurse:* You should be. How could anyone kill their mother?	The nurse belittles the patient. The patient will avoid the nurse.

BOX 9.3

Therapeutic Dialogue: Giving Advice Versus Recommendations

Ms. J has just received a diagnosis of phobic disorder and has been given a prescription for fluoxetine (Prozac). She was referred to the home health agency because she does not want to take her medication. She is fearful of becoming suicidal. Two approaches are given in the following section.

INEFFECTIVE COMMUNICATION (ADVICE)

Nurse: Ms. J, the doctor has ordered the medication because it will help with your anxiety.

Ms. J: Yes, but I don't want to take the medication. I'm afraid it will make me suicidal. Some psychiatric medication does that. I haven't had any attacks for 2 weeks, and it seems too risky since I'm doing better. I'm scared of the side effects.

Nurse: This medication has rarely had that side effect. You should try it and see if you have any suicidal thoughts.

Ms. J: [Remains silent for a while, crosses her legs, and looks away from the nurse and down at her feet] Okay.

(The nurse leaves, and Ms. J decides not to take the medication. Within 1 week, Ms. J is taken to the emergency room with a panic attack.)

EFFECTIVE COMMUNICATION

Nurse: Ms. J, how have you been doing?

Ms. J: So far, so good. I haven't had any attacks for 2 weeks.

Nurse: I understand that the doctor gave you a prescription for medication that may help with the panic attacks.

Ms. J: Yes, but I don't want to take it. I'm afraid of becoming suicidal. Some of this psychiatric medication does that. I don't really want to take a needless risk since I've been feeling better.

Nurse: Those worries are understandable. Have you ever had feelings of hurting yourself?

Ms. J: Not yet.

Nurse: If you took the medication and had thoughts like that, what would you do?

Ms. J: I don't know, that's why I'm scared.

Nurse: I think I see your dilemma. This medication may help with your panic attacks, but if the medication produces suicidal thoughts, then it might compromise your progress and that's a pretty serious risk. Is that correct?

Ms. J: Yeah, that's it.

Nurse: What are the circumstances under which you would feel more comfortable trying the medication?

Ms. J: If I knew that I would not have suicidal thoughts. If I could be assured of that.

Nurse: I can't guarantee that, but perhaps we could create an environment in which you would feel safe. I could call you every few days to see if you are having any of these thoughts and, if so, I could help you deal with them and make sure you see the doctor to review the medication.

Ms. J: Oh, that helps. If you do that, then I think that I will be alright.

(Ms. J successfully takes the medication.)

CRITICAL THINKING CHALLENGE

1. Contrast the communication in the first scenario with that in the second.
2. What therapeutic communication techniques did the second nurse use that may have contributed to a better outcome?
3. Are there any cues in the first scenario that indicate that the patient will not follow the nurse's advice? Explain.

explore alternative ways of viewing the patient's world. The patient can then reach their own conclusions about the best approaches to use.

EFFECTIVE COMMUNICATION AND RELATIONSHIPS

When the nurse is interacting with patients, the quality of communication is critical. This section describes the importance of **rapport**, **empathy**, recognition of **empathic linkages**, the role of **boundaries** and body space, and recognition of defense mechanisms in nurse–patient interactions.

Rapport

Rapport is the development of interpersonal harmony characterized by understanding and respect. Rapport is important in developing a trusting, therapeutic relationship. When rapport develops, a patient feels comfortable with the nurse and finds self-disclosure easier. People living with psychiatric conditions often feel alone and isolated. Establishing rapport helps lessen feelings of being alone. Nurses establish rapport by demonstrating interpersonal warmth, understanding, and a nonjudgmental attitude. A skilled nurse establishes rapport that alleviates the patient's anxiety in discussing issues and underlying needs.

Empathy

The use of **empathy** in a therapeutic relationship is central to psychiatric–mental health nursing. Empathy is sometimes confused with sympathy, which is the expression of compassion and kindness. Empathy is the ability to experience, in the present, a situation as another did at some point in the past. The nurse does not actually need to have had the experience for themselves but must be able to imagine the feelings associated with it. For empathy to develop, there must be a "giving of the self" to the other individual as well as a reciprocal desire to know each other personally. The process involves the nurse receiving information from the patient with open, nonjudgmental acceptance and communicating their understanding of the patient's experience and emotions, so the patient feels understood. Lack of empathy can cause distrust, alienation, and miscommunication (Dinoso & Baudoin, 2023).

Recognition of Empathic Linkages

Although empathy is essential, it is important for the nurse to be aware of **empathic linkages**, or the *direct* communication of feelings (Peplau, 1952, 1992). This can commonly occur with anxiety. For example, a nurse may be speaking with a patient who is talking rapidly while experiencing anxiety, and the nurse may notice that their own speech is becoming more rapid in tandem with the patient's, or the nurse may have subjective feelings of anxiety. It may be difficult for the nurse to determine if the anxiety was communicated interpersonally or if the nurse had a personal reaction to some content of the conversation. However, being aware of one's own feelings, and having the ability to analyze them, is critical to determining the source of the feelings and addressing any associated issues.

Biopsychosocial–Spiritual Boundaries and Body Space Zones

Boundaries are the defining limits of individuals, objects, or relationships. Boundaries mark territory, distinguishing what is "mine" from what is "not mine." Human beings have many different types of boundaries. Material boundaries, such as fences around property, artificially imposed state lines, and bodies of water, define territory as well as provide security and order. Personal boundaries can be conceptualized within the biopsychosocial model as including physical, psychological, and social dimensions. Physical boundaries are those established in terms of physical closeness to others—who we allow to touch us or how close we want others to stand near us.

Psychological boundaries are established in terms of emotional distance from others—how much of our innermost feelings and thoughts we want to share. Social boundaries, such as norms, customs, and roles, help us establish our closeness and place within the family, culture, and community. Boundaries are not fixed but dynamic. When boundaries are involuntarily infringed upon, the individual feels threatened and responds to the perceived threat. The nurse must elicit permission before implementing interventions that invade the patient's personal space.

Spiritual boundaries protect the right to believe what an individual wants to believe, worship as they choose, and practice their spiritual or religious beliefs. In providing care, nurses should support patients' spirituality but should not share personal religious and spiritual beliefs.

Personal Boundaries

Every individual is surrounded by four different body zones that provide varying degrees of protection against unwanted physical closeness during interactions. These were identified by Hall (1990) as the intimate zone (e.g., for whispering and embracing), the personal zone (e.g., for close friends), the social zone (e.g., for acquaintances), and the public zone (usually for interacting with strangers) (Fig. 9.4). The actual sizes of the different zones vary according to culture. Some cultures define the intimate zone narrowly and the personal zones widely; thus, friends in these cultures may stand and sit close while

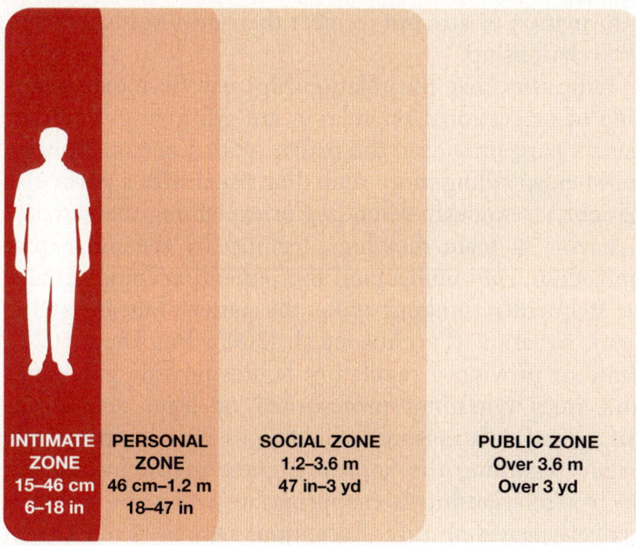

FIGURE 9.4 Body space zones.

interacting. Other cultures define the intimate zone widely; people of those cultures are uncomfortable when others stand close to them.

The variability of intimate and personal zones has implications for nursing. For a patient to be comfortable with a nurse, the nurse needs to protect the intimate zone of that individual. The patient usually will allow the nurse to enter the personal zone but will express discomfort if the nurse breaches the intimate zone. For the nurse, the difficulty lies in differentiating the personal zone from the intimate zone for each patient. The nurse should be especially careful when communicating through touch, especially with patients who have experienced trauma. Although touch can be therapeutic, the nurse should use their best judgment and always seek permission from the patient first (Dinoso & Baudoin, 2023).

The nurse's awareness of their own need for intimate and personal space is another prerequisite for therapeutic interaction with the patient. It is important that a nurse feels comfortable while interacting with patients. Establishing a comfort zone may well entail fine tuning the size of body zones. Recognizing this will help the nurse understand occasional inexplicable reactions to the proximity of patients.

Professional Boundaries in a Nurse–Patient Relationship

For nurses, professional boundaries are also essential to consider in the context of the nurse–patient relationship. Patients often enter such relationships at a very vulnerable point, and nurses need to be aware of professional boundaries to avoid exploitation of the patient. For example, in a friendship, there is a two-way sharing of personal information and feelings, but in nurse–patient relationship interactions, the focus is on the patient's needs, and the nurse generally does not share personal information or attempt to meet their own needs through the relationship.

Indicators that the relationship may be moving outside of professional boundaries are gift giving on either party's part, providing the patient with a personal phone number, spending more time than usual with a particular patient, strenuously defending or explaining the patient's behavior in team meetings, feelings by the nurse that only they truly understand the patient, keeping secrets, or frequently thinking about the patient outside of the work situation (Forchuk et al., 2006; Pinckney, 2021). State or provincial regulatory bodies provide guidelines and rules regarding professional or legal restrictions for sexual relationships. Guidelines are comparatively vague regarding the appropriateness of friendship, but such a relationship is inappropriate when the nurse is actively providing care. Exceptions may be when a relationship preceded the nursing context and another nurse is unavailable to provide care, such as in a rural area. Therapeutic relationships that meet the nurse's needs are also a breach of professional boundaries. When concerns arise related to therapeutic boundaries, the nurse must immediately seek clinical supervision or transfer the care of the patient.

Defense Mechanisms

When communicating with patients, it is also important for the nurse to be aware of the defense mechanisms that patients may use. **Defense mechanisms**, also known as coping styles, are psychological mechanisms that help an individual respond to and cope with difficult situations, emotional conflicts, and external stressors. Although defense mechanisms might seem to indicate the existence of problematic mental state, this is not true. Healthy individuals in many different contexts use defense mechanisms. The use of defense mechanisms may be conscious or unconscious. Some defense mechanisms (e.g., projection, splitting, acting out) are mostly maladaptive. Others (e.g., suppression, denial) may be either maladaptive or adaptive depending on the context in which they occur. The use of defense mechanisms becomes maladaptive when its persistent use interferes with the person's ability to function and their quality of life (see Table 9.4).

For example, responding to a difficult life event altruistically is very often a healthy way to recover. On the other hand, defense mechanisms such as acting out, autistic fantasies, projection, and splitting are rarely adaptive. A defense mechanism such as repression can be a natural way to react to a traumatic experience, specifically when used in appropriate moderation. However, the unchecked repression of difficult thoughts or feelings can keep someone from coming to terms with their experiences. In developing a successful therapeutic relationship, and in establishing open communication, such knowledge of defense mechanisms will prove invaluable.

As nurses develop communication skills, they will recognize their patients using defense mechanisms. With experience, the nurse will evaluate the purpose of a defense mechanism and then determine whether it should be discussed with the patient. For example, if a patient is using humor to alleviate an emotionally intense situation, that may be very appropriate. On the other hand, if someone continually rationalizes antisocial behavior, the use of the defense mechanism should be discussed.

NCLEXNOTE When studying defense mechanisms, focus on mechanisms and coping styles that are similar. For example, displacement versus devaluation versus projection should be differentiated. Identify these mechanisms in your process recordings.

TABLE 9.4 SPECIFIC DEFENSE MECHANISMS AND COPING STYLES

The following defense mechanisms and coping styles are commonly used when the individual deals with emotional conflict or stressors (either internal or external).

Defense Mechanism	Definition	Example
Acting out	Using actions rather than reflections or feelings during periods of emotional conflict	A teenager gets mad at their parents and begins staying out late at night.
Affiliation	Turning to others for help or support (sharing problems with others without implying that someone else is responsible for them)	An individual has a fight with their spouse and turns to their best friend for emotional support.
Altruism	Dedicating life to meeting the needs of others (receives gratification either vicariously or from the response of others)	After being rejected by their partner, a young adult joins the Peace Corps.
Anticipation	Experiencing emotional reactions in advance or anticipating consequences of possible future events and considering realistic, alternative responses or solutions	A parent cries for 3 weeks before their last child leaves for college.
Autistic fantasy	Excessive daydreaming as a substitute for human relationships, more effective action, or problem-solving	A young adult sits in their room all day and dreams about being a rock star instead of attending a baseball game with a friend.
Denial	Refusing to acknowledge some painful aspect of external reality or subjective experience that would be apparent to others (*Psychotic denial* is used when there is gross impairment in reality testing.)	A teenager's best friend moves away, but the adolescent says they do not feel sad.
Devaluation	Attributing exaggerated negative qualities to self or others	A teenager is rejected by their long-time partner. They tell friends that they now realize the partner is stupid and ugly.
Displacement	Transferring a feeling about, or a response to, one object onto another (usually less threatening) substitute object	A person has an argument with their boss. They come home from work and yell at their children.
Dissociation	Experiencing a breakdown in the usually integrated functions of consciousness, memory, perception of self or the environment, or sensory and motor behavior	An adult relates severe sexual abuse experienced as a child but does it without feeling. They say that the experience was as if they were outside their body watching the abuse.
Help-rejecting complaining	Complaining or making repeated requests for help that disguise covert feelings of hostility or reproach toward others, which are then expressed by rejecting the suggestions, advice, or help that others offer (Complaints or requests may involve physical or psychological symptoms or life problems.)	A college student asks a teacher for help after receiving a bad grade on a test. Every suggestion the teacher has is rejected by the student.
Humor	Emphasizing the amusing or ironic aspects of the conflict or stressor	A person makes a joke right after experiencing an embarrassing situation.
Idealization	Attributing exaggerated positive qualities to others	An adult falls in love and fails to see the negative qualities in the other person.
Intellectualization	Excessive use of abstract thinking or the making of generalizations to control or minimize disturbing feelings	After rejection in a romantic relationship, the rejected person explains the relationship dynamics to a friend.
Isolation of affect	Separation of ideas from the feelings originally associated with them	The individual loses touch with the feelings associated with rape while remaining aware of the details.
Omnipotence	Feeling or acting as if one possesses special powers or abilities and is superior to others	An individual tells a friend about personal expertise in the stock market and the ability to predict the best stocks.
Passive aggression	Indirectly and unassertively expressing aggression toward others. There is a facade of overt compliance masking covert resistance, resentment, or hostility.	An employee who dislikes another employee secretly steals their milk from the office refrigerator. The other employee is unaware of their coworker's hostile feelings.

(*continued*)

TABLE 9.4 SPECIFIC DEFENSE MECHANISMS AND COPING STYLES (*Continued*)

Defense Mechanism	Definition	Example
Projection	Falsely attributing to another one's own unacceptable feelings, impulses, or thoughts	A child is very angry at a parent but accuses the parent of being angry.
Projective identification	Falsely attributing to another one's own unacceptable feelings, impulses, or thoughts. Unlike simple projection, the individual does not fully disavow what is projected. Instead, the individual remains aware of their own affect or impulses but misattributes them as justifiable reactions to the other person. Frequently, the individual induces the very feelings in others that were first mistakenly believed to be there, making it difficult to clarify who did what to whom first.	A child is mad at a parent, who in turn becomes angry at the child but may be unsure of why. The child then feels justified at being angry with the parent.
Rationalization	Concealing the true motivations for one's own thoughts, actions, or feelings through the elaboration of reassuring or self-serving but incorrect explanations	A person is rejected by their partner but explains to friends that the breakup is for the best because the partner was beneath them socially and would not be liked by their family.
Reaction formation	Substituting behavior, thoughts, or feelings that are diametrically opposed to one's own unacceptable thoughts or feelings (this usually occurs in conjunction with their repression)	A person finds out about their spouse's extramarital affairs and tells friends that they think the affairs are perfectly appropriate. They truly do not feel, on a conscious level, any anger or hurt.
Repression	Expelling disturbing wishes, thoughts, or experiences from conscious awareness (The feeling component may remain conscious, detached from its associated ideas.)	A person does not remember the experience of being raped in the basement of a certain house but does feel anxious when going into that house.
Self-assertion	Expressing feelings and thoughts directly in a way that is not coercive or manipulative	An individual reaffirms that going to a ball game is not what they want to do.
Self-observation	Reflecting feelings, thoughts, motivation, and behavior and responding to them appropriately	An individual notices they are irritated at their friend's late arrival and decides to tell the friend of the irritation.
Splitting	Compartmentalizing opposite affect states and failing to integrate the positive and negative qualities of the self or others into cohesive images	Self and object images tend to alternate between opposites: exclusively loving, powerful, worthy, nurturing, and kind or exclusively bad, hateful, angry, destructive, rejecting, or worthless. One friend is wonderful and another former friend, who was at one time viewed as being perfect, is now believed to be an evil person.
Sublimation	Channeling potentially maladaptive feelings or impulses into socially acceptable behavior	A teenager is very angry with their parents. On the football field, they tackle someone very forcefully.
Suppression	Intentionally avoiding thinking about disturbing problems, wishes, feelings, or experiences	A student is anxiously awaiting test results but goes to a movie to stop thinking about it.
Undoing	Words or behavior designed to negate or to make amends symbolically for unacceptable thoughts, feelings, or actions	A person has sexual fantasies about their spouse's sibling. The person takes their spouse away for a romantic weekend.

COMMUNICATION CONSIDERATIONS FOR PEOPLE WITH MENTAL HEALTH CHALLENGES

For patients with specific, known mental health issues or illnesses, the nurse must consider how these issues may impact communication and be prepared to analyze the content of nurse–patient interactions.

Specific Mental Health Issues

It is important to consider the individual's mental health challenges when selecting specific communication strategies. For example, patients with increased levels of anxiety may have poor communication, requiring the nurse to use shorter and simpler statements or questions. Patients who are experiencing depression may have difficulty articulating their feelings, or their thinking and responses may be slowed. The nurse will frequently use silence and empathic techniques throughout this interaction. People who are depressed may also use communication styles such as overgeneralizing ("This always happens to me.... Everything always turns out for the worse."). The nurse can assist patients by asking them to be more specific (e.g., asking about a specific time or a specific exception).

Patients with schizophrenia may exhibit symptoms such as hallucinations or delusions. For people having auditory hallucinations (hearing sounds that are imagined), the nurse's voice may be one of several voices being heard. Clear, short sentences may assist in focusing the patient's attention on the nurse's voice. People experiencing delusions may use pronouns vaguely ("they" did it) or other forms of vague or unclear communication. Asking patients to be more specific may help in clarifying thinking as well as communication.

As you read through the chapters on various psychiatric disorders, consider how the signs and symptoms of each illness could have an impact on communication and the evolving therapeutic relationship.

Analyzing Interactions

Many patients with psychiatric disorders have difficulty communicating. They may have perceptual, cognitive, and information-processing deficits that interfere with their ability to express ideas, understand concepts, and accurately perceive the environment (Clarke et al., 2023). Because of the complexity of communication, mental health professionals monitor their interactions with patients using various methods, including audio recording, video recording, and **process recording**, which entails writing a verbatim transcript of the interaction. A video or audio recording of an interaction provides the most accurate monitoring but is cumbersome to use. Process recording, one of the easiest methods to use, is adequate in most situations. Nurses should use it when first learning therapeutic communication and during times when communication becomes a problem. In a process recording, the nurse records, from memory, the verbatim interaction immediately after the communication (Table 9.5). Nonverbal communication, by both the patient and the nurse, should also be recorded.

The nurse then analyzes the content of the interaction in terms of the words and their meaning for both the

TABLE 9.5 PROCESS RECORDING

Setting: The living room of Mr. S's home. Mr. S is 23 years old and was hospitalized for 2 weeks. His diagnosis is bipolar mood disorder, and he is recovering from a depressive episode. His parents are in the room but cannot hear the conversation. Mr. S is sitting on the couch, and the nurse is sitting on a chair. This is the nurse's first visit after Mr. S's discharge from the hospital.

Patient	Nurse	Interpretation/Analysis
	How are you doing, Mr. S? (smiles and offers hand to shake)	*Plan:* Initially develop a sense of trust and initiate a therapeutic relationship.
I'm fine. It's good to be home (looking at floor, takes nurse's hand to briefly shake). I really don't like the hospital (shakes his head while still looking at floor).	You didn't like the hospital?	Interpretation: Validating assumption that Mr. S does not want to return to hospital. Nonverbal communication may indicate sadness or low self-esteem. This needs further exploration.
No. The nurses lock you up (maintains eye contact with nurse, frowning, arms crossed). Are you a nurse?		Patient validates assumption regarding hospital, but nonverbal behavior indicates there may be further concerns.
	I'm a nurse. I'm wondering if you think that I will lock you up (maintains eye contact and open posture).	Interpretation: Mr. S may be wondering what my role is and whether I will put him back in the hospital. This assumption needs to be validated, and my role needs clarification.
You could tell my mom to put me back in the hospital (maintains eye contact with nurse).	Any treatment that I recommend will be thoroughly discussed with you first. I am here to help you stay out of the hospital. I will not discuss anything with your mother unless you give me permission to do so (nurse maintains eye contact and open posture).	Use interpretation to clarify Mr. S's thinking. Mr. S is wondering about my relationship with his mother. Explain my role and confidentiality.
(Patient maintains eye contact and uncrosses arms.)		Patient's nonverbal communication appears to indicate he is more comfortable with this clarification.

patient and the nurse. The analysis is especially important because the ability to communicate is often compromised in people with mental disorders. Because words may not have the same meaning for the patient as they do for the nurse, clarification of meaning becomes especially important. The analysis can identify symbolic meanings, **content themes**, and blocks in communication.

Symbolism

Symbolism, the use of a word or phrase to represent an object, event, or feeling, is used universally. For example, automobiles are named for wild animals that represent speed, prowess, and beauty. In people with mental disorders, the use of words to symbolize events, objects, or feelings is often idiosyncratic, and they cannot explain their choices. For example, a person who is feeling scared and anxious may tell the nurse that bombs and guns are exploding. It is up to the nurse to make the connection between the bombs and guns and the patient's feelings and then to validate this with the patient. Because of the patient's cognitive limitations, the individual may express feelings only symbolically. Another example is found in Table 9.6.

Some patients, for example, those with developmental disabilities or organic brain difficulties, may have difficulty with abstract thinking and symbolism. Conversations may be interpreted literally. For example, in response to the question "What brings you to the hospital?" a patient might reply, "The ambulance." In these situations, the nurse must be cautious to avoid using symbols or metaphors. Concrete language, that is, language reflecting what can be observed through the senses, will be more easily understood.

Content Themes

Verbal behavior is also interpreted by analyzing **content themes**. Patients often express concerns or feelings repeatedly in several different ways. After a few sessions, a common theme emerges. Themes may emerge symbolically, as in the case of the patient who constantly talks about the "guns and bombs." Alternatively, a theme may simply be identified as a recurrent thread of a story that a patient retells at each session. For example, one patient often discussed early abandonment by their family. This led the nurse to hypothesize that they had an underlying fear of rejection. The nurse was then able to test whether there was an underlying fear and to develop strategies to help the patient explore the fear (Box 9.4). It is important to involve patients in analyzing themes so they may learn this skill. Within the therapeutic relationship, the person who does the work is the one who develops the competencies, so the nurse must be careful to share this opportunity with the patient (Peplau, 1952, 1992).

Communication Blocks

Communication blocks are identified by topic changes that either the nurse or the patient makes. Topics are changed for various reasons. A patient may change the topic from one that does not interest them to one that

TABLE 9.6 USE OF SYMBOLISM

Setting: Mr. A has been diagnosed with schizophrenia and expresses himself through the use of television characters. A nurse observed another patient shoving him against the wall. As the nurse approached the two patients, the other patient ran, leaving Mr. A noticeably shaking. The nurse checked to see if Mr. A was all right.

Patient	Nurse	Interpretation/Analysis
	Mr. A, are you OK? (approaches patient)	
Robin Hood saved the day. (trembling, arms crossed)		Mr. A could not say, "Thank you for helping me." Instead, he could only describe a fictional character's response.
	You feel that you are saved?	The nurse focused on what Mr. A must be feeling if he felt that he had been rescued.
It's a glorious day in Sherwood Forest! (trembling decreases; smiles at nurse)		He seems to be happy now.
	Mr. A, are you hurt anywhere? (Eyes scan over patient, using concerned tone of voice.)	The nurse wanted to check whether the patient had been hurt when pushed against the wall.
The angel of mercy put out the fire (continues to smile and extends hand to shake hands with nurse).		The patient is apparently not hurting now.

BOX 9.4

Themes and Interactions

Session 1: Patient discusses the death of a parent at a young age.
Session 2: Patient explains that their sister is now married and never visits.
Session 3: Patient says that their best friend in the hospital was discharged, and the patient really misses them.
Session 4: Patient cries about a lost kitten.
Interpretation: Theme of loss is pervasive in several sessions.

they find more meaningful. However, an individual usually changes the topic because they are uncomfortable with a particular subject. When a topic change is identified, the nurse or patient hypothesizes the reason for it. If the nurse changes the topic, they need to determine why. The nurse may find that they are uncomfortable with the topic or may not be listening to the patient. Novice mental health nurses, who are uncomfortable with silences or trying to elicit specific information from the patient, often change topics. When communication blocks are recognized, the nurse should attempt to redirect the conversation back to the topic at hand unless the topic is too uncomfortable for the patient at that point in time.

The nurse must also record and interpret the patient's nonverbal behavior in light of the verbal behavior. Is the patient communicating one thing verbally and another nonverbally? Is the behavior consistent with the patient's cultural norms? For example, if a patient denies any issues but is affectionate and physically demonstrative (which is antithetical to their the traditionally stoic beliefs and behaviors of their culture), the nonverbal behavior is inconsistent with what is typical behavior for that person. Further exploration is needed to determine the meaning of the culturally atypical behavior.

THE NURSE–PATIENT RELATIONSHIP

The nurse–patient relationship is a dynamic process that changes with time. It can be viewed in steps or phases with characteristic behaviors for both patient and nurse. This text uses an adaptation of Hildegarde Peplau's model, which she introduced in her seminal work, *Interpersonal Relations in Nursing* (1952, 1992). Emerging evidence suggests that a well-developed nurse–patient relationship positively affects patient care.

Introduction

The nurse–patient relationship begins with the initial introduction. Nurses initiate the introduction by simply explaining their role and their task—an initial assessment or an invitation to a group. It is very important to introduce oneself. The language used is also very important. The nurse should be sensitive to using patient-centered and gender-neutral language. When first meeting a patient, do not assume gender or sexual orientation by clothing or appearance. If you are unsure of the patient's gender but must use pronouns, the terms "they/them/their" are preferable to terms that make patients select either a male or female category (Braybrook et al., 2022; Reeves et al., 2024).

Phases

The nurse–patient relationship is conceptualized in three overlapping phases that evolve with time: **orientation phase**, **working phase**, and **resolution phase**. The orientation phase is the phase during which the nurse and patient get to know each other. During this phase, which can last from a few minutes to several months, the patient develops a sense of trust in the nurse. The second is the working phase, in which the patient uses the relationship to examine specific problems and learn new ways of approaching them. The final stage, resolution phase, is the termination stage of the relationship and lasts from the time the problems are resolved to the close of the relationship. The relationship does not evolve as a simple linear relationship. Instead, the relationship may be predominantly in one phase, but reflections of all phases can be seen in each interaction (Table 9.7).

KEYCONCEPT The nurse–patient relationship is a dynamic process that changes with time. It can be viewed in steps or phases with characteristic behaviors for both the patient and the nurse.

Orientation Phase

The orientation phase begins when the nurse and patient meet and ends when the patient begins to identify the problems to be examined. During the orientation phase, the nurse discusses the patient's expectations, explains the purpose of the relationship and its boundaries, and facilitates the development of the relationship. It is natural for the nurse to be nervous during the first few sessions. The goal of the orientation phase is to develop trust and security within the nurse–patient relationship. During this initial phase, the nurse listens intently to the patient's history and perception of problems and begins to understand the patient and identify themes. The use of empathy facilitates the development of a positive therapeutic relationship.

First Meeting

During the first meeting, outlining both nursing and patient responsibilities is important. The nurse is responsible for providing guidance throughout the therapeutic

TABLE 9.7 PHASES OF THE NURSE–PATIENT RELATIONSHIP

	Orientation	Working	Resolution
Patient	Seeks assistance Identifies needs Commits to a therapeutic relationship During the later part, begins to test relationship	Discusses problems and underlying needs Uses emotional safety of relationship to examine personal issues Tests new ways of solving problems Feels comfortable with nurse May use transference	May express ambivalence about the relationship and its termination Uses personal style to say "good-bye"
Nurse	Actively listens Establishes boundaries of the relationship Clarifies expectations Identifies countertransference issues Uses empathy Establishes rapport	Supports development of healthy problem-solving Encourages patient to prepare for the future	Avoids returning to patient's initial problems Encourages independence Promotes positive family interactions

relationship, protecting confidential information, and maintaining professional boundaries. The patient is responsible for attending agreed-upon sessions, interacting during the sessions, and participating in the nurse–patient relationship. The nurse should also explain clearly to the patient meeting times, handling of missed sessions, and the estimated length of the relationship. Issues related to recording information and how the nurse will work within the interdisciplinary team should also be made explicit.

Usually, both the nurse and the patient feel anxious at the first meeting. The nurse should recognize the anxieties and attempt to alleviate them before the meeting. The patient's behavior during this first meeting may indicate to the nurse some of the patient's issues in interpersonal relationships. For example, a patient may talk nonstop for 15 minutes or may brag of sexual conquests. What the patient chooses to tell or not to tell is significant. What a patient first does or says may not accurately indicate their true feelings or the situation. In the beginning, patients may deny issues or employ various forms of defense mechanisms or prevent the nurse from getting to know them. The patient is usually nervous and insecure during the first few sessions and may exhibit behavior reflective of these emotions, such as rambling. Typically, by the third session, the patient can focus on a topic.

Confidentiality in Treatment

Ideally, nurses include people who are important to the patient in planning and implementing care. The nurse and patient should discuss the issue of confidentiality in the first session. The nurse should be clear about any information that is to be shared with anyone else. The nurse shares significant assessment data and patient progress with a supervisor, team members, and a provider. Most patients expect the nurse to communicate with other mental health professionals and are comfortable with this arrangement. Restrictions regarding what can be shared and with whom are also covered by state or provincial mental health acts and health information acts.

Testing the Relationship

This first part of the orientation phase, called the "honeymoon phase," is usually pleasant. However, the therapeutic team typically hits rough spots before completing this phase. The patient begins to test the relationship to become convinced that the nurse will really accept them. Typical "testing behaviors" include forgetting a scheduled session or being late. Patients may also express anger at something a nurse says or accuse the nurse of breaking confidentiality. Another common pattern is for the patient to first introduce a relatively superficial issue as if it is the major issue. The nurse must recognize that these behaviors are designed to test the relationship and establish its parameters, not to express rejection or dissatisfaction with the nurse. The student nurse often feels personally rejected during the patient's testing and may even become angry with the patient. If the nurse simply accepts the behavior and continues to be available and consistent to the patient, these behaviors usually subside. Testing needs to be understood as a typical way that human beings develop trust.

Working Phase

When the patient begins identifying problems to work on, the working phase of the relationship has started. Problem identification can yield a wide range of issues, such as managing symptoms of a mental disorder, coping with chronic pain, examining issues related to sexual abuse, or dealing with problematic interpersonal relationships. Through the relationship, the patient begins to explore the identified problems and develop strategies to resolve them. By the time the working phase is reached, the patient has developed enough trust that they can examine the identified problems within the security of the therapeutic relationship. In the working phase, the nurse can use various verbal and nonverbal techniques to help the patient examine problems and to support the patient through the healing process.

Transference (unconscious assignment to others of the feelings and attitudes that the patient originally associated with important figures) and **countertransference** (the provider's emotional reaction to the patient based on personal unconscious needs and conflicts) become important issues in the working phase. For example, a patient could be hostile to a nurse because of underlying resentment of authority figures; the nurse, in turn, could respond defensively because of earlier experiences of anger. The patient uses transference to examine problems. During this phase, the patient is psychologically vulnerable and emotionally dependent on the nurse. The nurse needs to recognize countertransference and prevent it from eroding professional boundaries.

Often, nurses are eager to implement rehabilitation plans. However, this cannot be done until the patient trusts the nurse and identifies what issues they wish to work on in the context of the relationship.

Resolution Phase

The final stage of the nurse–patient relationship is resolution, which begins when the actual problems are resolved and ends with the termination of the relationship. During this phase, the patient is redirected toward a life without this specific therapeutic relationship. The patient connects with community resources, solidifies a newly found understanding, and practices new behaviors. The patient takes responsibility for follow-up appointments and interacts with significant others in new ways. New problems are not addressed during this phase except in terms of what was learned during the working stage. The nurse assists the client in strengthening relationships, making referrals, and recognizing and understanding signs of future relapse.

Termination begins on the first day of the relationship, when the nurse explains that this relationship is time limited and has been established to resolve the patient's issues and help them handle their problems. Because a therapeutic relationship is dependent, the nurse must constantly evaluate the patient's level of dependence and continually support the patient's move toward independence. Termination is usually stressful for the patient, who must sever ties with the nurse who has shared thoughts and feelings and given guidance and support over many sessions.

Depending on previous experiences with terminating relationships, some patients may not handle their emotions well during termination. Some may not show up for the last session at all to avoid their feelings of sadness and separation. Many patients display anger about the relationship's ending. Patients may express anger toward the nurse or displace it onto others. For example, a patient may shout obscenities at another patient after being told that the patient's therapeutic relationship with the nurse will end in a few weeks. One of the best ways to handle anger is to help the patient acknowledge it, to explain that anger is a typical emotion when a relationship is ending, and to reassure the patient that it is acceptable to feel angry. The nurse should also reassure the patient that anger subsides after the relationship is over.

Another typical termination behavior is raising old problems that have already been resolved. The nurse may feel frustrated if patients in the termination phase present resolved issues as if they were new. The nurse may feel that the sessions were unsuccessful. In reality, patients are attempting to prolong the relationship and avoid its ending. Nurses should avoid addressing these issues. Instead, they should reassure patients that they already covered those issues and learned methods to control them. They should explain that the patient may be feeling anxious about the relationship's ending and redirect the patient to newly found skills and abilities in forming new relationships, including support groups and social groups. The final meeting should focus on the future (Box 9.5). The nurse can reassure the patient that the nurse will remember them, but the nurse should not agree to see the patient outside the relationship.

Nontherapeutic Relationships

Although it is hoped that all nurse–patient relationships will go through the phases of the relationship described earlier, this is not always the case. In a **nontherapeutic relationship**, the nurse and the patient both feel very frustrated and keep varying their approach with each other to establish a meaningful relationship. This is different from a prolonged orientation phase in that the efforts are not sustained; rather, they vary constantly.

The nurse may try longer meetings, shorter meetings, being directive, and varying the therapeutic stance from warm and friendly to aloof. Patients in this phase may try to talk about the past but then change to discussions of the "here and now." They will try talking about their family and in the next meeting talk about their work goals. Both *grapple and struggle* to come to a common ground, and both become increasingly frustrated with each other.

Eventually, the frustration becomes so great that the pair gives up on each other and moves to a phase of *mutual withdrawal*. The nurse may schedule a visit with this patient at the end of the shift and "run out of time" so the meeting never happens. The patient will leave the unit or otherwise be unavailable during scheduled meeting times. If a meeting does occur, the nurse will try to

BOX 9.5

Research for Evidence-Based Practice: Transitional Discharge Model

Forchuk, C., Martin, M. L., Sherman, D., Corring, D., Srivastava, R., O'Regan, T., Gyamfi, S., & Harerimana, B. (2020). Healthcare professionals' perceptions of the implementation of the transitional discharge model for community integration of psychiatric clients. International Journal of Mental Health Nursing, *29(3), 498–507.*

THE QUESTION: The transitional discharge model (TDM) facilitates a safe and effective discharge from the hospital to the community, in part, through the development and maintenance of therapeutic and peer-based relationships. In this study, the researchers asked: (1) What are the experiences and perceived roles of health care professionals in the implementation of TDM? (2) What are health care professionals' perceptions regarding the effectiveness of TDM? (3) What are health care professionals' perspectives for the sustainability of the TDM implementation?

METHODS: This qualitative component of a focused ethnographic study was part of a broader participatory action research project to examine the effectiveness and sustainability of implementing the TDM in Ontario, Canada. Research staff conducted focus groups with 216 health professionals across 9 hospitals in Ontario, including 14 psychiatric units. Focus group participants met at 6- and 12-month timepoints to discuss their perspectives on implementing the TDM and recommendations for its sustainability. Data were analyzed for descriptors, similarities, and differences according to the process of Leininger (1985).

FINDINGS: Health professionals assumed a variety of roles to identify patients who were suitable for the TDM intervention and to facilitate their discharge to the community. They found the TDM provided a helpful framework to support discharge planning. However, issues with interprofessional communication, insufficient staffing and peer support, and concerns about providers' record liability posed challenges. To sustain implementation of the TDM, participants suggested enhancing active interprofessional communication, standardizing the TDM practice by distributing informational resources across units, and outlining clear roles for members of the team.

IMPLICATIONS FOR NURSING: Patients are vulnerable during times of transition. Discharge planning should begin at the point of hospital admission to enhance continuity of care after discharge. Health professionals also need to facilitate the development of peer relationships early in hospitalization and implement effective communication strategies with hospital staff, patients, and peer supporters through regular discussions about discharge priorities and postdischarge progress.

keep it short, thinking, "What's the point—we just cover the same old ground anyway." The patient will attempt to keep it superficial and stay on safe topics ("You can always ask about your medications—nurses love to health teach, you know.").

A **deteriorating relationship** is also nontherapeutic and has been shown to have predictable phases (Coatsworth-Puspoky et al., 2006). This relationship starts in the *withholding* phase, during which the nurse is perceived as "withholding" nursing support. The nurse fails to recognize that the patient is a person with an illness or health needs. The patient feels uncomfortable, anxious, frustrated, and guilty about being ill and does not develop a sense of trust. A barrier exists between the patient and the nurse.

The middle phase of a deteriorating relationship consists of two subphases: *avoiding* and *ignoring*. The patient begins to avoid the nurse and perceives that the nurse is avoiding them. The patient abides by the rules because they do not want to cause problems. The nurse is perceived as rude and condescending. The nurse ignores and avoids the patient's requests for help; in turn, the patient becomes more anxious, frustrated, and fearful. Patients experiencing this phase report feelings of wanting to give up, being rejected, not being cared for, and not being listened to.

The end phase is named *struggling with and making sense* of. In the final phase of a nontherapeutic, deteriorating relationship, the patient struggles with and tries to understand the unsatisfactory relationship. The patient feels hopeless and frustrated because of the lack of support received by the nurse. In a deteriorating relationship, the patient and nurse begin as strangers and end as enemies.

Obviously, no therapeutic progress can be made in a nontherapeutic or deteriorating relationship. The nurse may be hesitant to ask for a therapeutic transfer, assuming that a relationship would similarly fail with another nurse. However, each relationship is unique, and difficulties in one relationship do not predict difficulties in the next. Clinical supervision early on may assist the development of the relationship, but often a therapeutic transfer to another nurse is required.

THERAPEUTIC RELATIONSHIP STRATEGIES

Motivational Interviewing

Motivational interviewing (MI) is a clinical method intended to engage a patient's own decision-making ability. By focusing and reinforcing the client's own arguments for change, MI can be used to achieve positive outcomes. This is a collaborative process involving directed counseling and focused discussions between the care provider and the patient. As a result, MI is inherently exploratory and adaptive (Miller, 2023; Miller & Rollnick, 2023).

MI and similar interventions can have varying degrees of efficacy (Schwenker et al., 2023). Because much of the success of MI depends on the quality of interaction between the care provider and the patient, good communication practices are essential for effective implementation of MI. Acknowledging the patient's culture (Self et al., 2023), building a trusting relationship with the patient, adapting the MI strategy for the patient, and incorporating the patient's values to the change outcome can contribute to successful outcomes in MI.

Because the success of MI is, in part, dependent on contingent factors, care providers require frequent instruction and feedback. Strong communication in the context of therapeutic relationships as discussed in this chapter, especially self-awareness, empathic linkages, active listening, and the avoidance of unhelpful varieties of defense mechanisms, requires ongoing training and will affect therapeutic outcomes. Although challenging to successfully implement, MI has produced positive health outcomes in many different settings (Driedger et al., 2023; Jamison et al., 2022; Kumar et al., 2022). Every particular use of MI is likely to vary according to patient needs; Miller and Moyers (2006) have identified eight features of MI that should appear in every application of this technique:

1. Openness to collaboration with clients' own expertise,
2. Proficiency in client-centered counseling, including accurate empathy,
3. Recognition of key aspects of client speech that guides the practice of MI,
4. Eliciting and strengthening client change talk,
5. Rolling with resistance,
6. Negotiating change plans,
7. Consolidating client commitment, and
8. Switching flexibly between MI and other intervention styles.

Transitional Relationship Model/ Transitional Discharge Model

The Transitional Relationship Model (TRM; Forchuk et al., 2012, 2013) is theoretically grounded in the work of Hildegard Peplau; healing occurs in relationships. Therapeutic relationships can be formed with either professionals or peer supporters. The TRM was first developed to ease the transition from hospital to community, but its use has now been expanded to a variety of transitional care processes. There are two essential components of the TRM:

1. The therapeutic relationship should be extended until a new relationship with another care provider is established (continuing relationships formed in the hospital until new therapeutic relationships in the community are formed).
2. Trained peer support (often through a group of people who currently or formerly sought mental health services) from a person who has now successfully transitioned to the community.

In addition to producing positive therapeutic outcomes, the TRM also reduces time spent in hospital and costs to the health care system (Forchuk et al., 2019a) (see Box 9.6).

Technology and the Therapeutic Relationship

As technology develops and becomes increasingly accessible, traditional face-to-face communication can be replaced with technologic interactions. Situations such as the coronavirus disease 2019 (COVID-19) pandemic have quickly accelerated mental health services moving to a virtual environment. Telehealth modalities can include phone and video conferencing, mental health apps, and internet-delivered programs. Studies have found telephone or video conferencing to be effective alternatives, when appropriate, to standard in-person treatment for a variety of mental health disorders, particularly depression and anxiety disorders (Hatami et al., 2022). Telehealth is a useful alternative for individuals living in rural and other underserved areas, those perceiving stigma associated with going to a provider's office, and those lacking reliable transportation (Goldin et al., 2021; Williamson & Jillian, 2024). Patients report many advantages to receiving virtual care, including accessibility, convenience, cost effectiveness, and privacy (Crawford et al., 2024). However, currently, face-to-face therapy is reportedly still patients' preferred means of interaction, making it difficult to determine which telehealth modality is best suited for each mental health disorder (Crunelle et al., 2023; Hatami et al., 2022).

There are barriers to telehealth. Establishing a therapeutic relationship can take longer due to a lack of physical presence. Nonverbal communication, such as gestures, mannerisms, and tone, is more difficult to assess when not communicating in person. Misinterpretation of body language and behavioral manifestations may result in an inaccurate assessment of the patient (Goldin et al., 2021). There are concerns that the impersonal nature of telehealth may impact the therapeutic relationship between provider and patient (Galvin et al., 2022). Telepsychiatry is not appropriate when a patient's safety is an imminent risk. It is also less effective in individuals with severe mental illness who have diminished cognitive abilities and impaired insight (Lipschitz et al., 2023). Lack of technology, comfort with using

BOX 9.6

Therapeutic Dialogue: The Last Meeting

INEFFECTIVE APPROACH

Ms. J: Why did the other nurses bring you flowers and cards today?

Nurse: Well, that's because today is my last day; I'm transferring to the new hospital, across town.

Ms. J: Oh, um. I was just thinking, I need to talk to you about something important.

Nurse: What is it?

Ms. J: I have been worrying about my medication again.

Nurse: Oh, have you had any side effects?

Ms. J: No, but I might.

Nurse: I think you should tell the new nurse.

Ms. J: She is too new. She won't understand and you helped me last time. I feel so worried about your leaving. Is there any way you can stay? You said that you would check in, remember?

Nurse: Well, I could check on you tomorrow?

Ms. J: Oh, would you? I would really appreciate it if you would give me your new telephone number and that way I can tell you if anything happens.

Nurse: I don't know what the number will be, but you might be able to find it online.

EFFECTIVE APPROACH

Ms. J: Why did the other nurses bring you flowers and cards today?

Nurse: Oh, hello Ms. J. Do you remember? Today is my last day.

Ms. J: Oh, yes. Well, I need to talk to you about something important.

Nurse: We talked about that. Anything "important" needs to be shared with the new nurse.

Ms. J: But I want to tell you. You really made me feel better last time.

Nurse: Thank you but remember that you improved a lot because you know what to do to continue progressing. Saying goodbye can be very hard.

Ms. J: I'll miss you.

Nurse: Your feelings are very typical when relationships are ending. I will remember you in a very special way.

Ms. J: Can I please have your telephone number in case I need to talk to you?

Nurse: No, I can't give that to you. It is important that we say goodbye today. And remember, you can always talk to the new nurse about your concerns.

Ms. J: Okay, I know. Goodbye. Good luck.

Nurse: Goodbye.

CRITICAL THINKING CHALLENGE

1. What were some of the mistakes the nurse in the first scenario made?
2. In the second scenario, how does therapeutic communication in the termination phase differ from effective communication in the working phase?

technology, or unreliable internet access is another barrier (Galvin et al., 2022). It is critical for communication over the internet to be HIPAA compliant and secure to maintain confidentiality. Many cheaper hardware devices may have "bloatware" that tracks information, and similarly "free" or cheap software may sell information to third parties. Hospital firewalls can be useful in establishing such connections (Forchuk et al., 2019b). One must always be aware of a community agency, hospital, or research site's policies and best practices regarding communication online. Some commonly used platforms for online communication, such as Facebook Messenger, cannot meet privacy standards and should not be used in communication with patients. However, the internet is an invaluable resource for educational and research purposes.

SUMMARY OF KEY POINTS

- To deal therapeutically with the emotions, feelings, and issues of patients, nurses must understand their own values and beliefs and interpersonal strengths and limitations.

- The nurse–patient relationship is built on therapeutic communication, including verbal and nonverbal interactions between the nurse and the patient. Some communication skills include active listening, positive body language, appropriate verbal responses, and the ability of the nurse to interpret appropriately and analyze the patient's verbal and nonverbal behaviors.
- Two of the most important communication concepts are empathy and rapport.
- In the nurse–patient relationship, as in all types of relationships, certain physical, emotional, and social boundaries and limitations need to be observed.
- The therapeutic nurse–patient relationship consists of three major and overlapping stages or phases: the orientation phase, in which the patient and nurse meet and establish the parameters of the relationship; the working phase, in which the patient identifies and explores problems; and the resolution phase, in which the patient learns to manage the problems and the relationship is terminated.
- The nontherapeutic relationship consists of three major and overlapping phases: the orientation phase, the grappling and struggling phase, and the phase of mutual withdrawal. A deteriorating relationship begins with a withholding phase, continues through the phases of avoiding and ignoring, and finally ends unsatisfactorily with a phase named "struggling with and making sense of."

DEVELOPING CLINICAL JUDGMENT

1. Your patient was recently admitted to the inpatient psychiatric unit following a suicide attempt. When you begin your initial assessment, the patient starts to cry, saying, "I should have died. There is absolutely no reason for me to be on this earth. I have nothing left to live for!" How do you respond?
2. Your patient who is depressed does not seem inclined to talk about their depression. Describe the measures you would take to initiate a therapeutic interaction with them.
3. A patient is in the resolution phase of a therapeutic relationship with the nurse and is preparing for discharge. Although they had been adherent to all treatment recommendations over the past couple of weeks, they are very late for their appointment and announce they are no longer going to take their medication. Discuss patient behaviors that could occur during the resolution phase of the nurse–patient relationship.
4. Think of a time that you worked with a patient whose values and beliefs differed from yours. What is the best approach in developing a therapeutic relationship?

MOVIES, TV, OR STREAMING PROGRAMS

Good Will Hunting: 1997. Robin Williams plays a therapist, Dr. Sean Maguire. His patient, Will Hunting (Matt Damon), is a self-taught mathematics genius who was recently paroled and is working as a janitor at MIT. Through a strong relationship, Will begins to realize his potential. This film deals with intense blocks to communication, as well as issues around justice system use and class.

Viewing Points:

1. Will Hunting initially met with two other therapists before working with Dr. Maguire. Why were the first two not successful, and what features contributed to a therapeutic relationship with Dr. Maguire?
2. After Dr. Maguire's first meeting with Will, he arranged the second meeting to be held at a local park. Why did he change locations?
3. Was Dr. Sean Maguire's use of self-disclosure appropriate?
4. Will Hunting demonstrates many defense mechanisms in order to reduce his anxiety associated with his traumatic childhood and resulting circumstances. Provide examples of these.

Unfolding Patient Stories: Sharon Cole • Part 1

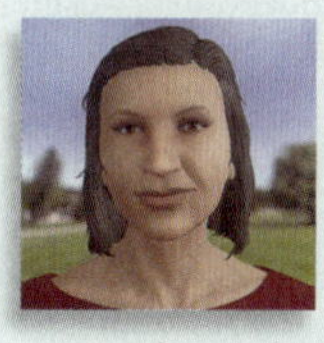

Sharon Cole, a 31-year-old diagnosed with bipolar 1 disorder, had a surgical repair of an ankle fracture sustained in a fall during a manic episode. The nurse needs to manage Sharon's physiological postsurgery needs while Sharon is still in a manic state. What interventions and communication techniques might the nurse consider to help develop a therapeutic relationship with Sharon and manage her manic behavior? What approaches can block effective communication? (Sharon Cole's story continues in Chapter 26.)

Care for Sharon Cole and other patients in a realistic virtual environment: ***vSim** for Nursing* (thepoint.lww.com/vSimMentalHealth). Practice documenting these patients' care in DocuCare (thepoint.lww.com/DocuCareEHR).

REFERENCES

Bhugra, D., Smith, A., Liebrenz, M., Ventriglio, A., Gnanapragasam, S. N., Buadze, A., Pemberton, M., & Poulter, D. (2023). "Otherness", otherism, discrimination, and health inequalities: entrenched challenges for modern psychiatric disciplines. *International Review of Psychiatry, 35*(3-4), 234–241.

Braybrook, D., Bristowe, K., Timmins, L., Roach, A., Day, E., Clift, P., Rose, R., Marshall, S., Johnson, K., Sleeman, K. E., & Harding, R. (2023). Communication about sexual orientation and gender between clinicians, LGBT+ people facing serious illness and their significant others: a qualitative interview study of experiences, preferences and recommendations. *BMJ Quality & Safety*, *32*, 109–120. https://doi.org/10.1136/bmjqs-2022-014792

Clark, A., Rose, T. A., & Meredith, P. J. (2023). Language skills and interpersonal trust in adolescents with and without mental illness. *International Journal of Speech-Language Pathology*, *25*(4), 589–607.

Coatsworth-Puspoky, R., Forchuk, C., & Ward-Griffin, C. (2006). Nurse–client processes in mental health: recipient's perspectives. *Journal of Psychiatric and Mental Health Nursing*, *13*(3), 347–355.

Crawford, J., Haffar, S., Fernando, S., Stephens, H., Harvey, S. B., & Black, M. (2024). Client perspectives: Telehealth for mental health services. *Australasian Psychiatry, 33(1), 96–102.*

Crunelle, C. L., Van Daele, T., Van Laere, S., Blancke, S., Vanderbruggen, N., & Matthys, F. (2023). Remote consultations for mental health: Patient experiences. *Journal of Community Health*, *48*(2), 347–352.

Dinoso, L., & Baudoin, C. (2023). Using principles of therapeutic communication to enhance trauma-informed care in the critical care setting to promote positive encounters. *Critical Care Nursing Clinics of North America*, *35*, 235–246.

Driedger, S. M., Kirby, S., Maier, R., Süss, R., Thorlacius, L., Saranchuk, J. W., Bohm, E., & Singer, A. (2023). Strategies used in managing conversations about prostate-specific antigen (PSA) testing among family physicians (FPs): A qualitative study. *BMJ Open*, *13*(4), e073415. https://doi.org/10.1136/bmjopen-2023-073415

Forchuk, C., Carmichael, K., Golea, G., Johnston, N., Martin, M. L., Patterson, P., Ray, K., Robinson, T., Sogbein, S. A., Srivastava, R., & Skov, T. (2006). *Nursing best practice guideline: Establishing therapeutic relationships (revision)*. Registered Nurses Association of Ontario.

Forchuk, C., Martin, M. L., Corring, D., Sherman, D., Srivastava, R., Harerimana, B., & Cheng, R. (2019a). Cost-effectiveness of the implementation of a transitional discharge model for community integration of psychiatric clients: Practice insights and policy implications. *International Journal of Mental Health*, *48*(3), 236–249.

Forchuk, F., Martin, M. L., Jensen, E., Ouseley, S., Sealy, P., Beal, G., Reynolds, W., Sharkey, S. (2012). Integrating the transitional relationship model into clinical practice. *Archives of Psychiatric Nursing*, *26*(5), 374–381.

Forchuk, C., Martin, M. L., Jensen, E., Ouseley, S., Sealy, Pl, Beal, G., Reynolds, W., Sharkey, S. (2013). Integrating an evidence-based intervention into clinical practice: 'transitional relationship model.' *Journal of Psychiatric and Mental Health Nursing*, *20*(7), 584–594.

Forchuk, C., Serrato, J., Rudnick, A., Corring, D., Mann, R., & Frampton, B. (2019b). An interconnected smart technology system for individuals with mental illness living in the community and transitional hospital apartments [Paper presentation]. In J. Pagan, M. Mokhtari, H. Aloulou, B. Abdulrazak, & M. Cabrera (Eds.), *How AI impacts urban living and public health, International Conference on Smart Homes and Health Telematic* (pp. 131–142). International Conference on Smart Homes and Health Telematics.

Galvin, E., Desselle, S., Gavin, B., Quigley, E., Flear, M., Kilbride, K., McNicholas, F., Cullinan, S., & Hayden, J. (2022). Patient and provider perspectives of the implementation of remote consultations for community-dwelling people with mental health conditions: a systematic mixed studies review. *Journal of Psychiatric Research*, *156*, 668–678. https://doi.org/10.1016/j.jpsychires.2022.10.051

Goldin, D., Maltseva, T., Scaccianoce, M., & Brenes, F. (2021). Cultural and practical implications for psychiatric telehealth services: a response to COVID-19. *Journal of Transcultural Nursing*, *32*(2), 186–190.

Hall, E. T. (1990). *The hidden dimension*. Anchor Books.

Hatami, H., Deravi, N., Danaei, B., Zangiabadian, M., Shahidi Bonjar, A. H., Kheradmand, A., & Nasiri, M. J. (2022). Tele-medicine and improvement of mental health problems in COVID-19 pandemic: a systematic review. *International Journal of Methods in Psychiatric Research*, *31*(3), e1924–n/a. https://doi.org/10.1002/mpr.1924

Jamison, K. C., Ahmed, A. H., Spoerner, D. A., & Kinney, D. (2022). Best shot: a motivational interviewing approach to address vaccine hesitancy in pediatric outpatient settings. *Journal of Pediatric Nursing*, *67*, 124–131. https://doi.org/10.1016/j.pedn.2022.08.012

Kumar, R., Sahu, M., & Tamar, R. (2022). Efficacy of Motivational Interviewing and Brief Interventions on tobacco use among healthy adults: a systematic review of randomized controlled trials. *Investigación y educación en enfermería*, *40*(3), e03. https://doi.org/10.17533/udea.iee.v40n3e03

Kwame, A., & Petrucka, P. M. (2021). A literature-based study of patient-centered care and communication in nurse-patient interactions: barriers, facilitators, and the way forward. *BMC Nursing*, *20*(1), 158. https://doi.org/10.1186/s12912-021-00684-2

Lipschitz, J. M., Connolly, S. L., Van Boxtel, R., Potter, J. R., Nixon, N., & Bidargaddi, N. (2023). Provider perspectives on telemental health implementation: lessons learned during the COVID-19 pandemic and paths forward. *Psychological Services*, *20*(Suppl 2), 11–19.

Miller, W. R. (2023). The evolution of motivational interviewing. *Behavioural and Cognitive Psychotherapy*, *51*(6), 616–632. https://doi.org/10.1017/S1352465822000431

Miller, W. R., & Moyers, T. B. (2006). Eight stages in learning motivational interviewing. *Journal of Teaching in the Addictions*, *5*(1), 3–17.

Miller, W. R., & Rollnick, S. (2023). *Motivational interviewing: Helping people change and grow* (4th ed.). The Guilford Press.

Orlando, I. (1961). *Orlando's dynamic nurse-patient relationship: Function, process and principles*. G. P. Putman's Sons.

Peplau, H. E. (1952, 1992). *Interpersonal relations in nursing*. G. P. Putnam's Sons.

Pinckney, M. Y. (2021). Examining the moral and ethical expectations of the nurse/patient relationship. *JOCEPS: The Journal of Chi Eta Phi Sorority*, 1–14.

Reeves, K., Job, S., Blackwell, C., Sanchez, K., Carter, S., & Taliaferro, L. (2024). Provider cultural competence and humility in healthcare interactions with transgender and nonbinary young adults. *Journal of Nursing Scholarship*, *56*(1), 18–30.

Schwenker, R., Dietrich, C. E., Hirpa, S., Nothacker, M., Smedslund, G., Frese, T., & Unverzagt, S. (2023). Motivational interviewing for substance use reduction. *The Cochrane Database of Systematic Reviews*, *12*, CD008063. https://doi.org/10.1002/14651858.CD008063.pub3

Self, K. J., Borsari, B., Ladd, B. O., Nicolas, G., Gibson, C. J., Jackson, K., & Manuel, J. K. (2023). Cultural adaptations of motivational interviewing: A systematic review. *Psychological Services*, *20*(Suppl 1), 7–18. https://doi.org/10.1037/ser0000619

Williamson Yarbrough, J. R. (2024). Telehealth: Measurement for best outcomes in support of rural residents. *Online Journal of Rural Nursing & Health Care*, *24*(1), 7–28. https://doi.org/10.14574/ojrnhc.v24i1.743

Wright, K.M., (2021). The therapeutic relationship in nursing theory and practice. *Mental Health Practice*, *24*(8).

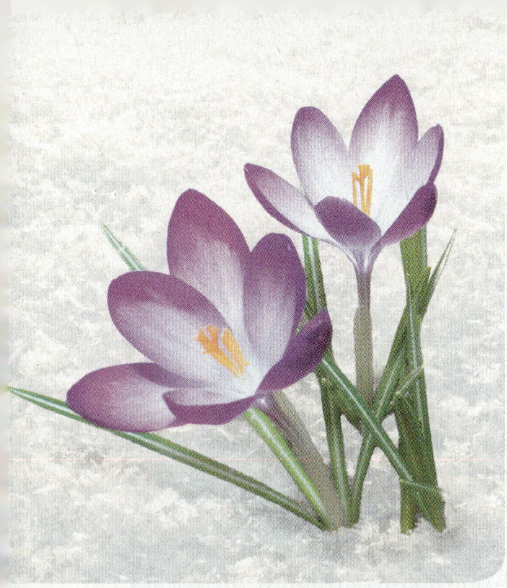

10

Clinical Judgment Nursing Care Planning in Psychiatric–Mental Health

Mary Ann Boyd

KEYCONCEPTS

- assessment
- biopsychosocial-spiritual framework
- clinical judgment
- clinical judgment measurement model
- mental status examination
- outcomes
- recovery-oriented nursing interventions
- spirituality

LEARNING OBJECTIVES

After studying this chapter, you will be able to:

1. Discuss the use of standards in psychiatric–mental health (PMH) nursing practice.
2. Discuss the relationship between the biopsychosocial–spiritual, wellness and recovery models used as frameworks for PMH nursing practice.
3. Using a clinical judgment model, define person-centered, recovery-oriented care planning in PMH nursing.
4. Recognize relevant cues in prioritizing assessment information.
5. Analyze cues in determining mental health needs, concerns, and problems.
6. Prioritize hypotheses (problems) of greatest significance for the plan of nursing care.
7. Develop recovery-oriented goals and outcomes in collaboration with the patient.
8. Apply person-centered, recovery-oriented interventions by supporting patient strengths and applying nursing actions that address prioritized mental health issues and mental disorders.
9. Collaborate with the patient in evaluating patient outcomes.

KEY TERMS

• affect • behavior modification • bibliotherapy • biologic component • body image • clarification • cognition • conflict resolution • containment • counseling • critical thinking • cultural brokering • decision-making • de-escalation • distraction • dysphoric • emotional well-being • environmental well-being • euphoric • euthymic • explicit bias • financial well-being • gender identity • guided imagery • health teaching • home visits • implicit bias • insight • intellectual well-being • judgment • labile • milieu therapy • mood • occupational well-being • open communication • patient observation • personal identity • physical well-being • psychoeducation • psychological component • reflection • registered nurses • reminiscence • risk factors • scope • self • self-care • self-concept • self-esteem • social component • social well-being • spiritual assessment • spiritual component • spiritual support • standards • structured interaction • token economy • validation

INTRODUCTION

Psychiatric–mental health (PMH) nursing practice is based on a comprehensive, holistic understanding of the people and communities in nurses' care. These nurses are licensed to practice nursing and are recognized as **registered nurses**. PMH nurses consider the physical, psychological, social, and spiritual dynamics that influence mental health and accept the challenge of including mental health promotion and wellness approaches as part of their ethical and professional obligation.

THE BIOPSYCHOSOCIAL-SPIRITUAL FRAMEWORK

The **biopsychosocial-spiritual framework** (Fig. 10.1) is a holistic model for organizing patient care. Each of the model's components—biologic, psychological, social, and spiritual—has an independent knowledge and focus but interacts and is mutually interdependent with the other components. Each component (described in the following sections) influences an individual's mental health and is useful in organizing relevant assessment information and nursing care approaches (Van Denend et al., 2022).

KEYCONCEPT The **biopsychosocial-spiritual framework** consists of four separate but interdependent components: biologic, psychological, social, and spiritual. Each component has an independent knowledge and treatment focus but interacts and is mutually interdependent with the other components.

Biologic Component

The **biologic component** is concerned with the physiologic aspects of all health conditions, including the biologic aspects of mental health conditions or disorders. Biologic theories and concepts include functional health patterns, which are essential when assessing an individual's mental health; these are exercise, elimination patterns, sleep, and nutrition. Neurobiologic theories serve as a basis for understanding and administering pharmacologic agents (see Chapters 7 and 11).

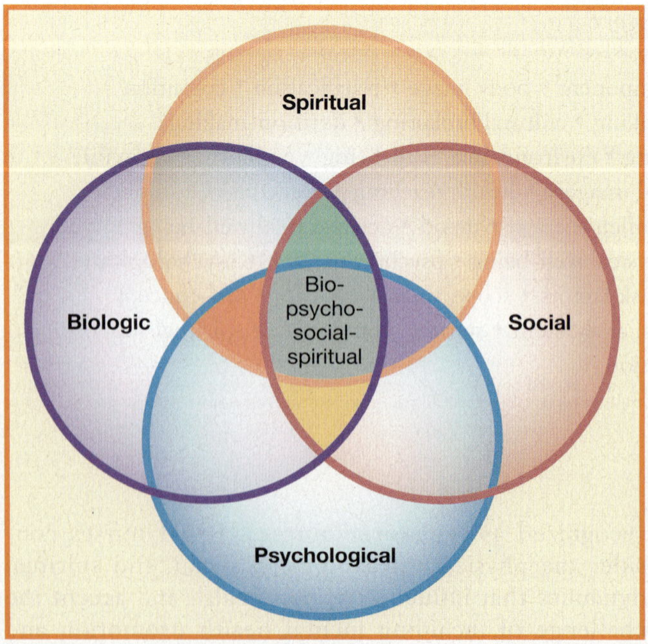

FIGURE 10.1 The biopsychosocial-spiritual model.

Psychological Component

The **psychological component** involves the theoretical basis of the psychological processes—thoughts, feelings, and behavior (intrapersonal dynamics) that influence one's emotion, cognition, and behavior. Communication and the development of a collaborative, therapeutic relationship is an important aspect of the psychological component. Psychological and nursing sciences generate theories and research critical to a nurse's understanding and assessment of patients' mental health symptoms and responses to treatment. Although some mental disorders have a neurobiologic basis, symptoms are experienced and observed as psychological. For example, even though manic behavior is caused by dysfunction in the brain, there are no laboratory tests to confirm a diagnosis, only a pattern of behavior.

Social Component

The **social component** includes theories that describe the influence of social forces on the patient, family, and community within cultural settings. Social and nursing sciences illustrate how social connections within families and communities influence mental health, treatment, and recovery. Mental disorders are not caused by social factors, but their manifestations and treatment can be significantly affected by the society in which a patient lives. For example, the presence of social and family support often improves treatment outcomes. Moreover, families of origin, extended families, or other significant relationships can positively influence or complicate a patient's mental health condition and treatment outcomes. Community forces, including cultural and ethnic groups within larger communities, shape the patient's manifestation of disorders, response to treatment, and overall view of mental illness.

Spiritual Component

The **spiritual component** focuses on the meaning of life, belief in a higher power, and connectedness with self-others and nature. Views of mental health and illnesses are shaped by the spiritual component. Mental health is influenced by spirituality and in turn spiritual beliefs and connections influence the experience of mental health.

SELF AND REFLECTION

The most important tool of psychiatric nursing is the **self**. Through relationship building, patients learn to trust the nurse who guides, teaches, and advocates for quality care and treatment. This text emphasizes the primary importance of the patient–nurse relationship. See Chapter 9.

Reflection involves ongoing self-evaluation through observing, monitoring, and judging one's own and others' behaviors with the goal of providing effective and meaningful nursing care. Reflective skills are used to enhance all aspects of PMH nursing practice, including self-awareness, nurse–patient interactions, and evaluating systems of care.

One of the biggest challenges facing nurses is examination of explicit and implicit biases. An **explicit bias** is a prejudice or negative attitude toward groups; the individual is consciously aware of this type of bias. Everyone has explicit biases; they develop from our childhoods and are steeped in our cultural attitudes toward others. An **implicit bias** is an unconscious prejudice or negative attitude toward a certain group. Biases easily lead to discriminatory behavior and microaggressions.

Both biases need to be acknowledged as problematic to quality patient care. The first step in reducing biases is recognizing and owning them as personal biases. One of the most effective ways of reducing bias is frequent contacts with group members.

HOLISTIC PLANS OF CARE

As with patients receiving treatment for a physical condition, patients receiving PMH services also have holistic plans of care. The patient and family (or member of the patient's support system) should participate in the development of the plan. Any planning should be soundly based in evidence-based practice (see Chapter 1). Planning is guided by recovery principles and practices (see Chapters 2 and 8), legal and ethical guidelines (see Chapter 4), and scope and standards of practice.

The **scope** of nursing practice is defined within a legislative and regulatory framework and delineates the services (procedures, actions, levels of care) and educational preparation that a qualified health professional is competent to perform and permitted to undertake. The **standards** of PMH nursing practice describe the responsibilities for which the nurse is accountable (American Nurses Association [ANA], American Psychiatric Nurses Association [APNA], & International Society of Psychiatric-Mental Health Nurses [ISPN), 2022; Fornili & Fogger, 2022). Scope and standards for PMH nursing care are developed by several organizations including the ANA, APNA, ISPN, International Nurses Society on Addictions (INSA), state practice acts, agency policies and procedures, and federal regulations. Nurses are held accountable to these standards and assure the public that safe, competent care is provided. All nurses should make sure that their practice is consistent with the appropriate scope and standards of practice.

CLINICAL JUDGMENT AND THE CLINICAL JUDGMENT MEASUREMENT MODEL

Sound clinical judgment depends on critical thinking skills and reflection. **Critical thinking** is an ongoing process that undergirds safe, ethical, and effective PMH nursing care. Using the critical thinking skills of problem-solving and decision-making, nurses analyze, evaluate, explain, infer, and interpret assessment information. **Decision-making** is a collaborative process of making an informed, rational decision about care. Some critical thinking activities in nursing assessments occur in an orderly fashion, over a period of time. Some clinical judgments, especially those made in response to an emergency, occur quickly, such as deciding whether a patient can leave a unit or whether a patient in crisis should receive a medication.

> **KEYCONCEPT Clinical judgment** is an iterative decision-making process that uses nursing knowledge to observe and assess presenting situations, identify a prioritized patient concern, and generate the best possible evidence-based solutions to deliver safe client care.

In this text, planning nursing care is based on the **Clinical Judgment Measurement Model (CJMM),** developed by the National Council of State Boards of Nursing (NCSBN).

> **KEYCONCEPT** The **Clinical Judgment Measurement Model** consists of six cognitive skills: recognizing cues, analyzing cues, prioritizing the hypotheses (problems), generating solutions, taking action, and evaluating outcomes.

The CJMM is consistent with the nursing process model that is based on assessment, diagnosis, outcomes identification, planning, implementation, and evaluation. See Figure 10.2.

RECOGNIZING CUES: RELEVANT ASSESSMENT INFORMATION

Assessment is the collection and interpretation of patient information related to specific health concerns, general health, wellness, strengths, and functional status. Assessment involves recognizing cues and analyzing the information that will be used in prioritizing patient problems (developing hypotheses) and generating solutions for nursing interventions.

Assessment is not an isolated activity. Rather, it is a systematic and ongoing process that occurs throughout the nurse's care of the patient. The PMH nursing assessment (Box 10.1) is a basic guide to collecting assessment data. Assessment information is entered into the patient's written or computerized record, which

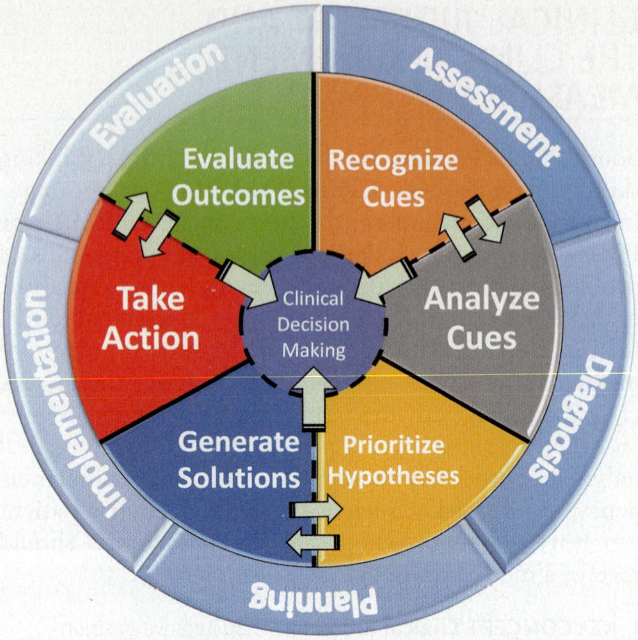

FIGURE 10.2 The Clinical Judgment Measurement Model and how it relates to the steps of the nursing process. (Reprinted with permission from Brenton, A., & Petersen, E. K. [2019]. *Next generation NCLEX® [NGN] Educator Webinar Part I*. National Council of State Boards of Nursing [NCSBN®].)

may be presented in several different formats, including forms, checklists, narratives, and problem-oriented notes.

KEYCONCEPT Assessment is the deliberate and systematic collection and interpretation of information to determine current and past health, wellness, strengths, functional status, and mental health issues, both actual and potential.

Assessment begins with the first contact with the patient, when a collaborative relationship is initiated. Legal consent must be given by the patient, and the nurse must follow the Health Insurance Portability and Accountability Act of 1996 guidelines (see Chapter 4). Patients must develop a sense of trust before they will be comfortable revealing intimate life details. It is of paramount importance that nurses have a healthy knowledge of themselves as well (Box 10.2). The nurse's own biases and values, which may be different from those of the patient, can influence the nurse's interpretation of assessment information. A careful self-assessment helps the nurse interpret the data objectively.

One of the challenges of conducting an assessment is recognizing important health and mental health cues and differentiating significant signs and symptoms from those that may not be relevant to the patient's concern. For example, a history of type 2 diabetes may not be relevant to the patient's current suicidal ideation. Safety issues are always relevant and need to be assessed.

Patient Interviews

The interview should begin with the nurse initiating introductions that include name and pronouns. For example, "Hello, my name is Jane Smith. I use she/her/hers pronouns. How may I help you today?" Note that pronouns may vary depending on the patient's **gender identity** (see Chapter 3) and that because gender identity is not an external expression, clothes, grooming, or speech may not correspond to the person's gender identity. Including pronouns helps create an inclusive environment and encourages patients to share their own pronouns, especially when patients are less comfortable with their pronouns or may have previously felt uncomfortable or unsafe sharing them. Even if the patient does not respond with pronouns, the nurse is providing a safe and inclusive interpersonal environment (Bhatt et al., 2022).

The assessment interview usually involves direct questions to obtain facts, clarify perceptions, validate observations, interpret the meanings of facts, or compare information. The specific questions may take different forms. The nurse must clearly state the purpose of the interview and, if necessary, modify the interview process, so that both the patient and the nurse agree on its purpose. The nurse may choose to use open- or closed-ended questions. Open-ended questions are most helpful when beginning the interview because they allow the nurse to observe how the patient responds verbally and nonverbally. They also convey caring and interest in the person's well-being, which helps to establish rapport. Nurses should use closed-ended questions when they need specific information. For example, "How old are you?" asks for specific information about the patient's age. These types of questions limit the individual's response but often serve as good follow-up questions for clarification of thoughts or feelings expressed.

Questions such as "How did you come to this clinic today?" allow patients to describe their experience in their own way. Some patients may answer this question concretely by saying, "I took a taxi" or "I came by car." Others may address this question by responding, "My family thought I should come, so they brought me" or "Well, I got up this morning…I took a shower, got dressed…and then, well you know, it's difficult sometimes to decide." Each of these answers helps the nurse assess the patient's thinking process as well as evaluate the content of the response.

Clarification is extremely important during the assessment process. Words do not have the same meaning to all people. Education, language, culture, history, and experience may influence the meaning of words. Sometimes, simple and direct questioning provides clarification. In other situations, the nurse may clarify by providing a specific example for a more global thought the patient is trying to express. For example, a patient may say, "Things have been so strange since the children left." The nurse

BOX 10.1

Psychiatric–Mental Health Nursing Assessment

I. **Major reason for seeking help** ______

II. **Initial information**

Name ______

Age ______ **Marital status** ______ **Gender** ______ **Ethnic identification** ______

III. **Present and past health status** ______ (Include ht., wt., BMI) ______

Summary of strengths and wellness related to physical health

	Adequate	Treated	Untreated
Physical functions: System review	☐	☐	☐
Elimination	☐	☐	☐
Activity/exercise	☐	☐	☐
Sleep	☐	☐	☐
Appetite and nutrition	☐	☐	☐
Hydration	☐	☐	☐
Sexuality	☐	☐	☐
Self-care	☐	☐	☐
Neurologic status (head trauma, movement disorder)	☐	☐	☐
Existing physical illnesses	☐	☐	☐
Medications (prescription and over the counter)	Dosage	Side effects	Frequency
Significant laboratory tests	Values	Usual range	

IV. **Mental health issues**

Major concerns regarding mental health issue ______

Recovery goals ______

Major loss/change in past year: No ______ Yes ______

Fear of violence: No ______ Yes ______

Past abuse or trauma: No ______ Yes ______

Strategies for managing issues/disorder ______

Substance Use: No ______ Yes ______

Amount ______ Frequency ______ Pattern of use ______

Need for additional screening No ______ Yes ______

V. **Mental status examination**

General observations (appearance, psychomotor activity, attitude) ______

Orientation (time, place, person) ______

Mood, affect, emotions ______

Speech (verbal ability, speed, correct use of words) ______

Thought processes (tangential, logic, repetition, rhyming of words, loose connections, disorganized) ______

Cognition and intellectual performance ______

Attention and concentration ______

Abstract reasoning and comprehension ______

Memory (recall, short term, recent, and remote) ______

Judgment and insight ______

VI. **Significant behaviors (psychomotor, agitation, aggression, withdrawn)** ______

VII. **Self-concept (body image, self-esteem, personal identity)** ______

VIII. **Stress and coping patterns** ______

IX. **Risk assessment**

Suicide: High ______ Low ______ Assault/homicide: High ______ Low ______

Suicidal thoughts or ideation: No ______ Yes ______

Current thoughts of harming self ______

Intention ______

Behavior ______

Lethality ______

Assault/homicide thoughts: No ______ Yes ______

What do you do when angry with a stranger? ______

What do you do when angry with family or partner? ______

Have you ever hit or pushed anyone? No ______ Yes ______

Have you ever been arrested for assault? No ______ Yes ______

Current thoughts of harming others ______

X. **Functional status**

Changes in functioning (work, school, home) ______

XI. **Social systems**

Family assessment

Family members ______

Members important to patient ______

Decision makers, family roles, supportive members ______

Cultural assessment

Self-identified Cultural group ______

What cultural rules do you try to live by? ______

Important cultural foods ______

Community resources ______

XII. **Spiritual assessment**

XIII. **Economic status**

XIV. **Legal status**

XV. **Quality of life**

XVI. **SUMMARY OF PSYCHOSOCIAL–SPIRITUAL STRENGTHS:**

Summary of significant data that can be used in prioritizing patient needs.

SIGNATURE/TITLE ______ Date ______

BOX 10.2

Self-Concept Awareness

Self-awareness is important in any interaction. To understand a patient's self-concept, the nurse must be aware of their own self-concept. By answering these questions, nurses can evaluate self-concept components and increase their self-understanding. The more comfortable nurses are with themselves, the more effective they can be in each patient interaction.

BODY IMAGE

- How do I feel about my body?
- How important is my physical appearance?
- How does my body measure up to my ideal body? (How would I like to appear?)
- What is positive about my body?
- What would I like to change about my body?
- How does my body image affect my self-esteem?

SELF-ESTEEM

- When do I feel confident and good about myself?
- When do I feel unimportant?
- What do I do when I feel good about myself? (Call friends, socialize?)
- What do I do when I have negative feelings about myself? (Withdraw, dress poorly?)
- When do I make negative statements?
- Am I able to correct my negative self-statements?

PERSONAL IDENTITY

- How do I describe myself?
- What three adjectives describe who I am?
- Do I identify with a particular cultural group, family role, or place of residence?
- What would I like to have on my tombstone?

COMFORT LEVEL

- How comfortable am I in caring for people with mental disorders?
- How comfortable am I in caring for people from different cultures than mine?
- How comfortable am I in caring for people with gender identities and/or sexual orientations that are different from mine?
- If I am uncomfortable caring for people in certain populations, what is my plan for becoming more comfortable?

BIASES

- What are my explicit biases?
- How can I examine my implicit biases?
- What is my plan for reducing my biases?

BOX 10.3

Assessment Interview Behaviors

The following behaviors carried out by the nurse will enhance the effectiveness of the assessment interview:

- *Exhibiting empathy*—to show empathy to the patient, the nurse uses phrases such as "That must have been upsetting for you" or "I can understand your hurt feelings."
- *Giving recognition*—the nurse gives recognition by listening actively: verbally encouraging the patient to continue and nonverbally presenting an open, interested demeanor.
- *Demonstrating acceptance*—note that acceptance does not mean agreement or nonagreement with the patient but is a neutral stance that allows the patient to continue.
- *Restating*—the nurse tries to clarify what the patient is trying to say by restating it.
- *Reflecting*—the nurse presents the patient's last statement as a question. This gives the patient a chance to expand on the information.
- *Focusing*—the nurse attempts to bring the conversation back to the questions at hand when the patient goes off on a tangent.
- *Using open-ended questions*—general questions give the patient a chance to speak freely.
- *Presenting reality*—the nurse presents reality when the patient makes unrealistic or exaggerated statements.
- *Making observations*—the nurse says aloud what patient behaviors are observed to give the patient a chance to speak to those behaviors. For example, the nurse may say, "I notice you are twisting your fingers; are you nervous about something?"

may respond with, "Sometimes, parents and caregivers feel sad and empty when their children leave home. They don't know what to do with their time." Frequently summarizing what has been said allows the patient the opportunity to correct the nurse's interpretation. For example, verbalizing a sequence of events that the patient has reported may help to identify omissions or inconsistencies. Restating information or reflecting feelings that the patient has described also allows the opportunity for clarification. It is essential that nurses understand exactly what patients are attempting to communicate before beginning to intervene. Box 10.3 provides a summary of other behaviors that enhance the effectiveness of an assessment interview.

Many psychiatric symptoms are beyond a patient's awareness. Family members, friends, and other health care professionals are important sources of information. Before seeking information from others, the nurse must obtain permission from the patient. The nurse needs to provide the patient with a clear explanation of why the information is needed and how it will be used. The nurse should explain that the strength-based assessment will include questions about wellness and strengths as well as mental health issues because these are all related to well-being.

Telehealth

There is an emerging trend to use virtual health technology (i.e., telehealth) in the assessment and treatment of mental health issues. The need for social distancing due to the COVID-19 pandemic escalated the use of digital tools. Limiting face-to-face contact is especially important for vulnerable populations such as the older adult. Virtual health care increases access to care in those areas where there is a shortage of services.

Telehealth presents challenges in maintaining confidentiality, securing informed consent, documenting, and transmitting information. In telehealth, all PMH guidelines and evidence-based practice are followed. Because telehealth can cross state and national boundaries, the nurse must practice according to applicable state, national, and international standards.

Mobile technologies, cell phones, and other devices are becoming increasingly popular and useful throughout the care process. Consistent with patient-centered care, use of mobile health applications (*mHealth*) is useful for history taking, interviewing, assessment, and treatment as well as clinician support for decision-making and up-to-date treatment (Tsanas et al., 2021).

It is important that nurses assess their patients' use of virtual devices. These devices can be incorporated into their care based on patient preference, skill, and need. There are some risks related to using virtual technology, such as privacy breaches, unnecessary self-disclosure, and cyberbullying.

Physical Health

Many mental disorders produce physical symptoms, such as the lack of appetite and weight loss associated with depression. Physical health can also affect mental health and illness, producing a recurrence or increase in symptoms. Many physical disorders may present first with symptoms considered to be psychiatric. For example, hypothyroidism often presents with feelings of lethargy, decreased concentration, and depressed mood. For these reasons, physical health information about the patient is always considered.

Current and Past Health Status

Beginning with a history of the patient's general medical condition, the nurse should consider the following:

- Availability of, frequency of, and most recent medical evaluation, including test results
- Past hospitalizations and surgical procedures
- Vision and hearing impairments
- Cardiac problems, including cerebrovascular accidents (strokes), myocardial infarctions (heart attacks), and childhood illnesses
- Respiratory problems, particularly those that result in a lack of oxygen to the brain
- Neurologic problems, particularly head injuries, seizure disorders, or any losses of consciousness
- Endocrine disorders, particularly unstable diabetes or thyroid or adrenal dysfunction
- Immune disorders, particularly human immunodeficiency virus (HIV) and autoimmune disorders
- Use, exposure, misuse, or dependence on substances, including alcohol, tobacco, prescription drugs, illicit drugs, and herbal preparations

Physical Examination

Body Systems Review

After the nurse obtains historical information, they should examine physiologic systems to evaluate the patient's current physical condition. The psychiatric nurse should pay special attention to various systems that treatment may affect. For example, if a patient is being treated with antihypertensive medication, the dosage may need to be adjusted if an antipsychotic medication is prescribed. If a patient is overweight or has diabetes, some psychiatric medications can affect these conditions. Patients with compromised immune function (HIV, cancer) may experience mood alterations.

Neurologic Status

Particular attention is paid to recent head trauma; episodes of hypertension; and changes in personality, speech, or the ability to handle activities of daily living (ADLs). Cranial nerve dysfunction, reflexes, muscle strength, and balance are included in a thorough assessment. The nurse routinely assesses and documents movement disorders using tools such as the Abnormal Involuntary Movement Scales (see Chapter 24 and Appendix).

Laboratory Results

The nurse reviews and documents any available laboratory data, especially any anomalies. Hepatic, renal, or urinary anomalies are particularly important to document because these systems metabolize or excrete many psychiatric medications. In addition, the nurse notes unusual white blood cell and electrolyte levels. Laboratory data are especially important, particularly if the nurse is the only member of the mental health team who has a "medical" background (Table 10.1).

Physical Functions

Physical functions is a broad category that includes activities that are important in daily living including activities and systems that support a positive outcome.

Self-Care

Self-care is the ability to perform ADLs successfully. Often, a patient's ability to care for themselves or to carry out ADLs, such as washing and dressing, are indicative of their psychological state. For example, a depressed patient may not have the energy to change into clean clothes. This

TABLE 10.1 SELECTED HEMATOLOGIC MEASURES AND THEIR RELEVANCE TO PSYCHIATRIC DISORDERS

Test	Possible Results	Possible Cause or Meaning
Complete Blood Count		
Leukocyte (WBC) count	Leukopenia—decrease in leukocytes (WBCs)	May be produced by phenothiazine, clozapine, carbamazepine
		Lithium causes a benign mild to moderate increase (11,000–17,000/μL)
	Agranulocytosis—decrease in number of granulocytic leukocytes	NMS can be associated with increases of 15,000–30,000/mm^3 in about 40% of cases
	Leukocytosis—increase in leukocyte count above usual limits	
WBC differential	"Shift to the left"—from segmented neutrophils to band forms	Shift often suggests a bacterial infection but has been reported in about 40% of cases of NMS
RBC count	Polycythemia—increased RBCs	Primary form—true polycythemia caused by several disease states
		Secondary form—compensation for decreased oxygenation, as in chronic pulmonary disease
		Blood is more viscous, and the patient should not become dehydrated
	Decreased RBCs	Decrease may be related to some types of anemia, which requires further evaluation
Hct	Elevations	Elevation may be caused by dehydration
	Decreased Hct	Anemia may be associated with a wide range of mental status changes, including asthenia, depression, and psychosis
		In the United States, 20% of people assigned female at birth who are of childbearing age have iron-deficiency anemia
Hb	Decreased	Another indicator of anemia; further evaluation of source requires review of erythrocyte indices
Erythrocyte indices such as RDW	Elevated RDW	Finding suggests a combined anemia, as in that from chronic alcohol use disorder, resulting from both vitamin B_{12} and folate acid deficiencies and iron deficiency
		Oral contraceptives also decrease vitamin B_{12}
Other Hematologic Measures		
Vitamin B_{12}	Deficiency	Neuropsychiatric symptoms, such as psychosis, paranoia, fatigue, agitation, marked personality change, dementia, and delirium may develop
Folate	Deficiency	The use of alcohol, phenytoin, oral contraceptives, and estrogens may be responsible
Platelet count	Thrombocytopenia—decreased platelet count	Some psychiatric medications, such as carbamazepine, phenothiazine, or clozapine, or other nonpsychiatric medications may cause thrombocytopenia
		Several medical conditions are other causes
Serum Electrolytes		
Sodium	Hyponatremia—low serum sodium	Significant mental status changes may ensue. Condition is associated with Addison disease, SIADH, and polydipsia (water intoxication) as well as carbamazepine use
Potassium	Hypokalemia—low serum potassium	Produces weakness, fatigue, ECG changes; paralytic ileus and muscle paresis may develop
		Common in individuals with bulimic behavior or psychogenic vomiting and use or misuse of diuretics; laxative misuse may contribute; can be life-threatening
Chloride	Elevation	Chloride tends to increase to compensate for lower bicarbonate
	Decrease	Binging–purging behavior and repeated vomiting may be causes
Bicarbonate	Elevation	Causes may be binging and purging in eating disorders, excessive use of laxatives, or psychogenic vomiting
	Decrease	Decrease may develop in some patients with hyperventilation syndrome and panic disorder

TABLE 10.1 SELECTED HEMATOLOGIC MEASURES AND THEIR RELEVANCE TO PSYCHIATRIC DISORDERS (*Continued*)

Test	Possible Results	Possible Cause or Meaning
Renal Function Tests		
BUN	Elevation	Increase is associated with mental status changes, lethargy, and delirium Cause may be dehydration Potential toxicity of medications cleared via the kidney, such as lithium and amantadine, may increase
Serum creatinine	Elevation	Level usually does not become elevated until about 50% of nephrons in the kidney are damaged
Serum Enzymes		
Amylase	Elevation	Level appears to increase after binging and purging behavior in eating disorders and declines when these behaviors stop
ALT—formerly SGPT	ALT > AST Elevation	Disparity is common in acute forms of viral and drug-induced hepatic dysfunction Mild elevations are common with use of sodium valproate
AST—formerly SGOT	AST > ALT	Severe elevations in chronic forms of liver disease and postmyocardial infarction may develop
CPK	Elevations of the isoenzyme related to muscle tissue	Muscle tissue injury is the cause Level is elevated in NMS Level is also elevated by repeated intramuscular injections (e.g., antipsychotics)
Thyroid Function		
Serum triiodothyronine (T_3)	Decrease	Hypothyroidism and nonthyroid illness cause decrease Individuals with depression may convert less T_4 to T_3 peripherally but not out of the usual range. Medications such as lithium and sodium valproate may suppress thyroid function, but clinical significance is unknown
	Elevations	Hyperthyroidism, T_3, and toxicosis may produce mood changes, anxiety, and symptoms of mania
Serum thyroxine (T4)	Elevations	Hyperthyroidism is a cause
TSH or thyrotropin	Elevations	Hypothyroidism—symptoms may appear very much like those of depression except for additional physical signs of cold intolerance, dry skin, hair loss, bradycardia, and so on Lithium—may also cause elevations
	Decrease	Considered nondiagnostic—may be hyperthyroidism, pituitary hypothyroidism, or even euthyroid status

ALT, alanine aminotransferase; AST, aspartate aminotransferase; BUN, blood urea nitrogen; CPK, creatine phosphokinase; ECG, electrocardiogram; Hb, hemoglobin; Hct, hematocrit; NMS, neuroleptic malignant syndrome; RBC, red blood cell; RDW, red cell distribution width; SGPT, serum glutamic pyruvic transaminase; SGOT, serum glutamic oxaloacetic transaminase; SIADH, syndrome of inappropriate secretion of antidiuretic hormone; TSH, thyroid-stimulating hormone; WBC, white blood cell.

information (i.e., whether a patient can carry out ADLs) may also help the nurse to determine actual or potential obstacles to a patient's adherence with a treatment plan.

Elimination

The nurse should inquire about and document the patient's daily urinary and bowel habits. Various medications can affect bladder and bowel functioning, so a baseline must be noted. For example, diarrhea and frequency of urination can occur with the use of lithium carbonate. Anticholinergic effects of antipsychotic medication can cause constipation and urinary hesitancy or retention.

Activity and Exercise

The patient's daily methods and levels of activity and exercise must be queried and documented. Activities are important interventions, and baseline information is needed to determine what the patient already enjoys or dislikes and whether they are getting sufficient exercise or adequate recreation. A patient may have altered activity or exercise in response to medication or therapies. In addition, many psychiatric medications cause weight gain, and nurses need to develop interventions that assist the patient in increasing activities to counteract the weight gain.

Sleep

Changes in sleep patterns often reflect changes in a patient's emotions and are symptoms of disorders. If the patient responds positively to a question about changes in sleep patterns, it is important to clarify just what those changes are. For example, "difficulty falling asleep" means different things to different people. For people who usually fall right to sleep, it could mean that it takes 10 extra minutes to fall asleep. For others who usually take 35 minutes to fall asleep, it could mean that it takes 90 minutes to do so.

Appetite and Nutrition

Changes in appetite and nutritional intake are assessed and documented because they can indicate changes in moods or relapse. For example, a patient who is depressed may not notice hunger or even that they do not have the energy to prepare food. Others may handle stressful emotions by eating more than usual. This information also provides valuable clues to possible eating disorders and problems with body image.

Obesity is one of the major health issues of many Americans, but it is particularly problematic for people with mental disorders. Many of the medications are associated with weight gain. A baseline body mass index should be determined as treatment is initiated.

Hydration

Gaining perspective on how much fluid patients usually drink and how much they are drinking now provides important data. Some medications can cause retention of fluids, and others can cause diuresis; thus, the patient's current fluid status must be understood.

Sexuality

Questioning a patient on issues involving sexuality requires comfort with one's own sexuality. The nurse should also note the patient's comfort with their sexual orientation and gender identity; issues involving these aspects that are unsettled in a patient or between a patient and a family member may cause anxiety, shame, or discomfort. It is necessary to explore how comfortable the patient is with their sexuality and sexual functioning. Asking the patient's preference for pronouns can begin a discussion about gender identity. These questions should be asked in a matter-of-fact but gentle and nonjudgmental manner. Initiating the topic of sexuality may begin with a question such as "Are you sexually active?" Birth control medications may also alter mood. Changes in sexual activity are important to assess.

History of Trauma

During the assessment, the nurse should listen for any clues of trauma including physical, emotional, or social events. If an individual has been hospitalized for any mental health issue, it is important to understand the meaning of the experience to the individual. Psychiatric hospitalizations can be traumatic and can contribute to posttraumatic stress disorders. Any abuse or mistreatment should be identified in the assessment (see Chapters 23 and 29).

Medication Assessment

The review of systems serves as a baseline from which the nurse may judge whether the initiation of a medication exacerbates symptoms or causes new ones to develop. It is important to determine which medications the patient takes now or has taken in the past. These include over-the-counter, herbal, or nonprescription medications as well as prescribed medications. This assessment is important for reasons other than serving as a baseline. It helps target possible drug interactions, determines whether the patient has already used medications that are being considered, and identifies whether medications may be causing psychiatric symptoms.

Substance Use

Substances are widely used, and information about use should always be collected in a nursing assessment. The nurse should ask about the use of illegal substances purchased on the street or internet, over-the-counter drugs, prescribed medications that are used for a nonprescribed purpose, and legal recreational substances such as alcohol and cannabis. The amount, frequency, and patterns of use should be included in the assessment. There are several screening tools that can be used to identify patterns of use such as the Alcohol Use Disorder Identification Test (AUDIT) (see Chapter 31).

Psychological Cues

Psychological concerns are the emphasis of the PMH nursing assessment. Mental disorders and emotional problems are manifested through psychological symptoms related to mental status, moods, thoughts, behaviors, and interpersonal relationships. Psychological strengths, psychological growth, and development are important parts of this assessment as well as wellness and emotional and intellectual well-being.

Mental Health Issues

Concerns regarding mental health issues or their consequences are collected in the mental health assessment.

A mental disorder, like any other illness, affects patients and families in many ways. It is safe to say that a mental disorder changes an individual's life, and the nurse should identify what the changes are and their meaning to the patient and family members. Many patients experience specific fears, such as losing their job, family, or safety. Because the nurse will be supporting coping strategies, it is important to identify current coping strategies or behaviors the patient uses. A simple question such as "How do you deal with your voices when you are with other people?" may initiate a discussion about responses to the mental disorder or emotional problem.

Mental Status Examination

The mental status examination establishes a baseline, provides a snapshot of where the patient is at a moment, and creates a written record. Areas of assessment include general observations, orientation, mood and affect, speech, thought processes, and cognition. Box 10.4 provides a narrative note of the results from a patient's mental status examination.

> **KEYCONCEPT** The **mental status examination** is an organized systematic approach to the assessment of an individual's current psychiatric condition.

General Observations

At the beginning of the interview, the nurse should record their initial impressions of the patient. These general observations include the patient's appearance, affect, psychomotor activity, and overall behavior. How is the patient dressed? Is the dress appropriate for the weather and setting? What is the patient's affect (emotional expression)? What behaviors is the patient displaying? For example, the same nurse assessed two male patients with depression. At the beginning of the mental status examination, the differences between these two men were very clear. The nurse described the first patient as "a large, well-dressed man who is agitated and appears angry, shifts in his seat, and does not maintain eye contact. He interrupts often in the initial explanation of mental status." The nurse described the other patient as a "small, unshaven, disheveled man with a strong body odor who appears withdrawn. He shuffles as he walks, speaks very softly, appears sad, and avoids direct eye contact."

> **BOX 10.4**
>
> **Narrative Mental Status Examination Note**
>
> M. J. is a 65-year-old widowed patient assigned male at birth who is slightly disheveled. He is cooperative with the interviewer and judged to be an adequate historian. His mood and affect are depressed and anxious. He becomes tearful throughout the interview when speaking about his wife. His flow of thought is hesitant but coherent when he is speaking about his wife. He is oriented to time, place, and person. He shows good recent and remote memory. He can recall several items given to him by the interviewer. He shows poor insight and judgment regarding his sadness since the loss of his wife. He repeatedly says, "Mary wouldn't want me to be sad. She would want me to continue with my life."

Orientation

The nurse can determine the patient's orientation by asking the date, time, and current location of the interview setting. If a patient knows the year but not the exact date, the interviewer can ask the season. An individual's orientation tells the nurse the extent of confusion. If a patient does not know the year or the place of the interview, they are exhibiting considerable confusion.

Mood and Affect

Mood refers to the prominent, sustained, overall emotions that the person expresses and exhibits. Mood may be sustained for days or weeks, or it may fluctuate during the day. For example, some patients with depression have a diurnal variation in their mood. They experience their lowest mood in the morning, but as the day progresses, their depressed mood lifts and they feel somewhat better in the evening. Terms used to describe mood include **euthymic** (typical), **euphoric** (elated), **labile** (changeable), and **dysphoric** (depressed, disquieted, and restless).

Affect refers to the capacity to vary outward emotional expression. Affects fluctuate with thought content and can be observed in facial expressions, vocal fluctuations, and gestures. During the assessment, the patient may exhibit anger, frustration, irritation, apathy, and helplessness while their overall mood remains unchanged.

Affect can be described in terms of range, intensity, appropriateness, and stability. Range can be full or restricted. An individual who expresses several different emotions consistent with the stated feelings and content being expressed is described as having a *full range* of affect that is congruent with the situation. An individual who expresses few emotions has a restricted affect. For example, a patient could be describing the recent tragic death of a loved one in a monotone with little expression. In determining whether this response is typical, the nurse compares the patient's emotional response with the cultural norm for that particular response. *Intensity* can be increased, flat, or blunted. The nurse determines whether the emotional response is *appropriate* for the situation. For example, an inappropriate response is shown by a patient who has an extreme reaction to the death of the children of the Uvalde elementary school shooting tragedy in 2022, as if the victims were personal friends. Another patient said that their life stopped in 2001 when the Twin Towers of the World Trade Center in New York

City collapsed due to a terrorist attack. They could not eat or sleep for weeks afterward. *Stability* can be mobile (typical) or labile. If a patient reports feeling happy one minute and reduced to tears the next, the person probably has an unstable mood. During the interview, the nurse should look for rapid mood changes that indicate lability of mood. A patient who exhibits intense, frequently shifting emotional extremes has a labile affect.

Speech

Speech provides clues about thoughts, emotional patterns, and cognitive organization. Speech may be pressured, fast, slow, or fragmented. Speech patterns reflect the patient's thought patterns, which can be logical or illogical. To check the patient's comprehension, the nurse can show a patient an object (e.g., pen, watch) and ask the person to name them. During the conversation, the nurse assesses the fluency and quality of the patient's speech. The nurse listens for repetition or rhyming of words.

Thought Processes

The nurse assesses the patient for rapid change of ideas; inability or taking a long time to get to the point; loose or no connections among ideas or words; rhyming or repetition of words, questions, or phrases; or use of unheard-of words. Any of these observations indicates anomalous thought patterns. The content of what the patient says is also important. What thought is the patient expressing? The nurse listens for unusual and unlikely stories, fears, or behaviors, for example, "The FBI is tracking me" or "I am afraid to leave my house."

Cognition and Intellectual Performance

The nurse can assess for **intellectual well-being** by determining the extent that the patient recognizes their creative abilities and is able to learn new knowledge and skills. To assess the patient's **cognition**, that is, the ability to think and know, the nurse uses memory, calculation, and reasoning tests to identify specific areas of impairment. The cognitive areas include (1) attention and concentration, (2) abstract reasoning and comprehension, (3) memory, and (4) insight and judgment.

Attention and Concentration

To test attention and concentration, the nurse asks the patient, without pencil or paper, to start with 100 and subtract 7 until reaching 65 or to start with 20 and subtract 3. The nurse must decide which is most appropriate for the patient considering education and understanding. Subtracting 3 from 20 is the easier of the two tasks. Asking a patient to spell "world" backward is also useful in determining attention and concentration.

Abstract Reasoning and Comprehension

To test abstract reasoning and comprehension, the nurse gives the patient a proverb to interpret. Examples include "People in glass houses shouldn't throw stones," "A rolling stone gathers no moss," and "A penny saved is a penny earned."

Recall, Short-Term, Recent, and Remote Memory

There are four spheres of memory to check: recall, or immediate, memory; short-term memory; recent memory; and long-term, or remote, memory. To check immediate and short-term memory, the nurse gives the patient three unrelated words to remember and asks them to recite them right after telling them and at 5- and 15-minute intervals during the interview. To test recent memory, the nurse may question about a holiday or world event within the past few months. The nurse tests long-term or remote memory by asking about events years ago. If they are personal events and the answers seem incorrect, the nurse may check them with a family member.

Insight and Judgment

Insight and judgment are related concepts that involve the ability to examine thoughts, conceptualize facts, solve problems, think abstractly, and possess self-awareness. **Insight** is an individual's awareness of their own thoughts and feelings and the ability to compare them with the thoughts and feelings of others. It involves an awareness of how others view one's behavior and its meaning. For example, many patients do not believe that they have mental illness. They may have delusions and hallucinations or be hospitalized for bizarre and sometimes dangerous behavior, but they are completely unaware that their behavior is unusual or atypical. During an interview, a patient may adamantly proclaim that nothing is wrong or that they do not have a mental illness. Even if a problem is recognized, the patient may lack insight regarding issues related to care.

Judgment is the ability to reach a logical decision about a situation and to choose a course of action after examining and analyzing various possibilities. Throughout the interview, the nurse evaluates the patient's ability to make logical decisions. For example, some patients may continually choose partners who are abusive. The nurse could logically conclude that these patients have poor judgment in selecting partners. Another way to examine a patient's judgment is to give a simple scenario and ask the person to identify the best response. An example of such a scenario is asking, "What would you do if you found a bag of money outside a bank on a busy street?" If the patient responds with "Run with it," their judgment is questionable.

Behavior

Throughout the assessment, the nurse observes any behavior that may have significance in understanding the patient's response or symptoms of the mental disorder or emotional problem. For example, a depressed patient may be tearful throughout the session, whereas an anxious patient may twist or pull their hair, shift in the chair, or be unable to maintain eye contact. The nurse may find that whenever a topic is addressed, the patient's behavior changes. The nurse needs to relate patterned behaviors to significant events by connecting behaviors with the assessment data. For example, a patient may change jobs frequently, causing family distress and financial problems. Exploration of the events leading up to job changes may elicit important information regarding the patient's ability to solve problems.

Self-Concept

Self-concept, which develops over a lifetime, represents the total beliefs about three interrelated dimensions of the self: body image, self-esteem, and personal identity. The importance of each of these dimensions varies among individuals. For some, beliefs about themselves are strongly tied to body image; for others, personal identity is most important. Still others develop personal identity from what others have told them over the years. The nurse carrying out an assessment must keep in mind that self-concept and its components are dynamic and variable. For example, a person may have a consistent self-concept until their first pregnancy. At that time, the many physiologic changes of pregnancy may cause a change in body image. The person may be comfortable and enjoy the "glow of pregnancy" or may feel like a "bloated cow." Suddenly, body image is the most important part of their self-concept, and how they handle it can increase or decrease self-esteem or sense of personal identity. Thus, all the components are tied together, and each one affects the others.

Self-concept is assessed through eliciting patients' thoughts about themselves, their ability to navigate in the world, and their nonverbal behaviors. A disheveled sloppy physical appearance outside cultural norms is an indication of poor self-concept. Negative self-statements, such as "I could never do that," "I have no control over my life," and "I'm so stupid," reveal poor views of self. The nurse's own self-concept can shape the nurse's view of the patient. For example, a nurse who is self-confident and feels inwardly scornful of a patient who lacks such confidence may intimidate the patient through unconscious, judgmental behaviors, or inconsiderate comments.

A useful approach to measuring self-concept is asking the patient to draw a self-portrait. For many patients, drawing is much easier than writing and serves as an excellent technique for monitoring changes. Interpretation of self-concept from drawings focuses on size, color, level of detail, pressure, line quality, symmetry, and placement. Low self-esteem is expressed by small size, lack of color variation, and sparse details in the drawing. Powerlessness and feelings of inadequacy are expressed through a lack of a head, a mouth, arms, or feet in the drawing. A lack of symmetry (placement of figure parts or entire drawings off center) represents feelings of insecurity and inadequacy. As self-esteem builds, size increases, color tends to become more varied and brighter, and more details appear. Figure 10.3 shows a self-portrait of a patient at the beginning of treatment for depression and another drawn 3 months later.

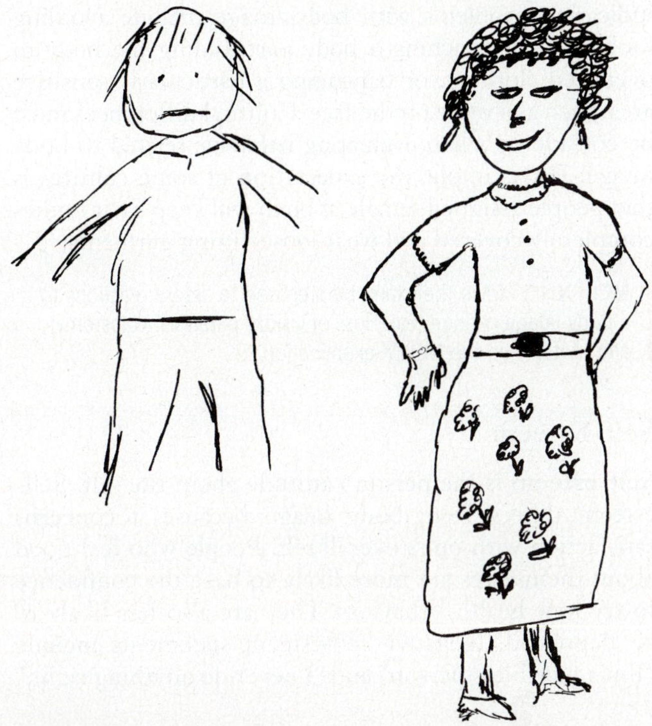

FIGURE 10.3 **Left.** Self-portrait of a 52-year-old woman at first group session following discharge from hospital for treatment of depression. **Right.** Self-portrait after 3 months of weekly group interventions.

Body Image

Body image represents an individual's beliefs and attitudes about their body and includes such dimensions as size (large or small) and attractiveness (pretty or ugly). People who are satisfied with their body have a more positive body image than those who are not satisfied. Generally, women attach more importance to their body image than do men (Gualdi-Russo et al., 2022).

Patients express body image beliefs through statements about their bodies. Statements such as "I feel so ugly," "I'm so fat," and "No one will want to have sex with me" express negative body images. Nonverbal behaviors indicating problems with body image include avoiding looking at or touching a body part; hiding the body in oversized clothing; or bandaging a particularly sensitive area, such as a mole on the face. Cultural differences must be considered when evaluating behavior related to body image. For example, the expectation of some cultures is that people assigned female at birth will keep their bodies completely covered and wear loose-fitting garments.

NCLEXNOTE On the exam, be prepared to assess reactions to a body image change (e.g., loss of vision, paralysis, colostomy, amputation) on the NCLEX examination.

Self-Esteem

Self-esteem is the person's attitude about the self. Self-esteem differs from body image because it concerns satisfaction with one's overall self. People who feel good about themselves are more likely to have the confidence to try new health behaviors. They are also less likely to be depressed. Negative self-esteem statements include "I'm a worthless person" and "I never do anything right."

Personal Identity

Personal identity is knowing "who I am." Every life experience and interaction contributes to knowing oneself better. Personal identity allows people to establish boundaries and understand personal strengths and limitations. In some psychiatric disorders, individuals cannot separate themselves from others, which shows that their personal identity is not strongly developed. A problem with personal identity is difficult to assess. Statements such as "I'm just like my mother, and she was always in trouble," "I become whatever my current boyfriend wants me to be," and "I can't make a decision unless I check it out first" are all statements that require further exploration into the person's view of self.

Stress and Coping Patterns

Everyone has stress (see Chapter 19). One of the dimensions of wellness is **emotional well-being** or the ability to cope with stress through skills and strategies. Sometimes, the experience of stress contributes to the development of mental disorders. Identification of major stresses in a patient's life helps the nurse understand the person and support the use of successful coping behaviors in the future. The nurse should explore how the patient deals with stress and identify successful coping mechanisms to encourage their use.

NCLEXNOTE Every assessment should focus on stress and coping patterns. Identifying how a patient copes with stress can be used as a basis of care in all nursing situations. Include content from Chapter 19 when studying these concepts.

Risk Assessment

Risk factors are characteristics, conditions, situations, or events that increase the patient's vulnerability to threats to safety or well-being. Throughout this text, the sections concerning risk factors focus on the following:

- Risks to the patient's safety
- Risks for developing psychiatric disorders
- Risks for increasing, or exacerbating, symptoms and impairment in an individual who already has a psychiatric disorder

Consideration of risk factors involving patient safety should be included in each assessment. Examples of these risks include the risk for suicide and violence toward others or the risk for events, such as falling, seizures, allergic reactions, or elopement (unauthorized absence from health care facility). Nurses assess factors on a priority basis. For example, threats of violence or suicide take priority.

Suicide Screening

Every mental health nursing assessment should include a suicide screening. During the assessment, the nurse needs to listen closely to whether the patient describes or mentions thinking about self-harm. If the patient does not openly express ideas of self-harm, it is necessary to ask straightforward questions related to suicide.

The Columbia Suicide Severity Rating Scale (C-SSRS) is a commonly used, evidence-based measure used to identify and assess individuals at risk for suicide (Posner et al., 2011). This instrument measures severity of suicidal ideation, intensity of ideation, suicidal behavior, and lethality. It is appropriate for use over the telephone or in telehealth. C-SSRS screening toolkits are available for specific settings such as health care, correctional facilities, primary care, and police officers. All the C-SSRS screening tools consist of six questions. The C-SSRS for health care providers is a good place for nurses to learn the questions and how to respond (Box 10.5).

Two questions should be included in the screening. "Have you wished you were dead or wished you could go to sleep and not wake up?" and "Have you actually had any thoughts about killing yourself?" If the answer is "no" to both questions, the nurse should ask one more, "Have you done anything, started to do anything, or prepared to do anything to end your life?" If the answer is "no" to the third question, the nurse can assume that the person most likely is not suicidal.

If the answer is "yes" to any of these three questions, the nurse should ask the following three questions: "Have you thought about how you might do this?" "Have you had any intention of acting on these thoughts of killing yourself, as opposed to you have the thoughts but you

BOX 10.5

How to Use the Columbia Suicide Severity Rating Scale

	Past Month	
1) Have you wished you were dead or wished you could go to sleep and not wake up?		
2) Have you actually had any thoughts about killing yourself?		
If **YES** to 2, answer questions 3, 4, 5, and 6 If **NO** to 2, go directly to question 6		
3) Have you thought about how you might do this?		
4) Have you had any intention of acting on these thoughts of killing yourself, as opposed to you have the thoughts but you definitely would not act on them?	**High Risk**	
5) Have you started to work out or worked out the details of how to kill yourself? Do you intend to carry out this plan?	**High Risk**	
Always Ask Question 6	**Life-time**	**Past 3 Months**
6) Have you done anything, started to do anything, or prepared to do anything to end your life? *Examples:* Collected pills, obtained a gun, gave away valuables, wrote a will or suicide note, held a gun but changed your mind, cut yourself, tried to hang yourself, etc.		**High Risk**

NATIONAL SUICIDE PREVENTION LIFELINE™
1-800-273-TALK(8255)
suicidepreventionlifeline.org

Any YES indicates that someone should <u>seek a behavioral health referral.</u> However, if the answer to 4, 5, or 6 is YES, seek <u>immediate help:</u> go to the emergency room, call 1-800-273-8255, text 741741, or call 911 and <u>STAY WITH THEM</u> until they can be evaluated.

Reprinted with permission from The Columbia Lighthouse Project. (2016). About the Protocol: Using the Columbia Protocol. https://cssrs.columbia.edu/the-columbia-scale-c-ssrs/about-the-scale/

would definitely not act on them?" and "Have you done anything, started to do anything, or prepared to do anything to end your life?" If the answer is "yes" to any of these questions, the nurse should seek a referral to an advanced practice nurse, psychologist, or other mental health clinicians trained to complete a comprehensive assessment. The nurse should notify the supervisor and clearly document the patient responses and nursing follow-up. The nurse should not leave the patient alone and should explore the details of the intention and behavior. If a nurse and patient are not face-to-face, but on the telephone or other virtual means, the nurse should keep the patient talking and follow agency policy. The National Suicide Prevention Lifeline 988 or 1-800-273-8255 is a resource that can provide support and direction to the nurse as well as the patient.

To assess the patient's ability to cope with suicidal thoughts, the nurse can ask the patient to identify strategies that were used in resisting suicidal urges and actions. For example, one patient reported calling a family member to talk when the suicidal urges were strong. The nurse can encourage the patient to use these strategies in the future. This information will be helpful in the development of a safety plan (see Chapter 22).

Assaultive or Homicidal Ideation

When assessing a patient, the nurse also needs to listen carefully to any delusions or hallucinations that the patient shares. If the patient gives any indication that they must or are being told to harm someone, the nurse must first think of self-safety and institute assaultive precautions as indicated by the facility protocols. General questions to ascertain assaultive or homicidal ideation follow:

- Do you intend to harm someone? If yes, who?
- Do you have a plan? If yes, what are the details of the plan?
- Do you have the means to carry out the plan? (If the plan requires a weapon, is it readily available?)

Social Cues

The nurse collects information on the patient's social support and networks. The nurse elicits cues about interactions with others in the family and community (work, church, or other organizations); parents/caregivers and their marital relationship; place in birth order; and relationships with spouse, siblings, and children. The nurse also assesses work and education history and community activities. The nurse observes how the patient relates to any family or friends who may be in attendance. This component of the assessment helps the nurse anticipate how the patient may get along with other patients in an inpatient setting. It also allows the nurse to plan for any anticipated difficulties.

Functional Status

An important aspect of the assessment is determining the functioning of the patient (i.e., Is an adult working and living independently? Is a student attending classes?). How the patient copes with strangers and those with whom they do not get along is also important information.

Social Systems

A significant component of the patient's life involves the social systems in which they may be enmeshed. **Social well-being** involves developing a sense of connection and a well-developed support system. The social systems to examine include the family, the culture to which the patient belongs, and the community in which they live.

Family Assessment

How the patient fits in with and relates to their family is important to know. General questions to ask include the following:

- Who do you consider family?
- How important to you is your family?
- How does your family make decisions?
- What are the roles in your family, and who fills them?
- Where do you fit in your family?
- With whom in your family do you get along best?
- With whom in your family do you have the most conflict?
- Who in your family is supportive of you?

Cultural Assessment

Culture can profoundly affect an individual's worldview (see Chapter 3). Culture helps people frame beliefs about life, death, health and illness, and roles and relationships. During cultural assessment, the nurse must consider factors that influence the manifestations of the current mental disorder. For example, a patient mentions "speaking in tongues." The nurse may identify this experience as a hallucination when, in fact, the patient was having a religious experience common within some branches of Christianity. In this instance, knowing and understanding such religious practices will prevent a misinterpretation of the symptoms.

The nurse can elicit important cultural information by asking the following questions:

- To what cultural group do you belong?
- Were you raised in an ethnic community?

- How do you define health?
- How do you define illness?
- How do you define good and evil?
- What do you do to get better when you are physically ill? Mentally ill?
- Whom do you see for help when you are physically ill? Mentally ill?
- By what cultural rules or taboos do you try to live?
- Do you eat special foods?

Community Support and Resources

Many patients are connected to community resources, and the nurse needs to assess what they are and the patterns of usage. For example, a patient who is homeless may know of a church where they can sleep but may go there only on cold nights. Or a patient may go to the community center daily for lunch to be with other people. Examining the environment is a part of the individual's assessment. **Environmental well-being** involves living in pleasant, stimulating environments that support a healthy lifestyle.

Occupational Status

Occupational well-being involves personal satisfaction and enrichment derived from one's work. The nurse should document the occupation the patient is now in as well as a history of jobs. If the patient has changed jobs frequently, the nurse should ask about the reasons. Perhaps the patient has faced such problems as an inability to focus on the job at hand or to get along with others. If so, such issues require further exploration.

Economic Status

Finances are very private for many people; thus, the nurse must ask questions about economic status carefully. However, **financial well-being** is satisfaction with present and future situations. What the nurse needs to ascertain is not specific dollar amounts but whether the patient feels stressed by finances and has enough for basic needs.

Legal Status

Because of laws governing people with mental illness, ascertaining the patient's correct age, marital status, and any legal guardianship is important. The nurse may need to check the patient's medical records for this information.

Quality of Life

The patient's perspective on quality of life (QoL) means how the patient rates their life. Does a patient feel their life is poor because they cannot purchase everything they want? Does another patient feel blessed because the sun is shining today? Listening carefully to the patient's discussion of their life and how they measure the quality of that life provides important information about self-concept, coping skills, desires, and dreams.

Spiritual Assessment

> **KEYCONCEPT Spirituality** "Spirituality is a dynamic and intrinsic aspect of humanity thought which persons seek ultimate meaning, purpose, and transcendence and experience relationship to self, family, others, community, society, nature, and the significant or sacred. Spirituality is expressed through beliefs, values, traditions, and practices" (Puchalski et al., 2014).

Several studies show that spirituality and religion are important in coping with mental disorders through providing hope, comfort, and meaning of life and serve as a resource for coping with symptoms, substance misuse, and protection against suicide (Clark & Emerson, 2021; Rosmarin et al., 2021). Nurses must be clear about their own spirituality to be sure it does not interfere with assessment of the patient's spirituality. Nurses also need to work within their area of competence and recognize the importance of referring patients to a health care chaplain or other spiritual care support.

The purpose of a nursing **spiritual assessment**, which is often the responsibility of the nurse, is to identify specific spiritual care needs and include these in a care plan. A nursing spiritual assessment is usually included in the general nursing assessment, even when there are chaplains available (Toney-Butler & Unison-Pace, 2022). *The Joint Commission* requires that spiritual care assessment and spiritual care delivery be directed to the patient or the patient's family but does not identify specific disciplines of the personnel who will conduct the assessment (The Joint Commission, 2022).

The spiritual assessment is based on an individual's needs, which are discovered within an open, trusting dialogue. It is important that the nurse does not self-disclose personal values and beliefs during the assessment. The following questions can serve to initiate the assessment:

- How important is spirituality and/or religion in your life and coping with an illness?
- Are you involved in a religious or faith community?
- Would you like to address these issues in your mental health care?
- If yes, with whom would you like to address these issues?

Spiritual assessment questions need to correspond to the patient's readiness to discuss this topic. Patients and clinicians agree that it may take time for the patient to feel comfortable and ready to discuss spirituality. It is essential that questions are asked that focus on a patient's strengths. For example, asking the question "Was there a time in your life where you felt great peace and joy and maybe not so stressed out?" is less judgmental than the question "What were your sources of deep meaning, peace, joy, and strength during your times of stress?" The latter statement has an implied expectation that there should be sources (religious, spiritual) that exist.

Examples of questions that could help patients examine past or current spiritually related strengths and resources include the following (Gomi et al., 2014):

- Was there a time in your life when you really felt at peace?
- What do you do to get through the tough times (pray, meditate, visit nature, family)?
- When do you feel most positive about yourself?
- What brings inspiration to your life?

Questions that can help the individual connect spiritual goals to recovery goals (if that is a goal of the person) include the following (Gomi et al., 2014):

- What helps you feel good or hopeful about your life?
- Is spirituality something you want to connect with in your recovery?
- Based on what you said, how would you say your spirituality could support your recovery?

Strengths and Wellness Assessment

During the assessment, the nurse should identify areas of strength and wellness including **physical well-being** or positive sleep patterns, healthy diet, or motivation to engage in healthy behaviors. Does the patient recognize the need for physical activity, diet, and nutrition? Recognition of this wellness dimension can help motivate the individual to improve these behaviors. A description of these areas should be validated with the patient and documented in the patient's record.

ANALYZING CUES AND DEVELOPING HYPOTHESES

Once the nurse collects the assessment cues, the next step is analyzing the information and identifying the patient's needs, concerns, or problems. Analyzing cues ideally is carried out with the patient who participates in the analysis process. For example, based on a patient's responses, appearance, nonverbal communication, and behavior, the nurse suggests that the patient is depressed. The patient then can agree or disagree with the nurse's analysis.

When analyzing assessment cues, the following questions can be used:

- Why did the patient seek out mental health help?
- What is the most critical health issue?
- Are there any signs of a medical crisis such as hypoglycemia, hypertensive crisis?
- Are there any signs of a mental health crisis such as suicidal or homicidal thoughts?
- Is there confusion or psychosis that would result in a fall or poor judgment?

PRIORITIZING HYPOTHESES AND CONCERNS

The nurse needs to be able to hypothesize the patient's health care priorities. In a collaborative process, the patient and nurse prioritize the patient's concerns and generate solutions. There will be times when the patient and nurse are at odds about the top priority. For example, a nurse may identify the treatment of psychosis as a priority and the patient may want a place to stay. Using evidence that supports the patient's request, the nurse generates a plan to find housing before the patient considers medications. In another instance, a patient has a credible suicide plan, and the nurse insists that safety is the top priority and is a life-or-death situation.

Safety is always the first priority to be considered. Is the patient suicidal or homicidal? If the patient is thinking about self-harm or hurting others, this concern is a priority. In prioritizing other concerns, the nurse could start with Maslow's hierarchy of needs (see Chapter 6). Does the patient need shelter, food, rest, physical health care? These basic needs should be addressed before higher-level needs are met.

Typical mental health needs and concerns include thought disorders, mood-related problems, and anxiety. Self-esteem, self-worth, and identity are important considerations. These concerns can be prioritized according to the problems that most interfere with the patient's ability to function and QoL.

With experience, the nurse can cluster the assessment data to identify two or three immediate health or mental health issues related to promotion of health and well-being, prevention of illness, reduction of risks, or treatment of health care problems.

GENERATING SOLUTIONS: PLANNING RECOVERY AND WELLNESS GOALS

Mutually agreed-upon goals flow from the prioritization of needs and provide guidance in determining appropriate interventions. As the nurse guides the development of the plan, the impact of trauma should be considered. It may be necessary to address the triggers surrounding a traumatic event before focusing on enhancing self-esteem. For example, until the beliefs underlying self-blame for interpersonal violence are changed, the goal of increasing self-esteem is not realistic.

Nursing is not only concerned about mental health needs and problems, but also enhancing wellness activities. Goals are monitored and evaluated throughout the care process. For example, no longer hearing voices is a short-term goal for someone with schizophrenia, but a long-term goal is returning to meaningful activities such as work or school.

KEYCONCEPT Outcomes are results and consequences of interventions that are attributed to nursing care at a given point in time to address specific concerns, problems, or symptoms as reported by the patient or observed by the nurse.

An expected outcome is concise, measurable, stated in few words and in neutral terms. Measuring outcomes not only demonstrates clinical effectiveness but also helps to promote rational clinical decision-making and is reflective of the nursing interventions. Outcomes can be expressed in terms of the patient's actual responses (no longer reports hearing voices) or the health or mental health changes after the implementation of nursing interventions (see Table 10.2 for example outcomes).

Interdisciplinary Care

Nurses are accountable for documenting patient outcomes, nursing interventions, and any changes in health status or care plan, or both. The nurse also collaborates with other professionals, patients, and family members in all settings. In the hospital, a patient may see a psychiatrist or psychiatric nurse practitioner who treats the symptoms and prescribes the medication; a case manager who coordinates care; a psychiatric social worker for individual psychotherapy; a psychiatric nurse for management of responses related to the mental disorder, administration of medication, and monitoring side effects; and an occupational therapist for transition into the workplace. In a community clinic, patients may meet weekly with a therapist, monthly with a mental health provider who prescribes medication, and twice a week with a group leader in a day treatment program. An interdisciplinary group of professionals bring specialized skills to the patient's care.

When professionals from other disciplines provide services to the same patient, as in a hospital or outpatient treatment facility, an interdisciplinary treatment plan may be used with or instead of a traditional nursing care plan. When an interdisciplinary plan is used, nurses should make sure the nursing components of the plan are easily identified and take responsibility for implementation and team input. The nurse provides care within the PMH nurse's scope of practice, so a traditional nursing care plan may or may not be used, depending on institutional policies.

Both nursing care plans and interdisciplinary treatment plans are individualized, based on the patient's needs and strengths. It is important for the nurse to understand the complete treatment plan and the nurse's role when working with other disciplines. At times, third-party payers, who reimburse the costs of the service, review, and approve the plan.

This text places an emphasis on developing nursing care plans because they serve as a basis of nursing practice and can also be used in a multidisciplinary or interdisciplinary individual treatment plan.

TABLE 10.2 EXAMPLE OUTCOMES

Concern	Outcome	Intervention
Socially isolated on unit	Interact with other patients	Using a contract format, ask patient to commit to interacting with two people each day.
	Attend group meetings	Ask patient to identify groups of interest and commit to attending at least two each day.

TAKING ACTION: RECOVERY-ORIENTED NURSING INTERVENTIONS

Recovery-oriented nursing interventions are autonomous actions within the scope of nursing practice. Some nursing interventions, such as administering medication, require provider orders to initiate. In both instances, the nurse is held to a standard of nursing care.

KEYCONCEPT Recovery-oriented nursing interventions are nursing actions or treatment, selected based on clinical judgment and mutual decision-making with the patient, that are designed to achieve patient, family, or community outcomes. Interventions can be direct or indirect and can target specific symptoms, health needs, and strengths (Box 10.6).

There are several nursing intervention systems, including the Nursing Interventions Classification (Wagner et al., 2024), the Clinical Care Classification system (Saba, 2012), and the Omaha System nursing model (Martin, 2005; Muehlbauer et al., 2023; Schleder Goncalves et al., 2024). All these systems are recognized by the ANA. In this text, the *Psychiatric-Mental Health Nursing: Scope and Standards of Practice* (3rd ed.) and the *Addictions Nursing: Scope and Standards of Practice* guide the use of interventions (ANA, APNA, & ISPN, 2022; Fornili & Fogger, 2022). Some are adapted from classification systems and others from the PMH nursing literature.

BOX 10.6

Research for Evidence-Based Practice: Recovery-Oriented Interventions

Tamayo, N., & Lane, A. (2022). Effective nursing recovery-oriented interventions for individuals with substance use disorder. Journal of Addictions Nursing, *33(4), 233–246. https://doi.org/10.1097/JAN.0000000000000489*

THE QUESTION: What are the effective nursing interventions, actions, and behaviors that support the recovery of individuals with substance use disorder (SUD)?

METHODS: CINAHL, PsychIINFO, Academic Search Complete, Sage Journals, ScienceDirect, SocINDEX, and MEDLINE databases were searched using keywords "interventions" or "actions", or "behavior", and "recovery" and "substance use" or "addiction", and "nurs." Seventeen studies were found that included nurses who provided care to adults with SUD. All studies used a qualitative data collection methodology.

FINDINGS: Three themes and subthemes emerged from these studies including person-centered care, empowerment, and enhancing supports and capability. Subthemes that emerged included maintaining the humanness of the person, collaboration and promotion of autonomy, sustaining hope and future orientation, listening and stimulating reflections, and skill acquisition.

IMPLICATIONS FOR NURSING: These results support the use of the recovery model in caring for individuals with SUDs.

Trauma-Informed Approaches

During the implementation of nursing interventions, the nurse must be sensitive to the impact of the trauma on the individual. For example, if a patient was abused as a child, interventions that remind the patient of the abuse should be avoided. Before touching a patient, the nurse should ask permission. Other patients may be uncomfortable in the presence of another patient or staff member who reminds the patient of the person who abused them. Nurses should recognize that psychiatric hospitalization is a traumatizing experience.

Cultural Humility

Cultural humility is a core PMH nursing standard (see Chapter 3). Self-evaluation and personal critique are inherent in caring for any patient, but especially those with highly stigmatized mental health issues such as schizophrenia or bipolar disorder. When caring for culturally diverse individuals, it is important to assess personal biases through self-reflection. The nurse needs to recognize the power imbalance between the nurse, who has access to private health information, and the patient who is at the mercy of the mental health system—often on a locked unit in a hospital. Promotion of respectful, nonpaternalistic partnerships help challenge any power imbalances experienced by the patient.

Gender-Sensitive Care

The health and mental health disparities of LGBTQ+ patients are well documented with transgender individuals, who experience greater challenges and disparities due to societal norms, institutionalized discrimination, prejudice, and violence (Bhatt et al., 2022). Nursing care should be provided within an inclusive, gender-affirming atmosphere. See Chapter 3.

Physical Care

Biologic interventions focus on physical functioning and are directed toward the patient's self-care, activities and exercise, sleep, nutrition, relaxation, hydration, and thermoregulation as well as pain management and medication management. All these activities are important to mental health and wellness. The nurse should always consider enhancing the mental health of all patients. The following discussion focuses on the care of people with mental health issues.

Promotion of Self-Care Activities

Many patients with PMH issues can manage ADLs or self-care activities such as bathing, dressing appropriately, selecting adequate nutrition, and sleeping regularly. Others cannot manage such self-care activities, either because of their symptoms or because of the side effects of medications.

In the inpatient setting, the nurse structures the patient's activities, so that basic self-care activities are completed. During acute phases of psychiatric disorders, the inability to attend to basic self-care tasks, such as getting dressed, is very common. Thus, the ability to complete personal hygiene activities (e.g., dental care, grooming) is monitored, and patients are assisted in completing such activities. In a psychiatric facility, patients are encouraged and expected to develop independence in completing these basic self-care activities. In the community, monitoring these basic self-care activities is always a part of the nursing visit or clinic appointment.

Activity and Exercise Interventions

In some psychiatric disorders (e.g., schizophrenia), people become sedentary and appear to lack the motivation to complete ADLs. This lack of motivation is part of the disorder and requires nursing intervention. In addition, side effects of medication often include sedation and lethargy. Encouraging regular activity and exercise can improve general well-being and physical health. In some instances, exercise behavior becomes an exaggerated focus of attention, as may be observed in some patients with anorexia nervosa.

When assuming the responsibility of direct care provider, the nurse can help patients identify realistic activities and exercise goals. As a leader or manager of a psychiatric unit, the nurse can influence ward routine. Alternatively, the nurse can delegate activity and exercise interventions to nurses' aides. Some institutions have other professionals (e.g., recreational therapists) available for the implementation of exercise programs. As a case manager, the nurse should consider the activity needs of individuals when coordinating care.

Sleep Interventions

Many psychiatric disorders and medications are associated with sleep disturbances. Sleep is also disrupted in patients with dementia; such patients may have difficulty falling asleep or may frequently awaken during the night. In dementia of the Alzheimer type, individuals may reverse their sleeping patterns by napping during the day and staying awake at night.

Nonpharmacologic interventions are always used first because of the side-effect risks associated with the use of sedatives and hypnotics (see Chapter 11). Sleep interventions to communicate to patients include the following:

- Go to bed only when tired or sleepy.
- Establish a consistent bedtime routine.
- Avoid stimulating foods, beverages, or medications.
- Avoid naps in the late afternoon or evening.
- Eat lightly before retiring and limit fluid intake.
- Use your bed only for sleep or intimacy.
- Avoid emotional stimulation before bedtime.
- Use behavioral and relaxation techniques.
- Limit distractions.

Nutrition Interventions

Psychiatric disorders and medication side effects can affect eating behaviors. For varying reasons, some patients eat too little, but others eat too much. For instance, patients with mental illnesses who are homeless have difficulty maintaining adequate nutrition because of their deprived lifestyle. Substance misuse also interferes with maintaining adequate nutrition, either through stimulation or suppression of appetite or through neglecting nutrition because of drug-seeking behavior. Thus, nutrition interventions should be specific and relevant to the individual's circumstances and mental health. In addition, recommended daily nutritional allowances are important in the promotion of physical and mental health, and nurses should consider them when planning care.

Some psychiatric symptoms involve changes in perceptions of food, appetite, and eating habits. If a patient believes that food is poisonous, they may eat sparingly or not at all. Interventions are then necessary to address the suspiciousness as well as to encourage adequate intake of recommended daily allowances. Allowing patients to examine foods, participate in preparations, and test the safety of the meal by eating slowly or after everyone else may be necessary. For patients who are paranoid, it is sometimes helpful to serve prepackaged foods.

Relaxation Interventions

Relaxation promotes comfort, reduces anxiety, alleviates stress, eases pain, and prevents aggression. It can diminish the effects of hallucinations and delusions. The many different relaxation techniques used as mental health interventions range from simple deep breathing to biofeedback to hypnosis. Although some techniques, such as biofeedback, require additional training and, in some instances, certification, nurses can easily apply simple relaxation, distraction, and imagery techniques.

Simple relaxation techniques encourage and elicit relaxation to decrease undesirable signs and symptoms. **Distraction** is the purposeful focusing of attention away from undesirable sensations, and **guided imagery** is the purposeful use of imagination to achieve relaxation or direct attention away from undesirable sensations (Box 10.7).

Relaxation techniques that involve physical touch (e.g., back rubs) usually are not used for people with mental disorders. Touching and massaging usually are not appropriate, especially for those who have a history of physical or sexual abuse. Such patients may find touching too stimulating or misinterpret it as being sexual or aggressive.

Hydration Interventions

Assessing fluid status and monitoring fluid intake and output are often important interventions. Over- or underhydration can be a symptom of a disorder. For example, some patients with psychotic disorders experience chronic fluid imbalance. Many psychiatric medications affect fluid and electrolyte balance (see Chapter 11). For example, when taking lithium carbonate, patients must have adequate fluid intake and pay special attention to testing serum sodium levels. Interventions that help patients understand the relationship of medications to fluid and electrolyte balance are important in their overall care.

Thermoregulation Interventions

Many psychiatric disorders can disturb the body's typical temperature regulation. Thus, patients cannot sense

BOX 10.7

Relaxation Techniques: Descriptions and Implementation

RELAXED BREATHING

The goal of this exercise is to slow down your breathing, especially your exhaling.

STEPS

1. Choose a word that you associate with relaxation such as calm, relax, or peaceful.
2. Inhale through your nose and exhale slowly through your mouth. Take usual breaths, not deep ones.
3. While you exhale, say the relaxing word you have chosen. Say it very slowly, like this: "c-a-a-a-a-a-a-l-m" or "r-e-e-e-l-a-a-a-x."
4. Pause after exhaling before taking your next breath. If it is not too distracting, count to 4 before inhaling each new breath.
5. Repeat the entire sequence 10 to 15 times.

MUSCLE RELAXATION

The goal of this technique is to gently stretch your muscles to reduce stiffness and tension. The exercises start at your head and work down to your feet. You can do these exercises while sitting in a chair.

STEPS

1. *Neck rolls.* Drop your head to one side. Gently roll it around in a wide circle. Repeat three to five times. Then reverse directions, and gently roll your head in a wide circle the other way. Repeat three to five times.
2. *Shoulder shrugs.* Lift both shoulders in a shrugging motion. Try to touch your ears with your shoulders. Let your shoulders drop down after each shrug. Repeat three to five times.
3. *Overhead arm stretches.* Raise both arms straight above your head. Interlace your fingers, like you are making a basket, with your palms facing down (toward the floor). Stretch your arms toward the ceiling. Then, keeping your fingers interlaced, rotate your palms to face upward (toward the ceiling). Stretch toward the ceiling. Repeat three to five times. If it is not comfortable to do this step with your arms overhead, try it with your arms reaching out in front of you.
4. *Knee raises.* Reach down and grab your right knee with one or both hands. Pull your knee up toward your chest (as close to your chest as is comfortable). Hold your knee there for a few seconds, before returning your foot to the floor. Reach down and grab your left knee with one or both hands and bring it up toward your chest. Hold it there for a few seconds. Repeat the sequence three to five times.
5. *Foot and ankle rolls.* Lift your feet and stretch your legs out. Rotate your ankles and feet, three to five times in one direction, then three to five times in the other direction.

Reprinted from Substance Abuse and Mental Health Services Administration. (2009). *Illness management and recovery: Practitioner guides and handouts.* HHS Pub. No. SMA-09-4462. Center for Mental Health Services, Substance Abuse and Mental Health Services Administration, U.S. Department of Health and Human Services.

temperature increases or decreases and consequently cannot protect themselves from extremes of hot or cold. This problem is especially difficult for people who are homeless or live outside the protected environments of institutions and boarding homes. In addition, many psychiatric medications affect the ability to regulate body temperature.

Interventions include educating patients about the problem of thermoregulation, identifying potential extremes in temperatures, and developing strategies to protect the patient from the adverse effects of temperature changes. For example, reminding patients to wear coats and sweaters in the winter or to wear loose, lightweight garments in the summer may prevent frostbite or heat exhaustion, respectively.

Pain Management

Psychiatric nurses are more likely to provide care to patients experiencing chronic pain than acute pain. However, a single intervention is seldom successful for relieving chronic pain. In some instances, pain is managed by medication; in other instances, nonpharmacologic strategies, such as simple relaxation techniques, distraction, or imagery, are used. Indeed, relaxation is one of the most widely used cognitive and behavioral approaches to pain. Education, stress management techniques, hypnosis, and biofeedback are also used in pain management. Physical agents include heat and cold therapy, exercise, and transcutaneous nerve stimulation.

The key to managing pain is identifying how it disrupts the patient's personal, social, professional, and family life. Education focusing on the pain, use of medications for treatment, and development of cognitive skills are important pain management components. In some cases, redefining treatment success as improvement in functioning, rather than alleviation of pain, may be necessary. The interaction between stress and pain is important; that is, increased stress leads to increased pain. Patients can better manage their pain when stress is reduced.

Wellness Interventions

Several of the interventions that the nurse and patient agree upon can be considered wellness interventions such as exercise, healthy food choices, and sleep. The nurse should emphasize the importance of these interventions as a lifestyle choice that should continue once the mental disorder is in remission.

Medication Interventions

The nurse administers many psychiatric medications to help patients maintain therapeutic regimens. **Medication intervention** involves more than the actual administration of medications. Nurses also assess medication effectiveness and side effects and consider drug–drug interactions. Monitoring the amount of lethal prescription medication is particularly important. For example, check if patients have old prescriptions of tricyclic antidepressants in their medicine cabinets. Treatment with psychopharmacologic agents can be lengthy because of the chronic nature of many disorders; many patients remain on medication regimens for years and manage their own medications. Thus, medication education is an ongoing intervention that requires careful documentation. Medication follow-up may include home visits as well as telephone calls.

Psychological Interventions

A major emphasis in PMH nursing is the psychological component: emotion, behavior, and cognition. The basis of nursing care is establishing a therapeutic relationship with the patient. Because the therapeutic relationship was extensively discussed in Chapter 9, it is not covered in this chapter. This section does cover cognitive interventions, counseling, conflict resolution, bibliotherapy, reminiscence, behavior therapy, psychoeducation, health teaching, and spiritual interventions. Chapter 6 presents the theoretic basis for many of these interventions.

Cognitive Interventions

Evidence-based cognitive interventions are used in a variety of practice settings (in- and outpatient). The knowledge and skills inherent in cognitively based interventions have been extensively studied, and their effectiveness has been demonstrated for a variety of psychiatric disorders, especially depression (see Chapter 25) and anxiety and related disorders (see Chapters 27 and 28).

Cognitive interventions are based on the concept of cognition. Cognition can be defined as an internal process of perception, memory, and judgment through which an understanding of self and the world is developed.

Cognitive interventions aim to change or reframe an individual's automatic thought patterns that have developed over time and that interfere with the individual's ability to function optimally. The skills and techniques developed based on cognitive theory result in a new view of self and the environment.

Counseling Interventions

Counseling interventions are interactions between a nurse and a patient, family, or group experiencing immediate or ongoing difficulties related to their health or well-being. Counseling is usually short term and focuses on stabilizing symptoms, supporting personal recovery goals, improving coping abilities, reinforcing healthy behaviors, fostering positive interactions, or preventing illness and disability. Counseling strategies are discussed throughout the text. Psychotherapy, which differs from counseling, is generally a long-term approach aimed at improving or helping patients regain previous health status and functional abilities. Mental health specialists, such as advanced practice nurses, use psychotherapy.

Conflict Resolution and Cultural Brokering

Conflict resolution is a process that two or more individuals, families, and groups use to find a peaceful solution to a problem. Conflict can be positive if individuals see the problem as solvable and providing an opportunity for growth and interpersonal understanding. The nurse may be in the position of teaching family members how to resolve their own conflicts positively. Key elements of any conflict resolution process are collaboration, motivation to seek a solution, and the ability to see the other person's point of view. Conflict resolution strategies are commonly taught to adolescents who are experiencing cyberbullying and to adults in marital or romantic relationships (Bickham et al., 2021; Craft et al., 2021; Moyano et al., 2023). Nurses are often in leadership positions and use conflict resolution skills to settle employee disputes.

At times, patients who are politically and economically powerless find themselves in conflict with the health care system. Differences in cultural values and languages among patients and health care organizations contribute to feelings of powerlessness. For example, immigrant families, migrant farm workers, people who are homeless, and people who need to make informed decisions under stressful conditions may be unable to navigate the health care system. The nurse can help to resolve such conflicts through **cultural brokering**, the act of bridging, linking, or mediating messages, instructions, and belief systems between groups of people of differing cultural systems to reduce conflict or produce change (Kayrouz et al., 2021).

For the "nurse as broker" to be effective, the nurse establishes and maintains a sense of connectedness or relationship with the patient. In turn, the nurse also establishes and cultivates networks with other health care facilities and resources. Cultural sensitivity enables the nurse to be aware of and sensitive to the needs of patients from a variety of cultures. Cultural humility is necessary for the brokering process to be effective.

Bibliotherapy and Social Media

Bibliotherapy, sometimes referred to as bibliocounseling, is the reading of selected written materials to express feelings or gain insight under the guidance of a health care provider. The provider assigns and discusses with the patient a book, story, or article. The provider makes the assignment because they believe that the patient can receive therapeutic benefit from the reading. (It is assumed that the provider who assigned the reading has also read it.) The provider needs to consider the patient's reading level before making an assignment. If a patient has limited reading ability, the provider should not use bibliotherapy.

Literary works serve as a projective screen through which people see themselves in the story. Literature can help patients identify with characters and vicariously experience their reality. The use of bibliotherapy has been shown to reduce suicidal thoughts (Franz et al., 2022). It can also expose people to situations that they have not personally experienced—the vicarious experience allows growth in self-knowledge and compassion (Davis et al., 2023). Bibliotherapy can also support recovery through reading books written in first person (Brewster & McNicol, 2021). Through reading, patients can enrich their lives in the following ways:

- *Catharsis:* expression of feelings stimulated by parallel experiences
- *Problem-solving:* development of solutions to problems in the literature from practical ideas about problem-solving
- *Insight:* increased self-awareness and understanding as the reader explores personal meaning from what is read
- *Anxiety reduction:* use of self-help written materials that can reduce concerns about a diagnosed problem and treatment

Using the internet can be helpful to patients, but it also has drawbacks. Some websites can help patients gain insight into their problems through acquiring new knowledge and interacting with others in the privacy of their own surroundings. Web materials and chat groups are variable in quality and accuracy. Nurses should carefully evaluate the quality of the website.

Reminiscence

Reminiscence, the thinking about or relating of past experiences, is used as a nursing intervention to enhance life review in older patients. Reminiscence encourages patients, either in individual or in group settings, to discuss their past and review their lives. Through reminiscence, individuals can identify past coping strategies that can support them in current stressful situations. Patients can also use reminiscence to maintain self-esteem, stimulate thinking, and support the natural healing process of life review. Activities that facilitate reminiscence include writing an account of past events, making an audio recording and playing it back, explaining pictures in old family albums, drawing a family tree, and writing to old friends.

Behavior Therapy

Behavior therapy interventions focus on reinforcing or promoting desirable behaviors or altering undesirable ones. The basic premise is that because most behaviors are learned, new functional behaviors can also be learned. Behaviors—not internal psychic processes—are the targets of the interventions. The models of behavioral theorists serve as a basis for these interventions (see Chapter 6).

Behavior Modification

Behavior modification is a specific, systematized behavior therapy technique that can be applied to individuals, groups, or systems. The aim of behavior modification is to reinforce desired behaviors and extinguish undesired ones. Desired behavior is rewarded to increase the likelihood that patients will repeat it, and over time, replace the problematic behavior with it. Behavior modification is used for various problematic behaviors, such as dysfunctional eating, alcohol or substance use disorders, anger management, and impulse control and often is used in the care of children and adolescents.

Token Economy

Used in inpatient settings and in group homes, a **token economy** applies behavior modification techniques to multiple behaviors. In a token economy, patients are rewarded with tokens for selected desired behaviors. They can use these tokens to purchase meals, leave the unit, watch television, or wear street clothes. In less restrictive environments, patients use tokens to purchase additional privileges, such as attending social events.

Token economy systems have been especially effective in reinforcing positive behaviors in people who are developmentally disabled or have severe and persistent mental illnesses. The strategy has been helpful for reducing aggression in children (Yassine & Tipton-Fisler, 2022) and in increasing daily living skill acquisition for people with disabilities (Beahm et al., 2023).

There is evidence that the use of token economy for behavior and symptom management is effective in adults who are hospitalized, but there is no standardized token economy program that varies from facility to facility (Fernandez et al., 2023). More research is needed to show that the changes that occur as a result of a token economy intervention are generalizable to everyday life.

Complementary Therapies

Use of complementary and integrative therapies is one of the PMH nurse's practice standards (see Chapter 12).

BOX 10.8

Research for Evidence-Based Practice: Psychoeducation Program for People With Schizophrenia

Alhadidi, M., Hadid, L. A. R. A., Danaee, M., Abdullah, K. L., & Yoong, T. L. (2023). Effects of psychoeducation on people with schizophrenia in long-term care: An intervention study. Journal of Psychosocial Nursing and Mental Health Services, *61(2), 9–18. https://doi.org/10.3928/02793695-20220613-02*

THE QUESTION: What is the effect of a psychoeducation intervention on knowledge, insight, and internalized stigma among people with schizophrenia in a long-term care facility?

METHODS: The study was based on a cluster randomization pre- and posttest design. Seven sessions were given to an intervention group ($n = 66$) over a 3-week period. A control group ($n = 56$) received care as usual.

FINDINGS: The intervention group significantly improved knowledge (15.5%) and insight (22.5%) and reduced stigma (18%) compared to the control group (2.6%, 4.7%, and 3.6%, respectively).

IMPLICATIONS FOR NURSING: Psychiatric–mental health nurses can use psychoeducation programs in care for people with schizophrenia in long-term care facilities.

These therapies include meditation, yoga, acupuncture, Reiki, Health Touch, nutrition, physical exercises, dietary supplement, aromatherapy, herbology, art, and music (ANA, APNA, & ISPN, 2022). To use these therapies, the nurse should apply the current research findings to guide nursing actions. The nurse may need additional credentialing to implement these therapies.

Psychoeducation

Psychoeducation uses educational strategies to teach patients the skills they lack because of a psychiatric disorder. The goal of psychoeducation is a change in knowledge and behavior. Nurses use psychoeducation to meet the educational needs of patients by adapting teaching strategies to their disorder-related deficits (Box 10.8). As patients gain skills, functioning improves. Some patients may need to learn how to maintain their morning hygiene. Others may need to understand their illness and cope with hearing voices that others do not hear.

Specific psychoeducation techniques are based on adult learning principles, such as beginning at the point where the learner is currently and building on their current experiences. Thus, the nurse assesses the patient's current skills and readiness to learn. From there, the nurse individualizes a teaching plan for each patient. They can conduct such teaching in a one-to-one situation or in a group format.

Psychoeducation is a continuous process of assessing, setting goals, developing learning activities, and evaluating for changes in knowledge and behavior. Nurses use it with individuals, groups, families, and communities. Psychoeducation serves as a basis for psychosocial rehabilitation, a service delivery approach for those with severe and persistent mental illness (see Chapter 24).

NCLEXNOTE Apply knowledge from social sciences to help patients manage responses to psychiatric disorders and emotional problems.

Health Teaching

Health teaching is one of the standards of care for psychiatric nurses. Teaching methods should be appropriate to the patient's development level, learning needs, readiness, ability to learn, language preference, and culture. Teaching can be conducted in an individual or group setting (see Chapter 14). Based on principles of learning, health teaching involves transmitting new information to the patient and providing constructive feedback and positive rewards, practice sessions, homework, and experimental learning. Health teaching is the integration of principles of teaching and learning with the knowledge of health and illness (see Fig. 10.4).

Thus, in health teaching, the psychiatric nurse attends to potential health care problems other than mental disorders and emotional problems. For example, if an individual has diabetes mellitus and is taking insulin, the nurse provides health care teaching related to diabetes and the interaction of this problem with the mental disorder.

Spiritual Interventions

Spiritual interventions are based on an assessment of the patient's spiritual needs. Some interventions require actions such as listening, requesting a chaplain's presence, or providing spiritual or meaningful readings; other interventions involve use of personal abilities and characteristics such as the use of the therapeutic relationship in supporting patient well-being. A nonjudgmental relationship and just "being with" (not doing for) the patient are key spiritual interventions. To assist people in spiritual distress, the nurse should know and understand the beliefs and practices of various spiritual groups. **Spiritual support,** which is assisting patients to feel balance and connection within their relationships, involves listening to expressions of loneliness, using empathy, and if available, providing patients with desired spiritual articles (McLean, 2022).

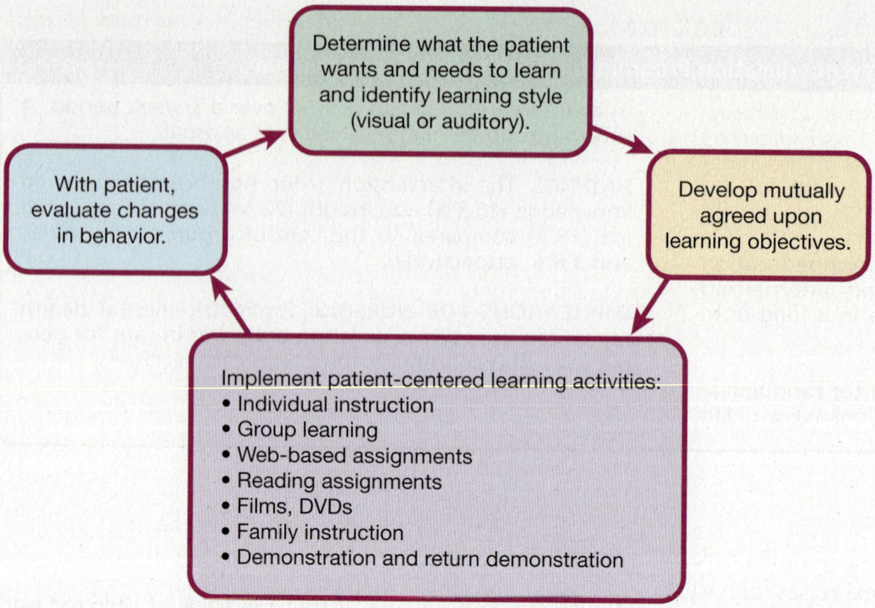

FIGURE 10.4 Teaching evaluation model.

Social Interventions

The social component includes the individual's environment and its effect on their responses to mental disorders and distress. Interventions within the social component are geared toward couples, families, friends, and large and small social groups, with special attention given to ethnicity and community interactions. In some instances, nurses design interventions that affect a patient's environment, such as helping a family member decide to admit a loved one to a long-term care facility. In other instances, the nurse modifies the environment to promote positive behaviors. Group interventions are discussed in Chapter 14.

Social Behavior and Privilege Systems in Inpatient Units

In psychiatric units, unrelated strangers who have problems interacting live together in close quarters, sometimes with two to four people sharing bedrooms and bathrooms. For this reason, most psychiatric units develop a list of behavioral expectations called unit rules that staff members post and explain to patients upon admittance. Their purpose is to facilitate a comfortable and safe environment; they have little to do with the patients' reasons for admission. Getting up at certain times, showering before breakfast, making the bed, and not visiting others' rooms are typical expectations. It is usually the nurse manager who oversees the operation of the unit and the implementation of privilege systems.

Most psychiatric facilities use a privilege system to protect patients and to reinforce unit rules and other appropriate behavior (also see the previous section discussing token economies). The more appropriate the behavior, the more privileges of freedom the person has. Privileges are based on the assessment of a patient's risk of harming self or others and ability to follow treatment regimens. For example, a patient with few privileges may be required to stay on the unit and eat only with other patients. A patient with full privileges may have freedom to leave the unit and go outside the hospital and into the community for short periods.

Milieu Therapy

Milieu therapy provides a stable and coherent social organization to facilitate an individual's treatment. (The terms *milieu therapy* and *therapeutic environment* are often used interchangeably.) In **milieu therapy**, the design of the physical surroundings, structure of patient activities, and promotion of a stable social structure and cultural setting enhance the setting's therapeutic potential. A therapeutic milieu facilitates patient interactions and promotes personal growth. Milieu therapy is the responsibility of the nurse in collaboration with the patient and other health care providers. The key concepts of milieu therapy include containment, validation, structured interaction, and open communication.

Containment

Containment is the process of providing safety and security and involves the patient's access to food and shelter. In a well-contained milieu, patients feel safe from their illnesses and protected against social stigma. The physical surroundings are also important in this process and should be clean and comfortable, with special attention paid to promoting a noninstitutionalized environment. Pictures on walls, comfortable furniture, and soothing colors help patients relax. Most facilities encourage patients and nursing staff to wear street clothes, which helps decrease the formalized nature of hospital settings and promote nurse–patient relationships.

Therapeutic milieus emphasize patient involvement in treatment decisions and operation of the unit; nurses should encourage freedom of movement within the contained environment. Patients participate in maintaining the quality of their physical surroundings, assuming responsibility for making their own beds, attending to their own belongings, and keeping an acceptable living area. Families are viewed as a part of the patient's life, and ties are maintained. In most inpatient settings, specific times are set for family interaction, education, and treatment. Family involvement is often a criterion for admission for treatment, and the involvement may include regular family attendance at therapy sessions.

Validation

In a therapeutic environment, **validation** is another process that affirms patient individuality. Staff–patient interactions should constantly reaffirm the patient's humanity and human rights. All interaction a staff member initiates with a patient should reflect their respect for that patient. Patients must believe that staff members truly like and respect them.

Structured Interaction

One of the most interesting milieu concepts is **structured interaction,** which is purposeful interaction that allows patients to interact with others in a useful way. For instance, the daily community meeting provides structure to explain unit rules and consequences of violations. Ideally, patients who either are elected or volunteer for the responsibility assume leadership for these meetings. In the meeting, the group discusses behavioral expectations, such as making beds daily, appropriate dress, and rules for leaving the unit. Usually, there are other rules, such as no fighting or name calling.

In some instances, the treatment team assigns structured interactions to specific patients as part of their treatment. Specific attitudes or approaches are directed toward individual patients who benefit from a particular type of interaction. Nurses consistently assume indulgence, flexibility, passive or active friendliness, matter-of-fact attitude, casualness, watchfulness, or kind firmness when interacting with specific patients. For example, if a patient is known to overreact and dramatize events, the staff may provide a matter-of-fact attitude when the patient engages in dramatic behavior.

Open Communication

In **open communication,** the staff and patient willingly share information. Staff members invite patient self-disclosure within the support of a nurse–patient relationship. In addition, they provide a model of effective communication when interacting with one another as well as with patients. They arrange an environment to facilitate optimal interaction and resocialization. Support, attention, praise, and reassurance given to patients improve self-esteem and increase confidence. Patient education is also a part of this support, as are directions to foster coping skills.

Milieu Therapy in Different Settings

Milieu therapy is applied in various settings. In long-term care settings, the therapeutic milieu becomes essential because patients may reside there for months or years. These patients typically have schizophrenia or developmental disabilities. Structure in daily living is important to the successful functioning of the individuals and the overall group but must be applied within the context of individual needs. For example, if a patient cannot get up one morning in time to complete assigned tasks (e.g., showering or making a bed) because of a personal crisis the night before, the nurse should consider the situation compassionately and flexibly, not applying the "consequences" rule or taking away the patient's privileges. In turn, the nurse must weigh individual needs against the collective needs of all the patients. For a patient who is consistently late for treatment activities, the nurse should apply the rules of the unit even if it means taking away privileges.

Concepts of milieu therapy have been applied to short-term inpatient and community settings. In acute care inpatient settings, nursing actions provide limits to and controls on patient behavior and provide structure and safety for the patients. Milieu treatments are based on the individual needs of the patients and include relaxation groups, discussion groups, and medication groups. Spontaneous and planned activities are possible on a short-term unit as well as in a long-term setting. In the community, it is possible to apply milieu therapy approaches in day treatment centers, group homes, and single dwellings.

Promoting Safety

Although the use of social rules of conduct and privilege systems can enhance smooth operation of a unit, some potentially serious problems can be associated with these practices. The most critical aspect of PMH nursing is the promotion of patient safety, especially in inpatient units.

Observation

Patient observation is the ongoing assessment of the patient's mental status to identify and subvert any potential problem. An important process in all nursing practice, observation is particularly important in psychiatric nursing. In psychiatric settings, patients are ambulatory and thus more susceptible to environmental hazards. In addition, judgment and cognition impairment are symptoms of many psychiatric disorders. Often, patients are admitted because they pose a danger to themselves or others. In psychiatric nursing, observation is more than just "seeing" patients. It means continually monitoring them for any indication of harm to themselves or others.

All patients who are hospitalized for psychiatric reasons are continually monitored. The intensity of the observation depends on their risk to themselves and others. Some patients are merely asked to "check in" at different times of the day, but others have a staff member assigned to only them, as in instances of potential suicide. Often "sharps," such as razors, are locked up and given to patients at specified times. Mental health facilities and units all have policies that specify levels of observation for patients of varying degrees of risk.

De-escalation

De-escalation is an interactive process of calming and redirecting a patient who has an immediate potential for violence directed toward self or others. This intervention involves assessing the situation and preventing it from escalating to one in which injury occurs to the patient, staff, or other patients. After the nurse has assessed the situation, the nurse calmly calls to the patient and asks the individual to leave the situation. The nurse must avoid rushing toward the patient or giving orders (see Chapter 20). Nurses can use various interventions in this situation, including distraction, conflict resolution, and cognitive interventions.

Home Visits

Patients usually have been hospitalized or have received treatment for acute psychiatric symptoms before they are referred to psychiatric home service. The goal of **home visits**, the delivery of nursing care in the patient's living environment, is to maximize the patient's functional ability within the nurse–patient relationship and with the family or partner as appropriate. The psychiatric nurse who makes home visits needs to be able to work independently, is skilled in teaching patients and families, can administer and monitor medications, and uses community resources for the patient's needs.

Home visits are especially useful in certain situations, including helping patients who are reluctant to enter therapy, conducting a comprehensive assessment, strengthening a support network, and maintaining patients in the community when their condition deteriorates. Home visits are also useful in helping individuals adhere to the medication regimen. The home visit process consists of three steps: the previsit phase, the home visit, and the postvisit phase. During previsit planning, the nurse sets goals for the home visit based on data received from other health care providers or the patient. In addition, the nurse and patient agree on the time of the visit. As the nurse travels to the home, the nurse should assess the neighborhood for access to services, socioeconomic factors, and safety.

The actual visit can be divided into four parts. The first is the greeting phase, in which the nurse establishes rapport with family members. Greetings, which are usually brief, establish the communication process and the atmosphere for the visit. Greetings should be friendly but professional. In cultures that consider greetings important, this phase may involve more formal interactions, such as eating food or drinking tea with family members. The next phase establishes the focus of the visit. Sometimes, the purpose of the visit is medication administration, health teaching, or counseling. The patient and family must be clear regarding the purpose. The implementation of the service is the next phase and should use most of the visit time. If the purpose of the visit is problem-solving or decision-making, the family's cultural values may determine the types of interaction and decision-making approaches. Closure is the last phase, the end of the home visit. It is a time to summarize and clarify important points. The nurse should also schedule any additional visits and reiterate patient expectations between visits. Usually, the nurse is the only provider to see the patient regularly. The nurse should acknowledge family members on leaving if they were not a part of the visit.

The postvisit phase includes documentation, reporting, and follow-up planning. This is also when the nurse meets with the supervisor and presents data from the home visit at the team meeting.

Community Action

Nurses have a unique opportunity to promote mental health awareness and support humane treatment for people with mental disorders. Activities range from being an advisor to support groups to participating in the political process through lobbying efforts and serving on community mental health boards. These unpaid activities are usually outside the realm of a job. However, an important role of professionals is to provide community service in addition to service through income-generating positions.

Evaluating Outcomes

Evaluation of patient outcomes involves answering the following questions:

- What is the cost-effectiveness of the intervention?
- What benefits did the patient receive?
- What was the patient's level of satisfaction?
- Was the outcome specific or nonspecific to the patient's need?

Outcomes can be measured immediately after the nursing intervention or after time passes. For example, a patient may be able to resolve the acute depression and demonstrate confidence and improved self-esteem during a hospital stay. In various cases, it may be several months before the person can engage in positive interpersonal relationships.

SUMMARY OF KEY POINTS

- Assessment is the deliberate and systematic collection of information or data to determine current and past health, mental health, wellness, strengths, functional status, and present and past coping patterns.
- Self-knowledge and the use of reflection underlie the development of cultural humility and the use of gender-neutral language.
- Trauma shapes the significance of mental health symptoms and the ability to participate in care. Sensitivity to the impact of trauma forms the basis of quality mental health nursing care.
- Physical cues include current and past health status; physical examination with review of body systems; review of physical functions; and pharmacologic, substance use, strengths, and wellness status.
- Psychological cues include the mental status examination, behavioral responses, and risk factor assessment.
- The mental status examination includes general observation of appearance, psychomotor activity, and attitude; orientations; mood; affect; emotions; speech; and thought processes.
- Behavioral responses are assessed, as are self-concept and current and past coping patterns.
- Risk factor assessment includes ascertaining whether the patient has any suicidal, assaultive, or homicidal ideation.
- Psychological strengths and wellness attributes are summarized.
- Social cues include functional status; social systems; occupational, economic, and legal status; QoL; social strengths; and wellness attributes.
- Spiritual assessment is an important aspect of understanding the person from a holistic perspective.
- Once information is collected, the nurse analyzes the information, generates hypotheses including establishing priorities, and planning with the patient for mutually agreeable outcomes. Anticipated patient outcomes provide direction for PMH nursing interventions.
- Nurses take action through the integration of interventions focusing on biologic (self-care, activity and exercise, sleep, nutrition, thermoregulation, and pain and medication management); psychological (counseling, conflict resolution, bibliotherapy, reminiscence, behavior therapy, psychoeducation, health teaching, and spiritual interventions); social (safety interventions, behavior therapy and modification, milieu therapy, and various home and community interventions) and spiritual (assisting patients to feel balanced, connected through use of empathy, listening) concerns. Complementary and integrative therapies are used to address all these concerns.
- Evaluation of patient outcomes involves assessing cost-effectiveness of the interventions, benefits to the patient, and the patient's level of satisfaction. Outcomes should be measurable, either immediately after intervention or after some time.

DEVELOPING CLINICAL JUDGMENT

1. A 23-year-old person assigned female at birth is admitted to an acute psychiatric setting for depression. This is the patient's first admission, but they have had bouts of depression since early adolescence. The patient and their partner have just ended their wedding engagement and moved into separate apartments. The patient's parents had told the couple that they were "living in sin" and that living together before marriage was against God's will. The patient wants to "end it all!" From this scenario, develop three important assessment questions related to physical health and safety.
2. Identify usual laboratory values for sodium, blood urea nitrogen, liver enzymes (ALT and AST), leukocyte count, and thyroid functioning. Why are these values important to know?
3. Write a paragraph on your self-concept, including all three components: body image, self-esteem, and personal identity. Explore the type of patient situations in which your self-concept can help your interactions with patients. Explore the types of patient situations in which your self-concept can hinder your interactions with patients.
4. Tom, age 25, has schizophrenia. He lives with his parents, who want to retire and move to Florida. Tom goes to work each day but relies on his parents for meals, laundry, and reminders to take his medication. Tom believes that he can manage the home, but his parents are concerned. They ask the nurse for advice about leaving their son to manage on his own. What approach would you use?
5. Joan, a 35-year-old married person assigned female at birth, is admitted to an acute psychiatric unit for stabilization of her mood disorder. Joan is extremely depressed but refuses to consider a recommended medication change and asks the nurse what to do.

Using a nursing intervention, explain how you would approach Joan's problem.

6. A nurse reports to work for the evening shift. The unit is chaotic. The television in the day room is loud; two patients are arguing about the program. Visitors are mingling in patients' rooms. The temperature of the unit is high. One patient is running up and down the hall yelling, "Help me, help me." Using a milieu therapy approach, what would you do to calm the unit?

REFERENCES

American Nurses Association (ANA), American Psychiatric Nurses Association, & International Society of Psychiatric-Mental Health Nurses. (2022). *Psychiatric-mental health nursing: Scope and standards of practice* (3rd ed.). ANA.

Beahm, L. A., Ingvarsson, E. T., Funk, N., Haskins, L., & Frazier, J. (2023). Using an App-based token economy to increase engagement in daily living and vocational tasks with adults with developmental disabilities. *Behavior Analysis in Practice, 16*(4), 1–14. https://doi.org/10.1007/s40617-023-00774-4

Bhatt, N., Cannella, J., & Gentile, J. P. (2022). Gender-affirming care for transgender patients. *Innovations in Clinical Neuroscience, 19*(4–6), 23–32.

Bickham, D. S., Moukalled, S., Inyart, H. K., & Zlokower, R. (2021). Evaluating a middle-school digital citizenship curriculum (screenshots): Quasi-experimental study. *JMIR Mental Health, 8*(9), e26197. https://doi.org/10.2196/26197

Brewster, L., & McNicol, S. (2021). Bibliotherapy in practice: A person-centred approach to using books for mental health and dementia in the community. *Medical Humanities, 47*(4), e12. https://doi.org/10.1136/medhum-2020-011898

Clark, M., & Emerson, A. (2021). Spirituality in psychiatric nursing: A concept analysis. *Journal of the American Psychiatric Nurses Association*, 27(1), 22–32. https://doi.org/10.1177/1078390320902834

Craft, A. L., Perry-Jenkins, M., & Newkirk, K. (2021). The implications of early marital conflict for children's development. *Journal of Child and Family Studies, 30*(1), 292–310. https://doi.org/10.1007/s10826-020-01871-6

Davis, P., Corcoran, R., Billington, J., & Frank, A. (2023). Editorial: Reading, literature, and psychology in action. *Frontiers in Psychology, 13*, 1068030. https://doi.org/10.3389/fpsyg.2022.1068030

Fernandez, N., Argueta, T., & DeLeon, I. G. (2023). Common practices used to establish and implement token economies in clinical and instructional settings: A Survey of BACB certificants. *Behavior Analysis in Practice, 16*(4), 1151–1162. https://doi.org/10.1007/s40617-023-00800-5

Fornili, K., & Fogger, S. (Eds.). (2022). *Addictions nursing: Scope and standards of practice* (3rd ed.). American Nurses Association & International Nurses Society on Addictions.

Franz, P. J., Mou, D., Kessler, D. T., Stubbing, J., Jaroszewski, A. C., Ray, S., Cao-Silveira, V. B., Bachman, S., Schuster, S., Graupensperger, D., Alpert, J. E., Porath, M., & Nock, M. K. (2022). Digital bibliotherapy as a scalable intervention for suicidal thoughts: A randomized controlled trial. *Journal of Consulting and Clinical Psychology, 90*(8), 626–637. https://doi.org/10.1037/ccp0000752

Gomi, S., Starnino, V. R., & Canda, E. R. (2014). Spiritual assessment in mental health recovery. *Community Mental Health Journal, 50*(4), 447–453.

Gualdi-Russo, E., Rinaldo, N., Masotti, S., Bramanti, B., & Zaccagni, L. (2022). Sex differences in body image perception and ideals: Analysis of possible determinants. *International Journal of Environmental Research and Public Health, 19*(5), 2745. https://doi.org/10.3390/ijerph19052745

Kayrouz, R., Schofield, C., Nielssen, O., Karin, E., Staples, L., & Titov, N. (2021). A review and clinical practice guideline for health professionals working with indigenous and culturally and linguistically diverse (CALD) populations during COVID-19. *Frontiers in Public Health, 9*, 584000. https://doi.org/10.3389/fpubh.2021.584000

Martin, K. S. (2005). *The Omaha system: A key to practice, documentation, and information management* (2nd ed.). Elsevier Saunders.

McLean G. (2022). Spiritual health support for individuals with serious mental illness in the community. *The Journal of Pastoral Care & Counseling: JPCC, 76*(2), 129–138. https://doi.org/10.1177/15423050221092318

Moyano, N., Sánchez-Fuentes, M. D. M., Parra-Barrera, S. M., & Granados de Haro, R. (2023). Only "yes" means "yes": Negotiation of sex and its link with sexual violence. *Journal of Interpersonal Violence, 38*(3–4), 2759–2777. https://doi.org/10.1177/08862605221102483

Muehlbauer, M., Bradley, C., Marquard, J., & Monsen, K. A. (2023). Clinical judgment and informatics: Encoding simulations using the Omaha System. *Journal of Nursing Education, 62*(4), 237–239. https://doi.org/10.3928/01484834-20230208-07

Posner, K., Brown, G. K., Stanley, B., Brent, D. A., Yershova, K. V., Oquendo, M. A., Currier, G. W., Melvin, G. A., Greenhill, L., Shen, S., & Mann, J. J. (2011). The Columbia-Suicide Severity Rating Scale: Initial validity and internal consistency findings from three multisite studies with adolescents and adults. *The American Journal of Psychiatry, 168*(12), 1266–1277. https://doi.org/10.1176/appi.ajp.2011.10111704

Puchalski, C. M., Vitillo, R., Hull, S. K., & Reller, N. (2014). Improving the spiritual dimension of whole person care: reaching national and international consensus. *Journal of Palliative Medicine, 17*(6), 642–656. https://doi.org/10.1089/jpm.2014.9427

Rosmarin, D. H., Pargament, K. I., & Koenig, H. G. (2021). Spirituality and mental health: Challenges and opportunities. *The Lancet Psychiatry, 8*(2), 92–93. https://doi.org/10.1016/S2215-0366(20)30048-1

Saba, V. K. (2012). *Clinical care classification (CCC) system (version 2.5) (User's Guide)* (2nd ed.). Springer Publishing Company.

Schleder Goncalves, L., Picanco, G. S., Dipp, H. M., & da Silva, C. S. (2024). Omaha System: An integrative literature review from 2012 to 2022. *Studies in Health Technology and Informatics, 315*, 600–601. https://doi.org/10.3233/SHTI240235

The Joint Commission Standards. (2022). *Spiritual beliefs and preferences—evaluating a patient's spiritual needs*. https://www.jointcommission.org/standards/standard-faqs/home-care/provision-of-care-treatment-and-services-pc/000001669

Toney-Butler, T. J., & Unison-Pace, W. J. (2022). Nursing admission assessment and examination. In *StatPearls*. StatPearls Publishing. www.ncbi.nlm.nih.gov/books/NBK493211

Tsanas, A., Little, M. A., & Ramig, L. O. (2021). Remote assessment of Parkinson's Disease symptom severity using the simulated cellular mobile telephone network. *IEEE Access: Practical Innovations, Open Solutions, 9*, 11024–11036. https://doi.org/10.1109/ACCESS.2021.3050524

Van Denend, J., Ford, K., Berg, P., Edens, E. L., & Cooke, J. (2022). The body, the mind, and the spirit: Including the spiritual area in mental health care. *Journal of Religion & Health, 61*(5), 3571–3588. https://doi-org.libproxy.siue.edu/10.1007/s10943-022-01609-2

Wagner, C. M., Butcher, H. K., Bulechek, G. M., Dochterman, J. M., & Clark, M. F. (2024). *Nursing interventions classification (NIC)* (8th ed.). Elsevier.

Yassine, J., & Tipton-Fisler, L. A. (2022). Independent contingency and token economy at recess to reduce aggression. *Contemporary School Psychology, 26*(4), 481–491. https://doi.org/10.1007/s40688-021-00364-7

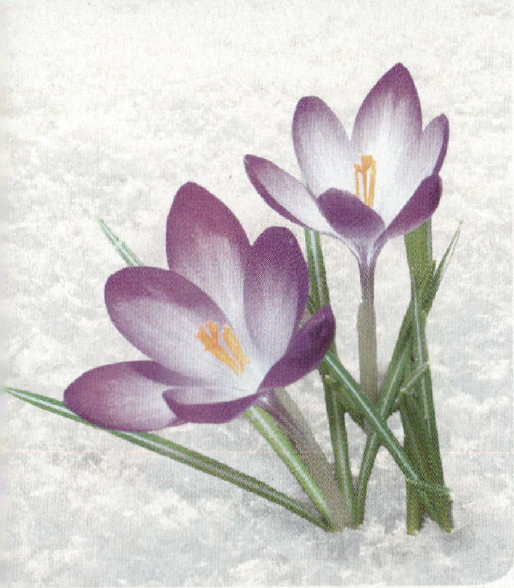

11 Psychopharmacology and Biologic Interventions

Mary Ann Boyd

KEYCONCEPTS

- agonists
- antagonists
- pharmacodynamics
- pharmacokinetics

LEARNING OBJECTIVES

After studying this chapter, you will be able to:

1. Differentiate target symptoms from side effects.
2. Identify nursing interventions for common side effects of psychiatric medications.
3. Explain the role of the government regulatory process in the approval of medication and the use of other biologic interventions.
4. Discuss the pharmacodynamics of psychiatric medications.
5. Discuss the pharmacokinetics of psychiatric medications.
6. Explain the major classifications of psychiatric medications.
7. Identify nursing interventions related to the administration of psychiatric medications.
8. Analyze the potential benefits of other forms of somatic treatments, electroconvulsive therapy, light therapy, transcranial magnetic stimulation, and vagus nerve stimulation.
9. Evaluate the significance of nonadherence and discuss strategies supportive of medication adherence.

KEY TERMS

• absorption • adherence • adverse reactions • affinity • akathisia • atypical antipsychotics • augmentation • bioavailability • biotransformation • boxed warning • carrier protein • chronic syndromes • clearance • conventional antipsychotics • cytochrome P450 (CYP450) system • desensitization • distribution • dosing • drug–drug interaction • dystonia • efficacy • enzymes • ethnopsychopharmacology • excretion • extrapyramidal symptoms • first-pass effect • half-life • hypnotics • inducer • inhibitor • intrinsic activity • metabolism • metabolites • partial agonists • pharmacogenomics • phototherapy • polypharmacy • poor metabolizer • potency • prescribing information • protein binding • pseudoparkinsonism • rapid metabolizer • receptors • relapse • sedative–hypnotics • sedatives • selectivity • serotonin syndrome • side effects • solubility • steady state • substrate • tardive dyskinesia • target symptoms • therapeutic index • tolerance • toxicity • transcranial magnetic stimulation • uptake receptors • vagus nerve stimulation (VNS)

INTRODUCTION

Recent scientific and technologic developments have opened the door for the development of new medications that treat mental disorders. Nurses administer these medications, monitor their effectiveness, and manage side effects; they also have an important role in educating patients about their medications. Psychiatric medications are increasingly prescribed in primary care settings, and nurses practicing in nonpsychiatric settings now need an in-depth knowledge of them.

This chapter presents an overview of the pharmacodynamics and pharmacokinetics of selected psychiatric medications. Medications used to treat substance use disorders are discussed in Chapter 31. Included in this chapter are the major classes of psychopharmacologic drugs and a discussion of herbal supplements and nutritional therapies. In addition, other biologic treatments are discussed, including electroconvulsive therapy (ECT), light therapy, transcranial magnetic stimulation (TMS), and vagus nerve stimulation (VNS).

PSYCHIATRIC MEDICATIONS

As with any drug, psychiatric medications are designated for use in certain conditions for specific symptoms. The nurse quickly realizes that these symptoms are present in several conditions, leading to many medications being prescribed for different diagnoses. Because medications can have both desirable and undesirable effects, it is important for the nurse to understand these factors to help ensure patient safety.

Target Symptoms and Side Effects

Psychiatric medications and other biologic interventions are indicated for **target symptoms**, which are specific measurable symptoms expected to improve with treatment. Legal regulations, standards of care, and facility policies guide nurses in monitoring and documenting the effects of medications and other biologic treatments on target symptoms.

Yet, no drug has been developed that is so specific it affects only its target symptoms; instead, drugs usually act on several other organs and sites within the body. Even drugs with a high affinity and selectivity for a specific neurotransmitter will cause some responses in the body that are not related to the target symptoms. These unwanted effects of medications are called side effects. If unwanted effects have serious physiologic consequences, they are considered **adverse reactions**. The nurse monitors, documents, and reports the appearance of side effects and adverse reactions and implements nursing interventions for relief of medication side effects (Table 11.1).

Drug Regulation and Use

The U.S. Food and Drug Administration (FDA) is responsible for ensuring the safety, efficacy, and security of human and veterinary drugs, biologic products, medical devices, nation's food supply, cosmetics, and products that emit radiation (www.FDA.gov). The FDA approves the labeling of medications and other biologic treatments after a thorough review of efficacy and safety data (Box 11.1). Nurses administering medications are responsible for knowing the labeling content, which is found in each medication's package insert or **prescribing information (PI)** and includes approved indications for the medication, side effects, adverse reactions, contraindications, and other important information. If the FDA identifies serious adverse reactions that can occur with the use of a specific medication, it may issue a warning found in a **boxed warning** in the PI. The nurse should be aware of these boxed warnings and monitor for the appearance of adverse reactions. If a PI is not readily available, the labeling information is easily found on the FDA's website and in most pharmacy departments.

BOX 11.1

Testing New Drugs for Safety and Efficacy

PHASES OF NEW DRUG TESTING

- Phase I: Testing defines the range of dosages tolerated in healthy individuals.
- Phase II: Effects of the drug are studied in a limited number of people with the disorder. This phase defines the range of clinically effective dosage.
- Phase III: Extensive clinical trials are conducted at multiple sites throughout the country with larger numbers of patients. Efforts focus on corroborating the efficacy identified in phase II. Phase III concludes with a new drug application being submitted to the FDA.
- Phase IV: Drug studies continue after FDA approval to detect new or rare adverse reactions and potentially new indications. During this period, adverse reactions from the new medication should be reported to the FDA.

IMPLICATIONS FOR MENTAL HEALTH NURSES

- Throughout the phases, side effects and adverse reactions are monitored closely. The studies are tightly controlled, and strict regulations are enforced at each step.
- To prove drug effectiveness, diagnoses must be accurate, strict guidelines are followed, and subjects are not usually taking other medications and do not have complicating illnesses.
- A newly approved drug is approved only for the indications for which it has been tested.

PSYCHOPHARMACOLOGY

A comparatively small amount of medication can have a significant and large impact on cell function and resulting behavior. When tiny molecules of medication are compared with the vast amount of cell surface in the human body, the fraction seems disproportionate. Yet, the drugs used to treat mental disorders often have profound effects on behavior. To understand how this occurs, one needs to understand both where and how drugs work. The following discussion highlights important concepts relevant to psychiatric medications.

Pharmacodynamics: Where Drugs Act

Drug molecules act at specific sites, not on the entire cell surface. Psychiatric medications primarily target the central nervous system (CNS) at the cellular, synaptic

TABLE 11.1 MANAGING COMMON SIDE EFFECTS OF PSYCHIATRIC MEDICATIONS

Side Effect or Discomfort	Intervention
Blurred vision	Reassurance (generally subsides in 2–6 weeks)
Dry eyes	Artificial tears may be required; increased use of wetting solutions for those wearing contact lens Alert ophthalmologist; no eye examination for new glasses for at least 3 weeks after a stable dose
Dry mouth and lips	Frequent rinsing of mouth, good oral hygiene, sucking sugarless candies or lozenges, lip balm, lemon juice, and glycerin mouth swabs
Constipation	High-fiber diet; encourage bran, fresh fruits, and vegetables Metamucil (must consume at least 16 oz of fluid with dose) Increase hydration Exercise; increase fluids Mild laxative
Urinary hesitancy or retention	Monitor frequently for difficulty with urination, including changes in starting or stopping stream Notify prescriber if difficulty develops A cholinergic agonist, such as bethanechol, may be required
Nasal congestion	Nose drops, moisturizer, *not* nasal spray
Sinus tachycardia	Assess for infections Monitor pulse for rate and irregularities Withhold medication and notify prescriber if resting rate exceeds 120 bpm
Decreased libido, anorgasmia, ejaculatory inhibition	Reassurance (reversible); change to another medication
Postural hypotension	Frequently monitor lying-to-standing blood pressure during dosage adjustment period, immediate changes and accommodation, and measure pulse in both positions; consider change to less antiadrenergic drug Advise patient to get up slowly, sit for at least 1 minute before standing (dangling legs over side of bed), and stand for 1 minute before walking or until light-headedness subsides Increase hydration, avoid caffeine Elastic stockings if necessary Notify prescriber if symptoms persist or significant blood pressure changes are present; medication may have to be changed if patient does not have impulse control to get up slowly
Photosensitivity	Protective clothing Dark glasses Use of sun block; remember to cover all exposed areas
Dermatitis	Stop medication usage Consider medication change; may require a systemic antihistamine Initiate comfort measures to decrease itching
Impaired psychomotor functions	Advise patients to avoid dangerous tasks, such as driving Avoid alcohol, which increases this impairment
Drowsiness or sedation	Encourage activity during the day to increase accommodation Avoid tasks that require mental alertness, such as driving May need to adjust dosing schedule or, if possible, give a single daily dose at bedtime May need cholinergic medication if sedation is the problem Avoid driving or operating potentially dangerous equipment May need to change to less sedating medication Provide quiet and decreased stimulation when sedation is the desired effect
Weight gain and metabolic changes	Exercise and diet teaching Caloric control
Edema	Check fluid retention Reassurance May need a diuretic
Irregular menstruation or amenorrhea	Reassurance (reversible) May need to change class of drug Reassurance and counseling (does not indicate lack of ovulation) Instruct patient to continue birth control measures
Vaginal dryness	Instruct in use of lubricants

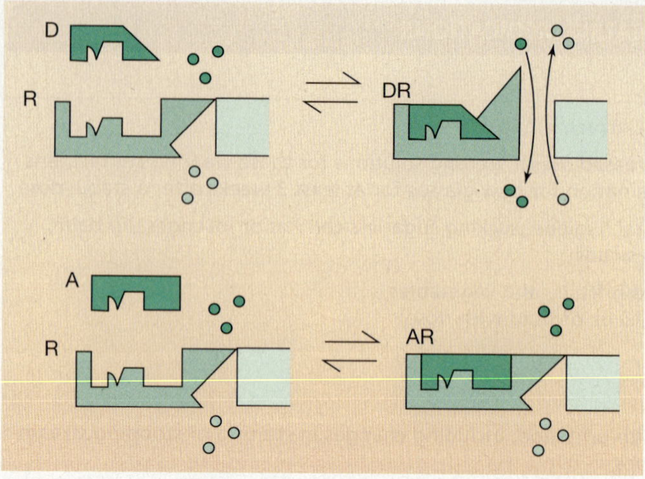

FIGURE 11.1 Agonist and antagonist drug actions at a receptor site. This schematic drawing represents drug–receptor interactions. **Top:** Drug D has the correct shape to fit receptor R, forming a drug–receptor complex, which results in a conformational change in the receptor and the opening of a pore in the adjacent membrane. Drug D is an agonist. **Bottom:** Drug A also has the correct shape to fit the receptor, forming a drug–receptor complex, but in this case, there is no conformational change and therefore no response. Drug A is, therefore, an antagonist.

level at four sites: receptors, ion channels, enzymes, and carrier proteins.

> **KEYCONCEPT Pharmacodynamics** is the action or effect of drugs on living organisms.

Receptors

Receptors are specific proteins intended to respond to a chemical (i.e., neurotransmitter) present in blood or tissues (see Chapter 7). Receptors also respond to drugs with similar chemical structures. When drugs attach to a receptor, they can act as **agonists**—substances that initiate the same response as the chemicals naturally found in the body—or as **antagonists**—substances that block the response of a given receptor. Figure 11.1 illustrates the action of an agonist and an antagonist drug at a receptor site. A drug's ability to interact with a given receptor type may be judged by three properties: selectivity, affinity, and intrinsic activity.

> **KEYCONCEPT Agonists** (mimic the neurotransmitter) have all three properties: selectivity, affinity, and intrinsic activity.
> **Antagonists** (block the receptor) have only selectivity and affinity properties; they do not have intrinsic activity because they produce no biologic response by attaching to the receptor.

Some drugs are referred to as **partial agonists** because they have some intrinsic activity (although weak). Because there are no "pure" drugs affecting only one neurotransmitter, most drugs have multiple effects. A drug may act as an agonist for one neurotransmitter and an antagonist for another. Medications that have both agonist and antagonist effects are called mixed agonist–antagonists.

Selectivity

Selectivity is the ability of a drug to be specific for a receptor. If a drug is highly selective, it will interact only with its specific receptors in the areas of the body where these receptors occur and therefore not affect tissues and organs where its receptors do not occur. Using a "lock-and-key" analogy, only a specific, highly selective key will fit a given lock. The more selective or structurally specific a drug is, the more likely it will affect only the specific receptor for which it is meant. The less selective the drug, the more receptors are affected and the more likely there will be unintended effects or side effects.

Affinity

Affinity is the degree of attraction or strength of the bond between the drug and its biologic target. Affinity is strengthened when a drug has more than one type of chemical bond with its target. If a cell membrane contains several receptors to which a drug will adhere, the affinity is increased. The weaker the chemical bond, the more likely a drug's effects are reversible. Most drugs used in psychiatry adhere to receptors through weak chemical bonds; but some drugs, specifically the monoamine oxidase inhibitors (MAOIs; discussed later), have a different type of bond, called a covalent bond. A covalent bond is formed when two atoms share a pair of electrons. This type of bond is stronger and irreversible at usual temperatures. The effects of the drugs that form covalent bonds are often called "irreversible" because they are long lasting, taking several weeks to resolve. Knowledge of a medication's affinity for receptors and subtypes of receptors may give some indication of the likelihood that specific target symptoms might improve and what side effects might be predicted.

Intrinsic Activity

A drug's ability to interact with a given receptor is its **intrinsic activity**, or the ability to produce a response after it becomes attached to the receptor. Some drugs have selectivity and affinity but produce no response. An important measure of a drug is whether it produces a change in the cell containing the receptor.

Ion Channels

Some drugs directly block the ion channels of the nerve cell membrane. For example, the antianxiety benzodiazepine drugs, such as diazepam, bind to a region of the gamma aminobutyric acid (GABA) receptor–chloride channel complex, which helps to open the chloride ion channel. In turn, the activity of GABA is enhanced.

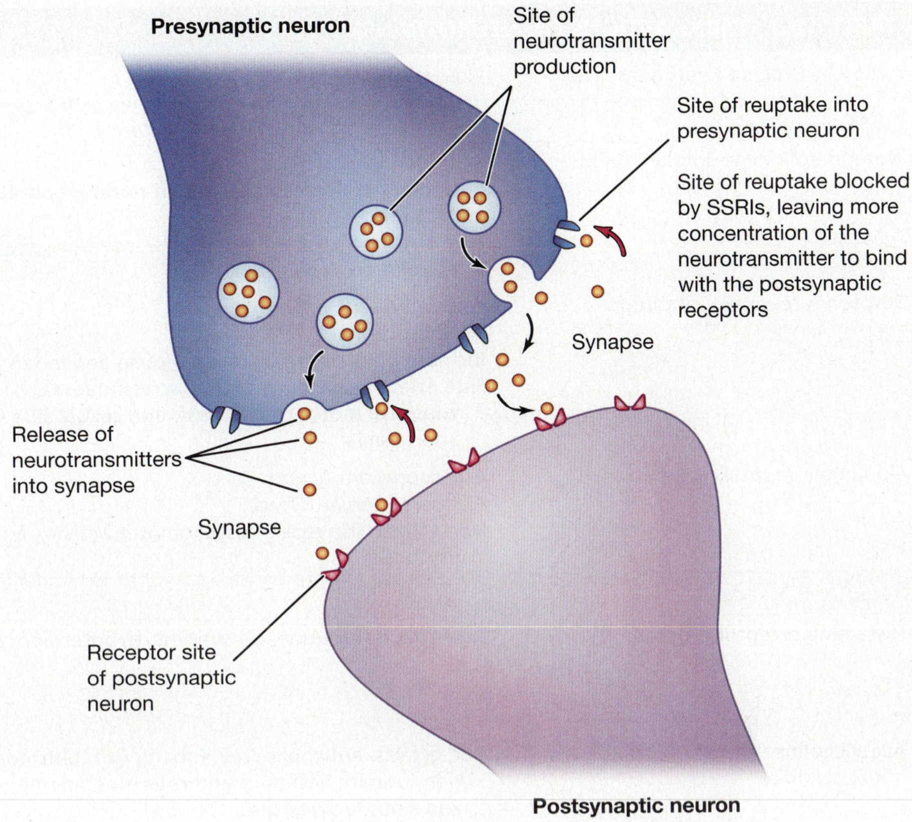

FIGURE 11.2 Reuptake blockade of a carrier molecule for serotonin by a selective serotonin reuptake inhibitor. SSRI, selective serotonin reuptake inhibitor.

Enzymes

Enzymes are usually proteins that act as catalysts for physiologic reactions and can be targets for drugs. For example, monoamine oxidase (MAO) is an enzyme required to break down neurotransmitters associated with depression (norepinephrine, serotonin, and dopamine). MAOI antidepressants inhibit this enzyme, resulting in more neurotransmitter activity.

Carrier Proteins: Uptake Receptors

A **carrier protein** is a membrane protein that transports a specific molecule across the cell membrane. Carrier proteins (also referred to as **uptake receptors**) recognize sites specific to the type of molecule to be transported. When a neurotransmitter is removed from the synapse, specific carrier molecules return it to the presynaptic nerve, where most of it is stored to be used again. Medications specific for this site block or inhibit this transport and therefore increase the activity of the neurotransmitter in the synapse. Figure 11.2 illustrates the reuptake blockade.

Clinical Concepts

Efficacy is the ability of a drug to produce a response and is considered when a drug is selected. The degree of receptor occupancy contributes to the drug's efficacy, but a drug may occupy many receptors and not produce a response. Table 11.2 provides a brief summation of possible physiologic effects from drug actions on specific neurotransmitters. This information should serve only as a guide in predicting side effects because many physical outcomes or behaviors resulting from neural transmission are controlled by multiple receptors and neurotransmitters.

Potency refers to the dose of drug required to produce a specific effect. One drug may be able to achieve the same clinical effect as another drug but at a lower dose, making it more potent. Although the drug given at the lower dose is more potent because both drugs achieve similar effects, they may be considered to have equal efficacy.

In some instances, the effects of medications diminish with time, especially when they are given repeatedly, as in the treatment of chronic psychiatric disorders. This loss of effect is most often a form of physiologic adaptation that may develop as the cell attempts to regain homeostatic control to counteract the effects of the drug. There are many reasons for decreased drug effectiveness (Box 11.2).

Desensitization is a rapid decrease in drug effects that may develop in a few minutes of exposure to a drug. This reaction is rare with most psychiatric medications but can occur with some medications used to treat serious side effects (e.g., physostigmine, sometimes used to relieve

TABLE 11.2 DRUG ACTIONS ON NEUROTRANSMITTERS

Action by Drug on Neurotransmitter	Physiologic Effects	Example of Drugs
Reuptake Inhibition		
Norepinephrine reuptake inhibition	Antidepressant action Potentiation of pressor effects of norepinephrine Interaction with guanethidine Side effects: tachycardia, tremors, insomnia, erectile, and ejaculation dysfunction	Desipramine Venlafaxine
Serotonin reuptake inhibition	Antidepressant action Antiobsessional effect Increase or decrease in anxiety (dose dependent) Side effects: gastrointestinal distress; nausea; headache; nervousness; motor restlessness; and sexual side effects, including anorgasmia	Fluoxetine Fluvoxamine
Dopamine reuptake inhibition	Antidepressant action Antiparkinsonian effect Side effects: increase in psychomotor activity, aggravation of psychosis	Bupropion
Receptor Blockade		
Histamine receptor blockade (H1)	Side effects: sedation, drowsiness, hypotension, and weight gain	Quetiapine Imipramine Clozapine Olanzapine
Acetylcholine receptor blockade (muscarinic)	Side effects: anticholinergic (dry mouth, blurred vision, constipation, urinary hesitancy and retention, memory dysfunction) and sinus tachycardia	Imipramine Amitriptyline Olanzapine
Norepinephrine receptor blockade (α1 receptor)	Potentiation of antihypertensive effect of prazosin and terazosin Side effects: postural hypotension, dizziness, reflex tachycardia, sedation	Amitriptyline Clomipramine Clozapine
Norepinephrine receptor blockade (α2 receptor)	Increased sexual desire (yohimbine) Interactions with antihypertensive medications, blockade of the antihypertensive effects of clonidine Side effect: priapism	Amitriptyline Clomipramine Clozapine Trazodone Yohimbine
Norepinephrine receptor blockade (β1 receptor)	Antihypertensive action (propranolol) Side effects: orthostatic hypotension, sedation, depression, sexual dysfunction (including impotence and decreased ejaculation)	Propranolol
Serotonin receptor blockade ($5\text{-}HT_{1A}$)	Antidepressant action Antianxiety effect Possible control of aggression	Trazodone Risperidone Ziprasidone
Serotonin receptor blockade ($5\text{-}HT_2$)	Antipsychotic action Some antimigraine effect Decreased rhinitis Side effects: hypotension, ejaculatory problems	Risperidone Clozapine Olanzapine Ziprasidone
Dopamine receptor blockade (D_2)	Antipsychotic action Side effects: extrapyramidal symptoms, such as tremor, rigidity (especially acute dystonia and parkinsonism); endocrine changes, including elevated prolactin levels	Haloperidol Ziprasidone

severe anticholinergic side effects). A rapid decrease can also occur with some drugs because of immediate transformation of the receptor when the drug molecule binds to the receptor. Other drugs cause a decrease in the number of receptors or exhaust the mediators of neurotransmission.

Tolerance is a gradual decrease in the action of a drug at a given dose or concentration in the blood. This decrease may take days or weeks to develop and results in loss of therapeutic effect of a drug. For therapeutic drugs, this loss of effect is often called *treatment refractoriness*. In the use of substances such as alcohol

BOX 11.2

Mechanisms Causing Decrease in Medication Effects

- Change in receptors
- Loss of receptors
- Exhaustion of neurotransmitter supply
- Increased metabolism of the drug
- Physiologic adaptation

or cocaine, tolerance is related to the use of these substances (see Chapter 31).

Toxicity generally refers to the point at which concentrations of the drug in the bloodstream are high enough to become harmful or poisonous to the body. Individuals vary widely in their responses to medications. Some patients experience adverse reactions more easily than others. The **therapeutic index** is the ratio of the maximum nontoxic dose to the minimum effective dose. A high therapeutic index means that there is a large range between the dose at which the drug begins to take effect and a dose that would be toxic to the body. Drugs with a low therapeutic index have a narrow range.

This concept of toxicity has some limitations. The range can be affected by drug tolerance. For example, when tolerance develops, the person increases their dosage, which makes them more susceptible to accidental suicide. The therapeutic index of a medication also may be greatly changed by the coadministration of other medications or drugs. For example, alcohol consumed with most CNS-depressant drugs will have added depressant effects, greatly increasing the likelihood of toxicity or death.

Pharmacokinetics: How the Body Acts on the Drugs

The field of pharmacokinetics studies the process of how drugs are acted on by the body through absorption, distribution, metabolism (biotransformation), and excretion. Pharmacokinetics for specific medications is always explained in a drug's PI. Together with the principles of pharmacodynamics, this information is helpful in monitoring drug effects and predicting behavioral response.

KEYCONCEPT Pharmacokinetics is the process by which a drug is absorbed, distributed, metabolized, and eliminated by the body.

Absorption and Routes of Administration

The first phase of **absorption** is the movement of the drug from the site of administration into the plasma. The usual routes of administration of psychiatric medications include oral (tablet, capsule, and liquid), deltoid and gluteal intramuscular (IM; short- and long-acting agents), and intravenous (IV; rarely used for treatment of the primary psychiatric disorder but instead for rapid treatment of adverse reactions). A transdermal patch antidepressant and nasal inhalation are also available. The advantages and disadvantages of each route and the subsequent effects on absorption are listed in Table 11.3.

Drugs taken orally are usually the most convenient for the patient; however, this route is also the most variable because absorption can be slowed or enhanced by several factors. Taking certain drugs orally with food or antacids may slow the rate of absorption or change the amount of the drug absorbed. For example, antacids containing aluminum salts decrease the absorption of most antipsychotic drugs; thus, antacids must be given at least 1 hour before administration or 2 hours after.

Oral preparations are absorbed from the gastrointestinal tract into the bloodstream through the portal vein and then to the liver. They may be metabolized within the gastrointestinal wall or liver before reaching the rest of the body. This is called the **first-pass effect**. The consequence of the first-pass effect is that only a fraction of the drug reaches systemic circulation. Oral dosages are adjusted for the first-pass effect. That is, the dose of the oral form is significantly higher than the IM or IV formulations.

Bioavailability describes the amount of the drug that reaches systemic circulation unchanged. The route by which a drug is administered significantly affects bioavailability. With some oral drugs, the amount of drug entering the bloodstream is decreased by first-pass metabolism, and bioavailability is lower. On the other hand, some rapidly dissolving oral medications have increased bioavailability.

Concept Mastery Alert

First-pass effect refers to the metabolism that a drug undergoes within the gastrointestinal wall or liver before reaching the rest of the body. Bioavailability describes the amount of a drug that reaches the systemic circulation unchanged.

Distribution

Distribution of a drug is the amount of the drug found in various tissues, particularly the target organ at the site of drug action. Factors that affect distribution include the size of the organ; amount of blood flow or perfusion within the organ; solubility of the drug; plasma protein binding (the degree to which the drug binds to plasma proteins); and anatomic barriers, such as the blood–brain barrier, that the drug must cross. A psychiatric drug may have rapid absorption and high bioavailability, but if it

TABLE 11.3 SELECTED FORMS AND ROUTES OF PSYCHIATRIC MEDICATIONS

Preparation and Route	Examples	Advantages	Disadvantages
Oral tablet	Basic preparation for most psychopharmacologic agents, including antidepressants, antipsychotics, mood stabilizers, anxiolytics, and so on	Usually most convenient	Variable rate and extent of absorption, depending on the drug May be affected by the contents of the intestines May show first-pass metabolism effects May not be easily swallowed by some individuals
Oral liquid	Also known as concentrates The antipsychotic risperidone The antidepressant fluoxetine Antihistamines, such as diphenhydramine Mood stabilizers, such as lithium citrate	Ease of incremental dosing Easily swallowed In some cases, more quickly absorbed	More difficult to measure accurately Depending on drug: • Possible interactions with other liquids such as juice, forming precipitants • Possible irritation to mucosal lining of mouth if not properly diluted
Rapidly dissolving tablet	Atypical antipsychotics, such as olanzapine, risperidone, asenapine	Dissolves almost instantaneously in mouth	Patient needs to remember to have completely dry hands and to place tablet in mouth immediately Tablet should not linger in the hand Handy for people who have trouble swallowing or for patients who let medication linger in the cheek for later expectoration Can be taken when water or other liquid is unavailable
Intramuscular	Some antipsychotics, such as ziprasidone, olanzapine, haloperidol, and chlorpromazine Anxiolytics, such as lorazepam Anticholinergics, such as benztropine mesylate No antidepressants No mood stabilizers	More rapid acting than oral preparations No first-pass metabolism	Injection-site pain and irritation Some medications may have erratic absorption if heavy muscle tissue at the site of injection is not in use
Intramuscular depot (or long acting)	Risperidone, paliperidone palmitate, olanzapine, aripiprazole, aripiprazole lauroxil, haloperidol decanoate, fluphenazine decanoate	Better adherence to medication regime	Pain at injection site
Intravenous	Anticholinergics, such as diphenhydramine, benztropine mesylate Anxiolytics, such as diazepam, lorazepam, and chlordiazepoxide	Rapid and complete availability to systemic circulation	Inflammation of tissue surrounding site Often inconvenient for patient and uncomfortable Continuous dosage requires use of a constant rate IV infusion
Subcutaneous (abdominal)	Risperidone	More convenient than oral regime; injection in abdomen may be preferable to the gluteus	Pain at injection site
Transdermal patch	Antidepressant, selegiline	Avoid daily oral ingestion of medication	Skin irritation
Oral inhalation	Conventional antipsychotic, loxapine	Rapidly absorbed to treat psychomotor agitation	Bronchospasm
Intranasal spray	Antidepressant, esketamine	Rapidly absorbed to treat severe depression	Nasal discomfort Oropharyngeal pain Throat irritation

IV, intravenous.

TABLE 11.4 FACTORS AFFECTING DISTRIBUTION OF A DRUG

Factor	Effect on Drug Distribution
Size of the organ	Larger organs require more drug to reach a concentration level equivalent to other organs and tissues.
Blood flow to the organ	The more blood flow to and within an organ (perfusion), the greater the drug concentration. The brain has high perfusion.
Solubility of the drug	The greater the solubility of a drug within a tissue, the greater its concentration.
Plasma protein binding	If a drug binds well to plasma proteins, particularly to albumin, it will stay in the body longer but have a slower distribution.
Anatomic barriers	Both the gastrointestinal tract and the brain are surrounded by layers of cells that control the passage or uptake of substances. Lipid-soluble substances are usually readily absorbed and pass the blood–brain barrier.

does not cross the blood–brain barrier to reach the CNS, it is of little use. Table 11.4 provides a summary of how some significant factors affect distribution. Two of these factors, solubility (ability of a drug to dissolve) and protein binding, warrant additional discussion about how they relate to psychiatric medications.

Solubility

Substances may cross a membrane in several ways, but passive diffusion is by far the simplest. To do this, the drug must dissolve in the structure of the cell membrane. Therefore, the **solubility** of a drug is an important characteristic. Being soluble in lipids allows a drug to cross most of the membranes in the body, and the tissues of the CNS are less permeable to water-soluble drugs than are other areas of the body. Most psychopharmacologic agents are lipid soluble and easily cross the blood–brain barrier. However, this characteristic means that psychopharmacologic agents also cross the placenta; consequently, most are contraindicated during pregnancy.

Protein Binding

Of considerable importance is the degree to which a drug binds to plasma proteins. Only unbound or "free" drugs act at the receptor sites. High **protein binding** reduces the concentration of the drug at the receptor sites. However, because the binding is reversible, as the unbound drug is metabolized, more drug is released from the protein bonds. Drugs are also released from storage in the fat depots. These processes can prolong the duration of action of the drug. When patients stop taking their medication, they often do not experience an immediate return of symptoms because they continue to receive the drug as it is released from storage sites in the body.

Metabolism

Metabolism, also called **biotransformation**, is the process by which a drug is altered and broken down into smaller substances, known as metabolites. Most metabolism occurs in the liver, but it can also occur in the kidneys, lungs, and intestines. Phase I includes oxidation, hydrolysis, and reduction reactions. In most cases, **metabolites** are inactive but in some psychiatric drugs, such as norfluoxetine (metabolite of fluoxetine), they are also active. Phase II reactions or conjugation combines a drug or metabolite with other chemicals. Through the phases of biotransformation, lipid-soluble drugs eventually become more water soluble so they may be readily excreted.

Cytochrome P450

Phase I oxidation reactions are carried out by the **cytochrome P450 (CYP450) system,** a set of microsomal enzymes (usually hepatic) referred to as CYP1, CYP2, and CYP3. Within each CYP family, there are enzyme subgroups identified by a number–letter sequence (i.e., 1A2 or 3A4). There are more than 50 enzymes, but most of the metabolism occurs in only a few of them. A **substrate** is a drug or compound that is identified as a target of an enzyme. For example, clozapine is the substrate for the CYP1A2 enzyme.

The functioning of these enzymes is influenced by drugs and other chemical substances. An **inhibitor** of a CYP enzyme slows down metabolism, which in turn decreases the clearance of the substrate and elevates its plasma level. An **inducer** speeds up metabolism, which in turn increases the clearance of the substrate and decreases its plasma level. For example, cigarette smoke is a potent inducer of CYP1A2, which in turn speeds up the clearance of clozapine and decreases its plasma level. A patient who smokes will clear clozapine faster than a patient who does not smoke, even though both take the same dose.

Drug–Drug Interaction

A **drug–drug interaction** can occur if one substance inhibits an enzyme system. For example, nortriptyline (an antidepressant with a narrow therapeutic index) is the substrate of the CYP2D6 enzyme. By adding paroxetine (a selective serotonin reuptake inhibitor [SSRI] antidepressant and an inhibitor of the CYP2D6 enzyme), the 2D6 enzyme is inhibited, and the level of nortriptyline in the blood increases. Toxicity can easily develop because of a low therapeutic index. The PI informs the nurse which drugs should not be given together.

Each human CYP450 enzyme is an expression of a unique gene. The science of pharmacogenomics blends pharmacology with genetic knowledge and is concerned with understanding and determining an individual's specific CYP450 makeup and then individualizing medications to match the person's CYP450 profile. Genetically (inherited as an autosomal recessive trait), some individuals are poor metabolizers, and others may be rapid metabolizers. Whereas **poor metabolizers** are more likely to have adverse reactions, **rapid metabolizers** may not allow certain drugs to reach therapeutic levels. Research has suggested that there are variations among ethnic groups with poor metabolizers accounting for up to 7% of White individuals for CYP2D6 and up to 25% of East Asians for CYP2C19. Knowing whether patients are poor or rapid metabolizers is important because most psychiatric medications are metabolized by these enzymes. DNA laboratory tests are available for patients who have a personal or family history of adverse drug reactions to medications metabolized by 2D6 and 2D19 to confirm the presence of genotypes that affect metabolism. Enzyme CYP2D6 is important in the metabolism of many antidepressants and antipsychotics, and CYP2C19 is important for some antidepressant metabolism (Bousman et al., 2023).

Excretion

Excretion refers to the removal of drugs from the body either unchanged or as metabolites. **Clearance** refers to the total volume of blood, serum, or plasma from which a drug is completely removed per unit of time to account for the excretion. The half-life of a drug provides a measure of the expected rate of clearance. **Half-life** refers to the time required for plasma concentrations of the drug to be reduced by 50%. For most drugs, the rate of excretion slows, but the half-life remains unchanged. It usually takes four half-lives or more of a drug in total time for more than 90% of a drug to be eliminated.

Drugs bound to plasma proteins do not cross the glomerular filter freely. These lipid-soluble drugs are passively reabsorbed by diffusion across the renal tubule and thus are not rapidly excreted in the urine. Because many psychiatric medications are protein bound and lipid soluble, most of their excretion occurs through the liver, where they are excreted in the bile and delivered into the intestine. Lithium and gabapentin, mood stabilizers, are notable examples of renal excretion. Any impairment in renal function or renal disease may lead to toxic symptoms.

Dosing refers to the administration of medication over time so that therapeutic levels may be achieved or maintained without reaching toxic levels. In general, it is necessary to give a drug at intervals no greater than the half-life of the medication to avoid excessive fluctuation of concentration in the plasma between doses. With repeated dosing, a certain amount of the drug is accumulated in the body.

Steady-state plasma concentration, or simply **steady state,** occurs when absorption equals excretion and the therapeutic level plateaus. The rate of accumulation is determined by the half-life of the drug. Drugs generally reach steady state in four to five times the elimination half-life. However, because elimination or excretion rates may vary significantly in any individual, fluctuations may still occur, and dose schedules may need to be modified.

Individual Variations in Drug Effects

Many factors affect drug absorption, distribution, metabolism, and excretion. These factors may vary among individuals, depending on their age, genetics, and ethnicity.

Age

Pharmacokinetics is significantly altered at the extremes of the life cycle. Gastric absorption changes as individuals age. Gastric pH increases, and gastric emptying decreases. Gastric motility slows and splanchnic circulation is reduced. Usually, these changes do not significantly impair oral absorption of a medication, but addition of common conditions, such as diarrhea, may significantly alter and reduce absorption. Malnutrition, cancer, and liver disease decrease the production of the primary protein albumin. More free drug is circulating in the system, producing higher blood levels of the medication with potentially toxic effects. The activity of hepatic enzymes also slows with age. As a result, the ability of the liver to metabolize medications may slow as much as a fourfold decrease between the ages of 20 and 70 years. Production of albumin by the liver generally declines with age. Changes in the parasympathetic nervous system produce a greater sensitivity in older adults to anticholinergic side effects, which are more severe with this age group.

Creatinine clearance in a young adult is 100 to 120 mL/min, but this rate declines with age (Shahbaz et al., 2024). Medical illnesses, such as diabetes and hypertension, may contribute to further decline of renal function. When creatinine clearance falls below 30 mL/min, the excretion of drugs by the kidneys is significantly impaired, and potentially toxic levels may accumulate.

Pharmacogenetics and Ethnopsychopharmacology

Pharmacogenomics is the study of how a person's genetic makeup affects their response to drugs. There are important genetic variations that influence the metabolism and action of psychotropic drugs in different ethnic groups. Various tests are used to predict genetic responses to drugs and the potential for adverse effects. For example, studies show that selecting antidepressants according to genetic profile can improve treatment outcomes for people with depression and anxiety (Nicholson et al., 2021).

Overlapping pharmacogenetics is the field of **ethnopsychopharmacology,** the study of how culture and genetic differences in human groups determine and influence the response to medications. Ethnopsychopharmacology focuses on the impact of cultural practices, such as consuming foods or ingesting beverages, on genetic variations in metabolism, on complementary and alternate health care practices, and on herbal substances.

Although ethnic and racial groups are genetically heterogeneous, there are population differences in disease susceptibility (All of Us Research Program Genomics Investigators, 2024). For example, some individuals of Asian descent produce higher concentrations of acetaldehyde with alcohol use than do those of European descent, resulting in a higher incidence of adverse reactions such as flushing and palpitations (Yokoyama et al., 2021). Asian individuals often require lower doses of antipsychotics and antidepressants than White individuals (Flanagan et al., 2023). In African populations, there is a high degree of variability in the dosage of many medications (Marazziti et al., 2021).

PHASES OF DRUG TREATMENT AND THE NURSE'S ROLE

Phases of drug treatment include initiation, stabilization, maintenance, and discontinuation of the medication. The following explains the role of the nurse in these phases.

Initiation Phase

Before the initiation of medications, patients must undergo several assessments.

- A psychiatric evaluation to determine the diagnosis and target symptoms.
- A nursing assessment that includes cultural beliefs and practices (see Chapter 10).
- Physical examination and indicated laboratory tests—often including baseline determinations such as a complete blood count (CBC), liver and kidney function tests, electrolyte levels, urinalysis, and possibly thyroid function tests and electrocardiography (ECG)—to determine whether a physical condition may be causing the symptoms and to establish that it is safe to initiate use of a particular medication.

During the initiation of medication, the nurse assesses, observes, and monitors the patient's response to the medication; teaches the patient about the action, dosage, frequency of administration, and side effects; and develops a plan for ongoing contact with clinicians. The first medication dose should be treated as if it were a "test" dose. Patients should be monitored for adverse reactions such as changes in blood pressure, pulse, or temperature; changes in mental status; allergic reactions; dizziness; ataxia; or gastric distress. If any of these symptoms develop, they should be reported to the prescriber.

Stabilization Phase

During stabilization, the prescriber adjusts or titrates the medication dosage to achieve the maximum amount of improvement with a minimum of side effects. Psychiatric–mental health (PMH) nurses assess for improvements in the target symptoms and for the appearance of side effects. If medications are being increased rapidly, such as in a hospital setting, nurses must closely monitor temperature, blood pressure, pulse, mental status, common side effects, and unusual adverse reactions.

In the outpatient setting, nurses focus on patient education, emphasizing the importance of taking the medication, expected outcomes, and potential side effects. Patients need to know how and when to take their medications, how to minimize any side effects, and which side effects require immediate attention. A plan should be developed for patients and their families to clearly identify what to do if adverse reactions develop. The plan, which should include emergency telephone numbers or available emergency treatment, should be reviewed frequently.

Therapeutic drug monitoring is most important in this phase of treatment. Many medications used in psychiatry improve target symptoms only when a therapeutic level of medication has been obtained in the individual's blood. Some medications, such as lithium, have a narrow therapeutic range and must be monitored frequently and accurately. Nurses must be aware of when and how these levels are to be determined and assist patients in learning these procedures. Because of protein binding and lipid solubility, most medications do not have obtainable plasma levels that are clinically relevant. However, plasma levels of these medications may still be requested to evaluate further such issues as absorption and adverse reactions.

Sometimes, the first medication chosen does not adequately improve the patient's target symptoms. In such cases, use of the medication will be discontinued, and treatment with a new medication will be started. Medications may also be changed when adverse reactions or seriously uncomfortable side effects occur, or these effects substantially interfere with the individual's quality of life. Nurses should be familiar with the pharmacokinetics of both drugs to be able to monitor side effects and possible drug–drug interactions during this change.

At times, an individual may show only partial improvement from a medication, and the prescriber may try an

augmentation strategy by adding another medication. For example, a prescriber may add a mood stabilizer, such as lithium, to an antidepressant to improve the effects of the antidepressant. **Polypharmacy,** using more than one group from a class of medications, is increasingly being used as an acceptable strategy with most psychopharmacologic agents to match the drug action to the neurochemical needs of the patient. Nurses must be familiar with the potential effects, side effects, drug interactions, and rationale for the treatment regimen.

Maintenance Phase

After the individual's target symptoms have improved, medications are usually continued to prevent **relapse** or return of the symptoms. In some cases, this may occur despite the patient's continued use of the medication. Patients must be educated about their target symptoms and have a plan of action if the symptoms return. In other cases, the patient may experience medication side effects. The PMH nurse has a central role in assisting individuals to monitor their own symptoms, identify emerging side effects, manage psychosocial stressors, and avoid other factors that may cause the medications to lose effect.

Discontinuation Phase

Some psychiatric medications will be discontinued; others will not. Some require a tapered discontinuation, which involves slowly reducing dosage while monitoring closely for re-emergence of the symptoms. Some psychiatric disorders, such as mild depression, respond to treatment and do not recur. Other disorders, such as schizophrenia, usually require lifetime medication. Discontinuance of some medications, such as controlled substances, produces withdrawal symptoms; discontinuance of others does not.

MAJOR PSYCHOPHARMACOLOGIC DRUG CLASSES

Major classes of psychiatric drugs include antipsychotics, mood stabilizers, antidepressants, antianxiety and sedative–hypnotic medications, and stimulants.

Antipsychotic Medications

Antipsychotic medications can be thought of as "newer" and "older" medications. Newer or **atypical antipsychotics** appear to be equally or more effective but have fewer side effects than the traditional older agents. The term *typical or* **conventional antipsychotics** identifies the older antipsychotic drugs. Table 11.5 provides a list of selected antipsychotics.

Indications and Mechanism of Action

Antipsychotic medications are indicated for schizophrenia, mania, and autism and to treat the symptoms of psychosis, such as hallucinations, delusions, bizarre behavior, disorganized thinking, and agitation. (These symptoms are described more fully in later chapters.) These medications also reduce aggressiveness and inappropriate behavior associated with psychosis. Within the typical antipsychotics, haloperidol and pimozide are approved for treating patients with Tourette syndrome, reducing the frequency and severity of vocal tics. Some of the typical antipsychotics, particularly chlorpromazine, are used as antiemetics or for postoperative intractable hiccoughs.

The atypical antipsychotic medications differ from the typical antipsychotics in the various approaches to dopamine. For example, risperidone binds to serotonin receptors in addition to dopamine; clozapine has a very low affinity to dopamine, and aripiprazole is a partial agonist to dopamine. The differences between the mechanisms of action of the typical and atypical antipsychotics help to explain their differences in terms of effect on target symptoms and in the degree of side effects they produce.

The research on dopamine as the primary target of medication action is expanding to other neurotransmitter systems in hopes that they will have better efficacy and less side effects. Serotonin and glutamate are identified as being involved in brain processes that are likely candidates (Saha & González-Maeso, 2023).

Pharmacokinetics

Antipsychotic medications administered orally have a variable rate of absorption complicated by the presence of food, antacids, smoking, and even the coadministration of anticholinergics, which slow gastric motility. Clinical effects begin to appear in about 30 to 60 minutes. Absorption after IM administration is less variable because this method avoids the first-pass effects. Therefore, IM administration produces greater bioavailability. It is important to remember that IM medications are absorbed more slowly when muscles are not used. Usually, the deltoid is used more than the gluteal muscles, which may account for faster absorption of medication, and which has better blood perfusion.

Metabolism of these drugs occurs almost entirely in the liver except for paliperidone, which is not extensively metabolized by the liver but is excreted largely unchanged through the kidney, and lurasidone, which is excreted through the urine and feces. Most antipsychotics are subject to the effects of other drugs that induce or inhibit the liver enzymes described earlier (see Table 11.6). Careful observance of concurrent medication use, including prescribed, over the counter, and

TABLE 11.5 ANTIPSYCHOTIC MEDICATIONS

Generic Drug Name	Usual Dosage Range	Half-Life	Route of Administration
Atypical Antipsychotics			
Aripiprazole	10–30 mg/day	75–94 hours	Oral tablets, injection, disintegrating tablet
Aripiprazole LAI	200–400 mg	29.9–46.6 days	Injection
Aripiprazole lauroxil	441–882 mg monthly	29.2–34.9 days	Injection
Asenapine	5–10 mg bid	24 hours	Sublingual tablet
Brexpiprazole	0.5–1.0 mg/day	86–91 hours	Oral tablet
Cariprazine	1.5–6.0 mg/day	2–4 days 1–3 weeks (metabolite)	Oral capsule
Clozapine	300–900 mg/day	4–12 hours	Oral tablet, disintegrating tablet, oral suspension
Iloperidone	6–12 mg bid	18–33 hours	Oral tablet
Lurasidone	40 mg/day	18 hours	Oral tablet
Lurasidone HCl	40–80 mg	18 hours	Oral tablet
Olanzapine	5–15 mg/day 2.5–10 mg/day IM	21–54 hours	Oral tablet, disintegrating tablet Injection
Olanzapine LAI	150–300 mg q2–4 weeks	30 days	Injection
Olanzapine/samidorphan	5 mg/10 mg–15 mg/10 mg once daily	Similar to olanzapine	Tablet
Paliperidone extended release	3–12 mg once daily in AM	23 hours	Oral
Paliperidone LAI	117 mg monthly	29–49 days	Injection
Pimavanserin	34 mg once daily	57 hours for 17 mg	Oral tablet
Quetiapine fumarate	150–750 mg/day	7 hours	Oral tablet
Risperidone	2–8 mg/day	20 hours	Oral tablet, oral solution, disintegrating tablet
Risperdal LAI	25–50 mg q2wks	3–6 days	IM injection
Risperidone SQ	90 or 120 mg once monthly	9–11 days	Abdominal subcutaneous injection
Ziprasidone HCl	40–160 mg/day 10–20 mg/day IM	7 hours	Oral capsule, oral suspension Injection
Conventional (Typical) Antipsychotics			
Chlorpromazine	50–1,200 mg/day	2–30 hours	Oral tablet
Fluphenazine	2–20 mg/day	4.5–15.3 hours	Oral elixir, oral tablet, injection
Fluphenazine decanoate	12.5–25 mg q3wks		Injection
Haloperidol	2–20 mg/day	21–2 hours	Oral tablet, oral concentration, injection
Haloperidol decanoate	50–100 mg q3wks	3 weeks	Injection
Loxapine	10 mg/day	7 hours	Oral inhalation with inhaler
Molindone	50–400 mg/day	1.5 hours	Oral tablets
Perphenazine	12–64 mg/day	Unknown	Oral tablet
Pimozide	10 mg/day	55 hours	Oral tablets
Trifluoperazine	5–40 mg/day	47–10 hours	Oral tablet
Thiothixene	5–60 mg/day	3 hours	Oral capsule

IM, intramuscular; LAI, long-acting injection; SQ, subcutaneous.

TABLE 11.6 CYP450 METABOLISM OF COMMONLY USED ANTIPSYCHOTICS

Drug	How Metabolized	Induces	Inhibits
Aripiprazole	2D6, 3A4	None	None
Clozapine	1A2, 2C19, 2D6, 3A4	None	None
Haloperidol	1A2, 2D6, 3A4	None	2D6
Iloperidone	3A4, 2D6	None	3A
Lurasidone	3A4 Eliminated in urine and feces	None	None
Olanzapine	1A2, 2D6	None	None
Paliperidone	<10% 2D6, 3A4; primarily renal elimination	None	None
Quetiapine	3A4	None	None
Risperidone	2D6	None	Mild 2D6
Ziprasidone	1A2, 3A4	None	None

Note: Information based on prescribing information of each medication.

substances of misuse, is required to avoid drug–drug interactions. For example, atypical antipsychotic concentrations may be affected by CYP450-inhibiting drugs such as paroxetine and fluoxetine.

Excretion of these substances tends to be slow. Most antipsychotics have a half-life of 24 hours or longer, but many also have active metabolites with longer half-lives. These two effects make it difficult to predict elimination time, and metabolites of some of these agents may be found in the urine months later. When a medication is discontinued, the adverse reactions may not immediately subside. The patient may continue to experience and sometimes need treatment for the adverse reactions for several days. Similarly, patients who discontinue their antipsychotic drugs may still derive therapeutic benefit for several days to weeks after drug discontinuation.

High lipid solubility, accumulation in the body, and other factors have also made it difficult to correlate blood levels with therapeutic effects. Table 11.5 shows the therapeutic ranges available for some of the antipsychotic medications. The potency of the antipsychotics also varies widely and is of specific concern when considering typical antipsychotic drugs.

Long-Acting Preparations

Currently, in the United States, atypical and conventional antipsychotics are available in long-acting forms. These antipsychotics are administered by injection once every 2 weeks to 3 to 6 months. Long-acting injection (LAI) medications maintain a constant blood level between injections. Because they bypass problems with gastrointestinal absorption and first-pass metabolism, this method may enhance therapeutic outcomes for the patient. The use of these medications is expected to increase the likelihood of adhering to a prescribed medication regimen.

Nurses should be aware that each LAI has specific manufacturer recommendations for injection techniques. Nurses should carefully read the PI that accompanies the medication. In some instances, special training is needed to give the LAI correctly. For any LAI, the injection site may become sore and inflamed if certain precautions are not taken. The oil-based injections (fluphenazine and haloperidol) are viscous liquids. For these injections, a large gauge needle (at least 21 gauges) should be used. Manufacturer recommendations should be followed.

Side Effects, Adverse Reactions, and Toxicity

Various side effects and interactions can occur with antipsychotics, with the conventional (typical) antipsychotics producing different side effects than the atypical antipsychotics. The side effects vary largely based on their degree of attraction to different neurotransmitter receptors and their subtypes.

Cardiovascular Side Effects

Cardiovascular side effects include orthostatic hypotension and prolongation of the QTc interval (a marker indicating an anomalous electrocardiogram that could cause serious irregular heart rhythms). Orthostatic hypotension is very common and depends on the degree of blockade of α-adrenergic receptors. Typical and atypical antipsychotics have been associated with prolonged QTc intervals and should be used cautiously in patients who have increased QTc intervals or are taking other medications that may prolong the QTc interval. People assigned female at birth and older adults are more likely to experience QTc prolongation (Du et al., 2023). Other cardiovascular side effects from typical antipsychotics have been rare, but occasionally they cause ECG changes that have a benign or undetermined clinical effect.

Anticholinergic Side Effects

Anticholinergic side effects resulting from blockade of acetylcholine are other common side effects associated with antipsychotic drugs. Dry mouth, slowed gastric motility, constipation, urinary hesitancy or retention, vaginal dryness, blurred vision, dry eyes, nasal congestion, and confusion or decreased memory are examples of these side effects. Interventions for decreasing the impact of these side effects are outlined in Table 11.1.

This group of side effects occurs with many of the medications used for psychiatric treatment. Using more than one medication with anticholinergic effects often increases the symptoms. Older patients are often most susceptible to a potential toxicity that results from high blockade of acetylcholine. This toxicity is called an *anticholinergic crisis* and is described more fully, along with its treatment, in Chapter 24.

Weight Gain

Weight gain is a common side effect of the atypical antipsychotics, particularly clozapine and olanzapine, which can cause a weight gain of up to 20 lb within 1 year. Weight gain is associated with an increase in dosage (Sabé et al., 2023). Ziprasidone, aripiprazole, and lurasidone are associated with little to no weight gain. If a patient becomes overweight or obese, switching to another antipsychotic is often considered and weight control interventions implemented.

Diabetes

One of the more serious side effects is the risk of type II diabetes. The FDA has determined that all atypical antipsychotics increase the risk for type II diabetes. Nurses should routinely assess for emerging symptoms of diabetes and alert the prescriber of these symptoms (see Box 11.3).

BOX 11.3

Recommended Assessments Before and During Antipsychotic Therapy

- Weigh all patients and track BMI during treatment
- Determine if overweight (BMI 25–29.9) or obese (BMI ≥30)
- Monitor BMI monthly for the first 3 months; then quarterly
- Obtain baseline personal and family history of diabetes, obesity, dyslipidemia, hypertension, and cardiovascular disease
- Get waist circumference (at umbilicus)
- People assigned male at birth: >40 in (102 cm)
- People assigned female at birth: >35 in (88 cm)
- Monitor BP, fasting plasma glucose, and fasting lipid profile within 3 months and then annually (more frequently for patients with diabetes or who have gained >5% of initial weight)
- Prediabetes (fasting plasma glucose 100–125 mg/dL)
- Diabetes (fasting plasma glucose >126 mg/dL)
- Hypertension (BP >140/90 mm Hg)
- Dyslipidemia (increased total cholesterol [>200 mg], decreased HDL, and increased LDL)

BMI, body mass index; BP, blood pressure; HDL, high-density lipoprotein; LDL, low-density lipoprotein.

Sexual Side Effects

Sexual side effects result primarily from the blockade of dopamine in the tuberoinfundibular pathways of the hypothalamus. As a result, blood levels of prolactin may increase, particularly with risperidone and the typical antipsychotics. Increased prolactin causes breast enlargement and rare but potential galactorrhea (milk production and flow), decreased sexual drive, amenorrhea, menstrual irregularities, and increased risk for growth in preexisting breast cancers. Other sexual side effects include retrograde ejaculation (backward flow of semen), erectile dysfunction, and anorgasmia.

Blood Disorders

Blood dyscrasias are rare but have received renewed attention since the introduction of clozapine. Agranulocytosis is an acute reaction that causes the individual's white blood cell count to drop to very low levels often related to neutropenia, a drop in neutrophils. In the case of antipsychotics, the medication suppresses the bone marrow precursors to blood factors. The exact mechanism by which the drugs produce this effect is unknown. The most notable symptoms of this disorder include high fever, sore throat, and mouth sores. Although benign elevations in temperature have been reported in individuals taking clozapine, no fever should go uninvestigated. Untreated neutropenia can be life threatening. Although severe neutropenia can occur with any of the antipsychotics, the risk with clozapine is greater than with the other antipsychotics. Therefore, prescription of clozapine requires regular monitoring of absolute neutrophil count. If sore throat or fever develops, medications should be withheld until a leukocyte count can be obtained. Hospitalization, including reverse isolation to prevent infections, is usually required. Severe neutropenia is more likely to develop during the first 18 weeks of treatment (Novartis, 2023).

Neuroleptic Malignant Syndrome

Neuroleptic malignant syndrome (NMS) is a serious complication that may result from antipsychotic medications. Characterized by rigidity and high fever, NMS is a rare condition that may occur abruptly with even one dose of medication. Temperature must always be monitored when administering antipsychotics, especially high-potency medications. This condition is discussed more fully in Chapter 24.

Other Side Effects

Photosensitivity reactions to antipsychotics, including severe sunburns or rash, most commonly develop with the use of low-potency typical medications. Sun block must be worn on all areas of exposed skin when taking these drugs. In addition, sun exposure may cause pigmentary deposits to develop, resulting in discoloration of exposed areas, especially the neck and face. This discoloration may progress from a deep orange color to a blue gray. Skin exposure should be limited, and skin tone changes reported to the prescriber. Pigmentary deposits, retinitis pigmentosa, may also develop on the retina of the eye.

Antipsychotics may also lower the seizure threshold. Patients with an undetected seizure disorder may experience seizures early in treatment. Those who have a preexisting condition should be monitored closely.

Medication-Related Movement Disorders

Medication-related movement disorders are side effects or adverse reactions that are commonly caused by typical antipsychotic medications but less commonly with atypical antipsychotic drugs. These disorders of anomalous motor movements can be divided into two groups: acute **extrapyramidal symptoms (EPS)**—which develop early during treatment (sometimes after just one dose), and chronic syndromes—which develop from longer exposure to antipsychotic drugs.

Acute Extrapyramidal Symptoms

Acute EPS are acute unusual movements that include dystonia, pseudoparkinsonism, and akathisia. They develop early in treatment, sometimes from as little as one dose. Although these movements are treatable, they are at times dramatic and frightening, causing physical and emotional impairments that often prompt patients to stop taking their medication. EPS occur when there is an imbalance of acetylcholine, dopamine, and GABA in the basal ganglia because of blocking dopamine.

Dystonia, sometimes referred to as an *acute dystonic reaction*, is impaired muscle tone that generally is the first EPS to occur, usually within a few days of initiating use of an antipsychotic. Acetylcholine is overactive because one of its modulators, dopamine, is blocked. Dystonia is characterized by involuntary muscle spasms that lead to unusual postures, especially of the head and neck muscles. Acute dystonia occurs most often in young people assigned male at birth, adolescents, and children. Patients usually first report a thick tongue, tight jaw, or stiff neck. Dystonia can progress to a protruding tongue, oculogyric crisis (eyes rolled up in the head), torticollis (muscle stiffness in the neck, which draws the head to one side with the chin pointing to the other), and laryngopharyngeal constriction. Unusual postures of the upper limbs and torso may be held briefly or sustained. In severe cases, the spasms may progress to the intercostal muscles, producing more significant breathing difficulty for patients who already have respiratory impairment from asthma or emphysema. The treatment is the administration of a medication such as the anticholinergic agents that inhibit acetylcholine and thereby restore the balance of neurotransmitters (Table 11.7).

Drug-induced parkinsonism is sometimes referred to as **pseudoparkinsonism** because its presentation is identical to Parkinson disease. The difference is that the activity of dopamine is blocked in pseudoparkinsonism, and in Parkinson disease, the cells of the basal ganglia are destroyed. Older patients are at the greatest risk for experiencing pseudoparkinsonism (Baizabal-Carvallo & Morgan, 2022). Symptoms include the classic triad of rigidity, slowed movements (akinesia), and tremors. The rigid muscle stiffness is usually seen in the arms. Akinesia can be observed by the loss of spontaneous movements, such as the absence of the usual relaxed swing of the arms while walking. In addition, mask-like facies or loss of facial expression and a decrease in the ability to initiate movements also are present. Usually, tremor is more pronounced at rest, but it can also be observed with intentional movements, such as eating. If the tremor becomes severe, it may interfere with the patient's ability to eat or maintain adequate fluid intake. Hypersalivation is possible as well. Pseudoparkinsonism symptoms may occur on one or both sides of the body and develop abruptly or subtly but usually within the first 30 days of treatment. The treatment is the reduction in dosage or a change of antipsychotic that has less affinity for the dopamine receptor. Anticholinergic medication is sometimes given.

Akathisia is characterized by an inability to sit still or restlessness and is more common in middle-aged patients. The person will pace, rock while sitting or standing, march in place, or cross and uncross their legs. All these repetitive motions have an intensity that is frequently beyond the explanation of the individual. In addition, akathisia may be present as a primarily subjective experience without obvious motor behavior. This subjective experience includes feelings of anxiety, jitteriness, or the inability to relax, which the individual may or may not be able to communicate. It is extremely uncomfortable for a person experiencing akathisia to be forced to sit still or be confined. These symptoms are sometimes misdiagnosed as agitation or an increase in psychotic symptoms. If an antipsychotic medication is given, the symptoms will not abate and will often worsen. Differentiating akathisia from agitation may be aided by knowing the person's symptoms before the introduction of medication. Whereas psychotic agitation does not usually begin abruptly after antipsychotic medication use has been started, akathisia may occur after administration. In addition, the nurse may ask the patient if the experience is felt primarily in the muscles (akathisia) or in the mind or emotions (agitation).

TABLE 11.7 DRUG THERAPIES FOR ACUTE MEDICATION-RELATED MOVEMENT DISORDERS

Agents	Typical Dosage Ranges	Routes Available	Common Side Effects
Anticholinergics			
Benztropine	2–6 mg/day	PO, IM, IV	Dry mouth, blurred vision, slowed gastric motility causing constipation, urinary retention, increased intraocular pressure; overdose produces toxic psychosis
Biperiden	2–8 mg/day	PO	Fewer peripheral anticholinergic effects Euphoria and increased tremor may occur
Trihexyphenidyl	4–15 mg/day	PO	Same as benztropine, plus gastrointestinal distress Older adults are most prone to mental confusion and delirium
Antihistamines			
Diphenhydramine	25–50 mg QID to 400 mg daily	PO, IM, IV	Sedation and confusion, especially in older adults
Dopamine Agonists			
Amantadine	100–400 mg daily	PO	Indigestion, decreased concentration, dizziness, anxiety, ataxia, insomnia, lethargy, tremors, and slurred speech may occur with higher doses Tolerance may develop on fixed dose
β-Blockers			
Propranolol	10 mg TID to 120 mg daily	PO	Hypotension and bradycardia Must monitor pulse and blood pressure Do not stop abruptly because doing so may cause rebound tachycardia
Benzodiazepines			
Clonazepam	1–4 mg/day	PO	Tolerance and withdrawal are potential problems
Diazepam	2–5 mg TID	PO, IV	Most side effects are rare and will disappear if dose is decreased
Lorazepam	1–2 mg IM 0.5–2 mg PO	PO, IM	All may cause drowsiness, lethargy, and general sedation or paradoxical agitation Confusion and disorientation in older adults

IM, intramuscular; IV, intravenous.

Akathisia is the most difficult acute medication-related movement disorder to relieve. It does not usually respond well to anticholinergic medications. Rapid initiation of antipsychotics can increase the onset of akathisia (Yang et al., 2022). The pathology of akathisia may involve more than just the extrapyramidal motor system. It may include serotonin changes that also affect the dopamine system. The usual approach to treatment is to change or reduce the antipsychotic. Several medications are used to reduce symptoms, including β-adrenergic blockers, anticholinergics, antihistamines, and low-dose antianxiety agents with limited success. Current evidence supports the use of propranolol (β-blocker) and mirtazapine (antidepressant) (Thippaiah et al., 2021).

Several nursing interventions reduce the impact of these syndromes. Individuals with acute EPS need frequent reassurance that this is not a worsening of their psychiatric condition but instead is a treatable side effect of the medication. They also need validation to ensure that what they are experiencing is real and that the nurse is concerned and will be responsive to changes in these symptoms. Physical and psychological stress appears to increase the symptoms and further frighten the patient; therefore, decreasing stressful situations becomes important. These symptoms are often physically exhausting for the patient, and the nurse should ensure that the patient receives adequate rest and hydration. Because tremors, muscle rigidity, and motor restlessness may interfere with the individual's ability to eat, the nurse may need to assist the patient with eating and drinking fluids to maintain nutrition and hydration.

Risk factors for acute EPS include previous episodes of EPS. The nurse should listen closely when patients say they are "allergic" or have had "bad reactions" to antipsychotic medications. Often, they are describing one of the medication-related movement disorders, particularly dystonia, rather than a rash or other allergic symptom.

Chronic Syndromes: Tardive Dyskinesia

Chronic syndromes develop from long-term use of antipsychotics. They are serious and affect about 20%

of the patients who receive typical antipsychotics for an extended period. These conditions are usually irreversible and cause significant impairment in self-image, social interactions, and occupational functioning. Early symptoms and mild forms may go unnoticed by the person experiencing them.

Tardive dyskinesia, the most well-known of the chronic syndromes, involves irregular, repetitive involuntary movements of the mouth, face, and tongue, including chewing, tongue protrusion, lip smacking, puckering of the lips, and rapid eye blinking. Unusual finger movements are common as well. In some individuals, the trunk and extremities are also involved, and in rare cases, irregular breathing and swallowing lead to belching and grunting noises. These symptoms usually begin no earlier than after 6 months of treatment or when the medication is reduced or withdrawn. Once thought to be irreversible, considerable controversy now exists as to whether this is true.

The risk for experiencing tardive dyskinesia increases with age. Although the prevalence of tardive dyskinesia averages 15% to 20%, the rate rises to 50% to 70% in older patients receiving antipsychotic medications. The risk of probable tardive dyskinesia is three times lower in older adults receiving atypical antipsychotics compared to conventional antipsychotics (Sajatovic et al., 2022). People assigned female at birth are at higher risk than people assigned male at birth. Anyone receiving antipsychotic medication can develop tardive dyskinesia. Risk factors are summarized in Box 11.4.

The causes of tardive dyskinesia remain unclear, but a widely accepted theory is that when dopamine antagonists block dopamine receptors over time, a hypersensitivity of dopamine develops that is associated with the emergence of tardive dyskinesia. The vesicular monoamine transporter 2 (VAMT2) is a presynaptic protein that regulates the release of dopamine and other monoamines from neuronal vesicles into the synapse. When the VAMT2 is inhibited, the symptoms of tardive dyskinesia improve (Golsorkhi et al., 2024). Two VAMT2 inhibitors—valbenazine and deutetrabenazine—are approved by the FDA for the treatment of tardive dyskinesia.

The best approach to treatment remains avoiding the development of the chronic syndromes. Preventive measures include use of atypical antipsychotics, using the lowest possible dose of typical medication, minimizing use of as-needed (PRN) medication, and closely monitoring individuals in high-risk groups for development of the symptoms of tardive dyskinesia. Modifiable factors should be addressed such as diabetes, smoking, substance use, and anticholinergic medications. All members of the mental health treatment team who have contact with individuals taking antipsychotics for 1 to 6 months must be alert to the risk factors and earliest possible signs of chronic medication-related movement disorders (Vasan & Padhy, 2023).

Monitoring tools, such as the Abnormal Involuntary Movement Scale (see Appendix), should be used routinely to standardize assessment and provide the earliest possible recognition of the symptoms. Standardized assessments should be performed at a minimum of 3- to 6-month intervals. The earlier the symptoms are recognized, the more likely they will resolve if the medication can be changed, or its use discontinued. Newer, atypical antipsychotic medications have a much lower risk of causing tardive dyskinesia and are increasingly being considered first-line medications for treating patients with schizophrenia. Other medications are under development to provide alternatives that limit the risk for tardive dyskinesia.

BOX 11.4

Risk Factors for Tardive Dyskinesia

- Age older than 50 years
- Being a person assigned female at birth
- Affective disorders, particularly depression
- Brain damage or dysfunction
- Increased duration of treatment
- Standard antipsychotic medication
- Possible higher doses of antipsychotic medication

Mood Stabilizers (Antimanic Medications)

Mood stabilizers, or antimanic medications, are psychopharmacologic agents used primarily for stabilizing mood swings, particularly those of mania in bipolar disorders. Lithium, the oldest, is the gold standard of treatment for acute mania and maintenance of bipolar disorders. Not all respond to lithium, and increasingly, other drugs are being used as first-line agents. Anticonvulsants, calcium channel blockers, adrenergic blocking agents, and atypical antipsychotics are used for mood stabilization.

Lithium

Lithium, a naturally occurring element, is effective in about 40% of patients with bipolar disorder. Although lithium is not a perfect drug, a great deal is known regarding its use—it is inexpensive, it has restored stability to the lives of thousands of people, and it remains the gold standard of bipolar pharmacologic treatment.

Indications and Mechanisms of Action

Lithium is indicated for symptoms of mania characterized by rapid speech, flight of ideas (jumping from topic to topic), irritability, grandiose thinking, impulsiveness, and agitation. Because it has mild antidepressant effects, lithium is used in treating depressive episodes of bipolar illness. It is also used as augmentation in patients experiencing major depression that has only partially responded to antidepressants alone. Lithium also has been shown to be helpful in reducing impulsivity and aggression in certain psychiatric patients.

The exact action by which lithium improves the symptoms of mania is unknown, but it is thought to exert multiple neurotransmitter effects, including enhancing serotonergic transmission, increasing synthesis of norepinephrine, and blocking postsynaptic dopamine. It has also been suggested that lithium's mood-stabilizing effects are related to the fact that it acts on cellular targets and exerting neuroprotective effects (Ghanaatfar et al., 2023).

Lithium is actively transported across cell membranes, altering sodium transport in both nerve and muscle cells. It replaces sodium in the sodium–potassium pump and is retained more readily than sodium inside the cells. Conditions that alter sodium content in the body, such as vomiting, diuresis, and diaphoresis, also alter lithium retention. The results of lithium influx into the nerve cell lead to increased storage of catecholamines within the cell, reduced dopamine neurotransmission, increased norepinephrine reuptake, increased GABA activity, and increased serotonin receptor sensitivity. Lithium also alters the distribution of calcium and magnesium ions and inhibits second messenger systems within the neuron. The mechanisms by which lithium improves the symptoms of mania are complex and interrelated, involving the sum of all or part of these actions and more.

Pharmacokinetics

Lithium carbonate is available orally in capsule, tablet, and liquid forms. Slow-release preparations are also available. Lithium is readily absorbed in the gastric system and may be taken with food, which does not impair absorption. Peak blood levels are reached in 1 to 4 hours, and the medication is usually completely absorbed in 8 hours. Slow-release preparations are absorbed at a slower, more variable rate.

Lithium is not protein bound, and its distribution into the CNS across the blood–brain barrier is slow. The onset of action is usually 5 to 7 days and may take as long as 2 weeks. The elimination half-life is 8 to 12 hours and is 18 to 36 hours in individuals whose blood levels have reached steady state and whose symptoms are stable. Lithium is almost entirely excreted by the kidneys but is present in all body fluids. Conditions of renal impairment or decreased renal function in older patients decrease lithium clearance and may lead to toxicity. Several medications affect renal function and therefore change lithium clearance. See Chapter 26 for a list of these and other medication interactions with lithium. About 80% of lithium is reabsorbed in the proximal tubule of the kidney along with water and sodium. In conditions that cause sodium depletion, such as dehydration caused by fever, strenuous exercise, hot weather, increased perspiration, and vomiting, the kidneys attempt to conserve sodium. Because lithium is a salt, the kidneys retain lithium as well, leading to increased blood levels and potential toxicity. Significantly increasing sodium intake causes lithium levels to fall.

Lithium is usually administered in doses of 300 mg two to three times daily. Because it is a drug with a narrow therapeutic range or index, blood levels are monitored frequently during acute mania, and the dosage is increased every 3 to 5 days. These increases may be slower in older adult patients or patients who experience uncomfortable side effects. Blood levels should be monitored 12 hours after the last dose of medication. In the hospital setting, nurses should withhold the morning dose of lithium until the serum sample is drawn to avoid falsely elevated levels. Individuals who are at home should be instructed to have their blood drawn in the morning about 12 hours after their last dose and before they take their first dose of medication. During the acute phases of mania, blood levels of 0.8 to 1.4 mEq/L are usually attained and maintained until symptoms are under control. The therapeutic range for lithium is narrow, and patients in the higher end of that range usually experience more uncomfortable side effects. During maintenance, the dosage is reduced, and dosages are adjusted to maintain blood levels of 0.4 to 1 mEq/L.

Lithium clears the body relatively quickly after discontinuation of its use. Withdrawal symptoms are rare, but occasional anxiety and emotional lability have been reported. It is important to remember that almost half of the individuals who discontinue lithium treatment abruptly experience a relapse of symptoms within a few weeks. Some research suggests that if a person stops taking lithium, the drug will be less effective when the medication is restarted. Patients should be warned of the risks in abruptly discontinuing their medication and should be advised to consider the options carefully in consultation with their prescriber.

Side Effects, Adverse Reactions, and Toxicity

At lower therapeutic blood levels, side effects from lithium are relatively mild. These reactions correspond with peaks in plasma concentrations of the medication after administration and most subside during the first few weeks of therapy. Frequently, individuals taking lithium complain of excessive thirst and an unpleasant metallic-like taste. Sugarless throat lozenges may be useful in minimizing this side effect. Other common side effects include increased frequency of urination, fine head tremor, drowsiness, and mild diarrhea. Weight gain occurs in about 20% of the individuals taking lithium. Nausea may be minimized by taking the medication with food or by use of a slow-release preparation. However, slow-release forms of lithium increase diarrhea.

Muscle weakness, restlessness, headache, acne, rashes, and exacerbation of psoriasis have also been reported. See Chapter 26 for a summary of selected nursing interventions to minimize the impact of common side effects associated with lithium treatment. Patients most frequently discontinued their own medication use because of concerns with mental slowness, poor concentration, and memory problems.

As blood levels of lithium increase, the side effects of lithium become more numerous and severe. Early signs of lithium toxicity include severe diarrhea, vomiting, drowsiness, muscular weakness, and lack of coordination. Lithium should be withheld, and the prescriber consulted if these symptoms develop. Lithium toxicity can easily be resolved in 24 to 48 hours by discontinuing the medication, but hemodialysis may be required in severe situations. See Chapter 26 for a summary of the side effects and symptoms of toxicity associated with various blood levels of lithium.

Monitoring of creatinine concentration, thyroid hormones, and CBC every 6 months during maintenance therapy helps to assess the occurrence of other potential adverse reactions. Kidney damage is considered an uncommon but potentially serious risk of long-term lithium treatment. This damage is usually reversible after discontinuation of the lithium use. A gradual rise in serum creatinine and decline in creatinine clearance indicate the development of renal dysfunction. Individuals with preexisting kidney dysfunction are susceptible to lithium toxicity.

Lithium may alter thyroid function, usually after 6 to 18 months of treatment. About 30% of the individuals taking lithium exhibit elevations in thyroid-stimulating hormone, but most do not show suppression of circulating thyroid hormone. Thyroid dysfunction from lithium treatment is more common in people assigned female at birth, and some individuals require the addition of thyroxine to their care. During maintenance, thyroid-stimulating hormone levels may be monitored. Nurses should observe for dry skin, constipation, bradycardia, hair loss, cold intolerance, and other symptoms of hypothyroidism. Other endocrine system effects result from hypoparathyroidism, which increases parathyroid hormone levels and calcium. Clinically, this change is not significant, but elevated calcium levels may cause mood changes, anxiety, lethargy, and sleep disturbances. These symptoms may erroneously be attributed to depression if hypercalcemia is not investigated.

Lithium use must be avoided during pregnancy because it has been associated with birth defects, especially when administered during the first trimester. If lithium is given during the third trimester, toxicity may develop in a newborn, producing signs of hypotonia, cyanosis, bradykinesia, cardiac changes, gastrointestinal bleeding, and shock. Diabetes insipidus may persist for months. Lithium is also present in breast milk, and people should not breastfeed while taking lithium. Patients expecting to become pregnant should be advised to consult with a provider before discontinuing use of birth control methods.

Anticonvulsants

In the PMH area, anticonvulsants are commonly used to treat patients with bipolar disorder and are considered mood stabilizers. The following discussion highlights the use of anticonvulsants as mood stabilizers in the treatment of bipolar disorder.

Indications and Mechanisms of Action

Valproate (valproic acid) carbamazepine, and lamotrigine have FDA approval for the treatment of bipolar disorder, mania, or mixed episodes (see Chapter 26). In general, the anticonvulsant mood stabilizers have many actions, but their effects on ion channels, reducing repetitive firing of action potentials in the nerves, most directly decrease manic symptoms. Not all people with bipolar disorder respond to anticonvulsants. Research is emerging that genetic variability of the underlying mechanism may explain the variation in treatment outcomes (Spoelma et al., 2024).

Pharmacokinetics

Valproic acid is rapidly absorbed, but the enteric coating of divalproex sodium adds a delay of as long as 1 hour. Peak serum levels occur in about 1 to 4 hours. The liquid form (sodium valproate) is absorbed more rapidly and peaks in 15 minutes to 2 hours. Food appears to slow absorption but does not lower bioavailability of the drug.

Carbamazepine is absorbed in a somewhat variable manner. The liquid suspension is absorbed more quickly than the tablet form, but food does not appear to interfere with absorption. Peak plasma levels occur in 2 to 6 hours. Because high doses influence peak plasma levels and increase the risk for side effects, carbamazepine should be given in divided doses two or three times a day. The suspension, which has higher peak plasma levels and lower trough levels, must be given more frequently than the tablet form.

These medications cross easily into the CNS, move into the placenta as well, and are associated with an increased risk for birth defects. Carbamazepine, valproic acid, and lamotrigine are metabolized by the CYP450 system. However, one of the metabolites of carbamazepine is potentially toxic. If other concurrent medications inhibit the enzymes that break down this toxic metabolite, severe adverse reactions are often the result. Medications that inhibit this breakdown include erythromycin, verapamil, and cimetidine (now available in nonprescription form).

Teaching Points

Nurses need to educate patients about potential drug interactions, especially with nonprescription medications. Nurses can also inform other health care practitioners who may be prescribing medication that these patients are taking carbamazepine. It is important to note that oral contraceptives may become ineffective, and patients should be advised to use other methods of birth control.

Side Effects, Adverse Reactions, and Toxicity of Anticonvulsants

The most common side effects of carbamazepine are dizziness, drowsiness, tremor, visual disturbance, nausea, and vomiting. These side effects may be minimized by initiating treatment in low doses. Patients should be advised that these symptoms will diminish, but care should be taken when changing positions or performing tasks that require visual alertness. Giving the drug with food may diminish nausea. Adverse reactions include rare aplastic anemia, agranulocytosis, severe rash, rare cardiac problems, and syndrome of inappropriate secretion of the diuretic hormone caused by hyponatremia.

Valproic acid also causes gastrointestinal disturbances, tremors, and lethargy. In addition, it can produce weight gain and alopecia (hair loss). These symptoms are transient and should diminish with the course of treatment. Dietary supplements of zinc and selenium may be helpful to patients experiencing hair loss. Constipation and urinary retention occur in some individuals. Nurses should monitor urinary output and assist patients to increase fluid consumption to decrease constipation.

Benign skin rash, sedation, blurred or double vision, dizziness, nausea, vomiting, and other gastrointestinal symptoms are side effects of lamotrigine. In rare cases, lamotrigine produces severe, life-threatening rashes that usually occur within 2 to 8 weeks of treatment. This risk is highest in children. Use of lamotrigine should be immediately discontinued if a rash is noted.

Transient elevations in liver enzymes occur with both carbamazepine and valproic acid but symptoms of hepatic injury rarely occur. If the patient reports unusual pain or shows signs of jaundice, the prescriber should be notified immediately. Several blood dyscrasias are associated with carbamazepine, including aplastic anemia, agranulocytosis, and leukopenia. Patients should be advised to report fever, sore throat, rash, petechiae, or bruising immediately. In addition, patients should be advised of the importance of completing routine blood tests throughout treatment. The risks for aplastic anemia and agranulocytosis with carbamazepine use still require close monitoring of CBCs during treatment. Valproate and its derivatives have had a similar course of development.

Antidepressant Medications

Medications classified as antidepressants are used not only for the treatment of depression but also in the treatment of anxiety disorders, eating disorders, and other mental health states (Table 11.8). They are used very cautiously in people with bipolar disorder because of the possibility of precipitating a manic episode. The exact neuromechanism for the antidepressant effect is unknown in all of them. The onset of action also varies considerably and appears to depend on factors outside of steady-state plasma levels. Initial improvement with some antidepressants, such as the SSRIs, may appear within 7 days, but complete relief of symptoms may take several weeks. Antidepressants should not be discontinued abruptly because of uncomfortable symptoms that result. Discontinuance of the use of these medications requires slow tapering. Individuals taking these medications should be cautioned not to abruptly stop using them without consulting their prescriber. Antidepressant medications are well absorbed from the gastrointestinal system; however, some individual variations exist. Most of the antidepressants are metabolized by liver enzymes so that other drugs metabolized by these enzymes may increase or decrease blood levels of the antidepressants (see Table 11.9). All these medications have a "boxed warning" for increased risk of suicidal behavior in children, adolescents, and young adults.

Serotonin syndrome, or serotonin intoxication syndrome, can occur if there is an overactivity of serotonin or an impairment of the serotonin metabolism. Concomitant medications such as triptans used to treat migraines also can increase the serotonergic activity. With the advent of widely used antidepressants targeting the serotonergic systems, symptoms of this serious side effect should be assessed. Symptoms include mental status changes (hallucinations, agitation, coma), autonomic instability (tachycardia, hyperthermia, changes in blood pressure), neuromuscular problems (hyperreflexia, incoordination), and gastrointestinal disturbance (nausea, vomiting, diarrhea). Serotonin syndrome can be life threatening. The treatment for serotonin syndrome is discontinuation of the medication and symptom management.

Selective Serotonin Reuptake Inhibitors

The serotonergic system is associated with mood, emotion, sleep, and appetite and is implicated in the control of numerous emotional, physical, and behavioral functions (see Chapter 7). Decreased serotonergic neurotransmission has been proposed to play a key role in depression. In 1988, fluoxetine was the first of a class of drugs that acted "selectively" on serotonin, one group of neurotransmitters associated with depression. Other

TABLE 11.8 ANTIDEPRESSANT MEDICATIONS

Generic Drug Name	Usual Dosage Range (mg/day)	Half-Life (h)	Therapeutic Blood Level (ng/mL)
Selective Serotonin Reuptake Inhibitors			
Citalopram	20–50	35	Not available
Escitalopram	10–20	27–32	Not available
Fluoxetine	20–80	2–9 days	72–300
Fluvoxamine	50–300	17–22	Not available
Paroxetine	10–50	10–24	Not available
Sertraline	50–200	24	Not available
Serotonin Norepinephrine Reuptake Inhibitors			
Desvenlafaxine (extended release)	50	11	Not available
Duloxetine	40–60	8–17	Not available
Levomilnacipran	40–120	12	Not available
Nefazodone	100–600	2–4	Not available
Venlafaxine	75–375	5–11	100–500
Norepinephrine-Dopamine Reuptake Inhibitor			
Bupropion	200–450	8–24	10–29
α_2-Blocker Antagonist			
Mirtazapine	15–45	20–40	Not available
NMDA Antagonist			
Esketamine	56–84 titrated from twice a week to every other week	2–12 hours	Not available
Others			
Dextromethorphan/bupropion	45 /105 mg twice a day	22 hours	Not available
Trazodone	150–600	4–9	650–1,600
Vilazodone	10–40	25	Not available
Vortioxetine	5–20	66	Not available
Tricyclic Antidepressants			
Amitriptyline	50–300	31–46	110–250
Amoxapine	50–600	8	200–500
Clomipramine	25–250	19–37	80–100
Desipramine	25–300	12–24	125–300
Doxepin	25–300	8–24	100–200
Imipramine	30–300	11–25	200–350
Nortriptyline	30–100	18–44	50–150
Protriptyline	15–60	67–89	100–200
Tetracyclic			
Maprotiline	50–225	21–25	200–300
Monoamine Oxidase Inhibitors			
Isocarboxazid	20–60	Not available	Not available
Phenelzine	15–90	24 (effect lasts 3–4 days)	Not available
Selegiline	6–12 mg/24 hours	25–50% delivered in 24 hours	Not available
Tranylcypromine	10–60	24 (effect lasts 3–10 days)	Not available

NMDA, *N*-methyl D-aspartate.

TABLE 11.9 CYP450 METABOLISM OF COMMON ANTIDEPRESSANTS

Drug	How Metabolized	Induces	Inhibits
Bupropion	2B6	None	2D6
Citalopram	2C19, 2D6, 3A4	None	Mild 2D6
Desvenlafaxine	3A4	None	Mild 2D6
Duloxetine	1A2, 2D6	None	2D6
Escitalopram	2C19, 2D6, 3A4	None	Mild 2D6
Esketamine	2B6, 3A4, 2C9, 2C19	2B	3A4, 2D1
Fluoxetine	2C9, 2C19, 2D6, 3A4	None	2C19, 2D6 3A4, norfluoxetine
Fluvoxamine	1A2, 2D6	None	1A2, 2C9, 2C19, 3A4
Mirtazapine	1A2, 2D6, 3A4	None	None
Nefazodone	2D6, 3A4	None	3A4
Paroxetine	2D6	None	2D6, 2B6
Selegiline	2A6, 2C9, 3A4/5	None	2D6, 3A4/5
Sertraline	2B6, 2C9, 2D6, 3A4	None	2B6, 2C9, 2C19, 2D6, 3A4 (dosage >200 mg)
St. John's wort[a]	3A4	3A4	None
Trazodone	2D6, 3A4	None	None
Tricyclic antidepressants	2D6, others depending on drug	None	Mild 2D6
Venlafaxine	2D6	None	Mild 2D6
Vilazodone	3A4, 2C19, 2D6	None	2C8
Vortioxetine	2D6, 3A4/5, 2C9, 2A6, 2C8, 2B6	None	None

[a]Not a U.S. Food and Drug Administration–approved antidepressant.
Note: Information from the prescribing information of each medication.

similarly selective medications, sertraline, paroxetine, and fluvoxamine, soon followed. The newest SSRI is escitalopram oxalate.

All the SSRIs inhibit the reuptake of serotonin by blocking its transport into the presynaptic neuron, which in turn increases the concentration of synaptic serotonin. The concentration of synaptic serotonin is controlled directly by its reuptake; thus, drugs blocking serotonin transport have been successfully used for the treatment of depression and other conditions associated with serotonergic activity.

The SSRIs also have other properties that account for the common side effects, which include headache, anxiety, insomnia, transient nausea, vomiting, and diarrhea. Sedation may also occur, especially with paroxetine. Most often, these medications are given in the morning, but if daytime sedation occurs, they may be given in the evening. Higher doses, especially of fluoxetine, are more likely to produce sedation. Nausea and dizziness are common side effects which may subside within a few weeks. These side effects, along with sexual dysfunction, sedation, diastolic hypertension, and increased perspiration, tend to be dose dependent, occurring more frequently at higher doses. Other common side effects include insomnia, constipation, dry mouth, tremors, blurred vision, and asthenia or muscle weakness.

Sexual dysfunction is a relatively common side effect with most antidepressants. Erectile and ejaculation disturbances or anorgasmia may occur. This side effect is often difficult to assess if the nurse has not obtained a sexual history before initiation of use of the medication. Anorgasmia is particularly common with SSRIs and often goes unreported, frequently because nurses and other health care providers do not ask.

Serotonin Norepinephrine Reuptake Inhibitors

Decreased activity of the neurotransmitter norepinephrine is also associated with depression and anxiety disorders. Venlafaxine, nefazodone, duloxetine, and desvenlafaxine prevent the reuptake of both serotonin and norepinephrine at the presynaptic site and are classified as serotonin norepinephrine reuptake inhibitors (SNRIs). Desipramine is technically a tricyclic antidepressant (TCA) and is usually categorized as such. It works, however, on both serotonin and norepinephrine, so it can also be considered an SNRI.

The side effects are like those of the SSRIs; there is also a risk for an associated increase in blood pressure. Elevations in blood pressure have been described, and nurses should monitor blood pressure, especially in patients who have a history of hypertension. Venlafaxine has little effect on acetylcholine and histamine; thus, it creates only mild sedation and anticholinergic symptoms. This medication is often used if a depressed patient is sleeping excessively and reports little energy. The most common side effects of nefazodone include dry mouth, nausea, dizziness, muscle weakness, constipation, and tremor. It is unlikely to cause sexual disturbance. Nefazodone also has a "boxed warning" for hepatic failure and should not be used in those with acute liver disease.

Norepinephrine Dopamine Reuptake Inhibitors

Bupropion inhibits reuptake of norepinephrine, serotonin, and dopamine. Wellbutrin is indicated for depression and for nicotine dependency. Bupropion is given at a lower dose for smoking cessation than for depression. Bupropion has a chemical structure unlike any of the other antidepressants and somewhat resembles a few of the psychostimulants. Bupropion's activating effects may be experienced as agitation or anxiety by some patients. Others also experience insomnia and appetite suppression. For a few individuals, bupropion has produced psychosis, including hallucinations and delusions. Most likely, this is secondary to overstimulation of the dopamine system. Bupropion is contraindicated for people with seizure disorders and those at risk for seizures. The rate of seizures is similar to that with SSRIs and mirtazapine but is lower than the rate associated with the older antidepressants. Most importantly, bupropion has a lower incidence of sexual dysfunction and often is used in individuals who are experiencing these side effects with other antidepressants (GlaxoSmithKline, 2023; Ramli et al., 2021).

α_2-Antagonist

Mirtazapine boosts norepinephrine or noradrenaline and serotonin by blocking α_2-adrenergic presynaptic receptors on a serotonin receptor (5-HT_{2A}, 5-HT_{2C}, 5-HT_3). This is a different action than the other antidepressants. A histamine receptor is also blocked, which may explain its sedative side effect. Mirtazapine is indicated for depression. Side effects include sedation (at lower doses), dizziness, weight gain, dry mouth, constipation, and change in urinary functioning.

N-methyl D-aspartate Receptor Antagonist

In March 2019, the FDA approved a nasal spray formulation of esketamine for the treatment of resistant depression. Esketamine is a similar formulation to ketamine, an FDA-approved anesthetic. Esketamine is not approved as an anesthetic agent and ketamine is not approved for the treatment of depression, but it has been used off-label for rapid relief of severe depression. Ketamine also produces euphoria, dissociation, and hallucinations; has a high risk of misuse; and is a well-known street drug, Special K (see Chapter 31).

Esketamine is a nonselective, noncompetitive antagonist of *N*-methyl D-aspartate receptor, blocking glutamate. Esketamine reaches maximum plasma concentration in 20 to 24 minutes. Once administered, there is a rapid decline in plasma concentration within 4 to 8 hours. It is metabolized primarily in the liver and excreted in the urine (Buchmayer & Kasper, 2023).

Esketamine is given under direct supervision of a health care provider. The FDA recommends that esketamine be given in conjunction with an oral antidepressant. A treatment session consists of a nasal administration and postadministration observation. Blood pressure is assessed before and after treatment. The medication is given in two phases. During the induction phase (weeks 1 to 4), the medication is given twice a week; during maintenance phase (weeks 5 to 8), esketamine is given weekly; and after 9 weeks, it is given every 2 weeks. The medication has a boxed warning for sedation, dissociation, misuse, and suicidal thoughts and behavior. Other side effects include increase in blood pressure, short- and long-term cognitive impairment, impaired ability to drive and operate machinery, ulcerative or interstitial cystitis, and embryo–fetal toxicity (Buchmayer & Kasper, 2023; Feeney & Papkostas, 2023). Due to the possibility of nausea and vomiting after administration, patient should avoid food for at least 2 hours before administration and avoid drinking liquids at least 30 minutes prior to administration.

Other Antidepressants

Trazodone blocks serotonin 2A receptor potently and blocks the serotonin reuptake pump less potently. It is indicated for depression but is often used off-label for insomnia and anxiety. Sedation is a very common side effect. Other side effects include weight gain, nausea, vomiting, constipation, dizziness, fatigue, incoordination, and tremor.

Other newly FDA-approved antidepressants target other receptor sites. For example, vilazodone is a serotonin reuptake inhibitor and a partial agonist of 5-HT_{1A}; vortioxetine inhibits reuptake of serotonin and norepinephrine but is also a partial agonist to 5-HT_{1A}. These subtle differences translate into subtle clinical effects. In 2022, a combination of dextromethorphan (an NMDA receptor antagonist and sigma-1 receptor agonist) and bupropion (a CYP 2D6 inhibitor), was approved for the treatment of major depressive disorder (Chaki & Watanabe, 2023).

Tricyclic Antidepressants

The TCAs were once the primary medication used for treating depression. With the introduction of the SSRIs and other previously discussed antidepressants, the use of TCAs has significantly declined. In most cases, these medications are as effective as the other drugs, but they have more serious side effects and a higher lethal potential (see Table 11.9). The TCAs act on a variety of neurotransmitter systems, including the norepinephrine and serotonin reuptake systems.

Pharmacokinetics

The TCAs are highly bound to plasma proteins, which make the association between blood levels and therapeutic clinical effects difficult. However, some plasma ranges have been established (see Table 11.7). Most of the TCAs have active metabolites that act in as much the same manner as the parent drug. Most of these antidepressants may be given in a once-daily single dose. If the medication causes sedation, this dose should be given at bedtime.

Side Effects, Adverse Reactions, and Toxicity

Because the TCAs act on several neurotransmitters in addition to serotonin and norepinephrine, these drugs have many unwanted effects. With the TCAs, sedation, orthostatic hypotension, and anticholinergic side effects are the most common sources of discomfort for patients receiving these medications. Other side effects of the TCAs include tremors, restlessness, insomnia, nausea and vomiting, confusion, pedal edema, headache, and seizures. Blood dyscrasias may also occur, and any fever, sore throat, malaise, or rash should be reported to the prescriber. Interventions to assist in minimizing these side effects are listed in Table 11.1.

The TCAs have the potential for cardiotoxicity. Symptoms include prolongation of cardiac conduction that may worsen preexisting cardiac conduction problems. The TCAs are contraindicated with second-degree atrioventricular block and should be used cautiously in patients who have other cardiac problems. Occasionally, they may precipitate heart failure, myocardial infarction, arrhythmias, and stroke.

Antidepressants that block the dopamine (D_2) receptor, such as amoxapine, have produced symptoms of NMS. Mild forms of EPS and endocrine changes, including galactorrhea and amenorrhea, may develop.

Monoamine Oxidase Inhibitors

MAOIs, as their name indicates, inhibit MAO, an enzyme that breaks down the biogenic amine neurotransmitters serotonin, norepinephrine, and others. By inhibiting this enzyme, serotonin and norepinephrine activity is increased in the synapse. In the United States, there are three oral formulations—phenelzine, tranylcypromine, and isocarboxazid—and one that is available by a transdermal patch—selegiline. These are considered MAOIs because they form strong covalent bonds to block the enzyme MAO. The inhibition of this enzyme increases with repeated administration of these medications and takes at least 2 weeks to resolve after discontinuation of use of the medication.

The major problem with MAOIs is their interaction with tyramine-rich foods and certain medications that can result in a hypertensive crisis. All MAOIs have dietary modification except the 6 mg/24 hours dose of selegiline, which is delivered through the skin and is not absorbed in the gastrointestinal tract. The enzyme monoamine is important in the breakdown of dietary amines (e.g., tyramine). When the enzyme is inhibited, tyramine, a precursor for dopamine, increases in the nerve cells. Tyramine has a vasopressor action that induces hypertension. If the individual ingests food that contains high levels of tyramine while taking MAOIs, severe headaches, palpitation, neck stiffness and soreness, nausea, vomiting, sweating, hypertension, stroke, and, in rare instances, death may result. Patients who are taking MAOIs are prescribed a low-tyramine diet (Table 11.10).

In addition to food restrictions, many prescription and nonprescription medications that stimulate the sympathetic nervous system (sympathomimetic) produce the same risk for hypertensive crisis as do foods containing tyramine. The nonprescription medication interactions involve primarily diet pills and cold remedies. Patients should be advised to check the labels of any nonprescription drugs carefully for a warning against use with antidepressants, especially MAOIs, and then consult their prescriber before consuming these medications. In addition, symptoms of other serious drug–drug interactions may develop, such as coma, hypertension, and fever, which may occur when patients receive meperidine while taking an MAOI. Patients should notify other health care providers, including dentists, that they are taking an MAOI before being prescribed or given any other medication.

MAOIs frequently produce dizziness, headache, insomnia, dry mouth, blurred vision, constipation, nausea, peripheral edema, urinary hesitancy, muscle weakness, forgetfulness, and weight gain. Older patients are especially sensitive to the side effect of orthostatic hypotension and require frequent assessment of lying and standing blood pressures. They may be at risk for falls and subsequent bone fractures and require assistance in changing position. Sexual dysfunction—including decreased libido, impotence, and anorgasmia—also is common with MAOIs.

Antianxiety and Sedative–Hypnotic Medications

Sometimes called *anxiolytics*, antianxiety medications, such as buspirone and sedative–hypnotic medications, such as lorazepam come from various pharmacologic

TABLE 11.10 EXAMPLE OF A TYRAMINE-RESTRICTED DIET

Category of Food	Food With Tyramine	Food Allowed
Nonrefrigerated food	Spoiled foods or foods not refrigerated, handled, or stored properly	Food that is handled and stored properly
Cheese	All aged and mature cheeses, especially strong, aged, or processed cheeses such as American processed cheddar, Colby, blue, brie, mozzarella, and parmesan; yogurt, sour cream	Fresh cottage cheese, cream cheese, ricotta cheese
Meat, fish, and poultry	Air-dried, aged, and fermented meats; sausages and salamis Beef or chicken liver Dried and pickled herring Pepperoni Anchovies, meat extracts, meat tenderizers Meats prepared with tenderizers, improperly stored meat Spoiled or improperly stored animal liver	Fresh meat, poultry, and fish, including fresh processed meats (e.g., lunch meats, hot dogs, breakfast sausage, and cooked sliced ham)
Fruits and vegetables	Broad bean pods (Fava bean pods)	All other vegetables
Alcoholic beverages	All tap beers and other beers that have not been pasteurized; red wine, sherry, liqueurs; some alcohol-free and reduced alcohol beer	White wines may not contain tyramine
Miscellaneous foods	Marmite concentrated yeast extract Sauerkraut Soy sauce and other soybean condiments	Soy milk Pizzas from commercial chain restaurants with cheeses low in tyramine

Source: Parke-Davis. (2007). Retrieved August 24, 2024, from http://www.accessdata.fda.gov/drugsatfda_docs/label/2007/011909s038lbl.pdf

classifications, including barbiturates, benzodiazepines, nonbenzodiazepines, and nonbarbiturate sedative–hypnotic medications, such as chloral hydrate. These drugs represent some of the most widely prescribed medications today for the short-term relief of anxiety or anxiety associated with depression.

Benzodiazepines

Commonly prescribed benzodiazepines include alprazolam, lorazepam, diazepam, chlordiazepoxide, flurazepam, and triazolam. Although benzodiazepines are known to enhance the effects of the inhibitory neurotransmitter GABA, their exact mechanisms of action are not well understood. Of the various benzodiazepines in use to relieve anxiety (and treat insomnia), oxazepam and lorazepam are often preferred for patients with liver disease and for older patients because of their short half-lives.

Pharmacokinetics

The variable rate of absorption of the benzodiazepines determines the speed of onset. Table 11.11 provides relative indications of the speed of onset, from very fast to slow, for some of the commonly prescribed benzodiazepines. Whereas chlordiazepoxide and diazepam are slow, erratic, and sometimes incompletely absorbed when given intramuscularly, lorazepam is rapidly and completely absorbed when given intramuscularly.

All the benzodiazepines are highly lipid soluble and highly protein bound. They are distributed throughout the body and enter the CNS quickly. Other drugs that compete for protein-binding sites may produce drug–drug interactions. The degree to which each of these drugs is lipid soluble affects its duration of action. Most of these drugs have active metabolites, but the degree of activity of each metabolite affects duration of action and elimination half-life. Most of these drugs vary markedly in length of half-life. Oxazepam and lorazepam have no active metabolites and thus have shorter half-lives. Elimination half-life may also be sustained for obese patients when using diazepam and chlordiazepoxide.

Side Effects, Adverse Reactions, and Toxicity

The most commonly reported side effects of benzodiazepines result from the sedative and CNS depression effects of these medications. Drowsiness, intellectual impairment, memory impairment, ataxia, and reduced motor coordination are common adverse reactions. If prescribed for sleep, many of these medications, especially the long-acting benzodiazepines, produce significant "hangover" effects experienced on awakening. Older patients receiving repeated doses of medications such as flurazepam at bedtime may experience paradoxical confusion, agitation, and delirium, sometimes after the first dose. In addition, daytime fatigue, drowsiness, and cognitive impairments may continue while the person is

TABLE 11.11 ANTIANXIETY AND SEDATIVE–HYPNOTIC

Generic Drug Name	Usual Dosage Range (mg/day)	Half-Life (h)	Speed of Onset After Single Dose
Benzodiazepines			
Alprazolam	0.5–10	12–15	Intermediate
Chlordiazepoxide	15–100	50–100	Intermediate
Clonazepam	1.5–20	18–50	Intermediate
Clorazepate	15–60	30–200	Fast
Diazepam	4–40	30–100	Very fast
Halazepam	80–160	30–200	Slow intermediate
Lorazepam	2–8	10–20	Slow intermediate
Oxazepam	30–120	3–21	Slow intermediate
Prazepam	20–60	30–200	Very slow
Nonbenzodiazepine			
Buspirone	15–30	3–11	Very slow

awake. For most patients, the effects subside as tolerance develops; however, alcohol increases all these symptoms and potentiates the CNS depression. Individuals using these medications should be warned to be cautious when driving or performing other tasks that require mental alertness. If these tasks are part of the person's work requirements, another medication may be chosen. Administered intravenously, benzodiazepines often cause phlebitis and thrombosis at the IV sites, which should be monitored closely and changed if redness or swelling develops.

Because tolerance develops to most of the CNS depressant effects, individuals who wish to experience the feeling of "intoxication" from these medications may be tempted to increase their own dosage. Psychological dependence is more likely to occur when using these medications for a longer period. Abrupt discontinuation of the use of benzodiazepines may result in a recurrence of the target symptoms, such as rebound insomnia or anxiety. Other withdrawal symptoms appear rapidly, including tremors, increased perspiration, palpitations, increased sensitivity to light, abdominal discomfort or pain, and elevations in systolic blood pressure. These symptoms may be more pronounced with short-acting benzodiazepines, such as lorazepam. Gradual tapering is recommended for discontinuing use of benzodiazepines after long-term treatment. When tapering short-acting medications, the prescriber may switch the patient to a long-acting benzodiazepine before discontinuing the use of the short-acting drug.

Individual reactions to benzodiazepines appear to be associated with sensitivity to their effects. Some patients feel apathy, fatigue, tearfulness, emotional lability, irritability, and nervousness. Symptoms of depression may worsen. The PMH nurse should closely monitor these symptoms when individuals are receiving benzodiazepines as adjunctive treatment for anxiety that coexists with depression. Gastrointestinal disturbances, including nausea, vomiting, anorexia, dry mouth, and constipation, may develop. These medications may be taken with food to ease gastrointestinal distress.

Older patients are particularly susceptible to incontinence, memory disturbances, dizziness, and increased risk for falls when using benzodiazepines. Pregnant patients should be aware that these medications cross the placenta and are associated with increased risk for birth defects, such as cleft palate, intellectual disability, and pyloric stenosis. Infants born dependent on benzodiazepines often exhibit flaccid muscle tone, lethargy, and difficulties sucking. All the benzodiazepines are excreted in breast milk, and people who are breastfeeding should avoid using these medications. Infants and children metabolize these medications more slowly; therefore, more drug accumulates in their bodies.

Toxicity develops in overdose or accumulation of the drug in the body from liver dysfunction or disease. Symptoms include worsening of the CNS depression, ataxia, confusion, delirium, agitation, hypotension, diminished reflexes, and lethargy. Rarely do the benzodiazepines cause respiratory depression or death. In overdose, these medications have a high therapeutic index and rarely result in death unless combined with another CNS depressant drug, such as alcohol.

Nonbenzodiazepines: Buspirone

Buspirone, a nonbenzodiazepine, is effective in controlling the symptoms of anxiety but has no effect on panic disorders and little effect on obsessive-compulsive disorder (OCD).

Indications and Mechanisms of Actions

Nonbenzodiazepines are effective for treating anxiety disorders without the CNS depressant effects or the potential for misuse and withdrawal syndromes. Buspirone is indicated for treating generalized anxiety disorder; therefore, its target symptoms include anxiety and related symptoms, such as difficulty concentrating, tension, insomnia, restlessness, irritability, and fatigue. Because buspirone does not add to depression symptoms, it has been tried for treating anxiety that coexists with depression. In some instances, it is thought to potentiate the antidepressant actions of other medications.

Buspirone has no effect on the benzodiazepine–GABA complex but instead appears to control anxiety by blocking the serotonin subtype of receptor, 5-HT_{1A}, at both presynaptic reuptake and postsynaptic receptor sites. It has no sedative, muscle relaxant, or anticonvulsant effects. It also lacks potential for misuse.

Pharmacokinetics

Buspirone is rapidly absorbed but undergoes extensive first-pass metabolism. Food slows absorption but appears to reduce first-pass effects, increasing the bioavailability of the medication. Buspirone is given on a continual dosing schedule of three times a day because of its short half-life of 2 to 3 hours. Clinical action depends on reaching steady-state concentrations; taking this medication with food may facilitate this process.

Buspirone is highly protein bound but does not displace most other medications. However, it does displace digoxin and may increase digoxin levels to the point of toxicity. It is metabolized in the liver and excreted predominantly by the kidneys but also via the gastrointestinal tract. Patients with liver or kidney impairment should be given this medication with caution.

Buspirone cannot be used on a PRN basis; rather, it takes 2 to 4 weeks of continual use for symptom relief to occur. It is more effective in reducing anxiety in patients who have never taken a benzodiazepine.

Buspirone does not block the withdrawal of other benzodiazepines. Therefore, a switch to buspirone must be initiated gradually to avoid withdrawal symptoms. Nurses should closely monitor patients who are undergoing this change of medication for emergence of withdrawal symptoms from the benzodiazepines and report such symptoms to the prescriber.

Side Effects, Adverse Reactions, and Toxicity

Common side effects from buspirone include dizziness, drowsiness, nausea, excitement, and headache. Most other side effects occur at an incidence of less than 1%. There have been no reports of death from an overdose of buspirone alone. Older patients, pregnant people, and children have not been adequately studied. For now, buspirone can be assumed to cross the placenta and is present in breast milk; therefore, its use should be avoided in pregnant people, and individuals who are taking this medication should not breastfeed.

Antihistamines

Antihistamine, hydroxyzine, is increasingly used for the treatment of anxiety as a substitute for benzodiazepines which can lead to psychological dependence. Histamine can produce symptoms of itching or hives on the skin.

Indications and Mechanisms of Action

Even though hydroxyzine is primarily used for itching and nausea, it is also approved for anxiety, tension, and sleep. Hydroxyzine's metabolite, *cetirizine*, blocks the H1 histamine receptor and prevents symptoms that are caused by histamine activity on capillaries, bronchial smooth muscle, and gastrointestinal smooth muscle. It crosses the blood–brain barrier and acts on the H1 receptors in the CNS, which results in suppression of certain subcortical regions of the brain causing sedation and anticholinergic action.

Pharmacokinetics

Hydroxyzine is rapidly absorbed and distributed in oral and IM administration and is metabolized in the liver. The effects are observed within 1 hour of administration with a peak effect in 2 hours. The elimination half-life is around 20 hours in adults (Drugbank Online, 2024).

Side Effects, Adverse Reactions, and Toxicity

The side effects include deep sleep, incoordination, sedation, calmness, and dizziness as well as hypotension, tinnitus, and headaches. Due to the anticholinergic property, constipation and dry mouth can occur. There is some evidence that hydroxyzine can prolong the QTc interval. Hydroxyzine should be administered with caution in older adults (American Society of Health-System Pharmacists, 2024).

Sedative–Hypnotics

Sedatives reduce activity, nervousness, irritability, and excitability without causing sleep; but if given in large enough doses, they have a hypnotic effect. **Hypnotics** cause drowsiness and facilitate the onset and maintenance of sleep. These two classifications are usually referred to as **sedative–hypnotics**—drugs that have a calming

TABLE 11.12 HYPNOTICS FOR INSOMNIA

Generic Drug Name	Usual Dosage Range (mg/day)	Elimination Half-Life (h)	Speed of Onset After Single Dose
Benzodiazepine Hypnotics			
Estazolam	1	10–24	Fast
Flurazepam	15–30	47–100	Fast
Quazepam	0.75–15	39	Fast
Temazepam	15–30	9.5–20	Moderately fast
Triazolam	0.25–0.5	1.5–5	Fast
Nonbenzodiazepine Hypnotics			
Eszopiclone	2–3	6	Fast
Zaleplon	10	1	Fast
Zolpidem	5–10	2.6	Fast
Zolpidem CR	12.5	2.6	Fast
Melatonergic Hypnotics			
Melatonin	0.1–10	0.5–0.75	Fast
Ramelteon	8	1–2.6	Fast
Antihistamines			
Doxylamine	25	10	Fast
Hydroxyzine	50–100	20	Fast
Orexin Receptor Antagonist			
Suvorexant	10–20 mg	12	Fast

effect or depress the CNS. These medications include (1) benzodiazepines, (2) GABA enhancers, (3) melatonergic hypnotics, (4) antihistamines, and (5) the orexin receptor antagonist (Table 11.12). The benzodiazepines have been previously discussed. The GABA enhancers modulate GABA-A receptors. They do not cause a high degree of tolerance or dependence and are easier to discontinue than benzodiazepines. Melatonergic hypnotics are melatonin agonists, and antihistamines block histamines, causing sedation (Kim & Yang, 2022; Simone & Bobrin, 2023). The orexin receptor antagonists block the activity of orexins, neurotransmitters involved in wakefulness and arousal. These medications are discussed thoroughly in Chapter 34.

Stimulants and Wakefulness-Promoting Agents

Amphetamines were first synthesized in the late 1800s but were not used for psychiatric disorders until the 1930s. Initially, amphetamines were prescribed for a variety of symptoms and disorders, but their high misuse potential soon became obvious.

Currently, among the medications known as stimulants are methylphenidate, *d*-amphetamine, amphetamine/dextroamphetamine, dexmethylphenidate, and lisdexamfetamine. CNS stimulants modafinil and armodafinil are wakefulness-promoting agents used for narcolepsy and other sleep disorders.

Indications and Mechanisms of Action

Medical use of these stimulants is now restricted to a few disorders, including narcolepsy, attention-deficit hyperactivity disorder (ADHD), particularly in children, and obesity unresponsive to other treatments. However, stimulants are increasingly being used as an adjunctive treatment in depression and other mood disorders to address the fatigue and low energy common to these conditions.

Amphetamines indirectly stimulate the sympathetic nervous system, producing alertness, wakefulness, vasoconstriction, suppressed appetite, and hypothermia. Tolerance develops to some of these effects, such as suppression of appetite, but the CNS stimulation continues. Although the exact mechanism of action is not completely understood, stimulants cause a release of catecholamines, particularly norepinephrine and dopamine, into the synapse from the presynaptic nerve cell. They also block reuptake of these catecholamines. Methylphenidate is structurally like the amphetamines but produces a milder CNS stimulation. Psychostimulants should be used very cautiously in individuals who have a history of substance misuse.

Although the stimulant effects of these medications may seem logically indicated for narcolepsy, a disorder in which the individual frequently and abruptly falls asleep, the indications for childhood ADHD seem less obvious. The etiology and neurobiology of ADHD remain unclear, but psychostimulants produce a paradoxical calming of the increased motor activity characteristic of ADHD. Studies show that medication decreases disruptive activity during school hours, reduces noise and verbal activity, improves attention span and short-term memory, improves ability to follow directions, and decreases distractibility and impulsivity. Although these improvements have been well documented in the literature, the diagnosis of ADHD and subsequent use of psychostimulants with children remain matters of controversy (see Chapter 37).

Modafinil and armodafinil, wake-promoting agents, are used for treating excessive sleepiness associated with narcolepsy, sleep apnea, and residual sleepiness for shift work sleep disorder. Armodafinil is longer acting than modafinil. The mechanism of action is unclear, but it is hypothesized that they increase glutamate and suppress GABA in the hypothalamus, hippocampus, and thalamus. There is no evidence of direct effects on dopamine, but there may be action on a dopamine transport. These drugs may increase the risk of Stevens–Johnson syndrome (Greenblatt & Adams, 2023).

Pharmacokinetics

Psychostimulants are rapidly absorbed from the gastrointestinal tract and reach peak plasma levels in 1 to 3 hours. Considerable individual variations occur between the drugs in terms of their bioavailability, plasma levels, and half-lives. Table 11.13 compares the primary psychostimulants used in psychiatry. Some of these differences are age dependent because children metabolize these medications more rapidly, producing shorter elimination half-lives.

The psychostimulants appear to be unaffected by food in the stomach and should be given after meals to reduce the appetite-suppressant effects when indicated. However, changes in urine pH may affect the rates of excretion. Excessive sodium bicarbonate alkalizes the urine and reduces amphetamine secretion. Increased vitamin C or citric acid intake may acidify the urine and increase its excretion. Starvation from appetite suppression may have a similar effect. All these drugs are highly lipid soluble, crossing easily into the CNS and the placenta. Psychostimulants undergo metabolic changes in the liver, where they may affect, or be affected by, other drugs. They are primarily excreted through the kidneys; therefore, renal dysfunction may interfere with excretion.

Psychostimulants are usually begun at a low dose and increased weekly, depending on the improvement of symptoms and occurrence of side effects. Initially, children with ADHD are given a morning dose so their school performance may be compared from morning to afternoon. Rebound symptoms of excitability and over-talkativeness may occur when use of the medication is withdrawn or after dose reduction. These symptoms also begin about 5 hours after the last dose of medication, which may affect the dosing regimen for some individuals. The return of symptoms in the afternoon for children with ADHD may require that a second dose be given at school. Prescribers should work with parents/caregivers to implement other interventions after school and on weekends when the psychostimulants are not used. The severity of symptoms may require that the medications be continued during these times, but this dosing schedule should be determined after careful evaluation on an individual basis. Use of these medications should not be stopped abruptly, especially with higher doses, because the rebound effects may last for several days.

Modafinil is absorbed rapidly and reaches peak plasma concentration in 2 to 4 hours. Armodafinil reaches peak plasma concentration later and is maintained for 6 to 14 hours. Absorption of both may be delayed by 1 to 2 hours if taken with food. Modafinil is eliminated via liver metabolism with subsequent excretion of metabolites through renal excretion. They may interact with drugs that are metabolized by liver enzymes including phenytoin, diazepam, and propranolol. Concurrent use of modafinil or armodafinil and other drugs metabolized by the liver enzyme system may lead to increased circulating blood levels of the other drugs.

TABLE 11.13 PSYCHOSTIMULANT MEDICATIONS

Generic Drug Name	Usual Dosage Range (mg/day)	Elimination Half-Life
Amphetamine/dextroamphetamine	2.5 mg (3–5 years) 5 mg (6 years) 5–60 mg for narcolepsy	9–11 hours
Dexmethylphenidate extended release	5–40 mg	3 hours
Dextroamphetamine	5–40	Highly variable depending on urine pH
Lisdexamfetamine	30 mg	<1 hour
Methylphenidate	10–60	2.4 hours (children); 2.1 hours (adults)

Side Effects, Adverse Reactions, and Toxicity

Side effects associated with psychostimulants usually arise within 2 to 3 weeks after the use of the medication begins. From most to least common, these side effects include appetite suppression, insomnia, irritability, weight loss, nausea, headache, palpitations, blurred vision, dry mouth, constipation, and dizziness. Because of the effects on the sympathetic nervous system, some individuals experience blood pressure changes (both hypertension and hypotension), tachycardia, tremors, and irregular heart rates. Blood pressure and pulse should be monitored initially and after each dosage change.

Rarely, psychostimulants suppress growth and development in children. These effects are a matter of controversy, and research has produced conflicting results. Although suppression of height seems unlikely to some researchers, others have indicated that psychostimulants may have an effect on cartilage. Height and weight should be monitored several times annually for children taking these medications and compared with prior history of growth. Weight should be monitored, especially closely during the initial phases of treatment. These effects also may be minimized by drug "holidays," such as during school vacations.

Rarely, individuals may experience mild dysphoria, social withdrawal, or mild-to-moderate depression. These symptoms are more common at higher doses and may require discontinuation of the use of medication. Unusual movements and motor tics may also increase in individuals who have a history of Tourette syndrome. Psychostimulants should be avoided by patients with Tourette symptoms or with a positive family history of the disorder. In addition, dextroamphetamine has been associated with an increased risk for congenital anomalies. Because there is no compelling reason for a pregnant patient to continue to take these medications, patients should be informed and should advise their prescriber immediately if they plan to become pregnant or if pregnancy is a possibility.

Death is rare from overdose or toxicity of the psychostimulants, but a 10-day supply may be lethal, especially in children. Symptoms of overdose include agitation, chest pain, hallucinations, paranoia, confusion, and dysphoria. Seizures may develop, along with fever, tremor, hypertension or hypotension, aggression, headache, palpitations, rashes, difficulty breathing, leg pain, and abdominal pain. Toxic doses of dextroamphetamine are above 20 mg, with potential death resulting from a 400-mg dose. Parents/caregivers should be warned regarding the potential lethality of these medications and take preventive measures by keeping the medication in a safe place.

Side effects associated with modafinil and armodafinil include nausea, nervousness, headache, dizziness, and trouble sleeping. If the effects continue or are bothersome, patients should consult the prescriber. Modafinil and armodafinil are generally well tolerated with few clinically significant side effects. It is potentially habit forming and must be used with great caution in individuals with a history of substance misuse or dependence (Cephalon, 2017).

OTHER BIOLOGIC TREATMENTS

Although the primary biologic interventions remain pharmacologic, other somatic treatments have gained acceptance, remain under investigation, or show promise for the future. These include neurosurgery, ECT, phototherapy, and most recently repetitive transcranial magnetic stimulation (rTMS) and vagus nerve stimulation (VNS). The use of neurosurgery is very limited and outside the scope of this text.

Electroconvulsive Therapy

For hundreds of years, seizures have been known to produce improvement in some psychiatric symptoms. Camphor-induced seizures were used in the 16th century to reduce psychosis and mania. With time, other substances, such as inhalants, were tried, but most were difficult to control or produced adverse reactions, sometimes even fatalities. ECT was formally introduced in Italy in 1938. It is one of the oldest medical treatments available and remains safely in use today. It is one of the most effective treatments for severe depression but has been used for other disorders, including mania and schizophrenia, when other treatments have failed.

With ECT, a brief electrical current is passed through the brain to produce generalized seizures lasting 25 to 150 seconds. The patient does not feel the stimulus or recall the procedure. A short-acting anesthetic and a muscle relaxant are given before induction of the current. A brief pulse stimulus, administered unilaterally on the nondominant side of the head, is associated with less confusion after ECT. However, some individuals require bilateral treatment for effective resolution of depressive symptoms. Induction of a seizure is necessary to produce positive treatment outcomes. Because individual seizure thresholds vary, the electrical impulse and treatment method also may vary. In general, the lowest possible electrical stimulus necessary to produce seizure activity is used. Blood pressure and the ECG are monitored during the procedure. This procedure is repeated two or three times a week, usually for a total of 6 to 12 treatments. Because there is no difference in treatment efficacy and a twice-weekly regimen produces less accumulative memory loss, this treatment course is often chosen. After symptoms have improved, antidepressant medication may be used to prevent relapse. Some patients who cannot take or do not experience response to antidepressant treatment may continue to have ECT treatment. Usually, once-weekly treatments are gradually decreased in frequency to once monthly. The number and frequency vary depending on the individual's response.

Although ECT produces rapid improvement in depressive symptoms, its exact mechanism of antidepressant action remains unclear. It is known to downregulate β-adrenergic receptors in much the same way as antidepressant medications. However, unlike antidepressant therapy, ECT produces an upregulation in serotonin, especially 5-HT_2. ECT also has several other actions on neurochemistry, including increased influx of calcium and effects on second messenger systems.

Brief episodes of hypotension or hypertension, bradycardia or tachycardia, and minor arrhythmias are among the adverse reactions that may occur during and immediately after the procedure but usually resolve quickly. Common aftereffects from ECT include headache, nausea, and muscle pain. Memory loss is the most troublesome long-term effect of ECT. Many patients do not experience amnesia, but others report some memory loss for months or even years. Evidence is conflicting on the effects of ECT on the formation of memories after the treatments and on learning, but most patients experience no noticeable change. Memory loss occurring as part of the symptoms of untreated depression presents a confounding factor in determining the exact nature of the memory deficits from ECT. It is important to remember that patient surveys are positive, with most individuals reporting that they were helped by ECT, particularly older patients (Sauvaget et al., 2023).

ECT is contraindicated in patients with increased intracranial pressure. Risk also increases in patients with recent myocardial infarction, recent cerebrovascular accident, retinal detachment, or pheochromocytoma (a tumor on the adrenal cortex) and in patients at high risk for complications from anesthesia. Although ECT should be considered cautiously because of its specific side effects—added risks of general anesthesia, possible contraindications, and substantial social stigma—it is a safe and effective treatment.

PMH nurses are involved in many aspects of care for individuals undergoing ECT. Informed consent is required, and all treating professionals have a responsibility to ensure that the patient's and family's questions are answered completely. Available treatment options, risks, and consequences must be fully discussed. Sometimes, memory difficulties associated with severe depression make it difficult for patients to retain information or ask questions. Nurses should be prepared to restate or explain the procedure as often as necessary. Whenever possible, the individual's family or other support systems should be educated and involved in the consent process. Educational videos are available, but they should not replace direct discussions. Language should be in terms the patient and family members can understand. Other nursing interventions involve preparation of the patient before treatment, monitoring immediately after treatment, and follow-up. Many of these considerations are listed in Box 11.5.

BOX 11.5

Interventions for the Patient Receiving Electroconvulsive Therapy

- Discuss treatment alternatives, procedures, risks, and benefits with patient and family. Make sure that informed consent for ECT has been given in writing.
- Provide initial and ongoing patient and family education.
- Assist and monitor the patient who must take NPO after midnight, the evening before the procedure.
- Make sure that the patient wears loose, comfortable, nonrestrictive clothing to the procedure.
- If the procedure is performed on an outpatient basis, ensure that the patient has someone to accompany them home and stay with them after the procedure.
- Ensure that pretreatment laboratory tests are complete, including a CBC, serum electrolytes, urinalysis, ECG, chest radiography, and physical examination.
- Teach the patient to create memory helps, such as lists and notepads, before the ECT.
- Explain that no foreign or loose objects can be in the patient's mouth during the procedure. Dentures will be removed, and a bite block may be inserted.
- Insert an IV line and provide oxygen by nasal cannula (usually 100% oxygen at 5 L/min).
- Obtain emergency equipment and be sure it is available and ready if needed.
- Monitor vital signs frequently immediately after the procedure, as in every postanesthesia recovery period.
- When the patient is fully conscious and vital signs are stable, assist them to get up slowly, sitting for some time before standing.
- Monitor confusion closely; the patient may need reorientation to the bathroom and other areas.
- Maintain close supervision for at least 12 hours and continue observation for 48 hours after treatment. Advise family members to observe how the patient manages at home, provide assistance as needed, and report any problems.
- Assist the patient to keep or schedule follow-up appointments.

CBC, complete blood count; ECG, electrocardiogram; ECT, electroconvulsive therapy; IV, intravenous; NPO, nothing by mouth.

Light Therapy (Phototherapy)

Human circadian rhythms are set by time clues (*Zeitgebers*) inside and outside the body. One of the most powerful regulators of these body patterns is the cycle of daylight and darkness.

Research findings indicate that some individuals with certain types of depression may experience disturbance in these usual body patterns or of circadian rhythms, particularly those who experience a seasonal variation in their depression. These individuals are more depressed during the winter months, when there is less light; they improve spontaneously in the spring (see Chapter 25). These individuals usually have symptoms that are somewhat different from classic depression, including fatigue, increased need to sleep, increased appetite and weight gain, irritability, and carbohydrate craving. Sometimes, the symptoms appear in the summer, and some individuals have only subtle changes without developing the full pattern. Administering artificial light to these patients during winter months has reduced these depressive symptoms.

Light therapy, sometimes called **phototherapy,** involves exposing the patient to an artificial light source during winter months to relieve seasonal depression. Artificial light is believed to trigger a shift in the patient's circadian rhythm to an earlier time. The light source must be very bright, full-spectrum light, usually 2,500 lux, which is about 200 times brighter than usual indoor lighting. Harmful ultraviolet light is filtered out. Exposure to this light source has produced improvement and relief of depressive symptoms for significant numbers of seasonally and nonseasonally depressed individuals. Research remains ongoing (Huang et al., 2023).

Studies have shown that morning phototherapy produces a better response than either evening or morning and evening timing of the phototherapy session. Light banks with full-spectrum light may be put together by the individual or obtained from various companies now producing these light sources. Light visors (visors containing small, full-spectrum light bulbs that shine on the eyelids) have also been developed. The patient is instructed to sit in front of the lights at about 3 ft, engaging in a variety of other activities, but glancing directly into the light every few minutes. This should be done immediately on arising and is most effective before 8 AM. The duration of administration may begin with as little as 30 minutes and increase to 2 to 5 hours. One to 2 hours is usually sufficient, and the antidepressant response begins in 1 to 4 days, with the full effect usually complete after 2 weeks. Full antidepressant effect is usually maintained with daily sessions of 30 minutes.

Side effects of phototherapy are rare, but eye strain, headache, and insomnia are possible. An ophthalmologist should be consulted if the patient has a preexisting eye disorder. In rare instances, phototherapy has been reported to produce an episode of mania. Irritability is a more common complaint. Follow-up visits with the prescriber or therapist are needed to help manage side effects and assess positive results. Phototherapy should be implemented only by a provider knowledgeable in its use.

Transcranial Magnetic Stimulation

Transcranial magnetic stimulation (TMS) was introduced in 1985 as a noninvasive, painless method to stimulate the cerebral cortex. There are two types of TMS—the rTMS and the deep transcranial magnetic stimulation (dTMS). Both types are effective. Undergirding this procedure is the hypothesis that a time-varying magnetic field will induce an electrical field, which, in brain tissue, activates inhibitory and excitatory neurons, thereby modulating neuroplasticity in the brain. The low-frequency electrical stimulation from rTMS triggers lasting anticonvulsant effects in rats, and the therapeutic benefits of rTMS in humans are thought to be related to an action like that produced by anticonvulsant medication. The rTMS has been used for both clinical and research purposes. The rTMS stimulation of the brain's prefrontal cortex may help some depressed patients in much the same way as ECT but without its side effects (Tang et al., 2023). Thus, it has been proposed as an alternative to ECT in managing symptoms of depression. The rTMS treatment is administered daily for at least 1 week, much like ECT, except that subjects remain awake. Although proven effective for depression, rTMS does have some side effects, including mild headaches.

Vagus Nerve Stimulation

Vagus nerve stimulation (VNS) sends electrical impulses to the brain to improve depression. The vagus nerve has traditionally been considered a parasympathetic efferent nerve that was responsible only for regulating autonomic functions, such as heart rate and gastric tone. However, the vagus nerve (cranial X) also carries sensory information to the brain from the head, neck, thorax, and abdomen, and research has identified that the vagus nerve has extensive projections of its sensory afferent connections to many brain areas. Although the basic mechanism of action of VNS is unknown, incoming sensory, or afferent, connections of the left vagus nerve directly project into many of the very same brain regions implicated in neuropsychiatric disorders. These help us to understand how VNS is helpful in treating psychiatric disorders. VNS connections change levels of several neurotransmitters implicated in the development of major depression, including serotonin, norepinephrine, GABA, and glutamate, in the same way that antidepressant medications produce their therapeutic effect (Trifilio et al., 2023).

Approved by the FDA for the adjunctive treatment of severe depression for adults who are unresponsive to four or more adequate antidepressant treatments, VNS is a permanent implant. VNS is not a cure for depression, and patients must be seen regularly for assessment of mood states and suicidality.

THE ISSUE OF ADHERENCE

Medications and other biologic treatments work only if they are used. On the surface, **adherence** to a therapeutic routine, seems amazingly simple. However, following therapeutic regimens, self-administering medications as prescribed, and keeping appointments are amazingly complex activities that often prevent successful treatment. In recovery-oriented practice, the patient makes

BOX 11.6

Common Reasons for Not Taking Medications as Prescribed

- Medication is not working as expected
- Uncomfortable side effects and those that interfere with quality of life, such as work performance or intimate relationships
- Lack of awareness or denial of illness
- Stigma
- Feeling better
- Confusion about dosage or timing
- Difficulties in access to treatment
- Substance misuse

the decision to take medications. It is important that the patient does not feel coerced into taking the medication. The nurse's role is to support the patient's decision-making process and provide honest, evidence-based advice.

Adherence exists on a continuum and can be conceived of as full, partial, or nil. Partial adherence, whereby a patient either attempts to take medications but misses doses or takes more than prescribed, is by far the most common. Recent estimates indicate that on average, 50% or more of the individuals with schizophrenia taking antipsychotic medications stop taking the medications or do not take them as prescribed. It should be remembered that problems with adherence are an issue with many chronic health states, including diabetes and arthritis, not just psychiatric disorders. Box 11.6 lists some of the common reasons for nonadherence. PMH nurses should be aware that several factors contribute to the decision to discontinue medications.

The most often cited reasons for not taking medications as prescribed are the side effects. Medication side effects may interfere with work performance or other important aspects of the individual's life. For example, a construction worker cannot afford to be drowsy and sedated while operating a crane at a construction site, and a person in an intimate relationship may find anorgasmia intolerable. Even though symptom improvement may be observed by health care professionals, they may not be noticed by the patient. Nurses need to be sensitive to the patient's ability to tolerate side effects and to the impact that side effects have on the patient's life. Medication choice, dosing schedules, and prompt treatment of side effects may be crucial factors in helping patients continue with their treatment.

Cognitive deficits associated with some psychiatric disorders may make it difficult for the individual to self-monitor, develop insight, make choices, remember to fill prescriptions, or keep appointments. Forgetfulness, cost, and confusion regarding dosage or timing may also contribute to nonadherence. New advances in medication formulation are designed to address some of these issues. For example, long-acting injections are designed to reduce or eliminate the need to remember an oral medication regime. Recently, the FDA approved a tablet formulation of an antipsychotic aripiprazole embedded with a digital adherence-assessment device. The system consists of an ingestible sensor, a wearable sensor, and software applications that confirm adherence. More research is needed to confirm the practicality of using the device and its effectiveness in improving treatment adherence (Hadzi Boskovic et al., 2023).

Family members may have similar difficulties that influence the individual not to take the medication. They may misunderstand or deny the illness, thinking, for example, "My wife's better, so she doesn't need that medicine anymore." Family members may be distressed when observable side effects occur. Adherence concerns must not be dismissed as the patient's or family's problem. Nurses should actively address this issue. A positive therapeutic relationship between the nurse and patient and family must provide a strong sense of trust that side effects and other difficulties in treatment will be addressed and minimized. When individuals report experiencing distressing side effects, the nurse should immediately respond with assessment and interventions to reduce these effects. It is important to assess adherence often, asking questions in a nonthreatening, nonjudgmental manner. It also may be helpful to seek information from others who are involved with the patient.

Adherence can be improved by psychoeducation. This approach is most helpful if it addresses the individual's specific symptoms and concerns. For example, if the patient is having difficulty with understanding the purpose of the medication, it may be helpful to link taking it to reduction of specific unwanted symptoms or improved functioning, such as continuing to work. Family members should also be included in these discussions.

Other factors that interfere with adherence should also be assessed and plans developed to minimize their effect. For example, an individual who is being considered for clozapine therapy may have missed several appointments in the past. On assessment, the nurse may discover that it takes the individual 2 hours on three different buses each way to reach the clinic. The nurse can then assist with arranging for a home health nurse to visit the patient's apartment, draw blood samples for analysis, and assess side effects, thus decreasing the number of trips the patient must make to the clinic.

SUMMARY OF KEY POINTS

- Target symptoms and side effects of medications should be clearly identified. The FDA approves the use of medications for specific disorders and symptoms.
- Psychiatric medications primarily act on CNS receptors, ion channels, enzymes, and carrier proteins. Agonists mimic the action of a specific neurotransmitter; antagonists block the response.

- A drug's ability to interact with a given receptor type depends on three qualities: selectivity—the ability to interact with specific receptors while not affecting other tissues and organs; affinity—the degree of strength of the bond between drug and receptor; and intrinsic activity—the ability to produce a certain biologic response.
- Pharmacokinetics refers to how the human body processes the drug, including absorption, distribution, metabolism, and excretion. Bioavailability describes the amount of the drug that reaches circulation throughout the body. The wide variations in the way each individual processes any medication often are related to physiologic differences caused by age, genetic makeup, other disease processes, and chemical interactions.
- Antipsychotic medications are drugs used in treating patients with psychotic disorders, such as schizophrenia. They act primarily by blocking dopamine or serotonin postsynaptically. In addition, they have several actions on other neurotransmitters. Older typical antipsychotic drugs work on positive symptoms and are inexpensive but produce more side effects than the newer atypical antipsychotic drugs which work on positive and negative symptoms.
- Medication-related movement disorders are a particularly serious group of side effects that principally occur with the typical antipsychotic medications and that may be acute syndromes, such as dystonia, pseudoparkinsonism, and akathisia, or chronic syndromes, such as tardive dyskinesia.
- The mood stabilizers, or antimanic medications, are drugs used to control wide variations in mood related to mania, but these agents may also be used to treat patients with other disorders. Lithium and anticonvulsants are chemically unrelated and act in different ways to stabilize mood.
- Antidepressant medications are drugs used primarily for treating symptoms of depression. They act by blocking reuptake of one or more of the bioamines, especially serotonin and norepinephrine. These medications vary considerably in their structure and action. Newer antidepressants, such as SSRIs, have fewer side effects and are less lethal in overdose than the older TCAs.
- Antianxiety medications also include several subgroups of medications, but benzodiazepines and nonbenzodiazepines are those principally used in psychiatry. Benzodiazepines act by enhancing the effects of GABA, and the nonbenzodiazepine buspirone acts on serotonin. Benzodiazepines can be used on a PRN basis; but buspirone, the one available nonbenzodiazepine, must be taken regularly.
- Psychostimulants enhance neurotransmitter activity, acting at several sites in the nerves. These medications are most often used for treating symptoms related to ADHD and narcolepsy.
- ECT uses the application of an electrical pulsation to induce seizures in the brain. These seizures produce several effects on neurotransmission that result in the rapid relief of depressive symptoms.
- rTMS and VNS are two emerging somatic treatments for psychiatric disorders. They are both means to directly affect brain function through stimulation of the nerves that are direct extensions of the brain.
- Phototherapy involves the application of full-spectrum light in the morning hours, which appears to reset circadian rhythm delays related to seasonal affective disorder and other forms of depression. Nutritional therapies are in various stages of investigation.
- Adherence refers to the ability of an individual to self-administer medications as prescribed and to follow other instructions related to medication treatment. It can be full, partial, or nil. Nonadherence is related to factors such as medication side effects, stigma, and family influences. Nurses play a key role in educating patients and helping them to improve adherence.

DEVELOPING CLINICAL JUDGMENT

1. Discuss how you would go about identifying the target symptoms for a specific patient for the following medications: antipsychotic, antidepressant, and antianxiety drugs.
2. Obtain the PIs for the three atypical antipsychotics, two SSRIs, and one SNRI. Compare their boxed warnings, pharmacodynamics, pharmacokinetics, indications, side effects, and dosages.
3. Compare the oral and IM dose of lorazepam. Why are these doses similar?
4. T. J. has schizophrenia and was just prescribed an antipsychotic. The family wants to know the risk–benefits of the medication. How would you answer?
5. Identify the CYP450 enzyme(s) that metabolizes the following medications: risperidone, olanzapine, quetiapine, clozapine. Which medication is more likely to be associated with a drug–drug interaction? Please give rationale.
6. Explain the health issues associated with anticholinergic side effects of the antipsychotic medications.

7. Compare the type of movements that characterize tardive dyskinesia with those that characterize akathisia and dystonia and explore which one is easier for a patient to experience.
8. One patient is prescribed the MAOI selegiline, 6 mg/day; and another is taking another MAOI, phenelzine, 15 mg/day. Are the dietary restrictions different?
9. Two patients are getting their blood drawn. One patient is getting lithium and the other clozapine. What laboratory tests are being ordered?
10. Compare different approaches that you might use with a patient with schizophrenia who has decided to stop taking their medication because of intolerance to side effects.

MOVIES, TV, OR STREAMING PROGRAMS

Mysteries of Mental Illness: Episode 4; New Frontiers: 2021. This excellent PBS documentary is the fourth episode on mental illness. In this episode, new treatments for mental illness are presented in a case presentation format. One patient, Matthew, has a diagnosis of severe OCD; he is afraid that he will stop breathing and is completely incapacitated by this disorder. He has tried all the therapies and finally decided to have an experimental deep brain stimulation (not approved by the FDA for OCD). Cynthia has severe recurrent depression and has selected to have ECT for treatment. She has tried many treatment approaches including pharmacologic, nonpharmacologic, and complementary therapies. She received a series of ECT that successfully treated her symptoms. The last approach in the video is the use of psychedelics, MDMA, (not yet approved by the FDA) to treat posttraumatic stress disorder (PTSD). Laura is suffering with PTSD from being sexually assaulted in college. She became a lawyer and activist for people who are sexually abused. She tried 5 years of traditional therapy before trying MDMA, which improved her mental health and ability to deal with her trauma.

Viewing Points:

1. How did deep brain stimulation improve Matthew's quality of life?
2. How does the ECT treatment of today compare to the ECT treatment of the 1970s? The doctor describes the procedure as very quick and boring. Is that a realistic description of the procedure?
3. The use of psychedelics for the treatment of PTSD is not FDA approved. How does this program show how psychedelics could be used for treatment?

Unfolding Patient Stories: David Carter • Part 1

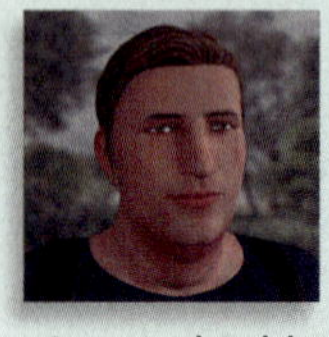

David Carter is a 28-year-old diagnosed with schizophrenia and major depression. He became violent with his mother and was brought to the emergency room with paranoid delusions and auditory hallucinations. His mother suspected that he stopped taking his medication olanzapine due to weight gain, and this medication cessation may have prompted an exacerbation of his symptoms. During admission, he was alternately agitated and withdrawn. Medications ordered include olanzapine, venlafaxine, lorazepam every 8 hours as needed for agitation, and haloperidol every 8 hours as needed for agitation. Describe the classification, action, dosing, and side effects for each medication. How will the nurse monitor the effectiveness and side effects of the medications? How will the nurse determine when to administer the as-needed medications? What client teaching should the nurse provide specific to the prescribed medications? (David's story continues in Chapter 19.)

Care for David Carter and other patients in a realistic virtual environment: ***vSim** for Nursing* (thepoint.lww.com/vSimMentalHealth). Practice documenting these patients' care in DocuCare (thepoint.lww.com/DocuCareEHR).

REFERENCES

All of Us Research Program Genomics Investigators. (2024). Genomic data in the All of Us Research Program. *Nature*, *627*(8003), 340–346. https://doi.org/10.1038/s41586-023-06957-x

American Society of Health-System Pharmacists (ASHP). (2024). Hydroxyzine. MedlinePlus. National Library of Medicine. Retrieved August 24, 2024 from https://medlineplus.gov/druginfo/meds/a682866.html#:~:text=Older%20adults%20should%20not%20usually,how%20this%20medication%20affects%20you

Baizabal-Carvallo, J. F., & Morgan, J. C. (2022). Drug-induced tremor, clinical features, diagnostic approach and management. *Journal of the Neurological Sciences*, *435*, 120192. https://doi.org/10.1016/j.jns.2022.120192

Bousman, C. A., Stevenson, J. M., Ramsey, L. B., Sangkuhl, K., Hicks, J. K., Strawn, J. R., Singh, A. B., Ruaño, G., Mueller, D. J., Tsermpini, E. E., Brown, J. T., Bell, G. C., Leeder, J. S., Gaedigk, A., Scott, S. A., Klein, T. E., Caudle, K. E., & Bishop, J. R. (2023). Clinical pharmacogenetics implementation consortium (CPIC) guideline for CYP2D6, CYP2C19, CYP2B6, SLC6A4, and HTR2A genotypes and serotonin reuptake inhibitor antidepressants. *Clinical Pharmacology and Therapeutics*, *114*(1), 51–68. https://doi.org/10.1002/cpt.2903

Buchmayer, F., & Kasper, S. (2023). Overcoming the myths of esketamine administration: Different and not difficult. *Frontiers in Psychiatry*, *14*, 1279657. https://doi.org/10.3389/fpsyt.2023.1279657

Cephalon. (2017). *Nuvigil (armodafinil) tablets*. Retrieved August 24, 2024, from https://www.accessdata.fda.gov/drugsatfda_docs/label/2017/021875s023lbl.pdf

Chaki, S., & Watanabe, M. (2023). Antidepressants in the post-ketamine era: Pharmacological approaches targeting the glutamatergic system. *Neuropharmacology*, *223*, 109348. https://doi.org/10.1016/j.neuropharm.2022.109348

Drugbank Online. (2024). Hydroxyzine. Retrieved August 23, 2024, from https://go.drugbank.com/drugs/DB00557

Du, W., Ge, M. W., Hu, F. H., Jia, Y. J., Zhao, D. Y., Cheng, Y. J., & Chen, H. L. (2023). QTc prolongation in patients with schizophrenia taking antipsychotics: Prevalence and risk factors. *Journal of Psychopharmacology*, *37*(10), 971–981. https://doi.org/10.1177/02698811231190864

Feeney, A., & Papakostas, G. I. (2023). Pharmacotherapy: Ketamine and esketamine. *The Psychiatric Clinics of North America*, *46*(2), 277–290. https://doi.org/10.1016/j.psc.2023.02.003

Flanagan, R. J., Hunter, S., Obee, S. J., & Reeves, S. (2023). Clozapine: Dose, sex, ethnicity, smoking habit, age, body weight, and plasma clozapine and N-desmethylclozapine (Norclozapine) concentrations in clinical practice. *Journal of Clinical Psychopharmacology*, *43*(2), 131–138. https://doi.org/10.1097/JCP.0000000000001653

Ghanaatfar, F., Ghanaatfar, A., Isapour, P., Farokhi, N., Bozorgniahosseini, S., Javadi, M., Gholami, M., Ulloa, L., Coleman-Fuller, N., & Motaghinejad, M. (2023). Is lithium neuroprotective? An updated mechanistic illustrated review. *Fundamental & Clinical Pharmacology*, *37*(1), 4–30. https://doi.org/10.1111/fcp.12826

GlaxoSmithKline. (2023). *Wellbutrin SR prescribing information*. https://www.accessdata.fda.gov/drugsatfda_docs/label/2022/020358s066lbl.pdf

Golsorkhi, M., Koch, J., Pedouim, F., Frei, K., Bondariyan, N., & Dashtipour, K. (2024). Comparative analysis of deutetrabenazine and valbenazine as VMAT2 inhibitors for tardive dyskinesia: A systematic review. *Tremor and Other Hyperkinetic Movements (New York, N.Y.)*, *14*, 13. https://doi.org/10.5334/tohm.842

Greenblatt, K., & Adams, N. (2023). Modafinil. In *StatPearls*. StatPearls Publishing. www.ncbi.nlm.nih.gov/books/NBK531476

Hadzi Boskovic, D., Liang, S., Parab, P., Wiggins, E., & Liberman, J. N. (2023). Real-world evidence of aripiprazole tablets with sensor: Treatment patterns and impacts on psychiatric healthcare resource utilization. *ClinicoEconomics and Outcomes Research*, *15*, 487–498. https://doi.org/10.2147/CEOR.S402357

Huang, X., Tao, Q., & Ren, C. (2023). A comprehensive overview of the neural mechanisms of light therapy. *Neuroscience Bulletin*, *40*(3), 350–362. https://doi.org/10.1007/s12264-023-01089-8

Kim, H. K., & Yang, K. I. (2022). Melatonin and melatonergic drugs in sleep disorders. *Translational and Clinical Pharmacology*, *30*(4), 163–171. https://doi.org/10.12793/tcp.2022.30.e21

Marazziti, D., Mucci, F., Avella, M. T., Palagini, L., Simoncini, M., & Dell'Osso, L. (2021). The increasing challenge of the possible impact of ethnicity on psychopharmacology. *CNS Spectrums*, *26*(3), 222–231. https://doi.org/10.1017/S1092852920000073

Nicholson, W. T., Formea, C. M., Matey, E. T., Wright, J. A., Giri, J., & Moyer, A. M. (2021). Considerations when applying pharmacogenomics to your practice. *Mayo Clinic Proceedings*, *96*(1), 218–230. https://doi.org/10.1016/j.mayocp.2020.03.011

Novartis. (2023). *Clozaril (prescribing information)*. https://www.accessdata.fda.gov/drugsatfda_docs/label/2023/019758s103lbl.pdf

Ramli, F. F., Azizi, M. H., & Syed Hashim, S. A. (2021). Treatments of sexual dysfunction in opioid substitution therapy patients: A systematic review and meta-analysis. *International Journal of Medical Sciences*, *18*(11), 2372–2380. https://doi.org/10.7150/ijms.57641

Sabé, M., Pallis, K., Solmi, M., Crippa, A., Sentissi, O., & Kaiser, S. (2023). Comparative effects of 11 antipsychotics on weight gain and metabolic function in patients with acute schizophrenia: A dose-response meta-analysis. *The Journal of Clinical Psychiatry*, *84*(2), 22r14490. https://doi.org/10.4088/JCP.22r14490

Saha, S., & González-Maeso, J. (2023). The crosstalk between 5-HT_{2A}R and mGluR2 in schizophrenia. *Neuropharmacology*, *230*, 109489. https://doi.org/10.1016/j.neuropharm.2023.109489

Sajatovic, M., Finkbeiner, S., Wilhelm, A., Barkay, H., Chaijale, N., Gross, N., & Gordon, M. F. (2022). Long-term safety and efficacy of deutetrabenazine in younger and older patients with tardive dyskinesia. *The American Journal of Geriatric Psychiatry*, *30*(3), 360–371. https://doi.org/10.1016/j.jagp.2021.08.003

Sauvaget, A., Bulteau, S., Galvao, F., Szekely, D., Fossati, P., & Poulet, E. (2023). ECT: An essential therapy in psychiatry. *L'Encephale*, *49*(1), 103–106. https://doi.org/10.1016/j.encep.2022.05.002

Shahbaz, H., Rout, P., & Gupta, M. (2024). Creatinine clearance. In *StatPearls*. StatPearls Publishing. www.ncbi.nlm.nih.gov/books/NBK544228

Simone, C. G., & Bobrin, B. D. (2023). Anxiolytics and sedative-hypnotics toxicity. In *StatPearls*. StatPearls Publishing. www.ncbi.nlm.nih.gov/books/NBK562309

Spoelma, M. J., Leidreiter, J., Bayes, A., Jebejian, A., & Parker, G. (2024). A naturalistic effectiveness study of maintenance therapies for the bipolar disorders. *Acta Psychiatrica Scandinavica*, *149*(2), 98–109. https://doi.org/10.1111/acps.13646

Tang, S. J., Holle, J., Dadario, N. B., Lesslar, O., Teo, C., Ryan, M., Sughrue, M., & Yeung, J. T. (2023). Personalized, parcel-guided rTMS for the treatment of major depressive disorder: Safety and proof of concept. *Brain and Behavior*, *13*(11), e3268. https://doi.org/10.1002/brb3.3268

Thippaiah, S. M., Fargason, R. E., & Birur, B. (2021). Struggling to find effective pharmacologic options for akathisia? B-CALM!. *Psychopharmacology Bulletin*, *51*(3), 72–78.

Trifilio, E., Shortell, D., Olshan, S., O'Neal, A., Coyne, J., Lamb, D., Porges, E., & Williamson, J. (2023). Impact of transcutaneous vagus nerve stimulation on healthy cognitive and brain aging. *Frontiers in Neuroscience*, *17*, 1184051. https://doi.org/10.3389/fnins.2023.1184051

Vasan, S., & Padhy, R. K. (2023). Tardive dyskinesia. In *StatPearls*. StatPearls Publishing. www.ncbi.nlm.nih.gov/books/NBK448207

Yang, H. J., Kim, S. G., Seo, E. H., & Yoon, H. J. (2022). Amisulpride withdrawal akathisia responding to aripiprazole with propranolol in first-onset psychosis: a case report. *BMC Psychiatry*, *22*(1), 74. https://doi.org/10.1186/s12888-022-03721-9

Yokoyama, A., Yokoyama, T., Kimura, M., Matsushita, S., & Yokoyama, M. (2021). Combinations of alcohol-induced flushing with genetic polymorphisms of alcohol and aldehyde dehydrogenases and the risk of alcohol dependence in Japanese men and women. *PLoS One*, *16*(7), e0255276. https://doi.org/10.1371/journal.pone.0255276

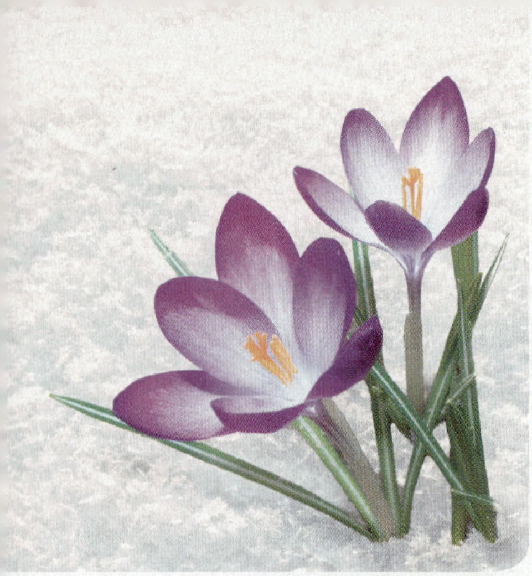

12 Complementary Therapies and Integrative Health

Rebecca Luebbert and Mary Ann Boyd

KEYCONCEPTS

- complementary therapies
- dietary supplements
- integrative health

LEARNING OBJECTIVES

After studying this chapter, you will be able to:

1. Distinguish between the concepts of complementary therapies and integrative health care.
2. Clarify the nursing role in the application of integrative and complementary therapies.
3. Apply complementary/integrative research findings that support mental health and wellness.
4. Discuss the use of complementary therapies for symptom management of mental health disorders.
5. Apply complementary intervention strategies to individuals with mental health and wellness needs.

KEY TERMS

• acupuncture • alternative therapies • aromatherapy • art therapy • asanas • autogenic training • brain–gut axis • carrier oil • chamomile • cinnamon • coherent breathing • curcumin • daily values • dance therapy • dense-nutrient foods • diaphragmatic breathing • dietary pattern • drama therapy • dyana • dysbiosis • essential oils • guided imagery • gut microbiota • herbal supplements • herbs • histidine • hypnotherapy • infused oils • kava • lecithin • massage therapy • meditation • melatonin • mindful breathing • mindfulness • mindfulness yoga • music therapy • pranayama • probiotics • progressive muscle relaxation • qi • qigong • recommended dietary allowances • relaxation exercises • saffron • short-chain fatty acids • spices • St. John's wort • tai chi • tryptophan • tyrosine • ultra-processed foods • valerian • Western diet • yoga

INTRODUCTION

Evidence-based complementary interventions can easily be included in nursing practice and contribute to patients' mental health and well-being. Incorporation of these interventions by psychiatric–mental health (PMH) nurses is supported by the *PMHN Scope and Standards of Practice* (ANA et al., 2022). These interventions are not typically included in conventional health care, and many have their origins outside Western health care. This chapter discusses complementary therapies and the evidence that supports their integration into nursing practice.

COMPLEMENTARY THERAPIES VERSUS INTEGRATIVE HEALTH CARE

The terms complementary and integrative are often used interchangeably. But these terms are conceptually different. If nonmainstream interventions are included with conventional practices, the term complementary therapies is used. When nonmainstream interventions are used in place of a conventional treatments, the term **alternative therapies** is used. For example, if yoga is used with antidepressants to treat depression, yoga is considered complementary therapy. If yoga is used in place of antidepressants, it is considered an alternative intervention (NCCIH, 2021).

> **KEYCONCEPT Complementary therapies** are nonmainstream interventions used with conventional approaches.

Integrative health is a term that includes both complementary therapies and conventional approaches/treatments in a coordinated manner (NCCIH, 2021). In integrative health, the care is well-coordinated among different providers and institutions. Integrative care focuses on the whole individual and is consistent with biopsychosocial–spiritual patient-centered model.

As a framework for practice, six principles of integrative nursing may guide patient care across populations and clinical settings. See Box 12.1 and Figure 12.1.

> **KEYCONCEPT Integrative health** treats the whole person by using two or more inventions that include conventional health care approaches (i.e., medications) and complementary interventions (i.e., acupuncture).

BOX 12.1

Principles of Integrative Nursing

1. Human beings are whole systems inseparable from and influenced by environments.
2. Human beings have an innate capacity for healing and well-being.
3. Integrative nursing is person-centered and relationship-based.
4. Nature has healing and restorative properties that contribute to health and well-being.
5. Integrative nursing is informed by evidence and uses a full range of conventional and integrative approaches, employing the least intensive intervention possible depending on the need and context.
6. Integrative nursing focuses on the health and well-being of caregivers as well as those they serve.

Reprinted with permission from Earl E. Bakken Center for Spirituality and Healing, University of Minnesota. (2024). Principles of integrative nursing. Retrieved May 5, 2024, from https://csh.umn.edu/academics/focus-areas/integrative-nursing/principles-integrative-nursing

NUTRITIONAL APPROACHES

Nutrition has long been the subject of interest in promoting mental health and well-being. Without adequate carbohydrates, proteins, fats, vitamins, and minerals, the body will be unable to function properly leading to pathologic states. Lack of necessary nutrients can lead to nutritional stress which in turn initiates an inflammatory response associated with mental health issues such as anxiety or mood disorders (Kunugi, 2023; Suárez-López et al., 2023).

Medications may also contribute to nutritional deficiencies that in turn worsen mental health symptoms. For example, drugs with strong anticholinergic properties often produce impaired or enhanced gastric motility, which may lead to generalized malabsorption of vitamins and minerals. In addition, many vitamin and mineral supplements have toxicities of their own when given in excess. For example, daily ingestion of more than 100 mg of pyridoxine (vitamin B_6) can produce neurotoxic symptoms, photosensitivity, and ataxia.

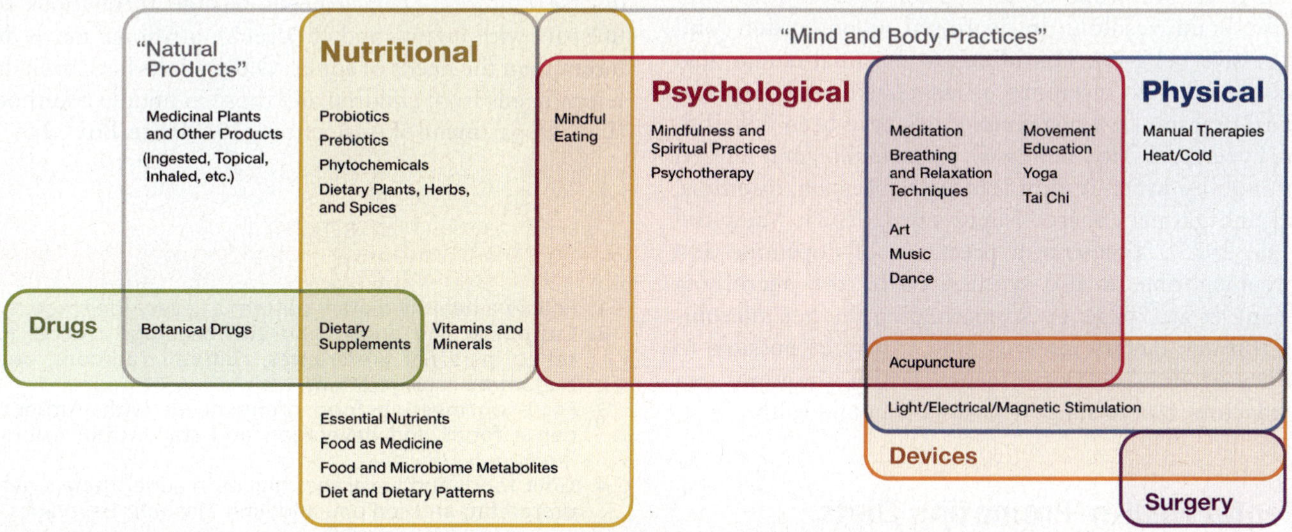

FIGURE 12.1 Examples of complementary health approaches: nutritional, psychological, and physical. (Reprinted from Complementary, Alternative, or Integrative Health: What's In a Name? [2021]. Retrieved May 18, 2024, from https://www.nccih.nih.gov/health/complementary-alternative-or-integrative-health-whats-in-a-name)

Gut Microbiota

The brain has the greatest metabolic demands of any organ, and the integrity of the **brain–gut axis** is dependent upon nutrients we eat. See Chapter 7. The **gut microbiota,** a complex system of microorganisms including bacteria, fungi, viruses, and other organisms, exists within the human digestive system and influences brain function through the production of neurotransmitters, immune signaling molecules, and metabolic substances. Some of these microorganisms protect mental functioning, whereas others contribute to development of mental disorders. The gut microbiota is implicated in several mental disorders including anxiety and depression (Xiong et al., 2023). The gut microbiota interacts with the brain through the neuroimmune, neuroendocrine, and vagus nerve pathways (Merlo et al., 2024).

It is especially important to maintain a healthy gut because the human microbiota is altered by dietary patterns. Diets rich in dietary fibers activate microbial enzymes that break down complex carbohydrates to **short-chain fatty acids** which engage in metabolism, cell differentiation, gene regulation, and the regulation of anti-inflammatory and proinflammatory cytokines. Diets containing ultraprocessed foods, sodium, saturated fats, trans-fat, and refined sugar can result in **dysbiosis,** a microbial imbalance that can lead to neuroinflammation associated with mental disorders and autoimmune disease.

Neurotransmitters are critical for brain functioning and many are produced through the brain–gut microbiota. **Tryptophan**, an essential amino acid and the dietary precursor for serotonin, is absorbed and regulated by the gut microbiota. Individuals who have low tryptophan levels are prone to have lower levels of serotonin in the brain, resulting in depressed mood, anxiety, and aggressive behavior. **Histidine**, an essential amino acid and precursor to histamine, is associated with sleep and sexual orgasm. Low histamine levels have been linked to gut hypersensitivity, increased permeability, and altered gut motility which in turn leads to depression, insomnia, and anorgasmia (Suárez-López et al., 2023; Vanuytsel et al., 2023). **Tyrosine**, a precursor of dopamine and norepinephrine, is also synthesized by the microbiota (Zhang et al., 2023). By strengthening the gut microbiota through dietary interventions, it may be possible to reduce or eliminate some mental health symptoms and risk factors, and to support positive mental health.

Mental Health–Promoting Diets

Western **dietary patterns** (food and beverage consumption over time) are linked to physical and mental health issues. A **Western diet** is a "modern dietary pattern characterized by high intake of pre-packaged foods, refined grains, red meat, processed meat, high-sugar drinks, candy and sweets, fried foods, conventionally raised animal products, high-fat dairy products, and high-fructose products" (Clemente-Suárez et al., 2023). High fried food consumption disturbs lipid metabolism and is associated with oxidative stress and neuroinflammation (Liu et al., 2023a). Frequent fried food consumption, especially potatoes, is strongly associated with higher risk of anxiety and depression (Wang et al., 2023).

Deficiencies in nutrients such as proteins, B vitamins, vitamin D, magnesium, selenium, iron, calcium, and omega-3 fatty acids negatively impact the brain and nervous system functioning (Zielińska et al., 2023). Inadequate intake of protein, fish (Omega 3 polyunsaturated fatty acids), vitamins (folate and vitamin D), and minerals (iron and zinc) increase the risk of depression. Energy overload (excessive calories), skipping breakfast, a Western diet, and inflammation-prone diets increase the risk of illness. Consumption of **ultra-processed foods** (industrial formulations extracted from foods or synthesized in laboratories) disturbs lipid metabolism and promotes neuroinflammation. Examples of ultra-processed foods include salty packaged snacks, energy drinks, instant soups and noodles, and flavored yogurts (Kunugi, 2023; Lane et al., 2024).

Dietary patterns that support mental health include those that contain unprocessed or minimally processed foods (fresh fruits, vegetables, grains, eggs, meats, poultry, fish and seafood, milk, yogurt without sugar, oils made from seed, nuts and fruits, honey, butter, refined or coarse salt) (Lane et al., 2024). See Box 12.2. Selection of **dense-nutrient foods** that contain vitamins, minerals, and other health-promoting ingredients with little or no added sugars and saturated fat can be customized for diverse cultures. Dietary needs change throughout the lifespan, with infant's and children's nutritional needs different than the needs of adults. Older adults have even different needs from children and those in middle adulthood (U.S. Department of Agriculture, 2020). See Box 12.3.

BOX 12.2

Guidelines for a Healthy Diet

1. Follow a healthy dietary pattern at every life stage.
2. Customize and enjoy food and beverage choices to reflect personal preferences, cultural traditions, and budgetary considerations.
3. Focus on meeting food group needs with nutrient-dense foods and beverages, and stay within calorie limits.
4. Limit foods and beverages higher in added sugars, saturated fat, and sodium, and limit alcoholic beverages.

Reprinted from U.S. Department of Agriculture and U.S. Department of Health and Human Services. (2020). *Dietary Guidelines for Americans, 2020–2025*. (9th Ed.). https://www.dietaryguidelines.gov/

BOX 12.3

Dietary Considerations Throughout the Life Span[a]

Age Group	Considerations	Recommendations
Infants and toddlers (0 to 23 months)	Consumption of small quantities of foods Make every bite count.	**For about the first 6 months of life,** exclusively feed infants human milk. Continue to feed infants human milk through at least the first year of life, and longer if desired. Feed infants iron-fortified infant formula during the first year of life when human milk is unavailable. • Provide infants with supplemental vitamin D beginning soon after birth. • **At about 6 months,** introduce infants to nutrient-dense complementary foods. • Introduce infants to potentially allergenic foods along with other complementary foods. • Encourage infants and toddlers to consume a variety of foods from all food groups. Include foods rich in iron and zinc, particularly for infants fed human milk. • Avoid foods and beverages with added sugars. • Limit foods and beverages higher in sodium. • As infants wean from human milk or infant formula, transition to a healthy dietary pattern.
Children and adolescents (2 to 18 years)	Transitions and the formation of dietary patterns Suboptimal intake patterns Consumption of sugar-sweetened beverages Underconsumption of potassium, calcium, and vitamin D	**In early childhood (ages 2 through 4),** females require about 1,000 to 1,400 calories per day and males require about 1,000 to 1,600 calories per day. With the transition to school-age (ages 5 through 8), females require about 1,200 to 1,800 calories per day and males require about 1,200 to 2,000 calories per day **Children and adolescents ages 9 through 13** In the late childhood and early adolescence stage, females require about 1,400 to 2,200 calories per day and males require about 1,600 to 2,600 calories per day. **Adolescents ages 14 through 18** Adolescent females require about 1,800 to 2,400 calories per day and males require about 2,000 to 3,200 calories per day.
Adults (19 to 59)	In the United States, 74% of adults are overweight or have obesity Inadequate intakes of dietary fiber, calcium, and vitamin D Excessive intake of saturated fats and sodium Overconsumption of sodium Excessive consumption of added sugars Overconsumption of alcoholic beverages	Examine attitudes, beliefs, and knowledge about healthy dietary patterns. Learn about healthy living and adopting a healthy dietary pattern. Develop a long-term strategy for weight loss and maintenance. Prepare and consume food at home. Be mindful of ingredients, preparation, and proportion of foods prepared by others. Increase dietary fiber by adding more fruits, vegetables, and whole grains. Increase calcium and vitamin D by adding dairy foods, fortified soy alternatives, and seafood. Substitute low-fat ingredients such as lean meats, low-fat cheese, avocados, nuts, or seeds for high-saturated fat meals. Limit consumption of sugars and alcoholic beverages.
Older adults (60 years and older)	Greater risk of chronic diseases Overweight from previous adult stage Inadequate protein intake Inability to absorb B_{12} Reduced intake of fluids (water)	Track and discuss all dietary supplement use with their health care provider. Note that beverage supplements should not replace regular food intake unless instructed by a health care professional. Keep in mind that sharing meals can increase enjoyment. Plan meals with a dietitian.

[a]Please note that in this box, "male" refers to an individual assigned male at birth, and "female" refers to an individual assigned female at birth.

Source: U.S. Department of Agriculture and U.S. Department of Health and Human Services. (2020). *Dietary guidelines for Americans, 2020–2025.* (9th ed.). https://www.dietaryguidelines.gov/sites/default/files/2021-03/Dietary_Guidelines_for_Americans-2020-2025.pdf

Nutrition becomes critical in reducing the risk of diabetes in patients with anxiety and depression and enhancing mental health in patient with diabetes. Research shows that there is an influential relationship between diabetes, anxiety, and depression. Anxiety and depression increase the risk of poor glycemic control increasing diabetes-related complications. Diabetes is also related to an increased risk of depression and anxiety (Basiri et al., 2023).

DIETARY SUPPLEMENTS

The use of dietary supplements to promote a healthy lifestyle is widespread. Dietary supplements can contain vitamins, minerals, herbs, spices, and other ingredients. They are classified as foods, not drugs, and are not regulated by the FDA.

> **KEYCONCEPT Dietary supplements**, products added to the diet for ingestion, contain dietary ingredients intended to supplement the diet. They are available over-the-counter and come in many forms including tablets, capsules, powders, liquids, gummies, and soft gels.

Melatonin, a naturally occurring hormone secreted from the pineal gland, is commonly used for treatment of circadian rhythm disorders, insomnia, and "jet lag" in air travelers (see Chapter 34). Since melatonin is considered a natural substance, the U.S. Food and Drug Administration (FDA) does not regulate the manufactured synthetic version. Melatonin is associated with headache, dizziness, nausea, and drowsiness. Exogenous melatonin has been extensively studied for other clinical conditions, but there is limited evidence for its effectiveness in these conditions. Relatively safe at appropriate amounts, the safety of melatonin in high doses has not been established (Boutin et al., 2023). Nurses should be cautious in recommending melatonin in high doses. Because melatonin can cause daytime drowsiness, operating cars or machinery should not occur within 5 hours of taking supplements (Pan et al., 2023).

Dietary supplements show improvement in cognitive functioning associated with Alzheimer disease, especially in combination with a pharmaceutical regime and healthy diet. **Lecithin**, a precursor to acetylcholine, is extracted from soybeans but contains little soy protein. Lecithin has been shown to improve memory, cognition, functioning, and mood in older adults (Ahmad et al., 2023).

Herbal versus Spice Supplements

The terms spice and herbs are often used interchangeably, but they come from various parts of the plant. **Herbs** are derived from the fresh part of the plant; whereas **spices** come from the dried root, dried stalk, seed, or dried fruit of the plant. Both spice and herbal supplements are used in the support of mental health and well-being. An in-depth discussion of these therapies is outside the scope of this text. Readers are encouraged to seek additional resources from the National Center for Complementary and Integrative Health within the National Institutes of Health.

Herbal and spice products are exempt from the FDA's efficacy and safety standards because they are considered food. Manufacturers and distributors are responsible for the evaluation of their safety and labeling of their products. Lack of regulation does not mean that these supplements are ineffective or unsafe. These substances can be effective and can also have adverse reactions and interact with prescribed medications. Nurses need to understand these potential interactions and assess their patients for the impact of these substances.

Herbal Supplements

Several **herbal supplements** are used in the treatment of mental disorders. For example, herbal supplements associated with improvement in Alzheimer disease include *ginkgo biloba*, *ginseng*, and *salvia officinalis* (Ahmad et al., 2023).

St. John's wort (SJW), derived from *Hypericum perforatum* L., is used for depression, pain, anxiety, insomnia, and premenstrual syndrome. SJW is believed to modulate serotonin, dopamine, and norepinephrine. The risk of developing serotonin syndrome is increased when taken with other serotonergic drugs. SJW has the potential to interact with other medications (i.e., birth control pills, digoxin) and should not be taken with prescribed antidepressants (National Center for Complementary and Integrative Health [NCCIH], 2024).

Chamomile, an herb derived from dried flowers of the Compositae family, is also known as German chamomile. Chamomile is promoted for sleeplessness, anxiety, and gastrointestinal symptoms. There is little research supporting the use of chamomile for sleeplessness, but side effects are uncommon. Chamomile has been reported to interact with cyclosporine and warfarin (NCCIH, 2024).

Kava, derived from the *Piper methysticum* plant, is used for anxiety reduction. Kava interacts with dopaminergic transmission, inhibits the monoamine oxidase B enzyme system, and modulates the GABA receptor. It may also inhibit uptake of noradrenaline. Kava is widely used by Pacific Islanders as a social and ceremonial tranquilizing drink. In 2002, the FDA issued warnings about the risk of severe liver injury associated with kava. Several countries have restricted its use. Thrombocytopenia, leukopenia, and hearing impairment have been reported with the use of kava-kava (Li & Wertheimer, 2023; NCCIH, 2024).

Valerian (*Valeriana officinalis*), a member of the Valerianaceae family, is a perennial plant native to Europe and Asia and naturalized to North America. Valerian is a common ingredient in products promoted for insomnia and nervousness. The evidence of its effectiveness is inconclusive. Valerian might have additive therapeutic and adverse effects if taken with sedatives and other herbs or dietary supplements with sedative properties. The mechanism of action is unclear. Side effects include headache, stomach upset, mental dullness, excitability, uneasiness, and heart disturbances. Some reports suggest hepatotoxicity in humans. The American Academy of Sleep Medicine recommended against using valerian for chronic insomnia (NCCIH, 2024; Sateia et al., 2017).

Curcumin (*Curcuma longa* [turmeric]) is used as both an herb and a spice. It is recognized as having anti-inflammatory, antimicrobial, antiproliferative, antitumoral, and antiaging properties. Studies have demonstrated the neuroprotective effect of curcumin in neurodegenerative diseases such as Alzheimer diseases and Parkinson disease. Research on curcumin is promising in the treatment of several diseases. Therapeutic use of curcumin is limited by its poor oral bioavailability due to its low solubility and rapid metabolism. Side effects and safety profiles have yet to be established (Benameur et al., 2021).

Spices

Spices found in many kitchens have medicinal properties, but research supporting effectiveness is limited. **Saffron**, a spice derived from the flower of the *crocus sativus*, has been shown to improve cognition. It has anti-inflammatory and antioxidant effects and may reduce symptoms of depression and anxiety (Ahmad et al., 2023). **Cinnamon** has been shown to have some hypolipic properties (Fateh & Amin, 2024). Other spices such as nutmeg, cloves, and ginger have not been shown to affect mental health and well-being (Mackonochie et al., 2023).

Vitamins and Minerals

The *Dietary Guidelines for Americans 2020–2025* recommends meeting vitamin and mineral requirements through a healthy eating pattern that includes nutrient-rich foods (U.S. Department of Agriculture & U.S. DHHS, 2020). The **Recommended Dietary Allowances** (RDA) for vitamins and minerals are set by the Institute of Medicine of the National Academy of Sciences and do not appear on food and supplement labels. The **Daily Values** (DV) are set by the FDA and the % DV is required by law to be listed. The nurse should be familiar with guidelines and educate patients to avoid excessive intake of vitamins and minerals, but also encourage a healthy diet. These RDA and DV guidelines are easily found on the website of the National Center for Complementary and Integrative Health (www.nccih.nih.gov).

Most Americans do not meet dietary guidelines especially in vitamin-rich fruit and vegetables. Many vitamin and mineral deficiencies may produce symptoms of psychiatric disorders. Fatigue, apathy, and depression are caused by deficiencies in iron, folic acid, pantothenic acid, magnesium, vitamin C, or biotin (Suárez-López et al., 2023). Logically, treating these deficiencies with dietary supplements should improve the psychiatric symptoms. The unanswered question becomes, can vitamin and mineral supplements improve psychiatric symptoms that are not the result of such deficiencies?

Supplementation with vitamins or minerals is not a primary treatment of mental disorders. Nutritional deficiencies are often present in patients with mental disorders, and supplementation is often used in their treatment. Thiamine (B_1) supplementation protects cognitive functioning for people with alcohol use disorder (Bonnet et al., 2023). Folate deficiency is associated with depression and is improved with folic acid supplementation (Liwinski & Lang, 2023).

More research is needed to identify the underlying mechanisms and relationships of dietary supplements and dietary precursors of the bioamines to mood and behavior and psychopharmacologic medications. For now, it is important for the PMH nurse to recognize that these issues may be potential factors in improvement of the patient's mental status and target symptoms.

Probiotics

Probiotics, beneficial live bacteria or other compounds that may influence gut neurotransmitters, are unregulated, but widely consumed for their physical and mental health benefits. Side effects of probiotics may be related to bacterial thickening in the small intestine that can lead to abdominal bloating, gas pain, poor judgment, impaired short-term memory, concentration difficulties, and mental confusion. Research findings are mixed, with some studies reporting positive effects and others negative. The specific strain of bacteria becomes crucial in determining effectiveness (Madabushi et al., 2023). Nurses are cautioned to carefully analyze marketing claims in light of emerging research.

PSYCHOLOGICAL AND PHYSICAL APPROACHES

Meditation and Mindfulness

The word **meditation** derives from the Latin word *meditari*, which means to reflect upon, contemplate, or consider. The practice of meditation dates back thousands of years and is rooted in Eastern traditions. Meditative practices focus on the integration of the mind and body with the intent of training the mind to regulate attention, with an overall purpose to cultivate mental well-being through improved concentration, compassion, or insight (U.S. Department of Veterans Affairs, 2024a). Meditation techniques generally include four features: a quiet environment, an auditory or visual stimulus to focus on, a passive attitude, and a comfortable position (Zisopoulou & Varvogli, 2023). Frequency of meditation sessions vary according to the individual's goals, and may range from once a week to daily, with a typical session lasting approximately 45 minutes.

Mindfulness is a form of meditation that is achieved through shifting attention from past ruminations, worries, and concerns and intentionally focusing on one's current, *moment-to-moment* experience in an accepting and nonjudgmental way. Through mindfulness, an individual becomes cognitively aware of what is happening at the present time, while simultaneously disengaging from other arising thoughts, emotions, and beliefs. The ultimate goal of mindfulness is to cultivate awareness of the present moment with acceptance and kindness (U.S. Department of Veteran Affairs, 2024a).

Mindfulness is achieved through both formal and informal strategies, and typically requires regular practice over several weeks (Giannou & Mantzios, 2023). When undergoing mindfulness meditation, the individual focuses on their breathing while also being aware of other internal and external stimuli (Semenenko et al., 2023; Tan et al., 2023b; Zisopoulou & Varvogli, 2023).

Although mindful behaviors are found to improve symptoms of anxiety and depression, meditation practices are not necessarily intended to be a therapy for a particular condition, rather an approach to improving overall well-being (Hatch et al., 2023; NIH NCCIH, 2022a; U.S. Department of Veterans Affairs, 2024a). Formal meditation and mindfulness practices enhance a sense of alliance, collaboration, and healing. While engaged in mindful behavior, an individual may be more cognizant of their thoughts, feelings, or perceptions as they arise. Through this enhanced state of awareness, the individual will be better positioned to identify their symptoms and can then develop skills to better manage their stress and regulate their emotions (Bello et al., 2023; Goldberg et al., 2023).

Relaxation

Relaxation exercises are practices to counter an individual's stress response by regulating the hypothalamus response to the parasympathetic nerves, generally resulting in slower breathing, lower heart rate, and reduced blood pressure. There are several different types of relaxation techniques, and they are often recommended in conjunction with other pharmacologic or nonpharmacologic therapies. Generally speaking, most relaxation techniques are low risk, cost effective, and can be practiced in a variety of settings, including in the comfort of an individual's own home. See Box 12.4. Some of the more common types of relaxation techniques include breathing exercises, guided imagery, progressive muscle relaxation (PMR), and autogenic training (NIH NCCIH, 2023a).

Breathing exercises promote respiratory and cardiovascular functioning by increasing parasympathetic activity and reducing sympathetic activity (Pathan et al., 2023; Zisopoulou & Varvogli, 2023). Breathing exercises include voluntary changes in the rate, pattern, and quality of breaths. There are many variations of breathing exercise in the literature. For example, *deep breathing*, also called **diaphragmatic breathing**, focuses on taking slow, deep breaths. This type of breathing is characterized by expansion of the abdomen when breathing rather than the chest. In **coherent breathing**, an individual inhales and exhales at equal length with only a slight pause in between. For example, inhalation for six seconds, followed by exhalation for six seconds. A breathing technique called "*moving the breath*" involves engaging the imagination to move one's breath throughout different parts of the body that may be tense. **Mindful breathing** is a guided breathing meditation practice that involves attention and focus on breathing patterns in order to regulate emotion and enhance body awareness (Zisopoulou & Varvogli, 2023).

In **guided imagery**, sometimes called *visualization*, an individual is directed to visualize pictures of pleasing objects, scenes, or events that are associated with

BOX 12.4

Research for Evidence-Based Practice: Relaxation and Education for Healing Trauma

Lu, W., Caldwell, B., Gao, N., Oursler, J., Wang, K., Beninato, J., Srijeyanthan, J., Kumi, C., Sawyer, J., Giacobbe, G., Chen, Y., Lin, K. W., & Mueser, K. T. (2023). Healing trauma while staying at home: Using telehealth to conduct a brief treatment program for posttraumatic stress disorder. Journal of Psychosocial Nursing and Mental Health Services, 1–11. *Advance online publication. https://doi.org/10.3928/02793695-20231205-01*

THE QUESTION: Can a three-session brief treatment program (brief relaxation, education, and trauma healing) help treatment of posttraumatic stress disorder (PTSD) and symptoms of trauma via telehealth?

METHODS: Thirty individuals with confirmed PTSD diagnoses participated in this telehealth program.

FINDINGS: Participants showed decreased PTSD symptoms, posttraumatic cognitions, depression, anxiety, overall psychiatric symptoms, and internalized stigma, and increased resiliency, at posttreatment and 3-month follow-up.

IMPLICATIONS FOR NURSING: Telehealth brief treatment program for PTSD symptoms is feasible and effective.

positive feelings and relaxation in an attempt for the individual to mimic that same feeling in their body. Guided imagery generally activates all senses and consists of three phases: body relaxation, imagery, and return to reality. First, the individual is guided to focus on their body and release body and muscle tension. The individual is then introduced to imagery of sights, sounds, smells, tastes, and feelings of a positive event or experience before then returning to the present time. The individual learns that they have the ability to return to that positive experience whenever they wish (Zisopoulou & Varvogli, 2023). Guided imagery can be led under the supervision of a professional or a recording or could be self-directed. Guided imagery is often used in conjunction with other relaxation strategies, for example, deep breathing or PMR, and has been found to reduce stress, anxiety, and depressive symptoms (Kumari & Patil, 2023).

Progressive muscle relaxation is a relaxation technique that involves purposeful tensing of the muscles, then a deliberate release of the muscle's tension. Often done simultaneously with deep breathing, different groups of muscles are contracted and relaxed sequentially until the whole body is relaxed. PMR generally involves muscle groups of the face, neck, shoulder, arm, forearm, back, abdomen, hip, leg, and foot (Seid et al., 2023). During PMR, the individual is often directed to inhale while tensing their muscles, then exhale when releasing the tension. The individual focuses on the contrast between the states of muscle tension and relaxation with the goal of eventually being able to relax their muscles without tensing first (Zisopoulou & Varvogli, 2023). With sessions generally lasting no longer than 20 minutes, PMR is one of the most commonly used relaxation techniques due to its low/no cost, low risk, and ease of use and is known to reduce stress, anxiety, and depression (Khir et al., 2024; Morikawa et al., 2023; Pathan et al., 2023; Talo & Turan, 2023).

Autogenic training utilizes autosuggestion to induce a relaxed state. It is a well-established self-relaxation strategy relying on passive concentration on bodily perceptions of heaviness and warmth that, in turn, elicits a psychophysiological response (Breznoscakova et al., 2023). Autogenic training encompasses six standard exercises, suggesting limb heaviness, limb warmth, reduced heart rate, reduced respiration rate, abdominal warmth, and forehead cooling. When undergoing autogenic training, the individual assumes a comfortable position, then listens to recorded instructions, silently repeating a specific self-suggestion (e.g., my right arm is heavy). As the individual focuses attention on the self-suggestion, they gravitate toward deep physical relaxation (Zisopoulou & Varvogli, 2023). Evidence supports the use of autogenic training to reduce symptoms of anxiety and depression (Breznoscakova et al., 2023).

Aromatherapy

Aromatherapy is the practice of inhaling or directly applying essential oils to achieve physical, psychological, and spiritual well-being. Administration usually involves the nasal cavity, skin, lung, and gastrointestinal tract. Aromatic smells from essential oils can stimulate the olfactory nerve to adjust brain function and regulate emotional states. Odor molecules participate in emotional expression, memory, discrimination, and neuroendocrine response. They also are part of the glutamate (excitation) and GABA (inhibition) responses. The essential oils can also enter the circulatory system through the skin and gastrointestinal tract and pass though the blood–brain barrier. Because of the small molecules, essential oils are easily absorbed through the skin to enter the blood system with little skin irritation. After oral administration, essential oils can enter systemic circulation through gastrointestinal metabolism and the brain–gut axis (Zhang et al., 2021).

Essential oils, also known as volatile oils, are concentrated plant extracts that retain the natural smell and flavor of their source that are easily evaporated at room temperature. They are packaged in dark glass bottles because they can be damaged by sunlight. They should not be applied directly to the skin unless they are diluted with a less volatile **carrier oil** (vegetable oil with little or no scent). Each essential oil has a unique composition of chemicals (National Institute of Environmental Health Science, 2022).

Infused oils are created when the plant matter is soaked (or infused) within an inexpensive oil base. They are less expensive than essential oils and can be applied directly to the skin and can be incorporated into massage therapy. They are packaged in either dark or light containers. Both essential and infused oils can be used for health and aromatherapy. They may also be used in combination.

Nurses should be aware of the benefits of essential oils but should carefully examine the evidence that supports their usage. Essential oils can complement nursing interventions. For example, lavender from the *Lavandula angustifolia* and *Lavandula intermedia* is one of the most widely used essential oil. It has been shown to promote sleep quality (Yang et al., 2023a), reduce anxiety (Amitani et al., 2023; Tan et al., 2023a), and treat depression (Zhang et al., 2021). Other essential oils that are used to promote well-being, but have limited studies include orange, peppermint, frankincense, Ylang Ylang, sandalwood, and cedarwood.

Hypnotherapy

Hypnotherapy, also known as clinical hypnosis, is an evidence-based complementary and integrative health approach that has been used extensively in both medical and mental health fields. Hypnotherapy is different than hypnosis which involves only triggering a trance state in an individual, generally with no therapeutic intent other than to increase a state of relaxation or to increase adherence. However, in hypnotherapy, after triggering a trance state, a trained provider will use that state to facilitate therapeutic cognitive, emotional, or physical healing responses (U.S. Department of Veterans Affairs, 2024b). Hypnotherapy provides a forum for patients to explore, discover, and learn, and generally includes three elements: absorption (the patient moves into an imaginative experience), dissociation from the environment, and suggestibility.

Hypnosis can facilitate the unconscious restructuring and reframing of dysfunctional thinking that is contributing to illness. During hypnosis, the patient's natural defense mechanisms are reduced, and they will be led to a heightened state of awareness where they may focus on subjective feelings and inner experiences (Chan et al., 2023; Flemons, 2024).

Hypnotherapy utilizes techniques including guided visualizations and relaxation to a state of peacefulness and relaxation, exploration of past experiences, and suggestion for behavior changes to aid in overcoming the issue. Through therapy sessions, the patient will learn cognitive-behavioral coping strategies to use when confronting anxiety or fears (Fritscher, 2023). While under hypnosis in the heightened state of awareness, a patient becomes more responsive to suggestions for behavior change from the therapist.

First introduced in the late 1700's, hypnotherapy has a long history in medicine. However, it is often misunderstood by the medical community, with some questioning its scientific merit (van Tilburg et al., 2024). Lack of knowledge and exposure, coupled with the negative portrayal of hypnosis in popular culture, contribute to perceptions and questions of its legitimacy (Szmaglinska et al., 2024). A common misconception of hypnotherapy is that an individual will lose their free will and be under the control of the hypnotist, potentially revealing information that they would not do under other circumstances. In reality, the individual under hypnosis does not become unconscious and remains fully awake and aware throughout the session. There is generally a substantial amount of brain activity during hypnosis, with the majority of individuals who undergo hypnosis remembering everything that occurred during the session (ACHS, 2024; Cavé, 2022; Fritscher, 2023).

Substantial evidence supporting the efficacy of clinical hypnosis has been made available over the past few decades. In mental health, hypnotherapy is particularly effective in treating anxiety disorders, depressive disorders, and posttraumatic stress disorder. Beyond its effectiveness in reducing clinical symptoms, hypnotherapy has also been found to build trust between patients and their health care providers. Additionally, individuals undergoing hypnotherapy report feeling empowered and more autonomous in their treatment plan (Chan et al., 2023; Rosendahl et al., 2024).

Massage Therapy

Massage therapy is the manipulation of soft and connective tissues for therapeutic benefit and has been practiced in both Eastern and Western cultures throughout history (NIH NCCIH, 2019). Massage is an effective noninvasive complementary therapy that has been used across all age groups. In mental health, massage therapy has been found to reduce stress and improve symptoms of anxiety and depression (Lin et al., 2023; Manard, 2022; Mitchinson et al., 2022; Sattayakhom et al., 2023; Yang et al., 2024).

Massage is effective for several reasons. The structured and purposeful way in which muscles and tissues are manipulated helps to reduce pain and improve body alignment. Some studies suggest that massage decreases stress chemicals, such as cortisol. Additionally, the effects of human touch contribute to its therapeutic effect, including the individual feeling comforted and cared for, having a sense of empowerment, and feeling connected to their massage therapist (Mayo Clinic, 2021).

Massage is usually performed in safe, quiet, and relaxed spaces. Music often accompanies the massage session. Aromatherapy is often used in conjunction with relaxation, including the use of essential oils during massage. Specifically, massage with lavender and geranium oils affect the autonomic nervous system and reduces blood pressure and heart rate. The use of lavender in massage has been shown to improve sleep. Lavendar, sweet orange, and bergamot in massage have been found to reduce symptoms of depression in older adults. To improve alertness and vigilance, peppermint, rosemary, grapefruit, and cinnamon oils have been used (Sattayakhom et al., 2023). To reduce risk for injury, a trained therapist should perform massage therapy. Additionally, consent for massage therapy is especially important due to the intimate nature of human touch (Kopf, 2021).

Yoga and Tai Chi

Rooted in Indian philosophy, **yoga** includes a holistic system of practices that promote both physical and mental health by uniting the body, mind, and spirit. Yoga emphasizes three key elements: physical postures (**"asanas"**), breathing techniques (**"pranayama"**), and mindfulness meditation (**"dyana"**) (Khunti et al., 2023; NIH NCCIH, 2023b). Although yoga has been practiced for thousands of years, it was not until the past two decades that the impact of yoga as a therapy has been studied. Evidence suggests that yoga practices result in improved muscular strength and flexibility, improved cardiovascular and respiratory function, and chronic pain. Several studies have demonstrated the effectiveness of yoga in reducing stress, anxiety, and depressive symptoms. Additionally, the practice of yoga has been found to increase self-esteem, self-compassion, and healthy behaviors. Studies of children find that yoga can allow them to redirect their energy in a more positive way and calm their minds and bodies, particularly during periods of anxiety. Cognitive functions of attention, memory, and executive function are also improved with yoga (Dutta et al., 2022; Kaligal et al., 2023; Khunti et al., 2023; Martinez-Calderon et al., 2023).

Mindfulness yoga is a combination of yoga and mindfulness practice, which teaches patients to practice yoga while simultaneously integrating awareness of their body and mind in the present moment. Mindfulness yoga differs from other forms of yoga styles due to its strong emphasis on meditation practices and mindful awareness in daily life. It is an effective complementary therapy for depression and for improving mental health (Miao et al., 2023; Yang et al., 2023b).

Yoga is considered a safe activity when performed properly and under the direction of a professional. Risks are minimal, with the most common injuries being minor sprains and strains, most often in the knee or lower leg. To minimize risk, yoga techniques should be introduced slowly, avoiding extreme practices such as headstands, shoulder stands, the lotus position, and forceful breathing until the individual is better experienced. Hot yoga, performing yoga under hot and humid conditions, results in excessive sweating has additional risks associated with overheating and dehydration (NIH NCCIH, 2023a).

Traditional yoga practice is often performed at a yoga studio, in a calm environment with dim lighting and clear space. The literature suggests that traditional yoga results in better outcomes than yoga completed more informally at home. However, yoga sessions are often not covered by insurance and can be cost prohibitive. There are disparities in individuals practicing yoga, with yoga practitioners being primarily middle adulthood, White women with a higher socioeconomic status. Financial barriers and logistical constraints limit access to traditional yoga therapy for some individuals. See Box 12.5. Because yoga is a low-risk complementary therapy that enhances overall mental well-being, it is important for yoga to be accessible. At home yoga, guided by videos, may be a practical alternative. Tele-yoga, used as an adjunct to in-person yoga, has gained popularity and gives patients a forum to practice yoga in a safe and familiar setting that is more convenient to them (Cole et al., 2022; Lagera et al., 2023).

Tai chi and **qigong**, two practices of Chinese origin, are considered "meditative movement" practices. Tai chi involves a series of slow gentle movements and physical postures, coupled with meditation, controlled breathing, and relaxation. Initially originating as a martial art, tai chi emphasizes continuous slow movements with small and large expressions of motions, shifts of body weight, and rotations of the head, trunk, and extremities, while incorporating deep breathing and relaxation. With greater focus on health promotion and rehabilitation, tai chi is an effective complementary therapy for symptoms of depression and anxiety, and for overall mental health (Jimenez et al., 2024; Yin et al., 2023).

BOX 12.5

Mental Health Inequities: Yoga-Based Interventions in Low-Income Groups

Research shows that most people engaged in yoga belong to a higher socioeconomic status (SES). A literature review was completed to better understand the feasibility and acceptability of yoga practices among individuals in low-income groups. To promote inclusivity and accessibility, practitioners should recognize the following as strategies to promote utilization:

- **Accessible psychoeducation:** Community-based seminars to provide education on what to expect would be beneficial for individuals with less familiarity with yoga. People should be told that yoga-specific clothing is not required, and that any comfortable clothing is okay to wear.
- **Cultural humility:** Practitioners should be mindful of differences in identity between themselves and community members, including race, SES, language, etc. Practitioners should be educated about the needs of the target community.
- **Cost barriers:** Costs for yoga therapy should be minimized when possible. For example, a reduction in session fees, provision of yoga mats, etc.
- **Yoga acceptability and accessibility:** Yoga practices should be accessible for all individuals new to yoga and should accommodate all experiences and abilities. Yoga should include trauma-informed practices.
- **Yoga delivery:** Yoga sessions should be held in locations with greater accessibility and offered at various times throughout the day to accommodate work and family obligations. Virtual or prerecorded classes could be made available for people to practice at their convenience and in their own setting.

Nagaswami, M. V., Saper, R. B., Streeter, C. C., Uebelacker, L., Ding, G., Dalvie, A., Norton, R., Mischoulon, D., & Neyer, M. B. (2024). Yoga-based interventions in low-income populations: A scoping review. *Journal of Integrative and Complementary Medicine, 30*(8), 735–752. https://doi.org/10.1089/jicm.2023.0479

Qigong, pronounced "chi gong," enhances the regulation of mind, body movement, posture, and breathing. General practices of qigong include slow, long, and deep breathing, alternating between abdominal breathing to breathing with speech sounds, gentle and smooth body movements, and mind regulation that includes focusing on attention and visualization (NIH NCCIH, 2022b).

Acupuncture

With roots in Chinese medicine, **acupuncture** has been practiced for thousands of years, and in medical practice in the United States for approximately 200 years. It was not until the mid-1990s that the FDA approved the acupuncture needle as a medical device. Although acupuncture is most often used for pain management, there is evidence supporting its use with other conditions as well, including management of chemo-induced nausea and vomiting, fatigue, hot flashes, xerostomia, neuropathy, anxiety, depression, and sleep disturbance (NIH, National Cancer Institute, 2024). Acupuncture may be effective as a stand-alone treatment or in conjunction with other treatments (U.S. Department of Veterans Affairs, 2024c).

Although several acupuncture styles exist, they are generally grounded in the following philosophy: (1) the human body must be perceived and treated as a whole and as part of nature, (2) health is the result of harmony among bodily functions and between the body and nature, and (3) when this harmony is disrupted, disease occurs. The overall intent of acupuncture is to restore the state of harmony by removing energy blockages and correcting the flow of energy or "**qi**" (pronounced chee) through meridians (pathways) of the body. This is accomplished by inserting fine needles in certain meridians of the body that are considered obstructed. The needles are inserted to various depths and usually do not cause discomfort. Typically, a treatment uses 5 to 20 needles. The needles may be manipulated manually by the provider by gently moving or twirling them or stimulated with small electrical currents, resulting in both central and peripheral physiologic effects.

In a typical treatment, the needles remain in place for 10 to 15 minutes. A typical treatment series may include one or two treatments a week up to 6 to 8 treatments (Mayo Clinic, 2024; NCCIH, 2022c; Verma, 2023). In addition to classical acupuncture techniques, some techniques focus on specific areas of the body, including the ear, scalp, face, hand, nose, foot, and wrist-ankle (NIH National Cancer Institute, 2024).

Acupuncture is safe and acceptable for both adults and children when practiced by a licensed practitioner. Most states have laws regulating acupuncture practice that rely on educational and license requirements. Not all insurance companies and federal payers cover acupuncture treatment.

Art Therapies

Creative art therapies are expressive, experiential therapies that provide a forum for individuals to express themselves in a way that does not rely on words. Art therapies is an umbrella term that includes art, drama, music, and dance therapies. Art therapies are especially beneficial for people challenged to fully express themselves verbally, as the individual is empowered to explore and communicate their thoughts, emotions, and experiences through artistic expression (Van Lith & Ettenberger, 2023). Through creativity, an individual is engaged in transformation, self-discovery, emotional healing, and personal growth (Van Lith & Ettenberger, 2023).

These therapies are provided in a safe and supportive environment where the individual can express themselves freely. A nonthreatening and nonjudgmental space allows the individual to explore their inner world, develop coping skills, enhance self-awareness, and build resilience (Van Lith & Ettenberger, 2023). Including art therapy as a complementary therapy has many benefits. It recognizes the individuality of each person, considering the individual's unique circumstances and background. It is flexible in that it can be provided in individual sessions or in larger groups, and is suitable for all age groups, ranging from young children to older adults (Cheng et al., 2023). Group art therapy programs enhance enjoyment and socialization, which contribute to overall well-being (Cheng et al., 2023; Galassi et al., 2022; Van Lith & Ettenberger, 2023).

Art therapy uses art media as its primary mode of communication and encompasses many different art forms, for example, drawing, painting, sculpture, clay, collage, and photography. Art making enables expression of emotions, distress, impulses, and individual identity (Abbing et al., 2023). Art therapy does not require an individual to have artistic skill or ability. It focuses on the creation and meaning of art, and not the quality of the art produced. Art therapy does not require extensive resources, as art can be created with minimal and inexpensive materials, such as plain paper and pencils (Cheng et al., 2023; Han et al., 2024). When practiced regularly, creative expression contributes to increased self-esteem and an enhanced relationship to self (Jay et al., 2022). Through art making, the individual may feel a sense of identity, empowerment, and self-control when they are undisturbed and allowed to self-direct the creation of their art. When sharing their art with others, the individual is able to reflect on the meaning of their creation (Abbing et al., 2023). Studies have shown that art therapy can be effective as a complementary therapy in reducing symptoms of depression and anxiety, agitation, cognitive impairment, schizophrenia, and autism (Hu et al., 2021; Liu et al., 2023b; Luo et al., 2023).

Drama therapy utilizes drama and theatrical techniques to achieve therapeutic goals and promote health.

This form of creative art therapy provides an opportunity for an individual to explore their feelings and thoughts through play. Drama interventions may include improvisation, role work, projection, story making, and images (Melvin et al., 2024). Role play and other drama techniques involve self-reflection, resulting in increased awareness of problematic behaviors and the development of problem-solving skills and improved self-esteem. Dramatizing past and present life situations through role play offers opportunities for self-expression that may lead to improved understanding and insight (Abbing et al., 2023). Drama therapy has been found to support individuals undergoing a process of change, developing new perspectives, improving relationships, making choices, and increasing self-understanding (Melvin et al., 2024).

Music therapy includes several activities, including music improvisation, songwriting, music performance, and listening to music. It is known to produce physical and mental benefit; however, the exact mechanism of action is not well understood. Music stimulates a variety of structures in the brain that engage in thinking, emotion, sensation, and movement. It can evoke emotions, memories, and feelings (NIH NCCIH, 2022d). Music has been found to increase levels of dopamine and endorphins, lower cortisol levels, and increase cerebral blood flow to areas of the brain associated with pleasing behaviors, leading to stress reduction, emotional regulation, and improved mood. Music promotes self-expression and exploring one's emotions. Music therapy can reduce social isolation and enhance social connections. In mental health, music therapy can be effective in reducing stress, anxiety, and agitation, as well as improving symptoms of depression and dementia (Abbing et al., 2023; Ma et al., 2024; Nobakht et al., 2023; Thompson et al., 2024). Because music can be associated with strong memories or emotional reactions, the music therapist should be mindful that exposure to certain types of music or specific pieces may be distressing (NIH NCCIH, 2022d).

Dance therapy is the therapeutic use of movement and dance to promote emotional, social, cognitive, and physical well-being. Dance therapy incorporates an individual's cognitive sphere (learning ability, attention, memory, coordination) with their creative and emotional sphere (movement improvisation, imagination, and sociability), resulting in both physical and mental health benefits (Tomaszewski et al., 2023). Participation in dance therapy contributes to improved motor skills, body awareness, and enhanced mind–body connection. Dance therapy provides a forum for an individual to identify, express, and externalize their emotions in a creative way. Individuals engaged in dance therapy report feeling rejuvenated, enjoyment of being in the present, empowered, and having increased self-confidence. Dance also contributes to therapeutic boundaries, interpersonal relationships, and socialization. Dance therapy is considered a useful complementary therapy for managing symptoms of stress, anxiety, depression, trauma, and chronic pain (Moratelli et al., 2023; Tomaszewski et al., 2023).

USE OF COMPLEMENTARY THERAPIES IN PSYCHIATRIC–MENTAL HEALTH NURSING

When standardized approaches are insufficient in addressing whole health needs, complementary and alternative therapies may be considered. Integrative care coordinates conventional and complementary therapies to provide a person-centered plan of care to optimize well-being. Taking an integrative, holistic approach to patient care is the responsibility of every nurse. Although some of the physical and psychological therapies require advanced education or certification to practice, all nurses should have a basic understanding of the complementary and alternative therapies that may benefit their patients. An integrative approach to care considers all contributing factors to illness and disruption in well-being. This includes completing an integrative assessment of needs, followed by identifying potential pharmacologic and nonpharmacologic interventions. When developing an individualized plan of care with the patient, the nurse should understand the evidence on the therapies being considered to better inform their practice (Voss et al., 2023).

SUMMARY OF KEY POINTS

- Complementary therapies are nonmainstream interventions that are incorporated into an integrative health care approach.
- The brain–gut axis is critical in healthy brain functioning and is dependent upon the nutrients consumed. Dietary fiber activates the enzymes that break down complex carbohydrates to short-chained fatty acids, which are important in neurotransmitter production.
- Western dietary patterns contribute to oxidative stress and neuroinflammation, which in turn lead to a higher risk of anxiety and depression.
- Dietary supplements can be useful in maintaining mental health and well-being. Herbs and spices are widely used to promote a healthy lifestyle. Nurses should carefully review the evidence related to specific supplements prior to recommending their use to patients.
- Although the *Dietary Guidelines for Americans 2020–2025* recommends meeting vitamin and mineral requirements through a healthy eating pattern, most Americans do not meet dietary guidelines, especially in fruit and vegetables. Vitamin and mineral deficiencies may produce psychiatric symptoms.

- Meditation techniques generally include a quiet environment, an auditory or visual stimulus, a passive attitude, and a comfortable position. Meditation cultivates mental well-being through improved concentration, compassion, or insight. Mindfulness is a form of meditation that focuses on moment-to-moment experiences.
- There are a variety of relaxation exercises including breathing exercises, guided imagery, PMR, and autogenic training.
- Aromatherapy involves the use of essential oils to achieve physical, psychological, and spiritual well-being. Several different essential oils are recommended for various effects. Nurses should be aware of the benefits of essential oils but should carefully examine the evidence for their use.
- Hypnotherapy provides a forum for patients to explore, discover, and learn cognitive-behavioral coping strategies when confronted with anxiety or fears. There is substantial evidence for its effectiveness.
- Massage is a noninvasive therapy used to reduce stress and improve symptoms of anxiety and depression. Consent for massage therapy is important because of the intimate nature of massage.
- Yoga from Indian philosophy emphasizes physical postures, breathing techniques, and mindfulness meditation. The practice of yoga reduces stress, anxiety, and depressive symptoms. It also increases self-esteem, self-compassion, and healthy behaviors.
- Tai chi and qigong from Chinese traditions are meditative movement practices incorporating slow gentle movements and physical postures with meditation and mindfulness, deep breathing, and relaxation. They target anxiety and depression, and improve mental well-being.
- Acupuncture is an ancient Chinese practice involving removing energy blockades by inserting fine needles in certain meridians of the body. The overall intent is to restore harmony and correct the flow of energy. Acupuncture is most often used for pain control.
- Creative art therapies provide a forum for nonverbal expression of thoughts and feelings. There are a variety of specialized therapies including art, music, dance, and drama.

DEVELOPING CLINICAL JUDGMENT

1. A 32-year-old patient is admitted to the mental health unit for depression and thoughts of suicide. During the assessment, the nurse asks about eating habits. The patient reports that a typical day includes coffee in the morning, cheese and crackers for lunch, and hamburger and French fries for dinner. Analyze the patient's diet. What interventions would support a healthy dietary intake?
2. A patient asks if the use of chamomile tea and melatonin will help with insomnia. How should the nurse respond?
3. A patient is extremely anxious and is asking about the benefits of yoga in reducing anxiety but is concerned that they do not have the correct yoga outfit for the activity. How should the nurse respond?
4. A nurse is asked to lead a progressive muscle relaxation group. The nurse questions whether leading a relaxation group is within the nurse's scope of practice.

MOVIES, TV, OR STREAMING PROGRAMS

Art Therapy: The Movie: **2016.** This documentary, directed by Alfonso Bui, explores the innovative ways that art therapy is used around the world. It features personal accounts of practicing art therapists and the clients they serve. Through various art media, people reflect on their inspirational journey of growth and healing.

Viewing Points:

1. The documentary features individuals of all ages, from varied backgrounds, and in diverse cultures worldwide. What does this say about the relevance and usefulness of art therapy?
2. What is the difference between "doing art that is therapeutic" and "art therapy"?
3. What are some of the challenges facing art therapy?
4. What is the role of an art therapist in a therapy session?

REFERENCES

Abbing, A., Haeyen, S., Nyapati, S., Verboon, P., & van Hooren, S. (2023). Effectiveness and mechanisms of the arts therapies in forensic care. A systematic review, narrative synthesis, and meta analysis. *Frontiers in Psychiatry, 14*, 1128252.

Ahmad, S., Ahmed, S. B., Khan, A., Wasim, M., Tabassum, S., Haider, S., Ahmed, F., Batool, Z., Khaliq, S., Rafiq, H., Tikmani, P., & Gilani, A. U. (2023). Natural remedies for Alzheimer's disease: a systematic review of randomized controlled trials. *Metabolic Brain Disease, 38*(1), 17–44. https://doi.org/10.1007/s11011-022-01063-9

American Nurses Association, American Psychiatric Nurse Association, & International Society of Psychiatric-Mental Health Nurses. (2022). *Psychiatric-mental health nursing: Scope and standards of practice* (3rd ed.). American Nurses Association.

American Society of Clinical Hypnosis (ASCH). (2024). *About hypnosis.* https://asch.net/about-hypnosis/

Amitani, H., Nishi, R., Sagiyama, K., Fukumoto, T., Funakoshi, K., Takayanagi, N., Watanabe, H., Hirose, M., Tagawa, K., Ota, K., Ito, Y. M., & Asakawa, A. (2023). The effect of lavender aroma for anxiety disorder: a study protocol for a multicenter, double-masked, randomized, placebo-controlled clinical trial. *BMC Complementary Medicine and Therapies, 23*(1), 397. https://doi.org/10.1186/s12906-023-04231-1

Basiri, R., Seidu, B., & Rudich, M. (2023). Exploring the interrelationships between diabetes, nutrition, anxiety, and depression: implications for treatment and prevention strategies. *Nutrients, 15*(19), 4226. https://doi.org/10.3390/nu15194226

Bello, C. M., Blagrave, A. J., & Lytle, R. K. (2023). Mindfulness-based practices in the classroom for stress and anxiety in students with disabilities. *Journal of Physical Education, Recreation and Dance, 94*(9), 29–38.

Benameur, T., Giacomucci, G., Panaro, M. A., Ruggiero, M., Trotta, T., Monda, V., Pizzolorusso, I., Lofrumento, D. D., Porro, C., & Messina, G. (2021). New promising therapeutic avenues of curcumin in brain diseases. *Molecules, 27*(1), 236. https://doi.org/10.3390/molecules27010236

Bonnet, U., Pohlmann, L., McAnally, H., & Claus, B. B. (2023). Further evidence of relationship between thiamine blood level and cognition in chronic alcohol-dependent adults: Prospective Pilot Study of an inpatient detoxification with oral supplementation protocol. *Alcohol (Fayetteville, N.Y.), 110*, 23–31. https://doi.org/10.1016/j.alcohol.2023.03.001

Boutin, J. A., Kennaway, D. J., & Jockers, R. (2023). Melatonin: facts, extrapolations and clinical trials. *Biomolecules, 13*(6), 943. https://doi.org/10.3390/biom13060943

Breznoscakova, D., Kovanicova, M., Sedlakova, E., & Pallayova, M. (2023). Autogenic training in mental disorders: What can we expect? *International Journal of Environmental Research and Public Health, 20*(5), 4344.

Cavé, J. (2022). The "new" brain-based approach: Hypnosis. *Mental Health Matters, 9*(5), 25–27.

Chan, N. A., Zhang, Z., Yin, G., Li, Z., & Ho, R. C. (2023). Update on hypnotherapy for psychiatrists. *BJ Psych Advances, 29*, 381–387.

Cheng, C., Elamin, M. E., May, H., & Kennedy, M. (2023). Drawing on emotions: the evolving role of art therapy. *Irish Journal of Psychological Medicine, 40*, 500–502.

Clemente-Suárez, V. J., Beltrán-Velasco, A. I., Redondo-Flórez, L., Martín-Rodríguez, A., & Tornero-Aguilera, J. F. (2023). Global impacts of Western diet and its effects on metabolism and health: a narrative review. *Nutrients, 15*(12), 2749. https://doi.org/10.3390/nu15122749

Cole, A. K., Pearson, T., & Knowlton, M. (2022). Comparing aerobic exercise with yoga in anxiety reduction: An integrative review. *Issues in Mental Health Nursing, 43*(3), 282–287.

Dutta, A., Aruchunan, M., Mukherjee, A., Metri, K. G., Ghosh, K., & Basu-Ray, I. (2022). A comprehensive review of yoga research in 2020. *Journal of Integrative and Complementary Medicine, 28*(2), 114–123.

Fateh, H. L., & Amin, S. M. (2024). Effects of cinnamon supplementation on lipid profile: A systematic review and meta-analysis of randomized controlled trials. *Clinical Nutrition Research, 13*(1), 74–87. https://doi.org/10.7762/cnr.2024.13.1.74

Flemons, D. (2024). Unraveling depression: Principles and practices of clinical hypnosis. *American Journal of Clinical Hypnosis, 66*(1), 6–19.

Fritscher, L. (2023). Hypnotherapy: How you can benefit from hypnosis with therapy. Retrieved May 11, 2024, from https://www.verywellmind.com/hypnotherapy-2671993

Galassi, F., Merizzi, A., D'Amen, B., & Santini, S. (2022). Creativity and art therapies to promote healthy aging: A scoping review. *Frontiers in Psychology, 13*, 906191.

Giannou, K., & Mantzios, M. (2023). Meditative and non-meditative mindfulness-based interventions for mind and body. *BMC Complementary Medicine and Therapies, 23*, 235.

Goldberg, S. B., Anders, C., Stuart-Maver, S. L., & Kivlighan III, D. M. (2023). Meditation, mindfulness, and acceptance methods in psychotherapy: a systematic review. *Psychotherapy Research, 33*(7), 873–885.

Han, B., Jia, Y., Hu, G., Bai, L., Gains, H., You, S., He, R., Jiao, Y., Huang, K., Cui, L., & Chen, L. (2024). The effects of visual art therapy on adults with depressive symptoms: a systematic review and meta-analysis. *International Journal of Mental Health Nursing, 33*(5), 1183–1196.

Hatch, S., Webber, J., Rej, S., Finlayson, M., & Kessler, D. (2023). The effectiveness of mindfulness-based meditation treatments for late life anxiety: a systematic review of randomized controlled trials. *Aging & Mental Health, 27*(6), 1045–1055.

Hu, J., Zhang, J., Hu, L., Yu, H., & Xu, J. (2021). Art therapy: a complementary treatment for mental disorders. *Frontiers in Psychology, 12*, 686005.

Jay, E. K., Patterson, C., Fernandez, R., & Moxham, L. (2022). Experiences of recovery among adults with a mental illness using visual art methods: a systematic review. *Journal of Psychiatric Mental Health Nursing, 30*, 361–374.

Jimenez, E. R., Juarez, J., Struwe, L., & Cohen, M. Z. (2024). Tai chi as a complementary therapy for depression and anxiety among U.S. veterans in a mental health inpatient setting. *Journal of the American Psychiatric Nurses Association, 30*(4), 778–784. https://doi.org/10.1177/10783903231201592

Kaligal, C., Kanthi, A., Mahadevappa, V., & Deepeshwar, S. (2023). Influence of yoga on cognitive functions in individuals with mental disorders: A systematic review of randomized controlled trials. *Integrative and Complementary Therapies, 29*(1), 15–24.

Khir, S. M., Unes, W. M. A. W. M., Mahmud, N., Wang, R., Panatik, S. A., Sukor, M. S. M., & Nordin, N. A. (2024). Efficacy of progressive muscle relaxation in adults for stress, anxiety, and depression: A systematic review. *Psychology Research and Behavior Management, 17*, 345–365.

Khunti, K., Boniface, S., Norris, E., De Oliveira, C. M., & Shelton, N. (2023). The effects of yoga on mental health in school-aged children: A systematic review and narrative synthesis of randomized control trials. *Clinical Child Psychology, 28*(3), 1217–1238.

Kopf, D. (2021). Massage and touch-based therapy. *Zeitschrift für Gerontologie und Geriatrie, 54*, 753–758.

Kumari, D., & Patil, J. (2023). Guided imagery for anxiety disorders: therapeutic efficacy and changes in quality of life. *Industrial Psychiatry Journal, 32*, S191–S195.

Kunugi, H. (2023). Depression and lifestyle: Focusing on nutrition, exercise, and their possible relevance to molecular mechanisms. *Psychiatry and Clinical Neurosciences, 77*(8), 420–433. https://doi.org/10.1111/pcn.13551

Lagera, P. G. D., Chan, S. R., & Yellowlees, P. M. (2023). Asynchronous technologies in mental health care and education. *Current Treatment Options in Psychiatry, 10*, 59–71.

Lane, M. M., Gamage, E., Du, S., Ashtree, D. N., McGuinness, A. J., Gauci, S., Baker, P., Lawrence, M., Rebholz, C. M., Srour, B., Touvier, M., Jacka, F. N., O'Neil, A., Segasby, T., & Marx, W. (2024). Ultra-processed food exposure and adverse health outcomes: umbrella review of epidemiological meta-analyses. *British Medical Journal, 384*, e077310. https://doi.org/10.1136/bmj-2023-077310

Li, W., & Wertheimer, A. (2023). Narrative review: The FDA's perfunctory approach of dietary supplement regulations giving rise to copious reports of adverse events. *Innovations in Pharmacy, 14*(1). https://doi.org/10.24926/iip.v14i1.4989

Lin, H. H., Shen, C. C., Ling, Y., & Lin, C. Y. (2024). Effect of traditional Chinese medicine massage on physical and mental health of middle-aged and elderly women. *Biotechnology and Genetic Engineering Reviews, 40*(1), 638–663.

Liu, X., Liu, X., Wang, Y., Zeng, B., Zhu, B., & Dai, F. (2023a). Association between depression and oxidative balance score: National Health and Nutrition Examination Survey (NHANES) 2005–2018. *Journal of Affective Disorders, 337*, 57–65. https://doi.org/10.1016/j.jad.2023.05.071

Liu, Q., Wang, F., Tan, L., Liu, L., Cheng, H., & Hu, X. (2023b). Comparative efficacy of various art therapies for patients with dementia: A network meta-analysis of randomized controlled trials. *Frontiers in Psychiatry, 14*, 1072066.

Liwinski, T., & Lang, U. E. (2023). Folate and its significance in depressive disorders and suicidality: A comprehensive narrative review. *Nutrients, 15*(17), 3859. https://doi.org/10.3390/nu15173859

Luo, X., Zhang, Z., Shi, X., He, C., Wang, J., Wu, Q., & Huang, G. (2023). Arts therapies for mental disorders in COVID-19 patients: A comprehensive review. *Frontiers in Public Health, 11*, 1289545.

Ma, Y. M., Yuan, M. D., & Zhong, B. L. (2024). Efficacy and acceptability of music therapy for post-traumatic stress disorder: A systematic review and meta-analysis of randomized trials. *European Journal of Pyschotraumatology, 15*(1), 2342739.

Mackonochie, M., Rodriguez-Mateos, A., Mills, S., & Rolfe, V. (2023). A scoping review of the clinical evidence for the health benefits of culinary doses of herbs and spices for the prevention and treatment of metabolic syndrome. *Nutrients, 15*(23), 4867. https://doi.org/10.3390/nu15234867

Madabushi, J. S., Khurana, P., Gupta, N., & Gupta, M. (2023). Gut biome and mental health: Do probiotics work? *Cureus, 15*(6), e40293. https://doi.org/10.7759/cureus.40293

Manard, M. B. (2022). Moms, massage, and mental health. *Massage Therapy Journal, 61*(3), 34–36.

Martinez-Calderon, J., Casuso-Holgado, M. J., Munoz-Fernandez, M. J., Garcia-Munoz, C., & Heredia-Rizo, A. M. (2023). Yoga-based interventions may reduce anxiety symptoms in anxiety disorders and depression symptoms in depressive disorders: A systematic review with meta-analysis and meta-regression. *British Journal of Sports Medicine, 57*, 1442–1449.

Mayo Clinic. (2021). The role of massage therapy for mental health. Retrieved May 26, 2024, from https://mcpress.mayoclinic.org/mental-health/mayo-clinic-explores-the-role-of-massage-therapy-for-mental-health/

Mayo Clinic. (2024). Acupuncture. Retrieved May 11, 2024, from https://www.mayoclinic.org/tests-procedures/acupuncture/about/pac-20392763

Melvin, E., Green, M., Keiller, E., Parmar, C., & Bourne, J. (2024). A systematic review of dramatherapy interventions used to support adults with psychosis. *Schizophrenia Research, 267*, 44–54.

Merlo, G., Bachtel, G., & Sugden, S. G. (2024). Gut microbiota, nutrition, and mental health. *Frontiers in Nutrition, 11*, 1337889. https://doi.org/10.3389/fnut.2024.1337889

Miao, C., Gao, Y., Li, X., Zhou, Y., Chung, J. W., & Smith, G. D. (2023). The effectiveness of mindfulness yoga on patients with major depressive disorder: A systematic review and meta-analysis of randomized controlled trials. *BMC Complementary Medicine and Therapies, 23*, 313.

Mitchinson, A., Fletcher, C. E., & Trumble, E. (2022). Integrating massage therapy into the health care of female veterans. *Federal Practitioner, 39*(2), 86–92.

Moratelli, J. A., Veras, G., Lyra, V. B., da Silveria, J., Colombo, R., & de Azevedo Guimaraes, A. C. (2023). Evidence of the effects of dance interventions on adults mental health: A systematic review. *Journal of Dance Medicine & Science, 27*(4), 183–193.

Morikawa, S., Newman, R., & Amanat, Y. (2023). Relaxation and guided imagery for adults living with and beyond breast cancer (2018–2022). *American Journal of Occupational Therapy*, 77(1), 1–2.

National Center for Complementary and Integrative Health (NCCIH). (2019). *Massage therapy: What you need to know*. National Institutes of Health. U.S. Department of Health and Human Services. Retrieved May 19, 2024, from https://www.nccih.nih.gov/health/massage-therapy-what-you-need-to-know

National Center for Complementary and Integrative Health (NCCIH). (2021). *Complementary, alternative, or integrative health: What's in a name?* National Institutes of Health. U.S. Department of Health and Human Services. Retrieved March 27, 2024, from https://www.nccih.nih.gov/health/complementary-alternative-or-integrative-health-whats-in-a-name

National Center for Complementary and Integrative Health (NCCIH). (2022a). *Meditation and mindfulness: What you need to know*. National Institutes of Health. U.S. Department of Health and Human Services. Retrieved May 18, 2024, from https://www.nccih.nih.gov/health/meditation-and-mindfulness-what-you-need-to-know

National Center for Complementary and Integrative Health (NCCIH). (2022b). *Qigong: What you need to know*. National Institutes of Health. U.S. Department of Health and Human Services. Retrieved May 18, 2024, from https://www.nccih.nih.gov/health/qigong-what-you-need-to-know

National Center for Complementary and Integrative Health (NCCIH). (2022c). *Acupuncture: Effectiveness and safety*. National Institutes of Health. U.S. Department of Health and Human Services. Retrieved March 23, 2025, from https://www.nccih.nih.gov/health/acupuncture-effectiveness-and-safety

National Center for Complementary and Integrative Health (NCCIH) (2022d). *Music and health. What you need to know*. National Institutes of Health. U.S. Department of Health and Human Services. Retrieved May 18, 2024, from https://www.nccih.nih.gov/health/music-and-health-what-you-need-to-know

National Center for Complementary and Integrative Health (NCCIH). (2023a). *Relaxation techniques: What you need to know*. National Institutes of Health. U.S. Department of Health and Human Services. Retrieved May 18, 2024, from https://www.nccih.nih.gov/health/relaxation-techniques-what-you-need-to-know

National Center for Complementary and Integrative Health (NCCIH). (2023b). *Yoga: What you need to know*. National Institutes of Health. U.S. Department of Health and Human Services. Retrieved May 12, 2024, from https://www.nccih.nih.gov/health/yoga-what-you-need-to-know

National Center for Complementary and Integrative Health (NCCIH). (2024). *Herbs at a glance*. National Institutes of Health. U.S. Department of Health and Human Services. https://www.nccih.nih.gov/health/herbsataglance

National Institute of Environmental Health Sciences (NIEHS). (2022). Essential oils. https://www.niehs.nih.gov/health/topics/agents/essential-oils#:~:text=Essential%20oils%2C%20which%20are%20obtained,and%20effects%20on%20the%20body

National Institute of Health National Cancer Institute (2024). Acupuncture (PDQ®). Retrieved May 11, 2024, from https://www.cancer.gov/about-cancer/treatment/cam/hp/acupuncture-pdq

Nobakht, N., Kamgar, M., Tavanaei, M., Bilder, R. M., & Nobakht, E. (2023). Music and medicine: Promoting harmony for health. *American Journal of Medicine, 137*, 92–98.

Pan, B., Ge, L., Lai, H., Hou, L., Tian, C., Wang, Q., Yang, K., Lu, Y., Zhu, H., Li, M., Wang, D., Li, X., Zhang, Y., Gao, Y., Liu, M., Ding, G., Tian, J., & Yang, K. (2023). The comparative effectiveness and safety of insomnia drugs: A systematic review and network meta-analysis of 153 randomized trials. *Drugs, 83*(7), 587–619. https://doi.org/10.1007/s40265-023-01859-8

Pathan, F. K. M., Pandian, J. S., Shaikh, A. I., Ahsan, M., Nuhmani, S., Iqbal, A., & Alghadir, A. H. (2023). Effect of slow breathing exercise and progressive muscle relaxation technique in the individual with essential hypertension: a randomized controlled trial. *Medicine, 102*(47), e35792.

Rosendahl, J., Alldredge, C. T., & Haddenhorst, A. (2024). Meta-analytic evidence on the efficacy of hypnosis for mental and somatic health issues: A 20-year perspective. *Frontiers in Psychology, 14*, 1330238.

Sateia, M. J., Buysse, D. J., Krystal, A. D., Neubauer, D. N., & Heald, J. L. (2017). Clinical practice guideline for the pharmacologic treatment of chronic insomnia in adults: an American Academy of Sleep Medicine Clinical Practice Guideline. *Journal of Clinical Sleep Medicine, 13*(2), 307–349. https://doi.org/10.5664/jcsm.6470

Sattayakhom, A., Wichit, S., & Koomhin, P. (2023). The effects of essential oils on the nervous system: a scoping review. *Molecules, 28*, 3771.

Seid, A. A., Mohammed, A. A., & Hasen, A. A. (2023). Progressive muscle relaxation exercises in patients with COVID-19: Systematic review and meta-analysis. *Medicine, 102*(14), e33464.

Semenenko, E., Banergee, S., Olver, I., & Ashinze, P. (2023). Review of psychological interventions in patients with cancer. *Supportive Care in Cancer, 31*, 210.

Suárez-López, L. M., Bru-Luna, L. M., & Martí-Vilar, M. (2023). Influence of nutrition on mental health: Scoping review. *Healthcare, 11*(15), 2183. https://doi.org/10.3390/healthcare11152183

Szmaglinska, M., Andrew, L., Massey, D., & Kirk, D. (2024). Exploring the underutilized potential of clinical hypnosis; A scoping review of healthcare professionals' perceptions, knowledge, and attitudes. *International Journal of Clinical and Experimental Hypnosis*, 72(2), 109–138.

Talo, B., & Turan, G. B. (2023). Effects of progressive muscle relaxation exercises on patients with epilepsy on level of depression, quality of sleep, and quality of life: A randomized controlled trials. *Seizure: European Journal of Epilepsy, 105*, 29–36.

Tan, L., Liao, F. F., Long, L. Z., Ma, X. C., Peng, Y. X., Lu, J. M., Qu, H., & Fu, C. G. (2023a). Essential oils for treating anxiety: a systematic review of randomized controlled trials and network meta-analysis. *Frontiers in Public Health, 11*, 1144404. https://doi.org/10.3389/fpubh.2023.1144404

Tan, L., Strudwick, J., Deady, M., Bryant, R., & Harvey, S.B. (2023b). Mind-body exercise interventions for prevention of post-traumatic stress disorder in trauma-exposed populations: A systematic review and meta-analysis. *British Medical Journal Open, 13*, e064758.

Thompson, N., Hsu, M. H., Odell-Miller, H., Underwood, B. R., & Wolverson, E. (2024). Characteristics, outcomes, facilitators, and barriers for psychosocial interventions on inpatient mental health wards: A systematic review. *BMC Geriatrics, 24*, 364.

Tomaszewski, C., Belot, R. A., Essadek, A., Onumba-Bessonnet, H., & Clesse, C. (2023). Impact of dance therapy on adults with psychological trauma: A systematic review. *European Journal of Psychotraumatology, 14*(2), 2225152.

U.S. Department of Agriculture and U.S. Department of Health and Human Services. (2020). *Dietary Guidelines for Americans, 2020–2025* (9th ed.). https://www.dietaryguidelines.gov/

U.S. Department of Veterans Affairs. (2024a). Whole health: Meditation. https://www.va.gov/WHOLEHEALTH/professional-resources/Meditation.asp

U.S. Department of Veterans Affairs. (2024b). Whole health: Clinical hypnosis. https://www.va.gov/wholehealth/professional-resources/Clinical_Hypnosis.asp

U.S. Department of Veterans Affairs. (2024c). Whole health: Acupuncture. https://www.va.gov/wholehealth/professional-resources/Clinical_Hypnosis.asp

Van Lith, T., & Ettenberger, M. (2023). Arts-based therapies, practices, and interventions in health. *BMC Complementary Medicine and Therapies, 23*, 351.

Van Tilburg, M. A. L., Monis, E. L., Braumann, R. E., Fleishman, K., & Lamm, K. (2024). Hypnotherapy as a medical treatment: Evidence-based or pseudoscience? *Complementary Therapies in Clinical Practice, 55*, 101841.

Vanuytsel, T., Bercik, P., & Boeckxstaens, G. (2023). Understanding neuroimmune interactions in disorders of gut-brain interaction: from functional to immune-mediated disorders. *Gut*, 72(4), 787–798. https://doi.org/10.1136/gutjnl-2020-320633

Verma, S. (2023). Substance use disorders and role of complementary and integrative medicine/functional medicine. *Child & Adolescent Psychiatric Clinics of North America, 32*, 217–241.

Voss, M. E., Sandquist, L., Otremba, K., & Kreitzer, M. J. (2023). Integrative nursing: A framework for whole-person mental health care. *Creative Nursing, 29*(1), 23–41.

Wang, A., Wan, X., Zhuang, P., Jia, W., Ao, Y., Liu, X., Tian, Y., Zhu, L., Huang, Y., Yao, J., Wang, B., Wu, Y., Xu, Z., Wang, J., Yao, W., Jiao, J., & Zhang, Y. (2023). High fried food consumption impacts anxiety and depression due to lipid metabolism disturbance and neuroinflammation. *Proceedings of the National Academy of Sciences of the United States of America, 120*(18), e2221097120. https://doi.org/10.1073/pnas.2221097120

Xiong, R. G., Li, J., Cheng, J., Zhou, D. D., Wu, S. X., Huang, S. Y., Saimaiti, A., Yang, Z. J., Gan, R. Y., & Li, H. B. (2023). The role of gut microbiota in anxiety, depression, and other mental disorders as well as the protective effects of dietary components. *Nutrients*, *15*(14), 3258. https://doi.org/10.3390/nu15143258

Yang, C. P., Yang, C. C., Tsai, I. J., Lin, T. H., Chiou, Y. L., Wang, H. F., Chang, C. M., & Yih, K. H. (2023a). The immediate effects of lavender-based essential oil inhalation on subsequent polysomnography in people with poor sleep quality. *Journal of the Chinese Medical Association: JCMA*, *86*(7), 665–671. https://doi.org/10.1097/JCMA.0000000000000932

Yang, Y., Cao, D., Lyu, T., & Gao, W. (2023b). Meta-analysis of a mindfulness yoga exercise intervention on depression-based on intervention studies in China. *Frontiers in Psychology*, *14*, 1283172.

Yang, J., Lim, K. H., Mohabbat, A. B., Fokken, S. C., Johnson, D. E., Calva, J. J., Do, A., Mueller, M. R., Chon, T. Y., & Bauer, B. A. (2024). Robotics in massage: a systematic review. *Health Services Research and Managerial Epidemiology*, *11*, 1–13.

Yin, J., Yue, C., Song, Z., Sun, X., & Wen, X. (2023). The comparative effects of Tai chi versus non-mindful exercise on measures of anxiety, depression and general mental health: A systematic review and meta-analysis. *Journal of Affective Disorders*, *337*, 202–214.

Zhang, H., Wang, Z., Wang, G., Song, X., Qian, Y., Liao, Z., Sui, L., Ai, L., & Xia, Y. (2023). Understanding the connection between gut homeostasis and psychological stress. *The Journal of Nutrition*, *153*(4), 924–939. https://doi.org/10.1016/j.tjnut.2023.01.026

Zhang, Y., Long, Y., Yu, S., Li, D., Yang, M., Guan, Y., Zhang, D., Wan, J., Liu, S., Shi, A., Li, N., & Peng, W. (2021). Natural volatile oils derived from herbal medicines: a promising therapy way for treating depressive disorder. *Pharmacological Research*, *164*, 105376. https://doi.org/10.1016/j.phrs.2020.105376

Zielińska, M., Łuszczki, E., & Dereń, K. (2023). Dietary nutrient deficiencies and risk of depression (Review article 2018–2023). *Nutrients*, *15*(11), 2433. https://doi.org/10.3390/nu15112433

Zisopoulou, T., & Varvogli, L. (2023). Stress management methods in children and adolescents: past, present, and future. *Hormone Research in Paediatrics*, *96*, 97–107.

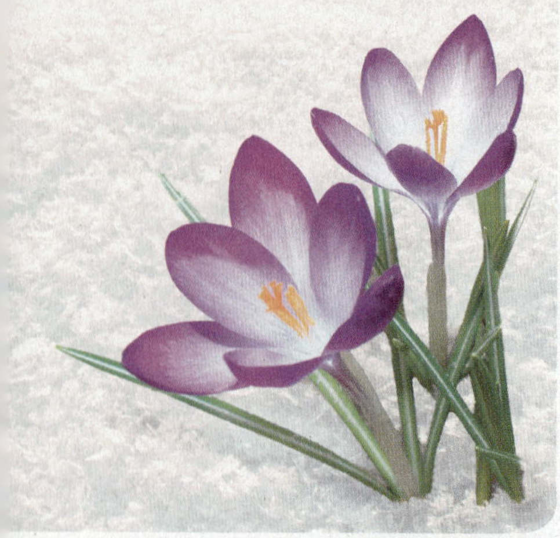

13 Cognitive Interventions in Psychiatric Nursing

Mary Ann Boyd

KEYCONCEPTS

- cognitive-behavioral therapy
- cultural adaptation
- rational emotive behavior therapy
- solution-focused brief therapy

LEARNING OBJECTIVES

After studying this chapter, you will be able to:

1. Discuss the history of cognitively based therapeutic interventions.
2. Identify the concepts underlying cognitive interventions.
3. Compare and contrast three forms of cognitively based therapies.
4. Apply cultural adaptation concepts to cognitive interventions.
5. Apply cognitive interventions in a clinical setting.
6. Describe the contexts in which psychiatric nurses use cognitive interventions.

KEY TERMS

• ABCDE • activating event • belief system • cognition • cognitive interventions • cognitive distortions • cognitive triad • compliments • dysfunctional consequences • exception questions • functional consequences • miracle questions • relationship questions • scaling questions • schema

INTRODUCTION

Psychiatric nurses use evidence-based cognitive interventions in a variety of practice settings (inpatient and outpatient). The knowledge and skills inherent in cognitively based interventions have been extensively studied and their effectiveness has been demonstrated for a variety of psychiatric disorders, especially depression (see Chapter 25) and anxiety disorders (see Chapter 27). Cognitive interventions are based on the concept of cognition.

Cognition can be defined as an internal process of perception, memory, and judgment through which an understanding of self and the world is developed. **Cognitive interventions** aim to change or reframe an individual's automatic thought patterns that have developed over time and which interfere with the individual's ability to function optimally. The skills and techniques that were developed on the basis of cognitive theory result in a new view of self and the environment.

Cognitive interventions had their beginnings in the long-term inpatient environment, but today they are a mainstay of psychiatric care in all settings and are used by all disciplines and at all levels of practice. Evidence from several studies, and as reinforced by meta-analysis of groups in the past decade, supports the use of cognitive therapies with a wide variety of psychological and psychiatric conditions, and it has been shown to be effective with diverse individuals in a variety of settings (Huey et al., 2023; Phiri et al., 2023). Cognitive therapies incorporate additional therapeutic modalities such as mindfulness and targeting for individuals with anxiety and depressive disorders (Hurwitz et al., 2023). The current chapter explains the theoretical perspectives and application of cognitive interventions.

DEVELOPMENT OF COGNITIVE THERAPIES

Cognitive therapy was first developed and implemented in the 1950s by Albert Ellis (1913–2007), a psychologist, who was uncomfortable with the nondirective Freudian and neo-Freudian approaches. According to Ellis, cognition, emotions, and behavior are integrated and holistic. From the 1950s until his death, Ellis continued to develop and refine his theory and therapeutic approach into what he calls rational emotive behavior therapy (REBT; Ellis et al., 2008).

Beginning in the 1960s, other cognitively based theories and therapeutic approaches were developed, the most prominent being cognitive-behavioral therapy (CBT) by Aaron Beck (see Chapter 6) (Beck, 2008). Steven de Shazer (1940–2005) and Insoo Kim Berg (1934–1997) developed solution-focused brief therapy (SFBT), an approach that is useful with individuals who have diagnoses such as substance use disorder, depression, obsessive–compulsive disorder, schizophrenia, and other psychiatric disorders (Franklin & Hai, 2021). These models will be discussed in the current chapter.

COGNITIVE THERAPY MODELS

Cognitive approaches are congruent with the standards of practice and are particularly effective in challenging care environments. Brief cognitive therapies offer approaches that can be applied within the therapeutic patient–nurse relationship and the nursing care plan. Patients undergoing cognitively based psychotherapy are frequently treated by an interdisciplinary team that supports this approach.

Cognitive-Behavioral Therapy

KEYCONCEPT Cognitive-behavioral therapy (CBT) is a highly structured psychotherapeutic method used to alter distorted beliefs and problem behaviors by identifying and replacing negative inaccurate thoughts and changing the rewards for behaviors.

In CBT, the relationship between thoughts, feelings, and behavior is examined and identified. CBT operates on the following assumptions:

- People are disturbed not by an event but by the perception of that event.
- Whenever and however a belief develops, the individual believes it.
- Work and practice can modify beliefs that create difficulties in living.

Figure 13.1 depicts the interaction of individual experiences, perception of these experiences, and the unique thoughts attached to these experiences that influence the development of beliefs (functional or dysfunctional). The individual develops an explanation of their relationship to their environment and to other people from these beliefs. Dysfunctional thinking develops from a variety of human experiences and can become the predominant way the world is viewed. To quote from Shakespeare's *Hamlet*, "For there is nothing either good or bad but thinking makes it so."

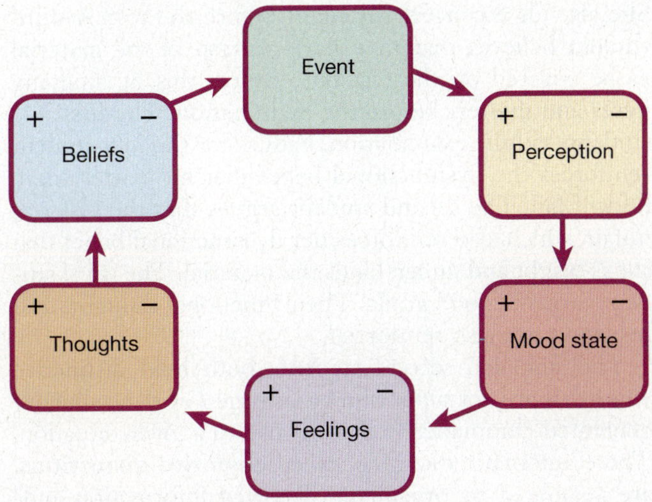

FIGURE 13.1 Model of perception, thoughts, and mood states: the cycle of cognition.

Thoughts have a powerful effect on emotion and behavior. By changing dysfunctional thinking, an individual can alter their emotional reaction to a situation and reinterpret the meaning of an event. That is, by identifying, analyzing, and changing thoughts and behaviors that are counterproductive, feelings such as helplessness, anxiety, and depression can be reduced. The goal of CBT is to restructure how an individual perceives events in their life to facilitate behavioral and emotional change.

Cognitive Processes

Three cognitive processes are involved in the development of common mental disorders: the cognitive triad, cognitive distortions, and schema.

The **cognitive triad** includes thoughts about oneself, the world, and the future. Accumulation of thoughts about oneself is reflected in spoken and unspoken beliefs and moods that grow out of these beliefs. Emotions and behavior reflect the strength of the accumulated beliefs. Dysfunctional thoughts about the self are usually overly negative or overly positive, whereas functional thoughts more closely reflect the reality of the perceived situation. For example, one student has the belief that learning is very difficult for him and that he will fail the examination no matter how hard he studies. He does not study for the examination because he believes that he will fail anyway. A second student believes that she is very bright, understands the material, and does not need to study.

She attends a concert the night before the test. A third student believes that they have a grasp of the material to be covered on the test but ensures this by studying notes and the text before the examination. The first two students fail the examination. Failure for the first student reinforces the dysfunctional belief that no matter what, he will fail. The second student argues that the test was unfair, which also reinforces her dysfunctional belief that she is bright and understands the material. The third student earned a good grade. Their functional thoughts and behaviors are also reinforced.

The first and second students both hold distinctive views that are not supported by empirical evidence but are generated automatically in response to a given situation. These automatic thoughts, called **cognitive distortions**, are generated by organizing distorted information and/or inaccurate interpretations of a situation. This "twisted thinking" occurs in a variety of ways such as *overgeneralization* (asserting that something general is always true about an event, situation, or group of people), *personalizing* (applying a general statement to oneself), *catastrophizing* (viewing or talking about an event as worse than it actually was), and *selective abstraction* (selectively abstracting negative information from stressful events) (see Box 13.1).

Schemas are the individual's life rules that function as a sieve or filter. They allow only information compatible with the internal picture of self and the world to be brought to the individual's awareness. Schemas develop in early childhood and become relatively fixed by middle childhood. Schemas are an accumulation of learning and experience from the individual's genetic makeup, family and school environments, peer relationships, and society as a whole. Ethnicity, culture, gender, and religious affiliation influence schema development, as well as the age of the individual at the time a given event occurs, the influence of the individuals or circumstances involved on how that event is perceived, and the relative strength of that influence. In the earlier example, the first student believes that he is not intelligent. This belief could have originated in early childhood if the student were constantly unfavorably compared with a sibling. This schema increases vulnerability in a host of interpersonal situations, particularly those that relate to scholarly endeavors. The second student was overly praised by parents and other relatives and developed a schema of being more accomplished than most. The third student was realistic about the amount of work needed to pass the test and did not demonstrate any cognitive distortions.

BOX 13.1

Clinical Judgment Vignette: Cognitive Distortions

Amy has been working on a group project with her classmates in a psychiatric nursing course. Part of the process for the group project is to provide anonymous peer evaluation of the work of each of the six group members. Amy received a score of 10/10 from four of the members, a 7/10 from another, and 5/10 from the sixth. Amy thinks, "I guess I did not do a good job on this project. I never do anything right. My classmates look down on me."

Building Clinical Judgment

1. What cognitive distortions does Amy exhibit?
2. How would you approach Amy's cognitive distortion?

Implementing Cognitive-Behavioral Therapy

The use of CBT is based on a collaborative therapeutic relationship in which mutual trust develops through promoting patients' strengths and control over their own lives. CBT assumes that individuals have the innate ability to solve their own problems; thus, the overarching treatment goal is for the patient to be able to engage in self-care, independent of professional assistance.

In CBT, goals are developed in partnership and supply a forward-looking focus on what "can be" in the future as opposed to "what happened" in the past. The present serves as a platform from which current perceptions of earlier events can be reexamined. Movement toward goals is facilitated by strategies designed to engage the patient in the service of their own mental health. Strategies emerge when nurse and patient develop a working conceptualization of the issue or problem as the patient sees it. The nurse educates the patient about the therapeutic approach. An agenda is mutually established for each therapeutic interaction. Techniques that focus on both cognition and behavior are used to promote patient growth.

Engagement and Assessment

The first step in CBT is engagement and assessment. In this phase, the therapist establishes rapport with the patient and develops the theme that problems are manageable. The patient's definition of the problem that brought them into treatment is explored through a series of open-ended questions. A problem list is developed and reframed into manageable goals that are prioritized. The prioritized list forms the agenda for the treatment plan and structures the content of each individual session. A contract is developed for a number of sessions (frequently 10–12). The therapist seeks information about the patient's strengths and successes on which to base reexamination and reframing of negative beliefs and to design interventions. During all sessions, the therapist summarizes issues identified and develops homework assignments that enhance and expand the work done during the sessions.

Intervention Framework

Specific interventions used with CBT, in addition to the interaction that takes place in the therapy sessions, revolve around carefully crafted homework assignments that the patient works on in the time between sessions. Subsequently, sessions may be scheduled regularly once or twice a month. Typical homework assignments include evaluating the accuracy of automatic thoughts and beliefs. It is important for the therapist to realize that the thoughts an individual has about a problem are not beliefs. In CBT, the therapist helps the patient identify the underlying belief, and then they:

- explore the evidence that supports or refutes the belief about the event,
- identify alterative explanations for the event, and
- examine the real implications if the belief is true. (e.g., "What is the worst thing that could happen?")

In the sessions, the therapist challenges negative beliefs and helps the patient examine the "self-talk" that helps to sustain these beliefs. Cognitive techniques focus on the patient's patterns of automatic thinking, first identifying what they are by examining the patient's recurrent patterns in everyday life and then testing the validity of these automatic thoughts.

Other tools that are used to help change the patient's self-perception include bibliotherapy (the use of books that offer alternative thoughts and responses), journaling, and keeping a diary focused on emotional and behavioral responses to upsetting situations that documents minor changes that might otherwise go unnoticed. The patient is also encouraged to make note of positive events and positive thoughts about themselves and their ability to cope with negative events. These positive thoughts and effective coping responses are reinforced in interactions with the therapist. As goals are developed at the beginning of each therapy session, the last few minutes are spent reviewing the progress toward the goals for that day.

Evaluation and Termination

Evaluation and termination begin with the original contract when patient and therapist determine the number of sessions. The patient's progress toward treatment goals is continually evaluated, and the patient is urged to become more self-reliant and independent. As progress is never a continuous upward process, therapists prepare the patient for setbacks by acknowledging that setbacks are normal and expected and crafting ways in which the patient can deal with them. It is common for the time between sessions to lengthen as the final session approaches. At the final session, the use of "booster" sessions is discussed. Frequently, a session is scheduled in 6 months to do a quick "check-up" and review continuing progress.

Strengths and Limitations of Cognitive-Behavioral Therapy

One of the strengths of CBT lies in the body of empirical evidence supporting the effectiveness of these interventions (Chand et al., 2023). Many studies show positive, sustained improvement in people treated with this form of intervention. Critics, however, identify some limitations. Chief among the limitations identified is the concern that the therapeutic relationship, long believed to be the main factor in patient improvement, may be forgotten in the rigid adherence to specific techniques. Others believe that change is dependent on the patient developing a clear understanding of their belief system and the origin of that system; thus, CBT may not be effective with individuals who have thought disorders and other issues that interfere with the ability to do so.

Rational Emotive Behavior Therapy

KEYCONCEPT Rational emotive behavior therapy (REBT) is a psychotherapeutic approach that proposes that unrealistic and irrational beliefs cause many emotional problems. It is a form of CBT with a primary emphasis on changing irrational beliefs that cause emotional distress into thoughts that are more reasonable and rational.

REBT is based on the assumption that people are born with the potential to be rational (self-constructive) and irrational (self-defeating). Ellis believes that highly cognitive, active, directive homework assignments and structured therapies are likely to be more effective in a shorter time than other therapies and that irrational thinking, self-damaging habituations, wishful thinking, and intolerance are exacerbated by culture and family groups (Ellis et al., 2008).

Rational Emotive Behavior Therapy Framework

The basic framework for REBT uses the acronym **ABCDE** (see Box 13.2). The **activating event** may be either external or internal and not necessarily an actual event, but it may also be an emotion or a thought/expectation. For example, an individual who is lonely and feels isolated but is uncomfortable in interpersonal situations may see a flyer advertising a gathering of people who are interested in discussing solutions to global warming and would really like to attend (**A**ctivating event).

BOX 13.2

The Rational Emotive Behavior Therapy ABCDE Framework

Activating event that triggers automatic thoughts and emotions
Beliefs that underlie the thoughts and emotions
Consequences of this automatic process
Dispute or challenge unreasonable expectations
Effective outlook developed by disputing or challenging negative belief systems

However, when this individual thinks about going to the gathering, they imagine going into the room where they do not know anybody and someone trying to engage them in conversation. Their imagination provides a picture of not being able to respond and leaving the room after suffering great embarrassment (**B**elief system: "I am a failure in social situations, and everybody can see what a loser I am."). They decide not to go (**C**onsequences of their belief system).

Belief systems are shaped by rationality, which is self-constructive, and irrationality, which is self-defeating. Rational beliefs are flexible and lead to reasonable evaluations of negative activating events. For example, after a low grade on an examination, instead of believing "I am stupid" or "that instructor is out to get me," student might conclude that "I earned a low grade on the test; I really need to work to develop a better understanding of the content," or "I think I need to get help with my test-taking skills." Other rational beliefs might be "I really didn't have time to study; so, I can accept this grade and just move on." In other words, "I don't like it, but I can live with it." Rational beliefs accept that human beings are fallible and reject absolutes such as always and never.

Irrational beliefs promote dysfunctional negative emotions that in turn lead to psychic pain and discomfort. Behaviors directed at relief of this pain tend to be self-defeating: "I can't fight the system; I will never succeed in this class." There are five themes common in irrational beliefs:

- A demand: "This *must* happen."
- Absolute thinking: "All or nothing at all."
- Catastrophizing: Exaggerating negative consequences of an event.
- Low frustration tolerance: Everything should be easy.
- Global evaluations of human worth: "People can be rated, and some are better than others."

Dysfunctional consequences of the interaction between A (activating event) and B (belief system) follow from absolute, rigid, and irrational beliefs whereas **functional consequences** follow from flexible and rational beliefs. For example, demands about self based on "musts" reinforce dysfunctional beliefs such as, "I must do well and be approved by significant others, and if I'm not, then it's awful." The consequences of these beliefs are often anxiety, depression, shame, and guilt that lead to the inability to develop or achieve life's goals or to develop satisfying interpersonal relationships. Self-regard that is dependent on the approval of others demands that others "treat me fairly and considerately; it's terrible I can't bear it when you don't." Thus, when fairness and consideration are not forthcoming, passive-aggressiveness, anger, rage, and violence may erupt. Demands that the world or life be exactly as one wants can also lead to self-pity as well as problems of self-discipline and addictive behaviors.

Rational Emotive Behavior Therapy Interventions

REBT uses role-playing, assertion training, desensitization, humor, operant conditioning, suggestion, support, and other interventions. According to Ellis, there are two basic forms of REBT: general and preferential. General REBT is synonymous with CBT and teaches patients rational and healthy behavior. Preferential REBT includes general REBT but also emphasizes a profound philosophic change. It teaches patients how to dispute irrational ideas and unhealthy behaviors and to become more creative, scientific, and skeptical thinkers (Ellis et al., 2008). The therapist uses the ABCDE model in a structured manner (Box 13.2). A major challenge for the therapist is to teach the patient the difference between thoughts and beliefs. Automatic thoughts are not irrational beliefs but are inferences about the belief. The focus of interventions during the therapy sessions (frequently several weeks or months apart) is on developing rational beliefs to replace those that are irrational and interfere with the patient's quality of life. Figure 13.2 examines the sequence of treatment used in REBT.

Solution-Focused Brief Therapy

KEYCONCEPT Solution-focused brief therapy (SFBT) focuses on solutions rather than problems. This approach does not challenge the existence of problems but proposes that problems are best understood in relation to their solutions. Solution-focused therapy assists the client in exploring life without the problem (De Shazer, 1985; Miller & Berg, 1995; Żak & Pękala, 2024).

Although SFBT is basically a cognitive approach, it differs in philosophy and approach from other cognitively based approaches. The primary difference is the de-emphasis on the patient's "problems," or symptoms, and an emphasis on what is functional and healthful. SFBT assists the patient in exploring life without the problem, and it asserts that what is expected to happen influences what the patient does. By discovering what future the client sees as worth striving for, the present becomes important to that future. Otherwise, there is no sense in the patient doing something different or seeing something in a different light. Empirical evidence exists that supports the use of solution-focused approaches (Jerome et al., 2023).

Solution-focused theory views the patient as an individual with a collection of strengths and successes as opposed to a diagnosis and collection of symptoms. The individual is the expert and becomes empowered through the therapeutic process. Solution-focused approaches emphasize the importance of collaboration and that change is inevitable and necessary for the individual to progress (Jerome et al., 2023).

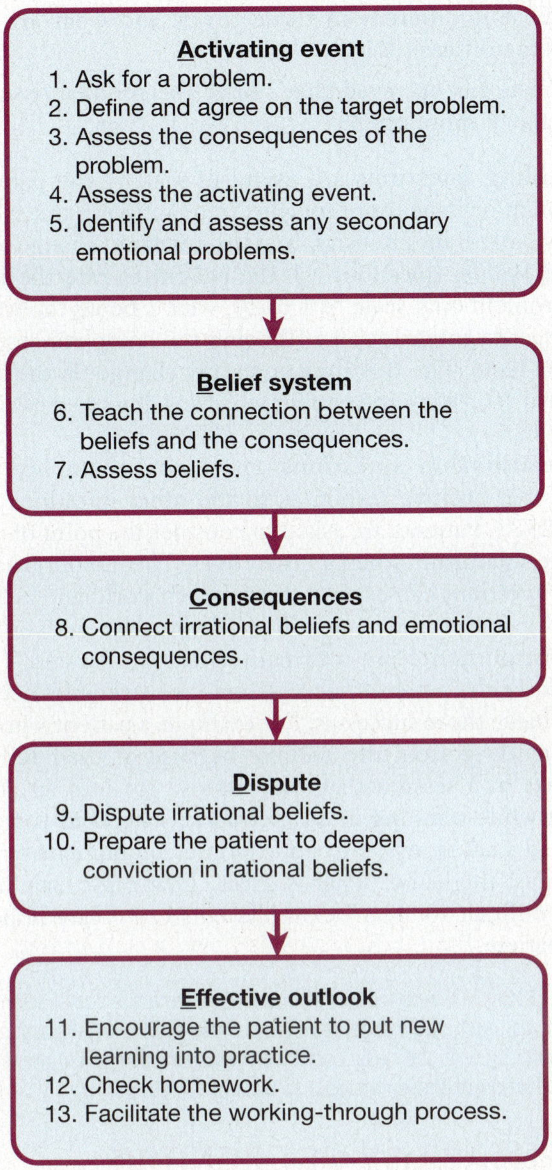

FIGURE 13.2 Rational emotive behavior therapy sequence of treatment (following the REBT framework's acronym, **ABCDE**).

Solution-Focused Behavior Therapy Assumptions

SFBT assumes that change is constant and inevitable. Everyone changes constantly and is never the same from 1 minute to the next. An individual interacts, if only in a minimal way, with a constantly changing environment. Minor changes can lead to larger changes, and the stimulus to change comes from a variety of sources. Constant change and its "ripple effect" direct the strategies and interventions used by the therapist. Both assumptions and strategies point the patient toward a positive, future-oriented change. Box 13.3 lists the assumptions that underlie this approach.

BOX 13.3

Solution-Focused Behavior Therapy Assumptions

1. People have the strengths and resources needed to solve their problems; therefore, the therapist's role is to recognize and emphasize these by amplifying them primarily through asking questions that enable a collaborative approach to constructing solutions.
2. It is not necessary to know a lot about the complaint and its origins or functions in order to resolve it.
3. Define and dissect the "problem" from the perspective of the patient and look for exceptions to the "problem" in the patient's life.
4. Even long-standing issues can be resolved in a relatively brief period of time.
5. There is no right or wrong way to see things.
6. Change is most likely to occur when the focus is on what is changeable.
7. The job of the therapist is to identify and amplify change and maintain a focus on the present and the future.
8. The therapist and patient cocreate reality, utilizing what the patient perceives is "truth," and develop small, concrete, specific, and reality-based goals that are realistic in the context of the patient's life.
9. The therapist expects change and movement and that expectation is inherent in the questions used and the attitude of the therapist.

Source: O'Hanlon, W. H., & Weiner-Davis, M. (2003). *In search of solutions: A new direction in psychotherapy*. W. W. Norton & Company.

Solution-Focused Behavior Therapy Interventions

In SFBT, the therapist takes a position of curiosity in learning about the patient, as opposed to an expert to whom the individual has come to be helped. This curiosity is manifested in the questions and techniques that are integral to this approach and enable the development of realistic goals at each session. Questions used in eliciting the "problem" (frequently referred to as the "issue(s)" to avoid focusing on the "problem") seek specific information. Examples of questioning in the initial session might include the following:

1. What brought you here today? What is going on that made you choose to seek help?
2. Give me a recent example of how that was demonstrated in your life.
3. Who was present when this happened? What did they say and do, and what did you say or do? And then what happened?
4. When does this kind of thing happen most often?
5. Where is it likely to occur?
6. Where is it least likely to occur?
7. Is there a particular time (of day, month, and year) when this is unlikely to happen?
8. How does this interfere with your life, your relationships, self-image, etc.?

If your partner/significant other/coworker were here now, how would they say that you were trying to solve the issue or problem?

Interventions in SFBT focus on the achievement of specific, concrete, and achievable goals developed in the collaboration between therapist and patient. These goals, formed using the patient's language, are specific and focus on strengths. Primary techniques used to facilitate progress toward goal attainment are skillfully crafted questions that include the use of the "miracle question," exceptions, scaling, relationship questions, as well as the use of feedback, with an emphasis on complimenting any small, goal-oriented change the patient makes. Feedback conveys to the patient that the therapist has listened carefully and recognizes that working toward a goal of change is difficult and requires hard work.

Miracle questions ask the patient to describe how life might be different for them if something miraculous happened (see Box 13.4 for a sample scenario and questions).

Other ways of facilitating a similar focus on what the solution would look like are to ask the patient to keep track of what goes well in their life that they would like to see happen again. The patient is encouraged to keep a written list of what they have noticed and bring it to the next session.

Exception questions are rooted in the belief that nothing is constantly present at the same level of intensity, so that there are fluctuations on how the patient experiences "the problem." Exception questions are used to help the patient identify times when they are not bothered by the issue or it causes less distress. The role of the therapist is then to amplify these times for the patient. Questions used to elicit exceptions may be as follows:

1. When do you not have that problem/issue?
2. How do you explain that the problem/issue does not happen then?
3. What is different in those times, and what are you doing differently?
4. What has occurred that causes the problem/issue to happen more often?

BOX 13.4

Miracle Questions

"I want you to pretend that tonight after you go to bed and are soundly asleep, a miracle occurs. The miracle is that the issues that have been bothering you and interfering in your life disappear. Since you have been asleep, you are not aware that the miracle has occurred when you wake up in the morning."

1. What would be your first clue that something was different for you?
2. How will your life be different?
3. What will you be doing instead of __________?
4. How will you be doing this?
5. Besides yourself, who will be the first to notice that there is something different about you?
6. What will that individual say or do?
7. How will you respond differently than you might if the issue or problem was still present?

Scaling questions are useful in making the patient's problem or issue more specific, in quantifying the exceptions noted in intensity, and in tracking change over time. Scaling questions ask the patient to rate the issue or problem on a scale of 1 to 10, with 1 being the worst, or greatest intensity, and 10 being the complete absence of the issue. The therapist notes any change on the scale toward 10, asking the patient what was done to make that happen.

Relationship questions are used to amplify and reinforce positive responses to the other questions (see Box 13.4). Patients are asked to consider the point of view of the significant others in their lives. The use of relationship questions can expand the patient's world and help to develop and maintain empathic relationships with others.

Compliments are affirmations of the patient. They reinforce the patient's successes and the strengths needed to achieve those successes. For example, a patient who has frequently gotten into trouble because of their temper reports in a session that they almost got into an argument while standing in a supermarket checkout lane but instead walked away. An appropriate compliment by the therapist might be "That is great. That must have been very difficult for you." Compliments can create hope in the patient.

NCLEXNOTE Application of knowledge from the social sciences such as psychology underlies many of the psychosocial questions. Familiarity with the basic cognitive therapy models strengthens the application of these concepts to patient situations.

APPLICABILITY OF COGNITIVE THERAPIES FOR DIVERSE POPULATIONS

Western cultural models of independence and assertiveness underlie cognitive-behavioral theory and practice, most likely because the research has focused on White populations. Independence and assertiveness may conflict with the patient's cultural values, such as interdependence and family control. For cognitive approaches to be relevant and accessible to individuals from underrepresented ethnic and cultural groups, they can be modified to consider language, culture, and context that is compatible with the patient's cultural patterns, meanings, and values (Huey et al., 2023).

KEYCONCEPT Cultural adaptation is systematic modification of an evidence-based practice or intervention to consider language, culture, and context that is compatible with cultural patterns, meanings, and values.

Family involvement, use of appropriate language terms, and an understanding of psychopathology from a culture viewpoint are important considerations when implementing cognitive approaches (Huey et al., 2023). Adaptations are dependent on a clinician's sound knowledge of the culture and the patient's degree of alignment with the culture. Recognizing and focusing on culturally relevant symptoms such as dizziness or insomnia creates credibility with the patient and family. In some cultures, there are catastrophic beliefs about symptoms. For example, dizziness may indicate a weak heart and an imminent heart attack. To alleviate stress and anxiety, it is important for the nurse to teach the patient about other causes of dizziness. The nurse should be familiar with and use cultural metaphors, stories, and analogies in conveying information. Cultural knowledge should extend to understanding and respecting religious traditions. Many cultures have certain methods of relieving stress and pain. Techniques from local traditions should be incorporated into care planning (Swihart et al., 2023).

USE OF COGNITIVE THERAPIES IN PSYCHIATRIC NURSING

The context of practice is evolving for psychiatric nurses. Cognitive interventions can be incorporated as a part of nursing care in any setting. Length of stay for patients in inpatient settings is becoming shorter every year. Patients admitted to inpatient settings are acutely ill and dealing with more complex issues than ever before. More psychiatric care occurs in prisons than in psychiatric hospitals. More and more the focus of practice is in the community, private homes, and primary care settings rather than in specialty hospitals.

Inpatient Settings

Solution-focused therapy is one of the brief cognitive therapies used by psychiatric nurses in acute inpatient psychiatric settings. SFBT's emphasis on strengths fits well with the values of psychiatric nurses, and the techniques used are well within their scope of practice. Solution-focused approaches have been effective with people who were experiencing mental health challenges (see Box 13.5).

Other cognitive therapeutic techniques used in inpatient settings include journaling and "homework" assignments that focus on education about diagnoses and medications, as well as on group process. These interventions seem to work well in conjunction with shortened length of stay in inpatient settings.

Primary Care Settings

Cognitive interventions in primary care settings are useful and cost-effective. For example, insomnia, depression, chronic pain, and anxiety in people who have had breast cancer have been successfully treated with CBT (Akkol-Solakoglu & Hevey, 2023; Bhattacharya et al., 2023; Crowther et al., 2023: Ploutarchou et al., 2023).

Community Settings

In community settings, cognitive approaches are used in combination with a broad array of interpersonal, behavioral, educational, and pharmacologic interventions. Cognitive interventions are used within a holistic evaluation of patients that includes a complete health history and physical examination and evaluation of possible co-occurring disorders such as depression and alcohol

BOX 13.5

Research for Evidence-Based Practice: Solution-Focused Brief Therapy (SFBT) Effects on Self-Care and Mental Health

Dong, H., Zhang, D., & Wang, T. (2024). The effects of solution-focused brief therapy on self-care and mental health among older adults at risk of coronary heart disease: a randomized controlled trial. Geriatric Nursing, 57, *11–16. https://doi.org/10.1016/j.gerinurse.2024.02.029*

THE QUESTION: Is a nursing approach based on SFBT effective in improving self-care and in alleviating anxiety and depression among older adults at risk for coronary artery disease (CHD)?

METHODS: A total of 120 older adults at risk of CHD living in the community were recruited for the study. The control group (n = 60) received the usual care including (1) health education lectures and pamphlets about CHD, (2) guidance on diet, alcohol consumption, and tobacco cessation, (3) guidance on exercise and daily activity, and (4) self-monitoring and guidance on psychological regulation. The intervention group attended 12 sessions implemented every 2 weeks for 6 months. Each session lasted 20 to 35 minutes. The content included (1) describing the problem (2 sessions), (2) establishing a constructive objective (2 sessions), (3) probing for exceptions (2 sessions), (4) providing feedback on implementation (3 sessions), and (5) evaluating the progress (2 sessions). Changes in self-care ability, depression, and anxiety were assessed with standardized, reliable instruments: Self-Care Ability Scale for the Elderly, Self-Rating Depression Scale, and Self-Rating Anxiety Scale. Parametric statistics were used for group comparisons.

FINDINGS: At the end of 6 months, the intervention group had significantly higher self-concept, self-skills, self-care awareness, and health knowledge than at baseline and compared to the control group (p values <0.05). The intervention group had significantly lower depression and anxiety scores at baseline and compared to the control group scores (all p values <0.05).

IMPLICATIONS FOR NURSING: SBFT can be considered as a possible intervention in helping patients at risk of CHD improve self-care and reduce depression and anxiety. More research is needed.

and other drug use or misuse. In particular, the use of questioning such as that integral to solution-focused approaches elicits strengths in a relatively brief time and can provide a means for the nurse to support positive coping. The focus on realistic goal development provides a means of evaluation of patient progress.

Home settings are also conducive to the implementation of cognitive techniques. Small, concrete, specific goals developed in a naturalistic setting such as the home can create meaningful change for the whole family. CBT and SFBT approaches are very effective in primary care settings where time with patients is short. Goal setting, use of scaling questions, and compliments can be done in a 15-minute interaction.

SUMMARY OF KEY POINTS

- Cognitive therapies have a long history in mental health care and have support as evidence-based interventions effective in several mental disorders.
- Psychiatric nurses use cognitive interventions in a variety of settings. Cognitive therapies serve as the framework for psychotherapy as well as interdisciplinary treatment.
- CBT focuses on dysfunctional thinking through the examination of the cognitive triad, cognitive distortions, and schema.
- REBT assumes that people are born with the tendency to be rational and irrational. Using the ABCDE framework, REBT focuses on identifying and changing irrational beliefs that lead to negative consequences.
- SFBT identifies the possible solutions before addressing the problem.

DEVELOPING CLINICAL JUDGMENT

1. Compare and contrast the three cognitive therapies (cognitive-behavioral therapy [CBT], rational emotive behavior therapy [REBT], and solution-focused brief therapy [SFBT]) in terms of emphasis.
2. A patient has recently been fired from their job, which is the third job loss within 1 year. The patient is depressed but denies suicidal thoughts. They tell you they are a failure and can never get and keep a job. Discuss how a therapist using each of the three cognitive therapies—CBT, REBT, and SFBT—would view and treat this patient.
3. A patient from an underrepresented group is admitted to a mental health unit for severe depression. The individual is highly aligned with a cultural belief that explains depression as a heart problem and is requesting heart medicine. How would the nurse approach this patient?
4. A nurse manager plans to use CBT as a theoretical model for an inpatient unit. Discuss the interventions that could be used on an inpatient unit that applies the CBT model.

REFERENCES

Akkol-Solakoglu, S., & Hevey, D. (2023). Internet-delivered cognitive behavioural therapy for depression and anxiety in breast cancer survivors: Results from a randomised controlled trial. *Psycho-oncology*, *32*(3), 446–456. https://doi.org/10.1002/pon.6097

Beck, A. T. (2008). The evolution of the cognitive model of depression and its neurobiological correlates. *American Journal of Psychiatry*, *165*(8), 969–977.

Bhattacharya, S., Goicoechea, C., Heshmati, S., Carpenter, J. K., & Hofmann, S. G. (2023). Efficacy of cognitive behavioral therapy for anxiety-related disorders: A meta-analysis of recent literature. *Current Psychiatry Reports*, *25*(1), 19–30. https://doi.org/10.1007/s11920-022-01402-8

Chand, S. P., Kuckel, D. P., & Huecker, M. R. (2023). Cognitive behavior therapy. In *StatPearls*. StatPearls Publishing. (nih.gov)

Crowther, M. E., Saunders, W. J., Sletten, T. L., Drummond, S. P. A., & Bei, B. (2023). Tailoring cognitive behavioural therapy for insomnia across contexts, conditions, and individuals: What do we know, where do we go? *Journal of Sleep Research*, e14023. https://doi.org/10.1111/jsr.14023

De Shazer, S. (1985). *Keys to solution in brief therapy*. W. W. Norton & Company.

Ellis, A., Abrams, M., & Lidia, D. A. (2008). *Personality theories: Critical perspectives*. Sage.

Franklin, C., & Hai, A. H. (2021). Solution-focused brief therapy for substance use: a review of the literature. *Health & Social Work*, *46*(2), 103–114. https://doi.org/10.1093/hsw/hlab002

Huey, S. J., Jr, Park, A. L., Galán, C. A., & Wang, C. X. (2023). Culturally responsive cognitive behavioral therapy for ethnically diverse populations. *Annual Review of Clinical Psychology*, *19*, 51–78. https://doi.org/10.1146/annurev-clinpsy-080921-072750

Hurwitz, C., Shiner, C. T., Sharrock, M. J., Millard, M., & Mahoney, A. (2023). Mindfulness-enhanced internet-based cognitive behavioural therapy for anxiety and depression: Outcomes in routine care. *Journal of Affective Disorders*, *341*, 1–7. https://doi.org/10.1016/j.jad.2023.08.073

Jerome, L., McNamee, P., Abdel-Halim, N., Elliot, K., & Woods, J. (2023). Solution-focused approaches in adult mental health research: a conceptual literature review and narrative synthesis. *Frontiers in Psychiatry*, *14*, 1068006. https://doi.org/10.3389/fpsyt.2023.1068006

Miller, S. D., & Berg, I. K. (1995). *The miracle method: A radically new approach to problem drinking*. W. W. Norton & Company.

Phiri, P., Clarke, I., Baxter, L., Zeng, Y. T., Shi, J. Q., Tang, X. Y., Rathod, S., Soomro, M. G., Delanerolle, G., & Naeem, F. (2023). Evaluation of a culturally adapted cognitive behavior therapy-based, third-wave therapy manual. *World Journal of Psychiatry*, *13*(1), 15–35. https://doi.org/10.5498/wjp.v13.i1.15

Ploutarchou, G., Savva, C., Karagiannis, C., Pavlou, K., O'Sullivan, K., & Korakakis, V. (2023). The effectiveness of cognitive behavioural therapy in chronic neck pain: A systematic review with meta-analysis. *Cognitive Behaviour Therapy*, *52*(5), 523–563. https://doi.org/10.1080/16506073.2023.2236296

Swihart, D. L., Yarrarapu, S. N. S., & Martin, R. L. (2023). Cultural religious competence in clinical practice. In *StatPearls*. StatPearls Publishing. https://www.ncbi.nlm.nih.gov/books/NBK493216

Żak, A. M., & Pękala, K. (2024). Effectiveness of solution-focused brief therapy: an umbrella review of systematic reviews and meta-analyses. *Psychotherapy*, 1–13. https://doi.org/10.1080/10503307.2024.2406540

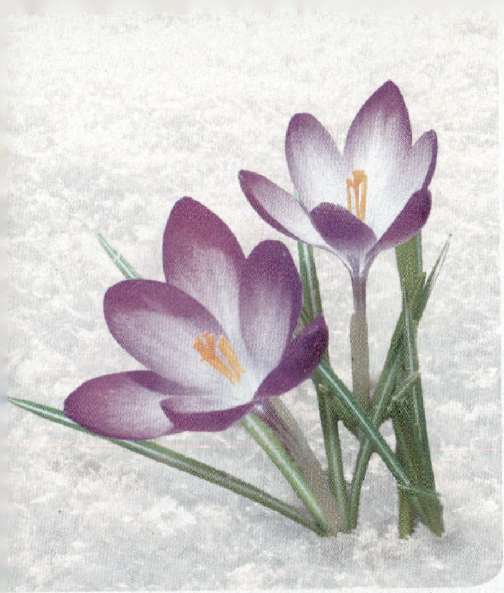

14 Group Interventions

Rita Tadych and Mary Ann Boyd

KEYCONCEPTS

- group
- group dynamics
- group process
- group counseling
- scope of practice

LEARNING OBJECTIVES

After studying this chapter, you will be able to:

1. Discuss concepts used in leading groups.
2. Compare the roles that group members can assume.
3. Identify important aspects of leading a group, such as member selection, leadership skills, seating arrangements, and ways of dealing with challenging behaviors of group members.
4. Distinguish types of groups: psychoeducation, support, psychotherapy, and self-help.
5. Describe common nursing intervention groups.

KEY TERMS

• closed group • cohesion • co-leadership • communication pathways • counseling • direct leadership • dyad • facilitate • formal group member roles • group leader • group themes • groupthink • indirect leadership • individual roles • informal group member roles • maintenance roles • open group • practice-based evidence (PBI) • task-related roles • triad

INTRODUCTION

Along with therapeutic interactions with individual patients, group counseling interventions are an added clinical nursing strategy in mental health promotion and recovery. Additional clinical strategies are available to the nurse using group work, but it is a complex therapeutic undertaking. There is more content, more dynamics, and more process.

A group experience has a social context that can help members enhance self-understanding, conquer unwanted thoughts and feelings, and learn new behaviors. In this multipatient treatment format, there are several pathways for members to learn from each other as well as from the leader. Additionally, group interventions are efficient because several patients can participate at one time and they can be used in a variety of health care delivery system settings.

Groups can vary in purpose from being a social group attending a local ball game to an intensive psychotherapy group. Group psychoeducation interventions, for example, are used in inpatient or outpatient settings and are delivered in formats such as face-to-face, virtual encounters, or mobile applications. Social media platforms are used by and with patients where engagement takes place via user-generated content, personalized profiles, likes, shares, comments, chats, and discussion with multiple others. This chapter discusses group concepts, considerations in group leadership, and types of groups that nurses commonly lead.

KEYCONCEPT A **group** is two or more people who develop interactive relationships and share at least one common goal or issue. As a system, *a group is more than the sum of its parts.* A group develops its own personality, patterns of interaction, and rules of behavior.

Ethnicity and Cultural Considerations

With an increasingly culturally and ethnically diverse population, nurses must focus attention on creating a physically and psychologically safe and equitable space for everyone in the group regardless of cultural origins. Multicultural groups are complex because members' diverse values and beliefs may generate insecurities in other members. A **group leader** needs the knowledge and skills to manage these insecurities (Honig & Martinez-Taboada Kurtz, 2022).

Recognizing the extent of one's own knowledge concerning the group's cultural mix—along with sensitivity to one's own values, prejudices, preconceived ideas, stereotypes, and personal limitations—is critical to engaging effectively as a trustworthy group leader. Nurses need to engage in strategies that demonstrate their lifelong journey toward cultural humility (see Chapter 3). These strategies involve using verbal and nonverbal communication skills that include, but are not limited to, being able to provide appropriate, effective, empathic, and inclusive care to patients with different backgrounds, traditions, values, beliefs, practices, and behaviors that will meet their biopsychosocial, multicultural, spiritual, and language needs. Use of peer and supervisor consultation when engaging in the art and skill of group work is an appropriate consideration for professional and personal development as a creative and skilled group leader.

Scope of Practice in Conducting Group Interventions With Patients

Nurses working with individuals, groups, couples, families, or communities should adhere to national professional standards and legal mandates (see Chapter 10). The *Scope and Standards of Practice: Psychiatric-Mental Health Nursing* (American Nurses Association [ANA], American Psychiatric Nurses Association [APNA], & International Society of Psychiatric-Mental Health Nurses [ISPN], 2022) differentiate **counseling** from psychotherapy interventions. *Standard 5H. Counseling and Psychotherapy* states: "The psychiatric-mental health registered nurse (PMH-RN) uses counseling interventions to assist patients/clients in their individual recovery journeys" (p. 76). According to this standard, the registered nurse's scope of practice does not include leading group psychotherapy. Individual and group psychotherapy are within the scope of practice of advanced practice nurses. Registered nurses conducting group interventions must also adhere to the *Code of Ethics for Nurses with Interpretive Statements (ANA, 2015).*

> **KEYCONCEPT Scope of practice** is the "services that an RN or APRN is deemed competent to perform, and is permitted to undertake, in keeping with the terms of their professional license" (ANA, APNA, ISPN, 2022, p. 101).

GROUP INTERVENTIONS: ONSITE (IN-PERSON) VERSUS ONLINE (VIRTUAL)

Both onsite (in-person) and online (virtual) group intervention strategies are viable care options. Each offers unique benefits as well as disadvantages.

Onsite (In-Person) Group Interventions

For onsite (in-person) group interventions, leaders select the location of the meetings, which can include choosing a space away from places where the patients live and work to support more neutral feelings and, thereby, comfort in sharing. Face-to-face onsite group interventions afford greater opportunities for direct, in-person individualized support actions, if needed, along with options to include art, music, and play as therapeutic measures that the members can do together. However, scheduling, accessibility, and cost are challenges or disadvantages to consider. Accessibility, or members' ability to get to and from group meetings, can be a major problem for some patients (McGee, 2022).

Online (Virtual) Group Interventions

Online (virtual) groups became more acceptable and common in 2020, when the social distancing requirements of the coronavirus pandemic sped up the general move toward telehealth, and as the availability and accessibility of video conferencing tools (e.g., Microsoft Teams, Zoom, Skype) increased. Connecting virtually preserved therapeutic person-to-person support and lowered social anxieties resulting from being socially isolated during the pandemic. For example, the virtual format often replaced in-person support and substance use groups during the pandemic (Patel et al., 2024).

Online, group interventions have the advantage of being efficient and convenient; in addition, patients are not seen going to an onsite location for meetings, which could be important to some patients. However, virtual meetings pose challenges for the provider when planning. For example, is the software new to members, or are they already using it? The software should be Health Insurance Portability and Accountability Act (HIPAA) compliant, which may necessitate purchase of new software. Do all the potential group members have access to the Internet? Even if everyone does have internet access, it is also important to recognize that strength and connectivity vary by location. What will it cost, and will the virtual group fit in with the provider's other work? For example, face-to-face inpatient groups require less preparation time because they do not involve time to prepare the technology.

Although convenient, it is important to remember that virtual group interventions may limit the ability to conduct assessments and interventions that are associated with onsite, in-person encounters. Additionally, in online interactions, some aspects of verbal and nonverbal communication between and among members and with the leader may be limited in depth of expression, understanding, and interpretation, as well as influenced by the environmental factors present wherever members and the leader are located.

PREPARING TO LEAD A GROUP

Thoughtful planning and preparation make for a successful group. Group interventions can be the primary therapy or an adjunct to one-to-one interventions. The following sections discuss important considerations when planning for group intervention treatment strategies.

Selecting a Leadership Style

Group preparation and interventions are formulated within the context of the group leader's theory-based background, leadership style, and the group's purpose and goals. For example, a leader with a cognitive-behavioral orientation may focus on working with patients within a mood disorders group by teaching members about cognitive distortions, exploring members' use of their identified negative or unhelpful thoughts, and then engaging them in supportive discussion about how to replace their negative or unhelpful thoughts with reality-based, healthier ones. Whatever a leader's theory-based orientation, their leadership style can be viewed on a continuum of direct to indirect.

Direct leadership style enables the leader to control the interaction by giving directions, instructions, and information and allowing little group discussion. The leader literally tells the members what to do. This leadership style may be warranted when time constraints are involved or when members are not motivated and need a leader's inspiration.

At the other end of the continuum is **indirect leadership** style, in which the leader primarily reflects the group members' discussion and offers guidance and support to enable members to make their own decisions. Sometimes, the group needs a more direct approach, such as in a psychoeducation class; other times, the group needs a leader who is indirect because enhancing members' motivation and coming up with creative solutions are congruent with the group's purpose, goals, and tasks.

The challenge of providing skillful leadership is to give sufficient direction to help the group meet its goals and develop its own group process but enough freedom to allow members to make mistakes and recover from their thinking errors in a supportive, caring, and learning environment. Being an effective group leader ultimately warrants the ability to move along the continuum in any group counseling session depending on what the group's dynamics and process require.

> **KEYCONCEPT Group counseling** is use of counseling interventions with a group experiencing difficulties related to health and well-being. Examples of topics used in nursing counseling groups include crisis intervention, stress management, interpersonal skill building, and relaxation techniques (ANA, APNA, ISPN, 2022).

Co-leadership involves two people sharing responsibility for leading the group. Though not as commonly used as single leadership in clinical environments where group counseling sessions with individuals are conducted, co-leadership is beneficial if the co-leaders attend all sessions, maintain open communication, and have a collaborative leadership style. Co-leadership works well when the co-leaders plan sessions together and meet before and after each session to discuss group dynamics and process. It is a leadership strategy that may be used in clinical learning and practice, and for registered nurse supervision of licensed practical nurses and unlicensed mental health workers.

Nurses lead a wide range of groups (see later discussion of Types of Groups). The purpose and goals of the group will dictate the amount of structure and types of activities. In all groups, nurse leaders must ensure members' informed consent to participate, preserve members' safety and the parameters of group confidentiality, and maintain professional boundaries with each member. Because some group activities are social in nature (unit parties, community trips), it is easy to forget that socialization is a treatment intervention. Nurses must remain vigilant to avoid meeting personal social needs within this context.

Using Evidence in Conducting Group Interventions

Group intervention strategies should be evidence based. Research literature should support the use of a particular strategy with a mental health issue. For example, if the goal of a group is to reduce fatigue, increase sleep quality, and increase self-efficacy, the approach should be evidence based, with measurement of fatigue, sleep quality, and self-efficacy to determine if intervention worked. See Box 14.1.

Another approach to conducting evidence-based practice is **practice-based evidence (PBE),** where group member feedback is systematically gathered by the leader and used to inform, guide, and evaluate treatment over the life of the group (Corey, 2023). For example, to determine the progress and satisfaction of group members, rating forms or standardized instruments to rate sessions

BOX 14.1

Research for Evidence-Based Practice: Nurse-Led Fatigue Management Group

Qomi, M., Rakhshan, M., Ebrahimi Monfared, M., & Khademian, Z. (2023). The effect of distance nurse-led fatigue management on fatigue, sleep quality, and self-efficacy in patients with multiple sclerosis: A quasi-experimental study. BMC neurology, *23(1), 71. https://doi.org/10.1186/s12883-023-03115-8*

THE QUESTION: What is the effect of a nurse-led virtual fatigue management group on fatigue, sleep quality, and self-efficacy in patients with multiple sclerosis?

METHODS: In a quasi-experimental design, a total of 60 patients were randomly assigned to either an 8-week nurse-led fatigue management intervention group (n = 30) or a usual care group (n = 30). One meeting was held every week which included the topics of energy conservation and storage strategies, sleep hygiene, relaxing breathing exercises, and exercise at home. Pre- and post-measurements included the Fatigue Severity Scale, the Pittsburgh Sleep Quality Index, and the Multiple Sclerosis Self-Efficacy Scale.

FINDINGS: The nurse-led fatigue management group improved sleep quality, reduced fatigue, and increased self-efficacy when compared to the control group.

IMPLICATIONS: Nurses have an important role in community-oriented care and can be effective in reducing fatigue, improving sleep quality, and improving self-efficacy.

or group leader can be completed by group members at the end of each session. Tallied data are used to supplement the clinical judgments. The data gathered from such outcome measurement tools may be beneficial, as well, in identifying and curtailing patients at risk before their exodus from group interventions and treatment. One assessment instrument that measures a patient's evaluation of the emotional positivity or negativity of a session is the *Session Evaluation Questionnaire (SEQ)*, reported to have good internal consistency (Stiles, 1987).

Selecting Members

Group interventions are used with diverse patient populations and for a variety of therapeutic or educational purposes or a combination of the two. Recruitment for group intervention as a treatment modality may occur through self-referral, clinician recommendation, or through a treatment team's determination that it be designated as part of a patient's treatment plan. The group leader, then, is responsible for screening and assessing each individual's readiness and suitability for assignment to a specific type of group best suited to their health care needs and goals. Not every individual is a good candidate for group interventions. A collaborative interview style with prospective group members is used to share and seek information from them. Other sources of information include clinical observation and judgments, information from ancillary resources, and other assessment tools and strategies for readiness and selection decision making. It is often easier to identify those individuals who should be excluded from engaging in group work than it is to identify those who should be included. However, some guidance for selection concerning an individual's suitability for a group can be based on addressing questions such as:

- Is the decision to join a particular type of group being made by the prospective member?
- Does the purpose and focus of the group match the needs and goals of the prospective member?
- Does the prospective member have the social skills and interpersonal functioning to work comfortably in a group?
- How is the prospective member likely to fit in with other members so the group can work effectively?
- Can the prospective member make a commitment to attending group meetings and honoring group agreements?

Forming an Open or Closed Group

In planning for a group, one of the early decisions is whether the group will be open or closed. In an **open group**, new members may join, and old members may leave the group at different sessions. Because the length of patient hospitalization is relatively short, open groups are typical of inpatient units. For example, a newly admitted patient may join an anger management group that is part of an ongoing program in an inpatient unit but leave when discharged several days later.

Open groups provide the advantage of allowing a diverse mix of members to interact with and learn from one another, but the group dynamics, or what goes on in each meeting with its changing membership, can be unpredictable. How to address members' comings and goings could be where leaders facilitate those part of the group longer to share with new members what their membership has meant to them. New members, in turn, can be asked to say something about what goals they hope to achieve from being in the group.

In a **closed group,** members begin the group at the same time and no new members are admitted for the predetermined duration of the group. If a member leaves, no replacement member is added. This policy offers stability, continuity, and supports **cohesion** among the members. In a closed group, participants get to know one another very well and can develop close relationships where contacts may continue after the group is over. Closed groups are more typical of outpatient groups and may have a sequential curriculum, such as an outpatient smoking cessation group or new parents group. These groups usually meet regularly for a specified period. One disadvantage of a closed group occurs if too many members drop out of the group so either the group process, the interaction between group members, is drastically affected, or the group itself must be disbanded.

Determining Composition

Another decision in planning a group's formation is the group size. The size of a group will depend on the overall group goals and patients' abilities. Other influencing variables include age(s) of the members, the type of group, the experience of the leader or leaders, and what the group's exploratory focus will be (Corey, 2023). Patients with challenging behaviors should be carefully screened and may be able to function in smaller rather than larger groups.

Small groups (usually no more than seven to eight members) become more cohesive, are less likely to form subgroups, and can provide a richer interpersonal experience than large groups (Leszcz & Yalom, 2005). A very small group is two people (**dyad**) or three (**triad**). Small groups function nicely with one group leader although small groups may be led by two people. Although small groups cannot easily withstand the loss of members, they are ideal for patients who are highly motivated to deal with complex emotional problems, such as sexual abuse, eating disorders, or trauma or for those who have cognitive dysfunction and require a more focused group environment with minimal distractions.

In leading a small group, the leader gets to know the members very well but strives to maintain objectivity, that is, being impartial or unbiased, in monitoring and responding to the group's dynamics. For example, observations are made for transference of participants' emotions or desires toward or onto the leader or other members. If a member becomes a "favorite patient" to the leader, then this leader has a responsibility to reflect upon any underlying personal countertransference issues (see Chapter 9).

> **NCLEXNOTE** Be prepared to select members and plan for a patient or family support group to help deal with the impact of mental disorders on the family lifestyle.

Large groups (more than 8 to 10 members) may be effective for specific problems or issues that require group psychoeducative interventions. Large groups are often used in the workplace for health promotion activities such as smoking cessation, healthy eating, stress management, exercise, and meditation. Conducted in an organization, group interventions create broader networking opportunities for more individuals to get to know one another. A large group can be open- or close-ended.

Leading large groups is challenging to their leaders because of the number of potential interactions and relationships that can form and the difficulty in visualizing all the members to monitor and process both verbal and nonverbal behaviors. As the size of the group increases, so does the potential for heightened disagreements. Eventually, these disagreements may lead to the formation of subgroups, in which members who have similar thoughts and feelings stick together in their mutual comfort zones.

It may be difficult to get everyone's attention and focus to begin a group session. Subgroups can form, making it difficult to develop a cohesive group. If subgroups form that are detrimental to the group, the leader can intervene by changing the structure and function of communication within the subgroups through rearranging seating and fostering the subgroup(s) to interact with the rest of the group.

The genders and ages of group participants can also make a difference in the success of the group. It is important to avoid making assumptions about the gender of your group members. Asking members for their personal pronouns will set the stage for gender-inclusive interactions. Age considerations may be significant in terms of the purpose and focus of the group being established.

Setting the Stage: Arranging Seating in an Onsite (In-Person) Group

Group sessions should be held in a quiet, pleasant room with adequate space and privacy. Holding a session in a room that is too large or too small inhibits communication. The sessions should be held in a private space that nonmembers cannot access to ensure the safety of the group members. Interruptions, such as members being removed for appointments with other providers or the door being accidentally opened by someone, are distracting and can also potentially compromise confidentiality. Arrangement of chairs should foster interaction and reduce communication barriers. Communication flows better when no physical barriers, such as tables, are between members. Tables in front of members are sometimes needed, though, such as during psychoeducation session note taking needs or when other therapeutic measures such as art are being used in the session. Group members should be able to see and hear each other. Arranging a group in a circle with chairs comfortably close to one another without a table enhances group work. No one should sit outside the group. If a table is necessary, a round table, if available, is better than a rectangular one, which implicitly increases the power of those who sit at the ends.

Group members tend to sit in the same places and, with choice rather than assigned seating, will sit next to someone who thinks like them or someone they work well with. Where a member sits in the group can influence the role sought or assumed. For example, those who sit next to the group leader may be seeking favor or protection from the group leader or may be looking for upward mobility and a bridge to power within the group.

Alternatively, sitting across from the group leader may be a strategic decision based on the member's feelings of competitiveness or defensiveness toward the leader. In all instances, members' seating positions provide valuable information for assessing dynamics within the group.

Setting the Stage: Arranging for an Online (Virtual) Group

An important requirement for a virtual group is that members have internet access and their devices are compatible with the platform. There should be a computer test prior to the group initiation. Group members should be able to see and hear each other. Because members can join from anywhere, the ground rules around privacy and distraction should be agreed upon in the beginning.

The leader should be prepared for unfolding or challenging technologic issues such as leader and/or member internet connection cut-outs, crashes, not being able to get back into the group, and camera or sound freezes (Pappas, 2023). Technologic issues can cause distress and influence the group dynamics (discussed later in this chapter). The leader should be prepared to address technologic issues as they arise as well as the distress in group members such issues may cause.

Planning the First Meeting

In planning for the first meeting, the leader needs to attend to "…preparing members to get the maximum benefit from their group experience" (Corey, 2023, p. 61). In the initial sessions, the leader sets the tone of the group through the varied planned strategies that will be implemented throughout the life of the group but are particularly vital during the first meeting.

The leader and members introduce themselves. The leader may ask participants to share some introductory information such as why they joined the group and what goals they hope to gain from the experience. The leader can share name, credentials for leading the group, and a brief statement about their experience. The leader should avoid self-disclosing personal information.

The first session is the time to explain the structure of group, including the purpose and group rules (Box 14.2). For example, it is important the group starts and ends at scheduled times; otherwise, members who tend to be late will not change their behavior, and those who are on time will resent waiting for the others. The leader can enlist a group timekeeper for each meeting, which makes starting and stopping on time a collaborative endeavor. The leader would also explain when and if new members can join the group as well as other areas already discussed that are pertinent to leadership considerations during the pregroup period.

BOX 14.2

Example of Group Guidelines

- Group sessions begin and end on time.
- All views are heard and respected. Cell phones are silenced; there are no side conversations.
- Only one individual speaks at a time. No interrupting.
- Emotion is acceptable; aggression is not. Disagreements should be expressed calmly and objectively.
- Everyone is expected to stay for the entire meeting.
- Who we see here, and what is said here, stay here.

LEADING A GROUP

During the early and ongoing group sessions, the leader begins and continues to assess the group dynamics, or interactions—both verbal and nonverbal. During the group sessions, these interactions will be important in understanding the group process and may determine the success of the group.

Group Dynamics

KEYCONCEPT Group dynamics are the verbal and nonverbal interactions that occur between and among members in the group

The theoretical basis of group dynamics is attributed to Kurt Lewin (1939) and proposes that by joining a group, one's interactions with the leader and fellow members change the individual and the other group members, consciously or unconsciously. When referring to group dynamics, it is essentially a view of the group processes in their totality; it is more than the sum of its parts. Specifically, the leader's and members' (a) internal and expressed thoughts and feelings, (b) their nonverbal communicative messages, and (c) the evolving relationships between and among the entire membership will be affected and influenced by the countless variations in process that occur over the course of the group's development.

As a group develops its unique characteristics, individual members' explorations facilitate members forming connections with one another as they discover commonalities or common bonds. Their efforts help everyone to look and seek their place in the group. Members finding commonalities is crucial to fostering motivation and building group cohesion, which are important influences, ultimately, to successful group processes and treatment outcomes.

For example, the group dynamics of initial sessions provide the leader with visibility into the group's personality, interactional patterns, evolving roles, and each individual member's characteristic behavioral patterns. These elements allow members to find an identity and inclusion in the group. Inclusion is a two-way street—that is, whether individual members are included in the group will depend on (1) how the group treats that individual, and (2) whether the individual is motivated to be included.

Group Process

A group leader is responsible for monitoring, facilitating, guiding, and shaping the group process, as well as focusing on the group content, which includes the literal conversational, content-based statements made by group members. The group process is more subjective and examines *how* the individuals are working together. For instance, if a group member is telling something about *what* happened to them (content), a group leader's process focus would be exploring *how* that member was affected by *what* happened to them (Parvez, 2022).

Although models of group development differ, most follow the distinctions of a beginning, middle, and ending phase (Table 14.1). These stages should not be viewed as a linear progression with one preceding the next but as a dynamic process that likely involves revisiting and reexamining group interactions and behaviors in earlier phases, as well as progressing forward to the next phase. Overlapping of stages is common in all groups. The group leader needs to be aware of the group's stage of development as well as leadership responsibilities.

KEYCONCEPT Group process is the development and culmination of the here-and-now session-to-session interactions of the members that move the group and its members toward successfully reaching their group and individual goals.

Stages of Group Development

Beginning Stage: The Honeymoon

In the beginning, the group leader will set the tone and shape the norms of the group by (a) facilitating members getting acquainted; (b) exploring group and members' goals and expectations; (c) listening to everyone's expressed concerns and clarifying misconceptions; (d) supporting interpersonal rapport and fostering the development of trust; and (e) communicating and clarifying essential group purpose and function parameters (Corey, 2023). To carry out these functions, the leader processes group interactions by staying objective and observing members' interactions as well as participating in the group. The leader reflects on, evaluates, and responds to interactions. Utilizing one's theory-based underpinnings and incorporating various techniques, the leader's ability to lead the group effectively and help the group and its members meet their goals are enhanced (Table 14.2).

During the beginning sessions, group members get to know one another and the group leader. The length of the beginning stage depends on the purpose of the group, the number of members, and the skill of the leader. It may last for only one or two sessions or several. Members often exhibit "a public image" such as polite, congenial behavior typical of those in new social situations. They are "good patients" and often intellectualize their problems—that is, these patients deal with emotional conflict or stress by excessively using abstract thinking or generalizations to minimize disturbing feelings. Members are usually anxious and sometimes display behavior that does not truly represent their feelings.

In this phase, members begin to test whether they can trust one another and the leader. Members may come late

TABLE 14.1 COMPARISON OF MODELS OF GROUP DEVELOPMENT

Phase	Robert Bales (1955)	William Schutz (1960)	Bruce Tuckman (1965)
Beginning	• *Orientation:* What is the problem?	• *Inclusion:* Deal with issues of belonging and being in and out of the group	• *Forming:* Get to know one another and form a group
Middle	• *Evaluation:* How do we feel about it?	• *Control:* Deal with issues of authority (who is in charge?), dependence, and autonomy	• *Storming:* Tension and conflict occur; subgroups form and clash with one another • *Norming:* Develop norms of how to work together • *Performing:* Reach consensus and develop cooperative relationships
Ending	• *Control:* What should we do about it?	• *Affection:* Deal with issues of intimacy, closeness, and caring versus dislike and distancing	• *Adjourning:* Task completion; good feelings about achievements; recognition occurs

Source: Bales, R. (1955). A set of categories for the analysis of small group interaction. *American Sociological Review*, 15, 257–263; Schutz, W. (1960). *FIRO: A three-dimensional theory of interpersonal behavior*. Holt, Rinehart & Winston; Tuckman, B. (1965). Developmental sequence in small groups. *Psychological Bulletin, 63*(6), 384–399; Tuckman, B. W., & Jensen, M. A. (1977). Stages of small-group development revisited. *Group and Organization Studies, 2*(4), 419–427.

TABLE 14.2 TECHNIQUES IN LEADING GROUPS

Technique	Purpose	Example
Support: Giving feedback that provides a climate of emotional support	Helps an individual or group continue with ongoing activities Informs group about what the leader thinks is important Creates a climate conducive to expressing unpopular ideas Helps the more quiet and fearful members speak up	"We really appreciate your sharing that experience with us. It looked like it was quite painful."
Confrontation: Challenging a participant (needs to be done in a supportive environment)	Helps individuals learn something about themselves Helps reduce some forms of disruptive behavior Helps members deal more openly and directly with one another	"Tom, this is the third time you have changed the subject when we have talked about spouse abuse. Is something going on?"
Advice and suggestions: Sharing expertise and knowledge that the members do not have	Provides information that members can use after they have examined and evaluated it Helps focus the group's task and goals	"The medication you are taking may be causing you to be sleepy."
Summarizing: Statements at the end of sessions that highlight the session's discussion, any problem resolution, and unresolved problems	Provides continuity from one session to the next Brings to focus still-unresolved issues Organizes the past in ways that clarify; brings into focus themes and patterns of interaction	"This session, we discussed Sharon's medication problems, and she will be following up with her providers."
Clarification: Restatement of an interaction	Checks on the meanings of the interaction and communication Avoids faulty communication Facilitates focus on substantive issues rather than allowing members to be sidetracked into misunderstandings	"What I heard you say was that you are feeling very sad right now. Is that correct?"
Probing and questioning: A technique for the experienced group leader that asks for more information	Helps members expand on what they are saying (when they are ready to) Gets a more extensive and wider range of information Invites members to explore their ideas in greater detail	"Could you tell us more about your relationship with your parents?"
Repeating, paraphrasing, highlighting: A simple act of repeating what was just said	Facilitates communication among group members Corrects inaccurate communication or emphasizes accurate communication	*Member:* "I forgot about my wife's birthday." *Leader:* "You forgot your wife's birthday."
Reflecting feelings: Identifying feelings that are being expressed	Orients members to the feelings that may lie behind what is being said or done Helps members deal with issues they might otherwise avoid or miss	"You sound upset."
Reflecting behavior: Identifying behaviors that are occurring	Gives members an opportunity to see how their behavior appears to others and to evaluate its consequences Helps members to understand others' perceptions and responses to them	"I notice that when the topic of sex is brought up, you look down and shift in your chair."

to the group or try to extend group time. Sometime after the initial sessions, group members usually experience a period of conflict, either among themselves or with the leader. This conflict is a usual part of group development, and many believe that conflict is necessary to move into any working phase. Sometimes, one or more group members become a scapegoat, or someone the group-as-a-whole blames for the conflict that really resides in the group itself. Such situations challenge the leader to guide the group during this period by avoiding taking sides and treating all members respectfully.

Working Stage: Realizing the Group's Purpose

The working stage of groups involves a real sharing of ideas and the development of closeness; the level of trust and cohesion is high during this stage, though also variable and fluid. A group personality may emerge that is distinct from the individual personalities of its members. The group develops norms, which are rules and standards that establish acceptable behaviors. Although some norms are formalized (such as beginning group on time), others are never really formalized (such as sitting in the same place each session). These normative standards encourage conformity and discourage behavioral deviations from the established norms. A member quickly learns the norms or is ostracized.

During this stage, the group realizes its purpose. If the purpose is education, the participants engage in learning new content or skills. If the aim of the group is to share feelings and experiences, these activities consume group meetings. During this phase, the group starts on time, and the members of the group are often so engrossed in the meetings that the leader needs to remind members when it is time to stop. It is common in the working stage for much less structure and fewer interventions be required of the leader than were needed during the beginning stage group sessions (Corey, 2023).

Termination Stage: Saying Goodbye

Termination can be difficult for a group, especially an effective one. Because of the challenges associated with this final stage, it is important to incorporate messages of when the group will end starting with the first group meeting.

During the final stages, members begin to grieve for the loss of the group's closeness and begin to reestablish themselves as individuals. As the saying goodbye meeting approaches, leaders can generate discussion about the impact of the group terminating. Members often terminate from groups in the same way they would from any relationship. One individual may not attend the last session, another individual may bring up issues that the group has already addressed, and others may demonstrate anger or hostility. Most members of successful groups are sad as the group terminates. During the last meetings, members may express their hopes and concerns for each other. They may plan for follow-up meetings after group. These plans rarely materialize or continue. Leaders should recognize these plans as part of the farewell process—separating and saying goodbye to the group.

In terminating a group, the leader discusses and summarizes the work of the group, including the accomplishments of members and how to use what they've learned in the group in their personal lives. The leader includes members sharing their own perspectives on these elements as well. The nurse focuses on ending the group and avoids being pulled into working stage issues. For example, when a patient brings up an issue that was once resolved, the nurse reinforces the skills and then reminds the member of the actions that will be taken after the group has ended.

Facilitating Group Communication

One of the responsibilities of the group leader is to **facilitate** both verbal and nonverbal communication to meet the treatment goals of the individual members and the entire group. Because of the number of people involved, developing trusting relationships within groups is more complicated than developing a single, one-to-one relationship with a patient. The communication techniques used in establishing and maintaining individual relationships are the same for groups, but the leader also attends to the communication patterns among the members.

Encouraging Interaction

The RN leads the group during each of the group stages by encouraging interaction among members and being responsive to their comments. Active listening enables the leader to process events and track interactions. The nurse can then formulate responses based on a true understanding of the discussion. A group leader who listens also models listening behavior for others, helping them improve their skills. Members may need to learn to listen to one another, track discussions without changing the subject, and not speak while others are talking. At the end of the session, the nurse summarizes the work of the session and identifies the work for the next meeting.

The group leader maintains a neutral, nonjudgmental style and avoids showing preference to one member over another. This may be difficult because some members may naturally seek out the leader's attention or ask for special favors. These behaviors are divisive to the group, and the leader should discourage them. Other important skills include providing everyone with an opportunity to contribute and respecting everyone's ideas. Leaders who truly want group participation and decision making do not reveal their beliefs.

Monitoring Verbal Communication

Group interaction can be viewed as a communication network that becomes patterned and predictable. In a group, verbal comments are linked in a chain formation. Monitoring verbal interactions and leading a group at the same time is difficult for one individual. If there are two group leaders, one may be the active leader of the group, and the other may sit outside the group and observe and record rather than participating. If all members provide written consent, the leader can use an audio or video recorder for reviewing interaction after the group session.

Interesting interaction patterns can be observed and analyzed (Fig. 14.1). By analyzing the content and patterns, the leader can determine the existence of **communication pathways**—who is most liked in the group, who occupies a position of power, what subgroups have formed, and who is isolated from the group. People who sit next to each other tend to communicate among themselves. Usually, those who are well liked, or display leadership abilities, tend to be chosen for interactions

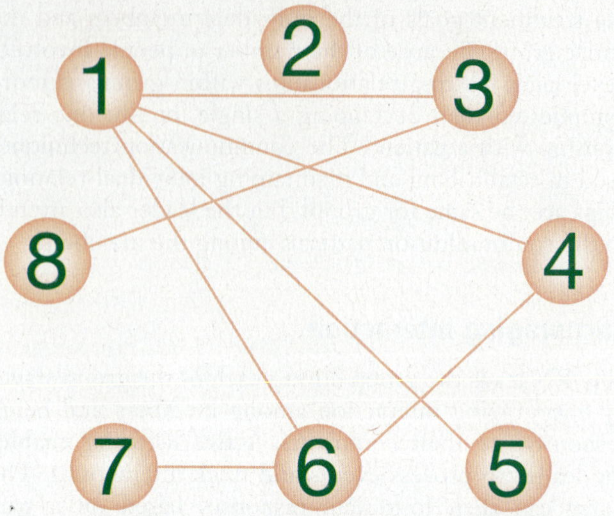

FIGURE 14.1 Sociometric analysis of group behavior. In this sociometric structure, response pattern was recorded during member interaction. Group members interacted with number **1** the most. Therefore, number **1** is the over-chosen individual. Numbers **5** and **7** are under-chosen. Number **2** is never chosen and is determined to be isolated.

more often than those who are not. The leader can also determine if there is a change of subject when a sensitive topic is introduced.

Deciphering Content Themes

Group themes are the collective conceptual underpinnings of a group and express members' underlying concerns or feelings regardless of the group's purpose. Themes that emerge in groups help leaders and members to understand group dynamics. Different groups have different themes. A grief group most likely would have a theme of loss or new beginnings, and an adolescent group may have a theme of independence seeking. Although some predictable themes occur in groups, the obvious or assumed themes at the beginning may wind up differing from themes that develop as the process continues. In one hospice support group, the members seemed to be focusing on the memories of their loved ones. However, upon examination of the content of their interactions, discussions were revolving around financial planning for the future. As another example, the theme of a symptom management group is on identifying symptoms that indicate an impending reemergence of psychotic symptoms, medication side effects, and managing the numerous symptoms that medication is not controlling; however, the theme of powerlessness emerges (see Box 14.3).

BOX 14.3

Group Themes

A large symptom management group is ongoing at a psychiatric facility. It is co-led by two nurses who are skilled in directing large groups and knowledgeable about the symptoms of mental disorders. Usually, 12 people attend. The usual focus of the group is on identifying symptoms that indicate an impending reemergence of psychotic symptoms, medication side effects, and managing the numerous symptoms that medication is not controlling.

The nurses identified the appearance of the theme of powerlessness based on the following observations:

- **Session 1:** T. L. expressed frustration at being unable to keep a job because of their symptoms. The rest of the group offered their own experiences of being unable to work.
- **Session 2:** C. R. is late to group and announces that they were late because the new bus driver forgot to tell them when to get off, so they missed their stop. They are irritated with the new driver.
- **Session 3:** N. T. is out of medication and says they cannot get more because they are out of money again. They ask the nurses to lend them some money and make arrangements to get free medication.
- **Session 4:** G. M. relies on family for all transportation and refuses to use public transportation.

In all of these sessions, participants expressed feelings that are consistent with loss of power.

Monitoring Nonverbal Communication

A substantial portion of one's communication with others is nonverbal. Thus, observing nonverbal communication, as well as verbal communication, contributes to understanding group dynamics. Members communicate nonverbally with each other, not only the group leader. Differences in eye contact, posture, facial expressions, voice tone, appearance, and body gestures of one member impact other members. For example, if group member A is explaining a painful experience and group member B looks away and tries to engage visually with group member C, the self-disclosing member A may feel devalued and rejected because member B's behavior is interpreted by member A as disinterest. If, on the other hand, the group leader interprets member B's looking away behavior as anxiety, possibly over the discussed painful topic experience, the group leader may use member B's looking away as a trigger to explore the impact in the group when hearing about painful stories.

Group leaders need to monitor the nonverbal behavior of group members during each session. Often, one or two people can set the overall mood of the group. Someone who comes to a session very sad or angry can set a tone of sadness or anger for the whole group. An astute group leader recognizes the effects of an individual's mood on the total group. If the purpose of the group is to deal with emotions, the group leader may choose to discuss the member's problem at the beginning of the session. The leader, thus, limits the mood to the one individual experiencing it. If the group's purpose is inconsistent with self-disclosure of personal problems, the nurse should acknowledge the individual member's distress and offer a private session after the group. In this instance, the nurse would not encourage repeated episodes of self-disclosure from that member or others.

Tracking Group Communication

The leader tracks the verbal and nonverbal interactions throughout the group sessions. Depending on the group's purpose, the leader may or may not share the observations with the group. For example, if the purpose of the group is psychoeducation, the leader may incorporate the information into a lesson plan without identifying any one individual. If the purpose of the group is to improve the self-awareness and interaction skills of members, the leader may point out the observations. The leader needs to be clear about the purpose of the group and tailor leadership intervention strategies accordingly.

Determining Roles of Group Members

There are two official or **formal group member roles**—the leader and the members. Both leadership and group member roles have a long history of being studied as part of group communication research. Within the roles and functions of group members, for example, members may exhibit important **informal group member roles** or positions which have implicit rights and duties that can, in the short or long term, either help or hinder the group's process. (Box 14.4.)

Ideally, one or more members assume **task-related roles** or functions. These individuals are concerned about the goal or purpose of the group and keep things on task. For example, the *information seeker* is the member who asks for clarification; the *coordinator* spells out relationships among ideas, and the *recorder* keeps the minutes.

Maintenance roles or functions are assumed by those who help keep the group together. Other members

BOX 14.4

Roles and Functions of Group Members

TASK ROLES

- *Initiator–contributor* suggests or proposes new ideas or a new view of the problem or goal.
- *Information seeker* asks for clarification of the values pertinent to the group activity.
- *Information giver* offers "authoritative" facts or generalizations or gives own experiences.
- *Opinion giver* states beliefs or opinions with emphasis on what should be the group's values.
- *Elaborator* spells out suggestions in terms of examples, develops meanings of ideas and rationales, and tries to deduce how an idea would work.
- *Coordinator* shows or clarifies the relationships among various ideas and suggestions.
- *Orienter* defines the position of the group with respect to its goals.
- *Evaluator–critic* measures the outcome of the group against some standard.
- *Energizer* attempts to stimulate the group to action or decision.
- *Procedural technician* expedites group movement by doing things for the group such as distributing copies and arranging seating.
- *Recorder* writes suggestions, keeps minutes, and serves as group memory.

MAINTENANCE ROLES

- *Encourager* praises, agrees with, and accepts the contributions of others.
- *Harmonizer* mediates differences among members and relieves tension in conflict situations.
- *Compromiser* operates from within a conflict and may yield status or admit error to maintain group harmony.
- *Gatekeeper* attempts to keep communication channels open by encouraging or facilitating the participation of others or proposes regulation of the flow of communication through limiting time.
- *Standard setter* expresses standards for the group to achieve.
- *Group observer* keeps records of various aspects of group processes and interprets data to group.
- *Follower* goes along with the movement of the group.

INDIVIDUAL ROLES

- *Aggressor* deflates the status of others; expresses disapproval of the values, acts, or feelings of others; attacks the group or problem; jokes aggressively; and tries to take credit for the work.
- *Blocker* tends to be negative and resistant, disagrees and opposes without or beyond "reason," and attempts to bring back an issue after group has rejected it.
- *Recognition seeker* calls attention to self through such activities as boasting, reporting on personal achievements, or acting in unusual ways.
- *Self-confessor* uses group setting to express personal, non–group-oriented feelings or insights.
- *Playboy* makes a display of lack of involvement in group's processes.
- *Dominator* tries to assert authority or superiority in manipulating the group or certain members of the group through flattery, being directive, or interrupting others.
- *Help-seeker* attempts to call forth sympathy from other group members through expressing insecurity, personal confusion, or depreciation of self beyond reason.
- *Special interest pleader* speaks for a special group, such as "grass roots," usually representing personal prejudices or biases.

Benne, K. D., & Sheats, P. (1948). Functional roles of group members. *Journal of Social Issues, 4*(2), 41–49.

assume maintenance roles and make sure that the group members get along with each other and try to make peace if conflict erupts. These individuals are as interested in maintaining the group's cohesiveness as focusing on the group's tasks. The *harmonizer*, *compromiser*, and *standard setter* are examples of maintenance roles.

Both task and maintenance functions are needed in an effective group. In selecting members and analyzing the progress of the group, the leader pays attention to the balance between the task and maintenance functions. If too many group members assume task functions and too few assume maintenance functions, the group may have difficulty developing cohesion, or sticking together. If too many members assume maintenance functions, the group may never finish its work.

Individual roles are played by members to meet personal needs, such as feeling important or being an expert on a subject. These roles have nothing to do with the group's purpose or cohesion and can divert attention from the group's tasks and detract from the group's overall functioning. Individual roles may be performed by different group members with varying degrees of frequency and intensity. If individual roles gain dominance, the group may become less successful or ineffective.

Dealing With Challenging Group Behaviors

Problematic behaviors occur in all groups and, if temporary, will be annoying. If intense or persistent, they can be challenging to the most experienced group leaders and frustrating to new leaders. In dealing with any problematic behavior or situation, the leader must remember to support the integrity of the individual members and the group as a whole. Overall, staying positive and being decisive in one's interventions as a group leader when dealing with challenging, disruptive group member behaviors are crucial. Seeking consultation with a seasoned peer or supervisor remains another important problem-solving strategy to use when complex group issues arise.

Monopolizer

Some people tend to monopolize a group by constantly talking or interrupting others. This behavior is common in the beginning stages of group formation and usually represents anxiety that the member displaying such behavior is experiencing. Within a few sessions, this individual usually relaxes and no longer attempts to monopolize the group. However, for some people, monopolizing discussions is part of their personality and will continue. Other group members usually find the behavior mildly irritating in the beginning and extremely annoying as time passes. Members may drop out of the group to avoid that individual. The leader needs to decide if, how, and when to intervene. The best-case scenario is when savvy group members remind the monopolizer to let others speak. The leader can then support the group in establishing rules that allow everyone the opportunity to participate. However, the group often waits for the leader to manage the situation. There are several ways to deal with the situation. The leader can interrupt the monopolizer by acknowledging the member's contribution and then redirecting the discussion to others, or the leader can become more directive and limit the discussion time per member. Another group management intervention is the use of a talking stick which is either picked up or passed to and held by the individual who speaks, and all others remain quiet and listen. The leader would have given directions to the group, at the onset of its use, as to how the talking stick would be used and passed on after an individual is finished speaking.

"Yes, But ..."

Some people have a patterned response to any suggestions from others. Initially, they agree with suggestions others offer them, but then they add "yes, but..." and give several reasons why the suggestions will not work for them. Leaders and members can easily identify this patterned response that suggests a member's resistance to different ideas. In such situations, it is best to avoid problem solving for the member and encourage the individual to develop their own solutions. The leader can serve as a role model of the problem-solving behavior for the other members and encourage them to let the member develop a solution that would work specifically for them.

Disliked Member

In some groups, members clearly dislike one member. This situation can be challenging for the leader because it can result in considerable tension and conflict. If the negative feelings are intense, this individual could become the group's scapegoat. The group leader may have made a mistake by placing the individual in this group, and another group may have been a better match. One solution may be to move the individual to a better matched group. Whether the individual stays or leaves, the group leader must stay neutral and avoid displaying negative verbal and nonverbal behaviors that indicate that they too dislike the group member or are displeased with the other members for their behavior. Often, the group leader can manage the situation by showing respect for the disliked member and acknowledging their contribution. In some instances, getting supervision from a more experienced group leader is useful. Defusing the situation may be possible by using conflict resolution strategies and discussing the underlying issues.

Silent Member

The engagement of a member who does not participate verbally in group discussion can be challenging. This member has had a lifetime of being "the quiet one" and is usually comfortable in the silent role. The leader should respect the individual's silent nature while, at the same time, observing this member's nonverbal behaviors for signs of involvement and investment in the group's process. For example, a silent member may show leaning in/forward or leaning out/backward postures while others are speaking, signaling interest or disinterest, respectively.

Like all the other group members, the silent member often gains a considerable amount of information and support without verbally participating. It is best for the group leader to get to know the member and understand the meaning of the silence before encouraging interaction.

Group Conflict

Within their development over time, most groups experience periods of disagreement and interpersonal conflict. Before conflict can be openly addressed and effectively and productively worked through, it must be recognized. Often there are efforts by leaders and group members to bypass or ignore conflict because of the belief it should be feared and avoided no matter what (Corey, 2023). When recognized, the leader first needs to decide whether the conflict is the natural and inevitable part of the group process or whether the group needs to address some issues.

Member-to-member conflict can be handled through conflict resolution. Leader-to-member conflict is more complicated because the leader has a formal position of power. In this instance, the leader can use conflict resolution strategies but should be sensitive to the power differential between the leader's role and the member's role. Ultimately, "the way conflict is recognized, accepted, and worked through is critical to the progress of the group" (Corey, 2023, p. 71) and reaching productive outcomes.

TYPES OF GROUPS

Psychoeducation Groups

Prior to the coronavirus pandemic, psychoeducation groups were originally a popular onsite (in-person) group intervention strategy used by clinicians; their popularity became virtual during the pandemic. Group mental health provider leaders now have the option to offer prospective clients these information-sharing and skill-building groups using either onsite or virtual methods. Virtual psychoeducational groups have the potential to reach patients who may otherwise not be able to attend onsite, in-person group offerings that would meet their mental health needs.

The purposes of psychoeducation groups are to enhance knowledge, improve skills, and solve problems. The intervention strategies used in psychoeducation groups focus on transmission of information necessary for making some type of change and providing a process for making the change. Psychoeducation groups are formally planned, and members are purposefully selected. The group leader develops a lesson plan for each session that usually includes objectives, content outline, references, and evaluation tools. These groups are time limited and usually last for only a few sessions. Ultimately, factors such as achieved group outcomes and postpsychoeducation member satisfaction may help to increase group members' interests in additional mental health care services.

Psychoeducation groups include recovery-oriented and mindfulness groups. Recovery-oriented groups facilitate consumer involvement in the educational process and build on the recovery principles (see Chapters 2 and 8). Examples of recovery-oriented groups include those that focus on how to manage a medication regimen or control angry outbursts. Psychoeducation groups have changed the perception of illness in people with bipolar disorder, leading to reduced occurrence of symptoms (Miklowitz et al., 2021). Mindfulness groups are helpful in stress reduction.

Task Groups

Task groups focus on completion of specific identified goal activities. An illustration of this would be a school nurse participating in a school personnel task group to develop a plan to assist students to receive certain services. Another example would be a community health RN being a member of a task group to assist disenfranchised individuals in the community with getting better access to valuable mental health care resources (Corey, 2023).

When members are strongly committed to completing a task and the leader encourages equal participation, cohesiveness promotes satisfaction and higher performance (Bae et al., 2023). To complete a task, group cohesiveness is especially important. Leaders can encourage cohesiveness by placing participants in situations that promote social interaction with minimal supervision, such as refreshment periods and team-building exercises.

Without cohesiveness, the group's true existence is questionable. In cohesive groups, members are committed to the existence of the group. In large groups, cohesiveness tends to be decreased, with subsequent poorer performance among group members in completing tasks. However, cohesiveness can be a double-edged sword. In very cohesive groups, members are more likely to transgress personal boundaries. Dysfunctional relationships may develop that are destructive to the group process and ultimately not in the best interests of individual members.

Decision-Making Groups

The psychiatric nurse often leads decision-making groups that plan activities, develop unit rules, and select learning materials. The nurse who is leading a decision-making group should observe the process for any signs of **groupthink**, the tendency of group members to avoid conflict and adopt a normative pattern of thinking that is often consistent with the ideas of the group leader (Janis, 1972, 1982). Group members form opinions consistent with the group consensus rather than critically evaluating the situation. Groupthink is more likely to occur if the leader is respected or persuasive. It can also occur if a closed leadership style is used and external threat is present, particularly with time pressure (DiPierro et al., 2022). Many catastrophes, such as the *Challenger* explosion and Bay of Pigs invasion, have been attributed to groupthink. The impact of groupthink on people's responses on social media to the COVID-19 pandemic is gaining interest by researchers who are examining the rapid transmission of misinformation (Joffe, 2021).

There may be instances where groupthink can lead to a reasonable decision: for example, a group decides to arrange a going-away party for another patient. In other situations, groupthink may inhibit individual thinking and problem solving. For example, a team is displaying groupthink if it decides that a patient should lose privileges based on the assumption that the patient is deliberately exhibiting bizarre behaviors. In this case, the team is failing to consider or examine other evidence that suggests the bizarre behavior is really an indication of psychosis.

Concept Mastery Alert

Groupthink is the tendency of group members to avoid conflict and adopt a normative pattern of thinking that is often consistent with the ideas of the group leader. Group cohesion is the ability of the group to stick together.

Support Groups

Support groups are usually less intense than psychotherapy groups and focus on helping individuals cope with similar issues, illnesses, and problems. Implementing support groups is one of the basic functions of the psychiatric RN. In conducting this type of group, the nurse focuses on helping members cope with situations that are common among the group members. Counseling strategies are used. Leadership of the group requires group management, understanding the impact of the group process, role modeling, awareness, willingness, agreeableness, and openness. For example, a group of patients with bipolar disorder whose illness is stable may discuss, at a monthly meeting, how to tell other people about their disorder or how to cope with a family member who seems insensitive to the illness. Through shared experiences, family caregivers of people with mental disorders benefit from the support and encouragement of the group, as well as getting practical, constructive, and helpful information about providing care for an ill family member.

Psychotherapy Groups

Psychotherapy groups treat emotional problems and can be implemented from various theoretic perspectives, including, but not limited to, psychoanalytic, behavioral, and cognitive depending on the psychotherapist's orientation. These groups focus on examining emotions and helping individuals face their life situations. At times, these groups can be extremely intense. Psychotherapy groups provide an opportunity for patients to examine and resolve psychological and interpersonal issues within a safe environment. Mental health specialists, such as PMH APRNs, psychologists, licensed professional counselors, or clinical social workers, who have a minimum of a master's degree and are trained in group psychotherapy lead such groups. Patients can be treated in psychotherapy and still be members of the nursing groups already discussed. If both nurses and other mental health specialists are providing group interventions to the same patients, collaborative exchanges between both providers are important for continuity of care.

One of the most respected approaches is Irvin D. Yalom's model of group psychotherapy. According to Leszcz and Yalom (2005), there are 11 primary factors through which therapeutic changes occur (Table 14.3). In this model, interpersonal relationships are very important because change occurs through a corrective emotional experience within the context of the group. The group is viewed as a social microcosm of the patients' psychosocial environment (Leszcz & Yalom, 2005).

Self-Help Groups

Self-help groups are a kind of support group in communities that are peer-led and free; they may be in-person or online, and many involve 12 steps. The people who lead these self-help groups are concerned about coping with a specific problem or life crisis. These groups do not explore psychodynamic issues in depth. Professionals usually do not attend these groups or serve as consultants. Examples of self-help groups include Alcoholics Anonymous, Overeaters Anonymous, and One Day at a Time (a grief group). Self-help groups have been formed to help individuals recover from substance use disorder, alcohol use disorder, gambling disorder, and compulsive sexual behavior.

TABLE 14.3 YALOM'S THERAPEUTIC FACTORS

Therapeutic Factors	Definition
Instillation of hope	Hope is required to keep patients in therapy
Universality	Finding out that others have similar problems
Imparting information	Didactic instruction about mental health, mental disorder, and so on
Altruism	Learning to give to others
Corrective recapitulation of the primary family group	Reliving and correcting early family conflicts within the group
Development of socializing techniques	Learning basic social skills
Imitative behavior	Assuming some of the behaviors and characteristics of the therapist
Interpersonal learning	Analog of therapeutic factors in individual therapy, such as insight, working through the transference, and corrective emotional experience
Group cohesiveness	Group members' relationship to therapist and other group members
Catharsis	Open expression of affect to purge or "cleanse" self
Existential factors	Patients' ultimate concerns of existence: Death, isolation, freedom, and meaninglessness

Source: Leszcz, M., & Yalom, I. (2005). *The theory and practice of group psychotherapy*. Basic Books.

Age-Related Groups

Group interventions for specific age groups require attention to the developmental needs of the group members, any physical and mental impairments, social ability, and cognitive level. Groups for children and adolescents should be structured to accommodate group members' intellectual and developmental functioning. Groups for older people should be adapted for age-related changes of the members (Box 14.5).

COMMON NURSING INTERVENTION GROUPS

Registered nurses lead groups of varying types that are geared toward a specific content area such as medication management, symptom management, anger management, and self-care skills. In addition, nurses' groups focus on other issues such as stress management, relaxation, and wellness. A competent leader integrates group leadership, knowledge, and skills with nursing interventions that fit a selected group. Most groups can be adapted to a virtual environment.

BOX 14.5

Working With Older People in Groups

SELF-ASSESSMENT

Because most group leaders do not have personal experience with the issues faced by older adults, the leaders should sensitize themselves to the positive and negative aspects of aging and the developmental issues facing older adults. If leaders have negative reactions to aging, they need to be aware of these and how they might affect their work.

COHORT EXPERIENCES

There is a wide variation in the experiences and history of older adults. Current 78- to 96-year-old adults grew up during World War II; 57- to 75-year-old adults (Baby Boomers) grew up during the Vietnam War era and during the political and sexual revolution of the 1960s.

TYPICAL THEMES IN GROUP MEETINGS

- **Continuity with the past:** Older adults enjoy recalling, reliving, and reminiscing about past accomplishments.
- **Understanding the modern world:** They often use groups to understand and adapt to the modern world.
- **Independence:** They worry about becoming dependent. Physical and cognitive impairments are threats to independence. Loss of family members and friends is also a threat. Leaders should be familiar with the grieving processes.
- **Changes in family relationships:** Family relationships, especially with children and grandchildren, are increasingly important as social roles change.
- **Changes in resources and environment:** Living on a fixed income focuses older people on the importance of their disposable income. They are more vulnerable to community and neighborhood changes because of their physical and financial limitations.
- **Changes in Technology:** Changes in technology can isolate older adults who may have limited resources to purchase, or knowledge to use, the latest device(s).

GROUP LEADERSHIP

- The pace of group meetings should be slowed. Speak to group members as fellow adults.
- Identify the main languages spoken by group members. When possible, match group with bilingual leader. Talk clearly and in a normal tone, but make sure group members can hear others. Encourage questions.
- Greater emphasis should be placed on using wisdom and experience rather than on learning new information. Provide written materials in patient's preferred language in an easily readable font size (at least 14-point font).
- Encourage the use of life review strategies such as autobiography and reminiscence.
- Teaching new coping skills should be placed within the context of previous attempts to resolve issues and problems.

Source: National Institute on Aging, 2023.

Medication Groups

Registered nurse-led medication groups are common in psychiatric nursing. Not all medication groups are alike, so the nurse must be clear regarding the purpose of each specific medication group (Box 14.6). A medication group

BOX 14.6

Medication Group Protocol

PURPOSE: Develop strategies that reinforce a self-medication routine.

DESCRIPTION: The medication group is an open, ongoing group that meets once a week to discuss topics germane to self-administration of medication. Members will not be asked to disclose the names of their medications.

MEMBER SELECTION: The group is open to any individual taking medication for a mental disorder or emotional problem who would like more information about medication, side effects, and staying on a regimen. Referrals from mental health providers are encouraged. Each individual will meet with the group leader before attending the group to determine if the group will meet the individual's learning needs.

STRUCTURE: The format is a small group, with no more than eight members and one psychiatric nurse group leader facilitating a discussion about the issues. Topics are rotated.

TIME AND LOCATION: 2:00 to 3:00 PM, every Wednesday at the Mental Health Center.

COST: No charge for attending.

TOPICS

- How Do I Know If My Medications Are Working?
- Side Effect Management: Is It Worth It?
- Hints for Taking Medications Without Missing Doses!
- Health Issue That Medications Affect.
- (Other topics will be developed to meet the needs of group members.)

EVALUATION: Short pretest and posttest for instructor's use only.

can be used primarily to transmit information about medications, such as action, dosage, and side effects, or it can focus on issues related to medications, such as adherence, management of side effects, and lifestyle adjustments. Many nurses incorporate both perspectives.

Assessing a member's medication knowledge is important before they join the group to determine what the individual would like to learn. People with mental disorders may have difficulty remembering new information, so assessment of cognitive abilities is important. Assessing attention span, memory, and problem-solving skills gives valuable information that nurses can use in designing the group. Importantly, the nurse should also determine the members' reading and writing skills to select effective patient education materials, as well as assessing the need for visual or auditory assistance.

An ideal group is one in which all members use the same medication or medication class, such as antipsychotics, antidepressants, anxiolytics, hypnotics, and mood stabilizers. This situation is rare. Usually, the group members are prescribed various medications. The nurse should know which medications each member is taking, but to avoid violating patient confidentiality, the nurse needs to be careful not to divulge that information to other patients. If group members choose, they can share the names of their medications with one another. A small, semistructured group format works best, and the more interaction built in, the better. Using a lecture method of teaching is less effective than involving the members in the learning process. The nurse should expose the members to various audio and visual educational materials, including workbooks, videotapes, and handouts. The nurse should ask members to write down information to help them remember and learn through various modes. Evaluation of the learning outcomes begins with the first class. Nurses can develop and give pretests and posttests, which, in combination, can measure learning outcomes.

Symptom Management Groups

Registered nurses often lead recovery-oriented groups that focus on helping patients deal with a severe and persistent mental disorders. Handling hallucinations, being socially appropriate, and staying motivated to complete activities of daily living are a few common topics. In symptom management groups, members also learn when a symptom indicates that relapse is imminent and what to do about it. Within the context of a symptom management group, patients can learn how to avoid relapse.

Anger Management Groups

Anger management is another common topic for a nurse-led group, often conducted in the inpatient setting. The purposes of an anger management group are to discuss the concept of anger, identify antecedents to aggressive behavior, and develop new strategies to deal with anger other than verbal and physical aggression (see Chapter 20). The treatment team refers individuals with histories of being verbally and physically abusive, usually to family members, to these groups to help them better understand their emotions and behavioral responses. Impulsiveness and emotional lability are problems for many of the group members. Anger management usually includes a discussion of associated stressful situations, events that trigger anger, feelings about the situation, and unmet personal needs.

Self-Care Groups

Another common nurse-led recovery-oriented psychiatric group is a self-care group. Although self-care is the foundation of health care (International Self-Care Foundation, 2024), people with psychiatric disorders often have self-care deficits and benefit from the structure that a group provides. These groups are challenging because members may or may not know how to perform certain self-care measures, such as processing basic health information; carrying out good hygiene measures or physical activity; eating healthy foods; avoiding or mitigating risks; or responsibly using products or services (International Self-Care Foundation, 2024). Their disorders may interfere with their organizational skills, cognitive capacity, or motivation to complete them. The RN leader not only reinforces the basic self-care skills but also, more importantly, facilitates identification of strategies that can motivate group members and provide structure to their daily lives.

Reminiscence Groups

Group-based reminiscence has been shown to be a valuable intervention for older clients. In this type of group, members are encouraged, using such things as pictures, music, and household objects of members' eras, to remember events from those past years. Such a group is easily implemented. Usually, a simple question about an important family holiday event will even spark memories.

Reminiscence groups have usually been associated with patients who have dementia or who are having difficulty with recent memory, but these recollection groups also assist older adults where the groups' social stimulation prevents their cognitive and/or physical decline or depressive symptoms (Hovey & Shropshire, 2023). Reminiscence groups can also be used as an intergenerational intervention with healthy older adults and children.

Seeking nonpharmacologic strategies as part of older adults' personalized, holistic health care is necessary. It has been shown that group-based reminiscence with older adults can preserve or improve their social, emotional, and mental well-being (Hovey & Shropshire, 2023).

SUMMARY OF KEY POINTS

- The definition of *group* can vary according to theoretic orientation. A general definition is that a group is two or more people who have at least one common goal or issue. Group dynamics are the interactions within a group that influence the group's development and process.
- With groups being increasingly diverse, the nurse must use intervention strategies based on a lifelong journey toward cultural humility to ensure a physically and psychologically safe and equitable space for everyone in the group.
- Registered nurses conducting group interventions must adhere to the *Scope and Standards of Practice: Psychiatric-Mental Health Nursing* and the *Code of Ethics for Nurses with Interpretive Statements.* The registered nurse's scope of practice does not include leading group psychotherapy.
- Group counseling intervention strategies should be carried out using evidence-based practice.
- Whatever a group leader's theory-based orientation, their leadership style can be designed to meet group goals, purposes, and membership needs using strategies that flow from the direct to indirect leadership continuum.
- In selecting members for group interventions, the group leader is responsible for screening and assessing each individual's readiness and suitability for assignment to a specific type of group tailored to their health care needs and goals, realizing that not every individual is a good candidate for group interventions.
- Groups can be open, with new members joining at any time, or closed, with members admitted only once. Either small or large groups can be effective, but dynamics change in different size groups.
- Online (virtual) applications have emerged as an important tool in leading groups. The group leader must adapt the technology to the purpose of the group and address issues of confidentiality, privacy, and safety when using the internet.
- The process of group development occurs in phases: beginning, middle, and termination. These stages are not fixed but dynamic. The process challenges the leader to guide the group effectively during each group stage. The leader should explain the structure of the group, including its purpose and rules, at the beginning of the group. During the working stage, the group addresses its purpose and members demonstrate real sharing. During the final stage of the group, members begin to grieve for the loss of what the group has meant to them and how the group has assisted meeting personal needs.
- During each group stage, leading a group involves many different functions, from obtaining and receiving information to testing and evaluating decisions. Quite significant over the course of a group's development is understanding the evolving difference between the group's process and its group dynamics.
- Verbal communication includes the communication network and group themes. Nonverbal communication is more complex and involves eye contact, body posture and gestures, facial expressions, voice tone, appearance, and the experienced mood of and when in the group. Decision-making groups can succumb to *groupthink*, which can have positive or negative outcomes. Groupthink research is ongoing.
- Seating arrangements can affect group interaction. The fewer physical barriers there are, such as tables, the better communication is. Everyone should be a part of the group, and no one should sit outside of it. In the most interactive groups, members face one another in a circle.
- Leadership skills involve active listening; tracking verbal and nonverbal behaviors; identifying evolving relationships among members; and maintaining a neutral, nonjudgmental style.

- Although there are only two formal group member roles, leader and member, there are many informal member group roles. These roles are usually categorized according to purpose—task functions, maintenance functions, and individual roles. Members who assume task functions encourage the group members to stay focused on the group's task. Those who assume maintenance functions worry more about the group working cohesively together than the actual task itself. Meeting personal needs through individual roles can either enhance or detract from the work of the group.
- The leader should address behaviors that challenge the leadership, group process, or other members to determine whether to intervene. In some instances, the leader redirects a member who is monopolizing the group; at other times, the leader lets the group deal with the behavior. Disagreements and interpersonal conflict occur in most groups and, importantly, must first be recognized and acknowledged before it can be addressed and effectively and productively worked through by the group.
- There are many different types of groups. Most types of groups can be adapted to either an onsite (in-person) or an online (virtual) platform. Most commonly, psychiatric nurses lead psychoeducation, task, decision-making, and support groups. Consumers lead self-help groups, and professionals assist only as requested.
- Leading age-related groups requires attention to the developmental, physical, social, and intellectual abilities of the participants. Themes of older adult groups include continuity with the past, understanding the modern world, independence, and changes in family and resources. Group leadership for older adult groups builds on participants' reminiscence about past experiences, as well as coping abilities in developing new coping skills.
- Medication, symptom management, anger management, and self-care groups are common nurse-led groups focused on specific interventions.

DEVELOPING CLINICAL JUDGMENT

1. Group members are very polite to one another and superficially discuss topics. Which phase would you assess this group is in, and why?
2. After three sessions of a support group, two members begin to share their frustration with having a mental disorder. The group is moving into which phase of group development? Explain your answer.
3. Identify the strengths and limitations of using online (virtual) technology.
4. Discuss the conditions that lead to *groupthink*. When is groupthink positive? When is groupthink negative? Explain.
5. List six behaviors that are important for a group leader, including one for age-related groups.
6. During the first meeting, one member seems very anxious and tends to monopolize the conversation. Discuss how you would assess the situation and whether you would intervene.
7. At the end of the fourth meeting, one group member angrily accuses another of asking too many questions. The other members look on quietly. How should the leader assess the situation? Should the leader intervene? Explain.

MOVIES, TV, OR STREAMING PROGRAMS

12 Angry Men: **1997.** In this excellent film, a 19-year-old stands accused of fatally stabbing his father. The ethnically and racially diverse all-male jury consisting is deciding whether the accused is guilty or not guilty. If guilty, the accused could receive the death sentence. The jury must reach a unanimous verdict. This jury is portrayed by an excellent cast, including Jack Lemmon (Juror 8), George C. Scott (Juror 3), Tony Danza (Juror 7), and Ossie Davis (Juror 2). The foreman is played by Courtney B. Vance. At first, the case appears to be "open and shut" with 11 votes to convict the accused. One juror (Juror 8) dissents because he wants to discuss the evidence in more detail. This film depicts an intense struggle to reach a verdict and is an excellent study of group process and group dynamics in a decision-making group.

Viewing Points:

1. Identify the formal and informal leaders of the group.
2. How does leadership change throughout the film?
3. Identify the roles and functions the jurors assumed in the deliberations.
4. Do you find any evidence of groupthink?
5. How does the group handle conflict?

Unfolding Patient Stories: Randy Adams • Part 2

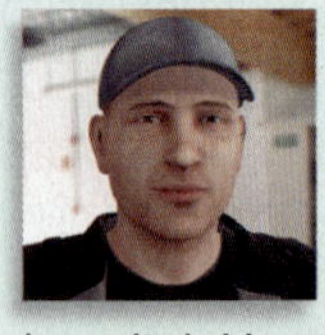

Recall from Chapter 6 **Randy Adams,** a veteran with symptoms of posttraumatic stress disorder (PTSD) and neurocognitive symptoms, which manifested after a recent car accident. He has resisted getting care from the Veterans Affairs hospital. How can he benefit from group therapy and be encouraged to attend? How can the nurse foster communication when Randy has decreased concentration and difficulty expressing his feelings?

Care for Randy Adams and other patients in a realistic virtual environment: ***vSim** for Nursing* (thepoint.lww.com/vSimMentalHealth). Practice documenting these patients' care in DocuCare (thepoint.lww.com/DocuCareEHR).

REFERENCES

American Nurses Association (ANA), American Psychiatric Nurses Association (APNA), & International Society of Psychiatric-Mental Health Nurses (ISPN). (2022). *Psychiatric-mental health nursing: Scope and standards of practice* (3rd ed.). nursesbooks.org.

American Nurses Association (ANA). (2015). *Code of ethics for nurses with interpretive statements*. nursesbooks.org.

Bae, S. H., Kim, S., & Myung, H. (2023). Mediating effects of workgroup processes on the relationship between nurse turnover and nurse outcomes in hospitals. *Frontiers in Public Health*, *11*, 1255983. https://doi.org/10.3389/fpubh.2023.1255983

Bales, R. (1955). A set of categories for the analysis of small group interaction. *American Sociological Review*, *15*(2), 257–263.

Benne, K. D., & Sheats, P. (1948). Functional roles of group members. *Journal of Social Issues*, *4*(2), 41–49.

Corey, G. (2023). *Theory & practice of group counseling* (10th ed.). Cengage.

DiPierro, K., Lee, H., Pain, K. J., Durning, S. J., & Choi, J. J. (2022). Groupthink among health professional teams in patient care: A scoping review. *Medical Teacher*, *44*(3), 309–318. https://doi.org/10.1080/0142159X.2021.1987404

Honig, M., & Martinez-Taboada Kutz, C. (2022). Working with cultural diversity in group therapy around the world. In C. Martinez-Taboada, & M. Honig (Eds.). *Cultural diversity, groups and psychotherapy around the world* (pp. 18–21). International Association for Group Psychotherapy and Group Process. https://www.iagp.com/wp-content/uploads/2024/03/Transcultural_2022_Ebook.pdf

Hovey, S., & Shropshire, M. (2023). Senior reminiscence therapy for older adults residing in assisted living environments: an intervention for social isolation. *The Nursing Voice*, *11*(1), 2023. https://www.healthecareers.com/nurse-resources/the-nursing-voice-june-2023/senior-reminiscence-therapy-for-older-adults-residing-in-assisted-living-environments-an-intervention-for-social-isolation

International Self-Care Foundation. (2024). *Measuring self-care*. Retrieved from https://isfglobal.org/what-is-self-care/measuring-self-care/

Janis, I. (1972). *Victims of groupthink*. Houghton Mifflin.

Janis, I. (1982). *Groupthink* (2nd ed.). Houghton Mifflin.

Joffe, A. R. (2021). COVID-19: rethinking the lockdown groupthink. *Frontiers in Public Health*, *9*, 625778. https://doi.org/10.3389/fpubh.2021.625778

Leszcz, M., & Yalom, I. (2005). *The theory and practice of group psychotherapy*. Basic Books.

Lewin, K. (1939). Experiments in social space. *Harvard Educational Review*, *9*, 21–32.

McGee, V. (2022). *Virtual therapy vs. in-person therapy*. Psychology.Org. https://www.psychology.org/resources/virtual-therapy-vs-in-person/

Miklowitz, D. J., Efthimiou, O., Furukawa, T. A., Scott, J., McLaren, R., Geddes, J. R., & Cipriani, A. (2021). Adjunctive psychotherapy for bipolar disorder: a systematic review and component network meta-analysis. *JAMA Psychiatry*, *78*(2), 141–150. https://doi.org/10.1001/jamapsychiatry.2020.2993

National Institute on Aging [NIA]. (2023). *Talking with your older patients*. National Institutes of health. U.S. Department of Health & Human Services. Retrieved October 16, 2024, from https://www.nia.nih.gov/health/health-care-professionals-information/talking-your-older-patients

Pappas, S. (2023). *Group therapy is as effective as individual therapy, and more efficient. Here's how to do it successfully*. American Psychological Association. https://www.apa.org/monitor/2023/03/continuing-education-group-therapy#:~:text=A%20recent%20survey%20indicated%20that,2%2C%202022)

Parvez, H. (2022). Process vs. content: Why it matters. *Psychology Concepts. PsychMechanics*. https://www.psychmechanics.com/process-vs-content/

Patel, E. U., Grieb, S. M., Winiker, A. K., Ching, J., Schluth, C. G., Mehta, S. H., Kirk, G. D., & Genberg, B. L. (2024). Structural and social changes due to the COVID-19 pandemic and their impact on engagement in substance use disorder treatment services: a qualitative study among people with a recent history of injection drug use in Baltimore, Maryland. *Harm Reduction Journal*, *21*(1), 91. https://doi.org/10.1186/s12954-024-01008-8

Schutz, W. (1960). *FIRO: A three-dimensional theory of interpersonal behavior*. Holt, Rinehart & Winston.

Stiles, W. B. (1987). Session evaluation questionnaire (SEQ). In K. Corcoran & J. Fischer (Eds.), *Measures for clinical practice: A sourcebook* (pp. 306–307). The Free Press

Tuckman, B. (1965). Developmental sequence in small groups. *Psychological Bulletin*, *63*(6), 384–399.

Tuckman, B. W., & Jensen, M. A. (1977). Stages of small-group development revisited. *Group and Organization Studies*, *2*(4), 419–427.

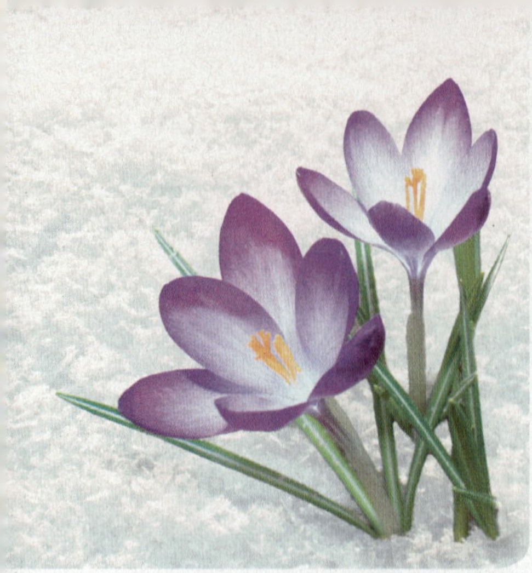

15 Family Assessment and Interventions

Rita Tadych and Mary Ann Boyd

KEYCONCEPTS

- comprehensive family assessment
- family
- family resilience
- family system

LEARNING OBJECTIVES

After studying this chapter, you will be able to:

1. Examine the changing family structure and mental health implications.
2. Discuss the impact of physical and psychological disorders on the family system.
3. Complete a genogram that depicts the family history, relationships, and physical and psychological disorders across at least three generations.
4. Develop a plan for a comprehensive family assessment.
5. Discuss nursing interventions that are useful strategies in family-centered care.

KEY TERMS

• boundaries • cohabitation • collateral informant • communication process • differentiation of self • dysfunctional • emotional cutoff • extended family • family belief system • family development • family life cycle • family projection process • family structure • genogram • identified patient • multigenerational transmission process • nuclear family emotional process • organizational patterns • sibling position • subsystems • transition times • triangles

INTRODUCTION

Over time and across cultures, many definitions of "family" have been envisioned, identified, and discussed in numerous reputable resources, including, but not limited to, nursing literature and practice. Defining "family" can be a challenge because of tendencies to base the definition on one's own family experience and expectations. For purposes of this chapter, a family is a group of people, connected emotionally or by blood, or both, that has developed patterns of interaction and relationships. Family members have a shared history and a shared future. Family includes the entire emotional system of three, four, or even five generations held together by blood, legal, emotional, and/or historical ties. As people move through life, their relationships with parents, siblings, and other family members go through transitions. (Please note that in this chapter, the term "parents" is used to encompass anyone caring for children, including guardians or caregivers.)

> **KEYCONCEPT Family** is a group of people, connected by emotions or blood, or both, that has developed patterns of interaction and relationships.

Family members have a shared history and a shared future (McGoldrick et al., 2016). The psychiatric–mental health nurse (PMH) interacts with families in several ways. Nursing care may begin with individual patients as the recipients of care and then expand to include members of their family. Because of the interpersonal and chronic nature of many mental disorders, PMH nurses often have frequent and long-term contact with families. Involvement may range from meeting family members only once or twice to treating the whole family as a patient.

> **KEYCONCEPT A family system** is an organized structure that consists of a group of people who are interrelated emotionally or by blood. A family system is more than the sum of its parts; social and interaction patterns of the family system shape the behavior of the individual family members who are interdependent, emotionally connected, and have a shared history.

Unlike a therapeutic group (see Chapter 14), the family system has a history and continues to function when the nurse is not there. The family reacts to past, present, and anticipated future relationships within at least a three-generation family system. Stressful life events and problems of individual patients affect the whole family as a unit. Family responses contribute to the adaptations to family dysfunctions (Roland & Walsh, 2023).

This chapter explains how to integrate important family concepts into the nursing assessment when providing nursing care to patients and their families experiencing mental health care needs.

CHARACTERISTICS OF FAMILIES

No matter their form, families play a significant role in people's lives and influence who and what they are. Families are a source of guidance, security, love, and understanding. For people experiencing mental illnesses and emotional problems, their family often assumes primary care for them and supports them through recovery. For patients, the family unit may provide their only constant support throughout their lives. Family characteristics such as size, member roles, mobility, and composition influence the strength of a family system.

Contemporary Roles

Over the last half-century, partners of all genders often work outside the home (in both single- and dual-income families) and participate in parenting. For employed partners in a relationship, the demands of paid work must be balanced against the family role responsibilities of caregiving, housework, and home maintenance, along with consideration for adult leisure activities. These tasks are not always divided equally between partners, which can contribute to family stress and strain (Aragão, 2023).

In a family system, roles shape how members interact with each other to create and maintain system balance. It is important to understand how roles assumed by members help or hurt the family as a whole or its individual members.

Mobility and Relocation

In today's world, families are mobile and may change residences frequently. Leaving familiar environments and readjusting to new surroundings and lifestyles stress the family system. For example, during the COVID-19 shutdowns (February 2020–December 2021), there were waves of changes in work and school environments. College students moved home because campuses closed; families were able to move from jobs in densely populated areas to suburbs because remote job opportunities increased. In some cases, such moves impose separation from the **extended family**, which traditionally has been a stabilizing force and a much-needed support system.

Family Size and Composition

According to the U.S. Census Bureau (2023), "size of family" includes the owner or renter of the housing unit (i.e., householder) and all other people in the living quarters who are related to the householder by birth, marriage, or adoption. The 2020 Census data reported that although one-person households had a minor increase in 2020 from 1990 (from 25% to 28%), family households remained the largest type of household (from 70.2% to 65.3%).

Types of families include married couples, unmarried couples, single-parent families, stepfamilies, families without children.

Married Couples

Married-couple households with their own children under 18 decreased by 6% from 1990 to 2020. This decrease was related to the aging of the U.S. population and the older age of couples at the birth of their first child (U.S. Census Bureau, 2023).

Unmarried Couples

Individuals living together in an intimate partnership relationship without legal marriage is referred to as **cohabitation**. The U.S. Census Bureau (2023) reports that cohabitating couples have become more prevalent, especially for young adults. Most such cohabitating couples do not have children living with them.

In general, unmarried couples living together have fewer legal rights than do married couples. For example, if one partner becomes incapacitated or dies, the other partner may not have the legal right to make health care decisions or claim property unless a preexisting legal contract is in place. The benefit of cohabitation is that unmarried partners can define the terms of their relationship and are not bound by marriage laws (Yeban, 2023a). The decision to live together without a legal contract provides the couple with the opportunity to evaluate their relationship compatibility, stability, strengths, and flexibility before considering further commitments. If cohabitation ceases to meet mutual needs, it is easier to end the relationship than if the couple had legally married.

Unmarried couples in the United States can create a legal contract that spells out their individual and collective rights and obligations to one another for their living arrangements. Like marital contracts, matters such as property, health care, and expenses can be specified. This legal contract is a cohabitation agreement, nonmarital contract, or living together contract (Yeban, 2023b). In the clinical environment, nurses who provide health care to someone who is in a cohabitation relationship need to be mindful of their legal boundaries.

Single-Parent Families

Single-parent family households have increased since the 1960s, impacted by factors such as changing notions about marriage and divorce, with single parenthood itself being more accepted. The predominant ethnicity of single parents is White non-Hispanic. The pandemic was especially difficult economically for single parents, with poverty levels being most challenging for Native American, African American, and Latina single mothers (Dionisi et al., 2023; National Academies of Sciences, Engineering, & Medicine, 2023).

Being a single divorced parent allows the custodial parent personal time when the children are with the other parent, but when the children return, there is the day-to-day, ongoing domestic load, discipline, and child-related responsibilities. Behavior issues of the children may be easier to address without two parents whose parental management styles may differ. If childcare is needed while the single parent works outside the home, there are household financial strains to bear. Higher levels of stress, anxiety, depression, and loneliness in single parents are common because single parenthood is not an easy family lifestyle (Dharani & Balamurugan, 2024). On the other hand, successfully taking on and enduring the day-to-day tasks of child-rearing alone, despite bumps along the way, serves as a role model of resilience and resourcefulness to one's children.

Stepfamilies

Most families are no longer composed of biologic mother, father, and children (Stepfamily Foundation, 2023). Stepfamilies (also called "blended families" or "remarried families") are becoming increasingly common, with one adult usually identified as the stepparent and the other as the biologic or legal parent. The former partner or former spouse of the biologic parent may or may not have legal visitation rights or informal contacts with their biologic children.

Making the transition from a single-parent family to a stepfamily takes a great deal of effort. This family type has a unique set of challenges. Each member has an array of thoughts and feelings about their new life and relationships.

Many parents find that stepparenting is much more difficult than parenting a biologic child. The bonding that occurs with biologic children rarely occurs with stepchildren, whose natural bond is with a parent not living with them. However, the stepparent often assumes a measure of financial and parental responsibility. The care and management of children often become the primary stressor to the adult partners. In addition, the children face multiple sets of parents, whose expectations may differ. The adults may also compete for the children's attention.

With new boundaries and rules in a stepfamily, the onset of any unexpected mental health needs can stress the family system. The nurse should assess and address the various relationship and communication complexities in the current stepfamily system, while also attending to custodial divorce legalities related to health care.

Families Without Children

Couples can be voluntarily without children (by choice) or involuntarily without children (because of infertility). As education and career opportunities for people assigned female at birth have increased, many people have chosen not to have children. A young couple may enjoy the socioeconomic advantages of having a dual income with no children. Child-free couples have the savings and highest median net worth of all types of family systems (Board of Governors of the Federal Reserve System, 2023). Personal benefits also include increased freedom and flexibility in the couple's daily life, such as advancing their careers and pursuing their interests, hobbies, and travel without having child-rearing responsibilities.

In the United States, about one in five married people assigned female at birth ages of 15 to 49 (19%) are unable to become pregnant after 1 year of trying. Another approximately one in four (26%) have difficulty getting pregnant or sustaining a pregnancy to term (Centers for Disease Control and Prevention, 2024). Fear, stress, anxiety, grief, and depression are some of the emotional consequences couples experiencing infertility may face. Such couples may believe that something is wrong with their bodies or that their bodies are failing them. The couple relationship may become strained as well, with the couple deciding whether to undergo infertility treatment, whether to continue or discontinue treatment, or whether to choose adoption or a surrogacy (Silver, 2023).

Families With Parents Who Are LGBTQ+

LGBTQ+ adults with their children face serious challenges securing basic health care and dealing with health disparities because of societal stigma and existing inequitable laws. Many LGBTQ+ adults continue to face discrimination in their personal lives, employment, housing, and health care, as well as in the public sphere. LGBTQ+

parents also experience bias and discrimination when accessing health care for their families. Many have negative experiences with mental health providers (Coulter-Thompson, 2023; Farr et al., 2024). There are as many as two million children living in lesbian, gay, bisexual, and transgender (LGBT) families (Movement Advancement Project, 2023).

FAMILY MENTAL HEALTH

A family can be viewed as a living system often consisting of several generations with multiple health care needs. In a mentally healthy family, members live in harmony among themselves and within society. These families support and nurture their members throughout their lives. However, stress and illnesses can negatively affect a family's overall mental health. Ideally, families can access health care services in an integrated system with primary health services and mental health care linked.

Family Dysfunction

A family becomes **dysfunctional** when interactions, decisions, or behaviors interfere with the positive development of the family and its individual members. Most families have periods of dysfunction such as during a crisis or stressful situation when the coping skills are not available. Families usually adapt and regain their mentally healthy balance. A family can be mentally healthy and at the same time have a member who has a mental illness. Conversely, a family can be dysfunctional and have no member with a diagnosable mental illness.

Effects of Illness and Mental Disorders on Family Functioning

The COVID-19 pandemic and the postpandemic period have made family-centered care a critical focus for all nurses. The long-term effects on families whose member(s) survived COVID-19 include more than 60 physical and psychological reported consequences (Konradsen, et al., 2023). Families with members who were hospitalized with COVID-19 suffered from anxiety, depression, and posttraumatic stress disorder (PTSD) (Laurent et al., 2023).

Families with mental health needs often require community support and resources. Social determinants of health are important for families with a member with a mental illness because of the heightened risk of comorbidities and cognitive and functional impairment (Jester et al., 2023). Caregivers often experience emotional and financial problems that affect their quality of life. A caregiver's age, sex assigned at birth, knowledge of the disorder, family status, income, time spent with the individual per day, and psychological stress can strain the caregiver's emotional and financial resources. The impact of the disorder on each family member is influenced by the individual member's age, sex assigned at birth, severity of illness, social functioning, and treatment adherence. Having a supportive social network, community services, and financial and educational support improves a family's resilience to provide support and direction for the member with a mental disorder (Sustrami et al., 2023).

Many adults with mental disorders live with their parents well into their 30s and beyond. For these adults with persistent mental illness, the family serves several functions that those without mental illness do not need. Such functions include the following:

- *Providing support.* People with mental illness have difficulty maintaining nonfamilial support networks and may rely exclusively on their families.
- *Providing information.* Families often have complete and continuous information about care and treatment over the years.
- *Monitoring services.* Families observe the progress of their relative and report concerns to those in charge of care.
- *Advocating for services.* Family groups advocate for money for residential care services.

The stigma associated with having a family member with a mental disorder underlies much of the burden and stress the caregivers experience. Families can become socially isolated; they may also become financially stressed because they lose employment opportunities as they struggle to care for their loved one. Frustration, anxiety, and low self-esteem may result (Manesh et al., 2023).

Conflicts can occur between parents and mental health workers who place a high value on independence. Members of the mental health care system may criticize families for being overly protective when the families actually have justified concerns that the patient with mental illness may face real barriers to independent living. Housing may be unavailable; when available, quality and conditions may be inadequate. The patient may fear leaving home, may be at risk for relapse if they do leave, or may be too comfortable at home to want to leave. When long-term caregivers, usually the parents, die, their adult children with mental illness experience housing disruptions and potentially traumatic transitions. Siblings who have other responsibilities expect to be less involved than their parents in the care and oversight of the sibling with mental illness. Siblings of the patient often suffer depressive symptoms, confusion about the mental disorder and the need to compensate, which in turn adds to the siblings' distress (Jayasinghe et al., 2023).

Nurses use an objective and rational approach when discussing independence and dependence of those with mental illness who live with aging parents. Family emotions often obscure the underlying issues, but nurses can diffuse such emotions, so that everyone can explore the alternatives comfortably. Although separation must eventually occur, the timing and process vary according to each family's particular situation. Parents may be highly anxious when their adult children first leave home, so they may need reassurance and support.

RECOGNIZING AND ANALYZING CUES: THE COMPREHENSIVE FAMILY ASSESSMENT

In a family assessment, the individual patient is viewed as the **identified patient** who is connected to the whole family as a living system. Family members are recognized as **collateral informants**. For healthy changes to be achieved, the family system and their set of relationships become a significant target for assessment and intervention strategies (Corey, 2024).

Because multiple family configurations exist, patients should define their family. The nurse can ask the patient to identify their family members by asking "Who is your family?" It is also important to clarify what the family means to the patient and who the current family is in their life today. Sometimes families view pets as family members. Through such collaborative exchanges, nurses can develop strategies for targeted patient-centered family assessments and interventions.

> **KEYCONCEPT A comprehensive family assessment** is the collection of all relevant cues related to family health, psychological well-being, and social functioning to identify problems for which the nurse can generate nursing interventions.

The assessment consists of a face-to-face interview with family members and can be conducted during several sessions. Nurses conduct a comprehensive family assessment when they care for patients and their families for an extended period. They also use them when a patient's mental health issues are so complex that family support is important for optimal care (Box 15.1).

Relationship Building

In preparing for a family-centered health care assessment, PMH nurses must concentrate on developing trust, rapport, and a safe therapeutic relationship with the family. Although necessary when working with any family, relationship development is particularly important when working with families from underrepresented groups. Because of the discrimination that those from these groups may experience, they may be less likely to trust those from outside their family or community, and communication may be hampered if the family does not speak English. Developing a healthy therapeutic relationship takes time, especially if working with more than one member of a family.

To develop a positive relationship with a family, nurses must establish credibility with the family system and address its immediate intervention needs. To establish credibility and secure a positive alliance, the nurse must be seen by the family as knowledgeable and skillful. Possessing nursing skills reflective of cultural humility and projecting a professional image are crucial to establishing credibility and a quality alliance with family members. The PMH nurse will make considerable progress in establishing a positive relationship with a family by helping members meet their immediate needs. A family that needs shelter or food is not ready to discuss a member's medication regimen until basic needs are met.

Genograms

Families possess various structural configurations (e.g., single-parent, multigenerational, same-gender relationships). The nurse can facilitate taking the family history by completing a **genogram**, which is a valuable multigenerational schematic depiction of family structure, ethnic heritage, health and social problems, legal issues, and relationship and interactive ties from generation to generation. A complete record includes at least three generations, which is especially important if caregiving for older adults is involved. The PMH nurse can use a genogram as a visual framework for exploring and assessing relationships and patterns of health and illness as a strategy for ascertaining needed family-centered health care interventions.

Creating Genograms

A multigenerational genogram includes the age and gender of each member. In detailed genograms, dates of marriage and death, and geographic location of each member, are also included. Specific symbols are used in the genogram and are defined in a legend. Horizontal lines represent marriages; dashed horizontal lines represent living together. Vertical lines connect biologic parents and children. Genograms can be particularly useful in understanding family history, composition, relationships, and illnesses (Fig. 15.1).

Genograms vary from simple to elaborate depending on the type of family system a patient is a member of. The patient's and family's assessment needs guide the level of detail. In a small family with limited issues, the genogram can be rather general. In a large family with multiple issues, the genogram should reflect these complexities. Thus, depending on the level of detail, PMH nurses collect various data. They can study major events such as marriages, divorces, deaths, and geographic movements.

BOX 15.1

Family Mental Health Assessment

I. Family members present

Name	Age	Relationship

II. Health status

Member	Disorder and current treatment

III. Mental health status

Member	Disorder and current treatment

IV. Impact of mental illness on family function
Describe the changes that occur in the family as a result of the family member's disorder. ______

V. Family life cycle
Describe the family life cycle phase and any transitions that are occurring. ______

VI. Communication patterns
Describe the family communication patterns in terms of usual times of communication (morning, dinner, etc.), which family members talk to each other, who communicates the family rules, who carries out discipline. Identify triangulated messages. ______

VII. Stress and coping
Identify current family stressful events and family coping mechanisms. ______

VIII. Problem-solving skills
Determine who solves problems in the family. Are the problem-solving skills of the family able to manage most family problems? ______

IX. Family system (from the genogram)
Family composition ______

Health and illness patterns ______

Relationship patterns ______

Social functioning patterns ______

Financial and legal status ______

Formal and informal network ______

X. Nursing diagnoses ______

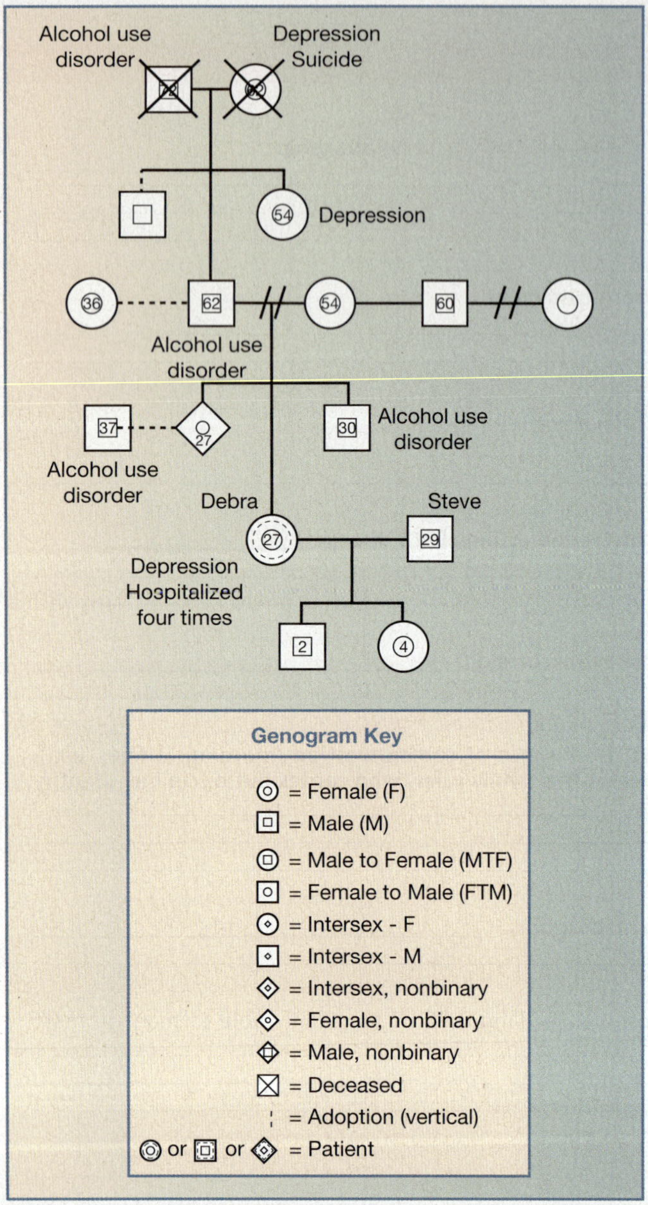

FIGURE 15.1 Analysis of genogram for a patient named Debra. Ages of the family members are shown inside the shapes. Horizontal lines represent marriages; dashed horizontal lines represent living together. Vertical lines connect biologic parents and children. Illness patterns are depression (paternal aunt, grandmother [suicide]) and alcohol use disorder (brother, father, grandfather). Relationship patterns show that the parents are divorced and neither sibling is married.

They can include cultural or religious affiliations, education and economic levels, and the nature of the work of each family member. PMH nurses should always include mental disorders and other significant health issues in the genogram but must not forget to focus on the family's strengths, as this is particularly important in constructing the family genogram. In the field of family therapy, there has been a major assessment and intervention shift from a deficit-based approach to a strengths-based approach; this involves collaborative attentiveness to family members with a focus on attaining and maintaining solutions to issues (Crisp & Gabbard, 2023).

It is important for the nurse to think about who in a family system will be interviewed for a genogram. Every family member may hold different information and different perspectives about their family's relationships, strengths, issues, problems, and perceived solutions to system dysregulation. Discrepancies are to be expected but can also be revealing in one's analysis of family dynamics. Knowing that bias and multicultural perspectives need to be considered, PMH nurses may deliberate over which family members might be key to gathering information for the family history.

Analyzing and Using Genograms

For a genogram to be useful in assessment, the PMH nurse needs to analyze the data for family composition, relationship issues, and mental health patterns. Nurses can begin with composition. How large is the family? Where do family members live? A large family whose members live in the same city is more likely to have support than a family in which distance separates members. Of course, this is not always the case. Sometimes even when family members live geographically close, they are emotionally distant from one another.

The PMH nurse should also study the genogram for relationship and illness patterns. For relationship patterns, the nurse may find a history of divorces or family members who do not stay connected with the rest of the family. The nurse can then explore the significance of these and other relationships. For illness patterns, alcohol use disorder, often seen across several generations, may be prevalent in individuals on one side of a family. The nurse can then hypothesize that alcohol use disorder, or substance misuse, is one of the mental health risks for the family system and collaborate with the patient to design interventions to reduce the risk.

Family Physical and Mental Health

The family system assessment includes a thorough picture of physical and mental health status and how the status affects family functioning. The family with multiple health issues, both physical and mental, must try to manage these issues as well as obtain the many financial and health care resources the family members need.

Physical Health Status

The family system health status includes the physical illnesses and disabilities of all members; the PMH nurse can record such information on the genogram and include the physical illnesses and disabilities of other

BOX 15.2

Research for Evidence-Based Practice: Parental Coping Strategies

Chin, W., Chang, H., & Chao, K. (2023). Exploring coping strategies of parents of children with autism spectrum disorder in Taiwan: A qualitative study. Journal of Nursing Research, *31(3), e278. https://doi.org/10.1097/jnr.0000000000000553.*

THE QUESTION: How do parents of children with autism spectrum disorder (ASD) cope with the stress of parenting in Taiwan?

METHODS: Using face-to-face semi-structured interviews, 14 parents answered questions related to the experiences of parenting a child with ASD. Questions were asked to gain an in-depth understanding of the stressful situations encountered by participants and their coping strategies. Interviews were audio recorded, transcribed, and analyzed using a thematic analysis approach.

FINDINGS: Parents coped with parenting by using communication (direct and indirect) for problem-solving with the child and support from outside resources to develop strategies. They worked to manage their child's stress by reminding (prompting the child), helping (explaining to children), and finding an outside helper. They also learned to accept their child's unique needs and adapted to the characteristics of the child.

IMPLICATIONS FOR NURSING: Nurses should evaluate how parents are coping with the stresses related to raising a child with ASD and consider cultural factors that may influence how they accept or adapt to parenting.

generations. Illnesses of family members are an indication not only of their physical status but also of the stress currently being placed on the family and its resources. The nurse should pay particular attention to any physical issues that affect family functioning. For example, if a member requires frequent visits to a provider or hospitalizations, the whole family will feel the effects of focusing excessive time and financial resources on that member. The nurse should explore how such situations specifically affect other members. See Box 15.2.

Mental Health Status

Detecting mental health disorders in families may be difficult because these disorders often are hidden, may go unrecognized, or are a "family secret." Very calmly, the nurse should ask family members to identify anyone who has experienced mental illness or mental health challenges, or an individual whose well-being is a concern. The nurse should record the information on the genogram as well as in the narrative. If family members do not know if anyone in the family had or has a mental illness, the nurse should ask if anyone was treated for "nerves" or had a "nervous breakdown." A good family history of mental illness across three generations helps the nurse understand the significance of mental illness or mental health challenges in the current generation. If one family member has a serious mental illness, the whole family will be affected. Usually, siblings of the member with the mental disorder receive less parental attention than the affected member.

Family's Psychological Domain

Assessment of the family's psychological domain focuses on the family's resilience, development and life cycle, communication patterns, stress, coping abilities, and problem-solving and decision-making skills. One aim of the family assessment is to understand the relationships within the family. Although family roles and structures are important, the true value of the family is in its relationships, which are irreplaceable. For example, if a parent leaves or dies, another person (e.g., stepparent, grandparent) can assume some parental functions but can never really replace the emotional relationship with the missing parent.

Family Resilience

Family resilience is a dynamic process in which individual members contribute to the adaptation of the whole family. Family resilience is important for families who are coping with stressors related to long-term health care (Kuang et al., 2023).

> **KEYCONCEPT Family resilience** is the ability of a family to cope and rebound from adversity and trauma. It includes adjusting and adapting to stressful situations. The family belief system interacts with the family's internal coping ability and external support systems to adapt to the crisis situation (Walsh, 2021).

When a family member has a physical and/or mental health disorder that requires complex care, maintaining family resilience can be challenging. Assessing family resilience can be conceptualized in three areas: Family belief systems, organizational patterns, and communication processes.

Family belief systems include the meaning of adversity, the outlook for the future (positive or negative), and transcendence or spirituality. It is likely that family members hold multiple, differing beliefs. A way to explore the family belief system is to focus on fears associated with the illness, the cause or cure of the illness, or attitude toward suffering.

A family's **organizational patterns** include *flexibility* to change, roles and cooperation, *connection* with each other (mutual support and respect), and *social and economic resources*. Organizational patterns involve the process of making the changes as they move through life. Watching members' small interactions in response to the illness, affecting the family, may provide cues for their organizational patterns and assist the nurse in supporting valuable system change.

A family's **communication processes** involve solving problems. Is there clarity in decision-making? Is emotional expression open, empathic, or closed? Do family members take responsibility for their feelings and behaviors? Is there collaborative problem solving with a focus on goals? The family's communication patterns are the glue in the family system. Identifying the communication processes used to solve problems helps in understanding how the family is coping with physical and/or mental health chronic illnesses (Prates et al., 2024).

Family Development

Family development is a broad term that refers to all the processes connected with the growth of a family system, including changes associated with work, geographic location, migration, acculturation, and serious illness. In optimal family development, family members are differentiated (capable of autonomous functioning) from one another, anxiety is low, and the parents have good emotional relationships with their own families of origin.

Family Life Cycle

The concept of **family life cycle** refers to a system evolving through phases based on significant events related to the arrival and departure of members, such as birth or adoption, child-rearing, departure of children from home, occupational retirement, and death. Identifying the family life cycle is helpful in assessing family relationships, roles, and stresses. The family life cycle is a process of expansion, contraction, and realignment of relationship systems to support the entry, exit, and development of family members (Table 15.1) (McGoldrick et al., 2016). A family's life cycle is conceptualized in terms of phases throughout the years. To move from one phase to the next, the family system undergoes changes. Structural and potential structural changes within phases can usually be managed by rearranging the family system (first-order changes), but transition from one phase to the next requires changes in the system itself (second-order changes). An example of a first-order change is when all the children are finally in school, and the stay-at-home parent returns to work. The system is rearranged, but the structure remains the same. In second-order changes, the family structure does change, such as when a member moves away from the family home to live independently.

NCLEXNOTE Apply family life cycle phases to a specific family with a member who has a mental health disorder. Identify the emotional transitions and the required family changes.

A family's life cycle is always evolving. As second marriages, career changes in midlife, and other life events occur, families are modified and redesigned to address contemporary structural and role changes. It is outside the scope of this text to present an exhaustive discussion of potential life cycles. Variations of the family life cycle are presented for divorcing and remarrying families (Table 15.2).

Transition times are the addition, subtraction, or change in status of family members. During transitions, family stresses are more likely to cause symptoms or dysfunction. Significant family events, such as the death of a member or the introduction of a new member, also affect the family's ability to function. During transitions, families may seek help from the mental health system.

Cultural Variations

The concept of "family" varies among cultures. In caring for families from diverse cultures, the nurse should examine whether the underlying assumptions and frameworks of the dominant life cycle models apply.

Work and Family Conflict

Although work can provide the economic security of a family, it can also cause stress. Parents are often torn between responsibilities of work and home. Conflict between two expectations can lead to additional family stress and poorer mental health.

Families in Poverty

Economic security programs like Social Security, Medicaid, Supplemental Nutrition Assistance Program (SNAP), tax credits, and housing assistance have been instrumental over the last half-century in reducing poverty and racial/ethnic inequities for families in the United States. One example of U.S. Government aid was the 2021 expansion of the American Rescue Plan's Child Tax Credit, along with the third round of stimulus payments and other measures of financial relief, such as expansions in unemployment insurance. The results demonstrated the largest percentage-point drop in child poverty on record, a statistic that involved a reduction in child poverty across racial and ethnic groups (Trisi, 2023). Nonetheless, barriers to the opportunity to thrive remain, and higher poverty rates for some racial and ethnic groups persist (Trisi, 2023; Trisi & Saenz, 2021).

In 2020 and 2021, during the COVID-19 pandemic, 54 million people were kept above the poverty line through support by the U.S. Government's pandemic economic security programs. Without these programs, there would have been an almost record increase in poverty. The government's assistance deterred a sharp poverty level rise "for all major racial and ethnic groups and narrowed differences in poverty rates between groups, yet wide inequities remain" (Trisi, 2023, p. 1).

TABLE 15.1 PHASES OF THE FAMILY LIFE CYCLE

Family Life Cycle Phase	Emotional Process of Transition: Key Prerequisite Attitudes	Changes in the System to Proceed Developmentally
Emerging young adults	Accepting emotional and financial responsibility for self	a. Differentiation of self in relation to family of origin b. Development of intimate peer relationships c. Establishment of self in respect to work and financial independence d. Establishment of self in community and larger society e. Establishment of one's worldview, spirituality, religion, and relationship to nature f. Parents shifting to consultative role in young adult's relationships
Couple formation: The joining of families	Commitment to new system	a. Formation of couple systems b. Expansion of family boundaries to include new partner and extended family c. Realignment of relationships with extended family, friends, and larger community to include new partners
Families with young children	Accepting new members into the system	a. Adjustment of couple system to make space for children b. Collaboration in child-rearing, financial, and housekeeping tasks c. Realignment of relationships with extended family to include parenting and grandparenting roles d. Realignment of relationships with community and larger social system to include new family structure and relationships
Families with adolescents	Increasing flexibility of family boundaries to permit children's independence and grandparents' frailties	a. Shift of parent–child relationships to permit adolescent to have more independent activities and relationships and to move more flexibility into and out of system b. Refocus on midlife couple and career issues c. Begin shift toward caring for older generation
Launching children and moving on at midlife	Accepting a multitude of exits from and entries into the system	a. Renegotiation of couple system as a dyad b. Development of adult-to-adult relationships between parents and grown children c. Realignment of relationships to include in-laws and grandchildren d. Realignment of relationships with community and larger social system to include new structure and constellation of family relationships e. Exploration of new interests or career given the freedom from child care responsibilities f. Dealing with care needs, disabilities, and death of parents (grandparents)
Families in late middle age	Accepting the shifting generational roles	a. Maintaining or modifying own and/or couple and social functioning and interests in face of physiologic decline: exploration of new familial and social role options b. Supporting more central role of middle generations c. Making room in the system for the wisdom and experience of older adults d. Supporting the older generation without overfunctioning for them
Families nearing the end of life	Accepting the realities of limitations and death and the completion of one cycle of life	a. Dealing with loss of spouse, siblings, and other peer b. Making preparations for death and legacy c. Managing reversed roles in caretaking between middle and older generations d. Realignment of relationships with larger community and social system to acknowledge changing life cycle relationships

McGoldrick, M., Garcia Preto, N., & Carter, B. (2016). Overview: The life cycle in its changing context: Individual, family and social perspectives. In M. McGoldrick, N. Garcia Preto, & B. Carter (Eds.), *The expanding family life cycle: Individual, family, and social perspectives* (5th ed., pp. 24–25). © 2016. Reprinted by permission of Pearson Education, Inc.

The family life cycle of those living in poverty may vary from those with adequate financial means. People living in poverty continue to struggle to make ends meet, and family members may face difficulties in meeting their own or other members' basic developmental needs. To experience poverty does not mean that a family system is automatically dysfunctional. But poverty is a key factor that can challenge the functioning of even the healthiest families.

Assessments and interventions with individuals and families must address the challenges faced by people in poverty. Because of poverty's effects on family members' health outcomes and disparities that exist across racial and ethnic groups, people of all ages from poor communities are at heightened risk for mental illness and early deaths, along with other life-threatening issues (Office of Disease Prevention and Health Promotion, n.d.). See Box 15.3.

TABLE 15.2 FAMILY LIFE CYCLE FOR THE DIVORCING AND REMARRYING FAMILIES

Phase and Task	Emotional Process	Developmental Issues
Divorce		
Decision to divorce	Acceptance of inability to resolve marital problems sufficiently to continue relationship	Acceptance of one's own part in the failure of the marriage
Planning the breakup of the system	Supporting viable arrangements for all parts of the system	a. Working cooperatively on problems of custody, visitation, and finances b. Dealing with extended family about the divorce
Separation	a. Willingness to continue cooperative coparental relationship and joint financial support of children b. Working on resolution of attachment to spouse	a. Mourning loss of intact family b. Restructuring marital and parent–child relationships and finances; adaptation to living apart c. Realignment of relationships with extended family; staying connected with spouse's extended family
Divorce	Working on emotional divorce: overcoming hurt, anger, guilt, and so on	a. Mourning loss of intact family; giving up fantasies of reunion b. Retrieving hopes, dreams, expectations from the marriage c. Staying connected with extended families
Postdivorce Family		
Single parent (custodial household or primary residence)	Willingness to maintain financial responsibilities, continue parental contact with ex-spouse, and support contact of children with ex-spouse and their family	a. Making flexible visitation arrangements with ex-spouse and family b. Rebuilding own financial resources c. Rebuilding own social network
Single parent (noncustodial)	Willingness to maintain financial responsibilities and parental contact with ex-spouse and to support custodial parent's relationship with children	a. Finding ways to continue effective parenting b. Maintaining financial responsibilities to ex-spouse and children c. Rebuilding own social network
Remarriage		
Entering new relationship	Recovery from loss of first marriage (adequate "emotional divorce")	Recommitment to marriage and to forming a family with readiness to deal with the complexity and ambiguity
Conceptualizing and planning new marriage and family	a. Accepting one's own fears and those of new spouse and children about forming a new family b. Accepting the need for time and patience for adjustment to complexity and ambiguity of the following: • Multiple new roles • Boundaries: space, time, membership, and authority • Affective issues: guilt, loyalty conflicts, desire for mutuality, unresolvable past hurts	a. Working on openness in the new relationships to avoid pseudomutuality b. Planning for maintenance of cooperative financial and coparental relationships with ex-spouses c. Planning to help children deal with fears, loyalty conflicts, and membership in two systems d. Realignment of relationships with extended family to include new spouse and children e. Plan maintenance of connections for children with extended family of ex-spouses
Remarriage and reconstruction of family	a. Resolution of attachment to previous spouse and ideal of "intact" family b. Acceptance of different models of family with permeable boundaries	a. Restructuring family boundaries to allow for inclusion of new spouse—stepparent b. Realignment of relationships and financial arrangements to permit interweaving of several systems c. Making room for relationships of all children with all parents, grandparents, and other extended family d. Sharing memories and histories to enhance stepfamily integration
Renegotiation of remarried family at all future life cycle transitions	Accepting evolving relationships of transformed remarried family	a. Changes as each child graduates, marries, dies, or becomes ill b. Changes as each spouse forms new couple relationship, remarries, moves, becomes ill, or dies

McGoldrick, M., Garcia Preto, N., & Carter, B. (2016). The remarriage cycle: Divorced, multinuclear and recoupled families. In M. McGoldrick, N. Garcia Preto, & B. Carter (Eds.), *The expanding family life cycle: Individual, family, and social perspectives* (5th ed., pp. 413–414).

BOX 15.3

Mental Health Inequities: Outpatient Mental Health Care by Socioeconomic Status

Families of lower socioeconomic status may not have the resources to provide mental health care to family members. Many parents struggle to find mental health care for their children, and many mental health clinicians do not accept insurance payments. In a descriptive cross-sectional analysis performed among youths ages 5 to 17 years in a 2018–2020 Medical Expenditure Panel survey, approximately 1 in 5 of 13,639 outpatient mental health specialist visits were self-pay. Use of self-pay is associated with higher income, but even families earning less than $28,000 a year utilized some self-pay services. The self-pay market potentially exacerbates inequities in access to care by burdening low-income families with high costs.

Overhage, L. N., Benson, N. M., Flores, M. W., & Cook, B. L. (2024). Self-pay outpatient mental health care for children and adolescents, by socioeconomic status. *Psychiatric Services, 75*(9), 833–838. https://doi.org/10.1176/appi.ps.20230524

Communication Patterns

Family system communication patterns develop over a lifetime and are essential information during an assessment. Some family members communicate more openly and honestly than others. In addition, family subgroups develop from their patterns of communication. Just as in any assessment interview, the nurse should observe the verbal and nonverbal communication of individual family members and the family unit. Using a family systems perspective and working from a multicultural framework, the nurse should be open minded and attend to families' cultural patterns in structures, processes, dynamics, and communication, which may not represent the traditional Western culture (Corey, 2024).

During an assessment, the nurse could consider some of the following. If a rectangular table is involved, who sits at the short end? Who sits next to each other or across from one another? Who looks at and/or talks to whom? Who gets "shut down" when communicating? Who answers most questions? Who volunteers information? Who changes the subject? Which subjects seem acceptable to discuss? Which topics are not discussed? Can spouses and children show affectionate nonverbal behavior with each other? What do family members' spoken voices communicate? What do family members nonverbally communicate? Are any family secrets revealed? Does nonverbal communication match the verbal communication? Who looks at or does not make eye contact with the PMH nurse interviewer? Nurses can use such information to guide identification of family issues, problems, and communication dysfunctions needing therapeutic intervention strategies to enhance family health and wellness.

PMH nurses should also assess the family system for its regular communication patterns. Identifying which family members confide in one another is a place to start examining ongoing communication. Other areas include how often children talk with parents, which child talks to which parent most, and who is most likely to discipline the children. Another question considers whether family members can express positive and negative feelings. In determining how open or closed the family is, the nurse explores the type of information the family shares with nonfamily members. For example, whereas one family member may tell people outside the family about a member's mental illness, another family may not discuss illnesses only with members of the family.

Stress and Coping Abilities

One of the most important assessment tasks is to determine how family members deal with major and minor stressful events and their available coping skills. Whereas some family systems seem able to cope with overwhelming stresses, such as the death of a family member, major illness, or severe conflict, other families are unable to cope with even relatively minor events. Some family caregivers of people with mental illness are resilient and recover or adjust to challenges over time. Some families not only survive the day-to-day stresses of caring for a family member with a serious mental health issue but also seem to grow stronger and healthier. It is important for the nurse to listen to which situation a family appraises as stressful and help the family identify their usual coping responses. The nurse can then evaluate these responses. On the other hand, if the family's responses are maladaptive (e.g., substance misuse, physical abuse), the nurse will discuss the need to develop coping skills that lead to family well-being (see Chapter 19).

NCLEXNOTE Identifying stressful events and coping mechanisms should be a priority in a family assessment.

Problem-Solving Skills

Nurses assess a family's problem-solving skills by focusing on the more recent problems the family system has experienced and determining the process that members used to solve them. The focus on assessing problem-solving skills helps in understanding family resilience discussed earlier in the chapter. For example, a child is sick at school and needs to go home. Which family member, caregiver, or babysitter receives the call from the school? Who then cares for the child? Underlying the ability to solve problems is the decision-making process. Who makes and implements decisions, particularly health care decisions? How does the family handle conflict? All these areas for data gathering and inquiry provide information regarding a family's problem-solving abilities and strengths. After family members' and family system abilities are identified, the PMH nurse can build on identified capacity and strengths in helping families deal with current and additional issues and problems.

Family Social Domain

An assessment of a family's social domain provides important data about the operation of the family as a system and its interaction within its environment. Areas of concern include the system itself, social and financial status, and formal and informal support networks.

Family Systems

Just as any group can be viewed as a living system, a family can be understood as a system with interdependent members. Family system theories view the family as an open system whose members interact with their environment as well as among themselves. One family member's change in thoughts or behavior can cause a ripple effect and change in everyone else's. For example, a parent who decides not to pick up their children's clothing from their bedroom floors anymore forces the children to deal with the cluttered rooms and dirty clothes in a different way than before.

One common scenario in the mental health field is the effect of a patient's improvement on the family system. With new medications and treatment, patients are more likely to be able to live independently, and this subsequently changes the responsibilities and activities of those who had assumed the role of family caregivers. Although on the surface members may seem relieved that their caregiving burden is lifted, they now must adjust their time and energies to fill the remaining void. This transition may not be easy because it is often less stressful to maintain familiar activities than to venture into uncharted territory.

Several system models are used in caring for families: the Wright Leahey Calgary model (Shajani & Snell, 2023); the Bowen family system (1975, 1976); and Minuchin, Lee, and Simon's (1996) structural family system.

Calgary Family Model

Lorraine M. Wright and Maureen Leahey developed the Calgary Family Assessment Model and the Calgary Family Intervention Model (CFIM). These nursing models are based on systems, cybernetics, and communication and change theories (Shajani & Snell, 2023). Families seek help when they have family health and illness issues, difficulties, and suffering. These two models are multidimensional frameworks that conceptualize the family into structural, developmental, and functional categories. Each assessment category contains several subcategories. Structure is further categorized into internal (e.g., family, gender, sexual orientation), external (i.e., extended family and larger systems), and context (i.e., ethnicity, race, social class, religion, spirituality, environment). Family developmental assessment is organized according to stages, tasks, and attachments. Functional assessment areas include instrumental (e.g., activities of daily living) and expressive (i.e., communication, problem-solving roles, beliefs).

The Calgary Family Assessment Model and the CFIM are built around four stages (Shajani & Snell, 2023):

- The *engagement* stage is the initial stage in which the family is greeted and made comfortable.
- In the *assessment* stage, issues are identified and relationships among family members and health providers develop. During this stage, the nurse opens space for the family members to tell their stories.
- The *intervention* stage is the core of the clinical work and involves providing a context in which the family can make changes.
- The *termination* phase refers to the process of ending the therapeutic relationship.

A recent systematic review regarding the use of the CFIM, derived from Leahey and Wright's Calgary Family Assessment Model published in 1994, concluded that it is an excellent tool for nurses to use to collaboratively work with and provide education to families and enable enhanced patient and family system outcomes (Mileski et al, 2022).

Family Systems Therapy Model

Murray Bowen (1913–1990) recognized the power of a system and believed that there is a balance between the family system and the individual. Bowen's emphasis on a multigenerational perspective laid the groundwork for his prominent colleagues, the renowned family therapists Monica McGoldrick and Betty Carter, to initiate their own developmental and multicultural family systems work, which included a focus on genograms, family life cycle, gender, and race (Corey, 2024). Bowen developed the following concepts that professionals often use today when working with families (Bowen, 1975, 1976; Bowen Center for the Study of the Family, 2024).

Differentiation of self involves two processes: intrapsychic and interpersonal. Intrapsychic differentiation means separating thinking from feeling: A differentiated individual can distinguish between thoughts and feelings and can consequently think through behavior. For example, an individual who has experienced intrapsychic differentiation, even though angry, will think through the underlying issue before acting. However, the feeling of the moment will drive the behavior of an undifferentiated individual. Interpersonal differentiation is the process of freeing oneself from the family's emotional chaos. That is, the individual can recognize the family turmoil but avoid reentering arguments and issues. For Bowen, the individual must resolve attachment to this chaos before they can differentiate into a mature, healthy personality.

Triangles: According to Bowen, the triangle is a three-person system and the smallest stable unit in human relations. Cycles of closeness and distance characterize a two-person relationship. When anxiety is high during periods of distance, one party "triangulates" a third person or thing into the relationship. For example, two partners may have a stable relationship when anxiety is low. When anxiety and tension rise, one partner may be so uncomfortable they confide in a friend instead of the other partner. In these cases, triangulating reduces the tension but freezes the conflict in place. In families, triangulating occurs when spouses diffuse tension by focusing on the children. To maintain the status quo and avoid the conflict, which tends to produce symptoms in the child (e.g., bed wetting, fear of school), one partner develops an overly intense relationship with one of the children.

Family projection process: Through this process, the triangulated member becomes the center of the family conflicts—that is, the family projects its conflicts onto the child or other triangulated person. Projection is an anxious, enmeshed concern. For example, a couple is having difficulty deciding how to spend money. One of their children is having difficulty with interpersonal relationships in school. Instead of the couple resolving their differences over money, one partner focuses on the child's needs and becomes intensely involved in the child's issues. The other partner then relates coolly and distantly to the involved partner.

Nuclear family emotional process: This concept describes four relationship patterns that guide the development of issues in the family. *Marital conflict pattern* is where each spouse focuses on what is wrong with the other, tries to control the other, and resists the other's attempt at control. *Dysfunction in a spouse pattern* is where one spouse yields to the pressure of the other spouse to think and act in certain ways. The subordinate spouse can become so anxious because of yielding so much self-control that a psychiatric, medical, or social dysfunction occurs. *Impairment of one or more children pattern* occurs when spouses focus anxieties on one or more of their children who acts out or internalizes family tensions. *Emotional distance* is a pattern where family members distance themselves emotionally from each other and risk becoming too isolated (Bowen Center for the Study of the Family, 2024).

Multigenerational transmission process: Bowen believed that one generation transfers its emotional processes to the next generation. Certain basic patterns among partners and children are replicas of those of past generations, and generations to follow will repeat them. The child who is the most involved with the family is least able to differentiate from their family of origin and passes on conflicts from one generation to another. For example, a partner may stay emotionally distant from their partner just as their parents were with each other.

Sibling position: Children often develop personality characteristics based on their sibling position in their families. For example, a first-born child may have more confidence and be more outgoing than the second-born child, who has grown up in the older child's shadow. Conversely, the second-born child may be more open to new experiences than the first-born child. These attitudinal and behavioral patterns may become parts of both children's personalities. Knowledge of these general personality characteristics is helpful in predicting the family's emotional processes and patterns. Although the other theoretical ideas of Bowen have not been supported by research, the general principle that birth order affects a child's personality has significant empirical support (McAndrew& Sbai, 2023).

Emotional cutoff: If a member cannot differentiate from their family, that member may just flee from the family, either by moving away or avoiding personal subjects of conversation.

In using the family systems therapy model, the nurse can observe family interactions to determine how differentiated family members are from one another. Are members autonomous in thinking and feeling? Do triangulated relationships develop during periods of stress and tension? Are family members interacting in the same manner as their parents or grandparents? How do the personalities of older siblings compare with those of younger siblings? Who lives close to one another? Does any family member live in another city? The Bowen model can provide a way of assessing the system of family relationships (Worch & Bartle-Haring, 2024).

Family Structure Model

Salvador Minuchin (1921–2017) emphasized the importance of family structure. In this model, the family consists of three essential components: Structure, subsystems, and boundaries.

Family structure is the organized pattern in which family members interact. As two adult partners come together to form a family, they develop the quantity of their interactions, or how much time they spend interacting. For example, a newly formed couple may establish their evening interaction pattern by talking to each other during dinner but not while watching television. The quality of the interactions also becomes patterned. Whereas some topics are appropriate for conversation during their evening walk (e.g., reciting daily events), controversial or emotionally provocative topics are relegated to other times and places (Minuchin et al., 1996).

Family rules are important influences on interaction patterns. For example, "family problems stay in the family" is a common rule. Both the number of people in the family and its development also influence the interaction pattern. For instance, the interaction between a single parent and their children changes when they remarry and introduces a stepparent. Over time, families repeat interactions, which develop into enduring patterns. For example, if the parent tells their child to straighten their room and the child refuses until their stepparent yells at the child, the family has initiated an interactional pattern. If this pattern continues, the child will come to see the stepparent as the disciplinarian and the parent as incompetent.

Subsystems develop when family members join together for various activities or functions. Minuchin et al. (1996) viewed each member, as well as dyads and other larger groups that form, as a subsystem. Groups could be parents and children, or family members of the same gender. Besides family members belonging to subgroups, they also can have different roles in the family. For example, a parent may also be a partner, sibling, and child of their parent. Sometimes, these roles can conflict. It may be acceptable for a person to be very firm as a disciplinarian in their role as a parent. However, in the role of sibling, partner, or child of their parent, similar behavior would provoke anger and resentment.

Boundaries are invisible barriers with varying permeabilities that surround each subsystem. They regulate the amount of contact an individual has with others and protect the autonomy of the family and its subsystems. If family members do not take telephone calls at dinner, they are protecting themselves from outside intrusion. When parents do not allow children to interrupt them, they establish a boundary between themselves and their children. According to Minuchin et al. (1996), the spouse subsystem must have a boundary that separates it from parents, children, and the outside world. A clear boundary between parent and child enables children to interact with their parents but excludes them from the spouse subsystem.

Boundaries vary from rigid to diffuse. If boundaries are too rigid and permit little contact from outside subsystems, disengagement results, and disengaged individuals are isolated. On the other hand, rigid boundaries permit independence, growth, and mastery within the subsystem, particularly if parents do not hover over their children, telling them what to do or fighting their battles. Enmeshed subsystems result when boundaries are diffuse. That is, when boundaries are too relaxed, parents may become too involved with their children, and the children learn to rely on the parents to make decisions, resulting in decreased independence. According to Minuchin et al. (1996), if children see their parents as friends and treat them as they would treat their peers, then enmeshment exists.

Autonomy and interdependence are key concepts, important both to individual growth and family system maintenance. Relationship patterns are maintained by universal rules governing family organization (especially power hierarchy) and mutual behavioral expectations. In a well-functioning family, boundaries are clear, and a hierarchy exists with a strong parental subsystem. Problems result when there is a malfunctioning of the hierarchical arrangement or boundaries, or if there is a maladaptive reaction to changing developmental or environmental requirements. Minuchin et al. (1996) believed in clear, flexible boundaries by which all family members can live comfortably.

In the family structural theory, what distinguishes well-functioning families is not the absence of problems but a functional family structure to manage them. Partners must learn to adjust to each other, rear their children, deal with their own parents, cope with their jobs, and fit into their communities. The types of struggles change with developmental stages and situational crises.

The PMH nurse with a structural family theoretical orientation assesses the family structure and the presence of subsystems, transactional rules, and boundaries. The nurse uses these data to determine how the subsystems, rules, and boundaries affect the family's functioning. For example, helping family members change a subsystem, such as including younger and older children together in family activities, may improve family functioning. The ultimate intervention goal would be to reduce symptoms of family dysfunction and enhance family system strengths by bringing about structural changes within the family system (Corey, 2024).

Social and Financial Status

Social status is often linked directly to financial status. Nurses should assess the occupations of the family members. Who works? Who is primarily responsible for the family's financial support? Families of low social status are more likely to have limited financial resources, which can place additional stresses on the family. Nurses can use information regarding the family's financial status to determine whether to refer the family to social services.

Formal and Informal Support Networks

Both formal and informal networks are important in providing support to individuals and families and should be identified in the family system assessments. These networks are the link among the individual, families, and the community. Assessing the extent of formal support (e.g., hospitals, agencies, licensed providers) and informal support (e.g., extended family, friends, and neighbors) gives a clearer picture of the availability of support. In assessing formal support, the nurse should ask about the family's involvement with government institutions and mental health self-help groups such as Twelve Step groups (e.g., Alcoholics Anonymous, Narcotics Anonymous), or other mental health self-help groups used by family members. Group involvement can be through either traditional in-person attendance or via online group attendance.

Assessing the informal network is particularly important in cultural groups with extended family networks or close friends because these individuals can be major sources of support to patients. If the PMH nurse does not ask about the informal network, these important people may be missed. Nurses can inquire whether family members volunteer at schools, local hospitals, or nursing homes. They can also ask whether the family attends religious services or group activities organized by their religious affiliations.

Family Spiritual Assessment

The importance of the spiritual assessment for an individual was discussed in Chapter 10. When caring for or interacting with the family of an individual with a mental health issue, the family spiritual assessment is also important (Kuckel et al., 2022). By asking family members if they are members of a religious group or a spiritual community, the nurse can begin to understand the significance of their faith or spiritual beliefs. They may not be affiliated with a particular religious group but may have spiritual beliefs and practices that have meaning to them. An important question to ask is if they would like to speak to a chaplain or a religious leader. Most health care organizations have relationships with a chaplaincy service.

TAKING ACTION: FAMILY INTERVENTIONS

Family interventions focus on supporting the integrity and functioning of the family as defined by its members. Although family therapy is reserved for licensed mental health specialists, the generalist PMH nurse can implement several interventions, such as counseling, promotion of self-care activities, supportive therapy, psychoeducation and health teaching, and the use of genograms.

In implementing any family intervention, flexibility is essential, particularly when working with culturally diverse groups. The nurse creates the context for change by making sure the therapeutic interventions are possible for the family (Shajani & Snell, 2023). For example, weekly appointments may be ideal but impossible for a busy family. To implement successful, culturally humble family interventions, nurses need to be open to modifying the structure and format of the sessions. Longer sessions are often useful, especially when there is a translator or interpreter. Nurses also need to respect and work with the changing composition of family and nonfamily participants (e.g., extended family members, intimate partners, friends and neighbors, community helpers) in sessions. Because of the stigma that some cultural groups associate with seeking help, PMH nurses may need to hold intervention sessions in community settings (e.g., places of worship and schools) or at the family's home. If adequate progress is made, the nurse should decrease the frequency of sessions and move toward termination. Families may move toward termination themselves if they recognize that improvement has occurred (Shajani & Snell, 2023).

Counseling

Counseling is a short-term problem-solving approach that addresses current issues. When engaging in counseling, the nurse should avoid taking sides by forming an alliance with one family member or subgroup (Shajani & Snell, 2023). If the assessment reveals complex, long-standing relationship issues, the nurse needs to refer the family to a family therapist. If the family is struggling with psychiatric issues of one or more family members, or if the family system is in a life cycle transition, the nurse should use short-term counseling strategies. Instead of giving advice, the counseling sessions should focus on specific issues or problems using sound group process theory (see Chapter 14). Usually, a problem-solving approach works well after an issue is identified (see Chapter 19).

Promoting Self-Care Activities

Families often need support in changing behaviors that promote self-care activities. For example, families may inadvertently reinforce a family member's dependency out of fear of the patient being taken advantage of in work or social situations. A nurse can help the family explore how to meet the patient's need for work and social activity and, at the same time, help alleviate the family's fears. It is important that nurses recognize that for self-care, patients can have some control over the decision-making process.

Caregiver distress or role strain can occur in families that are responsible for the care of members with long-term illness. Family interventions can help families deal with the burden of caring for members with psychiatric disorders.

Supporting Family System Functioning and Resilience

Supporting family system functioning involves various nursing approaches. In meeting with the family, the PMH nurse should identify and acknowledge its values. In developing rapport and a trusting relationship with the family, the nurse should confirm that all members have a sense of self and self-worth. Encouraging positive thinking and participation in support groups will contribute to the family's well-being. Supporting family subsystems (e.g., encouraging the children to play while meeting with the parents/caregivers) reinforces family boundaries. Based on assessment of the family system's operation and communication patterns, the PMH nurse can reinforce open, honest communication.

In communicating with the family, the nurse needs to observe boundaries constantly and avoid becoming triangulated into family issues. An objective, empathic leadership style can set the tone for the family sessions.

Psychoeducation and Health Teaching

One of the most important family interventions is psychoeducation and health teaching, particularly in families with mental illness. Families have a central role in the treatment of mental illnesses. Members need to learn about mental disorders, medications, actions, side effects, and overall treatment approaches and outcomes. For example, families may be reluctant to have members take psychiatric medications because they believe the medications will oversedate the patient or that the patient will become dependent on the medication. The family's beliefs about mental illnesses and treatment can affect whether patients will be able to manage their illness. Research shows that family psychoeducation interventions are effective in preventing relapse in schizophrenia (Rodolico et al., 2022). To initiate a family psychoeducation intervention, the nurse would first ask the patient what they think their family is doing to help them or what they feel is not helpful to them; the nurse would also ask which family member(s) the patient would want to attend the psychoeducation sessions.

Using Genograms

Besides being useful in assessment, genograms are also used as intervention strategies. PMH nurses can use genograms to help family members understand current feelings and emotions as well as the family's evolution over several generations. Genograms allow the family to view their family tree and examine relationships from a factual, objective perspective. Often, family members gain new insights and can begin to understand their problems within the context of their family system. For example, families may begin to view depression in an adolescent child with new seriousness when they see it as part of a pattern of several generations of adolescents who have struggled with depression. A partner, raised as an only child in a small Midwestern town, may better understand their feelings of being overwhelmed at gatherings of extended family of their partner's relatives after comparing their family structure with that of their partner, who comes from a large family of several generations living together in the urban Northeast (Box 15.4).

BOX 15.4

John and Judy Jones

John and Judy Jones were married 3 years ago after their graduation from a small liberal arts college in the Midwest. Judy's career choice required that she live in the Northeast, where she would be near her large family. John willingly moved with her and quickly found a satisfying position. After about 6 months of marriage, John became extremely irritable and depressed. He kept saying that his life was not his own. Judy was genuinely concerned but could not understand his feelings of being overwhelmed. His job was going well, and they had a busy social life, mostly revolving around her family, whom John loved. They decided to seek counseling and completed the following genogram:

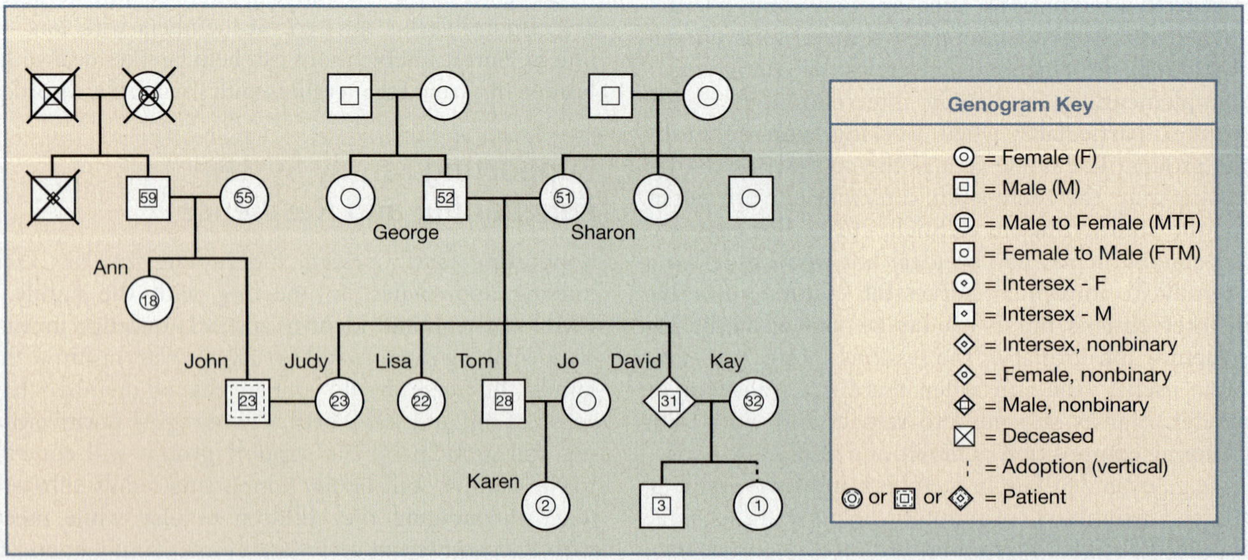

After looking at the genogram, both John and Judy began to realize that part of John's discomfort had to do with the number of family members from Judy's side of the family who participated in their lives. Judy and John began to redefine their social life, allowing more time with friends and each other.

SUMMARY OF KEY POINTS

- A family is a group of people who are connected emotionally, by blood, or both that has developed patterns of interactions and relationships. The family is an important societal unit that often is responsible for the care and coordination of treatment of members with mental disorders.
- Family characteristics such as size, member roles, mobility, and composition influence the strength of a family system. Traditional health care services will have to adapt to meet the mental health care needs of all types of families.
- Families come in various compositions, including unmarried couples, single-parent families, stepfamilies, families without children, and families with parents who are LGBTQ+. Cultural values and beliefs define family composition and roles.
- Nurses complete a comprehensive family assessment when they care for families for extended periods or if a patient has complex mental health issues.
- In building relationships with families, nurses must establish credibility and competence with the family. Unless the nurse addresses the family's immediate needs first, the family will have difficulty engaging in the challenges of caring for someone with a mental disorder.
- The genogram is an assessment and intervention tool that is useful in understanding health issues, relationship issues, and social functioning across several generations.
- In assessing the family, the nurse determines physical and mental health status of all family members and their effects on family functioning.
- Family members are often reluctant to discuss the mental disorders of family members because of the stigma associated with mental illness. In many instances, family members do not know whether mental illnesses were present in past generations.
- The family psychological assessment focuses on family development, the family life cycle, communication patterns, stress, coping abilities, and problem-solving skills. One assessment aim is to begin to understand family interpersonal relationships.
- The family life cycle is a process of expansion, contraction, and realignment of the relationship systems to support the entry, exit, and development of family members in a functional way. The nurse should determine whether a family fits any of the life cycle models.
- In assessing the family social domain, the nurse compiles data about the system itself, social and financial status, and formal and informal support networks.
- The family system model proposes that a balance should exist between the family system and the individual. An individual not only needs family connections but also needs to be differentiated as an individual. Important concepts include triangles, family projection process, nuclear family emotional process, multigenerational transmission, sibling position, and emotional cutoff.
- The family structure model explains patterns of family interaction. Subsystems develop that also influence interaction patterns. Boundaries can vary from rigid to relaxed. The rigidity of the boundaries affects family functioning.
- Family interventions focus on supporting the family's integrity and functioning as defined by its members. Family nursing interventions include counseling, promotion of self-care activities, supportive therapy, psychoeducation and health teaching, and the use of genograms. Mental health specialists, including psychiatric mental health advanced practice nurses, conduct family therapy.
- Psychoeducation of the family is one of the most useful interventions. Teaching the family about mental disorders, life cycles, family systems, and family interactions can help the family develop a new understanding of family functioning and the effects of mental disorders on the family.

DEVELOPING CLINICAL JUDGMENT

1. On what basis can a group of people who are unrelated by blood consider themselves a family?
2. A patient who is divorced with two small children reports that they are considering getting married again to someone they met 6 months ago. They ask for help in considering the advantages and disadvantages of remarriage. Using the remarried family formulations life cycle model, develop a plan for structuring the counseling session.
3. Discuss what happens to a family that has rigid boundaries.
4. A family is finding it difficult to provide transportation to a support group for an adult member with mental illness. The family is committed to the patient's treatment but is also experiencing severe financial stress because of another family illness. Using a problem-solving approach, outline a plan for helping the family explore solutions to the transportation problem.

MOVIES, TV, OR STREAMING PROGRAMS

My Big Fat Greek Wedding: 2002. This movie is about Fotoula "Toula" Portokalos, a Greek American woman who falls in love with a non-Greek protestant, Ian Miller. Toula is the only one in her family who has not met her family expectations of marrying a Greek person and having children. Toula is stuck working in the family business, a restaurant, whereas her sister married a Greek person and has children. Toula's father is adamantly opposed to Toula marrying a non-Greek person.

Viewing Points:

1. Discuss the stigma that faces Toula and Ian as they plan their life together.
2. How would you intervene if Toula approached you for help with her family?
3. Identify the cultural beliefs that are shaping and interfering with the wishes of the newly engaged couple.

REFERENCES

Aragão, C. (2023). Working husbands in U.S. have more leisure time than working wives do, especially among those with children. *Pew Research Center*, Retrieved January 17, 2024, from https://www.pewresearch.org/short-reads/2023/10/27/working-husbands-in-the-us-have-more-leisure-time-than-working-wives-do-especially-among-those-with-children

Board of Governors of the Federal Reserve System. (2023). *Survey of consumer finances (SCF)*. The Federal Reserve. https://www.federalreserve.gov/econres/scf/dataviz/scf/chart/#series:Net_Worth;demographic:famstruct;population:all;units:median;range:1989,2022

Bowen, M. (1975). Family therapy after twenty years. In S. Arieti, D. Freedman, & J. Dyrud (Eds.), *American handbook of psychiatry* (2nd ed., Vol. 5, pp. 379–391). Basic Books.

Bowen, M. (1976). Theory in the practice of psychotherapy. In P. Guerin (Ed.), *Family therapy: Theory and practice* (pp. 42–90). Gardner Press.

Bowen Center for the Study of the Family. (2024). *Nuclear family emotional process*. Retrieved October 18, 2024, from https://www.thebowencenter.org/nuclear-family-emotional-process

Centers for Disease Control. (2024). *Reproductive health*. Retrieved October 18, 2024, from https://www.cdc.gov/reproductive-health/infertility-faq/

Coulter-Thompson, E. I. (2023). Bias and discrimination against lesbian, gay, bisexual, transgender, and queer parents accessing care for their children: A literature review. *Health Education & Behavior*, *50*(2), 181–192. https://doi.org/10.1177/10901981221148959

Corey, G. (2024). *Theory and practice of counseling and psychotherapy*. Cengage.

Crisp, H., & Gabbard, G. O. (Eds.). (2023). *Gabbard's textbook of psychotherapeutic treatments* (2nd ed.). American Psychiatric Association Publishing.

Dharani, M. K., & Balamurugan, J. (2024). The psychosocial impact on single mothers' well-being – A literature review. *Journal of Education and Health Promotion*, *13*, 148. https://doi.org/10.4103/jehp.jehp_1045_23

Dionisi, A. M., Smith, C. J., & Dupré, K. E. (2023). Weathering the storm alone or together: Examining the impact of COVID-19 on sole and partnered working mothers. *Journal of Community Psychology*, *51*(6), 2408–2429. https://doi.org/10.1002/jcop.22829

Farr, R. H., Cashen, K. K., Siebenthaler, K. A., & Simon, K. A. (2024). Microaggression and discrimination experiences among diverse youth with LGBTQ+ parents in the United States. *Journal of Research on Adolescence*, *34*(2), 551–567. https://doi.org/10.1111/jora.12919

Jayasinghe, A., Wrobel, A., Filia, K., Byrne, L. K., Melvin, G., Murrihy, S., Moller, C., Berk, L., Berk, M., & Cotton, S. (2023). Distress, burden, and wellbeing in siblings of people with mental illness: a mixed studies systematic review and meta-analysis. *Psychological Medicine*, *53*(15), 6945–6964. https://doi.org/10.1017/S0033291723001733

Jester, D. J., Thomas, M. L., Sturm, E. T., Harvey, P. D., Keshavan, M., Davis, B. J., Saxena, S., Tampi, R., Leutwyler, H., Compton, M. T., Palmer, B. W., & Jeste, D. V. (2023). Review of major social determinants of health in schizophrenia-spectrum psychotic disorders: I. Clinical outcomes. *Schizophrenia Bulletin*, *49*(4), 837–850. https://doi.org/10.1093/schbul/sbad023

Konradsen, H., Brødsgaard, A., Østergaard, B., García-Vivar, C., Svavarsdottir, E. K., Dieperink, K. B., Imhof, L., Luttik, M. L. A., & Mahrer-Imhof, R. (2023). The COVID-19 post pandemic: Family nursing now more than ever. *Journal of Family Nursing*, *29*(1), 3–5. https://doi.org/10.1177/10748407221147965

Kuang, Y., Wang, M., Yu, N. X., Jia, S., Guan, T., Zhang, X., Zhang, Y., Lu, J., & Wang, A. (2023). Family resilience of patients requiring long-term care: A meta-synthesis of qualitative studies. *Journal of Clinical Nursing*, *32*(13–14), 4159–4175. https://doi.org/10.1111/jocn.16500

Kunkel, D. P., Jones, A. L., & Smith, D. K. (2022). The spiritual assessment. *American Family Physician*, *106*(4), 415–419.

Laurent, R., Correia, P., Lachand, R., Diconne, E., Ezingeard, E., Bruna, F., Guenier, P. A., Page, D., Périnel-Ragey, S., & Thiéry, G. (2023). Long-term outcomes of COVID-19 intensive care unit survivors and their family members: A one year follow-up prospective study. *Frontiers in Public Health*, *11*, 1236990. https://doi.org/10.3389/fpubh.2023.1236990

Manesh, A. E., Dalvandi, A., & Zoladl, M. (2023). The experience of stigma in family caregivers of people with schizophrenia spectrum disorders: A meta-synthesis study. *Heliyon*, *9*(3), e14333. https://doi.org/10.1016/j.heliyon.2023.e14333

McAndrew, F. T., & Sbai, Z. (2023). Perceptions of the personalities of namesaked children as a function of their sex and birth order. *Psychological Reports*, 332941231214166. https://doi.org/10.1177/00332941231214166

McGoldrick, M., Garcia Preto, N., & Carter, B. (2016). The life cycle in its changing context: individual, family and social perspectives. In M. McGoldrick, N. Garcia Preto, & B. Carter (Eds.), *The expanding family life cycle: Individual, family, and social perspectives* (5th ed.). Pearson.

Mileski, M., McClay, R. Heinemann, K., & Dray, G. (2022). Efficacy of the use of the Calgary Family Intervention Model in bedside nursing education: A systematic review. *Journal of Multidisciplinary Healthcare*, *15*, 1323–1347. https://doi.org/10.2147/JMDH.S370053.

Minuchin, S., Lee, W., & Simon, G. (1996). *Mastering family therapy: Journey of growth and transformation* (2nd ed.). John Wiley & Sons.

Movement Advancement Project. (2023). *Obstacles & opportunities: Health & wellness for LGBT families*. https://www.lgbtmap.org/policy-and-issue-analysis/obstacles-and-opportunities-ensuring-health-and-wellness-for-lgbt-families

National Academies of Sciences, Engineering, and Medicine. (2023). *Addressing the long-term effects of the COVID-19 pandemic on children and families*. The National Academies Press. https://doi.org/10.17226/26809.

Office of Disease Prevention and Health Promotion. (n.d.). *Healthy people 2030: Poverty*. Retrieved January 22, 2024, from https://health.gov/healthypeople/priority-areas/social-determinants-health/literature-summaries/poverty

Prates, P. E. G., Correa-Júnior, A. J. S., Russo, T. M. D. S., Paraizo-Horvath, C. M. S., Teles, A. A. D. S., & Sonobe, H. M. (2024). Effectiveness of family coping interventions in improving problem-solving skills in the care of children and adolescent cancer survivors during and after treatment: a scoping review. *Nursing Reports*, *14*(3), 2153–2178. https://doi.org/10.3390/nursrep14030161

Rodolico, A., Bighelli, I., Avanzato, C., Concerto, C., Cutrufelli, P., Mineo, L., Schneider-Thoma, J., Siafis, S., Signorelli, M. S., Wu, H., Wang, D., Furukawa, T. A., Pitschel-Walz, G., Aguglia, E., & Leucht, S. (2022). Family interventions for relapse prevention in schizophrenia: a systematic review and network meta-analysis. *The Lancet Psychiatry*, *9*(3), 211–221. https://doi.org/10.1016/S2215-0366(21)00437-5

Roland, J. S., & Walsh, F. (2023). Family therapy: systemic concepts and methods. In H. Crisp & G. O. Gabbard (Eds.), *Gabbard's textbook of psychotherapeutic treatments* (2nd ed., pp. 397–421). American Psychiatric Association Publishing.

Shajani, Z., & Snell, D. (2023). *Wright & Leahey's nurses and families: A guide to family assessment and intervention* (8th ed.). F. A. Davis.

Silver, N. E. (2023). What I tell my patients about mental health and infertility. *Expert view*. The American College of Obstetricians and Gynecologists. https://www.acog.org/womens-health/experts-and-stories/the-latest/what-i-tell-my-patients-about-mental-health-and-infertility

Sustrami, D., Yusuf, A., Fitryasari, R., Suhardiningsih, A. V. S., & Arifin, H. (2023). Determinants of burden in family caregivers of individuals with schizophrenia: A systematic review. *Journal of Psychosocial Nursing and Mental Health Services*, *61*(2), 38–43. https://doi.org/10.3928/02793695-20220804-02

The Stepfamily Foundation. (2023). *Stepfamily statistics*. https://www.stepfamily.org/stepfamily-statistics.html

Trisi, D. (2023). *Government's pandemic response turned a would-be poverty surge into a record poverty decline*. Center on Budget and Policy Priorities. Retrieved January 22, 2024, from https://www.cbpp.org/research/poverty-and-inequality/governments-pandemic-response-turned-a-would-be-poverty-surge-into

Trisi, D., & Saenz, M. (2021). *Economic security programs reduce overall poverty, racial and ethnic inequities*. Center on Budget and Policy Priorities. Retrieved January 22, 2024, from https://www.cbpp.org/research/poverty-and-inequality/more-than-4-in-10-children-in-renter-households-face-food-andor

United States Census Bureau. (2023). *Married couple households made up most of family households*. Retrieved from https://www.census.gov/library/stories/2023/05/family-households-still-the-majority.html

Walsh, F. (2021). Family resilience: a dynamic systemic framework. In M. Ungar (Eds.), *Multisystemic resilience: Adaptation and transformation in contexts of change*. (pp. 255–270). Oxford. https://doi.org/10.1093/oso/9780190095888.003.0015

Worch, S., & Bartle-Haring, S. (2024). Couple differentiation and health-related quality of life. *Family Process*, 10.1111/famp.12977. doi.org/10.1111/famp.12977

Yeban, J. (2023a). *Cohabitation: Background and legal issues*. FindLaw. Retrieved January 17, 2024, from https://www.findlaw.com/family/living-together/cohabitation-background-and-trends.html

Yeban, J. (2023b). *Cohabitation agreements*. FindLaw. https://www.findlaw.com/family/living-together/cohabitation-agreements.html

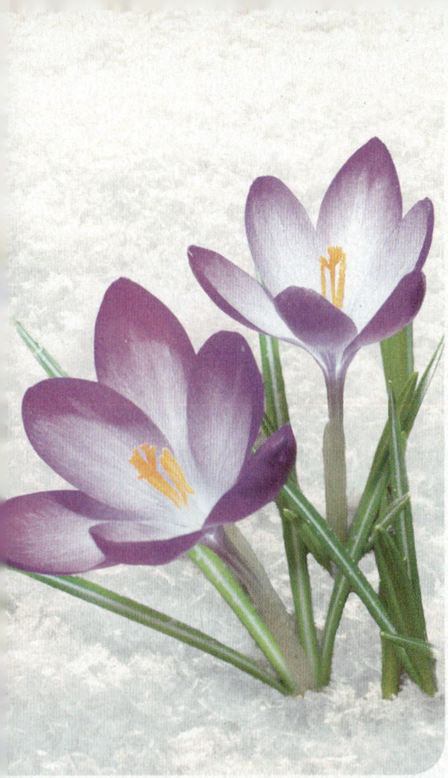

UNIT IV
Mental Health Across the Lifespan

16
Mental Health Promotion for Childhood and Adolescence

Catherine Gray Deering

KEYCONCEPTS

- emotional regulation
- egocentric thinking
- invincibility fable

LEARNING OBJECTIVES

After studying this chapter, you will be able to:

1. Describe common stressors for children and adolescents.
2. Identify risk factors for the development of psychopathology in childhood and adolescence.
3. Describe protective factors in the mental health promotion of children and adolescents.
4. Analyze the role of the nurse in mental health promotion for children and families.

KEY TERMS

• adverse childhood events • attachment • bullying • child abuse and neglect • developmental delays • early intervention programs • effortful control • executive functioning • family preservation • fetal alcohol syndrome • formal operations • normalization • protective factors • psychoeducational programs • relational aggression • resilience • risk factors • social skills training • temperament • vulnerable child syndrome

INTRODUCTION

Children and adolescents respond to the stresses of life in different ways according to their developmental levels. **Resilience** is the phenomenon by which some children at risk for psychopathology—because of genetic or experiential circumstances (or both)—attain good mental health, maintain hope, and achieve healthy outcomes (Flaskerud, 2022). This chapter examines specific determinants of childhood and adolescent mental health, discusses the effects of common childhood stressors, and identifies **risk factors** for psychopathology, or the characteristics that increase the likelihood of developing a disorder. This chapter also considers **protective factors**, or the characteristics that reduce the probability that a child will develop a disorder, and provides guidelines for mental health promotion and risk reduction. Over the past two decades, a large body of research on diverse populations has established a strong connection between **adverse childhood events** (e.g., abuse, neglect, domestic violence, household substance use and mental illness, parental separation or divorce, and incarceration of family members) and later physical and mental health issues (Abate et al., 2025). Nurses are in a key position to identify and intervene with children and adolescents at risk for psychopathology by virtue of their close contact with families in health care settings and their roles as educators. Knowing the difference between typical and atypical child development is crucial in helping parents to view their children's behavior realistically and to respond appropriately. (Please note that throughout this chapter, the term "parents" is used to refer to parents, guardians, or other caregivers who are caring for children.)

CHILDHOOD AND ADOLESCENT MENTAL HEALTH

Supportive social networks and positive childhood and adolescent experiences maximize the mental health of children and adolescents. Children are more likely to be mentally healthy if they have good physical health and positive social development. Their characteristic style of reactivity and self-regulation in adapting to environmental stress, defined as their **temperament**, is biologically based and evident from birth (Rothbart, 2012). An easy temperament allows the child to adapt to change without intense emotional reactions. Children's mental health is also closely linked to the quality of their **attachments** formed through the emotional bonds between them and their parents at an early age. A secure attachment style helps the child test the world without fear of rejection. These areas are considered in the mental health assessment of children (see Chapter 36). **Developmental delays** not only slow the child's progress but also can interfere with the development of a positive self-concept. A key developmental task of early childhood that continues into adolescence and young adulthood is the achievement of *emotional regulation* which allows for delay of gratification, self-soothing, healthy decision making, and positive socialization.

KEYCONCEPT Emotional regulation is a skill that develops with maturity but is the predominant developmental task for children aged 2 to 6 (Berger, 2023). By age 6 most children experience a full range of emotions and learn to regulate their reactions through practice and learning from their families and cultural norms. Emotional regulation depends on **effortful control** of intense reactions such as tantrums, as well as **executive functioning** of the brain through the development of the cerebral cortex continuing into adolescence, allowing for better planning and delay of gratification.

NCLEXNOTE Attachment, temperament, and emotional regulation are key concepts in the behavior of children and adolescents in any health care setting. Apply these concepts to any pediatric patient.

COMMON ISSUES IN CHILDHOOD

Children and adolescents are faced with many challenges while growing up. Loss is an inevitable part of life. All children experience significant losses, the most common being death of a grandparent, parental divorce, death of a pet, and loss of friends through moving or changing schools. Learning to mourn losses can lead to a renewed appreciation of the precious value of life and close relationships. Sibling rivalry, illness, and common adolescent risk-taking tendencies also may pose challenges for children as they grow and develop.

Death and Grief

Vast research shows that similar to adults, children who experience major losses are at risk for mental health issues, particularly if the natural grieving process is impeded. However, the grieving process differs somewhat between children and adults (Table 16.1).

Children's responses to loss reflect their developmental level. As early as age 3 years, children have some concept of death. For example, the death of a goldfish provides an opportunity for the child to grasp the idea that the fish will never swim again. However, not until about age 7 years can most children understand the permanence of death. Before this age, they may verbalize that someone has "died" but in the next sentence ask when the dead person will be "coming back." Some adolescents, aged 11 to 18, may believe they are immune to death and engage in risky behaviors, such as driving dangerously. This phenomenon is known as the *invincibility fable* because adolescents view themselves in an egocentric way, as unique and invulnerable to the consequences experienced by others.

KEYCONCEPT The **invincibility fable** is an aspect of **egocentric thinking** in adolescence that causes teens to view themselves as immune to dangerous situations, such as unprotected sex, driving over the speed limit, and substance use.

If the concept of death is difficult for adults to grasp, it is particularly important to be sensitive to children's struggle to understand and cope with it. Most children closely watch their parents' response to grief and loss and use fantasy to fill the gaps in their understanding. In many cases, family members take turns grieving, with children sensing that their parents are so overwhelmed by their own emotional pain that they cannot bear the children's grief. They also see adults taking turns being strong for each other.

Loss and Early Childhood

A child, aged 2 to 6, may react more to the parents' distress about a death than to the death itself. Young children who depend totally on their parents may be frightened when they see their parents upset. Anything the parent can do to alleviate their children's anxiety, such as reassuring them that the parent will be okay and continuing the child's routine (e.g., consistent bedtimes, snacks, play times), will help the child to feel secure (Worden, 2018). Because preschool-aged children have limited ability to

TABLE 16.1 GRIEVING IN CHILDHOOD, ADOLESCENCE, AND ADULTHOOD

Children	Adolescents	Adults
View death as reversible; do not understand that death is permanent until about age 7 years.	Understand that death is permanent but may flirt with death (e.g., reckless driving, unprotected sex) because of omnipotent feelings.	Understand that death is permanent; may struggle with spiritual beliefs about death.
Experiment with ideas about death by killing bugs, staging funerals, acting-out death in play.	May be fascinated by death, enjoy morbid books and movies, listen to rock music about death and suicide.	May try not to think about death, depending on cultural background.
Mourn through activities (e.g., mock funerals, playing with things owned by the loved one); may not cry.	Mourn by talking about the loss, crying, and reflecting on it, sometimes becoming dramatic (e.g., overidentifying with the lost person, developing poetic or romantic ideas about death).	Mourn through talking about the loss, crying, reviewing memories, and thinking privately about it.
May not discuss the loss openly but may instead express grief through regression, somatic complaints, behavior issues, or withdrawal.	Often withdraw when mourning or seek comfort through peer groups; may feel parents do not understand their feelings.	Usually discuss loss openly, depending on level of support available; may feel there is a "time limit" on how long it is socially acceptable to grieve.
Need repeated explanations to fully understand the loss; it may be helpful to read children's books that explain death.	Need permission to grieve openly because they may believe they should act strong or take care of the adults involved; need acceptance of their sometimes extreme reactions.	Need friends, family, and other supportive people to listen and allow them to mourn for however long it takes; need opportunities to review their feelings and memories.

verbalize their feelings, they may need to express them through fantasy play and activities, such as mock funerals. Books that explain death, such as *Charlotte's Web* by E. B. White, may also be helpful. Parents should take care not to use euphemisms that could fuel misconceptions of death, such as "They went to sleep." Young children may interpret these messages literally and fear going to sleep (because they might die) or focus their natural, grief-related anger on the irrational idea that the person deliberately has not returned. The best approach is to explain honestly that the person has died and is not coming back, elicit the child's understanding and questions about what has happened, and then repeat this process continually as the child gradually begins to grasp the reality of the situation. The decision of whether to take a young child to a funeral may be particularly complex. Figure 16.1 enumerates some factors to consider.

Loss and the Middle Childhood Years

Children, aged 6 to 11, understand the permanence of death more clearly than do younger children aged 2 to 6, but they may still struggle to articulate their feelings (Leming & Dickinson, 2021). Children in this age group, ages 6 to 11, may express their grief through somatic complaints, regression, behavior issues, withdrawal, and even anger toward their parents. They may think that others expect them to cry and react with immediate emotional intensity to the death; when they do not react this way, they feel guilty.

The death of a sibling can be a particularly difficult loss for both the child and the family. Common reactions to this are for the surviving child to feel guilt because of natural sibling rivalry and for the parents to unconsciously endow the surviving child with qualities of the lost sibling as if to fill the empty space in the family (Worden, 2018). Of course, the death of a parent can be even more devastating. The surviving parent's psychological functioning has a major impact on the child's adjustment to the loss (Donohue, 2024). Parents should provide grieving children with support, nurturance, continuity, and the opportunity to remember the lost person in concrete ways through photographs, stories, and family activities that allow the child to memorialize the loved one.

Loss and Adolescents

Adolescents who are in Piaget's stage of **formal operations**, characterized by the ability to use abstract reasoning to conceptualize and solve problems, can better understand death as an abstract concept (see Chapter 6). Because adolescents tend to be idealistic and to think in extremes, they may even have poetic or romantic notions about death. Many teenagers become fascinated with morbid rock music, movies, and books. Although they may be able to express their thoughts and feelings about death more clearly than younger children, they often are reluctant to do so for fear of being viewed as childish. Some adolescents assume a parental role in the family after a death, denying their own needs. School settings may be particularly helpful in providing group and individual support for grieving adolescents who may fear being viewed as different from their peers. Structured

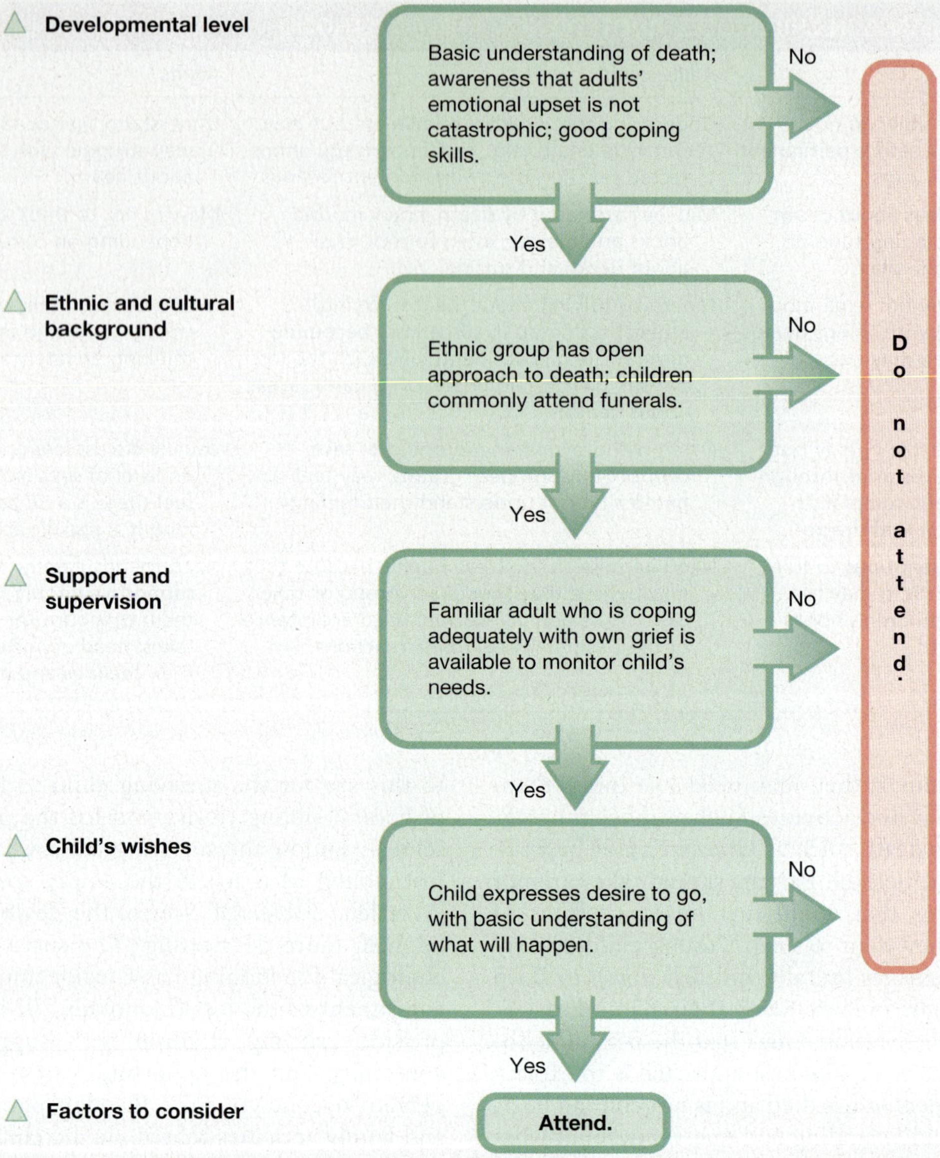

FIGURE 16.1 Decision tree: Should a child attend a funeral?

programs for children and adolescents can prevent complicated (pathologic) bereavement.

Separation and Divorce

Although many families adapt to separation and divorce without long-term negative effects for the children, youth often show at least temporary difficulties in dealing with this common stressor (Iqbal et al., 2021). Parental separation and divorce change the family structure, usually resulting in a substantial reduction in the contact that children have with one of their parents. The child's response to divorce is similar to the response to death. In some ways, divorce may be harder for the child to understand because the noncustodial parent is gone but still alive, and the parents have made a conscious choice to separate. Children of divorce are at increased risk for emotional, behavioral, and academic issues. However, the response to the loss that divorce imposes varies depending on the child's temperament; the parents' interventions; and the level of stress, change, and conflict surrounding the divorce (Kosher & Katz, 2022). A major change in socioeconomic status, such as moving from dual-earner status to single-parent family status, may account for much of the variation in levels of distress among divorcing families.

The first few years after the couple's breakup tend to be the most difficult. Typical childhood reactions include confusion, guilt, depression, regression, somatic symptoms, acting-out behaviors (e.g., stealing, disobedience), fantasies that the parents will reunite, fear of losing the custodial parent, and alignment with one parent against the other. After an initial adjustment period, children usually accept the reality of the situation and begin coping adaptively. Most divorced parents eventually remarry new partners, which often imposes another period of coping difficulties for the children. Children with stepparents and stepsiblings are at renewed risk for emotional and behavioral issues as they adjust to the new relationships (Browning & Artelt, 2014).

Protective factors against emotional issues in children of divorce and remarriage include a structured home and school environment with reasonable and consistent limit setting and a warm, supportive relationship with stepparents (Kelly, 2012). Helpful interventions for children of divorce include education regarding children's reactions; promotion of regular and predictable visitation; reduction of conflict between the parents through counseling, mediation, and clear visitation policies; continuance of usual routines; and family counseling to facilitate adjustment after remarriage (Cohen et al., 2016) (Table 16.2). It is also important to make it clear to children that the divorce was not caused by them. Egocentric thinking, which is typical for children, may cause children

TABLE 16.2 PLAY THERAPY WITH A 4-YEAR-OLD CHILD WHOSE PARENTS ARE DIVORCING

Patient Statement	Nurse Response	Analysis and Rationale
(Child smashes two cars together and makes loud, crashing sound.)	That's a loud crash. They really hit hard.	Child may be expressing anger and frustration nonverbally through play. Nurse attempts to establish rapport with child by relating at child's level using age-appropriate vocabulary.
Crrrash!	I know a boy who gets so mad sometimes that he feels like smashing something.	Child is engrossed in fantasy play, typical of preschoolers. Children often use toys as symbols of human figures (animism). Nurse uses indirect method of eliciting child's feelings because preschoolers often do not express feelings directly. Reference to another child's anger helps to normalize this child's feelings.
Yeah!	Sounds like you feel that way sometimes, too.	Child is beginning to relate to nurse and sense her empathy. Nurse reflects the child's feelings to facilitate further communication.
Yeah, when my mom and dad fight.	It's hard to listen to parents fighting. Sometimes, it's scary. You wonder what's going to happen.	Child is experiencing frustration and helplessness related to family conflict. Nurse expresses empathy and attempts to articulate child's feelings because preschool children have a limited ability to identify and label feelings.
My mom and dad are getting a divorce.	That's too bad. What's going to happen when they get the divorce?	Child has basic awareness of the reality of parents' divorce but may not understand this concept. Nurse expresses empathy and attempts to assess the child's level of understanding of the divorce.
Dad is not going to live in our house.	Oh, I guess you'll miss having him there all the time. It would be nice if you all could live together, but I guess that's not going to happen.	Preschool child focuses on the effects the divorce will have on him (egocentrism). Child seems to have a clear understanding of the consequences of the divorce. Nurse articulates the child's perspective and reinforces the reality of the divorce to avoid fueling child's possible denial and reconciliation fantasies.
(Silently moves cars across the floor.)	What do you think is the reason your parents decided to get a divorce?	Child expresses sadness nonverbally. Nurse further attempts to assess the child's understanding of the circumstances surrounding the divorce.
Because I did it.	What do you mean—you did it?	Child provides clue that he may be feeling responsible. Nurse uses clarification to fully assess child's understanding.
I made them mad because I left my bike in the driveway and Dad ran over it.	How? Do you think that is why they're getting the divorce?	Child uses egocentric thinking to draw conclusion that his actions caused the divorce. Nurse continues to clarify the child's thinking. The goal is to elicit the child's perceptions, so that misperceptions can be corrected.
Yeah, they had a big fight.	They may have been upset about the bike, but I don't think that is why they're getting a divorce.	The nurse goes on to explain why parents get divorced and to provide opportunities for the child to ask questions.
Why?	Because parents get divorced when they're upset with *each other*—when they can't get along—not when they're upset with their children.	

to believe that they are at the root of the problem. Some evidence shows that it is not the divorce itself but rather the continuing conflict between the parents that is most damaging to children (Cao et al., 2022). Parents manage divorce better if they can remember that children naturally idealize and identify with both parents and need to view both of them positively. Therefore, it is helpful for parents to guard against making negative statements about each other and focus on evidence of their former partner's love and respect for the child.

KEYCONCEPT In **egocentric thinking**, children naturally view themselves as the center of their own universe. Common examples of this are children looking out the car window at night and claiming that "the moon is following me" and children sitting in front of the television set, blocking the view for the parent, but believing that if they can see the television, the parent can, too. This kind of magical, self-focused thinking is charming, but it has a downside when children believe that they have caused a divorce or death in the family because of their own actions.

Sibling Relationships

Until recently, the role of siblings in children's development was underemphasized. A growing body of research shows that sibling relationships significantly influence personality development. Positive sibling relationships can be protective factors against the development of psychopathology (Fig. 16.2), particularly in troubled families in which the parents are emotionally unavailable (Bank & Kahn, 2014). Thus, nurses should emphasize to parents that minimizing sibling rivalry and maximizing cooperative behavior will benefit their children's social and emotional development throughout life.

Sibling rivalry begins with the birth of the second child. Often, this event is traumatic for the first child who, up until then, was the sole focus of the parents' attention (Nadelman & Begun, 2014). The older sibling usually reacts with anger and may reveal not-so-subtle fantasies of getting rid of the new sibling (e.g., "I dreamed that the new baby died."). Parents should recognize that these reactions are natural and allow the child to express feelings, both positive and negative, about the baby while reassuring the child that they have a very special place in the family. Allowing the older child opportunities to care for the baby and reinforcing any nurturing or affectionate behavior will promote positive bonding.

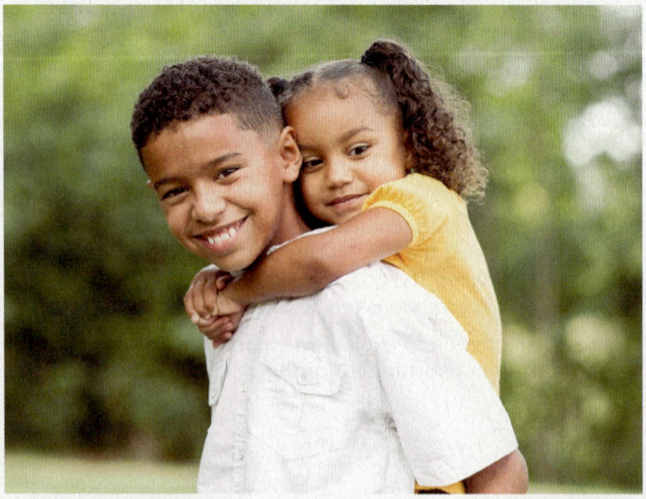

FIGURE 16.2 Sibling relationships significantly influence personality development.

Some sibling rivalry is natural and inevitable, even into adulthood. However, intense rivalry and conflict between siblings correlate with behavior issues in children. Positive temperament and effective, supportive coparenting can buffer against the negative outcomes associated with sibling conflict (Liu & Rahman, 2022). One factor that can exacerbate this sibling rivalry is differential treatment of children (Jensen et al., 2023). Although it is natural and appropriate for parents to use different methods to manage children with different personalities, parents must be sensitive to their children's perceptions of their behavior and emphasize each child's strengths. Helping each child to develop a separate identity based on unique talents and interests can minimize rivalry and perceptions of favoritism.

Children with siblings who have psychological disorders are also at increased risk for mental health issues. However, siblings may be an important source of support for children with mental health issues. Nurses should be alert to behavior issues of other family members and include siblings in family interventions, as they may also benefit from support (Jayasinghe et al., 2023).

Bullying

Children have experienced bullying throughout history and is a topic of widespread concern for mental health professionals.

Bullying is defined as repeated, deliberate attempts to harm someone, usually unprovoked. An imbalance in strength is a part of the pattern, with most people who experience bullying having difficulty defending themselves. Some studies suggest that children assigned female at birth are more likely to use **relational aggression**, which involves disrupting peer relationships by excluding or manipulating others and spreading rumors. Cyberbullying (spreading pictures, rumors, or smear campaigns via the Internet) has become an increasingly common phenomenon that can have devastating effects because of the speed and scope of its impact (Li et al., 2024).

Children who have insecure attachments, mental health issues, substance use, family dysfunction, exposure to violence, and who have a history of abuse are at risk for becoming bullies (Cuesta et al., 2021). On the other side, people who experience bullying often have low self-esteem and relationship difficulties, even into adulthood.

Nurses who work with children and adolescents should assess for the occurrence of bullying by asking direct questions because this problem is often hidden. Immediate intervention should involve a coordinated effort by the school, parents, bullies, and child experiencing the bullying because studies show that bullying does not occur in a vacuum. The most effective programs involve educating and changing the climate in the whole school (not just working with the bullies) (Bezerra et al., 2023).

Physical Illness

Many children experience a major physical illness or injury at some point during development. Hospitalization and intrusive medical procedures are acutely traumatic for most children. The likelihood of lasting psychological issues resulting from physical illness depends on the child's developmental level and previous coping mechanisms, the family's level of functioning before and after the illness, and the nature and severity of the illness. As with any major stressor, the perception of the event (i.e., meaning of the illness) will influence the family's ability to cope. One possible outcome of early childhood illness or injury is the phenomenon of **vulnerable child syndrome**, in which the family perceives the child as fragile despite current good health, causing them to be overprotective (Verbeek et al., 2021).

Common childhood reactions to physical illness include regression (e.g., loss of previous developmental gains in toilet training, social maturity, autonomous behavior), sleep and feeding difficulties, behavior issues (negativism, withdrawal), somatic complaints that mask attempts at emotional expression (e.g., headaches, stomach aches), and depression. Infants and children younger than school age are particularly vulnerable to separation anxiety during illness and may regress to earlier levels of anxiety about strangers, becoming fearful of health care providers. Young children often have magical thinking about the illness, and their tendency to process information in concrete terms may lead to misperceptions about the illness and treatment procedures (e.g., dye vs. die; stretcher vs. stretch her) (Navein et al., 2022). Adolescents may be concerned about body image and maintaining their sense of independence and control.

Nurses must remember that parents are the primary resource to the child and the experts who know the child's needs and reactions. Thus, nurses must maintain a collaborative approach in working with parents of physically ill children. If the child is a sick infant, nurses should take care to allow the expected attachment process between parents and the infant to unfold, despite health care professionals' efforts to assume some parenting functions.

Many parents react with guilt to their child's illness or injury, especially if the illness is genetically based or partially the result of their own behavior (e.g., drug or alcohol misuse during pregnancy). Parents may project their guilt onto each other or health care professionals, lashing out in anger and blame. Nurses should view this behavior as part of the grieving process and help parents to move forward in caring for their children and regaining competence. Teaching parents how to care for their children's medical issues and reinforcing their successes in doing so will help.

Chronic physical illness in childhood presents a unique set of challenges. Although most children with chronic illnesses and their families are remarkably resilient and adjust to the stressors and regimens involved in their care, children with chronic health conditions are significantly more likely to experience psychiatric symptoms than their healthy peers (Nibras et al., 2022). Conditions that affect the central nervous system (CNS) (e.g., infections, metabolic diseases, CNS malformations, brain and spinal cord trauma) are particularly likely to result in psychiatric difficulties. Nurses who understand pathophysiologic processes are in a unique position to assess the interaction between biologic and psychological factors that contribute to mental health issues in chronically ill children (e.g., lethargy from high blood sugar levels or respiratory issues, mood swings from steroid use). Inactivity and lack of sensory stimulation from hospitalization or bed rest may contribute to neurologic deficits and developmental delays.

The major challenge for a chronically ill child is to remain active despite the limitations of the illness and to become fully integrated into school and social activities. Children who view themselves as different or defective will experience low self-esteem and be more at risk for depression, anxiety, and behavior issues. Studies show that parental perceptions of the child's vulnerability predict greater adjustment issues (Gordo et al., 2022). Educating parents and helping them to foster maximum independence within the limitations of the child's health issue is the key. Nurses in primary care settings are in a good position to promote integrated mental health care to children with physical health issues.

Adolescent Risk-Taking Behaviors

Adolescence is a time of growing independence and, consequently, experimentation. Emotional extremes prevail. To adolescents, the world seems great one day and terrible the next; people are either for them or against them. Adolescents are struggling to consolidate their abilities to control their impulses and react to the many "crises" that may seem trivial to adults but are very important to teens. Biologic changes (e.g., onset of puberty, height and weight changes, hormonal changes), psychological changes (increased ability for abstract thinking), and social changes (dating, driving, increased autonomy) are all significant. Unevenness in adolescent brain development, specifically in the amygdala and frontal lobes, may contribute to difficulties with executive functioning and impulse control or the ability to "think twice" before acting (Steinberg, 2023).

Teenagers test different roles and struggle to find a peer group that fits their unfolding self-image. During this process, many adolescents experiment with risk–engaging in behaviors such as smoking, using alcohol and drugs, having unprotected sex, engaging in truancy or delinquent behaviors, and running away from home. Although most youths eventually become more responsible, some develop harmful behavior patterns and dependencies that endanger their mental and physical health. One recent trend is self-mutilation or cutting by adolescents who use this as a cry for help or a tension release (Miller et al., 2021). Adolescents whose psychiatric issues have already developed are particularly vulnerable to engaging in risky behaviors because they have limited coping skills, may attempt to self-medicate their symptoms, and may feel increased pressure to fit in with other teens.

Several approaches to mental health promotion with adolescents are recommended. First, intervening at the peer group level through education programs, alternative recreation activities, and peer counseling is most successful. Second, training in values clarification, problem solving, social skills, and assertiveness helps give adolescents the skills to cope with situations in which they are pressured by their peers. If just one person can find the strength to express an unpopular viewpoint in a group and decline to participate in a destructive activity, others will quickly follow. It takes enormous courage, as well as concrete knowledge and practice with assertiveness, to speak up in these situations. A third type of intervention is a program that uses team efforts by teachers, parents, community leaders, and teen role models. These programs help at-risk youth by building self-esteem, setting positive examples, and working to involve the youth in community activities.

Approaches that have not proved effective include mere education about dangerous activities without behavior training and programs that provide inadequate training for the professionals implementing them. In any intervention, it is also important to keep in mind that adolescents are skeptical of authority figures and tend to take cues from one another. Nurses working with teenagers find it helpful to use a discussion approach that encourages questioning and argument as opposed to talking down to or "talking at" teenagers.

RISK FACTORS FOR CHILDHOOD PSYCHOPATHOLOGY

Understanding the risk factors for psychopathology is vital in mental health promotion and the prevention of disorders. Any intervention must recognize and work to address these factors if it is to be successful.

Poverty and Housing Challenges

Children are born into their parents' socioeconomic class, and the effects of intergenerational poverty impact all aspects of their development (Saitadze & Lalayants, 2021). Lack of proper nutrition and lack of access to prenatal and infant care places children in poverty at risk for physical and mental health issues. Adolescence may be truncated when children from impoverished families are forced into adult roles as parents work long hours to meet basic needs (Axxe et al., 2022; see Chapter 15).

Although crime, drug misuse, gang activity, and teenage pregnancy are seen in adolescents from all socioeconomic backgrounds, children living in poverty may be more vulnerable to these issues because they may view their options as limited. Thus, they may have an increased need to maintain a tough image and struggle more for a sense of control over their environment. The obstacles inherent in overcoming the effects of poverty can seem insurmountable to young people.

A major focus of preventive nursing interventions for families who are economically disadvantaged involves simply forming an alliance that conveys respect and willingness to work as an advocate to help patients gain access to resources. In terms of Maslow need hierarchy, families living in poverty may be more focused on survival needs (e.g., food, shelter) than self-actualization needs (e.g., insight-oriented psychotherapy for themselves or their children). Unless the nurse can work as a partner with the family and address the issues that are most pressing for the family with an active, problem-solving approach, other types of intervention may be fruitless. At the same time, it is inappropriate to assume that poor families will be resistant to or unable to benefit from psychotherapy or other mental health interventions.

Additional risks arise for children and teens who are unhoused, which may result from loss of shelter for the entire family, running away, or being evicted from their homes (Box 16.1; see also Chapter 41). For youth who are without stable housing, there is an increased risk for physical health issues (e.g., nutrition deficiencies, infections, chronic illnesses), mental health issues (particularly developmental delays in language, fine or gross motor coordination, and social development; depression; anxiety; disruptive behavior disorders), and educational underachievement. Many youth experiencing homelessness have been physically and/or sexually abused, leading to elevated rates of mental disorders (Armoon et al., 2024). Adolescents who run away from an abusive home can find themselves living on the streets where staying alive and developing self-reliance are a daily struggle.

The living conditions of many shelters place children at risk for lead poisoning and communicable diseases and make the regular sleep, feeding, play, and bathing patterns important for typical development nearly impossible. Nurses working with families experiencing housing instability need to be aware of the effects of this lifestyle on children because they have a limited ability to speak for themselves and because their needs are often overlooked.

BOX 16.1

Research for Evidence-Based Practice: A Temperament Guidance Program for Parents of Infants

Iverson, S. L., Desmarais, E. E., Neumann, A.A., & Gartstein, M. A. (2020). New brief temperament program for parents of infants: A pilot evaluation. Journal of Child and Adolescent Psychiatric Nursing, *33, 38–48.*

THE QUESTION: Can a brief educational intervention increase biological mothers' knowledge about temperament and improve their responsiveness to their infants?

METHODS: Nurse researchers provided educational packets to biological mothers ($n = 35$) of infants 3 to 12 months of a ge during home visits and followed up a few weeks later with additional brochures containing information about differences in infant temperaments and the importance of goodness of fit (i.e., the match between parental expectations and the child's temperament profile). Nurses administered a quiz to measure gains in the mothers' knowledge, and they assessed changes in the mothers' responsiveness and flexibility in adapting to their infants by observing and recording their interactions with their infants while performing a learning task before and after the intervention.

FINDINGS: The mothers demonstrated increased knowledge of temperament and exhibited observable changes in their interactions with their infants following the intervention. An increase in sensitivity was evident as the mother–child interactions shifted from more parent-directed to more balanced and responsive. Changes were most evident for mothers of infants assigned male at birth and those who had higher levels of education.

IMPLICATIONS FOR NURSING: This study suggests that a simple, low-cost educational intervention using written materials can increase mastery in understanding and responding to differences in infant temperament. The mothers' increased sensitivity to their infants following the intervention is a promising result, as this interactional dynamic been shown to be a critical component of a healthy parent–child relationship and goodness of fit. The mothers' increased understanding of their infants' temperaments may have promoted the shift from more mother-directed to more balanced and responsive interaction. Other research suggests that sensitive and responsive parenting promotes greater autonomy and better developmental outcomes for children.

Child Abuse and Neglect

Early recognition and reduction of risk factors are the keys to preventing **child abuse and neglect**, which includes any actions that endanger or impair a child's physical, psychological, or emotional health and development. Risk factors for child abuse and neglect include high levels of family stress, drug or alcohol misuse, a partner who is unstable or unloving toward the child, and lack of social support for the parents (Mehta et al., 2023). In addition, young children (particularly those younger than 3 years) and children with a history of prematurity, medical issues, and severe emotional issues are at high risk because they place great demands on their parents. Abuse can have lifelong effects on development. Children who have been maltreated are more likely to enter aggressive relationships, misuse substances or alcohol to numb emotions, develop eating disorders, become depressed, and engage in self-destructive behavior (Kolko & Berkout, 2017).

Nurses are legally mandated to report any reasonable suspicion of abuse and neglect to the appropriate state authorities. Box 16.2 lists signs of physical and sexual abuse in children. Mandated reporting laws allow the state to investigate the possibility of abuse, provide protection to children, and link families with support and

BOX 16.2

Signs of Possible Child Abuse[a]

SEXUAL ABUSE

- Bruises or bleeding on the genitals or in the rectum
- Sexually transmitted infection (e.g., HIV, gonorrhea, syphilis, herpes genitalis)
- Vaginal or penile discharge
- Sore throats
- Enuresis or encopresis
- Foreign bodies in the vagina or rectum
- Pregnancy, especially in a young adolescent
- Difficulty in walking or sitting
- Engaging in inappropriate sexual behavior with siblings or peers
- Sophisticated knowledge of sexual activities
- Preoccupation with sexual ideas
- Somatic complaints, especially abdominal pain and constipation
- Sleep difficulties
- Hyperalertness to the environment
- Withdrawal
- Excessive daydreaming or seeming preoccupied
- Regressed behavior

PHYSICAL ABUSE

- Bruises or lacerations, especially in clusters on back, buttocks, thighs, or large areas of the torso
- Fractures inconsistent with the child's history
- Old and new injuries at the same time
- Unwilling to change clothes in front of others; wears heavy clothes in warm weather
- Identifiable marks from belt buckles, electrical cords, or handprints
- Cigarette burns
- Rope burns on arms, legs, face, neck, or torso from being bound and gagged
- Adult-size bite marks
- Bald spots interspersed with typical hair
- Shrinking at the touch of an adult
- Fear of adults, especially parents
- Apprehensive when other children cry
- Scanning the environment, staying very still, failing to cry when hurt
- Aggression or withdrawal
- Nondiscriminatory seeking of affection
- Defensive reactions when questioned about injuries
- History of being taken to many different clinics and emergency departments for different injuries

[a]Note: Because many injuries do not represent child abuse, a careful history must be taken.

services. Nurses are immune from liability for reporting suspected abuse, but they may be held legally accountable for not reporting it. The decision to report abuse sometimes poses an ethical dilemma for nurses as they try to balance the need to maintain the family's trust against the need to protect the child. This decision is further complicated by the knowledge that if temporary out-of-home placement is necessary, the quality of the placement may not be optimum, and the child and family may suffer in the process of the separation.

To minimize damaging the nurse–family relationship, experts recommend that nurses report abuse in the presence of the parents, preferably with the parent initiating the telephone call. The professional should explain that reporting is necessary to provide safety for the child and to obtain services for the family. If the parents cannot be present when the report is made, the nurse should, at minimum, notify the family that the report was made.

Preventing child abuse and neglect occurs with any intervention that supports the parents with physical, financial, mental health, and medical resources that will reduce stress within the family system. Early intervention and family support programs are considered the cornerstone of preventive efforts. A major protective factor against psychopathology stemming from abuse and neglect is the establishment of a supportive relationship with at least one adult who can provide empathy, consistency, and possibly, a corrective experience (e.g., a foster parent or other family member) for the child (Jackson et al., 2024).

Nurses working with children who are abused should resist the temptation to view the child as the only person deserving of empathy. Remembering that most abusive parents were abused as children and therefore may have limited coping mechanisms or little access to positive parental role models will help the nurse keep empathy toward the parents. After state agencies intervene to establish the child's safety, a family systems approach that is supportive of the whole family unit is most effective.

Substance Use Disorders in Families

Children whose parents use substances (see Chapter 31) live in an unpredictable family environment, coping with stress that may disrupt their ability to perform in school and lead to other emotional issues. The codependency movement, which emphasizes the effects of substance use disorders on family members and groups such as Adult Children of Alcoholics and Al-Anon, has brought increasing attention to the effects of parental substance use on child development.

Biologic factors affecting children of those with substance use disorders include **fetal alcohol syndrome**, nutritional deficits stemming from neglect, and neuropsychiatric dysfunction (Popova et al., 2024). Genetic factors are at least partly responsible for the well-documented increased risk for substance use among children whose parents have substance use disorders. Recent studies are beginning to link a family history of anxiety disorders and alcohol use disorders with genetically transmitted anxiety disorders, which may be a precursor to alcohol use disorders (Ummels et al., 2022). The precise mechanism of family transmission of alcohol use disorder is still unknown. Recent studies suggest that children of parents with substance use disorders may inherit a predisposition to a nonspecific form of biologic dysregulation that may be expressed either as alcohol use disorder or some other psychiatric disorder (e.g., hyperactivity, conduct disorder, depression), depending on the individual's developmental history (Jang et al., 2022).

Children of parents with substance use disorders are at high risk for both substance misuse and behavior disorders (McGovern et al., 2023). Moreover, other factors related to substance use disorder, such as family stress, violence, divorce, dysfunction, and other concurrent parental psychiatric disorders (e.g., depression, anxiety), further increase risk (Barrett et al., 2024). The experience of growing up in a family with substance use disorders is marked by unpredictability, fear, and helplessness because of the cyclic nature of addictive patterns.

Even for children who do not experience significant psychopathology, the experience of living with parents who have substance use disorders can lead to a poor self-concept when children feel responsible for their parents' behavior, become isolated, and learn to mistrust their own perceptions because the family denies the reality of the substance use disorder. The recent upsurge in opioid abuse has posed particular challenges for families. The experience of growing up with parents who use opioids has been characterized as living with ambiguous loss, as the parent may be physically present but psychologically absent due to preoccupation with obtaining and using the drug (Nayak et al., 2021).

Out-of-Home Placement

The tendency to blame parents and view out-of-home placement as a refuge for children has sharply declined in recent years. This change in attitudes results from public awareness of the deficiencies in the foster care system, greater support for parents' rights, and increased knowledge of the biologic basis for many of the disorders of parents and children that lead to out-of-home placement. **Family preservation** involves supporting and educating the family to secure the attachment between children and parents and to preserve the family unit and prevent the removal of children from their homes (LaBrenz et al., 2022). Today, children are removed from their homes only as a last resort. Family support services are designed to assist families with access to resources and education regarding child-rearing, monitor and facilitate the development of the bond between child

BOX 16.3

Mental Health Inequities: Disparities in Out-of-Home Placements for Black Children

Researchers investigated the disproportionately high number of children from Black families involved in out-of-home placements and the lower and slower rates of family reunification for these children in the child welfare system in a single urban county in the Midwest. This review included 58 participants plus another 15 case studies. The researchers found qualitative themes that the child welfare system is structured to the detriment of Black families with hypersurveillance, deficit-based investigations, and discriminatory policies and procedures that focus on issues and pathologies, with few efforts to honor families' strengths, protective factors, and culturally relevant contexts. The study underscores the need to provide resources and support to Black families in the child welfare system to prevent removal of their children.

Source: Wright, K., Becci, A., Byers, K., McCall, S., Alford, D., Parker, A., Clark, S., Shaw-Woody, N., Kline, M., Brown, N., Hill, E., Davis-Mays, S., Parham, W., & Rush, R. (2022). Using institutional analysis to examine the systemic sources of racial disproportionality and disparity: A case example. *Child Welfare*, *100*(2), 99–136.

and caregiver, and increase the caregiver's confidence in their abilities.

However, despite the latest trends toward family preservation, an increasing number of children are placed in foster homes, group homes, or residential treatment centers—in many cases for months to years (Jones et al., 2024), and a disproportionate number of children from families of color are in out-of-home placements (Box 16.3).

Factors leading to the increased number of children in out-of-home placement include greater willingness of the public and professionals to report child abuse and neglect; the epidemic proportions of substance use disorders; and the increasing number of families living in poverty. These situations may lead to abuse, neglect, and housing challenges. About 50% of children in out-of-home placement are adolescents, but the numbers of infants and young children are growing, particularly those with serious physical and emotional issues, who pose particular challenges for placement (Scribano, 2010). Infants who are abandoned by parents who misuse drugs and children with human immunodeficiency virus (HIV) whose parents are sick or deceased need permanent out-of-home placements, which are often difficult to find. When children with mental health needs are placed in foster care, a family support team is required to meet regularly, with the goal of providing holistic care, avoiding overuse of psychotropic medication, and moving toward a permanent placement that will provide stability (Simmel et al., 2025).

The adjustment to an out-of-home placement can be viewed through the conceptual framework of Bowlby's stages of coping with parental separation. According to Bowlby (1960), the child initially responds to separation from parents with protest (crying, kicking, screaming, pleading, and attempting to elicit the parent's return). The child then moves to a state of despair (listlessness, apathy, and withdrawal, which lead to some acceptance of caregiving by others but a reluctance to reattach fully). Finally, the child experiences detachment if the child and new parent cannot manage to form an emotional bond. Because children often experience multiple placements, the potential for a disrupted attachment may be great by the time the child faces the prospect of a permanent family. After repeatedly undergoing separation and mourning, the child learns that rejection is inevitable and may automatically maintain distance from a new caregiver.

Typical coping styles seen in children exposed to multiple placements include detachment, diffuse rage, chronic depression, antisocial behavior, low self-esteem, and chronic dependency or exaggerated demands for nurturing and support. Sometimes, these symptoms develop into attachment disorders that can be difficult to treat. It takes a very committed and resilient parent to continue caring for a child who does not reinforce attempts at caregiving and who exhibits these kinds of significant emotional and behavior issues.

INTERVENTION APPROACHES

The goal of health promotion and prevention interventions is to maximize the mental health of children and adolescents. The selected interventions should allow maximal autonomy for the child and family; keep the family unit intact, if possible; and provide the appropriate level of care to meet the needs of the child and family. A view of parents as partners is important to effective interventions. Interdisciplinary approaches are ideal in which the nurse acts as coordinator, case manager, and advocate to establish linkages with providers and nurse practitioners, teachers, speech and language specialists, social workers, and other professionals to develop and implement a comprehensive biopsychosocial plan of intervention (Box 16.4). Support groups are available for many stressors including substance use, death, divorce, and coping with a chronic illness. A continuum of modalities of care is available to children and families (Fig. 16.3).

Early intervention programs offer regular home visits, support, education, and concrete services to those in need. The assumption underlying these programs is that parents are the most consistent and important individuals in children's lives, and they should be afforded the opportunity to define their own needs and priorities. With support and education, parents are empowered to respond more effectively to their children. The effectiveness of these programs may be the key to preventing the placement of children outside the home (Ibabe et al., 2023).

BOX 16.4

Preventive Interventions With an Adolescent in Crisis

Ben and Rita were just transferred to a second foster home after being removed from their biological mother's care when she relapsed on cocaine and left them unattended. The plan is for the two children to return to their mother's home after she completes a 30-day drug treatment program. Ben, a high school freshman, is in the school nurse's office asking for aspirin for another headache.

The nurse notices that Ben's nose looks inflamed, he is sniffling, and he seems more "hyper" than usual. In a concerned tone of voice, she asks him if he has been using cocaine, and he snaps back, "Just because my mother's a coke head doesn't give you the right to suspect me!" When the nurse gently says, "Tell me about what's been happening with your mother; I had no idea," Ben responds less defensively and explains the situation about the foster home and his mother's drug issue. He says that if it weren't for Rita, his younger sister, he would have run away by now. His foster parents are "making him" go to school, but he's going to drop out as soon as he returns to live with his mother. The only thing that he likes about school is playing basketball, and the basketball coach, who is his physical education teacher, wants him on the team.

After a lengthy talk with Ben, the nurse finishes the assessment interview and concludes that he is at risk for substance use, running away, and dropping out of school. He is also showing symptoms of depression, which he may be attempting to medicate with cocaine. Protective factors for Ben include his strong attachment to his sister, his ability and willingness to express his thoughts and feelings, his interest in basketball, and a positive relationship with the basketball coach.

The nurse develops a plan with Ben to attend the weekly drug and alcohol discussion group at the school, so he can talk with other teens from families with members who have substance use disorders and learn coping skills to prevent substance misuse. The nurse contacts the basketball coach, who agrees to find a student mentor who can shoot hoops with Ben and to help him come up with a plan to stay in school, maybe find a part-time job, and join the basketball team. Ben agrees to check in regularly with the nurse to report how the plan is working and revise it if needed. The nurse feels optimistic that with support from his peers, coach, mentor, and herself, Ben can overcome what is probably a genetically based risk for depression and substance misuse. Ben shows signs of resilience. He is motivated to "keep his act together for Rita", capable of forming positive attachments, and willing to seek help when he knows where to find it.

WHAT DO YOU THINK?

1. If Ben "forgets" to check in regularly with the nurse, what would be the next course of action?
2. When are the times Ben is most susceptible to change his mind about staying in school and avoiding drugs? What action should be taken to avoid these times?

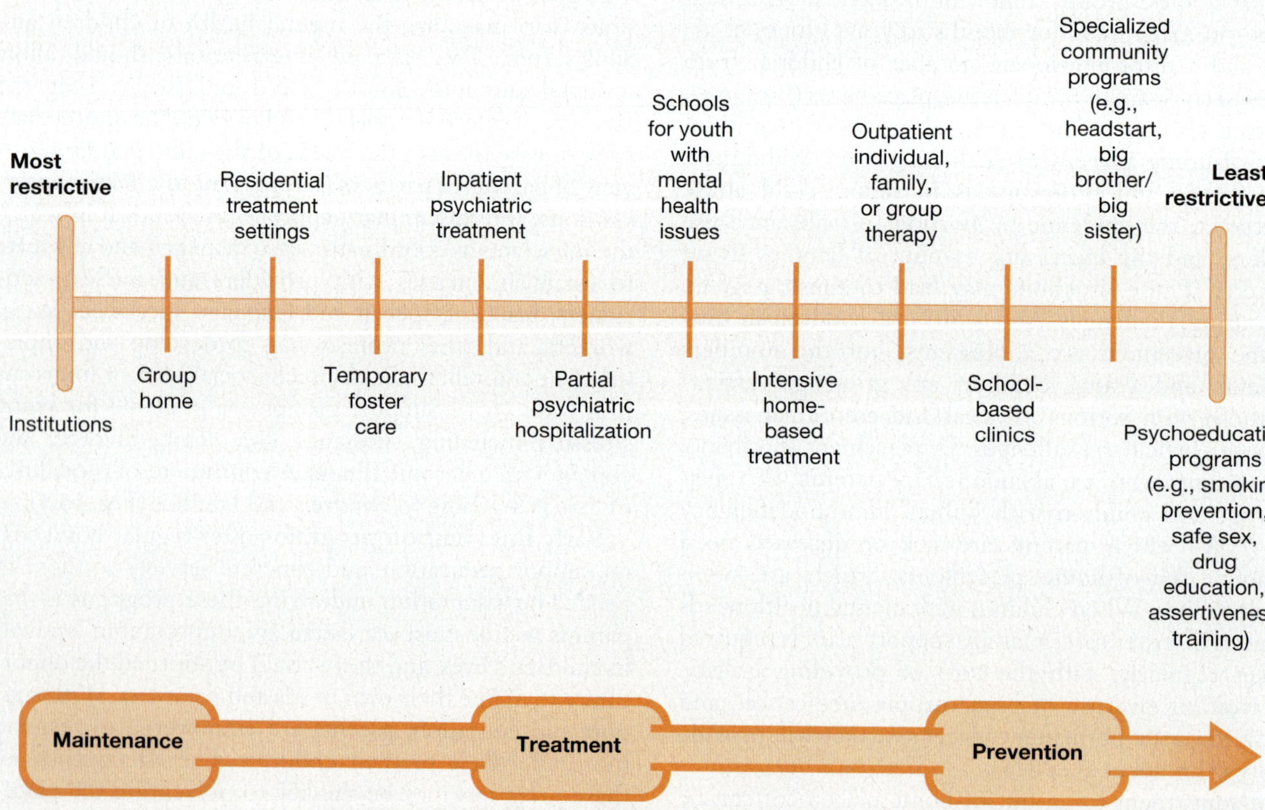

FIGURE 16.3 The continuum of mental health care for children and adolescents.

Psychoeducational programs designed to teach parents and children basic coping skills for dealing with various stressors are a particularly effective form of mental health intervention. By focusing on **normalization** (teaching families typical behaviors and expected responses) and providing families with information about typical child development and expected reactions to various stressors, families feel less isolated, know what to expect, and put their reactions into perspective. (See Box 16.1.) For example, if families learn that anger is a natural part of grieving, they will be less likely to view it as unusual and more likely to accept and cope with it constructively.

Social skills training is useful with youth who have low self-esteem or aggressive behavior (Bierman et al., 2017). Social skills training involves instruction, feedback, support, and practice with learning behaviors that help children to interact more effectively with peers and adults. When combined with assertiveness training, social skills training can be particularly helpful in providing children with coping skills to resist engaging in addictive or antisocial behaviors and to prevent social withdrawal under stress.

A wide variety of books are available to help children understand issues such as death, divorce, chronic illness, stepfamilies, adoption, and birth of a sibling. In addition, many mental health organizations and public health agencies have pamphlets designed to educate parents about various physical and psychological issues. By supplying concrete information and advice, these reading materials help to reduce anxiety by pointing out common reactions to the various stressors, so that families do not feel alone.

SUMMARY OF KEY POINTS

- Children who experience major losses, such as death or divorce, are at risk for developing mental health issues.
- Sibling relationships have significant effects on personality development. Positive sibling relationships can be protective factors against the development of mental health issues.
- Bullying is a severe problem that is often hidden yet can cause long-standing psychological harm; it must be addressed on a school-wide level.
- Medical issues in childhood and adolescence may cause psychological issues when illness leads to regression or lack of full participation in family, school, and social activities.
- Striving for identity and independence may lead adolescents to take part in high-risk activities (e.g., drug misuse, unprotected sex, smoking, delinquent behaviors) that may lead to mental health issues.
- Poverty, housing challenges, abuse, neglect, and parental substance use disorders all create conditions that undermine a child's ability to make typical developmental gains and contribute to vulnerability for various emotional and behavioral issues.
- Children who experience disrupted attachments because of out-of-home placements may have difficulty forming close relationships with their new parents and trusting others.
- Family support services and early intervention programs are designed to prevent removal of the child from the family because of abuse or neglect and to keep a strong, nurturing family system.
- Psychoeducational approaches, such as training opportunities, group experiences, and bibliotherapy, provide children and families with the information and skills to promote their own mental health.

DEVELOPING CLINICAL JUDGMENT

1. Analyze a case of a family that is grieving a loss and compare the parents' and children's reactions. Include an evaluation of how each child's reactions differ, depending on their developmental level.
2. Watch a movie or read a book that provides a child's view of death, divorce, or some other loss and consider how adults may be insensitive to the child's reactions.
3. Examine your own developmental history and pinpoint periods when stressful life events might have increased the risk for emotional issues for you or other family members. What protective factors in your own personality and coping skills and in the environment around you helped you to maintain your good mental health?
4. What aspects of life are more stressful for children than for adults (i.e., How is it different to experience life as a child)?
5. Examine how your own social and cultural background may either facilitate or create barriers to your ability to interact with families from other ethnic groups or those who are poor or experiencing homelessness.
6. Why is the process of normalization of feelings such a powerful intervention with children and families? How can nurses incorporate this kind of intervention into their practice roles?

MOVIES, TV, OR STREAMING PROGRAMS

***The Quiet Girl*: 2022.** This movie is set in rural Ireland where a young girl named Cait is growing up in a large, dysfunctional family living in poverty. One summer Cait is sent to live with relatives on a farm who show her love and help her develop confidence. This is a subtle but moving story that evokes the child's unique lens of experience.

Viewing Points:

1. Discuss the difference in the quality of attachment between Cait and her parents, as compared with the couple she stays with on the farm.
2. How do Cait's relatives exhibit a goodness of fit with Cait's temperament and what actions do they take to foster a secure attachment with her?
3. In the scene where Cait and her relatives attend a wake together, how do they respond to Cait's experience coping with death?
4. Do Cait's siblings seem to serve as a resource to buffer the stress in her life?

REFERENCES

Abate, B. B., Sendekie, A. K., Merchaw, A., Abebe, G. K., Azmeraw, M., Alamaw, A. W., Zemariam, A. B., Kitaw, T. A., Kassaw, A., Wodaynew, T., Kassie, A. M., Yilak, G., & Kassa, M. A. (2025). Adverse childhood experiences are associated with mental health problems later in life: An umbrella review of systematic review and meta-analysis. *Neuropsychobiology*, *84*(1), 48–64.

Armoon, B., Mohammadi, R., & Griffiths, M. D. (2024). The Global prevalence of non-suicidal self-injury, suicide behaviors, and associated risk factors among runaway and homeless youth: A meta-analysis. *Community Mental Health Journal*, *60*(5), 919–944.

Axxe, E., Hayford, S. R., & Eggum, N. D. (2022). Youth's family and non-family roles as predictors of subjective adulthood in three low-income agricultural settings. *Journal of Research on Adolescence · The Official Journal of the Society for Research on Adolescence*, *32*(4), 1546–1565.

Bank, S., & Kahn, M. D. (2014). Intense sibling loyalties. In M. E. Lamb, & B. Sutton-Smith (Eds.), *Sibling relationships: Their nature and significance across the lifespan*. Lawrence.

Barrett, S., Muir, C., Burns, S., Adjei, N., Forman, J., Hackett, S., Hirve, R., Kaner, E., Lynch, R., Taylor-Robinson, D., Wolfe, I., & McGovern, R. (2024). Interventions to reduce parental substance use, domestic violence and mental health problems, and their impacts upon children's well-being: A systematic review of reviews and evidence mapping. *Trauma, Violence & Abuse*, *25*(1), 393–412.

Berger, K.S. (2023). *The developing person through the lifespan*. (12th ed.). Worth Pub.

Bezerra, L. L., de A. L., Alves, D. L. G., Nunes, B. R., Stelko, P. A. C., Florêncio, R. S., & Gomes, I. L. V. (2023). Anti-bullying interventions with an emphasis on bystanders: A scoping review. *Journal of School Health*, *93*(11), 1036–1044.

Bierman, K. L., Greenberg, M. T., Coie, J. D., Dodge, K. A., Lochman, J. E., & McMahon, R. J. (2017). *Social & emotional skills training for children: The fast track friendship group manual*. Guilford Press.

Bloomquist, M. L. (2013). *The practitioner guide to skills training for struggling kids*. Guilford Press.

Bowlby, J. (1960). Grief and mourning in infancy and early childhood. *Psychoanalytic Study of the Child*, *15*, 9–52.

Browning, S., & Artelt, E. (2014). "Why are some stepfamilies vulnerable?" In S. Browning & E. Artelt (Eds.), *Stepfamily therapy: A 10-step clinical approach* (pp. 35–68). American Psychological Association.

Cao, H., Fine, M. A., & Zhou, N. (2022). The divorce process and child adaptation trajectory typology model: The shaping role of predivorce and postdivorce interparental conflict. *Clinical Child & Family Psychology Review*, *25*(3), 500–528. https://doi.org/10.1007/s10567-022-00379-3

Cohen, G. J., Weitzman, C. C., Yogman, M., Gambon, T. B., Lavin, A., Mattson, G., Rafferty, J. R., Wissow, L. S., Blum, N. J., Macias, M. M., Bauer, N. S., Bridgemohan, C., Goldson, E., & McGuinn, L. J. (2016). Helping children and families deal with divorce and separation. *Pediatrics*, *138*(6), e20163020. https://doi.org/10.1542/peds.2016-3020

Cuesta, I., Montesó, C. P., Metzler Sawin, E., Jiménez, H. M., Puig, L. M., Seabra, P., & Toussaint, L. (2021). Risk factors for teen suicide and bullying: An international integrative review. *International Journal of Nursing Practice*, *27*(3), e12930.

Donohue, E. (2024). Family coping with COVID-19: Unexpected parental loss and surviving parent coping, grief and posttraumatic Growth outcomes based on child age. Omega, 302228241272566.

Flaskerud, J. H. (2022). Resilience: Cultural values and support resources. *Issues in Mental Health Nursing*, *43*(8), 784–788.

Gordo, L., Elejalde, L. I., Martínez-Pampliega, A., & Iriarte Elejalde, L. (2022). Parental perception of child vulnerability in parents of young children. *Journal of Pediatric Psychology*, *47*(7), 850–857.

Ibabe, I., Arnoso, A., & Elgorriaga, E. (2023). Early intervention program in youth-to-parent aggression: Clinically relevant long-term changes. *Journal of Family Violence*, *38*(7), 1273–1285.

Iqbal, M., Khalid, M. S., Rehman, N., & Yanping, L. (2021). Parental divorce: Impact on socio-psychological behavior and academic performance of students in teacher's perception. *Journal of Divorce & Remarriage*, *62*(6), 475–492.

Jackson, A. L., Frederico, M., Cleak, H., & Perry, B. D. (2024). Interventions to support children's recovery from neglect—A systematic review. *Child Maltreatment*, *29*(4), 714–727.

Jang, S. K., Saunders, G., Liu, M., Jiang, Y., Liu, D. J., & Vrieze, S. (2022). Genetic correlation, pleiotropy, and causal associations between substance use and psychiatric disorder. *Psychological Medicine*, *52*(5), 968–978.

Jayasinghe, A., Wrobel, A., Filia, K., Byrne, L. K., Melvin, G., Murrihy, S., Moller, C., Berk, L., Berk, M., & Cotton, S. (2023). Distress, burden, and wellbeing in siblings of people with mental illness: A mixed studies systematic review and meta-analysis. *Psychological Medicine*, *53*(15), 6945–6964.

Jensen, A. C., Jorgensen-Wells, M. A., Andrus, L. E., Pickett, J. M., Leiter, V. K., Hadlock, M. E., & Dayley, J. (2023). Sibling differences and parents' differential treatment of siblings: A multilevel meta-analysis. *Developmental Psychology*, *59*(4), 644–654. https://doi.org/10.1037/dev0001406

Jones, D., Orsi-Hunt, R., Kim, H., Jonson-Reid, M., & Drake, B. (2024). Life-course trajectories of children through the U.S. foster care system. *Child Abuse & Neglect*, *153*, 106837.

Kelly, J. (2012). Risk and protective factors associated with child and adolescent adjustment following separation and divorce: Social science applications. In K. Kuehnle & L. Drozd (Eds.), *Parenting plan evaluations: Applied research for the family court* (pp. 49–84). Oxford University Press.

Kolko, D. J., & Berkout, O. V. (2017) Child physical abuse. In S. N. Gold (Ed.). *APA handbook of trauma psychology* (Vol. 1, Chap. 17, pp. 99–115). APA.

Kosher, H., & Katz, C. (2022). Impairment in parent–child relations in the context of high-intensity parental dispute: Practitioners' perceptions and experiences. *Children & Youth Services Review*, *132*, 106307.

LaBrenz, C. A., Childress, S., Robinson, E. D., Sieger, M. L., & Ontiberos, J. (2022). Reasonable efforts to preserve families? An examination of service utilization and child removal. *Child Abuse & Neglect*, *128*, 105631.

Leming, M. R., & Dickinson, G. E. (2021). *Understanding dying, death, and bereavement*. Cengage.

Li, C., Wang, P., Martin-Moratinos, M., Bella-Fernández, M., & Blasco-Fontecilla, H. (2024). Traditional bullying and cyberbullying in the digital age and its associated mental health problems in children and adolescents: A meta-analysis. *European Child & Adolescent Psychiatry*, *33*(9), 2895–2909.

Liu, C., & Rahman, M. N. A. (2022). Relationships between parenting style and sibling conflicts: A meta-analysis. *Frontiers in Psychology*, *13*, 936253.

McGovern, R., Bogowicz, P., Meader, N., Kaner, E., Alderson, H., Craig, D., Geijer, S. E., Jackson, K., Muir, C., Salonen, D., Smart, D., & Newham, J. J. (2023). The association between maternal and paternal substance use and child substance use, internalizing and externalizing problems: A systematic review and meta-analysis. *Addiction*, *118*(5), 804–818.

Mehta, D., Kelly, A. B., Laurens, K. R., Haslam, D., Williams, K. E., Walsh, K., Baker, P. R., Carter, H. E., Khawaja, N. G., Zelenko, O., & Matthews, B. (2023). Child maltreatment and long-term physical and mental health outcomes: An exploration of psychosocial determinants and implications for prevention. *Child Psychiatry & Human Development*, *54*, 421-435.

Miller, M. Redley, M., & Wilkinson, P. O. (2021). A qualitative study of understanding reasons for self-harm in adolescent girls. *International Journal of Environmental Research and Public Health*, *18*(7), 3361.

Nadelman, L., & Begun, A. (2014). The effect of the newborn on the older sibling: Mothers' questionnaire. In M. Lamb & B. Sutton-Smith (Eds.), *Sibling relationships: Their nature and significance across the lifespan*, pp. 13–37. Lawrence Erlbaum.

Navein, A., McTaggart, J., Hodgson, X., Shaw, J., Hargreaves, D., Gonzalez-Viana, E., & Mehmeti, A. (2022). Effective healthcare communication with children and young people: A systematic review of barriers and facilitators. *Archives of Disease in Childhood*, *107*(12), 1111–1116.

Nayak, S. M., Huhn, A. S., Bergeria, C. L., Strain, E. C., & Dunn, K. E. (2021). Familial perceptions of appropriate treatment types and goals for a family member who has opioid use disorder. *Drug and Alcohol Dependence*, *221*(10), 108649.

Nibras, S., Kentor, R., Masood, Y., Price, K., Schneider, N. M., Tenenbaum, R. B., & Calarge, C. (2022). Psychological and psychiatric comorbidities in youth with serious physical illness. *Children*, *9*(7), 1051.

Popova, S., Dozet, D., Faulkner, M.-R., Howie, L., & Temple, V. (2024). Prenatal exposures, diagnostic outcomes, and life experiences of children and youths with Fetal Alcohol Spectrum disorder. *Nutrients, 16*(11), 1655.

Rothbart, M. K. (2012). *Becoming who we are: Temperament and personality in development*. Guilford.

Saitadze, I., & Lalayants, M. (2021). Mechanisms that mitigate the effects of child poverty and improve children's cognitive and social-emotional development: A systematic review. *Child & Family Social Work, 26*(3), 289–308.

Scribano, P. V. (2010). Prevention strategies in child maltreatment. *Current Opinion in Pediatrics*, 22(5), 616–620.

Simmel, C., Bowden, C. F., Todd, S. N., Thorp, K., Hyde, J., & Crystal, S. (2025). Youth in foster care: Highlighting the importance of youth engagement in mental health treatment decisions. *Children and Youth Services Review*, 169.

Steinberg, L. (2023). *Adolescence* (13th ed.). McGraw-Hill.

Ummels, S. A., Seldenrijk, A., Bos, E. H., de Graaf, R., Batelaan, N. M., & Ten Have, M. (2022). The bidirectional relationship between anxiety disorders and alcohol use disorders in adults: Findings from a longitudinal population-based study. *Journal of affective disorders, 314*, 126–132.

Verbeek, I. N. E., van Onzenoort-Bokken, L., & Zegers, S. H. J. (2021). Vulnerable child syndrome in everyday paediatric practice: A condition deserving attention and new perspectives. *Acta Paediatrica, 110*(2), 397–399.

Worden, J. W. (2018). *Grief counseling and grief therapy: A handbook for the mental health practitioner* (5th ed.). Springer.

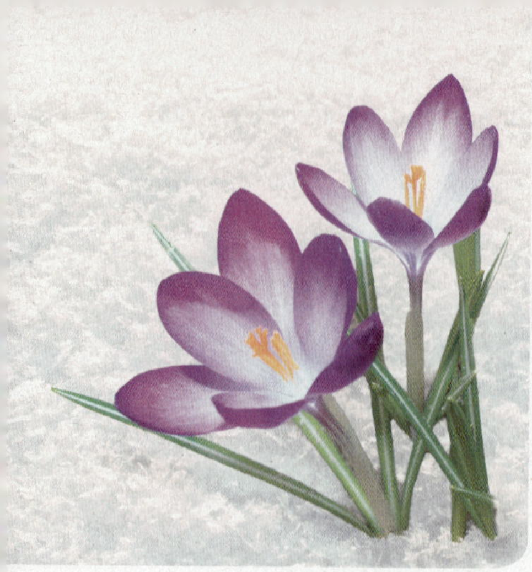

17 Mental Health Promotion for Young and Middle Adulthood

Mary Ann Boyd

KEYCONCEPTS

- middle adulthood
- young adulthood

LEARNING OBJECTIVES

After studying this chapter, you will be able to:

1. Describe psychosocial challenges common to young and middle adulthood.
2. Identify risk factors related to psychopathology in young and middle adulthood.
3. Describe protective factors in the mental health promotion of young and middle adulthood.
4. Analyze the role of the nurse in mental health promotion for young and middle adulthood.

KEY TERMS

• discrimination • empty nest • gray divorce • informal caregivers • minority stress • perceived discrimination • protective factors • risk factors • sandwich generation

INTRODUCTION

Young adulthood and middle adulthood are relatively new concepts. In 1900, life expectancy was age 47 (Centers for Diseases Control and Prevention [CDC], 2010). As life expectancy increased, the concepts of young and middle adulthood emerged. In 2020, life expectancy is averaging 77.0 years, ranging from 71.5 years for Black Americans to 77.9 years for Hispanic Americans (Kochanek et al., 2023).

Healthy lifestyles, medical advances, and economic success contribute to longevity. Many US families have achieved unprecedented economic stability that provides for prolonged periods of development. Technologic advances such as economic development, improved nutrition, public health control of infectious diseases, access to health care, and other modern developments have resulted in the lengthening of the life span chronologically in resource-abundant countries. This extended adulthood provides for an increased range of life choices, such as education, job selection; and lifestyle, including relationships, marriage, and family. Such advances do not exist worldwide because of the differences in the chronologic life span in different societies. In many resource-limited countries, the life span is characterized by a brief childhood followed by a mature adulthood that evolves quickly into old age.

MENTAL HEALTH IN YOUNG AND MIDDLE ADULTHOOD

Psychological changes in adulthood occur slowly and subtly with age and experience, not in a fixed stepwise manner. Until the late 1900s, adult development was viewed as a relatively stationary plateau with the rapid and complex changes of childhood and adolescence forming one steep side and the declining changes of old age on the other. Any rigid stage theory of adult life is oversimplifying young and middle adulthood development. Young and middle adulthood development is dynamic and multifaceted.

The developmental issues reported by young adults, midlife adults, and older adults are recurrent, taking new forms as their lives unfold. The developmental concepts of identity, intimacy, and generativity may have their initial blooming during adolescence, young adulthood, and middle adulthood, but they continue to be renegotiated in the face of life stresses such as unemployment and changes in family structure (see Chapter 6).

KEYCONCEPT The generally accepted age range for **young adulthood** is from 18 to 44 years. **Middle adulthood** spans the period from approximately 45 to 65 years.

Chronologic age is also losing its customary social meaning, resulting in a more fluid life cycle. Traditional notions of young adulthood as a time of leaving the parental home and establishing an independent career and family life, of college education taking place during late adolescence, or of the middle adulthood parents facing the **"empty nest"**—a home devoid of children and caregiving responsibilities—are being replaced with fewer age-defined life roles. (Please note that throughout this chapter, the term "parents" is used to refer to parents, guardians, or other caregivers who are caring for children.)

The timing of life events such as education, marriage, childrearing, career development, and retirement is becoming less regular, and more alternatives are embraced by Western society. Some people never marry, and others retire very early. Many young adults now remain in their parents' homes while they pursue their professional education rather than strike out on their own, as was customary in previous generations. Their middle adulthood parents are often already caring for their own parents, creating the **sandwich generation**, with its responsibilities toward the older generation above and two generations of children below them.

TABLE 17.1 MARITAL STATUS OF THE US ADULT POPULATION OVER THE AGE OF 15 YEARS

Marital Status	Males[a] (%)	Females[a] (%)
Married	49.3	46.3
Widowed	2.6	8.7
Divorced	9.5	12.1
Separated	1.6	2.2
Never married	37.0	30.7

[a]In this table, "males" refers to people assigned male at birth, and "females" refers to people assigned female at birth.
Source: U.S. Census Bureau. (2020). Marital status in the United States, https://www.census.gov/library/visualizations/interactive/marital-status-in-united-states.html

CHALLENGES IN YOUNG ADULTHOOD

Young adulthood is marked by many significant life events. Among them are leaving the primary family home for the first time or assuming a new household role, finding a permanent partner (or not), entering the work world, and taking on new caregiving responsibilities. Sometimes individuals choose to marry and establish a family and then return to finish their education or return to work when their children start school. See Table 17.1 for a breakdown of marital status in the US adult population. For young adults, health is related to parents' wealth as determined by parents' net worth. Young adults from wealthier families report higher levels of health when compared to young adults from less wealthy families (Sun et al., 2023).

Attachment Relationships

Young adulthood is a transitional period in which new ways of interacting with family members develop. This time can be stressful for the family members as well as the young adult (An et al., 2023). Stress is especially evident when the young adult's attachment needs conflict with family members' expectations. In some cultures, young adults are expected to leave their primary home and establish an independent living environment. If young adults who live independently are not ready to leave, attachment insecurity can occur. If parents are anxious about the change, they can easily become overinvolved or overly controlling. In other cultures, young adults are not expected to leave the primary home but are expected to assume a role of increasing responsibility within the family.

Loneliness

One of the outcomes of the COVID-19 pandemic was millions of children losing the opportunity to develop school-age friendships. The lost skills of face-to-face interactions along with the emphasis on social media and electronic communication led to a generation of young adults who report loneliness. The subjective feeling of loneliness can in turn lead to feeling disconnected and isolated. Other factors underlying loneliness include relationship breakups, moving from primary home or college to work, and feeling trapped while everyone else is improving. With an increasing use of social media, loneliness is exacerbated when young adults compare themselves to others who appear to be having fun and socializing (Fardghassemi & Joffe, 2022).

Loneliness can negatively impact physical and mental health. Loneliness is linked to immune deficiency, poor sleep, psychological stress, depression, and social anxiety. Research shows that social anxiety and depression are related to feelings of social isolation (Eres et al., 2023).

Minority Stress

Minority stress, or elevated level of stress experienced by members of stigmatized groups, can lead to chronic stress (see Chapter 19). It may be caused by poor social support, low socioeconomic status (SES), prejudice, and discrimination. Ethnic/racial and gender/sexual underrepresented groups are susceptible to minority stress, which can negatively impact their mental health and well-being. For example, chronic stress may be associated with an increase in drug-related health disparities in the African American individuals 18 to 25 years of age; evidence shows that skin conductivity levels, an indicator of autonomic nervous system function, is related to higher rates of alcohol and marijuana use in study participants with chronic race-related stress (Cavanagh & Obasi, 2022). Minority stress is prevalent in the LGBTQ+ community because of discrimination, which may lead to multiple mental health issues among LGBTQ+ individuals. Suicide risk is related to exposure to minority stress (Green et al., 2022).

CHALLENGES IN MIDDLE ADULTHOOD

Health, employment, and preparation for retirement are characteristic challenges of middle adulthood. The challenges of young adulthood do not disappear during middle adulthood, but often linger and impact middle adulthood also. For example, a young adult may resolve loneliness issues, but continue to experience the consequences of minority stress.

Physical Changes in Health

Health challenges become evident during middle adulthood. Health care access varies according to SES, with greater access among those with higher SES status. Health care access and health care experiences are worse for adults who are members of racial/ethnic or sexual underrepresented groups (Crenitte et al., 2022).

Excess body weight and obesity (defined as body mass index [BMI] = 30 or higher) are common, with obesity prevalence of 44.3% among Americans ages 40 to 59 years. Obesity can lead to type 2 diabetes, heart disease, and some cancers. Non-Hispanic Black adults have the highest age-adjusted prevalence of obesity (49.9%), followed by Hispanic adults (45.6%), non-Hispanic White adults (41.4%), and non-Hispanic Asian adults (16.1%) (CDC, 2022). Sexual and reproductive changes characterize middle adulthood. Sexual dysfunction, menopause, and other reproductive changes impact interpersonal relationships, sexual well-being, and general mental health.

COMMON CHALLENGES IN ADULTHOOD

There are many challenges that are common for young and middle adulthood. Although the challenges are often similar, there are different perspectives according to different ages.

Changes in Family Structure

The young adult and middle adulthood years are characterized by changes in family structures. Older adolescents finish school and often leave home, which alters the primary family structure. Marriage establishes new roles for adults who previously lived by themselves or their parents. The arrival of children changes the structure and dynamics of the newly formed family. These are all typical developmental events, but they can also lead to mental distress, physical issues, and social alienation.

Married adults are healthier than those in other non-married groups. Married adults are least likely to experience health issues and least likely to engage in risky health behaviors with one exception: middle adulthood married men have the highest rate of overweight or obesity. Widowed, divorced, or separated adults are more likely to experience serious psychological distress than married adults. In a dysfunctional marriage, problematic eating behaviors increase health issues (Huntington et al., 2022; Madani Civi et al., 2024; Skirbekk et al., 2023).

People are marrying later than in the 1990s. In 2019, the median age of men who marry for the first time was 30.6 and for women 28 years (Statista Research Department, 2023). People who marry in their teen years have the highest risk of divorce (Jones et al., 2024), whereas individuals with a higher education are more likely to be married. The percentage of couples who cohabitate decreases as education increases (Hemez et al., 2022).

There is an emerging trend for fewer women to marry and, at the same time, there is an increase in the percentage of women who cohabitate (Manning & Carlson, 2021). There are an increasing number of women who never marry. In 2020, nearly 19% of all pregnancies and 11% of first pregnancies were in individuals aged 35 years and older. The mean age of individuals having their first child has increased from 21.4 years in 1970 to 27.1 years in 2020 (Gantt et al., 2023).

Caring for Others

Based on the 2020 US Census, 73.2 million children (younger than the age of 18 years) resided in the United States, up from 64 million in 1990. Most of these children (70%) lived with two parents, and approximately 16% lived with only their mother, 5% lived with only their father, and another 3% lived in households with neither parent present. Within these numbers, there are further variations in ethnic groups. In 2022, the majority of White and Hispanic children lived in two-parent homes (75.6% and 67.5%, respectively), and 4 in 10 (43%) Black children lived in two-parent homes (U.S. Census Bureau, 2022).

Whether functioning in a two-parent or single-parent home, parents who work out of the home must provide for the care and safety of their children during their absence. Childcare outside the home is often disproportionately expensive compared to income and often is not available for parents who work evenings, nights, holidays, or weekends and during periods of illness and other crises. Federal support to single-parent families is limited. Working parents could formerly rely on their own parents and other family members to assist with childcare, but today many parents have no family available locally or are also serving as caretakers to family members in addition to their children.

In fact, **informal caregivers**, unpaid individuals who provide care, are the largest source of long-term care services in the United States. It is estimated that more than 53 million people provide care to an adult or child, with about 41.8 million of these Americans providing unpaid care to an adult aged 50 or older. Although men are increasingly becoming more involved in caregiving, women comprise the majority and perform the more difficult tasks of caregiving. The average age of a caregiver is 49.4 years, with 80% of caregivers being 64 years old and younger. The duration of caregiving spans from less than a year to more than 40 years, with an average duration of 4 to 5 years (AARP & National Alliance for Caregiving, 2020).

Caregivers are under considerable stress and often neglect their physical and mental health needs. Caregivers also report higher levels of loneliness, anxiety and depressive symptoms, and other mental health issues than noncaregiving peers. In turn, altered physical and mental health reduces the quality, satisfaction, and ability to cope with daily stresses related to caregiving (National Alliance for Caregiving, 2020).

Unemployment

Employment is an important societal value and thus serves as a source of economic, social, and emotional stability and self-esteem. For adults in a breadwinning role, the prospect of unemployment can also present a major life challenge that affects their ability to be effective in other life roles.

Young and middle-adulthood adults seek and maintain employment that maintains their lifestyle and provides for their children. In a society that is consumer driven, the ability to generate resources becomes critical. Yet shifts in the ownership and organizational structure of companies, downsizing, and the job market's ever-changing demands for workers with particular skills make employment stability questionable, both now and in the future. Career changes and the continuing necessity of training for new positions are now the norm.

In 2020, the United States faced an economic recession because of the COVID-19 pandemic. The unemployment rate jumped to over 14% in spring and by mid-2020, the rate dropped to over 10%, up 3.7% from a year earlier. Members of underrepresented groups were hit especially hard, with a combined unemployment rate of 18% for Black/African American individuals and Hispanics/Latinx individuals. Also severely affected were single parents who were employed in low-wage jobs, which disappeared; during the national shutdown of businesses, many people in this population lost their jobs. Then, as the restrictions on businesses eased with stay-at-home orders, these individuals were faced with the choice of returning to work or staying at home with their children, who were no longer in school or daycare.

By 2023, the unemployment rate in the United States had stabilized at 3.4%. Within the cohort of unemployed workers, the rate of unemployment is higher among US adults who have mental illness (7.4%). Generally, those with limited education and nonskilled workers remain at special risk for low wages and unemployment (NAMI, 2023; U.S. Bureau of Labor Statistics, 2023).

MENTAL DISORDERS IN YOUNG AND MIDDLE ADULTHOOD

Most people with mental illness experience their first diagnostic symptoms during late adolescence or early adulthood. By far, the highest rates of mental disorder occur among young adults. Late-life onset of mental disorder (older than age 40 years) is relatively rare, except for cognitive impairment, which typically occurs past the age of 70 years. Recent research suggests that 1 in 5 adults living in the United States will experience a mental disorder in their lifetime and that within a given year, 1 in 20 will experience serious mental illness (NAMI, 2023).

Changes in the biologic, psychological, and social domains can create a matrix of stress that may foster mental disorder. Most people with mental disorders do not come to the attention of the mental health system. In fact, fewer than half of those with mental disorders receive any kind of treatment from mental health professionals (NAMI, 2023).

RISK FACTORS FOR YOUNG AND MIDDLE ADULTHOOD PSYCHOPATHOLOGY

Mental health promotion and illness prevention are driven by cultivating an awareness of personal risk factors for mental illness and modifying those that can be changed. Specific **risk factors**, or characteristics that increase the likelihood of developing a disorder, can contribute to poor mental health and influence the development of a mental disorder. Risk factors do not cause the disorder or issue and are not symptoms of the illness but are factors that influence the likelihood that the symptoms will appear. The existence of a risk factor does not always mean the individual will get the disorder or disease; it just increases the chances. There are many kinds of risk factors, including genetic, biologic, environmental, cultural, and occupational. Even sex assigned at birth is a risk factor for some disorders (e.g., more people assigned female at birth experience depression than people assigned male at birth) (see Chapter 25). In general, sex assigned at birth, gender, age, unemployment, and lower education are risk factors associated with mental illness.

Biologic Risk Factors

The biologic functioning of young adults versus those in middle adulthood is a contrast between optimally running physiologic systems and those showing definite signs of wear and inefficiency. Of course, there are wide variations in the health of the various systems within each stage, with some young adults more physiologically and functionally compromised than their middle-adulthood counterparts. Most physical and mental systems have completed development by the time an individual reaches young adulthood. In general, the optimal health state of young adults begins to show changes around the age of 30 years. The perception of these physical changes often makes individuals aware of their aging process and may result in threats to bodily integrity and self-esteem. This section reviews the primary changes in the health of physiologic symptoms and possible mental health implications.

Skin

The most obvious change in physical appearance starts with the skin. Although the young adult's skin is smooth and taut, by late young adulthood, the skin begins to lose moisture and tone, and wrinkles develop. Self-esteem issues can erupt as the skin ages.

Cardiovascular and Respiratory Systems

Maximum cardiac output is reached between 20 and 30 years of age. Thereafter, blood pressure and cholesterol levels gradually increase. Although people assigned male at birth are especially prone to cardiovascular disease in middle adulthood because of testosterone levels, people assigned female at birth are not exempt from risk of heart disease. Similar to cardiovascular function, respiratory function decreases with age. After the age of 30 years, the maximum breathing capacity slowly decreases and may be reduced up to 75% compared with during young adulthood. Such changes are compounded if the individual smoked throughout adulthood. Alterations in cardiac and respiratory efficiency may result in limited energy for daily tasks and preference for lower activity levels, which makes exercise less of an enjoyable activity (Wagner et al., 2023).

Sensory Function

Sensory functions are also compromised as an individual moves from young into middle adulthood. Although the visual sense is at its peak in early young adulthood, the lenses of the eyes gradually lose their elasticity around the age of 30 years, and corrective lenses may be necessary. Such changes may result in issues regarding physical appearance that may affect self-esteem. Hearing is optimal in young adulthood, but middle adulthood brings changes in the bones of the inner ear and auditory nerve, resulting in the gradual inability to hear high-pitched tones and detect certain consonants. Such alterations in hearing may also present issues related to body integrity.

Neurologic System

In middle adulthood, brain structural changes are minimal. Although neurons are gradually being lost, changes in cognition are not evident. There may be some slowing of speed of reflexes because of slight changes in nerve conduction speed during middle adulthood.

Sexual and Reproductive Functioning

Concerns about changing physical appearance may also be tied to reactions to changes in sexual functioning. People whose sense of self was dependent on sexual characteristics or the level of sexual functioning typical of young adulthood may experience anxiety over such changes.

In middle adulthood adults assigned male at birth, testosterone production decreases, resulting in a lower sex drive, more time needed to achieve erection, and production of fewer sperm cells. Diminishing estrogen levels in midlife adults assigned female at birth result in the cessation of menses and capacity for pregnancy. The beginning of menopause may bring unpleasant symptoms such as hot flashes, night sweats, fatigue, and nausea. However, many people experience menopause as a relief from menses and the possibility of pregnancy.

Psychosocial Risk Factors

Any of the common challenges of adulthood previously discussed such as unemployment, changing family structure, and caregiving may serve as risks factors for mental disorders. These more general issues reveal underlying risk factors that have been shown to be common in the development of mental disorders. Also, risk factors rarely occur in isolation but tend to cluster because one may bring about another, and they influence each other.

Age

Most mental disorders occur among young adults and appear to be less common with increasing age. The first symptoms may occur in childhood but are usually evident in late adolescence and early middle adulthood. Such symptoms may be partially tied to the increasing demands for independence and social responsibility that Western society places on developing individuals. As some adults get older, they may experience decreasing stress because of learning to cope more efficiently.

Marital Status

Individuals who are happily married experience higher rates of both physical and mental health compared with those who are single, separated, or divorced. Marriage serves as a general marker for psychological health and the ability to connect with larger social networks. In contrast, an unhappy marriage has negative health effects. Unmarried individuals experience positive physical and mental health especially if they are not isolated from others and have support from a larger social system.

Recent data indicate that marital quality is declining in young and middle adulthood as evidenced by increasing divorce rates in these groups. The data show a doubling of **gray divorce** (divorce among individuals over the ago 50 years), which is a new phenomenon when compared to their counterparts 25 years ago. Expectations of self-fulfillment and happiness within marriage may be more important than in previous generations, when married couples stayed together for financial or family reasons. Middle adulthood dissatisfaction can lead to gray divorce. The erosion of marital quality prompts concerns about health and well-being of these individuals (Wright et al., 2023).

Unemployment and Other Job Stresses

In this consumer-oriented society, economic stability is a major value. Unemployment is a larger indicator of such socioeconomically related variables such as those experiencing poverty, lack of education, and the ability to obtain economic power within the larger social system. This creates an environment of stress that may contribute to the development of mental disorder or may indicate the negative effect that mental disorder has had on obtaining the education and independence necessary for obtaining job security and advancement. Employment rates for individuals with mental illnesses are notoriously low. Most adults with a mental disorder want to work and most can work with the proper supports.

Conversely, employment has its own set of stresses. Many people with low-paying jobs work two jobs, often going directly from one job to another. Shift work causes changes in circadian rhythms and sleep patterns, leading to an increase in stress. Interpersonal issues with coworkers can lead to emotional distress. Challenges even arise related to the different learning styles and career expectations of workers of different ages and backgrounds or who are reentering the workforce.

Sex Assigned at Birth

People assigned female at birth tend to come to the attention of the mental health system because of their greater awareness of health issues and willingness to seek interventions. People in this population are more prone to anxiety and depression, whereas people assigned male at birth tend to show issues with impulse control that result in alcohol use disorder and substance use disorder (Kirkbride et al., 2024).

LGBTQ+ and Gender Considerations

LGBTQ+ individuals are the subject of widespread discrimination, which may lead to psychological distress and trauma. They are also subject to minority stress. There is a higher prevalence of adverse childhood experiences among adults in gender-underrepresented groups than in cisgender adults (Tran et al., 2023).

History of Child Abuse

Being abused as a child increases the risk of a mental disorder as an adult. Data from multiple surveys indicate that there are long-term health and mental health consequences of early childhood abuse. Adults who experience severe childhood physical and sexual abuse are less likely to finish high school and more likely to live in poverty (Storrie et al., 2022).

Prior Mental Disorder

Mental illness tends to be a chronic disorder with symptoms manifesting early in life. Research has shown that mental illness arising in childhood and adolescence predicts further disorder in later years. Because most mental disorders are not completely understood, the existence of prior symptoms or full-blown disorder is a risk for mental illness at later periods in life. Increased stress provides the ground for the current emergence of symptoms of mental disorders that may have appeared to be in remission (Nudelman & Waltz, 2022).

Coping

Although the quality of coping is important in the reduction of stress, little is known about the continuity and changes in coping styles over the life span. Because past behavior is the best predictor of future behavior, coping styles used in the past would be repeated in the present time. The quality of such coping would determine how well stress is managed in the present and sets the stage for continued positive outcomes or more issues in the future.

There is an absence of epidemiologic studies that directly compare adult life stages according to mental health variables such as stress and coping. An exception is the Midlife Development in the United States (MIDUS) Study, which included more than 7,000 subjects between 25 and 74 years of age and those at midlife (defined as 40 to 60 years). The results of this study that compared

BOX 17.1

Research for Evidence-Based Practice: Responses to Daily Stressors and Physical Health according to Socioeconomic Status (SES)

Jiang, Y., Knauft, K. M., Richardson, C. M. E., Chung, T., Wu, B., & Zilioli, S. (2023). Age and sex differences in the associations among socioeconomic status, affective reactivity to daily stressors, and physical health in the MIDUS Study. Annals of Behavioral Medicine, *57(11), 942–950. https://doi.org/10.1093/abm/kaad034*

THE QUESTION: Do affective reactions from daily stress impact physical health of people in lower SES?

METHODS: The data were drawn from a MIDUS subsample of 1,522 midlife and older adults (34 to 83 years of age, 57.2% women, 83.5% White). SES data included education, household income, and indicators of financial distress. Affective reactivity was analyzed from the 8-day daily stress assessment and physical health was determined by self-report.

FINDINGS: Individuals from low SES backgrounds tend to experience poor physical health. They may be more vulnerable to stress exposure due to limited resources to cope with stress than people from higher SES. Among women, but not men, lower SES was related to increases in negative emotions to stress, which was related to chronic health conditions.

IMPLICATIONS FOR NURSING: Assessment of reactions to stress is important when caring for individuals from lower SES who are experiencing chronic health issues.

young and middle adulthood suggest that the process of coping improves in quality as life and satisfaction with life. A longitudinal follow-up of MIDUS respondents occurred over 2002 to 2006 and 2011 to 2016. The purposes of the follow-up were to repeat the assessments obtained in the original study and to expand into other areas of biologic and neurologic assessments. There are hundreds of research publications generated from this study. See Box 17.1 for an example.

Discrimination

Discrimination, unfair or prejudicial treatment of people and groups based on characteristics such as race/ethnicity, gender, age, or sexual orientation, is related to mental health and well-being. There are several groups in the United States such as sexual and gender underrepresented groups that experience discrimination, which may lead to chronic illness, emotional distress, and overall poor health and mental health outcomes. **Perceived discrimination**, the perception of differential and negative treatment because of membership in a particular group, is also associated with negative health and mental health outcomes. For example, lifetime and daily discrimination are related to an increased risk of mortality for African American adults in the United States (Obaoye et al., 2023).

Lack of Health Promotion Behaviors

People with mental disorders in young and middle adulthood appear to lack basic health promotion behaviors. This lack results in high rates of physical illness and premature mortality compared with the general population. This includes low levels of awareness about physical and mental health issues, smoking, poor quality diets, lack of exercise, lack of leisure activities and contact with friends, negative attitudes toward help seeking, and stigma associated with mental health issues (Fortuna et al., 2023).

NCLEXNOTE People with mental disorders frequently neglect their physical health and have premature mortality. Assessment of physical health and health-promoting activities is important in the care of people with mental disorders because of their high rate of smoking, lack of physical activity, and resistance to seeking help for physical concerns.

Parenting Stress

Young adults often find that the addition of children to the family, particularly the birth of the second child, tends to insulate the nuclear family from larger social networks. The responsibilities and time constraints involved in rearing small children may limit the couple's worldview to the home, and definitions of self may be constricted to the activities of the nuclear family. However, as children grow and create their own lives, the social connectedness of the parents tends to expand. By middle adulthood, couples may anticipate the emancipation of their children and may entertain more options for socializing with other people.

Factors Associated With Suicide

Suicide is a leading cause of death in the United States. Young and midlife adults are at risk for suicide, with the rates for both groups increasing (Curtin & Garnett, 2023; Garnett & Curtin, 2023). See Chapter 22. For young adults, alcohol use disorder, psychological distress, and hopelessness are related to suicidality (Kim et al., 2023). Lack of purpose, few positive relations with others, lack of personal growth, and negative affect are related to suicide, substance use disorder, and alcohol use disorder in White adults of lower SES (Song et al., 2023). The highest risk of suicide and deaths among racial/ethnic underrepresented groups occurs in young adulthood, with online racism increasing feelings of being a burden to society, which can trigger thoughts of suicide (Keum, 2023). Black and Asian individuals, and individuals who are members of sexual or gender-underrepresented groups, are at elevated risk for suicide ideation throughout all age groups (Cooley et al., 2023).

PROTECTIVE FACTORS

In contrast to risk factors, **protective factors** are characteristics that reduce the probability that an individual will develop a mental health disorder or issue or decrease the severity of existing issues. Common protective factors exist in multiple contexts—families, communities, and society. All these contexts should be considered when promoting mental health. For example, parental involvement can help combat drug misuse in their children, but a strong school policy is also needed. In addition, other community resources must be used to support the drug-free community environment. Targeting only one context is unlikely to make a lasting impact.

INTERVENTION APPROACHES

Many nursing interventions are effective in helping young and midlife adults achieve greater mental health. Whereas some are geared toward helping adults cope with the challenges typical of this period of life, others are more specifically designed toward preventing depression and suicide. Another aspect of intervention is helping adults overcome societal pressures that might prevent them from seeking care in the first place.

Mental Health Promotion

The psychiatric–mental health nurse supports the young and midlife adult through the developmental journey of life. Stresses associated with balancing the psychosocial demands and the adjustment to changes in the biologic, psychological, and social domains can be overwhelming. Validation and education are important interventions in helping these individuals cope with these changes (see Chapter 18).

An individual's mental health can be challenged by a variety of factors: Biologic changes or illnesses, psychological pressures, and interpersonal tensions are only a few. Developing coping strategies to eliminate or reduce the impact of these potentially destructive factors is a part of typical growth and development. In addition, sustaining positive health behaviors such as relaxation, proper nutrition, adequate sleep, regular exercise, and forming a network of trusting relationships can support one's mental health. Mental health promotion focuses on increasing the individual's physical, mental, emotional, and social competencies to increase well-being and actualize potential.

Social Support During Life Transitions

Young and midlife adults are prone to many life transitions: entrance into the workforce, job loss, career change, separation, divorce, the birth of children and their eventual leaving home, and changes in health status. Midlife adults are also subject to watching their parents' age and lose independence. Both young and middle adults can benefit from education about coping with the stresses involved with such transitions, linking with sources of social support, and anticipating the changes in role and adjustment.

Lifestyle Support

Although health may be at its maximum during the young adult years, changes in bodily appearance and function become evident by the age of 30 years and become more pronounced as middle adulthood begins. Although such changes are inevitable, their magnitude can be tempered by health promotion activities such as attention to regular exercise, good nutrition, adequate sleep, health screening, relaxation, leisure, and other forms of stress management. The young adult years are times of learning positive coping strategies for the stresses inherent to personal, marital, family, and occupational life. Such learning can be enhanced by a social support network consisting of people who are currently undergoing such stresses as well as older people who have the perspective and experience in managing these domains of life. These networks can be informal, such as regular contact with a circle of friends, or more formal, such as support groups sponsored by social, occupational, and religious organizations. A sense of belonging and availability of social support is important for the maintenance of health and recovery from illness of all kinds.

Self-Care Enhancement

The latter part of young adulthood and middle adulthood are times when chronic illnesses such as hypertension, heart disease, and arthritis may become evident. Symptoms of mental disorders may have arisen earlier in life but require continuous care because of their chronic and episodic nature. It is important for both young and midlife adults to be educated about the physiologic aspects of such disorders, the advances in medications used in treating them, possible side effects, the importance of medication adherence, lifestyle changes that can be instituted to control such disorders, and the possible use of complementary healing methods (e.g., massage, meditation). Such strategies require a good relationship with a health care provider as well as initiative from individuals to contributing to their own care through seeking and evaluating information available in the media, on the Internet, or from advocacy groups.

Prevention of Depression and Suicide

Suicide is the 12th leading cause of death for all ages in the United States but ranks as the 2nd leading cause of death for people of ages 10 to 34 and the 3rd leading cause for people of ages 35 to 54 (NAMI, 2023). The suicide rate is consistently higher for people assigned male at birth (hereinafter referred to in this section as "males") than for people assigned female at birth (hereinafter referred to in this section as "females"). Suicide rates are highest for American Indian, non-Hispanic males, followed by White, non-Hispanic males. Among females, the suicide rates are highest for American Indian, non-Hispanic females and White, non-Hispanic females. Suicide rates are increasing in most rural counties for both males and females (NIMH, 2023).

Symptoms of most psychiatric disorders have made their appearance by the time an individual enters young adulthood. Mood disorders may first arise during the young adult years and continue through middle adulthood and older adulthood. Because depression is a significant precipitating factor for suicide, early detection and intervention are critical for managing mood disorders and preventing suicide. Routine screening for depression and associated substance misuse is common in primary care settings.

Reducing the Stigma of Mental Health Treatment

Although mental disorders are common within the community and the rate of treatment has risen over the past 20 years, more than half of people do not receive mental health treatment of any kind. Part of this lack of attention is certainly because of the lack of available treatment in many communities (e.g., rural areas), but another major factor is the stigma that continues to be associated with mental illness and seeking help for mental health issues. Organizations such as the National Alliance on Mental Illness have spearheaded the movement toward viewing mental disorders as biologically based and devoid of moral implications, putting them on par with physical disorders. The National Alliance on Mental Illness is an important organization for obtaining information, support, and referrals for treatment for individuals with mental disorders as well as their families.

The Future of Mental Health for Young and Middle Adulthood

Young and middle adulthood can be some of the most productive periods in life. They can also be the most stressful and debilitating because of the rapid rate of social change and economic instability that society is currently experiencing. The division of adulthood into young and middle stages and the interest in adult development have paved the way for examining the challenges unique to these stages, in which individuals spend most of their lives. More needs to be known about the stresses of these stages, the ways that individuals cope, the changes that bring about increased life satisfaction, and the ways in which nurses can support adaptation and ensure health promotion. Such health-promoting interventions may serve as the foundation for future mental health.

Although more is known about childhood and older adults because of the more dramatic and time-dependent aspects of their development, the more subtle changes of adulthood also deserve consideration. Development does not end at childhood, and more needs to be known about the way young adults progress within their lives and achieve the satisfaction reported with middle adulthood.

Research also needs to examine the variables that promote and protect mental health as well as understanding risk factors. Researchers and clinicians often equate promotive or protective factors with the absence of risk factors. This is tantamount to equating health with the absence of illness. Models of thriving and flourishing in response to life's challenges have been proposed by theorists as a more appropriate model for mental health promotion rather than adequate functioning or the lack of criteria for a psychiatric disorder. Those who flourish do not merely lack psychiatric disorders; they also have lower risk for cardiovascular disease and other chronic physical illnesses, fewer health-related limitations, lower health care utilization, fewer missed days of work, and high resilience and intimacy. The adoption of such positive models has implications not only for prevention of mental illness but also for more proactive interventions that ensure continued wellness that progresses into older adulthood.

SUMMARY OF KEY POINTS

- Families in resource-abundant countries have achieved unprecedented economic stability that provides for prolonged periods of development and a range of choices in lifestyle.
- The periods of young and middle adulthood do not exist in resource-limited countries; a brief childhood progresses quickly into old age.
- Western society has recently shown greater flexibility in the timing of life events such as education, marriage, and childrearing.
- The periods of young and middle adulthood are characterized by changes in family structure caused by children leaving and returning home, marriage, and divorce.
- Caregiving for both children and older parents is a potential stress faced by both young and midlife adults.
- Most mental disorders usually begin during childhood or adolescence, with the first symptoms evident in late adolescence and young adulthood.
- As individuals progress from young to middle adulthood, they experience changes from optimally

running physiologic systems to those showing wear and inefficiency.

- Psychosocial risk factors for mental disorders include age, marital status, unemployment and job stresses, sex assigned at birth, gender, prior mental disorder, coping, discrimination, lack of health promotion behaviors, parenting stress, and factors associated with suicide.
- Despite decreases in the efficiency of physiologic functioning, young and midlife adults often lack health-promoting behaviors, especially if they have mental disorders.
- Suicide is a growing issue in young and middle adulthood. It requires early detection and treatment.
- Social support and stress management are important in helping people to cope with the stresses involved in life transitions.
- Fewer than half of individuals receive treatment for their mental health issues, and stigma and discrimination remain toward those experiencing issues.
- Mental health promotion in adulthood needs to embrace positive models of people who flourish in life rather than those who lack mental illness. Little is known about the factors that promote or protect mental health.

DEVELOPING CLINICAL JUDGMENT

1. A 19-year-old cisgender male visits the primary clinic with anxiety and insomnia. Currently living with parents, the student was told to pay rent for living at home or move out. His friends are telling him that his parents are being unfair and unrealistic. As a nurse, identify the generational views that are being expressed by the student and parents.
2. A nonbinary young adult is moving from a family home in an area of low socioeconomic status to an apartment in a middle-class neighborhood for work. Explain the challenges that the young adult could experience.
3. In middle adulthood, a nurse is working the night shift so that they can care for their mother with dementia during the day. The nurse's partner stays with the mother at night. What stresses will the nurse experience?
4. What factors do you think are protective or promotive of mental health? What kinds of interventions may promote both physical and mental health?

MOVIES, TV, OR STREAMING PROGRAMS

***The Kids Are All Right:* 2010.** This is a film about a same-sex couple and their adolescent daughter and son who were both conceived from the same anonymous donor via artificial insemination. The daughter, who is preparing to leave home for college, decides to initiate contact with her biologic father. The introduction of the father, although pleasant at first, reveals the strains in the family's relationships and functioning. This film illustrates the children negotiating the identity tasks of adolescence and ambivalently assuming initial responsibilities of young adulthood. The parents mirror their children's struggles in terms of renegotiating the roles played in their marriage, their identities, the level of independence given to their children, and acknowledging the imminent "empty nest."

Viewing Points:

1. Identify the life transitions faced by each of the family members in the film.
2. How does each member cope with the stresses they are experiencing?
3. How are the developmental issues the parents are facing similar to their children's?
4. How did the entrance of the father highlight the conflicts and change the dynamics in this family?

REFERENCES

AARP and National Alliance for Caregiving. (2020). *Caregiving in the United States 2020*. AARP. https://doi.org/10.26419/ppi.00103.001

An, D., Jager, J., Putnick, D. L., & Bornstein, M. H. (2023). Parenting stress and attachment insecurity in young adulthood: A social relations model. *Journal of Marriage and the Family*, *85*(2), 556–579. https://doi.org/10.1111/jomf.12893

Cavanagh, L., & Obasi, E. M. (2022). Chronic stress, autonomic dysregulation and prospective drug use among African American emerging adults. *Cultural Diversity & Ethnic Minority Psychology*, *28*(1), 91–102. https://doi.org/10.1037/cdp0000364

Centers for Diseases Control and Prevention. (2010). Table 22. Life expectancy at birth, at 65 years of age, and at 75 years of age, by race and sex: United States, selected years 1900–2007. https://www.cdc.gov/nchs/data/hus/2010/022.pdf

Centers for Diseases Control and Prevention. (2022). Adult and obesity facts. Data & Statistics. https://www.cdc.gov/obesity/adult-obesity-facts/index.html

Cooley, C. C., Zhang, Z. M., & Denney, J. T. (2023). Sexual orientation and age-related patterns of suicidal ideation among U.S. adults. *LGBT Health*, *11*(1), 38–46. https://doi.org/10.1089/lgbt.2021.0428

Crenitte, M. R. F., de Melo, L. R., Jacob-Filho, W., & Avelino-Silva, T. J. (2022). Transforming the invisible into the visible: Disparities in the access to health in LGBT+ older people. *Clinics*, *78*, 100149. https://doi.org/10.1016/j.clinsp.2022.1

Curtin, S. C., & Garnett, M. F. (2023). Suicide and homicide death rates among youth and young adults aged 10-24: United States, 2001–2021. *NCHS data brief*, (471), 1–8.

Eres, R., Lim, M. H., & Bates, G. (2023). Loneliness and social anxiety in young adults: The moderating and mediating roles of emotion dysregulation, depression and social isolation risk. *Psychology and Psychotherapy*, *96*(3), 793–810. https://doi.org/10.1111/papt.12469

Fardghassemi, S., & Joffe, H. (2022). The causes of loneliness: The perspective of young adults in London's most deprived areas. *PLoS One*, *17*(4), e0264638. https://doi.org/10.1371/journal.pone.0264638

Fortuna, K. L., Lebby, S., Geiger, P., Johnson, D., MacDonald, S., Chefetz, I., Ferron, J. C., St George, L., Rossom, R., Kalisa, J., Mestrovic, T., Nicholson, J., Pringle, W., Rotondi, A. J., Sippel, L. M., Sica, A., Solesio, M. E., Wright, M.,...Walker, R. (2023). Lived experience-led research agenda to address early death in people with a diagnosis of a serious mental illness: A consensus statement. *JAMA Network Open*, *6*(5), e2315479. https://doi.org/10.1001/jamanetworkopen.2023.15479

Gantt, A., Metz, T. D., Kuller, J. A., Louis, J. M., Cahill, A. G., Turrentine, M. A.; American College of Obstetricians and Gynecologists' Committee on Clinical Consensus-Obstetrics; Society for Maternal-Fetal Medicine; Society for Maternal-Fetal Medicine; American College of Obstetricians and Gynecologists. (2023). Obstetric Care Consensus #11, Pregnancy at age 35 years or older. *American Journal of Obstetrics and Gynecology*, *228*(3), B25–B40. https://doi.org/10.1016/j.ajog.2022.07.022

Garnett, M. F., & Curtin, S. C. (2023). Suicide mortality in the United States, 2001–2021. *NCHS Data Brief, No 464*. National Center for Health Statistics. https://dx.doi.org/10.15620/cdc:125705

Green, A. E., Price, M. N., & Dorison, S. H. (2022). Cumulative minority stress and suicide risk among LGBTQ youth. *American Journal of Community Psychology*, *69*(1–2), 157–168. https://doi.org/10.1002/ajcp.12553

Hemez, P., Guzzo, K. B., Eickmeyer, K., Brown, S., Manning, W., Westrick-Payne, K. (2022). Socioeconomic factors and differences in forming and maintaining marriages and cohabitations. *Child Trends*. Retrieved February 11, 2025, from https://www.childtrends.org/publications/socioeconomic-factors-and-differences-in-forming-and-maintaining-marriages-and-cohabitations

Huntington, C., Stanley, S. M., Doss, B. D., & Rhoades, G. K. (2022). Happy, healthy, and wedded? How the transition to marriage affects mental and physical health. *Journal of Family Psychology*, *36*(4), 608–617. https://doi.org/10.1037/fam0000913

Jones, A. M. W. (2024). *Age at first marriage and marital quality: Updating outdated social wisdom. Institute for Family Studies*. Retrieved February 11, 2025, from https://ifstudies.org/blog/age-at-first-marriage-and-marital-quality-updating-outdated-social-wisdom#:~:text=Most%20young%20adults%2C%20however%2C%20are,early%20marriage%20is%20curiously%20absent

Keum, B. T. (2023). Impact of online racism on suicide ideation through interpersonal factors among racial minority emerging adults: The role of perceived burdensomeness and thwarted belongingness. *Journal of Interpersonal Violence*, *38*(5–6), 4537–4561. https://doi.org/10.1177/08862605221117247

Kim, Y. J., Burlaka, V., & Yoon, S. (2023). Sex differences in suicidal ideation: Mediating effects of alcohol abuse/dependence on suicidal ideation through psychological distress and hopelessness. *Health & Social Work*, *48*(3), 179–187. https://doi.org/10.1093/hsw/hlad012

Kirkbride, J. B., Anglin, D. M., Colman, I., Dykxhoorn, J., Jones, P. B., Patalay, P., Pitman, A., Soneson, E., Steare, T., Wright, T., & Griffiths, S. L. (2024). The social determinants of mental health and disorder: Evidence, prevention and recommendations. *World Psychiatry*, *23*(1), 58–90. https://doi.org/10.1002/wps.21160

Kochanek, K. D., Murphy, S. L., Xu, J., Arias, E. (2023). Deaths: Final data for 2020. National Vital Statistics Reports, 72(10). National Center for Health Statistics. https://doi.org/10.15620/cdc:131355

Madani Civi, R., Mehranfar, S., Plunkett, R., Veenstra, G., & Conklin, A. I. (2024). A systematic review of social connections as determinants of obesity: Longitudinal evidence limited to marital transitions. *Obesity*, *25*(11), e13819. https://doi.org/10.1111/obr.13819

Manning, W. D., & Carlson, L. (2021). *Trends in cohabitation prior to marriage. Family Profiles, FP-21-04*. National Center for Family & Marriage Research. https://doi.org/10.25035/ncfmr/fp-21-04.

NAMI. (2023). *Mental health by the numbers. National Alliance on Mental Illness*. Retrieved on October 23, 2023, from NAMI https://www.nami.org/mhstats

National Institute of Mental Health [NIMH]. (2023). *Suicide. Mental health information statistics*. NIMH Information Resource Center. Retrieved October 28, 2023, from https://www.nimh.nih.gov/health/statistics/suicide

Nudelman, J. L., & Waltz, J. A. (2022). Acute and lifetime stress and psychotic illness: The roles of reward and salience networks. *Journal of Psychiatry and Brain Science*, 7(6), e220012. https://doi.org/10.20900/jpbs.20220012

Obaoye, J. O., Dawson, A. Z., Thakkar, M., Williams, J. S., & Egede, L. E. (2023). Understanding the relationship between perceived discrimination and mortality in United States adults. *Aging & Mental Health*, 27(2), 445–451. https://doi.org/10.1080/13607863.2022.2032593

Skirbekk, V., Bowen, C. E., Håberg, A., Jugessur, A., Engdahl, B., Bratsberg, B., Zotcheva, E., Selbæk, G., Kohler, H. P., Weiss, J., Harris, J. R., Tom, S. E., Krokstad, S., Stern, Y., & Strand, B. H. (2023). Marital histories and associations with later-life dementia and mild cognitive impairment risk in the HUNT4 70+ Study in Norway. *Journal of Aging and Health*, *35*(7–8), 543–555. https://doi.org/10.1177/08982643221131926

Song, J., Kang, S., & Ryff, C. D. (2023). Unpacking psychological vulnerabilities in deaths of despair. *International Journal of Environmental Research and Public Health*, *20*(15), 6480. https://doi.org/10.3390/ijerph20156480

Statista Research Department. (2023). *Estimated median age of Americans at their first wedding in the United States from 1998 to 2012, by sex*. https://www.statista.com/statistics/371933/median-age-of-us-americans-at-their-first-wedding/

Storrie, C. L., Kitissou, K., & Messina, A. (2022). The effects of severe childhood physical and sexual abuse on adult socioeconomic prosperity. *Journal of Child & Adolescent Trauma*, *16*(1), 55–68. https://doi.org/10.1007/s40653-022-00499-6

Sun, S., Lee, H., & Hudson, D. L. (2023). Racial/ethnic differences in the relationship between wealth and health across young adulthood. *SSM-population health*, *21*, 101313. https://doi.org/10.1016/j.ssmph.2022.101313

Tran, N. M., Mann, S., Cortez, M. G., Harrell, B., & Nettuno, L. (2023). Adverse childhood experiences (ACEs) and mental health by gender identity in the United States, 2019-2021. *Preventive Medicine*, *175*, 107705. https://doi.org/10.1016/j.ypmed.2023.107705

U.S. Bureau of Labor Statistics. (2023). *The employment situation–September 2023*. News Release. https://www.bls.gov/news.release/pdf/empsit.pdf

U.S. Census Bureau. (2022). Living arrangements of children under 18 years and marital status of parents, by age, sex, race, and Hispanic origin and selected characteristics of the child for all children: 2022. America's Families and Living Arrangements: 2022 (census.gov)

Wagner, J. U. G., Tombor, L. S., Malacarne, P. F., Kettenhausen, L. M., Panthel, J., Kujundzic, H., Manickam, N., Schmitz, K., Cipca, M., Stilz, K. A., Fischer, A., Muhly-Reinholz, M., Abplanalp, W. T., John, D., Mohanta, S. K., Weber, C., Habenicht, A. J. R., Buchmann, G. K., Angendohr, S., … Dimmeler, S. (2023). Aging impairs the neurovascular interface in the heart. *Science*, *381*(6660), 897–906. https://doi.org/10.1126/science.ade4961

Wright, M. R., Brown, S. L., & Manning, W. D. (2023). A cohort comparison of midlife marital quality: A quarter century of change. *Journal of Family Issues*, *44*(2), 538–559. https://doi.org/10.1177/0192513X211054466

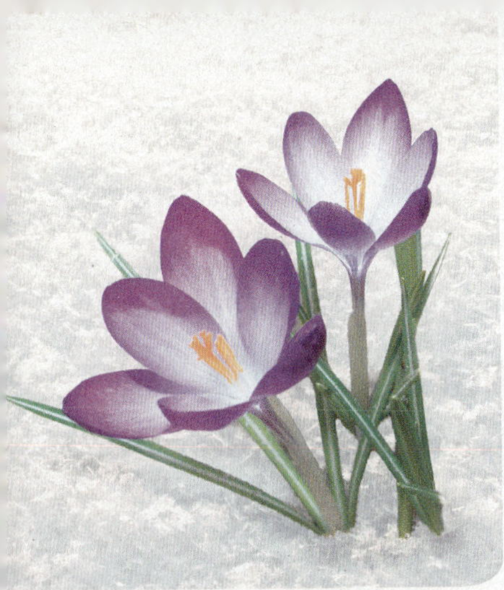

18 Mental Health Promotion for Older Adulthood

Mary Ann Boyd

KEYCONCEPTS

- cognitive health
- late adulthood
- positive mental health

LEARNING OBJECTIVES

After studying this chapter, you will be able to:

1. Describe the stages of late adulthood.
2. Discuss the importance of positive mental health for older adults.
3. Describe the biopsychosocial–spiritual changes that impact successful aging.
4. Analyze risk factors that challenge mental health status.
5. Analyze protective factors in the mental health promotion of older adults.
6. Apply mental health prevention and promotion interventions with older adults.

KEY TERMS

• biologic age • bridge employment • chronologic age • cognitive aging • cognitive reserve • cohabitation • crystallized intelligence • discrimination • financial exploitation • flourishing • fluid intelligence • functional status • gerotranscendence • life engagement • life satisfaction • middle–old adult • mindfulness • multigenerational caregiving • nonresidential caregiving • old–old adult • older adult mistreatment • polypharmacy • psychological resilience • skipped-generation custodial caregiving • spirituality • social determinants of health • social isolation • social support • working memory • young–old adult

INTRODUCTION

The number and proportion of older adults in the United States is rapidly increasing. By 2050, it is expected that Americans aged 65 and older will number nearly 83.7 million, more than double the number of older adults in the United States in 2012. The reason for the rapid growth in the aging population is that Americans are living longer lives (Arias et al., 2022).

Ninety percent of the US health care expenditures are for people with chronic and mental health conditions (CDC, 2024). Older adults are at somewhat greater risk than younger age groups for the development or recurrence of mental health issues. More than 20% of older adults aged 60 and older have a significant mental disorder, with depression, anxiety disorders, and dementia being among the most common (Alliance for Aging Research, 2025). There has been a significant increase in the use of antianxiety, sedative, and hypnotic medications in community-dwelling older adults as well as an increase in use of antidepressants in this group. Even with a high usage of psychotropic medications, depression often remains untreated in this population.

Yet, despite the high prevalence of psychiatric disorders and mental health issues in later life, older people remain vastly underserved by the current mental health system. This chapter explains the effects of aging on mental health and identifies risks and protective factors related to the mental health issues of older adults.

OLDER ADULT MENTAL HEALTH

Changing needs and personal development characterize older adulthood. This stage of life can be conceptualized in roughly three stages: **young–old** (ages 65 to 74 years), **middle–old** (ages 75 to 84 years), and **old–old** (age 85 years and older). The needs are different in the young–old than in the old–old. Generally, the young–old are challenged to develop new roles after retirement. This group of individuals may need programs and services that help them find meaningful activities. The old–old group tends to need supportive and protective services. However, the aging process is very individualized. Some young–old need supportive services and some in the old–old group are just beginning retirement (Min et al., 2023; Maltais et al., 2019).

KEYCONCEPT Late adulthood can be divided into three chronologic groups: young–old, middle–old, and old–old.

Chronologic Age versus Biologic Age

Aging can be considered from different perspectives. **Chronologic age** refers to the number of days living. **Biologic age,** however, reflects the time elapsed as well as biologic and physiologic factors such as genetics, lifestyle, nutrition, and comorbidities. Biologic age considers physiologic functioning relative to an average physiologic state at a specific chronologic age. For example, a 75-year-old individual with a biologic age of 80 has aged faster than a 75-year-old person with a biologic age of 73. The measure of biologic age provides a way of evaluating physiologic differences related to aging.

Positive Mental Health

The quality of the journey through older adulthood depends on many factors including biologic changes, psychosocial situations, and spiritual beliefs. When older adults retire from their lifelong work, they are challenged to establish a new meaning in life. There are now opportunities to do the things, such as traveling and visiting friends, which were impossible when work and family responsibilities took precedence. If there are health issues, financial limitations, or family issues, the person may not be able to pursue retirement opportunities.

Positive mental health helps older adults achieve a quality life and well-being. Positive mental health is related to happiness, which in turn fosters the development of positive resources that improve coping and resistance to daily stresses. Positive mental health is a crucial factor in recovery from mental disorders.

KEYCONCEPT Positive mental health is the existence of emotional, psychological, spiritual, and social well-being.

The individual's perception of aging also can impact late adulthood. For example, as once-dependent children grow into adulthood and become parents themselves, they no longer require close attention. No longer having dependent children is viewed positively by some who have more time to pursue personal interests and negatively by others who feel lonely and abandoned. The nurse can be instrumental in helping older adults consider the potential growth opportunities during this time.

COMMON CHALLENGES IN OLDER ADULTHOOD

Changes in vital biologic structures and processes occur gradually over decades and become evident in late adulthood. However, many older adults integrate profound decrements in physical capacity without significantly affecting their ability to function under typical conditions. It is only when functional reserves are needed, such as during an infection, that the absence of these reserves may be observed. Changes in health status, for example, can lead to loss in physical functioning and independence, which in turn can result in an unplanned change in residence. The risk of depression is increased as functional limitation increases and perceived physical health declines (Pearce et al., 2022).

Physical Changes

Many physical changes occur in older adults. Typically, body fat increases (18% to 24% in people assigned male at birth; 21% to 35% in people assigned female at birth), total body water decreases (10% to 15%), and muscle mass decreases. In the renal system, there is a predictable decline in glomerular filtration and tubular secretion. Although less efficient, the renal system without disease or injury can function adequately throughout late adulthood (Saxon et al., 2022). Liver function may be reduced because of decreases in blood flow and enzyme activity, resulting in increased blood and tissue concentrations of medications as well as half-life prolongation. Also, fat-soluble drugs may become sequestered in fatty tissue, rather than remaining in the circulating plasma, increasing the risk for drug accumulation and toxicity (see Chapter 11). Age-related changes in the brain are highly individual. For example, cortical thickness and anterior midcingulate cortex in some older adults (60 to 80 years) are indistinguishable from those in younger adults (Katsumi et al., 2022). For others, there may be a loss of neurons and a general atrophy of the brain (Saxon et al., 2022). Any of these changes over time can compromise the physiologic reserves to manage the everyday stresses of life.

Sensory Changes

All five senses gradually decline in acuity with age, usually beginning in the fourth and fifth decades of life, but these changes do not limit activity until the seventh and eight decades (Saxon et al., 2022). Visual and auditory losses can significantly impact independence, self-mastery, and

BOX 18.1

Research for Evidence-Based Practice: Hearing Loss and Social Participation

Prieur Chaintré, A., Couturier, Y., Nguyen, T. H. T., & Levasseur, M. (2024). Influence of hearing loss on social participation in older adults: Results from a scoping review. Research on Aging, *46(1), 72–90. https://doi.org/10.1177/01640275231174561*

THE QUESTIONS: How does hearing loss in older adults influence social participation? What individual and environmental factors influence the social participation of older adults with hearing loss?

METHODS: The Preferred Reporting Items for Systematic reviews and Meta-Analyses extension for Scoping Reviews was followed. Nine multidisciplinary databases in aging and health science were searched using 44 keywords related to social participation, older adults, and hearing loss. Of the 640 papers retrieved from the databases, 40 met the inclusion criteria. A thematic content analysis was conducted.

FINDINGS: Older adults with hearing loss have difficulty maintaining relationships and tend to withdraw from social activities that are important to them. Social support, engaged coping strategies, and the use of hearing aids facilitated social participation; however, greater hearing loss, communication difficulties, comorbidities, and reduced mental health impaired communication and participation in social activities. Stigma related to hearing loss and early detection of hearing loss are major challenges for improving social participation.

IMPLICATIONS FOR NURSING: Social participation is a key factor in the well-being of older adults. Early detection through expanding screening opportunities, holistic assessment, intervention, and interprofessional collaboration is needed to support healthy aging.

social participation (see Box 18.1). Taste, touch, and smell undergo a uniform dulling although the rate of decline is highly variable among individuals. Sensory decline is important to consider when assessing psychiatrically ill older adults because diminished senses may affect information processing, potentially affecting interpretation of standard mental status examinations. For example, patients who do not reveal hearing difficulty may be evaluated instead for dementia or depression.

Sexuality

Interest in and enjoyment of sexual activities can continue until one's death despite physical changes that affect sexual functioning. Health, a desire to remain sexually active, access to a partner, and a conducive environment contribute to positive sexual experiences. Physiologic changes in people assigned female at birth related to sexual functioning include decreasing estrogen levels, alterations in the structural integrity of the vagina (e.g., decreased blood flow, decreased flexibility, diminished lubrication, and diminished response during orgasm), and decreased breast engorgement during arousal (Saxon et al., 2022). Physiologic changes in people assigned male at birth include a decline in testosterone production, increased time to achieve erection, less firm erections, decreased urgency for ejaculation, decreased sperm production, and a longer refractory period (i.e., the amount of time before the another erection can be achieved). Issues with sexual performance in people in this population are usually centered around erectile dysfunction, which in turn affects self-esteem (Saxon et al., 2022).

The issue of sexuality in older adults is more complicated than just the physiologic changes. Sexual activity declines with age, with people assigned female at birth less likely to report being sexually active, but many people remain sexually active into their eighth and ninth decades (Steckenrider, 2023). Access to a conducive environment for sexual expression may be hindered if an older adult resides with an adult child or in a nursing home. Stigma associated with sexual activity in later life is also perpetuated by young adults' negative attitudes toward late-life sexuality and further contributes to lack of acceptance that sexual feelings and behaviors are expected at all ages. Lack of acceptance by others, particularly family members, and lack of privacy further contribute to a sense of isolation, loneliness, and poor social support, which are all associated with risks for depression. Individuals who are members of sexually underrepresented groups are at particularly elevated risk for stigma (Pereira, 2022).

Psychological Changes

Cognitive Health

Cognition includes several mental functions such as attention, thinking, understanding, learning, remembering, solving problems, and making decisions. Cognitive health, the maintenance of optimal cognitive function with age, is multidimensional and relies on several interrelated abilities that depend on brain anatomy and physiology. Many cognitive abilities (e.g., knowledge accumulated over a lifetime) are preserved or even enhanced during aging. Additionally, even though there are areas of cognitive decline beginning in middle adulthood, older adults can successfully use compensatory strategies to offset these changes and have a wealth of knowledge, skills, and experiences that younger adults may not have (Chilton & Schmitter-Edgecombe, 2023).

KEYCONCEPT Cognitive health is the maintenance of optimal cognitive function with age.

Cognitive aging is a process of gradual, ongoing, yet highly variable changes in cognitive functions that occur with age. Cognitive aging is a lifelong process beginning in utero. Typical aging does not impair consciousness, alertness, or attention. Health and environmental factors over a life span influence cognitive aging. Individual factors, including genetics, culture, medical comorbidities, acute illness, customary activity levels, socioeconomic status, education, and personality may modify the development or expression of age-related changes in cognition (Walhovd et al., 2023).

Mental Processing Speed and Reaction

Mental processing speed and reaction gradually decline in aging. Generally, it takes longer for older people to process information and give a response, which can lead to issues in reaction times (driving) and interactions with others. These changes may influence other cognitive operations such as working memory, speech processing, and attention. A person's ability to remember spoken word, attend to important information, or perform tasks may also be affected. Decline in processing speed may be offset by experience. For example, if older adults continue to engage in complex activities such as maintaining computer skills, they may not experience a significant decline in processing information. Communication with older adults requires paying special attention to verbal interactions and environmental influences. Hurrying older adults to answer questions may interfere with their ability to provide the correct answer (Saxon et al., 2022). Box 18.2 highlights many of the considerations necessary when interacting with older adults.

Memory

Older adults often worry about changes in memory as they age. Memory issues in later life are believed to result from encoding or retrieval issues (or both). There are many types of memory (measured by neuropsychologic tests); some remain stable, and others decline. **Working memory**, the ability to temporarily hold information in one's mind while it is processed, is central to many functions (see Chapter 7), such as remembering to take medication, processing language, solving problems, making decisions, and learning. Generally, working memory declines with age, especially for complex tasks. Despite these declines, performance of well-learned tasks often shows little decline. For example, there is little evidence that older workers are any less productive than younger workers. In most day-to-day tasks, older adults perform very well (Viviani et al., 2021; Zhao et al., 2023).

Other factors associated with memory changes include a lack of perceived relevance, sensory issues, not paying attention, a general failure to link the "to be remembered" information to existing knowledge through association, and a lack of using repetition to strengthen memory. The learning abilities of older people may be more selective, requiring motivation ("How important is this information?"), depend on meaningful content ("Why do I need to know this?"), and be related to familiarity with the idea or content. Level of education needs to be considered in evaluating responses on mental status examinations because lack of education may account for poor performance.

Although a decline in memory efficiency may be frustrating for the older individual, it does not necessarily hamper their ability to function daily. Threats to memory include medications, depression (impairs concentration and attention), poor nutrition, infection, heart and lung disease (lack of oxygen), thyroid issues (can cause symptoms of depression or confusion that mimic memory loss), alcohol use, and sensory loss (interferes with perception). However, it is important not to confuse memory decline with deficits in memory storage, such as those that are seen in dementia (see Chapter 39).

Intelligence

Intelligence includes both **crystallized intelligence**, knowledge such as language skills or knowledge about a particular topic, and fluid intelligence, that is, processing current or new information. **Fluid intelligence** involves thinking logically and solving problems. Crystallized intelligence remains fairly stable with modest declines in later life. Declines in fluid intelligence begin earlier and are more gradual throughout the life span (Zhao et al., 2023). Like other cognitive aspects, intelligence is impacted by other factors, including the environment, social context, knowledge, prior experience, health status, the demands of the task, and support.

Cognitive Reserve

The variability in cognitive aging can partially be explained by the concept of **cognitive reserve**, the

BOX 18.2
Communicating With Older Adults

- Focus the person's attention on the exchange of communication; the older adult may need extra time to begin to process information.
- Face the person when speaking to them.
- Minimize distractions in the room, including other people, objects in your hands, noise, and other activities.
- Reduce glare from room lighting by dimming too-bright lights. Conversely, avoid sitting in shadows.
- Speak slowly and clearly. Older adults may depend on lip reading, so ensure that the individual can see you. Speak loudly, but do not shout.
- Use short, simple sentences and be prepared to repeat or revise what you have said.
- Limit the number of topics discussed at one time to prevent information overload.
- Ask one question at a time to minimize confusion. Allow plenty of time for the person to answer and express ideas.
- Frequently summarize the important points of the conversation to improve understanding and comprehension.
- Avoid the urge to finish sentences.
- Consider factors such as fatigue and discomfort in structuring the communication.
- If the communication exchange is going poorly, postpone it for another time.

resistance to decline in the functioning of the brain. Factors that contribute to cognitive reserve include education, occupational attainment, physical activity, and engagement in intellectual and social activities. A deficit in early-life cognitive reserve is often related to socioeconomic status (Kim et al., 2024). Staying physically fit and maintaining an active social network can have positive effects in older adults (Amian et al., 2024; Jia et al., 2023).

Personality

Personalities and personality traits are generally believed to be stable throughout the life span. Some personality traits are associated with longevity, such as conscientiousness, responsibility, self-control, and traditionalism. Personality traits such as extroversion, openness to experience, agreeableness, and conscientiousness are related to successful aging. People who are assessed with low conscientiousness (low self-esteem, acting spontaneously without planning, showing little persistence in pursuing long-term goals, and not being driven by obligations of duty and responsibility) have a higher mortality rate than those with an average sense of conscientiousness. Characteristics of low conscientiousness may lead to unhealthy life choices and risk-taking behavior. Even though we generally believe that personalities are formed by the age of 30 years, evidence shows that personality traits are shaped by the environment and social experiences throughout life. Occupational and romantic experiences and other major life events influence the expression of personality traits in all age groups (Litwin & Levinsky, 2023).

Development

Late-life adult developmental phenomena are not well defined. Early developmental theorists viewed older adults as having the same psychological and social needs as when they were younger. They believed that as the aging person gave up their roles as employee and parent, the individual should replace the role losses with new roles and increase social interaction (Havighurst, 1961). The Disengagement Theory is similar but proposed that the aging individual and society mutually withdraw from each other to prepare the individual for an eventual exit from society (Cumming & Henry, 1960). Later, Erik Erikson identified "integrity versus despair" as a developmental task specific to late adulthood (Erikson & Erikson, 1997). He proposed that the primary task of the older adult is to reflect on their past experiences. If the individual is satisfied with their life, this eighth stage is resolved, and the person attains wisdom and acceptance of death.

Unlike the earlier theories, the Gerotranscendence Theory describes **gerotranscendence** as the continuation or progression toward maturation and shifting from a materialistic and pragmatic view of the world to a more cosmic view. For example, in young or middle adulthood, there is a focus on material possessions, but in older adulthood, there is a decreased focus on possessions and more emphasis on relationships and personal growth. The individual may experience personal growth in dimensions such as spirituality and inner strength with an emphasis on the meaning of life and making positive use of solitude (Tornstam, 2005). The concept of gerotranscendence may be used in establishing health promotion interventions. Gerotranscendence is also congruent with more recent research about mental health in late adulthood, which is more optimistic and addresses successful aging. This approach focuses on generation awareness, awareness of aging, the big picture of life, and a need for solitude (Abreu et al., 2023).

Emotional Health

Although personality is fairly stable across adulthood, emotional changes are small but generally positive. Aging adults tend to become more emotionally stable, more agreeable, and more conscientious, with a higher level of well-being. These positive changes are thought to be related to the development of better emotional regulation because of life experiences and involvement in meaningful activities, networks, and goals. Threats to emotional and physical well-being include limitations in daily activities, physical impairments, grief following loss of loved ones, caregiving or challenging living situations, or untreated mental illness such as depression and substance misuse.

Perception of Time

Older adults often comment that time seems to go faster than when they were younger. Experts have yet to agree on an explanation for this experience, but there are several factors that contribute to this change in time perception. The lives of older adults tend to be more stable than their younger counterparts as months, weeks, and years unfold with fewer life changes that demarcate periods of time. Life transitions of younger people are often dramatically different from each other, such as children growing up and leaving home, job changes, and relocation. Aging adults have less time left in life than younger people. Younger people often plan for their future, whereas time for older adults is limited.

Social Changes

Social determinants of health (SDOH) (conditions in the places where people live, learn, work, and play that affect a wide range of health risks and outcomes) significantly affect the health and well-being of older adults (see Chapter 3). Older adults with low incomes are more likely to have disabilities and die younger than those with higher incomes; in addition, if they become socially isolated and lonely, they are at increased risk of developing dementia and other health issues (U.S. Department of

Health and Human Services, 2024). Because most older adults have at least one chronic illness, access to health care becomes a priority. As mobility decreases with age, neighborhoods that are accessible, convenient, and safe, with access to grocery stores, are important (U.S. Department of Health and Human Services, 2024).

Functional Status

Functional status, the extent to which a person can independently conduct personal care, home management, and social functions in everyday life in a way that has meaning and purpose, often changes during the later years. Estimates of the prevalence of functional dependency vary, but in general, studies show that difficulty in performing activities of daily living and instrumental activities of daily living increases with advancing age and that cognitive impairment significantly predicts functional decline (Knoll et al., 2023). It is important to remember that most older adults live in the community and perceive that they are aging well despite chronic illnesses and some physical disability. A sense of control and self-efficacy contributes to an older person's sense of self-mastery despite limitations.

Retirement

Research shows an association between successful aging and a happy retirement. The ability to adapt to change and remain engaged and involved in life and social networks contributes to the successful negotiation of the retirement transition. Voluntary retirement is associated with postretirement well-being. For many, **bridge employment** (paid work for those receiving a pension) alleviates the negative consequences of retirement for those who are forced to retire involuntarily. On the other hand, changing roles and circumstances can cause stress and contribute to poorer mental health (Drazic et al., 2023).

Financial concerns certainly impact one's adjustment to retirement. Social Security Annuity continues to provide the largest single source of income for older adults, but retirement income security now often requires earnings from working in later life (Thompson & King, 2022). The traditional "three-legged stool" on which retirement rests—Social Security, pensions, and savings and investments—disproportionately excludes some groups, such as people of color, members of the LGBTQ+ community, women, and immigrants who have faced barriers to education, health, a stable work history, or financial stability. Many no longer have pensions or savings to sustain them in retirement (Tamborini & Kim, 2020).

Economic downturns have significant implications in terms of personal financial concerns; there is increased competition for jobs as well as a potential delay in retirement. Although mandatory retirement is becoming a thing of the past, older workers may be overlooked for promotions and employment opportunities because of their age and likelihood of retiring. Pensions are no longer the economic mainstay of retirement. The recent pandemic (COVID-19) accelerated unemployment and retirements of older workers who often had health issues, increasing their risks of contracting the deadly disease. Food insecurity became commonplace (Nicklett et al., 2023).

Leisure and Social Activities

As is the case with younger populations, participating in leisure activities is crucial in late adulthood. As age increases, participation in leisure and social activities decreases for many people. Health conditions such as depression, lung disease, and diabetes may prevent participation in home maintenance and leisure activities, especially walking, gardening, and active sports. Maintaining a positive mental attitude and participating in cognitively engaging, regularly scheduled leisure activities appear to exert a protective factor and are associated with a reduced risk of dementia even after adjusting for baseline cognitive status. Higher education levels are also associated with increased participation in both formal and informal activities (Klimecki et al., 2023).

Cultural Impact

With our communities increasingly becoming a reflection of multiple ethnic histories and values, the aging population is likewise becoming more diverse. Members of racial and ethnic underrepresented groups increased from 7.8 million in 2009 (20% of older Americans) to 14.5 million in 2022. Twenty-five percent of people aged 65 or older were members of racial or ethnic underrepresented groups (9% Hispanic origin, may be of any race; 9% African American; 5% Asian American; 0.6% American Indian and Alaska Native). Underrepresented groups face disparities in access to and provision of health care (Administration for Community Living, 2024). At the same time, they have higher-than-average health care needs (Farrell et al., 2022). Cultural variations also exist in family expectations of and responsibilities for older adults. For example, some groups highly value the experience and wisdom of older adults, and family members feel a responsibility for their care.

In the United States, racial and ethnic underrepresented groups are associated with accelerated biologic aging. Evidence shows that racial and ethnic underrepresented groups have biologic ages older than their chronologic age. Non-Hispanic Black individuals and Hispanic individuals have accelerated aging, and non-Hispanic White individuals have decelerated aging; these findings are strongly tied to educational attainment and socioeconomic factors (Farina et al., 2023).

Discrimination (unfair or differential treatment of people and groups based on characteristics such as race/ethnicity, gender, age, or sexual orientation) is known to negatively impact health outcomes. At least one-third of US adults have experience at least one major discriminatory event (i.e., denied residence in a neighborhood or unfairly fired from a job). Risk of mortality increases when discrimination is lifetime (experiencing a major discriminatory event that may affect socioeconomic status and life course) or daily unfair treatment. Examples of lifetime events related to mortality risk include being discouraged by a teacher from seeking higher education, not being hired for a job, and being denied a bank loan (Obaoye et al., 2023).

Family Relationship Changes

As family relationships change, interpersonal relationship strains can develop. Disappointments with the lifestyles of adult children and changes in caregiving responsibilities affect the quality of a long-term family relationship. In some instances, the young–old assume caregiving responsibilities for their old–old relatives.

There is a steady increase in grandparent caregiving. In the United States, 7.1 million grandparents (half of whom are over 60 years old) are living with their grandchildren under the age of 18, with 2.3 million of those grandparents responsible for their grandchildren. The increase in caregiving responsibilities by older adults is shown to be related to the recent COVID-19 pandemic (in which 140,000 children were orphaned) and the opioid epidemic (Baime, 2023).

The impact on the grandparents' health and well-being depends on the caregiving experience. Grandparent caregiving can be classified into three types: (1) **skipped-generation custodial caregiving** (grandparents raising minor grandchildren when parents are absent, (2) **multigenerational caregiving** (grandparents providing care to minor grandchildren while residing in a household with the children's parents), and (3) **nonresidential caregiving** (grandparents providing supplemental support to grandchildren while living elsewhere).

Health and well-being of the grandparents are associated with different caregiving situations. Caregiving responsibilities are particularly common among older adults who are members of underrepresented groups. African American grandparents are more likely than any other racial group to provide care in skipped-generation households. This group of grandparents is more likely to experience adverse health-related outcomes, including depression and poorer self-reported health when compared to noncaregiving grandparents. These adverse health-related outcomes may be related to the adverse circumstances that may result in grandparents caring for grandchildren, such as teen pregnancy, parental incarceration, substance use, mental illness, and death. These grandparents often experience food insecurity and financial distress adding more stress to an already stressful situation (Sneed & Chan, 2023).

For Hispanic grandparents, multigenerational caregiving is common, and they often face adverse conditions when caring for grandchildren. They may be caring for grandchildren whose parents are out of the country and share caregiving responsibility with adult children (not the parents). Nonresidential Asian-American grandparents often provide care to grandchildren while the parents are at work (Sneed & Chan, 2023).

Community Factors

Although most older adults live in their own homes, they may find themselves living in changing or deteriorating neighborhoods with inadequate social resources, such as places of worship and community, shopping, and health care centers. Relocating to smaller and more protective housing may be welcomed by some and fiercely resisted by others.

Residential Care

Residential care in foster care homes, family homes, personal care homes, residential care facilities, or assisted living arrangements provides the older adult with a protected environment. The quality of services and affordability of the arrangement need to be carefully evaluated to determine whether the older adult's needs and abilities match the care provided in that facility, including staff training and staffing patterns, medication supervision, approaches to behavior management, activities provided, services available (e.g., care management, family support, counseling, day care), safety and security issues, provision of personal care with attention to dignity and privacy, health and nutrition concerns, full disclosure of costs and funding, and payment issues.

Religious and Spiritual Changes

Older adults have time to reflect upon their religious and spiritual beliefs and often ponder the end of their lives. Religion and spirituality frame life and death expectations. Strong religious beliefs can reduce death anxiety, but some of those with doubts about their faith have greater death anxiety (Upenieks, 2023). Religion can be helpful during older adulthood but can also cause distress.

RISK FACTORS FOR OLDER ADULT MENTAL DISORDERS

Chronic Illnesses

Although the frequency of acute conditions declines with advancing age, nearly 95% of older adults have at least one chronic health condition; 80% have at least two. Poor physical health is associated with mental disorders both as a risk factor and as an outcome, with those with severe disabilities reporting lower levels of well-being (National Council on Aging, 2023). Common chronic conditions that cause activity limitation include arthritis, hypertension, heart disease, and respiratory disorders. Chronic illnesses can reduce physiologic capacity and consequently increase functional dependency. In addition, during acute episodes of illness, many older adults lose functional ability because they have limited reserves or cannot mobilize reserves to regain their premorbid performance levels.

Alcohol Use Disorder and Substance Use Disorder

Alcohol use disorder and substance use disorder are underestimated and undertreated. Substance use disorder is associated with poor health outcomes, higher health care utilization, and increased complexity of the course of the disorder. In addition, older adults with substance use disorder have increased disability and impairment, compromised quality of life, increased caregiver stress, increased mortality, and a higher risk of suicide. The prevalence of alcohol use disorder has increased among older adults, with a relative increase among women (Keyes, 2023). The majority of older adults with substance use disorder do not receive adequate treatment (Tampi et al., 2022).

Polypharmacy

More than 87% of older adults use prescription medication. The prevalence of **polypharmacy**, the use of five or more prescribed medications, is common in older adults who have more disease conditions requiring medications when compared to younger adults. Older adults also frequently use over-the-counter drugs and herbal and dietary supplements which may interact with prescribed drug therapies and lead to adverse events. The aging process affects pharmacokinetics and the strength and number of protein-binding sites (see Chapter 11). These changes place older adults at increased risk for adverse drug reactions (Delara et al., 2022; Rochon, 2023).

Difficulties in managing medications arising from memory impairment further compound the problem of medication misuse. Serious issues result when the treatment regimen and care delivery specific to prescribed medications are not coordinated. These issues are compounded when an older adult uses over-the-counter drugs, herbal remedies, and home or folk remedies without considering their potential interaction with prescribed drugs. Nurses can follow the principles delineated in Box 18.3 to improve drug therapy in the older adult population.

BOX 18.3

Drug Therapy Interventions

- Monitor the number of drugs that the patient uses. Alert providers if there are multiple prescribers. One-third of the residents in one long-term care facility received 8 to 16 drugs daily.
- Always consider alternatives among different drug classifications or dosage forms that are more suitable for older adult patients.
- Implement preventive measures to reduce the need for certain medications. Such prevention includes health promotion through proper nutrition, exercise, and stress reduction.
- Most age-dependent pharmacokinetic changes lead to potential accumulation of the drug; therefore, medication dosages should start low and go slow.
- Exercise caution when administering medication with a long half-life or in an older adult with impaired renal or liver function. Under these conditions, the time may be extended between doses.
- Be knowledgeable of each drug's properties, including such factors as half-life, excretion, and adverse effects (e.g., venlafaxine HCl, a structurally novel antidepressant that inhibits the reuptake of serotonin and norepinephrine, requires regular monitoring of the patient's blood pressure).
- Assess the patient's clinical history for physical issues that may affect excretion of medications.
- Monitor laboratory values (e.g., creatinine clearance) and urinary output in patients receiving medications eliminated by the kidneys.
- Monitor plasma albumin levels in patients receiving drugs that have high binding affinity to protein.
- Regularly monitor the patient's reaction to all medications to ensure a therapeutic response.
- Look for potential drug interactions that may complicate therapy. Antacids lower gastric acidity and may decrease the rate at which other medications are dissolved and absorbed.
- Instruct patients to consult with their providers before taking any over-the-counter medications.

Bereavement and Loss

Older adults experience many losses—friends and family members die, physical health can be compromised, choices and independence may be limited, and social status may diminish. Loss of one's partner, particularly when the relationship has been long and satisfying, constitutes a major life event. Survivors are at higher risk for depression and face financial issues after the death of a loved one. Because of differences in longevity, people assigned male at birth and those assigned female at birth usually experience life events at different ages. People assigned female at birth are more likely to lose their spouses and tend to be widowed at a younger age, so they have more time to adjust and to develop substitute social relationships to replace the partner. Conversely, people assigned male at birth tend to lose their partners at an older age, have fewer social networks to replace the partner, and express feelings of loneliness and abandonment. Health care professionals should collaborate closely with grieving survivors to help them understand that their lives will be displaced for some time. Support sessions on the grief process and financial and employment planning could become a standard part of care.

Poverty

Poverty is a risk for older adults' health, mental health, and wellness. Older adults living in poverty have inadequate resources for food, housing, basic needs, and medication. Many have to decide whether to buy food, pay rent, or buy medication. The number of older adults living in poverty has increased as the population has increased. In 2021, 5.8 million people aged 65 and older lived in poverty (Li & Dalaker, 2022). The percentage of non-Hispanic White older adults living in poverty was 8% compared to higher percentages of African American (17.8%), Asian American (13.3%), and Hispanic (18.7%) populations. Individuals aged 80 and older have the highest poverty rate, especially women; in this population, the percentage of those aged 80 and older living in poverty is 14.2% (Li & Dalaker, 2022).

Social Isolation

Social isolation, the relative absence of social relationships, is recognized as detrimental to quality of life and premature mortality. Meaningful interactions are important to the physical and mental health of older adults. Staying active, continuing to work, caring for others, and/or engaging with family, friends, and community contribute to the well-being of older people. Since the older adult population was very vulnerable to COVID-19 transmission, social isolation became a strategy to prevent transmission of the illness. Although social isolation protected many from physical illness, it led to negative consequences of loneliness and depression. As a result of the sheltering in place and other social distancing strategies, loneliness is higher than prior to the pandemic and associated with depression and suicidal ideation (Su et al., 2023).

Lack of Social Support and Suicide

Closely related to social isolation, a lack of social support is linked to transition into an institutional setting. When older adults can go to movies, dinner, or a casino and visit family and friends, they are more likely to live independently. Dissatisfaction with social life, lack of participation in organizations, and being distant from others are associated with a wish for death (O'Brien et al., 2023). Safety concerns are always a priority. Any suicidal ideation should be identified, and a safety plan developed (see Box 18.4).

BOX 18.4

Risk Factors for Suicide in Late Life (Age Older Than 65 Years)

- Depression
- Prior attempts at suicide
- Marked feelings of hopelessness; lack of interest in future plans
- Feelings of loss of independence or sense of purpose
- Medical conditions that significantly limit functioning or life expectancy
- Impulsivity due to cognitive impairment
- Social isolation
- Family discord or losses (i.e., recent death of a loved one)
- Inflexible personality or marked difficulty adapting to change
- Access to lethal means (i.e., firearms, other weapons, etc.)
- Daring or risk-taking behavior
- Sudden personality changes
- Alcohol or medication misuse
- Verbal suicide threats such as, "You'd be better off without me" or "Maybe I won't be around"
- Giving away prized possessions

Older Adult Mistreatment and Exploitation

Older adult mistreatment, intentional actions that cause harm or create a serious risk of harm to a vulnerable older adult by a caregiver or other person who stands in a trust relationship to the individual, has an estimated prevalence of 10%. Actual cases may be higher, with only 1 in 24 cases reported (U.S. Department of Justice, 2023). Clinical and empirical evidence suggests that a shared living arrangement increases the opportunities for contact that can lead to conflict and mistreatment. Abuse of older adults tends to take place where the individuals live—most often in the home, where people conducting the abuse are often adult children, other family members such as grandchildren, or spouses or partners of older adults. Institutional settings, especially long-term care facilities, can also be settings of abuse. The prevalence of mistreatment of older adults appears to be related to low income, poor health, and lack of social support. Race and ethnic differences have not been shown to play a role (Nyarko-Odoom et al., 2023).

Financial exploitation is a type of elder abuse that may occur with other forms of abuse (see Chapter 23). **Financial exploitation** is the illegal, unauthorized, or improper use of an older individual's resources by a caregiver or other person in a trusting relationship, for the benefit of someone other than the older individual. Examples include a caregiver using an older adult's money to pay for items without the person's permission, scams perpetrated through an imposter phone call or online contact, unexplained withdrawals from bank accounts, and property theft. Financial exploitation assessment should be included in nursing assessments.

PROTECTIVE FACTORS FOR MENTAL DISORDERS IN OLDER PEOPLE

Protective factors to minimize the occurrence of mental disorders in older adults are like those in younger adults. Protective factors include marriage, education and income level, psychological resilience, religion and spirituality, healthy lifestyle, nutrition, and exercise.

The Marriage Effect

It has long been thought that married people have lower mortality rates than unmarried at all ages. Many studies report that being part of a couple within a relationship is positively correlated with longevity and health,

FIGURE 18.1 Marriage/cohabitation is associated with positive physical and mental health. (Shutterstock/Rawpixel)

including cognitive and emotional function (Ma & Gu, 2023). **Cohabitation** (an arrangement where people live together, usually couples) of older adults may afford similar benefits (Zhou et al., 2025). There are several possible explanations for the marriage/cohabiting advantage. For example, married people may be less likely to engage in high-risk and health-damaging behaviors. They may also be more likely to receive care and support when needed. They have shared economic resources and a social network of relatives and friends who can provide vital support at older ages. Negotiating a partner relationship that presents ongoing social and emotional challenges may also contribute to higher functioning (see Fig. 18.1).

Education and Income

Education and income provide older adults with cognitive, economic, and coping reserves that support function and well-being and are related to physical activity and physical and cognitive function and disability. Education is the predominant indicator that has a causal effect on longevity. Lifestyles that result in smoking, obesity, and chronic diseases will partly decrease the education impact (Ye et al., 2023). Those with higher education and income are more likely to engage in physical activity and have the resources to provide care when needed. Higher levels of education are associated with higher levels of cognitive function as well as a lower risk of dementia (Dinius et al., 2023).

Psychological Resilience

Psychological resilience, having a meaning and purpose in life, social support, positive emotions, and coping skills, may be more important for well-being than physical health. The following factors contribute to psychological resilience: **life engagement** (finding enjoyment and meaning in activities), **life satisfaction** (feeling positive about physical health and mental health), **flourishing** (well-being factors such as self-esteem and meaningful relationships), and **mindfulness** (tendency to be conscientious of present experiences). Objective and subjective **social support** (number of active social roles, i.e., mother, child, friend, etc., number of people, and number of network groups) also contribute to psychological resilience. As older people engage in activities meaningful to them, their overall life satisfaction increases, which is associated with positive mental health outcomes. Flourishing is a well-being characteristic that includes successful relationships, self-esteem, purpose, and optimism. The more perceived success in these areas, the more likely there is life satisfaction. Mindfulness is related to physical health, sleep, positive affect, resiliency, and overall quality of life. Social support is a well-known factor related to global health status and positive mental health (O'Brien et al., 2023).

Religion and Spirituality

The relationship between religion/spirituality (R/S) and positive mental health is well documented. For older adults, R/S is highly related to positive mental health and well-being. Many older adults draw on R/S to provide meaning in life (Manoiu et al., 2023). Longevity and well-being are associated with R/S practices in many cultures. Collaboration of religious leaders in mental health care can strengthen the impact of R/S on positive mental health.

Healthy Lifestyle

A healthy lifestyle is important in preventing illness and promoting well-being at all ages, including in late adulthood. Such behaviors include not smoking; drinking alcohol in moderation; getting adequate rest and sleep; getting adequate hydration and nutrition, especially fruits and vegetables; exercising; and coping with stress (Jia et al., 2023).

Nutrition

Maintaining a healthy diet can be challenging for older adults. In the United States, the prevalence of obesity is 41.5% of all adults over the age of 60 (CDC, 2022). The prevalence of undernutrition is high in older adults, especially those living in institutionalized settings (Mostafa et al., 2023). Factors contributing to undernutrition include living alone, poor appetite, poor intake of fluid and nutritious foods, medications, malignancy, bereavement, and depression. Undernutrition can lead to anemia, inadequate wound healing, increased incidence of pressure sores, impaired elimination, impaired immunologic functions, weakness, fatigue, and mental issues (including depression, dementia, and agitation) (Saxon et al., 2022). Adequate nutrition is a crucial factor in maintaining mental health.

Physical Activity

Emerging evidence suggests that physical activity is related to positive mental health and may be a protective factor. There is a moderate amount of evidence that exercise can prevent the onset or worsening of depression.

Structured exercise programs enhance older people' overall physical functioning and well-being and reduce anxiety symptoms among sedentary adults with chronic illnesses (Galle et al., 2023).

PREVENTION INTERVENTIONS

Reducing the Stigma of Mental Health Treatment

The stigma of mental illness continues to interfere with the willingness of older adults to seek treatment. Older adults in America grew up during a time when institutionalization in asylums, electroconvulsive treatments, and other treatment approaches were regarded with fear. This fear can lead to denial of issues. Nurses can help reduce the stigma through educational interventions and facilitation of access to services.

Early Recognition of Depressive Symptoms and Suicide Risk

Depression is one of the most common mental disorders in older adults (see Chapter 25). Even with a high usage of psychotropic medications, depression remains untreated in this population (Uomoto, 2023). Because depression can be debilitating and can lead to suicide, recognition and early intervention are the keys to avoiding ongoing depressive episodes. Depressive symptoms among older adults are more likely to include vague somatic complaints, cognitive symptoms, hypersomnia, and appetite changes rather than complaints of depressed mood. Early indications of symptomatology can be identified in primary care settings using a screening tool such as the Geriatric Depression Scale (Yesavage et al., 1982). Several preventive interventions are helpful, such as grief counseling for widows and widowers, self-help groups, and physical and social activities.

Monitoring Medications

With the approval of new medications, older adults' health issues can be treated with pharmacologic agents that were not previously available. It is important to make sure that medications are being taken correctly as well as whether they are having the desired effects. Side effects and drug interactions should be carefully monitored to detect untoward symptoms and delirium. Dosages may need to be adjusted slowly. It is important to review all medications, including over-the-counter, natural, and alternative remedies.

Avoiding Premature Institutionalization

Although many people require nursing home care, integrated care in the community is effective and can delay nursing home placement. Home visits that focus on assessment of symptoms and coordination of health care needs can result in older adults receiving their mental health support within the community and, therefore, are able to stay in their current living arrangements. Older adults and those with disabilities prefer to receive community-based care, which to be most effective must include prevention and rehabilitation services as well as acute care.

MENTAL HEALTH PROMOTION INTERVENTIONS

Social Support Transitions

Compensating for loss of family by expanding friendship networks and employment may become an important method of establishing a network in late life. Older adults can be prepared for the transition by receiving information about internal developmental processes, sources of social support, and opportunities for personal growth and role supplementation. Interventions to support successful aging promote productive and social engagement, and effective coping groups can be particularly effective in developing a sense of community, decreasing isolation, and strengthening a safety network.

Cognitive Engagement

Frequent engagement in cognitive activities positively supports memory. Successful cognitive aging is supported not only by a cognitive reserve but also by development and use of compensatory strategies. For example, a nursing intervention is teaching the patient to write notes to self about upcoming events. Such compensatory strategies support cognitive functioning as well as a sense of personal control.

Lifestyle Support

Lifestyle interventions, such as exercise promotion and nutrition counseling, are particularly important in late life because a tendency to slow down and become more sedentary usually accompanies aging. For many, retirement provides an opportunity to restructure the time that was previously spent working. Developing regular exercise habits can help maintain physical and psychological well-being, especially if done with others. Self-help programs generally include components of exercise, nutrition, health screening, and health habits. Maintaining social support is an integral part of lifestyle support.

Self-Care Enhancement

Enhancing self-care is a major area for mental health promotion. Education of older adults and their families is crucial to ensuring adherence to agreed-upon care regimens. The nurse must consider the educational level, pace of learning, and visual and hearing deficits. The nurse should provide instructional aids, large-print labeling, and devices such as medication calendars that encourage adherence. Self-care enhancements assist older adults in the use of compensatory strategies and aid in their being as functionally independent for as long as possible. Supporting a sense of control and decisional capacity is critical to self-care.

Spiritual Support

Spirituality can be extremely important to older adults and can positively affect attitude, particularly as health declines. Participation in a community of faith is associated with better health outcomes and mental well-being (Lima et al., 2020). Supporting contact with spiritual leaders is important to the patient and is an ongoing mental health promotion intervention. The nurse can also support a patient's spiritual growth by exploring the meanings that a particular life change has for the patient. In late life, existential issues such as experiencing losses, redefining meanings in existence, and living in the present become the standard, replacing the performance and future orientation that characterize earlier adulthood.

Community Services

Community care options are needed that provide both sustenance and growth. Examples of supportive services that foster independent community living include information and referral services; transportation and nutrition services; legal and protective services; comprehensive older adult community centers; homemaker and handyman services; matching of older with younger individuals to share housing; and use of the supports available through places of worship, community groups, or mental health and other community agencies (e.g., area agencies on aging) to maintain older adults in the community for as long as possible. The availability and accessibility of these services vary greatly, and eligibility requirements may exist.

POSITIVE MENTAL AGING

There are many questions about the course of aging for future cohorts of older adults. It is probable that some of the losses and decrements associated with aging are in fact artifacts of a more sedentary, less healthy lifestyle over a lifetime. Furthermore, we must consider that positive mental aging is more than the absence of mental disorders and impairment but rather is more a reflection of resilience—the capacity to adapt, feel in control, and make decisions about care and life. Most important is to listen to older adults themselves. As nurses, it is incumbent upon us to help older adults to recognize and use their strengths to cope with and transcend losses and limitations. Recognizing and tapping into the wisdom accumulated over a lifetime may help older adults negotiate the many challenges faced in later life.

SUMMARY OF KEY POINTS

- Changes in vital biologic structures and processes occur, but older adults can sustain some structural losses without losing function.
- All five senses (sight, hearing, touch, taste, and smell) decline with age, which may affect information processing.
- Although older adults experience many physical changes, they have the desire to, and are able to, remain sexually active.
- Cognitive health is maintaining optimal cognitive function with age; cognitive aging is the gradual changes in cognitive function that occur with age.
- Threats to cognitive function in older adults include medication side effects, depression, poor nutrition, infection, heart and lung disease, thyroid issues, alcohol use, and sensory loss.
- Intelligence and personality are generally stable throughout the life span; however, reaction time slows with age.
- Gerotranscendence Theory is the leading theory that explains development of older adults and can be used to guide interventions.
- Major changes in social roles with aging include functional status, retirement, loss of partner, and changes in residence.
- Poverty and discrimination negatively affect ethnic and racial underrepresented groups. Caregiving responsibilities for grandchildren can negatively impact the health and well-being of grandparents.
- Polypharmacy is prevalent in older adults, particularly in nursing homes. Ongoing assessment of medications is needed to prevent inappropriate medication administration.
- Older people are at higher risk for poverty and social isolation.
- Older adults are vulnerable to mistreatment and exploitation.
- Mental health protective factors include marriage, education, psychological resilience, religion and spirituality, and healthy lifestyles (including nutrition and exercise).
- Interventions to prevent mental illness include reducing the stigma of mental health treatment, preventing depression and suicide, monitoring medications, and preventing premature institutionalization.
- Nurses can provide a number of interventions to promote mental health, addressing social support transitions, cognitive engagement, lifestyle support, self-care enhancement, spiritual support, and community-based services.

- Positive mental aging is more than the absence of mental disorders and impairment but is more a reflection of resilience, which is the capacity to adapt, feel in control, and be engaged, with a positive outlook.

DEVELOPING CLINICAL JUDGMENT

1. What is the difference between chronologic and biologic aging?
2. M.S., a 60-year-old African American assigned male at birth, reports being denied promotions at his job because of his race. He has difficulty seeking access to health care because of limited health insurance. He has diabetes, hypertension, and depression. What cues indicate that discrimination has impacted his health status and psychological well-being?
3. Using Gerotranscendence Theory, explain how life views change from middle adulthood to older adulthood.
4. A nursing assessment reveals that a 76-year-old individual who lives alone was admitted to an acute care facility for a suicide attempt. An astute nurse would look for which risk factors that underlie the suicide attempt?
5. A patient is admitted to the emergency department for confusion, memory issues, and a recent fall. The physical examination does not reveal any indications for an injury. What does the nurse want to include in the assessment?

MOVIE, TV, AND STREAMING PROGRAMS

Moving On: 2022. This American comedy film is about the reunion of Claire (Jane Fonda) and estranged friend Evelyn (Lily Tomlin) at long-time friend Joyce's funeral. Now that Joyce is dead, Claire can seek revenge on Claire's husband. Howard (Malcolm McDowell), who sexually assaulted her 50 years ago, derailing her life. This movie examines growing older and the impact of memories and regrets. Claire plots how to get revenge and finally gets to confront Howard. Evelyn is a retired musician who has her own secrets that come to life during the movie.

Viewing Points

1. Why did Claire not tell authorities that Howard sexually assaulted her? How did the sexual assault impact Claire's life?
2. Why was Evelyn's relationship with Joyce kept secret? What would have been the consequences of being open about their relationship in the 1960s?
3. How did the physical changes of aging affect Claire and Evelyn?
4. What emotions does Howard demonstrate in the movie?

REFERENCES

Abreu, T., Araújo, L., & Ribeiro, O. (2023). How to promote gerotranscendence in older adults? A scoping review of interventions. *Journal of Applied Gerontology*, *42*(9), 2036–2047. https://doi.org/10.1177/07334648231169082

Administration for Community Living. (2024). 2023 Profile of older Americans. Administration on Aging. U.S. Department of health and Human Services. https://acl.gov/sites/default/files/Profile%20of%20OA/ACL_ProfileOlderAmericans2023_508.pdf

Alliance for Aging Research. (2025). *Mental health*. Retrieved March 28, 2025, from https://www.agingresearch.org/aging-health/mental-health/

Amian, J. G., Fernandez-Portero, C., de la Bella, R., Arenilla-Villalba, M. J., López-Lluch, G., & Alarcon, D. (2024). Cognitive reserve and frontotemporal disorders: Exploring the relationship between education, physical activity, and cognitive dysfunction in older adults. *Perceptual and Motor Skills*, *131*(3), 720–736. https://doi.org/10.1177/00315125241241358

Arias, E., Tejada-Vera, M. S., & Ahmad, F. (2022). Provisional life expectancy estimates for 2021. National Vital Statistics Rapid Release. Centers for Diseases Control and Prevention Report No. 23. https://www.cdc.gov/nchs/data/vsrr/vsrr023.pdf

Baime, A. J. (2023). *When grandparents are called to parent–again*. AARP. Retrieved November 15, 2023, from https://www.aarp.org/home-family/friends-family/info-2023/grandparents-become-parents-again.html

Centers for Disease Control and Prevention. (2022). *Adult Obesity Facts*. National Center for Health Statistics. Retrieved December 3, 2023, from https://www.cdc.gov/obesity/data/adult.html

Centers for Disease Control and Prevention. (2024). *Fast facts: Health and economic costs of chronic conditions*. Retrieved March 28, 2025, from https://www.cdc.gov/chronic-disease/data-research/facts-stats/index.html

Chilton, R. L., & Schmitter-Edgecombe, M. (2023). Assessing functional ability of healthy adults with the Night Out Task. *The Clinical Neuropsychologist*, *37*(6), 1302–1320. https://doi.org/10.1080/13854046.2022.2096485

Cumming, E., & Henry, W. E. (1960). *Growing old: The process of disengagement*. Basic Books.

Delara, M., Murray, L., Jafari, B., Bahji, A., Goodarzi, Z., Kirkham, J., Chowdhury, M., & Seitz, D. P. (2022). Prevalence and factors associated with polypharmacy: a systematic review and Meta-analysis. *BMC Geriatrics*, *22*(1), 601. https://doi.org/10.1186/s12877-022-03279-x

Dinius, C. J., Pocknell, C. E., Caffrey, M. P., & Roche, R. A. P. (2023). Cognitive interventions for memory and psychological well-being in aging and dementias. *Frontiers in Psychology*, *14*, 1070012. https://doi.org/10.3389/fpsyg.2023.1070012

Drazic, I., Schermuly, C. C., & Büsch, V. (2024). Empowered to stay active: Psychological empowerment, retirement timing, and later life work. *Journal of Adult Development*, *31*, 261–278. https://doi.org/10.1007/s10804-023-09453-8

Erikson, E. H., & Erikson, J. M. (1997). *The lifecycle completed, extended version*. W.W. Norton & Company.

Farina, M. P., Kim, J. K., & Crimmins, E. M. (2023). Racial/ethnic differences in biological aging and their life course socioeconomic determinants: The 2016 Health and Retirement Study. *Journal of Aging and Health*, *35*(3–4), 209–220. https://doi.org/10.1177/08982643221120743

Farrell, T. W., Hung, W. W., Unroe, K. T., Brown, T. R., Furman, C. D., Jih, J., Karani, R., Mulhausen, P., Nápoles, A. M., Nnodim, J. O., Upchurch, G., Whittaker, C. F., Kim, A., Lundebjerg, N. E., & Rhodes, R. L. (2022). Exploring the intersection of structural racism and ageism in healthcare. *Journal of the American Geriatrics Society*, *70*(12), 3366–3377. https://doi.org/10.1111/jgs.18105

Galle, S. A., Deijen, J. B., Milders, M. V., De Greef, M. H. G., Scherder, E. J. A., van Duijn, C. M., & Drent, M. L. (2023). The effects of a moderate physical activity intervention on physical fitness and cognition in healthy elderly with low levels of physical activity: A randomized controlled trial. *Alzheimer's Research & Therapy*, *15*(1), 12. https://doi.org/10.1186/s13195-022-01123-3

Havighurst, R. J. (1961). Successful aging. *The Gerontologist*, *1*(1), 8–13.

Jia, J., Zhao, T., Liu, Z., Liang, Y., Li, F., Li, Y., Liu, W., Li, F., Shi, S., Zhou, C., Yang, H., Liao, Z., Li, Y., Zhao, H., Zhang, J., Zhang, K., Kan, M., Yang, S., Li, H., … Cummings, J. (2023). Association between healthy lifestyle and memory decline in older adults: 10 year, population based, prospective cohort study. *BMJ*, 380, e072691. https://doi.org/10.1136/bmj-2022-072691

Katsumi, Y., Wong, B., Cavallari, M., Fong, T. G., Alsop, D. C., Andreano, J. M., Carvalho, N., Brickhouse, M., Jones, R., Libermann, T. A., Marcantonio, E. R., Schmitt, E., Shafi, M. M., Pascual-Leone, A., Travison, T., Barrett, L. F., Inouye, S. K., Dickerson, B. C., & Touroutoglou, A. (2022).

Structural integrity of the anterior mid-cingulate cortex contributes to resilience to delirium in SuperAging. *Brain Communications*, *4*(4), fcac163. https://doi.org/10.1093/braincomms/fcac163

Litwin, H., & Levinsky, M. (2023). The interplay of personality traits and social network characteristics in the subjective well-being of older adults. *Research on Aging*, *45*(7–8), 538–549. https://doi.org/10.1177/01640275221113048

Keyes, K. M. (2023). Alcohol use in the older adult US population: Trends, causes, and consequences. *Alcohol*, *107*, 28–31. https://doi.org/10.1016/j.alcohol.2022.05.005

Kim, B., Yannatos, I., Blam, K., Wiebe, D., Xie, S. X., McMillan, C. T., Mechanic-Hamilton, D., Wolk, D. A., & Lee, E. B. (2024). Neighborhood disadvantage reduces cognitive reserve independent of neuropathologic change. *Alzheimer's & Dementia*, *20*(4), 2707–2718. https://doi.org/10.1002/alz.13736

Klimecki, O. M., Liebscher, M., Gaubert, M., Hayek, D., Zarucha, A., Dyrba, M., Bartels, C., Buerger, K., Butryn, M., Dechent, P., Dobisch, L., Ewers, M., Fliessbach, K., Freiesleben, S. D., Glanz, W., Hetzer, S., Janowitz, D., Kilimann, I., Kleineidam, L., ... DELCODE study group (2023). Long-term environmental enrichment is associated with better fornix microstructure in older adults. *Frontiers in Aging Neuroscience*, *15*, 1170879. https://doi.org/10.3389/fnagi.2023.1170879

Knoll, K., Rhee, Y., Hamm, J. M., Hammer, K. D. P., Heimbuch, H., Holloway, J., Jurivich, D., Lahr, P., McGrath, B., Parker, K., Robinson-Lane, S., Stover, E., Tomkinson, G. R., & McGrath, R. (2023). The prevalence and trends of instrumental activities of daily living impairments in the United States from 2008-2018. *Journal of Alzheimer's Disease Reports*, 7(1), 271–278. https://doi.org/10.3233/ADR-220107

Li, Z., & Dalaker, J. (2022). Poverty among Americans aged 65 and older. Congressional Research Service. R45791. https://crsreports.congress.gov

Lima, S., Teixeira, L., Esteves, R., Ribeiro, F., Pereira, F., Teixeira, A., & Magalhães, C. (2020). Spirituality and quality of life in older adults: A path analysis model. *BMC Geriatrics*, *20*(1), 259. https://doi.org/10.1186/s12877-020-01646-0

Ma, L., & Gu, D. (2023). The role of marriage in the life satisfaction and mortality association at older ages: age and sex differences. *Aging & Mental Health*, *27*(3), 612–620. https://doi.org/10.1080/13607863.2022.2039097

Maltais, M., Boisvert-Vigneault, K., Rolland, Y., Vellas, B., de Souto Barreto, P., & MAPT/DSA Study Group. (2019). Longitudinal associations of physical activity levels with morphological and functional changes related with aging: The MAPT study. *Experimental Gerontology*, *128*, 110758. https://doi.org/10.1016/j.exger.2019.110758

Manoiu, R., Hammond, N. G., Yamin, S., & Stinchcombe, A. (2023). Religion/spirituality, mental health, and the lifespan: Findings from a representative sample of Canadian adults. *Canadian Journal on Aging*, *42*(1), 115–125. https://doi.org/10.1017/S0714980822000162

Min, S. H., Lee, C., Scroggins, J. K., & Yang, Q. (2023). Transitions in social networks from young-old to old-old stage of life using latent transition analysis. *Journal of Aging and Health*, *36*(1–2), 110–119. https://doi.org/10.1177/08982643231177400

Mostafa, N., Sayed, A., Rashad, O., & Baqal, O. (2023). Malnutrition-related mortality trends in older adults in the United States from 1999 to 2020. *BMC Medicine*, *21*(1), 421. https://doi.org/10.1186/s12916-023-03143-8

National Council on Aging (NCOA). 2023. *The top 10 most common chronic conditions in older adults*. Retrieved November 21, 2023, from https://www.ncoa.org/article/the-top-10-most-common-chronic-conditions-in-older-adults

Nicklett, E. J., Cheng, G. J., & Morris, Z. A. (2023). Predictors of food insecurity among older adults before and during COVID-19 in the United States. *Frontiers in Public Health*, *11*, 1112575. https://doi.org/10.3389/fpubh.2023.1112575

Nyarko-Odoom, A., Lisha, N. E., Yank, V., Kotwal, A., Balogun, S., & Huang, A. J. (2023). Elder mistreatment experienced by older caregiving adults: Results from a national community-based sample. *Journal of General Internal Medicine*, *38*(7), 1709–1716. https://doi.org/10.1007/s11606-022-07981-9

Obaoye, J. O., Dawson, A. Z., Thakkar, M., Williams, J. S., & Egede, L. E. (2023). Understanding the relationship between perceived discrimination and mortality in United States adults. *Aging & Mental Health*, *27*(2), 445–451. https://doi.org/10.1080/13607863.2022.2032593

O'Brien, E., Whitman, K., Buerke, M., Galfalvy, H., & Szanto, K. (2023). Life-satisfaction, engagement, mindfulness, flourishing, and social support: Do they predict depression, suicide ideation, and history of suicide attempt in late life?. *The American Journal of Geriatric Psychiatry*, *31*(6), 415–424. https://doi.org/10.1016/j.jagp.2022.12.192

Pearce, M., Garcia, L., Abbas, A., Strain, T., Schuch, F. B., Golubic, R., Kelly, P., Khan, S., Utukuri, M., Laird, Y., Mok, A., Smith, A., Tainio, M., Brage, S., & Woodcock, J. (2022). Association between physical activity and risk of depression: A systematic review and meta-analysis. *JAMA Psychiatry*, *79*(6), 550–559. https://doi.org/10.1001/jamapsychiatry.2022.0609

Pereira, H. (2022). The impacts of sexual stigma on the mental health of older sexual minority men. *Aging & mental health*, *26*(6), 1281–1286. https://doi.org/10.1080/13607863.2021.1916883

Rochon, P.A. (2023). Drug prescribing for older adults. *Up To Date*. Retrieved November 27, 2023, from https://www.uptodate.com/contents/drug-prescribing-for-older-adults/print

Saxon, S. V., Etten, M. J., & Perkins, E. A. (2022). *Physical change and aging: A guide for the helping professions* (7th ed.). Springer.

Sneed, R. S., & Chan, A. C. Y. (2023). The implications of intergenerational relationships for minority aging: A review of recent literature. *Current Epidemiology Reports*, *10*(1), 44–50. https://doi.org/10.1007/s40471-023-00319-x

Steckenrider, J. (2023). Sexual activity of older adults: let's talk about it. *The Lancet. Healthy longevity*, *4*(3), e96–e97. https://doi.org/10.1016/S2666-7568(23)00003-X

Su, Y., Rao, W., Li, M., Caron, G., D'Arcy, C., & Meng, X. (2023). Prevalence of loneliness and social isolation among older adults during the COVID-19 pandemic: A systematic review and meta-analysis. *International Psychogeriatrics*, *35*(5), 229–241. https://doi.org/10.1017/S1041610222000199

Tamborini, C. R., & Kim, C. (2020). Are you saving for retirement? Racial/ethnic differentials in contributory retirement savings plans. *The Journals of Gerontology. Series B, Psychological Sciences and Social Sciences*, *75*(4), 837–848. https://doi.org/10.1093/geronb/gbz131

Tampi, R. R., Tampi, D. J., & Elson, A. (2022). Substance use disorders in the elderly. *The Psychiatric Clinics of North America*, *45*(4), 707–716. https://doi.org/10.1016/j.psc.2022.07.005

Thompson, D. & King, M.D. (2022). *Income sources of older households: 2017*. U.S. Department of Commerce. U.S. Census Bureau. Retrieved November 8, 2023, from https://www.census.gov/content/dam/Census/library/publications/2022/demo/p70br-177.pdf

Tornstam, L. (2005). *Gerotranscendence: A developmental theory of positive aging*. Springer Publishing Company.

Uomoto, K. E. (2023). Increasing identification and follow-up of older adult depression in primary care. *Journal of Primary Care & Community Health*, *14*, 21501319231152758. https://doi.org/10.1177/21501319231152758

Upenieks, L. (2023). Uncertainty in faith, fear of death? Transitions in religious doubt and death anxiety in later life. *Omega*, *87*(3), 814–837. https://doi.org/10.1177/00302228211029475

U.S. Department of Health and Human Services. (2024). Social determinants of health and older adults. Office of Disease Prevention and Health Promotion. Retrieved March 28, 2025, https://odphp.health.gov/our-work/national-health-initiatives/healthy-aging/social-determinants-health-and-older-adults

U.S. Department of Justice. (2023). Elder Abuse. Special Edition. Office of Justice Department Programs. Retrieved November 28, 2024, from Elder Abuse | Overview | Office of Justice Programs (https://www.ojp.gov/feature/elder-abuse/overview)

Viviani, C. A., Bravo, G., Lavallière, M., Arezes, P. M., Martínez, M., Dianat, I., Bragança, S., & Castellucci, H. I. (2021). Productivity in older versus younger workers: A systematic literature review. *Work*, *68*(3), 577–618. https://doi.org/10.3233/WOR-203396

Walhovd, K. B., Lövden, M., & Fjell, A. M. (2023). Timing of lifespan influences on brain and cognition. *Trends in Cognitive Sciences*, *27*(10), 901–915. https://doi.org/10.1016/j.tics.2023.07.001

Ye, C. J., Kong, L. J., Wang, Y. Y., Dou, C., Zheng, J., Xu, M., Xu, Y., Li, M., Zhao, Z. Y., Lu, J. L., Chen, Y. H., Ning, G., Wang, W. Q., Bi, Y. F., & Wang, T. G. (2023). Mendelian randomization evidence for the causal effects of socio-economic inequality on human longevity among Europeans. *Nature Human Behaviour*, 7(8), 1357–1370. https://doi.org/10.1038/s41562-023-01646-1

Yesavage, J. A., Brink, T. L., Rose, T. L., Lum, O., Huang, V., Adey, M., & Leirer, V. O. (1982). Development and validation of a geriatric depression screening scale: A preliminary report. *Journal of Psychiatric Research*, *17*(1), 37–49.

Zhao, S., Li, Y., Shi, Y., & Li, X. (2023). Cognitive aging: How the brain ages?. *Advances in Experimental Medicine and Biology*, *1419*, 9–21. https://doi.org/10.1007/978-981-99-1627-6_2

Zhou, Y., Sun, Y., Pan, Y., Dai, Y., Xiao, Y., & Yu, Y. (2025). Prevalence of successful aging in older adults: A systematic review and meta-analysis. *Archives of Gerontology and Geriatrics*, *128*, 105604. https://doi.org/10.1016/j.archger.2024.105604

UNIT V
Prevention of Mental Disorders

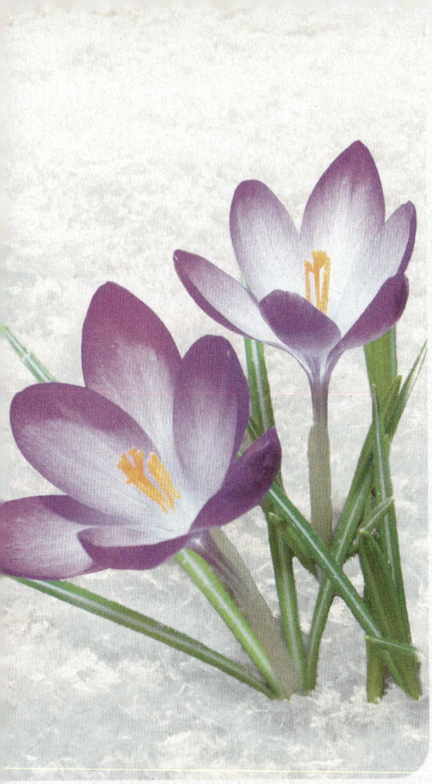

19
Stress and Mental Health

Kelley McGuire

KEYCONCEPTS

- appraisal
- adaptation
- allostatic load
- coping
- stress

LEARNING OBJECTIVES

After studying this chapter, you will be able to:

1. Discuss the concept of stress as it relates to mental health and mental illness.
2. Differentiate acute stress from chronic stress.
3. Discuss the factors that lead to allostatic load.
4. Discuss psychosocial factors that influence the experience of stress.
5. Discuss the variety of stress responses experienced by individuals.
6. Explain the role of coping and adaptation in maintaining and promoting mental health.
7. Apply clinical judgment skills to nursing care planning for people experiencing stress.

KEY TERMS

• acute stress • allostasis • chronic stress • diathesis • emotion-focused coping • emotions • general adaptation syndrome • homeostasis • problem-focused coping • reappraisal • social functioning • social network • social support • stress response • Transactional Stress Model

INTRODUCTION

Stress is a natural and complex concept in health and nursing. The term stress is used to describe the process of response to any stimuli. Stress is associated with the development or exacerbation of symptoms of mental illness. For example, a stressful event may precipitate a psychosis. Caregiver stress is a term used to describe the undesirable outcomes of providing direct care to a family member or friend who experiences a significant health event (Suntai et al., 2021). This stress occurs as the caregiver observes their family member or loved one receive undesirable diagnoses and be subjected to unpleasant treatments, and then sees their own role in the provision of care and responsibilities (Litzelman et al., 2023). Family caregivers can develop depression as they continually monitor their family member, cope with illness-related behaviors, and often witness deterioration of their partner (Litzelman et al., 2023).

Stress is approached from several overlapping theoretical perspectives—physiologic, psychological, and social. Consequently, there are many definitions of stress depending upon the theoretical perspective. This chapter provides an overview of the major evidence-based theories of stress and describes the applicability of the models in the practice of nursing.

BIOLOGIC PERSPECTIVES OF STRESS

Physiologic responses to stress are automatic and differ based on the event, duration, and intensity. During severe stress, some people draw on resources that they never realized they had and grow from those experiences. However, early childhood stress and trauma, unresolved stress, or chronic stress can have negative mental and physical health consequences.

Homeostasis versus Allostasis

The concept of **homeostasis**, which is the body's tendency to resist physiologic change and hold bodily functions relatively consistent, well-coordinated, and usually stable, was introduced by Walter Cannon in the 1930s. The body's internal equilibrium is regulated by physiologic processes such as blood glucose, pH, and oxygen; set points (usual reference ranges of physiologic parameters) are maintained (Cannon, 1932).

Allostasis is a term used to describe how the body adapts to maintain physiologic stability. Allostasis is a dynamic regulatory process involving functions of the autonomic nervous system, the hypothalamic–pituitary–adrenal (HPA) axis, and the cardiovascular, metabolic, and immune systems and how they respond to internal and external stimuli (McEwen, 2019).

Acute Stress

Acute stress, an intense biopsychosocial reaction to a threatening event, is time limited (usually less than a month) but can occur repeatedly. It is associated with the "fight-or-flight" response. When the brain (amygdala and hippocampus) interprets a stressor, the brain signals the hypothalamus and autonomic nervous system to secrete adrenaline, cortisol, and epinephrine to aid the body in adapting and maintaining optimal functioning (Chu et al., 2024). These hormones activate the sympathetic nervous system and physiologic stability is challenged. A "fight-or-flight" response occurs when the heart rate, blood pressure, and blood sugar increase. Energy is mobilized for survival. As the sympathetic system is activated, the parasympathetic nervous system is muted (Table 19.1). When the threat resolves the body returns to a state of homeostasis. When acute stressors occur frequently, or when a stressor persists, chronic stress occurs. Paradoxically, the same systems that are protective in acute stress can damage the body when activated by chronic stress. The benefits of the increase in circulating cortisol to the human body are initially adaptive, but if it continues, it can be damaging to both mental health (e.g., depression) and physical health (e.g., immune, cardiovascular, and metabolic issues) (Chu et al., 2024).

Chronic Stress

Chronic stress is an ongoing physiologic reaction to events resulting in "wear and tear" on the body and negatively impacts health and well-being. The adaptive physiologic changes that occur during acute stress become maladaptive when prolonged and contribute to the risk for illness. The relationship between chronic stress and

TABLE 19.1 FIGHT AND FLIGHT: PHYSIOLOGIC CHANGES

Sympathetic Nervous System Effect	Purpose	Parasympathetic Nervous System Conservation of Energy
Increased serum glucose	Increased energy	Decreased sexual and sex hormone activity
Increased cardiac output and blood pressure (increase in renin and angiotensin)	Increased blood flow	Decreased growth, repair, and maturation
Increased oxygen tension and hematocrit	Increased supply of oxygen in blood	Decreased digestion, assimilation, and whole food distribution
Other Physiologic Changes		
Effect	**Purpose**	
Increased immune responses	Reduced risk of infections	
Heightened vigilance in the brain	Increased decision-making attention and memory	
Hyperactivation of the hemostatic and coagulation system	Prevention of excessive bleeding from wounds	

Adapted from Hussain, L. S., Reddy, V., & Maani, C. V. (2023). Physiology, Noradrenergic Synapse. In StatPearls. StatPearls Publishing. https://www.ncbi.nlm.nih.gov/books/NBK540977 and Chu, B., Marwaha, K., Sanvictores, T., Awosika, A. O., & Ayers, D. (2024). Physiology, stress reaction. In StatPearls. StatPearls Publishing. https://www.ncbi.nlm.nih.gov/books/NBK541120/

BOX 19.1

Research for Evidence-Based Practice: Allostatic Load

Barry, L. E., O'Neill, S., Heaney, L. G., & O'Neill, C. (2021). Stress-related health depreciation: using allostatic load to predict self-rated health. Social Science & Medicine, 283, *114170. https://doi.org/10.1016/j.socscimed.2021.114170*

THE QUESTION: Is self-rated health (SRH) predicted by baseline allostatic load (AL)?

METHODS: A retrospective, secondary data analysis of 7,712 adults from the United Kingdom (UK) who participated in the UK Household Longitudinal Survey (Understanding Society survey) was conducted. AL index was composed of 12 physiologic markers and biomarkers. SRH was measured using the Short Form-12 (SF-12), which provides a score for physical health (PCS) and one for mental health (MCS). The authors also generated a combined variable to represent health-related quality of life.

FINDINGS: Participants with better baseline physical health and health-related quality of life demonstrated lower AL. This study confirms that higher AL may predict lower SRH.

IMPLICATIONS FOR NURSING: Indices and measures such as baseline AL may serve as important tools to motivate health-related behavior change. AL may be a valuable tool to predict long-term health.

illness was identified many years ago with the introduction of the general adaptation syndrome (GAS).

General Adaptation Syndrome

Hans Seyle, who is credited with initiation of the study of stress, defined stress as a nonspecific response to an irritant, a perceived danger, or a life threat. He called stress evoked by positive emotions or events *eustress* and stress evoked by negative feelings and events *distress* (Selye, 1973). He showed that corticosteroid secretion from the pituitary gland increased during stress and contributed to development of illnesses. Seyle described this process as **general adaptation syndrome (GAS)** (Selye, 1956, 1974). This early work set the stage for our understanding of the role of the HPA in chronic stress.

When the HPA axis is activated under conditions of stress, the hypothalamus secretes corticotropin-releasing hormone, causing the pituitary gland to increase secretion of adrenocorticotropic hormone (corticotropin), simultaneously stimulating adrenocortical secretion of cortisol. Over time, excessive exposure to cortisol contributes to the dysregulation of the autonomic nervous system.

Allostatic Load

Allostatic load (AL) is a term used to describe the wear and tear on an individual's body and brain resulting from chronic stress. The regulatory systems in our body are designed to be fluid and respond to critical, life-threatening stressors (fight-or-flight) followed by a longer period of relaxation (rest-and-digest); this is allostasis, the healthy equilibrium between stress response and relaxation. The cumulative changes of the biologic regulatory systems (cardiovascular, metabolic, and immune) are indicated by atypical laboratory values and may increase the risk of disease and illness. As wear and tear on the brain and body occurs, there is a corresponding increase in the AL. When an individual experiences AL, their body will respond in one of a few ways: failure to adapt, prolonged heightened stress response (regulatory systems remain activated and work in overdrive), or blunted response (regulatory systems inadequately respond) (Doan, 2021). The greater the AL, the greater the state of chronic stress, consequently leading to an increase in negative health outcomes (Chu et al., 2024; Guidi et al., 2021). See Box 19.1.

The worldwide response to the COVID-19 pandemic and the stress-related outcomes demonstrate AL. Seemingly countless stressors presented in near constant fashion, including countries' closing their borders to international travel; closing parks, beaches, and other public respite spaces; school closings; mask mandates; work-from-home orders; loss of employment and the financial repercussions that followed; and the immense and overwhelming grief that we collectively felt resulting from both the death of, and the loss of contact with loved ones, friends, and neighbors. The near-constant barrage of stressors experienced during the pandemic caused regulatory systems to repeatedly activate, leading to significant wear and tear on the body.

KEYCONCEPT Allostatic load is the consequence of the wear and tear on the body and brain and leads to ill health.

Consequences of Chronic Stress

In chronic stress, the immune system is suppressed. Cortisol is primarily immunosuppressive and contributes to reduction in lymphocyte numbers and function (primarily T-lymphocyte and monocyte subsets) and natural killer activities. The immune cells have receptors for cortisol and catecholamines that can bind with lymphatic cells and suppress the immune system. The continuous sustained activation of the sympathetic nervous system; HPA axis; cardiovascular, metabolic, and immune systems contribute to a hormonal overload, leading to impairment in memory, immunity, cardiovascular, and metabolic function (Chu et al., 2024).

Health disparities found in lower socioeconomic groups, racial and ethnic underrepresented groups, and older adults may be partly explained by the chronic stress they tend to experience. These groups have been found to have elevated AL (Cuevas et al., 2024). AL has been found to differ by race, with Black Americans displaying greater levels than White Americans (Zare et al., 2024). Further, in another study of young adults in the United States, Black women have higher AL scores than either Black men or White women. In fact, Black women were the only group of women who were disadvantaged compared to their male counterparts (Richardson et al., 2021).

Over time, chronic stress compromises health and increases susceptibility to illnesses. For example, the long-term outcomes of AL associated with the COVID-19 pandemic are now beginning to surface and include increased rates of mental health diagnoses such as anxiety and depression (Chen et al., 2025; World Health Organization, 2022). Elevation of white blood cell counts, and lower counts of T, B, and natural killer cells are found in those who face academic examinations, job strain, caregiving for a family member experiencing dementia, marital conflict, and daily stress (Gallagher et al., 2024; O'Toole et al., 2025). Altered parameters of immune function are present in those with negative moods (chronic hostility, depression, anxiety), social isolation, and marital disagreement (Ng et al., 2024). Antibody titers to herpes simplex viruses are also elevated in stressed populations (Boafo et al., 2023). If the stress is long term, the immune alteration continues (Chu et al., 2024). The relationship between stress and mental illness will be further discussed in the next section.

Chronic Stress and Mental Illness

When stress is associated with the development or exacerbation of a mental illness, the diathesis–stress model can be applied. A **diathesis** is a genetic predisposition that increases susceptibility of developing a disorder. This model describes how stress can trigger the development or exacerbation of an illness (Thomas-Odenthal et al., 2024). Exposure to childhood trauma can lead to negative long-term health consequences on mental and physical health throughout life (American Society for the Positive Care of Children, 2021); for example, consider an individual whose biologic parent had a long history of depression (indicating a genetic predisposition to mental disorders for the individual) and who was assaulted as they were leaving work, sustaining multiple injuries. The individual's first manic episode occurred within 2 months (see Chapter 22).

Stress reduction leads to positive mental health. Conversely, many patients attribute their first illness episode to a stressful event such as an assault, rape, or family tragedy.

PSYCHOSOCIAL PERSPECTIVES OF STRESS

The **Transactional Stress Model** describes the psychological experience of stress (Fig. 19.1) (Lazarus & Folkman, 1984). The external environment includes physical aspects such as air quality, cleanliness of food and water, temperature, and noise and social aspects such as living arrangements and personal contacts.

> **KEYCONCEPT Stress** is a process arising from real or perceived internal or external environmental demands that are appraised as threatening or benign (Lazarus & Folkman, 1984).

Appraisal

Appraisal is the individual perception of an event as either a threat or a challenge. A situation may be perceived as threatening to one person but not to another (Box 19.2). The more important or meaningful the event, the more vulnerable the person is to stress. For example, chest pain is threatening not only because of the immediate pain and incapacitation but also because the pain may mean a heart attack is occurring. The individual is afraid that they may not have the physiologic resources to survive the attack.

> **KEYCONCEPT Appraisal** is the process where potentially stressful events are evaluated for meaning and significance to individual well-being (Lazarus & Folkman, 1984).

Appraisal is a complex process that includes many aspects, namely the determination of importance or significance of the event and an assessment of the coping resources available (Rolin et al., 2021).

BOX 19.2

Clinical Judgment Vignette: Stress Responses to an Examination

Two students are preparing for the same examination. Susan is genuinely interested in the subject, prepares by studying throughout the semester, and reviews the content 2 days before test day. The night before the examination, she goes to bed early, gets a good night's sleep, and wakes refreshed but is slightly nervous about the test. She wants to do well and expects a difficult test but knows that she can retake it later if she does poorly.

In contrast, Joanne is not interested in the subject matter and does not study throughout the semester. She "crams" 2 days before the test date and does an "all-nighter" the night before. This is the last time that Joanne can take the examination, but she believes that she will pass because she has already taken it twice and is familiar with the questions. If she does not pass, she will not be able to return to school. On entering the room, Joanne is physically tired and somewhat fearful of not passing the test. As she looks at the test, she instantly realizes that it is not the examination she expected. The questions are new. She begins hyperventilating and tremoring. After yelling obscenities at the teacher, she storms out of the room. She is very distressed and describes herself as "being in a panic."

What Do You Think?

1. How are the students' experiences different? Are there any similarities?
2. What nursing interventions would be helpful to Joanne the next time she is faced with a similar situation?

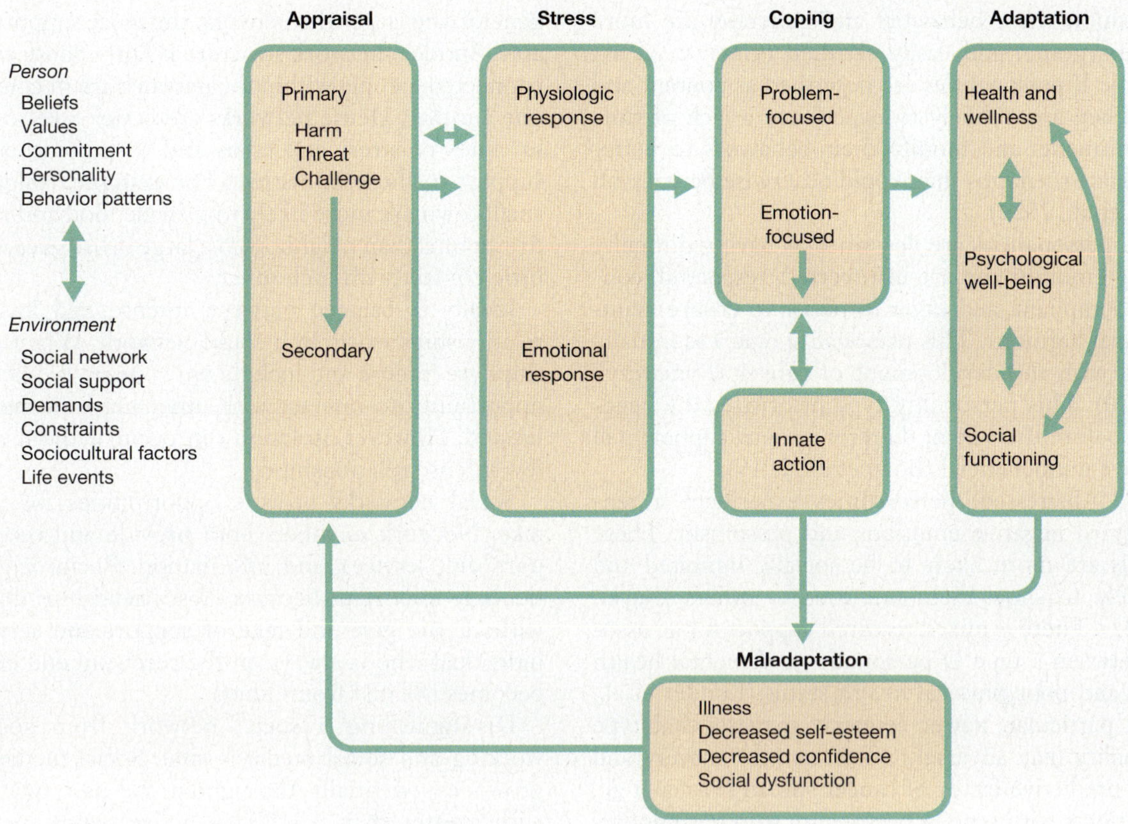

FIGURE 19.1 The Transactional Stress Model.

The appraisal process has two levels: primary and secondary. In a primary appraisal, an individual evaluates the events occurring in their life as a threat, harm, or challenge. During primary appraisal of an event, the person determines whether (1) the event is relevant, (2) the event is consistent with their values and beliefs, and (3) a personal commitment is present. In the clinical judgment vignette (Box 19.2), Susan's commitment to the goal of doing well on the test was consistent with her valuing the content, which in turn motivated her to study regularly and prepare carefully for the examination. She believed that the test would be difficult. Joanne had a commitment to pass the test but did not value the content. Unlike Susan, Joanne believed that the test would be relatively easy because she expected the questions to be the same as those on the previous examination.

In a secondary appraisal, the person determines if they possess the necessary coping mechanisms to overcome the event. In the example, Susan was nervous but took the test. Joanne's secondary appraisal of the test-taking situation began with the realization that she might not pass the test because the questions were different. She acted impulsively by blaming the teacher for giving a different examination and storming out of the room. She clearly did not cope effectively with a difficult situation.

Values and Goals

Cultural, ethnic, family, and religious values shape the significance and importance of the event. For example, one person may value a high-paying salary, and another may value the freedom to move around without the boundaries of material things.

If a goal (such as achieving a promotion) is important, an individual is more likely to do what it takes to reach the goal. The more important the goal or the more difficult the goal is to obtain, the greater the likelihood of stress. For example, students who earn mostly or all As often feel more stress about examinations than do students who earn Bs and Cs because the higher grade is more difficult to obtain.

Personality Types

Personality influences the appraisal process and the ability to cope with stress. The association of personality types to health or illness status has been studied for more than 50 years (Friedman & Rosenman, 1974). There are four general personality types. Type A personality is often characterized as high achieving and competitive as well as impatient and hostile. Owing to these characteristics, individuals with type A personality may also experience higher rates of burnout and lower job satisfaction (Lu et al., 2022). In contrast, type B personalities do not exhibit these behaviors and generally are more relaxed, easygoing, and easily satisfied (Garavan et al., 2022). Type B personalities are described as content and relaxed. They are unlikely to experience a lack of time for commitments and modify their behaviors to better accommodate scenarios that would otherwise be stressful (Garavan et al., 2022).

Type C personalities are described as having difficulty expressing emotion and are introverted, respectful, conforming, compliant, and eager to please to ensure maintained social harmony. This personality type was initially associated with the development of cancer (Rymarczyk et al., 2020). This personality type prioritizes the needs of others before their own; therefore, social support will likely prove nonbeneficial (Bozo et al., 2019).

Type D (distressed) personalities experience a tendency toward negative emotions and pessimism. These individuals are more likely to be socially inhibited and are unlikely to show their emotions to others (Raykh et al., 2022). There is mixed research support for an association between a type D personality and mental health disorders and poor physical health status (Lodder et al., 2021); in particular, newer research suggests that type D personality may adversely affect cancer recovery and may be a predictive factor of cancer spread (Pasha et al., 2022). Patients with type D personality who have undergone coronary artery bypass grafting (CABG) may also have poorer outcomes than their non–type D personality counterparts. Raykh et al. (2022) identified that patients with type D personality were more likely to experience negative outcomes 5 years after a CABG surgery (Raykh et al., 2022).

Social Networks

A **social network** consists of linkages among a defined set of people with whom an individual has personal contact. Social networks can serve as coping mechanisms for valuable support during stressful experiences, particularly if the relationships are strong and a sense of sufficient emotional support is present (Kneavel, 2021). Kneavel (2021) suggests that the quality of social support may be more instrumental than the quantity of social support in predicting stress.

Social networks vary in size and structure based largely on the degree of closeness between the members. The first level is considered the support groups. This consists of individuals close to the person who could be called upon for aid and assistance. Next is considered the sympathy group. This level consists of more people than the support group and is composed of relatives and friends. Finally, the outermost level is described as the social group. This group consists of members of the community, coworkers, and other acquaintances (Rollings et al., 2023).

Each person's social network is slightly different. Multiple contacts allow several networks to interact. In general, the larger the network, the more support is available. An ideal network structure is fairly dense and interconnected; people within the network are in contact with one another. Dense networks are better able to respond in times of stress and crisis and to provide emotional support to those in distress. For example, residents of a small town are more likely to provide food and shelter to fire victims than neighbors in a large urban area who have little contact with each other.

Ideally, a balance between intense and less intense relationships exists in a social network. When relationships are intense and include only one or two people, the opportunity to interact with other network members is limited. However, isolation can occur without at least a few intense relationships.

Social networks provide opportunities for give and take. Network members both provide and receive support, aid, services, and information. Reciprocity is particularly important because most friendships do not last without the give and take of support and services. An individual who is always on the receiving end eventually becomes isolated from others.

Distinguishing a social network from social networking and social media is vital. Social media use has grown exponentially throughout the past two decades, with greater than 4.3 billion active people per month on Facebook and Instagram combined (Herriman et al., 2023). Evidence supports that although people using social media may feel a temporary boost in self-esteem, the ability of people to digitally enhance and modify their content before posting creates impractical ideals for content that viewers may aspire to. Recent findings reveal that social media may cause decreased life satisfaction, body image concerns, dissatisfaction with relationships, and decreased well-being (Herriman et al., 2023).

Social Support

One of the important functions of the social network is to provide **social support**. Social support is particularly important in women, who frequently manage stress via "tend-and-befriend," where stress is reduced when a person perceives that they have high-quality relationships and feels sufficiently supported (Kneavel, 2021). Not all interpersonal interactions within a network are supportive. An individual can have a large, complex social network but little social support. Some life events, such as marriage, divorce, and bereavement, actually change the level of social support by adding to or subtracting from an individual's social network.

Social support serves three functions:

1. Emotional support contributes to an individual's feelings of being cared for or loved.
2. Tangible support provides an individual with additional resources.

TABLE 19.2 EXAMPLES OF FUNCTIONS OF SOCIAL SUPPORT

Function	Example
Emotional support	Attachment, reassurance, being able to rely on and confide in a person
Tangible support	Direct aid such as loans or gifts, services such as taking care of someone who is ill, doing a job or chore
Informational support	Providing information or advice, giving feedback about how a person is doing

Reprinted with permission from Springer Schaefer, C., Coyne, J. C., & Lazarus, R. S. (1981). The health-related functions of social support. *Journal of Behavioral Medicine*, *4*(4), 381–406. Copyright © 1981 Springer Nature.

3. Informational support helps an individual view situation in a new light (Table 19.2).

Social support enhances health outcomes and reduces mortality by helping members make needed behavior changes and buffering stressful life events. Perceived social support plays a key role in the evaluation of stressors and may have a positive impact on the coping strategies employed to manage or overcome the stress (Dai et al., 2021). In a supportive social environment, members feel helped, valued, and in personal control.

Cultural Factors and Ethnic Identity

Cultural expectations and role strain serve as both demands and constraints in the experience of stress. If an individual violates cultural group values to meet role expectations, stress occurs; for example, a person may stay in an abusive relationship to avoid the stress of violating a cultural norm that values lifelong marriage, no matter what the circumstances. The potential guilt associated with norm violation and the anticipated isolation from being ostracized seem worse than the physical and psychological pain caused by the abusive situation. Members of underrepresented groups may experience a phenomenon termed minority stress. This is described as the presence of chronic stress resulting from societal prejudice and stigma (Capriotti et al., 2022) and may apply to a broad range of underrepresented groups, including but not limited to racial, ethnic, and sexual and gender underrepresented groups (Capriotti et al., 2022; Hughes et al., 2022). Minority stress is driven by exposure to unique internal and external stimuli, including discrimination, internalized stigma, and negative perceptions of health and social services (Carden et al., 2022). Minority stress may increase the AL, increasing the future risk for negative health consequences (Capriotti et al., 2022; Carden et al., 2022). Social support and ethnic identification may represent protective buffers against negative outcomes of discrimination (Carden et al., 2022). Ethnic identity refers to the sense of belonging and community that exists among individuals of an ethnic group. A strong sense of ethnic identity has been linked to protective functions of stress coping. This concept suggests that when members of an underrepresented group concentrate their attention on the positive attributes of the group following a stressful encounter, it can lead to an improved sense of well-being (Oh et al., 2023).

Employment Factors

Employment is another highly valued cultural norm and provides social, psychological, and financial benefits. In all cultures, work is assigned significance beyond economic compensation. It is often the central focus of adulthood and, for many, a source of personal identity. Even if employment brings little real happiness, being employed implies financial needs are being met. Work offers status, regulates life activities, enables association with others, and provides a meaningful life experience. Although work is demanding, unemployment can be equally or more stressful because of the associated isolation, loss of social status, and potential financial strains.

Life Events

In 1967, Holmes and Rahe (1967) presented a psychosocial view of illness by pointing out the complex relationship between life changes and the development of illnesses. They hypothesized that people become ill after they experience major life events, such as marriage, divorce, and bereavement. The more frequent the changes, the greater the possibility of becoming sick. The investigators cited the events that they believed partially accounted for the onset of illnesses and began testing whether these life changes were actual precursors to illness. It soon became clear that not all events have the same effects. For example, the death of a spouse or partner is usually much more devastating and stressful than a change in residence. From their research, the investigators were able to assign relative weights to various life events according to the degree of associated stress. Rahe (1994) devised the Recent Life Changes Questionnaire (Table 19.3) to evaluate the frequency and significance of life-changing events. Numerous research studies subsequently demonstrated the relationship between a recent life change and the severity of near-future illness, illness progression, or the development of a new illness (Mwangwa et al., 2023; Rahe, 1994; Rahe et al., 2002). In response to the COVID-19 pandemic, people in all industries and representing all age distributions experienced a barrage of life changes. Studies indicate that physical and mental health have been negatively affected as a result (World Health Organization, 2022).

TABLE 19.3 RECENT LIFE CHANGES QUESTIONNAIRE

Life Changes	LCU Values[a]
Family	
Death of spouse	105
Marital separation	65
Death of close family member	65
Divorce	62
Pregnancy	60
Change in health of family member	52
Marriage	50
Gain of new family member	50
Marital reconciliation	42
Spouse begins or stops work	37
Adult child leaves home	29
In-law trouble	29
Change in number of family get-togethers	26
Personal	
Incarceration	56
Sexual difficulties	49
Death of a close friend	46
Personal injury or illness	42
Change in living conditions	39
Outstanding personal achievement	33
Change in residence	33
Minor violations of the law	32
Begin or end school	32
Change in sleeping habits	31
Revision of personal habits	31
Change in eating habits	29
Change in religious/spiritual-related activities	29
Vacation	29
Change in school	28
Change in recreation	28
Major holiday	26
Work	
Fired at work	64
Retirement from work	49
Trouble with boss	39
Business readjustment	38
Change to different line of work	38
Change in work responsibilities	33
Change in work hours or conditions	30
Financial	
Foreclosure of mortgage or loan	57
Change in financial state	43
Mortgage (e.g., home, car)	39
Mortgage or loan less than $20,000 (e.g., stereo)	26

[a]LCU, life-change unit. The number of LCUs reflects the average degree or intensity of the life change.
Adapted with permission from Rahe, R.J. (2000). *Recent Life Changes Questionnaire (RLCQ)*.

RESPONSES TO STRESS

A stress response includes simultaneous physiologic and emotional responses. The physiologic stress responses were previously discussed. Emotional responses to stress depend on the significance of the event experience. It is now known that people experience stress differently depending on their gender. Whereas men are more likely to respond to stress with a fight-or-flight response, women have less aggressive responses; they "tend and befriend" (Kneavel, 2021).

Emotional Responses

Emotions (psychophysiologic reactions that define an individual's mood) are usually ones of excitement or distress marked by strong feelings and usually accompanied by an impulse toward a definite action. If the emotions are intense, a disturbance in intellectual functions occurs. When the situation is viewed as a challenge, emotions are more likely to be positive. If the event is evaluated as threatening or harmful, negative emotions are elicited. Emotions can be categorized as follows:

- *Negative emotions* occur when there is a threat to, delay in, or thwarting of a goal or a conflict between goals: anger, fright, anxiety, guilt, shame, sadness, envy, jealousy, and disgust.
- *Positive emotions* occur when there is movement toward or attainment of a goal: happiness, pride, relief, and love.
- *Borderline emotions* are somewhat ambiguous: hope, compassion, empathy, sympathy, and contentment.
- *Nonemotions* describe emotional reactions that are too ambiguous to fit into any of the preceding categories: confidence, awe, confusion, and excitement (Lazarus, 2006).

Emotions are expressed as themes that summarize the dangers or benefits of each stressful situation. For instance, physical danger provokes fear; a loss leads to feelings of sadness (Table 19.4). Emotions have their

TABLE 19.4 CORE RELATIONAL THEMES FOR EACH EMOTION

Emotion	Relational Theme
Anger	A demeaning offense against me and mine
Anxiety	Facing an uncertain, existential threat
Compassion	Being moved by another's suffering and wanting to help
Disgust	Taking in or being too close to an indigestible object or idea (metaphorically speaking)
Envy	Wanting what someone else has
Fright	Facing an immediate, concrete, and overwhelming physical danger
Guilt	Having transgressed a moral imperative
Happiness	Making reasonable progress toward the realization of a goal
Hope	Fearing the worst but yearning for better
Jealousy	Resenting a third party for the loss of or a threat to another's affection
Love	Desiring or participating in affection, usually but not necessarily reciprocated
Pride	Enhancement of one's ego identity by taking credit for a valued object or achievement, either our own or that of someone or a group with whom we identify
Relief	A distressing goal/incongruent condition that has changed for the better or gone away
Shame	Having failed to live up to an ego ideal
Sadness	Having experienced an irrevocable loss

Adapted with permission from Oxford University Press from Lazarus, R. S. (1991). *Emotion and adaptation* (p. 122). Oxford University Press.

own innate responses that are automatic and unique; for example, anger may automatically provoke tremors in one person but both tremors and perspiration in another. Emotions often provoke impulsive behavior. For example, the first impulse of a young musician facing his first performance at Carnegie Hall who experiences stage fright is to run home. As he resists this impulse, he begins coping with his fears in order to perform.

COPING

Coping is a deliberate, planned, and psychological effort to manage stressful demands.

The coping process may inhibit or override the innate urge to act. Positive coping leads to adaptation, which is characterized by a balance between health and illness, a sense of well-being, and maximum social functioning. When a person does not cope well, maladaptations occur that can shift the balance toward illness, a diminished self-concept, and deterioration in social functioning.

KEYCONCEPT Coping is a deliberate, planned, and psychological effort to manage stressful demands.

There are two types of coping. In **problem-focused coping**, the person addresses the source of stress and solves the issue (eliminating it or changing its effects). In **emotion-focused coping**, the person reduces the stress by reinterpreting the situation to change its meaning (Boxes 19.3 and 19.4).

Different coping strategies will be needed for different situations. Over time, strategies become automatic and develop into patterns for each person. Some situations require a combination of strategies and activities. Ideally, a stressful situation is matched with the needed resources as the events are unfolding. Social support can be critical in helping people cope with difficult situations. Successful coping with life stresses is linked to quality of life and physical and mental health (Tracy et al., 2022).

As a part of the coping process, reappraisal is important because of the changing nature of the stressful situation. **Reappraisal**, which is the same as appraisal except that it happens after coping strategies are implemented, provides feedback about the outcomes and allows for continual adjustment and actions to new information.

BOX 19.3

Ways of Coping: Examples of Problem-Focused Versus Emotion-Focused Coping

PROBLEM-FOCUSED COPING

- When noise from the television interrupts a student's studying and causes the student to be stressed, the student turns off the television and eliminates the noise.
- An individual who experienced intimate partner violence is finally able to leave their partner because they realize that the abuse will not stop even though their partner promises never to hit them again.

EMOTION-FOCUSED COPING

- An individual is adamantly opposed to visiting their partner's relatives because the relatives keep dogs in their house. Even though the dogs are well cared for, their presence in the relative's home violates the individual's need for an orderly, clean house and causes the individual sufficient stress that they cope by refusing to visit. This becomes a source of conflict between the partners. One holiday, the individual is given a puppy and immediately becomes attached to the dog, who soon becomes a valued family member. This individual then begins to view their partner's relatives more positively and willingly visits their house more often.
- A caregiver is afraid that their adolescent has been in an accident because the teen did not come home after a party. Then, the individual remembers that they had given the teen permission to stay at a friend's house, and they immediately feel better.

BOX 19.4

Research for Evidence-Based Practice: Adaptive Coping

Tracy, E. L., Chin, B., Lehrer, H. M., Carroll, L. W., Buysse, D. J., & Hall, M. H. (2022). Coping strategies moderate the effect of perceived stress on sleep and health in older adults during the COVID-19 pandemic. Stress and Health, *38(4), 708–721. https://doi.org/10.1002/smi.3124*

THE QUESTION: How did perceived stress and coping impact older adult health outcomes—in particular, physical, mental, and sleep health—during the COVID-19 pandemic?

METHODS: A quantitative, descriptive study was conducted using retrospective and cross-sectional data. Data from a previous study on health outcomes, stress, and coping in order adults who had worked night-shifts was used as a baseline datapoint. The participants were contacted to participate in a follow-up study using the same variables after the onset of the pandemic. The sample included complete data from 115 older adults (58.3% women, mean age = 68.62 years). Data collection measures included: Perceived Stress Scale, Brief COPE, Pittsburgh Sleep Quality Index, Center for Epidemiologic Studies Depression Scale, and the RAND-12 Health Status Inventory.

FINDINGS: Stress experienced during the pandemic was associated with poorer sleep, decreased mental health, and increased depressive symptoms. Coping strategies were found to impact measures of health during the pandemic; however, they did not modify the relationship between perceived stress and sleep or mental health.

IMPLICATIONS FOR NURSING: Older adults most frequently applied problem-focused, meaning-focused social support, and acceptance as coping strategies during the pandemic. Perceived stress is a predictor of mental health outcomes. Stress management and stress reduction strategies may be beneficial for older adults.

ADAPTATION

Adaptation can be conceptualized as an individual's capacity to survive and flourish (Lazarus, 2006). Adaptation or lack of it affects three key areas: health, psychological well-being, and social functioning. A period of stress may compromise any or all of these areas. If an individual copes successfully with stress, they return to a previous level of adaptation. Successful coping results in an improvement in health, well-being, and social functioning. Unfortunately, coping strategies will not always be successful and maladaptation occurs.

> **KEYCONCEPT Adaptation** is an individual's capacity to survive and flourish. Adaptation affects three important areas: health, psychological well-being, and social functioning.

It is impossible to separate completely the adaptation areas of health, well-being, and social functioning. A maladaptation in any one area can negatively affect the others. For instance, the appearance of psychiatric symptoms can cause issues in performance in the work environment that, in turn, elicit a negative self-concept. Although each area will be discussed separately, the reader should realize that when one area is affected, most likely all three areas are affected.

Healthy Coping

Health can be negatively affected by stress when coping is ineffective, and the damaging condition or situation is not resolved or the emotional distress is not regulated. Examples of ineffective coping include using emotion-focused coping when a problem-focused approach is appropriate, such as if an individual reinterprets an abusive situation as their fault instead of getting help to remove themselves from the environment. In addition, if a coping strategy violates cultural norms and lifestyle, stress is often exaggerated. Some coping strategies actually increase the risk for mortality and morbidity, such as the excessive use of alcohol, drugs, or tobacco. Many people use overeating, smoking, or alcohol consumption to reduce stress. They may feel better temporarily but are actually increasing their risk for illness. For people whose behaviors exacerbate their illnesses, learning new behaviors becomes important. Healthy coping strategies such as exercising and obtaining adequate sleep and nutrition contribute to stress reduction and the promotion of long-term health.

Psychological Well-Being

An ideal outcome to a stress response is feeling good about how stress is managed. Outcome satisfaction for one person does not necessarily represent outcome satisfaction for another. For example, suppose that two students receive the same passing score on an examination. One may feel a sense of relief, but the other may feel anxious because they appraise the score as too low. Understanding an individual's emotional response to an outcome is essential to analyzing its personal meaning. People who consistently have positive outcomes from stressful experiences are more likely to have positive self-esteem and self-confidence. Unsatisfactory outcomes from stressful experiences are associated with negative mood states, such as depression, anger, or guilt, leading to decreased self-esteem and feelings of helplessness. Likewise, if the situation was appraised as challenging rather than harmful or threatening, increased self-confidence and a sense of well-being are likely to follow. If the situation was accurately appraised as harmful or threatening but viewed as manageable, the outcome may also be positive.

and generate solutions that address the priority hypotheses first. For example, if the patient reports stress-related deficits in sleep, the nurse should generate a solution targeting improved sleep first.

TAKING ACTION: NURSING INTERVENTIONS

People experiencing stress can often benefit from approaches supporting healthy behaviors. Activities of daily living may be interrupted, and the affected individuals often feel that they have no time for themselves. The person experiencing stress who is usually well groomed and dressed may appear disheveled and unkempt. Generating strategies to reinstate the daily routine of shaving or combing hair can improve the person's outlook on life and ability to cope with the stress.

Stress is commonly manifested in the areas of nutrition and activity. During stressful periods, an individual's eating patterns change. To cope with stress, an individual may either overeat or become anorexic. Both are ineffective coping behaviors and contribute to stress. Educating the patient about the importance of maintaining an adequate diet during the period of stress will highlight its importance. The nurse should also collaborate with the patient to set realistic goals and strategies to improve the behaviors.

Exercise can reduce the emotional and behavioral responses to stress. In addition to the physical benefits of exercise, a regular exercise routine can provide structure to an individual's life, enhance self-confidence, and increase feelings of well-being. People who are stressed are often not receptive to the idea of exercise, particularly if it has not been a part of their routine. Exploring the patient's personal beliefs about the value of activity and the activities that the patient finds most enjoyable will help to determine whether exercise is a reasonable activity for that person. Incorporating exercise and movement that provides joy and happiness first may help the patient establish a routine that includes more physical activity.

The person under stress tends to be tense, nervous, and on edge. Simple relaxation techniques help the person relax and may improve coping skills. If these techniques do not help the patient relax, distraction or guided imagery may be taught to the patient (see Chapter 10). In some instances, spiritually oriented interventions can be used. Referral to a mental health specialist for hypnosis or biofeedback should be considered for patients who have severe stress responses.

Psychosocial Nursing Interventions

Numerous interventions help reduce stress and support coping efforts. All the interventions are best conducted within the framework of a supportive nurse–patient relationship.

Problem Solving

Assisting patients to develop appropriate problem-solving strategies based on personal strengths and previous experiences is important in understanding and coping with stressful situations. Some aspects of any situation cannot be changed, such as a family member's illness or a death of a loved one, but usually there are areas within the patient's control that can be changed. For example, a caregiver cannot reverse the family member's disability but can arrange for short-term respite.

Encouraging patients to examine times when coping has been successful and examine aspects of that situation can help in identifying strengths and strategies for the current issue. For example, a young patient was completely overwhelmed with feelings of inadequacy after the birth of their third child. Further assessment revealed that the patient's parent had helped during the 6 weeks after the other children had been born. The patient's parent was not available for the third birth. First, the nurse acknowledged and validated that having three children could be overwhelming for anyone. The nurse also explained the postpartum hormonal changes that were occurring, validating that the patient's feelings were typical of many birthing parents. Finally, together, the nurse and the patient identified resources in her environment that could support her during the postpartum period.

Family Interventions

People who are coping with stressful situations can often benefit from interventions that facilitate family unit functioning and promote the health and welfare of all family members. To intervene with the total family, the stressed person must agree for the family members to be involved. If the data gathered from the assessment of supportive and unsupportive factors indicate that the family members are not supportive, the nurse should assist the patient to consider expanding their social network. If the family is the major source of support, the nurse should design interventions that support the functioning of the family unit. Parent/guardian education can also be effective in supporting family unit functioning. If family therapy is needed, the nurse should refer the family to an advanced practice specialist.

Evaluation and Treatment Outcomes

The treatment outcomes established in the initial plan of care guide the evaluation. Individual outcomes relate to improved health, well-being, and social function. Family outcomes may be related to improved communication or social support; for instance, caregiver stress is reduced when other members of the family help in the care of the ill member. Social network outcomes focus on modifying the social network to increase support for the individual.

SUMMARY OF KEY POINTS

- Stress affects everyone. Coping with stress can produce positive and negative outcomes. The person can learn and grow from the experience or maladaptation can occur.
- The concept of homeostasis is the body's tendency to resist physiologic change and hold bodily functions relatively consistent, well-coordinated, and usually stable.
- When the brain interprets an event as a threat, physiologic stability is challenged, and a "fight-or-flight" response occurs.
- Allostasis describes a dynamic regulatory process that maintains homeostasis through a process of adaptation. Physiologic stability is achieved when the autonomic nervous system, the hypothalamic–pituitary–adrenal (HPA) axis, and the cardiovascular, metabolic, and immune systems respond to internal and external stimuli. As wear and tear on the brain and body occur, there is a corresponding increase in the number of atypical biologic parameters called the allostatic load (AL). AL is an indication of chronic stress.
- **Stress** is a process arising from real or perceived internal or external environmental demands that are appraised as threatening or benign (Lazarus & Folkman, 1984).
- Stress responses are determined by the interaction with the environment and the individual's cognitive appraisal of the risks and benefits of a situation. Stress responses are simultaneously emotional and physiologic, leading to an innate tendency to act.
- Many personal factors, such as personality patterns, beliefs, values, and commitment to an outcome, interact with environmental demands and constraints that produce an individual–environment relationship.
- Effective coping can be either problem focused or emotion focused. The outcome of successful coping is adaptation through enhanced health, psychological well-being, and social functioning.
- Within the social network, social support can help an individual cope with stress.
- The overall goals in the nursing management of stress are to resolve the stressful person–environment situation, reduce the stress response, and develop positive coping skills.

DEVELOPING CLINICAL JUDGMENT

1. Compare and contrast the concepts of homeostasis and allostasis.
2. Discuss the impact of acute stress versus chronic stress. Why is chronic stress more of a concern than acute stress?
3. Explain why one person may experience the stress of losing a job differently from another.
4. An individual is experiencing being overweight, has hypertension and insomnia, smokes cigarettes, and was recently widowed. The doctor has told them to lose weight and quit smoking. The individual seeks your advice. Would you recommend a problem-focused or an emotion-focused approach?
5. An individual at the local shelter announced to the group that they were returning to their partner because it was partly their fault that they experienced abuse. Is this an example of problem-focused or emotion-focused coping? Justify your answer.

MOVIES, TV, OR STREAMING PROGRAMS

Inside Out: 2015. In this animated Disney film, Riley, an otherwise joy-filled adolescent, experiences the major stressor of her family moving from Minnesota to San Franscisco. At first, she copes with the stressors by focusing on happy memories; however, as the stressors continue to increase and compound, she succumbs to negative emotions such as anger, disgust, and fear. As the story progresses, Riley's emotions (who are each a personified animated character) reveal that it is important to embrace and acknowledge all emotions, including sadness, to achieve successful, healthy coping.

Viewing Points:

1. As Riley began to experience stressors related to the move, what problem-focused and emotion-focused coping strategies did you recognize?
2. What positive coping strategies could Riley have employed when she began to feel overwhelmed?
3. A primary focus in the movie is the importance of recognizing and feeling all of the emotions that people face. Rather than trying to hide sadness and anger, Riley could have allowed herself time to experience and share these emotions with the people she most trusted. In what ways did you observe the relationship between stress and health unfold?
4. Riley experiences signs of depression and ultimately makes the decision to steal money from her mother and run away. How would you help Riley recognize the cues of stress, and what priority interventions would you suggest?

Inside Out 2: 2024. The sequel to 2015's *Inside Out* features Riley 2 years later, when she is transitioning from childhood to adolescence and being challenged by new emotions. The initial five core emotions (joy, fear, sadness, anger, and disgust) are invaded by new confusing and ambiguous emotions: anxiety, envy, ennui (boredom), and embarrassment. (As with the first movie, each emotion is embodied by a different personified animated character.) These new, more complicated emotions take over Riley's life as she enters puberty. The story is about Riley and her two best friends, Bree and Grace; they attend a 3-day hockey camp after Riley discovers Bree and Grace will be attending a different school from Riley next year. Overwhelmed by emotion, Riley ignores her friends as she attempts to fit in with the older high school team members. Her emotions control her behavior, with the personified animated character Anxiety eventually taking control of Riley's behavior.

Viewing Points:

1. At what point in the film did anxiety begin to exert control over Riley?
2. What emotions complicated Riley's ability to cope with the loss of her friends?
3. Is Riley's experience with self-doubt and anxiety typical for an adolescent? Would she benefit from counseling? Explain.

Unfolding Patient Stories: David Carter • Part 2

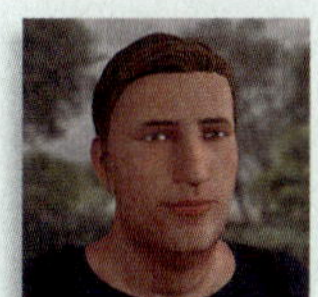

Recall from Chapter 11 David Carter, a 28-year-old diagnosed with schizophrenia and major depression who was hospitalized after a violent outburst toward his mother, involving paranoid delusions and auditory hallucinations. He lives with his mother and previously worked as a grocery clerk. How will the nurse assess improvements in psychotic symptoms? What can be contributing to his increased social isolation? What factors should the nurse consider when developing a plan of care for discharge to promote David's social functioning and lessen his isolation? How can the nurse collaborate with David to include his mother in discussions regarding his plan of care?

Care for David and other patients in a realistic virtual environment: ***vSim** for Nursing* (thepoint.lww.com/vSimMentalHealth). Practice documenting these patients' care in DocuCare (thepoint.lww.com/DocuCareEHR).

REFERENCES

American Psychiatric Association. (2022). *Diagnostic and statistical manual of mental disorders (5th ed., text rev.)*. Author.

American Society for the Positive Care of Children. (2021). *Get the facts: Adverse childhood experiences (ACES)*. https://americanspcc.org/get-the-facts-adverse-childhood-experiences/

Boafo, Y. S., Mostafa, S., & Obeng-Gyasi, E. (2023). Association of per- and polyfluoroalkyl substances with allostatic load stratified by herpes simplex virus 1 and 2 exposure. *Toxics*, *11*(9), 745. https://doi.org/10.3390/toxics11090745

Bozo, Ö., Ar, Y., & Eldoğan, D. (2019). Does marital adjustment mediate type C personality-depressive symptoms relation? A comparison between breast cancer patients and cancer-free women. *Current Psychology*, *38*(5), 1310–1317. https://doi.org/10.1007/s12144-017-9693-6

Cannon, W. B. (1932). *The wisdom of the body*. W. W. Norton & Company.

Capriotti, T., Constant, N., & Jucar, D. A. (2022). Minority stress and effects on cardiovascular health in African Americans. *MEDSURG Nursing*, *31*(5), 281–315.

Carden, K. D., McDuffie, D. L., Murry, K., Bui, C., & Allen, R. S. (2022). Minority stress process among older Black Americans: The role of age, perceived discrimination, and anxiety. *Aging & Mental Health*, *26*(4), 852–859. https://doi.org/10.1080/13607863.2021.1904380

Chen, B., Xie, M., Zhang, Y., Zhang, H., Yu, N. X., & Lin, D. (2025). Who still suffers? Effects of COVID-19 stressful experiences on somatic symptoms and anxious mood moderated by diurnal cortisol: A daily diary study. *Applied Psychology. Health and Well-Being*, *17*(1), e12638. https://doi.org/10.1111/aphw.12638

Chu, B., Marwaha, K., Sanvictores, T., Awosika, A. O., & Ayers, D. (2024). Physiology, stress reaction. In *StatPearls*. StatPearls Publishing. https://www.ncbi.nlm.nih.gov/books/NBK541120/

Cuevas, A. G., McSorley, A. M., Lyngdoh, A., Kaba-Diakité, F., Harris, A., Rhodes-Bratton, B., & Rouhani, S. (2024). Education, income, wealth, and discrimination in Black-White allostatic load disparities. *American Journal of Preventive Medicine*, *67*(1), 97–104. https://doi.org/10.1016/j.amepre.2024.02.021

Dai, Z., Liu, Q., Ma, W., & Yang, C. (2021). The influence of social support and ability perception on coping strategies for competitive stress in soccer players: The mediating role of cognitive assessment. *Frontiers in Psychology*, *12*. https://www.frontiersin.org/articles/10.3389/fpsyg.2021.554863

Doan, S. N. (2021). Allostatic load: developmental and conceptual considerations in a multi-system physiological indicator of chronic stress exposure. *Developmental Psychobiology*, *63*(5), 825–836. https://doi.org/10.1002/dev.22107

Friedman, M., & Rosenman, R. (1974). *Type A and your heart*. Knopf.

Gallagher, S., Grangel, A. B., Dempsey, A., & Howard, S. (2024). Caregiving, caring intensity, and allostatic load: A comparison of caring to others inside and outside the home. *Journal of Psychosomatic Research*, *187*, 111966. https://doi.org/10.1016/j.jpsychores.2024.111966

Garavan, T., Srivastava, S., Madan, P., O'Brien, F., & Matthews-Smith, G. (2021). Type A/B personality, work–family, and family–work conflict: The moderating effects of emotional intelligence. *Human Resource Development Quarterly*, *33*(3), 223–247. https://doi.org/10.1002/hrdq.21454

Guidi, J., Lucente, M., Sonino, N., & Fava, G. A. (2021). Allostatic load and its impact on health: A systematic review. *Psychotherapy and Psychosomatics*, *90*(1), 11–27. https://doi.org/10.1159/000510696

Herriman, Z., Taylor, A. M., & Roberts, R. M. (2023). Interventions to reduce the negative impact of online highly visual social networking site use on mental health outcomes: a scoping review. *Psychology of Popular Media*, *13*(1), 111–139. https://doi.org/10.1037/ppm0000455.supp

Holmes, T., & Rahe, R. (1967). The social readjustment patient scale. *Journal of Psychosomatic Research*, *11*(2), 213–218.

Hughes, T. L., Jackman, K., Dorsen, C., Arslanian-Engoren, C., Ghazal, L., Christenberry-deceased, T., Coleman, C. L., Mackin, M., Moore, S. E., Mukerjee, R., Sherman, A., Smith, S., & Walker, R. (2022). How can the nursing profession help reduce sexual and gender minority related health disparities: Recommendations from the National Nursing LGBTQ Health Summit. *Nursing Outlook*, *70*(3), 513–524. https://doi.org/10.1016/j.outlook.2022.02.005

Kneavel, M. (2021). Relationship between gender, stress, and quality of social support. *Psychological Reports*, *124*(4), 1481–1501. https://doi.org/10.1177/0033294120939844

Knowlton, C. N., & Nelson, K. G. (2021). PTSD telehealth treatments for veterans: Comparing outcomes from in-person, clinic-to-clinic, and home-based telehealth therapies. *Journal of Rural Mental Health*, *45*(4), 243–255. https://doi.org/10.1037/rmh0000190

Lazarus, R. S., & Folkman, S. (1984). *Stress, appraisal and coping*. Springer.

Lazarus, R. S. (2006). *Stress and emotion: A new synthesis*. Springer.

Litzelman, K., Berghoff, A., Stevens, J., & Kwekkeboom, K. (2023). Predictors of psychoneurological symptoms in cancer caregivers over time: Role of caregiving burden, stress, and patient symptoms. *Supportive Care in Cancer*, *31*(5), 274. https://doi.org/10.1007/s00520-023-07741-3

Lodder, P., Kupper, N., Antens, M., & Wicherts, J. M. (2021). A systematic review comparing two popular methods to assess a type D personality effect. *General Hospital Psychiatry*, *71*, 62–75. https://doi.org/10.1016/j.genhosppsych.2021.04.002

Lu, M., Zhang, F., Tang, X., Wang, L., Zan, J., Zhu, Y., & Feng, D. (2022). Do type A personality and neuroticism moderate the relationships of occupational stressors, job satisfaction and burnout among Chinese older nurses? A cross-sectional survey. *BMC Nursing*, *21*(1), 88. https://doi.org/10.1186/s12912-022-00865-7

McEwen, B. S. (2019). The good side of "stress." *Stress: The International Journal on the Biology of Stress*, *22*(5), 524–525. https://doi.org/10.1080/10253890.2019.1631794

Mwangwa, F., Charlebois, E. D., Ayieko, J., Olio, W., Black, D., Peng, J., Kwarisiima, D., Kabami, J., Balzer, L. B., Petersen, M. L., Kapogiannis, B., Kamya, M. R., Havlir, D. V., & Ruel, T. D. (2023). Two or more

significant life-events in 6-months are associated with lower rates of HIV treatment and virologic suppression among youth with HIV in Uganda and Kenya. *AIDS Care*, *35*(1), 95–105. https://doi.org/10.1080/09540121.2022.2052260
Na, H., Jo, M., Lee, C., & Kim, D. (2022). Development and evaluation: a behavioral activation mobile application for self-management of stress for college students. *Healthcare*, *10*(10), 1880. https://doi.org/10.3390/healthcare10101880
Ng, A. E., Gruenewald, T., Juster, R. P., & Trudel-Fitzgerald, C. (2024). Affect regulation and allostatic load over time. *Psychoneuroendocrinology*, *169*, 107163. https://doi.org/10.1016/j.psyneuen.2024.107163
Oh, S., Litam, S. D. A., & Chang, C. Y. (2023). Racism and stress-related growth among Asian internationals: Ethnic identity, resilience, and coping during Covid-19. *International Journal for the Advancement of Counselling*, *45*(2), 226–248. https://doi.org/10.1007/s10447-022-09494-w
O'Toole, T., Armitage, C. J., van Tongeren, M., & Dienes, K. A. (2025). Primary and secondary allostatic processes in the context of high-stress work: a multigroup moderation from the English longitudinal study of ageing. *Psychoneuroendocrinology*, *171*, 107193. https://doi.org/10.1016/j.psyneuen.2024.107193
Pasha, A., Bahrainian, S. A., & Farahani, H. (2022). The relationship between type D personality and the stress level of life events, personality traits and anxiety sensitivity in people with breast cancer. *Annales Médico-Psychologiques, Revue Psychiatrique*, *180*(6), 527–532. https://doi.org/10.1016/j.amp.2021.02.012
Rahe, R. H. (1994). The more things change. *Psychosomatic Medicine*, *56*(4), 306–307.
Rahe, R. H., Taylor, C. B., Tolles, R. L., Newhall, L. M., Veach, T. L., & Bryson, S. (2002). A novel stress and coping workplace program reduces illness and healthcare utilization. *Psychosomatic Medicine*, *64*(2), 278–286.
Raykh, O. I., Sumin, A. N., & Korok, E. V. (2022). The influence of personality type D on cardiovascular prognosis in patients after coronary artery bypass grafting: Data from a 5-year-follow-up study. *International Journal of Behavioral Medicine*, *29*(1), 46–56. https://doi.org/10.1007/s12529-021-09992-y
Richardson, L. J., Goodwin, A. N., & Hummer, R. A. (2021). Social status differences in allostatic load among young adults in the United States. *SSM—population health*, *15*, 100771. https://doi.org/10.1016/j.ssmph.2021.100771
Rolin, S. N., Flis, A., & Davis, J. J. (2021). Work coping, stress appraisal, and psychological resilience: reaction to the COVID-19 pandemic among health care providers. *Psychology & Neuroscience*, *15*(2), 131–146. https://doi.org/10.1037/pne0000257
Rollings, J., Micheletta, J., Van Laar, D., & Waller, B. M. (2023). Personality traits predict social network size in older adults. *Personality and Social Psychology Bulletin*, *49*(6), 925–938. https://doi.org/10.1177/01461672221078664
Rymarczyk, K., Turbacz, A., Strus, W., & Cieciuch, J. (2020). Type C personality: Conceptual refinement and preliminary operationalization. *Frontiers in Psychology*, *11*. https://www.frontiersin.org/articles/10.3389/fpsyg.2020.552740
Selye, H. (1956). *The stress of life*. McGraw-Hill.
Selye, H. (1973). The evolution of the stress concept. *American Scientist*, *61*(6), 692–699.
Selye, H. (1974). Stress without distress. *J. B. Lippincott*.
Suntai, Z., Laha-Walsh, K., & Albright, D. L. (2021). Effectiveness of remote interventions in improving caregiver stress outcomes for caregivers of people with traumatic brain injury. *Rehabilitation Psychology*, *66*(4), 415–422. https://doi.org/10.1037/rep0000402
Thomas-Odenthal, F., Ringwald, K., Teutenberg, L., Stein, F., Alexander, N., Bonnekoh, L. M., Brosch, K., Dohm, K., Flinkenflügel, K., Grotegerd, D., Hahn, T., Jansen, A., Leehr, E. J., Meinert, S., Pfarr, J. K., Renz, H., Schürmeyer, N., Stief, T., Straube, B., Thiel, K., … Kircher, T. (2024). Neural foundation of the diathesis-stress model: longitudinal gray matter volume changes in response to stressful life events in major depressive disorder and healthy controls. *Molecular Psychiatry*, *29*(9), 2724–2732. https://doi.org/10.1038/s41380-024-02526-4
Torné-Ruiz, A., Reguant, M., & Roca, J. (2023). Mindfulness for stress and anxiety management in nursing students in a clinical simulation: a quasi-experimental study. *Nurse Education in Practice*, *66*, 103533. https://doi.org/10.1016/j.nepr.2022.103533
Tracy, E. L., Chin, B., Lehrer, H. M., Carroll, L. W., Buysse, D. J., & Hall, M. H. (2022). Coping strategies moderate the effect of perceived stress on sleep and health in older adults during the COVID-19 pandemic. *Stress and Health*, *38*(4), 708–721. https://doi.org/10.1002/smi.3124
World Health Organization. (2022). *Mental health and COVID-19: Early evidence of the pandemic's impact: scientific brief.* World Health Organization.
Zare, H., Gilmore, D. R., Assari, S., Molina, I. B., Delarmente, B. A., Azadi, M., & Thorpe, R. J., Jr (2024). Income inequality, gender disparities, and ethnic differences: investigating allostatic load in American adults. *Journal of Racial and Ethnic Health Disparities*, https://doi.org/10.1007/s40615-024-02025-w

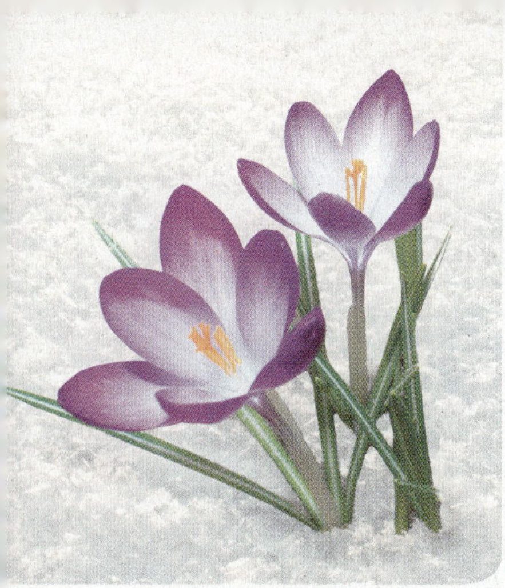

20 Safety and De-Escalation Practices

Mary Ann Boyd and Sandra P. Thomas

KEYCONCEPTS

- aggression
- anger
- de-escalation
- gender, culture, and ethnic differences
- impulsive aggression
- instrumental aggression
- intervention fit
- microaggression
- violence

LEARNING OBJECTIVES

After studying this chapter, you will be able to:

1. Discuss the significance of patient and nurse safety when caring for people with emotional issues and mental disorders.
2. Discuss the consequences of anger on thinking and behavior.
3. Discuss the role of implicit bias associated with response to anger and aggression.
4. Discuss the consequences of microaggression on self-esteem and behavior.
5. Discuss the factors that influence aggressive and violent behaviors.
6. Identify behaviors or actions that escalate violent behavior.
7. Generate options for de-escalating anger, aggression, and violent behaviors in clinical nursing practice.

KEY TERMS

• anger management • cultural humility • explicit bias • hostility • implicit bias • intermittent explosive disorder • inward directed anger • maladaptive anger • outward directed anger • problematic anger • suppression

INTRODUCTION

An important nursing role is keeping all patients safe. When caring for people with mental health issues, nurses are faced with unique safety challenges because of the risk of patients being violent, harming themselves, or attempting suicide. Contrary to a popular misconception, patients who have psychiatric issues are not more violent than other patients. However, they *might* become aggressive given a combination of known risk factors with specific environmental conditions. Patient and nurse safety are primary concerns. The purposes of this chapter are to present a spectrum of behavior related to anger, microaggression and violence, and to describe safety interventions including de-escalation techniques that protect patient and nurse from injury.

ANGER

Language pertaining to anger is imprecise and confusing. Some of the words used interchangeably with anger include *annoyance*, *frustration*, *temper*, *resentment*, *hostility*, *hatred*, and *rage*. Myths about anger abound (Box 20.1). One goal of this section is to dispel confusion between anger as an usual, healthy response to violation of one's integrity and maladaptive anger that is detrimental to one's mental and physical health.

Anger-Related Disorder

Because anger and aggression can be symptomatic of many underlying psychiatric or medical disorders, from posttraumatic stress disorder and bipolar disorder to

BOX 20.1

Cultural Myths About Anger

Myth: Anger is a knee-jerk reaction to external events.

Myth: Anger can be uncontrollable, resulting in crimes of passion such as "involuntary manslaughter."

Myth: Anger behavior in adulthood is determined by temperament and childhood experiences.

Myth: Men are angrier than women.

Myth: People must behave aggressively to get what they want.

toxicities and head injuries, any underlying disorder must be properly evaluated first. Only one anger-related disorder, **intermittent explosive disorder** (IED), appears in the *Diagnostic and Statistical Manual of Mental Disorders, fifth edition, text revision* (American Psychiatric Association [APA], 2022). This diagnosis is characterized by impulsive anger attacks that vary greatly in severity and consequences. These attacks are aimed at harming people or destroying property (Burke et al., 2024).

Once thought to be rare, more recent research has shown that IED is as common as many other psychiatric disorders. The disorder usually appears during the teen years and persists over the life course. Evidence suggests that the presence of childhood adversity and a chaotic environment are associated with IED. Genetic influence and injuries (traumatic brain injury) can also be related to the disorder. See Chapter 33 for further discussion of impulsive disorders (Shevidi et al., 2023).

Etiology of Anger

Biologic Factors

The physiology of anger involves the cerebral cortex, the sympathetic nervous system, the adrenal medulla (which secretes adrenaline and noradrenaline), the adrenal cortex (which secretes cortisol), the cardiovascular system, and even the immune system. From a biologic viewpoint, angry episodes may partially originate from developmental deficits, anoxia, malnutrition, toxins, tumors, neurodegenerative diseases, or trauma affecting the brain.

Psychosocial Factors

Anger is an internal affective state, usually temporary rather than an enduring hostile attitude. If expressed outwardly, anger behavior can be constructive or destructive. Whereas destructive anger alienates other people and invites retaliation, constructive anger can be a powerful force for asserting one's rights and achieving social justice.

KEYCONCEPT Anger is "a strong, uncomfortable emotional response to a provocation that is unwanted and incongruent with one's values, beliefs, or rights" (Thomas, 2001).

TABLE 20.1 STYLES OF ANGER EXPRESSION

Style	Characteristic Behaviors
Anger suppression	• Feeling anxious when anger is aroused • Acting as though nothing happened • Withdrawing from people when angry • Conveying anger nonverbally by body language • Sulking, pouting, or ruminating
Unhealthy outward anger expression	• Exploding in uncontrollable anger • Expressing anger in an attacking or blaming way • Yelling, saying nasty things • Calling the other individual names or using profanity • Using fists rather than words to express angry feelings
Constructive anger discussion	• Discussing the anger with a friend or family member even if the provocateur cannot be confronted at the time • Approaching the individual with whom one is angry and discussing the concern directly • Using "I" language to describe feelings and request changes in another's behavior

Anger is a signal that something is wrong in a situation; thus, the individual who is angry has the urge to act. The situation is more distressing than a minor annoyance such as a slow grocery line. An interpersonal offense such as unjust or disrespectful treatment (a spouse lying, a coworker taking advantage) often provokes anger. Within a couple relationship, anger in one partner can lead to an anger display in the other, which in turn increases cardiovascular reactivity in both (Meier et al., 2023).

The Expression of Anger

Although the physiologic arousal of anger is similar in all people, ways of expressing anger differ. The most common modes, or styles, of anger expression are listed in Table 20.1. Skillful anger control is essential to social and occupational success (Box 20.2). People with poor

BOX 20.2

Self-Awareness Exercise: Personal Experience of Anger

People's reactions differ when they experience anger. Some people report a sense of power, control, and calmness different from their usual experience; others report feeling shaky, tearful, and on the verge of collapse. Still others describe physical sensations of nausea and dizziness.

Think about the last time you felt angry. List the body sensations and other emotions that you experienced. Now ask a friend, colleague, or family member to do the same. Compare lists. What are the similarities and differences? How will awareness of these differences help you in your clinical practice?

anger control have more conflict at work, change jobs more frequently, take more unwise risks, and have more accidents than people with adaptive anger behavior (Liu et al., 2021; Petitta et al., 2021).

Suppression of anger, prolonged rumination about the grievance, and malevolent fantasies of revenge do not resolve a problem and may result in negative consequences later. Similarly, antagonistic anger toward an intimate partner or coworker only exacerbates the conflict (Meier et al., 2023). In contrast, if anger is expressed assertively, beneficial outcomes are possible. In Averill's classic study (1983) of everyday anger, 76% of those who were on the receiving end of someone else's anger reported that they recognized their own faults because of the anger incident. Contrary to popular misconception, the relationship with the individual who was angry was strengthened, not weakened.

Although much of this chapter focuses on people who need to *down*regulate anger, the reader must remember that anger suppressors have a need to *up*regulate their anger and express it more assertively. Learning to express legitimate angry feelings was a significant step in the trajectory of recovery for women who had experienced childhood abuse (Almeida et al., 2024; Thomas et al., 2012). Treatments should be tailored based on assessment data and patients' progress.

Maladaptive Anger

Although anger arousal is a reasonable response, anger becomes maladaptive when it is too frequent, too intense, or managed in unhealthy ways—excessive outward expression (losing temper, yelling) or **suppression** (seething inside and ruminating about grievances). **Maladaptive anger** is linked to psychiatric conditions as well as a plethora of medical conditions. For example, **outward directed anger** (toward others) and **hostility** (cynical attitudes, distrust, antagonism) are linked to coronary heart disease (Gaffey et al., 2023), type 2 diabetes (Mohseni et al., 2023), and myocardial infarction (Cai et al., 2023). **Inward directed anger** (toward oneself) leads to guilt and depression (Kaźmierczak et al., 2023). Suppressed anger is related to affective components of pain (Fernandez et al., 2022).

Culture and Gender Considerations

Anger is one of the six universal emotions (happiness, sadness, anger, fear, surprise, and disgust) with identifiable facial features and emotionally inflected speech. People across the globe experience the emotion of anger, along with the impulse to act when angry, but culture is perhaps the most important determinant of what people who are angry may do. Cultural differences in anger behavior can emanate from the historical trajectories, religions, languages, and customs of a group of people (Tamir et al., 2024). The same event can provoke very different emotional responses in people who are culturally different (e.g., a random act of greeting such as a smile by a stranger could be perceived as insulting by one individual but dismissed with a laugh by someone from another culture).

> **KEYCONCEPT** The meaning and expression of anger varies due to **gender, culture, and ethnic differences**.

Gender role socialization influences beliefs about the appropriateness of "owning" angry emotionality and revealing it to others. In Western cultures, aggressive behavior has traditionally been expected in men and more conciliatory behavior expected in women (Van Doren & Soto, 2021). Some Eastern cultures are also viewed as disapproving of anger in women. For example, one study suggests that suppression of anger by South Korean nurses (primarily women) contributed to their work stress and burnout (Lee et al., 2020).

Recent studies suggest anger expression that is viewed according to the East/West dichotomy may be better understood at the individual level. There is variation in emotion regulation in all countries with individuals who embrace harmony and collectivism (prioritizing group goals) are more likely to suppress emotion than those who embrace individualism (individual goals) (Klein et al., 2024).

EVIDENCE-BASED NURSING CARE OF PEOPLE WITH ANGER ISSUES

Both outward-directed anger (particularly the hostile, attacking form) and inward-directed anger (i.e., anger that is stifled despite strong arousal) produce adverse consequences, indicating a need for anger management intervention. Complicating matters, however, most people's anger styles cannot be neatly categorized as "anger-in" or "anger-out" because people behave differently in different environments (e.g., yelling at assistants in the office, stifling anger at a family member). Therefore, it is necessary to conduct a careful assessment of a patient's behavior pattern across various situations.

Recognizing Cues: Relevant Assessment Information

An anger assessment begins by asking the patient to describe anger episodes and their outcomes. The nurse can clarify the situations that provoke anger and determine the type of anger—inward, outward, or suppressed. Because anger is a subjective internal experience, a useful assessment tool is the evidence-based Spielberger State-Trait Anger Expression Inventory (Spielberger, 1999). This instrument measures the general temperamental proneness to be aroused to anger (trait anger) as well as current feelings (state anger) and several styles of anger expression, including anger-in, anger-out, and control through calming techniques.

The manner of anger expression is not the only important aspect of assessment. The difficulty in regulating the frequency and intensity of anger must also be assessed. **Problematic anger,** evident in clenched fists and readiness to burst when arguing, is associated with elevated generalized distress that interferes with functioning (Adler et al., 2022). The extent to which anger is creating issues at work or in intimate relationships should be evaluated, as well as the use of unhealthy coping techniques such as binge eating, drinking, or medicating their angry distress with over-the-counter or illicit drugs. An essential element in an assessment is exploration of what the patient learned about anger and its display in their culture and family of origin (the primary bearer of that culture). For example, research shows that some Black Americans learn to avoid discriminatory comments and actions for personal safety, but this coping strategy can lead to internalizing racial trauma that can, in turn, lead to depression, repressed anger, and self-destructive responses (Jacob et al., 2023). Traumatic events involving racism trigger several posttraumatic symptoms including anger (Dieujuste et al., 2023).

TAKING ACTION: NURSING INTERVENTION

Nurses may withdraw from patients who are angry, and they may try to hide their own anger because "good nurses" do not get angry at patients. Coldness and distancing on the part of staff are acutely painful to patients (Dil & Cam, 2024). What patients want are steady, dependable, and confident caregivers who will remain connected with them when they are angry.

Nurses' perceptions and beliefs about themselves as individuals and professionals influence their response to aggressive behaviors. For example, a nurse who considers any expression of anger inappropriate will approach a patient who is agitated differently from a nurse who considers agitated behavior to be meaningful. Understandably, nurses often shrink from patient anger when their own family backgrounds have been characterized by out-of-control anger or abuse. A nurse who has previously been assaulted by a patient is also more likely to have psychological reactions to assaults (Box 20.3).

Some patients have an uncanny ability to target a nurse's vulnerable characteristics. Although it is understandable to become defensive when feeling vulnerable, maintaining personal control is a must. If not, the potential for the nursing to become punitive toward the patient is greater. Threatening a patient who is agitated (e.g., "You are going to get an injection if you don't calm down.") will only escalate a volatile situation. Nurses must collaborate with other members of the treatment team when interacting with patients with particularly challenging behavior, obtaining consultation from supervisors if necessary.

Reducing Implicit Biases

Patient anger can provoke fear and frustration in the nurse. Cultural biases are sometimes exposed when nurses are threatened (see Chapter 3). An **implicit bias** is an unconscious attitude or stereotype that affects perceptions, decisions, and actions. With an **explicit bias,** an individual is aware of the negative attitudes and may allow these attitudes to affect their behavior. An implicit bias can lead to unequal treatment of people based on race, ethnicity, gender identity, sexual orientation, disability, and other characteristics.

We all have implicit biases; the challenge is to recognize our biases (so they are then explicit instead of implicit) and to then develop personal harm reduction

BOX 20.3

Research for Evidence-Based Practice: Workplace Assault Outcomes

Gillespie, G. L., & Berry, P. (2023). Qualitative analysis of workplace assault outcomes from the perspectives of emergency nurses. Journal of Emergency Nursing, *49(3), 450–460. https://doi.org/10.1016/j.jen.2022.09.015*

THE QUESTION: What are the negative consequences to emergency nurses who experience workplace assault?

METHODS: Based on the Ecological Occupational Health Model of Workplace Assault, this study used a descriptive qualitative design. Data from 167 emergency nurse participants who described an episode of workplace assault were analyzed using a content analysis method. The data collection tool was one open-ended question asking participants to describe the worst episode of assault or threat of assault in the last 30 days and to document the actions taken and consequences of the assault.

FINDINGS: The consequences to the patients included having limits set, being removed from the emergency department, being arrested, and having restraints used. Physical reactions were reported by 43 participants but more nurses described psychological reactions; however, only 2 participants received emotional support or debriefing. Most of the nurses had support from security personnel. Nurses also reported that nursing care to other patients was temporarily stopped or slowed while the event was being handled.

IMPLICATIONS FOR NURSING: Because assault can occur anywhere in patient care settings, all nurses need to be trained in de-escalation techniques.

TABLE 20.2 THE 5 R'S OF CULTURAL HUMILITY

Reflection	*Aim:* One will approach every encounter with humility and understanding that there is always something to learn from everyone. *Ask:* What did I learn from each individual in that encounter?
Respect	*Aim:* One will treat every individual with utmost respect and strive to preserve dignity and respect. *Ask:* Did I treat everyone involved in that encounter respectfully?
Regard	*Aim*: One will hold every individual in their highest regard while being aware of and not allowing unconscious biases to interfere in any interactions. *Ask:* Did unconscious biases drive this inter action?
Relevance	*Aim*: One will expect cultural humility to be relevant and apply this practice to every encounter. *Ask:* How was cultural humility relevant in this interaction?
Resiliency	*Aim:* One will embody the practice of cultural humility to enhance personal resilience and global compassion *Ask:* How was my personal resiliency affected by this interaction?

Adapted with permission from Robinson, D., Masters, C., & Ansari, A. (2021). The 5 Rs of cultural humility: A conceptual model for health care leaders. *The American Journal of Medicine, 134*(2), 161–163.

strategies. For example, the nurse who perceives older adults negatively may unconsciously provide less health education and have shorter patient interactions. To account for this bias and provide quality care, the nurse should deliberately devote more time to interactions with older patients. Another implicit bias may include perceptions regarding people from different ethnic groups. For example, Black, Latinx, and Indigenous patients may be treated abruptly or poorly by a White nurse. Finding things in common, expanding one's social network, and forming friendships with people of different groups are strategies that have been shown to reduce harm from implicit biases (Shah & Bohlen, 2023).

When caring for people who feel upset and angry, the **cultural humility** process of the "5 R's"—reflection, respect, regard, relevance, resiliency—can help reduce actions related to implicit biases. See Table 20.2 for more information on this process.

Anger Management: A Psychoeducational Intervention to Promote Wellness

Anger management is an effective intervention that nurses can use for people whose anger behavior is maladaptive in some way (i.e., interfering with success in work or relationships) but *not violent.* In recent years, there has been an increase in court-mandated "anger management" for people whose behavior is violent as opposed to angry. When these individuals do not greatly benefit, a conclusion may be drawn that anger management is ineffective. However, psychoeducational anger management courses cannot be expected to modify *violent* behavior. (Interventions designed for people who are aggressive and violent are presented later in the chapter.)

The desired outcomes of any anger management intervention are to teach people to (1) effectively modulate the physiologic arousal of anger, (2) alter any irrational thoughts fueling the anger, and (3) modify maladaptive anger behaviors (e.g., blaming, attacking, or suppressing) that prevent problem solving in daily living. Group work is valuable to anger management clients because they need to practice new behaviors in an interpersonal context that offers feedback and support. The leader of an anger management group functions as a teacher and coach, not as a therapist. Potential participants should be screened and referred to individual counseling or psychotherapy if their anger is chronic. Some people have deeper developmental issues that mitigate against their successful participation in anger management groups (Shepherd & Cant, 2020). Candidates for psychoeducational anger management classes must have some insight that their behavior is problematic and some desire to enlarge their behavioral repertoire.

Anger management includes both didactic and experiential components (Thomas, 2001). Educational handouts, videos, and workbooks are usually used. Ideally, participants commit to attendance for a series of weekly meetings, ranging from 4 to 10 weeks. Between the group meetings, participants are given homework assignments, such as keeping an anger diary and applying the lessons of the class in their homes and work sites. Fresh anger incidents can be brought to the class for role-plays and group discussions. Feedback from group members assists in reappraisal of situations in less hostile terms and permits practice of new anger behaviors in a supportive atmosphere. It may be useful to conduct gender-specific or culturally specific groups (Pebole et al., 2021). People can successfully reduce anger and foster forgiveness through religious/spiritual anger management strategies such as prayer, meditation, or yoga (Charzyńska, 2021; Ti et al., 2021).

Effectiveness of anger management has been demonstrated in numerous studies, including college students, drivers, veterans, and various medical and psychiatric outpatients who are angry, as well as parents/caregivers who have difficulty controlling anger toward their children (Lee & DiGiuseppe, 2018). Family members of patients with alcohol use disorder also can benefit from anger management.

Cognitive-Behavioral Therapy for Anger

Cognitive-behavioral therapy is often recommended for the treatment of uncontrollable anger. The first step is establishing a therapeutic alliance because some people who are angry are not in a state of readiness to change their behavior. Cognitive-behavioral therapy involves avoidance of provoking stimuli, self-monitoring regarding cues of anger arousal, stimulus control, response disruption, and guided practice of more effective anger behaviors. Relaxation or mindfulness training is often introduced early in the treatment because it strengthens the therapeutic alliance and convinces clients that they can indeed learn to calm themselves when angry. When the body relaxes, there is less physical impetus to act impulsively in a way that one will later regret.

MICROAGGRESSION

The concept of microaggression evolved from observations of the way cumulative proracist attitudes can motivate differential treatment of people of color (Pierce, 1970). Microaggression is commonly understood to involve any bias-driven, subtle, casual words and actions that are perceived as insulting to the targeted group.

Microaggressions may be unintentional and often are based on inherited biases from parents/caregivers, relatives, and others. These remarks or actions (such as avoiding the individual) are considered small, common, and sometimes ambiguous, but they are stressful for those on the receiving end. Consider the following example: Two professionally dressed executives attending a conference, one of whom is a member of an underrepresented group, stop by the coffee shop. Both are wearing conference name tags. Though the two executives are standing together, another attendee turns to the executive from the underrepresented group and says in a surly, condescending tone, "Don't you have any decaf?" This attendee has mistaken the executive from the underrepresented group for a coffee shop employee due to their biased assumption that people from that group are more likely to work in the service industry. Reactions to such experiences include confusion, anger, anxiety, helplessness, hopelessness, frustration, paranoia, and fear. Negative stereotypes and inequitable social norms are reinforced by these remarks or actions. Whether consciously or unconsciously motivated, microaggressions lead to discrimination and oppression that reinforces unjust power differentials between groups (Ehie et al., 2021; Williams et al., 2021).

Nurses are challenged to recognize and respond to microaggressions when caring for patients with mental health disorders. Self-awareness is essential to recognizing personal biases and identifying personal use of microaggression (Javier et al., 2022). It is important that everyone disarm the microaggressions, not just the individual who is targeted.

KEYCONCEPT Microaggression occurs when remarks, insults, or actions are made that intentionally or unintentionally express a prejudiced attitude toward a member of an underrepresented group (based on factors that include race, ethnicity, gender, and sexuality).

AGGRESSION

Aggression and violence command the attention of the criminal justice system as well as the mental health care system. During periods when people are a danger to others, they may be separated from the larger society and confined in prisons or locked psychiatric units. Because nurses frequently practice in these settings, management of aggressive and violent behavior is an essential skill.

Factors that Influence Aggressive and Violent Behavior

The individual who is violent may feel trapped, frightened, or desperate, perhaps at the end of their rope. The nurse must remember that many people who are violent have experienced childhood abandonment, physical brutality, or sexual abuse. Confinement that replicates earlier experiences of degrading treatment may provoke aggressive response, but humane care may kindle hope of recovery and rehabilitation. The response of the nurse may be critical in determining whether aggression escalates or diminishes. Aggressive or violent behavior does not occur in a vacuum. Both the patient and the context must be considered. Therefore, a multidimensional framework is essential for understanding and responding to these behaviors.

KEYCONCEPT Aggression involves overt or covert behavior intended to hurt, belittle, take revenge, or achieve domination and control. Aggression can be verbal (sarcasm, insults, threats) or physical (property damage, slapping, hitting). Mentally healthy people stop themselves from aggression by realizing the negative consequences to themselves or their relationships.

KEYCONCEPT Impulsive aggression occurs in situations of anger and anxiety when the individual lashes out. **Instrumental aggression** is a goal-directed aggressive behavior that is premeditated and unrelated to immediate feelings of frustration or threat; it is a means to secure a goal or reward.

KEYCONCEPT Violence is extreme aggression that involves the use of strong force or weapons to inflict bodily harm to another individual and, in some cases, to kill. Violence connotes greater intensity and destruction than aggression. All violence is aggressive, but not all aggression is violent.

Theories of Aggression and Violence

This section discusses some of the main theoretical explanations for aggression and violence. A single model or theory cannot fully explain aggression and violence;

instead, choose the most useful theories for explaining a patient's experience and for planning interventions.

Biologic Theories

The brain structures most frequently associated with aggressive behavior are the limbic system and the cerebral cortex, particularly the frontal and temporal lobes. Patients with a history of damage to the cerebral cortex are more likely to exhibit increased impulsivity, decreased inhibition, and decreased judgment than those who have not experienced such damage. The interaction of neurocognitive impairment and social history of abuse or family violence increases the risk for violent behavior, particularly for prepubescent people assigned male at birth (Thomas et al., 2023).

Differences in aggressive behavior depending on sex assigned at birth can partially be explained by neurobiology. Activation of the amygdala is correlated with higher anger scores in people assigned male at birth. When provoked, individuals in this population also have increased activation in the orbitofrontal cortex, rectal gyrus, and anterior cingulate cortex. Activation of these areas is associated with aggression (Bürger et al., 2023). Sex hormones also play a role in some aggressive behavior, with testosterone associated with aggression (Zhao & Gobrogge, 2023).

NCLEXNOTE In caring for a patient with the potential for aggression, the nurse should recognize that biochemical imbalance contributes to the individual's inability to control aggression.

Psychological Theories

Several psychological explanations exist for aggressive and violent behaviors. This section discusses selected theories and their treatment approaches.

Psychoanalytic/Psychodynamic Theories

Psychoanalytic theorists view emotions as instinctual drives. They view suppression of these drives as unhealthy and possible contributors to the development of psychosomatic or psychological disorders. Some psychoanalysts recommended the use of cathartic approaches to release patients' pent-up anger. Nurses in the mid-20th century often used interventions that directed the patient to "let it out" by pounding a pillow or ripping up telephone books. However, studies did not support the theory that catharsis reduces aggression.

Contemporary psychoanalysts do not adhere to any single explanatory model of aggression, often focusing on patients' tendencies to reenact old childhood conflicts or their defensive attempts to deny vulnerability. In working with patients who are angry, they focus on issues such as improved control over outbursts, heightened empathy for others, and repair of deficits in the personality structure. During analytic therapy, patients gradually achieve greater insight into unconscious processes (Town et al., 2021). Thus, they become aware of the reasons they developed maladaptive anger behaviors.

Behavioral Theories

As behavioral theories came into prominence, anger was viewed as a learned response to a stimulus rather than an instinctual drive. In the 1930s, the frustration–aggression hypothesis was advanced in which an individual may experience anger and act violently in response to interference with or blocking of a goal. The reality of everyday experience reveals the limitations of this theory. Not all situations in which one's goal is blocked lead to anger or violence.

Social Learning Theory

Social learning theory focuses on the role of learning and rewards in the expression of aggression and violence (see Chapter 6). Children's observations of aggressive behaviors among family members and violence in their communities foster a context for learning that aggressive behavior is an acceptable way of getting what they want. According to this view, people develop aggressive and violent behaviors by participating in an environment that rewards aggression, such as violent video games (Coyne et al., 2023).

General Aggression Model

The general aggression model is a framework that accounts for the interaction of cognition, affect, and arousal during an aggressive episode (Fig. 20.1) (He & Xiang, 2021; Kersten & Greitemeyer, 2024). In this model, an episode consists of *person and situation factors* in an ongoing *social interaction*. The episode is mediated through an individual's thoughts, feelings, and intensity of arousal. Within this context, the individual appraises the episode and then decides about a follow-up action. The outcome is either thoughtful or impulsive action. The *person factors* include characteristics such as gender, personality traits, beliefs and attitudes, values, goals, and behavior patterns. *Situational factors* include the actual provocation (insults, slights, verbal and physical aggression, interference with achieving goals) and cues that trigger memories of similar situations. *Cognition* includes hostile thoughts and scripts (previous behavior patterns and responses to similar episodes). Mood, emotion, and expressive motor responses (automatic reactions to specific emotions) represent the *affect component*. *Arousal* can be physiologic, psychological, or both. See Box 20.4.

EVIDENCE-BASED NURSING CARE OF PEOPLE WITH AGGRESSIVE BEHAVIOR

The paramount aims of psychiatric nurses, particularly those staffing inpatient facilities, are promoting safety and preventing aggression. The nurse works toward these

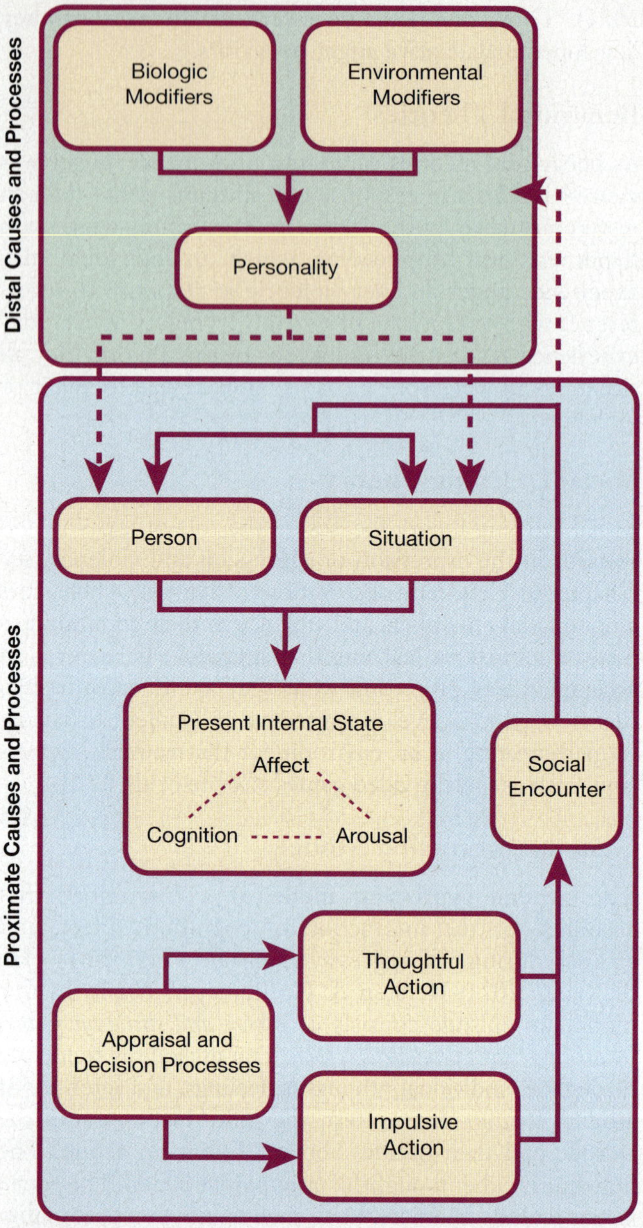

FIGURE 20.1 General aggression model overview. (Redrawn from Anderson, C. A., & Anderson, K. B. [2008]. Men who target women: Specificity of target, generality of aggressive behavior. *Aggressive Behavior*, *34*[6], 605–622. Copyright © 2008 Wiley-Liss, Inc. Reprinted by permission of John Wiley & Sons, Inc.)

goals by establishing therapeutic nurse–patient relationships, creating a therapeutic milieu, and de-escalation.

Recognizing Cues: Relevant Assessment Information

The patient's history is the most important predictor of potential for aggression and violence. Early life adverse circumstances, such as inadequate maternal nutrition, birth complications, traumatic brain injury, and lead exposure can contribute to risk for aggressive and criminal behaviors in adulthood (Koolschijn et al., 2023). Important markers in the patient's history include previous episodes of rage and violent behavior, escalating irritability, intruding angry thoughts, and fear of losing control.

Age, gender, and race are *not* good predictors, but several research reports suggest that particular characteristics are predictive of violent behaviors. Usually, but not always, there are some observable precursors to aggression and violence: staring or glaring in an intimating manner, raising voice tone or volume, making sarcastic or demanding comments, and pacing.

> **BOX 20.4**
>
> **Self-Awareness Exercise: Intensity of Anger**
>
> Imagine this scene: You are coming home late at night. You have been at the library studying for midterm examinations and are tired. As you come up the front walk, you trip over a skateboard, probably left by one of the neighborhood children. Before you know it, you are sprawled across the front step.
>
> What emotions threaten to overwhelm you at that moment? What contributes to the intensity of the anger that you feel?
>
> - The pain where you scraped your leg across the cement?
> - Your general state of tiredness?
> - The fact that you skipped dinner?
> - The five cups of coffee you had today?
> - The careless child who left a toy in your way?
>
> Now imagine that the same thing had happened when you were well-rested and feeling good. Would the feeling and the intensity be the same?

Impaired Communication

Impaired communication (including hearing loss and reduced visual acuity), disorientation, and depression have been found to be consistently associated with aggressive behavior among nursing home residents with dementia (Schnelli et al., 2021).

In patients with cognitive impairments, the anticipation of basic needs (e.g., thirst and hunger) is important, especially when working with adults and children who cannot readily express their needs. Similarly, the nurse needs to know when the patient last voided and the pattern of bowel movements. The urge to void can be a powerful stimulus to agitated behavior. Regular toileting routines are not just interventions to prevent incontinence. Other discomforts can arise from impaired communication, such as conditions like ingrown toenails and medication side effects.

Physical Health

The patient's physical condition contributes to the likelihood of aggression. Patients with long-standing poor dietary habits (e.g., patients who are indigent or those with alcohol use disorder) often have deficiencies of thiamine and niacin. Increased irritability, disorientation, and paranoia may result. Assessing overall dietary intake is relevant, particularly of good tryptophan sources, such as wheat, flour, corn, milk, and eggs. Intake of caffeine, a potent stimulant, should be assessed and limited as necessary.

Social Factors

The nurse should evaluate social factors, such as crisis conditions in the patient's home, family, or community, that could lead to aggression or violent episodes. If the assessment reveals stressful actions by family members, such as evicting the patient from the home, attention must be devoted to mobilizing resources for family and community support and alternative housing.

Are financial or legal troubles placing increased stress on the patient? Is the patient experiencing conflict with other patients on the unit or with certain staff? People reenact in new relationships the same behaviors that created problems in old ones. Thus, behavior in a mental health facility provides important clues to a patient's habitual responses to authority figures, peers of the same gender, and peers of other genders. Assessment data provide direction for interventions such as reassigning roommates or caregivers.

Milieu and Environmental Factors

Angry or out-of-control behavior is highly influenced by contextual factors. Successful psychiatric stabilization and treatment in a hospital often depend on the nature of the unit itself. A busy, noisy hospital unit can quickly provoke an aggressive episode. A rude comment or staff denial of a patient's request can trigger physical assault. Documented times of increased violence include meals, medication, and shift changes (Salzmann-Erikson & Yifter, 2020). Crowding and density during times of high patient census are also associated with patient aggression. Inadequate staffing has been identified as a contributing factor in units with a high incidence of assault.

Many characteristics of the unit culture and staff behavior, such as rigid rules and violation of boundaries, predict patient violence (Box 20.5). In units with a high incidence of violence, nurses should take steps to improve the milieu and staff–patient relationships. More skilled handling of "flashpoints," such as staff denial of patient requests, can avert crisis situations.

BOX 20.5

Characteristics of Unit Culture and Staff Behavior that Predict Patient Violence

- Rigid unit rules
- Lack of patient privacy or boundary violations
- Lack of patient autonomy (locked doors, restraints)
- Strict hierarchy of authority
- Lack of patient control over the treatment plan
- Denial of patient requests or privileges
- Lack of meaningful and predictable ward activities
- Insufficient help with activities of daily living and other needs from staff
- Patronizing behavior of staff
- Power struggles related to medications
- Failure of staff to listen, convey empathy

TAKING ACTION: NURSING INTERVENTIONS

Safety and de-escalation of the situation are priorities when tempers flare. Preventing injury to the patient and staff is the primary goal. When moving from anger to agitation, the patient loses the ability to think rationally, and intervention should focus on de-escalating the patient and the situation.

De-escalating Interventions

Both patients and staff have a right to safety in a psychiatric unit. De-escalation is a method to prevent potential violence.

> **KEYCONCEPT De-escalation** is the use of nonphysical interventions to stabilize or reduce the intensity of a potentially violent situation.

In de-escalation, the nurse uses communication techniques and cognitive interventions to calm the patient by providing the patient with the opportunity to gain control over intense emotions. The nurse's authentic engagement with the patient is the core component in therapeutic de-escalation. Creative, patient-centered strategies—not techniques of physical restraint—are of paramount importance. Individualizing interventions is important. With some patients, loudness and pacing can be ignored; with others, these behaviors indicate an escalation of agitation.

De-escalating potential aggression is always preferable to challenging or provoking a patient. De-escalating is a skill that every nurse can develop. Trying to clarify what has upset the patient is important, although not all patients are capable of articulating what provoked them, as in cases where violent acting out has been triggered by delusions or hallucinations (Haefner et al., 2021). Some analyses will have to take place after a crisis has been diffused. The nurse can use therapeutic communication techniques to prevent a crisis or diffuse a critical situation (Box 20.6).

Communication: First Step in De-escalation

Communicating with a patient who is becoming agitated follows the same principles discussed in Chapter 9.

BOX 20.6

Therapeutic Dialogue: The Patient With the Potential for Aggression

P.T. is a 23-year-old patient in the high observation area of an inpatient unit. The patient is pacing back and forth, pounding a fist into their other hand. In the past 24 hours, P.T. has been more cooperative and less agitated. However, the behavior the nurse is observing now is more like the agitated behavior the patient displayed 2 days ago. Yesterday, the psychiatrist agreed to grant the patient more freedom in the unit if the patient's behavior improved. Even after behavior improvement, the psychiatrist refused to change the restrictions.

INEFFECTIVE APPROACH

Nurse: P.T., I can understand this is frustrating for you.

P.T.: How can you understand? Have you ever been held like a prisoner?

Nurse: I do understand, P.T. Now you must calm down, or more privileges will be removed.

P.T. (voice gets louder): But I was told that calm behavior would mean more privileges. Now you're telling me calm behavior only gets me what I've got! Can't you talk to the doctor for me?

Nurse: No, P.T., I can't talk to the doctor. (P.T. appears more frustrated and agitated as the conversation continues.)

EFFECTIVE APPROACH

Nurse: P.T., you look upset (observation). What happened in your conversation with the psychiatrist? (Seeking information)

P.T.: Yesterday, the doctor said calmer behavior would mean more freedom in the unit. I've tried to be calmer and not to swear. You said you noticed the difference. But today, the doctor said "no" to more freedom.

Nurse: Some people might feel cheated if this happened to them (validation). Is that how you feel?

P.T.: Yeah, I feel really cheated. Nothing I do makes a difference. That's the way it is here, and that's the way it is when I am out of the hospital.

Nurse: It sounds like experiences like this leave you feeling powerless (validation).

P.T.: I don't have any power, anywhere. Sometimes, when I have no power, I get mean. At least then people pay attention to me.

Nurse: In this situation with your doctor, what would help you feel that you had some power? (Inviting patient partnership)

P.T.: Well, if the doctor would listen to me or read my chart.

Nurse: I'm a bit confused by the psychiatrist's decision. I won't make promises that your privileges will change, but would it be okay with you if I talk with the doctor?

P.T.: That would make me feel like someone is on my side.

CRITICAL THINKING CHALLENGE

- In the first scenario, how did the nurse escalate the situation?
- Compare the first scenario with the second. How are they different?

Agitation and aggression may be a way of communicating a need, especially if there are communication deficits. The following are general guidelines:

- When speaking to the patient, use a calm tone to demonstrate empathy.
- Avoid raising your voice.
- Speak slower than usual, which can be soothing to the patient.
- Be aware of emphasis on words that can have a negative connotation.
- Maintain a relaxed but alert stance to the side of the individual.
- Keep hands down, open, and visible.
- Maintain a neutral, nonjudgmental, and attentive expression.

Listening to the Patient's Illness Experience and Concerns

Development of the therapeutic nurse–patient relationship begins with listening. Many patients with persistent mental illness have had traumatic experiences related to previous hospitalizations. Understandably, they may harbor distrust of mental health clinicians and resentment being hospitalized again. Inviting patients and families to talk about their experiences with the health care system may highlight both their concerns and resources. Simply listening to patients' concerns and "being with" them is often as significant as "doing for" them (Box 20.6) (Sato & Kodama, 2021).

Validating

Patients who experience intense anger and rage can feel isolated and anxious. The nurse can acknowledge these intense feelings by reflecting, "This must be scary for you." Empathic responding can reduce emotional arousal because the patient feels understood and supported (see Chapter 9). By drawing on experience with other patients, the nurse can also reassure the patient that others have felt the same way.

Providing Choices

When possible, the nurse should provide the patient with choices, particularly patients who have little control over their situation because of their condition. Offering concrete choices is better than offering open-ended options. For example, a patient who is experiencing a manic episode and is confined to their room may have few options in their daily schedule. However, they may be allowed to make choices about food, personal hygiene, and which pajamas to wear.

Cognitive Interventions

Cognitive interventions are very useful in interacting with a patient with potential for aggression. These interventions are useful when the patient is in a nonaggressive state and willing to discuss the irrational thought process underlying aggressive episodes. These periods of interaction allow exploration of the patient's beliefs and provision of reassurance, support, and education.

> **NCLEXNOTE** The best time to teach the patient techniques for managing anger and aggression is when the patient is not experiencing the provoking event. Cognitive therapy approaches are useful and can be prioritized according to responses.

Providing Patient Education

Inpatient hospitalization offers opportunities for education of patients and families about a variety of topics. Nurses can seize "teachable moments" to convey important principles of anger management. For example, after an outburst of loud cursing by J., who mistakenly thought another patient, S., had stolen their cigarettes, the nurse helped them consider what they could have done differently in the situation. J. was more amenable to learning about calming techniques and problem-solving strategies at this time because their behavior had resulted in adverse consequences (estrangement from S., disruption of the dayroom during a popular bingo game, and cancellation of S.'s weekend pass). This incident could also be used for teaching in a subsequent group meeting of inpatients. Many units have daily meetings that permit the processing of such conflicts. S. could be invited to express feelings about being falsely accused of stealing. Other patients may reveal how distressed they were when J. was cursing loudly, providing their useful peer feedback about J.'s outburst. Together, group members could generate ideas for more appropriate behavior.

Developing Prevention Strategies

Although patients are not always aware of it, escalation of feelings, thoughts, and behavior from calmness to violence may follow a pattern. Disruption of the pattern can sometimes be a useful means for preventing escalation and helping the patient regain composure. Patients can learn to identify their own personal warning signs of aggression and develop aggression–prevention strategies. Both inpatients and outpatients benefit from nurse-led group therapy for aggressive behaviors. Group members can recognize their underlying feelings of helplessness and loss of control and then purposefully decrease their aggressive behaviors. Nurses can suggest a variety of strategies to interrupt patterns:

- Counting to 10
- Using a relaxation or breathing technique (see Chapter 10)
- Removing oneself from interactions or stimuli that may contribute to increased distress (voluntarily taking a "cooling-off walk" or "time-out")
- Doing something different (e.g., reading, listening to quiet music, watching television)

Milieu and Environmental Interventions

The inpatient environment can be modified proactively to decrease the potential of aggressive and violent behaviors (Box 20.7).

Reducing Stimulation

For people whose perceptions or thoughts are disordered from brain damage, degeneration, or other thought-processing difficulties, modification of the environment may be one of the main interventions. The patient with a brain injury, progressive dementia, or distorted vision may be experiencing intense and highly confusing stimulation even though the environment, from the nurse's or family's perspective, seems calm and orderly.

Likewise, introducing more structure into a chaotic environment can help decrease the risk for aggressive behavior. It is possible to make stimuli meaningful or to simplify and interpret the environment in many practical ways, such as by identifying people or equipment that may be unfamiliar, providing cues as to what is expected (e.g., posting signs with directions, putting a toothbrush

BOX 20.7

Environmental Management: Maintaining Patient Safety

DEFINITION

Maintaining patient safety includes identifying and eliminating environmental risks for people who are at risk of injuring self or others.

ACTIVITIES

- Search the environment routinely to make sure it is hazard free.
- Remove potential weapons (e.g., sharps, ropelike objects) from the environment.
- Search the patient and belongings for weapons or potential weapons.
- Monitor the safety of items that visitors bring to the environment.
- Instruct visitors and other caregivers about relevant patient safety issues.
- Limit patient use of potential weapons (e.g., sharps, ropelike objects).
- Monitor patient during use of potential weapons (e.g., razors).
- Place the patient with potential for self-harm with a roommate to decrease isolation and opportunity to act on self-harm thoughts, as appropriate.
- Assign a single room to the patient with potential for violence toward others.
- Place the patient in a bedroom located near a nursing station.
- Limit access to windows unless they are locked and shatterproof, as appropriate.
- Lock utility and storage rooms.
- Provide paper dishes and plastic utensils at meals.
- Place the patient in the least restrictive environment that still allows for the necessary level of observation.
- Provide ongoing surveillance of all patient access areas to maintain patient safety and therapeutically intervene, as needed.
- Remove other people from the vicinity of a patient who is violent or a patient who has the potential for violence.
- Maintain a designated safe area (e.g., seclusion room) for patient to be placed when violent.
- Provide plastic, rather than metal clothes hangers, as appropriate.

Adapted from the Mental Health Environment of Care Checklist. VHA National Center for Patient Safety, Department of Veterans Affairs. Version 06–01–2015. http://www.patientsafety.va.gov/professionals/onthejob/mentalhealth.asp

and toothpaste by the sink), and removing or silencing unnecessary stimuli (e.g., turning off paging systems).

Considering the environment from the patient's viewpoint is essential. For instance, if the surroundings are unfamiliar, the patient will need to process more information. Lack of a recognizable pattern or structure further taxes the patient's capacity to encode information. Appropriate interventions include clarifying the meaning and purpose of people and objects in the environment, enhancing the patient's sense of control and the predictability of the environment, and reducing other stimuli as much as possible.

Interventions for Managing Imminent Aggression and Violence

The nurse who works with patients with the potential for aggression should do so with respect and concern. The goal is to work with patients to find solutions, approaching these patients calmly, and empathizing with the patient's perspective. Offering a simple apology to a patient who is agitated can circumvent a power struggle (Rigamonti, 2022). In dealing with aggression, as in other aspects of nursing practice, at times the best intervention is silence. It is easy to equate intervention with activity, the sense that "I must do something." But offering quiet calmness may be enough to help a patient regain control of their behavior.

KEYCONCEPT Within the context of the therapeutic relationship, the nurse must be cognizant of **intervention fit**, or the appropriateness of the intervention used for the specific patient in the specific situation.

Interventions that are appropriate in early phases of escalation differ from those used when the patient's agitation is greater. The patient's affective, behavioral, and cognitive response to an intervention provides information about its effects and guides the nurse's next response. The following approaches are important in caring for patients who are aggressive or violent:

- Continuing to use nonthreatening body language
- Respecting the patient's personal space and boundaries
- Having immediate access to the door of the room in case you need to leave the room
- Choosing to leave the door open to an office while talking to a patient
- Knowing where colleagues are and making sure those colleagues know where you are
- Removing or not wearing clothing or accessories that could be used to harm you, such as scarves, necklaces, or dangling earrings

There are times when physical presence of other staff members helps de-escalate the situation and prevents the patient from injuring others or themselves. Some facilities use specially trained behavioral emergency response teams (BERTs) that de-escalate potentially violent situations.

Administering and Monitoring PRN Medications

Patients with potential for aggression and violence usually have a PRN (as-needed) medication order for agitation and aggression. If there is a provider or nurse practitioner PRN order for medication for agitation, administering a PRN medication is left to the discretion of the nurse, who makes a judgment about the patient after careful assessment. Antipsychotics and benzodiazepines are frequently used to reduce agitation. The medication can be administered orally if the patient is willing to take the medication. These medications are also administered intramuscularly (Wolfe & McCoin, 2024).

Avoiding the Use of Seclusion and Restraint

The use of seclusion and restraint is a traumatic experience for patients. Most patients with a mental disorder have already experienced traumas, usually in childhood. The act of placing an individual in seclusion or restraints retraumatizes the individual (Atdjian & Huckshorn, 2023). Many hospitals no longer use restraints as a form of behavioral management. Restraint-related injuries and deaths have prompted many facilities to ban their use entirely and train staff in alternative techniques.

In instances where seclusion and restraint are used, they should be the last resort to protect the patient or the staff. Seclusion and restraint have been used by nurses when patients need to be separated from other patients on the unit. The decision to use seclusion and restraint is a dynamic process involving evaluation of the risks to all who are present, as well as the need to maintain a therapeutic milieu. The decision is usually an interdisciplinary decision that follows ethical and legal standards as well as accrediting guidelines.

De-escalation interventions should be tried first and clearly documented in the patient's record. Seclusion or restraint must never be used for staff convenience or as punishment. The use of trauma-informed, recovery-oriented, person-centered care can prevent, reduce, and ultimately eliminate the use of seclusion and restraints (American Psychiatric Nurses Association, 2022).

American institutions that receive Medicare or Medicaid reimbursement must adhere to guidelines issued by the Centers for Medicare and Medicaid Services. These guidelines specify that a registered nurse must verify the need for restraint or seclusion and then contact the provider or other licensed practitioner; within 1 hour, that practitioner must examine the patient. Individual states have also enacted laws to regulate the use of restraints, and professional organizations released position statements on restraints as the last resort in an emergency (Centers for Medicare & Medicaid Services, 2010).

Sensory Modulation

Comfort or sensory rooms are becoming more widespread, providing an appealing alternative to coercive interventions by unit staff. These rooms can provide stimulation for sight, smell, hearing, touch, and taste in a demand-free environment that is controlled by the patient. The rooms may reduce patients' distress and agitation and reduce the need for seclusion and restraint. Some treatment facilities offer items such as weighted blankets, massage creams, and "squishy" balls to augment other de-escalation measures (Haig & Hallett, 2023).

Evaluation and Treatment Outcomes

Treatment outcomes can be considered at both individual and aggregate levels. The desired outcome at the individual level is for the patient to regain or maintain control over aggressive or potentially aggressive thoughts, feelings, and actions. The nurse may observe that the patient shows decreased psychomotor activity (e.g., less pacing), has a more relaxed posture, speaks more directly about feelings of anger and personal needs, requires less sedating medication, shows increased tolerance for frustration and the ability to consider alternatives, and makes effective use of other coping strategies.

If restraints or seclusion have been used, a debriefing occurs with the people involved in the incident, including the patient. This approach allows for a collaborative, community approach to preventing patient violence and avoids blaming one assailant for incidents provoked by a variety of contextual and interpersonal factors. The practice of prompt debriefing and reflection can ultimately transform a treatment setting to a learning community.

Evidence of a reduction in risk factors in the treatment setting includes decreased noise and confusion in the immediate environment; calmness on the part of nursing staff and others; and a climate of safety, clear expectations, and mutual acceptance and respect. In units, day hospitals, or group home settings, indicators of positive treatment outcomes include a reduction in the number and severity of assaults on staff and other patients, fewer incident reports, and increased staff competency in de-escalating potentially violent situations.

RESPONDING TO ASSAULT ON NURSES

Because nurses have extended contact with patients during highly stressful circumstances, there is always the risk that they may be the recipients of patient aggression. Assaults on nurses by patients can have both immediate and long-term consequences (see Table 20.3). Reported assaults range from verbal abuse or threats and minor altercations to severe injuries, rape, and murder. Any assault can produce severe consequences for the person who experiences the assault including posttraumatic stress disorder. After a violent incident, the nurse may avoid the patient or watch for any signs of patient remorse; the nurse's response differs depending on the nurse's feelings of safety and comfort with the patient. The nurse's interpretation of the assaultive behavior will depend on many factors such as experience with assault, the type of assault (impulsive or instrumental), and the nurse's injury.

Because patient aggression directed toward nurses is often downplayed or tolerated by nurses as "part of the

TABLE 20.3 NURSES' RESPONSES TO ASSAULT

Response Type	Personal	Professional
Affective	• Irritability • Depression • Anger • Anxiety • Apathy	• Erosion of feelings of competence, leading to increased anxiety and fear • Feelings of guilt or self-blame • Fear of patients with potential for violence
Cognitive	• Suppressed or intrusive thoughts of assault	• Reduced confidence in judgment • Consideration of job change
Behavioral	• Social withdrawal	• Possible hesitation in responding to other violent situations • Possible overcontrolling • Possible hesitation to report future assaults • Possible withdrawal from colleagues • Questioning of capabilities by coworkers
Physiologic	• Disturbed sleep • Headaches • Stomach aches • Tension	• Increased absenteeism because of somatic complaints

job," nurses seldom report attacks to the police or prosecute their attackers; however, such incidents should be reported to supervisors and possibly to legal authorities, depending on the circumstances. Aggression by patients must be addressed vigorously because it can threaten the other patients, other health care professionals, family members, and visitors, as well as the nursing staff. Reporting violent attacks increases public awareness and increases the likelihood that protective legislation will be enacted. The environment should be modified with the addition of security alarms, video monitors, and de-escalation teams.

All nurses must be provided with training programs in the prevention and management of aggressive behavior. These programs, like courses on cardiopulmonary resuscitation, impart both knowledge and skills, lessening the likelihood of emotional freezing in the presence of violent patient behavior. Like cardiopulmonary resuscitation training, the courses should be provided to undergraduate students and regularly offered to practicing nurses, so that they have opportunities to reinforce and update what they have learned. Some states have enacted legislation mandating workplace violence prevention programs; but the curricula vary, and the quality of training lacks systematic evaluation. Commercially marketed training programs have been criticized because they fail to consider the predatory aspect of some patients' violence and fail to cite nursing research.

COMMUNITY ROLE

There is a moral imperative for nurses to be involved in combating violence in the larger community. Lessening anger and violence in the workplace and home demands involvement of all mental health professionals. Nurses can share their expertise with parents/caregivers, children, teachers, and community agencies. Nurses are well positioned to teach health-promoting anger management classes in diverse practice settings, such as outpatient clinics, schools, and corporate sites. Classes for children and adolescents can be of great benefit because young people are forming the anger habits that will continue into adulthood. Youth who have high levels of anger are at risk for misuse of alcohol and other substances (Gamage et al., 2023) as well as interpersonal conflicts that hamper their educational and occupational success.

SUMMARY OF KEY POINTS

- Anger is an emotional state, usually temporary, that can be expressed constructively or destructively. Destructive anger alienates other people and invites retaliation.
- Anger, aggression, and violence should not be viewed as a continuum. The anger of ordinary people seldom progresses to aggression or violence. Anger does not necessarily lead to aggression or violence.
- Everyone has implicit biases that influence their interactions with others. Nurses need to be aware of implicit biases to prevent negative views from affecting patient care.
- Anger management is a useful psychoeducational intervention that is effective with a wide variety of people who are nonviolent. However, anger management is not designed to modify violent behavior.
- Several theories explain anger, aggression, and violence and include neurobiologic and psychosocial theories. These theories serve as the basis of assessment and interventions.
- The general aggression model accounts for the interaction of cognition, affect, and arousal during an aggressive episode.
- Microaggressions reinforce negative stereotypes and inequitable social norms.
- There is no one factor that predicts aggression or violence. Factors that have been observed to be precursors are staring and eye contact, tone and volume of voice, anxiety, and pacing.

- Nursing interventions can be affective, cognitive, behavioral, or sociocultural. A therapeutic milieu supports a nonviolent culture.
- Nurses who experience assault may experience changes in affective, cognitive, behavioral, and physiologic areas.
- Seclusion or restraints should be used only as a last resort.
- Patient aggression and violence are serious concerns for nurses in all areas of clinical practice. Training in policies and procedures for the prevention and management of aggressive episodes should be available in nursing education programs and all work settings.

DEVELOPING CLINICAL JUDGMENT

1. M.J., a 24-year-old, has just been admitted to an inpatient psychiatry unit; they were transferred from the emergency department after being treated for an intentional drug overdose. The patient is sullen when introduced to their roommate and refuses to answer the admission assessment questions. The nurse tells the patient that they will come back in 30 minutes to complete the assessment. A few minutes later, the patient approaches the nursing station and asks in a demanding tone to talk with someone because of being completely ignored.
   a. What theory can the nurse use to understand M.J.'s behavior?
   b. At this point in time, what data are available to develop a plan of care?
   c. What interventions might the nurse choose to use to help M.J. behave in a manner that is consistent with the norms of this inpatient unit?
2. Discuss the influence of gender and cultural norms on the expression of anger. When a nurse is caring for a patient from a culture that the nurse is not familiar with, what could the nurse ask to ensure that their expectations of the patient's behavior are consistent with the gender and cultural norms of the patient?
3. When a nurse minimizes verbally abusive behavior by a patient, family member, or health care colleague, what implicit message do they send?

MOVIES, TV, OR STREAMING PROGRAMS

***Hidden Figures:* 2016.** This movie takes place in 1961 in a segregated Virginia community during the Jim Crow period, in which racial segregation was legal. Three Black women mathematicians were instrumental in the development of American aviation and space technology. Based on true events, Katherine Goble (Taraji P. Henson), Dorothy Vaughn (Octavia Spencer), and Mary Jackson (Janelle Monáe) suffered microaggressions, prejudice, and discrimination because of their race and gender. The movie depicts how Black individuals, especially Black women, struggled to get an education, to get and maintain a job, and to gain respect in a White male-dominated world of NASA engineers.

Viewing Points:

1. The movie depicted multiple racial microaggressions. Identify verbal microaggressions in the film that could provoke an angry response from the recipient. In addition, speculate about why the recipient of the microaggressions did not respond with anger.
2. What environmental conditions maintained the White male dominance in the movie?
3. At what point did one of the women mathematicians express anger? Was it justified?
4. Reflect upon your interactions in the last week. Can you identify words spoken or actions undertaken, either consciously or unconsciously, that could be experienced by members of an underrepresented group as microaggressions?

REFERENCES

Adler, A. B., LeardMann, C. A., Yun, S., Jacobson, I. G., Forbes, D., & Millennium Cohort Study Team (2022). Problematic anger and economic difficulties: findings from the Millennium Cohort Study. *Journal of Affective Disorders*, *297*, 679–685. https://doi.org/10.1016/j.jad.2021.10.078

Alaka Mani, T. L., Omkar, S. N., Sharma, M. K., Choukse, A., & Nagendra, H. R. (2021). Development and validation of yoga module for anger management in adolescents. *Complementary Therapies in Medicine*, *61*, 102772. https://doi.org/10.1016/j.ctim.2021.102772

Almeida, T. C., Cardoso, J., Matos, A. F., Murça, A., & Cunha, O. (2024). Adverse childhood experiences and aggression in adulthood: the moderating role of positive childhood experiences. *Child Abuse & Neglect*, *154*, 106929.

American Psychiatric Association (APA). (2022). *Diagnostic and statistical manual of mental disorders* (5th ed., text rev.). Author.

American Psychiatric Nurses Association. (2022). *APNA Position: The Use of Seclusion and Restraint*. Author.

Atdjian, S., & Huckshorn, K. A. (2023). Toward the cessation of seclusion and mechanical restraint use in psychiatric hospitals: a call for regulatory action. *Psychiatric Services*, 75(1), 64–71. https://doi.org/10.1176/appi.ps.202100538

Averill, J. R. (1983). Studies on anger and aggression: Implications for theories of emotion. *American Psychologist*, *38*(11), 1145–1160.

Bürger, Z., Müller, V. I., Hoffstaedter, F., Habel, U., Gur, R. C., Windischberger, C., Moser, E., Derntl, B., & Kogler, L. (2023). Stressor-specific sex differences in amygdala-frontal cortex networks. *Journal of Clinical Medicine*, *12*(3), 865. https://doi.org/10.3390/jcm12030865

Burke, J.D., Butler, E. J., Shaughnessy, S., Karlovich, A. R., & Evans, S. C. (2024). Evidence-based assessment of DSM-5 disruptive, impulse control, and conduct disorders. *Assessment*, *31*(1), 75–93.

Cai, D., Fu, Y., Song, Y., Lin, H., Ba, Y., & Lian, J. (2023). A causal relationship between irritability and cardiovascular diseases: a Mendelian randomization study. *Frontiers in Cardiovascular Medicine*, *10*, 1174329. https://doi.org/10.3389/fcvm.2023.1174329

Centers for Medicare & Medicaid Service. (2010). *Condition of participation: Patient's rights. 482.13 Health & Human Services*. Retrieved on January 19, 2023, from https://www.govinfo.gov/content/pkg/CFR-2010-title42-vol5/pdf/CFR-2010-title42-vol5-sec482-13.pdf

Charzyńska, E. (2021). The effect of baseline patterns of spiritual coping, forgiveness, and gratitude on the completion of an alcohol addiction treatment program. *Journal of Religion and Health*, *60*(3), 1796–1817. https://doi.org/10.1007/s10943-021-01188-8

Coyne, S. M., Warburton, W., Swit, C., Stockdale, L., & Dyer, W. J. (2023). Who is most at risk for developing physical aggression after playing violent video games? An individual differences perspective from early adolescence to emerging adulthood. *Journal of Youth and Adolescence*, *52*(4), 719–733. https://doi.org/10.1007/s10964-023-01739-0

Dieujuste, N., Mekawi, Y., & Doom, J. R. (2024). Examination of race-based traumatic stress symptom networks in Black adults in the United States: A network analysis. *Journal of Traumatic Stress*, *37*(3), 397–409. https://doi.org/10.1002/jts.23003

Dil, S., & Çam, M. (2024). The mediator role of mindfulness in the relationship between the listening skills and anger management skills of emergency health care professionals. *International Emergency Nursing*, *75*, 101475. https://doi.org/10.1016/j.ienj.2024.101475

Ehie, O., Muse, I., Hill, L. & Bastien, A. (2021). Professionalism: Microaggression in the healthcare setting. *Current Opinion in Anaesthesiology*, *34*(2), 131–136.

Fernandez, E., Pham, T. M., Kolaparthi, K., Sun, R., Perez, B. S., Iwuala, E. C., Wu, W., & Shattuck, E. C. (2022). Parameters of anger as related to sensory-affective components of pain. *Scandinavian Journal of Pain*, *23*(2), 284–290. https://doi.org/10.1515/sjpain-2022-0131

Gaffey, A., Goldstein, C., Hays, M., Lee, S. & Gaalema, D. (2023). Psychological risk factors in cardiac rehabilitation. *Journal of Cardiopulmonary Rehabilitation and Prevention*, *43*(6), E20–E21. https://10.1097/HCR.0000000000000828

Gamage, N. M., Darker, C., & Smyth, B. P. (2023). Improvement in psychological wellbeing among adolescents with a substance use disorder attending an outpatient treatment programme. *Irish journal of psychological medicine*, *40*(3), 353–360. https://doi.org/10.1017/ipm.2021.6

Haefner, J., Dunn, I., & McFarland, M. (2021). A quality improvement project using verbal de-escalation to reduce seclusion and patient aggression in an inpatient psychiatric unit. *Issues in Mental Health Nursing*, *42*(2), 138–144. https://doi.org/10.1080/01612840.2020.1789784

Haig, S., & Hallett, N. (2023). Use of sensory rooms in adult psychiatric inpatient settings: A systematic review and narrative synthesis. *International Journal of Mental Health Nursing*, *32*(1), 54–75. https://doi.org/10.1111/inm.13065

He, N., & Xiang, Y. (2021). How child maltreatment impacts internalized/externalized aggression among Chinese adolescents from perspectives of social comparison and the general aggression model. *Child Abuse & Neglect*, *117*, 105024. https://doi.org/10.1016/j.chiabu.2021.105024

Jacob, G., Faber, S. C., Faber, N., Bartlett, A., Ouimet, A. J., & Williams, M. T. (2023). A systematic review of black people coping with racism: Approaches, analysis, and empowerment. *Perspectives on Psychological*, *18*(2), 392–415. https://doi.org/10.1177/17456916221100509

Javier, D., Solis L. G., Paul, M. F., Thompson, E. L., Maynard, G., Latif, Z., Stinson, K., Ahmed, T., & Vishwanatha, J. K. (2022). Implementation of an unconscious bias course for the National Research Mentoring Network. *BMC Medical Education*, *22*(1), 391.

Kaźmierczak, I., Zajenkowska, A., Rajchert, J., Jakubowska, A., & Abramiuk-Szyszko, A. (2023). The role of anger expression in unmet expectations and depressive symptoms. *Depression Research and Treatment*, *2023*, 8842805. https://doi.org/10.1155/2023/8842805

Kersten, R., & Greitemeyer, T. (2024). Human aggression in everyday life: An empirical test of the general aggression model. *British Journal of Social Psychology*, *63*(3), 1091–1111.

Klein, N. D., Bravo, A. J., Conway, C. C., Keough, M. T., Pilatti, A., Mezquita, M., & Cross-Cultural Addictions Study Team. (2024). Individualism, collectivism, and emotion regulation: a cross-cultural examination among young adults from seven countries. *Current Psychology*, *43*, 26007–26018. https://doi.org/10.1007/s12144-024-06226-8

Koolschijn, M., Janković, M., & Bogaerts, S. (2023). The impact of childhood maltreatment on aggression, criminal risk factors, and treatment trajectories in forensic psychiatric patients. *Frontiers in Psychiatry*, *14*, 1128020. https://doi.org/10.3389/fpsyt.2023.1128020

Lee, A., & DiGiuseppe, R. (2018). Anger and aggression treatments: A review of meta-analyses. *Current Opinion in Psychology*, *19*, 65–74.

Lee, E., Yeung, N., Xu, Z., Zhang, D., Yu, C. P., & Wong, S. (2020). Effect and acceptability of mindfulness-based stress reduction program on patients with elevated blood pressure or hypertension: A meta-analysis of randomized controlled trials. *Hypertension*, *76*(6), 1992–2001. https://doi.org/10.1161/HYPERTENSIONAHA.120.16160

Liu, Y., Wang, X., & Guo, Y. (2021). The moderating effects of emotions on the relationship between self-reported individual traits and actual risky driving behaviors. *Psychology Research and Behavior Management*, *14*, 423–447. https://doi.org/10.2147/PRBM.S301156

Meier, T., Stephens, J. E., & Haase, C. M. (2023). Feelings in words: Emotion word use and cardiovascular reactivity in marital interactions. *Emotion*. https://doi.org/10.1037/emo0001299

Mohseni, M., Lindekilde, N., Forget, G., Burns, R. J., Pouwer, F., Schmitz, N., & Deschênes, S. S. (2023). Trait anger, hostility, and the risk of type 2 diabetes and diabetes-related complications: A systematic review of longitudinal studies. *Current Diabetes Reviews*, *19*(4), e290322202789. https://doi.org/10.2174/1573399818666220329185229

Pebole, M. M., VanVoorhees, E. E., Chaudhry, N., Goldstein, K. M., Thompson, J., Parker, R., Caron, K. M., & Hall, K. S. (2021). Patient-centered behavioral services for women veterans with mental health conditions. *Translational Behavioral Medicine*, *11*(9), 1676–1681. https://doi.org/10.1093/tbm/ibab057

Petitta, L., Probst, T. M., Ghezzi, V., & Barbaranelli, C. (2021). The impact of emotional contagion on workplace safety: investigating the roles of sleep, health, and production pressure. *Current Psychology*, *42*, 2362–2376. https://doi.org/10.1007/s12144-021-01616-8

Pierce, C. M. (1970). Black psychiatry one year after Miami. *Journal of the National Medical Association*, *62*(6), 471–473.

Rigamonti, K. (2022). Effective compassionate communication and apology. *Journal of Radiology Nursing*, *41*(4), 331–333.

Salzmann-Erikson, M., & Yifter, L. (2020). Risk factors and triggers that may result in patient-initiated violence on inpatient psychiatric units: An integrative review. *Clinical Nursing Research*, *29*(7), 504–520. https://doi.org/10.1177/1054773818823333

Sato, K., & Kodama, Y. (2021). Nurses' educational needs when dealing with aggression from patients and their families: A mixed-methods study. *BMJ Open*, *11*(1), e041711. https://doi.org/10.1136/bmjopen-2020-041711

Schnelli, A., Ott, S., Mayer, H., & Zeller, A. (2021). Factors associated with aggressive behaviour in persons with cognitive impairments using home care services: A retrospective cross-sectional study. *Nursing Open*, *8*(3), 1345–1359. https://doi.org/10.1002/nop2.751

Shah, H. S., & Bohlen, J. (2023). *Implicit bias*. In *StatPearls*. StatPearls Publishing. (nih.gov).

Shepherd, G., & Cant, M. (2020). Difficult to change? The differences between successful and not-so-successful participation in anger management groups. *Counseling and Psychotherapy Research*, *20*, 214–223. https://doi.org/10.1002/capr.12276

Shevidi, S., Timmins, M. A., & Coccaro, E. F. (2023). Childhood and parental characteristics of adults with DSM-5 intermittent explosive disorder compared with healthy and psychiatric controls. *Comprehensive Psychiatry*, *122*, 152367. https://doi.org/10.1016/j.comppsych.2023.152367

Spielberger, C. D. (1999). Manual for the State-Trait Anger Expression Inventory-2. *Psychological Assessment Resources*.

Tamir, M., Ito, A., Miyamoto, Y., Chentsova-Dutton, Y., Choi, J. H., Cieciuch, J., Riediger, M., Rauers, A., Padun, M., Kim, M. Y., Solak, N., Qiu, J., Wang, X., Alvarez-Risco, A., Hanoch, Y., Uchida, Y., Torres, C., Nascimento, T. G., Afshar Jahanshahi, A., & Singh, R. (2024). Emotion regulation strategies and psychological health across cultures. *American Psychologist*, *79*(5), 748–764.

Thomas, A., Assari, S., Odukoya, E., & Caldwell, C. H. (2023). Efficacy to avoid violence and parenting: A moderated mediation of violence exposure for African American urban-dwelling boys. *Development and Psychopathology*, *35*(2), 838–849. https://doi.org/10.1017/S0954579422000098

Thomas, S. P. (2001). Teaching healthy anger management. *Perspectives in Psychiatric Care*, *37*(2), 41–48.

Thomas, S. P., Bannister, S. C., & Hall, J. M. (2012). Anger in the trajectory of healing from childhood maltreatment. *Archives of Psychiatric Nursing*, *26*(3), 169–180. https://doi.org/10.1016/j.apnu.2011.09.003

Town, J. M., Falkenström, F., Abbass, A., & Stride, C. (2021). The anger-depression mechanism in dynamic therapy: Experiencing previously avoided anger positively predicts reduction in depression via working alliance and insight. *Journal of Counseling Psychology*, *69*(3), 326–336. Advance online publication. https://doi.org.libproxy.siue.edu/10.1037/cou0000581

Van Doren, N., & Soto, J. A. (2021). Paying the price for anger: Do women bear greater costs? *International Journal of Psychology*, *56*(3), 331–337. https://doi.org/10.1002/ijop.12724

Williams, M. T., Skinta, M. D., & Martin-Willett, R. (2021). After Pierce and Sue: A revised racial microaggressions taxonomy. *Perspectives on Psychological Science*, *16*(5), 991–1007. https://doi.org/10.1177/1745691621994247

Wolfe, C., & McCoin, N. (2024). Management of the agitated patient. *Emergency Medicine Clinics of North America*, *42*(1), 13–29. https://doi.org/10.1016/j.emc.2023.06.010

Zhao, Z., & Gobrogge, K. (2023). Neurodevelopmental model explaining associations between sex hormones, personality, and eating pathology. *Brain Sciences*, *13*(6), 859. https://doi.org/10.3390/brainsci13060859

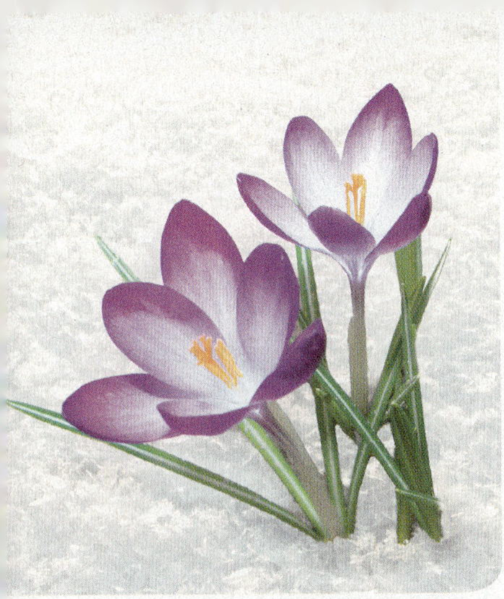

21 Crisis, Loss, Grief, Bereavement, and Disaster Management

Mary Ann Boyd

KEYCONCEPTS

- bereavement
- crisis
- disaster
- grief
- loss

LEARNING OBJECTIVES

After studying this chapter, you will be able to:

1. Describe the types of crises and their impact on mental health.
2. Discuss theoretical models explaining grief, uncomplicated bereavement, and complicated bereavement.
3. Discuss the impact of disasters on mental health.
4. Discuss nursing care for people experiencing crises, losses, grief, bereavement, and disasters.
5. Evaluate the effects of crises, losses, and disasters on lifestyle and survival.
6. Explain the psychological impact of crises, losses, and disasters on people who have experienced catastrophic events.

KEY TERMS

• ABCs of psychological first aid • acute grief • anticipatory grief • complicated bereavement • debriefing • developmental crisis • dual process model • experiential avoidance • integrated grief • loss-oriented coping • maturational crises • mourning • oscillation • prolonged grief disorder • restoration-oriented coping • rumination • situational crisis • traumatic crisis • traumatic grief • uncomplicated bereavement

INTRODUCTION

This chapter explores the concepts of crisis, loss, grief, bereavement, and disaster management; broadens the scope and understanding of the responses of people to crisis, loss, and disaster situations; and describes how nursing care planning can be used for people experiencing these events.

CRISIS

Adaptation and coping are a natural part of life (see Chapter 19). Crisis occurs when there is a perceived challenge or threat that overwhelms the capacity of the individual to cope effectively with the event at any age. Life is disrupted, and unexpected emotional (e.g., sadness, depression, anxiety) and biologic (e.g., nausea, vomiting, diarrhea, headaches) responses occur. Functioning can be severely impaired.

> **KEYCONCEPT Crisis** is a time-limited event that triggers adaptive or nonadaptive responses to maturational, situational, or traumatic experiences. A crisis results from stressful events for which previous coping mechanisms fail to provide adequate adaptive skills to address the perceived challenge or threat. Adaptation to crisis typically occurs in 6 weeks.

A crisis occurs when an individual is at a breaking point. A crisis can have either positive or negative outcomes. If positive, there is an opportunity for growth and change as new ways of coping are learned. If negative, suicide, homelessness, or depression can result. A crisis generally lasts no more than 4 to 6 weeks. At the end of that time, the individual in crisis should have begun to come to grip with the event and begun to harness resources to cope with its long-term consequences. By definition, there is no such thing as a chronic crisis. People who live in constant turmoil are not in crisis but in chaos.

Many events evoke a crisis, such as natural disasters (e.g., floods, tornadoes, earthquakes) and human-made disasters (e.g., wars, bombings, airplane crashes) as well as traumatic experiences (e.g., rape, sexual abuse, assault). In addition, interpersonal events (marriage, birth of a child) may create crises in the lives of any individual.

Feelings of fear, desperation, and being out of control are common during a crisis, but the precipitating event and circumstances are unusual or rare, perceived as a threat, and specific to the individual. For example, a disagreement with a family member may escalate into a crisis for one individual, but not another. If the individual is significantly distressed or social functioning is impaired, a diagnosis of acute stress disorder should be considered (American Psychiatric Association [APA], 2022). The individual with an acute stress disorder has dissociative symptoms and persistently reexperiences the event.

HISTORICAL PERSPECTIVES OF CRISIS

The psychiatrist Caplan (1961) defined a crisis as occurring when an individual faces a problem that cannot be solved by customary problem-solving methods. When the usual problem-solving methods no longer work, an individual's life balance or equilibrium is upset. During the period of disequilibrium, there is a rise in inner tension and anxiety, followed by emotional upset and an inability to function. This conceptualization of phases of a crisis is used today (Fig. 21.1). According to Caplan, during a crisis, an individual is open to learning new ways of coping to survive. The outcome of a crisis is governed by the kind of interaction that occurs between the individual and available key social support systems.

TYPES OF CRISES

Research has focused on categorizing types of crisis events, understanding responses to a crisis, and developing intervention models that support people through a crisis.

Developmental Crisis

While Caplan was creating his crisis model, Erik Erikson was formulating ideas about crisis and development. He proposed that **maturational crises** are a usual part of growth and development and successfully resolving a crisis at one stage allows one to move to the next. According to this model, the child develops positive characteristics after experiencing a crisis. If they develop fewer desirable traits, the crisis is not resolved (see Chapter 6). The concept of **developmental crisis** continues to be used today to describe significant maturational events, such as leaving home for the first time, completing school, and accepting the responsibility of adulthood.

Situational Crisis

A **situational crisis** occurs whenever a specific stressful event threatens an individual's physical and psychosocial integrity and results in some degree of psychological disequilibrium. The event can be an internal one, such as a disease process, or any number of external threats. A move to another city, a job promotion, or graduation from high school can initiate a crisis even though they are positive events. Graduation from high school marks the end of an established routine of going to school, participating in school activities, and doing homework assignments. When starting a new job after graduation, the former student must learn an entirely different routine and acquire new knowledge and skills. If an individual

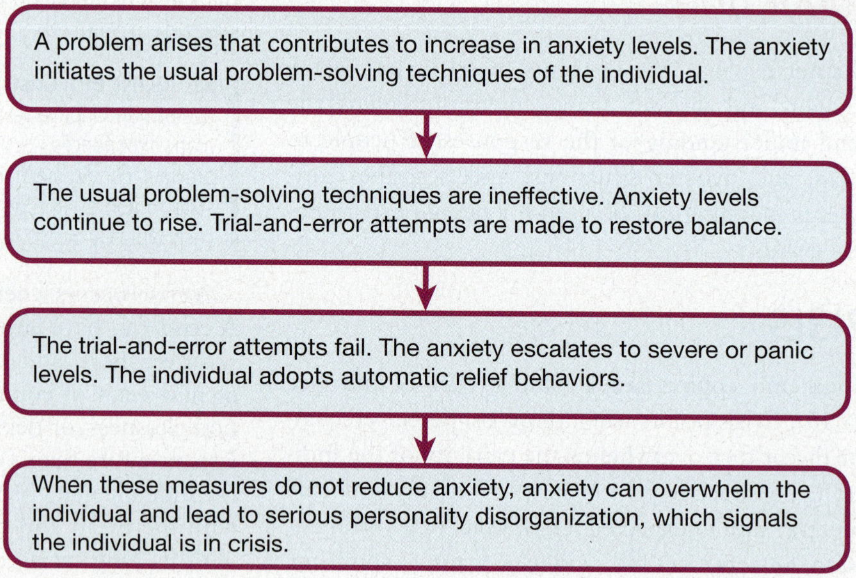

FIGURE 21.1 Phases of crisis.

enters a new situation without adequate coping skills, a crisis may occur.

Traumatic Crisis

A **traumatic crisis** is initiated by unexpected, unusual events that can affect an individual or a multitude of people. In such situations, people face overwhelmingly hazardous events that entail injury, trauma, destruction, or sacrifice. Examples of events include national disasters (e.g., racial persecutions, riots, war), violent crimes (e.g., rape, murder, kidnappings, and assault and battery), and environmental disasters (e.g., earthquakes, floods, forest fires, hurricanes).

RECOVERY-ORIENTED CARE FOR PEOPLE IN CRISIS

The goal for people experiencing a crisis is to return to the precrisis level of functioning. The role of the nurse is to provide a framework of support systems that guide the patient through the crisis and facilitate the development and use of positive coping skills.

Teamwork and Collaboration: Working Toward Recovery

During an environmental crisis that affects the well-being of many people, nursing interventions will be a part of the community's efforts to respond to the event (see later discussion of disasters for more detail). When a personal crisis occurs, however, the individual in crisis may have only the nurse to respond to their needs. After the assessment, the nurse must decide whether to provide the care needed or to refer the individual to a mental health specialist. Box 21.1 offers guidance in making this decision

Safety

Safety of the individual or groups is the first priority. The individuals may not be able to think logically about how to get to safety or stay safe. The nurse provides a logical approach such as calling for help, administering first aid, or removing unsafe items. A nurse should always be aware of personal safety while trying to provide a safe environment for others.

EMERGENCY CARE ALERT! It is important to be acutely aware that an individual in crisis may be at high risk for suicide or homicide. To determine the individual's level of effectiveness of coping capabilities, the nurse should complete a careful assessment for suicidal or homicidal risk. If an individual is at high risk for either, the nurse should consider referral for admission to the hospital.

BOX 21.1

Decision Tree for Determining Referral

Situation: A 35-year-old patient is being seen in a clinic because of minor burns they received during a house fire. Their home was completely destroyed. The patient is tearful, withdrawn, and complains of a great deal of pain from the minor burns. Biopsychosocial assessment is completed.

ASSESSMENT CUES	NURSING ACTION
Patient has psychological distress but believes that their social support is adequate. The patient would like to talk to a nurse when they return for the follow-up visit.	Provide counseling and support to the patient during the visit. Make an appointment for a return visit to the clinic for follow-up.
The patient is severely distressed. They have no social support and do not know how they will survive.	Refer the patient to a mental health specialist. The patient will need crisis intervention strategies provided by a mental health specialist.

NCLEXNOTE During a crisis, an individual's behaviors and verbalizations may provide data that are indicative of a mental illness. Nursing care should be prioritized according to the severity of responses. After the crisis has been resolved, assess whether those behaviors and verbalizations disappear.

EVIDENCE-BASED NURSING CARE OF PEOPLE IN CRISIS

Because the response to a crisis is individualized and differs from individual to individual, the nurse should make sure that a very complete assessment is done. The first priority is determining the extent of physical injury or trauma. The individual should receive medical care for any injuries. Once medically stable, changes in health practices following the crisis provide clues to the severity of the disruption in functioning.

RECOGNIZING CUES: RELEVANT ASSESSMENT INFORMATION

Physical Health and Functioning

Maintaining health is important because a crisis can be physically exhausting. Disturbances in sleep and eating patterns and the reappearance of physical or psychiatric symptoms are common. Changes in body function may include tachycardia, tachypnea, profuse perspiration, nausea, vomiting, dilated pupils, and extreme shakiness. Some people may exhibit loss of control and have total disregard for their personal safety. If sleep patterns are disturbed or nutrition is inadequate, the individual may not have the physical resources to deal with the crisis.

Emotional and Behavioral Responses

The mental health nursing assessment focuses on the individual's emotions and coping strengths. In the beginning of the crisis, the individual may report feelings of numbness and shock. Responses to psychological distress should be differentiated from symptoms of psychiatric illnesses that may be present. Later, as the reality of the crisis sinks in, the individual will be able to recognize and describe the felt emotions. The nurse should expect these emotions to be intense and be sure to provide some support during their expression.

Initially, the individual's thoughts and behaviors may be erratic and illogical. The nurse should assess for evidence of depression, confusion, uncontrolled weeping or screaming, disorientation, or aggression. The individual may be suffering from a loss of feelings of well-being and safety. In addition, panic responses, anxiety, and fear may be present. The ability to cope by problem solving may be disrupted. By assessing the individual's ability to solve problems, the nurse can evaluate whether they can cognitively cope with the crisis situation and determine the kind and amount of support needed.

Strengths and Coping Skills

Coping skills should be identified in an assessment of anyone undergoing a crisis. The coping skills of some people are sufficient to weather a crisis, but many skills are inadequate for the situation. Unusual behaviors may emerge that are ineffective. There may be evidence of self-mutilation activities or suicidal ideation.

The nurse should assess for strengths that will help to cope with the crisis. Is there a close family member that can be contacted? Is the individual young and relatively healthy? Are there resources that can be used during the crisis?

Religious/Spiritual Needs

During a crisis, the individual may want spiritual or religious support. During the assessment, the nurse should be alert to signs of needing religious or spiritual guidance. The crisis victim may verbally express a need for a higher power. The nurse should ask the individual if they are seeking spiritual help. If a referral is not possible, the nurse can offer a quiet moment or ask how they can help meet the individual's need.

Social Functioning and Support

It is critical to assess the individual's perception of the problem and the availability of support systems (emotional and financial). The extent of disruption of typical daily activities and routines is assessed to determine the need for additional support. The individual may not be shopping, paying bills, or cleaning the house. The nurse should identify the social network of family and friends who are available to provide help and support.

ANALYZING CUES AND DEVELOPING HYPOTHESES

Safety is a priority. Physical consequences of the crisis are the first priority. There may be tachycardia or hyperventilation. Reports of potential physical self-harm such as suicidal ideation or intention should be the focus of the next intervention. Body systems can change during a crisis. Diarrhea and urinary incontinence can occur. Food and shelter needs should be considered.

The emotional and psychological consequences of the crisis such as fear and extreme distress are also important to address. Any indication of a mental disorder should be monitored when developing a plan of care. A rapid crisis intervention plan can reduce the impact of the crisis on the individual's mental state.

PLANNING RECOVERY AND WELLNESS OUTCOMES: GENERATING SOLUTIONS

Immediate goals during a crisis may be providing first aid, preventing the individual from attempting suicide or homicide, arranging for food and shelter (if needed), and mobilizing social support. After safety needs are met, the individual can work toward recovery by addressing other goals such as reestablishing self-care routines and using positive coping strategies. Strengths supporting a healthy lifestyle prior to the crisis should be used to develop a plan of care. The individual may have exercised regularly and is ready to use exercise as a way of dealing with the stress, or the individual may have had a healthy diet before the crisis and is now ready to reengage in healthier eating choices. Guidelines for crisis intervention and examples are presented in Table 21.1. Individuals should be encouraged to report any depression, anxiety, or interpersonal difficulties during the recovery period.

During a mental health crisis such as an acute psychotic episode, the traumatic consequences of using extreme measures such as seclusion and restraint should be considered. Ideally, the mental health team trained in trauma-informed approaches can de-escalate the situation without involving security personnel.

THERAPEUTIC RELATIONSHIP

A nurse is often meeting the individual in crisis for the first time and will need to skillfully apply therapeutic communication techniques to meet the individual's immediate mental health needs. Patience, listening, and empathy are important tools that, along with a calm, nurturing approach, can help establish trust. In some instances, the

TABLE 21.1 GUIDELINES FOR CRISIS INTERVENTION

Approach	Rationale	Example
Support the expression (or nonexpression) of feelings according to cultural or ethnic practices.	Emotional support helps the individual face reality. The emotional expression by the victim may be culturally driven.	Ask the individual to actualize the loss using active and reflective listening. "Were you there when they died?" "Tell me how they died." "What special remembrances do you have?" If the individual is crying, sobbing, or angry, allow for the expression of their emotions. Sit quietly beside them. When they are done you can say, "I can tell how terribly sad or angry you are." Try to avoid handing a tissue. Wait for them to look for a tissue before you hand them one.
Help the individual think clearly and focus on one implication at a time.	Focusing on all the implications at once can be too overwhelming.	An individual left a partner because the partner abused them. At first, focus only on living arrangements and safety. You can say, "There are several things we need to focus on now for your safety." At another time, discuss the other implications of the separation.
Avoid giving false reassurances, such as "It will be all right" or "It is for the best."	Giving false reassurances blocks communication. It may not be all right.	Patient: "My doctor told me that I have a terminal illness." Nurse: Restatement: "Your doctor told you that you have a terminal illness. What does that mean to you?"
Clarify fantasies with facts.	Accurate information is needed to solve problems.	A young parent is holding their child who has died. The parent expresses disbelief that this has happened. Quietly sit beside them. The longer the parent holds their child, the realization of what has occurred will settle within them. You do not need to point out the obvious.
Link the individual and family with community resources, as needed.	Social support can ease the effect of the crisis or loss.	Provide information about the meeting of a support group such as that of the American Cancer Society, Alzheimer Support Groups; Compassionate Friends; resolve through sharing or other local bereavement support groups.

Adapted from Lazarus, R. (1991). *Emotion and adaptation (p. 122).* Oxford University Press; Worden, W. (1991). Grief counseling and grief therapy: A handbook for the mental health practitioner. Springer.

nurse has a relationship with the patient who reaches out during a crisis. In that instance, the nurse will have already established the therapeutic relationship and can quickly provide meaningful support and interventions. Be careful not to give unrealistic or false reassurances of positive outcomes over which you have no control. For example, it is not a good idea to reassure the individual that everything will be alright because things may get worse, not better.

NCLEXNOTE Individual responses to a crisis can be best understood by assessing the usual responses of the individual to stressful events. The response to the crisis will also depend on the meaning of the event to the individual. The use of therapeutic communication principles is a priority when caring for an individual who has experienced a crisis or disaster.

TAKING ACTION: NURSING INTERVENTIONS

Physical Care

An individual needs to eat and sleep in order to have the energy to cope with a crisis. Personal hygiene may be suffering. The nurse should encourage the individual to reestablish a healthy diet, practice sleep hygiene strategies, and attend to personal grooming. If the individual is unable to function, a referral can be made to other health care clinicians. Medication may be needed to help maintain a high level of psychophysical functioning.

Medications

Medication cannot resolve a crisis, but the judicious use of these agents can help reduce its emotional intensity. For example, the use of an antianxiety medication such as lorazepam may help the individual through the initial shock of the crisis (see Box 21.2).

Counseling

Counseling reinforces healthy coping behaviors and interaction patterns. Counseling, which focuses on identifying emotions and positive coping strategies, helps the individual integrate the effects of the crisis into a real-life experience. Responses to crisis differ with people. Some may present with behaviors that indicate transient disruptions in their ability to cope. Others may be totally devastated. At times, virtual counseling may provide the individual with enough help that face-to-face counseling is not necessary. If counseling strategies do not work, other stress reduction and coping enhancement interventions can be used (see Chapter 19). The nurse should refer anyone who cannot cope with a crisis to a mental health specialist for an evaluation.

BOX 21.2

Medication Profile: Lorazepam

DRUG CLASS: Benzodiazepine; antianxiety/sedative hypnotic agent

RECEPTOR AFFINITY: Acts mainly at the subcortical levels of the central nervous system (CNS), leaving the cortex relatively unaffected. Main sites of action may be the limbic system and reticular formation. It potentiates the effects of α-aminobutyric acid, an inhibitory neurotransmitter. The exact mechanism of action is unknown.

INDICATIONS: Management of anxiety disorders or for short-term relief of symptoms of anxiety or anxiety associated with depression (oral forms). Also used as preanesthetic medication in adults to produce sedation, relieve anxiety, and decrease recall of events related to surgery (parenteral form). Unlabeled parenteral uses for management of acute alcohol withdrawal.

ROUTE AND DOSAGE: Available in 0.5-, 1-, and 2-mg tablets; 2 mg/mL concentrated oral solution and 2 mg/mL and 4 mg/mL solutions for injection.

Adults: Usually 2–6 mg/day orally, with a range of 1–10 mg/day in divided doses, with the largest dose given at night. 0.05 mg/kg intramuscularly (IM) up to a maximum of 4 mg administered at least 2 hours before surgery. Initially 2 mg total or 0.044 mg/kg intravenously (IV) (whichever is smaller). Doses as high as 0.05 mg/kg up to a total of 4 mg may be given 15–20 minutes before the procedure to those benefiting by a greater lack of recall.

Geriatric patients: Dosage not to exceed adult IV dose. Orally, 1–2 mg/day in divided doses initially, adjusted as needed and tolerated.

Children: Drug should not be used in children younger than 12 years.

HALF-LIFE (PEAK EFFECT): 10–20 hours (1–6 hours [oral]; 60–90 minutes IM; 10–15 minutes IV).

SELECTED ADVERSE REACTIONS: Transient mild drowsiness, sedation, depression, lethargy, apathy, fatigue, light-headedness, disorientation, anger, hostility, restlessness, confusion, crying, headache, mild paradoxical excitatory reactions during first 2 weeks of treatment, constipation, dry mouth, diarrhea, nausea, bradycardia, hypotension, cardiovascular collapse, urinary retention, and drug dependence with withdrawal symptoms.

WARNINGS: Contraindicated in psychoses; acute narrow angle glaucoma; shock; acute alcoholic intoxication with depression of vital signs; and during pregnancy, labor and delivery, and while breastfeeding. Use cautiously in patients with impaired liver or kidney function and those who are debilitated. When given with theophylline, there is a decreased effect of lorazepam. When using the drug IV, it must be diluted immediately before use and administered by direct injection slowly or infused at a maximum rate of 2 mg/min. When giving narcotic analgesics, reduce its dose by at least half in patients who have received lorazepam.

SPECIFIC PATIENT AND FAMILY EDUCATION

- Take the drug exactly as prescribed; do not stop taking the drug abruptly.
- Avoid alcohol and other CNS depressants.
- Avoid driving and other activities that require alertness.
- Notify the prescriber before taking any other prescription or over-the-counter drug.
- Change your position slowly and sit at the edge of the bed for a few minutes before arising.
- Report to the prescriber any severe dizziness, weakness, drowsiness that persists, rash or skin lesions, palpitations, edema of the extremities, visual changes, or difficulty urinating.

Religious/Spiritual Interventions

If the patient is requesting spiritual or religious interventions, the nurse can provide support by including a chaplain (if available) in the care. If chaplaincy service is not available or not acceptable to the individual, the nurse can enlist the aid of community clergy to provide support. Many times, acknowledging the religious/spiritual need can provide the needed support.

Social Support Strategies

A crisis often disrupts an individual's social network, leading to changes in available social support. Development of a new social support network may help the individual cope more effectively with the crisis. Supporting the development of new support contacts within the context of available social networks can be done by contacting available local and state agencies for assistance as well as specific private support groups and religious groups.

Telephone Hotlines

Public and private funding and the efforts of trained volunteers permit most communities to provide crisis services to the public. For example, telephone hotlines for issues ranging from child abuse to suicide are a part of health delivery systems of most communities. Crisis services permit immediate access to the mental health system for people who are experiencing an emergency (such as threatened suicide) or for those who need help with stress or a crisis.

Residential Crisis Services

Many communities provide, as part of the health care network, residential crisis services for people who need short-term housing. The specific residential crisis services available within a community reflect the issues that the community members judge as particularly important. For example, some communities provide shelter for teenage runaways; others offer shelter for spouses who experience abuse. Still others provide shelter for people who would otherwise require acute psychiatric hospitalization. These settings provide residents with a place to stay in a supportive, home-like atmosphere. The people who use these services are linked to other community services such as financial aid.

Evaluation of Patient Outcomes

Outcomes developed in cooperation with the individual experiencing the crisis guide the evaluation. Once assessment data are clustered and prioritized and the outcomes are determined. Once interventions are developed and implemented in cooperation with the individual in crisis, the individual should come through the crisis with improved health, well-being, and social function. If complications occur, the nurse should make appropriate alterations in the entire nursing process or make appropriate referrals.

LOSS, GRIEF, AND BEREAVEMENT

Loss, grief, and bereavement are universal human experiences. The outcomes of loss, grief, and bereavement can range from an increase in psychosocial functioning to maladaptation, which can include death, illness, isolation, and/or mental illness. Nurses are important caregivers who are called upon to provide support and guidance during these difficult times. This section focuses on the loss of a loved one.

> **KEYCONCEPT Loss** can evoke minor to complex thoughts, feelings, and behaviors depending on the perceived relationship of the individual with the lost loved object or individual.

In death, the intensity of the loss is based on perceived relationship to the deceased and the circumstances of the loss. Death can be sudden and unexpected or after a long-term, chronic illness. Stigmatic losses (death associated with a stigmatized event or action such as abortion, acquired immunodeficiency syndrome [AIDS], homicide, and suicide) can also affect coping with and healing after a loss.

The first year after a loss is considered to be the most difficult as holidays, birthdays, anniversaries, and other important life events must be handled by the bereaved. Days surrounding the anniversary date of the death can be difficult for the bereaved.

> **KEYCONCEPT Grief** is a natural, intense, physical, emotional, social, or cognitive reaction to the death of a loved one (see Box 21.3). Spontaneous expressions of loss can include sobbing, crying, anger, and expressions of guilt.

Grief

There are commonalities in grief, but each grief experience is specific to the unique relationship that is lost. Although grief is usually associated with death, it can occur without a death and be unrecognized. **Anticipatory grief** occurs prior to a death, such as when a loved one has a terminal illness. The grief symptoms can be severe and are most likely to occur in caregivers of patients at the end of life, particularly patients with dementia. Higher anticipatory grief levels are associated with depressive symptoms, caregiver burden, and less communication within the family about dying. **Acute grief** occurs immediately after the death of a loved one and usually evolves to a permanent state of integrated grief after a process of adaptation. **Integrated grief** is a long-term process where there continues to be mild yearning and other painful emotions, thoughts, and memories, but they are not intrusive. Although occasional periods of grief intensity may occur, they do not interfere with ongoing life and the sense of well-being. Failure to adapt to the loss can lead to complicated bereavement or **prolonged grief disorder (PGD)** (intense longing for or persistent preoccupation with the deceased that lasts more than 6 months) (Hilberdink et al., 2023).

The grieving experience varies from culture to culture. Grief reactions considered typical in one culture may be considered atypical in others. Evidence shows that prolonged grief reactions are primarily recognized as Western symptoms, and PGD has not been established as a disorder in other cultures (Hilberdink et al., 2023).

Theories of Bereavement

Bereavement is shaped by cultural and social contexts. The bereaved express their grief through social acts and **mourning** (outward expression of grief) practices according to their cultural context. There are several bereavement theories; two approaches are discussed in this section.

> **KEYCONCEPT Bereavement** is the process of healing and learning how to cope with the loss. It begins immediately after the loss and can last months or years. Individual differences, age, religious and cultural practices, and social support influence grief and bereavement.

Stage Theories

There has been wide acceptance that bereavement follows stages: denial, anger, bargaining, depression,

BOX 21.3

Symptoms of Different Types of Reactions to Grief

Physical: stunned, weight gain/loss, insomnia, anorexia, exhausted, restless, aching arms, sleep difficulties, headaches, aching arms, feels ill, palpitations, breathlessness, sighing, lack of strength, blurred vision

Emotional: crying, sobbing, sadness, guilt, anger, sense of failure, irritability, resentment, bitterness, denial, frustration, shame, fear of own death, oversensitivity to environment, senses the presence of the deceased

Social: social withdrawal from typical activity, isolation from others

Cognitive: forgetful, difficulty in making decisions, disorganized, concentration is difficult, preoccupation with thoughts of the deceased, time confusion, short attention span, think they are out of touch with reality.

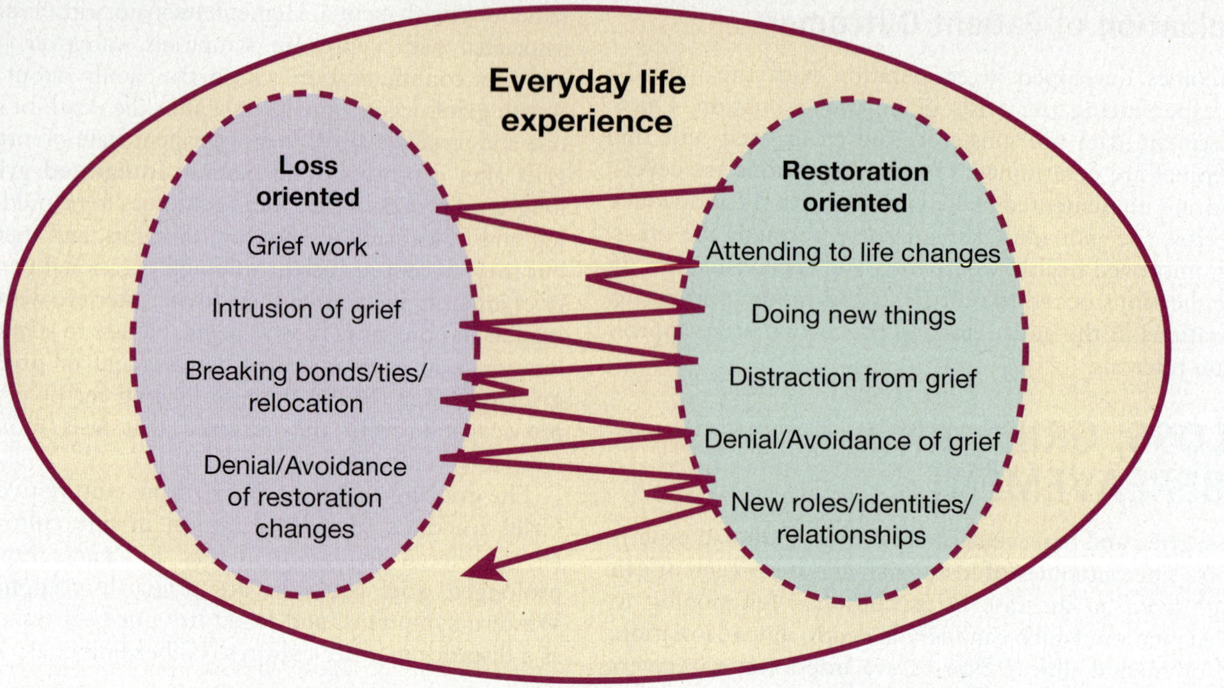

FIGURE 21.2 Dual process model of coping with bereavement. (Redrawn from Stroebe, M., & Schut, H. [1999]. The dual process model of coping with bereavement: Rationale and description. Death Studies, 23, 213. Used with permission from Taylor & Francis Ltd., https://www.tandfonline.com)

acceptance (Kübler-Ross, 1969; Kübler-Ross & Kessler, 2005). Although the stage theory of grief and bereavement remains unsupported by empirical evidence, it is ingrained in the public's mind and continues to be used by some health care professionals (Daniel, 2023).

Dual Process Model

The **dual process model (DPM)** offers a nonlinear explanation of how grieving individuals and families come to terms with their loss over time (Fiore, 2021; Stroebe et al., 2010; Stroebe & Schut, 2015). This model can be used to understand how bereaved people cope (Larsen et al., 2023). According to DPM, the individual adjusts to the loss by oscillating between **loss-oriented coping** (preoccupation with the deceased) and **restoration-oriented coping** (preoccupation with stressful events as a result of the death including financial issues, new identity as a widow[er]). **Oscillation** is the process of confronting (loss-oriented coping) and avoiding (restoration-oriented coping) the stresses associated with bereavement. At times, the bereaved individual is confronted with the loss and memories; and at other times, the individual will be distracted, and the thoughts and memories will be avoided. The bereaved experiences relief from the intense emotion associated with the loss by focusing on other things. For example, the bereaved individual may be recalling a special moment in the relationship such as a wedding or imagining what the individual would say about a current event but then switches to thinking about completing tasks that the deceased had previously undertaken (e.g., paying bills, cooking meals). In the loss-oriented coping mode, emotions relate to the relationship with the deceased individual; in the restoration-oriented coping, the bereaved individual's emotions relate to the stressful events associated with the responsibilities and changes as a result of the loss. Over time, after repeated confrontation with the loss, there is no longer a need to think about certain aspects of the loss. Restoration-oriented stressors vary and relate to coping and post-loss mental health (Eisma et al., 2021; Palm et al., 2023) (see Fig. 21.2).

Types of Bereavement

Uncomplicated Bereavement

Most bereaved people experience uncomplicated bereavement after the loss of a loved one. **Uncomplicated bereavement** is painful and disruptive; however, there is always movement. Questions surface such as "Why did the death happen?" "Why my loved one?" "Why me?" and "Why did God allow this to happen?"

The bereavement process is often applied to other situations in which a loss occurs, not necessarily the death of an individual. The "empty nest syndrome," divorce, birth of a child with a disability, and death of a pet are other examples of losses where there may be grief and bereavement.

Most bereaved people do not need clinical interventions and are able to find new meaning and purpose in their lives. Their self-esteem and sense of competency, although threatened, remain intact. They gradually accept the sense of loss as a reality and are able to move on with their lives. There is little evidence that they need or benefit from counseling or therapy. Those who experience suicidal thoughts with a plan and/or suicidal gestures should be evaluated for complicated grief (Ahn et al., 2023).

Traumatic Grief

Traumatic grief is a term that is used for a more difficult and prolonged grief. In traumatic grieving, external factors influence the reactions and potential long-term outcomes. For example, memories of the traumatic death of the deceased may lead to more traumatic memories including the violent death scene. The external circumstances of death associated with traumatic grief include (1) suddenness and lack of anticipation; (2) violence, mutilation, and destruction; (3) degree of preventability or randomness of the death; (4) multiple deaths (bereavement overload); and (5) mourner's personal encounter with death involving a significant threat to personal survival or a massive and shocking confrontation with the death (or mutilation) of others (Kokou-Kpolou et al., 2022).

The deaths of individuals with COVID-19 resulted in several million bereaved families and friends at high risk for traumatic grief. Funeral ceremonies were suspended. Families were deprived of assisting the dying individual because of the contagiousness of the disease. Families were unable to visit loved ones in the hospitals and intensive care units (ICUs), which led to feelings of guilt. As a result of these factors, an increase in traumatic grief and PGD, leading to possible bereavement overload, occurred (Denckla et al., 2023).

Complicated Bereavement

Complicated bereavement or PGD occurs in about 5% to 15% of bereaved people (Comtesse et al., 2024). The individual is frozen or stuck in a state of chronic mourning, which lasts for more than a month to 6 months after a loss. In other words, there is no movement in the thought processes in how the bereaved view and experience their loss. The individual may feel bitter over the loss and wish their life could revert to the time they were together.

Additionally, the individual may have trouble accepting the death, an inability to trust others since the death, excessive bitterness related to the death, and feeling that life is meaningless without the deceased individual. People who are more vulnerable for developing complicated bereavement are those who have experienced a sudden, unexpected loss, stigmatic loss, or death of a loved one after a long-term chronic illness as these situations have the potential to limit their social support.

Emotional disturbances are central to complicated bereavement. The literature shows that **experiential avoidance** (avoiding unwanted internal stimuli such as thoughts, physical sensations, or emotions) and **rumination** (repetitive thinking about the experience, causes, and consequences of the loss) are associated with persistent complicated bereavement. Positive thinking, cognitive reappraisal, problem solving, and mindfulness support adaptation and coping (Eisma & Strobe, 2021; Prigerson et al., 2023).

RECOVERY-ORIENTED CARE FOR PEOPLE WHO ARE GRIEVING

The individual with uncomplicated grief may not need mental health team intervention. When grief and bereavement become complicated with ongoing psychological and physical stress, mental health interventions can support an adaptive response to the loss.

Teamwork and Collaboration: Working Toward Recovery

Various professionals can provide support during grief. Chaplains are trained to provide spiritual support and their services should be offered to the bereaved. Mental health professionals can provide support and guidance for those experiencing uncomplicated grief as well as complicated bereavement or PGD.

Safety

A priority of concern is always safety. Are there thoughts of suicide? Is depression evident? The individual may need support from a psychiatrist, nurse, psychologist, social worker, counselor, or chaplain.

EVIDENCE-BASED NURSING CARE OF PEOPLE WHO ARE GRIEVING

Nurses will encounter patients and families grieving in all settings. It is important that nurses feel empowered to provide support and compassionate care to anyone experiencing grief (Box 21.4).

RECOGNIZING CUES: RELEVANT ASSESSMENT INFORMATION

The initial assessment determines whether the individual is experiencing anticipatory grief, acute grief, or complicated bereavement. In anticipatory grief, the loved one who is terminally ill is alive, but the caregiver has intense sadness, anger, and loneliness over the changes in the relationship with the patient, loss of shared activities, and plans for the future. In acute grief, there are bouts of yearning, sadness, and other painful emotions that are frequently intense. There may be intrusive thoughts

BOX 21.4

Research for Evidence-Based Practice: Compassionate Nursing Care

Younas, A., Porr, C., Maddigan, J., Moore, J., Navarro, P., & Whitehead, D. (2023). Implementation strategies to promote compassionate nursing care of complex patients: An exploratory sequential mixed methods study. Journal of Nursing Scholarship, *10.1111/jnu.12869. Advance online publication. https://doi.org/10.1111/jnu.12869*

THE QUESTION: What strategies enhance compassionate care for individuals with complex mental and physical health issues?

METHODS: Twenty-three individuals with multiple morbidities were interviewed about their perceptions of barriers to compassionate nursing care. The barriers were categorized and intervention frameworks were developed. Nurses, nurse managers, health care administrators, policymakers, and compassionate care experts ranked the intervention strategies.

FINDINGS: The patient perceived barriers were knowledge, intentions, skills, social influences, behavioral regulation, reinforcement, emotion, and environmental context and resources. The five highest ranked intervention strategies included facilitation, consultation with stress experts, involvement of patients and families, modeling compassion through shadowing, and utilizing implementation teams.

IMPLICATIONS FOR NURSING: Enhancing compassionate care in nursing practice requires support and modeling from other nurses and nurse managers.

and memories and heighted reaction to reminders of the loss. In complicated bereavement, the loss occurred at least 6 months prior, daily functioning is impaired with thoughts, yearning, and memories of the deceased with evidence of difficulty accepting the loss. Emotional pain exists longer than socially acceptable (Duffy & Wild, 2023).

Physical Health and Functioning

The status of physical health will provide clues to the intensity of the grief. Sleep difficulty, lack of appetite, and weight loss can indicate the severity of the grief. Substance use should be determined. One area to determine is how dependent the bereaved was on the deceased for physical care. Who prepared the meals, shopping, or house cleaning?

Cognitions

The thought process should be assessed for negative and maladaptive thoughts. If the individual is protesting the death (death should not have happened; it is not fair; could have prevented death) and has a negative view of the world (bad things happen; no one is safe), they are at risk of maladaptive thoughts that complicate bereavement. An example of other negative cognitions includes needing the individual (i.e., life is unbearable without the individual who died) (Duffy & Wild, 2023).

Emotional and Behavioral Responses

Assessing the individual's emotional state includes determining current mood and behavior. Poor grooming, disheveled appearance, or blank or tearful facial expressions could indicate depression. A suicide risk assessment should be conducted. By asking the question, "Have you wished that you were dead or wished that you could go to sleep and not wake up?", the nurse can determine if further suicide risk assessment should be completed, and the patient referred to a therapist (see Chapters 10 and 22).

Religious/Spiritual Needs

The assessment includes a discussion of the individual's spiritual needs. The nurse should inquire about the importance of spirituality and/or religion and if the bereaved individual is involved in a religious or faith community. The nurse should also ask if they would like these needs to be addressed and by whom (Martins et al., 2024).

Social Functioning and Support

Determining the presence of social support is important as well as determining the level of social functioning. Withdrawal from typical social activities or failure to resume previous activities may indicate the onset of depression.

ANALYZING CUES AND DEVELOPING HYPOTHESES

Patient safety is always a priority. If the patient answers "yes" to suicide risk questions, the individual should be referred to a suicide prevention professional or team. If there is no evidence of suicidal ideation, the nurse should analyze cues for prolonged grief disorder. If the symptoms are present, the nurse would consider PGD as a hypothesis. Other possible hypotheses include anticipatory or uncomplicated grief

PLANNING RECOVERY AND WELLNESS OUTCOMES: GENERATING SOLUTIONS

Once the nurse understands the bereaved's issues, the next step is collaborating with the bereaved and family for planning recovery. The ideal outcome is to resolve the grief and regain a quality life. There are several possible strategies, including referral to mental health professionals, if there is evidence of prolonged grieving. Chaplain support should always be considered and offered. Short-term counseling and community support groups should also be considered.

The nurse should consider physical health needs such as eating and sleeping. If there are changes in these areas, the nurse should consider the availability of food. For an older adult who has lost a spouse or partner, living arrangements could be considered. In many instances, grief may lead to depression because of social isolation and loneliness. Can the bereaved carry out activities of daily living and personal safety without the deceased? Helping the individual manage physical health needs is a priority.

THERAPEUTIC RELATIONSHIP

A positive therapeutic relationship is critical for the bereaved individual. The loss of attachment of a loved one leads to pain and emptiness that will take time to heal. A calm, empathic, and quiet approach of acceptance of the individual's level of pain will promote interaction. Providing an opportunity to share memories about the deceased is not only comforting but also helps to accept the loss. Listening is key. It is important to avoid giving reassurance that everything will be fine. It is appropriate to normalize the grief by reassuring the individual that sadness and yearning are typical. Keeping an open, nonjudgmental attitude will allow the individual to express feelings in a safe environment (Abel et al., 2023).

TAKING ACTION: NURSING INTERVENTIONS

The goal of bereavement interventions is to help the individual adapt and restabilize biopsychosocial–spiritual systems as the pain and sadness lessens with time. Adaptation involves accepting the reality of the loss and restoring a sense of well-being (Abel et al., 2023).

Physical Care

Self-care strategies can range from providing or arranging for physical care for the individual to suggesting resources. Adequate nutrition and sleep are critical to support the individual through bereavement. Strategies include recommending balanced meals and teaching sleep hygiene techniques.

Medications

Short-term reliance on antidepressants or sleep aids may be useful during acute grief. Careful monitoring of the use of medications is needed to prevent long-term use of these medications.

Counseling

Counseling is very beneficial to people experiencing a loss. The counseling goal is to foster adaptive coping and management of painful experiences. The focus of the counseling will be determined by the circumstances of the loss and the relationship of the bereaved to the deceased. If an individual is experiencing anticipatory grief, the nurse identifies the changes associated with the disease and fosters acceptance of the loved one's disease and symptoms. The nurse continues to monitor the health and well-being of the caregiver who may be unaware of the extent of their grief or the toll on their own health. For someone experiencing acute grief, in addition to normalizing the painful, sad feelings, the counseling approaches can encourage engagement with a natural support system or grief support group and focus on ways to live with the reminders of the loss. If prolonged grief is the primary characteristic with impaired functioning and preoccupation with thoughts of the deceased, the individual should be referred to a mental health specialist for further evaluation.

Religious/Spiritual Support

Social support by religious communities as well as religious practices can be important strategies to help the individual and family cope and adapt to the loss. The nurse should demonstrate an openness to the need for religious or spiritual support and facilitate referral to the appropriate religious or spiritual community.

Social Support Strategies

Bereavement can be a highly stressful time with increased physical and psychological demands. This is a time that the bereaved benefit from the support of family, friends, social–cultural, and religious communities. Typical life is suspended, and a new reality gradually evolves. Social support is especially needed after the busy time of planning a funeral or celebration of life is over and the social community gradually withdraws. Loneliness sets in and the full impact of the loss is realized. During this time, the individual is at high risk for suicide. Through social support, the individual can begin thinking about their future and focus on their own self-care and well-being.

The COVID-19 pandemic greatly complicated the grieving process for many because of the lack of face-to-face social support for the surviving family members. Not only were they unable to assist their loved one in dying, but they also did not have access to social support because of restrictions. The consequences of the isolation of the pandemic will be felt for several years.

Evaluation of Patient Outcomes

A positive outcome of bereavement is adaptation to a life without the deceased and learning to live with the reminders of the deceased. Other positive outcomes include attending to self-care and enjoying social and recreational activities again.

DISASTER AND TERRORISM

A disaster is a sudden ecologic or human-made phenomenon that is of sufficient magnitude to require external help to address the psychosocial needs as well as the physical needs of the victims. Acts of terrorism and pandemics present situations that mimic disasters and are categorized as disasters.

> **KEYCONCEPT** A **disaster** is a sudden, overwhelming, catastrophic event that causes great damage and destruction, that may involve mass casualties and human suffering requiring assistance from all available resources.

Although disasters can affect all members of a society, the most affected are the victims and survivors of the event, as well as nurses and others who are first to respond to the traumatic and life-threatening consequences of the event. The mental health of the survivors of disasters can be severely impacted by the event. Fear, anger, and distress elevate severe anxiety to the panic level, which can result in severe mental illnesses. Unresolved crises or disastrous events can lead to disorganized thinking. Postdisaster depression is a real risk (First, 2024). In addition, the victims may experience the development of acute stress disorder (which has a strong emphasis on dissociative symptoms) and posttraumatic stress disorder (PTSD).

HISTORICAL PERSPECTIVES OF DISASTERS IN THE UNITED STATES

Throughout history, disasters have been portrayed from a fatalistic perspective that humans have little control over catastrophic events. Some cultures contend that natural disasters are acts of God. Other cultures express their belief that natural disaster events can be attributed to gods dwelling within places such as volcanoes, with eruptions being an expression of the gods' anger. Although often caused by nature, disasters can have human origins. Wars and civil disturbances that destroy homelands and displace people are included among the causes of disasters. Other causes include a building collapse, blizzard, drought, earthquake, epidemic, explosion, famine, fire, flood, hazardous material or transportation incident (such as a chemical spill), hurricane, nuclear incident, terrorist attack, and tornado. Often, the unpredictability of such disasters causes fear, confusion, and stress that can have lasting effects on the health of affected communities and their sense of well-being.

TYPES OF DISASTERS

The types of disasters discussed in this chapter include natural disasters, terrorism, and the COVID-19 pandemic.

Natural Disasters

Climate change is a major threat to global public and mental health. The disastrous fires in the American West in 2023, Hurricane Ian in Florida (2022), Hurricane Maria in Puerto Rico in 2018, Hurricane Harvey in Texas in 2017, and the earthquake and tsunami in Indonesia in 2018 highlight the need for government attention to address climate change and the biologic threat of pandemics (Catton, 2023). In the United States, the lack of government response and breakdown in communication during Hurricanes Irma and Maria resulted in thousands of hurricane victims being displaced and injured. Many Puerto Ricans moved to Florida and experienced more emotional and psychological issues than those staying on the island (Purtle et al., 2023). The Japan earthquake disaster in 2011 became a cascade of disasters, resulting in the death of thousands of residents and contamination from the damaged nuclear site. Consequences of these disasters will still be occurring months and years after the initial events.

Terrorism

In recent history, we have experienced several attacks of violence and terrorism that are unprecedented in North America. Some examples are the Texas elementary school shooting in 2022; the Pittsburgh synagogue shooting in 2019, destruction of the World Trade Center in New York on September 11, 2001, the Sandy Hook school tragedy in 2012, and the Boston Marathon bombing in 2013, all of which shattered North Americans' sense of safety and security.

Since September 11, 2001, the emergency response planning of federal, state, and local agencies has focused on possible terrorist attacks with chemical, biologic, radiologic, nuclear, or high-yield explosive weapons. Before September 11, 2001, government agencies and public health leaders had not incorporated mental health into their overall response plans to bioterrorism. But in the aftermath of the mass destruction of human life and property in 2001, government and health care leaders are recognizing the need for monumental mental health efforts to be implemented during episodes of terrorism and disaster. The psychological and behavioral consequences of a terrorist attack are now included in most disaster plans.

COVID-19 Pandemic

In December 2019, the Wuhan Municipal Health Commission announced an outbreak of severe acute respiratory syndrome coronavirus 2 (SARS-CoV-2). The virus quickly spread globally and in 2020, World Health Organization (WHO) declared COVID-19 a pandemic and the United States declared a National Emergency. In the United States, an unprepared health care system was quickly overloaded with critically ill patients who needed ICU beds that did not exist. There was a lack of prepared health care workers who were quickly overwhelmed. Mortality rates were high, especially among people experiencing poverty, older adults, and those with comorbidities. Health care and public health care systems are trying to confront this disease around the globe (Boccellino, 2023).

Although classified as a disaster, COVID-19 is different from a natural disaster that is time limited. The physical and psychosocial consequences for the affected individuals, survivors, health care workers, and community are unprecedented. The effects will be felt for many years and societies will be forever changed.

PHASES OF DISASTER

Long-term mental health consequences are evident in most disasters. Natural and human-made disaster can be conceptualized in three phases:

1. *Prewarning of the disaster.* This phase entails preparing the community for possible evacuation of the environment, mobilization of resources, and review of community disaster plans. In some disasters, such as in the 2011 earthquake in Japan, there was very little warning. In other instances, such as the COVID-19 pandemic, there were unheeded warnings more than a decade before the disease appeared.
2. *A disaster event occurs.* In this phase, the rescuers provide resources, assistance, and support as needed to preserve the biopsychosocial functioning and survival of the victims. In large disasters, the rescuers and health care professionals also experience the traumatic event as both residents and health care providers. The victims experience the initial trauma and threats that occur immediately after the disaster such as confusion (communication breakdown), lack of safety (no available law enforcement), and lack of health care services.
3. *Recuperative effort.* In the third phase, the focus is on implementing strategies for healing sick and injured people, preventing complications of health issues, repairing damages, and reconstructing the community. The disruption effects can be traumatic to the community residents. The debris, lack of trust of the government, fragmentation of families, financial problems, lack of adequate housing, inadequate temporary housing, and fear of another disaster contribute to the long-term negative effects of disasters.

Responses to Disaster

Psychiatric nurses encounter three different types of disaster victims. The first category is the victims who may or may not survive. If they survive, the victims often experience severe physical injuries. The more serious the physical injury, the more likely the victim will experience a mental health issue such as PTSD, depression, anxiety, or other mental health issues (Kim & Lee, 2023). Victims and families need ongoing health care to prevent complications related to both their physical and mental health.

The second category of victims includes the professional rescuers. These are people who are less likely to experience physical injury but who often experience psychological stress. The professional rescuers, such as police officers, firefighters, nurses, and so on, have more effective coping skills than do volunteer rescuers who are not prepared for the emotional impact of a disaster. However, many professional responders report experiencing PTSD for many months after the traumatic event in which they were involved (Seidman et al., 2024).

The third category includes everyone else involved in the disaster. Psychological effects may be experienced worldwide by millions of people as they experience terrorism or disaster vicariously or as direct victims of the terrorism/disaster event. After an act of terrorism, most people will experience some psychological stress, including an altered sense of safety, hypervigilance, sadness, anger, fear, decreased concentration, and difficulty sleeping. Others may alter their behavior by traveling less, staying at home, avoiding public events, keeping children out of school, or increasing smoking and alcohol use. After Hurricane Maria, many were without electrical power, and more than half of the households sustained severe damage. In the aftermath, schools were closed, and jobs were lost. Families were subject to diseases, dependency on aid, and exposure to heat and humidity. Residents experienced an increase in the significant symptoms associated with depression, generalized anxiety, or posttraumatic stress (Stukova et al., 2023).

RECOVERY-ORIENTED CARE FOR PEOPLE EXPERIENCING DISASTER

Once a disaster occurs, health care workers respond to the emergency. The type of disaster (flood, fire, tornado, shooting) will determine the need for emergency health care workers.

Teamwork and Collaboration: Working Toward Recovery

In an acute disaster situation, the emergency response team takes the lead. Other helpers should allow the response team to direct the triage and work of health care workers. Security personnel will also be present to provide leadership to the response and rescue efforts.

Safety

Victims experiencing head injuries or psychic trauma after a disaster may have to be hospitalized. During a disaster, a victim with a mental illness may experience regression to their pretreatment condition. If community mental health facilities are available, individuals should be directed to seek assistance from mental health care professionals. The victims should receive follow-up care for the disaster response.

EVIDENCE-BASED NURSING CARE OF PEOPLE EXPERIENCING DISASTERS

As community members, nurses become a part of the disaster team. No matter the specialty, nurses are called to help with medical and mental health emergencies. They may assist with first-aid treatment or triage, or provide a high level of nursing care to support lifesaving activities and prevent additional casualties.

RECOGNIZING CUES: RELEVANT ASSESSMENT INFORMATION

The nurse should assess the kind and severity of a natural or human-made disaster or terrorist act to determine the capability of individuals and communities to respond in a supportive way. Assessment includes the ages of the victims, gender, their capability to participate in problem-solving activities related to the devastation left by the disaster, and their level of self-confidence or self-esteem. The nurse should maintain a calm demeanor, obtain and distribute information about the disaster and the victims, and reunite victims and their families. In addition, there is a need to monitor the news media's impact on the mental health of the victims of the crisis. Sometimes the persistence of the news media diminishes the ability of the survivors to achieve closure to the crisis. Constant rehashing of the disaster in the newspapers, television, and online can initiate feelings of anxiety and depression, or increase and prolong the severity of these feelings (Pfefferbaum et al., 2021).

People assigned female at birth exhibit higher levels of distress after a disaster than those assigned male at birth, especially those in this population who are pregnant or older adults (Howells et al., 2023; Ide-Okochi et al., 2024). Children are especially vulnerable to disasters and respond according to their ages and family experiences. Traumatized children and adolescents are high-risk victims of a wide range of behavioral, psychological, and neurologic issues after experiencing various traumatic events (Adu et al., 2023).

Physical Health and Functioning

The nurse should assess physical reactions that may involve many changes in body functions, such as tachycardia, tachypnea, profuse perspiration, nausea, vomiting, dilated pupils, and extreme shakiness. Virtually any organ may be involved. Some victims may exhibit panic reactions and loss of control and have a total disregard for their personal safety. The victims may be suicidal or homicidal and are at high risk for injuries that may include infection, trauma, and head injuries. During the rescue, medical care is a priority. Any medical or psychiatric disorders should be assessed, and information communicated to the rest of the health care team. Unexplained physical symptoms such as headache, fatigue, pain, chest pain, and gastrointestinal disturbances should be included in the assessment.

Mental Status

During a disaster, fear and hopelessness can immobilize victims. The victims may suffer from loss of feelings of well-being and various psychological issues, including panic responses, anxiety, and fear. Dissociation and fear are predictive of later developing PTSD and depressive symptoms. Victims witnessing others suffer are especially at high risk for future mental health issues and should be assessed for the details of the disaster (Lennon et al., 2023).

Emotional and Behavioral Responses

The survivors of the disaster may experience traumatic grief because of their feelings of guilt that they survived the disaster (Bistas & Grewal, 2023). Responses to psychological distress need to be differentiated from any psychiatric illness that the individual may be experiencing. The response to a disaster may leave the individual feeling overwhelmed, incapacitated, and disoriented.

The victims should be assessed for behaviors that indicate a depressed state, presence of confusion, uncontrolled weeping or screaming, disorientation, or aggressive behavior. Ideally, the nurse should assess the coping strategies the victim usually uses to manage stressful situations.

Social Functioning and Support

Cultural values and beliefs help define the significance and meaning of a disaster. In some instances, a disaster can slow physical and psychosocial development, but usually the customs, beliefs, and value systems remain the same. It is important that first responders and health care teams are sensitive to the cultural and religious beliefs of the community. In many instances, victims' spiritual beliefs and religious faith help them cope with the disaster.

In a disaster, the victims may experience economic distress because of job loss and loss of other resources. This may ultimately lead to psychological distress. In addition, acts of aggression and other mental health issues may emerge (Medina-Mora et al., 2023). Again, shelter, money, and food may not be available. The absence of basic human needs such as food, a place to live, or immediate transportation quickly becomes a priority that may precipitate acts of violence.

Religious/Spiritual Needs

During a disaster, spiritual needs are often paramount. Death, injury, and destruction of property leave individuals, families, and communities trying to find meaning and solace from the destruction. Religious and spiritual leaders may not be readily available. As the nurse conduct assessments, spiritual needs should be determined.

ANALYZING CUES AND DEVELOPING HYPOTHESES

Because the responses to disaster are so varied, assessment data are critical. What is the disaster—tsunami, terrorism, or pandemic? The nurse should be knowledgeable about the consequences of a particular disaster and identify the presence of expected symptoms or behaviors related to the disaster. The nurse then summarizes these symptoms, assuring the individual that they commonly occur during disasters.

PLANNING RECOVERY AND WELLNESS OUTCOMES: GENERATING SOLUTIONS

Priorities for people who are acutely affected include maintaining life systems and treating physical injuries. Depending on the long-term impact of the disaster and the type of disaster, the nurse will identify coping skills, support systems, and referral sources. The nurse should collaborate with the individual to seek assistance for physical and mental health disorders.

THERAPEUTIC RELATIONSHIP

Therapeutic communication is key to understanding the extent of the psychological responses to a disaster and to establishing a bridge of trust that communicates respect, commitment, and acceptance. Developing rapport with the victim communicates reassurance and support.

TAKING ACTION: NURSING INTERVENTIONS

The goals of care include helping the victims prioritize and match available resources with their needs, preventing further complications, monitoring the environment, disseminating information, and implementing disease-control strategies. People with preexisting mental health conditions should continue with their treatment plans during an emergency and monitor for any new symptoms (Centers for Disease Control and Prevention [CDC], 2023). Nursing interventions focus on the individual, family, and community.

Physical Care

Any physiologic issues or injuries should be treated quickly. During the emergency response, people will be triaged to the appropriate level of care. Victims who are primarily distressed and may have somatic symptoms will be treated after those suffering from exposure with critical injuries. The primary public health concern is clean drinking water, food, shelter, and medical care. In natural disasters, contaminated water and food and lack of shelter and medical care may worsen illnesses that already exist. In pandemics, the primary public health concern is stopping the spread of the disease, which means isolation of infected individuals and quarantine of contacts. For communities, a pandemic means mass home-confinement directives—new to Americans.

All patients, families, and communities need to be reassured of the caring and commitment of the nurse to their safety, comfort, and well-being throughout the triage process. Ideally, a mental health specialist is an integral member of the triage team. Many of the same interventions used for people experiencing stress or crisis will be used for these victims. See also Chapter 33 for discussion of somatization. Victims should be encouraged to do necessary chores and participate in decision making.

Medications

During the treatment process for the psychological consequences of the disaster, it may become necessary to administer an antianxiety medication or sedative, especially in the early phases of recovery.

Counseling

After the initial interventions, the nurse should support the development of resilience, coping, and recovery while providing technical assistance, training, and consultation. A useful model is the **ABCs of psychological first aid** that focuses on A (arousal), B (behavior), and C (cognition). When arousal is present, the intervention goal is to decrease excitement by providing safety, comfort, and consolation. When atypical or irrational behavior is present, survivors should be assisted to function more effectively in the disaster; and when cognitive disorientation occurs, reality testing and clear information should be provided. In the initial phases, the nurse should assist the victim in focusing on the reality of issues that are immediate, with specific goals that are consistent with available resources as well as the culture and lifestyle of the victim.

Debriefing (the reconstruction of the traumatic events by the victim) may be helpful for some. Long a common practice, debriefing was believed to be necessary in order for the individual to develop a healthy perspective of the event and ultimately prevent PTSD. However, debriefing is not useful for everyone. Additionally, cultural groups respond differently to traumatic events. Therefore, compulsory debriefing is not recommended. If the victim has symptoms of PTSD, referral to a mental health clinic for additional evaluation and treatment is important (see Chapter 29).

The nurse should prepare the victim for recovery by teaching about the effects of stress and helping the victim identify personal strengths and coping skills. Positive coping skills should be supported. The victims should be encouraged to report any depression, anxiety, or interpersonal difficulty during the recovery period. After most disasters, support groups are established that help victims and their families deal with the psychological effects of the disaster.

Psychoeducation

When the nurse explains anticipated reactions and behaviors, this helps the victims gain control and improve coping. For example, after a major disaster, they may have excessive worry, preoccupation with the event, and changes in eating and sleeping patterns. With time, counseling, and group work, these symptoms will lessen. Active coping strategies can be presented in multiple media forums, such as television and radio. After the initial shock, victims react by trying to do something to resolve the situation. When victims begin working to remedy the disaster situation, their physical responses become less exaggerated, and they are more able to work with less tension and fear.

Educating the public about the natural recovery process is important. Information gaps and rumors add to the anxiety and stress of the situation. Giving information and direction helps the public and victims to use the coping skills they already possess. Initially, the event may leave individuals and families in a stage of ambiguity with frantic, disorganized behavior. In addition, individuals and family members are concerned about their own physical and psychological responses to the disastrous event.

Religious/Spiritual Support

During a disaster, the nurse can offer comfort and hope. In some instances, the faith community may be prepared to respond to the disaster and religious leaders will be available. If spiritual or religious needs are identified, the nurse can request assistance from the chaplain or religious leader (if available). If neither is available, the nurse can express empathy and support interpersonal connections during this difficult period.

Community Care

Outreach is especially important because research shows that disaster victims do not access mental health systems. Peer-delivered mental health services are especially effective in identifying and connecting with victims, especially those with predisaster psychiatric issues (Kosoko et al., 2023).

Family support systems may need to be reestablished. The health care community should actively reach out to the media and keep the press engaged. Direct attention to stories that inform and help the public respond should be encouraged. Some federal agencies assist victims of disasters. This assistance is available for individuals, families, and communities. One of these agencies is the Federal Emergency Management Agency (FEMA). When a disaster occurs, FEMA sends a team of specialists who review the devastation of disaster. They provide counseling and mental health services and arrange for many of the victims to access other services needed for survival, including training programs. In addition, the Substance Abuse and Mental Health Services Administration (SAMHSA) of the Department of Health and Human Services is available to assist both victims of and responders to the disaster. When a disaster disrupts the victim's social network, other resources must be made available for social support.

The social support system provides an environment in which the victims experience respect and caring from the caregivers, the opportunity to ventilate and examine personal feelings regarding the tragedy, and the opportunity to begin the healing and recovery process. Supporting the development of more contacts within the social network can be done by organizing support groups within the area of the disaster that address grief and loss, trauma, psychoeducational needs, and substance misuse. In addition, the nurse may refer the victims to nearby support groups that are appropriate to meet their needs.

Evaluation of Patient Outcomes

To determine the effectiveness of nursing interventions, the nurse should evaluate the outcomes based on the success of resolution of the disaster. The outcomes will depend on the specific disaster and its meaning (appraisal) to the survivors. For example, are the survivors in a safe place? Are the victims able to cope with the disaster? Were the appropriate supports given, so that the victims could draw upon their own strengths?

SUMMARY OF KEY POINTS

- A crisis is a time-limited event that occurs when coping mechanisms fail to provide adaptive skills to address a perceived challenge or threat.
- Grief is a natural, intense physical, emotional, social, and cognitive response to loss, and bereavement is the process of healing after a loss. The variations in grief are influenced by the characteristics of the individual, perceived relationship to the deceased, and the type of loss.
- Stage theories propose that grief and bereavement follow stages/phases. Process models explain bereavement as nonlinear.
- For most people, bereavement is uncomplicated and there is no need for counseling. Complicated grief occurs in less than 16% of bereaved individuals. Interventions such as medication, counseling, and/or a support group may be required for this group.
- Interventions are designed to support people through crises by helping them understand the process of recovery and identify the resources they need and how to get them.
- Disaster is a sudden, overwhelming catastrophic event that causes great damage and may cause mass casualties and human suffering that require assistance from all available resources.
- Depending on the disaster, interventions are provided to individuals, families, and communities.

DEVELOPING CLINICAL JUDGMENT

1. An 18-year-old patient was admitted to the emergency department for a broken arm and jaw following a physical fight with their partner. The patient is now unhoused, estranged from their family, and has no money. The patient is crying that they will have no life now that they have been kicked out of the home shared with their partner. Once physical injuries are treated, what should be the nurse's next step?
2. A 24-year-old single individual with bipolar disorder moves into an apartment after the death of their mother. The individual continues to take their medication but feels sad about their mother's death. The individual is not adjusting well to living alone and tells the nurse that they no longer want to go to work and feels they would be better off joining their mother. The nurse generates the following hypothesis: Patient is grieving their mother and does not have a positive coping skill to address his grief. What are the nursing priorities for this patient? Outline a care plan for this patient.
3. Discuss the role of medication and counseling when used in crisis or bereavement.
4. Compare uncomplicated bereavement to complicated bereavement. How would you recognize the difference? When would it be appropriate to refer a bereaved individual to a support group or mental health specialist?
5. There is a terrorist threat in your community. A patient appears in the emergency department convinced that they are going to die. How would you proceed with assessing this patient?
6. A patient was recently diagnosed with COVID-19. The patient refused the vaccine because they do not believe in vaccines. The patient is showing fear about treatment and guilt about not taking the vaccine because they are afraid about transmitting the disease to her family. What is the first priority in providing care once the patient is medically stable?

MOVIES, TV, OR STREAMING PROGRAMS

Good Grief: **2023.** Marc's (Dan Levy) world shatters when his husband Oliver suddenly dies, sending him into a year of complicated grief. Marc's two best friends Sophie (Ruth Negga) and Thomas (Himesh Patel) provide unconditional support to him to help him deal with his grief. At the 1-year anniversary, Marc finally opens last year's Christmas card that contains a disturbing message. Marc, Sophie, and Thomas embark on a soul-searching trip to Paris that reveals some hard truths they each needed to face.

Viewing Points:

1. What makes Marc's bereavement complicated or prolonged grief disorder?
2. How was Marc's grief complicated by the message in the Christmas card?
3. How did the three friends grow emotionally after being honest with each other?

Unfolding Patient Stories: George Palo • Part 1

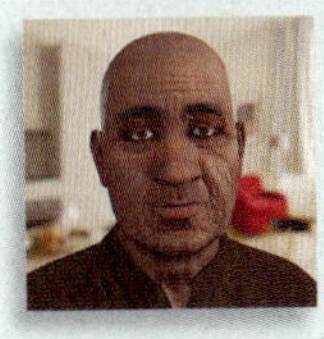

George Palo, age 90, was diagnosed 6 months ago with minor neurocognitive impairment, Alzheimer type. He lives independently in an apartment within a retirement community. His wife of 65 years died 3 years ago. He was managing well until the recent loss of his 13-year-old dog. How might the nurse assess his grieving and symptoms of depression? How can his grief complicate his cognitive disorder? What are the nurse's considerations in assessing George's cognition? How can the nurse develop a treatment plan to help George progress through grief and bereavement? (George Palo's story continues in Chapter 38.)

Care for George Palo and other patients in a realistic virtual environment: ***vSim** for Nursing* (thepoint.lww.com/vSimMentalHealth). Practice documenting these patients' care in DocuCare (thepoint.lww.com/DocuCareEHR).

REFERENCES

Abel, J., Kellehear, A., & Aoun, S. M. (2023). Bereavement care reimagined. *Annals of Palliative Medicine, 12*(4), 816–825. https://doi.org/10.21037/apm-23-24

Ahn, S. Y., Yu, S., Kim, J. E., & Song, I. H. (2023). The relationship between suicide bereavement and suicide ideation: Analysis of the mediating effect of complicated grief. *Journal of Affective Disorders, 331*, 43–49. https://doi.org/10.1016/j.jad.2023.03.008

Adu, M. K., Agyapong, B., & Agyapong, V. I. O. (2023). Children's psychological reactions to wildfires: A review of recent literature. *Current Psychiatry Reports, 25*(11), 603–616. https://doi.org/10.1007/s11920-023-01451-7

American Psychiatric Association (APA). (2022). *Diagnostic and statistical manual of mental disorders, fifth edition, text revision*. Washington, DC, Author.

Bistas, K., & Grewal, R. (2023). The intricacies of survivor's guilt: Exploring its phenomenon across contexts. *Cureus, 15*(9), e45703. https://doi.org/10.7759/cureus.45703

Boccellino, M. (2023). COVID-19 pandemic: Therapeutic strategies and vaccines. *International Journal of Molecular Sciences, 25*(1), 556. https://doi.org/10.3390/ijms25010556

Caplan, G. (1961). *An approach to community mental health*. Grune & Stratton.

Catton, H. (2023). Nursing our planet. *International Nursing Review, 70*(1), 7–9. https://doi.org/10.1111/inr.12825

Centers for Disease Control and Prevention. (2023). *Natural disasters and severe weather*. Retrieved February 11, 2024, from https://www.cdc.gov/disasters/index.html

Comtesse, H., Smid, G. E., Rummel, A. M., Spreeuwenberg, P., Lundorff, M., & Dückers, M. L. A. (2024). Cross-national analysis of the prevalence of prolonged grief disorder. *Journal of Affective Disorders, 350*, 359–365. https://doi.org/10.1016/j.jad.2024.01.094

Daniel, T. (2023). The stubborn persistence of grief stage theory. *Omega*, 302228221149801. https://doi.org/10.1177/00302228221149801

Denckla, C. A., Hahn, J., Cowden, R. G., Ho, S., Gao, K., Espinosa Dice, A. L., Jha, S. C., Kang, J. H., & Shear, M. K. (2023). Bereavement, memorial attendance, and mental health during the COVID-19 P\pandemic: Longitudinal results from the Nurses' Health Study. *The American Journal of Geriatric Psychiatry, 31*(12), 1045–1057. https://doi.org/10.1016/j.jagp.2023.06.012

Duffy, M., & Wild, J. (2023). Living with loss: A cognitive approach to prolonged grief disorder—incorporating complicated, enduring and traumatic grief. *Behavioural and Cognitive Psychotherapy, 51*(6), 645–658. https://doi.org/10.1017/S1352465822000674

Eisma, M. C., & Stroebe, M. S. (2021). Emotion regulatory strategies in complicated grief: A systematic review. *Behavior Therapy, 52*(1), 234–249. https://doi.org/10.1016/j.beth.2020.04.004

Eisma, M. C., de Lang, T. A., & Stroebe, M. S. (2022). Restoration-oriented stressors of bereavement. *Anxiety, Stress, and Coping, 35*(3), 339–353. https://doi.org/10.1080/10615806.2021.1957849

Fiore, J. (2021). A systematic review of the dual process model of coping with bereavement (1999–2016). *Omega, 84*(2), 414–458. https://doi.org/10.1177/0030222819893139

First, J. M. (2024). Post-traumatic stress and depression following disaster: Examining the mediating role of disaster resilience. *Frontiers in Public Health, 12*, 1272909. https://doi.org/10.3389/fpubh.2024.1272909

Hilberdink, C. E., Ghainder, K., Dubanchet, A., Hinton, D., Djelantik, A. A. A. M. J., Hall, B. J., & Bui, E. (2023). Bereavement issues and prolonged grief disorder: A global perspective. *Global Mental Health, 10*, e32. https://doi.org/10.1017/gmh.2023.28

Howells, M., Wander, K., Rivera, L., Arfouni, C., Benhelal, O., Galeano, M. A. O., Schultz, L., Flock, N., & Dancause, K. (2023). Maternal stress and hair cortisol among pregnant women following hurricane Florence. *American Journal of Human Biology, 35*(1), e23847. https://doi.org/10.1002/ajhb.23847

Ide-Okochi, A., He, M., Kanamori, Y., Samiso, T., Takamoto, K., & Murayama, H. (2024). Gender differences in the association between psychological distress and sociability among older adult survivors: Cross-sectional survey four years after the 2016 Kumamoto earthquake in Japan. *The Tohoku journal of experimental medicine, 262*(3), 143–155. https://doi.org/10.1620/tjem.2024.J003

Kim, Y., & Lee, E. (2023). The suicidal ideation of disaster victims: A nationwide cross-sectional study. *Psychology Research and Behavior Management, 16*, 905–914. https://doi.org/10.2147/PRBM.S405667

Kokou-Kpolou, C. K., Lenferink, L. I. M., Brunnet, A. E., Park, S., Megalakaki, O., Boelen, P., & Cénat, J. M. (2022). The ICD-11 and DSM-5-TR prolonged grief criteria: Validation of the Traumatic Grief Inventory-Self Report Plus using exploratory factor analysis and item response theory. *Clinical Psychology & Psychotherapy, 29*(6), 1950–1962. https://doi.org/10.1002/cpp.2765

Kosoko, A. A., Walia, S., & Huebinger, R. (2023). Emergency department virtual happy hour: A novel approach to peer group support during a pandemic. *Cureus, 15*(2), e35321. https://doi.org/10.7759/cureus.35321

Kübler-Ross, E. (1969). *On death and dying*. Macmillan Publishing Company.

Kübler-Ross, E., & Kessler, D. (2005). *On grief and grieving: Finding the meaning of grief through the five stages of loss*. Scribner.

Larsen, L. H., Guldberg, A., & Kring, V. (2023). A group therapy program for parentally bereaved young adults with grief complications: Rationale, method and case examples. *Omega, 86*(4), 1212–1234. https://doi.org/10.1177/0030222821997705

Lennon, T., Kemal, S., Heffernan, M. E., Bendelow, A., Sheehan, K., Davis, M. M., & Macy, M. L. (2023). Childhood exposure to firearm violence in Chicago and its impact on mental health. *Academic Pediatrics, 24*(6), 982–986. https://doi.org/10.1016/j.acap.2023.12.001

Martins, H., Romeiro, J., Casaleiro, T., Vieira, M., & Caldeira, S. (2024). Insights on spirituality and bereavement: A systematic review of qualitative studies. *Journal of Clinical Nursing, 33*(5), 1593–1603. https://doi.org/10.1111/jocn.17052

Medina-Mora, M. E., Kulis, S. S., Real, T., Nuño-Gutiérrez, B. L., Corona, M. D., Cutrín, O., & Marsiglia, F. F. (2023). The impact of major earthquakes on students' emotional distress and internalizing symptoms, externalizing behaviors, and coping during the implementation of keepin' it REAL-Mexico. *Prevention Science, 25*(2), 256–266. https://doi.org/10.1007/s11121-023-01542-0

Palm, S., Doering, B. K., Kubiak, T., Geschke, K., Fellgiebel, A., & Wuttke, A. (2023). Influence of loss- and restoration-oriented stressors on grief in times of COVID-19. *Scientific Reports, 13*(1), 19584. https://doi.org/10.1038/s41598-023-46403-6

Pfefferbaum, B., Palka, J. M., & North, C. S. (2021). Associations between news media coverage of the 11 September attacks and depression in employees of New York City area businesses. *Behavioral Sciences, 11*(3), 29. https://doi.org/10.3390/bs11030029

Prigerson, H. G., Singer, J., & Killikelly, C. (2023). Prolonged grief disorder: Addressing misconceptions with evidence. *The American Journal of Geriatric Psychiatry, 32*(5), 527–534. https://doi.org/10.1016/j.jagp.2023.10.020

Purtle, J., Rivera-González, A. C., Mercado, D. L., Barajas, C. B., Chavez, L., Canino, G., & Ortega, A. N. (2023). Growing inequities in mental health crisis services offered to indigent patients in Puerto Rico versus the US states before and after Hurricanes Maria and Irma. *Health Services Research, 58*(2), 325–331. https://doi.org/10.1111/1475-6773.14092

Seidman, A. J., Born, W., & Corriveau, E. (2024). First responders during COVID-19: Career calling, PTSD, and work self-efficacy. *American Journal of Preventive Medicine, 66*(6), 1017–1023. https://doi.org/10.1016/j.amepre.2024.01.001

Stroebe, M., & Schut, H. (2015). Family matters in bereavement: Toward an integrative intra-interpersonal coping model. *Perspectives on Psychological Science, 10*(6), 873–879.

Stroebe, M., Schut, H., & Boerner, K. (2010). Continuing bonds in adaptation to bereavement: Toward theoretical integration. *Clinical Psychology Review, 30*, 259–268.

Stukova, M., Cardona, G., Tormos, A., Vega, A., Burgos, G., Inostroza-Nieves, Y., & Carl, Y. (2023). Mental health and associated risk factors of Puerto Rico post-hurricane María. *Social Psychiatry and Psychiatric Epidemiology, 58*(7), 1055–1063. https://doi.org/10.1007/s00127-023-02458-4

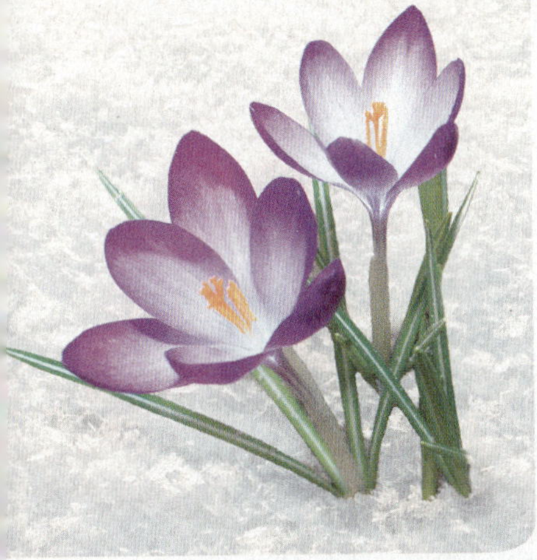

22 Suicide Prevention

Screening, Assessment, and Intervention*

Rebecca Luebbert

KEYCONCEPTS

- hopelessness
- lethality
- suicide

LEARNING OBJECTIVES

After studying this chapter, you will be able to:

1. Identify suicide as a major mental health issue worldwide.
2. Define *suicide, suicidality, suicide attempt*, and *suicidal ideation.*
3. Differentiate suicidality and nonsuicidal self-injury.
4. Describe population groups that have high rates of suicide.
5. Describe the individual, relationship, community, and social risk and protective factors associated with suicide.
6. Identify key factors associated with specific suicide acts.
7. Describe evidence-based interventions used to reduce imminent and ongoing suicide risk.
8. Explain the importance of documentation and reporting when caring for patients who may be at risk of suicide.

KEY TERMS

• acquired capability for suicide • case finding • commitment to treatment statement • ideation-to-action theories • nonsuicidal self-injury • perceived burdensomeness • suicidal ideation • suicidality • suicide attempt • suicide cluster • suicide contagion • thwarted belongingness

INTRODUCTION

Suicide is a major public health concern in the United States, accounting for a little over 48,000 deaths in 2021 (American Foundation for Suicide Prevention [AFSP], 2023). Suicide rates have steadily increased in the past 25 years, with a 37% increase in the total suicide rate from 2000 to 2018. Although rates decreased 5% between 2018 and 2020, they nearly returned to their peak in 2021 (Stone et al., 2023). The public health issue of suicidal behavior is so important that several goals identified in Healthy People 2030 directly target the reduction of deaths by suicide (U.S. Department of Health and Human Services [U.S. DHHS], n.d.).

Suicide is so rejected in contemporary society that people with strong suicidal thoughts often do not seek treatment for fear of being discriminated against or stigmatized by others. Reports and portrayals of suicide in the popular media and television further stigmatize those who consider or attempt suicide. Society's unwillingness to talk openly about suicide also contributes to the common misperceptions resulting in many myths regarding suicide (McGrath et al., 2023; Sufrate-Sorzano et al., 2023; Thomas et al., 2023). Table 22.1 presents several myths and facts about suicide.

Suicides are preventable deaths when immediate friends and family and health care providers identify symptoms and use effective interventions. All practicing nurses will come into contact with patients who are thinking about suicide and often can prevent suicides by identifying and intervening with those at risk. Through individual and public education, nurses also can do much to demystify suicide and reduce stigma for those at risk. To reduce the devastating public impact of suicide on those at risk and their families, nurses must be knowledgeable about

*In this chapter, "male" refers to a person assigned male at birth, and "female" refers to a person assigned female at birth.

TABLE 22.1 MYTHS AND FACTS ABOUT SUICIDE

Myth	Fact
Suicide affects only individuals with a mental health condition.	Many individuals with mental illness are not affected by suicidal thoughts, and not all people who attempt or die by suicide have mental illness.
Most suicides happen suddenly without warning.	Warning signs, verbally or behaviorally, precede most suicides.
People who die by suicide are selfish and take the easy way out.	Typically, people do not die by suicide because they do not want to live. People die by suicide because they want to end their suffering.
When people become suicidal, they will always be suicidal.	Active suicidal ideation is often short term and situation specific. Although suicidal thoughts can return, they are not permanent.
Talking about suicide will lead to and encourage suicide.	Talking about suicide not only reduces the stigma of talking about it but also allows individuals to seek help, rethink their opinions, and share their story with others.

Adapted with permission from Fuller, K. (2020). Five common myths about suicide debunked. https://nami.org/Blogs/NAMI-Blog/September-2020/5-Common-Myths-About-Suicide-Debunked

suicide and be able to implement effective preventive interventions. This chapter contains tools that can be used to reduce the broad effects of suicide and provide appropriate care for patients who are suicidal.

SUICIDE AND SUICIDE ATTEMPT

KEYCONCEPT Suicide is the voluntary act of killing oneself. It is a fatal, self-inflicted destructive act with explicit or inferred intent to die. It is sometimes called suicide completion.

This behavioral definition of suicide is limited and does not consider the complexity of potential underlying mental illness, personal motivations, and situational and family factors that provoke the suicide act. Except for the very young, suicide occurs in all age groups, social classes, and cultures (National Institute of Mental Health [NIMH], 2024).

The term **suicidality** refers to all suicide-related behaviors and thoughts of attempting or completing suicide and suicidal ideation. **Suicidal ideation** is thinking about and planning one's own death. In 2021, 4.8% of adults aged 18 and older had serious thoughts of suicide, with the highest prevalence among young adults aged 18 to 25 (13%) (NIMH, 2024). Population studies show that suicidal ideation varies depending on characteristics of the participants and the way suicidal ideation is measured. Although suicidal ideation often does not progress, having recurrent suicidal ideation is associated with poor mental health (Cantor et al., 2023).

A suicide attempt is a nonfatal, self-inflicted destructive act with explicit or implicit intent to die. In 2021, an estimated 1.7 million Americans attempted suicide, with adult females reporting an attempt 1.3 times more often than males (AFSP, 2023). Suicidal ideation, a previous suicide attempt, and psychiatric illness are significant predictors of a completed suicide (Favril et al., 2023).

Nonsuicidal self-injury (NSSI) is a voluntary, apparent attempt at suicide, commonly called a suicidal gesture or parasuicide, in which the aim is not death (e.g., taking a sublethal drug). NSSI behavior varies by intent. Some people truly wish to die, but others simply wish to feel nothing for a while. Still others want to send a message about their emotional state. NSSI behavior is never expected and should always be taken seriously.

KEYCONCEPT Lethality refers to the probability that a person will successfully complete suicide. Lethality is determined by the seriousness of the person's intent and the likelihood that the planned method of death will succeed. A plan to use an accessible firearm to die by suicide has greater lethality than a suicide plan that involves superficial cuts of the wrist.

Suicide is ranked as the 11th leading cause of death and accounts for 14 deaths per 100,000 population. On average, 132 Americans die by suicide each day, with a suicide occurring every 11 minutes in the United States. Mountain regions have the highest rate of suicide (Fig. 22.1). Its overall prevalence may be underestimated because suicide can be disguised as vehicular accidents or homicide, especially in young people (AFSP, 2023; Centers for Disease Control and Prevention [CDC], 2023).

Suicide Across the Life Span

Children, Adolescents, and Young Adults

Suicide is the second leading cause of death among those aged 10 to 14 and 25 to 34, and the third leading cause of death in individuals 15 to 24. Bullying, loneliness and anxiety, substance use, and weak family and social relationships all contribute to higher suicide risk in adolescents (Patra et al., 2023). The most recent Youth Risk and Behavior Survey found that in the preceding year 30% of female high school students seriously considered attempting suicide (14.3% of males), 23.6% made a suicidal plan (11.6% of males), and 13.3% made a suicide attempt (6.6% of males) (Gaylor et al., 2023). In the past 10 years, the proportion of mental health–related emergency room visits for children and adolescents has doubled, with a fivefold increase in suicide-related visits (Bommersbach et al., 2023).

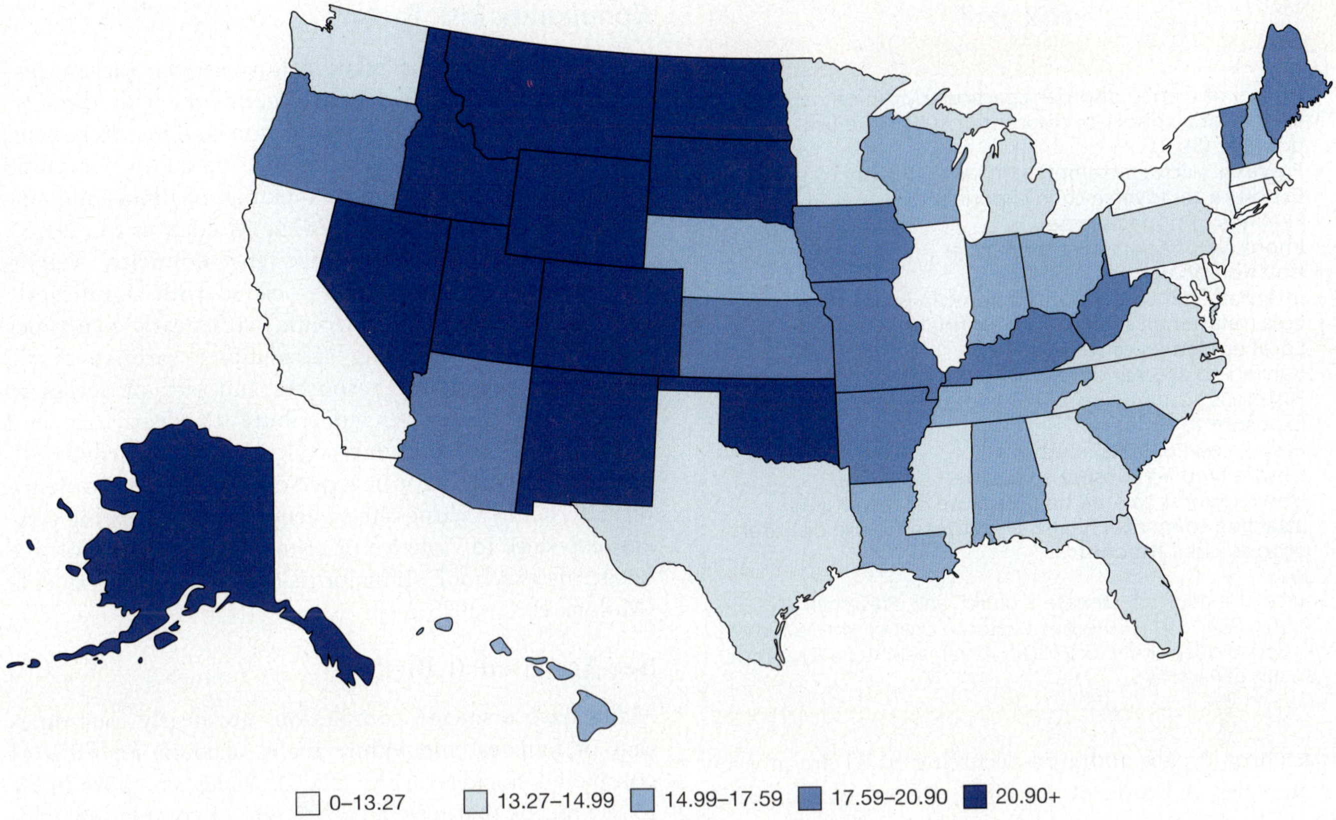

FIGURE 22.1 Number of deaths by state attributable to suicide in the United States per 100,000 population, 2022. (Reprinted from National Institute of Mental Health. Data courtesy of CDC. Retrieved on March 12, 2025, from https://www.nimh.nih.gov/health/statistics/suicide#part_154971)

Adults and Older Adults

Suicide is a major contributor to premature death in adults, ranking the fourth leading cause of death among adults aged 35 to 54. People ages 85 and older have the highest rates of suicide (CDC, 2023; NIMH, 2024). Physical illness, pain, cognitive decline, loss, loneliness, social isolation, bereavement, and disconnectedness are important precipitants to suicide in older adults (Dhole et al., 2023; Garnett et al., 2023).

Suicide disproportionally affects those who have served in the military, with suicide rates for Veterans 1.5 times the rate for non-Veterans and 2.1 times higher among female veterans compared to the general population. An estimated 18 veterans die by suicide per day (U.S. Department of Veterans Affairs, 2023). Mental health conditions, including depression, posttraumatic stress disorder (PTSD), and substance use disorder (SUD) are contributing factors to suicide for military members of all genders. Other contributing factors for suicide include combat exposure, access to lethal means, and homelessness and poverty. Military personnel and veterans often face major life disruptions that significantly impact their relationships and employment, oftentimes leading to isolation and social withdrawal. For females, military sexual trauma (MST) contributes to suicidal ideation and attempts, with MST reported in over 20% of females (Ruiz et al., 2023). Although suicide prevention is a top priority for the U.S. Department of Veterans Affairs, services available to veterans are significantly underutilized (U.S. Department of Veterans Affairs, 2023).

Epidemiology and Risk Factors

Suicidal behavior is complex and is rarely caused by one single factor. Although nearly half (46%) of people who die by suicide have a known mental health condition, many contributing factors can increase a person's risk for suicide, at individual, relationship, community, and societal levels (CDC, 2024; NAMI, 2023). Box 22.1 identifies risk factors for suicide (CDC, 2024).

Individual Risk Factors

History of mental illnesses, particularly depression, is associated with higher risk of suicide. SUD is also found to increase suicide risk, with adults with SUDs being nearly four times more likely to attempt suicide than those without SUD, and adolescents with SUD five times more likely (Jones et al., 2023). Serious physical illness and chronic pain that affect daily work and life activities are associated with higher suicide risk. Individuals

BOX 22.1

Suicide Risk Factors

- History of mental disorders, particularly clinical depression
- History of alcohol use disorder or substance use disorder (SUD)
- Previous suicide attempt(s) or family history of suicide
- Exposure to adverse child experiences
- Feelings of hopelessness
- Impulsive or aggressive tendencies
- Isolation or lack of belonging
- Interpersonal conflict or relationship issues
- Loss (relational, social, work, or financial)
- Local epidemics of suicide
- Barriers to accessing mental health treatment
- Historical trauma and discrimination
- Exposure to violence
- Easy access to lethal methods
- Unsafe media exposure to suicide
- Unwillingness to seek help because of the stigma attached to mental health and substance use disorders or to suicidal thoughts

Source: Centers for Disease Control and Prevention (CDC). (2024). *Risk and protective factors* [Online]. https://www.cdc.gov/suicide/risk-factors/?CDC_AAref_Val=https://www.cdc.gov/suicide/factors/

with chronic pain and a co-occurring SUD are at even greater risk (Cheatle et al., 2023; Rikard et al., 2023). Psychological pain, internal distress, low self-esteem, and interpersonal distress have long been associated with suicide (Wang et al., 2024). Exposure to adverse childhood experiences is linked to suicide and vulnerability to NSSI, particularly when the individual has poorer executive functioning and higher levels of impulsivity, anger, and reduced inhibition (Rogerson et al., 2023; Yarar et al., 2023; Zhou et al., 2024). Other individual risk factors for suicide include recent legal problems, loss of job or financial concerns, and unstable housing (Choi et al., 2024; Stanley et al., 2023).

Relationship Risk Factors

Social isolation and exclusion are primary risk factors for suicide. A significant portion of suicides are precipitated by intimate partner violence or other interpersonal conflict and relationship issues. Distress of divorce or the termination of a relationship contributes to risk (Choi et al., 2024). Lack of social support and bullying contribute to feelings of hopelessness and social isolation that may precipitate suicidality. Belongingness and social connection are associated with decreased risk of suicide, even if it consists of having just one important bond with another person (Silva et al., 2023). A suicide survivor, a person who has lost a family member or loved one to suicide, is at greater risk for suicide. This risk is highest when the family member of a person who died by suicide was a spouse, parent/caregiver, sibling, or child due to feelings of stigma, shame, responsibility, and guilt (Jang et al., 2022).

Community Risk Factors

Research has found a relationship between racism, discrimination, and suicidality. Experiences with discrimination can interfere with a person seeking treatment, and chronic experiences with discrimination over time can exacerbate stress and further risk of illness and suicidality (Marraccini et al., 2023; Molock et al., 2023). Discrimination based on race and ethnicity, weight, and sexual orientation are associated with significantly greater risk of suicide in youth, with nearly five times higher odds of reporting suicidality (Pearlman et al., 2023). Low economic resources and lack of access to mental health services contribute to disparities and increased risk. Community violence also contributes to suicide risk, whether it be a person experiencing violence directly, being a witness to violence, or experiencing general exposure to violence or crime. Exposure to violence occurring at school is a major risk factor for youth suicide (Molock et al., 2023).

Sex Assigned at Birth

Males have a suicide completion rate nearly four times that of females, and White males account for 70% of completed suicides (AFSP, 2023). Males are more likely to use means that have a higher rate of completion, with 60% of their suicide deaths by firearms (see Fig. 22.2). Males living in rural areas have a much higher risk of suicide than those in urban areas, and that gap is widening, perhaps attributable to the higher rates of gun ownership in rural areas (Ewell et al., 2024). Substance misuse, aggression, hopelessness, emotion-focused coping, social isolation, and feeling little purpose in life have been associated with suicidal behavior in males.

Females across age, racial, and ethnic groups are less likely to die from suicide than are males, but are more likely to attempt suicide; females make three attempts to every attempt by males. Among females, the suicide rate

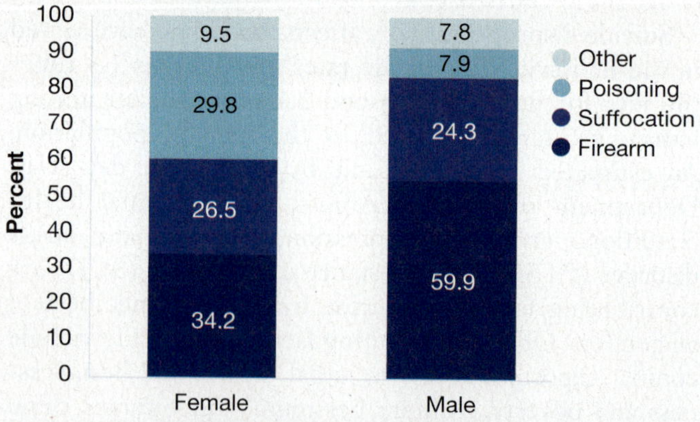

FIGURE 22.2 Suicide deaths by method in the United States, 2022. (Reprinted from National Institute of Mental Health. Data courtesy of CDC. Retrieved on March 12, 2025, from https://www.nimh.nih.gov/health/statistics/suicide#part_154971)

is highest for those aged 45 to 64 (NIMH, 2024). Females are less likely to complete suicide, partly because they are more likely to choose less lethal methods. Females with current or previous exposure to intimate partner violence are at an increased risk for suicidal behavior (Akinyemi et al., 2023).

Sexuality

Members of the LGBTQ+ community are at a higher risk for suicide than those of the heterosexual, cisgender population due to many individuals facing discrimination, prejudice, harassment, and rejection. This risk is exacerbated for individuals with intersecting racial or socioeconomic identities (National Alliance on Mental Illness [NAMI], 2024). LGBTQ+ youth are more than four times as likely to attempt suicide compared with heterosexual youth, with over 40% of LGBTQ+ youth seriously considering attempting suicide in the previous year, and 14% attempting it. Insufficient access to mental health care contributes to risk. LGBTQ+ youth report many reasons for not seeking care, including fear of talking with their parents/caregivers or a health care provider, concerns about not being taken seriously, lack of financial resources, lack of confidence that suicidal ideation is treatable, fear of disclosing their sexual identity, fear of looking weak, and not having permission by their parents/caregivers to pursue care (The Trevor Project, 2023).

There are high rates of suicidal ideation and suicide among transgender individuals as well, with transgender adults being nearly nine times more likely to attempt suicide at some point in their life compared to the general population (NAMI, 2024). A systematic review and meta-analysis of the prevalence of suicidal thoughts and attempts in the transgender population found that 50% of individuals had suicidal thoughts during their lifetime, with a prevalence rate of suicide attempt at nearly 30% (Kohnepoushi et al., 2023). Gender-based risk of exploitation, discrimination, bullying, violence, rejection by family, friends, and communities are risk factors associated with suicidal behavior (Small et al., 2024). Protective factors against self-harm in transgender populations include social support, connectedness, and school safety (Bird et al., 2024). Respecting a transgender or nonbinary person's preferred pronouns also contributes to lower rates of suicide attempts (Trevor Project, 2023).

Race and Ethnicity

There is considerable variation in the profile of suicide rates across racial/ethnic groups, including the age when rates are at their peak and the duration of high rates across several age groups. Understanding racial/ethnic differences is critical to providing more effective suicide prevention care. Disparities in access to culturally appropriate mental health care, as well as experiences of discrimination and historical trauma, contribute to risk (SPRC, 2024). Rates of suicide among American Indian/Alaska Native (AI/AN) and White populations are highest, at 24.0 and 16.8 per 100,000, respectively. Lower suicide rates are found among Asian/Pacific Island individuals (6.8 per 100,000), Hispanic individuals (7.5 per 100,000), and Black individuals (7.7 per 100,000) (SPRC, 2024).

Suicide rates among White populations steadily increase from age 15 to age 54, followed by a decrease. Rates then increase again from the age of 75 to over the age of 85. Completed suicides are highest for White individuals between the ages of 45 to 54. Suicide rates are more than three to four times higher in males than in females, with a rate of 29.0 (males) and 8.0 (females) per 100,000. The use of firearms is by far the most prominent method of suicide among White individuals (Liu et al., 2023). Access to firearms contributes to the risk of completed suicides. Firearm ownership is more prevalent in the United States than in any other country, with an estimated 1,205 firearms per 1,000 people (Pritchard et al., 2023).

Suicide rates among AI/AN populations are the highest of any racial/ethnic group in the United States. Rates in this population peak during adolescence and young adulthood, then decline (SPRC, 2024). Establishing true suicide rates in the AI/AN population is challenging because this population encompasses many ethnic and cultural groups, tribes, and traditions. It is recognized that tribes may have their own surveillance systems or definitions of suicide, tribes may be reluctant to share data for fear of misuse, and the concept of "suicide" may not be part of the cultural vocabulary (SPRC, 2024). AI/AN individuals engaged in suicidal behavior are more likely to have alcohol or substance use issues; additionally, individuals who have died by suicide were more likely to have been involved in a crisis with an intimate partner or had been exposed to recent suicide by family members or friends (Stone et al., 2023). For these reasons, community-level prevention strategies focusing on survivor support and substance use treatment are critical.

Suicide rates among Black or African American populations have steadily increased from 5.5 to 7.7 per 100,000 in the past 10 years; unlike the overall US population, suicide rates peak during adolescence and young adulthood in Black populations, then decline through age 85+ (SPRC, 2024). Suicide rates have increased dramatically among African American adolescents; depression and hopelessness contribute to increased risk (Whipple et al., 2023). Higher rates of suicide in young Black males may be associated with disparities in mental health treatment and social factors disproportionally affecting Black adolescents (Polanco-Roman et al., 2023). Barriers to accessing mental health care can be attributed to the person's experiences of bias, mental health stigma, mistrust of the health care system, and a shortage of providers who

BOX 22.2

Mental Health Inequities: Racial and Gender Disparities in Suicide and Mental Health Care Utilization

Electronic medical records of adolescents and young adults aged 8 to 20 in a large pediatric outpatient primary care center were reviewed. The analysis consisted of 24,547 patient records, with a mean patient age of 11.5 years. Black adolescent and young adult patients were less likely to have a documented diagnosis of anxiety or depression and were more likely to have underrecognition of a mental health disorder than White patients. Focusing on gender alone, females had higher odds of documented anxiety, depression, and suicide-related diagnoses as compared to males. However, females, especially Black females, had disproportionately high odds of unrecognized mental health needs as compared to White males, even though they had similar odds of having a suicide-related diagnosis.

Source: Prichett, L. M., Yolken, R. H., Severance, E. G., Young, A. S., Carmichael, D., Zeng, Y., & Kumra, T. (2024). Racial and gender disparities in suicide and mental health care utilization in a pediatric primary care setting. *Journal of Adolescent Health*, *74*(2), 277–282.

engage in cultural humility (SAMSA, 2023). Additionally, few suicide risk assessments are culturally tailored to communities of color, which contributes even further to disparities in assessment and subsequent treatment (Molock et al., 2023). See Box 22.2.

Even though the suicide rate for Hispanic individuals is just over half of the overall US rate, suicide is the second leading cause of death for Hispanic individuals, aged 15 to 34. Among Hispanic populations, suicide rates remain somewhat consistent across the life span, and the death rate for Hispanic males is three to four times the rate of Hispanic females. Suicide attempts by Hispanic adolescents were 30% greater than by non-Hispanic White adolescents (SPRC, 2024). Only just over a third of Hispanic and Latino Americans receive mental health services. Mental health stigma is a major barrier to accessing care. Additionally, language barriers, negative encounters with care providers, and lack of provider concordance contribute to unmet needs (Sweileh, 2024).

Although the suicide rate for Asian individuals or Pacific Island populations is approximately half of the overall suicide rate in the United States, the scant literature on suicide among Asian populations shows that suicidal ideation, plans, and attempts may be more common than popularly believed and vary within Asian ethnic groups (SPRC, 2024). The highest rates of suicide among Asian or Pacific Islander populations occur in those later in life, with the highest prevalence in those over 85 years old, and the suicide death rate for males is more than double that of females (SPRC, 2024). A study of racial/ethnic differences in youth having died by suicide found that Asian American/Pacific Islander youth had significantly lower rates of mental health treatment compared to White youth, consistent with research demonstrating disparities in mental health service utilization (Lee & Wong, 2020). Asian American, Native Hawaiians, and Pacific Islanders also face unique barriers to accessing mental health care. In addition to language barriers, mental health stigma, and cultural beliefs surrounding mental health limit help seeking (Sweileh, 2024).

Pandemic Impact

Although the full extent of the impact of coronavirus disease 2019 (COVID-19) on mental health will not be fully realized for quite some time, evidence of mental health challenges related to COVID-19–associated morbidity, mortality, and mitigation activities (including physical distancing and mandated stay-at-home orders) were noted within months of the outbreak in the United States. The outbreak of the pandemic was accompanied by profound physical, psychological, social, and economic consequences. Uncertainties about the future, and overwhelming fears and worries about health, contributed to distress, depression, and anxiety. Required quarantine periods contributed to loneliness and a disruption in interpersonal relationships. A rise in interpersonal conflict, intimate partner violence, and alcohol consumption was also seen. Financial strain and the inability for some to work compounded stress and uncertainty. With hopelessness, mental health issues, particularly depression and anxiety, socioeconomic status, and stressful life events being high predictors for suicide, suicide screening and prevention efforts were needed more than ever. Although a meta-analysis of studies examining suicide-related outcomes before and during the pandemic found that suicide completions have remained fairly stable, an upward trend of suicidal ideation and attempts was found; monitoring suicide risk as repercussions of the pandemic continue to be felt is essential, and prevention and intervention programs are critical (Yan et al., 2023). Additionally, trauma-informed, collaborative approaches are needed (Nicoll et al., 2023).

Societal Risk Factors

Social stigma negatively affects individuals living with mental illness or suicidality. This stigma often results in a person being less likely to reach out for help and disclose their suicidal thoughts due to fear of causing emotional distress to themselves or others, concern of burdening others, or a fear of being labeled, judged, or devalued (Oexle et al., 2022). Fears of being discriminated against also contribute to increased risk. An individual may fear that their disclosure of suicidal thoughts may negatively impact their employment or workplace culture and relationships (McGrath et al., 2023). Easy access to lethal means is another societal risk factor for suicide. Household firearm ownership is a known risk factor. Adolescent suicides by firearm are increasing in the United States, with nearly a third of adolescents reporting that they could access a loaded firearm within 5 minutes. Social media contributes to the adolescent gun culture (Bhatt et al., 2023). Whereas the media can raise awareness of mental health needs, unsafe media portrayal of suicide can be a risk factor for suicide. Studies have found that sensationalism, excessive detail about the site/location of suicide, explicit description of method, the inclusion of photographs, video footage or social media links, and repeating the news of suicide excessively contribute to increased risk of suicide (Sufrate-Sorzano et al., 2023).

Etiology

The convergence of biologic, psychological, and social factors can be directly linked to suicidal behavior. In genetically and physiologically vulnerable individuals, thoughts, feelings, and personality factors can interfere with personal problem solving, promote impulsivity, and support suicidal behavior. Poverty, unemployment, and social conflict also contribute to suicidal behavior in those at risk for suicide. Figure 22.3 depicts the prevalence of suicidal thoughts and behaviors among US adults.

Biologic Theories

Depression is linked to suicide, and those who have completed suicide have been noted to have a decrease in serotonin or in vitamin D levels. An increase in neuroinflammation in people who have died by suicide has also been found. Chronic stress and trauma contribute to suicide risk due to subsequent biologic adaptations. Hypothalamic–pituitary–adrenal (HPA) axis dysfunction and allostatic load are associated with both mental health issues, suicidal ideation, and suicide deaths (Bengoechea-Fortes et al., 2023; Herzog et al., 2023; Stacy & Schulkin, 2022). Although specific genetic markers of suicide have not yet been identified, a genetic link to suicide is evident (Li et al., 2023). Family history of mental illness and attempted suicide are risk factors for suicide (Favril et al., 2022). Family and twin studies point to a suicide heritability rate as large as 45% (Drago, 2024).

Psychological Theories

Cognitive Theories

Most evidence on the psychological contributions to suicidal behavior point to cognitive, affective, behavioral, and personality factors that intensify the experience of hopelessness and disconnection from others. Aaron Beck first identified the cognitive triad of hopelessness, helplessness, and worthlessness as integral to the experience of depression (Beck et al., 1979). Since then, a significant evidence base has been established linking hopelessness,

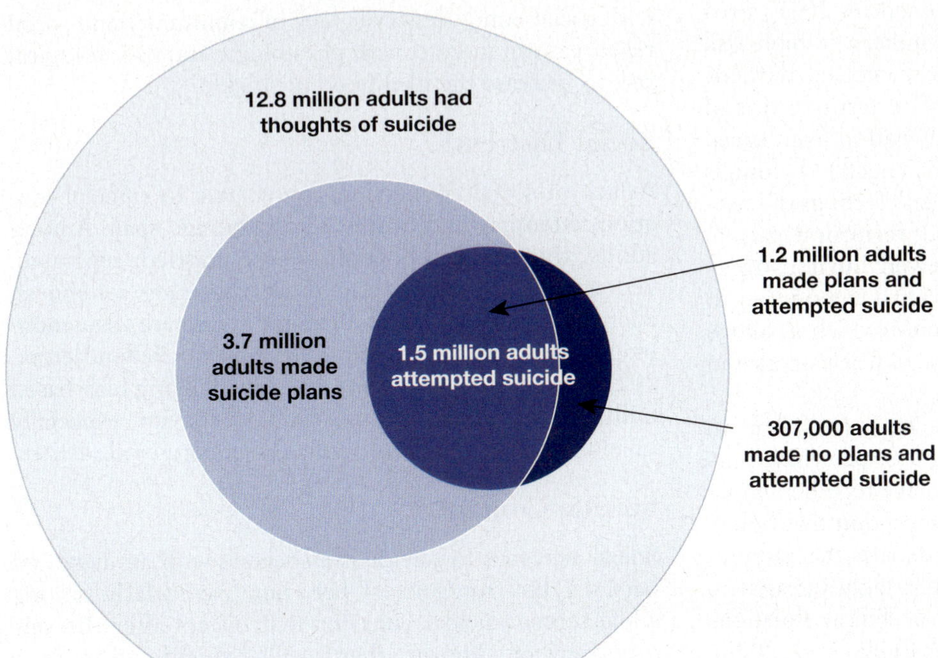

FIGURE 22.3 Past year suicidal thoughts and behaviors among U.S. adults, 2023. (Reprinted from National Institute of Mental Health. Data courtesy of SAMHSA. Retrieved on March 12, 2025, from https://www.nimh.nih.gov/health/statistics/suicide#part_154971)

loneliness, and other cognitive symptoms to suicidal ideation. Depressed people who are hopeless are more likely to consider suicide than those who are depressed but hopeful about the future (Riera-Serra et al., 2023).

KEYCONCEPT Hopelessness is the pervasive belief that undesirable events are likely to occur, coupled with the belief that one's situation is unlikely to improve.

Emotional and Personality Factors

Emotional factors and personality traits also play a role in suicidal behavior by enhancing perceptions of helplessness and hopelessness, contributing to poor self-esteem, and interfering with coping efforts. Shame, guilt, despair, and emotion-focused coping have been linked to suicidal behavior. Loss and grief are also important considerations. Emotional distress often is potentiated by personality traits that contribute to poor self-esteem, impulsivity, and suicidal behavior (Vidal-Ribas et al., 2024).

Ideation to Action Theories

Suicidal ideation does not necessarily lead to suicide attempts. Most people who think of suicide do not act on the idea, but the suicidal thoughts of those who do take lethal actions are often indistinguishable from those who do not (see Fig. 22.3). **Ideation-to-action theories** examine factors that identify those who are most likely to attempt suicide. These emerging theories, which are supported by research, provide a basis for discriminating between those who are only thinking about suicide versus those who are likely to engage in suicidal acts.

The *Interpersonal Psychological Theory of Suicidal Behavior (IPTS)*, introduced by Thomas Joiner in 2005, proposes that three interacting factors indicate a high risk of suicide—thwarted belongingness, perceived burdensomeness, and acquired capability. The term **thwarted belongingness** is used to describe alienation from social relationships or experiences; the human need to belong is not being met. It refers to an individual's feelings of loneliness and isolation, as well as a lack of reciprocal, caring, and meaningful relationships. **Perceived burdensomeness** is the perception that the individual is a burden to others. **Acquired capability for suicide**, which develops over time, involves a heightened sense of fearlessness and a high pain threshold (Joiner, 2005).

IPTS views the act of suicide as being very difficult to carry out. When thwarted belongingness, perceived burdensomeness, and acquired capability come together in one person, these beliefs lead to the misperception that others would be better off without them and the idea that sacrificing themselves is the appropriate action to take. Researchers are testing the theory in a variety of clinical situations (Calati et al., 2022; Chalker et al., 2022; Phillip et al., 2022).

Integrated Motivational–Volitional model proposes that feelings of entrapment contribute to suicidal ideation, and a set of motivational moderators may either facilitate or hinder the further development of suicidal behaviors. Motivational moderators may include factors such as attitudes, goals, social support, and thwarted belongingness (O'Connor & Kirtley, 2018). Reasons for living and life meaning are found to be protective roles against entrapment and suicidal thoughts (Moscardini et al., 2022). Positive mental health and psychological well-being also moderate the association between entrapment and suicidal thoughts (Souza et al., 2024).

The *Three-Step Theory (3ST)* explains progression from ideation to action in three steps. First, emotional pain and hopelessness cause the suicidal ideation. Second, thoughts of suicide become strong as the emotional pain exceeds connectedness. The third step involves the actual attempt when the person has the knowledge and capacity to carry out the suicide (Klonsky et al., 2021). Because psychological pain and fearlessness of death are associated with plans and preparations for suicide, in this model, suicide prevention focuses on reducing pain, increasing hope, improving connections, and reducing capacity to carry out the suicide (Tsai et al., 2021).

Social Theories

Before the turn of the 20th century, Emile Durkheim (1951[1897]) linked suicide to the social conditions in which people live. Both a lack of social connectedness and social conditions contribute to suicidal behavior. People who are socially connected are less likely to engage in suicidal behavior. When an individual has others they can depend on, suicide can be prevented, even among those at significant risk. Even among people with social bonds, however, lack of community and social resources can interact with physiologic and psychological risk to increase the likelihood of suicide.

Social Distress

A lack of social connection contributes to suicidal ideation, attempts, and deaths across the age span. Among adults, those who are single, never married, separated, widowed, living alone, and those reporting loneliness, alienation, and a lack of belongingness, are also more likely to engage in suicidal behavior (McClelland et al., 2023). Interpersonal conflict and experiencing bias-based bullying can contribute to suicidal behavior, especially in adolescents and young adults (Eisenberg et al., 2024).

Suicide Contagion

Social exposure to suicide is associated with an increased personal risk for suicidal behavior, particularly among adolescents. Suicidal behavior that occurs after the suicide death of a known other is called **suicide contagion**. Suicide contagion seems to work through modeling and is more likely to occur when the individual contemplating suicide is of the same age, gender, and background as the person who died. Contagion can be prompted by the suicide of a friend, an acquaintance, online social networking, or an idolized celebrity. Actions of peer groups, media reports of suicide, and even billboards with content about suicide can trigger suicidal behavior among adolescents. In the case of a celebrity suicide, the number of "copycat suicides" is proportional to the amount, duration, and prominence of media coverage. **Suicide clusters**, accounting for approximately 1% to 2% of teenage suicides, occur when a group of suicide attempts or completed suicides occur within a short period of time or geographic location. Point clusters occur within a time period in a specific location, for example, in a school or psychiatric inpatient setting. Mass clusters represent a higher number of suicides across a larger geographic region within a specified time period (Ballestero et al., 2024). Mental health practitioners and local and state health departments play an important role in leading community suicide prevention efforts (Ivey-Stephenson et al., 2024).

Economic Disadvantage

Poverty and economic disadvantage are associated with depression, suicidal ideation, and suicide mortality. Suicide risk is greater for adults in socially and materially deprived areas. Individuals who are financially stressed have been found to be almost 75% more likely to die by suicide (Roelfs & Shor, 2023). Individuals with extensive financial debt have been found to be nearly eight times more likely to die than those without debt (Stack, 2021). Housing insecurity and the lack of funds to cover basic needs also increase suicide risk (Choi et al., 2022; Elbogen et al., 2021).

In impoverished communities, particularly rural America, lack of access to quality education and employment opportunities leads to unemployment and loss of meaningful social roles. Access to health care is limited in these communities, and there is an increased exposure to others exhibiting suicidal behavior that enhances suicide risk (Edwards et al., 2023).

Family Response to Suicide

It is estimated that 50% of the US population is acquainted with one or more people who have died by suicide. Suicide has devastating effects on everyone it touches, especially family and close friends. One suicide is estimated to leave at least 25 individuals reporting being profoundly impacted by the loss. Family members of a person who has died by suicide experience more grief, anxiety and depression, guilt, shame, self-blame, and dysfunction than families whose loss was because of other reasons and the personal and familial disruption often lasts for years. Although recovery from a loved one's suicide is an ongoing task, survivors who are emotionally healthy before the suicide act and who have social support are able to manage the psychological trauma associated with suicide. Still, the intensity and duration of the postsuicide grief process for many survivors has led to the development of family intervention programs. Although the evidence base for these interventions is still small, strategies that support a positive sense of self, enhance problem solving, promote the formation of a suicide story, encourage social reintegration, reduce stigma, use journaling, or permit the survivor to debrief may be effective in reducing subjective distress and to resolve grief (Kircher & Niederkrotenthaler, 2024; Levi-Belz et al., 2021). These strategies may be most effectively delivered in survivor peer help groups.

Protective Factors

Protective factors buffer individuals from suicidal thoughts and behavior. Although identifying and understanding protective factors are very important, they have not been studied as extensively as risk factors. The CDC (2024) identifies some of the following individual, relationship, community, and societal protective factors:

- Individual protective factors:
  - Effective coping and problem-solving skills
  - Identified reasons for living (for example, family and friends)
  - An established cultural identity
- Relationship protective factors:
  - Supportive relationships with family and friends
  - Secured connections with others
- Community protective factors
  - Established connections within the community
  - Access to physical and mental health care
- Societal protective factors
  - Limited access to lethal means among people at risk
  - Cultural and religious beliefs that discourage suicide

TREATMENT AND NURSING CARE FOR SUICIDE PREVENTION

Interprofessional Treatment and Recovery

The challenges of preventing suicides and promoting healthy coping belong to all disciplines. An interprofessional treatment or recovery approach along with peer support is needed for managing the threats of suicide.

Clinical Judgment

Concept Mastery Alert

A true psychiatric emergency exists when an individual presents with one or more symptoms associated with imminent risk for suicidal behavior. Immediate and focused action is needed to prevent the patient's death.

The first priority is to provide for the patient's safety while initiating the *least* restrictive care possible. In contrast, an example of the *most* restrictive care is an outpatient who is admitted to a locked unit with one staff member who is assigned to observe the person at all times. Hospitalization should be reserved for those whose safety cannot be ensured in an outpatient environment.

Priority Care Issues: Preventing Suicide and Promoting Mental Health

Evidence-based care for people at risk for suicide includes a combination of approaches in preventing suicide and promoting long-term mental health: identification of those thinking about suicide (case finding), assessment to determine an imminent suicidal threat, intervening to change suicidal behavior associated with a specific suicidal threat, and institution of effective interventions to prevent future episodes of suicidal behavior (Mann et al., 2021).

Assessment

Case Finding

Case finding refers to identifying people who are at risk for suicide so proper treatment can be initiated. People who are contemplating suicide often do not share their ideation. This lack of disclosure often means that family, friends, and health professionals are unable to intervene until the suicidal ideation and planning have progressed. Yet early identification of suicidal ideation may reduce suicide deaths. Nurses can play important roles in suicide prevention by recognizing the warning signs. The Columbia Suicide Severity Rating Scale (C-SSRS) is a commonly used evidence-supported suicide risk assessment that measures severity of suicidal ideation, intensity of ideation, suicidal behavior, and lethality (see Chapter 10 for more information about the C-SSRS).

Case finding requires careful and concerned questioning and listening that make the patient feel valued and cared about (Box 22.3). Most standardized health questionnaires have questions about suicide thoughts. Many nurses are concerned that asking patients about their suicidal thoughts will provoke a suicide attempt. This belief simply is not true. The patient expressing suicidal ideation often has had these thoughts for some time and may feel more socially connected when another recognizes the seriousness of the situation. Under no circumstances should a patient be promised secrecy about suicidal thoughts, plans, or acts. Instead, tell patients that disclosure of suicidal intent will be shared with other interdisciplinary team members so the safety of the patient can be ensured.

Assessing Risk

After suicidal ideation has been established, the next step is to determine the risk for a suicide attempt. Suicide risk assessment is difficult and, whenever possible, should proceed only with the assistance of other members of the interprofessional treatment team. Assessing for risk includes determining the seriousness of the suicidal ideation, degree of hopelessness, disorders, previous attempt, suicide planning and implementation, and availability and lethality of suicide method. Risk assessment also includes the patient's resources, including coping skills and social supports, that can be used to counter suicidal impulses. Box 22.4 lists some questions that might be asked in assessing the risk for suicide.

The greatest predictor of a future suicide attempt is a previous attempt, partly because the individual already has broken the "taboo" around suicidal behavior. Repeated episodes of self-harm with or without suicidal intent also increase immediate risk because they increase an individual's capacity to complete suicide. Other important signs of high risk are the presence of suicide planning behaviors (detailed plan, availability of means, opportunity, and capability) and engaging in final acts, such as giving away prized possessions and saying goodbye to loved ones. Although the presence of a specific psychiatric disorder, such as depression, is an important consideration in risk assessment, anxiety, agitation, alcohol use, and impulsivity may be better indicators of immediate risk. However, support from important others, religious prohibitions, responsibility for young children, and employment may provide protection from suicidal impulses.

Ideally, an interprofessional team conducts suicide risk assessment in an emergency department or outpatient facility with multiple supports. Nurses practicing in more isolated situations should keep a list of contacts in settings that routinely conduct suicide risk assessments so the contacts may be consulted if a seriously suicidal individual appears in the nurse's setting.

NCLEXNOTE Suicide assessment is always considered a priority. Practice by asking patients about suicidal thoughts and plans. Develop a plan with a suicidal patient that focuses on resisting the suicidal impulse. Apply the assessment process that delineates the (1) intent to die, (2) severity of ideation, (3) availability of means, and (4) degree of planning.

Interventions for Imminent, Intermediate, and Long-Term Suicide Prevention

Interventions for Those at Imminent Risk

There are three urgent priorities in caring for a person who is at imminent risk for suicide: reconnecting the patient to other people and instilling hope, restoring emotional stability, and reducing suicidal behavior and ensuring safety. Reconnecting the patient interpersonally includes listening intently, and without judgment, to the patient's thoughts and feelings and validating their experience and suffering. This intervention directly

BOX 22.3

Therapeutic Dialogue: Suicide

When Caroline sought medical care for a cold from her nurse practitioner, the nurse observed more than a cough and runny nose. Caroline appeared downcast and extremely sad. As the nurse and patient talked, the subject of family life came up, whereupon Caroline began to cry softly. As words tumbled out, she said she had been unhappy at home for a long time. When she was very young, she recalled being happy, but things changed when her brother was born, 4 years after her. She says her father began to abuse her sexually, starting when Caroline was 5 years old and continuing until he moved out of the house when she was 12 years old. Caroline suspects her mother knew of the abuse, although she did nothing about it.

Two years ago, Caroline's father died by suicide. Caroline feels relieved about his death but frustrated that she never got a chance to tell him how angry she was with him. Caroline's relationship with her mother has not improved. Caroline says her mother favors her brother and is always telling Caroline she won't amount to anything. Caroline begins to cry harder.

INEFFECTIVE APPROACH

Nurse: Clearly, many things are troubling you. Don't you think that things seem worse now because you have a cold?

Caroline: Well, that could be. What are you going to do to make me feel better?

Nurse: Give you some medicine to help you sleep and clear your nose. I think you should see a psychiatrist, too.

Caroline: I don't need a psychiatrist. I came here for my cold.

Nurse: I know you did, but you seem to be depressed.

Caroline: What are you, some kind of social worker? I am just tired.

Nurse: I am a nurse, and you seem down to me. Are you thinking about suicide?

Caroline: I don't think you know what you're talking about. I want to go now. Could you give me my medicine?

EFFECTIVE APPROACH

Nurse: It seems as though many things have been piling up on you. Does it seem that way to you, too?

Caroline: It sure does. I've just been trying to get through 1 day at a time, but now with this cold and no sleep, I feel like I can't go on.

Nurse: When you say you can't go on, what does that mean to you?

Caroline: Lately, I have been thinking about running away to some place where I can't be found and maybe starting over. But then I think, where would I go? Where would I stay? Who would take care of me?

Nurse: When you think that your plan for escape won't work, what happens?

Caroline: (Starting to cry again.) Then I think that maybe it would be better if I just did what my father did. I really don't think anyone would miss me.

Nurse: So you think you might take your life, like your Dad did?

Caroline: Yeah, and what really scares me is lately I have been thinking about that a lot. I keep saying to myself, "You're just tired," but I am so exhausted now that I can't chase the thoughts away.

Nurse: So, do you think about suicide every day?

Caroline: It seems like I never stop thinking about it.

Nurse: Is there anything you can do to make the thoughts go away?

Caroline: Nothing. (Silence.)

Nurse: What would you do?

Caroline: I think I would get as many pills as I could find, drink a lot of alcohol, and maybe smoke some pot and just go to sleep.

Nurse: Do you have enough pills at home to kill yourself?

Caroline (wan smile): I was hoping that the sleeping medicine you would give me might do the job.

Nurse: It sounds like you need some help getting through this time in your life. Would you like some?

Caroline: I honestly don't know—I just want to sleep for a long time.

CRITICAL THINKING CHALLENGE

- In the first interaction, the nurse made two key blunders. What were they? What effect did they have on the patient? How did they interfere with the patient's care?
- What did Caroline do that might have contributed to the nurse's behavior in the first interaction?
- In the second interaction, the nurse did several things that ensured reporting of Caroline's suicidal ideation. What were they? What differences in attitude might differentiate the nurse in the first interaction from the nurse in the second?

BOX 22.4

Assessment of Suicidal Episode

INTENT TO DIE

1. Have you been thinking about hurting or killing yourself?
2. How seriously do you want to die?
3. Have you attempted suicide before?
4. Are there people or things in your life who might keep you from killing yourself?

SEVERITY OF IDEATION

1. How often do you have these thoughts?
2. How long do they last?
3. How much do the thoughts distress you?
4. Can you dismiss them, or do they tend to return?
5. Are they increasing in intensity and frequency?

DEGREE OF PLANNING

1. Have you made any plans to kill yourself? If yes, what are they?
2. Do you have access to the materials (e.g., gun, poison, pills) that you plan to use to kill yourself?
3. How likely is it that you could actually carry out the plan?
4. Have you done anything to put the plan into action?
5. Could you stop yourself from killing yourself?

challenges the patient's belief that no one cares. Using cognitive interventions can help the client regain hope and establish goals for the future.

Ensuring Patient Safety. Helping patients develop strategies for making safer choices when distressed is an important goal. Nurses caring for patients who are emerging from the initial hours and days of a suicide attempt can support the patient and focus on managing suicidal urges and developing protective strategies. As the nurse connects with the patient, together they can create a list of personal and professional resources that can be used when the individual is in crisis. With the nurse's help, the patient can visualize "emotional spaces that are safe places to go" when distressed.

For years, the no-suicide contract was a staple of psychiatric nursing practice and widely used across disciplines as a means of preventing suicide among those at risk. No-suicide contracts are verbal and written "contracts" between the individual at imminent risk for suicide and a health care provider that contain an agreement that the patient will not die by suicide during a specific time period. Careful evaluation of this practice has not established its efficacy in preventing suicidal behavior and suicide deaths. As a consequence, the nurse should avoid engaging in a no-suicide contract with a patient.

Inpatient Safety Considerations. When hospitalization is considered the best option to ensure the safety of the patient, the nurse has the responsibility for providing a safe, therapeutic environment in which human connection, instilling hope, and changing suicidal behavior can occur. Inpatient suicides do occur. Considered a sentinel event, roughly 1,500 suicides per year occur in a mental health institution, with approximately 70% by hanging (Gupta et al., 2022). Factors contributing to suicide deaths in the public mental health system include inappropriate or incomplete risk assessment, inadequate communication between treatment teams, poor execution of policies and procedures, insufficient guidelines for treatment, and patient access to means for self-harm (Wyder et al., 2020).

Removal of dangerous items and environmental hazards, continuous or intermittent observation of at-risk patients by hospital personnel trained in observation methods, and limitation of outpatient passes are the mainstays of hospital interventions. Observation procedures vary from facility to facility. For patients who require constant supervision, a staff member will be assigned only to the high-risk patient. For patients at a lower risk, observation may entail close or intermittent observations.

Observation is not, by itself, therapeutic. An observation becomes therapeutic when interaction occurs with the patient. Psychiatric intensive care of this kind and restriction of freedom can be very upsetting to the patient who is withdrawn and isolated. Nurses can help patients reestablish personal control by including them in decisions about their care and restricting their behavior only as necessary. Nurses can also reduce the patient's stress while ensuring the patient's safety by intruding as little as possible on the person's exercise of free will. Observational periods can be used to help patients express a broad range of feelings and strengthen their belief in their own abilities to keep themselves safe. During observation, the nurse can help the patient describe feelings and identify ways to manage safety needs (Box 22.5).

BOX 22.5

Psychoeducation Checklist: Suicide Prevention

When teaching the patient and family about suicide and its prevention, be sure to address the following topics:

- Importance of emotional connections to family and friends
- Importance of instilling hope
- Discouraging suicidal ideation, rumination, self-harming behaviors
- Self-validation
- Emotional distress management
- Finding alternatives to suicidal behavior
- Establishing and using a crisis management plan
- Reestablishing the social network of the patient
- Information about treatment of underlying psychiatric disorders

Interventions for Intermediate and Long-Term Risk

Patients who are suicidal may need ongoing preventive interventions. The risk varies with the genetic, psychiatric, and psychological profile of the patient and the extent of their social support. Discouragement and hopelessness often persist long past the suicidal episode. Episodes of hopelessness should be anticipated and planned for in the patient's care. Patients should be taught to expect setbacks and times when they are unable to see much of a future for themselves. They should be encouraged to think of times in their lives when they were not so hopeless and consider how they may feel similarly in the future. Helping patients review the goals they already have achieved and, at the same time, set goals that can be achieved in the immediate future can help them manage periods of discouragement and hopelessness.

Interventions for the Biologic Domain

Patients who have survived a suicide attempt often need physical care of their self-inflicted injury. Overdose, gunshot wounds, and skin wounds are common. There will be biologic interventions for the underlying psychiatric disorder (see Unit V).

Medication Management

Medication management focuses on treating the underlying psychiatric disorder. Currently, clozapine is the only U.S. Food and Drug Administration (FDA)–approved medication for suicide risk in individuals with schizophrenia. Studies showing reduced suicide risk in patients with bipolar disorder or major depression taking lithium are not conclusive. Ketamine is FDA approved for treatment-resistant depression and may have utility for short-term reduction of suicide risk. For depression, a nonlethal antidepressant, such as a selective serotonin reuptake inhibitor, usually will be prescribed (AFSP, 2024).

Electroconvulsive Therapy

Electroconvulsive therapy (ECT) has been used in both inpatient and outpatient settings to alleviate severe depression, especially in medically compromised groups, such as older adults, who may not tolerate conventional pharmacotherapy for depression (see Chapter 11). Rapid reduction in depression often leads to a decreased suicide drive. More research is needed to determine the role ECT may play in managing suicidal behavior. At this time, ECT is among several strategies used to decrease suicidal behavior over the long term (Griffiths et al., 2023).

Interventions for the Psychological Domain

The goals of treatment in the psychological domain include reducing the capacity for suicidal behavior, increasing tolerance for distress, expanding coping abilities, and developing effective crisis management strategies. During the early part of a hospitalization, the most important way to reduce stress is to help the patient feel more secure and hopeful. The nurse should be empathetic and engage in active listening and validate the patient's struggle with their suicidality. As patients become more comfortable in their environment, the nurse can provide education about emotions, help patients explore and link presuicidal beliefs to a positive and hopeful future, support the application of new skills in managing negative thoughts, and help develop effective problem-solving skills.

Challenging the Suicidal Mindset

Teaching patients to distract themselves when thinking about suicide or engaging in negative self-evaluation can help to diminish suicidal ideation, dysfunctional thinking, and emotional reactivity. Simple distracting techniques such as reminding oneself to think of other things or engaging in other activities such as talking on the telephone, reading, or watching a movie are excellent temporary means of distracting the patient from negative cognitive states (see Box 22.5).

Validating the patient and teaching the patient to self-validate are powerful means of reducing suicidal thinking. Patients can learn that everyone experiences emotional distress and can begin to recognize it as a routine event. To manage emotional distress and increase tolerance for it, patients can be taught simple anxiety management strategies such as relaxation and visualization. The patient can be encouraged to write about their emotional experiences.

When negative thoughts and emotions coexist, they reinforce each other and contribute to suicidal ideation. Individuals who are suicidal often believe they are a burden to their family, who would be better off without them and do not feel connected to others. Nurses can challenge negative beliefs, especially the patient's idea that they are a burden to others. Ask the patient to describe the events that led to specific suicidal behavior so the patient can be engaged in developing alternative solutions. For each event, work with the patient to identify specific strategies that could be used to manage their distress, sense of disconnection, extreme focus on suicidal ideas, and other experiences that led the person to believe they had no option other than to die.

Developing New Coping Strategies

Preventing suicidal behavior requires that patients develop crisis management strategies, generate solutions to difficult life circumstances other than suicide, engage in effective interpersonal interactions, and maintain hope. The nurse can help the patient develop a written plan that can be used as a blueprint for action when the patient feels that they are losing control. The plan should include strategies that the patient can use to self-soothe; friends and family members that could be called, including multiple phone numbers where they can be reached; self-help groups and services such as suicide hotlines; and professional resources, including emergency departments and outpatient emergency psychiatric services.

Commitment to Treatment

Patients are usually ambivalent about wanting to die. **The commitment to treatment statement** (CTS) directly addresses ambivalence about treatment by asking the patient to engage in treatment by making a commitment to try new approaches. Different from the no-suicide contract, the CTS does not restrict the patient's rights regarding the option of suicide. Instead, the patient agrees to engage in treatment and access emergency services if needed. Underlying the CTS is the expectation that the patient will communicate openly and honestly about all aspects of treatment, including suicide. This commitment is written and signed by the patient. The efficacy of this approach has yet to be established by systematic research. Whether using the CTS or other means, be observant for lapses in the patient's participation in treatment and discuss them with the patient and other members of the interdisciplinary team.

Interventions for the Social Domain

Poor social skills may interfere with the patient's ability to engage others. The nurse should assess the patient's social capability early in treatment and make necessary provisions for social skills training. The interpersonal relationship with the nurse is an ideal place to begin shaping social behaviors that will help the patient establish a social network that will sustain them during periods of discouragement or crisis. Participation in support networks, such as recovery groups, clubhouses, drop-in centers, self-help groups, or other therapeutic social engagement, will help the patient become connected to others.

Patients need to anticipate that even some of the people closest to them will feel uncomfortable with their suicidal behavior. Helping the patient to anticipate the stigmatizing behavior of others and how to manage it will go far in reintegrating the patient into a supportive social community. The nurse can also explore the patient's participation in specific social activities, such as attending church or community activities.

Evaluation and Treatment Outcomes

The most desirable treatment outcome is the patient's recovery with no future suicide attempts. Short-term outcomes include maintaining the patient's safety, averting suicide, and mobilizing the patient's resources. Whether the patient is hospitalized or cared for in the community, their emotional distress must be reduced. Long-term outcomes must focus on maintaining the patient in psychiatric treatment, enabling the patient and family to identify and manage suicidal crises effectively, and widening the patient's support network.

Continuum of Care

Whether the suicide prevention plan is instituted in the hospital or in an outpatient setting, the patient cannot be released home until a workable plan of care is in place. The care plan includes scheduling an appointment for outpatient treatment, providing for continuing somatic treatments until the first outpatient treatment visit, ensuring postrelease contact between the patient and significant other, providing for access to emergency psychiatric care, and arranging the patient's environment so it provides both structure and safety.

At the first follow-up visit, the patient and health care provider can establish a plan of care that specifies the intensity of outpatient care. Patients who are very unstable may need frequent supervision (e.g., telephone or face-to-face meetings or both) in the early days after hospitalization to maintain the patient's safety in the community. These contacts often can be short; their purpose is to convey the ongoing concern and caring of professionals involved in the patient's care. In arranging outpatient care, be certain to refer the patient to a provider who can provide the intensity of care the patient may need.

The patient's outpatient environment should be made as safe as possible before discharge. The nurse must share the care plan with family members so they can remove any objects in the patient's environment that could be used to engage in self-harm. The nurse should explain this measure to the patient to reinforce their sense of self-control. It is important to be reasonable in deciding what to remove from the environment. Patients who are truly determined to kill themselves after discharge will succeed in doing so, using whatever means are available.

Documentation and Reporting

The nurse must thoroughly document encounters with patients who are suicidal. This action is for the patient's ongoing treatment and the nurse's protection. Lawsuits for malpractice in psychiatric settings often involve completed suicides. The medical record must reflect that the nurse took every reasonable action to provide for the patient's safety.

The record should describe the patient's history, assessment, and interventions agreed upon by the patient and nurse. The nurse should document the presence or absence of suicidal thoughts, intent, plan, and available means to illustrate the patient's current and ongoing suicide risk. If the patient denies any suicidal ideation, it is important that the denial is documented. Documentation must include any recent use of substances, alcohol, or prescription medications by the patient. It should include the use of antidepressants that are especially lethal (e.g., tricyclics), as well as any medication that might impair the patient's judgment (e.g., a sleep medication). Notes should reflect the level of the patient's judgment and ability to be a partner in treatment.

The documentation should reflect if any medications were prescribed, the dosages, and the number of pills dispensed. Notes should reflect the plan for ongoing treatment, including the time of the next appointment with the provider, instructions given to the patient about obtaining emergency care if needed, and the names of family members and friends who will act as supports if the patient needs them.

IMPORTANCE OF NURSES' REFLECTION

Caring for patients who are suicidal is highly stressful and can lead to secondary trauma for the nurse. Nurses who care for patients who are suicidal must regularly share their experiences and feelings with one another. Talking about how the situations or actions of patients make them feel will help alleviate symptoms of stress. Some nurses find outpatient therapy helpful because it enhances their understanding of what situations are most likely to trigger secondary trauma. By demonstrating how to effectively manage the stressors in their own lives, nurses can be powerful role models for their patients.

SUMMARY OF KEY POINTS

- Suicide is a common and major public health issue.
- Suicide completion is more common in White males, especially older males.
- Nonsuicidal self-injury is more common among females than males.
- People who attempt suicide and fail are likely to try again without treatment.
- Suicidal behavior has genetic, biologic, and psychosocial origins.
- Suicide is associated with feelings of being a burden and not belonging.
- Acquired capability for suicide means that the person is fearless about death and has a high pain threshold.
- A suicide assessment focuses on the intention to die, hopelessness, available means, previous attempts and self-harm behavior, and degree of planning.
- Patients who are in crisis, are depressed, or use substances are at risk for suicide.
- The major objectives of brief hospital care are to maintain the patient's safety, reestablish the patient's biologic equilibrium, help the patient reconnect to others, instill hope, strengthen the patient's cognitive coping skills, and develop an outpatient support system.
- The nurse who cares for patients who are suicidal is vulnerable to secondary trauma and must take steps to maintain personal mental health.

DEVELOPING CLINICAL JUDGMENT

1. A person who lives with their spouse and three children comes to see their primary care provider. They are tearful and very depressed. What factors should be investigated to determine this person's risk for suicide and need for hospitalization?
2. A person experiencing poverty with no insurance is hospitalized after their third suicide attempt. Antidepressant medication is prescribed. What kinds of treatment will be most effective in preventing future suicidal behavior?
3. A young adult enters their workplace inebriated and carrying a gun. They do not threaten anyone but say they must end it all. Assuming the person can be disarmed, what civil rights must be considered in taking further action in managing their suicidal risk?
4. How should the nurse respond to a distressed teen who asks what causes suicidal ideation and wonders if it is treatable?

MOVIES, TV, AND STREAMING PROGRAMS

A Man Called Otto: 2022. In this film, Tom Hanks portrays a widower (Otto) who becomes cynical and grumpy after several major life events, including losing his wife to cancer. Believing he has nothing to live for, Otto attempts suicide on several occasions, with each attempt being ultimately disrupted. Living in a small, gated community, he is forced to interact with neighbors who ultimately build a community in which he finds meaning and purpose.

Viewing Points:

1. Name some of Otto's risk factors for suicide.
2. Over time, Otto builds relationships with his neighbors. How does this built sense of community become a protective factor for Otto?
3. Aside from Otto's renewed purpose for living, what other protective factors for suicide developed through the course of the film?

REFERENCES

Akinyemi, O., Ogundare, T., Oladunjoye, A. F., Nasef, K. E., Lipscombe, C., Akinbote, J. A., & Bezold, M. (2023). Factors associated with suicide/self-inflicted injuries among women aged 18–65 years in the United States: A 13-year retrospective analysis of the National Inpatient Sample database. *PloS One, 18*(10), e0287141.

American Foundation of Suicide Prevention (AFSP). (2023). *Suicide Statistics*. https://afsp.org/suicide-statistics

American Foundation of Suicide Prevention (AFSP). (2024). *Treatment for suicide and suicide attempts*. https://afsp.org/medications-as-a-part-of-the-treatment-plan/

Ballesteros, M. F., Ivey-Stephenson, A. Z., Trinh, E., & Stone, D. M. (2024). Background and rationale—CDC guidance for communities assessing, investigating, and responding to suicide clusters, United States, 2024. *MMWR Supplements*, *73*(2), 1–7.

Beck, A. T., Rush, A. J., Shaw, B. F., & Emery, G. (1979). *Cognitive therapy of depression*. The Guilford Press.

Bengoechea-Fortes, S. P., Ramírez-Expósito, M. J., & Martínez-Martos, J. M. (2023). Suicide, neuroinflammation and other physiological alterations. *European Archives of Psychiatry and Clinical Neuroscience*, *274*(5), 1037–1049. https://doi.org/10.1007/s00406-023-01584-z

Bhatt, A., Gonzales, H., Pallin, R., & Barnhorst, A. (2023). Rising rates of adolescent firearm suicide and the clinician's role in addressing firearms. *Journal of the American Academy of Child and Adolescent Psychiatry*, *62*(6), 614–617.

Bird, K., Arcelus, J., Matsagoura, L., O'Shea, B. A., & Townsend, E. (2024). Risk and protective factors for self-harm thoughts and behaviours in transgender and gender diverse people: A systematic review. *Heliyon*, *10*(5), e26074.

Bommersbach, T. J., McKean, A. J., Olfson, M., & Rhee, T. G. (2023). National trends in mental health-related emergency department visits among youth, 2011–2020. *JAMA*, *329*(17), 1469–1477.

Calati, R., Romano, D., Magliocca, S., Madeddu, F., Zeppegno, P., & Gramaglia, C. (2022). The interpersonal-psychological theory of suicide and the role of psychological pain during the COVID-19 pandemic: A network analysis. *Journal of Affective Disorders*, *302*, 435–439.

Cantor, N., Kingsbury, M., Warner, E., Landry, H., Clayborne, Z., Islam, R., & Colman, I. (2023). Young adult outcomes associated with adolescent suicidality: A meta-analysis. *Pediatrics*, *151*(3), e2022058113.

Centers for Disease Control and Prevention (CDC). (2024). Risk and protective factors for suicide [Online]. https://www.cdc.gov/suicide/risk-factors/?CDC_AAref_Val=https://www.cdc.gov/suicide/factors/

Centers for Disease Control and Prevention (CDC). (2023). *Suicide prevention* [Online]. https://www.cdc.gov/suicide/index.html

Chalker, S. A., Parrish, E. M., Cano, M., Kelsven, S., Moore, R. C., Granholm, E., Pinkham, A., Harvey, P. D., & Depp, C. A. (2022). Childhood trauma associations with the interpersonal psychological theory of suicide and social cognitive biases in psychotic disorders. *Journal of Nervous & Mental Disease*, *210*(6), 432–438.

Cheatle, M. D., Giordano, N. A., Themelis, K., & Tang, N. K. Y. (2023). Suicidal thoughts and behaviors in patients with chronic pain, with and without co-occurring opioid use disorder. *Pain Medicine*, *24*(8), 941–948.

Choi, N. G., Marti, C. N., & Choi, B. Y. (2022). Job loss, financial strain, and housing problems as suicide precipitants: Associations with other life stressors. *SSM—Population Health*, *19*, 101243.

Choi, N. G., Marti, C. N., & Choi, B. Y. (2024). Suicide from intimate partner and other relationship conflicts: Demographic and clinical correlates'. *Journal of Mental Health*, *33*(1), 84–91.

Dhole, A. R., Petkar, P., Choudhari, S. G., & Mendhe, H. (2023). Understanding the factors contributing to suicide among the geriatric population: A narrative review. *Cureus*, *15*(10), e46387.

Drago, A. (2024). Genetic signatures of suicide attempt behavior: Insights and applications. *Expert Review of Proteomics*, *21*(1–3) 41–53.

Durkheim, E. (1951 [1897]). *Suicide*. The Free Press.

Edwards, A., Hung, R., Levin, J. B., Forthun, L., Sajatovic, M., & McVoy, M. (2023). Health disparities among rural individuals with mental health conditions: A systematic literature review. *Rural Mental Health*, *47*(3), 163–178.

Eisenberg, M. E., Lawrence, S. E., Eadeh, H.-M., Suresh, M., Rider, G. N., & Gower, A. L. (2024). Emotional distress disparities across multiple intersecting social positions: The role of bias-based bullying. *Pediatrics*, *153*(2), 1–10.

Elbogen, E. B., Lanier, M., Blakey, S. M., Wagner, H. R., & Tsai, J. (2021). Suicidal ideation and thoughts of self-harm during the COVID-19 pandemic: The role of COVID-19-related stress, social isolation, and financial strain. *Depression and Anxiety*, *38*(7), 739–748. https://doi.org/10.1002/da.23162

Ewell Foster, C., Derwin, S., Bornheimer, L. A., Magness, C., Kahsay, E., Eis, M., Verdugo, J. L., Smith, T., Massey, L., Rivara, F. P., & King, C. A. (2024). Firearm safe storage in rural families: Community perspectives about ownership and safety messaging. *Health Promotion Practice*, *25*(1), 33–48.

Favril, L., Yu, R., Geddes, J. R., & Fazel, S. (2023). Individual-level risk factors for suicide mortality in the general population: an umbrella review. *The Lancet. Public Health*, *8*(11), e868–e877.

Favril, L., Yu, R., Uyar, A., Sharpe, M., & Fazel, S. (2022). Risk factors for suicide in adults: Systematic review and meta-analysis of psychological autopsy studies. *Evidence-Based Mental Health*, *25*(4), 148–155.

Garnett, M. F., Spencer, M. R., & Weeks, J. D. (2023). Suicide among adults age 55 and older, 2021. *NCHS Data Brief*, *483*, 1–8.

Gaylor, E. M., Krause, K. H., Welder, L. E., Cooper, A. C., Ashley, C., Mack, K. A., Crosby, A. E., Trinh, E., Ivey-Stephenson, A. Z., & Whittle, L. (2023). Suicidal thoughts and behaviors among high school students—Youth Risk Behavior Survey, United States, 2021. *MMWR Supplements*, *72*(1), 45–54.

Griffiths, J. J., Zarate, C. A. Jr, & Rasimas, J. J. (2023). Existing and novel biological therapeutics in suicide prevention. *Focus (American Psychiatric Publishing)*, *21*(2), 225–232.

Gupta, M., Moll, J., & Gupta, N. (2022). Smart doors: innovative idea for reducing inpatient and institutional suicides: Focus on safe suicide-proof architecture. *Suicide & Life-Threatening Behavior*, *52*(4), 828–831.

Herzog, S., Galfalvy, H., Keilp, J. G., Mann, J. J., Sublette, M. E., Burke, A., Oquendo, M. A., & Stanley, B. H. (2023). Relationship of stress-reactive cortisol to suicidal intent of prior attempts in major depression. *Psychiatry Research*, *327*, 115315.

Ivey-Stephenson, A. Z., Ballesteros, M. F., Trinh, E., Stone, D. M., & Crosby, A. E. (2024). CDC guidance for community response to suicide clusters, United States, 2024. *MMWR Supplements*, *73*(2), 17–26.

Jang, J., Park, S. Y., Kim, Y. Y., Kim, E. J., Lee, G., Seo, J., Na, E. J., Park, J.-Y., & Jeon, H. J. (2022). Risks of suicide among family members of suicide victims: A nationwide sample of South Korea. *Frontiers in Psychiatry*, *13*, 995834.

Joiner, T. (2005). *Why people die by suicide*. Harvard University.

Jones, A. A., Hard, G., Gray, J., Apsley, H. B., & Santos-Lozada, A. R. (2023). The role of substance use disorders on suicidal ideation, planning, and attempts: A nationally representative study of adolescents and adults in the United States, 2020. *Substance Abuse: Research & Treatment*, *17*, 11782218231216233.

Kirchner, S., & Niederkrotenthaler, T. (2024). Experiences of suicide survivors of sharing their stories about suicidality and overcoming a crisis in media and public talks: A qualitative study. *BMC Public Health*, *24*(1), 142.

Klonsky, E. D., Pachkowski, M. C., Shahnaz, A., & May, A. M. (2021). The three-step theory of suicide: Description, evidence, and some useful points of clarification. *Preventative Medicine*, *152*, 106549.

Kohnepoushi, P., Nikouei, M., Cheraghi, M., Hasanabadi, P., Rahmani, H., Moradi, M., Moradi, G., Moradpour, F., & Moradi, Y. (2023). Prevalence of suicidal thoughts and attempts in the transgender population of the world: A systematic review and meta-analysis. *Annals of General Psychiatry*, *22*(1), 28.

Lee, C. S., & Wong, Y. J. (2020). Racial/ethnic differences in the antecedents of youth suicide. *Cultural Diversity and Ethnic Minority Psychology*, *26*(4), 532–543.

Levi-Belz, Y., Krysinska, K., & Andriessen, K. (2021). "Turning personal tragedy into triumph": A systematic review and meta-analysis of studies on posttraumatic growth among suicide-loss survivors. *Psychological Trauma: Theory, Research, Practice and Policy*, *13*(3), 322–332.

Li, Q. S., Shabalin, A. A., DiBlasi, E., Gopal, S., Canuso, C. M., Palotie, A., Drevets, W. C., Docherty, A. R., & Coon, H.; FinnGen, International Suicide Genetics Consortium. (2023). Genome-wide association study meta-analysis of suicide death and suicidal behavior. *Molecular Psychiatry*, *28*(2), 891–900.

Liu, G. S., Nguyen, B. L., Lyons, B. H., Sheats, K. J., Wilson, R. F., Betz, C. J., & Fowler, K. A. (2023). Surveillance for violent deaths—National Violent Death Reporting System, 48 states, the district of Columbia, and Puerto Rico, 2020. *MMWR Surveillance Summaries*, *72*(5), 1–38.

Mann, J. J., Michel, C. A., & Auerbach, R. P. (2021). Improving suicide prevention through evidence-based strategies: A systematic review. *American Journal of Psychiatry*, *178*(7), 611–624.

Marraccini, M. E., Lindsay, C. A., Griffin, D., Greene, M. J., Simmons, K. T., & Ingram, K. M. (2023). A trauma—and justice, equity, diversity, and inclusion (JEDI)- informed approach to suicide prevention in school: Black boys' lives matter. *School Psychology Review*, *52*(3), 292–315.

McClelland, H., Evans, J. J., & O'Connor, R. C. (2023). The association of family, social and romantic loneliness in relation to suicidal ideation and self-injurious behaviours. *Journal of Psychiatric Research*, *158*, 330–340.

McGrath, M. O., Krysinska, K., Reavley, N. J., Andriessen, K., & Pirkis, J. (2023). Disclosure of mental health problems or suicidality at work: A systematic review. *International Journal of Environmental Research and Public Health*, *20*(8), 5548.

Molock, S. D., Boyd, R. C., Alvarez, K., Cha, C., Denton, E.-G., Glenn, C. R., Katz, C. C., Mueller, A. S., Meca, A., Meza, J. I., Miranda, R., Ortin-Peralta, A., Polanco-Roman, L., Singer, J. B., Zullo, L., & Miller, A. B. (2023). Culturally responsive assessment of suicidal thoughts and behaviors in youth of color. *The American Psychologist*, *78*(7), 842–855.

Moscardini, E. H., Oakey-Frost, D. N., Robinson, A., Powers, J., Aboussouan, A. B., Rasmussen, S., Cramer, R. J., & Tucker, R. P. (2022). Entrapment and suicidal ideation: The protective roles of presence of life meaning and reasons for living. *Suicide & Life-threatening Behavior*, *52*(1), 14–23.

National Alliance on Mental Illness (NAMI). (2023). *LGBTQI* [Online]. https://www.nami.org/Your-Journey/Identity-and-Cultural-Dimensions/LGBTQI

National Institute of Mental Health (NIMH). (2024). *Suicide*. https://www.nimh.nih.gov/health/statistics/suicide.shtml

Nicoll, G., Vincent, J., Gajaria, A., & Zaheer, J. (2023). A trauma-informed approach to suicide prevention for the COVID-19 pandemic. *Psychiatry Research*, *327*, 115407.

O'Connor, R. C., & Kirtley, O. J. (2018). The integrated motivational-volitional model of suicidal behaviour. *Philosophical Transactions of the Royal Society of London. Series B, Biological Sciences*, *373*(1754), 20170268.

Oexle, N., Puschner, N., Votruba, N., Rüsch, N., & Mayer, L. (2022). Perceived determinants of disclosing suicide loss. *Crisis*, *44*(6), 470–476. https://doi.org/10.1027/0227-5910/a000891

Patra, B. N., Sen, M. S., Sagar, R., & Bhargava, R. (2023). Deliberate self-harm in adolescents: A review of literature. *Industrial Psychiatry Journal*, *32*(1), 9–14.

Pearlman, A. T., Murphy, M. A., Raiciulescu, S., Johnson, N., Klein, D. A., Gray, J. C., & Schvey, N. A. (2023). Longitudinal associations between perceived discrimination and suicidality in youth. *Journal of Pediatrics*, *262*, 113642.

Phillip, A., Pellechi, A., DeSilva, R., Semler, K., & Makani, R. (2022). A plausible explanation of increased suicidal behaviors among transgender youth based on the Interpersonal Theory of Suicide (IPTS): Case series and literature review. *Journal of Psychiatric Practice*, *28*(1), 3–13.

Polanco-Roman, L., Williams, S. Z., & Ortin-Peralta, A. (2023). Study preregistration: Does state-level structural racism impact risk for suicidal thoughts and behaviors among US adolescents across race and ethnicity? *Journal of the American Academy of Child and Adolescent Psychiatry*, *62*(7), 829–830.

Pritchard, C., Hansen, L., Dray, R., & Sharif, J. (2023). USA suicides compared to other western countries in the 21st century: Is there a relationship with gun ownership? *Archives of Suicide Research: Official Journal of the International Academy for Suicide Research*, *27*(1), 135–147.

Riera-Serra, P., Navarra-Ventura, G., Castro, A., Gili, M., Salazar-Cedillo, A., Ricci-Cabello, I., Roldán-Espínola, L., Coronado-Simsic, V., García-Toro, M., Gómez-Juanes, R., & Roca, M. (2023). Clinical predictors of suicidal ideation, suicide attempts and suicide death in depressive disorder: A systematic review and meta-analysis. *European Archives of Psychiatry and Clinical Neuroscience*, *274*(7), 1543–1563. https://doi.org/10.1007/s00406-023-01716-5

Rikard, S. M., Strahan, A. E., Schmit, K. M., & Guy, G. P. Jr. (2023). Chronic pain among adults: United States, 2019–2021. *MMWR. Morbidity and Mortality Weekly Report*, *72*(15), 379–385.

Roelfs, D. J., & Shor, E. (2023). Financial stress, unemployment, and suicide: A meta-analysis. *Crisis*, *44*(6), 506–517.

Rogerson, O., Baguley, T., & O'Connor, D. B. (2023). Childhood trauma and suicide. *Crisis*, *44*(5), 433–441.

Ruiz, F., Burgo-Black, L., Hunt, S. C., Miller, M., & Spelman, J. F. (2023). A practical review of suicide among veterans: Preventive and proactive measures for health care institutions and providers. *Public Health Reports*, *138*(2), 223–231. https://doi.org/10.1177/00333549221085240

Silva, C., McGovern, C., Gomez, S., Beale, E., Overholser, J., & Ridley, J. (2023). Can I count on you? Social support, depression and suicide risk. *Clinical Psychology & Psychotherapy*, *30*(6), 1407–1415.

Small, L. A., Godoy, S. M., Lau, C., & Franke, T. (2024). Gender-based violence and suicide among gender-diverse populations in the United States. *Archives of Suicide Research: Official Journal of the International Academy for Suicide Research*, *28*(1), 107–122.

Souza, K., Sosu, E. M., Thomson, S., & Rasmussen, S. (2024). A systematic review of the studies testing the integrated motivational-volitional model of suicidal behaviour. *Health Psychology Review*, *18*(4), 698–722.

Stack, S. (2021). Contributing factors to suicide: Political, social, cultural and economic. *Preventative Medicine*, *152*(Pt 1), 106498.

Stacy, M., & Schulkin, J. (2022). Suicide: Allostatic regulation and resilience. *Psychoneuroendocrinology*, *139*, 105691.

Stanley, A. R., Aguilar, T., Holland, K. M., & Orpinas, P. (2023). Precipitating circumstances associated with intimate partner problem-related suicides. *American Journal of Preventive Medicine*, *65*(3), 385–394.

Stone, D. M., Mack, K. A., & Qualters, J. (2023). Notes from the field: Recent changes in suicide rates, by race and ethnicity and age group—United States, 2021. *Morbidity and Mortality Weekly Report*, *72*(6), 160–162.

Sufrate-Sorzano, T., Di Nitto, M., Garrote-Cámara, M. E., Molina-Luque, F., Recio-Rodríguez, J. I., Asión-Polo, P., Durante, Á., Gea-Caballero, V., Juárez-Vela, R., Pérez, J., & Santolalla-Arnedo, I. (2023). Media exposure of suicidal behaviour: An umbrella review. *Nursing Reports*, *13*(4), 1486–1499.

Suicide Prevention Resource Center (SPRC). (2024). *Racial and ethnic disparities* [Online]. https://sprc.org/about-suicide/scope-of-the-problem/racial-and-ethnic-disparities/

Sweileh, W. (2024). Analysis and mapping of research on barriers to mental health service utilization in minority and underserved groups (1993–2022). *Mental Health & Social Inclusion*, *28*(6), 1000–1013.

The Trevor Project. (2023). *2023 U.S. national survey on the mental health of LGBTQ young people*. https://www.thetrevorproject.org/survey-2023/assets/static/05_TREVOR05_2023survey.pdf

Thomas, S., Hummel, K. V., Schäfer, J., Wittchen, H.-U., & Trautmann, S. (2023). Harassment and its association with depressive symptoms and suicidal behavior: The role of perceived stigma and nondisclosure. *Psychological Services*, *20*(1), 84–93.

Tsai, M., Lari, H., Saffy, S., & Klonsky, E. D. (2021). Examining the Three-Step Theory (3ST) of suicide in a prospective study of adult psychiatric inpatients. *Behavior Therapy*, *52*(3), 673–685.

United States Department of Health and Human Services. (n.d.). *Healthy people 2030* [Online]. Healthy People 2030 | health.gov. https://health.gov/healthypeople

United States Department of Veterans Affairs, Office of Mental Health and Suicide Prevention (2023). 2023 National Veteran Suicide Prevention Annual Report. [Online]. https://www.mentalhealth.va.gov/docs/data-sheets/2023/2023-National-Veteran-Suicide-Prevention-Annual-Report-FINAL-508.pdf

Vidal-Ribas, P., Govender, T., Yu, J., Livinski, A. A., Haynie, D. L., & Gilman, S. E. (2024). The developmental origins of suicide mortality: A systematic review of longitudinal studies. *European Child & Adolescent Psychiatry*, *33*(7), 2083–2110. https://doi.org/10.1007/s00787-022-02092-6

Wang, T., Yang, L., Yang, L., Liu, B.-P., & Jia, C.-X. (2024). The relationship between psychological pain and suicidality in patients with major depressive disorder: A meta-analysis. *Journal of Affective Disorders*, *346*, 115–121.

Whipple, C. R., Robinson, W. L., Flack, C. E., Jason, L. A., & Keenan, K. (2023). Longitudinal patterns and predictors of suicidal ideation in African American adolescents. *American Journal of Community Psychology*, *71*(3–4), 453–464.

Wyder, M., Ray, M. K., Roennfeldt, H., Daly, M., & Crompton, D. (2020). How health care systems let our patients down: A systematic review into suicide deaths. *International Journal for Quality in Health Care: Journal of the International Society for Quality in Health Care*, *32*(5), 285–291.

Yan, Y., Hou, J., Li, Q., & Yu, N. X. (2023). Suicide before and during the COVID-19 pandemic: A systematic review with meta-analysis. *International Journal of Environmental Research and Public Health*, *20*(4), 3346.

Yarar, E. Z., Bulut, B. P., & Demirbaş, H. (2023). Does gender really matter: Childhood trauma, trait anger, and suicide risk in early adulthood. *Journal of Interpersonal Violence*, *38*(1–2), NP1222–NP1238.

Zhou, J., Hu, T., Xue, S., Dong, Z., & Tang, W. (2024). The association of childhood trauma with suicidality in adult psychiatric patients: The mediating role of NSSI and the moderating role of self-esteem. *Journal of Clinical Psychology*, *80*(3), 664–677.

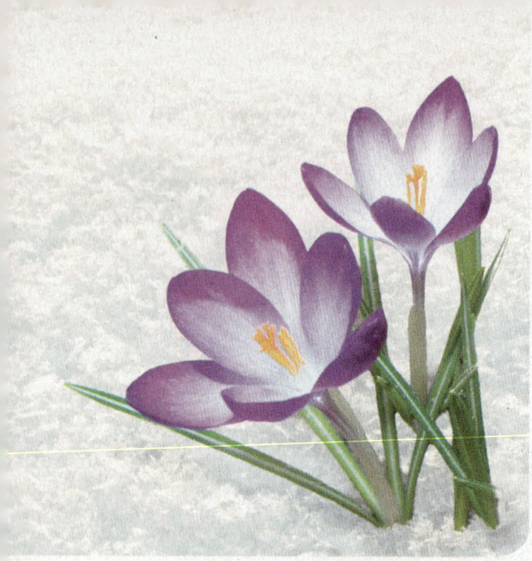

23 Mental Health Care for People Who Have Experienced Violence*

Beverly Baliko and Rachel S. Bush

KEYCONCEPTS

- intimate partner violence
- psychological abuse
- sexual violence
- teen partner abuse
- gaslighting
- Basic Needs

LEARNING OBJECTIVES

After studying this chapter, you will be able to:

1. Describe types of violence and abuse, including intimate partner violence, stalking, rape and sexual assault, child abuse and neglect, and elder abuse.
2. Describe selected theories of violence.
3. Compare the reasons some people become abusive and why some people who experience violence remain in violent relationships.
4. Discuss the formation of a therapeutic relationship with an individual who has experienced violence.
5. Formulate nursing care plans for people who have experienced violence and abuse.
6. Describe treatment for people perpetrating abuse.

KEY TERMS

• adverse childhood experiences • batterer intervention programs • body map • child abuse • child neglect • cycle of violence • Danger Assessment Screen • elder abuse • gaslighting • human trafficking • intergenerational transmission of violence • mandatory reporting • rape • revictimization • sexual assault nurse examiner (SANE) • social–ecologic model of violence prevention • stalking • trauma-informed approach

INTRODUCTION

Violence in the form of abuse of intimate partners, children, and older adults is a national health issue. This type of violence permanently changes the reality and meaning of life for the individual who has experienced violence. It wounds deeply, endangering core beliefs about the self, others, and the world. Without intervention, it can damage or destroy the self-esteem and sense of security of the individual who has experienced violence.

Nurses encounter people who have experienced violence and abuse in all health care settings. For this reason, being knowledgeable about abuse risk factors, indicators, causes, assessment techniques, and effective nursing interventions is a must. This chapter presents evidence that can shape contemporary nursing practice in caring for people who have experienced violence and abuse, and their families.

TYPES OF VIOLENCE AND ABUSE

The most common type of abuse occurs as a result of domestic (family) violence; that is, the individual perpetrating the abuse is or formerly was a loved and trusted partner or family member. When this kind of violence occurs, the world and home are no longer safe in the

*In this chapter, "woman," "man," "girl," "boy," "female," and "male" refer to people who identify as these genders.

eyes of the individual who has experienced violence. This chapter includes a discussion of intimate partner violence (IPV), child abuse and neglect, and elder abuse, with emphasis on IPV.

Intimate Partner Violence

IPV is a significant public health issue in the United States, and across the world. Behaviors that constitute IPV include physical, sexual, and psychological (emotional) abuse or a combination of these perpetrated by a current or former spouse, significant other, or dating partner.

The prevalence of IPV can only be estimated because much abuse goes unreported. The most recent data available suggest that during their lifetimes, 1 in 4 women and nearly 1 in 10 men experience adverse psychological or physical consequences related to physical or sexual violence perpetrated by an intimate partner (Centers for Disease Control and Prevention [CDC], 2021). Economic costs associated with acute and chronic medical and mental health services for people who have experienced violence, lost productivity, and criminal justice activities create a substantial ongoing societal burden (CDC, 2021). In its most extreme form, IPV is fatal. The vast majority (89%) of female homicide victims are murdered by someone they know, most often a current or former intimate partner (Violence Policy Center, 2023).

KEYCONCEPT Intimate partner violence involves physical violence, sexual violence, stalking, and psychological aggression (including coercive acts) by a current or former intimate partner. IPV occurs on a continuum from psychological abuse to lethal violence.

Physical Abuse

Physical abuse involves any act of aggression, with or without the use of an object or a weapon, that results in injury, pain, or impairment to another. Examples include striking, kicking, shoving, choking, and burning. Frequently, this behavior becomes a pattern that increases in severity over time. Physical abuse not only causes immediate injuries but also contributes to health issues that may persist long after the abuse ends. Although people of any gender can perpetrate or experience physical abuse, women are far more likely than men to be seriously injured or killed by an intimate partner.

Psychological Abuse

KEYCONCEPT Psychological abuse (also referred to as emotional abuse) involves threats, intimidation, or destructive behaviors used as a means of manipulating someone, asserting dominance, or causing fear. Psychological abuse includes behaviors such as criticizing, insulting, humiliating, or ridiculing someone in private or in public. People perpetrating abuse may destroy property, threaten or harm pets, control or monitor spending and daily activities, or isolate an individual from family and friends.

Gaslighting is a form of psychological abuse in which the individual experiencing the gaslighting is made to question their own judgment and perceptions. People perpetrating abuse downplay the consequences of their behavior, deny abusive intent, or argue that actions are somehow justified. They often blame the individual they abuse for provoking or otherwise causing the abuse, leaving the individual experiencing the abuse with feelings of guilt or responsibility. About one-third of adults report experiencing psychological abuse by an intimate partner during their lifetime (CDC, 2021).

Whereas physical violence may be episodic, psychological abuse is frequently more unrelenting. Over time, psychological abuse is devastating to an individual's self-esteem and self-confidence and can lead to psychiatric and physical disorders resulting from chronic stress. The varieties of abuse used to exert power and control over romantic partners are represented in Figure 23.1.

KEYCONCEPT Teen partner abuse refers to violence experienced by teens within an intimate relationship. Teens and adults are often not aware of the frequency with which teen dating violence occurs. In a national survey of adolescents in the United States, 1 in 11 female and 1 in 14 male high school students reported having experienced physical violence by a dating partner in the last year (CDC, 2021). Sexual violence is also prevalent, reported by 1 in 8 female and 1 in 26 male students. Conflict or relationship issues with parents/caregivers and peers may be predictors of teen partner abuse. Teens who experience violence in intimate relationships are more likely to develop issues such as depression, substance misuse, eating disorders, and thoughts of suicide. School performance may suffer. Dating violence places youths at higher risk for experiencing abuse during college and in subsequent relationships throughout adulthood.

Comorbidities

Besides injuries and death, people who have experienced violence suffer multiple conditions directly caused by IPV or the chronic stress associated with it. Anxiety disorders, depression, posttraumatic stress disorder (PTSD), and substance use disorders are all associated with family violence. Examples of health issues associated with IPV include asthma, gastrointestinal conditions, cardiovascular issues, bladder infections, migraines, joint pain, gynecologic disorders, and sexually transmitted infections (STIs) (Office on Women's Health, 2021). Strangulation can cause airway obstruction and damage to blood vessels, and blows to the head can cause traumatic brain injuries that have lasting effects on cognition and functioning.

Risk Factors for Intimate Partner Violence

IPV occurs across all demographics and socioeconomic levels. Younger women, women who are divorced or separated, and Native American and Alaska Native women are at the highest risk (National Center for Victims of Crime, n.d.). Although women are disproportionately affected, men can also experience IPV. LGBTQIA+ couples

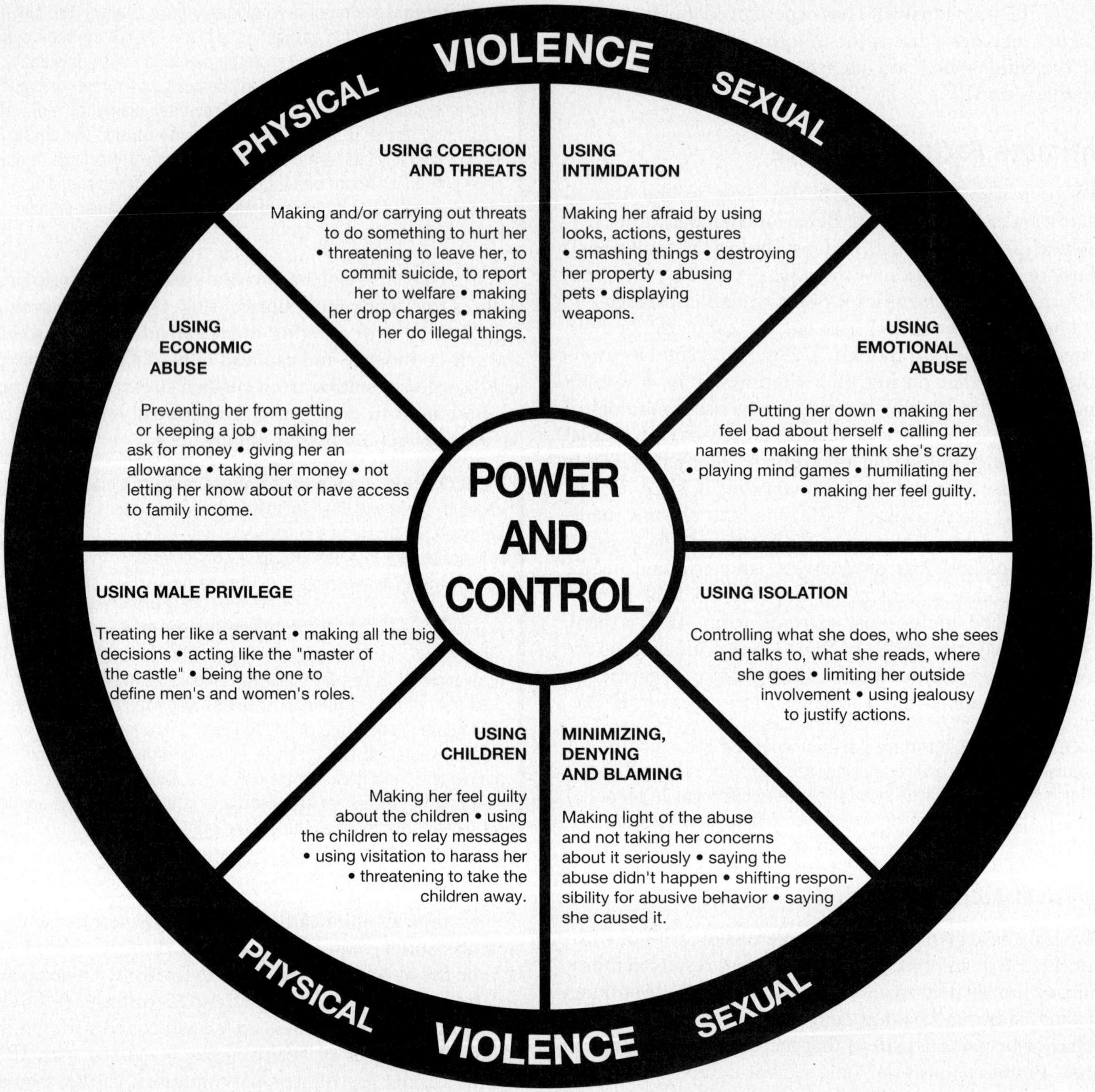

FIGURE 23.1 Power and control wheel. (Courtesy of Domestic Abuse Intervention Programs, 202 East Superior Street, Duluth, MN 55802. www.theduluthmodel.org)

experience IPV at rates similar to heterosexual couples, but people in this population often receive less support because of social stigma associated with nontraditional relationships. Within any type of relationship, frequent conflicts, jealousy, and possessiveness are associated with an increased risk of violence.

Individual characteristics such as low self-esteem, emotional insecurity, antisocial or borderline personality traits, disorders such as depression and PTSD, or a history of violence increase the likelihood of perpetration of violence (CDC, 2021). There is a strong association of substance use, especially alcohol use disorder, with family violence. The presence of firearms in the home increases the risk of lethal violence.

Personal stressors, such as low income and unemployment, and external stressors, such as natural disasters or economic crises, may challenge individual and family coping, resulting in violence (CDC, 2021). In unstable families, violence sometimes begins or escalates when a pregnancy occurs. Abuse during pregnancy is associated with fetal and maternal complications prenatally and postnatally (Alhusen et al., 2023). Pregnancy is a window of opportunity for health care providers to screen pregnant patients for IPV and refer patients to the appropriate services.

Impact of the COVID-19 Pandemic

The onset of the COVID-19 pandemic saw a global escalation in gender-based violence that had a pervasive negative impact on women's mental health and perceptions of safety (U.N. Women, 2021). Pandemic lockdowns resulted in significant psychosocial, health, and economic stressors; decreased contact with social support networks; and disruptions to services. In families at risk for violence, extended time in contact with each other, school closures, fewer leisure outlets, and changes in employment contributed to heightened family stress and conflict. Reaching out for assistance was more challenging, and resources and support systems were less readily available. During the most acute phase of the pandemic, access to health care was reduced, while calls to domestic violence hotlines and violent incidents increased. Job loss, economic hardship, and a diagnosis of COVID-19 in one or both partners were associated with an increase in prevalence and severity of IPV (McNeil et al., 2023). Preexisting vulnerabilities combined with pandemic-related stressors to increase the risk of family violence, while the pandemic reduced access to resources that were already struggling to meet community needs.

KEYCONCEPT Sexual violence includes any form of nonconsenting sexual activity, ranging from verbal threats to penetration.

Sexual Violence

Sexual violence is any type of sexual activity inflicted on a nonconsenting individual. Sexual violence can include acts that are not identified as illegal but that are nevertheless traumatic or harmful in that the individual experiencing the violence feels objectified, unsafe, or without choice. **Rape** and sexual assault are criminal acts. Sexual assault covers a range of nonconsensual sexual contact, whereas rape specifically refers to penetration of a bodily orifice (FindLaw, 2022). In most states, the gender and relationship of the individual perpetrating the abuse and the individual experiencing the abuse are not relevant to the legal definition of rape. The important factor is the lack of consent. People who rape may use physical force, coercion, or threats to gain control over the individual who is raped. Rape is a crime of violence and domination, with sexuality used as a weapon. Sexual activity that occurs with an individual who is unable to consent because of age, mental status, or impairment is considered sexual assault. When the individual experiencing the violence is a minor, sexual assault is often referred to as sexual abuse. Most sexual assaults are perpetrated by someone known to the individual experiencing the violence. Children are most likely to be sexually abused by family members, caregivers, or others close to them, as are older adults and adults with disabilities. Adolescents and young adults are especially vulnerable to drug-facilitated assault by acquaintances, which involves the use of "date-rape" drugs, often combined with alcohol, to make an individual incapable of resistance. It is common for sexual assault to occur in conjunction with IPV, as an additional means of intimidation and humiliation. Nonconsensual sex within a marriage was exempt from rape laws until the 1970s, and it was not until 1993 that all states had removed that exemption (England, 2020).

Stalking

Stalking is a pattern of repeated unwanted contact, attention, and harassment that often increases in frequency. Stalkers harass and terrorize people they target with behavior that causes fear or substantial emotional distress. Stalking may include such behaviors as following someone, showing up at the individual's home or workplace, vandalizing property, using technology to track or harass someone (cyberstalking), or sending unwanted gifts. One in 6 women and 1 in 19 men experience stalking at some point in their lifetime (CDC, 2021). Stalking can be prolonged and takes a tremendous toll on the health and functioning of the people being stalked.

Human Trafficking

Human trafficking involves the use of force, fraud, or coercion to obtain some type of labor or commercial sex act. Human trafficking affects an estimated 27.6 million people globally, including in the United States (U.S. Department of State, n.d.), though actual prevalence is difficult to determine. People of color, LGBTQIA+ youth, and others who experience systemic oppression are at particularly high risk. However, people experiencing human trafficking may be of any age, race/ethnicity, gender, or nationality. Traffickers often prey on people who are psychologically, emotionally, or financially vulnerable. Some are forced into sexual acts or physical labor through violence or manipulation. Others are exploited after being lured by false promises of money, jobs, or romantic relationships. Language barriers, fear of law enforcement or immigration authorities, dependence on the people perpetrating abuse for basic needs, or fear of retribution by traffickers can keep people experiencing abuse from seeking help. Under U.S. law, inducing minors under age 18 to participate in sexual acts for pay is considered trafficking. In the United States in 2021, the approximately 200 convictions for trafficking primarily involved sex trafficking (U.S. Department of State, n.d.). However, there is evidence that many labor trafficking cases in the United States are not identified or prosecuted. It is not always apparent that trafficking is occurring. Unexplained injuries, malnourishment, poor health and dental care, lack of identification documents, and reluctance to speak to providers are warning signs.

Child Abuse and Neglect

Child abuse includes acts of commission and acts of omission. Acts of commission are intentional harmful behaviors directed toward a child and include physical, sexual, and psychological abuse. **Child neglect** is an act of omission, which occurs when a child's basic physical, emotional, educational, and health care needs are not met. Failure to protect a child from harm, inadequate supervision, or exposure to violence are other forms of neglect (CDC, 2021). Neglect is the most common form of child abuse.

Children who are younger than 4 years of age, who are products of unwanted pregnancies, or who have developmental or physical disabilities are at highest risk of abuse (CDC, 2021). Young parents/caregivers who lack social support, resources, and knowledge of typical childhood development are at increased risk of abusing their children. Multiple stressors, emotional or substance misuse issues, and the use of harsh punishment are additional parental risk factors.

Children who are abused or neglected may develop physical, emotional, and behavioral issues (CDC, 2021). Their cognitive development may be impaired, and they may exhibit academic difficulties. Abuse leads to issues getting along with or trusting others. People who have experienced child abuse are at increased risk for depression, anxiety, low self-esteem, and substance misuse. **Adverse childhood experiences (ACEs)** have a negative impact on health and well-being throughout life (CDC, 2023).

A child who is emotionally or psychologically abused does not have visible injuries to alert others. Nevertheless, psychological abuse severely affects a child's self-esteem and often leaves permanent emotional scars. For many people who have experienced childhood abuse, emotional abuse is worse than physical abuse. Psychological abuse frequently co-occurs with other types of abuse and can take various forms. Children often believe the abuse is their fault.

Sexual abuse occurs to children of all ages and is frequently perpetrated by someone the child knows and trusts. Sexual abuse affects about 1 in 4 girls and 1 in 13 boys at some point in their childhood (American Academy of Child & Adolescent Psychiatry [AACAP], 2023). To maintain their silence, children may be threatened or told that they will not be believed if they disclose the abuse. No child is psychologically prepared to cope with repeated sexual stimulation. A child who experiences prolonged sexual abuse will develop low self-esteem, a feeling of worthlessness, and a distorted view of sex. The child may become withdrawn, distrustful, or suicidal. Other characteristics of children who have been sexually abused include an unusual interest or avoidance of sexually related content, nightmares, seductiveness, refusal to go to school, conduct issues, secretiveness, and unusual aggressiveness (AACAP, 2023).

Abuse of Older Adults

Older adults and adults who have mental or physical disabilities are vulnerable to abuse. Older individuals may experience physical, psychological, or sexual abuse. The most common type of elder abuse is financial abuse, in which older adults may be manipulated by family or caregivers to give up control of their money and are vulnerable to scams and fraud perpetrated by outsiders.

Elder abuse is increasingly recognized as a serious problem in the United States and other countries. As the population continues to age, it is likely that the problem will worsen. The actual prevalence of elder abuse is uncertain, as most abuse is unreported, and relatively little research has focused on this population. An estimated 1 in 10 people over age 60 who live at home suffer some type of abuse, including neglect and exploitation (CDC, 2021). The abuse usually occurs at the hands of a caregiver or an individual the older adult trusts but is a significant issue in nursing homes and assisted living facilities as well.

Individuals who are isolated, have poor support systems, or have mental or physical impairments that foster dependency on others are more vulnerable to harm. Older people may be reluctant to report maltreatment by those they love or on whom they depend, or cognitive deficits may prevent them from being able to articulate their situation. In addition to the obvious physical issues (e.g., injuries, pressure sores, malnutrition) that can result from abuse or neglect, older adults can experience worsening of existing medical conditions and emotional issues such as depression, anxiety, and fearfulness (CDC, 2021).

Risk factors for those who are more likely to abuse older adults include using drugs or alcohol, high levels of stress, lack of social support, emotional or financial dependence on the older adult, lack of training in taking care of older adults, and depression (CDC, 2021). Caring for a dependent older adult can be overwhelming. It is important for the nurse to listen to and assess both older adults and their caregivers to help prevent abuse and neglect in this population.

THEORIES OF VIOLENCE

No single cause is sufficient to explain the phenomenon of family violence. The neurobiologic and psychological factors that contribute to anger and poor impulse control (as outlined in Chapter 20) are relevant to the use of aggression in the home. However, the ability of many people perpetrating abuse to refrain from angry outbursts and violence in public settings suggests that their behavior toward family members is not solely attributable to poor self-control. The risk factors discussed in previous sections increase the likelihood of violence occurring but do not cause it. Many people share the same risks but do not engage in violence. Outlined below are a few prominent theories among the many researchers that attempt to explain IPV and other types of violence in the family. Individual characteristics such as genetics and temperament likely intersect with risk factors to produce behavior that is learned and reinforced in families, communities, and society.

Social Learning Theory (Intergenerational Transmission of Violence)

Experiencing childhood abuse is one of the strongest predictors of violence as an adult. Children in violent homes learn that violent behavior is an acceptable and legitimate way to solve issues and to cope with conflict. Social learning or **intergenerational transmission of violence** theory posits that children who witness or experience violence, including harsh physical discipline, in their homes are more likely to perpetuate violent behavior or experience violence within their own families (Zhang et al., 2023). Positive environmental influences such as healthy support systems can introduce more adaptive coping strategies to children who have experienced violence, reducing the likelihood that these children will engage in violence as adults.

Community and Sociologic Influences

The **social–ecologic model of violence prevention** places individual and family characteristics within a larger community and societal context, taking into account the resources, relationships, values, and beliefs in an individual's environment that encourage or inhibit violence (CDC, 2021). Communities that are less economically advantaged, cohesive, and nurturing tend to exert less social control over violent behavior. In such communities, a lack of resources to support individuals experiencing violence may contribute to family isolation and delayed intervention. From a societal perspective, family violence, particularly within intimate relationships, has increasingly been viewed as a manifestation of broader gender-based imbalances of social and economic power.

Gender-Based Influences

Feminist theorists point out that patriarchal societies—or those in which authority and control is held predominantly by men—have historically tolerated, if not sanctioned, men's use of violence to maintain a dominant status in relationships, with negligible legal penalties for doing so (De Coster & Heimer, 2021). Many people continue to endorse traditional gender roles, often bolstered by religious views or cultural norms. Despite awareness and advocacy efforts, most sexual assaults are unreported and criminal justice responses remain weak. Inequities in expectations and attitudes surrounding sexual behaviors often result in an emphasis on actions of the individual experiencing abuse (e.g., reducing vulnerability) rather than accountability of the individual perpetrating the abuse.

Cycle of Violence

Many, but not all, cases of IPV reflect a recognized **cycle of violence**. The cycle consists of three recurring phases that often increase in frequency and severity. The cycle is fully described in Figure 23.2.

Factors Influencing Leaving Versus Staying in a Violent Relationship

Many people who experience IPV do not report abuse, fearing retaliation against themselves or their children. Often, they continue to hold strong feelings for their partners despite the abuse. When medical care is required, injuries may be attributed to other causes; health care providers may be reluctant to inquire about abuse. Provision of assistance to those who are involved in violent intimate relationships can pose unique issues; seeking support can be dangerous to the people experiencing the violence if their activities are discovered by the abusive partner. Therefore, the challenge for health care providers is twofold—ensuring that support is both available and safely accessible, whether or not it is accepted at a given time. Even though it might be difficult to understand why an individual would stay in an abusive relationship, it is critical to be nonjudgmental and to realize that there are valid reasons for deciding to remain in a potentially harmful environment.

Leaving an abusive relationship is a process that can be quite complex. Many people leave and return several times as they learn new coping skills and build support networks before ending the relationship permanently. When abuse is intermittent and strong emotional and psychological ties to the abusive partner persist, people experiencing violence continue to hope that the behavior will change. People who lack job skills, financial resources, and support systems may stay because of economic dependence on their partner. Some are concerned about losing custody of their children if they are unable to provide for them independently.

Fear is another important factor in deciding whether to leave or stay in a violent relationship. Some people stay because of threats not only against themselves but also against other family members or pets. There is a valid concern that leaving may not stop the violence. If people experiencing violence attempt to leave or actually do leave the relationship, the people perpetrating the abuse

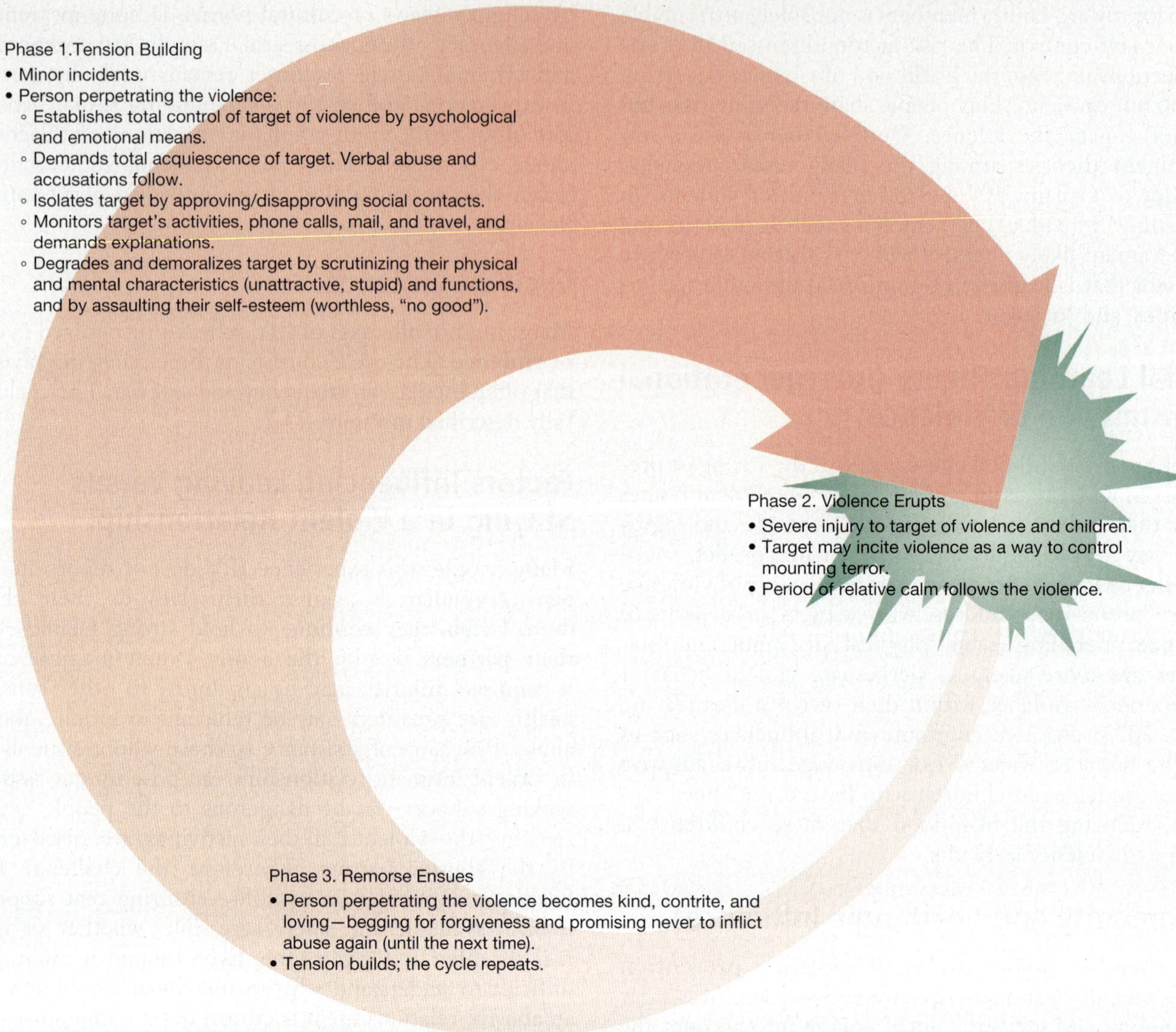

FIGURE 23.2 The cycle of violence.

often escalate their violence, stalk their partners, and may even kill them, which makes leaving the time of greatest risk in an abusive relationship (National Coalition against Domestic Violence [NCADV], n.d.).

Safety Issues and Mandatory Reporting

Health care providers, including nurses, are mandated reporters. This means that they must report known or suspected abuse in specific circumstances. Some states require reporting of injuries sustained as a result of abuse. **Mandatory reporting** for IPV is controversial because it may act as a barrier to disclosure or seeking care (U.S. Department of Justice, 2023). Concerns center around triggering involvement with the legal system that can result in removal of children from custody, loss of economic support, or retaliation from the individual perpetrating the abuse. Immigrants, especially those who are undocumented, may fear that discussing IPV will lead to contacts with immigration authorities and deportation or separation from their children.

All states require reporting of known or suspected abuse involving children and vulnerable adults. It is important for nurses to be familiar with the laws of the state in which they practice and with the policies of their organization. Removing children and older adults from their families or caregivers may be necessary to ensure their immediate safety. In most settings, nurses do not have to make this decision alone; rather, they involve other professionals to assist with assessment and alternate placement if the current living situation of a child or older adult who is abused or neglected cannot be made safe. When an older adult's decision making is not impaired (*competence* is the legal term), they must be allowed to participate in deciding how to manage the issue (Saghafi et al., 2019).

THE ROLE OF TECHNOLOGY IN CARING FOR PEOPLE WHO HAVE EXPERIENCED INTIMATE PARTNER VIOLENCE

For people who have experienced violence, technology can be a weapon or a lifeline. People perpetrating abuse can use technology to monitor their partner's activities or threaten to post compromising photos or confidential information on a public forum as a means of control. More often, the internet is a valuable source of information and support when using reliable sources such as hotlines, particularly for people who have experienced violence who are not emotionally ready for in-person meetings or who do not have ready access to nearby services. For those who are in abusive relationships, websites, 24-hour hotlines, and chats provide resources for safety planning (The Domestic Violence Hotline, n.d.). Most websites and chats designed for people who have experienced IPV have escape features to disconnect quickly if necessary. people who have experienced violence are warned to clear their search histories if there is a risk they are being checked. Technology extends the reach of services for people who have experienced violence in rural and underserved locations via virtual therapy and consultations, and peer support can come through online groups and texts and messaging apps.

When connecting with an individual who has experienced violence online, confidentiality is crucial. Therapists are careful to use secure platforms that cannot be tracked or monitored. Telemedicine providers should be aware of risks when incorporating screening questions into the visit. Yes or no questions can be used to ensure that the client is alone, and it is safe to speak. If an individual who has experienced violence is at risk, messages can be moved to password-protected health portals. When language is a barrier, it is important to utilize certified interpreters who are not family members. Virtual access to services and health care became critical when controlling the spread of the new coronavirus, which required social distancing and limitation of in-person services. These situations increased safety risks for people who have experienced IPV, and expanded use of technology created opportunities to reduce isolation. In all cases, effective use of technology requires Internet or mobile access, which is not universally available.

THERAPEUTIC RELATIONSHIP

Establishing a trusting nurse–patient relationship is one of the most important steps in caring for any individual experiencing violence (McCarthy & Bianchi, n.d.). Disclosing abuse for the first time is a moment of increased vulnerability. To establish rapport and put the individual who has experienced violence at ease, start an interview with the least sensitive areas and progress to more sensitive topics. Patients are unlikely to disclose sensitive information unless they perceive the nurse to be trustworthy and nonjudgmental. Important considerations in establishing open communication are ensuring confidentiality, disclosing any mandatory reporting responsibilities, and providing a quiet, private place in which to interact. A supportive, empathetic approach is most effective. The nurse must continually monitor personal reactions to prevent negative feelings from influencing the nurse–patient relationship in a way that could retraumatize the patient. Understand and accept that not everyone is going to be willing to talk about their situation. Convey belief in patients' disclosures and acceptance of their responses to inquiries. Provide them with information necessary to support decision making about next steps.

EVIDENCE-BASED NURSING CARE WITH PEOPLE EXPERIENCING VIOLENCE

Nurses encounter people who have experienced violence and abuse in many health care settings, not just in mental health settings. Abuse may be disclosed or discovered by providers in urgent care clinics, primary care settings, obstetrics and gynecology settings, pediatric units, well-child clinics, geriatric units, schools, and nursing homes, among others.

RECOGNIZING CUES: RELEVANT ASSESSMENT INFORMATION

Conducting a Safety Assessment First

Once physiologic stability is established, the nurse should determine whether the people who have experienced violence are in danger for their life, either from homicide or suicide, and, if children or other dependents are in the home, whether they are in danger. Trauma may trigger suicidal ideation or exacerbate pre-existing mental health conditions that place the individual who has experienced violence at risk. Suicide precautions should be initiated if indicated.

The **Danger Assessment Screen** is a useful tool for assessing the risk that IPV will end in homicide (Danger Assessment, 2025) (Box 23.1). This assessment may help people who have experienced violence recognize the serious nature of the violence they routinely experience. An abbreviated version of this tool, the Danger Assessment-5 (Messing et al., 2017), can be used for brief screening. The brief screening highlights five key factors that increase the risk for violence to ultimately result in homicide.

Screening for Violence and Abuse

Because of the prevalence of IPV, the U.S. Preventive Services Task Force recommends universal screening

BOX 23.1

Danger Assessment

Several risk factors have been associated with homicides (murders) of both people perpetrating abuse and people experiencing abuse in research that has been conducted after the killings have taken place. We cannot predict what will happen in your case, but we would like you to be aware of the danger of homicide in situations of severe battering and to see how many of the risk factors apply to your situation.

1. Has the physical violence increased in frequency during the past year?
2. Has the physical violence increased in severity during the past year, or has a weapon or threat with weapon been used?
3. Does your partner ever try to choke you?
4. Is there a gun in the house?
5. Has your partner ever forced you to have sex when you did not wish to do so?
6. Does your partner use drugs? By drugs, I mean "uppers" or amphetamines, speed, angel dust, cocaine, "crack," street drugs, heroin, or mixtures.
7. Does your partner threaten to kill you, or do you believe they are capable of killing you?
8. Is your partner drunk every day or almost every day? (In terms of quantity of alcohol.)
9. Does your partner control most or all of your daily activities? For instance, do they tell you who you can be friends with, how much money you can take with you for shopping, or when you can take the car?
10. Has your partner ever beaten you while you were pregnant? (If never pregnant by them, check here ________.)
11. Is your partner violently and constantly jealous of you? (For instance, do they say, "If I can't have you, no one can.")
12. Have you ever threatened or tried to commit suicide?
13. Have they ever threatened or tried to commit suicide?
14. Is your partner violent toward the children?
15. Is your partner violent outside the home?

TOTAL YES ANSWERS: ________

Thank you. Please talk to your nurse, advocate, or counselor about what the danger assessment means in terms of your situation.

Adapted from Campbell, J., & Humphreys, J. (Eds.). (1993). *Nursing care of survivors of family violence* (p. 259). Mosby. Copyright © 1993 Elsevier. With permission.

for all women of childbearing age (Alhusen et al., 2023). However, actual rates of screening in most settings are low. Providers cite uncertainty about how to approach the topic and how to help, concerns about reporting policies, and time constraints as barriers to routine screening. People who have experienced violence may be reluctant to report abuse because of shame, embarrassment, fear of not being believed, or fear of retaliation. People who have experienced violence who depend on the people perpetrating the abuse for care or financial support may be concerned about the consequences of disclosure. If the individual suspected of perpetrating the abuse is present, it is important to speak to the survivor alone.

Validated screening tools are readily accessible (Center for Justice Innovation, 2025). Asking specific abuse screening questions substantially increases the detection of abuse. For that reason, nurses must develop a repertoire of age-appropriate, culturally sensitive abuse-related questions. Avoid using terms such as *abuse* and *rape*, because those labels may not be consistent with an individual's perception of their experience. See Boxes 23.2 and 23.3.

Other questions that might be useful in eliciting disclosure are as follows:

- "When there are fights at home, have you ever been hurt or afraid?"
- "It looks like someone has hurt you. Tell me about it."
- "Some individuals have described issues like yours. If this is happening to you, can we talk about it?"

When patients are disclosing abuse, they need privacy and time to tell their story. The nurse should listen attentively without offering unsolicited advice or making judgmental remarks about the possible abuse or the individual perpetrating the abuse. Use validating messages to convey that the people who have experienced violence are believed and that the nurse is concerned for their safety and well-being. Examples of such messages include the following:

- "I'm really sorry this happened to you."
- "I'm glad you told me."
- "It sounds like a frightening experience."
- "It was not your fault."

People who have experienced IPV may deny the abuse, make excuses for the behavior of the individual perpetrating the abuse, or attribute an injury to an unlikely cause. Avoid pressuring or confronting them, but carefully document a description of the patient's account of how

BOX 23.2

Abuse Assessment Screen

1. Have you ever been emotionally or physically abused by your partner or someone important to you?	YES	NO
2. Within the past year, have you been hit, slapped, kicked, or otherwise physically hurt by someone? If YES, by whom: ________ Number of times: ________ Mark the area of injury on body map.	YES	NO
3. Within the past year, has anyone forced you to have sexual activities? If YES, who: ________ Number of times: ________	YES	NO
4. Are you afraid of your partner or anyone you listed above?	YES	NO

BOX 23.3

Burgess-Partner Abuse Scale for Teens

Directions: During the past 12 months, you and one of your partners may have had a fight. Following is a list of things one of your partners may have done to you. Please circle the number of how often this partner did these things to you. This is not a test and there are no right or wrong answers. Remember, having a partner(s) does not mean you are having sex with the partner(s).

If you have not had a partner in the past 12 months, do not fill this form out.

	Never	Once	A few times	More than a few times	Routinely or a lot
1. My partner doesn't let me go out with my friends.	0	1	2	3	4
2. My partner tells me what to wear.	0	1	2	3	4
3. My partner says if I don't have sex with them, then I don't love them.	0	1	2	3	4
4. My partner says they will hurt me if I talk to another guy/girl.	0	1	2	3	4
5. My partner calls me bad names like bitch.	0	1	2	3	4
6. My partner says they will hurt me with a weapon.	0	1	2	3	4
7. My partner forces me to have sex.	0	1	2	3	4
8. My partner tells me I am stupid or dumb.		1	2	3	4
9. My partner follows me when I do things with my friends or family.	0	1	2	3	4
10. My partner hits or kicks something when they get mad at me.	0	1	2	3	4
11. My partner kicks me.	0	1	2	3	4
12. My partner says they can have sex with other people even though they said I can't.	0	1	2	3	4
13. My partner gives me sexually transmitted infections.	0	1	2	3	4
14. My partner hurts me using a weapon.	0	1	2	3	4
15. My partner forces me to use drugs even though I don't want to.	0	1	2	3	4
16. My partner beats me up so bad.	0	1	2	3	4
17. My partner says they will hurt my family if I don't do what they say.	0	1	2	3	4
18. My partner tells me what school activities I can and can't do.	0	1	2	3	4
19. My partner tells me what friends I can hang out with.	0	1	2	3	4
20. My partner chokes me if they get mad at me.	0	1	2	3	4
21. My partner yells at me if they don't know where I am.	0	1	2	3	4
22. My partner says we can't break up even though I want to.	0	1	2	3	4

How many partners have you had in the past 12 months?___________

Reprinted with permission from Burgess, S. E., & Tavakoli, A. (2005). Psychometric assessment of the Burgess-Partner Abuse Scale for Teens (B-PAST). *Aquichan, 5*, 96–107.

the injury happened, using the individual's own words. Remain supportive even if the patient is not ready to accept assistance at the time. By introducing options and resources, the nurse opens the door to future intervention. Be aware of resources for shelter, protective orders, and law enforcement involvement.

After assessment is completed in a health care agency and abuse is evident, the nurse should offer the adult patient use of the telephone. This may be the only time that the individual can make calls in private to family, who might offer support, or to the police, lawyers, or shelters. Scheduling future appointments may provide the patient with a legitimate reason to leave the individual perpetrating the abuse and to continue to explore options.

Physical Health Assessment

Documentation of abuse or suspected abuse includes a complete history and physical examination. Note vital signs, sleep and appetite disturbances, exaggerated startle responses, flashbacks, and nightmares that may suggest PTSD or depression. Assess for injuries in need of immediate attention. Documentation should include a detailed history of how injuries occurred and a careful description of the injuries. A **body map** may be used to indicate location, size, and type of injuries. The nurse's documentation may become evidence if there are legal consequences related to the violence, even if the people who have experienced violence declines to file a report at the time of the incident. People experiencing the violence experience physical consequences that range in severity. Mild injuries may include bruises and abrasions of the head, neck, face, trunk, and limbs. People who are chronically abused may have multiple bruises in various stages of healing. Severe injuries include multiple traumas, major fractures, major lacerations, and internal injuries (including chest and abdominal injuries and subdural hematomas). Loss of vision and hearing can result from blows to the head. It is critical to include an assessment for strangulation even if there are no visible injuries. Patients should be notified that strangulation, a common occurrence in domestic assault, increases the risk of homicide 750%. Damage can occur within seconds, and life-threatening complications can occur days to weeks later from trauma to structures and blood vessels in the throat (U.S. Department of Justice, 2023).

Physical or sexual violence may result in head injuries that can produce changes in cognition, affect, motivation, and behavior. People who have experienced sexual abuse may have vaginal and perineal trauma. Anorectal injuries may also be present, including disruption of anal sphincters, retained foreign bodies, and mucosal lacerations. Determine the need for emergency contraception, or prophylactic treatment for human immunodeficiency virus (HIV) or STIs. Sexual assault examination involves evidence gathering, careful documentation, and attention to psychosocial needs and emotional distress. When possible, a specially trained registered nurse, known as a ***s**exual **a**ssault **n**urse **e**xaminer* **(SANE)**, or another provider trained in forensic examination should conduct the examination (Gaines, n.d.) (see Box 23.4 for additional considerations).

Healthy child development and deviations that may be related to abuse or neglect are critical components of the nursing assessment of children. Assessing developmental

BOX 23.4

Special Concerns for People Who Have Experienced Sexual Assault

ASSESSMENT FOCUS

The history and physical examination of the people who have experienced sexual assault differ significantly from other assessment routines because the evidence obtained may be used in prosecuting the individual who perpetrated the abuse. Therefore, the purpose is twofold:

- To assess the patient for injuries
- To collect evidence for forensic evaluation and proceedings

Usually, someone with appropriate training, such as a nurse practitioner who has taken special courses, examines an individual who has experienced rape or sexual assault. Generalist nurses may be involved in treating the injuries that result from the assault, including genital trauma (e.g., vaginal and anal lacerations) and extragenital trauma (e.g., injury to the mouth, throat, wrists, arms, breasts, thighs).

KEY INTERVENTIONS

Nursing intervention to prevent short- or long-term psychopathology after sexual assault is crucial. Psychological trauma after rape and sexual assault includes immediate anxiety and distress and the development of PTSD, depression, panic, and substance use disorder.

Key interventions include the following:

- Early treatment because initial levels of distress are strongly related to later levels of posttraumatic stress disorder, panic, and anxiety.
- Supportive, caring, and nonjudgmental nursing interventions during the forensic rape examination are also crucial. This examination often increases the immediate distress because of people who have experienced violence they must recount the assault in detail and submit to an invasive pelvic or anal examination.
- Anxiety-reducing education, counseling, and emotional support, particularly regarding unwanted pregnancies and sexually transmitted infections, including HIV. All people who have experienced violence should be tested for these possibilities. Treatment may include terminating a pregnancy; administering medications to treat gonorrhea, chlamydia, trichomoniasis, and syphilis; and administering medications that may decrease the likelihood of contracting HIV infection.
- Interventions that are helpful for people who have experienced domestic violence; these also apply to survivors of sexual assault.

milestones, school history, and relationships with siblings and friends is important. Intracranial hemorrhage in an infant in the absence of an obvious cause, such as a motor vehicle accident, may suggest shaken baby syndrome. Infants do not begin to move or ambulate on their own prior to the age of 6 months, when they begin to crawl; therefore, any bruises on an infant before the age of 6 months is cause for suspicion. Any discrepancies between the history and physical examination and implausible explanations for injuries and other symptoms should be an alert to the possibility of abuse (CDC, 2021). Children and adolescents who wear clothing that covers parts of the body in a manner inconsistent with the season may be hiding bruises, abrasions, or burns caused by cigarettes or boiling water. Other circumstances that should heighten the suspicion of childhood abuse include multiple fractures or types of fractures (such as spiral fractures) that would only occur in an abusive situation. Other injuries such as bite marks or injuries to the genitals or anus always require further investigation.

For reference, when assessing older adults, become familiar with typical aging and signs and symptoms of common illnesses to distinguish those conditions from abuse. Observe for signs of malnutrition or inattention to activities of daily living (ADLs). As with children, bruises, lacerations, and other injuries are suspicious if they are inconsistent with a description of how they occurred. Some older adults are unable to communicate effectively because of dementia or other cognitive impairment. Evidence that excessive medications or physical restraints are being used to control an older adult's behavior should be investigated. Box 23.5 lists indicators of actual or potential abuse that need to be thoroughly assessed for all people who have experienced violence.

BOX 23.5

History and Physical Findings Suggestive of Abuse

PRESENTING PROBLEM

- Vague information about cause of the problem
- Delay between occurrence of injury and seeking of treatment
- Inappropriate reactions of significant other or family
- Denial or minimizing of seriousness of injury
- Discrepancy between history and physical examination findings

FAMILY HISTORY

- Past family violence
- Physical punishment of children
- Children who are fearful of parent(s) or caregivers
- Parent or caregiver who demands unquestioning obedience
- Alcohol or substance use disorder
- Violence outside the home
- Unemployment or underemployment
- Financial difficulties or poverty
- Use of older adult's finances for other family members
- Finances rigidly controlled by one member

HEALTH AND PSYCHIATRIC HISTORY

- Fractures at various stages of healing
- Spontaneous abortions
- Injuries during pregnancy
- Multiple visits to the emergency department
- Elimination disturbances (e.g., constipation, diarrhea)
- Multiple somatic complaints
- Eating disorders
- Substance use disorder
- Depression
- Posttraumatic stress disorder
- Self-mutilation
- Suicide attempts
- Feelings of helplessness or hopelessness
- Low self-esteem
- Chronic fatigue
- Apathy
- Sleep disturbances (e.g., hypersomnia, hyposomnia)
- Psychiatric hospitalizations

PERSONAL AND SOCIAL HISTORY

- Feelings of powerlessness
- Feelings of being trapped
- Lack of trust
- Traditional values about home, partner, and children's behavior
- Major decisions in a family controlled by one individual
- Few social supports (isolated from family, friends)
- Little activity outside the home
- Unwanted or unplanned pregnancy
- Dependency on caregivers
- Extreme jealousy by partner
- Difficulties at school or work
- Short attention span
- Running away
- Promiscuity
- Child who has knowledge of sexual matters beyond that appropriate for age
- Sexualized play with self, peers, dolls, toys
- Masturbation
- Excessive fears and clinging in children
- Verbal aggression
- Themes of violence in artwork and schoolwork
- Distorted body image
- History of chronic physical or psychological disability
- Inability to perform activities of daily living
- Delayed language development

PHYSICAL EXAMINATION FINDINGS

General Appearance

- Fearful, anxious, hyperactive, hypoactive
- Watching partner, parent, or caregiver for approval of answers to your questions
- Poor grooming or inappropriate dress
- Malnourishment
- Signs of stress or fatigue
- Flinching when approached or touched
- Inappropriate or anxious nonverbal behavior
- Wearing clothing inappropriate to the season or occasion to cover body parts

(continued)

BOX 23.5 (*Continued*)

Vital Statistics
- Elevated pulse or blood pressure
- Other signs of autonomic arousal (e.g., exaggerated startle response, excessive sweating)
- Underweight or overweight

Skin
- Bruises, welts, edema, or scars
- Burns (cigarette, immersion, friction from ropes, pattern like an electric iron or stove)
- Subdural hematoma
- Missing hair
- Poor skin integrity: dehydration, pressure injuries, untreated wounds, urine burns, or excoriation

Eyes
- Orbital swelling
- Conjunctival hemorrhage
- Retinal hemorrhage
- Black eyes
- No glasses to accommodate poor eyesight

Ears
- Hearing loss
- No prosthetic device to accommodate poor hearing

Mouth
- Bruising
- Lacerations
- Missing or broken teeth
- Untreated dental issues

Abdomen
- Abdominal injuries during pregnancy
- Intra-abdominal injuries

Genitourinary System or Rectum
- Bruising, lacerations, bleeding, edema, tenderness
- Untreated infections

Musculoskeletal System
- Recent fractures or old fractures in various stages of healing
- Dislocations
- Limited range of motion in extremities
- Contractures

Neurologic System
- Difficulty with speech or swallowing
- Hyperactive reflexes
- Developmental delays
- Areas of numbness
- Tremors

Mental Status
- Anxiety, fear
- Depression
- Suicidal ideation
- Difficulty concentrating
- Memory loss

Medications
- Medications that are not indicated by physical condition
- Overdose of drugs or medications (prescribed or over the counter)
- Medications not taken as prescribed

Communication Patterns and Relations
- Verbal hostility, arguments
- Negative nonverbal communication, lack of visible affection
- One individual answers questions and looks to other individual for approval
- Extreme dependency of family members

Psychosocial Cues

Fear

Living with an abusive partner, parent/guardian, or caregiver means living with constant fear and uncertainty. Because people experiencing violence never know what might precipitate an incident of violence, they are constantly hypervigilant and fearful. The back-and-forth nature of the relationship, that is, alternating between love and violence, is confusing, so the people who have experienced violence may try to do everything possible to please the individual perpetrating the violence in an effort to prevent another violent episode.

Low Self-Esteem

Experiencing abuse is devastating to healthy self-esteem (feelings of self-acceptance, self-worth, self-love, and self-nurturing). Emotional abuse may be particularly devastating. People who experience emotional abuse are criticized, rejected, devaluated, and ignored. Over time, people begin to internalize the negative messages and may come to believe the abuse is deserved. Low self-esteem has been linked to physical and mental health issues, problems with relationships, and may affect people's ability to achieve financial independence.

Guilt and Shame

A history of abuse is often associated with guilt and shame. People who have experienced violence are ashamed of being manipulated and violated and for having put themselves in such a situation. Abusive partners tell them that the abuse is their fault, and many people experiencing violence believe that. Feelings of humiliation and shame prevent people who have experienced violence from seeking medical care and other forms of support and reporting abuse to authorities. The experience of being battered is so degrading and humiliating that people who have experienced violence are often afraid to disclose it to anyone. Many fear that they will not be taken seriously or will be blamed for inciting the abuse or for staying with the people perpetrating the abuse. Keeping their circumstances secret and maintaining a front of normality places enormous tension and pressure on people who have experienced violence.

Issues With Intimacy

Abused children, especially those who have experienced child sexual abuse, experience intrusion, abandonment, devaluation, or pain in the relationship with the individual perpetrating the abuse instead of the closeness and nurturing that are typical for intimate relationships (AACAP, 2023). Consequently, intimacy is associated with shame and fear rather than warmth and caring and with concerns about dominance and submission rather than mutuality. Shame, in turn, is associated with being submissive, feeling devalued, and the desire to retaliate against an individual who is seen as the source of humiliation. In adulthood, unresolved feelings of shame, as well as symptoms of PTSD or depression, may disrupt the development of intimacy and interfere with the ability to develop and sustain healthy relationships.

Conversely, some people who have experienced child abuse and child sexual abuse may engage in risky sexual behavior such as early sexual activity (before age 15 years), promiscuity, and prostitution (AACAP, 2023). These behaviors place people who have experienced violence at risk for developing STIs and HIV. People who engage in this type of behavior may have learned that sexual activity is a means for securing affection, intimacy, or material rewards such as money or drugs.

Revictimization

Many people who have experienced childhood trauma are revictimized later in life. Numerous factors are related to **revictimization**, including symptoms of PTSD, dissociation, boundary issues, and feelings of self-blame and shame. Internalized stigma, statements blaming the individual who has experienced the violence, and past negative social reactions from others affect the self-perception and willingness of people who have experienced violence to disclose subsequent abuse (Latiff et al., 2024). People with abuse histories frequently have difficulty with boundaries. During childhood abuse, they experienced frequent boundary violations and associate those violations with intimate relationships. Excessive use of alcohol and other drugs by people who have experienced violence makes them less able to defend themselves and more vulnerable to revictimization.

Social Networks

An evaluation of social networks provides additional clues of psychological abuse and controlling behavior. Having supportive family or friends is crucial in short-term planning for developing a safety plan and is also important to long-term recovery. An individual cannot leave an abusive situation with nowhere to go. Supportive family and friends may be willing to provide shelter and safety, as well as emotional support. As part of safety planning, people experiencing violence can set up code words to make contacts aware that help is needed or ask friends to keep belongings or documents that they may require if they leave home quickly.

Social Isolation

Many people perpetrating abuse isolate their family from all social contacts, including other relatives. Some people who have experienced violence isolate themselves because they are ashamed of the abuse or fear nonsupportive responses. Nurses can assess restrictions on freedom that may suggest abuse and control by asking such questions as “Are you free to go where you want?” “Is staying home your choice?” and “Is there anything you would like to do that you cannot?”

Economic and Emotional Dependency

Women who have young children and depend on the individual perpetrating the abuse financially may believe that they cannot leave the abusive relationship. Those who are emotionally dependent on the individual perpetrating the abuse may experience an intense grief reaction that further complicates their leaving. Older adults and children often depend on the individual perpetrating the abuse and cannot leave the abusive situation without workable alternatives.

ANALYZING CUES AND DEVELOPING HYPOTHESES

Violence and abuse are critical situations that need to be addressed immediately. The nurse should prioritize the most serious threats to the individual’s well-being, including ensuring physiological stability by identifying and treating acute injuries, and addressing the safety of the individual and others who might be vulnerable to harm. Individuals who do not wish to return to the unsafe environment may require assistance identifying support systems and obtaining resources to meet basic needs.

TAKING ACTION: NURSING INTERVENTIONS

The goals of all nursing interventions in cases of violence are to prevent injury, stop the violence, ensure the patient’s safety, and restore health.

As appropriate concerning age and ability, nursing interventions should empower people who have experienced violence to act on their own behalf. This must be done in a collaborative partnership. Strong psychological and economic bonds tie many people experiencing violence to the people perpetrating the violence. Moreover, adult people experiencing violence who are capable of making decisions are the experts about their situations. They are the best judges to determine the safest and most appropriate time to leave a relationship. Interventions that are nonjudgmental, individually tailored, and sensitive to patient privacy and autonomy are the most successful (Alhusen et al., 2023).

Intervention strategies for older adults depend on whether the individual accepts or refuses assistance and whether they can make decisions. If the individual refuses treatment, it is important to remain nonjudgmental and provide information about available services and emergency contact information. If the older adult appears incapable of making decisions, then guardianship, foster care, or nursing home placement may be needed. The nurse should initiate a referral to a case manager or others who can facilitate further intervention.

Safety Planning

Leaving or planning to leave is a dangerous time for people in violent relationships. One of the most important interventions when caring for individuals who are in an ongoing abusive relationship is to help people experiencing violence develop a safety plan (Domestic Violence Resource Center, 2023). The first step in developing such a plan is helping the patient recognize the signs of danger. Changes in tone of voice, substance use, and increased criticism may indicate that the individual perpetrating the abuse is losing control. Detecting early warning signs helps people experiencing violence to escape before violence begins.

The next step is to devise an escape. For families at risk for violence, this may involve mapping the house for an escape route. The individual who has experienced IPV needs to have a bag packed and hidden but readily accessible that includes what is needed to get away. Important things to pack are clothes, a set of car and house keys, bank account numbers, birth certificate, insurance policies and numbers, marriage license, valuable jewelry, important telephone numbers, and money. If children are involved, the adult individual experiencing violence should make arrangements to get them out safely. That might include arranging a signal to indicate when it is safe for them to leave the house and to meet at a prearranged place.

A safety plan for a child or dependent older adult might include safe places to hide and important telephone numbers, including 911, and those of the police and fire departments, and other family members and friends.

Physical Health Interventions

Treatment of trauma symptoms may include cleaning and dressing burns or other wounds and assisting with setting and casting broken bones. Malnourished and dehydrated children and older adults may require nursing interventions such as intravenous therapy or nutritional supplements that alleviate the alteration in nutrition and fluid and electrolyte imbalances. People who have experienced sexual assault require additional considerations (see Box 23.5).

> **KEYCONCEPT** Individuals who are experiencing IPV need their basic needs met (e.g., safety, housing, food, childcare) before their psychological traumas can be addressed.

Promoting Healthy Daily Activity

Teaching sleep hygiene (i.e., practices conducive to healthy sleep patterns) and promoting exercise, leisure time, and nutrition will help people who have experienced violence regain a healthy physical state and self-care activities. Taking care of themselves may be difficult for people who have spent years trying to separate themselves from their bodies (dissociate) to endure abuse. Techniques such as going to bed and arising at consistent times, avoiding alcohol and caffeine, and engaging in relaxing activities before retiring may be useful in promoting sleep (Newsom, 2021). The sleep environment should be one in which people who have experienced violence feel safe and comfortable. Aerobic exercise is a useful technique for relieving anxiety and depression and promoting sleep.

Trauma-Informed Approach

A trauma-informed approach is widely used among health care providers based on the understanding that most people have experienced some form of trauma that impacts them in different ways (Center for Health Care Strategies, 2021). The focus is on what has happened to people rather than what is wrong with them. The aim of this approach is to create an environment that is safe, sensitive, inclusive, and supportive by building trust, respecting autonomy, and collaborating with people in their own care. See Chapter 2. Sensitivity includes being aware of triggers that can reawaken trauma-related stress responses and attempting to avoid retraumatization of people in the process of providing care.

People who have experienced abuse and sexual assault, and those in abusive relationships, may experience depression, anxiety, and posttraumatic stress. These disorders interfere with cognitive processes—including judgment, decision making, and problem solving—and impede healing even after the patient is in a safe environment. Trauma-informed therapy specifically targeting psychological consequences of IPV is an effective treatment for people who have experienced violence (Ragucci et al., 2024). Refer the patient to a qualified mental health provider for treatment.

Patients who have a substance use disorder need referral to a treatment center for such disorders. The treatment center should utilize a trauma-informed approach that addresses the special needs of people who have experienced violence. Patients who are impaired by substance use are at increased risk for HIV infection and other infectious diseases. If patients do not know their HIV status, they should be encouraged to get tested.

Psychosocial Interventions

Several issues must be addressed for people who have experienced violence, including guilt, shame, and stigmatization. These issues can be approached in several ways. Assisting patients to verbalize their experience in an accepting, nonjudgmental atmosphere is the first step. Directly challenging attributions of self-blame for the abuse and feelings of being dirty and different is another. Helping patients to identify their strengths and validating thoughts and feelings may help to increase their self-esteem.

Working With Children

Children may need to learn a "violence vocabulary" that allows them to talk about their abuse and assign responsibility for abusive behavior. Children also need to learn that violence is not okay, and it is not their fault. Allowing children to discuss their abuse in the safety of a supportive, caring relationship may alleviate anxiety and fear. Respond to children's disclosures with sensitivity, belief, and a calm demeanor. Avoid pressuring children to talk or share details if they are uncomfortable (Ramamoorthy & Myers-Walls, 2021).

Reenacting the abuse through play is another technique that may be helpful in assisting children to express and work through their anxiety and fear. Play therapy uses dolls, human or animal figures, video games, or puppets to work through anxiety or fears. Other techniques include reading stories about recovery from abusive experiences (literal or metaphoric), using art or music to express feelings, and using psychodrama to reenact the abusive episode. In addition, teaching strategies to manage fear and anxiety, such as relaxation techniques, coping skills, and imagery, may give the children an added sense of mastering their fear (National Child Traumatic Stress Network, n.d.).

Managing Anger

Anger and rage are part of the healing process for people who have experienced violence. Expression of intense anger is uncomfortable for many nurses. However, anger expression should be expected from the patient, so it is necessary to develop comfortable ways to respond. Moreover, an important nursing intervention is teaching and modeling anger expression appropriately. Inappropriate expressions of anger might drive supportive people away. Anger management techniques include appropriately recognizing and labeling anger and expressing it assertively rather than aggressively or passive-aggressively. Assertive ways of expressing anger include owning the feeling by using "I feel" statements and avoiding blaming others. Teaching anger management and conflict resolution may be especially important for children who have seen nothing but violence to resolve issues.

Coping With Anxiety

Anxiety management is a crucial intervention for all people who have experienced violence. A high comorbidity exists involving trauma, PTSD, and anxiety disorders. During treatment, patients experience situations and memories that provoke intense anxiety and must know how to soothe themselves when they experience painful feelings. Moreover, most people who have experienced violence struggle with control issues, especially involving their bodies. Anxiety management skills offer one way to maintain some control over their bodies and choices. See Chapter 27.

Finding Strength and Hope

Providing hope and a sense of control is fundamental for people who have experienced trauma. Help patients find hope by assisting them identify specific strengths and aspects of their lives that are under their control. This type of intervention may empower patients to find options other than remaining in an abusive relationship. Interventions that focus on empowerment encourage and create opportunities for patients to make decisions about their lives, thereby restoring a sense of autonomy and competence lost in the abusive environment (SAMHSA, 2024).

Psychoeducation

Other nursing interventions include teaching self-protection skills, healthy relationship skills, and healthy sexuality (Box 23.6). Again, this teaching may be especially important for children who have no role models for healthy relationships. Children also need to know what constitutes controlling and abusive behavior and how to

BOX 23.6

Abuse

When caring for the patient who has been abused, be sure to address the following topics in the teaching plan:

- Cycle of violence
- Access to shelters
- Legal services
- Government benefits
- Support network
- Symptoms of anxiety, dissociation, and PTSD
- Safety or escape plan
- Relaxation
- Adequate nutrition and exercise
- Sleep hygiene
- HIV testing and counseling

get help for abuse. People who have experienced violence also need information about resources, such as shelters, legal services, government benefits, and support networks. Before giving the patient any written material, first discuss the possibility that if the individual perpetrating the abuse were to find the information in the patient's possession, they might use it as an excuse for further violence.

Family Interventions

There are many evidence-based interventions designed to promote family cohesion and improve the well-being of children and their parents or other caregivers. Interventions that include trauma-specific components are concerned with the reduction of traumatic stress symptoms in children who have experienced child abuse or witnessed violence in their families (National Child Traumatic Stress Network, n.d.). Intervention strategies focus on bolstering children's coping resources and making their environments safer by working with parents or other caregivers. Parental support and positive family functioning are protective factors for children who have been exposed to violence, whereas parental distress or impairment increases the risk for poor trauma-related outcomes. Parenting interventions typically provide parents or caregivers with a network of support and training to enhance positive parenting skills, reduce negative parenting practices, and reduce parental stress. Parental mental health is a key factor in promoting positive parent–child interactions.

Community Involvement

Nurses may be involved in interventions to reduce violence at the community level. Developing support networks may help reduce stress and therefore, reduce abuse. Community contacts vary for each individual perpetrating the abuse and individual experiencing violence but might include crisis hotlines, support groups, and education classes.

Nurses may also make home visits. Home visits provide support to families and provide them with knowledge about stress and management. Abuse of any kind creates a volatile situation, so nurses may be putting themselves or the individual who experiencing violence in danger if they do make home visits. Carefully assess this possibility before proceeding. If necessary, arrange a safe place to meet the patient instead.

Evaluation and Patient Outcomes

Evaluation and outcome criteria depend on the setting for interventions. For instance, if an individual who has experienced violence is encountered in the emergency department, successful outcomes might be that injuries are appropriately managed, and the patient's immediate safety is ensured. For long-term care, outcome criteria and evaluation might center on ending abusive relationships and addressing the emotional and physical consequences of trauma. Examples of other outcome criteria that would indicate successful nursing interventions are recognizing that one is not to blame for the violence, demonstrating knowledge of strengths and coping skills, and reestablishing social networks.

Evaluation of nursing care for children who have been abused depends on attaining goals mutually set with the parents or guardians. An end to all violence is the optimal outcome criterion; however, attainment of smaller goals indicates progress toward that end. Outcomes such as increased problem-solving and communication skills within the family, increased self-esteem in both children and parents/guardians, and increased use of nonphysical forms of discipline may all indicate progress toward the total elimination of child abuse.

Follow-up efforts are important in evaluating the outcomes of older individual abuse. The optimal outcome is to end all abuse and keep the older adults in their own living environment, if appropriate. Although the abuse may have been resolved temporarily, it may flare up again. Ongoing support for the caregiver and assistance with caregiving tasks may be necessary if the older adult is to remain at home. Nursing home or assisted living may be the only desirable option if the burden is too great for the family and the likelihood of ongoing abuse or neglect is high.

Another important outcome of nursing intervention with people who have experienced violence is appropriate treatment of any disorder resulting from abuse (e.g., acute stress disorder, PTSD, anxiety disorders, dissociative identity disorder [DID], major depression, substance use disorder). Follow-up nursing assessments should monitor symptom reduction or exacerbation, adherence to any medication regimen, and side effects of medication. The ultimate outcome is to end violence and enable the individual who has experienced violence to return to a more productive, safe, and nurturing life without being continually haunted by memories of the abuse.

Nurses must become accustomed to measuring gains in small steps when working with people who have experienced violence. Making any changes in significant relationships has serious consequences and can be done only when the adult patient is ready. It is easy to become frustrated or discouraged when working with people who have experienced violence, so it is important not to allow responses to interfere with the nurse–patient relationship. Discussing such feelings with other staff provides a way of dealing with them appropriately and regaining perspective. In such discussions with supervisors or other staff, it is imperative to protect the confidentiality of the individual who has experienced violence by discussing feelings around issues, not particular individuals, to ensure that patients cannot be identified. Recognize that recovery from trauma is not a linear process and that healing may be challenging for people who have experienced violence.

TREATMENT FOR THE INDIVIDUAL PERPETRATING ABUSE

In cases of IPV, people perpetrating the abuse are often court-ordered to engage in **batterer intervention programs** (BIPs) with the goal of preventing further violence. Therefore, participants are present only because the treatment is mandated, which may affect receptivity to intervention. Programs are often outpatient groups that meet weekly for an extended period, averaging about 8 months (Voith et al., 2020). The recent emergence of online options may increase program accessibility. BIPs use varying approaches based on cognitive behavioral, power and control, or psychoeducational frameworks, with few programs tailoring interventions to individual participant needs. Components of treatment include understanding the definition of abuse, accepting responsibility, and teaching alternatives to violent behavior. Most BIPs do not account for the multiple factors that affect use of violence against others, including sociocultural factors, co-occurring mental illness, and a personal history of trauma. Some programs include concurrent substance use treatment when applicable, and a few programs employ a trauma-informed approach to intervention, with promising initial results. Critics of trauma-informed approaches are concerned that a focus on personal history provides people perpetrating the abuse with an "excuse" for their behavior. Despite widespread implementation, there is little reliable evidence to support the efficacy of BIPs in general, particularly on a long-term basis. It is difficult to determine how many people who have perpetrated abuse repeat their abuse, because so many incidents are unreported. Misplaced confidence in the ability of BIPs to promote safety can put people experiencing violence who choose to return to the relationship at risk. It is important to pursue high-quality evidence to determine which strategies successfully prevent recurrence of violent behavior, and then to invest resources in their implementation.

SUMMARY OF KEY POINTS

- The most common type of abuse results from domestic violence.
- IPV is a significant public health issue; it includes physical violence, sexual violence, stalking, and psychological aggression.
- IPV crosses all ethnic, racial, and socioeconomic lines. Women are more likely to be injured or killed by current or former intimate partners than by any other people.
- Stalking is repeated unwanted contact, attention, and harassment that increase in frequency.
- Child maltreatment includes child abuse (i.e., overt actions that cause harm, potential or threat of harm) and child neglect (i.e., failure to provide needs or to protect from harm or potential harm).
- Older adults may also be physically, emotionally, and sexually abused or neglected. The most common type of elder abuse is economic.
- Among the many theories that have been proposed to explain violence are neurologic issues, psychopathology, alcohol use disorder and substance use disorder, intergenerational transmission of violence, and economic and community factors.
- A well-documented cycle of violence consists of three phases of increasing frequency and severity.
- Nurses need to be familiar with signs and symptoms of abuse and to be vigilant when assessing patients.
- Nurses need to be nonjudgmental when caring for an individual who has experienced abuse. There are many reasons an individual might remain in an abusive situation.
- Nursing interventions include physical health interventions and psychosocial interventions that focus on helping people who have experienced abuse identify their strengths and validate thoughts and feelings.

DEVELOPING CLINICAL JUDGMENT

1. A 40-year-old female is admitted to the emergency department secondary to a fall. When the admitting nurse enters the room to initiate the admission assessment, the patient does not make eye contact and responds to questions with her head down. When taking vital signs, the nurse notices that the patient has a black eye and bruising around the neck.
   a. What is the first step the nurse should undertake before asking questions about the patient's injuries?
   b. What observation would be most concerning to the nurse and why?
   c. Using the symptom cues, what priority assessment questions would likely generate helpful solutions for this patient? (Provide three possibilities.)
   d. The patient does eventually share with the nurse that her partner has been physically abusing her. The nurse does not immediately confront her with instructions on how to leave the individual perpetrating the abuse but responds with validating messages such as "It sounds like you have had a frightening experience, and I am glad you

trusted me enough to share." This is based on the understanding that_____.

e. The patient states that she does not know what to do. The nurse is concerned about her safety. What other information would the nurse need to develop a plan of care? How might the nurse gain relevant information to assess the patient's risk?

f. The nurse determines there are no immediate risks to children in the home. The patient acknowledges anxiety, a history of depression, and denies suicidal or homicidal ideation either past or present. She has a part-time job and a small group of friends who are unaware of the abuse she is experiencing. What possible solutions could the nurse offer this patient?

g. The patient signs a consent for photographs but declines to report the incident. She decides she wants to return home for now and consider her next steps, because her partner is typically remorseful and treats her well for some time after an abusive incident. What should the nurse include in her plan of care?

h. After the patient is discharged, the nurse talks with a trusted colleague who assisted with the patient's care that evening. She expresses her ongoing concerns for the patient's safety and wonders whether she did enough since the patient did not make a commitment to leave. If you were this colleague, what points might you include in your response to the nurse?

MOVIES, TV, OR STREAMING PROGRAMS

***Big Little Lies*: 2017.** In this miniseries, Nicole Kidman plays the role of Celeste, a retired lawyer who lives in a beautiful home with an attentive husband (Perry) and young twin sons. She appears to live an ideal life and is the envy of many in her community. Her story eventually reveals that she is enduring physical, sexual, and emotional abuse from the man who claims to love her. Celeste appears confident, assured, and professional when with her friends, but becomes fearful and powerless when facing her husband's abuse. Despite the danger she is in with her husband, she is emotionally conflicted and finds it difficult to leave him. She only gains the strength to face the truth after discovering that her young son has been physically abusive to a girl at school. After she is away from the violence, Celeste continues to struggle with trauma and shares her conflicted emotions during therapy sessions. She shares feelings of grief over missing her husband. It takes Celeste a long time to fully acknowledge the extent of abuse that she suffered.

Viewing Points:

1. What were some of Perry's behaviors that were indicators of domestic violence?
2. What characteristics of a partner who is abused did Celeste display?
3. How was the cycle of violence demonstrated in Celeste's marriage?
4. What were some of the factors that kept Celeste from leaving her marriage?
5. What is the significance of her son's aggression toward his female schoolmate?
6. What explains Celeste's feelings of grief and sadness about losing her husband?

***Wild Indian*: 2021.** The movie *Wild Indian* (2021) tells the story of a troubled Native American teenager (Makwa) who grows up in poverty on a reservation in Wisconsin. His life shows the plight of reservation life as he suffers abuse from his father, who has alcohol use disorder, and neglect from his mother, who did not protect him from his father. Fueled by his derision of the White Catholic school he attends, Makwa grows more hateful and emotionally detached. He is bullied and has only one friend, his cousin, Teddo. He develops a crush on a girl at school and becomes envious of another schoolmate (James) who seems to have her affection. One day while hanging out with Teddo in the woods, Makwa sees James and impulsively shoots and kills him. Afraid of the repercussions, Teddo helps Makwa hide the body. Years later, Makwa, now called Michael, has left reservation life and is living in California, married to a beautiful White woman. He no longer appears troubled but is confident, successful, and obsessed with power and a good life. His private life, however, reveals duplicity and violence as he fights violent urges, with one scene showing him choking a stripper. Ultimately, he is confronted by his past when his old friend Teddo shows up. Makwa feels threatened and kills Teddo to preserve his façade of well-being and respectability.

Viewing Points:

1. What were the cues that teenage Makwa was experiencing abuse at home?
2. What evidence can you find in this film that may reflect intergenerational transmission of violence?
3. In what ways do you think that culture influences occurrence and response to family violence?
4. After James' death, Makwa's behavior starts to change. When his father attempts to hit him, Makwa bites his hand. He then goes out and urinates on the burial site. What is happening to Makwa?
5. Does Makwa's past as an child who was abused sufficiently account for Makwa's mindset and violent behaviors? Why or why not?
6. What early interventions might have resulted in different outcomes in Makwa's life?

Unfolding Patient Stories: Sandra Littlefield • Part 2

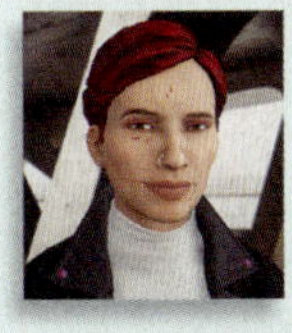

Recall from Chapter 2 **Sandra Littlefield** with borderline personality disorder. She has a history of unstable relationships, several divorces, prostitution, poor impulse control, substance use disorder, anxiety, cutting, and suicide attempts. The nurse ascertains that Sandra was sexually abused as a child. What factors in her history are suggestive of abuse? How does the nurse start to think about setting limits with Sandra and maintaining a safe environment in the clinic? What nursing interventions and education can help promote her mental health stability?

Care for Sandra Littlefield and other patients in a realistic virtual environment: ***vSim** for Nursing* (thepoint.lww.com/vSimMentalHealth). Practice documenting these patients' care in DocuCare (thepoint.lww.com/DocuCareEHR).

REFERENCES

Alhusen, J., McDonald, M., & Emery, B. (2023). Intimate partner violence: A clinical update. *The Nurse Practitioner*, *48*(9), 40–46. https://doi.org/10.1097/01.NPR.0000000000000088

American Academy of Child & Adolescent Psychiatry (AACAP). (2023). *Sexual abuse*. https://www.aacap.org/AACAP/Families_and_Youth/Facts_for_Families/FFF-Guide/Child-Sexual-Abuse-009.aspx

Center for Healthcare Strategies. (2021). *What is trauma-informed care?* https://www.traumainformedcare.chcs.org/what-is-trauma-informed-care/

Center for Justice Innovation. (2025). *Domestic violence resource for increasing safety and connection (DV RISC). Intimate partner violence risk assessments and models*. https://dvrisc.org/domestic-violence-homicide-prevention-tools-strategies-assessments/

Centers for Disease Control and Prevention (CDC). (2021). *Violence prevention*. https://www.cdc.gov/violenceprevention/index.html

Centers for Disease Control and Prevention (CDC). (2023). *Adverse childhood experiences*. https://www.cdc.gov/violenceprevention/aces/

Danger Assessment. (2025). Dangerassessment.org.

De Coster, S., & Heimer, K. (2021). Unifying theory and research on intimate partner violence: A feminist perspective. *Feminist Criminology*, *16*(3), 286–303. https://doi.org/10.1177/1557085120987615

Domestic Violence Resource Center. (2023). *Safety planning*. https://www.dvrc-or.org/safety-planning/

England, D. C. (2020). *The history of marital rape laws*. Criminal Defense Lawyer. https://www.criminaldefenselawyer.com/resources/criminal-defense/crime-penalties/marital-rape.htm

FindLaw. (2022). *Rape crimes defined, common defenses and rape penalties*. Thomson Reuters. Retrieved March 18, 2022, from https://www.findlaw.com/criminal/criminal-charges/rape.html

Gaines, K. (n.d.). *SANE nurse*. Nurse.org. https://nurse.org/resources/SANE-nurse/

Latiff, M. A., Fang, L., Goh, D. A., & Fan, L. J. (2024). A systematic review of factors associated with child sexual abuse. *Child Abuse and Neglect*, 147, 106564. https://www.sciencedirect.com/science/article/pii/S0145213423005525

McCarthy, J., & Bianchi, A. (n.d.). *The CARE approach: Supporting women who disclose intimate partner violence*. https://www.nursingcenter.com/ce_articleprint?an=00152258-201909000-00008

McNeil, A., Hicks, L., Yalcinoz-Ucan, B., & Browne, D. (2023). Prevalence & Correlates of Intimate Partner Violence During COVID-19: A Rapid Review. *Journal of Family Violence*, (38), 241–261. https://doi.org/10.1007/s10896-022-00386-6

Messing, J. T., Campbell, J. C., & Snider, C. (2017). Validation and adaptation of the Danger Assessment-5: A brief intimate partner violence risk assessment. *Journal of Advanced Nursing*, *73*(12), 3220–3230.

National Center for Victims of Crime. (n.d.). *2018 NCVRW Resource Guide: Intimate Partner Violence Fact Sheet*. https://ovc.ojp.gov/sites/g/files/xyckuh226/files/ncvrw2018/info_flyers/fact_sheets/2018NCVRW_IPV_508_QC.pdf

National Child Traumatic Stress Network. (n.d.). *Interventions*. https://www.nctsn.org/what-is-child-trauma/trauma-types/intimate-partner-violence/interventions

National Coalition against Domestic Violence (NCADV). (n.d.). *Why do victims stay?* https://ncadv.org/why-do-victims-stay

Newsom, R. (2021). *Trauma and sleep*. https://www.sleepfoundation.org/mental-health/trauma-and-sleep

Office on Women's Health, U.S. Department of Health and Human Services. (2021). *Relationships and safety: Effects of violence against women*. https://www.womenshealth.gov/relationships-and-safety/effects-violence-against-women

Ragucci, F., Dragan, M., Cuomo, A., Fagiolini, A., & Pozza, A. (2024). Psychological interventions for post-traumatic stress disorder in women survivors of intimate partner violence: A systematic review and meta-analysis. *Journal of Affective Disorders Reports*, *17*, 100802. https://doi.org/10.1016/j.jadr.2024.100802

Ramamoorthy, S., & Myers-Walls, J. A. (2021). *Talking to a child who has been abused*. Family Nurturing Center. https://familynurture.org/resources-from-family-nurturing-center/talking-child-abused/

Saghafi, A., Bahramnezhad, F., Poormollamirza, A., Dadgari, A., & Navab, E. (2019). Examining the ethical challenges in managing elder abuse: a systematic review. *Journal of Medical Ethics and History of Medicine*, *12*, 7.

SAMHSA. (December 3, 2024). Trauma-informed approaches and programs. https://www.samhsa.gov/mental-health/trauma-violence/trauma-informed-approaches-programs

The National Domestic Violence Hotline (n.d.). https://thehotline.org

U.N. Women. (2021). *Measuring the shadow pandemic: Violence against women during COVID-19*. https://data.unwomen.org/publications/vaw-rga

U.S. Department of Justice Office on Violence Against Women. (2023). *A national protocol for intimate partner violence medical forensic examinations*. https://www.safeta.org/wp-content/uploads/2023/05/IPVMFEProtocol.pdf

U.S. Department of State. (n.d.). *2022 trafficking in persons report: United States*. https://www.state.gov/reports/2022-trafficking-in-persons-report/united-states/

Violence Policy Center. (2023). *When men murder women: An analysis of 2020 homicide data*. https://vpc.org/when-men-murder-women

Voith, L. A., Logan-Greene, P., Strodthoff, T., & Bender, A. E. (2020). A paradigm shift in batterer intervention programming: A need to address unresolved trauma. *Trauma, Violence, & Abuse*, *21*(4), 691–705.

Zhang, L., Mersky, J. P., Gruber, A. M. H., & Kim, J. Y. (2023). Intergenerational transmission of parental adverse childhood experiences and children's outcomes: A scoping review. *Trauma, violence & abuse*, *24*(5), 3251–3264. https://doi.org/10.1177/15248380221126186

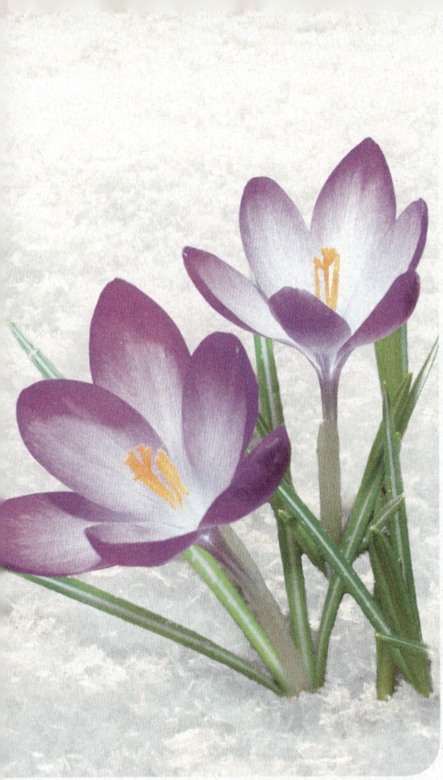

UNIT VI
Care and Recovery for People With Mental Disorders

24 Schizophrenia and Related Disorders

Nursing Care of People With Thought Disorders

Andrea C. Bostrom

KEYCONCEPTS

- delusions
- disorganized symptoms
- hallucinations
- negative symptoms
- neurocognitive impairment
- positive symptoms
- psychosis

LEARNING OBJECTIVES

After studying this chapter, you will be able to:

1. Examine the role of psychosis in schizophrenia.
2. Relate the primary theories of schizophrenia spectrum disorders to clinical symptoms and the course of the disorder.
3. Evaluate the significance of trauma in the appearance of schizophrenia symptoms.
4. Examine the relationship between social determinants of health and schizophrenia disorder.
5. Select strategies to establish a therapeutic relationship with people with schizophrenia disorder.
6. Using a clinical judgment model, formulate a person-centered, recovery-oriented nursing care plan for people with schizophrenia disorder.
7. Identify medications that are used to treat people with schizophrenia disorder and evaluate their effectiveness.
8. Develop wellness strategies for people with schizophrenia disorder.
9. Compare and contrast mental health care provided in emergency, inpatient, community, and virtual settings.
10. Support the integration of health care and mental health care for people with schizophrenia disorder.
11. Compare and contrast schizophrenia and other common schizophrenia spectrum disorders.

KEY TERMS

• affective lability • aggression • agitation • agranulocytosis • akathisia • alexithymia • alogia • ambivalence • anhedonia • anosognosia • anticholinergic crisis • apathy • autistic thinking • avolition • catatonia • catatonic excitement • cholinergic rebound • circumstantiality • clang association • command hallucinations • concrete thinking • confused speech and thinking • echolalia • echopraxia • extrapyramidal side effects • flight of ideas • gut–brain axis • hypervigilance • hypofrontality • illusions • loose associations • metonymic speech • neologisms • neuroleptic malignant syndrome • oculogyric crisis • paranoia • pressured speech • prodromal period • referential thinking • regressed behavior • religious coping • retrocollis • self-disturbance • stereotypy • stilted language • tangentiality • tardive dyskinesia • torticollis • verbigeration • waxy flexibility • word salad

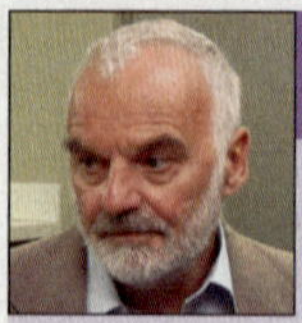

Case Study: Arnold

Arnold, a 53-year-old who was diagnosed with paranoid schizophrenia at an early age, had been living on the family farm for the last 30 years with his mother after his father died. After his mother's death, the farm was to be sold and the proceeds divided among the siblings, who arranged for Arnold to move to town. Arnold became agitated and threatening and refused to believe that his parents had died and that he would have to leave the farm.

INTRODUCTION

Schizophrenia spectrum disorders have confounded scientists and philosophers for centuries. Schizophrenia spectrum disorders are among the most severe mental illnesses; they are found in all cultures, races, and socioeconomic groups. Their symptoms have been attributed to possession by demons, considered punishment by gods for evils done, or accepted as evidence of the inhumanity of its sufferers. Historically, these explanations have resulted in enduring stigma for people diagnosed with these disorders. Today, the stigma has less to do with demonic possession than with society's unwillingness to shoulder the costs associated with housing, treatment, and rehabilitation.

SCHIZOPHRENIA SPECTRUM DISORDERS OVERVIEW

The schizophrenia spectrum disorders include schizophrenia, schizoaffective disorder (SAD), delusional disorder, schizotypal disorders (discussed in Chapter 30), schizophreniform disorder, brief psychotic disorder, and substance medication–induced psychotic disorder (American Psychiatric Association [APA], 2022). Schizophrenia is the highlighted disorder in this chapter because it has a broad range of symptoms that are found in other schizophrenia spectrum disorders. A discussion of other schizophrenia spectrum disorders follows the content on schizophrenia.

Central to understanding the issues of people with schizophrenia spectrum disorders is the concept of **psychosis,** a term used to describe a state in which an individual experiences positive symptoms of schizophrenia, also known as psychotic symptoms (e.g., **hallucinations; delusions;** disorganized thoughts, speech, or behavior) where an individual has difficulty recognizing what is real or not real. Although psychosis may be present in other diagnoses, this is the hallmark experience of schizophrenia.

> **KEYCONCEPT Psychosis**, a state in which an individual experiences hallucinations, delusions, or disorganized thoughts, speech, or behavior, is the key diagnostic factor in schizophrenia spectrum disorders.

SCHIZOPHRENIA

In the late 1800s, Emil Kraepelin first described the course of the disorder he called *dementia praecox* because of its early onset and notable changes in an individual's cognitive functioning. In the early 1900s, Eugen Bleuler renamed the disorder *schizophrenia*, meaning *split minds*, and began to determine that there was not just one type of schizophrenia but rather a group of schizophrenias. More recently, Kurt Schneider differentiated behaviors associated with schizophrenia as "first rank" symptoms (e.g., psychotic delusions, hallucinations) and "second rank" symptoms (i.e., all other experiences and behaviors associated with the disorder). These pioneering physicians had a great influence on the current diagnostic conceptualizations of schizophrenia that emphasize the heterogeneity of the disorder in terms of symptoms, course of illness, and positive and negative symptoms.

CLINICAL COURSE

Schizophrenia robs people of mental health and imposes social stigma. People with schizophrenia struggle to maintain control of their symptoms, which affect every aspect of their lives. An individual with schizophrenia displays various interrelated symptoms and experiences and cognitive deficits in several areas.

Because schizophrenia is a disorder of thoughts, perceptions, and behavior, it is sometimes not recognized as an illness by the individual experiencing the symptoms. Many people with thought disorders sincerely do not believe that they have a mental illness. They experience **anosognosia** or lack of awareness of their symptoms or illness even when they are presented with evidence of their condition. Their anosognosia and the need for treatment poses issues for the family and clinicians. Ideally, in lucid moments, patients recognize that their thoughts are really delusions, that their perceptions are hallucinations, and that their behavior is disorganized. In reality, many patients do not believe that they have a mental illness but agree to treatment to please family and clinicians.

The natural progression of schizophrenia is usually described as a chronic illness that deteriorates over time and with an eventual plateau in the symptoms. Only for older adults with schizophrenia has it been suggested that improvement might occur. In reality, no one really knows what the course of schizophrenia would be if patients were able to adhere to a treatment regimen throughout their lives. Only recently have medications become relatively effective, with manageable side effects. The clinical picture of schizophrenia is complex; individuals differ from one another, and the experience for a single individual may vary from episode to episode.

Prodromal Period

A **prodromal period** (stage of early changes that are a precursor to the disorder) may begin in early childhood. More than half of patients report the following prodromal symptoms: tension and nervousness, lack of interest in eating, difficulty concentrating, disturbed sleep, decreased enjoyment and loss of interest, restlessness, forgetfulness, depression, social withdrawal from friends, feeling laughed at, more thinking about religion, feeling bad for no reason, feeling too excited, and hearing voices or seeing things (Baeza et al., 2024). The benefit of discovering the presence of symptoms early, before they have solidified into a major disorder, is that treatment might be initiated earlier.

Acute Illness

Initially, the behaviors of this illness may be both confusing and frightening to the individual and the family. The symptoms of acute illness usually occur in late adolescence or early adulthood. The behaviors may be subtle; however, at some point they become so disruptive or bizarre that they can no longer be overlooked. These might include episodes of staying up all night for several nights, incoherent conversations, or aggressive acts against oneself or others. For example, one patient's parents reported the patient walking around the apartment for several days holding their arms and hands as if they were a machine gun, pointing them at their parents and siblings, and saying "rat-a-tat-tat, you're dead." Another caregiver described their teenager's first delusional–hallucinatory episode as so convincing that it was frightening. The teen began visiting cemeteries and said they were making "mind contact" with the deceased; they also saw their deceased grandmother walking around in the home and was certain that pipe bombs were hidden in objects in the home.

As symptoms worsen, patients are less and less able to care for their basic needs (e.g., eating, sleeping, bathing). Substance use is common. Functioning at school or work deteriorates. Dependence on family and friends increases, so those individuals recognize the patients' need for treatment. In the acute phase, individuals afflicted by schizophrenia are at high risk for suicide due to delusional thinking or feelings of desperation because of isolation and misunderstanding. Patients may be hospitalized to protect themselves or others.

Initial treatment focuses on alleviation of symptoms through beginning therapy with medications, decreasing the risk of suicide through safety measures, normalizing sleep, and reducing substance use. Functional deficits persist during this period, so the patient and family must begin to learn to cope with these deficits. Emotional blunting diminishes the ability and desire to engage in hobbies, vocational activities, and relationships. Limited participation in social activities spirals into numerous skill deficits, such as difficulty engaging others interpersonally. Cognitive deficits lead to issues recognizing patterns in situations and transferring learning and behaviors from one circumstance to a similar one.

Stabilization

After the initial diagnosis of schizophrenia and initiation of treatment, stabilization of symptoms becomes the focus. Symptoms become less acute but may still be present. Treatment is intense during this period as medication regimens are established, and patients and their families begin to adjust to the idea of a family member having a long-term severe mental illness. Ideally, the use of substances is eliminated. Socialization with others begins to increase, so that rehabilitation can begin.

Recovery

The ultimate goal is recovery. For individuals with a severe mental illness such as schizophrenia, this will entail learning to live as well as possible with the illness and its symptoms. Medication generally diminishes the symptoms and allows the individual to work toward recovery. However, no medication will cure schizophrenia. As with any chronic illness, following a therapeutic regime will help the individual to live as well as possible with the illness. Living well with schizophrenia requires the patient, family, and providers to work toward acceptance of the illness while offering hope for the best possible outcomes, encouraging autonomy with personal and reasonable goal setting, decreasing self-stigma while creating a positive self-image, finding ways to extract pleasure from life, and creating and maintaining social connections with families and peers (Vita et al., 2023). This can be partially obtained by maintaining a healthy lifestyle, managing the stresses of life, and developing meaningful interpersonal relationships. Family support and involvement are extremely important at this time. After the initial diagnosis has been made, patients and families must be educated to anticipate and expect relapse and know how to cope with it.

Relapses

Relapses can occur at any time during treatment and recovery. They are very detrimental to the successful management of this disorder. Relapse is not inevitable; however, it occurs with sufficient regularity to be a major concern in the treatment of schizophrenia. With each relapse, a longer period of time is needed to recover. Combining medications and psychosocial treatment greatly diminishes the severity and frequency of recurrent relapses (Tandon et al., 2024).

One major reason for relapse is failure to take medication consistently. Even with newer medications, adherence continues to be a challenge. Discontinuing medications will almost certainly lead to a relapse. Lower relapse rates are found, for the most part, among groups who carefully follow a treatment regimen (Rivelli et al., 2024).

Many other factors trigger relapse. Impairment in cognition and coping leaves patients vulnerable to stressors. Limited accessibility of community resources, such as public transportation, housing, entry-level and low-stress employment, and limited social services, leaves individuals without access to social support. Income supports that can buffer the day-to-day stressors of living may be inadequate. The degree of stigmatization that the community holds for mental illness attacks the self-concept of patients. Social isolation and the level of responsiveness from family members, friends, and supportive others (e.g., peers and professionals) when patients need assistance also have an impact (Smit et al., 2024).

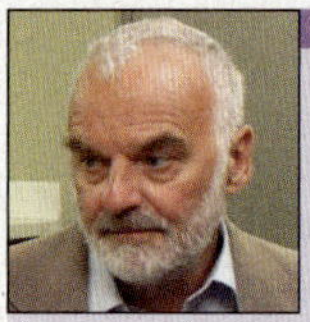

Consider Arnold

Recall that Arnold's relapse was triggered by his mother's death and being forced to leave the family farm.

DIAGNOSTIC CRITERIA

Schizophrenia is characterized by positive and negative symptoms that are present for a significant portion of a 1-month period but with continuous signs of disturbance persisting for at least 6 months (APA, 2022). **Positive symptoms** are defined as hallucinations and delusions, and **negative symptoms** as diminished emotional expression and **avolition** (lack of interest or motivation in goal-directed behavior, such as getting dressed and going to work or school). See Key Diagnostic Characteristics 24.1.

Positive Symptoms of Schizophrenia

Positive symptoms can be thought of as excessive or distorted thoughts and perceptions that occur within the individual but are not experienced by others. Hallucinations and delusions are positive symptoms of schizophrenia and the primary evidence of psychosis in people with schizophrenia. An easy way to remember the difference between hallucinations and delusions is that hallucinations involve one or more of the five senses. Delusions involve only thoughts.

KEY DIAGNOSTIC CHARACTERISTICS 24.1

***DSM-5-TR* DIAGNOSTIC CRITERIA: Schizophrenia**

A. Two (or more) of the following, each present for a significant portion of time during a 1-month period (or less if successfully treated). At least one of these must be (1), (2), or (3):
   1. Delusions
   2. Hallucinations
   3. Disorganized speech (e.g., frequent derailment or incoherence)
   4. Grossly disorganized or catatonic behavior
   5. Negative symptoms (i.e., diminished emotional expression or avolition)

B. For a significant portion of the time since the onset of the disturbance, level of functioning in one or more major areas, such as work, interpersonal relations, or self-care, is markedly below the level achieved prior to the onset (or when the onset is in childhood or adolescence, there is failure to achieve expected level of interpersonal, academic, or occupational functioning).

C. Continuous signs of the disturbance persist for at least 6 months. This 6-month period must include at least 1 month of symptoms (or less if successfully treated) that meet Criterion A (i.e., active-phase symptoms) and may include periods of prodromal or residual symptoms. During these prodromal or residual periods, the signs of the disturbance may be manifested by only negative symptoms or by two or more symptoms listed in Criterion A present in an attenuated form (e.g., odd beliefs and unusual perceptual experiences).

D. Schizoaffective disorder and depressive or bipolar disorder with psychotic features have been ruled out because either (1) no major depressive or manic episodes have occurred concurrently with the active-phase symptoms or (2) if mood episodes have occurred during active-phase symptoms, they have been present for a minority of the total duration of the active and residual periods of the illness.

E. The disturbance is not attributable to the physiologic effects of a substance (e.g., a drug of abuse, a medication) or another medical condition.

F. If there is a history of autism spectrum disorder or a communication disorder of childhood onset, the additional diagnosis of schizophrenia is made only if prominent delusions or hallucinations, in addition to the other required symptoms of schizophrenia, are also present for at least 1 month (or less if successfully treated).

A fairly common hallucination is a command hallucination, that is, an auditory hallucination instructing the patient to act in a certain way, because voices are telling the individual to do something. **Command hallucinations** range from innocuous (eat all of your dinner) to very serious (hurt someone or jump in front of a bus).

KEYCONCEPT Positive symptoms reflect an excess or distortion of expected functions, including delusions and hallucinations.

KEYCONCEPT Hallucinations are perceptual experiences that occur without actual external sensory stimuli. They can involve any of the five senses, but they are usually *visual* or *auditory*. Auditory hallucinations are more common than visual ones. For example, the patient may hear voices carrying on a discussion about their own thoughts or behaviors.

KEYCONCEPT Delusions are erroneous, fixed, false beliefs that cannot be changed by reasonable argument. They usually involve a misinterpretation of experience. For example, the patient believes someone is reading their thoughts or plotting against them.

Common types of delusions include the following:

- *Grandiose:* the belief that one has exceptional powers, wealth, skill, influence, or destiny
- *Nihilistic:* the belief that one is dead, or a calamity is impending
- *Persecutory:* the belief that one is being watched, ridiculed, harmed, or plotted against
- *Somatic:* beliefs about irregularities in bodily functions or structures

Negative Symptoms of Schizophrenia

The term *negative symptoms* is used to describe emotions and behaviors that should be present but are diminished in people with schizophrenia. Negative symptoms are not as dramatic as positive symptoms, but they can interfere greatly with the patient's ability to function day to day. People with schizophrenia often experience **alexithymia** or difficulty in identifying, expressing, or describing emotion. Because expressing emotion is difficult for them, people with schizophrenia laugh, cry, and get angry less often. Their affect is flat; they show little or no emotion when personal loss occurs. They also experience **ambivalence,** which is the concurrent experience of equally strong opposing feelings so that it is impossible to make a decision. Avolition may be so profound that simple activities of daily living (ADLs), such as dressing or combing hair, may not get done. **Anhedonia** prevents the individual with schizophrenia from enjoying activities. People with schizophrenia may have limited speech and difficulty saying anything new or carrying on a conversation. These negative symptoms cause the individual with schizophrenia to withdraw and experience feelings of severe isolation.

KEYCONCEPT Negative symptoms reflect a lessening or loss of expected functions, such as restriction or flattening in the range and intensity of emotion (diminished emotional expression), reduced fluency and productivity of thought and speech (**alogia**), withdrawal and inability to initiate and persist in goal-directed activity (avolition), and inability to experience pleasure (anhedonia).

Neurocognitive Impairment

Neurocognitive impairment exists in people with schizophrenia and may be independent of positive and negative symptoms. Neurocognition includes memory (short and long term); vigilance or sustained attention; verbal fluency or the ability to generate new words; and executive functioning, which includes volition, planning, purposeful action, and self-monitoring behavior. Working memory is a concept that includes short-term memory and the ability to store and process information.

KEYCONCEPT Neurocognitive impairment in memory, vigilance, and executive functioning is related to poor functional outcomes in schizophrenia.

This impairment is independent of the positive symptoms. That is, cognitive dysfunction can exist even if the positive symptoms are in remission. Not all areas of cognitive functioning are impaired. Long-term memory and intellectual functioning are not necessarily affected. However, low intellectual functioning is common and may be related to a lack of educational experiences and opportunities due to the age of illness onset. Neurocognitive dysfunction is often manifested in disorganized symptoms (Karyakina & Shmukler, 2021).

KEYCONCEPT Disorganized symptoms of schizophrenia are findings that make it difficult for the individual to understand and respond to the ordinary sights and sounds of daily living. These include **confused speech and thinking,** and disorganized behavior.

Disorganized Thinking

The following are examples of confused speech and thinking patterns:

- **Echolalia**—repetition of another's words that is parrot-like and inappropriate
- **Circumstantiality**—extremely detailed and lengthy discourse about a topic
- **Loose associations**—absence of the expected connectedness of thoughts, ideas, and topics; sudden shifts without apparent relationship to preceding topics
- **Tangentiality**—the topic of conversation is changed to an entirely different topic that is a logical progression but causes a permanent detour from the original focus

- **Flight of ideas**—the topic of conversation changes repeatedly and rapidly, generally after just one sentence or phrase
- **Word salad**—stringing together words that are not connected in any way
- **Neologisms**—words that are made up that have no common meaning and are not recognizable
- **Paranoia**—suspiciousness and guardedness that are unrealistic and often accompanied by grandiosity
- **Referential thinking**—a belief that neutral stimuli have special meaning to the individual, such as a television commentator who is speaking directly to the individual
- **Autistic thinking**—restricts thinking to the literal and immediate so that the individual has private rules of logic and reasoning that make no sense to anyone else
- **Concrete thinking**—lack of abstraction in thinking; inability to understand punch lines, metaphors, and analogies
- **Verbigeration**—purposeless repetition of words or phrases
- **Metonymic speech**—use of words with similar meanings interchangeably
- **Clang association**—repetition of words or phrases that are similar in sound but in no other way, for example, "right, light, sight, might"
- **Stilted language**—overly and inappropriately artificial formal language
- **Pressured speech**—speaking as if the words are being forced out

Disorganized perceptions often create oversensitivity to colors, shapes, and background activities. **Illusions** occur when the individual misperceives or exaggerates stimuli that actually exist in the external environment. This is in contrast to hallucinations, which are perceptions in the absence of environmental stimuli. Ancillary symptoms that may accompany schizophrenia include anxiety, depression, and hostility.

Disorganized Behavior

Disorganized behavior (which may manifest as very slow, rhythmic, or ritualistic movement), coupled with disorganized speech, makes it difficult for the individual to partake in daily activities. Examples of disorganized behavior include the following:

- **Aggression**—behaviors or attitudes that reflect rage, hostility, and the potential for physical or verbal destructiveness (usually comes about if the individual believes someone is going to do them harm)
- **Agitation**—inability to sit still or attend to others, accompanied by heightened emotions and tension
- **Catatonia**—psychomotor disturbances, such as stupor, mutism, posturing, or repetitive behavior
- **Catatonic excitement**—a hyperactivity characterized by purposeless activity and unexpected movements, such as grimacing and posturing
- **Echopraxia**—involuntary imitation of another individual's movements and gestures
- **Regressed behavior**—behaving in a manner of a less mature life stage; childlike and immature behavior
- **Stereotypy**—repetitive purposeless movements that are idiosyncratic to the individual and to some degree outside of the individual's control
- **Hypervigilance**—sustained attention to external stimuli as if expecting something important or frightening to happen
- **Waxy flexibility**—posture held in an odd or unusual fixed position for extended periods of time

Disruption in Sense of Self

Many of the symptoms observed in schizophrenia may be attributable to brain deficiencies that affect the individual's experience of "self." The self is difficult to define but is often used to describe who we are: self-concept, self-consciousness, self-awareness, and, for people with schizophrenia, **self-disturbance**. This self-disturbance leads to significant difficulty determining what thoughts and experiences are internal versus external to the individual. Delusions and hallucinations can be explained by this, as can the individual's failures of insight, self-awareness, and self-monitoring (Gruber et al., 2023; Parnas & Sandsten, 2024). Self-disturbance also suggests ways that adolescents and young adults may be identified during the prodromal period of the illness by their difficulties in integrating self-experiences.

Treatment that focuses on self-disturbance aims to help clients to become active agents in their own care. This can be done by helping them to develop concepts of themselves in the world and creating narratives of how their experiences have developed and can be managed in the future in their own unique way (Green & Jimenez, 2022). Treatment that helps to develop a sense of "self" is possible and integral to recovery (Lysaker, 2021). This may be facilitated by creating a milieu that encourages therapeutic relationships for developing an individual's sense of self versus the self of others and to help develop skills for mastering self-care (Hasson-Ohayon et al., 2021).

SCHIZOPHRENIA ACROSS THE LIFESPAN

Although schizophrenia is usually diagnosed in late adolescence, it can be diagnosed in children and older adults.

Children

The diagnosis of schizophrenia is rare in children before adolescence. When it does occur in children aged 5 or 6 years, the symptoms are essentially the same as in adults. In this age group, hallucinations tend to be visual, and delusions less developed. Because disorganized speech and behavior may be explained better by other disorders that are more common in childhood, those disorders should be considered before applying the diagnosis of schizophrenia to a child.

However, recent studies suggest that the likelihood of children later experiencing schizophrenia can be predicted. Developmental irregularities in childhood, including delays in attainment of speech and motor development, issues s in social adjustment, and poorer academic and cognitive performance, have been found to be present in individuals who experience schizophrenia in adulthood. Adults who had childhood cognitive, social, behavioral, and emotional impairments may be at higher risk of developing schizophrenia (Correll et al., 2024).

Older Adults

Some people develop schizophrenia in late life. For older patients who have had schizophrenia since young adulthood, this may be a time in which they experience some improvement in symptoms or decrease in relapse fluctuations. There is some evidence that suggests that older adults with schizophrenia may be more likely to develop cognitive impairment than those without mental disorders (Yang et al., 2023). However, their lifestyle is probably dependent on the effectiveness of earlier treatment, the support systems that are in place (including relationships with family members and professionals), and the interaction between environmental stressors and the patient's functional impairments. The cost of caring for older patients with schizophrenia remains high because many are no longer cared for in institutions and because community-based treatment has developed more slowly for this age group than for younger adults.

EPIDEMIOLOGY AND RISK FACTORS

Schizophrenia is found in all cultures and countries. It is prevalent in the worldwide population (ranging from 0.29% to 0.72%) and is listed within the top 20 illnesses for life lost resulting from premature death and years lived in less than full health (GBD 2021 Diseases and Injuries Collaborators, 2024; Solmi et al., 2023). Its economic costs are enormous. Direct costs include treatment expenses; indirect costs include lost wages, premature death, and involuntary commitment. In addition, employment among people with schizophrenia is one of the lowest of any group with disabilities. The costs of schizophrenia in terms of individual and family suffering are inestimable.

People with schizophrenia tend to cluster in the lowest social classes in industrialized countries and urban communities. The symptoms of the illness are so pervasive that it is difficult for these individuals to maintain any type of gainful employment (Venkataraman et al., 2024). Housing challenges are often problematic for people with severe mental illness (e.g., schizophrenia or bipolar illness). People with schizophrenia who relapse are more likely to remain unhoused with few opportunities for employment (Martins et al., 2023).

Internal and External Risk Factors

Genetic factors related to cognitive and brain function and brain structure are known risks for schizophrenia. Early neurologic issues, stressful life events, and nonhereditary genetic factors also contribute to the likelihood of developing the disorder. Environmental factors related to schizophrenia include migrant status, having an older biologic father, *Toxoplasma gondii* antibodies, prenatal famine, lifetime cannabis use, obstetric complications, urban rearing, and winter or spring birth (Robinson et al., 2024; Steen et al., 2023).

Age of Onset

Schizophrenia is usually diagnosed in late adolescence and early adulthood. People assigned male at birth tend to be diagnosed between the ages of 18 and 25 years, and people assigned female at birth between the ages of 25 and 35 years. The earlier the diagnosis and the longer the psychosis remains untreated, the more severe the disorder becomes. Conversely, the earlier the psychosis is recognized and treated within an evidence-based comprehensive program, the better the outcomes (Zhan et al., 2023).

Sex Assigned at Birth

People assigned male at birth tend to be diagnosed earlier and have a poorer prognosis than those assigned female at birth. This may be a sex-linked outcome, but it may also reflect the poorer prognosis for any individual who develops the disorder at an early age (Giordano et al., 2021). When patients assigned female at birth are diagnosed early, they are at higher risk for physical comorbidities than those assigned male at birth (Esposito et al., 2024).

When considering treatment for people who identify as LGBTQ+ and are diagnosed with schizophrenia, we must first recognize that schizophrenia is neither a cause nor an effect of gender identities. However, we may need to consider the effects of trauma and stress for those who identify as LGBTQ+, especially those who are transgender and develop schizophrenia. Second, it is important to realize that the health care system has not always been welcoming to these individuals and care must be given to show respect and acceptance by using the patient's requested name and pronoun and recognizing their specified significant others. Third, we must recognize that during treatment, whether it is inpatient or in the community, safety is a vital consideration. Many individuals within the LGBTQ+ community (especially transgender individuals) have experienced discrimination and violence, which can also occur in mental health treatment settings. It is also important to recognize that peers within the LGBTQ+ community may be frightened by mental health diagnoses and may express discomfort and stigma toward an LGBTQ+ community member with a severe mental illness such as schizophrenia (Nolan et al., 2023).

Ethnicity and Culture

Increasingly, efforts are being made to consider culture and ethnic origin when diagnosing and treating individuals with schizophrenia. Racial groups may have varying diagnostic rates of schizophrenia. However, it is not clear whether these findings represent correct diagnosis or misdiagnosis of the disorder based on the cultural bias of the clinician. For instance, schizophrenia has been consistently overdiagnosed among African Americans (Fashaw-Walters et al., 2021). African American and Latinx individuals with bipolar disorder are more likely to have misdiagnoses of schizophrenia than are White individuals with bipolar disorder. Serious mental disorders may be underreported by Asian American individuals because of the mistrust of the mental health system by some individuals in those communities (Lim et al., 2021).

Familial Differences

First-degree biologic relatives (e.g., children, siblings, parents) of an individual with schizophrenia have a 10 times estimated greater risk for schizophrenia than the general population (Ohi et al., 2021). Other relatives may have an increased risk for related disorders, such as SAD and schizotypal personality disorder (Saarinen et al., 2024).

COMORBIDITY

Several somatic and psychological disorders coexist with schizophrenia. A genome-wide study shows that anxiety disorders, bipolar disorder, major depressive disorder, suicidal ideation or attempt, and tobacco use disorder are genetically related to schizophrenia (Mulugetta et al., 2023).

Physical health conditions and illnesses to which people with schizophrenia are particularly susceptible include tuberculosis, human immunodeficiency disease, hepatitis B and C, osteoporosis, poor dentition, impaired lung function, altered (reduced) pain sensitivity, sexual dysfunction, obstetric complications, cardiovascular issues, hyperpigmentation, obesity, diabetes, metabolic syndrome with hyperlipidemia, polydipsia, thyroid dysfunction, and hyperprolactinemia (Castle & Li, 2023; Halstead et al., 2024).

This susceptibility to certain diseases results in significant morbidity and mortality for people with schizophrenia, with individuals who have this diagnosis dying up to 20 years earlier than individuals in the general population. Neurocognitive dysfunction in the areas of immediate verbal memory and executive functioning is related to lower life-expectancy (Mohn et al., 2023). Early mortality may be from natural causes (cardiovascular, cancer, chronic obstructive pulmonary disease, diabetes, and influenza and pneumonia) or unnatural causes (suicide, substance and alcohol misuse, and legal interventions) (Yung et al., 2023). Several health system factors contribute to this, including barriers to obtaining primary care and the primary care providers' lack of preparation and discomfort addressing mental health issues and conditions, the insufficient preparation of mental health practitioners in managing physical illness, the tendency for mental health providers to fail to ask about physical health, and the absence of standards of care that include screening and monitoring medical issues.

COVID-19

People living with schizophrenia are at an increased risk of COVID-19 and have worse outcomes (including mortality) than the general population (Barlati et al., 2021). Their symptoms, such as delusions, hallucinations, disorganized behavior, cognitive impairment, and poor insight, make it harder for adequate infection control. Furthermore, long-term chronic health conditions (multi-morbidities) and health care access inequities related to socio-economic status and discrimination increase the vulnerability of people with schizophrenia (Impara et al., 2022). Many people with schizophrenia live in congregate housing, which compounds the likelihood of infection. People with schizophrenia may be less distressed by the social restrictions required during a pandemic than others because these may cause minimal change to daily routines for those with this disorder (Benedyk et al., 2023).

Substance Use and Depression

Among the behavioral comorbidities, substance use is common. Depression may also be observed in patients with schizophrenia. This is an important symptom for several reasons. First, depression may be evidence that the diagnosis of a mood disorder is more appropriate. Second, depression is not unusual in chronic stages of schizophrenia and deserves attention. Third, 50% of people with schizophrenia attempt suicide, and 10% to 15% die by suicide. The suicide rate for people with schizophrenia is 4.5 times higher than it is in the general US population (Olfson et al., 2021). Risk factors for suicide are untreated psychosis, history of suicide attempt, age younger than 28 years, severity of depression, and substance misuse (Cernika & Vrublevska, 2024; Miola et al., 2023).

Diabetes and Obesity

In the 19th century, an association was established between glucose regulation and psychiatric disorders, suggesting that people with schizophrenia may be more prone to type 2 diabetes than the general public (Franzen, 1970; Schimmelbusch et al., 1971). Evidence that supports this view includes a higher rate of type 2 diabetes in first-degree relatives of people with schizophrenia and higher rates of impaired glucose tolerance and insulin resistance among people with schizophrenia. However, obesity, which is associated with type 2 diabetes, is a growing issue in the United States in general, and is complicated in schizophrenia treatment by the tendency of individuals to gain weight after their disease is managed with antipsychotic medications. Weight gain in some individuals may be attributed to a return to a healthier living situation, in which regular meals are available and symptoms that interfere with obtaining food regularly (e.g., delusions) are decreased. For others, weight gain may be a medication side effect (Mizuki et al., 2021).

ETIOLOGY

Schizophrenia is believed to be caused by the interaction of a biologic predisposition or vulnerability and environmental stressors (see the diathesis-stress model discussed in Chapter 19). See Box 24.1 for deficits related to vulnerability in schizophrenia. Environmental stressors include pregnancy or obstetric complications and social adversity, such as migration, unemployment, urban living, childhood abuse, and social isolation or absence of close friends (Kotsakis Ruehlmann et al., 2023; Peralta et al., 2024).

BOX 24.1

Issues that Cause Vulnerability in Schizophrenia

COGNITIVE ISSUES

- Processing complex information
- Maintaining attention
- Inability to distinguish between relevant and irrelevant stimuli
- Difficulty in abstract thinking
- Impaired working memory

PSYCHOPHYSIOLOGICAL ISSUES

- Deficits in sensory inhibition
- Poor control of autonomic responsiveness

SOCIAL SKILLS ISSUES

- Processing interpersonal stimuli, such as eye contact or assertiveness
- Conversational capacity
- Initiating activities
- Experiencing pleasure

Source: Cummings, M. A., Arias, A. W., & Stahl, S. M. (2024). What is the neurobiology of schizophrenia? *CNS Spectrums*, 1–6. https://doi.org/doi.org/10.1017/S1092852924000518; Redlich Bossy, M., Müller, D. R., Niedermoser, D. W., Burrer, A., Spiller, T. R., Vetter, S., Seifritz, E., & Egger, S. T. (2024). Impact of psychopathology on day-to-day living in patients with schizophrenia: A network analysis. *Comprehensive Psychiatry*, *133*, 152501. https://doi.org/10.1016/j.comppsych.2024.152501

Biologic Theories

Neuroanatomic Findings

The lateral and third ventricles are somewhat larger, and total brain volume is somewhat less in people with schizophrenia compared with those without schizophrenia. The thalamus and the medial temporal lobe structures, including the hippocampus, and superior temporal and prefrontal cortices, tend to be smaller also (Gangadin et al., 2021; Liloia et al., 2021).

Genetic Associations

Genetic associations have been identified in a number of regions of the brain, and some have already been tied to neuropathways related to cognitive deficits. The future of treatment of schizophrenia will rely heavily on the outcome of ongoing research (Tandon et al., 2024).

Neurodevelopment

The neurodevelopmental hypothesis explains the etiology of schizophrenia as pathologic processes caused by genetic and environmental factors that begin before the brain reaches its adult state. Evidence suggests that in utero during the first or second trimester, genes involved with cell migration, cell proliferation, axonal outgrowth, and myelination may be affected by neurologic insults, such as viral infections. That is, early neurodevelopmental insults may lead to dysfunction of specific networks that become obvious at adolescence during the expected loss of some neuronal plasticity and synapse development (Reckziegel et al., 2022).

Neurotransmitters, Pathways, and Receptors

Positron emission tomography (PET) scan findings suggest that in schizophrenia, brain metabolism is generally reduced, with a relative hypermetabolism in the left side of the brain and in the left temporal lobe. Irregularities exist in specific areas of the brain in the frontal, temporal, and cingulate regions. These findings support further exploration of differential brain hemisphere function in people with schizophrenia. Other PET studies show **hypofrontality**, or a reduced cerebral blood flow and glucose metabolism in the prefrontal cortex of people with schizophrenia and hyperactivity in the limbic area (Buchsbaum, 1990; Hazlett et al., 2019; Rooy et al., 2021).

Dopamine Dysregulation

A long-standing explanation of the neurobiologic symptoms of schizophrenia is the dopamine hypothesis. Because conventional antipsychotics blocked dopamine and treated the positive symptoms of schizophrenia—specifically, hallucinations and delusions—it was reasoned that *hyperactivity* in the mesolimbic tract at the D2 receptor site in the striatal area (where memory and emotion are regulated) was responsible for these symptoms. Conversely, chronic low levels of dopamine in the prefrontal cortex were thought to underlie cognitive dysfunction in schizophrenia.

Today, research focuses on several of the molecular links to dopamine synthesis and increased release of dopamine. Dopamine has a role in the pathogenesis of schizophrenia, but it is more complicated than previously thought. Dopamine activity is related to other disorders, cortical functioning, and stress (Howes et al., 2024).

Role of Other Receptors

Other receptors are also involved in dopamine neurotransmission, especially serotonergic receptors. It is becoming clear that schizophrenia does not result from dysregulation of a single neurotransmitter or biogenic amine (e.g., norepinephrine, dopamine, or serotonin). Investigators are also hypothesizing a role for glutamate and gamma-aminobutyric acid (GABA) because of the complex interconnections of neuronal transmission and the complexity and heterogeneity of schizophrenia symptoms. The *N*-methyl-D-aspartate class of glutamate receptors is being studied because of the actions of phencyclidine (PCP) at these sites and because of the similarity of the psychotic behaviors that are produced when someone takes PCP.

Gut Microbiota

The **gut–brain axis** (the two-way communication system that connects the gut with the brain) is involved with the intestinal microbiome, neuroendocrine (hypothalamus–pituitary–adrenal axis), immune, and nervous systems. The gut microbiota communicates with the central nervous system (CNS) through the vagus nerve. Emerging research is linking the gut microbiota to the development of mental disorders through the gut–brain axis. It is hypothesized that irregularities in the gut microbiota increase inflammatory cytokines that may cause neuronal damage, cell death, and unusual brain development. Gut microbiota alterations are observed in people with schizophrenia. It is hypothesized that these alterations may account for the biologic alterations in psychosis (Li et al., 2024).

BOX 24.2

Clinical Judgment Vignette: Graduate Student in Peril

B.G.W., born in 1993, spent most of his teenage years using drugs and alcohol, behavior that started when he was 11 years old. He failed 8th grade, repeated it, and made it to 10th grade. He was removed permanently from school at the age of 16 years. His dress included a dirty denim jacket or Army fatigues, torn tee shirts with rock band logos, and tight-fitting jeans. At age 16, he was hospitalized for a psychotic episode initiated by lysergic acid diethylamide (LSD); it was the scariest moment of his life. His mind had been getting fuzzier every day; he had dabbled with black magic and Satanism. Later, he admitted that for years he had been trapped in a fantasy land, only partially explained by his drug use.

Years of treatment followed; even with abstinence from drugs, his mental status fluctuated. After antipsychotic agents were prescribed, he began to feel like himself. He was motivated to complete his General Education Diploma (GED) and entered college. He kept his mental illness a secret. While in graduate school, his thoughts, feelings, and behaviors began to change. His thinking became delusional, his moods unpredictable, and his behaviors illogic. Finally, he was hospitalized again, and his condition was stabilized with medication. Currently, he is reapplying to graduate school, and this time he vows to keep people close to him aware of his mental status.

Building Clinical Judgment

1. What role did stigma play in the treatment process?
2. What information should B.G.W. share with his social network about his mental illness and treatment?

Psychosocial Theories

Social factors can contribute to the changes in brain function that result in schizophrenia and add to the day-to-day challenges of living with a mental illness. Childhood trauma, living in an urban environment, and being a member of an underrepresented group are all associated with psychotic syndromes. They can also create barriers to obtaining necessary treatment and recovery (Tandon et al., 2024). One of the major social stressors is the social stigma that surrounds all mental illnesses (see Chapter 2). The clinical vignette in Box 24.2 describes the impact of living with a stigmatizing illness. Another social stressor is the absence of good, affordable, and supportive housing in many communities. With 2010's enactment of insurance parity for mental illness in the Affordable Care Act, it was hoped that quality and continuity of care would be enhanced; however, this Act has been inconsistently implemented based on individual state insurance policies. Finally, the mental health service delivery system is fragmented; its quality and types of services vary from community to community, based in part on state legislative and mental health department funding differences.

FAMILY RESPONSE TO DISORDER

Initially, families usually experience disbelief, shock, and fear, along with concern for the family member. Families

BOX 24.3

Research for Evidence-Based Practice: Family Functioning of Caregivers of Patients With Schizophrenia

Hsiao, C. Y., Hsieh, M. H., Chung, F. C., Chiu, S. C., Chang, C. W., & Tsai, Y. F. (2023). Changes in family functioning among primary family caregivers of patients with schizophrenia. Journal of Nursing Scholarship, *55(5), 967–976. https://doi.org/10.1111/jnu.12887*

THE QUESTION: What changes occur in the family functioning in primary family caregivers of individuals with schizophrenia over a 6-month postdischarge period?

METHODS: In a longitudinal study, data from 58 primary family caregivers of patients with schizophrenia were collected four times including 1 week before hospital discharge and at 1-, 3-, and 6-month intervals postdischarge. Demographic and clinical questionnaires, affiliate stigma (self-stigma of family caregivers), family empowerment, and general function scales were used.

FINDINGS: Family function was viewed by most caregivers (59.6% to 77.6%) as unhealthy during the 6-month period. In these families, affiliate stigma increased, empowerment decreased, and family functioning declined. Primary caregivers who viewed their family functioning as healthy experienced a decrease in self-stigma during the first month but returned to their baseline score at 6 months. Their empowerment score increased throughout the 6-month period.

IMPLICATIONS FOR NURSING: Nurses should recognize the importance of family functioning to support the recovery of people with schizophrenia. Anti-stigma interventions and family education can support healthy family functioning.

may attribute the episode to taking illicit drugs or to extraordinary stress or fatigue and hope that this is an isolated or transient event. They may be fearful of the behaviors and respond to patient's anger and hostility with fear, confusion, and anxiety. They may deny the severity and chronicity of the illness and only partially engage in treatment. As families begin to acknowledge the disorder and the long-term care nature of recovery, they themselves may feel overwhelmed, angry, and depressed. In many instances, parents/guardians become caregivers as the individual transitions into adulthood. As caregivers for their adult children, these individuals face many challenges accessing health care and resources (Girdhar & Patil, 2023; Kadakia et al., 2021). See Box 24.3.

RECOVERY-ORIENTED CARE FOR PEOPLE WITH SCHIZOPHRENIA

Teamwork and Collaboration: Working Toward Recovery

The most effective approach to treatment for individuals with schizophrenia involves various disciplines, including nursing (both generalist and advanced practice psychiatric nurses), psychiatry, psychology, social work, occupational and recreational therapy, and pastoral counseling. Individuals with general education in psychology, sociology, and social work often serve as case managers, nursing aides, technicians, and other support personnel in hospitals and community treatment agencies. Peer counselors are increasingly used in community agencies and offer support and hope for a better future.

Patients need help in accepting and understanding their illness, setting goals, and developing a support system that encourages their recovery. Recovery-oriented strategies can address hopelessness associated with suicide attempts or withdrawal from relationships with others and encourage an independent lifestyle. Medication management is central to the treatment of schizophrenia and is the responsibility of the patient, physicians, nurses, and pharmacists. Psychosocial interventions can be implemented by all members of the mental health team and may include cognitive-behavioral, music, vocational, mindfulness, and support therapies. These varied professionals and paraprofessionals are important because of the complex nature of the symptoms, the long-term nature of the disorder, and the need for health promotion support. Complementary and alternative therapies, such as yoga, breathing exercises, relaxation, meditation and mindfulness, and aerobic exercise, may be helpful as adjunctive to the usual care.

Safety Issues

Several special concerns exist when working with people with schizophrenia. A suicide assessment should always be completed when an individual is experiencing a psychotic episode. In an inpatient unit, patient safety concerns extend to potentially aggressive actions toward staff and other patients during episodes of psychosis. During times of acute illness, a priority of care is treatment with antipsychotic medications and, in some instances, hospitalization.

Nurses should assess the individual's risk for suicide because of the high suicide and attempted suicide rates among people with schizophrenia. One challenge is to distinguish among the displayed behaviors to determine if the individual is displaying negative symptoms, side effects of antipsychotic medications, or actual depression and demoralization as a result of this illness. Does the patient speak of suicide, or have delusional thinking that could lead to dangerous behavior, or have command hallucinations telling them to harm self or others? Does the patient have homicidal ideations? Does the patient lack social support and the skills to be meaningfully engaged with other people or a vocation? Does the patient express feelings of not belonging to a social group or being a burden to loved ones? Substance-related disorders are also common among patients with schizophrenia, so that nurses should assess for substance use.

EVIDENCE-BASED NURSING CARE OF PEOPLE WITH SCHIZOPHRENIA

Recovery is a long-term journey requiring various nursing interventions at different times. During exacerbation of symptoms, many patients are hospitalized for safety and medication adjustment. During periods of relative stability, the nurse and patient collaborate in developing recovery-oriented strategies that include maintaining a healthy lifestyle, developing positive coping skills, and seeking meaningful relationships. Schizophrenia research is ongoing, and the results are leading to new treatment approaches. It is critical that nurses continually seek out evidence-based strategies through accessing the best possible sources of evidence and formulating clinical questions. See Clinical Judgment Nursing Care Plan 24.1, which sets forth a plan of care for Arnold, the case study patient in this chapter.

RECOGNIZING CUES: RELEVANT ASSESSMENT INFORMATION

The nursing assessment should include the biologic, psychological, social, and spiritual areas because schizophrenia affects all aspects of the individual's life. Not only are symptoms assessed, but strengths are also important in the assessment process.

Physical Health

The nurse should first determine whether any underlying medical disorders are present, particularly those associated with schizophrenia, such as diabetes, hypertension, and cardiac disease, or a family history of such disorders. Usually, a medical examination is conducted by primary

CLINICAL JUDGMENT NURSING CARE PLAN 24.1

The Patient With Schizophrenia

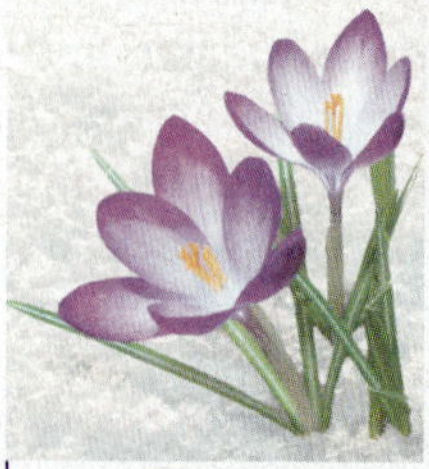

Arnold, age 53 years, assigned male at birth, has a history of schizophrenia with multiple hospitalizations. He was admitted per mental health court order to the inpatient mental health unit accompanied by the county sheriff. Arnold was given antipsychotic and antianxiety medication in the emergency room for the safety of himself and others after he attempted to strike an emergency room nurse. Arnold had become agitated and threatening while being removed from his family's farm, where he lived with his mother for the past 30 years. Arnold refused to acknowledge that his parents had died.

Setting: Psychiatric Intensive Care Unit

Assessment Cues: Arnold is dressed in a suit and dress shirt. On admission, he was also wearing a tie, which is his habit whenever he leaves his home. His tie, shoes, and belt were removed after arriving on the unit from the emergency room for safety reasons. Arnold wears his hair short, and he has been completing ADL. Arnold is watchful with a worried and anxious expression. He has a small stack of slightly used paper napkins stored between his shirt and suit jacket and holds a small stack of flattened single-serving milk cartons in his hand.

Arnold states that he is not ill and that his previous hospitalizations were attempts by multinational corporations to keep him from following his parents' wishes. Even though he attended both parents' funerals, he continues to say they are merely away for a while. He denies suicidal thoughts. Denies using alcohol or illegal drugs. He has been taking his prescribed medications sporadically.

Arnold is 5 ft 11 in, weighs 180 lb, BMI 25, BP 140/80, P 78, R 16. Laboratory values are expected.

Associated Psychiatric Diagnosis

Schizophrenia, multiple episode, currently in acute episode

Medications

Risperidone, 2 mg BID
Lorazepam, 2 mg PO for agitation PRN

Priority Hypothesis: Changes in Thought Process

Important Characteristics

- Delusional thinking (believes there is conspiracy against family by multinational corporations, and parents not really deceased)
- Auditory hallucinations (parents talking to him)
- Suspiciousness (refuses to use telephone or other technology)

Associated Considerations

- Uncompensated alterations in brain activity

Clinical Judgment Nursing Care Plan 24.1 Continued

Planning Recovery and Wellness Outcomes

Initial

- Decreased delusional thinking through accurate interpretation of environment
- Expresses less suspiciousness about family
- Decreased frequency of hearing voices
- Able to participate in activities of increasing length and complexity (e.g., sitting through group and group activities, able to make projects that require increased concentration and contain more steps)

Long Term

- Able to identify, monitor, and recognize delusional thinking and hallucinations
- Able to use coping mechanisms that will help to minimize or control symptoms of delusions and hallucinations
- Able to develop a reasonable medication routine
- Reestablish self-care activities

Taking Action: Nursing Interventions

Interventions	Rationale	Ongoing Assessment
• Initiate a nurse–patient relationship by using an accepting, nonjudgmental approach.	• A therapeutic relationship will provide support as Arnold begins to deal with his life change.	• Determine the extent to which Arnold is willing to trust and engage in a relationship.
• Be patient.	• Be patient because his brain is not processing information normally.	• Determine the length of time Arnold can attend to conversation or activity with others.
• Administer risperidone as prescribed. Observe for affect, side effects, and adverse effects. Begin teaching about the medication and its importance after symptoms subside.	• Risperidone is a D2 and 5-HT2A antagonist and is indicated for the treatment of schizophrenia.	• Make sure Arnold swallows pills. Monitor for relief of positive symptoms using a standardized measure such as the SAPS. Assess side effects, especially extrapyramidal. Monitor blood pressure for orthostatic hypotension and body temperature increase (NMS).
• During hallucinations and delusional thinking, assess significance (what feelings is Arnold experiencing; what actions do the voices or his thoughts suggest he accomplish?). Reassure Arnold that you will keep him safe and that you are aware that his experiences are very real to him even though you may not be having the same experiences (Do not try to convince Arnold that his delusions are not true.) Redirect Arnold to here-and-now activities and experiences.	• It is important to understand the experience and context of the hallucinations and delusions to be able to provide appropriate interventions and redirect the patient to more reality-based activities. By avoiding arguments about the content of the patient's delusional beliefs or the experiences of patient's hallucinations, the nurse will enhance communication. Arguing about delusional thoughts or hallucinatory experiences just places the patient in a position to defend his beliefs.	• Assess the meaning of the hallucinations or delusions of the patient. Monitor whether he is a danger to himself or others. Determine whether patient can be directed to a more reality-based activity.
• Assess ability for self-care activities.	• Disturbed thinking may interfere with Arnold's ability to carry out ADLs.	• Continue to assess: Determine whether Arnold can manage his own self-care.

Priority Hypothesis: Lack of Recognition of Illness and Consequences

Important Characteristics

- Displaces fear of impact of losing parents and home
- Does not perceive personal relevance to behavior
- Unable to admit impact of schizophrenia on life pattern

Associated Considerations

- Anxiety about leaving home
- Lack of control of life situation
- Threat of unpleasant reality

Planning Recovery and Wellness Outcomes

Initial

- Avoid hurting self or assaulting other patients or staff.
- Decreased anxiety.

Long Term

- Recognize that parents have died.
- Develop coping skills to address moving to a new house.

Continued

Clinical Judgment Nursing Care Plan 24.1 Continued

Taking Action: Nursing Interventions

Interventions	Rationale	Ongoing Assessment
• Acknowledge patient's anxiety about parents' absence and loss of family home.	• Beginning with the facts that Arnold accepts as true helps establish a supportive, communication alliance.	• Assess the patient's ability to hear you and respond appropriately to your comments and requests; assess the patient's ability to concentrate on what is being said and happening around him.
• Be genuine and empathic.	• Arnold will benefit from your ability to understand his experience and express that understanding while presenting reality.	• Assess for evidence that the client is less frightened with less potential for striking out.
• Prioritize goals by including maintaining safety, learning about prescribed medication, and participation in treatment activities.	• By having choices, he will begin to develop a sense of control over his behavior.	• Observe the patient's nonverbal communication for evidence of increased agitation.
• Use medications to help the patient relax and maintain more calm: administer lorazepam, 2 mg, for agitation. The PO route is preferable to injection, so offer the patient this choice long before he has lost control.	• Exact mechanisms of action are not understood, but medication is believed to potentiate the inhibitory neurotransmitter GABA, relieving anxiety and producing sedation.	• Observe for a decrease in agitated behavior. • Offering this to the patient early, as fear and agitation are beginning to become evident, prevents the potential for the patient to lose control.

Evaluation

Outcomes	Revised Outcomes	Interventions
• Arnold gradually decreased agitated behavior. • Lorazepam was given regularly for first 2 days.	• Demonstrate control of behavior when discussing realistic discharge plans.	• Problem-solve possible scenarios for discharge.

ADL, activity of daily living; BID, twice a day; GABA, gamma-aminobutyric acid; NMS, neuroleptic malignant syndrome; PO, oral; SAPS, Scale for the Assessment of Positive Symptoms.

care providers prior to initiation of mental health care. People with schizophrenia have a higher mortality rate from physical illness and often have smoking-related illnesses, such as emphysema as well as other pulmonary and cardiac issues (Pizzol et al., 2023).

Nutrition

A nutritional history should be completed to determine baseline eating habits and preferences. Taking baseline measures for metabolic syndrome is highly recommended and should include weight, waist circumference, cholesterol, and blood sugar (Morris et al., 2024). A healthy diet is important in managing the illness. Medications can alter expected nutrition, leading to excessive consumption of calories.

Sleep

Sleep patterns are often disrupted during all the periods of the illness, likely caused by the severity of positive symptoms and changes in circadian rhythms. Insomnia has been associated with higher risk of suicide (Miller & McCall, 2023). Sleep patterns should be regularly assessed. Sleep hygiene methods should be taught. Medications help to manage positive symptoms. The degree to which antipsychotic medications help with sleep as opposed to too much sleep should be assessed as well.

Physical Functioning

Physical abilities can be a strength; the potential to maintain optimal physical health should be assessed. Self-care often deteriorates in schizophrenia. Information regarding physical functioning may best be collected from family members.

History of Trauma

Explorations of social determinants of health have identified early life adversities and trauma as contributing to the development of psychosis (Jester et al., 2023) and to

BOX 24.4

Social Determinants of Health Related to Schizophrenia-Spectrum Psychotic Disorders

- Early-life adversities/adverse childhood experiences (ACEs)
- Social disconnection (a small or absent social network)
- Racism (racial/ethnic discrimination)
- Disadvantaged neighborhoods (urbanicity and lower socioeconomic status)
- Migration (immigrants, refugees, asylees)
- Social fragmentation—(neighborhood instability in relationships)
- Homelessness/unhoused
- Food insecurity
- Incarceration
- Positive social determinants of health include resilience, positive attitude, compassion

Source: Jester, D. J. Thomas, M. L., Sturm, E. T., Harvey, P. D., Keshavan, M., Davis, B. J., Saxena, S., Tampi, R., Leutwyler, H., Compton, M. T., Palmer, B. W., & Jeste, D. V. (2023). Review of major social determinants of health in schizophrenia-spectrum psychotic disorders: I. Clinical outcomes. *Schizophrenia Bulletin, 49*(4), 837–850.

the development of health and metabolic disorders associated with stress responses (Balaji & Sankaranarayanan, 2023). Early-life adversities include emotional abuse, physical abuse, sexual abuse, and neglect, with emotional abuse having the strongest association with psychosis (Jester et al., 2023). Emotional abuse is often more constant in a child's life compared to episodic sexual or physical abuse, which may account for the substantial impact of emotional abuse (Dokuz et al., 2022). See Box 24.4.

Other sources of trauma for people with schizophrenia are related to their vulnerability. For instance, individuals who are unhoused may find themselves attacked for their possessions or medications, or they may be vulnerable to exploitation, including rape. Further, nurses should be aware of the trauma that may accompany treatment interventions when a patient with schizophrenia is brought to a hospital and treated against their will or has been incarcerated prior to hospitalization. Sensitive assessment of these sources of trauma will help the nurse to develop a comprehensive plan of care.

Medication

The nurse should obtain a complete list of medications the patient is taking, including over-the-counter (OTC) agents and herbal supplements. Before initiation of psychiatric medications, standardized assessment of motor movements should be conducted using one of several assessment tools designed for that purpose, such as the Abnormal Involuntary Movement Scale (AIMS) (see Appendix), the Dyskinesia Identification System (DISCUS) (Sprague & Kalachnik, 1991), or the Simpson-Angus Rating Scale (Simpson & Angus, 1970), which is designed for Parkinson symptoms.

Substance Use (Alcohol, Illicit Drugs, Tobacco)

The nurse should ask specific questions about alcohol, drug, and tobacco use. The use of these substances is common with people with schizophrenia and will significantly influence the treatment approach (Neyra et al., 2024).

Psychosocial Cues

The individual who is in an acute phase may be unable to provide an accurate history of early psychosocial issues. Family members' reports help in detailing occurrences of psychotic symptoms of delusions and hallucinations; however, onset of negative symptoms may be more difficult to date. In fact, negative symptoms vary from a slight deviation from expected to a clear impairment. Negative symptoms probably occur earlier than positive symptoms but are less easily recognized. Several assessment scales have been developed to help evaluate clusters of positive and negative symptoms (see Box 24.5).

Mental Status and Appearance

The patient may look eccentric or disheveled or have poor hygiene and bizarre dress. The patient's posture may suggest lethargy or stupor.

Mood and Affect

Patients with schizophrenia often display altered mood states. In some cases, they may show heightened emotional activity; others may display severely limited emotional responses. Affect, the outward expression of mood, is categorized on a continuum: flat (i.e., emotional expression entirely absent), blunted (i.e., expression of emotions is present but greatly diminished), and full range of expression. Inappropriate affect is marked by incongruence between the emotional expression and the thoughts expressed (e.g., laughing when telling a sad story). Other common emotional symptoms include the following:

- **Affective lability**—abrupt, dramatic, unprovoked changes in type of emotions expressed
- **Ambivalence**—the presence and expression of two opposing feelings, leading to inaction
- **Apathy**—little emotional expression, diminished interest and desire

Speech

Thought content and other mental processes are expressed in speech. The nurse should assess both content and speech patterns. Speech content may include obvious obsessions or delusions, loose associations, or flight of ideas. In some instances, as already noted, patients make

BOX 24.5

Rating Scales for Use With Schizophrenia

SCALE FOR THE ASSESSMENT OF NEGATIVE SYMPTOMS (SANS)

Available from Nancy C. Andreasen, MD, PhD, Department of Psychiatry, College of Medicine, The University of Iowa, Iowa City, IA 52242. Copyright 1984.

SCALE FOR THE ASSESSMENT OF POSITIVE SYMPTOMS (SAPS)

Available from Nancy C. Andreasen (see above).

POSITIVE AND NEGATIVE SYNDROME SCALE (PANSS)

Kay, S. R., Fiszbein, A., & Opler, L. A. (1987). The Positive and Negative Syndrome Scale (PANSS) for Schizophrenia. *Schizophrenia Bulletin*, *13*(2), 261–276.

ABNORMAL INVOLUNTARY MOVEMENT SCALE (AIMS)

Guy, W. (1976). ECDEU: Assessment manual for psychopharmacology (DHEW Publication No. 76–338). Department of Health, Education, and Welfare, Psychopharmacology Branch.

BRIEF PSYCHIATRIC RATING SCALE (BPRS)

Overall, J. E., & Gorham, D. R. (1988). The Brief Psychiatric Rating Scale (BPRS): Recent developments in ascertainment and scaling. *Psychopharmacology Bulletin*, *24*, 97–99.

DYSKINESIA IDENTIFICATION SYSTEM: CONDENSED USER SCALE (DISCUS)

Sprague, R. L., & Kalachnik, J. E. (1991). Reliability, validity, and a total score cutoff for the Dyskinesia Identification Scale System: Condensed User Scale (DISCUS) with mentally ill and mentally retarded populations. *Psychopharmacology Bulletin*, *27*(1), 51–58.

SIMPSON-ANGUS RATING SCALE

Simpson, G. M., & Angus, J. W. (1970). A rating scale for extrapyramidal side effects. *Acta Psychiatrica Scandinavica*, *212*, 11–19. Copyright 1970 Munksgaard International Publishers, Ltd.

up their own words (neologisms). Speech may be pressured (words seem to rapidly jump out without pauses) or slow. The nurse should note any difficulty in articulating words (dysarthria) or difficulty in swallowing (dysphagia) as indicators of medication-related side effects.

Thought Process

Thought process assessment includes determining if any hallucinations, delusions, disorganized communication, or cognitive impairments are present. Because thought process assessment is critical in the nursing assessment, each area is discussed separately in the following sections.

Hallucinations

Hallucinations are the most common example of disturbed sensory perception observed in patients with schizophrenia. Hallucinations are experienced in the sensory modalities (visual, auditory, gustatory, tactile, olfactory); however, auditory hallucinations are the most common type in schizophrenia. Some specific hallucinations may be sufficient to diagnose schizophrenia, such as hearing voices, hearing voices conversing with each other, or carrying on a discussion with someone who is not there. Because most individuals will not spontaneously share their hallucinatory experiences with an interviewer, the nurse may need to rely on indirect evidence in the patient's behavior, such as (1) pauses during conversations in which the individual seems preoccupied or appears to be listening to someone other than the interviewer, (2) looking toward the perceived source of a voice, or (3) responding to the voices in some manner. Although patients may not spontaneously share their hallucinations, many validate observations of the examiner or admit to a history of hallucinations when asked (see Box 24.6). If a patient has command hallucinations, it is important for the safety of the individual and others to know what the voices are telling the patient to do.

Delusions

Delusions are different from strongly held beliefs. Delusions do not change even though strong evidence contradicts the belief. The individual continues to hold the belief despite contradictory evidence (APA, 2022). An individual's culture must be considered when evaluating delusions. Delusional beliefs are those not sanctioned or held by a cultural or religious subgroup.

Bizarre delusions are those beliefs that are impossible, illogic, and not derived from ordinary life experiences. Bizarre delusions often include delusions of control (that some outside force controls thoughts and actions), thought broadcasting (that others can read or hear one's thoughts), thought insertion (that someone has placed thoughts into one's mind), and thought withdrawal (that someone is removing thoughts from one's mind). For example, a patient who has been seeing a hypnotist for 2 months reports that the hypnotist continued to read his mind and was "picking his brain away piece by piece." Another patient was convinced that a computer chip was placed in her vagina during a gynecologic examination and that this somehow directly influenced her physical movements and her thoughts.

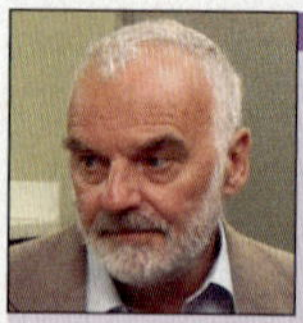

Remember Arnold?

He believes that his parents are still alive and that they will return. He refuses to leave the farm and insists that everything be left as it is.

Nonbizarre delusions generally have themes of jealousy and persecution and are derived from life experiences. For example, an individual believes that their

BOX 24.6

Therapeutic Dialogue: The Patient With Hallucinations

The following conversation took place in Arnold's room during the night checks. The nurse observed that Arnold was talking with someone, but no one else was in the room.

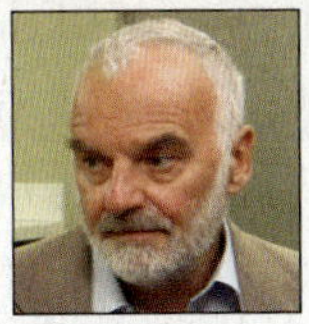

INEFFECTIVE APPROACH

Nurse: Arnold?

Arnold: Yeah?

Nurse: Who are you talking to?

Arnold: My mother visits me at night. I am telling her about my day.

Nurse: You know, Arnold, you are having a hallucination. Your mother died a few weeks ago.

Arnold: She did not. She is away for a while, but she will be back soon.

Nurse: Arnold. (Looks at nurse.) You're going to have to accept that your mother is gone.

Arnold: Oh yeah? What do you know?

Nurse: Well, we can talk about it in the morning.

Arnold: You don't know what you're talking about.

EFFECTIVE APPROACH

Nurse: Arnold?

Arnold: Yeah?

Nurse: Are you talking to someone?

Arnold: Yes, she visits me at night.

Nurse: Oh, does she talk to you?

Arnold: Yes, she asks me about my day. She visits in the evening.

Nurse: Is there anything else you talk about?

Arnold: No, she leaves after I tell her.

Nurse: OK, how do you feel when she visits you?

Arnold: A little sad, but I like to tell her about my day.

Nurse: A little sad?

Arnold: Yeah, I wish I could see her more.

Nurse: Sounds like you are lonely.

Arnold: Yeah, it's nice when you talk with me.

Nurse: I can do that. If you're not asleep when I finish rounds, we can talk more.

CRITICAL THINKING CHALLENGE

1. How did the nurse's impatience translate into Arnold's response in the first scenario?
2. What effective communication techniques did the nurse use in the second scenario?

partner, from whom they have recently separated, is trying to poison them, or an individual believes that members of the Mafia are trying to kill them because, when they were in high school, this individual reported to the principal that several of their classmates were selling drugs at school.

Assessing and judging the content of the delusion and exploring other aspects of the delusional experience are helpful in understanding the significance of these false beliefs. The underlying feeling that accompanies the delusion (i.e., fear or inflated self-esteem) should be explored. Other aspects to consider include the conviction with which the delusion is held; the extent to which other aspects of the individual's life are incorporated or affected by the delusion; the degree of internal consistency, organization, and logic evidenced in the delusion; and evaluating the amount of pressure (in terms of preoccupation and concern) individuals feel in their lives as a result of the delusion (Box 24.7).

Disorganized Communication

Abrupt shifts in the focus of conversation, which are often altered in schizophrenia, are typically symptomatic of disorganized thinking. Impaired verbal fluency (i.e., ability to produce spontaneous speech) is commonly present. The most severe shifts in focus may occur after only one or two words (i.e., word salad), after one or two

BOX 24.7

Therapeutic Dialogue: The Patient With Delusions

John joined the nurse in a game of pool. The following conversation occurred as they played.

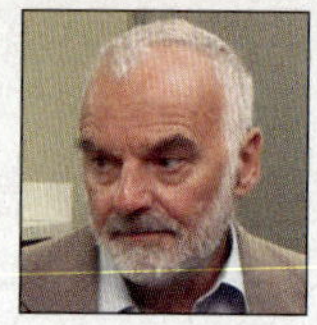

INEFFECTIVE APPROACH

John: The CIA put a transmitter in my molar, here (points to his right cheek).

Nurse: No one would put a transmitter in your tooth; come on, the CIA is not looking for you.

John: Yeah, they want to monitor me while I'm here. I know that they have a real spy here in the hospital. They are trying to get the President to intervene with the Michigan Militia. Mark from Michigan told me that.

Nurse: The spy is not here. I can guarantee you that the President is not interested in anyone here.

John: Maybe—but there are imposters. They're just trying to keep people from knowing what they're doing.

Nurse: John, the President is not looking for anyone here. I would know it because I work here.

John: (With anger) You don't know anything! You're probably working for the CIA too. I have nothing else to say to you.

EFFECTIVE APPROACH

John: The CIA put a transmitter in my molar, here (points to his right cheek).

Nurse: Oh. Which balls are mine?

John: You get the striped ones. Yeah, they want to monitor me while I'm here. I know that they have a real spy here in the hospital. They are trying to get the President to intervene with the Michigan Militia. Mark from Michigan told me that.

Nurse: Well, I don't know anything about that, but I want you to know that we will keep you safe.

John: Maybe...

Nurse: You sound a little overwhelmed with all the information you have.

John: No, no. I can handle it. The CIA can't do anything to me. I'll never talk.

Nurse: I thought you said they could hear you when you talk to me.

John: Huh? Oh, that transmitter is so that they can send me misinformation. They send a tower of babble to my brain. They are trying to confuse me so that I stay away from the President. They all think they can keep me from my mission.

Nurse: Who are they?

John: Everyone in the government. The CIA, FBI, ATF, IRS—all those alphabets.

Nurse: So, you believe that everyone in the government is trying to get to you?

John: Well, maybe not everybody. Just the ones that care about money and the militia. I don't think they care about me much in Commerce or Health and Human Services. Although they'd care too if they knew.

Nurse: I would think that's pretty frightening to have all these people out looking for you. You must be scared a lot.

John: It's scary, but I can handle it. I've handled it all my life.

Nurse: You've been in scary situations all your life?

John: Yeah. I don't know. Maybe not scary, just hard. I never seemed to be able to do as well as my parents wanted—or as I wanted.

CRITICAL THINKING CHALLENGE

1. How did the nurse's argumentative responses cause the patient to react in the first scenario?
2. What effective communication techniques did the nurse use in the second scenario?

phrases or sentences (i.e., flight of ideas or loose associations), or somewhat less severely as a shift that occurs when a new topic is repeatedly suggested and pursued from the current topic (i.e., tangentiality).

Cognitive Impairments

Mental status assessment focuses on eliciting indications of cognitive impairments associated with schizophrenia. Although these impairments vary widely from patient to patient, several primary features have been identified (Vita et al., 2024):

- Increased, sustained attention on external stimuli over a period of time (hypervigilance).
- Quick speed of processing information leading to inappropriate or illogic conclusions from available observations and information.
- Issues with visual and verbal memory, and with working memory.

- Problems with executive function leading to difficulty in planning, conceptualization, cognitive flexibility.

Cognitive impairments are not easy to recognize. By relying only on clinical assessment, the nurse can miss the extent of the impairment. Using a standardized instrument can provide a screening measurement of cognitive function (see Chapter 10). If impairment exists, neuropsychological testing by a qualified psychologist may be necessary.

Memory and Orientation

Impairment in orientation, memory, and abstract thinking is often present. Orientation to time, place, and person may remain relatively intact unless the patient is particularly preoccupied with delusions and hallucinations. Although all aspects of memory may be affected in schizophrenia, registration or the ability to recall within seconds of newly learned information may be particularly diminished. This affects the individual's short- and long-term memory. The ability to engage in abstract thinking may be impaired (see Box 24.8).

Insight and Judgment

Insight and judgment are closely related to each other. Individuals display insight when they recognize that their hallucinations or delusions are symptoms of a mental disorder. Judgment is the ability to decide or act about a situation. If judgment is poor, the individual may not recognize personal vulnerabilities and consequently engages in detrimental behavior. For example, the individual may be taken advantage of by others or fail to realize a potentially dangerous situation.

BOX 24.8

Arnold's Cognitive Symptoms

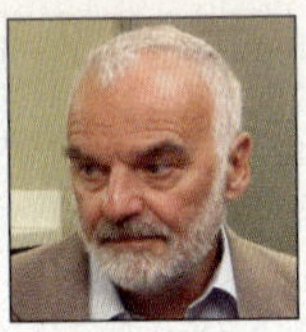

Arnold's symptoms of schizophrenia began long before he was actually diagnosed. Throughout school, he had difficulty learning new material. His teachers would describe him as being "slow" or "inattentive." Because he appeared to be functioning as expected, his teachers and family attributed his poor academic behavior to lack of interest. His father would often get frustrated with him because he would spend many hours in his bedroom and would not help out on the farm. When prodded to complete schoolwork or a household task, he would often get distracted before finishing the tasks. Family members and teachers quickly learned to provide several prompts for Arnold to complete a task. As he progressed to high school, he was labeled as a "slow learner" and assigned to less demanding classes.

The reality was that Arnold was experiencing unrecognized prodromal cognitive symptoms of schizophrenia. He was having difficulty remembering his assignments. He was having difficulty grasping concepts that other students seemed to easily understand. He was becoming frustrated with his difficulty and retreated to his room. He waited for specific directions that he could easily process. His thinking was concrete, and he had difficulty expressing himself. When he was bombarded with several directions at once, he could not process any of the directions. In his frustration, he would throw objects, frightening others. His family was very concerned with the changes that were occurring with their once easygoing son.

Behavioral Responses

During periods of psychosis, unusual or bizarre behavior often occurs. These behaviors can usually be understood within the context of the patient's disturbed thinking. The nurse needs to understand the significance of the behavior to the individual. For example, one patient moved the family furniture into the yard because he thought that evil spirits were hiding in the furniture. His bizarre behavior was an attempt to protect his family. Another patient painted a sequence of numbers on his bedroom walls. He said that the numbers were the language of the angels. His delusional thoughts were the basis of his behavior.

Because of the negative symptoms, specifically avolition, patients may not seem interested or organized enough to complete expected daily activities. They may stay in bed most of the day or refuse to take a shower. Many times, they agree to get up in the morning and go to work, but they never get around to it. Several specific behaviors are associated with schizophrenia, including stereotypy (i.e., idiosyncratic, repetitive, purposeless movements); echopraxia (i.e., involuntary imitation of others' movements); and waxy flexibility (i.e., posture held in odd or unusual fixed positions for extended periods). In some cases, certain behaviors need to be evaluated carefully to distinguish them from movements that are associated with medication-related side effects, such as grimacing, stereotypical behavior, or agitation.

Self-Concept

In schizophrenia, self-concept is usually poor. Patients often are aware that they are hearing voices that others do not hear. They recognize that they are different from others and are often scared they are "going crazy." Many are aware of their own loss of expectations for their future achievements. The pervasive stigma associated with having a mental illness contributes to the poor self-concept. Body image can be disturbed, especially during periods of hallucinations or delusions. For example, a patient believes that their body is infected with germs, and she can feel them eating away their insides.

Stress and Coping Patterns

Stressful events are often linked to psychiatric symptoms. It is important to determine stresses from the patient's perspective because a stressful event for one may not be stressful for another. It is also important to determine typical coping patterns, especially negative coping strategies, such as the use of substances or showing aggressive behavior.

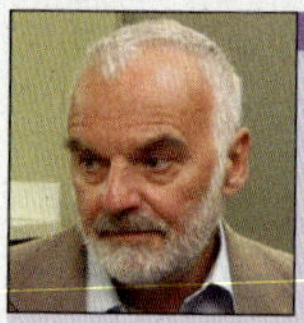

Consider This

Recall Arnold's symptoms? They appeared after the stress of his mother's death.

Social Network

Several difficulties involving social functioning occur in schizophrenia. As the disorder progresses, individuals can become increasingly socially isolated. On a one-to-one basis, this occurs as the individual seems unable to connect with people in their environment. Several aspects of symptoms already discussed can contribute to this. For example, emotional blunting and anhedonia (the inability to experience pleasure) result in an experience of not being engaged in activities and relationships.

Interpretation of facial expressions and affect displayed by others is often problematic for people with schizophrenia. Cognitive deficits affect social relationships when individuals are unable to recall past interactions and have issues with decision making and judgment. Other behaviors that affect social relationships are poverty of speech and language and the inability to complete ADLs, which results in poor hygiene, malnutrition, and social isolation.

Functional Status

Functional status of patients with schizophrenia should be assessed initially and at regular intervals. Level of independence, ability to work, ability to maintain an independent living environment, and self-care should be evaluated.

Support Systems

In schizophrenia, support systems become especially important in maintaining the patient in the community. The individual may become socially isolated if the treatment and management occur in long-term care facilities and group homes, away from family and friends. One challenge is to identify and maintain the patient's links with family and significant others. Assessment of the formal support (e.g., family, health care providers) and informal support (e.g., neighbors, friends) should be conducted.

Spiritual Assessment

Determining spiritual needs enhances the nursing assessment and helps the nurse provide holistic care (see Chapter 10). Even though delusions sometime have religious content, an astute nurse will be able to differentiate delusional thoughts (such as the patient believing they are a deity) from the patient's spiritual needs. For example, the nurse could ask if a higher power is important or what gives the patient meaning in life. The nurse should focus on the patient's spirituality and avoid disclosing personal beliefs. Asking the patient to reflect on spiritual questions can increase the nurse's understanding of the patient's needs as well as enhance therapeutic relationships.

Quality of Life

People with schizophrenia often have a poor quality of life (QoL), especially older people, who may have spent many years in long-term hospitals. The nurse should assess the patient's QoL and how it could be improved. Simple changes, such as arranging for a different roommate or improving access to social activities by meeting transportation needs, can greatly improve a patient's QoL.

Strengths Assessment

An important part of recovery is identification of personal and family strengths. Because schizophrenia is usually diagnosed at a young age, the individual may be physically fit with little evidence of chronic illness. As the assessment is completed, strengths will emerge. Family support is critical for an individual with schizophrenia. Intellectual ability and coping with stress are areas that can be strengths. The following questions are examples that can be used in assessing strengths.

- What do you do for relaxation, fun?
- How do you manage stressful events?
- How do you cope with the voices, thoughts, or impulses?
- Who do you talk with when you are upset?
- Are you hopeful about the future, and if so, what gives you hope for the future?

ANALYZING CUES AND DEVELOPING HYPOTHESES

People with schizophrenia have a variety of nursing care needs because of the complexity of this chronic and difficult-to-treat illness. These needs emerge at different times and in different manifestations of the illness. In identifying relevant cues and prioritizing hypotheses, nurses need to consider the point in time during the progression of schizophrenia, the acceptability of its treatment to the individual, and the availability of community resources. In many ways, treatment needs should be considered through a matrix of factors including (1) the stage of the illness (prodromal, acute, stable, and recovering); (2) the type, mixture, and intensity of symptoms; (3) the medication effects and side effects; (4) the method and availability of treatment; and (5) sources of social support and recovery-based care. For example, during an episode of psychosis, a nurse needs to be aware of the symptoms that affect the patient's safety. Hallucinatory voices may be telling the individual to self-injure or injure others. Delusional thinking may result in suspicion or isolation. General functioning and basic care may be compromised: sleep patterns may be severely disrupted; the individual may be undernourished due to inability to obtain food or fear of eating. There may be hygiene issues that interfere with the individual's ability to engage in social activities. An acute psychotic episode early in the disease may be accompanied by grief and loss due to changes in the expectations of the individual and their family.

Mood disturbances, specifically depression, may be a priority later in the course of the disorder and may require a significant plan to avoid suicide. Motivation may be an issue during the course of the illness: early on as the individual and family wrestle with the implications of the illness and later as the chronicity of the symptoms continues. Medication management requires different assessments over the course of the illness. Early on, patients need considerable encouragement to continue taking medications that do not always make them feel comfortable and are not always believed to be necessary. In order to help patients take medications to control symptoms, dosage regimens need to be convenient and easy to follow; medications need to be sufficient to control symptoms without burdening the patient with unpleasant side effects. Long-acting injectable antipsychotic medications may be an answer to the issues of convenience and help to avoid relapse.

Late in the illness, medication management needs to be a mutual process, particularly for patients who have managed their illness well. Community resources differ based on funding and location: rural versus urban; state priorities versus county and city policies. For many individuals with schizophrenia, the course of their illness is not just dependent on their symptoms but also on the availability of resources to help them manage their illness. A very careful and ongoing assessment of needs and issues is important throughout recovery.

NCLEXNOTE When assessing a patient with schizophrenia, the nurse should prioritize the severity of the current responses to the disorder. If hallucinations are impairing function, then managing hallucinations is a priority, and medications are needed immediately. If hallucinations are not an issue, however, coping with negative symptoms becomes a priority.

PLANNING RECOVERY AND WELLNESS OUTCOMES

Nurses should aim to help their patients with schizophrenia to maximize their health, given this chronic illness. Goals need to take into consideration the symptoms that accompany schizophrenia, as well as the side effects of the medications used to treat schizophrenia. Helping people to recover and feel the best they can physically with this chronic illness includes the development of healthy day-to-day habits around hygiene, exercise, and nutrition. Nurses also need to be aware of specific issues that can arise for people who have schizophrenia around temperature regulation and fluid and electrolyte balance.

Another aspect of recovery and wellness is to help patients with schizophrenia maintain and/or develop relationships with family and peers, as well as with the various providers of care with whom they come in contact. Trauma experiences may be an issue in some of these relationships. With family relationships, the challenge for nurses is to recognize trauma as an issue without blaming and to examine ways of developing interventions to help families at risk. A trauma-informed approach suggests the need to recognize traumatic experiences and strive to develop transparency, trust, safety, collaboration, and empowerment for the patient with schizophrenia to heal from traumatic experiences. See Box 24.9.

THERAPEUTIC RELATIONSHIP

Development of the therapeutic nurse–patient relationship centers on developing trust, accepting the individual as a worthy human being, and infusing the relationship with hope. People with schizophrenia are often reluctant to engage in any relationship because of previous rejection and, in some instances, an underlying suspiciousness, which is a part of the illness. They are often trying to trust their own thoughts and perceptions, so interactions with another human being may prove to be too overwhelming. If they are hallucinating, their images of other people may be distorted and frightening as well.

The nurse should approach the patient in a calm and caring manner. Engaging the patient in a relationship may take time, but it begins with the first encounter. Short time-limited interactions are best for a patient who is experiencing psychosis. Being consistent in interactions and following through on promises will help establish trust within the relationship.

Establishing a therapeutic relationship is crucial, especially with patients who deny that they are ill. Patients are more likely to agree to and continue treatment if these recommendations are made within the context of a safe, trusting relationship. Even if some patients deny having mental illness, they may take medication and attend treatment activities because they trust the nurse (Howe et al., 2023).

Furthermore, for long-term care and outcomes, recovery-oriented relationships are important. Using the recovery model, all efforts should be made to individualize treatment. Care should be person-centered through

BOX 24.9

Trauma-Informed Approaches: Bodily Self-Disturbance and Trauma

Background

Depression, guilt, and positive symptoms of schizophrenia were shown to be directly associated with bodily self-disturbance that occurs as a result of childhood trauma. Bodily self-disturbances consist of unclear body boundaries, feelings of unreality or estrangement of the body, feelings of deterioration of one's body parts, perceptions of the change of size of one's body parts, and changes in appearance of the body. Bodily self-disturbance is an early marker of schizophrenia and is considered one of its core experiences. Researchers suggest that bodily self-disturbance might activate hallucinations and delusions in individuals with a history of childhood trauma, especially sexual trauma.

Interventions

Bodily disturbances can be considered prodromal symptoms of schizophrenia indicating a need for early intervention. These disturbances can indicate that the child is experiencing or has experienced sexual trauma. Within a trusting relationship, a trauma-informed approach addressing bodily disturbances may reduce the impact on the positive symptoms of schizophrenia.

Source: Torregrossa, L. J., Liu, J., Armstrong, K., Heckers, S., & Sheffield, J. M. (2024). Interplay between childhood trauma, bodily self-disturbances, and clinical phenomena in schizophrenia spectrum disorders: A network analysis. *Schizophrenia Research*, *266*, 107–115. https://doi.org/10.1016/j.schres.2024.02.034

partnering with the patient in all aspects of care and encouraging self-direction. Although long-term therapeutic relationships become important to the patient and the nurse, the nurse should respect patient confidentiality when seeing a patient outside the therapeutic setting (see Box 24.10). Treatment should be focused on strengths and the empowerment of the individual. Patients need encouragement to see that although their diagnosis may seem devastating, recovery is possible (Thongsalab et al., 2024).

TAKING ACTION: NURSING INTERVENTIONS

Priorities of Care

Safety is always the first priority for people with schizophrenia. In people who are experiencing hallucinations and delusions, safety priorities focus on preventing self-harm or harm to others. Agitation can quickly escalate into aggression and violent behavior. For people who are currently taking medication, adverse effects such as neuroleptic malignant syndrome (NMS; discussed later in chapter) should be considered.

BOX 24.10

Reflection of a Nurse: Maintaining Confidentiality

Incident

Sally, a recent nursing graduate, was entering the venue for a local art fair. Bill, a participant in a local clubhouse where Sally had been assigned as a student nurse, approached her from the opposite direction. As was typical, his appearance and behaviors were unusual. He immediately recognized her and said "Hey, you're the nurse!" Sally greeted him back, acknowledging that she was indeed, and asked: "How are you doing, Bill?" He said "Fine" and continued on his way.

Reflection

Sally realized that responding to Bill with a usual greeting acknowledged his personhood and demonstrated for the people around her a nonstigmatizing response.

1. Who should initiate a greeting or conversation in a public space when a nurse encounters a patient?
2. How important is it for nurses to minimize stigma and fear in members of the public?

Physical Care

For many people with schizophrenia, the plan of care will include specific interventions to enhance self-care, nutrition, and overall health knowledge. Negative symptoms commonly leave patients unable to initiate these seemingly simple activities. Developing a daily schedule of routine activities (e.g., showering, shaving) can help the patient structure the day. Most patients actually know how to perform self-care activities (e.g., hygiene, grooming) but lack motivation (avolition) to carry them out consistently. Interventions include developing a schedule with the patient for various hygiene-related activities and emphasizing the importance of maintaining appropriate self-care. Given the issues related to attention and memory in people with schizophrenia, education about these areas requires careful planning.

Activity, Exercise, and Nutritional Interventions

Encouraging activity and exercise is necessary, not only to maintain a healthy lifestyle but also to counteract the side effects of psychiatric medications that cause weight gain. Because the diagnosis is usually made in late adolescence or early adulthood, it is possible to establish solid exercise patterns early.

During episodes of acute psychosis, patients are sometimes unable to focus on eating. Often when patients begin antipsychotic medication, expected satiety and hunger responses change, and overeating or weight gain can become an issue. Patients report that their appetites increase and cravings for food develop when some medications are initiated. Promoting and maintaining healthy nutrition is a key intervention. Monitoring calorie intake is also important because of the effect many medications have on eating habits.

Weight gain is one of the reasons some patients stop taking their medications. Increased weight places patients at greater risk for several health issues, such as type 2 diabetes and early death. Monitoring for diabetes and managing weight are important activities for all health care providers. Patients should be screened for risk factors of diabetes, such as family history, obesity as indicated by a body mass index (BMI) exceeding or equal to 27, and age older than 45 years. Patients' weight should be measured at regular intervals and the BMI calculated. Blood pressure readings should be taken regularly. Laboratory findings for triglycerides, high-density lipoprotein cholesterol, and glucose level should be monitored and reviewed regularly. All health care providers should be alert to the development of hyperglycemia, particularly in patients known to have diabetes who begin taking second-generation antipsychotic agents. A program to address weight gain should be initiated at the earliest sign of weight gain (probably between 5 and 10 lb over desired body weight). Reduced caloric intake may be accomplished by increasing the patient's access to affordable, healthful, and easy-to-prepare foods. Behavioral management of weight gain includes keeping a food diary, diet teaching, and support groups. Setting small goals and offering a lot of encouragement can lead to some success (Fitzgerald et al., 2024). Innovative programs of health education, mentoring, and monitoring using smart phone applications might be useful tools to enhance health (Daniel et al., 2024).

Thermoregulation Interventions

Patients with schizophrenia may have disturbed body temperature regulation. In winter, they may seem to be oblivious to cold weather. In the heat of summer, they may dress for winter. Observing patients' responses to environmental temperatures helps in identifying issues in this area. In patients who are taking psychiatric medications, body temperature needs to be monitored, and the patient needs to be protected from extremes in temperature.

Fluid Balance

Some people with schizophrenia develop disturbed fluid and electrolyte balance. Nurses should observe for polydipsia (frequently drinking an excessive amount of fluids) or frequent incontinence. These individuals are obsessed with drinking water and compulsively consume fluids. For people with schizophrenia who demonstrate polydipsia, regulation of their fluid intake is disturbed, resulting in an unusually low serum sodium level, which can lead to severe water intoxication and delirium, a medical emergency.

Nursing interventions include teaching and assisting the patient to develop self-monitoring skills. Fluid intake and weight gain should be monitored to control fluid intake and reduce the likelihood of developing water intoxication. Patients with mild polydipsia are easily treated in outpatient settings and benefit from educational programs that teach them to monitor their own urine's specific gravity and daily weight gains. Patients with moderate polydipsia may respond well to education but still have a more difficult time controlling their own fluid intake, which requires more careful monitoring of intake and weight throughout the day. Patients with severe polydipsia require considerable assistance, probably in an inpatient unit, to restrict their continual water-seeking behavior. These patients may create disruption on the unit, so they are best managed by one-on-one observation to redirect their behavior.

Wellness Challenges

The challenges to the overall wellness of people with schizophrenia include the symptoms of schizophrenia, the effects of medication treatment, and the circumstances around where they live, and their social connections. One example: addressing a goal related to a healthy diet and exercise. Symptoms of schizophrenia that must be considered are ambivalence, avolition, and lack of motivation. Effects and side effects of medication treatment may include weight gain and sleepiness. Living and social circumstances may include living in group homes with limited access to consistently healthy food, limited funds to purchase healthy food, or living in food deserts in cities or at great distances from food markets in rural towns and communities. These living and social circumstances may limit exercise interventions because housing locations may not be in the safest areas of a city or town.

Wellness goals need to be manageable and specific. Creating goals that focus on small steps is less overwhelming. For instance, selecting a goal to lose 25 lb may be overwhelming. More manageable goals could be to eat French fries only twice a week and to walk 10 minutes twice a day around the yard of the adult foster care home. Supporting these goals would include conversations around the accomplishment of these activities, as well as measuring outcomes such as weight, blood pressure, and hemoglobin A1c, if indicated. Goals can be revised based on levels of success.

Medication Interventions: Antipsychotics

Antipsychotic medications are the treatment of choice for patients with psychosis. Antipsychotic drugs are used because they have the general effect of blocking dopamine transmission, leading to a decrease in psychotic symptoms (see Chapter 11). Some medications also block receptors of other neurotransmitters to varying degrees (see Table 24.1).

TABLE 24.1 SELECTED ANTIPSYCHOTIC DRUGS

Second-Generation Antipsychotics	Dosage Range for Adults (mg/d)
Aripiprazole	10–15
Asenapine	10–20
Brexpiprazole	0.5–3
Cetirizine	1.5–6
Clozapine	200–600
Lumateperone	42
Lurasidone	40–80
Olanzapine	10–20
Paliperidone	3–12
Primavanserin	34
Quetiapine	300–400
Risperidone	4–16
Ziprasidone	40–160
New (2024) Class Antipsychotic Drug Used to Treat Schizophrenia	
Xanomeline and trospium chloride 125 mg/30 mg	
Selected First-Generation Antipsychotic Drugs Used to Treat Psychosis in the United States	
Chlorpromazine	30–800
Fluphenazine	0.5–20
Haloperidol	1–15
Loxapine	20–250
Perphenazine	4–32
Pimozide	1–10
Thiothixene	5–25
Trifluoperazine	5–25

The prescription of first-generation antipsychotics (e.g., haloperidol, chlorpromazine) decreased dramatically with the introduction of second-generation antipsychotics. However, it is important that medication choice be individualized based on each patient's experience and preference, as well as the side effect profiles of selected drugs rather than to limit drug selection to one type or class of antipsychotic medication. This is particularly true during the acute phase of the illness for people with schizophrenia who are known to respond to treatment.

Second-generation antipsychotic drugs including risperidone, olanzapine, quetiapine, paliperidone, ziprasidone, aripiprazole, iloperidone, asenapine, lurasidone, cariprazine, and lumateperone, brexpiprazole, and pimavanserin are available in a variety of formulations. See Box 24.11 for more information about risperidone. Second-generation antipsychotic drugs are effective in treating both negative and positive symptoms. These drugs also target other neurotransmitter systems, such as serotonin and glutamate. This is believed to contribute to their antipsychotic effectiveness.

A new antipsychotic, xanomeline (a muscarine agonist) and trospium chloride (a muscarinic antagonist) was approved by the FDA for the treatment of schizophrenia in adults in 2024. Clinical trials showed a reduction in positive and negative symptoms. The mechanism of action is unclear, but it is thought to be due to agonist activity at M_1 and M_4 receptors. Trospium chloride antagonizes the muscarinic receptors primarily in peripheral tissues. The medication is formulated in a capsule and is administered orally 1 hour before meals twice a day. Heart rate, liver enzymes and bilirubin should be assessed prior to initiation and during treatment. Patients should be assessed for hepatic impairment and for anticholinergic side effects including for urinary retention. Xanomeline and trospium can increase the heart rate. Nausea, dyspepsia, constipation, vomiting, and diarrhea are common side effects (Bristol Myers Squibb, 2024).

Administering Medications

Nursing interventions during the initial acute phase of schizophrenia include prompt, safe, and informed administration of antipsychotic medications. In general, it takes about 1 to 2 weeks for antipsychotic drugs to effect a change in symptoms. During the stabilization period, the selected drug should be given an adequate trial, generally 6 to 12 weeks, before considering a change in the drug prescription. For maximum absorption, ziprasidone and lurasidone should be given with food. Specifically, for lurasidone, 350 calories should be eaten when administering this (Pfizer, 2022). If treatment effects are not seen, a different antipsychotic agent may be tried. Clozapine is used when no other second-generation antipsychotic is effective; see Box 24.12 for more information about clozapine.

Adherence to a prescribed medication regimen is the best approach to prevent relapse. Unfortunately, adherence to the second-generation antipsychotic agents is not improved from the first-generation antipsychotic. The use of long-acting injectables has improved adherence outcomes (Lee & Schwartz, 2021). Box 24.13 provides evidence related to interventions that promote medication adherence for patients with schizophrenia.

Patients with schizophrenia generally need to take antipsychotic medications for their entire lifetime. Rarely is discontinuation of medications prescribed; however, many patients stop taking medications on their own. Some conditions do require the cessation of medication use, such as NMS (see the discussion later in this chapter), agranulocytosis (i.e., a dangerously low level of circulating neutrophils), or drug reaction with eosinophilia and systemic symptoms (DRESS) (i.e., fever with a rash and/or swollen lymph glands). Discontinuation is also an

BOX 24.11

Medication Profile: Risperidone

DRUG CLASS: Atypical antipsychotic

RECEPTOR AFFINITY: Antagonist with high affinity for dopamine D2 and serotonin 5-HT_2, also histamine (H1) and α_1-, α_2-adrenergic receptors, weak affinity for D1 and other serotonin receptor subtypes; no affinity for acetylcholine or β-adrenergic receptors

INDICATIONS: Treatment of schizophrenia; short-term treatment of acute manic or mixed episodes associated with bipolar I disorder; and irritability associated with autistic disorder in children and adolescents, including symptoms of aggression toward others, deliberate self-injuriousness, temper tantrums, and quickly changing moods

ROUTES AND DOSAGE: 0.25-, 0.5-, 1-, 2-, 3-, and 4-mg tablets and liquid concentrate (1 mg/mL); orally disintegrating tablets, 0.5, 1, 2, 3, and 4 mg

Adult: Schizophrenia: Initial dose: typically, 1 mg BID. Maximal effect at 6 mg/day. Safety not established above 16 mg/day. Use lowest possible dose to alleviate symptoms.

Bipolar mania: 2 to 3 mg/day

Geriatric: Initial dose, 0.5 mg/day; increase slowly as tolerated

Children: 0.25 mg/day for patients <20 kg and 0.5 mg/day for patients >20 kg

HALF-LIFE (PEAK EFFECT): Mean, 20 hours (1 hour; peak active metabolite = 3–17 hours)

SELECT SIDE EFFECTS: Insomnia, agitation, anxiety, extrapyramidal symptoms, headache, rhinitis, somnolence, dizziness, headache, constipation, nausea, dyspepsia, vomiting, abdominal pain, hypersalivation, tachycardia, orthostatic hypotension, fever, chest pain, coughing, photosensitivity, weight gain

BOXED WARNING: Increased mortality in older patients with dementia-related psychosis

WARNING: Rare development of NMS. Observe frequently for early signs of tardive dyskinesia. Use caution with individuals who have cardiovascular disease; risperidone can cause electrocardiographic changes. Avoid use during pregnancy or while breastfeeding. Hepatic or renal impairments increase plasma concentration.

SPECIFIC PATIENT/FAMILY EDUCATION

- Notify your prescriber if tremor, motor restlessness, unusual movements, chest pain, or other unusual symptoms develop.
- Avoid alcohol and other CNS depressant drugs.
- Notify your prescriber if pregnancy is possible or if planning to become pregnant. Do not breastfeed while taking this medication.
- Notify your prescriber before taking any other prescription or OTC medication.
- May impair judgment, thinking, or motor skills; avoid driving or potentially other hazardous tasks.
- During titration, the individual may experience orthostatic hypotension and should change positions slowly.
- Do not abruptly discontinue.

BID, twice a day; CNS, central nervous system; OTC, over the counter.

option when tardive dyskinesia develops. Discontinuation of medications, other than in the circumstances of a medical emergency, should be achieved by gradually lowering the dose over time. This diminishes the likelihood of withdrawal symptoms.

Monitoring Extrapyramidal Side Effects

In some patients, the use of antipsychotic drugs can cause **extrapyramidal side effects** such as parkinsonism, dystonic reactions, akathisia, tardive dyskinesia, tardive dystonia, and tardive akathisia.

Parkinsonism

Parkinsonism, which is more common in older patients who take antipsychotic drugs, is identical in appearance to the symptoms of Parkinson disease. The symptoms are believed to be caused by the blockade of dopamine D2 receptors in the basal ganglia, which throws off the balance between acetylcholine and dopamine in this area of the brain and effectively increases acetylcholine transmission. The symptoms are managed by reducing dosage and thereby increasing dopamine activity or adding an anticholinergic drug, such as benztropine or trihexyphenidyl, thus decreasing acetylcholine activity.

Dystonic Reactions

As with parkinsonism, *dystonic reactions* are believed to result from the imbalance of dopamine and acetylcholine, with the latter dominant. Young people assigned male at birth seem to be more vulnerable to this particular extrapyramidal side effect. This side effect, which develops rapidly and dramatically, can be very frightening for patients as their muscles tense and their body contorts. The experience often starts with **oculogyric crisis**, in which the muscles that control eye movements tense and pull the eyeball so that the patient is looking toward the ceiling. This may be followed rapidly by **torticollis**, in which the neck muscles pull the head to the side, or **retrocollis**, in which the head is pulled back, or orolaryngeal–pharyngeal hypertonus, in which the patient has extreme difficulty in swallowing. The patient may also experience contorted limbs. These symptoms generally occur early in antipsychotic drug treatment, when the patient may still be enduring psychotic symptoms, which compounds the patient's fear and anxiety and requires a quick response. The immediate treatment is to administer benztropine 1 to 2 mg, or diphenhydramine, 25 to 50 mg, intramuscularly or intravenously. This is followed by daily administration of anticholinergic drugs and, possibly, by a decrease in dosage of the antipsychotic

BOX 24.12

Medication Profile: Clozapine

DRUG CLASS: Atypical antipsychotic

RECEPTOR AFFINITY: D1 and D2 blockade, antagonist for 5-HT2, histamine (H1), α-adrenergic, and acetylcholine. These additional antagonist effects may contribute to some of its therapeutic effects. Produces fewer extrapyramidal effects than standard antipsychotics with lower risk for tardive dyskinesia.

INDICATIONS: Severely ill individuals who have schizophrenia and have not responded to standard antipsychotic treatment; reduction in risk of recurrent suicidal behavior in schizophrenia or SADs.

ROUTES AND DOSAGE: Available only in tablet form, 25- and 100-mg doses.

Adult Dosage: Initial dose 25 mg PO twice or four times daily, may gradually increase in 25 to 50 mg/day increments, if tolerated, to a dose of 300 to 450 mg/day by the end of the second week. Additional increases should occur no more than once or twice weekly. Do not exceed 900 mg/day. For maintenance, reduce dosage to lowest effective level.

Children: Safety and efficacy with children younger than 16 years have not been established.

HALF-LIFE (PEAK EFFECT): 12 hours (1 to 6 hours)

SELECT ADVERSE REACTIONS: Drowsiness, dizziness, headache, hypersalivation, tachycardia, hypo- or hypertension, constipation, dry mouth, heartburn, nausea or vomiting, blurred vision, diaphoresis, fever, weight gain, hematologic changes, seizures, tremor, akathisia

BOXED WARNING: Agranulocytosis, defined as a granulocyte count of <500 mm^3, occurs at about a cumulative 1-year incidence of 1.3%, most often within 4 to 10 weeks of exposure, but may occur at any time; WBC count before initiation, and weekly WBC counts while taking the drug and for 4 weeks after discontinuation.

Seizures, myocarditis, and other adverse cardiovascular and respiratory side effects (i.e., orthostatic hypotension).

WARNING: Increased mortality in older patients with dementia-related psychosis; rare development of NMS; *hyperglycemia and diabetes, tardive dyskinesia*, cases of sudden, unexplained death have been reported; avoid use during pregnancy and while breastfeeding.

PRECAUTIONS: Fever, pulmonary embolism, hepatitis, anticholinergic toxicity, and interference with cognitive and motor functions.

SPECIFIC PATIENT/FAMILY EDUCATION

- Need informed consent regarding risk for agranulocytosis. Weekly or biweekly blood draws are required. Notify your prescriber immediately if lethargy, weakness, sore throat, malaise, or other flu-like symptoms develop.
- You should not take clozapine if you are taking other medicines that may cause the same serious bone marrow side effects.
- Inform the patient of risk of seizures, hyperglycemia and diabetes, and orthostatic hypotension. It may potentiate the hypotensive effects of antihypertensive drugs and anticholinergic effects of atropine-like drugs.
- Administration of epinephrine should be avoided in the treatment of drug-induced hypotension.
- Notify your prescriber if pregnancy is possible or if you are planning to become pregnant. Do not breastfeed while taking this medication.
- Notify your prescriber before taking any other prescription or OTC medication. Avoid alcohol or other CNS depressant drugs.
- May cause drowsiness and seizures; avoid driving or other hazardous tasks.
- During titration, the individual may experience orthostatic hypotension and so should change positions slowly.
- Do not abruptly discontinue.

CNS, central nervous system; NMS, neuroleptic malignant syndrome; OTC, over-the-counter; WBC, white blood cell.

BOX 24.13

Research for Evidence-Based Practice: Treatment Attitudes and Adherence

Nyanyiwa, S., Peters, K., & Murphy, G. (2022). A scoping review: Treatment attitudes and adherence for adults with schizophrenia. Journal of Clinical Nursing, *Online ahead of print. https://doi.org/10.1111/jocn.16219*

THE QUESTIONS: What is the relationship between treatment attitudes and adherence in adults diagnosed with schizophrenia? What are the gaps in the literature concerning attitudes to treatment and adherence in people experiencing schizophrenia?

METHODS: The focus of the review was determining the key concepts, gaps in evidence, and a synthesis of the research related to attitudes toward treatment and adherence. A five-step structured process was used in conducting a scoping review; it included identifying the research question, identifying relevant studies, selecting the studies, charting and collating the data, and summarizing and reporting the results. Ten papers met the quality assessment criteria.

FINDINGS: The review validated that family, health care professionals, and subjective factors such as quality of life, psychosocial functioning, perceived illness, severity of side effects, and satisfaction with medication mediated the individual's attitude toward adherence in adults experiencing schizophrenia. Positive influences on attitudes were associated with greater adherence, and people who did not adhere to treatment were influenced by negative attitudes toward treatment.

IMPLICATIONS FOR NURSING: Treatment adherence is complex. Nurses should empower and promote adherence rather than use coercive approaches that force people to adhere. Nurses should avoid viewing adherence as the treatment objective and instead embrace empowering strategies to recognize and respect an individual's decision-making role in treatment.

BOX 24.14

Medication Profile: Benztropine Mesylate

DRUG CLASS: Antiparkinsonism agent

RECEPTOR AFFINITY: Blocks cholinergic (acetylcholine) activity, which is believed to restore the balance of acetylcholine and dopamine in the basal ganglia.

INDICATIONS: Used in psychiatry to reduce extrapyramidal symptoms (acute medication-related movement disorders), including pseudoparkinsonism, dystonia, and akathisia (but not tardive syndromes) caused by neuroleptic drugs such as haloperidol. Most effective with acute dystonia.

ROUTES AND DOSAGE: Available in tablet form, 0.5-, 1-, and 2-mg doses, also injectable 1 mg/mL

Adult Dosage: For acute dystonia, 1 to 2 mg IM or IV usually provides rapid relief. No significant difference in onset of action after IM or IV injection. Treatment of emergent symptoms may be relieved in 1 or 2 days, with 1 to 2 mg PO two to three times a day. Maximum daily dose is 6 mg/day. After 1 to 2 weeks, withdraw drug to see if continued treatment is needed. Medication-related movement disorders that develop slowly may not respond to this treatment.

Geriatric: Older adults and very thin patients cannot tolerate large doses.

Children: Do not use in children younger than 3 years. Use with caution in older children.

HALF-LIFE: 12 to 24 hours; very little pharmacokinetic information is available.

SELECT SIDE EFFECTS: Dry mouth, blurred vision, tachycardia, nausea, constipation, flushing or elevated temperature, decreased sweating, muscular weakness or cramping, urinary retention, urinary hesitancy, dizziness, headache, disorientation, confusion, memory loss, hallucinations, psychoses, and agitation in toxic reactions, which are more pronounced in older adults and occur at smaller doses.

WARNING: Avoid use during pregnancy and while breastfeeding. Give with caution in hot weather because of possible heatstroke. Contraindicated with angle-closure glaucoma, pyloric or duodenal obstruction, stenosing peptic ulcers, prostatic hypertrophy or bladder neck obstructions, myasthenia gravis, megacolon, and megaesophagus. May aggravate the symptoms of tardive dyskinesia and other chronic forms of medication-related movement disorder. Concomitant use of other anticholinergic drugs may increase side effects and risk for toxicity. Coadministration of haloperidol or phenothiazines may reduce serum levels of these drugs.

SPECIFIC PATIENT/FAMILY EDUCATION

- Take with meals to reduce dry mouth and gastric irritation.
- Dry mouth may also be alleviated by sucking sugarless candies, maintaining adequate fluid intake, and good oral hygiene; increase fiber and fluids in diet to avoid constipation; stool softeners may be required. Notify your prescriber if urinary hesitancy or constipation persists.
- Notify your prescriber if rapid or pounding heartbeat, confusion, eye pain, rash, or other side effects develop.
- May cause drowsiness, dizziness, or blurred vision; use caution driving or performing other hazardous tasks requiring alertness. Avoid alcohol and other CNS depressants.
- Do not abruptly stop this medication because a flu-like syndrome may develop.
- Use with caution in hot weather. Ensure adequate hydration. May increase susceptibility to heat stroke.

CNS, central nervous system; IM, intramuscular; IV, intravenous; PO, oral.

medication. See Box 24.14 for more information about benztropine.

Akathisia

Akathisia also appears to be caused by the same biologic mechanism as other extrapyramidal side effects (i.e., an imbalance of dopamine and acetylcholine). Patients are restless and report they feel driven to keep moving. They are extremely uncomfortable. Frequently, this response is misinterpreted as anxiety or increased psychotic symptoms, so that the patient may inappropriately be given increased dosages of an antipsychotic drug, which perpetuates the side effect. If possible, the dose of antipsychotic drug should be reduced. A β-adrenergic blocker such as propranolol, 20 to 120 mg, may be required. An anticholinergic medication may not be helpful. Failure to manage this side effect is a leading cause of patients ceasing to take antipsychotic medications (see Chapter 11).

Tardive Dyskinesia, Tardive Dystonia, and Tardive Akathisia

Tardive dyskinesia, *tardive dystonia*, and *tardive akathisia* are less likely to occur than other extrapyramidal side effects but still may appear in individuals taking second-generation, rather than first-generation, antipsychotics. Table 24.2 describes these and associated motor irregularities. The term *tardive* means late-appearing; thus, all of these movements appear after an individual has taken these drugs for a period of time, usually a few months. Thus, **tardive dyskinesia** is late-appearing unexpected involuntary movements. It can be viewed as the opposite of parkinsonism, both in observable movements and in etiology. Whereas muscle rigidity and absence of movement characterize parkinsonism, constant movement characterizes tardive dyskinesia. Typical movements involve the mouth, tongue, and jaw and include lip smacking, sucking, puckering, tongue protrusion, the "bonbon sign" (where the tongue rolls around in the mouth and protrudes into the cheek as if the patient is sucking on a piece of hard candy), athetoid (worm-like) movements of the tongue, and chewing. Other facial movements, such as grimacing and eye blinking, may also be present.

Movements in the trunk and limbs are frequently observable with tardive dyskinesia. These include rocking from the hips, athetoid movements of the fingers and toes, jerking movements of the fingers and toes,

TABLE 24.2 EXTRAPYRAMIDAL SIDE EFFECTS OF ANTIPSYCHOTIC DRUGS

Side Effect	Period of Onset	Symptoms
Acute Motor Irregularities		
Parkinsonism or pseudoparkinsonism	5–30 d	Resting tremor, rigidity, bradykinesia or akinesia, masklike face, shuffling gait, decreased arm swing
Acute dystonia	1–5 d	Intermittent or fixed unusual postures of the eyes, face, tongue, neck, trunk, and limbs
Akathisia	1–30 d	Obvious motor restlessness evidenced by pacing, rocking, shifting from foot to foot; subjective sense of not being able to sit or be still; these symptoms may occur together or separately
Late-Appearing Motor Irregularities		
Tardive dyskinesia	Months to years	Unusual dyskinetic movements of the face, mouth, and jaw; choreoathetoid movements of the legs, arms, and trunk
Tardive dystonia	Months to years	Persistent sustained unusual postures in the face, eyes, tongue, neck, trunk, and limbs
Tardive akathisia	Months to years	Persistent unabating sense of subjective and objective restlessness

Source: D'Souza, R. S., & Hooten, W. M. (2023). Extrapyramidal Symptoms. In *StatPearls*. StatPearls Publishing. https://www.ncbi.nlm.nih.gov/books/NBK

guitar-strumming movements of the fingers, and foot tapping. The long-term health issues for people with tardive dyskinesia are choking, associated with loss of control of muscles used for swallowing, and compromised respiratory function, leading to infections and possibly respiratory alkalosis.

Because the movements resemble the dyskinetic movements of some patients who have idiopathic Parkinson disease and who have received long-term treatment with L-dopa (a direct-acting dopamine agonist that crosses the blood–brain barrier), the suggested hypothesis for tardive dyskinesia includes the supersensitivity of the dopamine receptors in the basal ganglia.

An effective treatment for tardive dyskinesia has been elusive. However, antipsychotic drugs mask the movements of tardive dyskinesia and have periodically been suggested as a treatment. This is counterintuitive because these drugs cause the disorder. Second-generation antipsychotic drugs, such as clozapine, may be less likely to cause it; however, recent interest suggests that the tardive dyskinesia is still prevalent but at a lesser rate (Citrome et al., 2021). Two medications, deutetrabenazine and valbenazine, are approved by the US Food and Drug Administration (FDA) and appear to ameliorate the movements of tardive dyskinesia by decreasing the transport of dopamine into storage vesicles (via inhibition of vesicular monoamine transporter 2—VMAT2) and therefore reducing the overall availability of dopamine (Warren et al., 2022). However, the best management remains prevention through using the lowest possible dose of an antipsychotic drug over time that minimizes the symptoms of schizophrenia as well as regular evaluation of movements using tools like the DISCUS (see Box 24.5).

Monitoring Other Side Effects

Orthostatic Hypotension

Orthostatic hypotension is a common side effect of antipsychotic drugs. Primarily an antiadrenergic effect, decreased blood pressure may be generalized or orthostatic. Patients may be protected from falls by teaching them to rise slowly and by monitoring blood pressure before giving the medication. The nurse should monitor and document lying, sitting, and standing blood pressures when any antipsychotic drug therapy begins.

Hyperprolactinemia

Another possible side effect of antipsychotic drugs is *hyperprolactinemia*, in which higher-than-expected levels of prolactin are found in the blood. When dopamine is blocked in the tuberoinfundibular tract, it can no longer repress prolactin, the neurohormone that regulates lactation and mammary function. The prolactin level increases, and, in some individuals, side effects appear. Gynecomastia (i.e., enlarged breasts) can occur in people of all genders and is understandably distressing to individuals who may be experiencing delusional or hallucinatory body image disturbances. Galactorrhea (i.e., lactation) may also occur. Menstrual irregularities and sexual dysfunction are possible. If these symptoms appear, the medication should be reduced or changed to another antipsychotic agent. Hyperprolactinemia is associated with the use of haloperidol and risperidone.

Sedation

Sedation is another possible side effect of antipsychotic medication and a frequent reason that patients discontinue medications. Patients should be monitored for the sedating effects of antipsychotic agents. In older patients, sedation can be associated with falls.

Weight Gain and Increased Appetite

Weight gain and increased appetite are related to antipsychotic agents, especially olanzapine and clozapine. Patients may gain as much as 20 or 30 lb within 1 year. Such increased appetite and weight gain are distressing to patients. Diet teaching and monitoring may have some effect. Another solution is to increase the accessibility of healthful easy-to-prepare food. Simple exercise routines may be helpful.

New-Onset Diabetes

New-onset diabetes should be assessed in patients taking antipsychotic drugs. An association has been found between new-onset diabetes and the administration of second-generation antipsychotic agents, especially after weight gain. Patients should be monitored for clinical symptoms of diabetes. Fasting blood glucose tests and hemoglobin A1c monitoring are commonly ordered for these individuals.

Cardiac Arrhythmias

Cardiac arrhythmias may also occur in patients taking antipsychotic medication. Prolongation of the QTc interval is associated with torsade de pointe (polymorphic ventricular tachycardia) or ventricular fibrillation. The potential for drug-induced prolonged QT interval is associated with many drugs. Ziprasidone is more likely than other second-generation antipsychotics to prolong the QT interval and thus change the heart rhythm. For these patients, baseline electrocardiograms may be ordered. Nurses should observe these patients for cardiac arrhythmias.

Agranulocytosis

Agranulocytosis is a reduction in the number of circulating granulocytes and decreased production of granulocytes in the bone marrow, which limits one's ability to fight infection. Agranulocytosis can develop with the use of all antipsychotic drugs, but it is most likely to develop with clozapine use. Although laboratory values below 500 cells/mm^3 are indicative of agranulocytosis, often granulocyte counts drop to below 200 cells/mm^3 with this syndrome.

Patients taking clozapine should have regular blood tests. White blood cell and granulocyte counts should be measured before treatment is initiated and at least weekly or twice weekly after treatment begins. Initial white blood cell counts should be above 3,500 cells/mm^3 before treatment initiation; in patients with counts of 3,500 and 5,000 cells/mm^3, cell counts should be monitored three times a week if clozapine is prescribed. Anytime the white blood cell count drops below 3,500 cells/mm^3 or granulocytes drop below 1,500 cells/mm^3, use of clozapine should be stopped, and the patient should be monitored for infection.

However, a faithfully implemented program of blood monitoring should not replace careful observation of the patient. It is not unusual for blood cell counts to drop precipitously over a period of 2 to 3 days. This may not be discovered when the patient is on a strict weekly blood monitoring schedule. Any reported symptoms that suggest a bacterial infection (e.g., fever, pharyngitis, weakness) should be cause for concern, so immediate evaluation of blood count status should be undertaken. Because patients are frequently discharged before the critical period of risk for agranulocytosis, patient education about these symptoms is also essential so that they will report these symptoms, obtain blood monitoring, and reduce their potential exposure to infections. In general, granulocyte levels return to expected within 2 to 4 weeks after discontinuation of use of the medication.

DRESS

DRESS (drug rash with eosinophilia and systemic symptoms) is a very rare, potentially life-threatening, drug-induced hypersensitivity reaction recently associated with antipsychotic therapy. Symptoms include skin eruption, hematologic irregularities (e.g., eosinophilia, atypical lymphocytosis), lymphadenopathy, and internal organ involvement (e.g., liver, kidney, lung). Skin assessment, to look for any sign of skin rashes, is important (Mallaro & Rosenthal, 2023).

Preventing Drug–Drug Interactions

Antipsychotic medications have the potential to interact with other medications, nicotine, and grapefruit juice. For example, olanzapine and clozapine have the potential to interact with some antidepressants. Some antipsychotics are metabolized faster in people who smoke than in people who don't smoke (Reeves et al., 2024). Conversely, issues with increased side effects from slower drug metabolism can occur when smoking cessation programs are initiated. Before giving medication, the nurse should check all medications for potential interactions.

Teaching Points

Nonadherence to the medication regimen is a key factor in relapse; the family must be made aware of the importance of the patient's taking medications consistently. Medication education should cover the association between medications and the amelioration of symptoms, side effects and their management, and interpersonal skills that help the patient and family report medication effects.

Management of Complications

Neuroleptic Malignant Syndrome

Neuroleptic malignant syndrome (NMS) is a life-threatening condition that can develop in reaction to antipsychotic medications. The primary symptoms of NMS are *mental status changes, severe muscle rigidity*, and *autonomic changes*, including elevated temperature (usually between 101°F and 103°F), tachycardia, and blood pressure lability. These mental status changes and severe muscle rigidity occur usually within the first week of initiation of antipsychotic therapy and can include two or more of the following: hypertension, tachycardia, tachypnea, prominent diaphoresis, incontinence, mutism, leukocytosis, and laboratory evidence of muscle injury (e.g., elevated creatinine phosphokinase). The incidence of NMS ranges from 0.01% to 3.2% of patients taking neuroleptic medications. The incidence is decreasing, probably because of increased awareness of symptoms, use of second-generation antipsychotics, and earlier interventions, such as stopping the offending medication (Simon et al., 2023). As many as 5% to 15% of affected patients may die as a result of the syndrome. In the past, NMS was probably underreported and may have accounted for unexplained emergency department deaths of patients taking these drugs because their symptoms did not seem serious.

The most important aspects of nursing care for patients with NMS relate to recognizing symptoms early, withholding any antipsychotic or any other dopamine antagonist (e.g., gastric reflux medications), and initiating supportive nursing care (Fig. 24.1). In any patient with muscle rigidity, fluctuating vital signs, abrupt changes in levels of consciousness, or any of the symptoms presented in Box 24.15, NMS should be suspected. The nurse should be especially alert for early signs and symptoms of NMS in high-risk patients, such as those who are agitated, physically exhausted, or dehydrated or who have an

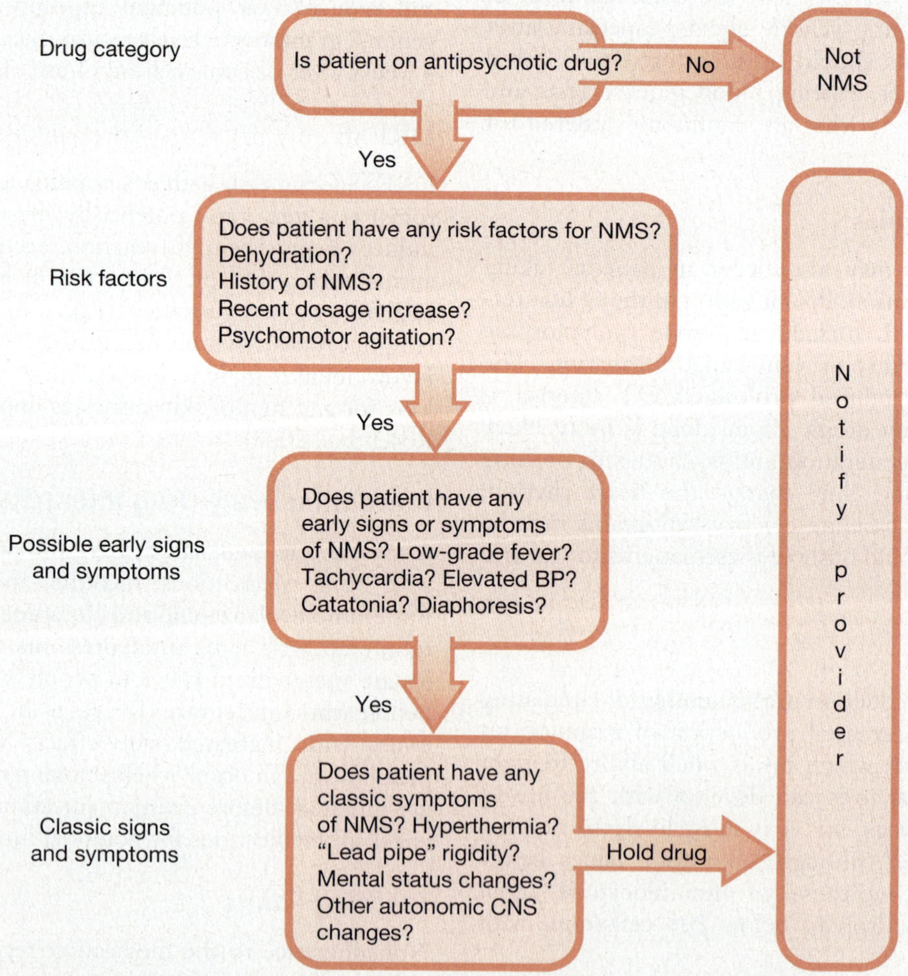

FIGURE 24.1 Action tree for "holding" an antipsychotic drug because of suspected neuroleptic malignant syndrome. *BP*, blood pressure; *CNS*, central nervous system; *NMS*, neuroleptic malignant syndrome.

BOX 24.15

Recognizing Neuroleptic Malignant Syndrome

Onset: 2 weeks after initiation of antipsychotic treatment or change in dosage

Risk factors: Assigned male at birth, preexisting medical or neurologic disorders, depot injection administration, and high ambient temperature

IMMINENT INDICATORS

- Mental status changes
- Muscle rigidity
- Hyperthermia
- Tachycardia
- Hypertension or hypotension
- Tachypnea or hypoxia
- Diaphoresis or sialorrhea
- Tremor
- Incontinence
- Creatinine phosphokinase elevation or myoglobinuria
- Leukocytosis
- Metabolic acidosis

Source: Neuroleptic malignant syndrome. Retrieved February 20, 2021, from https://rarediseases.org/rare-diseases/neuroleptic-malignant-syndrome/

existing medical or neurologic illness. See Box 24.16 for Building Clinical Judgment with SBAR. Patients receiving parenteral or higher doses of neuroleptic drugs or lithium concurrently must also be carefully assessed. The nurse should carefully monitor fluid intake, and fluid and electrolyte status.

NCLEXNOTE Recognition of side effects, including movement disorders, tardive dyskinesia, and weight gain, should lead to interventions. NMS is a medical emergency.

Medical treatment focuses on symptom management and includes administering dopamine agonist drugs, such as bromocriptine (modest success), and muscle relaxants, such as dantrolene or benzodiazepine. Antiparkinsonism drugs are not particularly useful. Some patients experience improvement with electroconvulsive therapy (ECT).

The nurse must frequently monitor vital signs of the patient with symptoms of NMS. In addition, it is important to check the patient's laboratory results for increased creatine phosphokinase, an elevated white blood cell count, elevated liver enzymes, or myoglobinuria. The nurse must be prepared to initiate supportive measures or anticipate emergency transfer of the patient to a medical-surgical or an intensive care unit.

Treating fever (which frequently exceeds 103°F) is an important priority for these patients. High body temperature may be reduced with a cooling blanket and acetaminophen therapy. Because many of these patients experience diaphoresis, temperature elevation, or dysphagia, it is important to monitor hydration. Another

BOX 24.16

Building Clinical Judgment With SBAR: Nurse Communication With Provider Regarding a Patient With Schizophrenia

SBAR

S: Situation

Bruce is a 26-year-old assigned male at birth who is diagnosed with schizophrenia. He was admitted 6 days ago and started on risperidone 2 mg twice a day on admission. Risperidone Consta 25 mg was given IM 2 days ago. He has been wandering aimlessly on the unit today, looking flushed and a little confused. When asked, he says he feels a little nauseated.

B: Background

This is Bruce's second hospitalization in the past 8 months. He was discharged on risperidone but quit taking it when the prescription ran out. The decision was made to use a long-acting antipsychotic to stabilize Bruce's symptoms and avoid a relapse.

A: Assessment

- Physical Health: Ht. 6′1″, Wt. 150
- Vital Signs: BP 90/60, P 106, R 32, T 102.3 F
- Oriented only to person
- Increased risk of neuroleptic malignant syndrome

R: Recommendations

- Treat this as an emergency; call provider immediately
- Get Bruce to sit down or lie down
- Place ice packs on neck, underarms, and groin
- Obtain order for blood draw for CPK
- Hold next dose of oral risperidone
- Be prepared to transport to emergency room or ICU

Building Clinical Judgment

1. What symptoms are atypical for a patient receiving an antipsychotic?
2. Did the nurse overreact by holding the next dose of risperidone, ordering blood work, and preparing patient for transfer to the emergency room or ICU?

important aspect of care for patients with NMS is safety. Joints and extremities that are rigid or spastic must be protected from injury. The treatment of these patients depends on the facility and availability of medical support services. In general, patients in psychiatric inpatient units that are separated from general hospitals are transferred to medical-surgical settings for treatment.

Cholinergic Rebound

If patients are prescribed an anticholinergic agent, such as benztropine, for movement disorders and they abruptly stop taking it, they could experience **cholinergic rebound** symptoms including vomiting, excessive sweating, and altered dreams and nightmares. Cholinergic rebound can be especially problematic if patients discontinue other medications with anticholinergic properties (e.g., antipsychotics, antidepressants, antibiotics) at the same time. Medications with anticholinergic properties should be reduced gradually (tapered) over several days. Table 24.3 lists anticholinergic side effects and several antipsychotic medications and interventions to manage them.

Anticholinergic Medication Effects and Misuse

The potential exists for misuse of anticholinergic drugs. Some patients may find the anticholinergic effects of these drugs on mood, memory, and perception pleasurable.

TABLE 24.3 NURSING INTERVENTIONS FOR ANTICHOLINERGIC SIDE EFFECTS

Effect	Intervention
Dry mouth	Provide sips of water, hard candies, and chewing gum (preferably sugar free).
Blurred vision	Avoid dangerous tasks; teach patient that this side effect will diminish in a few weeks.
Decreased lacrimation	Use artificial tears if necessary.
Mydriasis	May aggravate glaucoma; teach patient to report eye pain.
Photophobia	Wear sunglasses.
Constipation	High-fiber diet; increased fluid intake; take laxatives as prescribed.
Urinary hesitancy	Privacy; run water in sink; warm water over perineum
Urinary retention	Regular voiding (at least every 2–3 h) and whenever urge is present; catheterize for residual urine; record intake and output; evaluate for benign prostatic hypertrophy.
Tachycardia	Evaluate for preexisting cardiovascular disease.

Although at toxic dosages, patients may experience a mild to moderate delirium with disorientation and hallucinations, lesser doses may cause patients to experience greater sociability and euphoria.

Anticholinergic Crisis

An **anticholinergic crisis** is a potentially life-threatening medical emergency caused by an overdose of or sensitivity to drugs with anticholinergic properties. This syndrome (also called anticholinergic delirium) may result from an accidental or intentional overdose of anticholinergic drugs, including atropine, scopolamine, or belladonna alkaloids, which are present in numerous prescription drugs and OTC medicines. The syndrome may also occur in psychiatric patients who are not only receiving therapeutic doses of anticholinergic drugs but also taking other drugs with anticholinergic properties. As a result of either drug overdose or sensitivity, these anticholinergic substances may produce acute delirium or a psychotic reaction resembling schizophrenia. Severe anticholinergic effects may occur in older patients, even at therapeutic levels (Oudewortel et al., 2021).

The signs and symptoms of anticholinergic crisis are dramatic and physically uncomfortable (Box 24.17). This disorder is characterized by fever, parched mouth, burning thirst, hot dry skin, decreased salivation, decreased bronchial and nasal secretions, widely dilated eyes (bright light becomes painful), decreased ability to accommodate visually, increased heart rate, constipation, difficulty urinating, and hypertension or hypotension. The face, neck, and upper arms may become flushed because of reflexive blood vessel dilation. In addition to peripheral symptoms, patients with anticholinergic psychosis may experience neuropsychiatric symptoms of anxiety, agitation, delirium, hyperactivity, confusion, hallucinations (especially visual), speech difficulties, psychotic symptoms, or seizures. The acute psychotic reaction that is produced resembles schizophrenia.

In general, episodes of anticholinergic crisis are self-limiting, usually subsiding in 3 days. However, if left untreated, the associated fever and delirium may progress to coma or cardiac and respiratory depression. Although

BOX 24.17

Signs and Symptoms of Anticholinergic Crisis

- **Neuropsychiatric signs:** confusion; recent memory loss; agitation; dysarthria; incoherent speech; pressured speech; delusions; ataxia; periods of hyperactivity alternating with somnolence, paranoia, anxiety, or coma
- **Hallucinations:** accompanied by "picking," plucking, or grasping motions; delusions; or disorientation
- **Physical signs:** nonreactive dilated pupils; blurred vision; hot, dry, flushed skin; facial flushing; dry mucous membranes; difficulty swallowing; fever; tachycardia; hypertension; decreased bowel sounds; urinary retention; nausea; vomiting; seizures; or coma

rare, death is generally caused by hyperpyrexia and brain stem depression. After use of the offending drug is discontinued, improvement usually occurs within 24 to 36 hours.

A specific and effective antidote, physostigmine, a reversible inhibitor of cholinesterase, is frequently used to treat and diagnose anticholinergic crisis. Administration of this drug rapidly reduces both behavioral and physiologic symptoms. However, the usual adult dose of physostigmine is 1 to 2 mg, intravenously given slowly during a period of 5 minutes because rapid injection of physostigmine may cause seizures, profound bradycardia, or heart block. Physostigmine is relatively short acting, so it may need to be given several times during the course of treatment. This drug provides relief from symptoms for a period of 2 to 3 hours. In addition to receiving physostigmine, patients who intentionally overdose on large amounts of anticholinergic drugs are treated by gastric lavage, administration of charcoal, and catharsis.

It is important for the nurse to be alert for signs and symptoms of anticholinergic crisis, especially in older and pediatric patients, who are much more sensitive to the anticholinergic effects of drugs, and in patients who are receiving multiple medications with anticholinergic effects. If signs and symptoms of the syndrome occur, the nurse should discontinue use of the offending drug and notify the provider immediately.

Electroconvulsive Therapy

ECT is suggested as a feasible alternative when the patient's schizophrenia is not being successfully treated by medication alone. For the most part, this modality is not indicated unless the patient is catatonic or has depression that is not treatable by other means. In general, ECT is not used often for the treatment of schizophrenia, but it may be useful for those people who are medication resistant, assaultive, and psychotic (Karl et al., 2024).

Psychosocial Interventions

Psychosocial interventions, such as counseling, conflict resolution, behavior therapy, and cognitive interventions, are appropriate for patients with schizophrenia. The following discussion focuses on applying these interventions.

Therapeutic Interactions

Although antipsychotic medications may relieve positive symptoms, they do not always eliminate hallucinations and delusions. The nurse must continue helping the patient develop creative strategies for dealing with these sensory and thought disturbances. Information about the content of the hallucinations and delusions is necessary, not only to determine whether the medications are effective but also to assess safety and the meaning of these thoughts and perceptions to the patient. In caring for a patient who is experiencing hallucinations or delusions, nursing actions should be guided by three general patient outcomes:

- Decrease the frequency and intensity of hallucinations and delusions.
- Recognize that hallucinations and delusions are symptoms of a brain disorder.
- Develop strategies to manage the recurrence of hallucinations or delusions.

When interacting with a patient who is experiencing hallucinations or delusions, the nurse must remember that these experiences are real to the patient. It is important for the nurse to understand the content and meaning of the hallucinations, particularly those involving command hallucinations.

On the one hand, the nurse should never tell a patient that these experiences are not real. Discounting the experiences blocks communication. On the other hand, it is also dishonest for the nurse to tell the patient that the nurse is having the same hallucinatory experience. It is best to validate the patient's experiences and identify the meaning of these thoughts and feelings to the patient. For example, a patient who believes that they are under surveillance by the Federal Bureau of Investigation probably feels frightened and suspicious of everyone. By acknowledging how frightening it must be to always feel like you are being watched, the nurse focuses on the feelings that are generated by the delusion, not the delusion itself. The nurse can then offer to help the patient feel safe within this environment. The patient, in turn, begins to feel that someone understands them.

Enhancing Cognitive Functioning

After identifying deficits in cognitive functioning, the nurse and patient can develop interventions that target specific deficits. The most effective interventions usually involve the whole treatment team and the patient. If the ability to focus or maintain attention is an issue, patients can be encouraged to select activities that improve attention, such as computer games. For memory issues, patients can be encouraged to make lists and to write down important information.

Executive functioning issues are the most challenging for these patients. Patients who cannot manage daily problems may have planning and problem-solving impairments. For these patients, developing interventions that closely simulate real-world problems may help. Through coaching, the nurse can teach and support the development of problem-solving skills. For example, during hospitalizations, patients are given medications and reminded to take them on time. They are often instructed in a classroom setting but rarely have an opportunity to practice self-medication and figure out what to do if their prescription expires, the medications are lost, or they forget to take their medications. Even so, when discharged, patients are expected to take medication at the prescribed dose at the prescribed time. Interventions designed to have patients actively engage in problem-solving behaviors focused on real problems are needed.

Other approaches to helping patients solve problems and learn new strategies for dealing with problems include solution-focused therapy, which focuses on the strengths and positive attributes that exist within each individual, and cognitive-behavioral therapy (Giacco et al., 2021), which focuses directly on collaboratively determined symptoms and strategies to address them. These therapies involve years of training to master, but certain techniques can be used. For example, the nurse can ask patients to identify the most important issue from their perspective. This focuses the patient on a critical issue pertinent to them.

Using Behavioral Interventions

Behavioral interventions can be highly effective in helping patients improve motivation and organize routine, daily activities, such as maintaining a regular schedule and completing activities. Reinforcement of positive behaviors (getting up on time, completing hygiene, going to treatment activities) can easily be included in a treatment plan. In the hospital, patients gain unit privileges by following an agreed-on treatment plan. In the community, a behavioral intervention is more likely to be combined with other approaches or used for a specific behavior such as smoking (McDonagh et al., 2022).

Complementary Therapies

Complementary therapies can be helpful to people with the symptoms of schizophrenia. Art and music therapies improve cognitive functioning and decrease positive and negative symptoms (Stone & Short, 2024; Utas-Akhan et al., 2024). Art therapy has been shown to improve expression of feelings, and music therapy can improve sleep (Box 24.18).

Mindfulness-based interventions and yoga are being explored for their feasibility and effectiveness for treating people with schizophrenia. Yoga has been shown to improve positive and negative symptoms, and mindfulness may help to improve positive symptoms and decrease depression (Böge et al., 2021; Su et al., 2024). Yoga as a form of exercise can be modified to match the physical abilities of participants. It can help with relaxation and self-care, increased body awareness, and spiritual comfort. When held in a group setting, yoga can help individuals to feel connected to others (Töbelmann et al., 2023).

Spiritual Interventions

Patients should be given the opportunity to have a spiritual or religious consultation. Religious beliefs are deeply embedded in many cultures. **Religious coping,** which involves engaging in behaviors that strengthen the belief in a benevolent higher power, is associated with positive well-being and mental health. If a patient has a spiritual or religious belief in a higher power, it is important to determine if the higher power is viewed as benevolent or belligerent. If the higher power is considered benevolent, encouraging patients to engage in religious coping behaviors such as attending religious services or praying can instill hope, comfort and meaning in life, as well as reducing depression, anxiety, and suicidality (Lopez et al., 2023).

Psychoeducation

Teaching Strategies

Cognitive deficits (e.g., difficulty in processing complex information, maintaining steady focus of attention,

BOX 24.18

Research for Evidence-Based Practice: Efficacy of Music Therapy and Predictors of Sleep Disturbance Among Patients With Chronic Schizophrenia: A Prospective Study

Lu, M. J., Chen, W. Y, & Li, D. J. (2022). Efficacy of music therapy and predictors of sleep disturbance among patients with chronic schizophrenia: A prospective study. Archives of Psychiatric Nursing, *40, 1–7.*

THE QUESTIONS: What is the efficacy of music therapy on sleep disturbance in patients with schizophrenia compared to a control group? What predictors are related to the treatment outcome for sleep disturbance?

METHODS: Volunteer subjects were recruited from two chronic wards which were randomly selected from five chronic wards and then randomly assigned to an intervention or control ward. Thirty-one patients volunteered in the control ward and 35 from the intervention ward. The Pittsburgh Sleep Quality Index (PSQI) was used to assess sleep prior to the intervention and one month later at the completion of the intervention. The intervention group was taken to an activity room from 9:00 to 10:00 pm for 4 weeks during which time nurses played a variety of music pre-selected for its slow beat of 60 to 80 beats per minute.

FINDINGS: As measured by the PSQI, the intervention group had significant improvement in sleep quality as a result of the intervention. Patients with chronic medical conditions and who reported little religious affiliation had greater improvement on the PSQI.

IMPLICATIONS FOR NURSING: Offering a quiet space with quiet music is a simple and inexpensive method to prepare patients for sleep and to incorporate into a sleep hygiene practice for individuals with a mental illness like schizophrenia. People with mental illness can also learn from encounters where they are expected to respond and follow social norms.

distinguishing between relevant and irrelevant stimuli, and forming abstractions) may challenge the nurse planning educational activities. Evidence indicates that people with schizophrenia may learn best in an errorless learning environment (Allott et al., 2020; Kern et al., 2018). That is, they are directly given correct information and then encouraged to write it down. Errorless learning is an educational intervention based on the principle of operant conditioning that learning is stronger and more likely to last if it occurs in the absence of errors. Asking questions that encourage guessing is not as effective in helping patients retain information. Trial-and-error learning is avoided.

Teaching and explaining should occur in an environment with minimal distractions. Terminology should be clear and unambiguous. Visual aids can supplement verbal information, but these materials should have simple information stated in simple language. The nurse takes care not to overcrowd the visual material or incorporate images that draw attention away from important content. Teaching should occur in small segments with frequent reinforcement. Most importantly, teaching should occur when the patient is ready. Regular assessments of cognitive abilities with standardized instruments can help determine this readiness. These suggestions can be adapted for teaching during any phase of the illness.

Teaching About Symptoms

Teaching patients that hallucinations and delusions are part of the disorder becomes easier after the medication begins working. When patients believe and acknowledge that they have a mental illness and that some of their thoughts are delusions and some of their perceptions are hallucinations, they can develop strategies to manage their symptoms.

Patients benefit greatly by learning recovery strategies of self-regulation, symptom monitoring, and relapse prevention. By monitoring events, time, place, and stimuli surrounding the appearance of symptoms, the patient can begin to predict high-risk times for symptom recurrence. Cognitive-behavioral therapy is often used in helping patients monitor and identify their emerging symptoms to prevent relapse (Bighelli et al., 2024).

Another important nursing intervention is to help the patient identify to whom and where to talk about delusional or hallucinatory material. Because self-disclosure of these symptoms immediately labels someone as having a mental illness, patients should be encouraged to evaluate the environment for negative consequences of disclosing these symptoms. For example, it may be fine to talk about it at home but not at the grocery store.

Teaching How to Cope With Stress

Developing skills to cope with personal, social, and environmental stresses is important to everyone but particularly to those with a severe mental illness. Stresses can easily trigger symptoms that patients are trying to avoid. Establishing regular counseling sessions to support the development of positive coping skills is helpful for both hospitalized patients and those living in the community.

Wellness Strategies

Wellness strategies require providers to consider multiple aspects of what is considered a well-lived life. As with recovery, it is important to establish what "living well with mental illness" means to the individual with schizophrenia. Within the limitations of the illness and its treatment, providers need to collaborate with the individual to define wellness. Wellness should be defined beyond just the best physical health possible and includes positive social relationships, engaging leisure and work activities, and spiritual connections, to name a few. To varying degrees, evidence supports interventions such as (1) cognitive training and remediation that focus on cognitive impairments and social functioning (Martini et al., 2024) and could incorporate new methodologies that use virtual reality (Bogie et al., 2024); (2) support that provides information about the illness, addresses emotional needs, acknowledges the challenges of the illness, encourages the individual, and provides guidance (Stewart et al., 2024); and (3) goal setting with the individual that uses methodologies like the "Choose-Get-Keep" model that supports client goals over the imposition of provider goals (Stewart et al., 2021).

Social Skills Training

Social skills training, provided either individually or in groups, is also useful when collaborating with patients who have schizophrenia. This training teaches patients specific behaviors needed for social interactions. The skills are taught by lecture, demonstration, role-playing, and homework assignments. Nurses may be team members and be involved in case management or provision of services. Furthermore, efforts to offer supportive employment experiences that incorporate patient preferences, rapid job search and employment, and ongoing job supports have shown effectiveness. Although long-term self-sufficiency has not necessarily been achieved, supportive employment has been the most effective vocational rehabilitation method (Barlati et al., 2024).

Skill-training interventions should be designed to compensate for cognitive deficits. To help patients learn to process complex activities, such as catching a bus, preparing a meal, or shopping for food or clothing, nurses should break the activity into small parts or steps and list them for the patient's reference, for example:

- Leave your apartment with your keys in hand.
- Make sure you have correct bus fare in your pocket.
- Close the door.

- Walk to the corner.
- Turn right and walk three blocks to the bus stop.

Concept Mastery Alert

If the patient has active psychosis, with symptoms such as hallucinations and social withdrawal, wait until a lucid period to begin social skills training. When a patient is in active psychosis, it is not a good time to introduce additional stressors.

Providing Family Education

Because having a family member with schizophrenia is a life-changing event for the family and friends who provide care and support, educating patients and their families is crucial. It is a primary concern for the psychiatric–mental health nurse. Family support is crucial to help patients maintain treatment. Education should include information about the disease course, treatment regimens, support systems, and life management skills (Box 24.19). The most important factor to stress during patient and family education is the consistent taking of medication.

Promoting Safety

Although violence is not a consistent behavior of people with schizophrenia, it is always a concern during the initial phase, when hallucinations or delusions may put patients at risk for harming themselves or others. Nonviolent patients who are experiencing hallucinations and delusions can also be at risk for violence by more aggressive patients. The patient who is hallucinating needs to be protected; this may include increased staff monitoring and, if necessary, a safer environment in a secluded area.

Identifying patient risk factors for violence, such as a history of violence, can alert the nursing staff of a potential for the patient to engage in aggressive behavior, but careful assessment and management of the immediate environment and treating the psychiatric symptoms are more important in avoiding aggression. The nurse's best approach to avoiding violence or aggression is to demonstrate respect for the patient and the patient's personal space, assess and monitor for signs of fear and agitation, and use preventive interventions before the patient loses control. Patients should be encouraged to discuss their anger and to be involved in their treatment decisions. Medications should be administered as ordered. Because most antipsychotic and antidepressant medications take 1 to 2 weeks to begin moderating behavior, the nurse must be vigilant during this period of acute illness.

If the patient loses control and is a danger to self or others, restraints and seclusion may be used as a last resort. Health Care Financing Administration guidelines and hospital policy must be followed (see Chapter 4), and staff should be trained in the proper use of seclusion and restraints. In addition, staff need to hold sessions after all incidents of violence or physical management to analyze the event, allowing clinicians to learn how better to manage these situations and evaluate patients' cues. With sensitive leadership, these sessions can help health care workers to learn more about the interaction of patient and staff characteristics that can contribute to these incidents.

BOX 24.19

Psychoeducation Checklist: Schizophrenia

When caring for the patient with schizophrenia, be sure to include the caregiver during planning as appropriate and address the following topic areas in the teaching plan:

- Psychopharmacologic agents, including drug action, dosage, frequency, and possible side effects; stress the importance of adherence to the prescribed regimen
- Management of hallucinations
- Recovery strategies
- Coping strategies (e.g., self-talk, getting busy with something)
- Management of the environment
- Community resources

Convening Support Groups

People with mental illness benefit from support groups that focus on daily issues and the stress of dealing with a mental illness. These groups are useful throughout the continuum of care and help reduce the risk of suicide. In the hospital setting, the focus of the group can be simply sharing the experience of living with a mental illness. In the community, a regular support group can provide interaction with people with similar issues. Friendships often develop from these groups. Using peer counseling and support groups is a component of recovery-oriented care, but research is needed to understand these groups' impact on care (Roelandt et al., 2024).

Implementing Milieu Therapy

Individuals with schizophrenia may be hospitalized or may live in group homes for an extended period of time. The challenge is helping people who are unable to live with family members to live harmoniously with strangers who have similar interpersonal difficulties. *Milieu therapy*, which is arranging the treatment environment to encourage therapeutic relationships is crucial to the rehabilitation of the patient.

Developing Recovery-Oriented Rehabilitation Strategies

Rehabilitation strategies are used to support the individual's recovery and integration into the community (see Box 24.20).

BOX 24.20

Perspective of a Brother of a Patient With Schizophrenia

A sibling describes his brother with schizophrenia and the importance of both medications and relationships.

In 1998, at the age of 40 years, Robert was admitted to a psychiatric hospital. His brother was told at the time that Robert would never be able to live independently, and even if discharged, would only be repeatedly hospitalized. Robert had a long history of treatment and in 1998 he had received various types of antipsychotic medications, but he had not received any of the "new atypical variety." He was prescribed one of these drugs, and within months, the staff who had predicted the most discouraging of outcomes told Robert's brother that he was in the midst of a miraculous recovery—his thinking was clear and free from delusions, and they were preparing Robert's discharge.

A few weeks into the discharge planning, Robert called his brother; Robert was distressed because his social worker, whom Robert had known for years from a prior hospitalization, was leaving. The social worker had been abruptly transferred to another hospital. Robert deteriorated rapidly into tantrums, hallucinations, and dangerous behaviors. His discharge was put on hold. Robert's brother's rhetorical question was, "What was the difference between Robert on the same medication on Monday, when he was all right, and Tuesday, when he no longer was?" The answer to this question was the loss of an important relationship.

Robert is now living in a community-based home where the dedicated staff members have shown that they can maintain rehospitalization rates below 3%.

Robert's brother has interviewed many former psychiatric patients for a book. He found that every one of his interviewees, although attributing their recovery to medications or finding God, or a particular program, also identified an important relationship with one human being who believed in their ability to recover. Most of the time, this individual was a professional, such as a social worker, a nurse, or a doctor. Sometimes, however, it was a member of the clergy or a family member.

Robert's brother concluded, "Let's provide a range of medications, and let's study their effectiveness, but let's remember that the pill is the ultimate downsizing. Let's find resources to give people afflicted with mental illness what all of us need: fellow human beings upon whom we can depend on to help us through our dark times and, once through, to emerge into gloriously imperfect lives."

For nurses, it is important to remember that it is not what we do *to* people that is the most important, but rather what we do *with* people: give hope, listen to their dreams, help them find ways to get as close to recovery as they can.

Source: Neugeboren, J. (2006). Meds alone couldn't bring Robert back. Newsweek. National Empowerment Center. Retrieved February 21, 2022, from http://power2u.org/meds-alone-couldnt-bring-robert-back/

Factors that have been shown to promote recovery include the following:

- Adjustment, coping, and reappraisal
- Responding to the illness
- Social support, close relationships, and belonging

Factors that have a negative impact on the process of recovery include (1) self-stigma, (2) economic barriers, and (3) depression and hopelessness (Huxley et al., 2021; Ociskova et al., 2023; Sari et al., 2021). Community-based psychosocial rehabilitation programs usually offer long-term intensive case management services to adults with schizophrenia. Programs provide a continuum of services to meet the changing needs of people with psychiatric disabilities. Patients set rehabilitation goals, and services are then provided to help "clients" (most programs do not use the term *patients*) reach their goals. Services range from daily home visits to providing transportation, occupational training and supported employment, and group support. Assertive community treatment (ACT) is one example of these types of services and has a solid base of evidence to support its use (Munch Nielsen et al., 2023).

Evaluation of Patient Outcomes

Outcome research related to schizophrenia has redefined previous ways of thinking about the course of the disorder. Schizophrenia was formerly considered to have a progressively long-term and downward course, but it is now known that schizophrenia can be successfully treated, and recovery is possible (Huxley et al., 2021). In one older but significant study, the researchers interviewed patients 20 to 25 years after diagnosis and found that 50% to 66% experienced significant improvement or recovery (Harding et al., 1987). This study is important because it occurred before the development of second-generation antipsychotic agents and the international focus on recovery. Today, we can be hopeful that even more people can experience improvement or recover from schizophrenia.

Continuum of Care

Continuity of care has been identified as a primary strategy for recovery because individuals with schizophrenia are at risk for becoming "lost" to services if left alone after discharge. Discharge planning encourages follow-up care in the community. In fact, many state mental health systems require an outpatient appointment before discharge. Treatment of people with schizophrenia occurs across a variety of settings. Not only inpatient hospitalization but also partial hospitalization, day treatment, and crisis stabilization can be used effectively.

Emergency Care

Emergency care ideally takes place in a hospital emergency department, but often the crisis occurs in the home. Patients are usually relapsing and do not recognize their bizarre or aggressive behaviors as symptoms. A specially trained crisis team is sent to assess the emergency and recommend further treatment. In the emergency department, patients are brought not only because of relapse but also because of medication side effects or water intoxication. Nurses should refer to the previous discussion for nursing management. Crisis stabilization units are proposed as another alternative to provide more psychiatric emergency care in the community (Mark et al., 2024).

Inpatient-Focused Care

Inpatient hospitalizations are brief and focus on stabilization. Many times, patients are involuntarily admitted for a brief period (see Chapter 4). During the stabilization period, the status is changed to voluntary admission, whereby the patient agrees to treatment.

Community Care

Most of the care of people with schizophrenia is provided in the community through publicly supported recovery-oriented mental health delivery systems. The recovery journey can be long and require a variety of services such as ACT, outpatient therapy, case management, and psychosocial rehabilitation, including clubhouse programs. While the patient is in the community, their health care should be integrated with physical health care. Nurses should be especially vigilant that patients with mental illnesses receive proper primary and medical health care.

NCLEXNOTE Priorities in the patient with acute symptoms of schizophrenia include managing psychosis and keeping the patient safe and free from harming themselves or others. In the community, the priorities are preventing relapse, maintaining psychosocial functioning, engaging in psychoeducation, improving quality of life, and instilling hope.

In some cases, it is not the disorder itself that threatens the mental health of the individual with schizophrenia but the stresses of trying to receive care and services. Health care systems are complex and are often at the mercy of outdated policies. Development of assertiveness and conflict resolution skills can help the individual in negotiating access to systems that will provide services. Developing a positive support system for stressful periods helps promote a positive outcome.

Virtual Mental Health Care

Telehealth is being used more broadly for many conditions. It is helpful in circumstances in which physical distance can be a barrier to treatment, such as in some rural communities or in other circumstances, such as when physical distancing was needed during the COVID-19 pandemic. People with schizophrenia who require supportive regular contacts with provider services for counseling, medication and side effect reviews, and assertive community engagement can benefit from telephone or computer-based conferencing. In addition, cellphone applications can help people to monitor health-related activities such as exercise and diet, and they can provide education and interventions such as cognitive-behavioral treatment or mindfulness activities. However, the effectiveness of providing care to people with schizophrenia over distances and with mobile applications needs ongoing evaluation to determine to whom these services accrue the most value.

Integration With Primary Care

Traditionally, mental disorders were treated separately from medical disorders. We now know that an individual cannot successfully recover unless physical and mental health care are integrated. The medical needs of people with schizophrenia are significant and require treatment. There should be a systematic coordination of general and behavioral health. Ideally, the patient would have one record where all care would be documented.

Treatment interventions for mental disorders impact the general health status of the individual. Frequent communication with primary care providers allows monitoring and adjustment of medical treatment. Medication interactions are a concern when patients are receiving medications from several different clinicians.

OTHER SCHIZOPHRENIA SPECTRUM DISORDERS

SCHIZOAFFECTIVE DISORDER (SAD)

SAD, a complex and persistent psychiatric illness, is characterized by periods of intense symptom exacerbation alternating with periods of adequate psychosocial functioning. This disorder is at times marked by psychosis, at other times, by mood disturbance. Patients with SAD are more likely to exhibit persistent psychosis than are patients with a mood disorder. They feel that they are on a "chronic roller coaster ride" of symptoms that are often difficult to manage (Arndtzén & Sandlund, 2022).

The long-term outcome of patients with SAD is generally better than that of schizophrenia but worse than that of a mood disorder (Preda & Bota, 2024). These patients resemble the mood disorder group in work function (see Chapter 25) and the schizophrenia group in social function. People with SAD usually have higher functioning than those with schizophrenia with severe negative symptoms and early onset of illness (Arndtzén & Sandlund, 2022).

Patients with SAD are at risk for suicide. The risk for suicide in patients with psychosis is increased by the presence of depression. Risk factors for suicide increase with the use of alcohol or substances, cigarette smoking, previous suicide attempts, and hospitalizations. Lack of regular social contact may be a factor that confers a long-term risk for suicidal behavior. This risk may be reduced by treatments designed to enhance social networks and contacts, and those focused on helping patients protect themselves against environmental stressors (Defayette et al., 2024).

DELUSIONAL DISORDER

Delusional disorder is characterized by stable and well-systematized delusions that occur in the absence of other psychiatric disorders. Delusions are the primary symptom of this disorder. Apart from the direct impact of the delusion, psychosocial functioning is not markedly impaired. Examples of delusions include being followed, poisoned, infected, loved at a distance, or deceived by a spouse or lover (Joseph & Siddiqui, 2023).

The course of delusional disorder varies. The onset can be acute, or the disorder can occur gradually and become chronic. Patients usually live with delusions for years, rarely receiving psychiatric treatment unless their delusion relates to their health (somatic delusion), or they act on the basis of their delusion and violate legal or social rules. Full remissions can be followed by relapses. Behavior is not unusual except when the patient focuses on the delusion. At that time, thinking, attitudes, and mood may change abruptly. Personality does not usually change, but the patient is gradually and progressively involved with the delusional concern.

Delusional disorder is relatively uncommon in clinical settings (Joseph & Siddiqui, 2023).

SCHIZOPHRENIFORM DISORDER

The essential features of schizophreniform disorder are identical to those of schizophrenia, with the exception of the duration of the illness, which can be less than 6 months. Symptoms must be present for at least 1 month to be classified as a schizophreniform disorder. About one third of the individuals recover, with the other two thirds developing schizophrenia (APA, 2022).

BRIEF PSYCHOTIC DISORDER

In brief psychotic disorder, the length of the episode is at least 1 day but less than 1 month. The onset is sudden and includes at least one of the positive symptoms of schizophrenia. The individual generally experiences emotional turmoil or overwhelming confusion and rapid, intense shifts of affect. Although episodes are brief, impairment can be severe, and supervision may be required to protect the individual. Suicide is a risk, especially in younger patients (Fusar-Poli et al., 2022).

SUBSTANCE MEDICATION–INDUCED PSYCHOTIC DISORDER

Patients with a psychotic disorder attributed to a substance present with prominent hallucinations or delusions that are the direct physiologic effects of a substance (e.g., drug use, toxin exposure). During intoxication, symptoms continue as long as the use of the substance continues. Withdrawal symptoms can last for several weeks. Differential diagnosis is recommended (Baldaçara et al., 2023).

SUMMARY OF KEY POINTS

- Schizophrenia displays a complex of symptoms typically categorized as positive symptoms (i.e., those that exist but should not), such as delusions or hallucinations, and disorganized thinking and behavior, and negative symptoms (i.e., characteristics that should be there but are lacking), such as alogia, avolition, anhedonia, and diminished emotional expression.
- The clinical course of schizophrenia begins with a prodromal period in childhood that is usually not recognized as a precursor to schizophrenia. An acute illness usually occurs in late adolescence and may require hospitalization when medication and recovery-oriented care are initiated. In recovery-oriented care, the nurse instills hope and partners with the individual with schizophrenia to develop strategies to recover and lead a meaningful life.
- The cause of schizophrenia is thought to be related to genetic, neurodevelopmental, and neurotransmission dysfunction. Environmental stress can trigger acute episodes.
- Nursing assessment begins with the development of the therapeutic relationship and includes biologic, psychological, social, and spiritual areas.
- Risk for self-injury or injury to others should always be included in the assessment. Establishment of baseline health information should be done before any medications are administered. Several standardized assessment tools are available to help assess characteristic unexpected motor movements.
- In general, the antipsychotic drugs used to treat patients with schizophrenia not only block dopamine transmission in the brain but also cause some troublesome and sometimes serious side effects, primarily anticholinergic side effects and extrapyramidal side effects (i.e., motor irregularities). Newer second-generation antipsychotic agents block serotonin, as well as dopamine. The nurse should be familiar with these drugs, their possible side effects, and the interventions required to manage or control side effects.

- Extrapyramidal side effects of antipsychotic drugs may appear early in drug treatment or after months or years of treatment. These side effects include acute parkinsonism or pseudoparkinsonism, acute dystonia, and akathisia. The primary example of late-appearing extrapyramidal side effects is tardive dyskinesia, which is a severe syndrome involving unusual motor movements of the mouth, tongue, jaw, trunk, fingers, and toes.
- Health promotion and wellness interventions are important for overall well-being. People with schizophrenia spectrum disorders have special challenges because their medications can produce a negative impact on their physical health. Nurses can provide education and guidance for positive activity, exercise, and nutrition strategies that can counteract the effect of the medications and symptoms.
- Because schizophrenia is a lifetime disorder and patients require the continued support and care of mental health professionals and family or friends, one of the primary nursing interventions is ensuring that patients and families are properly educated regarding the course of the disorder, importance of drug maintenance, and need for consistent care and support. Positive interaction between patients and their families is key to the success of long-term treatments and outcomes.
- Other schizophrenia spectrum disorders (e.g., schizoaffective, delusional, and schizotypal disorders, brief psychotic disorder, schizophreniform disorder, and substance medication–induced psychotic disorder) have symptoms similar to those of schizophrenia. Nursing care should be individualized based on a nursing assessment and current evidence related to care.

DEVELOPING CLINICAL JUDGMENT

1. Describe steps the nurse should take to ensure an assessment considers the cultural basis of a patient's hallucinations and delusions.
2. A patient asks you to explain the difference between "positive" and "negative" symptoms. Develop an answer in "lay" terms for the question.
3. What steps might the nurse take to develop trust in a patient who has hallucinations and delusions and is frightened of other people?
4. Given that a patient with mental illness requires extra efforts at confidentiality and that patients with schizophrenia are often suspicious of their family members, explain ways you can help families and patients develop positive interactions.
5. A patient tells you that they have nothing to live for and everyone would be better off without them. You recognize that the patient may be having suicidal thoughts. What assessment questions would you ask? How would you help the patient develop a safety plan?
6. Discuss how therapeutic communication might have to change when collaborating with an individual with schizophrenia who is displaying primarily negative symptoms. How will you deal with the individual's diminished response to you (both verbally and emotionally) when you are teaching or giving instructions for activities? How will you help the individual compensate for some of their cognitive deficits?
7. An individual with schizophrenia is admitted during a relapse. The patient says they did not want to take haloperidol anymore because it made them shake. The provider prescribes olanzapine. Develop a medication education plan that includes a comparison between olanzapine and haloperidol.
8. Mr. J. has just received a diagnosis of schizophrenia. During a recent outpatient visit, he confides to a nurse that he just has stress and does not think that he really has any psychiatric issues. Identify assessment areas that should be pursued before the patient leaves his appointment. How would you confront the patient's anosognosia?
9. A patient says their medication is not working. The patient is taking ziprasidone 40 mg twice a day. The patient tells you that they take 40 mg before breakfast and 40 mg before bed. What interventions are needed to increase the effectiveness of the drug?
10. Ms. J. was prescribed olanzapine for schizophrenia 1 month ago. Since her last monthly visit, she has gained 15 lb. She is considering discontinuing her medication regimen because of the weight gain. Develop a plan to address her weight gain and her intention to discontinue her medication regimen.
11. An older adult in a nursing home has a delusion that their spouse is having an affair with their sibling. Discuss nonpharmacologic nursing interventions that should be implemented with this patient. How would you explain the patient's delusion to their spouse? Develop a plan for clinical management, focusing on psychiatric nursing care, for a patient experiencing this condition.
12. A patient is taking clozapine and asks you to explain the purpose of the regular blood draws.

MOVIES, TV, OR STREAMING PROGRAMS

A Beautiful Mind: **2001.** This Academy Award-winning movie starring Russell Crowe is based on the biography by Sylvia Nasar of the mathematician and Nobel Laureate John Nash, Jr. It presents the life and experiences of this individual as he dealt with schizophrenia. It shows how his life and work were altered and the effects on his relationships with family and colleagues. The movie depicts how this man came to terms with his illness.

Viewing Points:

1. How does the treatment John Nash received in the 1950s differ from treatment today?
2. How would you classify his symptoms according to the *DSM-5-TR*?
3. What is typical or problematic about Mr. Nash's relationship with the medications prescribed for him?
4. How did the film show the impact of public stigma on Mr. Nash?

***The Soloist:* 2009.** Based on a true story, this movie portrays the experience of a reporter/novelist named Steve Lopez (played by Robert Downey, Jr.) when he befriends Nathaniel Anthony Ayers, "the soloist" (played by Jamie Fox), who has severe, persistent, and untreated schizophrenia—and more importantly, exceptional musical talent. Formerly a student at the prestigious Julliard School of Music in New York City, Ayers now lives on the streets of Los Angeles playing his two-string violin. See also the book by the same title.

Viewing Points:

1. What were the risks and rewards of Steve Lopez taking on such an intense personal relationship with Nathaniel?
2. What were the symptoms of schizophrenia that Nathaniel Aryes exhibited when Steve Lopez met him?
3. How best can nurses advocate for individuals with severe mental illness (and their family and friends) when community resources are inadequate?

REFERENCES

Allott, K., van-der-El, K., Bryce, S., Parrish, E. M., McGurk, S. R., Hetrick, S., Bowie, C. R., Kidd, S., Hamilton, M., Killackey, E., & Velligan, D. (2020). Compensatory interventions for cognitive impairments in psychosis: A systematic review and meta-analysis. *Schizophrenia Bulletin, 46*(4), 869–883. https://doi.org/10.1093/schbul/sbz134

American Psychiatric Association. (2022). *Diagnostic and statistical manual of mental disorders* (5th ed. text revision). Author.

Arndtzén, M., & Sandlund, M. (2022). To live with a schizoaffective disorder. *Journal of Psychiatric and Mental Health Nursing, 29*(1), 4–8. https://doi.org/10.1111/jpm.12708

Baeza, I., de la Serna, E., Mezquida, G., Cuesta, M. J., Vieta, E., Amoretti, S., Lobo, A., González-Pinto, A., Díaz-Caneja, C. M., Corripio, I., Valli, I., Puig, O., Mané, A., Bioque, M., Ayora, M., Bernardo, M., Castro-Fornieles, J., & PEPs Group.(2024). Prodromal symptoms and the duration of untreated psychosis in first episode of psychosis patients: what differences are there between early vs. adult onset and between schizophrenia vs. bipolar disorder?. *European Child & Adolescent Psychiatry, 33*(3), 799–810. https://doi.org/10.1007/s00787-023-02196-7

Balaji, S., & Sankaranarayanan, A., (2023). The association between adverse childhood experiences and metabolic syndrome in severe mental illness: A literature review. *Australasian Psychiatry, 31*(3), 381–388.

Baldaçara, L., Ramos, A., & Castaldelli-Maia, J. M. (2023). Managing drug-induced psychosis. *International Review of Psychiatry, 35*(5–6), 496–502. https://doi.org/10.1080/09540261.2023.2261544

Barlati, S., Nibbio, G., & Vita, A. (2021). Schizophrenia during the COVID-19 pandemic. *Current Opinion in Psychiatry, 34*(3), 203–210. https://doi.org/10.1097/YCO.0000000000000702

Barlati, S., Nibbio, G., & Vita, A. (2024). Evidence-based psychosocial interventions in schizophrenia: A critical review. *Current Opinion in Psychiatry, 37*(3), 131–139. https://doi.org/10.1097/YCO.0000000000000925

Benedyk, A., Moldavski, A. Reichert, M., Reinhard, I., Lohr, S., Schwarz, K., Berhe, O., Höflich, A., Lautenbach, S., von der Goltz, C., Ebner-Priemer, U., Zipf, A., Tost, H., & Meyer-Lindenberg, A. (2023). Initial response to the COVID-19 pandemic on real-life well-being, social contact and roaming behavior in patients with schizophrenia, major depression and healthy controls: A longitudinal ecological momentary assessment study. *European Neuropsychopharmacology, 69*, 79–83.

Bighelli, I., Çıray, O., Salahuddin, N. H., & Leucht, S. (2024). Cognitive behavioural therapy without medication for schizophrenia. *The Cochrane Database of Systematic Reviews, 2*(2), CD015332. https://doi.org/10.1002/14651858.CD015332.pub2

Böge, K., Hahne, I., Bergmann, N., Wingenfeld, K., Zierhut, M., Thoma, N., Ta, T. M. T., Bajbouj, M., & Hahn, E. (2021). Mindfulness-based group therapy for in-patients with schizophrenia spectrum disorders—Feasibility, acceptability, and preliminary outcomes of a rater-blinded randomized controlled trial. *Schizophrenia Research, 228*, 134–144.

Bogie, B. J. M., Noël, C., Gu, F., Nadeau, S., Shvetz, C., Khan, H., Rivard, M. C., Bouchard, S., Lepage, M., & Guimond, S. (2024). Using virtual reality to improve verbal episodic memory in schizophrenia: A proof-of-concept trial. *Schizophrenia Research. Cognition, 36*, 100305. https://doi.org/10.1016/j.scog.2024.100305

Bristol Myers Squibb. (2024). Prescribing information. Retrieved December 30, 2024, from https://packageinserts.bms.com/pi/pi_cobenfy.pdf

Buchsbaum, M. S. (1990). The frontal lobes, basal ganglia, and temporal lobes as a site for schizophrenia. *Schizophrenia Bulletin, 16*(3), 377–387.

Castle, D., & Li, A. (2023). Physical health monitoring for people with schizophrenia. *Australian Prescriber, 46*(4), 75–79. https://doi.org/10.18773/austprescr.2023.024

Cernika, K., & Vrublevska, J. (2024). The impact of adverse childhood experiences on depression and suicidality in patients with schizophrenia. *Psychiatria Danubina, 36*(Suppl 2), 61–67.

Citrome, L., Isaacson, S. H., Larson, D., & Kremens, D. (2021). Tardive dyskinesia in older persons taking antipsychotics. *Neuropsychiatric Disease and Treatment, 17*, 3127–3134. https://doi.org/10.2147/NDT.S328301

Correll, C. U., Arango, C., Fagerlund, B., Galderisi, S., Kas, M. J., & Leucht, S. (2024). Identification and treatment of individuals with childhood-onset and early-onset schizophrenia. *European Neuropsychopharmacology: The Journal of the European College of Neuropsychopharmacology, 82*, 57–71. https://doi.org/10.1016/j.euroneuro.2024.02.005

Daniel, D. G., Cohen, A. S., Harvey, P. D., Velligan, D. I., Potter, W. Z., Horan, W. P., Moore, R. C., & Marder, S. R. (2024). Rationale and challenges for a new instrument for remote measurement of negative symptoms. *Schizophrenia Bulletin Open, 5*(1), sgae027. https://doi.org/10.1093/schizbullopen/sgae027

Defayette, A. B., Silverstein, S. M., & Pisani, A. R. (2024). Social network structure as a biopsychosocial suicide prevention target for young people at clinical high-risk for psychosis. *Schizophrenia Research, 270*, 63–67. https://doi.org/10.1016/j.schres.2024.06.006

Dokuz, G., Kani, A. S., Uysal, Ö. & Kuşcu, M. K. (2022). The impact of childhood trauma and daily life experiences on emotional and psychotic symptom intensity in psychosis: An experience sampling study. *Psychiatry Research, 317*, 114872. https://doi.org/10.1016/j.psychres.2022.114872

Esposito, C. M., De Cagna, F., Caldiroli, A., Capuzzi, E., Ceresa, A., Di Paolo, M., Auxilia, A. M., Capellazzi, M., Tagliabue, I., Cirella, L., Clerici, M., Brondino, N., Barkin, J. L., Politi, P., & Buoli, M. (2024). Gender differences in clinical and biochemical parameters among patients hospitalized for schizophrenia: towards precision medicine. *European Archives of Psychiatry and Clinical Neuroscience, 274*(5), 1093–1103. https://doi.org/10.1007/s00406-023-01644-4

Fashaw-Walters, S. A., McCreedy, E., Bynum, J. P. W., Thomas, K. S., & Shireman, T. I. (2021). Disproportionate increases in schizophrenia diagnoses among Black nursing home residents with ADRD. *Journal of the American Geriatrics Society, 69*(12), 3623–3630. https://doi.org/10.1111/jgs.17464

Fitzgerald, I., Crowley, E. K., Ní Dhubhlaing, C., O'Dwyer, S., & Sahm, L. J. (2024). Informing the development of antipsychotic-induced weight gain management guidance: Patient experiences and preferences—qualitative descriptive study. *BJPsych Open, 10*(5), e136. https://doi.org/10.1192/bjo.2024.725

Franzen, G. (1970). Plasma free fatty acids before and after an intravenous insulin injection in acute schizophrenic men. *British Journal of Psychiatry, 116*(531), 173–177.

Fusar-Poli, P., Salazar de Pablo, G., Rajkumar, R. P., López-Díaz, Á., Malhotra, S., Heckers, S., Lawrie, S. M., & Pillmann, F. (2022). Diagnosis, prognosis, and treatment of brief psychotic episodes: A review and research agenda. *The Lancet Psychiatry, 9*(1), 72–83. https://doi.org/10.1016/S2215-0366(21)00121-8

Gangadin, S. S., Cahn, W., Scheewe, T. W., Hulshoff Pol, H. E., & Bossong, M. G. (2021). Reduced resting state functional connectivity in the hippocampus-midbrain-striatum network of schizophrenia patients. *Journal of Psychiatric Research, 138*, 83–88. https://doi.org/10.1016/j.jpsychires.2021.03.041

GBD 2021 Diseases and Injuries Collaborators (2024). Global incidence, prevalence, years lived with disability (YLDs), disability-adjusted life-years (DALYs), and healthy life expectancy (HALE) for 371 diseases and injuries in 204 countries and territories and 811 subnational locations, 1990–2021: a systematic analysis for the Global Burden of Disease Study 2021. *Lancet*, S0140-6736(24)00757-8. Advance online publication. https://doi.org/10.1016/S0140-6736(24)00757-8

Giacco, D., Chevalier, A., Patterson, M., Hamborg, T., Mortimer, R., Feng, Y., Webber, M., Xanthopoulou, P., & Priebe, S. (2021). Effectiveness and cost-effectiveness of a structured social coaching intervention for people with psychosis (SCENE): Protocol for a fizerzed controlled trial. *BMJ Open, 11*(12), e050627. https://doi.org/10.1136/bmjopen-2021-050627

Giordano, G. M., Bucci, P., Mucci, A., Pezzella, P., & Galderisi, S. (2021). Gender differences in clinical and psychosocial features among persons with schizophrenia: A mini review. *Frontiers in Psychiatry, 12*, 789179. https://doi.org/10.3389/fpsyt.2021.789179

Girdhar, A., & Patil, R. (2023). Caregivers' burden in patients with bipolar disorder and schizophrenia and its relationship with anxiety and depression in caregivers: a narrative review. *Cureus, 15*(10), e47497. https://doi.org/10.7759/cureus.47497

Green, M. F., & Jimenez, A. M. (2022). Clinical observations and neuroscientific evidence tell a similar story: Schizophrenia is a disorder of the self-other boundary. *Schizophrenia Research, 22*, 45–48. https://doi.org/10.1016/j.schres.2021.12.032

Gruber, M., Alexopoulos, J., Doering, S., Feichtinger, K., Friedrich, F., Klauser, M., Hinterbuchinger, B., Litvan, Z., Mossaheb, N., Parth, K., Wininger, A., & Blüml, V. (2023). Personality functioning and self-disorders in individuals at ultra-high risk for psychosis, with first-episode psychosis and with borderline personality disorder. *BJPsych Open, 9*(5), e150. https://doi.org/10.1192/bjo.2023.530

Halstead, S., Cao, C., Høgnason Mohr, G., Ebdrup, B. H., Pillinger, T., McCutcheon, R. A., Firth, J., Siskind, D., & Warren, N. (2024). Prevalence of multimorbidity in people with and without severe mental illness: a systematic review and meta-analysis. *The Lancet Psychiatry, 11*(6), 431–442. https://doi.org/10.1016/S2215-0366(24)00091-9

Harding, C. M., Zubin, J., & Strauss, J. S. (1987). Chronicity in schizophrenia: Fact, partial fact or artifact? *Hospital and Community Psychiatry, 38*(5), 477–486.

Hasson-Ohayon, I., Cheli, S., & Lysaker, P. H. (2021). Emerging psychotherapeutic approaches to addressing self-experience in schizophrenia spectrum disorders. *Journal of Clinical Psychology*, 77(8), 1781–1785. https://doi.org/10.1002/jclp.23223

Hazlett, E. A., Vaccaro, D. H., Haznedar, M. M., & Goldstein, K. E. (2019). F-18 Fluorodeoxyglucose positron emission tomography studies of the schizophrenia spectrum: The legacy of Monte S. Buchsbaum, M. D. *Psychiatry Research, 271*, 535–540. https://doi.org/10.1016/j.psychres.2018.12.030

Howe, J., MacPhee, M., Duddy, C., Habib, H., Wong, G., Jacklin, S., Oduola, S., Upthegrove, R., Carlish, M., Allen, K., Patterson, E., & Maidment, I. (2023). A realist review of medication optimisation of community dwelling service users with serious mental illness. *BMJ Quality & Safety*, bmjqs-2023-016615. https://doi.org/10.1136/bmjqs-2023-016615

Howes, O. D., Bukala, B. R., & Beck, K. (2024). Schizophrenia: from neurochemistry to circuits, symptoms and treatments. *Nature Reviews Neurology, 20*(1), 22–35. https://doi.org/10.1038/s41582-023-00904-0

Huxley, P., Krayer, A., Poole, R., Prendergast, L., Aryal, S., & Warner, R. (2021). Schizophrenia outcomes in the 21st century: A systematic review. *Brain and Behavior, 11*(6), e02172. https://doi.org/10.1002/brb3.2172

Impara, E., Bakolis, I., Bécares, L., Dasch, H., Dregan, A., Dyer, J., Hotopf, M., Stewart, R.J., Stuart, R., Ocloo, J., & Das-Munshi, J. (2022). COVID-19 ethnic inequalities in mental health and multimorbidities: Protocol for the COVEIMM study. *Social Psychiatry and Psychiatric Epidemiology, 57*, 2511–2521. https://doi.org/10.1007/s00127-022-02305-y

Jester, D. J. Thomas, M. L., Sturm, E. T., Harvey, P. D., Keshavan, M., Davis, B. J., Saxena, S., Tampi, R., Leutwyler, H., Compton, M. T., Palmer, B. W., & Jeste, D. V. (2023). Review of major social determinants of health in schizophrenia-spectrum psychotic disorders: I. Clinical outcomes. *Schizophrenia Bulletin, 49*(4), 837–850.

Joseph, S. M., & Siddiqui, W. (2023). Delusional disorder. In *StatPearls*. StatPearls Publishing. https://pubmed.ncbi.nlm.nih.gov/30969677/

Kadakia, A., Fan, Q., Shepherd, J., Bailey, H., Dembek, C., Walker, C., & Williams, G. R. (2021). Point-in-time survey of healthcare resource utilization, employment, quality of life and caregiver status by disease severity in patients with schizophrenia in the US. *Current Medical Research and Opinion, 38*(3), 469–478. https://doi.org/10.1080/03007995.2021.2007690

Karl, S., Sartorius, A., & Aksay, S. S. (2024). Catatonia and ECT across the lifespan. *Schizophrenia Research, 263*, 246–251. https://doi.org/10.1016/j.schres.2023.04.004

Karyakina, M., & Shmukler, A. (2021). Network analysis of cognitive deficit in patients with schizophrenia spectrum disorders. *Schizophrenia Research Cognition, 26*, 100213. https://doi.org/10.1016/j.scog.2021.100213

Kay, S. R., Fiszbein, A., & Opler, L. A. (1987). The Positive and Negative Syndrome Scale (PANSS) for schizophrenia. *Schizophrenia Bulletin, 13*(2), 261–276.

Kern, R. S., Zarate, R., Glynn, S. M., Turner, L. R., Smith, K. M., Mitchell, S. S., Sugar, C. A., Bell, M. D., Liberman, R. P., Kopelowicz, A., & Green, M. F. (2018). Improving work outcome in supported employment for serious mental illness: Results from 2 independent studies of errorless learning. *Schizophrenia Bulletin, 44*(1), 38–45. https://doi.org/10.1093/schbul/sbx100

Kotsakis Ruehlmann, A., Sammallahti, S., Cortés Hidalgo, A. P., Bakulski, K. M., Binder, E. B., Campbell, M. L., Caramaschi, D., Cecil, C. A. M., Colicino, E., Cruceanu, C., Czamara, D., Dieckmann, L., Dou, J., Felix, J. F., Frank, J., Håberg, S. E., Herberth, G., Hoang, T. T., Houtepen, L. C., … Brunst, K. J. (2023). Epigenome-wide meta-analysis of prenatal maternal stressful life events and newborn DNA methylation. *Molecular Psychiatry, 28*(12), 5090–5100. https://doi.org/10.1038/s41380-023-02010-5

Lee, S., & Schwartz, S. (2021). Adherence and persistence to long-acting injectable dopamine receptor blocking agent therapy in the United States: A systematic review and meta-analysis of cohort studies. *Psychiatry Research, 306*, 114277. https://doi.org/10.1016/j.psychres.2021.114277

Li, Z., Tao, X., Wang, D., Pu, J., Liu, Y., Gui, S., Zhong, X., Yang, D., Zhou, H., Tao, W., Chen, W., Chen, X., Chen, Y., Chen, X., & Xie, P. (2024). Alterations of the gut microbiota in patients with schizophrenia. *Frontiers in Psychiatry, 15*, 1366311. https://doi.org/10.3389/fpsyt.2024.1366311

Liloia, D., Brasso, C., Cauda, F., Mancuso, L., Nani, A., Manuello, J., Costa, T., Duca, S., & Rocca, P. (2021). Updating and characterizing neuroanatomical markers in high-risk subjects, recently diagnosed and chronic patients with schizophrenia: A revised coordinate-based meta-analysis. *Neuroscience and Biobehavioral Reviews, 123*, 83–103. https://doi.org/10.1016/j.neubiorev.2021.01.010

Lim, C., Hernandez, M., Gaona, L., & Barrio, C. (2021). Recruitment of Asian Americans with schizophrenia spectrum disorder for research participation: Barriers, strategies, and outcomes. *Community Mental Health Journal, 57*(3), 490–501. https://doi.org/10.1007/s10597-020-00670-z

Lopez, D., Escalante, G. S., & de Mamani, A. W. (2023). The role of religious coping on suicidality among Latinx and Black/African American individuals with schizophrenia spectrum disorders. *Spirituality in Clinical Practice, 10*(3), 219–232. https://doi.org/10.1037/scp0000317

Lysaker, P. H. (2021). Schizophrenia, the self and psychotherapy: Is there really anything new under the sun?. *Journal of Clinical Psychology*, 77(8), 1865–1870. https://doi.org/10.1002/jclp.23234

Mallaro, H. L., & Rosenthal, L. J. (2023). DRESS syndrome: quetiapine associated case report and literature review. *International Clinical Psychopharmacology, 38*(5), 356–360. https://doi.org/10.1097/YIC.0000000000000474

Mark, T. L., Henretty, K., Gibbons, B. J., & Zarkin, G. A. (2024). Association of Arizona's implementation of a behavioral health crisis response system with suicide hospitalizations. *Psychiatric Services, 75*(2), 148–154. https://doi.org/10.1176/appi.ps.20220628

Martini, F., Spangaro, M., Bechi, M., Agostoni, G., Buonocore, M., Sapienza, J., Nocera, D., Ave, C., Cocchi, F., Cavallaro, R., & Bosia, M. (2024). Improving outcome of treatment-resistant schizophrenia: effects of cognitive remediation therapy. *European Archives of Psychiatry and Clinical Neuroscience, 274*(6), 1473–1481. https://doi.org/10.1007/s00406-023-01731-6

Martins, R., Kadakia, A., Williams, G. R., Milanovic, S., & Connolly, M. P. (2023). The lifetime burden of schizophrenia as estimated by a government-centric fiscal analytic framework. *The Journal of Clinical Psychiatry, 84*(5), 22m14746. https://doi.org/10.4088/JCP.22m14746

McDonagh, M. S., Dana, T., Kopelovich, S. L., Monroe-DeVita, M., Blazina, I., Bougatsos, C., Grusing, S., & Selph, S. S. (2022). Psychosocial interventions for adults with schizophrenia: An overview and update of systematic reviews. *Psychiatric Services*, *73*(3), 299–312. https://doi.org/10.1176/appi.ps.202000649

Miller, B. J. & McCall, W. V. (2023). Meta-analysis of insomnia, suicide, and psychopathology in schizophrenia. *Current Opinion Psychiatry*, *36*(3), 156–165.

Miola, A., Gardea-Reséndez, M., Ortiz-Orendain, J., Nunez, N. A., Ercis, M., Coombes, B. J., Salgado, M. F., Gruhlke, P. M., Michel, I., Bostwick, J. M., McKean, A. J., Ozerdem, A., & Frye, M. A. (2023). Factors associated with suicide attempts in the antecedent illness trajectory of bipolar disorder and schizophrenia. *International Journal of Bipolar Disorders*, *11*(1), 38. https://doi.org/10.1186/s40345-023-00318-3

Mizuki, Y., Sakamoto, S., Okahisa, Y., Yada, Y., Hashimoto, N., Takaki, M., & Yamada, N. (2021). Mechanisms underlying the comorbidity of schizophrenia and type 2 diabetes mellitus. *The International Journal of Neuropsychopharmacology*, *24*(5), 367–382. https://doi.org/10.1093/ijnp/pyaa097

Mohn, C., Olsson, A. K., van Dijk Härd, I., & Helldin, L. (2023). Neurocognitive function and mortality in patients with schizophrenia spectrum disorders. *Schizophrenia Research. Cognition*, *33*, 100284. https://doi.org/10.1016/j.scog.2023.100284

Morris, A., Reed, T., McBride, G., & Chen, J. (2024). Dietary interventions to improve metabolic health in schizophrenia: A systematic literature review of systematic reviews. *Schizophrenia Research*, *270*, 372–382. https://doi.org/10.1016/j.schres.2024.06.056

Mulugeta, A., Suppiah, V., & Hyppönen, E. (2023). Schizophrenia and co-morbidity risk: Evidence from a data driven phenomewide association study. *Journal of Psychiatric Research*, *162*, 1–10. https://doi.org/10.1016/j.jpsychires.2023.04.010

Munch Nielsen, C., Hjorthøj, C., Arnfred, B. T., & Nordentoft, M. (2023). Patient outcomes of flexible assertive community treatment compared with assertive community treatment. *Psychiatric Services*, *74*(7), 695–701. https://doi.org/10.1176/appi.ps.20220235

Neyra, A., Parro-Torres, C., Ros-Cucurull, E., Carrera, I., Echarri, E., & Torrens, M. (2024). Management of schizophrenia and comorbid substance use disorders: expert review and guidance. *Annals of General Psychiatry*, *23*(1), 40. https://doi.org/10.1186/s12991-024-00529-7

Nolan, C. J., Roepke, T. A., & Perreault, M. L. (2023). Beyond the binary: Gender inclusivity in schizophrenia research. *Biological Psychiatry*, *94*(7),543–549. https://doi.org/10.1016/j.biopsych.2023.03.018

Ociskova, M., Prasko, J., Holubova, M., Latalova, K., Sollar, T., Zatkova, M., Slepecky, M., & Bocek, J. (2023). Self-stigma in patients with schizophrenia: Impact and management. *Neuro Endocrinology Letters*, *44*(6), 368–383.

Ohi, K., Nemoto, K., Kataoka, Y., Sugiyama, S., Muto, Y., Shioiri, T., & Kawasaki, Y. (2021). Alterations in hippocampal subfield volumes among schizophrenia patients, their first-degree relatives and healthy subjects. *Progress in Neuro-psychopharmacology & Biological Psychiatry*, *110*, 110291. https://doi.org/10.1016/j.pnpbp.2021.110291

Olfson, M., Stroup, T. S., Huang, C., Wall, M. M., Crystal, S., & Gerhard, T. (2021). Suicide risk in Medicare patients with schizophrenia across the life span. *JAMA Psychiatry*, *78*(8), 876–885. https://doi.org/10.1001/jamapsychiatry.2021.0841

Oudewortel, L., van der Roest, H. G., Onder, G., Wijnen, V. J. M., Liperoti, R., Denkinger, M., Finne-Soveri, H., Topinková, E., Henrard, J. C., & van Gool, W. A. (2021). The association of anticholinergic drugs and delirium in nursing home patients with dementia: Results from the SHELTER Study. *Journal of the American Medical Directors Association*, *22*(10), 2087–2092. https://doi.org/10.1016/j.jamda.2021.05.039

Parnas, J., & Sandsten, K. E. (2024). The phenomenological nature of schizophrenia and disorder of selfhood. *Schizophrenia Research*, *270*, 197–201. https://doi.org/10.1016/j.schres.2024.06.032

Peralta, V., García de Jalón, E., Moreno-Izco, L., Peralta, D., Janda, L., Sánchez-Torres, A. M., & Cuesta, M. J.; SEGPEPs group.(2024). The association of adverse childhood experiences with long-term outcomes of psychosis: A 21-year prospective cohort study after a first episode of psychosis. *Psychological Medicine*, *54*(11), 3099–3108. https://doi.org/10.1017/S0033291724001223

Pfizer. (2022). GEODON U.S. Physician prescribing information including patient summary of information. Retrieved January 26, 2022, from ShowLabeling.aspx (fizer.com).

Pizzol, D., Trott, M., Butler, L., Barnett, Y., Ford, T., Neufeld, S. A., Ragnhildstveit, A., Parris, C. N., Underwood, B. R., López Sánchez, G. F., Fossey, M., Brayne, C., Fernandez-Egea, E., Fond, G., Boyer, L., Shin, J. I., Pardhan, S., & Smith, L. (2023). Relationship between severe mental illness and physical multimorbidity: a meta-analysis and call for action. *BMJ Mental Health*, *26*(1), e300870. https://doi.org/10.1136/bmjment-2023-300870

Preda, A., & Bota, R. G. (2024). Schizoaffective disorder. *BMJ Best Practice*. Retrieved November 20, 2024, from https://bestpractice.bmj.com/topics/en-us/1199#:~:text=Patients%20have%20a%20better%20prognosis,medications%20than%20patients%20with%20schizophrenia

Reckziegel, R., Czepielewski, L. S., Hasse-Sousa, M., Martins, D. S., de Britto, M. J., Lapa, C. O., Schwartzhaupt, A. W., & Gama, C. S. (2022). Heterogeneous trajectories in schizophrenia: Insights from neurodevelopment and neuroprogression models. *Brazilian Journal of Psychiatry*, *44*(1), 74–80. https://doi.org/10.1590/1516-4446-2020-1670

Reeves, S., Bertrand, J., Obee, S. J., Hunter, S., Howard, R., & Flanagan, R. J. (2024). A population pharmacokinetic model to guide clozapine dose selection, based on age, sex, ethnicity, body weight and smoking status. *British Journal of Clinical Pharmacology*, *90*(1), 135–145. https://doi.org/10.1111/bcp.15691

Rivelli, A., Fitzpatrick, V., Nelson, M., Laubmeier, K., Zeni, C., & Mylavarapu, S. (2024). Real-world predictors of relapse in patients with schizophrenia and schizoaffective disorder in a large health system. *Schizophrenia*, *10*(1), 28. https://doi.org/10.1038/s41537-024-00448-2

Robinson, N., Ploner, A., Leone, M., Lichtenstein, P., Kendler, K. S., & Bergen, S. E. (2024). Environmental risk factors for schizophrenia and bipolar disorder from childhood to diagnosis: a Swedish nested case-control study. *Psychological Medicine*, *54*(9), 2162–2171. Advance online publication. https://doi.org/10.1017/S0033291724000266

Roelandt, J. L., Vinet, M. A., Delissen, S., Askevis-Leherpeux, F., & Chevreul, K. (2024). Impact of follow-up by peer support workers on mental health service users' global functioning and self-stigmatisation. *Encephale*, *50*(4), 416–420. https://doi.org/10.1016/j.encep.2023.08.011

Rooy, M., Lazarevich, I., Koukouli, F., Maskos, U., & Gutkin, B. (2021). Cholinergic modulation of hierarchical inhibitory control over cortical resting state dynamics: Local circuit modeling of schizophrenia-related hypofrontality. *Current Research in Neurobiology*, *2*, 100018. https://doi.org/10.1016/j.crneur.2021.100018

Saarinen, A., Hietala, J., Lyytikäinen, L. P., Hamal Mishra, B., Sormunen, E., Lavonius, V., Kähönen, M., Raitakari, O., Lehtimäki, T., & Keltikangas-Järvinen, L. (2024). Polygenic risk for schizophrenia predicting social trajectories in a general population sample. *Psychological Medicine*, *54*(8), 1589–1597. Advance online publication. https://doi.org/10.1017/S003329172300346X

Sari, S. P., Agustin, M., Wijayanti, D. Y., Sarjana, W., Afrikhah, U., & Choe, K. (2021). Mediating effect of hope on the relationship between depression and recovery in persons with schizophrenia. *Frontiers in Psychiatry*, *12*, 627588. https://doi.org/10.3389/fpsyt.2021.627588

Schimmelbusch, W. H., Mueller, P. S., & Sheps, J. (1971). The positive correlation between insulin resistance and duration of hospitalization in untreated schizophrenia. *British Journal of Psychiatry*, *118*(545), 429–436.

Simon, L. V., Hashmi, M. F., & Callahan, A. L. (2023). Neuroleptic Malignant Syndrome. In *StatPearls*. StatPearls Publishing. https://www.ncbi.nlm.nih.gov/books/NBK482282

Simpson, G. M., & Angus, J. W. (1970). A rating scale for extrapyramidal side effects. *Acta Psychiatrica Scandinavica Suppl*, *212*, 11–19.

Smit, R., Luckhoff, H. K., Phahladira, L., Du Plessis, S., Emsley, R., & Asmal, L. (2024). Relapse in schizophrenia: The role of factors other than non-adherence to treatment. *Early Intervention in Psychiatry*, *18*(9), 710–719. Advance online publication. https://doi.org/10.1111/eip.13510

Solmi, M., Seitidis, G., Mavridis, D., Correll, C. U., Dragioti, E., Guimond, S., Tuominen, L., Dargél, A., Carvalho, A. F., Fornaro, M., Maes, M., Monaco, F., Song, M., Il Shin, J., & Cortese, S. (2023). Incidence, prevalence, and global burden of schizophrenia—data, with critical appraisal, from the Global Burden of Disease (GBD) 2019. *Molecular Psychiatry*, *28*(12), 5319–5327. https://doi.org/10.1038/s41380-023-02138-4

Sprague, R. L., & Kalachnik, J. E. (1991). Reliability, validity, and a total score cutoff for the Dyskinesia Identification Scale System: Condensed User Scale (DISCUS) with mentally ill and mentally retarded populations. *Psychopharmacology Bulletin*, *27*(1), 51–58.

Steen, N. E., Rahman, Z., Szabo, A., Hindley, G. F. L., Parker, N., Cheng, W., Lin, A., O'Connell, K. S., Sheikh, M. A., Shadrin, A., Bahrami, S., Karthikeyan, S., Hoseth, E. Z., Dale, A. M., Aukrust, P., Smeland, O. B., Ueland, T., Frei, O., Djurovic, S., & Andreassen, O. A. (2023). Shared genetic loci between schizophrenia and white blood cell counts suggest genetically determined systemic immune abnormalities. *Schizophrenia Bulletin*, *49*(5), 1345–1354. https://doi.org/10.1093/schbul/sbad082

Stewart, K., Hancock, N., Chapparo, C., & Stancliffe, E. R. J. (2024). Supports that help me to live well in the community: experiences of people living with schizophrenia. *Australian Occupational Therapy Journal*, *71*(2), 340–351. https://doi.org/10.1111/1440-1630.12919

Stewart, V., McMillan, S. S., Roennfeldt, H., El-Den, S., Ng, R., & Wheeler, A. J. (2021). Exploring goal planning in mental health service delivery: A systematic review protocol. *BMJ Open*, *11*(5), e047240. https://doi.org/10.1136/bmjopen-2020-047240

Stone, T., & Short, A. (2024). Can music therapy help adults with schizophrenia improve their cognitive skills? A scoping review. *Issues in Mental Health Nursing*, *45*(1), 55–65. https://doi.org/10.1080/01612840.2023.2266851

Su, Y., Pan, X., Li, H., & Zhang, G. (2024). Effects of mind-body therapies on schizophrenia: A systematic review and network meta-analysis. *Schizophrenia Research*, *264*, 236–247. https://doi.org/10.1016/j.schres.2023.12.030

Tandon, R., Nasrallah, H., Akbarian, S., Carpenter, W. T., Jr, DeLisi, L. E., Gaebel, W., Green, M. F., Gur, R. E., Heckers, S., Kane, J. M., Malaspina, D., Meyer-Lindenberg, A., Murray, R., Owen, M., Smoller, J. W., Yassin, W., & Keshavan, M. (2024). The schizophrenia syndrome, circa 2024: What we know and how that informs its nature. *Schizophrenia Research*, *264*, 1–28. https://doi.org/10.1016/j.schres.2023.11.015

Thongsalab, J., Yunibhand, J., & Uthis, P. (2024). Navigating personal recovery: multinomial logistic regression analysis of schizophrenia outcomes in community-dwelling individuals. *General Psychiatry*, *37*(2), e101325. https://doi.org/10.1136/gpsych-2023-101325

Töbelmann, L., Hahne, I., Schulze, T., Bergmann, N., Fuchs, L., Zierhut, M., Hahn, E., & Böge, K. (2023). Mechanisms of action and processes of yoga-based group intervention for inpatients with schizophrenia spectrum disorders—A longitudinal qualitative study. *Frontiers in Psychiatry*, *14*, 1086468. https://doi.org/10.3389/fpsyt.2023.1086468

Utas-Akhan, L., Avci, D., & Basak, I. (2024). Art Therapy as a Nursing Intervention for Individuals With Schizophrenia. *Journal of psychosocial nursing and mental health services*, *62*(5), 29–38. https://doi.org/10.3928/02793695-20231025-02

Venkataraman, S., Hazan, H., Li, F., Ferrara, M., Harper, A., Ma, J., Shah, J., Musket, C., Levine, N., Keshavan, M. S., & Srihari, V. (2024). Role of early psychosis detection in the relationship between personal income and duration of untreated psychosis. *Psychiatric Services*, *75*(5), 427–433. https://doi.org/10.1176/appi.ps.20230239

Vita, A., Barlati, S., Deste, G., Nibbio, G., Penn, D. L., Pinkham, A. E., McIntyre, R. S., & Harvey, P. D. (2023). Life engagement in people living with schizophrenia: predictors and correlates of patient life engagement in a large sample of people living in the community. *Psychological Medicine*, *53*(16), 7943–7952. https://doi.org/10.1017/S0033291723002106

Vita, A., Nibbio, G., & Barlati, S. (2024). Conceptualization and characterization of "primary" and "secondary" cognitive impairment in schizophrenia. *Psychiatry Research*, *340*, 116126. https://doi.org/10.1016/j.psychres.2024.116126

Warren, B., Vanderhoef, D., & Johnson, J. (2022). VMAT2 Inhibitors for the treatment of tardive dyskinesia. *Issues in Mental Health Nursing*, *43*(1), 22–31. https://doi.org/10.1080/01612840.2021.1948643

Yang, V. X., Sin Fai Lam, C. C., & Kane, J. P. M. (2023). Cognitive impairment and development of dementia in very late-onset schizophrenia-like psychosis: a systematic review. *Irish Journal of Psychological Medicine*, *40*(4), 616–628. https://doi.org/10.1017/ipm.2021.48

Yung, N. C. L., Wong, C. S. M., Chan, J. K. N., & Chang, W. C. (2023). Mortality rates in people with first diagnosis of schizophrenia-spectrum disorders: A 5-year population-based cohort study. *The Australian and New Zealand Journal of Psychiatry*, *57*(6), 854–864. https://doi.org/10.1177/00048674221121575

Zhan, N., Sham, P. C., So, H. C., & Lui, S. S. Y. (2023). The genetic basis of onset age in schizophrenia: evidence and models. *Frontiers in Genetics*, *14*, 1163361. https://doi.org/10.3389/fgene.2023.1163361

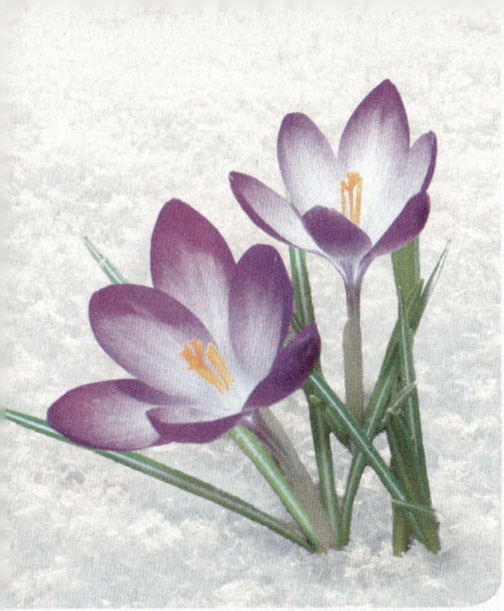

25 Depression

Nursing Care of People With Depressive Moods and Suicidal Behavior

Barbara Jones Warren and Mary Ann Boyd

KEYCONCEPTS

- depression
- mood
- suicidal behavior

LEARNING OBJECTIVES

After studying this chapter, you will be able to:

1. Examine the roles of mood and depression in depressive disorders.
2. Relate the primary theories of major depressive disorder to clinical symptoms and the course of the disorder.
3. Evaluate the significance of trauma in the appearance of depression symptoms.
4. Examine the relationship between social determinants of health and major depressive disorder.
5. Select strategies to establish a therapeutic relationship with people with major depressive disorder.
6. Using a clinical judgment model, formulate a person-centered, recovery-oriented nursing care plan for people with major depressive disorder.
7. Identify medications that are used to treat people with major depressive disorder and evaluate their effectiveness.
8. Develop wellness strategies for people with major depressive disorder.
9. Compare and contrast mental health care provided in emergency, inpatient, community, and virtual settings.
10. Support the integration of health care and mental health care for people with major depressive disorder.
11. Compare and contrast depression and other depressive disorders.

KEY TERMS

• affect • anhedonia • antenatal depression • cognitive-behavioral therapy • cytokines • depressive disorders • disruptive mood dysregulation disorder • esketamine • glucocorticoids • gut–brain axis • insomnia • interpersonal therapy • interpersonal trauma • major depressive disorder • medical home model • microaggression • perinatal depression • persistent depressive disorder • postpartum depression • premenstrual dysphoric disorder • racism • resilience • self-concept • self-esteem • serotonin syndrome • social determinants of health • suicidal ideation • suicidality

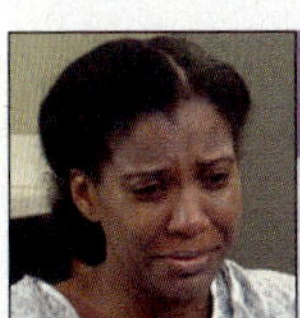

Case Study: Louise

Louise, age 31, was admitted voluntarily to an inpatient mental health unit with depression with suicidal ideation. Louise and her husband, Brian, have three children ages 9, 5, and 3 years.

INTRODUCTION

Most people have bad days or times of feeling sad and overwhelmed. When depressed feelings interfere with daily activities and relationships, however, this mood can impair judgment and contribute to negative views of the world. In some instances, depression is a symptom of a depressive disorder. This chapter discusses mood and depression, depressive disorders, and the related serious issue of suicidal behavior. Major depressive disorder is highlighted.

MOOD AND DEPRESSION

Usual variations in mood occur in response to life events. Normal mood variations (e.g., sadness, euphoria, and anxiety) are time-limited and are not usually associated with significant functional impairment. Normal range of mood or affect varies considerably both within and among different cultures (Umucu et al., 2024).

> **KEYCONCEPT Mood** is a pervasive and sustained emotion that influences one's perception of the world and how one functions.

Affect, or outward emotional expression, is related to the concept of mood. Affect provides clues to the individual's mood. For example, in depression, people often have limited facial expression. Several terms are used to describe affect, including the following:

- *Blunted:* significantly reduced intensity of emotional expression
- *Bright:* smiling, projection of a positive attitude
- *Flat:* absent or nearly absent affective expression
- *Inappropriate:* discordant affective expression accompanying the content of speech or ideation
- *Labile:* varied, rapid, and abrupt shifts in affective expression
- *Restricted or constricted:* mildly reduced in the range and intensity of emotional expression

Depression is the primary mood of depressive disorders. Depression can be overwhelming. Unless appropriately treated, depression persists over time, has a significant negative effect on quality of life (QoL), and increases the risk of suicide (Qaseem et al., 2024; Won et al., 2021).

> **KEYCONCEPT Depression** is a common mental state characterized by sadness, loss of interest or pleasure, feelings of guilt or low self-worth, disturbed sleep or appetite, low energy, and poor concentration associated with changes in neurobiologic functioning (American Psychiatric Association [APA], 2022; World Health Organization [WHO], 2023).

DEPRESSIVE DISORDERS OVERVIEW

When a sad mood interferes with daily life, a depressive disorder may exist that will benefit from treatment. In **depressive disorders**, a sad, irritable, or empty mood is present with somatic and cognitive changes that interfere with functioning. Depressive disorders are differentiated according to duration, timing, or cause (APA, 2022). These disorders include major depressive disorder, persistent depressive disorder (dysthymia), premenstrual dysphoric disorder, disruptive mood dysregulation disorder, and substance/medication-induced depressive disorder, and other specified depressive and unspecified depressive disorders (APA, 2022).

Depressive disorders are complex, dynamic, biopsychosocial-spiritual processes. The clinical symptoms and course of these disorders vary throughout the life span according to cultural values and beliefs. People with depressive disorders experience a lower QoL and are at greater risk for development of physical health issues than those who are not depressed. Depressive disorders are so widespread that they are generally diagnosed and treated in the primary care setting. Every nurse will have an opportunity to impact this global health concern.

Depressive disorders are characterized by severe and debilitating depressive episodes and are associated with high levels of impairment in occupational, social, and physical functioning. They cause as much disability and distress to patients as chronic medical disorders. Frequently, they are undetected and untreated. Because suicide is a significant risk, these disorders are associated with premature death, especially in those individuals who have been hospitalized for depression (GBD 2021 Diseases and Injuries Collaborators, 2024).

MAJOR DEPRESSIVE DISORDER

CLINICAL COURSE

Major depressive disorder is usually a progressively recurrent illness. With time, episodes tend to occur more frequently, become more severe, and are of a longer duration. Onset of depression may occur at any age. Even though the initial onset may occur in puberty; the most common onset occurs in people in their 20s (APA, 2022). Recurrences of depression are related to age of onset, increased intensity and severity of symptoms, and presence of psychosis, anxiety, and/or personality features. The risk for relapse is higher in people who have experienced initial symptoms at a younger age and incur other mental disorders (O'Connor et al., 2023).

DIAGNOSTIC CRITERIA

The primary diagnostic criterion for major depressive disorder is one or more moods, which is either a

KEY DIAGNOSTIC CHARACTERISTICS 25.1

***DSM-5-TR* DIAGNOSTIC CRITERIA: Major Depressive Disorder**

A. Five (or more) of the following symptoms have been present during the same 2-week period and represent a change from previous functioning; at least one of the symptoms is either (1) depressed mood or (2) loss of interest or pleasure.

Note: Do not include symptoms that are clearly attributable to another medical condition.

1. Depressed mood most of the day, nearly every day, as indicated by either subjective report (e.g., feels sad, empty, hopeless) or observation made by others (e.g., appears tearful). (**Note:** In children and adolescents, can be irritable mood.)
2. Markedly diminished interest or pleasure in all, or almost all, activities most of the day, nearly every day (as indicated by either subjective account or observation).
3. Significant weight loss when not dieting or weight gain (e.g., a change of more than 5% of body weight in a month) or decrease or increase in appetite nearly every day. (**Note:** In children, consider failure to make expected weight gain.)
4. Insomnia or hypersomnia nearly every day.
5. Psychomotor agitation or retardation nearly every day (observable by others, not merely subjective feelings of restlessness or being slowed down).
6. Fatigue or loss of energy nearly every day.
7. Feelings of worthlessness or excessive or inappropriate guilt (which may be delusional) nearly every day (not merely self-reproach or guilt about being sick).
8. Diminished ability to think or concentrate, or indecisiveness, nearly every day (either by subjective account or as observed by others).
9. Recurrent thoughts of death (not just fear of dying), recurrent suicidal ideation without a specific plan, or a suicide attempt or a specific plan for committing suicide.

B. The symptoms cause clinically significant distress or impairment in social, occupational, or other important areas of functioning.

C. The episode is not attributable to the physiologic effects of a substance or to another medical condition.

Note: Criteria A to C represent a major depressive episode (MDE).

Note: Responses to a significant loss (e.g., bereavement, financial ruin, losses from a natural disaster, a serious medical illness, or disability) may include the feelings of intense sadness, rumination about the loss, insomnia, poor appetite, and weight loss noted in Criterion A, which may resemble a depressive episode. Although such symptoms may be understandable or considered appropriate to the loss, the presence of an MDE in addition to the normal response to a significant loss should also be carefully considered. This decision inevitably requires the exercise of clinical judgment based on the individual's history and the cultural norms for the expression of distress in the context of loss.

D. At least one MDE is not better explained by schizoaffective disorder and is not superimposed on schizophrenia, schizophreniform disorder, delusional disorder, or other specified and unspecified schizophrenia spectrum and other psychotic disorders.

E. There has never been a manic episode or a hypomanic episode.

Note: This exclusion does not apply if all of the manic-like or hypomanic-like episodes are substance induced or are attributable to the physiologic effects of another medical condition.

depressed mood or a loss of interest or pleasure in nearly all activities for at least 2 weeks. Four of seven additional symptoms must be present: disruption in sleep, appetite (or weight), concentration, or energy; psychomotor agitation or retardation; excessive guilt or feelings of worthlessness; and suicidal ideation (Key Diagnostic Characteristics 25.1).

The incidence of misdiagnosis is often greater for people who are treated by someone from a population that is culturally and ethnically different from the patient's. The clinician's explanation of symptomatology may be expressed using unfamiliar terminology, or the patient may feel uncomfortable with a clinician from a different culture (Dorsey Holliman et al., 2024).

DEPRESSIVE DISORDERS ACROSS THE LIFE SPAN

Children and Adolescents

Children with depressive disorders have symptoms similar to those seen in adults with a few exceptions. They are more likely to have anxiety symptoms, such as fear of separation, and somatic symptoms, such as stomach aches and headaches. They may have less interaction with their peers and avoid play and recreational activities that they previously enjoyed. Mood may be irritable, rather than sad, especially in adolescents. See Chapter 37 for discussion of mental health disorders in children and adolescents.

The risk of suicide, which peaks during the midadolescent years, is very real in children and adolescents. Mortality from suicide, which increases steadily through the teens, is the third leading cause of death for that age group. Findings from research indicate that experiencing chronic bullying increases the risk for depression and suicidal ideation and attempts (Kennedy & Brausch, 2024). The use of substances intensifies depressive symptomatology and the risk of suicide (Oladunjoye et al., 2023).

The COVID-19 pandemic presented psychological challenges to children and adolescents. Virtual learning during community lockdowns meant children could not engage in normal childhood socialization. College students spent weeks in isolation either at home or in a college dormitory. Learning suffered, and suicidal ideation and attempts increased during the pandemic (Danzo et al., 2024). See Chapter 16 for further discussion of suicide in children and adolescents.

Older Adults

Depression in older adults is often undetected or inadequately treated (Brasileiro et al., 2024). The prevalence of major depressive disorder in adults aged 65 and older ranges from 6% to 9%. Significant depressive symptoms are present in approximately 15% of older adults (Sekhon et al., 2023). Depression in older adults is often associated with chronic illnesses, such as heart disease, stroke, and cancer; symptoms may have a more somatic focus. Depressive symptomatology in this group may be confused with symptoms of bipolar, dementia, or cerebrovascular accidents. Hence, differential diagnosis may be required to ascertain the root and cause of symptoms. See Chapter 39 for further discussion of mental health disorders in older adults.

COVID-19 negatively affected the psychological well-being of many older adults. Social isolation due to sheltering-in-place was associated with greater loneliness and depression. Relationships with family and friends often changed, sometimes permanently. Pandemic-related stressors included confinement and restrictions, concern about other family members, and feelings of loneliness and isolation (Ahmadi et al., 2023).

Suicide is a very serious risk for older adults, especially for those assigned male at birth. Suicide rates peak during middle age, but a second peak occurs in those aged 75 years and older (Garnett et al., 2023). During the COVID-19 pandemic, there was concern among mental health experts that many older adults felt that if they contracted the disease they would need more care than younger people and therefore might believe they would place a burden on society. This belief, combined with lack of access to mental health care caused by COVID-19 social restrictions, increased older adults' risk of suicide during the pandemic (Sadek et al., 2024). See Box 25.1 and Chapter 22.

EPIDEMIOLOGY AND RISK FACTORS

The prevalence of major depressive disorder within the U.S. population is approximately 8.3% within a 12-month time period, with a lifetime prevalence of 20.6%. Individuals between the ages of 18 and 29 years have a higher prevalence rate than do people aged 65 and older. The prevalence of adults with a major depressive disorder was highest among individuals aged 18 to 25 (18%). Episodes typically last more than 6 months. The prevalence of depression is highest among non-Hispanic White adults (21.9%), followed by non-Hispanic Black or African-American (16.2%), non-Hispanic Native Hawaiian or other Pacific Islander (14.6%), Hispanic or Latino (14.6%), and non-Hispanic Asian (7.3%) adults (Lee et al., 2023). In 2021, 14.7% of adolescents aged 12 to 17 years experienced at least one major depressive episode (MDE) with impairment (NIMH, 2023).

The prevalence of major depressive disorder among cultural and ethnic groups is unclear. Although some studies show that Non-Hispanic Black individuals have lower prevalence of major depression compared to non-Hispanic White individuals, researchers suggest that measurement scales for depression may not be culturally adapted to identify symptoms in certain racial and ethnic groups; additionally, as a result of stigma and lack of trust of the health care system, fewer Black people than White people access mental health services (Pederson, 2023).

Data from the WHO indicate that depression is the leading cause of years lost because of disability. More than 50% of people who recover from an initial episode of depression experience another episode within 5 to 10 years (WHO, 2023).

Risk factors for the development of depression include the following:

- Prior episode of depression
- Family history of depressive disorder
- Lack of social support
- Lack of coping abilities
- Presence of life and environmental stressors
- Current substance use or misuse
- Medical and/or mental illness comorbidity

BOX 25.1

Clinical Judgment Vignette: Depression in an Older Adult

Bob, age 75, lost his wife to cancer 18 months ago. Since his wife's death, he continued to live in their family home with his dog. His dog died 2 weeks ago, and he has been despondent since then. His children found him sitting on the side of his bed with a loaded gun. He had already written a note stating he did not want to be a burden and that his children would be better off without him. His family brought him to the emergency department for evaluation.

Building Clinical Judgment

1. What is the likelihood that Bob would actually kill himself?
2. What do you think the next recovery-oriented strategy should be for Bob and his family?

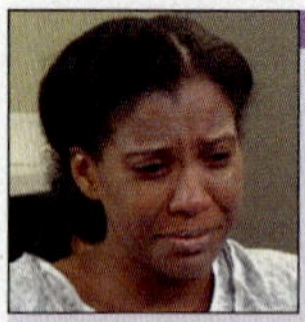

Consider Louise

Louise's sister died as a result of drowning 2 months ago. She has been telling her husband that she just wants to go to sleep and not wake up. What risk factors do you recognize?

Sex Assigned at Birth

Throughout the life cycle, people assigned female at birth have a higher rate of depression than those assigned male at birth. There are a variety of explanations for this occurrence; people assigned female at birth are more likely to experience abuse and trauma during childhood, setting the stage for depression in later life (Canatan et al., 2024); in addition, endocrine changes associated with depression that occur across their reproductive lifestyle are well documented (Hantsoo et al., 2023).

Depression is associated with low-income living (Corcoran et al., 2021). White people assigned female at birth (8.9%) are more likely than White people assigned male at birth (7.1%) to live in poverty. Other groups have even higher rates, with 18.8% of Black, 17.0% of Latinx, 10.0% of Asian, and 21% of Native American people assigned female at birth living in poverty (Sun, 2023). People assigned female at birth living in poverty are more likely to be the sole parent, leading to food insecurity, inadequate nutrition, and unstable housing (Smith & Mazure, 2021).

Pregnancy

Perinatal depression is conceptualized as **antenatal depression** (depression during pregnancy) and **postpartum depression** (depression that occurs up to a year after delivery). Perinatal depression occurs in one of four pregnancies, and rates are higher in vulnerable populations (Al-Abri et al., 2023). Antenatal depression can lead to pre-term births, low-birth weight, gestational diabetes, substance use, ambivalence about pregnancy, and overall poor health. Infants can be exposed to elevated maternal cortisol and inflammation. Postpartum depression can lead to poor infant–parent bonding and delayed infant development including lower IQ, slower language development, and behavioral issues. It is important for perinatal depression to be recognized and treated (Stewart & Payne, 2023).

LGBTQ+ Individuals and Depressive Disorders

The prevalence of depression in LGBTQ+ individuals is higher than in non-LGBTQ+ people. Individuals who identify as LGBTQ+ face discrimination and stigmatization in school, work, and social settings. In many instances they are rejected by their own family members. These factors predispose them to depression at higher rates than their non-LGBTQ+ peers (Cai et al., 2024). It is estimated that LGBTQ+ youth (ages 13 to 24) make up 20% to 40% of the unhoused population (Mitsdarffer et al., 2023). The circumstances of the COVID-19 pandemic—such as lack of social support, social isolation leading to loneliness, and lack of access to mental health services—further exacerbated the risk for depression and suicide (Kneale & Bécaresm, 2024; Mejova & Homadova, 2023).

Ethnicity and Culture

Mental Health Inequities

Culture and ethnic identity are related to mental health disparities in mental health access and treatment (Cook et al., 2024). **Social determinants of health** (environmental conditions where people are born, live, work, learn, play, worship, and age) are recognized as contributing factors to disparities in various cultural and ethnic groups in the outcomes of depressive disorders; see Box 25.2. (For more information on social determinants of health, see Chapter 3.)

Cultural Communication of Symptoms

People from culturally and ethnically diverse populations may formulate and describe their depressive

BOX 25.2

Mental Health Inequities: Social Determinants of Health and Depression

In a large sample of 30,762 U.S. adults (49.2% of whom identified as male), 8.7% showed depressive symptoms. The majority were non-Hispanic White (44.5%) individuals, followed by non-Hispanic Black (21.4%) individuals, and then by people of other races (18.7%), and then by Mexican American individuals (15.3%). The mean age was 47.25 (SE = 0.26) years. In this sample, there was a higher prevalence of racial/ethnic and gender disparities in depression symptoms. People assigned female at birth and non-Hispanic Black individuals with unfavorable social determinants of health (SDOH) were more prone to depression symptoms compared to individuals in other groups. Adults aged 20 to 59 years had higher odds of depression when exposed to unfavorable SDOHs than older adults (i.e., those 60 years of age or older).

Individuals exhibiting depressive symptoms were more likely to be associated with various SDOHs including unemployment, poverty, food insecurity, education level below high school, lack of health insurance or having government coverage, and not being married or cohabiting with a partner. The severity of depressive symptoms was associated with an increase in the number of SDOHs. Cumulative inequality in SDOHs had a significant impact on depression symptoms. Individuals with 6 or more unfavorable SDOHs were four times more likely to experience depression compared to those with no unfavorable SDOHs.

Source: Liang, J. H., Liu, M. L., Pu, Y. Q., Huang, S., Jiang, N., Bao, W. W., Hu, L. X., Zhang, Y. S., Gui, Z. H., Pu, X. Y., Huang, S. Y., & Chen, Y. J. (2024). Cumulative inequality in social determinants of health in relation to depression symptom: An analysis of nationwide cross-sectional data from U.S. NHANES 2005–2018. *Psychiatry Research*, *336*, 115894. https://doi.org/10.1016/j.psychres.2024.115894

symptoms differently than the clinical language used for diagnosis. In some cultures, somatic symptoms, rather than sadness or guilt, may predominate. Individuals from various cultural groups may have complaints of weakness, tiredness, or imbalance. Culturally distinctive experiences should be assessed to differentiate depression from an expected cultural emotional response (Sik, 2021).

COMORBIDITY

Major depressive disorders often co-occur with other psychiatric disorders including those that are substance related. Depression often is associated with a variety of chronic medical conditions, particularly endocrine disorders, cardiovascular disease, and neurologic disorders (Basiri et al., 2023; Lee et al., 2024).

ETIOLOGY

The etiology of depression is complex and evolving. Once thought to be only psychologically based, we now know that there are multiple neurobiologic changes that underlie depression.

Biologic Theories

The following discussion summarizes current understanding of biologic theories of depression.

Genetic Factors

Family, twin, and adoption studies demonstrate that genetic influences undoubtedly play a substantial role in the etiology of mood disorders. Major depressive disorder tends to run in families and has a heritable component. Major research efforts are focused on developing a more accurate paradigm regarding the contribution of genetic factors to the development of major depressive disorder (Nguyen et al., 2023).

Neurobiologic Hypotheses

Neurobiologic theories of the etiology of depression emerged in the 1950s. These theories posit that major depression is caused by a deficiency or dysregulation in central nervous system (CNS) concentrations of the neurotransmitters norepinephrine, dopamine, serotonin, and glutamate, or in their receptor functions. These hypotheses arose in part from observations that some pharmacologic agents elevate mood; subsequent studies identified their mechanisms of action. All antidepressants currently available have their therapeutic effects on these neurotransmitters or receptors. Current research continues to focus on the role of neurotransmitters and the neurobiology of depression (Cui et al., 2024).

Neuroendocrine and Neuropeptide Hypotheses

Major depressive disorder is associated with multiple endocrine alterations, specifically of the hypothalamic–pituitary–adrenal (HPA) axis, the hypothalamic–pituitary–thyroid (HPT) axis, the hypothalamic–growth hormone axis, and the hypothalamic–pituitary–gonadal axis. High HPA activity with the release of glucocorticoids is among the most typical neurobiologic alterations in people who are depressed. **Glucocorticoids** are harmful to neurons in various brain regions. In addition, mounting evidence indicates that components of neuroendocrine axes (e.g., neuromodulatory peptides such as corticotropin-releasing factor) may themselves contribute to depressive symptoms. Evidence also suggests that the secretion of these hypothalamic and growth hormones is controlled by many of the neurotransmitters implicated in the pathophysiology of depression (Cui et al., 2024).

Cytokine Hypothesis

Psychoneuroimmunology is a recent area of research into a diverse group of proteins known as *chemical messengers* between immune cells. These messengers, called **cytokines**, signal the brain and serve as mediators between immune and nerve cells. The brain is capable of influencing immune processes, and conversely, immunologic response can result in changes in brain activity. Increased cytokine levels are associated with depression and cognitive impairment indicating that inflammatory reactions are involved in the development of some mental health disorders including depression (Cui et al., 2024).

Gut–Brain Axis

A new pathway being studied to understand major depressive disorder is the **gut–brain axis**, which communicates in complex and bidirectional ways. See Chapter 7. Research shows that individuals with major depressive disorders have altered gut microbiota. Stress disturbs the microbiota balance, leading to increased inflammation, which in turn is thought to affect depressive mood and behavior. The benefits of probiotics are currently being studied for the improvement of depressive moods (Carlessi et al., 2021; Cui et al., 2024).

Psychosocial Theories

Psychological theories that serve as a basis for nursing practice for people with a mental health disorder are explained in Chapter 6. Depression is one of the disorders treated from a psychological perspective. The following discussion identifies theoretical models often used in nursing care.

Psychodynamic Factors

Most psychodynamic theorists acknowledge some debt to Freud's original conceptualization of the psychodynamics of depression, which ascribes the cause to an early lack of love, care, warmth, and protection and resultant anger, guilt, helplessness, and fear regarding the loss of love. The ensuing conflict between wanting to be loved and fear of rejection engenders pathologic self-punishment (also conceptualized as aggression turned inward), self-rejection, low self-esteem, and depressive symptoms (see Chapter 6).

Behavioral Factors

Behavioral psychologists hold that depression primarily results from a severe reduction in rewarding activities or an increase in unpleasant events in one's life. The subsequent depression then leads to further restriction of activity, thereby decreasing the likelihood of experiencing pleasurable activities, which, in turn, intensifies the mood disturbance. Affected individuals often self-criticize and believe that they do not have the coping skills to deal with life's stresses. If family members believe that the individual is "sick" and lacks the necessary coping skills, they inadvertently reinforce the hopeless self-view of the person who is depressed.

Cognitive Factors

The cognitive approach maintains that irrational beliefs and negative distortions of thought about the self, the environment, and the future engender and perpetuate depressive effects (see Chapter 13). These depressive cognitions can be learned socially from family members or lack of experience in developing coping skills. These individuals think differently than nondepressed individuals and view their environment and themselves in negative ways. They blame themselves for any misfortunes that occur and see situations as being much worse than they are.

Developmental Factors

Developmental theorists posit that depression may result from the loss of a parent/caregiver through death or separation, or through lack of emotionally adequate parenting. These factors may delay or prohibit the realization of appropriate developmental milestones.

Social Theories

Social theories include family and environmental factors.

Family Factors

Family theorists ascribe maladaptive patterns in family interactions as contributing to the onset of depression, particularly in the onset and occurrence of depression in younger individuals. A family becomes dysfunctional when interactions, decisions, or behaviors interfere with the positive development of the family and its individual members. Most families have periods of dysfunction, such as during a crisis or stressful situation when coping skills are not available. Unhealthy interactions within a family system can have a negative impact on one or more family members who do not have the coping skills to deal with the situation.

Environmental Factors

Depression has long been understood as a multifactorial disorder that occurs when environmental factors (e.g., death of family member) interact with the biologic and psychological makeup of the individual. Major depression may follow adverse or traumatic life events, especially those that involve the loss of an important human relationship or role in life. Social isolation, deprivation, and financial deprivation are associated with depression (Chau et al., 2021).

Discrimination and **microaggression** (subtle, ambiguous slights, and actions that are perceived as insulting to targeted groups) are associated with depression and anxiety (Rastogi et al., 2024). **Racism** (a multifaceted system of oppression) disproportionately harms adults and children of color. Racism occurs when access to services and opportunities is based on racial group membership and is maintained through systems such as laws and policies, culture, and discrimination. Research shows that racism is a traumatic experience and can result in depression. When mothers of color experience racism and then develop depression, their children are also likely to develop depression, leading to intergenerational transmission of depression (Mekawi et al., 2023).

FAMILY RESPONSE TO DISORDER

Depression in one family member affects the whole family. Spouses/partners, children, parents/caregivers, siblings, and friends experience frustration, guilt, and anger when a family member is immobilized and cannot function. It is often hard for others to understand the depth of the mood and how disabling it can be. Financial hardship can occur when the affected family member cannot work and instead spends days in bed. The lack of understanding and difficulty of living with a person who is depressed can lead to abuse. People assigned female at birth between the ages of 18 and 45 years constitute the majority of those experiencing depression.

Depression can affect these individuals' ability not only to have productive lives and take care of themselves but also to take care of their children or other family members for whom they may have responsibility. Moreover, research indicates that the incidence of depression may be higher in children whose mothers experience depression (Wu, 2024).

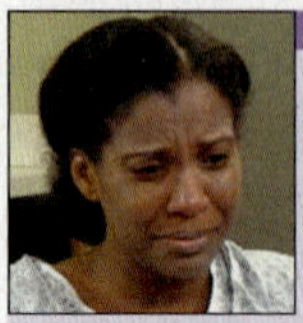

Remember Louise?

According to her husband, Louise has neglected her self-care and that of her children since her sister's death. Brian is very understanding and supportive of Louise's need to grieve, but he is concerned that this is more than grief. Brian says that he is afraid to leave Louise alone and that the children are suffering. What recommendations would you suggest to Louise's husband? Are there indications that Louise's grief is developing into depression?

RECOVERY-ORIENTED CARE FOR PEOPLE WITH MAJOR DEPRESSIVE DISORDER

Teamwork and Collaboration: Working Toward Recovery

Although depressive disorders are the most commonly occurring mental disorders, they are usually treated within the primary care setting rather than psychiatric setting. Individuals with depression enter mental health settings when their symptoms become so severe that hospitalization is needed, usually after suicide attempts, or if they self-refer because of incapacitation. Antidepressants are indicated for depression and are discussed later in this chapter. Interdisciplinary treatment of these disorders, which is often lifelong, needs to include a wide array of health professionals in all areas. The specific goals of treatment are:

- Reduce or control symptoms and, if possible, eliminate signs and symptoms of the depressive syndrome.
- Improve occupational and psychosocial function as much as possible.
- Reduce the likelihood of relapse and recurrence through recovery-oriented strategies.

Cognitive and Interpersonal Therapies

Recent studies suggest that for mild depression, short-term cognitive and interpersonal therapies may be as effective as pharmacotherapy. In many instances, **cognitive-behavioral therapy (CBT)** is an effective strategy for preventing relapse in patients who have had only a partial response to pharmacotherapy alone (Strawn et al., 2022). CBT is implemented in individual or group therapy by a trained clinician.

Interpersonal therapy seeks to recognize, explore, and resolve the interpersonal losses, role confusion and transitions, social isolation, and deficits in social skills that may precipitate depressive states. It maintains that losses must be mourned and related affects appreciated, role confusion and transitions must be recognized and resolved, and social skills deficits must be overcome.

Combination Therapies

For patients with severe or recurrent major depressive disorder, the combination of psychotherapy (including interpersonal, cognitive-behavioral, behavior, brief dynamic, or dialectical behavioral therapies) and pharmacotherapy has been found to be superior to treatment using a single modality. Clinical practice guidelines suggest that the combination of medication and psychotherapy is particularly useful in more complex situations (e.g., depression in the context of concurrent, chronic general-medical or other psychiatric disorders, or in patients who fail to experience complete response to either treatment alone). Psychotherapy in combination with medication is also used to address collateral issues, such as medication adherence or secondary psychosocial issues (Gaddey et al., 2024). If medications and psychotherapy are not effective, other options are available: electroconvulsive therapy (ECT), light therapy, and repetitive transcranial magnetic stimulation (TMS) discussed later in the chapter.

Safety Issues

The overriding concern for people with major depressive disorder is safety because these individuals may experience self-destructive thoughts and suicidal ideation. Hence, the assessment of possible suicide risk should be routinely conducted for any person who is depressed (see Chapter 22).

EVIDENCE-BASED NURSING CARE OF PEOPLE WITH A MAJOR DEPRESSIVE DISORDER

An awareness of the risk factors for depression, a comprehensive and culturally competent mental health nursing assessment, history of illness, and past treatment are key to formulating a treatment or recovery plan and to evaluating outcomes. Interviewing a family member or close friend about the patient's day-to-day functioning and specific symptoms may help determine the course of the illness, current symptoms, and level of functioning. The family's level of support and understanding of the disorder should be assessed. See Clinical Judgment Nursing Care Plan 25.1, which sets forth a plan of care for Louise, the case study patient in this chapter.

RECOGNIZING CUES: RELEVANT ASSESSMENT INFORMATION

The mental health nursing assessment focuses on the physical consequences of the depression as well as the psychosocial aspects. The symptoms of depression are similar to those of some medical issues or medication side effects. Often, the psychiatric-mental health nurse is the only clinician who provides holistic care to an individual with depression. Throughout the assessment, the nurse should demonstrate cultural humility in discussing patient values and beliefs. See Chapter 3.

Physical Health

The nursing assessment should include a physical systems review and a thorough history of medical issues, with special attention to CNS function, endocrine function, anemia, chronic pain, autoimmune illness, diabetes mellitus, or menopause. Additional medical history includes surgeries; medical hospitalizations; head injuries; episodes of loss of consciousness; and pregnancies, childbirths, miscarriages, and abortions. A complete list of prescribed and over-the-counter (OTC) medications and herbal supplements should be compiled, including the reason a medication was prescribed, or its use discontinued. A physical examination is recommended with baseline vital signs and baseline laboratory tests, including a comprehensive blood chemistry panel, complete blood counts, liver function tests, thyroid function tests, urinalysis, and electrocardiograms (see Chapter 10).

The following symptoms are characteristics of depression and should be assessed:

- *Appetite and weight changes*: In major depression, changes from baseline include a decrease or increase in appetite with or without significant weight loss or gain (i.e., a change of more than 5% of body weight in 1 month). Weight loss occurs when the individual is not dieting. Older adults with moderate-to-severe depression need to be assessed for dehydration as well as weight changes.
- *Sleep disturbance*: The most common sleep disturbance associated with major depression is **insomnia**, which is broken into three categories: initial insomnia (difficulty falling asleep), middle insomnia (waking up during the night and having difficulty returning to sleep), and terminal insomnia (waking too early and being unable to return to sleep). Less frequently, the sleep disturbance is hypersomnia (i.e., prolonged sleep episodes at night or increased daytime sleep). The individual with either insomnia or hypersomnia complains of not feeling rested on awakening.
- *Tiredness, decreased energy, and fatigue*: Fatigue associated with depression is a subjective experience of feeling tired regardless of how much sleep or physical activity an individual has had. Even the smallest tasks require substantial effort.

NCLEXNOTE In determining the severity of depressive symptoms, nursing assessment should explore physical changes in appetite, sleep patterns, and energy level. Remember these three major assessment categories. A question on the exam may state several patient symptoms and expect the student to recognize that the patient being described is depressed.

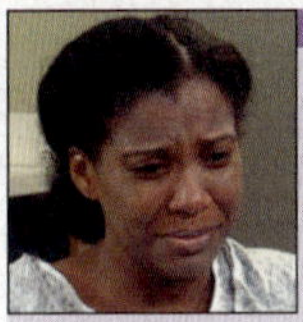

Consider This:

Recall that Louise has not been eating because she is not hungry; she has lost 15 lb over the last 6 weeks. She is also not sleeping well. She wakes up during the middle of the night and cannot go back to sleep. What symptoms of depression is Louise experiencing?

Physical Functioning

Changes in physical functioning (mobility and activities of daily living) may be an indication of the severity of the mood disturbance. The nurse should assess any changes and the rate of change in physical functioning over time. Other areas to assess include the presence of excessive sleepiness or falling asleep, sleep apnea, and sudden lapses into sleeping throughout the day.

History of Trauma

Assessing the history of trauma is important in everyone with depression because depressive states are linked to trauma. Childhood trauma is associated with depression in youths and adults. Multiple traumas and interpersonal and sexual trauma in childhood are associated with worsening depression. **Interpersonal trauma** (child maltreatment, physical and sexual assault, witnessing of violence) in childhood is associated with suicidality (Goodman et al., 2024).

Encouraging people who identify as LGBTQ+ to self-identify gender status will allow the nurse to gather trauma history cues. LGBTQ+ people have high rates of lifetime trauma exposure that is linked to depression and

CLINICAL JUDGMENT NURSING CARE PLAN 25.1

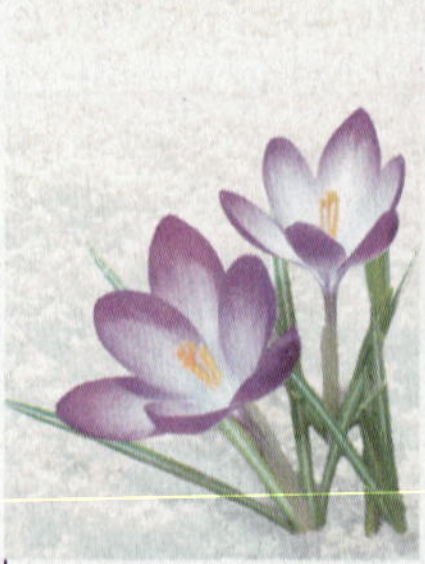

The Individual With Depressive Disorder

Louise is a 31-year-old female assigned at birth with a diagnosis of major depressive disorder with suicidal ideation. She feels hopeless, helpless, and worthless. She is grieving the loss of her sister and also feels that she has failed her. She believes her family would be better off without her. She has lost interest and pleasure in everything that she used to enjoy. She lacks energy to get out of bed or do basic self-care. Her thoughts are negative and distorted. Her facial expression is sad and restricted. She has difficulty smiling or seeing humor in a situation.

Setting: Intensive Care Psychiatric Unit in a General Hospital

Baseline Assessment: Louise is oriented to time, place, and person. She is dressed in a sweatshirt and sweatpants. Her appearance is disheveled, she has a slight body odor, and her hair is not combed. Her physical care plan reveals a recent 15 lb weight loss, insomnia, and loss of appetite. Her vital signs and laboratory values are within normal limits. She denies having a suicidal plan but says she wants to go to sleep and not wake up. Her husband said he is very worried about her because "she is physically there but not available to any of us."

Associated Psychiatric Diagnosis	Medications
Major depressive disorder	Initiated escitalopram (Lexapro) 20 mg/day

Priority Hypothesis Safety and Suicide Prevention

Important Characteristics

Feelings of hopelessness
Expresses desire to die
Lethal means available

Associated Considerations

Recently lost sister
Believes she is a burden to family

Planning Recovery and Wellness Outcomes

Initial

1. Remain free from self-harm.
2. Identify factors that led to suicidal intent and methods for managing suicidal impulses if they return.
3. Accept treatment of depression by trying the SSRI antidepressants and psychotherapy.

Discharge

1. Agrees to continue with outpatient therapy.
2. Agrees to take antidepressant.
3. Agrees that family can remove gun(s) from home.

Taking Action: Nursing Interventions

Interventions	Rationale	Ongoing Assessment
Initiate a nurse–patient relationship by demonstrating an acceptance of Louise as a worthwhile human being through the use of nonjudgmental statements and behavior.	A sense of worthlessness often underlies suicidal ideation. The positive therapeutic relationship can support hopefulness.	Assess the stages of the relationship and determine whether a therapeutic relationship is actually being formed. Identify indicators of trust.
Initiate suicide precautions per hospital policy.	Safety of the individual is a priority with people who have suicidal ideation.	Determine intent to harm self—plan and means.
Discuss with family members removal of lethal weapons from home.	Suicidal behavior is often impulsive. Removing means of suicide may prevent people from acting on impulsive thoughts.	Follow-up with the patient and family member about removing lethal weapons.

Evaluation

Outcomes	Revised Outcomes	Interventions
Has not harmed herself.	Identify strategies to resist suicide attempts in the future.	Discuss antecedents that led to the suicide attempt. Discuss initiation of an antidepressant.

Clinical Judgment Nursing Care Plan 25.1 Continued

Priority Hypothesis Hopelessness

Important Characteristics	Associated Considerations
Decreased affect Decreased appetite Insomnia Lack of initiative States she has no reason to live	Loss of sister

Planning Recovery and Wellness Outcomes

Initial	Discharge
Accept support through the nurse–patient relationship. Identify hopelessness as a pervasive feeling.	Express feelings of being hopeful for the future.

Taking Action: Nursing Interventions

Interventions	Rationale	Ongoing Assessment
Establish a trusting therapeutic relationship.	Therapeutic relationships are effective in instilling hope.	Observe verbal and nonverbal cues that increase communications.
Enhance Louise's sense of hope by being attentive, validating your interpretation of what is being said or experienced, and helping him verbalize what she is expressing nonverbally.	By showing respect for the patient as a human being who is worth listening to, the nurse can support and help build the patient's sense of self.	Determine whether the patient confirms interpretation of situation and if she can verbalize what she is expressing nonverbally.
Assist to reframe and redefine negative statements ("not a burden but missing your sister").	Reframing an event positively rather than negatively can help the patient view the situation in an alternative way.	Assess whether Louise is feeling more hopeful.
Participate in a recovery group focusing on hope.	Group support can be very effective in discussing hope and identifying strategies to establish hopefulness.	Determine if the patient is attending group sessions and participating in discussions.

Evaluation

Outcomes	Revised Outcomes	Interventions
Able to discuss future events in a positive manner. Attending recovery group regularly.	Discuss specific plans for future events. None.	Continue with cognitive approaches when discussing future events.

SSRI, selective serotonin reuptake inhibitor.

other mental disorders. Many can associate their trauma directly to their gender identity. The trauma and depression of individuals in this population are also linked to suicidality (Hammer et al., 2024). See Box 25.3.

Medication

In addition to a physical assessment, an assessment of current medications should be completed. The frequency and dosage of prescribed medications, OTC medications, and use of herbal or culturally related medication treatments should be explored. When treating a patient with depression, the nurse must always assess the possible lethality of the medication the patient is taking. For example, if a patient has sleeping medications at home, the individual should be further questioned about the number of pills in the bottle.

A patient's use of herbal substances should be determined because of the potential for drug–drug interactions. For example, patients taking antidepressants that affect serotonin regulation could also be taking St. John's wort (*Hypericum perforatum*) to fight depression. The combined drug and herb could interact to cause serotonin syndrome (altered mental status, autonomic dysfunction, and neuromuscular abnormalities). SAMe (*S*-adenosyl-L-methionine) is another herbal preparation that patients may be taking. Patients need to be advised of possible adverse side effects of SAMe taken with any prescribed antidepressant because the exact action of this herb remains unclear. (See Chapters 11 and 12.)

BOX 25.3

Trauma-Informed Approaches: Childhood Trauma and Psychological Distress for LGBTQ+ Individuals

Background

People who identify as LGBTQ+ experience discrimination, prejudice, microaggressions, and internalized stigma. They are at risk of experiencing a mental disorder, self-injury, and suicidal thoughts. They experience high rates of trauma exposure and posttraumatic stress disorder.

Interventions

- Recognize the impact of identity-based trauma on cognition, emotion, development, behavior, and perception.
- Provide physical and emotional safety.
- Communicate safety procedures.
- Create a predictable environment.
- Demonstrate respect and empathy in interactions in a nonjudgmental approach.

Source: Hammer, L. A., Fergerson, A. K., & Bonfils, K. A. (2024). Recommendations for the assessment of sexual and gender minority status in serious mental illness research and clinical care. *Psychological Services*, *21*(3), 417–425. https://doi.org/10.1037/ser0000852

Substance Use

A significant proportion (25%) of people with a major depressive disorder also have a substance use disorder (Rao et al., 2023). Patients should be assessed for their use of alcohol, marijuana, and other mood-altering medications. Alcohol use disorder increases the risk of a depressive disorder more than fourfold (Hassan & Le Foll, 2021). Self-medicating with substances as a coping strategy for dysphoria and stress is well documented (Seager et al., 2024). Not only can substance use lead to dependency, but self-medicating can heighten inflammation and lead to dysregulation of the brain circuitry (Nusslock et al., 2024). These co-occurring disorders have an adverse impact on both mood and substance use outcomes.

Psychosocial Cues

The psychosocial assessment for people who have major depressive disorder includes the mental status (mood and affect, thought processes and content, cognition, memory, and attention), coping skills, developmental history, psychiatric family history, patterns of relationships, quality of support system, education, work history, and impact of physical or sexual abuse on interpersonal function. See Chapter 10. The nurse should identify the individual's strengths, as well as problem areas, by asking the patient to describe their thoughts, feelings, and behaviors before the current depressive episode. Including a family member or close friend in the assessment process can be helpful. The following discussion identifies key assessment areas for people who are depressed.

Mental Status and Appearance

Mood and Affect

The individual with major depressive disorder has a sustained period of feeling depressed, sad, or hopeless and may experience **anhedonia** (loss of interest or pleasure). The patient may report "not caring any more" or not feeling any enjoyment in activities that were previously considered pleasurable. In some individuals, this may include a decrease in or loss of libido (i.e., sexual interest or desire) and sexual function. In others, irritability and anger are signs of depression, especially in those who deny being depressed. Individuals often describe themselves as depressed, sad, hopeless, discouraged, or "down in the dumps." If individuals complain of feeling "blah," having no feelings, constantly tired, or feeling anxious, a depressed mood can sometimes be inferred from their facial expression and demeanor (APA, 2022).

Numerous assessment scales are available for assessing depression. Easily administered self-report questionnaires can be valuable detection tools. These questionnaires cannot be the sole basis for making a diagnosis of MDE, but they are sensitive to depressive symptoms. The following are five commonly used self-report scales:

- General Health Questionnaire (GHQ)
- Center for Epidemiological Studies Depression Scale (CES-D)
- Beck Depression Inventory (BDI)
- Zung Self-Rating Depression Scale (SDS)
- PRIME-MD

Clinician-completed rating scales may be more sensitive to improvement in the course of treatment, can assess symptoms in relationship to the depressive diagnostic criteria, and may have a slightly greater specificity than do self-report questionnaires in detecting depression. These include the following:

- Hamilton Rating Scale for Depression (HAM-D)
- Montgomery–Asberg Depression Rating Scale (MADRS)
- National Institute of Mental Health Diagnostic Interview Schedule (DIS)

Thought Content

Depressed individuals often have an unrealistic negative evaluation of their worth or have guilty preoccupations or ruminations about minor past failings. Such individuals often misinterpret neutral or trivial day-to-day events as evidence of personal defects. They may also have an exaggerated sense of responsibility for untoward events. As a result, they feel hopeless, helpless, worthless, and powerless. The possibility of disorganized thought processes (e.g., tangential or circumstantial thinking) and perceptual disturbances (e.g., hallucinations, delusions) should also be included in the assessment.

Cognition and Memory

Many individuals with depression report an impaired ability to think, concentrate, or make decisions. They may appear easily distracted or complain of memory difficulties. In older adults with major depression, memory difficulties may be the chief complaint and may be mistaken for early signs of dementia (pseudodementia) (APA, 2022). When the depression is fully treated, the memory issue often improves or fully resolves.

Behavioral Responses

Changes in patterns of relating (especially social withdrawal) and changes in level of occupational functioning are commonly reported. These changes may represent a significant deterioration from baseline behavior. Increased use of "sick days" may occur.

Self-Concept

A negative **self-concept** (beliefs about self) with low **self-esteem** (self-value) is associated with several health issues such as obesity, cardiovascular events, and depression (Segal & Gunturu, 2024; Yavari et al., 2023). Assessing self-esteem helps in establishing goals and direction for treatment.

Stress and Coping Patterns

The individual should be assessed for coping patterns and **resilience** (the ability to adapt successfully to stress, trauma, or chronic adversity). How does the individual cope with the everyday stresses of life? How does the individual cope with the depression and how does the depression impact the individual's ability to cope with daily stressors? The nurse helps the patient identify positive coping patterns such as meditating, talking to a loved one, and negative coping patterns such as overeating and using alcohol or nonprescribed drugs.

Suicidal Behavior

Patients with major depressive disorder are at increased risk for suicide. The development of suicide behavior is a complex phenomenon because symptoms are often hidden or veiled by somatic symptoms.

> **KEYCONCEPT Suicidal behavior** is the occurrence of persistent thought patterns and actions that indicate an individual is thinking about, planning, or enacting suicide.

Suicidal ideation includes thoughts that range from a belief that others would be better off if the individual were dead, or thoughts of death (passive suicidal ideation), to actual specific plans for suicide (active suicidal ideation). See Chapter 22. The frequency, intensity, and lethality of these thoughts can vary and can help to determine the seriousness of intent. The more specific the plan and the more accessible the means, the more serious becomes the intent. The risk for suicide needs to be initially assessed in patients when diagnosed with depressive disorders as well as reassessed throughout the course of treatment.

Suicidal ideation is not an ordinary reaction to stress. People who express any suicidal ideation need immediate mental health assessment regarding the depth of their thoughts and intentions. Risk factors for suicidal ideation include lack of availability and inadequacy of social supports; family violence, including physical or sexual abuse; past history of suicidal ideation or behavior; presence of psychosis or substance use or misuse; and decreased ability to control suicidal impulses. See Chapter 22.

Differences exist regarding suicidal behavior.

- Sex Assigned at Birth: People assigned male at birth often use firearms, whereas those assigned female at birth often use pills or other poisonous substances to attempt suicide.
- Age: Children often use suffocation to attempt suicide.
- Ethnicity: Data on suicide completion rates are reported highest in people of Native American, Alaskan Native, and non-Hispanic White descent. These rates are lowest for people of Hispanic, non-Hispanic Black, and Asian and Pacific Islander descent (Stone et al., 2023).
- Veterans: Ongoing research regarding suicide in veterans indicates that they have a higher risk than people in the general population (VA Suicide Prevention, 2023). Psychological stress and previously diagnosed psychiatric disorders are major risk factors for veterans.

> **NCLEXNOTE** With patients who are depressed, the possibility of suicide should always be a priority for the nurse. Assessment and documentation of suicide risk should always be included in patient care.

Social Network

Assessment and documentation of patients' social network, social systems, and functional status always need to be a component of patient care. It is important to determine how the patient defines their social network. A network of connections on social media will not provide the needed support that family and friends can provide.

An astute nurse will determine the number of friends and family members that make up the patient's social network. Fewer members in the social network increases the risk for depression. Emotional support from the social network is critical in supporting a patient with depression (Li et al., 2023).

Quality of Life

A poor QoL often occurs with an individual who is depressed. They no longer seek out friends and families and experience extreme loneliness. They often forget or neglect to carry out routine activities of daily living such as bathing, eating, and cleaning. As the lack of social contacts continues, loneliness increases, and QoL continues to decrease (Fadipe et al., 2023).

Spiritual Assessment

The spiritual assessment is especially important for people experiencing depression and suicidal ideation. Assessing the individual's spiritual or religious beliefs helps the nurse view the patient from a holistic perspective and provides the patient the opportunity to explain their perspective on the meaning of life and their views on medical or psychiatric treatment. For example, a religious belief may prevent a patient from taking certain medications. By discussing the patient's religious/spiritual beliefs, the nurse can understand how the patient copes with being sick (Henry & Gilley, 2024).

Strength Assessment

Throughout the assessment, the nurse should be observing for strengths such as positive physical health status, coping skills, and social support. A positive self-concept is protective for the development of severe depression. The following questions may be used to determine an individual's strength:

- When you have been depressed before, how did you cope with the feelings?
- What do you do to relax?
- Do you reach out to anyone when you are feeling down?
- When you are not depressed, what makes you feel good?

ANALYZING CUES AND DEVELOPING HYPOTHESES

Several symptoms and effects of depression could potentially require nursing care. In collaboration with the patient, the nurse can discuss hypotheses and establish priorities of care. Suicidal thoughts and behaviors are always the first priority and should be considered. If a patient does not have suicidal thoughts, the nurse can focus on the physical impact of the depression such as lack of sleep, loss of appetite, and lack of energy to carry out daily routines. Feelings of hopelessness and low self-esteem are usually present and need attention. Many people who are depressed have difficulty making decisions. As the priorities are established, the results of the strength assessment should be discussed and included in the determining approaches to care. These strengths will help the individual recover from the depressed state.

PLANNING RECOVERY AND WELLNESS OUTCOMES: GENERATING SOLUTIONS

Nursing intervention selection is a collaborative process between the patient and the nurse. As goals and interventions are agreed on by both the nurse and the patient, the individual's strengths (e.g., motivation to get better, resources, family support) should be emphasized in making treatment choices.

THERAPEUTIC RELATIONSHIP

One of the most effective tools for caring for any person with a mental disorder is the therapeutic relationship. For an individual who is depressed, there are a number of effective approaches:

- Establishment and maintenance of a supportive relationship based on the incorporation of culturally competent interventions and strategies
- Support in times of crisis
- Vigilance regarding danger to self and others
- Education about the illness and treatment goals
- Encouragement and feedback concerning progress
- Guidance regarding the patient's interactions with the personal and work environment
- Realistic goal setting and monitoring
- Support of individual strengths in treatment choices

Interacting with individuals who are depressed is challenging because they tend to be withdrawn and have difficulty expressing feelings and engaging in interpersonal interactions. The therapeutic relationship can be strengthened through the use of cognitive interventions as well as the nurse's ability to win the patient's trust through the use of culturally competent strategies in the context of empathy (Box 25.4).

Nurses should avoid approaching patients with depression with an overly cheerful attitude. This "cheerleading" blocks communication and can be quite irritating to

BOX 25.4

Therapeutic Dialogue: Approaching the Patient Who Is Depressed

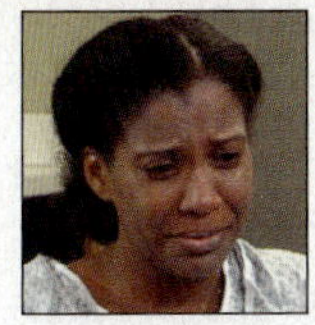

Louise is severely depressed and has not left her hospital room since admission to the mental health unit. She has missed breakfast and is not interested in taking a shower or getting dressed.

INEFFECTIVE APPROACH

Nurse: Hello, Louise. My name is Sally. How are you feeling today?

Louise: I didn't sleep last night and need to rest. Please go away.

Nurse: Sorry, but it is time to get up. You've already missed breakfast. You have to take a quick shower now to get to group on time.

Louise: I have no interest in taking a shower or going to group.

Nurse: Why are you here if you don't want to be treated?

Louise: Go away. I don't want you in this room.

EFFECTIVE APPROACH

Nurse: Good morning. My name is Sally. I am your nurse today.

Louise: I didn't sleep last night and need to rest. Please go away.

Nurse: You didn't sleep well last night?

Louise: No, I can't remember when I was able to sleep through the night.

Nurse: Oh, I see. Is that why you missed breakfast?

Louise: I'm just not hungry. I have no energy.

Nurse: Lack of appetite and lack of energy are very common when people are depressed.

Louise: Really?

Nurse: Yes, so let's take one step at time. I'd like to help you get up.

Louise: Ok, I might be able to sit up.

Nurse: (Helps her sit up). Now, let's walk to the bathroom.

Louise: (Walks to the bathroom). Now what?

Nurse: Let's work on your AM care.

CRITICAL THINKING CHALLENGE

1. What ineffective techniques did the nurse use in the first scenario and how did they impair communication?
2. What effective techniques did the nurse use in the second scenario, and how did they facilitate communication?

patients who are depressed. Instead, a calm, supportive empathic approach keeps communication open.

> **NCLEXNOTE** Establishing the patient–nurse relationship with an individual who is depressed requires an empathic, quiet approach that is grounded in the nurse's understanding of the cultural needs of the patient.

TAKING ACTION: NURSING INTERVENTIONS

Priorities of Care

Safety is a priority for anyone with a depressive disorder. The nurse should frequently ask the patient if they have any suicidal thoughts or intentions. The nurse should continue to monitor mood and behavior for any changes that indicate a change in suicidal ideation. (See Box 25.5.) Another priority is helping the patient engage in the therapeutic process and plan of care.

Physical Care

Because weeks or months of disturbed sleep patterns and nutritional imbalance only worsen depression, one of the first nursing interventions is helping the individual re-establish normal sleep patterns and healthy nutrition. Supporting self-care management by encouraging patients to practice positive sleep hygiene and eat well-balanced meals regularly helps the patient move toward remission or recovery.

Activity and exercise are important for improving depressed mood state (Noetel et al., 2024). Many people find that regular exercise is hard to maintain, and people who are depressed may find it impossible. When teaching about exercise, it is important to start with the current level of patient activity and increase it slowly. For example, if the patient is spending most of the time in bed, encouraging the patient to get dressed every day and walk for 5 or 10 minutes may be all that the patient can tolerate.

BOX 25.5

Building Clinical Judgment With SBAR: Nurse Communication With Provider Regarding Suicide Precautions

SBAR

S: Situation

Harper is a 45-year-old patient admitted to a mental health unit at 10:00 pm for depression. There is no order for suicide precautions.

B: Background

This is the second admission for Harper, who had a recent breakup from a long-time partner. Harper has a history of depression, substance use, childhood abuse, loss of social support, and discrimination.

A: Assessment

- Suicide screen is positive for ideation (thoughts of killing self) and plan (loaded gun at home).
- Has a history of previous suicide attempts.

R: Recommendation

- Notify supervisor that Harper is a suicide risk, and implement one-to-one observation protocol.
- Harper needs to remain on observation until suicide is no longer considered a risk.

BUILDING CLINICAL JUDGMENT

1. Why did the nurse screen the patient for suicide?
2. Should the nurse have contacted the provider before placing Harper on one-to-one observation?

Gradually, patients should be encouraged to establish a regular exercise program and to slowly increase their food intake. These activities are consistent with wellness goals.

Wellness Challenges

Depression robs the individual of energy to carry out simple activities. Previous wellness activities from physical activities, nutrition and stress management often disappear during depression. The side effects of the antidepressants may actually interfere with normal wellness activities. The nurse should work with the individual to re-establish these activities. The individual may not feel like doing anything, but through the nurse–patient relationship, the nurse should seek commitment to gradually incorporate wellness activities. See Table 25.1.

Medication Interventions

Antidepressant medications have proven effective in all forms of major depression. To date, controlled trials have shown no single antidepressant drug to have greater efficacy in the treatment of major depressive disorder. See Chapter 11 for a list of antidepressant medications, usual dosage range, half-life, and therapeutic blood levels.

An antidepressant is selected based primarily on an individual patient's target symptoms; genetic factors; responses related to cultural, racial, and ethnic influences; and a pharmacologic agent's side-effect profile. Other factors that may influence choice include prior medication response, drug interactions and contraindications, concurrent medical and psychiatric disorders, patient age, and cost of medication. Selecting medications on the basis of pharmacogenetic properties improves symptom remission (Vest et al., 2023).

TABLE 25.1 WELLNESS CHALLENGES AND COPING STRATEGIES FOR THE INDIVIDUAL WITH DEPRESSION

Challenge	Coping Strategies
To cope effectively with lack of energy and sadness	Start with the easiest—take a walk after dinner; talk to a friend
To manage stress	Say "no" to being a perfectionist; consider a massage; meditation
To decrease feelings of worthlessness	Keep a list of accomplishments, help others; keep busy
To understanding the stigma of depression	Educate yourself and others about depression; join a support group
To recognize the need for physical activity, healthy foods, and sleep	Track physical activity, diet, and sleep in a journal
To develop a sense of connection, belonging, and a support system	Contact at least one friend, attend religious service
To expand a sense of purpose and meaning in life	Pray, meditate, help others, volunteer

BOX 25.6

Medication Profile: Escitalopram Oxalate

DRUG CLASS: Antidepressant

RECEPTOR AFFINITY: A highly SSRI with low affinity for 5-HT1–7 or α- and β-adrenergic, dopamine D_{1-5}, histamine H_{1-3}, muscarinic M_{1-5}, and benzodiazepine receptors or for Na^+, K^+, Cl^-, and Ca^{++} ion channels that have been associated with various anticholinergic, sedative, and cardiovascular side effects.

INDICATIONS: Treatment of major depressive disorder, generalized anxiety disorder

ROUTES AND DOSAGES: Available as 5-, 10-, and 20-mg oral tablets

Adults: Initially 10 mg once a day. May increase to 20 mg after a minimum of 1 week. Trials have not shown greater benefit at the 20-mg dose.

Geriatric: 10-mg dose is recommended. Adjust dosage related to the drug's longer half-life and the slower liver metabolism of older adult patients.

Renal Impairment: No dosage adjustment is necessary for mild-to-moderate renal impairment.

Children: Safety and efficacy have not been established in this population.

HALF-LIFE (PEAK EFFECT): 27 to 32 hours (4 to 7 hours)

SELECTED ADVERSE REACTIONS: Most common adverse events include insomnia, ejaculation disorder, diarrhea, nausea, fatigue, increased sweating, dry mouth, somnolence, dizziness, and constipation. Most serious adverse events include ejaculation disorder in men; fetal abnormalities and decreased fetal weight in pregnant patients; and serotonin syndrome if coadministered with MAOIs, St. John's wort, or SSRIs, including citalopram (Celexa), of which escitalopram (Lexapro) is the active isomer.

BOXED WARNING: Suicidality in children, adolescents, and young adults

WARNING: There is potential for interaction with MAOIs. Lexapro should not be used in combination with an MAOI or within 14 days of discontinuing an MAOI.

SPECIFIC PATIENT AND FAMILY EDUCATION

- Do not take in combination with citalopram (Celexa) or other SSRIs or MAOIs. A 2-week washout period between escitalopram and SSRIs or MAOIs is recommended to avoid serotonin syndrome.
- Families and caregivers should be advised of the need for close observation and communication with the prescriber.
- Notify your prescriber if pregnancy is possible or being planned. Do not breastfeed while taking this medication.
- Use caution driving or operating machinery until you are certain that escitalopram does not alter your physical abilities or mental alertness.
- Notify your prescriber of any OTC medications, herbal supplements, and home remedies being used in combination with escitalopram.
- Ingestion of alcohol in combination with escitalopram is not recommended, although escitalopram does not seem to potentiate mental and motor impairments associated with alcohol.

MAOI, monoamine oxidase inhibitor; OTC, over-the-counter; SSRI, selective serotonin reuptake inhibitor.

The newer antidepressants, selective serotonin reuptake inhibitors (SSRIs), serotonin-norepinephrine reuptake inhibitors (SNRIs), and the norepinephrine-dopamine reuptake inhibitor (NDRI) are used most often because these drugs selectively target the neurotransmitters and receptors thought to be associated with depression and minimize side effects. See Boxes 25.6 and 25.7. Individualizing dosages is usually done by fine-tuning medication dosage based on patient feedback. See Box 25.8. The tricyclic antidepressants (TCAs) and monoamine oxidase inhibitors (MAOIs) are being used less often than the other agents. Given their dietary restrictions, MAOIs usually are reserved for patients whose depression fails to respond to other antidepressants or patients who cannot tolerate typical antidepressants. See Chapter 11.

Ketamine, a noncompetitive *N*-methyl-D-aspartate receptor (NMDAR) antagonist, has recently been approved by the FDA to treat severe depression or treatment resistant depression. The use of ketamine, a clinical anesthetic, is significant because of its rapid antidepressant effects (Kim et al., 2024). Patients feel the effects immediately and do not have to wait for weeks for the antidepressant relief. Currently, **esketamine** nasal spray is the only ketamine formulation that is approved by the FDA for the treatment of depression. The side effects include sedation, loss of consciousness, dissociation, and respiratory depression.

NCLEXNOTE Patients may be reluctant to take prescribed antidepressant medications or may self-treat depression based on their cultural beliefs and values (Leung, 2023). A plan for culturally competent nursing care and teaching needs to address the importance of adherence to a medication regimen and emphasize any potential drug–drug interactions.

Administering Medications

Antidepressants are available in oral form and should be taken as prescribed. See Box 25.8. Even after complete remission of symptoms, medication should be continued for at least 6 months to 1 year after the patient achieves. If the patient experiences a recurrence after tapering the first course of treatment, the regimen should be reinstituted for at least another year, and if the illness reoccurs, medication should be continued indefinitely (DeBattista & Schatzberg, 2024).

Esketamine is administered twice per week initially and then once weekly or every 2 weeks after the induction. Nurses should receive instruction on the operation of the nasal device prior to administration. Some

BOX 25.7

Medication Profile: Mirtazapine

DRUG CLASS: Antidepressant

RECEPTOR AFFINITY: Believed to enhance central noradrenergic and serotonergic activity antagonizing central presynaptic α_2-adrenergic receptors. Mechanism of action is unknown

INDICATIONS: Treatment of depression

ROUTES AND DOSAGE: Available as 15- and 30-mg tablets

Adults: Initially, 15 mg/day as a single dose preferably in the evening before sleeping. Maximum dosage is 45 mg/day.

Geriatric: Use with caution; reduced dosage may be needed.

Children: Safety and efficacy have not been established.

HALF-LIFE (PEAK EFFECT): 20 to 40 hours (2 hours)

SELECTED ADVERSE REACTIONS: Somnolence, increased appetite, dizziness, weight gain, elevated cholesterol or triglyceride and transaminase levels, malaise, abdominal pain, hypertension, vasodilation, vomiting, anorexia, thirst, myasthenia, arthralgia, hypoesthesia, apathy, depression, vertigo, twitching, agitation, anxiety, amnesia, increased cough, sinusitis, pruritus, rash, urinary tract infection, mania (rare), agranulocytosis (rare)

BOXED WARNING: Suicidality in children, adolescents, and young adults

WARNING: Contraindicated in patients with known hypersensitivity. Use with caution in older adults, patients who are breastfeeding, and patients with impaired hepatic function. Avoid concomitant use with alcohol or diazepam, which can cause additive impairment of cognitive and motor skills.

SPECIFIC PATIENT AND FAMILY EDUCATION

- Take the dose once a day in the evening before sleep.
- Families and caregivers should be advised of the need for dose observation and communication with the prescriber.
- Avoid driving and performing other tasks requiring alertness.
- Notify your prescriber before taking any OTC or other prescription drugs.
- Avoid alcohol and other CNS depressants.
- Notify your prescriber if pregnancy is possible or planned.
- Monitor temperature and report any fever, lethargy, weakness, sore throat, malaise, or other "flu-like" symptoms.
- Maintain medical follow-up, including any appointments for blood counts and liver studies.

CNS, central nervous system; OTC, over-the-counter.

state statutes require nurse to complete an instructional program and have supervised clinical practice prior to administration. Blood pressure should be taken prior to administration and the provider should be notified for baseline blood pressure >140 mm Hg systolic or >90 mm Hg diastolic. Patients should be monitored for at least 2 hours after administration. Blood pressure should be reassessed at approximately 40 minutes after administration. Patients should be monitored for signs of misuse (Janssen Pharmaceutical Companies, 2024).

BOX 25.8

Guidelines for Administering and Monitoring Antidepressant Medications

Nurses should do the following in administering and monitoring antidepressant medications:

- Observe the patient for cheeking or saving medications for a later suicide attempt.
- Monitor vital signs (such as orthostatic vital signs and temperature): Obtain baseline data before the initiation of medications.
- Monitor periodically results of liver and thyroid function tests, blood chemistry, and complete blood count as appropriate and compare with baseline values.
- Monitor the patient symptoms for therapeutic response and report inadequate response to the prescriber.
- Monitor the patient for side effects and report to the prescriber serious side effects or those that are chronic and problematic for the patient. (Table 25.3 indicates pharmacologic and nonpharmacologic interventions for common side effects.)
- Monitor drug levels as appropriate. (Therapeutic drug levels for antidepressants are listed in Chapter 11.)
- Monitor dietary intake as appropriate, especially with regard to MAOI antidepressants.
- Inquire about patient use of other medications, alcohol, "street" drugs, OTC medications, and herbal supplements that might alter the desired effects of prescribed antidepressants.

MAOI, monoamine oxidase inhibitor; OTC, over-the-counter.

Monitoring Medications

Patients should be carefully observed for therapeutic effects and side effects of the antidepressants. In the depths of depression, saving medication for a later suicide attempt is quite common. If there are minimal therapeutic effects, the nurse can suspect the patient is saving medications and ask the patient about this possibility. If the patient has been saving medications, the nurse should retrieve the medications and closely observe the patient for suicide attempts.

During antidepressant treatment, the nurse should monitor and document vital signs, plasma drug levels (as appropriate), liver and thyroid function tests, complete blood counts, and blood chemistry to make sure that patients are receiving a therapeutic dosage and are adherent to the prescribed regimen. Results of these tests also can help the nurse evaluate for toxicity (see Chapter 11 for therapeutic blood levels).

Baseline orthostatic vital signs should be obtained before initiation of any medication, and in the case of medications known to have an impact on vital signs (such as TCAs, MAOIs, or SNRIs), vital signs should be monitored on a regular basis. If these medications are administered to children or older adults, the dosage should be lowered to accommodate the physiologic state of the individual.

Managing Side Effects

Many people stop taking the prescribed antidepressants because of the side effects. (See Table 25.2.) Ideally, side effects are minimal and can be alleviated by nonpharmacologic interventions. For example, if a patient is having difficulty falling asleep, avoiding caffeinated products may help (Table 25.3). SSRIs tend to be safer and have fewer side effects than the older medications. The most common reason individuals stop taking their SSRIs is gastrointestinal side effects including diarrhea, cramping, and heartburn. The most common side effects associated with TCAs are the antihistaminic side effects (e.g., sedation and weight gain) and anticholinergic side effects (potentiation of CNS drugs, blurred vision, dry mouth, constipation, urinary retention, sinus tachycardia, and decreased memory).

For the MAOIs, the most common side effects are headache, drowsiness, dry mouth and throat, constipation, blurred vision, and orthostatic hypotension. Additional adverse effects of MAOIs include insomnia, nausea, agitation, dizziness, asthenia, weight loss, and postural hypotension. Although priapism was not reported during clinical trials, the MAOIs are structurally similar to trazodone, which has been associated with priapism (prolonged painful erection). For those taking MAOIs, close attention to dietary restrictions should be given. See Chapter 11 for tyramine-restricted diets.

EMERGENCY CARE ALERT If coadministered with food or other substances containing tyramine (e.g., aged cheese, beer, red wine), MAOIs can trigger a hypertensive crisis that may be life threatening. Symptoms include a sudden, severe pounding, or explosive headache in the back of the head or temples, racing pulse, flushing, stiff neck, chest pain, nausea and vomiting, and profuse sweating.

Management of Complications

Suicidality

Suicidality is highlighted as a boxed warning on all antidepressants for an increased risk of suicide in children, adolescents, and young adults with major depressive or other psychiatric disorders. After the age of 24 years, the suicidality risk does not increase when taking an antidepressant, and after age 65, the risk of suicide decreases when taking an antidepressant. The SSRIs are the least lethal of the antidepressants, but fatalities due to suicide have been reported (DeBattista & Schatzberg, 2024).

EMERGENCY CARE ALERT If possible, TCAs should not be prescribed for patients at risk for suicide. Lethal doses of TCAs are only three to five times the therapeutic dose, and more than 1 g of a TCA is often toxic and may be fatal. Death may result from cardiac arrhythmia, hypotension, or uncontrollable seizures.

Serum TCA levels should be evaluated when overdose is suspected. In acute overdose, almost all symptoms develop within 12 hours. Anticholinergic effects are prominent and include dry mucous membranes, warm and dry skin, blurred vision, decreased bowel motility, and urinary retention. CNS suppression (ranging from drowsiness to coma) or an agitated delirium may occur. Basic overdose treatment includes induction of emesis, gastric lavage, and cardiorespiratory supportive care.

MAOIs are more lethal in overdose than are the newer antidepressants and thus should be prescribed with caution if the patient's suicide potential is elevated (see Chapter 11). An MAOI generally is given in divided doses to minimize side effects.

Serotonin Syndrome

Serotonin syndrome is a potentially serious side effect caused by drug-induced excess of intrasynaptic serotonin, 5-hydroxytryptamine (5-HT). See Box 25.9. First reported in the 1950s, it was relatively rare until the introduction of SSRIs. Serotonin syndrome is most often reported in patients taking two or more medications that increase CNS serotonin levels by different mechanisms. The most common drug combinations associated with serotonin syndrome involve the MAOIs, the SSRIs, and the TCAs (Simon et al., 2024).

Although serotonin syndrome can cause death, it is mild in most patients, who usually recover with supportive care alone. Unlike neuroleptic malignant syndrome, which develops within 3 to 9 days after the introduction of neuroleptic medications (see Chapter 24), serotonin syndrome tends to develop within hours or days after starting or increasing the dose of serotonergic medication. Symptoms include altered mental status, autonomic dysfunction, and neuromuscular abnormalities. At least three of the following findings must be present for a diagnosis: Mental status changes, agitation, myoclonus, hyperreflexia, fever, shivering, diaphoresis, ataxia, and diarrhea. In patients who also have peripheral vascular disease or atherosclerosis, severe vasospasm, and hypertension may occur in the presence of elevated serotonin levels. In addition, in a patient who is a slow metabolizer of SSRIs, higher-than-normal levels of these antidepressants may circulate in the blood. Medications that are not usually considered serotonergic, such as ciprofloxacin and fluconazole have been associated with the syndrome (Simon et al., 2024).

TABLE 25.2 ANTIDEPRESSANTS AND COMMON SIDE EFFECTS IN TREATING DEPRESSION

Medications	Common Side Effects
Selective Serotonin Reuptake Inhibitors (SSRIs)	
Fluoxetine Sertraline Paroxetine Fluvoxamine Citalopram Escitalopram	Gastrointestinal distress Sedation Anticholinergic effects Weight gain or loss in some people Sexual dysfunction Dizziness Diaphoresis
Serotonin-Norepinephrine Reuptake Inhibitors (SNRIs)	
Desvenlafaxine Duloxetine Levomilnacipran Milnacipran Venlafaxine	Gastrointestinal distress Anticholinergic effects Insomnia or sedation Decreased appetite Sexual dysfunction Unusual dreams Dizziness Jitteriness Hypertension Irritability Photosensitivity
Norepinephrine-Dopamine Reuptake Inhibitor (NDRI)	
Bupropion	Anticholinergic effects Headache Agitation Gastrointestinal distress Insomnia Anorexia Anxiety Weight loss Diarrhea and flatulence
Alpha$_2$ Antagonist	
Mirtazapine	Sedation Anticholinergic effects Appetite increase Weight gain Hypercholesterolemia Weakness and lack of energy Dizziness Hypertriglyceridemia
Other Antidepressants	
Trazadone	Sedation Anticholinergic effects Headache Dizziness Nausea/vomiting
Vilazodone	Diarrhea Nausea Dizziness Dry mouth Insomnia Unusual dreams
Vortioxetine	Nausea Diarrhea Dizziness Dry mouth Constipation Vomiting
Tricyclic Antidepressants	
Amitriptyline Amoxapine Clomipramine Imipramine Desipramine Doxepin Nortriptyline Protriptyline	Drowsiness Anticholinergic effects Orthostatic hypotension Palpitations Tachycardia Impaired coordination Increased appetite Diaphoresis Weakness Disorientation Sexual side effects (impotence, changes in libido)
Tetracyclic Antidepressants	
Maprotiline	Blurred vision Dizziness Lightheadedness Sedation Dry mouth Libido changes Impotence Weight changes
Monoamine Oxidase Inhibitors	
Isocarboxazid	Dizziness Headache Nausea Dry mouth Constipation Drowsiness Sleep disturbance Orthostatic hypotension
Phenelzine	Orthostatic hypotension Edema Dizziness Headache Drowsiness Sleep disturbance
Tranylcypromine	Orthostatic hypotension Dizziness Headache Drowsiness Sleep disturbance Restlessness Central nervous system stimulation
Selegiline	Application site reaction Headache Insomnia Diarrhea Dry mouth Orthostatic hypotension Dyspepsia

TABLE 25.3 INTERVENTIONS TO RELIEVE SIDE EFFECTS OF ANTIDEPRESSANTS

Side Effect	Pharmacologic Intervention	Nonpharmacologic Intervention
Dry mouth, caries, inflammation of the mouth	Bethanechol 10–30 mg tid Pilocarpine drops	Sugarless gum Sugarless lozenges 6–8 cups of water per day Toothpaste for dry mouth
Nausea, vomiting	Change medication	Take medication with food Soda crackers, toast, tea
Weight gain	Change medication	Nutritionally balanced diet Daily exercise
Urinary hesitation	Bethanechol 10–30 mg tid	6–8 cups of water per day
Constipation	Stool softener	Bulk laxative Daily exercise 6–8 cups of water per day Diet rich in fresh fruits, vegetables, and whole grains
Diarrhea	OTC antidiarrheal	Maintain fluid intake
Orthostatic hypotension		Increase hydration Sit or stand up slowly
Drowsiness	Shift dosing time Lower medication dose Change medication	One caffeinated beverage at strategic time Do not drive when drowsy No alcohol or other recreational drugs Plan for rest time
Fatigue	Lower medication dose Change medication	Daily exercise
Blurred vision	Bethanechol 10–30 mg tid Pilocarpine eye drops	Temporary use of magnifying lenses until body adjusts to medication
Flushing, sweating	Terazosin 1 mg once daily Lower medication dose Change medication	Frequent bathing Lightweight clothing
Tremor	β-Blockers Lower medication dose	Reassure the patient that tremor may decrease as the patient adjusts to medication. Notify the caregiver if tremor interferes with daily functioning.

OTC, over-the-counter; tid, three times a day.

BOX 25.9

Serotonin Syndrome

CAUSE: Excessive intrasynaptic serotonin

HOW IT HAPPENS: Combining medications that increase CNS serotonin levels, such as SSRIs + MAOIs; SSRIs + St. John's wort; or SSRIs + diet pills; dextromethorphan or alcohol, especially red wine; or SSRI + street drugs, such as LSD, MMDA, or ecstasy

SYMPTOMS: Mental status changes, agitation, ataxia, myoclonus, hyperreflexia, fever, shivering, diaphoresis, diarrhea

TREATMENT

- Assess all medications, supplements, foods, and recreational drugs ingested to determine the offending substances.
- Discontinue any substances that may be causative factors. If symptoms are mild, treat supportively on an outpatient basis with propranolol and lorazepam and follow-up with the prescriber.
- If symptoms are moderate to severe, hospitalization may be needed with monitoring of vital signs and treatment with intravenous fluids, antipyretics, and cooling blankets.

FURTHER USE: Assess on a case-by-case basis and minimize risk factors for further medication therapy.

CNS, central nervous system; LSD, lysergic acid diethylamide; MAOI, monoamine oxidase inhibitor; MMDA, 3-methoxy-4,5-methylenedioxyamphetamine; SSRI, selective serotonin reuptake inhibitor.

EMERGENCY CARE ALERT The most important emergency interventions are stopping use of the offending drug, notifying the prescriber, and providing necessary supportive care (e.g., intravenous fluids, antipyretics, cooling blanket). Severe symptoms have been successfully treated with antiserotonergic agents, such as cyproheptadine (Simon et al., 2024).

Monitoring for Drug Interactions

Several potential drug interactions are associated with antidepressants. Alcohol consumption should be avoided when taking any antidepressant because SSRIs are metabolized in the liver, and other substances (such as alcohol) that are also metabolized in the liver by the same enzyme can cause an increase in drug levels, leading to toxicity and serotonin syndrome. For example, if migraine medications known as "triptans" are given with the SSRIs, serotonin syndrome can occur. Bupropion cannot be given at the same time as an MAOI. Grapefruit should not be consumed while taking trazodone. It is beyond the scope of this text to review drug–drug interactions in detail. Nurses should check with pharmacy resources for any drug–drug interactions when administering medications.

Teaching Points

If depression goes untreated or is inadequately treated, episodes can become more frequent, more severe, longer in duration, and can lead to suicide. Patient education involves explaining this pattern and the importance of continuing medication use after the acute phase of treatment to decrease the risk for future episodes. Patient concerns regarding long-term antidepressant therapy need to be assessed and addressed. All teaching points need to be developed and delivered using a culturally competent approach to enhance patient adherence.

Patients should also be advised not to take herbal substances such as St. John's wort or SAMe if they are also taking prescribed antidepressants. St. John's wort also should not be taken if the patient is taking nasal decongestants, hay fever and asthma medications containing monoamines, amino acid supplements containing phenylalanine, or tyrosine. The combination may cause hypertension.

Other Somatic Therapies

Electroconvulsive Therapy

Although its therapeutic mechanism of action is not completely understood, ECT is an effective treatment for patients with severe depression. It is generally reserved for patients whose disorder is refractory or intolerant to initial drug treatments such as older adults or for those who are so severely ill that rapid treatment is required (e.g., patients with malnutrition, catatonia, or suicidality). Older age is associated with a favorable response to ECT, but the effectiveness and safety in this group has not been shown (Sarma et al., 2024).

ECT is contraindicated for patients with increased intracranial pressure. Other high-risk patients include those with recent myocardial infarction, recent cerebrovascular accident, retinal detachment, or pheochromocytoma (a tumor in the cells of the adrenal gland) and those at risk for complications of anesthesia.

The role of the nurse in the care of the patient undergoing ECT is to provide educational and emotional support for the patient and family, assess baseline or pretreatment levels of function, prepare the patient for the ECT process, monitor and evaluate the patient's response to ECT, provide assessment data with the ECT team, and modify treatment as needed. The actual procedure, possible therapeutic mechanisms of action, potential adverse effects, contraindications, and nursing interventions are described in detail in Chapter 11.

Light Therapy (Phototherapy)

Light therapy is described in Chapter 11. Given current research, light therapy is an option for well-documented mild-to-moderate seasonal, nonpsychotic, winter depressive episodes in patients with recurrent major depressive disorders, including children and adolescents. Evidence also indicates that light therapy can modestly improve symptoms in nonseasonal depression, especially when administered during the first week of treatment in the morning for those experiencing sleep deprivation (Chen et al., 2024).

Repetitive Transcranial Magnetic Stimulation

Repetitive transcranial magnetic stimulation (rTMS) is FDA approved for the treatment of patients with mild treatment-resistant depression. In rTMS, a magnetic coil placed on the scalp at the site of the left motor cortex releases small electrical pulses that stimulate the site of the left dorsolateral prefrontal cortex in the superficial cortex. This rapidly changing magnetic field stimulates the brain sufficiently to depolarize neurons and exert effects across synapses. These pulses (similar in type and strength as a magnetic resonance imaging machine) easily pass through the hair, skin, and skull, requiring much less electricity than ECT. The patient is awake, reclining in an rTMS chair during the procedure, and can resume normal activities immediately after the procedure. Because anesthesia is not required, no risks are associated with sedation. Treatment of depression typically consists of 20 to 30 sessions, lasting 37 minutes each over 4 to 6 weeks. Depending on the level of practice and training, the nurse's role in the use of the rTMS varies from patient education, pre- and postprocedure care to performing the procedure (Oberman & Benussi, 2024).

Psychosocial Interventions

Therapeutic Interactions

Individuals experiencing depression often withdraw from daily activities, such as engaging in family activities, attending work, and participating in community functions. During hospitalization, patients often withdraw to their rooms and refuse to participate in unit activity. Nurses help the patient balance the need for privacy with the need to return to normal social functioning. Explain to patients that attending social activities, even though they do not feel like it, will promote the recovery process and help them achieve their goals. Even though patients who are depressed should not be approached in an overly enthusiastic, cheerful manner, they should be encouraged to set realistic goals to reconnect with their families and communities. Nurses should help the patient identify personal strengths and encourage them to use their strengths to reduce their depressive feelings.

Enhancing Cognitive Functioning

Cognitive interventions such as thought stopping and positive self-talk can dispel irrational beliefs and distorted attitudes and in turn reduce depressive symptoms during the acute phase of major depression. Nurses should consider using cognitive approaches when caring for people who are depressed. The use of cognitive interventions in the acute phase of treatment combined with medication is now considered first-line treatment for mildly to moderately depressed outpatients. See Chapter 13.

NCLEXNOTE A cognitive therapy approach is recommended for helping people restructure the negative thinking processes related to an individual's concept of self, others, and the future. This approach should be included in most nursing care plans for patients with depression.

Using Behavioral Interventions

Behavioral interventions are effective in the acute treatment of patients with mildly to moderately severe depression, especially when combined with pharmacotherapy. Therapeutic techniques include activity scheduling, social skills training, and problem solving. Behavioral therapy techniques are described in Chapter 6.

Complementary Therapies

Alternative or complementary therapies are often used in the treatment of depression. Acupuncture, yoga or tai chi, meditation, guided imagery, and massage therapy are a few therapies that may be helpful to palliate depression. Music or art therapy is also used often in conjunction with medication or psychotherapy (Zhao et al., 2023).

Spiritual Intervention

Spiritual well-being can reduce depression and anxiety. There are several interventions that lead to improved spiritual well-being. For example, reminiscence therapy has been shown to relieve anxiety and depression in stoke patients and their spouse caregivers (Zhang et al., 2024a). Other interventions that support spiritual well-being include spiritual counseling, prayer, worship, and religious rituals. Interventions associated with specific religious practices should be conducted by a religious or spiritual expert specific to that belief system.

Psychoeducation

Teaching About Symptoms

Patients with depression and their significant others often incorrectly believe that their illness is their own fault and that they should be able to "pull themselves up by their bootstraps and snap out of it." People from some cultural groups believe that the symptoms of depression may be a result of someone placing a hex on the affected person because the individual has done something evil. It is vital to be culturally competent to be effective in teaching patients and their families about the treatment modalities for depression.

Patients need to know the full range of suitable treatment options before consenting to participate in treatment. Information empowers patients to ask questions, weigh risks and benefits, and make the best treatment choices. The nurse can provide opportunities for patients to question, discuss, and explore their feelings about past, current, and planned use of medications and other treatments. Developing strategies to enhance adherence and to raise awareness of early signs of relapse can be important aids to increasing treatment efficacy and promoting recovery (Box 25.10).

Wellness Strategies

The patient needs to be able to incorporate wellness strategies to support recovery and resilience processes. The nurse needs to assess what the patient may be doing now for their wellness and support current wellness strategies, as well as provide new strategies. Sleep hygiene, healthy nutritional choices, leisure activities, relaxation, exercise, and positive interactions should be encouraged. For example, the nurse suggests walking 5 to 10 minutes 1 or 2 days a week and gradually increasing to 20 minutes a day three to four times per week. Nurses should encourage multiple strategies to help patients understand how to improve their resilience and recovery in conjunction with everyday functioning. The nurse should support any positive health approaches that the patient is incorporating into their daily life.

BOX 25.10

Psychoeducation Checklist: Major Depressive Disorder

When caring for the patient with a major depressive disorder, be sure to include the following topic areas in the teaching plan:

- Psychopharmacologic agents, including drug action, dosing frequency, and possible side effects
- Risk factors for recurrence; signs of recurrence
- Adherence to therapy and treatment program
- Recovery strategies
- Nutrition
- Sleep measures
- Self-care management
- Goal setting and problem solving
- Social interaction skills
- Follow-up appointments
- Community support services

Providing Family Education

The family needs education and support during and after the treatment of family members. Because major depressive disorder is a recurring disorder, the family needs information about specific antecedents to a family member's depression and what therapeutic steps to take. For example, one patient may routinely become depressed during the fall of each year, with one of the first symptoms being excessive sleepiness. For another patient, a major loss, such as a child going to college or the death of a pet, may precipitate a depressive episode. Families of older adults need to be aware of the possibility of depression and related symptoms, which often occur after the deaths of friends and relatives. Families of children who are depressed often misinterpret depression as behavioral issues.

Promoting Safety

For patients who are admitted to the psychiatric hospital because of a suicide attempt, suicidality should continually be evaluated, and the patient should be protected from self-harm (see Chapter 22). During the depths of depression, patients may not have the energy to complete a suicide. As patients begin to feel better and have increased energy, they therefore may be at a greater risk for suicide. If a patient who was previously depressed appears to have become energized overnight, they may have decided to die by suicide and thus may be relieved that the decision is finally made. The nurse may misinterpret the mood improvement as a positive move toward recovery; however, this patient may be very intent on suicide. These individuals should be carefully monitored to maintain their safety.

Convening Support Groups

Individuals who are depressed can receive emotional support in groups and learn how others deal with similar issues. As group members serve as role models for new group members, they also benefit as their self-esteem increases, which strengthens their ability to address their own issues (see Chapter 14). Group interventions are often used to help an individual cope with depression associated with bereavement or chronic medical illness. Group interventions are also commonly used to educate patients and families about their disorder and medications.

Nurses are exceptionally well positioned to engage patients and their families in the active process of improving daily functioning, increasing knowledge and skill acquisition, and increasing independent living. Consumer-oriented support groups can help to enhance the self-esteem and the support network of participating patients and their families. Advice, encouragement, and the sense of group camaraderie may make an important contribution to recovery. Organizations providing support and information include the Depression and Bipolar Support Network (DBSA), National Alliance on Mental Illness (NAMI), and the Mental Health Association and Recovery, Inc. (a self-help group).

Implementing Milieu Therapy

While hospitalized, milieu therapy (see Chapter 10) helps patients who are depressed maintain socialization skills and continue to interact with others. When depressed, people are often unaware of the environment and withdraw into themselves. On a psychiatric unit, patients who are depressed should be encouraged to attend and participate in unit activities. These individuals have decreased energy levels and thus may be moving more slowly than others; however, their efforts should be praised.

Family Interventions

Patients who perceive high family stress are at risk for greater future severity of illness, higher use of health services, and higher health care expense. Marital and family issues are common among patients with mood disorders; comprehensive treatment requires that these issues be assessed and addressed. They may be a consequence of the major depression but may also predispose people to develop depressive symptoms or inhibit recovery and resilience processes. Family and friends of people who attempt or die by suicide should be provided counseling and supportive services because they may experience feelings of grief, guilt, anger, depression, and confusion.

Research suggests that marital and family therapy may reduce depressive symptoms and the risk for relapse in patients with marital and family issues (Salinger et al., 2021). The depressed spouse's depression has a significant impact on the marital adjustment of the nondepressed spouse. It is recommended that treatment approaches be designed to help couples be supportive of each other, to adapt, and to cope with the depressive symptoms within the framework of their ongoing marital relations.

Counseling and supportive services should be provided to family and friends of people who attempt or die by suicide because family and friends may experience feelings of grief, guilt, anger, and confusion.

Many family nursing interventions may be used by the psychiatric nurse in providing targeted family-centered care. These include:

- Monitoring patient and family for indicators of stress
- Teaching stress management techniques

- Counseling family members on coping skills for their own use
- Providing necessary knowledge of options and support services
- Facilitating family routines and rituals
- Assisting the family to resolve feelings of guilt
- Assisting the family with conflict resolution
- Identifying family strengths and resources with family members
- Facilitating communication among family members

Developing Recovery-Oriented Rehabilitation Strategies

Nurses should incorporate recovery and resilience concepts into inpatient settings as these strategies help to improve the QoL, help the transition to outpatient care, and decrease hospital readmission rates (Aggestrup et al., 2024). The guiding principles for recovery include a strength-based, self-directed approach so patients can feel a sense of hope, gain an understanding of their disorder, decrease the effects of trauma, and increase their ability to become more resilient in dealing with their everyday life situations.

Evaluation of Patient Outcomes

The major goals of treatment are to help the patient to be as independent as possible and to achieve stability, remission, and recovery from major depression. These goals are often a lifelong struggle. To monitor outcomes of treatment, ongoing evaluation of the individual's symptoms, functioning, and QoL should be carefully documented in the patient's record.

Continuum of Care

Mild-to-moderate depression is often first recognized in primary care settings. Primary care nurses should be able to recognize depression in these patients and make appropriate interventions or referrals.

Emergency Care

Those with more severe depressive symptoms or thoughts of suicide will be directly admitted to inpatient and outpatient mental health settings or emergency departments.

Inpatient-Focused Care

Although most patients with major depression are treated in outpatient settings, brief hospitalization may be required if the patient is suicidal, a danger to others, or experiencing psychosis. Nurses working on inpatient units provide a wide range of direct services, including administering and monitoring medications and target symptoms; conducting psychoeducational groups; and more generally, structuring and maintaining a therapeutic environment.

Community Care

The continuum of care beyond primary care and hospital settings may include partial hospitalization or day treatment programs; individual, family, or group psychotherapy; and home visits. Nurses providing home care have an excellent opportunity to detect undiagnosed depressive disorders and make appropriate referrals.

Virtual Mental Health Care

Virtual mental health care or telehealth is an important resource that has emerged as an efficacious option for assessing and treating depression and depressive disorders (Kelber et al., 2024). The use of video and audio formats can closely mimic in-person interactions and psychotherapy sessions. Although more research is needed regarding patient satisfaction and treatment effectiveness, studies support the use of telehealth for individuals who are depressed and have a chronic disease, are homebound, need a physically safe environment, or have transportation issues (Wu et al., 2024). Internet-based CBT for depression can be a cost-effective intervention and is showing efficacy in treating major depression (Newby et al., 2024).

Telehealth is becoming an important tool in suicide prevention. National hotline numbers, texting sites, and suicide alert systems imbedded in telehealth psychotherapy programs have the potential to reduce communication barriers for individuals with suicidal ideation or intention (Shoib et al., 2024).

Integration with Primary Care

Comprehensive services require a coordinated ongoing interaction among patients, families, and health care providers. This includes using the complementary skills of both psychiatric and medical care colleagues for forming overall goals, plans, and decisions and for providing continuity of care as needed. Collaborative care between the primary care provider and mental health specialist is also key to achieving remission of symptoms and physical well-being, restoring baseline occupational and psychosocial functioning, and reducing the likelihood of relapse or recurrence.

Depression is often treated in the primary care setting with readily available antidepressants. Ideally, mental health services are integrated into primary health care settings. See Box 25.11. Many individuals need more than

BOX 25.11

Research for Evidence-Based Practice: Mental Health Integration in a Nurse Home Visiting Program

Beeber, L. S., Gasbarro, M., Knudtson, M., Ledford, A., Sprinkle, S., Leeman, J., McMichael, G., Zeanah, P., & Mosqueda, A. (2024). A mental health innovation for nurse home visiting program shows effectiveness in reducing depressive symptoms and anxiety. Prevention Science, *25(1), 126–136. https://doi.org/10.1007/s11121-023-01574-6*

THE QUESTION: Is a mental health intervention within a nurse-delivered home visiting program for first-time mothers effective in increasing mental health screenings and referral to mental health services?

METHODS: The Mental Health Innovation (MHI) program prepares nurses to assess, refer, manage crises, and intervene using evidence-based approaches including mindful cognitive-behavioral approaches, social support mobilization, advance directives, activity amplification. Two versions of the MHI were evaluated. The *standard* intervention provided online learning modules, team meeting education modules, and clinical resources to Nurse Family Partnership (NFP) agencies nationwide. The *enhanced* intervention provided the standard intervention with periodic consultations with experts in mental health care to a subset of NFP teams.

A pre/postlaunch comparison of 356 teams randomized to standard versus enhanced intervention was analyzed for an increase in screenings and enrollment in NFP services. Six teams (42 nurses and 6 supervisors) were randomized to the enhanced intervention.

FINDINGS: There was a significant increase in enrollment of patients with a mental health diagnosis or positive screen for depression from pre- to postlaunch MHI. The enhanced group served more patients with a mental health diagnosis or positive depression screen.

IMPLICATION FOR NURSING: This study supports the use of mental health screenings in a nurse home visiting program for first-time mothers who are experiencing a mental disorder or screen positively for depression.

medication, but do not access mental health services for a variety of reasons such as stigma, fear of being labeled as mentally ill, and lack of resources. There are also several medical issues associated with depression such as hypothyroidism (Zhou et al., 2024). Pain is a common issue for individuals who are depressed (Tesic et al., 2023). It is important to communicate with the primary care provider to coordinate care.

The **medical home model** is becoming widely accepted in the United States. If a patient is cared for within a medical home model, all of their health and mental health needs are coordinated by one health provider. Meaningful long-term relationships can be developed. The advantage of a medical home is the recognition and coordination of all health care needs. This model is helpful when many of comorbid disorders requiring multiple providers. This model reduces expensive care and enhances continuity of care (Fakeye et al., 2023).

OTHER DEPRESSIVE DISORDERS

Other depressive disorders with similar symptoms are treated similarly to the major depressive disorders. Nursing care should be individualized and based on their patients' mental health needs and strengths.

PERSISTENT DEPRESSIVE DISORDER

In **persistent depressive disorder** (*dysthymia*), major depressive disorder symptoms last for at least 2 years for an adult and 1 year for children and adolescents. These individuals are depressed for most of each day. A major depressive disorder may precede the persistent depressive disorder or co-occur with it (Patel et al., 2024).

PREMENSTRUAL DYSPHORIC DISORDER

Premenstrual dysphoric disorder is diagnosed when there are clinically significant somatic and psychological manifestation (mood swings, feelings of sadness, or sensitivity to rejection) that occur consistently during the luteal phase of the menstrual cycle and negatively impact functioning and lifestyle. The mood begins to improve a few days after menses begins. Stress, history of interpersonal trauma, seasonal changes are associated with this disorder (Mishra et al., 2023).

DISRUPTIVE MOOD DYSREGULATION DISORDER

Disruptive mood dysregulation disorder is characterized by severe irritability and outbursts of temper. The onset of disruptive mood dysregulation disorder begins before the age of 10, when children have verbal rages and/or are physically aggressive toward others or property. These outbursts are outside of the normal temper tantrums children display. They are more severe than what would be expected developmentally and occur frequently (i.e., two or three times a week). This behavior disrupts family functioning as well as the child's ability to succeed in school and social activities. This disorder can co-occur with attention-deficit/hyperactivity disorder. See Chapter 37.

Disruptive mood dysregulation disorder is similar to pediatric bipolar disorder, but the *DSM-5-TR* differentiates it from bipolar disorder. Children with this disorder have similar deficits in recognition of emotion through facial expression, decision-making, and control as those with bipolar disorder. More research is needed in understanding this disorder (Zhang et al., 2024b).

SUMMARY OF KEY POINTS

- Moods influence perception of life events and functioning. Depressive disorders are characterized by persistent or recurring disturbances in mood that cause significant psychological distress and functional impairment (typified by feelings of sadness, hopelessness, loss of interest, and fatigue).
- Risk factors include a family history of depressive disorders, prior depressive episodes; lack of social support; stressful life events; substance use; and medical issues, particularly chronic or terminal illnesses.
- Pregnant patients and people who are subjects of discrimination, such as people of color and people who identify as LGBTQ+, are at high risk for depression and being unhoused.
- Treatment of major depressive disorder primarily includes antidepressant medication, psychotherapy, or a combination of both. ECT, light therapy, and rTMS are also used.
- Nurses must be knowledgeable regarding culturally competent related to the use of antidepressant medications, pharmacologic therapeutic effects and associated side effects, toxicity, dosage ranges, and contraindications. Nurses must also be familiar with ECT protocols and associated interventions. Patient education and the provision of emotional support during the course of treatment are also nursing responsibilities.
- Many symptoms of depression (e.g., weight and appetite changes, sleep disturbance, decreased energy, fatigue) are similar to those of medical illnesses. Assessment includes a thorough medical history and physical examination to detect or rule out medical or psychiatric comorbidity.
- Suicide assessment and prevention are priorities in caring for people with depression.
- Mental health nursing assessment includes assessing physical health and functioning; mood; speech patterns; thought processes and content; suicidal or homicidal thoughts; cognition and memory; spirituality and social factors, such as patterns of relationships, quality of support systems, and changes in occupational functioning. Several self-report scales are helpful in evaluating depressive symptoms.
- Establishing and maintaining a therapeutic culturally competent nurse–patient relationship is key to successful outcomes. Nursing interventions based on cultural humility that foster the therapeutic relationship include being available in times of crisis, providing understanding and education to patients and their families regarding goals of treatment, providing encouragement and feedback concerning the patient's progress, providing guidance in the patient's interpersonal interactions with others and work environment, spiritual interventions, and helping to set and monitor realistic goals.
- Psychosocial interventions for depressive disorders include self-care management, cognitive therapy, behavior therapy, interpersonal therapy, patient and family education regarding the nature of the disorder and treatment goals, marital and family interventions, and group interventions that include medication maintenance support groups and other consumer-oriented support groups.

DEVELOPING CLINICAL JUDGMENT

1. Describe how you would do a suicide assessment on a patient who comes into a primary care office and is distraught, expressing concerns about their ability to cope with the current situation.
2. Describe how you would approach a patient who does not want to talk with you.
3. Describe how you would approach a patient who is expressing concern that the diagnosis of depressive disorder will negatively affect personal social and work relationships.
4. If a patient is depressed and does not seem inclined to talk about their depression, what measures would you take to initiate a therapeutic relationship?
5. Compare the primary side effects of the SSRIs, TCAs, and MAOIs.
6. Think about all the above situations and relate them to people from a specific cultural or ethnic underrepresented group (e.g., people of African, Latinx, or Asian descent; individuals who practice Judaism or who are Jehovah's Witnesses; individuals across the life span, from children to older adult populations).

MOVIES, TV, OR STREAMING PROGRAMS

***The Holdovers:* 2023.** In the 1970s, five students at a prestigious New England boys' boarding school are unable to leave school for their Christmas break. One of the boys, Angus Tully (Dominic Sessa), is unable to leave school because his mother unexpectedly canceled their family vacation at the last minute in order to be with her new husband. Angus is often in trouble and is not well liked by his peers. Faculty member Paul Hunham (Paul Giamatti) is forced to stay and supervise the boys with the cafeteria manager, Mary Lamb, whose son was recently killed in Vietnam. (Da'Vine Joy Randolph won the 2024

Best Supporting Actress Oscar for her portrayal of Mary Lamb.) Professor Hunham is a cranky, depressed, stern middle-aged teacher of the classics who is determined to maintain a strict schedule for the boys. When one of the students' fathers arrives to take the boys on a skiing trip, all of the boys are able to go except Angus, who is unable to reach his mother for permission to go on the trip. The story unfolds as the three distraught people left at the school try to make the best of the situation.

Paul, Mary, and Angus have symptoms of depression from trauma. Paul's career has been derailed, and he is fearful of losing his teaching position. Mary is grieving the death of her only son. Angus is dealing with being abandoned by his father and rejected by his mother.

Viewing Points:

1. Identify the traumas that Paul, Mary, and Angus experienced.
2. How does each character exhibit and cope with their depression?
3. How could these three diverse people manage to experience a meaningful holiday? Give an example.
4. Identify the medication that Angus was prescribed. Would that medication be the best treatment for his depression today?

Unfolding Patient Stories: Li Na Chen • Part 2

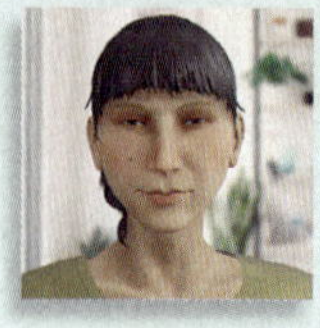

Recall from Chapter 3 **Li Na Chen**, who was hospitalized with a diagnosis of recurrent major depressive disorder after a suicide attempt by overdose. Her treatment plan includes transitioning to a partial hospitalization program before fully transitioning home. Her husband is concerned about their two children, ages 12 and 14, and his ability to collaborate with Li Na in the management of her treatment when she is home. How can the nurse further assess the husband's concerns? How may Li Na's depression and attempted suicide affect her husband and children? The nurse includes the pharmacologic plans for Li Na's care in discharge planning. What nonpharmacologic interventions need to be considered in discharge planning for Li Na as well as for her husband and children?

Care for Li Na and other patients in a realistic virtual environment: ***vSim** for Nursing* (thepoint.lww.com/vSimMentalHealth). Practice documenting these patients' care in DocuCare (thepoint.lww.com/DocuCareEHR).

REFERENCES

Aggestrup, A. S., Martiny, F., Lund Henriksen, L., Davidsen, A. S., & Martiny, K. (2024). Interventions promoting recovery from depression for patients transitioning from outpatient mental health services to primary care: A scoping review. *PLoS One*, *19*(5), e0302229. https://doi.org/10.1371/journal.pone.0302229

Ahmadi, A., Allahverdipour, H., Valiee, S., Pashazadeh, F., Ghassab-Abdollahi, N., Abdoli, F., & Matlabi, H. (2023). COVID-19 stress and coping strategies among older adults: a systematic review of qualitative evidences. *BMC Psychology*, *11*(1), 333. https://doi.org/10.1186/s40359-023-01382-1

Al-Abri, K., Edge, D., & Armitage, C. J. (2023). Prevalence and correlates of perinatal depression. *Social Psychiatry and Psychiatric Epidemiology*, *58*(11):1581–1590. https://doi.org/10.1007/s00127-022-02386-9

American Psychiatric Association (APA). (2022). *Diagnostic and statistical manual of mental disorders, fifth edition, text revision*. Author.

Basiri, R., Seidu, B., & Rudich, M. (2023). Exploring the interrelationships between diabetes, nutrition, anxiety, and depression: Implications for treatment and prevention strategies. *Nutrients*, *15*(19), 4226. https://doi.org/10.3390/nu15194226

Brasileiro, L. E. E., Dantas, A. A. G., Linhares, D. B., Vale, H. A., Terradas-Monllor, M., Ochandorena-Acha, M., Paiva, A. L. M., de Medeiros, M. Y. D., Jerez-Roig, J., & de Souza, D. L. B. (2024). Incidence of depression among community-dwelling older adults: A systematic review. *Psychogeriatrics*, *24*(2), 496–512. https://doi.org/10.1111/psyg.13081

Cai, H., Chen, P., Zhang, Q., Lam, M. I., Si, T. L., Liu, Y. F., Zheng, W. Y., Su, Z., Cheung, T., Jackson, T., Ungvari, G. S., Ren, Z., Li, X., Li, X. H., & Xiang, Y. T. (2024). Global prevalence of major depressive disorder in LGBTQ+ samples: A systematic review and meta-analysis of epidemiological studies. *Journal of Affective Disorders*, *360*, 249–258. https://doi.org/10.1016/j.jad.2024.05.115

Canatan, S. D., Arifoğlu, B., & Yatmaz, G. (2024). Adverse childhood events of individuals and its relationship with resilience. *Archives of Psychiatric Pursing*, *51*, 114–119. https://doi.org/10.1016/j.apnu.2024.05.003

Carlessi, A. S., Borba, L. A., Zugno, A. I., Quevedo, J., & Réus, G. Z. (2021). Gut microbiota-brain axis in depression: The role of neuroinflammation. *The European Journal of Neuroscience*, *53*(1), 222–235. https://doi.org/10.1111/ejn.14631

Chau, R., Kissane, D. W., & Davison, T. E. (2021). Risk factors for depression in long-term care: A prospective observational cohort study. *Clinical Gerontologist*, *44*(2), 112–125. https://doi.org/10.1080/07317115.2019.1635548

Chen, G., Chen, P., Yang, Z., Ma, W., Yan, H., Su, T., Zhang, Y., Qi, Z., Fang, W., Jiang, L., Chen, Z., Tao, Q., & Wang, Y. (2024). Increased functional connectivity between the midbrain and frontal cortex following bright light therapy in subthreshold depression: A randomized clinical trial. *The American Psychologist*, *79*(3), 437–450. https://doi.org/10.1037/amp0001218

Cook, B. L., Rastegar, J., & Patel, N. (2024). Social risk factors and racial and ethnic disparities in health care resource utilization among Medicare advantage beneficiaries with psychiatric disorders. *Medical Care Research and Review*, *81*(3), 209–222. https://doi.org/10.1177/10775587231222583

Corcoran, J., Marinescu, I., Vogelsang, C., Kim, J. C., & Morgan, S. (2021). Prevalence of depression in women with low income living in developed countries. *Depression and Anxiety*, *38*(10), 1046–1053. https://doi.org/10.1002/da.23208

Cui, L., Li, S., Wang, S., Wu, X., Liu, Y., Yu, W., Wang, Y., Tang, Y., Xia, M., & Li, B. (2024). Major depressive disorder: Hypothesis, mechanism, prevention and treatment. *Signal Transduction and Targeted Therapy*, *9*(1), 30. https://doi.org/10.1038/s41392-024-01738-y

Danzo, S., Kuklinski, M. R., Sterling, S. A., Beck, A., Braciszewski, J. M., Boggs, J., Briney, J. S., Charvat-Aguilar, N., Eisenberg, N., Kaffl, A., Kline-Simon, A., Loree, A. M., Lyons, V. H., Morse, E. F., Morrison, K. M., Negusse, R., & Scheuer, H. (2024). Anxiety, depression, and suicidal ideation among early adolescents during the COVID-19 pandemic. *Journal of Adolescence*, *96*(6), 1379–1387. https://doi.org/10.1002/jad.12333

DeBattista, C., & Schatzberg, A. F. (2024). *Schatzberg's manual of clinical psychopharmacology* (10th ed.). American Psychiatric Association Publishing.

Dorsey Holliman, B., Dieujuste, N., Yost, E., & Allison, M. A. (2024). A qualitative inquiry into nurse-family partnership black client perspectives. *Prevention Science*, *25*, 1143–1152. https://doi.org/10.1007/s11121-024-01709-3

Fadipe, M. F., Aggarwal, S., Johnson, C., & Beauchamp, J. E. S. (2023). Effectiveness of online cognitive behavioural therapy on quality of life in adults with depression: A systematic review. *Journal of Psychiatric and Mental Health Nursing*, *30*(5), 885–898. https://doi.org/10.1111/jpm.12924

Fakeye, O. A., Hsu, Y. J., Weiner, J. P., & Marsteller, J. A. (2023). Impact of the patient-centered medical home on consistently high-cost patients. *The American Journal of Managed Care*, *29*(12), 680–686. https://doi.org/10.37765/ajmc.2023.89467

Gaddey, H. L., Mason, B., & Naik, A. (2024). Depression: Managing resistance and partial response to treatment. *American Family Physician*, *109*(5), 410–416.

Garnett, M. F., Spencer, M. R., & Weeks, J. D. (2023). Suicide among adults age 55 and older, 2021. NCHS Data Brief, No. 483. Hyattsville, MD:

National Center for Health Statistics. https://www.cdc.gov/nchs/data/databriefs/db483.pdf

GBD 2021 Diseases and Injuries Collaborators. (2024). Global incidence, prevalence, years lived with disability (YLDs), disability-adjusted life-years (DALYs), and healthy life expectancy (HALE) for 371 diseases and injuries in 204 countries and territories and 811 subnational locations, 1990–2021: A systematic analysis for the Global Burden of Disease Study 2021. *Lancet*, *403*(10440), 2133–2161. https://doi.org/10.1016/S0140-6736(24)00757-8

Goodman, L. C., Elmore, J. S., Mayes, T. L., Minhajuddin, A., Slater, H., Blader, J. C., Liberzon, I., Baronia, R. B., Bivins, E. J., LaGrone, J. M., Jackson, S., Martin, S. L., Brown, R., Soares, J. C., Wakefield, S. M., & Trivedi, M. H. (2024). Linking trauma to mental health in the statewide Texas Youth Depression and Suicide Research Network (TX-YDSRN). *Psychiatry Research*, *331*, 115620. https://doi.org/10.1016/j.psychres.2023.115620

Hammer, L. A., Fergerson, A. K., & Bonfils, K. A. (2024). Recommendations for the assessment of sexual and gender minority status in serious mental illness research and clinical care. *Psychological Services*, *21*(3), 417–425. https://doi.org/10.1037/ser0000852

Hantsoo, L., Jagodnik, K. M., Novick, A. M., Baweja, R., di Scalea, T. L., Ozerdem, A., McGlade, E. C., Simeonova, D. I., Dekel, S., Kornfield, S. L., Nazareth, M., & Weiss, S. J. (2023). The role of the hypothalamic-pituitary-adrenal axis in depression across the female reproductive lifecycle: Current knowledge and future directions. *Frontiers in Endocrinology*, *14*, 1295261. https://doi.org/10.3389/fendo.2023.1295261

Hassan, A. N., & Le Foll, B. (2021). Survival probabilities and predictors of major depressive episode incidence among individuals with various types of substance use disorders. *The Journal of Clinical Psychiatry*, *82*(5), 20m13637. https://doi.org/10.4088/JCP.20m13637

Henry, N. L., & Gilley, N. (2024). Spiritual assessment. In *StatPearls*. StatPearls Publishing. www.ncbi.nlm.nih.gov/books/NBK599554

Janssen Pharmaceuticals, Inc. (2024). Spravato prescribing information. Retrieved December 31, 2024, from https://www.accessdata.fda.gov/drugsatfda_docs/label/2024/211243s015lbl.pdf

Kelber, M. S., Smolenski, D. J., Boyd, C., Shank, L. M., Bellanti, D. M., Milligan, T., Edwards-Stewart, A., Libretto, S., Parisi, K., Morgan, M. A., & Evatt, D. P. (2024). Evidence-based telehealth interventions for posttraumatic stress disorder, depression, and anxiety: A systematic review and meta-analysis. *Journal of Telemedicine and Telecare*, 1357633X231224491. https://doi.org/10.1177/1357633X231224491

Kennedy, A., & Brausch, A. M. (2024). Emotion dysregulation, bullying, and suicide behaviors in adolescents. *Journal of Affective Disorders Reports*, *15*, 100715. https://doi.org/10.1016/j.jadr.2023.100715

Kim, J. W., Suzuki, K., Kavalali, E. T., & Monteggia, L. M. (2024). Ketamine: Mechanisms and relevance to treatment of depression. *Annual Review of Medicine*, *75*, 129–143. https://doi.org/10.1146/annurev-med-051322-120608

Kneale, D., & Bécares, L. (2024). The influence of a hostile environment on a syndemic of depression, stress and chronic limiting illness among LGBTQ+ people during the COVID-19 pandemic. *Sociology of Health & Illness*, *46*(1), 114–136. https://doi.org/10.1111/1467-9566.13689

Lee, B., Wang, Y., Carlson, S. A., Greenlund, K. J. Lu, H., Liu, Y., Croft, J. B., Eke, P. I., Town, M., & Thomas, C. W. (2023). National, state-level, and county-level prevalence estimates of adults aged ≥18 years self-reporting a lifetime diagnosis of depression—United States, 2020. *MMWR Morbidity Mortality Weekly Report*, 72, 644–650. http://dx.doi.org/10.15585/mmwr.mm7224a1

Lee, W., Shin, H. J., Min, I. K., Kim, C. S., Kim, K. M., Heo, K., & Chu, M. K. (2024). Shared comorbidity of depression, migraine, insomnia, and fibromyalgia in a population-based sample. *Journal of Affective Disorders*, *354*, 619–626. https://doi.org/10.1016/j.jad.2024.03.077

Leung, J. G. (2023). Ethnopsychopharmacology: Clinical and scientific writing pearls. *The Mental Health Clinician*, *13*(6), 276–288. https://doi.org/10.9740/mhc.2023.12.276

Li, G., Li, Y., Lam, A. I. F., Tang, W., Seedat, S., Barbui, C., Papola, D., Panter-Brick, C., van der Waerden, J., Bryant, R., Mittendorfer-Rutz, E., Gémes, K., Purba, F. D., Setyowibowo, H., Pinucci, I., Palantza, C., Acarturk, C., Kurt, G., Tarsitani, L., Morina, N.,…Hall, B. J. (2023). Understanding the protective effect of social support on depression symptomatology from a longitudinal network perspective. *BMJ Mental Health*, *26*(1), e300802. https://doi.org/10.1136/bmjment-2023-300802

Mejova, Y., & Lu, A. H. (2023). Self-disclosure of loneliness by LGBTQ+ twitter users during COVID-19. *Journal of Homosexuality*, 1–28. https://doi.org/10.1080/00918369.2023.2263801

Mekawi, Y., Ishiekwene, M. N., Jimenez, A. N., Ware, M., Carter, S. E., Stenson, A. F., Jovanovic, T., Bradley-Davino, B., & Powers, A. (2023). Intergenerational transmission of depression: Examining the roles of racism and trauma among Black mothers and youth. *Journal of the American Academy of Child and Adolescent Psychiatry*, *62*(10), 1147–1156. https://doi.org/10.1016/j.jaac.2023.04.016

Mishra, S., Elliott, H., & Marwaha, R. (2023). Premenstrual dysphoric disorder. In *StatPearls*. StatPearls Publishing. www.ncbi.nlm.nih.gov/books/NBK532307

Mitsdarffer, M. L., McColl, R., Nescott, E., Bianchetta, J., Layland, E. K., & Tőth, T. (2023). LGBTQ+ Youth homelessness in Delaware: Building a case for targeted surveillance and assessment of LGBTQ+ youth needs and experiences. *Delaware Journal of Public Health*, *9*(2), 80–86. https://doi.org/10.32481/djph.2023.06.014

National Institute of Mental Health (NIMH). (2023). Major depression. Retrieved August 28, 2024, from https://www.nimh.nih.gov/health/statistics/major-depression#part_2563

Newby, J. M., Upton, E., Mason, E., & Black, M. (2024). Technology-based cognitive behavioral therapy interventions. *The Psychiatric Clinics of North America*, *47*(2), 399–417. https://doi.org/10.1016/j.psc.2024.02.004

Nguyen, T. D., Kowalec, K., Pasman, J., Larsson, H., Lichtenstein, P., Dalman, C., Sullivan, P. F., Kuja-Halkola, R., & Lu, Y. (2023). Genetic contribution to the heterogeneity of major depressive disorder: Evidence from a sibling-based design using Swedish national registers. *The American Journal of Psychiatry*, *180*(10), 714–722. https://doi.org/10.1176/appi.ajp.20220906

Noetel, M., Sanders, T., Gallardo-Gómez, D., Taylor, P., Del Pozo Cruz, B., van den Hoek, D., Smith, J. J., Mahoney, J., Spathis, J., Moresi, M., Pagano, R., Pagano, L., Vasconcellos, R., Arnott, H., Varley, B., Parker, P., Biddle, S., & Lonsdale, C. (2024). Effect of exercise for depression: Systematic review and network meta-analysis of randomised controlled trials. *British Medical Journal*, *384*, e075847. https://doi.org/10.1136/bmj-2023-075847

Nusslock, R., Alloy, L. B., Brody, G. H., & Miller, G. E. (2024). Annual research review: Neuroimmune network model of depression: A developmental perspective. *Journal of Child Psychology and Psychiatry, and Allied Disciplines*, *65*(4), 538–567. https://doi.org/10.1111/jcpp.13961

Oberman, L. M., & Benussi, A. (2024). Transcranial magnetic stimulation across the lifespan: Impact of developmental and degenerative processes. *Biological Psychiatry*, *95*(6), 581–591. https://doi.org/10.1016/j.biopsych.2023.07.012

O'Connor, S. J., Hewitt, N., Kuc, J., & Orsini, L. S. (2023). Predictors and risk factors of treatment-resistant depression: A systematic review. *The Journal of Clinical Psychiatry*, *85*(1), 23r14885. https://doi.org/10.4088/JCP.23r14885

Oladunjoye, A. F., Li, E., Aneni, K., & Onigu-Otite, E. (2023). Cannabis use disorder, suicide attempts, and self-harm among adolescents: A national inpatient study across the United States. *PLoS One*, *18*(10), e0292922. https://doi.org/10.1371/journal.pone.0292922

Patel, R. K., Aslam, S. P., & Rose, G. M. (2024). Persistent depressive disorder. In *StatPearls*. StatPearls Publishing. www.ncbi.nlm.nih.gov/books/NBK541052

Pederson, A. B. (2023). Management of depression in Black people: Effects of cultural issues. *Psychiatric Annals*, *53*(3), 122–125. https://doi.org/10.3928/00485713-20230215-01

Qaseem, A., Andrews, R. A., Campos, K., Goldzweig, C. L., MacDonald, S., McLean, R. M., Powell, R. E., Fitterman, N., Performance Measurement Committee of the American College of Physicians; Basch, P., Choi, E., Chou, R., Hamori, C. J., Mount, C. A., & Campos, K. (2024). Quality indicators for major depressive disorder in adults: A review of performance measures by the American College of Physicians. *Annals of Internal Medicine*, 177(4), 507–513. https://doi.org/10.7326/M23-3077

Rao, V., Lanni, S., Yule, A. M., DiSalvo, M., Stone, M., Berger, A. F., & Wilens, T. E. (2023). Diagnosing major depressive disorder and substance use disorder using the electronic health record: A preliminary validation study. *Journal of Mood and Anxiety Disorders*, *2*, 100007. https://doi.org/10.1016/j.xjmad.2023.100007

Rastogi, R., Woolverton, G. A., Lee, R. M., Yip, T., Stevens, C., Chen, J. A., & Liu, C. H. (2024). Microaggression and discrimination exposure on young adult anxiety, depression, and sleep. *Journal of Affective Disorders*, *363*, 141–151. https://doi.org/10.1016/j.jad.2024.07.083

Sadek, J., Diaz-Piedra, B., Saleh, L., & MacDonald, L. (2024). A narrative review: Suicide and suicidal behaviour in older adults. *Frontiers in Psychiatry*, *15*, 1395462. https://doi.org/10.3389/fpsyt.2024.1395462

Salinger, J. M., Whisman, M. A., Randall, A. K., & Hilpert, P. (2021). Associations between marital discord and depressive symptoms: A cross-cultural analysis. *Family Process*, *60*(2), 493–506. https://doi.org/10.1111/famp.12563

Sarma, S., Zeng, Y., Barreiros, A. R., Dong, V., Massaneda-Tuneu, C., Cao, T. V., Waite, S., McCosker, L. K., Branjerdporn, G., Loo, C. K., & Martin, D. M. (2024). Clinical outcomes of electroconvulsive therapy (ECT) for depression in older old people relative to other age groups across the adult life span: A CARE network study. *International Journal of Geriatric Psychiatry, 39*(8), e6133. https://doi.org/10.1002/gps.6133

Seager, M. J., Bolton, S. L., Bolton, J. M., Mota, N. P., Afifi, T. O., Sareen, J., & Enns, M. W. (2024). Coping style as a risk factor for future alcohol use disorder: A 16-year longitudinal study in a Canadian military sample. *Drug and Alcohol Dependence, 262*, 111408. https://doi.org/10.1016/j.drugalcdep.2024.111408

Segal, Y., & Gunturu, S. (2024). Psychological issues associated with obesity. In *StatPearls*. StatPearls Publishing. www.ncbi.nlm.nih.gov/books/NBK603747

Sekhon, S., Patel, J., & Sapra, A. (2023). Late-life depression. In *StatPearls*. StatPearls Publishing. www.ncbi.nlm.nih.gov/books/NBK551507.

Shoib, S., Shaheen, N., Anwar, A., Saad, A. M., Mohamed Akr, L., Saud, A. I., Kundu, M., Nahidi, M., Chandradasa, M., Swed, S., & Saeed, F. (2024). The effectiveness of telehealth interventions in suicide prevention: A systematic review and meta-analysis. *The International Journal of Social Psychiatry, 70*(3), 415–423. https://doi.org/10.1177/00207640231206059

Sik, D. (2021). From lay depression narratives to secular ritual healing: An online ethnography of mental health forums. *Culture, Medicine and Psychiatry, 45*(4), 751–774. https://doi.org/10.1007/s11013-020-09702-5

Simon, L. V., Torrico, T. J., & Keenaghan, M. (2024). Serotonin syndrome. In *StatPearls*. StatPearls Publishing. www.ncbi.nlm.nih.gov/books/NBK482377

Smith, M. V., & Mazure, C. M. (2021). Mental health and wealth: Depression, gender, poverty, and parenting. *Annual Review of Clinical Psychology, 17*, 181–205. https://doi.org/10.1146/annurev-clinpsy-071219-022710

Stewart, A. L., & Payne, J. L. (2023). Perinatal depression: A review and an update. *The Psychiatric Clinics of North America, 46*(3), 447–461. https://doi.org/10.1016/j.psc.2023.04.003

Stone, D. M., Mack, K. A., & Qualters J. (2023). Notes from the field: Recent changes in suicide rates, by race and ethnicity and age group—United States, 2021. *MMWR Morbidity Mortality Weekly Report*, 72, 160–162. http://dx.doi.org/10.15585/mmwr.mm7206a4

Strawn, J. R., Mills, J. A., Suresh, V., Peris, T. S., Walkup, J. T., & Croarkin, P. E. (2022). Combining selective serotonin reuptake inhibitors and cognitive behavioral therapy in youth with depression and anxiety. *Journal of Affective Disorders, 298*(Pt A), 292–300. https://doi.org/10.1016/j.jad.2021.10.047

Sun, S. (2023). *National snapshot: Poverty among women & families*. National Women's Law Center. https://nwlc.org/wp-content/uploads/2023/02/2023_nwlc_PovertySnapshot-converted.pdf

Tesic, I., Pigoni, A., Moltrasio, C., Brambilla, P., & Delvecchio, G. (2023). How does feeling pain look like in depression: A review of functional neuroimaging studies. *Journal of Affective Disorders, 339*, 400–411. https://doi.org/10.1016/j.jad.2023.07.083

Umucu, E., Gooding, D. C., Granger, T., Wyman, M., Lambrou, N., Summers, M., Strong, L., Martin, W., Carter, F., Bouges, S., Johnson, A., & Gleason, C. E. (2024). Ethno-racial differences in depressive symptom endorsement: Evaluation of brief forms of the Geriatric Depression Scale in older adults. *Journal of Affective Disorders, 364*, 274–278. https://doi.org/10.1016/j.jad.2024.08.063

VA Suicide Prevention. (2023). *2023 National Veteran suicide Prevention Annual Report*. Office of mental Health and Suicide Prevention. U.S. Department of Veterans Affairs. https://www.mentalhealth.va.gov/docs/data-sheets/2023/2023-National-Veteran-Suicide-Prevention-Annual-Report-FINAL-508.pdf

Vest, B. M., Wray, L. O., Thase, M. E., Brady, L. A., Chapman, S. R., & Oslin, D. W. (2023). Providers' use of pharmacogenetic testing to inform antidepressant prescribing: Results of qualitative interviews. *Psychiatric Services, 74*(12), 1270–1276. https://doi.org/10.1176/appi.ps.20220537

Won, M. R., Choi, E. J., Ko, E., Um, Y. J., & Choi, Y. J. (2021). The mediating effect of life satisfaction and the moderated mediating effect of social support on the relationship between depression and suicidal behavior among older adults. *International Journal of Geriatric Psychiatry, 36*(11), 1732–1738. https://doi.org/10.1002/gps.5593

World Health Organization (WHO). (2023). *Depression*. Retrieved August 28, 2024, from https://www.who.int/news-room/fact-sheets/detail/depression

Wu, M., Li, C., Hu, T., Zhao, X., Qiao, G., Gao, X., Zhu, X., & Yang, F. (2024). Effectiveness of Telecare interventions on depression symptoms among older adults: Systematic review and meta-analysis. *JMIR Mhealth and Uhealth, 12*, e50787. https://doi.org/10.2196/50787

Wu, Q. (2024). Fluctuations in maternal depressive symptoms, anxiety, and anger and children's depression risks in middle childhood. *Research on Child and Adolescent Psychopathology, 52*(8), 1247–1260. https://doi.org/10.1007/s10802-024-01201-0

Yavari, S., Radfar, M., Faraji, N., Goli, R., Bagherzadi, A., Atharifar, R., Kazemi, S., & Dadashi, M. (2023). Self-esteem and optimism in patients with major depression disorder: A cross-sectional study. *Annals of Medicine and Surgery, 85*(11), 5379–5383. https://doi.org/10.1097/MS9.0000000000001263

Zhang, L., Li, X., Wang, J., & Liu, Y. (2024a). Reminiscence therapy relieves anxiety, depression and boosts spiritual well-being in both stroke patients and their spouse caregivers: A randomized, controlled study: Reminiscence therapy in stroke patients/caregivers. *Irish Journal of Medical Science, 193*(1), 407–415. https://doi.org/10.1007/s11845-023-03451-1

Zhang, Y., Zhang, W., & Yu, E. (2024b). Systematic review and meta-analysis: Pharmacological and nonpharmacological interventions for disruptive mood dysregulation disorder. *Journal of Child and Adolescent Psychopharmacology, 34*(5), 217–225. https://doi.org/10.1089/cap.2024.0013

Zhao, F. Y., Xu, P., Zheng, Z., Conduit, R., Xu, Y., Yue, L. P., Wang, H. R., Wang, Y. M., Li, Y. X., Li, C. Y., Zhang, W. J., Fu, Q. Q., & Kennedy, G. A. (2023). Managing depression with complementary and alternative medicine therapies: A scientometric analysis and visualization of research activities. *Frontiers in Psychiatry, 14*, 1288346. https://doi.org/10.3389/fpsyt.2023.1288346

Zhou, H., Zhu, H., Wang, J., Gao, X., & Jiang, C. (2024). Association between hypothyroidism subtypes and major depression: A two-sample Mendelian randomization study. *Journal of Affective Disorders, 351*, 843–852. https://doi.org/10.1016/j.jad.2024.02.006

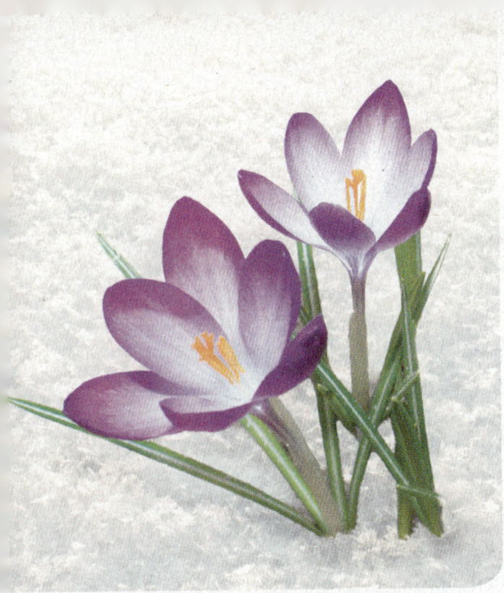

26

Bipolar and Related Disorders

Nursing Care of People With Mood Lability

Mary Ann Boyd

KEYCONCEPTS

- mania
- mood lability

LEARNING OBJECTIVES

After studying this chapter, you will be able to:

1. Examine the roles of mania and mood lability in bipolar disorder.
2. Relate the primary theories of bipolar disorder to clinical symptoms and the course of the disorder.
3. Evaluate the significance of trauma in the appearance of bipolar symptoms.
4. Examine the relationship between social determinants of health and bipolar disorder.
5. Select strategies to establish a therapeutic relationship with people with bipolar disorder.
6. Using a clinical judgment model, formulate a person-centered, recovery-oriented nursing care plan for people with bipolar disorder.
7. Identify medications that are used to treat people with bipolar disorder and evaluate their effectiveness.
8. Develop wellness strategies for people with bipolar disorder.
9. Compare and contrast mental health care provided in emergency, inpatient, community, and virtual settings.
10. Support the integration of health care and mental health care for people with bipolar disorder.
11. Compare and contrast bipolar disorder and related disorders.

KEY TERMS

• allostatic load • bipolar I disorder • bipolar II disorder • carbamazepine • cyclothymic disorder • divalproex sodium • elation • euphoria • expansive mood • flight of ideas • grandiosity • hypomania • imagery-based treatment • irritable mood • lamotrigine • lithium • mixed episode • racing thoughts • rapid cycling • social rhythm disruption theory

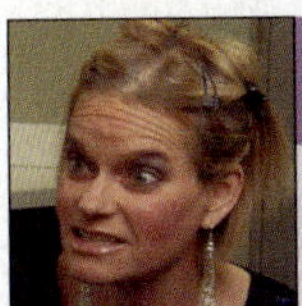

Case Study: Christine

Christine, age 34 years, assigned female at birth, has a history of bipolar I disorder. She is brought to the emergency room by the police from the airport, where she was demanding a plane ticket to Hawaii. She became very belligerent when she did not get her ticket. She is wearing an evening dress with several pieces of expensive jewelry. How would you document Christine's behavior and appearance? Was her belligerent behavior at the airport excessive considering the circumstances? How would you support her?

INTRODUCTION

Everyone has ups and downs. Mood changes are a part of everyday life; expression of feeling is integral to communication. But when moods are so pervasive that they cloud reasoning and judgment, they become problematic and interfere with interpersonal relationships. In some instances, extreme moods such as mania are symptoms of mental disorders. This chapter discusses bipolar disorders that are characterized by severe mood changes, with bipolar I disorder highlighted.

MANIA

Mania is one of the primary symptoms of bipolar disorders. It is recognizable by an elevated, expansive, or **irritable mood**. Mania is easily recognized by the cognitive changes that occur. Elevated self-esteem is expressed as **grandiosity** (exaggerating personal importance) and may range from unusual self-confidence to grandiose delusions. Speech is pressured (push of speech); the individual is more talkative than usual and, at times, is difficult to interrupt. There is often a **flight of ideas** (illogical connections between thoughts) or **racing thoughts** and distractibility increases.

KEYCONCEPT Mania is primarily characterized by an unusual and persistently elevated, expansive, or irritable mood.

In mania, the need for sleep is decreased and energy is increased. The individual often remains awake for extended periods or wakes up several times at night full of energy. Initially, there is an increase in goal-directed activity that is purposeful (e.g., cleaning the house), but it deteriorates into hyperactivity, agitation, and disorganized behavior. Social activities, occupational functioning, and interpersonal relationships are eventually impaired. There can be excessive involvement in pleasurable activities with little regard for painful consequences (e.g., excessive spending, risky sexual behavior, drug or alcohol misuse). People with mania are often hospitalized to prevent self-harm. See Box 26.1.

Even though mania is primarily associated with bipolar disorders, other psychiatric disorders, including schizophrenia, schizoaffective disorder, anxiety disorders, some personality disorders (borderline personality disorder and histrionic personality disorder), substance misuse involving stimulants, and adolescent conduct disorders, may have symptoms that mimic a manic episode. Mania can also be caused by medical disorders or their treatments, certain metabolic anomalies, neurologic disorders, central nervous system (CNS) tumors, and medications.

Mood lability is the term used for the rapid shifts in moods that often occur in bipolar disorder. One month an individual is happy, and the next month they are in the depths of depression. These mood shifts leave everyone around the individual confused and interfere with social interaction.

BOX 26.1

Clinical Judgment Vignette: The Patient With Mania

George was a day trader in the stock market. Initially, he was quite successful and, as a result, upgraded his lifestyle with a more expensive car; a larger, more luxurious house; and a boat. When the value of his stock portfolio declined dramatically, George continued to trade, saying that if he could just find the "right" stock he could earn back all of the money he had lost. He spent his days and nights in front of his computer screen, taking little or no time to eat or sleep. He defaulted on his mortgage and car and boat payments and was talking nonstop to his wife. She brought him to the hospital for evaluation.

Building Clinical Judgment

1. What behavioral symptoms of mania does George exhibit?
2. What cognitive symptoms of mania does George exhibit?

KEYCONCEPT Mood lability is alterations in moods with little or no change in external events.

Rapid cycling is an extreme form of mood lability that can occur in bipolar disorders. In its most severe form, rapid cycling includes continuous cycling between subthreshold mania and depression or hypomania and depression.

BIPOLAR DISORDERS OVERVIEW

Bipolar and related disorders are characterized by periods of mania or hypomania that alternate with depression. These disorders are further classified as bipolar I, bipolar II, and cyclothymic disorders, depending on the severity of the manic and depressive symptoms. Bipolar disorder may also be related to substance misuse, prescription use, or a medical condition.

BIPOLAR I DISORDER

Bipolar I disorder is the classic manic–depressive disorder with mood swings alternating from depressed to manic. Although the depression component is similar to that experienced in a major depressive disorder, in this disorder there is also a distinct period (of at least 1 week or less if hospitalized) of unusual and persistently elevated, expansive, or irritable mood with unusually increased goal-directed behavior or energy (American Psychiatric Association [APA], 2022). An elevated mood can be expressed as **euphoria** (exaggerated feelings of well-being) or **elation** (feeling "high," "ecstatic," "on top of the world," or "up in the clouds"). An **expansive mood** is characterized by lack of restraint in expressing feelings; an overvalued sense of self-importance; and a constant and indiscriminate enthusiasm for interpersonal, sexual, or occupational interactions.

For some people, an irritable mood instead of an elevated mood is pervasive during mania. Such individuals are easily annoyed and provoked to anger, particularly when their wishes are challenged or thwarted. Maintaining social relationships during these episodes is difficult.

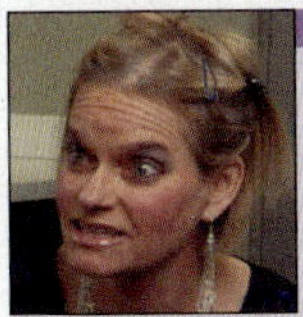

Consider Christine

When Christine is brought to the hospital, she is experiencing grandiose delusions. She believes that she is starting a business. She has spent a large amount of money over a brief period of time on clothes and jewelry. Her neighbors reported that she was selling household goods in her yard. Her mood is labile. She is loud and condescending toward staff members. She has pressured speech and flight of ideas. What behaviors are characteristic of bipolar disorder?

CLINICAL COURSE

Bipolar I disorder is a chronic multisystemic cyclic disorder. Those with an earlier onset have more frequent episodes than people who develop the illness later in life. Bipolar disorder is a progressive condition with prodromal, symptomatic, and residual states. The progressive nature of this disorder can be arrested with an early diagnosis, proper treatment, and individually tailored management An early onset and a family history of illness are associated with multiple episodes or continuous symptoms. Symptoms of the illness can be unpredictable and variable. Bipolar I disorder can lead to severe functional impairment, such as alienation from family, friends, and coworkers; indebtedness; job loss; divorce; and other problems of living (Nierenberg et al., 2023).

DIAGNOSTIC CRITERIA

To be diagnosed with bipolar I disorder, at least one manic episode or mixed episode and a depressive episode have to occur. See Key Diagnostic Characteristics 26.1. The term **mixed episode** is used when mania and depression occur at the same time, which leads to extreme anxiety, agitation, and irritability. These individuals are clearly miserable and are at high risk for suicide.

BIPOLAR I DISORDER ACROSS THE LIFE SPAN

Children and Adolescents

Only recently has bipolar disorder been recognized in children. Although it has not been well studied, depression usually appears first. Somewhat different than in adults, the hallmark of childhood bipolar disorder is intense rage. Children may display seemingly unprovoked rage episodes for as long as 2 to 3 hours. The symptoms of bipolar disorder reflect the developmental level of the child. Children younger than 9 years exhibit more irritability and emotional lability; older children exhibit more classic symptoms, such as euphoria and grandiosity. The first contact with the mental health system often occurs when the behavior becomes disruptive, possibly 5 to 10 years after its onset. These children often have other psychiatric disorders, such as attention-deficit hyperactivity disorder or conduct disorder (Long et al., 2024). See Chapter 37.

Older Adults

The onset of bipolar disorder can also occur in older adults. Symptoms are similar to the earlier onset bipolar disorder, but the incidence of mania decreases with age. Older adults with bipolar disorder have more neurologic anomalies and cognitive disturbances (confusion and disorientation) than younger patients (Montejo et al., 2024). See Chapter 39.

EPIDEMIOLOGY AND RISK FACTORS

Risk factors for bipolar disorders include a family history of mood disorders, prior mood episodes, substance use, stressful life events, and medical issues, particularly chronic or terminal illnesses (Bach et al., 2021). People with bipolar I disorder have a higher prevalence of hypertension and 10-year cardiovascular risk which correlate with the number of episodes and the duration of the illness (Aguglia et al., 2022).

Age of Onset

Bipolar disorders have an estimated prevalence of 2.4% (Jain & Mitra, 2023). The onset of the majority of cases occurs in early life, from the ages of 14 to 21 years, with fewer cases occurring after 40 years of age. There is emerging evidence that there is an early, mid, and late onset of bipolar disorders, with the early onset the more heritable form of bipolar disorder than late onset (Nierenberg et al., 2023).

Sex Assigned at Birth

Recent analysis of large clinical studies discovered a higher rate of people assigned female at birth diagnosed with bipolar disorder than those assigned male at birth (Zhang & Swaab, 2024). Being a person assigned female at birth is associated with higher rates of rapid cycling, dysphoria, lifetime prevalence of depression and suicide attempts, and with reduced quality of life. These results

KEY DIAGNOSTIC CHARACTERISTICS 26.1

DSM-5-TR DIAGNOSTIC CRITERIA: Bipolar I Disorder

For a diagnosis of bipolar I disorder, it is necessary to meet the following criteria for a manic episode. The manic episode may have been preceded by and may be followed by hypomanic or major depressive episodes.

Manic Episode

A. Distinct period of abnormally and persistently elevated, expansive, or irritable mood and abnormally and persistently increased activity or energy, lasting at least 1 week and present most of the day, nearly every day (or any duration if hospitalization is necessary).

B. During the period of mood disturbance and increased energy or activity, three (or more) of the following symptoms (four if the mood is only irritable) are present to a significant degree and represent a noticeable change from usual behavior:
   1. Inflated self-esteem or grandiosity.
   2. Decreased need for sleep (e.g., feels rested after only 3 hours of sleep).
   3. More talkative than usual or pressure to keep talking.
   4. Flight of ideas or subjective experience that thoughts are racing.
   5. Distractibility (i.e., attention too easily drawn to unimportant or irrelevant external stimuli), as reported or observed.
   6. Increase in goal-directed activity (either socially, at work or school, or sexuality) or psychomotor agitation (i.e., purposeless non–goal-directed activity).
   7. Excessive involvement in activities that have a high potential for painful consequences (e.g., engaging in unrestrained buying sprees, sexual indiscretions, or foolish business investments).

C. The mood disturbance is sufficiently severe to cause marked impairment in social or occupational functioning or to necessitate hospitalization to prevent harm to self or others, or there are psychotic features.

D. The episode is not attributable to the physiologic effects of a substance (e.g., a drug of abuse, a medication, other treatment) or to another medical condition.

Note: A full manic episode that emerges during antidepressant treatment (e.g., medication, electroconvulsive therapy) but persists at a fully syndromal level beyond the physiological effect of that treatment is sufficient evidence for a manic episode and, therefore, a bipolar I diagnosis.

Note: Criteria A–D constitute a manic episode. At least one lifetime manic episode is required for the diagnosis of bipolar I disorder.

Hypomanic Episode

A. A distinct period of abnormally and persistently elevated, expansive, or irritable mood and abnormally and persistently increased activity or energy, lasting at least 4 consecutive days and present most of the day, nearly every day.

B. During the period of mood disturbance and increased energy and activity, three (or more) of the following symptoms (four if the mood is only irritable) have persisted, represent a noticeable change from usual behavior, and have been present to a significant degree:
   1. Inflated self-esteem or grandiosity.
   2. Decreased need for sleep (e.g., feels rested after only 3 hours of sleep).
   3. More talkative than usual or pressure to keep talking.
   4. Flight of ideas or subjective experience that thoughts are racing.
   5. Distractibility (i.e., attention too easily drawn to unimportant or irrelevant external stimuli), as reported or observed.
   6. Increase in goal-directed activity (either socially, at work or school, or sexually) or psychomotor agitation.
   7. Excessive involvement in activities that have a high potential for painful consequences (e.g., engaging in unrestrained buying sprees, sexual indiscretions, or foolish business investments).

C. The episode is associated with an unequivocal change in functioning that is uncharacteristic of the individual when not symptomatic.

D. The disturbance in mood and the change in functioning are observable by others.

E. The episode is not severe enough to cause marked impairment in social or occupational functioning or to necessitate hospitalization. If there are psychotic features, the episode is, by definition, manic.

F. The episode is not attributable to the physiological effects of a substance (e.g., a drug of abuse, a medication, other treatment) or another medical condition.

Note: A full hypomanic episode that emerges during antidepressant treatment (e.g., medication, electroconvulsive therapy) but persists at a fully syndromal level beyond the physiological effect of that treatment is sufficient evidence for a hypomanic episode diagnosis. However, caution is indicated so that one or two symptoms (particularly increased irritability, edginess, or agitation following antidepressant use) are not taken as sufficient for diagnosis of a hypomanic episode, nor necessarily indicative of a bipolar diathesis.

Note: Criteria A–F constitute a hypomanic episode. Hypomanic episodes are common in bipolar I disorder but are not required for the diagnosis of bipolar I disorder.

Major Depressive Episode

A. Five (or more) of the following symptoms have been present during the same 2-week period and represent a change from previous functioning; at least one of the symptoms is either (1) depressed mood or (2) loss of interest or pleasure.

Note: Do not include symptoms that are clearly attributable to another medical condition.
   1. Depressed mood most of the day, nearly every day, as indicated by either subjective report (e.g., feels sad, empty, or hopeless) or observation made by others (e.g., appears tearful). (**Note:** In children and adolescents, can be irritable mood.)
   2. Markedly diminished interest or pleasure in all, or almost all, activities most of the day, nearly every day (as indicated by either subjective account or observation).
   3. Significant weight loss when not dieting or weight gain (e.g., a change of more than 5% of body weight in a month), or decrease or increase in appetite nearly every day. (**Note:** In children, consider failure to make expected weight gain.)
   4. Insomnia or hypersomnia nearly every day.
   5. Psychomotor agitation or retardation nearly every day (observable by others, not merely subjective feelings of restlessness or being slowed down).
   6. Fatigue or loss of energy nearly every day.
   7. Feelings of worthlessness or excessive or inappropriate guilt (which may be delusional) nearly every day (not merely self-reproach or guilt about being sick).
   8. Diminished ability to think or concentrate, or indecisiveness, nearly every day (either by subjective account or as observed by others).

KEY DIAGNOSTIC CHARACTERISTICS 26.1 (*Continued*)

9. Recurrent thoughts of death (not just fear of dying); recurrent suicidal ideation without a specific plan; a specific suicide plan; or a suicide attempt.

B. The symptoms cause clinically significant distress or impairment in social, occupational, or other important areas of functioning.

C. The episode is not attributable to the physiological effects of a substance or another medical condition.

Note: Criteria A–C constitute a major depressive episode. Major depressive episodes are common in bipolar I disorder but are not required for the diagnosis of bipolar I disorder.

Note: Responses to a significant loss (e.g., bereavement, financial ruin, losses from a natural disaster, a serious medical illness or disability) may include the feelings of intense sadness, rumination about the loss, insomnia, poor appetite, and weight loss noted in Criterion A, which may resemble a depressive episode. Although such symptoms may be understandable or considered appropriate to the loss, the presence of a major depressive episode in addition to the normal response to a significant loss should also be carefully considered. This decision inevitably requires the exercise of clinical judgment based on the individual's history and the cultural norms for the expression of distress in the context of loss.

Bipolar I Disorder

A. Criteria have been met for at least one manic episode (Criteria A–D under "Manic Episode" above).

B. At least one manic episode is not better explained by schizoaffective disorder and is not superimposed on schizophrenia, schizophreniform disorder, delusional disorder, or other specified or unspecified schizophrenia spectrum and other psychotic disorder.

can be improved with better recognition of this disorder in this population, which in turn can set the stage for more adequate treatment (Zhang & Swaab, 2024).

Ethnicity and Culture

Although there is a general belief that no significant racial and ethnic differences related to bipolar disorder exist, most of the research is based on White individuals who have not experienced a disparity in access to health care. A lack of representation from ethnic/racial underrepresented groups makes it difficult to determine the impact of race and ethnicity on the morbidity of people with bipolar disorder. Also, African American individuals with bipolar disorder are more likely to be misdiagnosed as having schizophrenia, schizoaffective, or major depressive disorders; the incidence of bipolar disorder in older African American individuals might be underreported because these patients are more likely to use general medical services for treatment than mental health services (Li et al., 2023). See Box 26.2.

COMORBIDITY

The most frequent comorbid mental disorders are anxiety disorders (panic disorder most common), substance use disorders, and disruptive, impulse-control, and conduct disorder (Léda-Rêgo et al., 2024). About 20% of people with bipolar disorder also meet the criteria for borderline personality disorder (Temes et al., 2024). Individuals with a comorbid anxiety disorder are more likely to experience a more severe course. A history of substance use further complicates the course of illness and results in less chance for remission and poorer treatment adherence (Bareis et al., 2024). Bipolar disorder is associated with several medical conditions, such as asthma, dementia, Parkinson disease, diabetes, hypertension, cardiovascular disease, and thyroid dysfunction (Kang et al., 2024; Song et al., 2023).

ETIOLOGY

The etiology of mood disorders is unknown, but the current thinking is that bipolar disorder results when

BOX 26.2

Mental Health Inequities: Demographic and Clinical Features of Bipolar Disorder in People of African and European Ancestry

The results of a study comparing demographic and clinical features of bipolar disorder in people of African ancestry (AA) and European ancestry (EUR) showed that the AA participants were more likely to have a history of posttraumatic stress disorder (PTSD) (39.7% vs. 26.2%), cocaine use disorder (24.2% vs. 11.9%), and tardive dyskinesia (7.1% vs. 3%). Consistent with other genetic studies, there is a low rate of AA participants ($n = 65$ or 3.5%) compared to EUR participants ($n = 1{,}800$). The authors conclude that these differences in rates of trauma, substance use, and tardive dyskinesia may represent health disparities among individuals of African ancestry, such as limited medication formularies and limited access to health care.

Source: Taylor-Desir, M. J., Balls-Berry, J. E., McElroy, S. L., Bond, D. J., Vallender, E. J., Ladner, M., Coombes, B. J., Jackson, L., Arceo, D., Caples, F. V., Colby, C., Patten, C. A., Biernacka, J. M., & Frye, M. A. (2023). Comparison of demographic and clinical features of bipolar disorder in persons of African and European Ancestry. *Journal of Racial and Ethnic Health Disparities*, *10*(1), 367–372. https://doi.org/10.1007/s40615-022-01228-3

an interaction occurs among genetic, epigenetic, neurochemical, and environmental factors such as abuse or trauma (Jain & Mitra, 2023). Childhood trauma including physical, sexual, and verbal abuse, as well as family conflict and emotional and physical neglect, are associated with early-onset bipolar disorder (Chauhan et al., 2023). Substance use, decreased socioeconomic status, sleep disturbances, and comorbid vascular conditions are more likely associated with mid- and late-onset bipolar disorder (Bolton et al., 2021).

Biologic Theories

Chronobiologic Theories

Sleep disturbance is common in individuals with bipolar disorder, especially mania. Sleep patterns appear to be regulated by an internal biologic clock center in the hypothalamus. Artificially induced sleep deprivation is known to precipitate mania in some patients with bipolar disorder. It is possible that circadian dysregulation underlies the sleep–wake disturbances of bipolar disorder. Seasonal changes in light exposure also trigger affective episodes in some patients, typically depression in winter and hypomania in the summer in the northern hemisphere (Scott & McClung, 2023).

Genetic Factors

Results from family, adoption, and twin studies indicate that bipolar disorder is highly heritable. Studies of monozygotic twins show risks from 40% to 70% of acquiring the illness if their identical twin has the disorder (Song et al., 2024). No one gene or sequence of genes is responsible for the pathology of bipolar disorder. Evidence suggests that the genetic etiologies of schizophrenia and bipolar disorders overlap (Dines et al., 2024).

Chronic Stress and Inflammation

The role of an **allostatic load** or wear and tear on the body (see Chapter 19) is thought to contribute to cognitive impairment, comorbidity, and eventual mortality of those with bipolar disorder. As the allostatic load increases, the number of mood episodes increases, which, in turn, increases physical and mental health issues. An interaction between stress and brain development is viewed as dynamic; individuals have different kinds of stress adaptation depending on their neurobiologic responses (Cordeiro et al., 2023).

The characteristic mood dysregulation of bipolar I disorder is associated with a decrease in serum brain-derived neurotrophic factor, oxidative stress resulting in DNA damage, and inflammation. Proinflammatory cytokines bind to neuronal death receptors, leading to cell death. In some patients with repeated episodes, there is a decrease in hippocampal volume and reduction in prefrontal grey matter (Poletti et al., 2024).

Psychosocial Theories

Psychosocial theories are useful in planning recovery-oriented interventions that focus on reducing environmental stress and trauma in genetically vulnerable individuals. It is now generally accepted that psychosocial and environmental events contribute to the severity of the disorder and the frequency of the mood episodes.

The **social rhythm disruption theory** is consistent with the research on circadian rhythm dysregulation. According to this theory, there are environmental factors that set the circadian clock, such as the rising and setting of the sun. There are also social cues or social rhythms that can set the circadian clock, such as the time we get out of bed, our first contact with an individual in the morning, when we start our day, have dinner, and go to bed. These are patterned social events. Individuals with bipolar disorder have fewer regular social rhythms than those without bipolar disorder. This theory suggests that when patterned social events are disrupted, mood swings are more likely to appear (Yeo et al., 2024).

FAMILY RESPONSE TO DISORDER

Bipolar disorder can devastate families, who often feel that they are on an emotional merry-go-round, particularly if they have difficulty understanding the mood shifts. A major issue for family members is dealing with the consequences of impulsive behavior during manic episodes, such as taking on excessive debt, assault charges, and sexual infidelities.

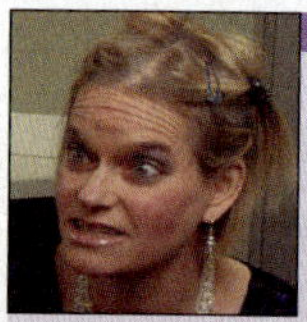

Remember Christine?

She has been married for 2 years to Karl, who was unaware of her bipolar disorder. He believed that she used to take antidepressants but that she no longer needed them. Her episode at the airport occurred when he was out of town. He is concerned about her health and their new financial obligations. How do you explain that Karl was unaware of Christine's illness? How would you explain Christine's illness to her husband?

RECOVERY-ORIENTED CARE FOR PEOPLE WITH BIPOLAR DISORDER

Teamwork and Collaboration: Working Toward Recovery

An important recovery goal is to minimize or prevent both manic and depressive episodes, which tend to accelerate over time. The fewer the episodes, the more likely the individual can live a fully productive life. A trauma-informed approach is important in people with bipolar disorder because many have experienced trauma. See Chapter 2.

Patients with bipolar disorder have a complex set of issues and have the best chance of recovery by collaborating with an interdisciplinary team. Nurses, providers, social workers, psychologists, and activity therapists all have valuable expertise. For children with bipolar disorder, schoolteachers and counselors are included in the team. For older adult patients, the primary care provider becomes part of the team. Helping the patient and family learn about the disorder and managing it throughout a lifetime is critical for recovery.

The primary treatment modalities are medications, psychotherapy, education, and support. Mood stabilizers and antipsychotics are the mainstay medications in the treatment of bipolar disorders. Mood stabilizers are discussed later in this chapter. Antipsychotics are discussed in Chapter 24. Long-term psychotherapy may help prevent symptoms by reducing the stresses that trigger episodes and increasing the patient's acceptance of the need for medication. Patients should be encouraged to keep their appointments with the therapist, be honest and open, do the assigned homework, and give the therapist feedback on whether the treatment is effective.

Safety Issues

Risk of suicide is always present for those having a depressive or manic episode (Arnone et al., 2024). During a depressive episode, the patient may believe that life is not worth living. During a manic episode, the patient may believe that they have supernatural powers, such as the ability to fly.

During a manic episode, poor judgment and impulsivity lead to risk-taking behaviors that can have dire consequences for the patient and family. For example, when one patient gambled all of his family's money away, he blamed his partner for letting him have access to the money. A physical confrontation with the partner resulted.

As patients recover from a manic episode, they may be so devastated by the consequences of their impulsive behavior and poor judgment that suicide seems like the only option.

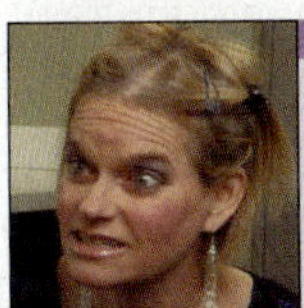

Consider This:

Consider Christine's history of poor judgment during a manic episode. She left her first husband and their two children during her third manic episode. At that time, Christine went to Hawaii and stayed there for several months without informing her family of her whereabouts. She was unhoused most of the time. Once Christine is stable, what interventions will support long-term remission of bipolar disorder?

EVIDENCE-BASED NURSING CARE OF PEOPLE WITH BIPOLAR DISORDER

In general, the behavior of patients with bipolar disorder is unremarkable between mood episodes. The nurse's first contact with the patient is usually during a manic or depressive episode.

RECOGNIZING CUES: RELEVANT ASSESSMENT INFORMATION

Recovery-oriented nursing care begins with the initial assessment through engaging the patient in a partnership and empowering them to make decisions in setting overall goals of care. During acute episodes, the patient's judgment may be impaired, but as the manic or depressive symptoms subside, they will be able to participate in care decisions.

Physical Health and Functioning

The physical health assessment should follow the process explained in Chapter 10. Target assessment symptoms include the changes and severity of activity, eating, and sleep patterns. The patient may not sleep, resulting in irritability and physical exhaustion. Diet and body weight usually change during a manic or depressive episode. Laboratory studies, such as thyroid function and electrolytes, should be completed to detect evidence of malnutrition and fluid imbalance. Atypical thyroid functioning can be responsible for mood and behavioral disturbances. In mania, patients often become hypersexual and engage in risky sexual practices. Changes in sexual practices should be included in the assessment.

History of Trauma

People with bipolar disorder experience trauma at much higher rates than the general population. As the number of traumatic events increases, the severity of the symptoms increases (Rowe et al., 2024). The extent of childhood and adult traumas should be determined to help gauge the best approach to recovery (see Box 26.3). The cumulative effects of the trauma could result in posttraumatic stress disorder (Russell et al., 2024).

Medication

A careful assessment of current medications is important in determining physical status. Many times, manic or depressive episodes occur after patients stop taking their medication. Exploring reasons for discontinuing the medication will help in planning adherence strategies in the future. Some stop taking their medications because of side effects; others do not believe they have a mental disorder. In some instances, patients have been taking an antidepressant as prescribed for depression without realizing that a bipolar disorder existed.

BOX 26.3

Trauma-Informed Approaches: Childhood Trauma and Bipolar Disorder in People Assigned Female at Birth

Background

People assigned female at birth who have bipolar disorder often suffer from childhood trauma. If they also do not have adequate social support in childhood, they are more likely to consider suicide. People in this population who are engaged in treatment with medications are more likely to have social support, more likely to have higher cognitive functioning, and less likely to consider suicide.

Interventions

Trauma-informed approaches targeting social support and access to treatment for people assigned female at birth can help improve treatment outcomes and reduce caregiver burden.

Source: Yang, M., Li, J., Fu, Y., Wang, G., Liu, M., Chen, J., & Liu, J. (2024). Association of childhood trauma, social support, cognition, and suicidality in females with bipolar disorder. *BMC Psychiatry*, *24*(1), 243. https://doi.org/10.1186/s12888-024-05672-9

Substance Use

The use of alcohol and other substances should be carefully assessed. When a patient has a manic episode, it is difficult to determine whether the symptoms are related to the mania of bipolar disorder or to intoxication. During an episode of depression, it is important to determine when and what substance was used to rule out a suicidal event. Usually, a drug screen is ordered.

Psychosocial Assessment

The psychosocial assessment should follow the process explained in Chapter 10. Individuals with bipolar disorder can usually participate fully in this part of the assessment.

Mental Status and Appearance

Mood

By definition, bipolar disorder is a disturbance of mood. If the patient is depressed, using an assessment tool for depression may help determine the severity of depression. If mania predominates, evaluating the quality of the mood (e.g., elated, grandiose, irritated, or agitated) becomes important. Usually, mania is diagnosed by clinical observation.

Cognition

In a depressive episode, an individual may not be able to concentrate enough to complete cognitive tasks, such as those called for in a mental status assessment. During the acute phase of a manic or depressive episode, mental status may be atypical, and in a manic phase, judgment is impaired by extremely rapid, disjointed, and distorted thinking. Moreover, feelings such as grandiosity can interfere with executive functioning. See Box 26.4.

Thought Disturbances

Psychosis commonly occurs in patients with bipolar disorder, especially during acute episodes of mania. Auditory hallucinations and delusional thinking are part of the clinical picture. In children and adolescents, however, psychosis is not so easily disclosed.

Behavioral Responses

Behavior varies according to mood. In periods of mania and poor judgment, there may be episodes of uncharacteristic behaviors such as excessive spending, impulsive gambling, or sexual activities. Behaviors during a manic episode can lead to life-long relationships or legal issues. During periods of depression, remorse for the consequences of poor judgment and behavior contributes to the negative mood state. See Chapter 25.

BOX 26.4

Clinical Judgment Vignette: Cognitive Functioning in Mania

Sam, age 35, was diagnosed with bipolar disorder 10 years ago. He is now being successfully treated and has insight into his disorder. In a recent discussion with his close friend, he describes his personal experience of mania as follows:

"At first, I started having more energy and felt happy most of the time. I decided to date a couple of other women because I thought my girlfriend was rather boring. Within a couple of weeks, I started sleeping less, but I thought that meant I could do more things. I decided to go back to school to be a scientist—thought I could save the world. I started to apply to graduate school and became very upset when I was told that I did not have the prerequisites for biochemistry. I was so mad that I started threatening the admissions counselor, who, in turn, called the police. My family was called. They convinced the police that I would not bother the school again. After that, I started drinking and smoking pot. I had periods of confusion, and my family said I became disoriented. There is a lot I don't remember. Eventually, I was hospitalized and started on medication."

Building Clinical Judgment

1. At what point could an early intervention have prevented Sam from progressing to a major manic episode?
2. Why does Sam not remember the complete manic episode?

Self-Concept

The self-concept of an individual with bipolar disorder is generally consistent with others who have stigmatized mental disorders. Even though bipolar disorder is less stigmatized than schizophrenia, the behaviors that are characteristic of people with these disorders are often not recognized as symptoms of a disorder, but as a character flaw. Consequently, even in periods of mania, self-esteem is severely impaired.

Stress and Coping Patterns

Stress and coping are critical assessment areas for an individual with bipolar disorder. A stressful event often triggers a manic or depressive episode. In some instances, no particular stressors preceded the episode, although it is important to discuss the possibility. Determining the patient's usual coping skills for stresses lays the groundwork for developing interventional strategies. Negative coping skills, such as substance use or aggression, should be identified because these behaviors can be targeted in the recovery plan.

Social Network

Cultural views of mental illness influence the patient's acceptance of the disorder. During illness episodes, patients often behave in ways that jeopardize their social relationships. Losing a job and going through a divorce are common events. When performing an assessment of the social area, the nurse should identify changes resulting from a manic or depressive episode, such as no longer engaging in favorite activities.

Functional Status

Symptoms of bipolar disorder can interfere with daily functioning. Sleep, nutrition, and hygiene often suffer during manic or depressive episodes. The individuals are often unable to maintain usual functioning and activities of daily living.

Support Systems

The nurse should assess the available support systems. Individuals who have been symptomatic may have destroyed their support networks as a result of their depressive or manic behavior. The nurse should determine if there are any positive support systems that can help the individual toward recovery.

Risk Assessment

People with bipolar disorder are at high risk for injury to themselves and others, with up to 60% of those with bipolar disorder attempting suicide at some time, and suicide fatalities occurring in 5% to 20% of adults with bipolar disorder. People with bipolar disorder account for 3.4% to 14% of all suicide deaths, with self-poisoning and hanging being the most common methods (Tondo et al., 2021). Child abuse, spouse abuse, or other violent behaviors may occur during severe manic or depressive episodes; thus, patients should be assessed for suicidal or homicidal risks. In addition, they are at elevated risk for comorbid mental disorders, such as substance use and anxiety disorders. Significant risks for cardiovascular and metabolic diseases also occur in this group (Léda-Rêgo et al., 2024; Kang et al., 2024). Smoking is also a major health hazard and is associated with suicidal behavior in people with bipolar disorder (Pietschnig et al., 2024).

Several risk factors associated with bipolar disorders make patients more vulnerable to relapses and resistant to recovery. Among these are high rates of nonadherence to medication therapy, obesity, marital conflict, separation, divorce, unemployment, and underemployment. Even those who take their medication regularly are likely to experience recurrences and may have difficulty keeping jobs and maintaining significant relationships.

Social Determinants of Health

People with bipolar disorder are negatively impacted by the social determinants of health (SDOH) (see Chapter 2), as are most individuals with a mental disorder. But, for people with bipolar disorder, educational attainment and higher income are shown to be protective factors (Baranova et al., 2024). Compared to people with higher incomes, patients who have lower income, less education, and live in rural or small towns are less likely to have access to mental health care (Teigland et al., 2024). Level of education and income are important data to collect and can be used in planning for recovery.

Social and Occupational Functioning

One of the tragedies of bipolar disorder is its effect on social and occupational functioning. Individuals with this disorder are often employed, but when unrecognized symptoms erupt, their job is often jeopardized. Manifestations of their symptoms often result in being excluded from social and occupational groups.

Spiritual Assessment

The spiritual assessment found in Chapter 10 can be used for the spiritual assessment of people with bipolar disorder. Depending on their mood state, the individual may be attracted to or distanced from their spiritual beliefs and values (van Nieuw Amerongen-Meeuse et al., 2024). Determining baseline spiritual/religious beliefs and practices can be helpful in identifying coping strategies for future recovery interventions.

Quality of Life

The quality of life for someone with bipolar disorder depends upon their ability to manage their symptoms, maintain meaningful employment, and engage in positive relationships. Some individuals are able to manage their symptoms, adhere to a treatment plan, and live productive lives. Others struggle with symptoms that interfere with their ability to work and maintain meaningful, supportive relationships.

Strengths Assessment

The nurse should always be listening for thoughts, feelings, or behaviors that could be identified as strengths. For example, one patient recognized an increase in drinking alcohol as a sign of the beginning of a manic episode and made an appointment with a health care provider. The following questions may be used to determine an individual's strength:

- What healthy behaviors do you routinely practice?
- Are there any cues that a manic or depressive episode will occur?
- Who provides emotional support to you?
- What do you do to relax? Manage stress?
- What makes you feel good when you are on medication?
- How do you remember to take your medications?

ANALYZING CUES AND DEVELOPING HYPOTHESES

The priority of nursing care is always patient safety. Is the patient likely to self-injure or hurt another person? (see Chapter 20). After the patient's safety is established, the nurse analyzes the assessment data for other priorities. For example, sleep deprivation, inadequate nutrition, and dehydration may be imminent needs. The individual may be depressed or manic and unable to function socially. Their coping skills may not be effective, and their job may be in jeopardy.

GENERATING SOLUTIONS: PLANNING RECOVERY AND WELLNESS OUTCOMES

The individual with a bipolar disorder has emotional ups and downs with periods of poor judgment and erratic behavior. However, there are many periods (months to years) during which few symptoms occur. The periods of stable mental health are perfect times to focus on stress reduction, illness management, and relapse prevention. During these relatively quiet periods, it is possible to establish recovery and wellness goals. Goals focus on managing long-term illness and supporting well-being. Recovery and wellness goals are interrelated. For example, preventing relapse includes managing stress (wellness strategies) that can trigger erratic behavior (mental health goals).

THERAPEUTIC RELATIONSHIP

Interacting with an individual with mania is interesting and, at times, exhausting. The individual often quickly jumps from subject to subject and is usually unable to sit still. When in a manic state, the individual can be very engaging and intense. Their stories may be very grandiose. The nurse should acknowledge the verbal content but recognize that many of the thoughts, feelings, and behaviors are symptomatic of mania and then try to refocus the patient. If an individual is in a depressive state, the nurse should use the same approach as when caring for an individual with a depressed disorder as discussed in Chapter 25.

People with mania are typically impatient with others and may express irritability at someone's perceived incompetence and lack of understanding of their special powers. When interacting with an individual with bipolar disorder, the nurse should remain calm and avoid any arguments. This is not the time to confront the individual about their unrealistic perceptions of their status. For example, one agitated person was convinced that they owned a hotel. The nurse acknowledged how difficult it must be to have such responsibilities. The person agreed with the nurse and subsequently became less agitated. See Box 26.5.

In some instances, an individual who has mania cannot sit still long enough to have a meaningful interaction. The nurse can initiate a conversation while walking with the patient, but there will be times when the nurse needs to give the patient space to avoid increasing agitation.

A therapeutic relationship can be instrumental in preventing a relapse. When an individual is in the depths of a depression or the height of mania, a therapeutic connection is critical in helping them take steps toward recovery. However, since there are often long periods of time between acute episodes, the individual may not seek out care on a regular basis and rely only on medication prescription refills.

BOX 26.5

Interacting With an Individual With Mania

- Use a calm, nonthreatening approach.
- Be direct and use simple commands (e.g., time for lunch, let's go to group).
- Avoid open-ended sentences; redirect conversation if flight of ideas occurs; avoid confrontation and arguments.
- Limit interaction time and recognize the patient's need for space and movement.
- Do not place demands on patients that they cannot meet.

TAKING ACTION: NURSING INTERVENTIONS

Physical Care

In a state of mania, the patient's physical needs are rest, adequate hydration and nutrition, and reestablishment of physical well-being. Self-care has usually deteriorated. For a patient unable to sit long enough to eat, snacks and high-energy foods that can be eaten while moving should be provided. Consumption of alcohol should be avoided. Sleep hygiene is a priority but may not be realistic until medications have taken effect. Limiting stimuli can be helpful in decreasing agitation and promoting sleep.

NCLEXNOTE Protection of patients with mania is always a priority. Ongoing assessment should focus on irritability, fatigue, and the potential for harming self or others.

After the patient's mood stabilizes, the nurse should focus on monitoring changes in physical functioning in sleep or eating behavior and teaching patients to identify antecedents to mood episodes such as a family argument or a financial issue. Strategies for dealing with future events can then be identified. The patient can begin to problem solve the best approach for future episodes.

A regular sleep routine should be maintained if possible. High-risk times for manic episodes, such as changes in work schedule (day to night), should be avoided if possible. Patients should be encouraged to monitor the amount of their sleep each night and report decreases in sleep of longer than 1 hour per night because this may be a precursor to a manic episode.

Highlighting the recovery concept of hope will support the individual who has had multiple episodes and is frustrated with the impact of several episodes (Box 26.6). In educating people with bipolar disorder, the nonlongitudinal nature of the disorder should be emphasized.

BOX 26.6

Therapeutic Dialogue: Instilling Hope

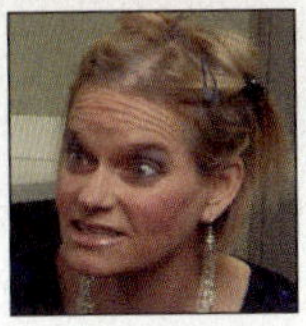

Christine is sitting in the dayroom of an inpatient unit with tears in her eyes. She acknowledges that she has bipolar disorder and wishes that she had been taking her medication and told her husband about her previous relapses.

INEFFECTIVE APPROACH

Nurse: Christine, I am glad that you realize that you have bipolar disorder and want to take your medication. You must commit to staying on your medicine, or you will lose your second husband.

Christine: No one understands what it is like to have this problem. I don't quite understand how this little pill and seeing a shrink will help.

Nurse: Well, medication and therapy will help.

Christine: You don't know what I am talking about.

EFFECTIVE APPROACH

Nurse: Christine, I hope that you are feeling better.

Christine: No one understands what it is like to have this problem. I don't quite understand how this little pill and seeing a shrink will help.

Nurse: Let's talk about it. What does it feel like to have bipolar disorder?

Christine: Sometimes it is wonderful—on top of the world, but after the mood goes away, having this problem is terrible. The bad times outweigh the good feelings.

Nurse: Other people have said the same thing. Many people decide to take their medication and "check in" with a mental health provider in order to stay on track and avoid the bad times that can happen after a manic period.

Christine: Really?

Nurse: There are many successful people with bipolar disorder who find that taking medication helps keep order in their life. I can give you information about a support group.

Christine: Ok, I'm willing to try.

Nurse: Now, what about this medication? Are you willing to try it also? This medication is an effective treatment for bipolar disorder and has helped others to control moods.

Christine: Okay, but I want to know more about this medication.

Nurse: It's a deal. We can spend some time talking about your medications after dinner.

CRITICAL THINKING CHALLENGE

1. How did the nurse block communication with Christine in the first scenario? Did she seem hopeful after the interaction?
2. How did the nurse instill hope in Christine in the second scenario?

Wellness Challenges

As people with bipolar disorder manage their mood swings, they are also challenged to develop wellness skills. Their impulsivity during a manic episode and sense of hopelessness during a depressive episode can easily interfere with well-meaning plans to exercise, eat healthy meals, and get adequate sleep. Interpersonal relationships can be fractured during a manic or depressive episode, requiring extra attention on rebuilding relationships during periods of stability. These individuals appear to be more sensitive to life events than people without the disorder. The stress of daily life can easily interfere with wellness activities. If the individuals can strengthen their coping skills, they may be less sensitive to stressful life events. See Table 26.1.

TABLE 26.1 WELLNESS CHALLENGES AND COPING STRATEGIES

Challenge	Coping Strategies
To reduce emotional responses to daily stresses	• Reframe experiences • Use problem-focused coping techniques and relaxation
To support positive circadian rhythms consistent with relapse prevention needs	• Establish sleep hygiene and eating routines
To establish a healthy diet with reducing substance use	• Eat at regular times • Maintain a healthy diet
To seek pleasant environments that support well-being	• Seek comfortable, relaxing living arrangements • Explore community resources that support people with bipolar disorder
To satisfy current and future financial situations	• Seek financial counseling • Protect resources during periods of relapses
To engage in satisfying and enriching work	• Select job opportunities that are consistent with health promotion activities
To recognize the need for physical activity, healthy foods, and sleep	• Encourage regular physical activity • Discuss healthy diets • Encourage establishing healthy sleep hygiene routines
To develop a sense of connection, belonging, and a support system	• Explore expanding a positive support system
To expand a sense of purpose and meaning in life	• Focus on goals, values, and beliefs • Read inspiring stories or essays

Medication Interventions

Medications are essential in bipolar disorder to achieve two goals: rapid control of symptoms and prevention of future episodes or, at least, reduction in their severity and frequency.

Mood-Stabilizing Drugs

The mainstays of pharmacotherapy are the mood-stabilizing drugs, including lithium carbonate, divalproex sodium, carbamazepine, and lamotrigine. Antidepressant therapy is not recommended in people with bipolar depression because of a risk of switching from depression to mania.

Lithium Carbonate

Lithium is the most widely used mood stabilizer (Box 26.7). Combined response rates from five studies

BOX 26.7

Medication Profile: Lithium Carbonate

DRUG CLASS: Mood stabilizer

RECEPTOR AFFINITY: Alters sodium transport in nerve and muscle cells, increases norepinephrine uptake and serotonin receptor sensitivity, slightly increases intraneuronal stores of catecholamines, and delays some second messenger systems. Mechanism of action is unknown.

INDICATIONS: Treatment and prevention of manic episodes in bipolar affective disorder.

ROUTES AND DOSAGE: 150-, 300-, and 600-mg capsules, 300-mg slow-release tablets; 450-mg controlled-release tablets; lithium citrate, 300-mg/5 mL liquid form.

Adults: In acute mania, optimal response is usually 600 mg TID or 900 mg BID. Obtain serum levels twice weekly in acute phase. Do not rely on serum levels alone. Maintenance: Use lowest possible dose to alleviate symptoms and maintain serum level of 0.6 to 1.2 mEq/L. In uncomplicated maintenance, obtain serum levels every 2 to 3 months. Monitor patient's side effects.

Geriatric: Increased risk for toxic effects; use lower doses; monitor frequently.

Children: 6 to 12 years: 15 to 60 mg/kg/day in 3 to 4 divided doses.

HALF-LIFE (PEAK EFFECT): Mean, 24 hours (peak serum levels in 1 to 4 hours). Steady state reached in 5 to 7 days.

SELECTED ADVERSE REACTIONS: Weight gain.

WARNING: Avoid use during pregnancy or while breastfeeding. Hepatic or renal impairments increase plasma concentration.

SPECIFIC PATIENT AND FAMILY EDUCATION

- Avoid alcohol and other CNS depressant drugs.
- Notify your prescriber if pregnancy is possible or planned. Do not breastfeed while taking this medication.
- Notify your prescriber before taking any other prescriptions, OTC medications, or herbal supplements.
- May impair judgment, thinking, or motor skills; avoid driving or other hazardous tasks.
- Do not abruptly discontinue use.

BID, twice a day; CNS, central nervous system; OTC, over-the-counter; TID, three times a day.

TABLE 26.2 LITHIUM BLOOD LEVELS AND ASSOCIATED SIDE EFFECTS

Plasma Level	Side Effects or Symptoms of Toxicity
<1.5 mEq/L Mild side effects	Metallic taste in mouth Fine hand tremor (resting) Nausea Polyuria Polydipsia Diarrhea or loose stools Muscular weakness or fatigue Weight gain Edema Memory impairments
1.5–2.5 mEq/L Moderate toxicity	Severe diarrhea Dry mouth Nausea and vomiting Mild to moderate ataxia Incoordination Dizziness, sluggishness, giddiness, vertigo Slurred speech Tinnitus Blurred vision Increasing tremor Muscle irritability or twitching Asymmetric deep tendon reflexes Increased muscle tone
>2.5 mEq/L Severe toxicity	Cardiac arrhythmias Blackouts Nystagmus Coarse tremor Fasciculations Visual or tactile hallucinations Oliguria, renal failure Peripheral vascular collapse Confusion Seizures Coma and death

demonstrate that 70% of patients experienced at least partial improvement with lithium therapy. However, for many patients, lithium is not a fully adequate treatment for all phases of the illness, and particularly during the acute phase, supplemental use of antipsychotics and benzodiazepines is often beneficial (Table 26.2).

NCLEXNOTE Monitoring blood levels of lithium carbonate and divalproex sodium is an ongoing nursing assessment for patients receiving these medications. Side effects of mood stabilizers vary.

Lithium is a salt; the interaction between lithium levels and sodium levels in the body and the relationship between lithium levels and fluid volume in the body remain crucial issues in its safe, effective use. The higher the sodium levels, the lower the lithium level will be and vice versa. Thus, changes in dietary sodium intake can affect lithium blood levels that, in turn, may affect therapeutic results or increase the incidence and severity of side effects. The same principle applies to fluid volume. If body fluid decreases significantly because of hot weather, strenuous exercise, vomiting, diarrhea, or drastic reduction in fluid intake for any reason, then lithium levels can rise sharply, causing an increase in side effects, progressing to lethal lithium toxicity. The key is to start with a lower dose and then increase it slowly to maximize the therapeutic response and avoid overshooting the therapeutic window. See Table 26.3 for lithium interactions with other drugs. See Chapter 11 for further discussion of lithium's possible mechanisms of action, pharmacokinetics, side effects, and toxicity.

Lithium toxicity can range from mild to severe, requiring immediate medical attention and prompt intervention. *Mild toxicity* symptoms include lethargy, drowsiness, coarse hand tremor, muscle weakness, nausea, vomiting, and diarrhea. *Moderate toxicity* is associated with confusion, dysarthria, nystagmus, myoclonic twitches, and ECG changes. *Severe toxicity* is life threatening and associated with grossly impaired consciousness, increased deep tendon reflexes, seizures, syncope, renal insufficiency, coma, and death.

Lithium toxicity can be caused by an overdose (ingesting a large amount at one time) or by other effects of concomitant medications that increase blood concentrations of lithium, such as loop diuretics, angiotensin-converting enzyme (ACE) inhibitors, or nonsteroidal anti-inflammatory drugs (NSAIDs). Chronic kidney disease increases the risk of toxicity, and use of lithium increases the risk of chronic kidney disease. Renal function generally declines with long-term use of lithium. Treatment includes maintaining airway, managing changes in consciousness, inserting a nasogastric tube, and performing gastric lavage. Hemodialysis may be necessary (Hedya et al., 2023). See Box 26.8.

EMERGENCY CARE ALERT If symptoms of moderate or severe toxicity (e.g., cardiac arrhythmias, blackouts, tremors, seizures) are noted, withhold additional doses of lithium, immediately obtain a blood sample to analyze the lithium level, and push fluids if the patient can take fluids. Contact the provider for further direction about relieving the symptoms.

Mild side effects tend to subside or can be managed by nursing measures (Table 26.4).

Concept Mastery Alert

Fine tremors are mild side effects of lithium. They are made worse by stress, so the nurse should assist the client in minimizing exposure to stressors. Lithium therapy can continue unless the tremors interfere with the client's quality of life.

Divalproex Sodium

Divalproex sodium, an anticonvulsant, has a broader spectrum of efficacy and has about equal benefit for patients with pure mania as for those with other forms of

TABLE 26.3 LITHIUM INTERACTIONS WITH MEDICATIONS AND OTHER SUBSTANCES

Substance	Effect of Interaction
ACE inhibitors, such as: • Captopril • Lisinopril • Quinapril	Increase serum lithium; may cause toxicity and impaired kidney function
Acetazolamide	Increases renal excretion of lithium; decreases lithium levels
Alcohol	May increase serum lithium level
Caffeine	Increases lithium excretion; increases lithium tremor
Carbamazepine	Increases neurotoxicity despite expected serum levels and dosage
Fluoxetine	Increases serum lithium levels
Haloperidol	Increases neurotoxicity despite expected serum levels and dosage
Loop diuretics, such as furosemide	Increase lithium serum levels but may be safer than thiazide diuretics; potassium-sparing diuretics (e.g., amiloride, spironolactone) are safest
Methyldopa	Increases neurotoxicity without increasing serum lithium levels
NSAIDs, such as: • Diclofenac • Ibuprofen • Indomethacin • Piroxicam	Decrease renal clearance of lithium Increase serum lithium levels by 30–60% in 3–10 days Aspirin and sulindac do not appear to have the same effect
Osmotic diuretics, such as: • Urea • Mannitol • Isosorbide	Increase renal excretion of lithium and decreases lithium levels
Sodium chloride	High sodium intake decreases lithium levels; low sodium diets may increase lithium levels and lead to toxicity
Thiazide diuretics, such as: • Chlorothiazide • Hydrochlorothiazide	Promote sodium and potassium excretion; increase lithium serum levels; may produce cardiotoxicity and neurotoxicity
TCAs	Increases tremor; potentiates pharmacologic effects of tricyclic antidepressants

ACE, angiotensin-converting enzyme; NSAID, nonsteroidal anti-inflammatory drug; TCA, tricyclic antidepressant.

BOX 26.8

Building Clinical Judgment With SBAR: Hand-Off Communication During Change of Shift

SBAR

S: Situation

S.J. is a 46-year-old person assigned male at birth with a diagnosis of bipolar disorder who was admitted today for depression.

B: Background

S.J. was diagnosed with bipolar I disorder 20 years ago and has been working as a truck driver. His last hospitalization was 15 years ago. Since then, he has been treated as an outpatient and has adhered to the prescribed lithium carbonate; his lithium levels have been stable. He was recently divorced and moved out of his house. He has lost weight and is not sleeping well. His family reports that he has been depressed since the divorce.

A: Assessment

S.J. is oriented to person and date, but not to place. He thinks he is at a hotel. His vital signs are stable. He reports nausea and diarrhea. He has hand tremors and has difficulty walking without help. An ECG and lab tests are ordered. He has been taking lithium carbonate 1,200 mg per day. His next dose of lithium is due in 2 hours.

R: Recommendation

S.J. has clinical symptoms of lithium toxicity. Do not give lithium until lithium level is determined. Notify the provider of the lithium and ECG results. Continue to observe for deterioration of mental status and changes in vital signs, and seizures.

Building Clinical Judgment

1. Why does the nurse hypothesize that S.J. could be experiencing lithium toxicity?
2. Why does the nurse prioritize the assessment for lithium toxicity instead of the depression?

TABLE 26.4 INTERVENTIONS FOR LITHIUM SIDE EFFECTS

Side Effect	Intervention
Edema of feet or hands	Monitor intake and output of water; check for possible decreased urinary output Monitor sodium intake Patient should elevate legs when sitting or lying Monitor weight
Fine hand tremor	Provide support and reassurance if it does not interfere with daily activities Tremor worsens with anxiety and intentional movements; minimize stressors Notify prescriber if tremor interferes with patient's work so that adherence may be an issue More frequent smaller doses of lithium may also help
Mild diarrhea	Take lithium with meals Provide for fluid replacement Notify prescriber if it worsens; may need a change in medication preparation or may be early sign of toxicity
Muscle weakness, fatigue, or memory and concentration difficulties	Provide support and reassurance; this side effect will usually pass after a few weeks of treatment. Short-term memory aids such as lists or reminder calls may be helpful Notify prescriber if side effect becomes severe or interferes with the patient's desire to continue treatment
Metallic taste	Suggest sugarless candies or throat lozenges Encourage frequent oral hygiene
Nausea or abdominal discomfort	Consider dividing the medication into smaller doses or giving it at more frequent intervals Give medication with meals
Polydipsia	Reassure patient that this is a typical mechanism to cope with polyuria
Polyuria	Monitor intake and output Provide reassurance and explain the nature of this side effect Explain that this side effect causes no physical damage to the kidneys
Toxicity	Withhold medication Notify prescriber Use symptomatic treatments

bipolar disorder (i.e., mixed mania, rapid cycling, comorbid substance misuse, and secondary mania) (Box 26.9). The recommended initial dose is 750 mg daily, increases as rapidly as possible to achieve therapeutic response or desired plasma level. The maximum recommended dosage is 60 mg/kg/day (Divalproex Prescribing Information, 2024). Divalproex is usually initiated at 250 mg twice a day or lower. In the inpatient setting, it can be initiated in baseline liver function tests and a complete blood count with platelets should be obtained before starting therapy,

BOX 26.9

Medication Profile: Divalproex Sodium

DRUG CLASS: Antimanic agent.

RECEPTOR AFFINITY: Thought to increase level of inhibitory neurotransmitter, GABA, to brain neurons. Mechanism of action is unknown.

INDICATIONS: Mania, epilepsy, migraine.

ROUTES AND DOSAGE: Available in 125-mg delayed-release capsules, and 125-, 250-, and 500-mg enteric-coated tablets.

Adult Dosage: Dosage depends on symptoms and clinical picture presented; initially, the dosage is low and gradually increased, depending on the clinical presentation.

HALF-LIFE (PEAK EFFECT): 6 to 16 hours (1 to 4 hours).

SELECTED ADVERSE REACTIONS: Sedation, tremor (may be dose related), nausea, vomiting, indigestion, abdominal cramps, anorexia with weight loss, slight elevations in liver enzymes, hepatic failure, thrombocytopenia, transient increases in hair loss.

BOXED WARNING: Hepatotoxicity, teratogenicity, pancreatitis.

WARNING: Use cautiously during pregnancy and lactation. Contraindicated in patients with hepatic disease or significant hepatic dysfunction. Administer cautiously with salicylates; may increase serum levels and result in toxicity.

SPECIFIC PATIENT AND FAMILY EDUCATION

- Take with food if gastrointestinal upset occurs.
- Swallow tablets or capsules whole to prevent local irritation of mouth and throat.
- Notify your prescriber before taking any other prescription or OTC medications or herbal supplements.
- Avoid alcohol and sleep-inducing OTC products.
- Avoid driving or performing activities that require alertness.
- Do not abruptly discontinue use.
- Keep appointments for follow-up, including blood tests to monitor response.

GABA, gamma-aminobutyric acid; OTC, over-the-counter.

and patients with known liver disease should not be given divalproex sodium. The boxed warning notes hepatotoxicity. Optimal blood levels appear to be in the range of 50 to 150 ng/mL. Levels should be obtained weekly until the patient is stable and then every 6 months. Divalproex sodium is associated with increased risk for birth defects. Cases of life-threatening pancreatitis have been reported in adults and children receiving valproate, both initially and after several years of use. Some cases were described as hemorrhagic, with a rapid progression from onset to death. If pancreatitis is diagnosed, valproate use should be discontinued (Divalproex Sodium Prescribing Information, 2024).

Carbamazepine

Carbamazepine, an anticonvulsant, also has mood-stabilizing effects. Data from various studies suggest that it may be effective in patients who experience no response to lithium. The most common side effects of carbamazepine are dizziness, drowsiness, nausea, and vomiting, which may be avoided with slow incremental dosing. Carbamazepine has a boxed warning for aplastic anemia and agranulocytosis, but frequent clinically unimportant decreases in white blood cell counts also occur. Estimates of the rate of severe blood dyscrasias vary from 1 in 10,000 patients treated to a more recent estimate of 1 in 125,000 (DeBattista & Schatzberg, 2024). Mild, nonprogressive elevations of liver function test results are relatively common. Carbamazepine is associated with increased risk for birth defects.

In patients older than 12 years, carbamazepine is begun at 200 mg once or twice a day. The dosage is increased by no more than 200 mg every 2 to 4 days, to 800 to 1,000 mg a day or until therapeutic levels or effects are achieved. It is important to monitor for blood dyscrasias and liver damage. Liver function tests and complete blood counts with differential are the minimal pretreatment laboratory tests, and they should be repeated about 1 month after initiating treatment and at 3 months, 6 months, and yearly. Other yearly tests assessments should include electrolytes, blood urea nitrogen, thyroid function tests, urinalysis, and eye examinations. Carbamazepine levels are measured monthly until the patient is on a stable dosage. Studies suggest that blood levels in the range of 8 to 12 ng/mL correspond to therapeutic efficacy. See Table 26.5 for carbamazepine's interactions with other drugs. See Chapter 11 for further discussion of carbamazepine's possible mechanisms of action, pharmacokinetics, side effects, and toxicity.

EMERGENCY CARE ALERT Both valproate and carbamazepine may be lethal if high doses are ingested. Toxic symptoms appear in 1 to 3 hours and include neuromuscular disturbances, dizziness, stupor, agitation, disorientation, nystagmus, urinary retention, nausea and vomiting, tachycardia, hypotension or hypertension, cardiovascular shock, coma, and respiratory depression.

TABLE 26.5 SELECTED MEDICATION INTERACTIONS WITH CARBAMAZEPINE

Interaction	Drug Interacting With Carbamazepine
Increased carbamazepine levels	Erythromycin Calcium channel blockers (verapamil) Cimetidine Danazol Diltiazem Fluoxetine Isoniazid Nicotinamide Propoxyphene
Decreased carbamazepine levels	Phenobarbital Phenytoin Primidone
Drugs whose levels are decreased by carbamazepine	Acetaminophen: increased metabolism but also increased risk for hepatotoxicity Divalproex sodium Doxycycline Haloperidol Oral contraceptives Theophylline Tricyclic antidepressants Warfarin, oral anticoagulants

Lamotrigine

For a depressive episode, mood stabilizers such as **lamotrigine** which requires a dose titration are frequently prescribed (Box 26.10). Lamotrigine is approved by the U.S. Food and Drug Administration (FDA) for the maintenance treatment of bipolar disorder. It may be particularly effective for rapid cycling and in the depressed phase of bipolar illness. If lamotrigine is given with valproic acid the dose should be reduced. Valproic acid decreases the clearance of lamotrigine. Lamotrigine does have an FDA boxed warning for rash. Nurses should be especially vigilant for the appearance of any rash. If a rash does appear, it is most likely benign. However, it is not possible to predict whether the rash is benign or serious (Stevens–Johnson syndrome).

Antipsychotics

Several atypical antipsychotics that were primarily developed for the treatment of schizophrenia are also FDA approved for treatment of various symptoms of bipolar disorder. See Table 26.6. The dosages for the treatment of patients with bipolar disorder are generally lower than for those for schizophrenia. Recently, these agents have become a mainstay of treatment because they provide some of the broadest efficacy and are more likely used as the only medication to treat bipolar disorder than the mood stabilizers. Complications such as neuroleptic malignant syndrome can occur if antipsychotics are used in treating the mood disorder. An overview of

BOX 26.10

Medication Profile: Lamotrigine

DRUG CLASS: Antiepileptic

RECEPTOR AFFINITY: Lamotrigine has a weak inhibitory effect on the serotonin 5-HT3 receptor. It does not exhibit high-affinity binding: adenosine A_1 and A_2; adrenergic α_1, α_2, and β; dopamine D_1 and D_2; GABA-A and -B; histamine H1; kappa opioid; muscarinic acetylcholine; and serotonin 5-HT_2.

INDICATIONS: Epilepsy, bipolar disorder (acute mood with standard therapy).

ROUTES AND DOSAGE: Available in tablets: 25, 100, 150, and 200 mg scored.

CHEWABLE DISPERSIBLE TABLETS: 2, 5, and 25 mg.

HALF-LIFE (PEAK EFFECT): 32 hours but can be increased if taking valproate.

SELECTED ADVERSE REACTIONS: Dizziness, somnolence, and other symptoms and signs of CNS depression.

BOXED WARNING: Lamotrigine can cause serious rashes requiring hospitalization and discontinuation of treatment. The incidence of these rashes, which have included Stevens–Johnson syndrome, is approximately 0.3% to 0.8% in pediatric patients (aged 2 to 17 years) and 0.08% to 0.3% in adults receiving LAMICTAL.

WARNING: Hypersensitivity reaction, multiorgan failure, blood dyscrasias, and suicidal behavior and ideation have occurred.

SPECIFIC PATIENT AND FAMILY EDUCATION

- Do not drive a car or operate other complex machinery until you have gained sufficient experience taking lamotrigine.
- Lamotrigine may cause a serious rash that may cause you to be hospitalized or to stop taking lamotrigine; it may rarely cause death.

CNS, central nervous system; GABA, gamma-aminobutyric acid.

antipsychotics is presented in Chapter 11, and they are discussed in detail in Chapter 24.

Administering and Monitoring Medications

During acute mania, patients may not believe that they have a psychiatric disorder and may refuse to take medication. Because their energy level is still high, they can be highly creative in avoiding medication. Through patience and the development of a trusting relationship, patients will more likely begin to participate in a shared decision-making process. It is important for patients to have a sense of empowerment and participation in treatment even during the most acute episodes. After patients

TABLE 26.6 FOOD AND DRUG ADMINISTRATION–APPROVED ANTIPSYCHOTICS FOR THE TREATMENT OF SYMPTOMS OF BIPOLAR DISORDER

Antipsychotic Agent	FDA Indication for Bipolar Disorder	Adult Dosage
Aripiprazole	Acute treatment of manic and mixed episodes associated with bipolar disorder	10–30 mg/day
Aripiprazole lauroxil	Maintenance monotherapy for treatment for bipolar I disorder in adults	300 mg monthly (extended-release, injectable suspension)
Asenapine	Acute treatment of manic or mixed episodes associated with bipolar I disorder as monotherapy or adjunctive treatment to lithium or valproate	5–10 mg BID
Cariprazine	Acute treatment of manic or mixed episodes associated with bipolar I disorder in adults	3–6 mg/day
Lurasidone	Depressive episodes associated with bipolar I disorder as monotherapy or as adjunctive treatment to lithium or valproate	20–120 mg daily with food (comprising 350 calories)
Olanzapine	Acute treatment of manic or mixed episodes associated with bipolar I disorder (monotherapy and in combination with lithium or valproate) and maintenance treatment of bipolar I disorder	10–15 mg daily
Quetiapine	Bipolar I disorder, manic or mixed episodes; bipolar disorder, depressive episodes	300–800 mg daily
Risperidone	Bipolar mania, combination of risperidone with lithium or valproate for short-term treatment of acute manic or mixed episodes associated with bipolar I disorder	2–6 mg daily
Risperidone injection	Monotherapy or adjunctive to lithium or valproate for maintenance treatment of bipolar I disorder	25–50 mg every 2 weeks (extended-release, injectable suspension)
Ziprasidone	Acute manic or mixed episodes associated with bipolar disorder, with or without psychotic features	40–80 mg with food (comprising 500 calories)

FDA, U.S. Food and Drug Administration.

begin to take medications, symptom improvement should be evident. If a patient is very agitated, a benzodiazepine may be given for a brief period.

Monitoring Side Effects

Patients with bipolar disorder are usually treated with several medications. In addition, patients may be taking other "nonpsychiatric" medications. In some instances, one agent is used to augment the effects of another, such as supplemental thyroid hormone to boost antidepressant response in depression. Possible side effects for each medication should be listed and cross-referenced. When a side effect appears, the nurse should document the side effect and notify the prescriber so that further evaluation can be made. In some instances, medications should be changed.

Management of Complications

It is a well-established practice to combine mood stabilizers with antidepressants or antipsychotics. The previously discussed drug interactions should be considered when caring for an individual with bipolar disorder. One big challenge is monitoring alcohol, prescription drugs, over-the-counter (OTC) medications, and herbal supplements. A complete list of all medications should be maintained and evaluated for any potential interaction.

Promoting Adherence

Adherence to a complex medication regimen over months to years is difficult. Yet one of the primary reasons that acute symptoms reappear is because of discontinuation of medications. It is important to recognize that taking medication as prescribed over time is difficult. Nurses can help patients and families incorporate taking medications into their lifestyles by developing realistic plans. The use of pillboxes, reminders, and other cues will increase the likelihood of adherence.

Teaching Points

For patients who are taking lithium, it is important to explain that a change in dietary salt intake can affect the therapeutic blood level. If salt intake is reduced, the body will naturally retain lithium to maintain homeostasis. This increase in lithium retention can lead to toxicity. After the patient has been stabilized on a lithium dose, salt intake should remain constant. This is fairly easy to do, except during the summer when excessive perspiration can occur. Patients should increase salt intake during periods of perspiration, increased exercise, and dehydration. Most mood stabilizers and antidepressants can cause weight gain. Patients should be alerted to this potential side effect and should be instructed to monitor any changes in eating, appetite, or weight. Weight-reduction techniques may need to be instituted. Patients should also be clearly instructed to check with the nurse or provider before taking any OTC medications, herbal supplements, or other complementary and alternative treatment approaches.

Other Somatic Therapies

Electroconvulsive therapy (ECT) may be a treatment alternative for patients with severe mania who exhibit unremitting, frenzied physical activity. Other indications for ECT are acute mania that is unresponsive to antimanic agents or high suicide risk. ECT is safe and effective in patients receiving antipsychotic drugs. Use of valproate or carbamazepine will elevate the seizure threshold, requiring some adjustments in treatment.

Transcranial magnetic stimulation is another option for bipolar depression. Most of the research has focused on depressive phase rather than the mania episode. There may be cognitive benefits, such as improvement in verbal fluency, memory, and executive functioning. The research is ongoing (Taniguchi et al., 2024).

Psychosocial Interventions

Medications are necessary for the treatment of bipolar disorder, but it is only one aspect of recovery. Psychosocial strategies are critical in successful treatment and prevention of relapse.

Therapeutic Interactions

Through therapeutic interaction, treatment and recovery strategies are developed. It is also important to help the patient understand the disorder and manage the mood lability and dysfunctional thoughts that are often precursors to a manic or depressive episode. The nurse partners with the patient in developing strategies to remember to take medications, identify therapeutic and side effects, and know when and how to contact a clinician. Particularly important are enhancing social and occupational functioning, improving quality of life, increasing the patient and family's acceptance of the disorder, and reducing suicide.

Enhancing Cognitive and Behavioral Functioning

Individual cognitive-behavioral therapy, individual interpersonal therapy, and adjunctive therapies (such as those for substance use) are all recommended psychotherapeutic approaches.

There is emerging evidence supporting the use of interpersonal and social rhythm therapy and sleep/light manipulation targeting social rhythms to promote mood stability. The goals of this approach are to stabilize daily social rhythms that impact circadian rhythms, understand the link between mood and regularity of social rhythms, and develop self-awareness of bipolar disorder, early warning signs, and effective actions to take (Orhan et al., 2024).

BOX 26.11

Research for Evidence-Based Practice: Spirituality and Recovery

Sawab, S., Yusuf, A., Fitryasari, R., & Arifin, H. (2024). Spirituality and recovery from severe mental disorders: A systematic review. Journal of Psychosocial Nursing and Mental Health Services, *62(8), 11–17. https://doi.org/10.3928/02793695-20240227-01*

THE QUESTION: What is the impact of spirituality and recovery interventions among individuals with severe mental illness?

METHODS: A comprehensive search across six databases (Scopus, ScienceDirect, ProQuest, SpringerLink, PubMed, and CINAHL) elicited 651 relevant articles. There were 16 that met inclusion criteria.

FINDINGS: Spirituality significantly contributed to the recovery of individuals with severe mental disorders. Spirituality enhanced the overall quality of life by fostering the development of self-confidence, self-control, strength, and hope.

IMPLICATIONS FOR NURSING: Spirituality is an essential element in the recovery of individuals with severe mental health disorders. Psychiatric–mental health nurses could easily include assessment of spiritual needs and provide support to patients in meeting these needs.

Complementary Therapies

Various complementary therapies are helpful for people with bipolar disorder. Relaxation techniques can enhance sleep quality and reduce aggression in people with bipolar disorder (Gharehbaghi et al., 2024). A promising therapy to improve emotion regulation and anxiety is **imagery-based treatment,** which focuses on changing negative mental images (a sensory experience of visualizing scenarios or images in one's mind) such as suicide plans or traumatic childhood events (Elkington et al., 2024). Yoga has been shown to improve mood in depression suggesting an enhancement of GABA functioning (Reddy et al., 2024).

Spiritual Interventions

For patients with a religious/spiritual belief system, the bipolar symptoms can be especially challenging. During manic or depressive episodes, individuals may engage in behaviors that violate their usual values. Follow-up with a religious counselor can help patients view the behavior from a spiritual perspective (van Nieuw Amerongen-Meeuse et al., 2024). It is important for the nurse to maintain a nonjudgmental approach when discussing any religious struggles that the patient is having. See Box 26.11.

Psychoeducation

Teaching Strategies

Psychoeducation is designed to provide information on bipolar disorder and its successful treatment and recovery. The nurse provides information about the illness and obstacles to recovery. In the interest of improved medication adherence, listening carefully to the patient's concerns about the medication, dosing schedules and dose changes, and side effects helps individualize teaching approaches. Resistance to accepting the illness and taking medication, the symbolic meaning of medication taking, and worries about the future are discussed openly. See Box 26.12.

Teaching About Symptoms

Helping the patient recognize warning signs and symptoms of relapse, cope with residual symptoms, and improve functional impairments are important interventions. Watching for early warning signs and triggers can mean early treatment. Family members should be included in developing an emergency plan for recognizing and intervening if relapse symptoms occur. See Box 26.13.

Wellness Strategies

Many self-care interventions that prevent or delay symptoms are also wellness strategies. For example, individuals with bipolar disorder who relapse often describe a stressful life event that led to the manic episode. Mental health promotion activities should be the focus during remissions. During this period, patients have an opportunity to learn new coping skills that promote positive mental health. Stress management and relaxation techniques can be practiced for use when needed. A plan for managing emerging symptoms can also be developed during this period.

Social Skills Training

Social skills training may or may not be needed for the individual with bipolar disorder. Even though their

BOX 26.12

Psychoeducation Checklist: Bipolar I Disorder

When caring for the patient with a bipolar I disorder, be sure to include the following topic areas in the teaching plan:

- Psychopharmacologic agents, including drug action, dosage, frequency, and possible side effects
- Medication regimen adherence
- Recovery plan
- Relapse prevention plan
- Strategies to decrease agitation and restlessness
- Safety measures
- Self-care management
- Follow-up laboratory testing
- Support services

BOX 26.13

Relapse Prevention and Emergency Plan

COMMON INDICATORS FOR RELAPSE

Mania

- Reading several books or newspapers at once
- Cannot concentrate on one topic
- Talking faster than usual
- Feeling irritable
- Hungry all the time
- Friends remark on changes in mood
- More energy than usual

Depression

- Quit cooking, cleaning, daily chores
- Avoid people
- Crave foods (e.g., chocolate)

Headaches

- Do not care about other people
- Sleeping more or restless sleep
- People are irritating to be around

EMERGENCY PLAN

- Keep a list of emergency contacts (primary health care provider, close family members)
- Keep a current list of all medications, including their dosages
- Information about other health issues
- Symptoms that indicate others need to take responsibility for care
- Treatment preferences (who, where, medications, advanced directive location)

social skills will be impaired during periods of mania or depression, once symptoms are controlled, the individual should return to previous level of functioning. There are instances when an individual does need help with social skills, such as learning to listen to others, taking time to finish projects, and organizing daily living demands of cooking, cleaning, and shopping. For these individuals, a social skills group is useful.

Providing Family Education

Family psychoeducation strategies are particularly useful in decreasing the risk of relapse and hospitalization. Family needs may vary, with some families needing education about bipolar disorder and others needing more information about resource availability (Zauszniewski et al., 2024). The sooner the education is begun, the more effective this approach is (Mousavi et al., 2021). Marital and family interventions are often needed at different periods in the life of an individual with bipolar disorder. For the family with a child with this disorder, additional parenting skills are needed to manage the behaviors. The goals of family interventions are to help the family understand and cope with the disorder. Interventions may range from occasional counseling sessions to intensive family therapy.

Promoting Safety

The safety issues previously discussed should be addressed with the individual and family before a manic or depressive episode emerges. The nurse can help the individual and family identify specific thoughts and behaviors associated with unsafe situations. For example, during manic episodes, one patient would often threaten airlines and government officials. Within a therapeutic relationship, the nurse and patient agreed that the first call would be to the nurse or another family member who, in turn, would seek more intensive treatment, such as a medication adjustment.

The individual should keep a safety plan for suicidal ideations nearby to be used when thoughts occur. Firearms, weapons, and unused lethal medication should be removed from the environment.

Convening Support Groups

Support groups are helpful for people with this disorder. Participating in groups allows the individual to meet others with the same disorder and to learn management and preventive strategies. Support groups also are helpful in dealing with the stigma associated with mental illness.

Implementing Milieu Therapy

In the hospital or treatment setting, a calm, therapeutic milieu is usually the responsibility of the nurse. An overly stimulating environment can result in behavior escalation for people with mania. A noisy unit, frequent demands for group and individual participation, and lack of privacy cause an escalation in behavior. See Box 26.14.

Developing Recovery-Oriented Rehabilitation Strategies

The recovery plan should be developed with the patient and should include treatment for the disorder, mental health promotion strategies, and wellness activities. Building on the individual's strengths and resilience will foster a healthy lifestyle and well-being.

Evaluation of Patient Outcomes

Desired treatment outcomes are stabilization of mood and enhanced quality of life. Primary tools for evaluating outcomes are nursing observation and patient self-report. (See Clinical Judgment Nursing Care Plan 26.1, which sets forth a plan of care for Christine, the case study patient in this chapter.)

Continuum of Care

In today's health care climate, with efforts to reduce hospitalization, most patients with bipolar disorder are treated in a community setting. Hospitalizations are

BOX 26.14

Reflection of a Nurse: De-Escalation

Incident

A patient with mania who is agitated enters the day room to watch television. The inpatient unit is very busy. The patient who is agitated accuses another patient of taking their favorite seat. The nurse wants to de-escalate the situation and asks the patient who is seated to get up and move to another chair. That patient quietly moves to a different chair, and further confrontation is avoided.

Reflection

Upon evaluation of the intervention, the nurse realizes that by asking the patient to move, the accusatory behavior of the patient with mania was reinforced.

1. How could the nurse avoid reinforcing the behavior of the patient with mania without escalating the situation?
2. What other interventions could that nurse implement to calm the unit?

usually brief; recovery is emphasized, and medication regimen promotes adherence. Psychoeducation helps in understanding and managing the disorder, and supportive psychotherapy helps these individuals move toward recovery. Patients need extended and continued follow-up to monitor medication trials and side effects, reinforce self-care management, and provide continued psychosocial support.

Emergency Care

Emergency care is necessary during periods of depression or mania, when there are safety issues such as suicidal or homicidal ideation. Agitation and aggression in an emergency department are not unusual, and staff are usually well prepared to de-escalate the situation. Another critical situation is when an individual is unwillingly brought to the hospital for treatment. Assaults in the emergency departments can lead to patient and staff injuries (Keslar, 2024).

CLINICAL JUDGMENT NURSING CARE PLAN 26.1

The Patient With Bipolar I Disorder

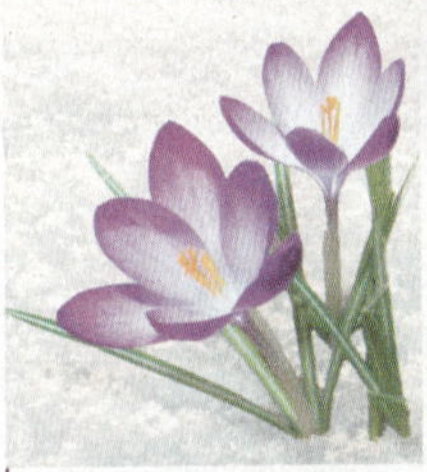

Christine, age 34, is admitted involuntarily to the inpatient unit, following an altercation at the airport when she became loud and belligerent and caused a ruckus. She believes that she has special powers over others and has a direct connection to God. She stated she needed to leave town because of the "three men" in her house, who are chasing her. She is accompanied by her mother and husband, Karl. She believes that she is being taken to a safe place, which can protect her from the men who were chasing her.

Her mother stated that Christine was first diagnosed with bipolar disorder at age 22, after her first child was born. She received treatment for 2 years. After her second pregnancy, she refused to take her medication. During her third manic episode, she left her husband and children. She was reunited with her parents 4 years later and reinitiated treatment. After her marriage to Karl, she stopped her medication. Karl believed that Christine had a history of depression but did not realize that she had bipolar disorder. He wants to be supportive and help her.

Setting: Intensive Care Psychiatric Unit in a General Hospital

Assessment Cues: A 34-year-old person assigned female at birth who is flamboyantly dressed in a cocktail dress with several pieces of expensive jewelry. She is oriented to time, place, and person, but she believes she has special powers. She states that she is "not suicidal—I have a mission." She is displaying a pressured speech and flight of ideas. She is hyperverbal and hyperactive. It is difficult to interrupt her thoughts. She states she has not slept for several days and does not need to sleep because she is gifted. She is not taking any medications and denies substance use except for an occasional marijuana joint. She admits to taking mood stabilizers in the past but states that they made her gain weight. She does not want to take that medication again. BP 130/70, P 70, R 18, Ht. 5'5', Wt 125 (BMI 20.8).

Associated Psychiatric Diagnosis	Medications
Bipolar I disorder	Ziprasidone 40 mg PO BID (give with a full meal) Lorazepam 1 mg PO q4h as needed for anxiety or agitation

Priority Hypothesis: Lack of Problem-Solving Ability

Important Characteristics	Associated Considerations
Denial of problems obvious to others Projection of blame or responsibility for problems	Biochemical/neurophysiologic imbalance

Continued

Clinical Judgment Nursing Care Plan 26.1 Continued

Planning Recovery and Wellness Outcomes

Initial	Discharge
1. Increase problem-solving ability 2. Identify factors that led to current manic episode 3. Accept treatment of bipolar disorder	4. Agree to continue medication and follow-up 5. Attend support group

Taking Action: Nursing Interventions

Interventions	Rationale	Ongoing Assessment
Initiate a nurse–patient relationship by demonstrating an acceptance of Christine as a worthwhile human being through the use of nonjudgmental statements and behavior	The positive therapeutic relationship can maintain the patient's dignity and open communication	Assess the stages of the relationship, and determine whether a therapeutic relationship is actually being formed. Identify indicators of trust
Administer ziprasidone 40 mg BID per health care provider order (Christine refused mood stabilizers because of side effects.) Teach Christine the therapeutic and side effects of medication Instruct her to take medication with a full meal	Most new antipsychotics are indicated for mood disorders. Best absorption of ziprasidone occurs when taken with a full meal	Determine effectiveness of medication. Observe for side effects

Evaluation

Outcomes	Revised Outcomes	Interventions
Increased ability to problem solve Is dressing appropriately for situation Taking medication as prescribed after discharge Considering attending support groups	Take medication as prescribed	Continue to encourage Christine to attend support groups

Priority Hypothesis: Unable to Cope With Life Stressors

Important Characteristics	Associated Considerations
Asking for help Reported difficulty with life stressors Inability to problem solve Insufficient access to social support Destructive behavior toward self Frequent illnesses Substance misuse	Altered mood (mania) caused by changes secondary to body chemistry (bipolar disorder) Sensory overload secondary to excessive activity

Planning Recovery and Wellness Outcomes

Initial	Discharge
1. Accept support through the nurse–patient relationship 2. Identify areas of ineffective coping 3. Examine the current efforts at coping 4. Identify areas of strength 5. Learn new coping skills	6. Practice new coping skills 7. Focus on strengths

Clinical Judgment Nursing Care Plan 26.1 Continued

Taking Action: Nursing Interventions

Interventions	Rationale	Ongoing Assessment
Identify the current stresses in Christine's life, including bipolar disorder	When areas of concern are verbalized by the patient, she will be able to focus on one issue at a time. If she identifies the mental disorder as a stressor, she will more likely be able to develop strategies to deal with it	Determine whether Christine is able to identify problem areas realistically. Continue to assess for suicidality
Identify Christine's strengths in dealing with past stressors	By focusing on past successes, she can identify strengths and build on them in the future	Assess whether Christine can identify any previous successes in her life
Assist Christine in discussing, selecting, and practicing positive coping skills (e.g., jogging, yoga, thought stopping)	New coping skills take a conscious effort to learn and will at first seem strange and unnatural. Practicing these skills will help the patient incorporate them into her coping strategy repertoire	Assess whether Christine follows through on learning new skills
Assist patient in coping with bipolar disorder, beginning with education about it	A mood disorder is a major stressor in a patient's life. To manage the stress, the patient needs a knowledge base	Determine Christine's knowledge about bipolar disorder
Administer lorazepam as needed for anxiety or agitation	Benzodiazepine helps decrease anxiety and calm the patient	Assess for target action, side effects, and toxicity

Evaluation

Outcomes	Revised Outcomes	Interventions
Christine is easily engaged in a therapeutic relationship. She examined the areas in her life where she coped ineffectively	Establish a therapeutic relationship with a therapist at the mental health clinic	Refer to mental health clinic
She identified her strengths and how she coped with stressors and especially her illness in the past. She is willing to try medications again, in hopes of not gaining weight	Continue to view illness as a potential stressor that can disrupt life	Seek advice immediately if there are any problems with medications
She learned new problem-solving skills and reported that she learned a lot about her medication. She is committed to adhering to her medication regimen. She identified new coping skills that she could realistically do. She will focus on strengths	Continue to practice new coping skills as stressful situations arise	Discuss with therapist the outcomes of using new coping skills. Attend bipolar support group

Inpatient-Focused Care

Inpatient hospitalization is necessary for patients who are severely psychotic or who are an immediate threat to themselves or others. In acute mania, nursing interventions focus on patient safety because patients are prone to injury because of hyperactivity and are often unaware of injuries they sustain. Distraction may also be effective when a patient is talking or acting inappropriately. Removal to a quieter environment may be necessary if other interventions have not been successful, but the patient should be carefully monitored. During acute mania, patients are often impulsive, disinhibited, and interpersonally inappropriate, so the nurse should avoid direct confrontations or challenges.

During manic phases, patients usually violate others' boundaries. For example, roommate selection for patients requiring hospital admittance needs to be carefully considered. If possible, a private room is ideal because patients with bipolar disorder tend to irritate others, who quickly tire of the intrusiveness. These patients may miss the cues indicating anger and aggression from others. The nurse should protect the patient who is manic from self-harm, as well as harm from other patients.

The length of stay in an inpatient unit will be relatively short, 3 to 5 days. The plan of care will focus on medication management, including control of side effects, initiation or revision of a recovery plan, psychoeducation, and promotion of self-care. Nurses should be familiar with drug–drug interactions and with interventions to help control side effects.

Intensive Outpatient Programs

Intensive outpatient programs for several weeks of acute-phase care during a manic or depressive episode are used when hospitalization is not necessary or to prevent or shorten hospitalization. These programs are usually called partial hospitalization. Close medication monitoring and milieu therapies that foster restoration of a patient's previous adaptive abilities are the major nursing responsibilities in these settings.

Setting up frequent office visits and crisis telephone calls are additional nursing interventions that can help shorten or prevent hospitalization during the acute phase of a manic episode. Family sessions or psychoeducation that includes the patient are alternatives. Severely and persistently ill patients may need ongoing intensive treatment, but the frequency of visits can be decreased for patients whose conditions stabilize and who enter the continuation or the maintenance phase of treatment.

Community Care

People with bipolar disorder are treated throughout the continuum of care. When symptoms are acute, hospitalization may be necessary. Other times, minimal interaction with the mental health providers is needed. The individual will need to be seen regularly to monitor symptoms and medications.

Virtual Mental Health Care

The use of telemedicine can be highly effective for people with bipolar disorder during periods of remission. Telephone text contacts are a useful strategy for monitoring medication adherence (Chen & Hilliard, 2024). The use of telephones is relatively inexpensive and widespread. The use of smartphones allows frequent reminders of medication dosage and is unobtrusive. They can also be used for texting and voice-based mobile interventions. Video teleconferencing is feasible and acceptable for adolescents and young adults who grew up using digital technology (Sankar et al., 2021).

Integration With Primary Care

There are several reasons that coordination of care is especially important for people with bipolar disorder. A substantial proportion of people with bipolar disorder are treated in the primary care setting. There may be an average of 6 to 8 years between the onset of symptoms and diagnosis. Because there may be several episodes of depression before there is a manic episode, bipolar disorder is often misdiagnosed as depression in primary care, leading to a delay in treatment. If antidepressants are prescribed for someone with a bipolar disorder, these medications may precipitate a manic episode. The need exists to improve the health of this population. Collaborative care of mental health with primary care increases the likelihood that an individual would be screened for bipolar disorder, resulting in an early diagnosis and effective treatment (Cerimele & Fortney, 2023). Patients with bipolar disorder frequently require primary care management for comorbidities, such as cardiovascular and metabolic disorders.

OTHER BIPOLAR AND RELATED DISORDERS

BIPOLAR II DISORDER

In **bipolar II disorder**, the individual is mostly depressed, which can severely affect their social and occupational life. Even though there are brief periods of elevated, expansive, or irritable moods, bipolar II disorder is not as easily recognized as bipolar I disorder because the symptoms are less dramatic. **Hypomania**, a mild form of mania, is characteristic of bipolar II disorder. Judgment remains fundamentally intact.

CYCLOTHYMIC DISORDER

In a **cyclothymic disorder**, hypomanic symptoms occur alternating with numerous periods of depressive symptoms. However, these symptoms are less severe than bipolar disorders. To be diagnosed with this disorder, numerous periods of hypomanic symptoms have to be present for at least 2 years.

OTHER CAUSES OF MANIC-LIKE BEHAVIOR

Illicit drugs, prescription medications, and some medical conditions such as changes in thyroid functioning can be responsible for manic-like behavior. These symptoms cause significant distress and impairment in social functioning.

SUMMARY OF KEY POINTS

- Bipolar and related disorders are characterized by one or more manic episodes or mixed mania (co-occurrence of manic and depressive states) that cause marked impairment in social activities, occupational functioning, and interpersonal relationships and may require hospitalization to prevent self-harm.

- In bipolar and related disorders, there are periods of mania or hypomania that alternate with depression. These disorders are classified as bipolar I disorder, bipolar II disorder, or cyclothymic disorder, depending on the severity of the manic and depressive symptoms. Bipolar disorder may also be related to substance misuse, prescription drug use, or a medical condition.
- Manic episodes are periods in which the individual experiences unusual and persistently elevated, expansive, or irritable mood characterized by inflated self-esteem, decreased need to sleep, excessive energy or hyperactivity, racing thoughts, easy distractibility, and an inability to stay focused. Other symptoms can include hypersexuality and impulsivity.
- Bipolar disorders are underreported and are often misdiagnosed. Bipolar I disorder is more dramatic than bipolar II disorder, so it is easier to diagnose.
- Genetics plays a role in the etiology of bipolar disorders. Risk factors include a family history of mood disorders, prior mood episodes, lack of social support, stressful life events, substance use, and medical issues, particularly chronic or terminal illnesses.
- Mental health nursing assessment includes assessing mood; speech patterns; thought processes and thought content; suicidal or homicidal thoughts; cognition and memory; and social factors, such as patterns of relationships, quality of support systems, and changes in occupational functioning. Several self-report scales are helpful in evaluating depressive symptoms.
- Many symptoms of bipolar depression, such as weight gain and appetite changes, sleep disturbance, decreased energy, and fatigue, are similar to those of medical illnesses. Assessment includes a thorough medical history and physical examination to detect or rule out medical or psychiatric comorbidity.
- Establishing and maintaining a therapeutic nurse–patient relationship is key to successful outcomes. Shared decision making with the patient leads to positive outcomes. Recovery-oriented nursing interventions that foster the therapeutic relationship include being available in times of crisis, providing understanding and education to patients and their families regarding goals of treatment and recovery, providing encouragement and feedback concerning the patient's progress, providing guidance in the patient's interpersonal interactions with others and work environment, and helping to set and monitor realistic goals.
- Pharmacotherapy includes mood stabilizers used alone or in combination with antipsychotics or benzodiazepines to treat psychosis, agitation, or insomnia. ECT is a valuable alternative for patients with severe mania that does not respond to other treatments.
- Recent major advances in bipolar disorder treatment research validate the efficacy of integrated psychosocial and pharmacologic treatment involving family or couple therapies, psychoeducational programs, and individual cognitive-behavioral or interpersonal therapies.
- Psychosocial interventions for bipolar disorders include self-care management, cognitive therapy, behavioral therapy, interpersonal therapy, patient and family education regarding the nature of the disorder and treatment goals, marital and family therapy, and group therapy that includes medication maintenance support groups and other consumer-oriented support groups.
- The use of virtual health care strategies can be highly effective in monitoring medication adherence and providing virtual therapy and psychoeducation.

DEVELOPING CLINICAL JUDGMENT

1. A patient tells you that they no longer need medication because they have special powers that protect them from evil forces. The patient says sleep is no longer needed and they can see things that others do not see. What approaches would you use to help the patient to consider taking medication?
2. Describe how you would approach a patient who is expressing concern that the diagnosis of bipolar disorder will negatively affect their social and work relationships.
3. Your patient with mania is experiencing physical hyperactivity that is interfering with their sleep and nutrition. Describe the actions you would take to meet the patient's needs for rest and nutrition.
4. Prepare a hypothetical discussion with a patient with potential bipolar disorder concerning the advantages and disadvantages of lithium versus divalproex sodium for treatment of bipolar disorder.

MOVIES, TV, OR STREAMING PROGRAMS

The Year Between: 2022. This film, an American independent dramedy, follows a young woman recently diagnosed with bipolar disorder and her struggle to understand and accept her diagnosis, and begin her recovery journey. The film opens as Clemence (Alex Heller), a college sophomore, is acting aggressively and bullying her roommate during a manic bout. Even though her family is unprepared for her return, Clemence's mother, Sherri, takes her home from college and assigns Clemence the unfurnished basement as her bedroom. Clemence is taken to a psychiatrist, who diagnoses her with bipolar disorder and prescribes medications including lithium. Clemence's father, Don, is a school teacher who avoids family conflict and assumes a passive, disengaged, but loving role in the family. Clemence's sister, Carlin, and brother, Neil, have difficulty adjusting to Clemence's presence and behavior. Carlin is afraid that she will also develop a mental illness.

This movie is a realistic portrayal of the life of a young individual with bipolar disorder who is struggling to learn about and cope with the disorder. Viewers can see the day-to-day struggle of self-acceptance and responsibility for treatment.

Viewing Points:

1. Identify the symptoms of bipolar disorder that Clemence exhibits.
2. Why does Clemence stop her medication?
3. How does the illness shape Clemence's views of herself?
4. How does the family impact Clemence's struggle with managing her disorder?

Unfolding Patient Stories: Sharon Cole • Part 2

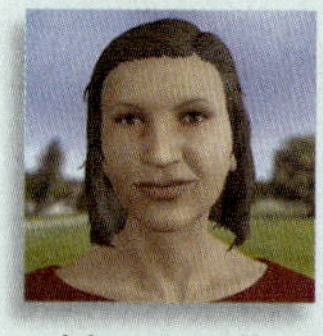

Recall from Chapter 9 **Sharon Cole,** diagnosed with bipolar disorder, who is admitted to the orthopedic unit following surgery for a fractured ankle from a fall during a manic episode. She is exhibiting manic behavior postoperatively with grandiose thoughts, irritability, poor judgment, and wanting to leave the hospital. What are the benefits of having a sitter at her bedside? What education would the nurse provide to a sitter without prior experience caring for a client with manic behavior? How might the nurse plan interventions to promote the safety of Sharon and the staff caring for her? How might the nurse attend to Sharon's postoperative needs while her behavior remains manic?

Care for Sharon Cole and other patients in a realistic virtual environment: ***vSim** for Nursing* (thepoint.lww.com/vSimMentalHealth). Practice documenting these patients' care in DocuCare (thepoint.lww.com/DocuCareEHR).

REFERENCES

Aguglia, A., Salvi, V., Amerio, A., Gari, G., Dragogna, F., Mencacci, C., Volpe, U., Serafini, G., & Amore, M. (2022). Number of episodes and duration of illness associated with hypertension and 10-year cardiovascular risk in patients with bipolar disorder type I. *Psychiatry Research*, *308*, 114344. https://doi.org/10.1016/j.psychres.2021.114344

American Psychiatric Association. (2022). *Diagnostic and statistical manual of mental disorders (5th ed., text rev.)*. Author.

Arnone, D., Karmegam, S. R., Östlundh, L., Alkhyeli, F., Alhammadi, L., Alhammadi, S., Alkhoori, A., & Selvaraj, S. (2024). Risk of suicidal behavior in patients with major depression and bipolar disorder—A systematic review and meta-analysis of registry-based studies. *Neuroscience and Biobehavioral Reviews*, *159*, 105594. https://doi.org/10.1016/j.neubiorev.2024.105594

Bach, S. L., Cardoso, T. A., Moreira, F. P., Mondin, T. C., Simjanoski, M., Kapczinski, F. P., Frey, B. N., Souza, L. D. M., da Silva, R. A., & Jansen, K. (2021). Risk factors for new-onset bipolar disorder in a community cohort: A five-year follow up study. *Psychiatry Research*, *303*, 114109. https://doi.org/10.1016/j.psychres.2021.114109

Baranova, A., Cao, H., & Zhang, F. (2024). Exploring the influences of education, intelligence and income on mental disorders. *General Psychiatry*, *37*(1), e101080. https://doi.org/10.1136/gpsych-2023-101080

Bareis, N., Olfson, M., Dixon, L. B., Chwastiak, L., Monroe-Devita, M., Kessler, R. C., Gibbons, R. D., Edlund, M., Guyer, H., Kreski, N. T., Graupensperger, S., Winans, K. S., & Stroup, T. S. (2024). Clinical characteristics and functioning of adults with bipolar I disorder: evidence from the mental and substance use disorders prevalence study. *Journal of Affective Disorders*, *366*, 317–325. https://doi.org/10.1016/j.jad.2024.08.133

Bolton, S., Warner, J., Harriss, E., Geddes, J., & Saunders, K. (2021). Bipolar disorder: Trimodal age-at-onset distribution. *Bipolar Disorders*, *23*(4), 341–356. https://doi.org/10.1111/bdi.13016

Cerimele, J. M., & Fortney, J. C. (2023). Bipolar disorder assessment and monitoring measures in clinical care: Updates from a large randomized controlled trial in primary care. *Bipolar Disorders*, *25*(8), 708–710. https://doi.org/10.1111/bdi.13382

Chauhan, V. S., Sharma, M., Chatterjee, K., Prakash, J., Srivastava, K., & Chaudhury, S. (2023). Childhood trauma and bipolar affective disorder: Is there a linkage?. *Industrial Psychiatry Journal*, *32*(Suppl 1), S9–S14. https://doi.org/10.4103/ipj.ipj_206_23

Chen, C. J., & Hilliard, W. (2024). Text message reminders for long-acting injectable antipsychotics in patients with schizophrenia spectrum disorders. *Journal of the American Psychiatric Nurses Association*, *30*(4), 828–833. https://doi.org/10.1177/10783903231183918

Cordeiro, R. C., Lima, C. N. C., Fries, G. R., Zunta-Soares, G., Soares, J. C., Quevedo, J., & Scaini, G. (2023). Mitochondrial health index correlates with plasma circulating cell-free mitochondrial DNA in bipolar disorder. *Molecular Psychiatry*, *28*(11), 4622–4631. https://doi.org/10.1038/s41380-023-02249-y

DeBattista, C., & Schatzberg, A. F. (2024). *Schatzberg's Manual of clinical psychopharmacology* (10th ed.). American Psychiatric Association Publishing

Dines, M., Kes, M., Ailán, D., Cetkovich-Bakmas, M., Born, C., & Grunze, H. (2024). Bipolar disorders and schizophrenia: discrete disorders? *Frontiers in Psychiatry*, *15*, 1352250. https://doi.org/10.3389/fpsyt.2024.1352250

Divalproex Sodium Prescribing Information. (March 2024). [Online]. Accessed October 4, 2024. Available at: label (fda.gov)

Elkington, S., Brown, M., Wright, K., Regan, J., Pattarnaraskouwski, K., Steel, C., Hales, S., Holmes, E., & Morant, N. (2024). Experiences of imagery-based treatment for anxiety in bipolar disorder: A qualitative study embedded within the image based emotion regulation feasibility randomised controlled trial. *Psychology and Psychotherapy: Theory, Research and Practice*, *97*(3), 531–548. https://doi.org/10.1111/papt.12538

Gharehbaghi, M., Mirhosseini, S., Minaei-Moghadam, S., Salari, M., Grimwood, S., & Vaghee, S. (2024). Benson relaxation technique to address sleep quality and aggression among patients with bipolar type I disorder: A randomized clinical trial study. *Heliyon*, *10*(9), e30648. https://doi.org/10.1016/j.heliyon.2024.e30648

Hedya, S. A., Avula, A., & Swoboda, H. D. (2023). Lithium toxicity. In *StatPearls*. StatPearls Publishing. www.ncbi.nlm.nih.gov/books/NBK499992

Jain, A., & Mitra, P. (2023). Bipolar disorder. In *StatPearls*. StatPearls Publishing. www.ncbi.nlm.nih.gov/books/NBK558998.

Kang, J., Lee, H., Park, J., Kim, H. J., Kwon, R., Kim, S., Fond, G., Boyer, L., Rahmati, M., Smith, L., Nehs, C. J., Son, Y., Kim, S., Lee, H., Lee, J., Kim, M. S., Kim, T., & Yon, D. K. (2024). Comorbid physical health outcomes in patients with bipolar disorder: An umbrella review of systematic reviews and meta-analyses. *Asian Journal of Psychiatry*, *99*, 104138. https://doi.org/10.1016/j.ajp.2024.104138

Keslar R. (2024). Emergency nurses' perspectives on mental health boarders: An integrative review. *International Emergency Nursing*, *75*, 101463. https://doi.org/10.1016/j.ienj.2024.101463

Léda-Rêgo, G., Studart-Bottó, P., Abbade, P., Rabelo-Da-Ponte, F. D., Casqueiro, J. S., Sarmento, S., Dallalana, C., Troesch, M., Prates, S., & Miranda-Scippa, Â. (2024). Lifetime prevalence of psychiatric comorbidities in patients with bipolar disorder: A systematic review and meta-analysis. *Psychiatry Research*, *337*, 115953. https://doi.org/10.1016/j.psychres.2024.115953

Li, K., Richards, E., & Goes, F. S. (2023). Racial differences in the major clinical symptom domains of bipolar disorder. *International Journal of Bipolar Disorders*, *11*(1), 17. https://doi.org/10.1186/s40345-023-00299-3

Long, Y., Pan, N., Yu, Y., Zhang, S., Qin, K., Chen, Y., Sweeney, J. A., DelBello, M. P., & Gong, Q. (2024). Shared and distinct neurobiological bases of bipolar disorder and attention-deficit/hyperactivity disorder in children and adolescents: A comparative meta-analysis of structural abnormalities. *Journal of the American Academy of Child and Adolescent Psychiatry*, *63*(6), 586–604. https://doi.org/10.1016/j.jaac.2023.09.551

Montejo, L., Retuerto, M., Solé, B., Martín, S., Ruiz, A., Clougher, D., Bort, M., Sánchez-Moreno, J., Martínez-Arán, A., Vieta, E., & Torrent, C. (2024). Facing life in old age: exploring resilience in older adults with bipolar disorder. *Journal of Clinical Medicine*, *13*(13), 3942. https://doi.org/10.3390/jcm13133942

Mousavi, N., Norozpour, M., Taherifar, Z., Naserbakht, M., & Shabani, A. (2021). Bipolar I disorder: a qualitative study of the viewpoints of the family members of patients on the nature of the disorder and pharmacological treatment non-adherence. *BMC Psychiatry*, *21*(1), 83. https://doi.org/10.1186/s12888-020-03008-x

Nierenberg, A. A., Agustini, B., Köhler-Forsberg, O., Cusin, C., Katz, D., Sylvia, L. G., Peters, A., & Berk, M. (2023). Diagnosis and treatment of bipolar disorder: A review. *JAMA*, *330*(14), 1370–1380. https://doi.org/10.1001/jama.2023.18588

Orhan, M., Korten, N., Mans, N., van Schaik, D., Kupka, R., Stek, M., Steenhuis, D., van Dijk, M., Swartz, H. A., van Oppen, P., & Dols, A. (2024). Feasibility and acceptability of group interpersonal and social rhythm therapy for recurrent mood disorders: A pilot study. *American Journal of Psychotherapy*, 77(1), 1–6. https://doi.org/10.1176/appi.psychotherapy.20220067

Pietschnig, J., Oberleiter, S., & Köhler, M. D. (2024). Smoking behavior is associated with suicidality in individuals with psychosis and bipolar disorder: A systematic quantitative review and meta-analysis. *Frontiers in Psychology*, *15*, 1369669. https://doi.org/10.3389/fpsyg.2024.1369669

Poletti, S., Mazza, M. G., & Benedetti, F. (2024). Inflammatory mediators in major depression and bipolar disorder. *Translational Psychiatry*, *14*(1), 247. https://doi.org/10.1038/s41398-024-02921-z

Reddy, P. V., Basavaraju, R., Sanjay, T. N., Ramesh, A., Chowdhury, P., Mehta, U. M., Venkatasubramanian, G., Thirthalli, J., & Kesavan, M. (2024). Investigational applications of transcranial magnetic stimulation (TMS) in mood disorders: Studies from a tertiary care center in India. *Asian journal of psychiatry*, *97*, 104054. https://doi.org/10.1016/j.ajp.2024.104054

Rowe, A. L., Perich, T., & Meade, T. (2024). Bipolar disorder and cumulative trauma: A systematic review of prevalence and illness outcomes. *Journal of Clinical Psychology*, *80*(3), 692–713. https://doi.org/10.1002/jclp.23650

Russell, S. E., Wrobel, A. L., Lotfaliany, M., Ashton, M. M., Kaur, R., Yocum, A. K., Duval, E. R., Diaz-Byrd, C., Ehrlich, T. J., Marshall, D. F., Berk, M., McInnis, M. G., Dean, O., & Turner, A. (2024). Trauma and comorbid post-traumatic stress disorder in people with bipolar disorder participating in the Heinz C. Prechter Longitudinal Study. *Journal of Affective Disorders*, *348*, 275–282. https://doi.org/10.1016/j.jad.2023.12.058

Sankar, A., Panchal, P., Goldman, D. A., Colic, L., Villa, L. M., Kim, J. A., Lebowitz, E. R., Carrubba, E., Lecza, B., Silverman, W. K., Swartz, H. A., & Blumberg, H. P. (2021). Telehealth social rhythm therapy to reduce mood symptoms and suicide risk among adolescents and young adults with bipolar disorder. *American Journal of Psychotherapy*, *74*(4), 172–177. https://doi.org/10.1176/appi.psychotherapy.20210011

Scott, M. R., & McClung, C. A. (2023). Bipolar disorder. *Current Opinion in Neurobiology*, *83*, 102801. https://doi.org/10.1016/j.conb.2023.102801

Song, X., Feng, Y., Yi, L., Zhong, B., & Li, Y. (2023). Changes in thyroid function levels in female patients with first-episode bipolar disorder. *Frontiers in Psychiatry*, *14*, 1185943. https://doi.org/10.3389/fpsyt.2023.1185943

Song, J., Pasman, J. A., Johansson, V., Kuja-Halkola, R., Harder, A., Karlsson, R., Lu, Y., Kowalec, K., Pedersen, N. L., Cannon, T. D., Hultman, C. M., & Sullivan, P. F. (2024). Polygenic risk scores and twin concordance for schizophrenia and bipolar disorder. *JAMA Psychiatry*, e242406. https://doi.org/10.1001/jamapsychiatry.2024.2406

Taniguchi, K., Kaneko, N., Wada, M., Moriyama, S., Nakajima, S., Mimura, M., & Noda, Y. (2024). Neurophysiological profiles of patients with bipolar disorders as probed with transcranial magnetic stimulation: A systematic review. *Neuropsychopharmacology Reports*, *44*(3), 572–584. https://doi.org/10.1002/npr2.12458

Teigland, C., Mohammadi, I., Agatep, B. C., Boskovic, D. H., & Sajatovic, M. (2024). Relationship between social determinants of health and hospitalizations and costs among patients with bipolar disorder 1. *Journal of Managed Care & Specialty Pharmacy*, *30*(1), 72–85. https://doi.org/10.18553/jmcp.2024.30.1.72

Temes, C. M., Boccagno, C., Gold, A. K., Kobaissi, H., Hsu, I., Montinola, S., & Sylvia, L. G. (2024). Comorbidity of bipolar disorder and borderline personality disorder: Phenomenology, course, and treatment considerations. *Bipolar Disorders*, 26(6), 548–555. https://doi.org/10.1111/bdi.13465

Tondo, L., Vázquez, G. H., & Baldessarini, R. J. (2021). Prevention of suicidal behavior in bipolar disorder. *Bipolar Disorders*, *23*(1), 14–23. https://doi.org/10.1111/bdi.13017

van Nieuw Amerongen-Meeuse, J. C., Braam, A. W., Westerbroek, G., Ouwehand, E., Anbeek, C., & Schaap-Jonker, H. (2024). Varieties of religious and spiritual struggles by type of mental disorder: a qualitative approach. *Psychopathology*, *57*(1), 27–38. https://doi.org/10.1159/000531027

Yeo, H., Lee, J., Jeon, S., Hwang, Y., Kim, J., Lee, S., & Kim, S. J. (2024). Moderating effect of shift work on sleep and depression in individuals at high risk of bipolar disorder. *Journal of Affective Disorders*, *359*, 206–214. https://doi.org/10.1016/j.jad.2024.05.090

Zauszniewski, J. A., Burant, C. J., Almutairi, R., Juratovac, E., Sweetko, J. S., Jeanblanc, A., Larsen, C., Colon-Zimmerman, K., & Sajatovic, M. (2024). Family caregivers of persons with bipolar disorder: caregiver demographics and need and preference for intervention. *Issues in Mental Health Nursing*, 1–7. https://doi.org/10.1080/01612840.2024.2393866

Zhang, L., & Swaab, D. F. (2024). Sex differences in bipolar disorder: The dorsolateral prefrontal cortex as an etiopathogenic region. *Frontiers in Neuroendocrinology*, 72, 101115. https://doi.org/10.1016/j.yfrne.2023.101115

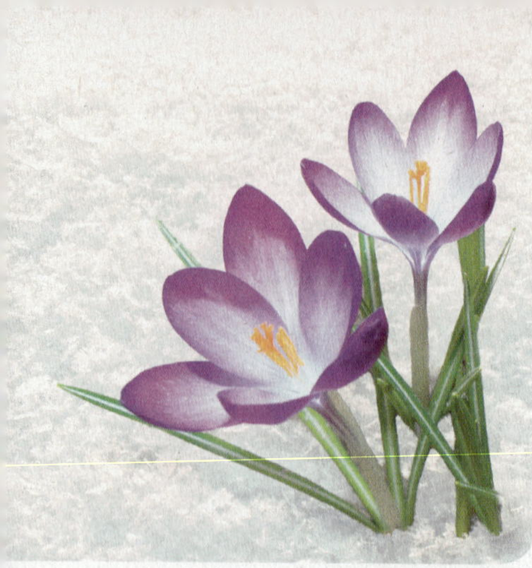

27 Anxiety Disorders

Nursing Care of People With Anxiety, Panic, and Phobia

Mary Ann Boyd

KEYCONCEPTS

- anxiety
- panic
- phobia
- physical symptoms

LEARNING OBJECTIVES

After studying this chapter, you will be able to:

1. Examine the roles of anxiety, panic, and phobia in mental disorders.
2. Relate the primary theories of anxiety and panic disorders, including phobias, to clinical symptoms and the course of the disorder.
3. Evaluate the significance of trauma in the appearance of anxiety symptoms.
4. Examine the relationship between social determinants of health and panic disorder.
5. Select strategies to establish a therapeutic relationship with people with panic disorder.
6. Using a clinical judgment model, formulate a person-centered, recovery-oriented nursing care plan for people with panic disorder.
7. Identify medications that are used to treat people with panic disorder and evaluate their effectiveness.
8. Develop wellness strategies for people with panic disorder.
9. Compare and contrast mental health care provided in emergency, inpatient, community, and virtual settings.
10. Support the integration of health care and mental health care for people with panic disorder.
11. Compare and contrast anxiety disorders and related disorders.

KEY TERMS

• agoraphobia • anxiety disorders • blood injection injury phobia • cognitive processes • coping strategies • defense mechanisms • depersonalization • expected anxiety • expected anxiety response • exposure therapy • flooding • generalized anxiety disorder • implosive therapy • interoceptive conditioning • panic attacks • panic control treatment • panic disorder • physiologic arousal • positive self-talk • reframing • selective mutism • separation anxiety disorder • social anxiety disorder • specific phobia disorder • systematic desensitization

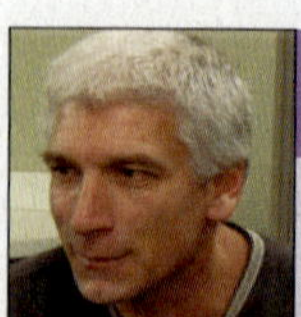

Case Study: Doug

Doug, age 50, lives with his wife Norma and two sons: Greg, a sophomore in college, and Leon, a high school student. Norma was recently laid off from her job and has been unable to find employment. The family is now experiencing financial and marital issues. Leon was recently expelled from school for drug and alcohol use. Doug had an argument with his boss and was afraid that he would lose his job. He appears at the emergency department for chest pain and is convinced he is having a heart attack. All lab test results are expected. Consider how the nurse can help Doug deal with his health issues.

INTRODUCTION

Anxiety is part of many emotional issues and mental disorders. At one time, most mental conditions with anxiety aspects were categorized as "anxiety disorders," but today anxiety disorders have been redefined. Trauma–stressor-related disorder and obsessive-compulsive disorder, both previously identified as anxiety disorders, are now categorized as separate disorders (American Psychiatric Association [APA], 2022). Trauma- and stressor-related disorders, as well as dissociative disorders, are discussed in Chapter 29. Obsessive-compulsive disorders are discussed in Chapter 28. In this chapter, panic disorder is highlighted.

EXPECTED VERSUS EXAGGERATED ANXIETY RESPONSE

Anxiety is an unavoidable human condition that takes many forms and serves different purposes. Anxiety can be positive and can motivate one to act, or it can produce paralyzing fear, causing inaction. **Expected anxiety** is anxiety that is realistic for the situation (Peplau, 1989). An **expected anxiety response** is a response to the anxiety-provoking situation that is appropriate and can be used to help identify the underlying issue that caused the anxiety.

> **KEYCONCEPT Anxiety** is an uncomfortable feeling of apprehension or dread that occurs in response to internal or external stimuli; it can result in physical, emotional, cognitive, and behavioral symptoms.

During a perceived threat, rising anxiety levels cause physical and emotional changes in all individuals. An expected emotional response to anxiety consists of three parts: physiologic arousal, cognitive processes, and coping strategies. **Physiologic arousal,** or the fight-or-flight response, is the signal that an individual is facing a threat. **Cognitive processes** decipher the situation and decide whether the perceived threat should be approached or avoided. **Coping strategies** are used to resolve the threat. Box 27.1 summarizes many physical, affective,

BOX 27.1

Symptoms of Anxiety

PHYSICAL SYMPTOMS

Cardiovascular

Sympathetic

- Palpitations
- Heart racing
- Increased blood pressure

Parasympathetic

- Actual fainting
- Decreased blood pressure
- Decreased pulse rate

Respiratory

- Rapid breathing
- Difficulty getting air
- Shortness of breath
- Pressure of chest
- Shallow breathing
- Lump in throat
- Choking sensations
- Gasping
- Spasm of bronchi

Neuromuscular

- Increased reflexes
- Startle reaction
- Eyelid twitching
- Insomnia
- Tremors
- Rigidity
- Spasm
- Fidgeting
- Pacing
- Strained face
- Unsteadiness
- Generalized weakness
- Wobbly legs
- Clumsy motions

Skin

- Flushed face
- Pale face
- Localized sweating (palm region)
- Generalized sweating
- Hot and cold spells
- Itching

Gastrointestinal

- Loss of appetite
- Revulsion about food
- Abdominal discomfort
- Diarrhea
- Abdominal pain
- Nausea
- Heartburn
- Vomiting

Eyes

- Dilated pupils

Urinary Tract Parasympathetic

- Pressure to urinate
- Increased frequency of urination

AFFECTIVE SYMPTOMS

- Edgy
- Impatient
- Uneasy
- Nervous
- Tense
- Wound-up
- Anxious
- Fearful
- Apprehensive
- Scared
- Frightened
- Alarmed
- Terrified
- Jittery
- Jumpy

COGNITIVE SYMPTOMS

Sensory-Perceptual

- Mind is hazy, cloudy, foggy, dazed
- Objects seem blurred or distant
- Environment seems different or unreal
- Feelings of unreality
- Self-consciousness
- Hypervigilance

Thinking Difficulties

- Cannot recall important things
- Confused
- Unable to control thinking
- Difficulty concentrating
- Difficulty focusing attention
- Distractibility
- Blocking
- Difficulty reasoning
- Loss of objectivity and perspective
- Tunnel vision

Conceptual

- Cognitive distortion
- Fear of losing control
- Fear of not being able to cope
- Fear of physical injury or death
- Fear of mental disorder
- Fear of negative evaluations
- Frightening visual images
- Repetitive fearful ideation

BEHAVIORAL SYMPTOMS

- Inhibited
- Tonic immobility
- Flight
- Avoidance
- Speech disfluency
- Impaired coordination
- Restlessness
- Postural collapse
- Hyperventilation

Adapted from Beck, A. T., & Emery, C. (1985). *Anxiety disorders and phobias: A cognitive perspective* (pp. 23–27). Basic Books.

TABLE 27.1 DEGREES OF ANXIETY

Degree of Anxiety	Effects on Perceptual Field and on Ability to Focus Attention	Observable Behavior
Mild	Perceptual field widens slightly. Able to observe more than before and to see relationships (make connection among data). Learning is possible.	Is aware, alert, sees, hears, and grasps more than before. Usually able to recognize and identify anxiety easily.
Moderate	Perceptual field narrows slightly. Selective inattention: does not notice what goes on peripheral to the immediate focus but can do so if attention is directed there by another observer.	Sees, hears, and grasps less than previously. Can attend to more if directed to do so. Able to sustain attention on a particular focus; selectively inattentive to contents outside the focal area. Usually able to state, "I am anxious now."
Severe	Perceptual field is greatly reduced. Tendency toward dissociation: to not notice what is going on outside the current reduced focus of attention; largely unable to do so when another observer suggests it.	Sees, hears, and grasps far less than previously. Attention is focused on a small area of a given event. Inferences drawn may be distorted because of the inadequacy of observed data. May be unaware of and unable to name anxiety. Relief behaviors generally used.
Panic (e.g., terror, horror, dread, uncanniness, awe)	Perceptual field is reduced to a detail, which is usually "blown up," that is, elaborated by distortion (exaggeration), or the focus is on scattered details; the speed of the scattering tends to increase. Massive dissociation, especially of contents of self-system. Felt as an enormous threat to survival. Learning is impossible.	Says, "I'm in a million pieces," "I'm gone," or "What is happening to me?" Perplexity, self-absorption. Feelings of unreality. Flights of ideas or confusion. Fear. Repeats a detail. Many relief behaviors used automatically (without thought). The enormous energy produced by panic must be used and may be mobilized as rage. May pace, run, or fight violently. With dissociation of contents of self-system, there may be a very rapid reorganization of the self, usually going along pathologic lines (e.g., a "psychotic break" is usually preceded by panic).

Adapted with permission from Peplau, H. (1989). Theoretical constructs: Anxiety, self, and hallucinations. In A. O'Toole & S. Welt (Eds.), Interpersonal theory in nursing practice: Selected works of Hildegarde E. Peplau. Springer.

cognitive, and behavioral symptoms associated with anxiety. The factors that determine whether anxiety is a symptom of a mental disorder include the intensity of anxiety relative to the situation, the trigger for the anxiety, and the particular symptom clusters that manifest the anxiety. Table 27.1 describes the four degrees of anxiety and associated perceptual changes and patterns of behavior. Anxiety is a component of all the disorders discussed in this chapter.

Exaggerated Anxiety Response: Phobia

KEYCONCEPT Phobia is an irrational fear of an object, individual, or situation that leads to a compelling avoidance.

The development of a phobia may be the outcome of extreme anxiety. Phobias are often present in anxiety disorders but may also develop into a specific phobia disorder (see the "Phobias" section later in this chapter).

DEFENSE MECHANISMS AND ANXIETY

Defense mechanisms are used to reduce anxiety by preventing or diminishing unwanted thoughts and feelings. See Chapter 9 for definitions. Defense mechanisms can be helpful in coping with everyday issues, but they become problematic when overused. The first step is identifying an individual's use of defense mechanisms. The next step is determining whether the reasons the defense mechanisms are being used support healthy coping or are detrimental to an individual's health. What may be healthy for one individual may be unhealthy for another. See Table 27.2.

OVERVIEW OF ANXIETY DISORDERS

The primary symptoms of anxiety disorders are fear and anxiety. Even though symptoms of anxiety disorders can be found in healthy individuals, an anxiety disorder is diagnosed when the fear or anxiety is excessive or out of proportion to the situation. An individual's ability to work and interpersonal relationships may be impaired. Anxiety disorders are differentiated by the situation or objects that provoke fear, anxiety, or avoidance behavior and related cognitive thoughts (APA, 2022).

Anxiety disorders are the most common of the mental disorders treated by health care providers. Approximately 40 million American adults (older than 18 years old) or about 18.1% of this age group within a given year have an anxiety disorder. Direct and indirect costs of treating anxiety disorders amount to tens of billions of dollars. Women experience anxiety disorders more often than men by a 2:1 ratio. Anxiety disorders may also be

TABLE 27.2 CONSEQUENCES OF DECREASING ANXIETY USING DEFENSE MECHANISMS

Defense Mechanism	Positive Consequences	Negative Consequences
Altruism	Satisfies internal needs through helping others	Prevents examination of underlying fears or concerns
Denial	Avoids feelings associated with recognizing an issue	Avoidance of major issue that should be addressed
Displacement	By taking out frustrations on an unsuspecting or vulnerable individual, animal, or object, anxiety is reduced and the individual is protected from anticipated retaliation from the source of the frustration	Does not deal with issue and inappropriately expresses feelings toward a more vulnerable individual or object
Intellectualization	Able to analyze events in a distant, objective, analytical way	Inability to acknowledge feelings that may be interfering with relationships
Projection	By assigning unwanted thoughts, feelings, or behaviors to another individual or object, the individual does not have to acknowledge undesirable or unacceptable thoughts or feelings	Does not acknowledge undesirable or unwanted feelings or thoughts and can act on inaccurate interpretation of the other individual's thoughts and behaviors
Rationalization	Avoids anxiety by explaining an unacceptable or disappointing behavior or feeling in a logical, rationale way. May protect self-esteem and self-concept	Avoids the reality of a situation, which may be detrimental to the individual
Reaction Formation	Reduces anxiety by taking the opposite feeling. Hides true feelings, which may be appropriate in many situations	Unable to acknowledge personal feelings about others, which leads to negative consequences
Regression	When stressed, abandons effective coping strategies and reverts to behaviors used earlier in development. These strategies are comfortable and may be effective	May reengage in detrimental behaviors such as smoking, drinking, or inappropriate interpersonal responses leading to ineffective coping
Repression	Avoids unwanted thoughts and anxiety by blocking thoughts, experiences from conscious awareness	Cannot recall traumatic events that should be addressed to be healthy (i.e., rape)
Sublimation	Avoids anxiety and channels maladaptive feelings or impulses into socially acceptable behaviors. Maintains socially acceptable behavior	By not recognizing maladaptive feelings, the individual cannot address underlying feelings
Suppression	Reduces anxiety by intentionally avoiding thinking about disturbing issues, wishes, feelings, or experiences. Useful in many situations such as test-taking situations	Avoiding problem situation prevents finding a solution to the issue

associated with other mental or physical comorbidities, such as heart disease, respiratory disease, and mood disorders (Han et al., 2024). The relationship between depression and anxiety disorders is particularly strong. A single patient may concurrently have more than one anxiety disorder or other mental disorders as well.

Anxiety disorders tend to be chronic and persistent, with full recovery more likely among those who do not have other mental or physical disorders (Remmerswaal et al., 2024). The first episode of an anxiety disorder tends to appear in late adolescence or young adult.

Anxiety Disorders Across the Lifespan

Prompt identification, diagnosis, and treatment of individuals with anxiety disorders may be difficult for special populations such as children and older adult patients. Often, the symptoms suggestive of anxiety disorders may go unnoticed by caregivers or are misdiagnosed because they mimic cardiac or pulmonary pathology rather than a psychological disturbance. Children and adolescents are discussed in Chapter 37; older adults are discussed in Chapter 39.

Children and Adolescents

Anxiety disorders are among the most common conditions of children and adolescents. If left untreated, symptoms persist and gradually worsen and sometimes lead to suicidal ideation and suicide attempts, early parenthood, drug and alcohol dependence, and educational underachievement later in life (McEvoy et al., 2023).

Separation anxiety disorder (i.e., excessive fear or anxiety concerning separation from home or attachment figures) usually first occurs in childhood. Affected children experience extreme distress when separated from home or attachment figures, worry about them when separated from them, and worry about untoward events (i.e., getting lost) and what will happen to them. This disorder is discussed in Chapter 37.

A rare disorder typically seen in childhood is **selective mutism**, in which children do not initiate speech or respond when spoken to by others (APA, 2022). Children with this disorder are often very anxious when asked to speak in school or read aloud. They may suffer academic impairment because of their inability to communicate with others.

Older Adults

The prevalence of anxiety disorders typically declines with age. However, in the older adult population, rates of anxiety disorders are as high as mood disorders, which commonly co-occur. This combination of depressive and anxiety symptoms has been shown to decrease social functioning, increase somatic (physical) symptoms, and increase depressive symptoms (Atchison et al., 2024). Chronic pain is associated with anxiety. Detecting and treating anxiety is an important component of pain management (Docherty et al., 2023). Because the older adult population is at risk for suicide, special assessment of anxiety symptoms is essential.

LGBTQ+ Population

Anxiety and depression are significantly higher in LGBTQ+ groups than in non-LGBTQ+ populations. LGBTQ+ people experience significant health disparities especially in access to mental health care. Widespread discrimination and unemployment contribute to the health inequity and mental health conditions of these individuals (Kempinski, 2024). Negative media depiction is associated with clinically significant symptoms of depression, anxiety, posttraumatic stress disorder (PTSD), and psychological distress (Gonzales & McKay, 2024).

PANIC DISORDER

Panic is an extreme, overwhelming form of anxiety often experienced when an individual is placed in a real or perceived life-threatening situation. Panic is expected during periods of threat but is unexpected when it is continuously experienced in situations that pose no real physical or psychological threat. Some people experience heightened anxiety because they fear experiencing another panic attack. This type of panic interferes with the individual's ability to function in everyday life and is characteristic of **panic disorder**.

> **KEYCONCEPT Panic** is an extremely overwhelming form of anxiety, often experienced when an individual is placed in a real or perceived life-threatening situation.

CLINICAL COURSE

The onset of panic disorder is typically between 20 and 24 years of age. The disorder usually surfaces in childhood but may not be diagnosed until later. Panic disorder is treatable, but studies have shown that even after years of treatment, many people remain symptomatic. In some cases, symptoms may even worsen (APA, 2022).

Panic Attacks

Panic attacks are characteristic of panic disorder. A **panic attack** is a sudden, discrete period of intense fear or discomfort that reaches its peak within a few minutes and is accompanied by significant physical discomfort and cognitive distress (APA, 2022). Panic attacks usually peak in about 10 minutes but can last as long as 30 minutes before returning to baseline functioning. The physical symptoms include palpitations, chest discomfort, rapid pulse, nausea, dizziness, sweating, paresthesia (burning, tickling, pricking of skin with no apparent reason), trembling or shaking, and a feeling of suffocation or shortness of breath. Cognitive symptoms include disorganized thinking, irrational fears, **depersonalization** (being detached from oneself), and a decreased ability to communicate. Usually, feelings of impending doom or death, fear of going crazy or losing control, and desperation ensue.

The physical symptoms can mimic those of a heart attack. Individuals often seek emergency medical care because they feel as if they are dying, but most have negative cardiac workup results. People experiencing panic attacks may also believe that the attacks stem from an underlying major medical illness (APA, 2022). Even with medical testing and assurance of no underlying disease, they often remain unconvinced.

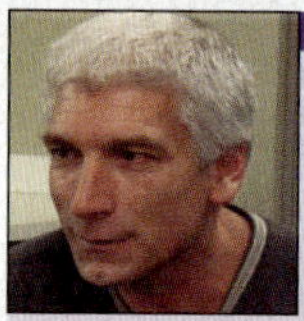

Remember Doug?
He had chest pains and believed he was having a heart attack. How can you help Doug recognize that even though he is not having a heart attack, his symptoms are serious and that his panic attack could indicate an underlying anxiety disorder? Why wouldn't you tell him that everything is fine?

> **KEYCONCEPT Physical symptoms** of panic attack are similar to cardiac emergencies. These symptoms are physically taxing and psychologically frightening to patients. Recognition of the seriousness of panic attacks should be communicated to the patient.

In a panic disorder, recurrent unexpected panic attacks are followed by persistent concern about experiencing subsequent panic attacks. Because of fear of future attacks, these affected individuals modify their usual behaviors to avoid future attacks (APA, 2022). Panic attacks are either expected with an obvious cue or trigger or unexpected with no such obvious cue. The first panic attack is usually associated with an identifiable cue (e.g., anxiety-provoking medical conditions, such as asthma, or in initial trials of illicit substance use), but subsequent attacks are often

BOX 27.2

Clinical Judgment Vignette: The Patient With Panic Disorder

Susan, age 22, has experienced several life changes, including a recent engagement, loss of her father to cancer and heart disease, graduation from college, and entrance into the workforce as a computer programmer in a large inner-city company. Because of her active lifestyle, her sleep habits have been poor. She frequently uses sleeping aids at night and now drinks a full pot of coffee to start each day. She continues to smoke to "relieve the stress." While sitting in heavy traffic on the way to work, she suddenly experienced chest tightness, sweating, shortness of breath, feelings of being "trapped," and foreboding that she was going to die. Fearing a heart attack, she went to an emergency department, where her discomfort subsided within a half hour. After several hours of testing, the doctor informed her that her heart was healthy. During the next few weeks, she experienced several episodes of feeling trapped and slight chest discomfort on her drive to work. She fears future "attacks" while sitting in traffic and while in her crowded office.

Building Clinical Judgment

1. What risk factors does Susan have that might contribute to the development of panic attacks?
2. What lifestyle changes do you think would help Susan reduce stress?

unexpected without any obvious cue. See Box 27.2. Panic attacks not only occur in panic disorders but can also occur in other mental disorders such as depression, bipolar disorder, eating disorders, and some medical conditions such as cardiac or respiratory disorders (APA, 2022).

DIAGNOSTIC CRITERIA

Panic disorder is a chronic condition that has several exacerbations and remissions during the course of the disease. Disabling panic attacks often lead to other symptoms, such as phobias.

Other diagnostic symptoms include palpitations, sweating, shaking, shortness of breath or smothering, sensations of choking, chest pain, nausea or abdominal distress, dizziness, derealization or depersonalization, fear of going crazy, fear of dying, paresthesia, and chills or hot flashes (APA, 2022) (see Key Diagnostic Characteristics 27.1).

PANIC DISORDER ACROSS THE LIFESPAN

Children

Panic disorder is more likely to occur in adolescents than in younger children. It is estimated that panic disorder is experienced by 1% to 3% of adolescents aged 15 to 19. Children and adolescents with panic disorder are most likely experiencing another anxiety or mood disorder. Panic disorder has a significant impact on social and academic functioning and expected development (Baker et al., 2022).

Older Adults

Panic disorder occurs in older adults, but it is an understudied disorder. It is unclear whether the disorder was

KEY DIAGNOSTIC CHARACTERISTICS 27.1

***DSM-5-TR* DIAGNOSTIC CRITERIA: Panic Disorder**

A. Recurrent unexpected panic attacks. A panic attack is an abrupt surge of intense fear or intense discomfort that reaches a peak within minutes, and during which time four (or more) of the following symptoms occur:
   Note: The abrupt surge can occur from a calm state or an anxious state.
   1. Palpitations, pounding heart, or accelerated heart rate.
   2. Sweating.
   3. Trembling or shaking.
   4. Sensations of shortness of breath or smothering.
   5. Feelings of choking.
   6. Chest pain or discomfort.
   7. Nausea or abdominal distress.
   8. Feeling dizzy, unsteady, lightheaded, or faint.
   9. Chills or heat sensations.
   10. Paresthesia (numbness or tingling sensations).
   11. Derealization (feelings of unreality) or depersonalization (being detached from oneself).
   12. Fear of losing control or "going crazy."
   13. Fear of dying.
   Note: Culture-specific symptoms (e.g., tinnitus, neck soreness, headache, uncontrollable screaming, or crying) may be seen. Such symptoms should not count as one of the four required symptoms.
B. At least one of the attacks has been followed by 1 month (or more) of one or both of the following:
   1. Persistent concern or worry about additional panic attacks or their consequences (e.g., losing control, having a heart attack, "going crazy").
   2. A significant maladaptive change in behavior related to the attacks (e.g., behaviors designed to avoid having panic attacks, such as avoidance of exercise or unfamiliar situations).
C. The disturbance is not attributable to the physiological effects of a substance (e.g., a drug of abuse, a medication) or another medical condition (e.g., hyperthyroidism, cardiopulmonary disorders).
D. The disturbance is not better explained by another mental disorder (e.g., the panic attacks do not occur only in response to feared social situations, as in social anxiety disorder; in response to circumscribed phobic objects or situations, as in specific phobia; in response to obsessions, as in obsessive-compulsive disorder; in response to reminders of traumatic events, as in posttraumatic stress disorder; or in response to separation from attachment figures, as in separation anxiety disorder).

present, but undiagnosed in early or middle adulthood, or had its onset in the later years. In the older adult, panic disorder is associated with significant functional impairment, which compounds any functional issues associated with other comorbid disorders such as dementia (Pace et al., 2021).

EPIDEMIOLOGY AND RISK FACTORS

Panic disorder has a moderately high lifetime prevalence in the general population with 1% to 2% 1-year prevalence rate and 2% to 4% lifetime rate (Forstner et al., 2021). Increased risk is associated with being a person assigned female at birth, middle adulthood, of low socioeconomic status, and widowed, separated, or divorced. The estimates of isolated panic attacks may affect 22.7% of the population. Panic disorder occurs in several cultures, but the panic symptoms may be experienced differently across racial/ethnic groups (Tunnell et al., 2024).

Family history, alcohol use disorder and substance and stimulant use disorders, smoking tobacco, and severe stressors are risk factors for panic disorder. People who have several anxiety symptoms and those who experience separation anxiety during childhood often develop panic disorder later in life (Tunnell et al., 2024). Early-life traumas and adverse events, self-stigma, a history of physical or sexual abuse, socioeconomic or personal disadvantages, and behavioral inhibition have also been associated with an increased risk for anxiety disorders in children (Holubova et al., 2021).

COMORBIDITY

People with a panic disorder may experience other anxiety disorders, depression, eating disorder, substance use disorder, or bipolar disorder (Barbuti et al., 2021; Gros et al., 2023; Oh et al., 2021; Surace et al., 2024). Although people with panic disorder are thought to have more somatic complaints than the general population, panic disorder does correlate with some medical conditions, including vertigo, cardiac disease, gastrointestinal disorders, asthma, and those related to cigarette smoking (Tunnell et al., 2024).

ETIOLOGY

Biologic Theories

There appears to be a substantial familial predisposition to panic disorder with an estimated heritability of 40% (Cackovic et al., 2023). Studies show unexpected changes in the brain's "fear network" (amygdala, hippocampus, thalamus, midbrain, pons, medulla, and cerebellum) and changes in volume in different brain areas (Shi et al., 2024).

Serotonin and Norepinephrine

Serotonin and norepinephrine are both implicated in panic disorder. Norepinephrine acts on those systems that are most affected by a panic attack—the cardiovascular, respiratory, and gastrointestinal systems. Serotonergic neurons are distributed in central autonomic and emotional motor control systems regulating anxiety states and anxiety-related physiologic and behavioral responses (Moraes et al., 2024).

Gamma-Aminobutyric Acid

Gamma-aminobutyric acid (GABA) is the most abundant inhibitory neurotransmitter in the brain. GABA receptor stimulation causes several effects, including neurocognitive effects, reduction of anxiety, and sedation. GABA stimulation also results in increased seizure threshold. Dysfunction in the benzodiazepine–GABA–chloride ion channel complex has been implicated in panic disorder (Moraes et al., 2024).

Hypothalamic–Pituitary–Adrenal Axis

The hypothalamic–pituitary–adrenal (HPA) axis is involved in a panic disorder (Moraes et al., 2024). In panic disorder, the microbiome–gut–brain axis is altered due to an inflammatory response in which proinflammatory cytokines are increased. This inflammatory response involves the HPA axis and is thought to influence the intensity of anxiety (MacKay et al., 2024). That is, an increase in proinflammatory cytokine activity causes an inflammatory response. Stress hormones are then activated, anxiety increases, and a panic attack occurs. See Chapter 19.

Psychosocial Theories

Psychoanalytic and Psychodynamic Theories

Psychodynamic theories examine panic disorder that develops after adverse childhood experiences (ACEs), but the empirical evidence remains inadequate for a psychodynamic explanation. Therapy based on psychodynamic and psychoanalytic theories is helpful in treating a panic disorder when there is a history of trauma or ACEs (Nowak et al., 2023).

Cognitive-Behavioral Theories

Learning theory underlies most cognitive-behavioral explanations of panic disorder. Classic conditioning theory suggests that one learns a fear response by linking an adverse or fear-provoking event, such as a car accident, with a previously neutral event, such as crossing a bridge. One becomes conditioned to associate fear with crossing a bridge. Applying this theory to people with panic disorder has limitations. Phobic avoidance is not always developed secondary to an adverse event.

Further development of this theory led to an understanding of **interoceptive conditioning**, an association between physical discomforts, such as dizziness or palpitations, and an impending panic attack. For example, during a car accident, the individual may experience rapid heartbeat, dizziness, shortness of breath, and panic. Subsequent experiences of dizziness or palpitations, unrelated to an anxiety-provoking situation, incite anxiety and panic. Furthermore, people with panic disorder may misinterpret mild physical sensations (e.g., sweating, dizziness) as being catastrophic, causing panic because of learned fear (catastrophic interpretation). Some researchers hypothesize that individuals with a low sense of control over their environment or with a particular sensitivity to anxiety are vulnerable to misinterpreting expected stress. Controlled exposure to anxiety-provoking situations and cognitive countering techniques have proven successful in reducing the symptoms of panic (Alcan et al., 2024).

FAMILY RESPONSE TO DISORDER

People with panic disorder may inadvertently cause excessive fears, phobias, or excessive worry in other family members. Families may limit social functions to prevent panic attacks. Those affected need a tremendous amount of support and encouragement from significant others.

RECOVERY-ORIENTED CARE FOR PEOPLE WITH PANIC DISORDER

Teamwork and Collaboration: Working Toward Recovery

Nurses are pivotal in providing a safe and therapeutic inpatient environment and teaching strategies for managing anxiety and fears. The nurse also administers prescribed medication, monitors its effects, and provides medication education. Advanced practice nurses, licensed clinical social workers, or licensed counselors provide individual psychotherapy sessions as needed. Often, a clinical psychologist gives psychological tests and interprets the results to assist in diagnosing and treating panic disorder.

Panic Control Treatment

Panic control treatment involves intentional exposure (through exercise) to panic-invoking sensations such as dizziness, hyperventilation, tightness in the chest, and sweating. Identified patterns become targets for treatment. Patients are taught to use breathing training and cognitive restructuring to manage their responses and are instructed to practice these techniques between therapy sessions to adapt the skills to other situations.

Exposure Therapy

Exposure therapy is the treatment for phobias (see the "Phobias" section later in this chapter). and posttraumatic disorder (see Chapter 29). The patient is repeatedly exposed to real or simulated anxiety-provoking situations until they become desensitized, and anxiety subsides (Roth-Rawald et al., 2023). **Implosive therapy** is a provocative exposure technique useful in treating panic disorder and agoraphobia in which the therapist identifies phobic stimuli for the patient and then presents highly anxiety-provoking imagery to the patient, describing the feared scene as dramatically and vividly as possible. **Flooding** is a technique used to desensitize the patient to the fear associated with a particular anxiety-provoking stimulus. Desensitizing is done by presenting feared objects or situations repeatedly without session breaks until the anxiety dissipates. For example, a patient with ophidiophobia (i.e., a morbid fear of snakes) might be presented with a real snake repeatedly until the patient's anxiety decreases.

Systematic desensitization, another exposure method used to desensitize patients, exposes the patient to a hierarchy of feared situations that the patient has rated from least to most feared. The patient is taught to use muscle relaxation as levels of anxiety increase through multisituational exposure. Planning and implementing exposure therapy require special training. Exposure therapy is delivered in an in-person or virtual setting (Schröder et al., 2023).

Cognitive-Behavioral Therapy

Cognitive-behavioral therapy (CBT) is a highly effective tool for treating individuals with panic disorder. It is considered a first-line treatment for those with panic and other anxiety disorders and is often used in conjunction with medications, including selective serotonin reuptake inhibitors (SSRIs) (Bandelow et al., 2023). The goals of CBT include helping the patient manage their anxiety and correcting anxiety-provoking thoughts through interventions, including cognitive restructuring, breathing training, and psychoeducation.

Safety Issues

Panic attack symptoms mimic a heart attack—chest pain, palpitations, dyspnea. It is important to rule out any cardiac issues prior to diagnosing and treating a panic attack. Research shows that people with panic disorder have higher oxidative stress due to impaired serotonin metabolism, which is related to heart disease (Quagliato & Nardi, 2023).

Panic disorder is associated with an increased risk of suicide. Suicidal ideation is especially related to experiencing childhood physical trauma (Kim et al., 2023).

EVIDENCE-BASED NURSING CARE OF PEOPLE WITH PANIC DISORDER

Individuals often first seek help in the emergency department for their physical symptoms, but they are told that there are no life-threatening cardiac or neurologic causes for the severe physical symptoms. Although no laboratory tests exist to confirm anxiety disorders, a careful clinical assessment will reveal the presence of an anxiety disorder. See Clinical Judgment Nursing Care Plan 27.1, which sets forth a plan of care for Doug, the case study patient in this chapter.

RECOGNIZING CUES: RELEVANT ASSESSMENT INFORMATION

A comprehensive nursing assessment includes overall physical and mental status, suicidal tendencies and thoughts, cognitive thought patterns, avoidance behavior patterns, and family and cultural factors. Patients can be encouraged to keep a daily log of the severity of anxiety and the frequency, duration, and severity of panic episodes. This log will be a basic tool for monitoring progress as symptoms decrease.

Panic Attack Assessment

The assessment of the individual with a panic disorder focuses on identifying the characteristics of the panic attack and the individual's strengths and issues. If the panic attack occurs in the presence of the nurse, direct assessment of the symptoms should be made and documented. Questions to ask the patient might include the following:

- What were you doing when the panic attack occurred?
- What did you experience before and during the panic episode, including physical symptoms, feelings, and thoughts?
- When did you begin to feel that way? How long did it last?
- Do you have an explanation for what caused you to feel and think that way?
- Have you experienced these symptoms in the past? If so, under what circumstances?

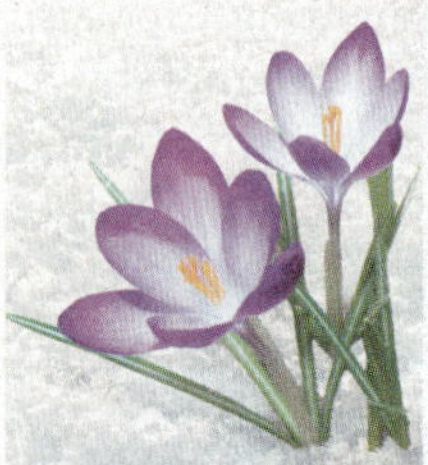

CLINICAL JUDGMENT NURSING CARE PLAN 27.1

The Patient With Panic Disorder

Douglas, age 50, is being evaluated in the emergency department by a nurse from the mental health crisis team. Doug was brought into the emergency department by his wife after experiencing chest pain early in the evening. He arrived in a state of severe level of anxiety and believed that he was having a heart attack. An ECG and laboratory values were usual.

Setting: Day Treatment Program, Adult Psychiatric Services

Assessment Cues: Doug arrived at the ED trembling, dizzy, pale, experiencing tachycardia, nausea, and feelings of dread. He could not follow directions and responded poorly to redirection. His attention and thoughts are scattered.

Associated Psychiatric Diagnosis	Medications
Panic disorder History of hypertension	Paroxetine CR 12.5 mg every day Lisinopril 20 mg daily Lorazepam 1 mg q6h PRN for extreme anxiety

Priority Hypothesis: Anxiety

Important Characteristics	Associated Considerations
Trembling, increased pulse Fearful, irritable, scared, worried Apprehensive	Impending panic attacks Panic attacks

Planning Recovery and Wellness Outcomes

Initial	Long term
Develop skills to decrease impact of panic attack	Carry out usual daily living and social activities outside of the house

Clinical Judgment Nursing Care Plan 27.1 Continued

Taking Action: Nursing Interventions

Interventions	Rationale	Ongoing Assessment
Meet daily with Doug to assess whether he has had a panic attack within the last 24 hours.	Asking Doug to monitor panic attacks will provide data regarding potential antecedents to attacks.	Determine whether Doug has had a panic attack.
Using a calm reassuring approach, encourage verbalization of feelings, perceptions, and fears. Identify periods of time when anxiety level is at its highest.	Discussing the experience of anxiety will help the patient notice when his anxiety increases.	Explore the antecedents and determine whether he was able to practice techniques from education programs.
Teach Doug how to perform relaxation techniques.	Having strategies to deal with impending panic attack will decrease the intensity of the experience.	Observe effectiveness of his technique and changes in anxiety/panic episodes.
Teach Doug about the actions and side effects of paroxetine. Explain the purposes of the medication. Track the number of PRN medications that are used for anxiety. Also, monitor for use of alcohol and herbal supplements.	Panic attacks are neurobiologic occurrences that respond to medications.	Determine whether panic attacks decrease over time and whether there are side effects. Determine his commitment to living a more typical life.

Evaluation

Outcomes	Revised Outcomes	Interventions
Doug's panic attacks decreased to once a week. Attended day treatment program every day. Able to go to grocery store.	Increase social activity outside of house.	Meet with Doug twice a week to monitor progress. Continue to reinforce the use of strategies in managing anticipatory anxiety.

- Has anyone in your family ever had similar experiences?
- What do you do when you have these experiences to help you to feel safe?
- Have the feelings and sensations ever gone away on their own?

Physical Health

Key assessment areas of physical health that could have precipitated the panic attack include nutrition, sleep patterns/physical activity, history of trauma, medication, and substance use.

Nutrition

A nutritional assessment is important because eating disorders are often comorbid with panic disorder. Additionally, some foods and drinks contain stimulants that contribute to the severity of the panic attacks. The assessment is especially important in women, who are more likely to have a comorbid eating disorder than men (Crisp & Grant, 2024). The nurse should inquire about the food and drink intake on a typical day and also include questions about binge or fasting behavior.

Sleep Patterns and Physical Activity

Sleep is often disturbed in panic disorder. In fact, panic attacks can occur during sleep, so the patient may fear sleep for this reason (Smith et al., 2022). Nurses should closely assess the impact of sleep disturbance because fatigue may increase anxiety and susceptibility to panic attacks. Panic disorder can be improved through active participation in a routine exercise program. If the patient does not exercise routinely, define the barriers to it. If exercise is avoided because of chronic muscle tension, poor muscle tone, muscle cramps, general fatigue, exhaustion, or shortness of breath, the symptoms may indicate poor physical health.

History of Trauma

Trauma history is important to elicit for an individual with panic disorder because the initial panic attack may be related to a trauma. See Box 27.3. If the trauma was physical abuse that occurred during childhood, not only does it affect the severity of the panic disorder, but early trauma is related to an increased risk for suicidal ideation (Kim et al., 2023).

BOX 27.3

Trauma-Informed Approaches: Childhood Trauma and Panic Disorder

Background

Suffering childhood trauma can increase the vulnerability for the development of panic disorder (Hong et al., 2023). Trauma may change the fear network circuitry of the brain so that the individual is more sensitive to external events, leading to fear and arousal.

Interventions

Fears of patients with history of trauma should be recognized as important cues that could trigger panic attacks.

Source: Hong, A., Zhou, S., Yang, C., Liu, X., Su, S., & Wang, Z. (2023). Impact of childhood trauma on the abnormal functional connectivity of brain regions in the fear network model of panic disorder. *Journal of Affective Disorders*, *329*, 500–510. https://doi-org.libproxy.siue.edu/10.1016/j.jad.2023.02.128

Medication

Several medications can cause anxiety. Bronchodilators, oral contraceptives, amphetamines (i.e., methylphenidate), steroids, thyroid medication, and several other medications can increase anxiety. In addition, medicines that contain caffeine, such as some pain and anti-inflammatory agents, decongestants (i.e., phenylephrine), and some illegal drugs (cocaine), also increase anxiety. Many over-the-counter (OTC) herbal remedies contain substances that may induce panic by increasing the heart rate, basal metabolic rate, blood pressure, and sweating (see Chapter 11).

Substance Use

Caffeine, pseudoephedrine, amphetamines, cocaine, or other stimulants are associated with panic disorder and may stimulate a panic attack. Tobacco use can also contribute to the risk of panic symptoms. Many individuals with panic disorder use alcohol or central nervous system (CNS) depressants to self-medicate anxiety symptoms; withdrawal from CNS depressants may produce symptoms of panic.

Other Physical Assessment Areas

Recent changes in physical status should be assessed. For example, pregnant patients should be assessed carefully for an underlying panic disorder. Although pregnancy may protect the patient from developing panic symptoms, postpartum onset of panic disorder requires particular attention. During a time that tremendous effort is spent on family, postpartum onset of panic disorder negatively affects lifestyle and decreases self-esteem in affected patients, leading to feelings of overwhelming personal disappointment.

Psychosocial Cues

A psychosocial assessment includes the patient's report of the symptoms and a careful cognitive, behavioral, and social assessment. The assessment should include the following behavioral responses, self-concept, stress and coping patterns, social network, functional status, and support systems. See Chapter 10.

Self-Report Scales

Self-evaluation is difficult in panic disorder. Often, the memories of the attack and its triggers are irretrievable. Several tools are available to characterize and rate the patient's state of anxiety. Examples of these symptoms and behavioral rating scales are provided in Box 27.4. All these tools are self-report measures and as such are limited by the individual's self-awareness and openness. However, the Hamilton Rating Scale for Anxiety, provided in Table 27.3, is an example of a scale rated by the clinician (Hamilton, 1959). This 14-item scale reflects both psychological and somatic aspects of anxiety.

Mental Status Examination

During a mental status examination, individuals with panic disorder may exhibit anxiety symptoms, including restlessness, irritability, poor concentration, and apprehensive behavior. Disorganized thinking, irrational fears, and a decreased ability to communicate often occur during a panic attack. Assess by direct questioning whether the patient is experiencing suicidal thoughts, especially if they are misusing substances or taking antidepressant medications.

Cognitive Thought Patterns

Catastrophic misinterpretations of trivial physical symptoms can trigger panic symptoms. After they have been identified, these thoughts should serve as a basis for individualizing patient education to counter such false beliefs. Table 27.4 presents a scale to assess catastrophic misinterpretations of the symptoms of panic.

Individuals who feel a sense of control have less severe panic attacks. Individuals who fear loss of control during a panic attack often make the following type of statements:

- "I feel trapped."
- "I'm afraid others will know or that I'll hurt someone."
- "I feel alone. I can't help myself."
- "I'm losing control."

BOX 27.4

Rating Scales for Assessment of Panic Disorder and Anxiety Disorders

PANIC SYMPTOMS

Panic-Associated Symptom Scale (PASS)
Argyle, N., Delito, J., Allerup, P., Maier, W., Albus, M., Nutzinger, D., Rasmussen, S., Ayuso, J. L., & Bech, P. (1991). The panic-associated symptom scale: Measuring the severity of panic disorder. *Acta Psychiatrica Scandinavica*, *83*(1), 20–26.

Acute Panic Inventory
Dillon, D. J., Gorman, J. M., Liebowitz, M. R., Fyer, A. J., & Klein, D. F. (1987). Measurement of lactate-induced panic and anxiety. *Psychiatry Research*, *20*(2), 97–105.

National Institute of Mental Health Panic Questionnaire (NIMH PQ)
Scupi, B. S., Maser, J. D., & Uhde, T. W. (1992). The National Institute of Mental Health Panic Questionnaire: An instrument for assessing clinical characteristics of panic disorder. *Journal of Nervous and Mental Disease*, *180*(9), 566–572.

COGNITIONS

Anxiety Sensitivity Index
Reiss, S., Peterson, R. A., Gursky, D. M., & McNally, R. J. (1986). Anxiety sensitivity, anxiety frequency, and the prediction of fearfulness. *Behaviour Research and Therapy*, *24*(1), 1–8.

Agoraphobia Cognitions Questionnaire
Chambless, D. L., Caputo, G. C., Bright, P., & Gallagher, R. (1984). Assessment of fear in agoraphobics: The body sensations questionnaire and the agoraphobic cognitions questionnaire. *Journal of Consulting and Clinical Psychology*, *52*(6), 1090–1097.

Body Sensations Questionnaire
Chambless, D. L., Caputo, G. C., Bright, P., & Gallagher, R. (1984). Assessment of fear in agoraphobics: The body sensations questionnaire and the agoraphobic cognitions questionnaire. *Journal of Consulting and Clinical Psychology*, *52*(6), 1090–1097.

PHOBIAS

Mobility Inventory for Agoraphobia
Chambless, D. L., Caputo, G. C., Jasin, S. E., Gracely, E., & Williams, C. (1985). The mobility inventory for agoraphobia. *Behavior Research and Therapy*, *23*(1), 35–44.

Fear Questionnaire
Marks, I. M., & Matthews, A. M. (1979). Brief standard self-rating for phobic patients. *Behaviour Research and Therapy*, *17*(3), 263–267.

ANXIETY

State-Trait Anxiety Inventory (STAI)
Spielberger, C. D., Gorsuch, R. L., & Luchene, R. E. (1976). Manual for the State-Trait Anxiety Inventory. *Consulting Psychologists Press*.

Penn State Worry Questionnaire (PSWQ)
16 items developed to assess the trait of worry. Meyer, T. J., Miller, M. L, Metzger, R. L., & Borkovec, T. D. (1990). Development and validation of the Penn State Worry Questionnaire. *Behaviour Research and Therapy*, *28*(6), 487–495.

Beck Anxiety Inventory
21 items rating the severity of symptoms on a 4-point scale. Beck, A. T., Epstein, N., Brown, G., & Steer, R. A. (1988). An inventory for measuring clinical anxiety: The Beck Anxiety Inventory. *Journal of Consulting and Clinical Psychology*, *56*(6), 893–897.

These individuals also tend to show low self-esteem, feelings of helplessness, demoralization, and overwhelming fears of experiencing panic attacks. They may have difficulty with assertiveness or expressing their feelings.

Behavioral Responses

People with panic disorder are often fearful of having additional panic attacks. If the panic attack is associated with a specific situation, such as a crowded room, the individual may avoid places associated with the attack. The nurse can gain cues as to how the panic disorder impacts the patient's behavior by assessing any behavior changes because of the panic attacks.

Stress and Coping Patterns

People with panic disorder are highly susceptible to perceived stressful situations. It is important to identify stress and coping patterns, especially in catastrophic situations. When they believe that a catastrophe is imminent, they often draw conclusions on limited information and make impulsive decisions without considering other alternatives (Öğüt, 2024). For example, an individual who is short of breath is immediately convinced that they are dying from a heart attack rather than considering alternative explanations for shortness of breath.

Social Network

Marital and parental/caregiver functioning can be adversely affected by panic disorder. During the assessment, the nurse should try to grasp the patient's understanding of how panic disorder with or without severe avoidance behavior has affected their life, along with that of the family. Pertinent questions include the following:

- How has the disorder affected your family's social life?
- What limitations related to travel has the disorder placed on you or your family?
- What coping strategies have you used to manage symptoms?
- How has the disorder affected your family members or others?

TABLE 27.3 HAMILTON RATING SCALE FOR ANXIETY

Max Hamilton designed this scale to help clinicians gather information about anxiety states. The symptom inventory provides scaled information that classifies anxiety behavior and assists the clinician in targeting behaviors and achieving outcome measures. Provide a rating for each indicator based on the following scale:

0 = None
1 = Mild
2 = Moderate
3 = Severe
4 = Severe, grossly disabling

Item	Symptoms	Rating
Anxious mood	Worries, anticipation of the worst, fearful anticipation, irritability	
Tension	Feelings of tension, fatigability, startle response, moved to tears easily, trembling, feelings of restlessness, inability to relax	
Fear	Of dark, strangers, being left alone, animals, traffic, crowds	
Insomnia	Difficulty in falling asleep, broken sleep, unsatisfying sleep, and fatigue on waking; dreams, nightmares, night terrors	
Intellectual (cognitive)	Difficulty concentrating, poor memory	
Depressed mood	Loss of interest, lack of pleasure in hobbies, depression, early waking, diurnal swings	
Somatic (sensory)	Tinnitus, blurring of vision, hot and cold flushes, feelings of weakness, prickly sensation	
Somatic (muscular)	Pains and aches, twitching, stiffness, myoclonic jerks, grinding of teeth, unsteady voice, increased muscular tone	
Cardiovascular symptoms	Tachycardia, palpitations, pain in chest, throbbing of vessels, fainting feelings, missing beat	
Respiratory symptoms	Pressure or constriction in chest, choking feelings, sighing, dyspnea	
Gastrointestinal symptoms	Difficulty in swallowing, gas, abdominal pain, burning sensation, abdominal fullness, nausea, vomiting, looseness of bowels, loss of weight, constipation	
Genitourinary symptoms	Frequency of micturition, urgency of micturition, amenorrhea, menorrhagia, development of frigidity, premature ejaculation, loss of libido, impotence	
Autonomic symptoms	Dry mouth, flushing, pallor, tendency to sweat, giddiness, tension headache, raising of hair	
Behavior at interview	Fidgeting, restlessness or pacing, tremor of hands, furrowed brow, strained face, sighing or rapid respiration, facial pallor, swallowing, belching, brisk tendon jerks, dilated pupils, exophthalmos	

Reprinted with permission from Hamilton, M. (1959). The assessment of anxiety states by rating. *British Journal of Medical Psychology*, *32*(1), 50–55.

Cultural Factors

Cultural humility calls for cultural awareness and the use of cultural assessment skills and practices. Cultural differences must be considered in the assessment of panic disorder. Different cultures interpret sensations, feelings, or understandings differently. For example, symptoms of anxiety might be seen as witchcraft or magic (APA, 2022). Several cultures do not have a word to describe *anxiety* or *anxious* and instead may use words or meanings to suggest physical complaints (López-Cepero et al., 2024). In some cultures, anxiety is experienced as fear or dread; in others, it may be experienced as physical symptoms such as heart palpitations or dizziness.

Social Support and Social Determinants of Health

The identification of support systems moves the assessment from the family to a broader context including consideration of the social determinants of health (SDOH). Gaps in income between upper-income and middle- and lower-income households are increasing. Share of wealth in middle-income households is decreasing, resulting in a greater number of young adults experiencing financial stress. Student debt has become a burden and a barrier, especially for lower-income individuals pursuing further education. The availability and cost of housing have worsened over the past decade (Brunette et al., 2023). Because greater severity of mental health symptoms is reported by those experiencing financial and other stressors, the impact of the patient's SDOH should be determined. See Box 27.5.

Quality of Life

People with panic disorder have a reduced quality of life because of the underlying anxiety and fear of a spontaneous panic attack. Instead of fully participating in social, educational, and occupational activities, they are more likely to restrict activity and social engagement, which can

TABLE 27.4 PANIC ATTACK COGNITIONS QUESTIONNAIRE

Rate each of the following thoughts according to the degree to which you believe each thought contributes to your panic attack.

1 = Not at all; 3 = Quite a lot;
2 = Somewhat; 4 = Very much

I'm going to die.	1	2	3	4
I'm going insane.	1	2	3	4
I'm losing control.	1	2	3	4
This will never end.	1	2	3	4
I'm really scared.	1	2	3	4
I'm having a heart attack.	1	2	3	4
I'm going to pass out.	1	2	3	4
I don't know what people will think.	1	2	3	4
I won't be able to get out of here.	1	2	3	4
I don't understand what is happening to me.	1	2	3	4
People will think I am crazy.	1	2	3	4
I'll always be this way.	1	2	3	4
I am going to throw up.	1	2	3	4
I must have a brain tumor.	1	2	3	4
I'll choke to death.	1	2	3	4
I'm going to act foolish.	1	2	3	4
I'm going blind.	1	2	3	4
I'll hurt someone.	1	2	3	4
I'm going to have a stroke.	1	2	3	4
I'm going to scream.	1	2	3	4
I'm going to babble or talk funny.	1	2	3	4
I'll be paralyzed by fear.	1	2	3	4
Something is physically wrong with me.	1	2	3	4
I won't be able to breathe.	1	2	3	4
Something terrible will happen.	1	2	3	4
I'm going to make a scene.	1	2	3	4

Adapted from Clum, G. A. (1990). *Panic attack cognitions questionnaire. Coping with panic: A drug-free approach to dealing with anxiety attacks.* Brooks/Cole. Reprinted with permission from Dr. George A. Clum.

lead to depression. In addition, they are at higher risk of alcohol use disorder and substance use compared to the general population (Cackovic et al., 2023).

Spiritual Assessment

Exploring the significance of spirituality to the patient will facilitate inclusion of interventions that support spiritual well-being. The nurse should follow the spiritual assessment guidelines presented in Chapter 10.

BOX 27.5

Mental Health Inequities: Men's Depression and Anxiety

Men living in urban, ethnically/racially diverse, and impoverished neighborhoods are disproportionately affected by depression and anxiety compared to men from more affluent neighborhoods. Men living in such neighborhoods identified factors that contributed to anxiety and depression in their community and barriers to mental health interventions. In this qualitative study of 6 focus groups of 6 to 12 men each, the men's responses for modifiable factors that contributed to anxiety and depression were categorized into three themes: cognitive health behaviors, economic conditions, and social and community context. *Cognitive health behaviors* included negative thoughts, dwelling in the past, and fear of the unknown. *Economic conditions* included not having a job, losing a job, and a lack of financial education. *Social and community context* included issues at school, lack of opportunities in their communities, and systemic racism. The barrier that all focus groups identified was stigma associated with mental health care. The other barriers identified included a lack of resources and a lack of knowledge of mental disorders.

Source: Molewyk Doornbos, M., & Zandee, G. L. (2024). Men's depression and anxiety: Contributing factors and barriers to intervention. *Journal of the American Psychiatric Nurses Association*, *30*(2), 199–209. https://doi.org/10.1177/10783903241226718

Strengths Assessment

During the assessment, the patient's strengths will emerge. For example, a patient may tell you that they do not drink alcohol or use tobacco. Another may relate that they would like to exercise. Still another patient's strength is a supportive partner or family member. The nurse should build on these strengths in the plan of care.

ANALYZING CUES AND DEVELOPING HYPOTHESES

Suicide prevention is the first priority when caring for an individual with a panic disorder. People with panic disorder are often depressed and consequently are at high risk for suicide. Adolescents with panic disorder are at higher risk for suicidal thoughts or may attempt suicide more often than other adolescents. Panic symptoms in early adolescence predict high risk for late adolescent depression and suicidal ideation (Kim et al., 2023).

Once the nurse establishes that there is no indication of a risk of suicide, the nurse assesses whether the individual may be depressed, lonely, and socially isolated. Panic attacks may be unpredictable, leading the individual to be fearful of another attack. Self-esteem may be low as feelings of powerlessness emerge. The patient may be experiencing physical panic symptoms, such as dizziness and hyperventilation. Because the whole family is affected by one member's symptoms, the family's needs may need to be considered.

The patient's strengths should be considered in planning care. For example, the individual may be motivated to gain more control through making lifestyle changes. There may be evidence of family support. Outcomes will depend upon the particular health care issue and the interventions that are agreed upon by the patient and nurse.

PLANNING RECOVERY AND WELLNESS OUTCOMES: GENERATING SOLUTIONS

The course of panic disorder culminates in phobic avoidance as the affected individual attempts to avoid situations that increase panic. Even though identifying and avoiding anxiety-provoking situations are important during therapy, drastically changing lifestyle to avoid situations does not aid recovery. Goals and interventions that focus on developing a healthy lifestyle, supporting a sense of accomplishment and control, and reducing anxiety and panic are particularly helpful in reducing the number and severity of the attacks.

The history of trauma should be considered when planning goals. If the panic disorder is associated with an early trauma, any interventions should be sensitive to results of physical or sexual abuse that occurred.

THERAPEUTIC RELATIONSHIP

The therapeutic relationship is a critical aspect of helping the individual work toward recovery. These individuals may appear to be very nervous or anxious throughout the interaction. The nurse should help the patient relax and be comfortable with discussing fears and anxiety. A calm, understanding approach in a comfortable environment will help the individual relax and be willing to engage in a therapeutic relationship.

TAKING ACTION: NURSING INTERVENTIONS

Trauma-Informed Approaches

For those individuals who have experienced trauma, nursing interventions should be implemented within a trauma-informed approach. The nurse can begin by reminding the patient that they are in a safe place and that the nurse will maintain any physical or emotional boundaries that the patient needs to feel safe and secure.

Physical Care

Physical distancing may exacerbate the feeling of seclusion and lead to detrimental, prolonged health effects. Quarantine and social isolation can easily prevent an individual with panic disorder from following up with medical issues, such as changes in cardiac functioning. For example, fears of being infected may prevent the individual from picking up regular medications from the local pharmacy or grocery shopping.

Psychiatric–mental health nurses who make home visits often provide the individual with both medical and mental health care. Nurses should consider providing care that is usually given by other nurses.

Breathing Control

Hyperventilation is common. Often, people are unaware that they take rapid shallow breaths when they become anxious. See Box 27.6.

Teaching patients breathing control can be helpful. Focus on breathing and help them to identify the rate, pattern, and depth. If the breathing is rapid and shallow, reassure the patient that exercise and breathing practice can help change this breathing pattern. Then, assist the patient in practicing abdominal breathing by performing the following exercises:

- Instruct the patient to breathe deeply by inhaling slowly through the nose. Have them place a hand on the abdomen just beneath the rib cage.
- Instruct the patient to observe that when one is breathing deeply, the hand on the abdomen will rise.
- After the patient understands this process, ask them to inhale slowly through the nose while counting to five, pause, and then exhale slowly through pursed lips.
- While the patient exhales, direct attention to feeling the muscles relax, focusing on "letting go."
- Have the patient repeat the deep abdominal breathing for 10 breaths, pausing between each inhalation and

BOX 27.6

Reflection of a Nurse: Panic Attack

Incident

On an inpatient unit, a patient with a diagnosis of an anxiety disorder begins hyperventilating after reading a text from a close friend. The patient cannot sit still and begins pacing the room. A nurse intervenes by encouraging the patient to disregard the text, but this suggestion only increases the hyperventilation.

Reflection

Upon evaluation of the intervention, the nurse realizes that by encouraging the patient to disregard the text, hyperventilation increased, and the patient's anxiety increased.

1. What cues make it evident that the patient was experiencing a panic attack?
2. What interventions would be more effective to help the patient manage their anxiety?

exhalation. Count slowly. If the patient complains of lightheadedness, reassure them that this is an expected feeling while deep breathing. Instruct the patient to stop for 30 seconds, breathe regularly, and then start again.

- The patient should stop between each cycle of 10 breaths and monitor breathing for 30 seconds.
- This series of 10 slow abdominal breaths followed by 30 seconds of regular breathing should be repeated for 3 to 5 minutes.
- Help the patient establish a time for daily practice of abdominal breathing.
- Abdominal breathing may also be used to interrupt an episode of panic as it begins. After patients have learned to identify their own early signs of panic, they can learn the four-square method of breathing, which helps divert or decrease the severity of the attack. Patients should be instructed as follows:
  - Advise the patient to practice during calm periods and to begin by inhaling slowly through the nose, count to four, and then hold the breath for a count of four.
  - Direct the patient to exhale slowly through pursed lips to a count of four and then rest for a count of four (no breath).
- Finally, the patient may take two regular breaths and repeat the sequence.
- After patients practice the skill, the nurse should assist them in identifying the physical cues that will alert them to use this calming technique.

Nutritional Planning

Maintaining regular and balanced eating habits reduces the likelihood of hypoglycemic episodes, lightheadedness, and fatigue. To help teach the patient about healthful eating and ways to minimize physical factors contributing to anxiety:

- Advise the patient to reduce or eliminate substances in the diet that promote anxiety and panic, such as food coloring, monosodium glutamate, and caffeine (withdrawal from which may stimulate panic). Patients need to plan to reduce caffeine consumption and then eliminate it from their diet. Many OTC remedies are now used to boost energy or increase mental performance; some of these contain caffeine. A thorough assessment should be made of all OTC products used to assess the potential of anxiety-provoking ingredients.
- Instruct the patient to check each substance consumed and note whether symptoms of anxiety occur and whether the symptoms are relieved by not consuming the product.

Relaxation Techniques

Teaching the patient relaxation techniques is another way to help individuals with panic and anxiety disorders. Some are unaware of the tension in their bodies and first need to learn to monitor their own tension. Isometric exercises and progressive muscle relaxation are helpful methods to learn to differentiate muscle tension from muscle relaxation. This method of relaxation is also useful when patients have difficulty clearing the mind, focusing, or visualizing a scene, which are often required in other forms of relaxation, such as meditation. Box 27.7 provides one method of progressive muscle relaxation.

BOX 27.7

Teaching Progressive Muscle Relaxation

Ask clients to follow these steps to teach progressive muscle relaxation:

1. Choose a quiet, comfortable location where you will not be disturbed for 20 to 30 minutes. Your position may be lying or sitting, but all parts of your body should be supported, including your head. Wear loose clothing, taking off restrictive items, such as glasses and shoes.
2. Begin by closing your eyes and clearing your mind. Moving from head to toe, focus on each part of your body and assess the level of tension. Visualize each group of muscles as heavy and relaxed.
3. Take two or three slow abdominal breaths, pausing briefly between each breath. Imagine the tension flowing from your body.
4. Each muscle group listed subsequently should be tightened (or tensed isometrically) for 5 to 10 seconds and then abruptly released; visualize this group of muscles as heavy, limp, and relaxed for 15 to 20 seconds before tightening the next group of muscles. There are several methods to tighten each muscle group, and suggestions are provided subsequently.

   Each muscle group may be tightened two to three times until relaxed. Do not overtighten or strain. You should not experience pain.
   - Hands: tighten by making fists
   - Biceps: tighten by drawing forearms up and "making a muscle"
   - Triceps: extend forearms straight, locking elbows
   - Face: grimace, tightly shutting mouth and eyes
   - Face: open mouth wide and raise eyebrows
   - Neck: pull head forward to chest and tighten neck muscles
   - Shoulders: raise shoulders toward ears
   - Shoulders: push shoulders back as if touching them together
   - Chest: take a deep breath and hold for 10 seconds
   - Stomach: suck in your abdominal muscles
   - Buttocks: pull buttocks together
   - Thighs: straighten legs and squeeze muscles in thighs and hips
   - Calves: pull your toes carefully toward you, avoid cramps
   - Feet: curl toes downward and point toes away from your body
5. Finally, repeat several deep abdominal breaths and mentally check your body for tension. Rest comfortably for several minutes, breathing regularly, and visualize your body as warm and relaxed. Get up slowly when you are finished.

Physical Activity

Physical exercise can effectively decrease the occurrence of panic attacks by reducing muscle tension, increasing metabolism, increasing serotonin levels, and relieving stress. Exercise programs reduce many of the precipitants of anxiety by improving circulation, digestion, endorphin stimulation, and tissue oxygenation. In addition, exercise lowers cholesterol levels, blood pressure, and weight. After assessing contraindications to physical exercise, assist the patient in establishing a routine exercise program. Engaging in 10- to 20-minute sessions on treadmills or on stationary bicycles two to three times weekly is ideal during the winter months. Casual walking or bike riding during warmer weather promotes health. Help the patient to identify community resources that promote exercise.

Wellness Challenges

Many of the strategies that promote wellness are the same as those used to treat anxiety. The individual who is anxious or fearful may be more comfortable with a gradual incorporation of the strategies. Many wellness strategies for the individual who is anxious should focus on physical health. See Table 27.5.

TABLE 27.5 WELLNESS CHALLENGES AND COPING STRATEGIES FOR THE INDIVIDUAL WITH ANXIETY

Challenge	Coping Strategy
To cope effectively with daily stresses without excessive worry	• Develop a daily schedule • Allow time to relax • Avoid trying to multitask • Practice deep breathing and mindfulness
To have satisfying and enriching work	• Choose activities that are consistent with your skills and knowledge • Consider other possibilities if a job is too stressful.
To incorporate physical activity, healthy foods, and adequate sleep into daily life	• Schedule regular physical activity • Make a weekly menu of healthy meals • Establish healthy sleep hygiene routines
To develop a sense of connection, belonging, and a support system	• Join a support group • Seek out recreational activities with friends and families
To expand a sense of purpose and meaning in life	• Focus on goals, values, and beliefs • Read inspiring stories or essays

Medication Interventions

Some antidepressants (e.g., SSRIs and serotonin–norepinephrine reuptake inhibitors [SNRIs]) and antianxiety medication (e.g., benzodiazepines) are approved by the US Food and Drug Administration for treating people with panic disorder (see Table 27.6).

Selective Serotonin Reuptake Inhibitors (SSRIs)

SSRIs are recommended as the first drug option in the treatment of patients with panic disorder. They have the best safety profile, and if side effects occur, they tend to be present early in treatment before the therapeutic effect takes place. Hence, the SSRIs should

TABLE 27.6 MEDICATION FOR PANIC DISORDER

Medication	Starting Dose (mg/day)	Therapeutic Dose	Side Effects
SSRIs			Class effects: nausea, anorexia, tremors, anxiety, sexual dysfunction, jitteriness, insomnia, suicidality
Fluoxetine	10	20–60	Class effects
Sertraline	25	50–200	Class effects, loose stools
Paroxetine	10	10–60	Class effects, drowsiness, fatigue
Paroxetine (controlled release)	12.5	12.5–75	Class effects
SNRIs			Class effects: nausea, sweating, dry mouth, dizziness, insomnia, somnolence, sexual dysfunction, hypertension
Venlafaxine (extended release)	37.5	75–300	Class effects
Benzodiazepines			Class effects: sedation, cognitive slowing, physical dependence
Clonazepam	0.25 TID	0.5–2.0 BID	Class effects
Alprazolam	0.25 TID	0.5–1.5 TID	Class effects

BID, two times a day; SNRIs, serotonin–norepinephrine reuptake inhibitors; SSRIs, selective serotonin reuptake inhibitors; TID, three times a day.

BOX 27.8

Building Clinical Judgment With SBAR: Nurse Communication With Provider

SBAR

S: Situation

Taylor is a 32-year-old person assigned female at birth who is diagnosed with panic disorder. She was admitted last night following a severe panic attack after an argument with her partner. She was treated in the ED with lorazepam 2 mg with orders for lorazepam 1 mg every 4 hours as needed for anxiety. Sertraline 25 mg once a day is to be started today. Did not tell provider about the use of herbal supplements.

B: Background

This is the first inpatient admission for Taylor, who has a history of panic attacks and has been treating them with stress management interventions and St. John's wort. She recently doubled her usual dose of St. John's wort because of increasing fear of panic attacks.

A: Assessment

- Physical health: Ht. 5′5′, Wt. 135
- Vital signs: BP 130/70, HR 85, R 12
- Oriented X 4; reports dizziness, diarrhea
- Herbal supplement with St. John's wort

R: Recommendation

- Closely monitor patient for serotonin syndrome.
- Hold sertraline until discussion with provider about the patient's use of St. John's wort.

Building Clinical Judgment

1. Why did the nurse associate the patient's use of St. John's wort with sertraline?
2. Why did the nurse recommend monitoring serotonin syndrome and hold sertraline?

be started at low doses and titrated every 5 to 7 days. Antidepressant therapy is recommended for long-term treatment of the disorder and antianxiety as adjunctive treatment (Cackovic et al., 2023). The SSRIs produce anxiolytic effects by increasing the transmission of serotonin by blocking serotonin reuptake at the presynaptic cleft. The initial increase in serotonergic activity with SSRIs may cause temporary increases in panic symptoms and even panic attacks. After 4 to 6 weeks of treatment, anxiety subsides, and the antianxiety effect of the medications begins (see Chapter 11). Increased serotonin activity in the brain is believed to decrease norepinephrine activity. This decrease lessens cardiovascular symptoms of tachycardia and increased blood pressure, which are associated with panic attacks. See Chapter 25 for administration and monitoring side effects. See Box 27.8.

NCLEXNOTE Psychopharmacologic treatment is almost always needed. Antidepressants are the medications of choice. Antianxiety medication is used only for short periods of time.

Serotonin–Norepinephrine Reuptake Inhibitors (SNRIs)

The SNRIs increase levels of both serotonin and norepinephrine by blocking their reuptake presynaptically. Classified as antidepressants, the SNRIs are also used in anxiety disorders. Venlafaxine is the most commonly used SNRI. See Table 27.6. These medications have been shown to reduce the severity of panic and anticipatory anxiety. Similar to the SSRIs, they should not be abruptly discontinued (see Chapter 11).

Benzodiazepine Therapy

The high-potency benzodiazepines have produced antipanic effects; their therapeutic onset is much faster than that of antidepressants (see Table 27.6). Therefore, benzodiazepines are tremendously useful in treating intensely distressed patients. Alprazolam, lorazepam, and clonazepam are widely used for panic disorder. They are well tolerated but carry the risk for withdrawal symptoms upon discontinuation of use. See Box 27.9. The benzodiazepines are still commonly used for panic disorder even though the SSRIs are recommended for first-line treatment of panic disorder. In people with substance use disorder, gabapentin and mirtazapine are recommended instead of benzodiazepines to avoid dependency (Cackovic et al., 2023).

Administering and Monitoring Benzodiazepines

Treatment may include administering benzodiazepines concurrently with antidepressants for the first 4 weeks and then tapering the benzodiazepine to a maintenance dose. This strategy provides rapid symptom relief but avoids the complications of long-term benzodiazepine use. Benzodiazepines with short half-lives do not accumulate in the body, but benzodiazepines with half-lives

BOX 27.9

Medication Profile: Alprazola

DRUG CLASS: Antianxiety agent

RECEPTOR AFFINITY: Exact mechanism of action is unknown; believed to increase the effects of γ-aminobutyrate.

INDICATIONS: Management of anxiety disorders, short-term relief of anxiety symptoms or depression-related anxiety, panic attacks with or without agoraphobia.

ROUTES AND DOSAGES: Available in 0.25-, 0.5-, 1-, and 2-mg scored tablets.

Adults: For anxiety: Initially, 0.25 to 0.5 mg PO TID titrated to a maximum daily dose of 4 mg in divided doses. For panic disorder: Initially, 0.5 mg PO TID increased at 3- to 4-day intervals in increments of no more than 1 mg/day.

Geriatric Patients: Initially, 0.25 mg BID to TID, increased gradually as needed and tolerated.

HALF-LIFE (PEAK EFFECT): 12 to 15 hours (1 to 2 hours).

SELECTED ADVERSE REACTIONS: Transient mild drowsiness, initially; sedation, depression, lethargy, apathy, fatigue, lightheadedness, disorientation, anger, hostility, restlessness, headache, confusion, crying, constipation, diarrhea, dry mouth, nausea, and possible drug dependence.

WARNINGS: Contraindicated in patients with psychosis, acute narrow-angle glaucoma, shock, acute alcohol intoxication with depressed vital signs, pregnancy, labor and delivery, and breastfeeding. Use cautiously in patients with impaired hepatic or renal function and severe debilitating conditions. Risk for digitalis toxicity if given concurrently with digoxin. Increased CNS depression if taken with alcohol, other CNS depressants, and propoxyphene (Darvon).

SPECIFIC PATIENT AND FAMILY EDUCATION

- Avoid using alcohol, sleep-inducing drugs, and other OTC drugs.
- Take the drug exactly as prescribed, and do not stop taking the drug without consulting your primary health care provider.
- Take the drug with food if gastrointestinal upset occurs.
- Avoid driving a car or performing tasks that require alertness if drowsiness or dizziness occurs.
- Report any signs and symptoms of adverse reactions.
- Notify your primary health care provider if severe dizziness, weakness, or drowsiness persists or if rash or skin lesions, difficulty voiding, palpitations, or swelling of extremities occurs.

BID, two times a day; CNS, central nervous system; OTC, over the counter; PO, oral; TID, three times a day.

of longer than 24 hours tend to accumulate with long-term treatment, are removed more slowly, and produce less intense symptoms on discontinuation of use (see Chapter 11).

Short-acting benzodiazepines, such as alprazolam, are associated with rebound anxiety, or anxiety that increases after the peak effects of the medication have decreased. Medications with short half-lives (alprazolam, lorazepam) should be given in three or four doses spaced throughout the day, with a higher dose at bedtime to allay anxiety-related insomnia. Clonazepam, a longer-acting benzodiazepine, requires less frequent dosing and has a lower risk for rebound anxiety.

Because of their depressive CNS effects, benzodiazepines should not be used to treat patients with comorbid sleep apnea. In fact, these drugs may decrease the rate and depth of respirations. Exercise caution in older adult patients for these reasons. Discontinuing medication requires a slow taper during a period of several weeks to avoid rebound anxiety and serious withdrawal symptoms. Benzodiazepines are not indicated in the chronic treatment of patients with substance use disorder but can be useful in quickly treating anxiety symptoms until other medications take effect.

Symptoms associated with withdrawal of benzodiazepine therapy are more likely to occur after high doses and long-term therapy. They can also occur after short-term therapy. Withdrawal symptoms manifest in several ways, including psychological (e.g., apprehension, irritability, agitation).

Monitoring Side Effects

SSRIs should not be given with monoamine oxidase inhibitors (MAOIs) because of potential drug interaction. Drugs that interact with benzodiazepines include the tricyclic antidepressants (TCAs) and digoxin; interaction may result in increased serum TCA or digoxin levels. Alcohol and other CNS depressants, when used with benzodiazepines, increase CNS depression. Their concomitant use is contraindicated. Histamine-2 blockers (e.g., cimetidine) used with benzodiazepines may potentiate sedative effects. Monitor closely for effectiveness in patients who smoke; cigarette smoking may increase the clearance of benzodiazepines.

Management of Complications

The side effects of benzodiazepine medications generally include headache, confusion, dizziness, disorientation, sedation, and visual disturbances. Sedation should be monitored after beginning medication use or increasing the dose. The patient should avoid operating heavy machinery until the sedative effects are known.

Concurrent use of SSRIs and MAOIs is contraindicated. These antidepressants should not be given together.

Teaching Points

Warn patients to avoid alcohol because of the chance of CNS depression. In addition, warn them not to operate heavy machinery until the sedative effects of the medication are known.

Psychosocial Interventions

Therapeutic Interactions

Peplau (1989) devised general guidelines for nursing interventions that might be successful in treating patients with anxiety. These interventions continue to be relevant today and help patients attend to and react to input other than the subjective experiences of anxiety. They are designed to help patients focus on other stimuli and cope with anxiety in any form (Box 27.10; Table 27.7). These general interventions apply to all anxiety disorders and therefore are not reiterated in subsequent sections.

Enhancing Cognitive and Behavioral Functioning

Distraction

After patients can identify the early symptoms of panic, they may learn to implement distraction behaviors that take the focus off the physical sensations. Some activities include initiating conversation with a nearby individual or engaging in physical activity (e.g., walking, gardening, or housecleaning). Performing simple repetitive activities such as snapping a rubber band against the wrist, counting backward from 100 by 3s, or counting objects along the roadway might also deter an attack.

TABLE 27.7 NURSING INTERVENTIONS BASED ON DEGREES OF ANXIETY

Degree of Anxiety	Nursing Interventions
Mild	Assist patient to use the energy anxiety provides to encourage learning.
Moderate	Encourage patient to talk: to focus on one experience, to describe it fully, and then to formulate the patient's generalizations about that experience.
Severe	Allow relief behaviors to be used but do not ask about them. Encourage the patient to talk: ventilation of random ideas is likely to reduce anxiety to a moderate level.
Panic	Stay with the patient. Allow pacing and walk with the patient. No content inputs to the patient's thinking should be made by the nurse. (They burden the patient, who will distort them.) Be direct with the fewest number of words: e.g., "Drink this" (give liquids to replace lost fluids and to relieve dry mouth); "Say what's happening to you," "Talk about yourself," or "Tell what you feel now" (to encourage ventilation and externalization of inner, frightening experience). Pick up on what the patient says, for example, Patient: "What's happening to me—how did I get here?" Nurse: "Say what you notice." Use short phrases to the point of the patient's comment. Do not touch the patient; patients experiencing panic are very concerned about survival, are experiencing a grave threat to self, and usually distort intentions of all invasions of their personal space.

Adapted from Peplau, H. (1989). Theoretical constructs: Anxiety, self, and hallucinations. In A. O'Toole & S. Welt (Eds.), *Interpersonal theory in nursing practice: Selected works of Hildegarde*. E Springer.

Reframing

Reframing is a cognitive technique that can change the way a situation, event, or individual is viewed and reduce the impact of anxiety-provoking thoughts. People with anxiety disorders often view themselves negatively and use "should statements" and "negative labels." Should statements lead to rigid rules and unrealistic expectations? By encouraging patients to avoid the use of should statements and reframe their views, they can change their beliefs to be more realistic. For example, if a patient says, "I should be a better parent" or "I'm a useless failure," the nurse could ask the individual to identify the positive aspects of parenting and other successes.

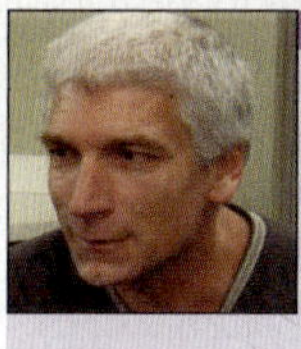

Consider This:
Could distraction and reframing help Doug reduce his anxiety and frequency of his panic attacks? What interventions would you recommend and why?

Positive Self-Talk

During states of increased anxiety and panic, individuals can learn to counter fearful or negative thoughts by using another cognitive approach. Positive self-talk involves planning and rehearsing positive coping statements "This is only anxiety, and it will pass," "I can handle these symptoms," and "I'll get through this" are examples of positive self-talk. These types of positive statements can give the individual a focal point and reduce fear when panic symptoms begin. Handheld cards that offer positive statements can be carried in a purse or wallet so the individual can retrieve them quickly when panic symptoms are felt.

NCLEXNOTE Cognitive interventions give patients with anxiety a sense of control over the recurring threats of panic and obsessions.

Complementary Therapies

Complementary therapies are used as adjuncts to standard care (psychological and pharmacologic interventions). Daily yoga along with standard care has been shown to reduce anxiety and improve quality of life for those with panic disorder when compared to a similar group not engaging in yoga practice (Yadla et al., 2024). Other complementary therapies such as music

BOX 27.10

Therapeutic Dialogue: Panic Disorder

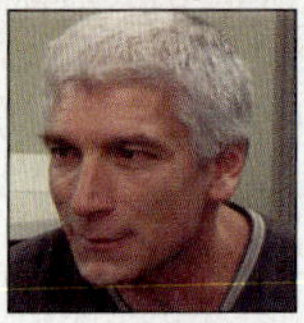

Doug is admitted to an inpatient unit following another severe panic attack. He had an argument with his high school son, who continues to use alcohol and marijuana. Financial issues are also escalating.

INEFFECTIVE APPROACH

Nurse: Oh.... Why are you crying?

Doug: (Looks up, gives a nervous chuckle.) Obviously, because I'm upset. I am tired of living this way. I just want to be normal again. I can't even remember what that feels like.

Nurse: You look fine to me. Everyone has bad days. It'll pass.

Doug: I've felt this way longer than you've been alive. I've tried everything, and nothing works.

Nurse: You're not the first depressed individual that I've taken care of. You just need to go to groups and stay out of your room more. You'll start feeling better.

Doug: (Angrily) Oh, it's just that easy. You have no idea what I'm going through! You don't know me! You're just a kid.

Nurse: I can help you if you help yourself. The group starts in 5 minutes, and I'd like to see you there.

Doug: I'm not going to no damn group! I want to be alone so I can think!

Nurse: (Looks about anxiously.) Maybe I should come back after you've calmed down a little.

EFFECTIVE APPROACH

Nurse: Doug, I noticed that you are staying in your room more today. What's troubling you?

Doug: (Looks up) I feel like I've lost complete control of my life. I'm so anxious, and nothing helps. I'm tired of it.

Nurse: I see. That must be difficult. Can you tell me more about what you are feeling right now?

Doug: I feel like I'm going crazy. I worry all the time about having panic attacks. They make me scared I'm going to die. Sometimes I think I'd be better off dead.

Nurse: (Remains silent, continues to give eye contact.)

Doug: Do you know what it's like to be a prisoner to your emotions? I can't even go to work sometimes, and when I do, it's terrifying. I don't know what to think anymore.

Nurse: Doug, you have lived with this disorder for a long time. You say that the medications do not work to your liking, but what has helped you in the past?

Doug: Well, I learned in relaxation group that panic symptoms are probably caused by chemicals in my brain that are not working correctly. I learned that medications can help, but they don't work well for me. I tried an exposure plan and relaxation techniques to deal with my fears of leaving the house and my chronic anxiety. That did help some, but it's scary to do.

Nurse: It sounds like you have learned a lot about your illness, one that can be treated, so that you don't always have to feel this way.

Doug: This is easier to say right now when I'm here and can get help if I need it. It's hard to remember this when I'm in the middle of a panic attack and think I'm dying.

Nurse: It's harder when you're alone?

Doug: Much harder! And I'm alone so much of the time.

Nurse: Let's talk about some ways you can manage your panics when you're alone. Tell me some of the techniques you've learned.

CRITICAL THINKING CHALLENGE

1. What tone is established by the nurse's opening question in the first scenario?
2. Which therapeutic communication techniques did the nurse use in the second scenario to avoid the pitfalls encountered in the first scenario?
3. What information was uncovered in the second scenario that was not touched on in the first?
4. What predictions can you make about the interpersonal relationship likely to develop between the nurse and the patient in each scenario?

BOX 27.11

Research for Evidence-Based Practice: Group Music Therapy for Anxiety and Depression for People With Dementia

Feng, X., Dang, W., & Apuke, O. D. (2024). How does group music therapy help in combating the anxiety and depression of dementia patients? A quasi-experimental investigation. Archives of Psychiatric Nursing, 52, *83–88. https://doi.org/10.1016/j.apnu.2024.07.010*

THE QUESTION: What impact does music therapy have on anxiety and depression symptoms of dementia?

METHODS: A quasiexperimental design was used with participants randomly allocated to the control group or music group. The sample consisted of 130 people over the age of 65 years who had lived in a nursing home for at least 1 month. The Hospital Anxiety and Depression questionnaire was used to measure the level of patients' anxiety and depression. Data were collected preintervention, 2 days after the intervention, and after 3 months. The intervention consisted of 12 hour-long sessions, each with 10 minutes of warm up, 40 minutes spent listening to and rehearsing live music performances on a variety of instruments, and 10 minutes of storytelling.

FINDINGS: There were no statistical differences in the anxiety and depression scores at the beginning of the study. Following the intervention, the anxiety and depression scores in the music group were significantly decreased. There were no changes in the control group.

IMPLICATIONS FOR NURSING: Music therapy is an effective, nonpharmacologic treatment for anxiety and depression in people with dementia living in nursing homes. Music therapy could easily be included in long-term care facilities.

therapy, meditation, aromatherapy, and biofeedback are being studied for their effectiveness in reducing anxiety (Amitani et al., 2023; Cho et al., 2024; Seetharaman et al., 2024). See Box 27.11.

Spiritual Interventions

Patients can use prayer, worship, and religious ritual to bring meaning and fulfillment to their lives. Complementary therapies can also be used to enhance spiritual well-being. For example, meditation can be used to focus on staying in the moment and slowing down inner thoughts, which in turn can promote a sense of peace.

Psychoeducation

Psychoeducation programs help to teach patients and families about the symptoms of panic. Individuals with panic disorder legitimately fear going crazy, losing control, or dying because of their physical symptoms. Attempting to convince a patient that such fears are groundless only heightens anxiety and impedes communication. Information and physical evidence (e.g., electrocardiogram results, laboratory test results) should be presented in a caring and open manner that demonstrates acceptance and understanding of their situation.

Box 27.12 suggests topics for individual or small-group discussion. It is especially important to cover such topics as the differences between panic attacks and heart attacks, the difference between panic disorder and other mental disorders, and the effectiveness of various treatment methods.

Wellness Strategies

Individuals with panic disorder, especially those with significant anxiety sensitivity, may need assistance in reevaluating their lifestyle. Time management can be a useful tool. In the workplace or at home, underestimating the time needed to complete a chore or being overly involved in several activities at once increases stress and anxiety. Procrastination, lack of assertiveness, and difficulties with prioritizing or delegating tasks intensify these issues.

Writing a list of chores to be completed and estimating the time to complete them provides concrete feedback to the individual. Crossing out each activity as it is completed helps the patient to regain a sense of control and accomplishment. Large tasks should be broken into a series of smaller tasks to minimize stress and maximize sense of achievement. Rest, relaxation, and family time—frequently omitted from the daily schedule—must be included.

Providing Family Education

In addition to learning the symptoms of panic disorder, nurses should have information sheets or pamphlets available concerning the disorder and any medications prescribed. Parents/caregivers, especially single parents, will need assistance in child rearing and may benefit from services designed to provide some respite. Moreover, the entire family will need support in adjusting to the

BOX 27.12

Psychoeducation Checklist: Panic Disorder

When caring for a patient with panic disorder, be sure to include the following topic areas in the teaching plan:

- Psychopharmacologic agents (anxiolytics or antidepressants) if ordered, including drug action, dosage, frequency, and possible adverse effects
- Breathing control measures
- Nutrition
- Exercise
- Progressive muscle relaxation
- Distraction behaviors
- Exposure therapy
- Time management
- Positive coping strategies

disorder. A referral for family therapy is indicated, because involving the entire family in the therapy process is imperative. Families experience the symptoms, treatments, clinical setbacks, and recovery from chronic mental illnesses as a unit. Misunderstandings, misconceptions, false information, and the stigma of mental illness, singly or collectively, impede recovery efforts.

Convening Support Groups

Participation in supportive groups is helpful in managing anxiety and fears (Vickery, 2022). People with a panic disorder are usually comfortable in groups with individuals who have other mental disorders and issues. As they participate in a group, they are able to share their fears of an impending panic attack and identify strategies to deal with their fears.

Developing Recovery-Oriented Rehabilitation Strategies

Recovery begins with an understanding of the components of recovery discussed in Chapters 2 and 8. As the components of recovery are explained, the nurse should continue to engage the individual in a collaborative decision-making process. The nurse's role in developing recovery-oriented strategies is to negotiate the most effective, evidence-based strategies. The nurse should encourage healthy behaviors supporting wellness as well as strategies directed toward illness management. Empowering the individual to make choices that best match the individual's lifestyle increases the likelihood of treatment adherence and recovery. It will also foster a feeling of hopefulness. Treatment recommendations for one individual may not be appropriate for another. For example, some people will attend support groups, but others only respond to individual psychotherapy. The nurse should encourage the patient to commit to as many recovery strategies that are realistic.

Evaluation and Treatment Outcomes

Although many researchers consider panic disorder a chronic, long-term condition, the positive results from outcome studies should be shared with patients to provide encouragement and optimism that patients can learn to manage these symptoms. Outcome studies have demonstrated success with panic control treatment, CBT therapy, exposure therapy, and various medications specific to certain symptoms.

Continuum of Care

Emergency Care

Because individuals with panic disorder are likely to first present for treatment in an emergency department or primary care setting, nurses working in these settings should be involved in early recognition and referral. Consultation with a psychiatrist or mental health professional by the primary care provider can decrease both costs and overall patient symptoms. Several interventions may be useful in reducing the number of emergency department visits related to panic symptoms. Psychiatric consultation and nursing education can be provided in the emergency department to explore other avenues of treatment. Remembering that the patient experiencing a panic attack is in crisis, nurses can take several measures to help alleviate symptoms, including the following:

- Stay with the patient and maintain a calm demeanor. (Anxiety often produces more anxiety, and a calm presence will help calm the patient.)
- Reassure the patient that you will not leave, that this episode will pass, and that they are in a safe place. (The patient often fears dying and cannot see beyond the panic attack.)
- Give clear concise directions using short sentences. Do not use medical jargon.
- Walk or pace with the patient to an environment with minimal stimulation. (The patient in panic has excessive energy.)
- Administer PRN (i.e., as-needed) anxiolytic medications as ordered and appropriate. (Pharmacotherapy is effective in treating those patients with acute panic attack.)
- After the panic attack has been resolved, allow the patient to vent their feelings. This often helps the patient in clarifying their feelings.

Inpatient-Focused Care

Inpatient settings provide control for the stabilization of the acute panic symptoms and initiation of recovery-oriented strategies. Medication use is often initiated here because patients who show initial panic symptoms require in-depth assessment to determine the cause. As recovery begins, crisis stabilization, medication management, milieu therapy, and psychotherapies are introduced, and outpatient discharge linkage appointments are set.

Community Care

Most individuals with panic disorder are treated on an outpatient basis. Referral lists of community resources and support groups are useful in this setting. A discussion about the recovery and the importance of the 10 components helps healing begin (see Chapters 2 and 8). Nurses are more directly involved in treatment, conducting psychoeducation groups on relaxation and breathing techniques, symptom management, and anger management. Advanced practice nurses conduct CBT and individual and family psychotherapy. In addition, medication monitoring groups reemphasize the role of medications, monitor for side effects, and enhance treatment adherence overall.

As with any disorder, a continuum of patient care across multiple settings is crucial. Patients are treated in the least restrictive environment that will meet their safety needs. As the patient progresses through treatment, the environment of care changes from an emergency or inpatient setting to outpatient clinics or individual therapy sessions.

Virtual Mental Health Care

Virtual mental health services are more important now because of their positive impact during the coronavirus pandemic. Virtual treatment is ideal for those who fear transmission of infections. Most therapies discussed in this chapter are available in a virtual format. The patient should be cautioned about selecting services that are credible. Support groups such as the National Alliance on Mental Illness and the Anxiety and Depression Association of America are easily accessed online and provide resources for clinicians and patients.

Integration With Primary Care

Coordination of care between mental health and primary care leads to safer management of anxiety disorders. Some groups are more likely to seek out care in primary care rather than in mental health clinics. People with anxiety disorders are often treated in the primary care environment, particularly those who experience panic disorder. Because panic attacks mimic cardiac difficulties, it is important that the patient continues to seek health care monitoring with medical clinicians. Anxiety can be related to physical health issues, such as immune, metabolic, and cardiovascular issues. Many prescription and nonprescription drugs can cause anxiety, such as asthma, blood pressure, steroid, and thyroid medications. Without coordination of care, the clinicians will not be able to make a meaningful assessment, which could lead to the wrong treatment.

GENERALIZED ANXIETY DISORDER

Patients with **generalized anxiety disorder** (GAD) typically feel frustrated, disgusted with life, demoralized, and hopeless. They may state that they cannot remember a time when they did not feel anxious. They experience a sense of ill-being and uneasiness and fear of imminent disaster. Over time, they may recognize that their chronic tension and anxiety are unreasonable.

CLINICAL COURSE

The onset of GAD is insidious. Many patients complain of being chronic worriers. GAD affects individuals of all ages. About half of individuals with GAD report an onset in childhood or adolescence, although onset after 20 years of age is also common. Adults with GAD often worry about matters such as their job, household finances, health of family members, or simple matters (e.g., household chores or being late for appointments). The intensity of the worry fluctuates, and stress tends to intensify the worry and anxiety symptoms (APA, 2022).

Patients with GAD may exhibit mild depressive symptoms, such as dysphoria. They are also highly somatic, with complaints of multiple clusters of physical symptoms, including muscle aches, soreness, and gastrointestinal ailments. In addition to physical complaints, patients with GAD often experience poor sleep habits, irritability, trembling, twitching, poor concentration, and an exaggerated startle response. People with this disorder often are seen in a primary care setting with somatic symptoms (Khazanov et al., 2024).

DIAGNOSTIC CRITERIA

GAD is characterized by excessive worry and anxiety (apprehensive expectation) for at least 6 months. Anxiety does not usually pertain to a specific situation; rather, it concerns several real-life activities or events. Ultimately, excessive worry and anxiety cause great distress and interfere with the patient's daily personal or social life.

NURSING CARE

Nursing care for the individual with GAD is similar to the care of the individual with a panic disorder. In many instances, antidepressants and an antianxiety agent will be prescribed. Nursing interventions should focus on helping the individual target specific areas of anxiety and reducing the impact of the anxiety. See Box 27.13.

BOX 27.13

Psychoeducation Checklist: Generalized Anxiety Disorder

When caring for the patient with GAD, be sure to include the following topic areas in the teaching plan:

- Psychopharmacologic agents (benzodiazepines, antidepressants, nonbenzodiazepine anxiolytics, β-blockers) if ordered, including drug action, dosage, frequency, and possible adverse effects
- Breathing control
- Nutrition and diet restriction
- Sleep measures
- Progressive muscle relaxation
- Time management
- Positive coping strategies

PHOBIAS

As mentioned earlier in this chapter, a phobia is an irrational fear of an object, individual, or situation that leads to a compelling avoidance; phobias have anxiety as their defining feature. Phobias include generalized phobia, agoraphobia, specific phobias, and social anxiety disorder (social phobia).

AGORAPHOBIA

Agoraphobia is fear or anxiety triggered by about two or more situations, such as using public transportation, being in open spaces, being in enclosed places, standing in line, being in a crowd, or being outside of the home alone. When these situations occur, the individual believes that something terrible might happen and that escape may be difficult. The individual may experience panic-like symptoms or other embarrassing symptoms (e.g., vomiting, diarrhea) (APA, 2022). Agoraphobia leads to avoidance behaviors. Such avoidance interferes with routine functioning and eventually renders the individual afraid to leave the safety of home. Some affected individuals continue to face feared situations but with significant trepidation (i.e., going in public only to pay bills or to take children to school). Agoraphobia may occur with panic disorder, but is considered a separate disorder.

SPECIFIC PHOBIA DISORDER

Specific phobia disorder is marked by persistent fear of clearly discernible, circumscribed objects or situations, which often leads to avoidance behaviors. Phobic objects can include animals (e.g., spiders, snakes), natural environment (e.g., heights, storms), blood injection injury (e.g., fear of blood, injections), and situational (e.g., elevators, enclosed spaces). The 12-month community prevalence estimate ranges from 8% to 12%, and the disorder generally affects women twice as much as men (APA, 2022). It has a bimodal distribution, peaking in childhood and then again in the 20s. The focus of the fear in a specific phobia may result from the anticipation of being harmed by the phobic object. For example, dogs are feared because of the chance of being bitten, or automobiles are feared because of the potential of crashing. The focus of fear may likewise be associated with concerns about losing control, panicking, or fainting on exposure to the phobic object.

Anxiety is usually felt immediately on exposure to the phobic object; the level of anxiety is usually related to both the proximity of the object and the degree to which escape is possible. For example, anxiety heightens as a cat approaches an individual who fears cats and lessens when the cat moves away. At times, the level of anxiety escalates to a full panic attack, particularly when the individual must remain in a situation from which escape is deemed to be impossible. Fear of specific objects is common, and the diagnosis of specific phobia is not made unless the fear significantly interferes with functioning or causes marked distress. Assessment differentiates simple phobia from other diagnoses with overlapping symptoms. Box 27.14 provides a list of common phobias. Among adult patients who are seen in clinical settings, typical phobias are situational phobias, natural environment phobias, blood injection, injury phobia, and animal phobias (APA, 2022).

BOX 27.14

Common Phobias

- Acrophobia: fear of heights
- Agoraphobia: fear of open spaces
- Ailurophobia: fear of cats
- Algophobia: fear of pain
- Arachnophobia: fear of spiders
- Brontophobia: fear of thunder
- Claustrophobia: fear of closed spaces
- Cynophobia: fear of dogs
- Entomophobia: fear of insects
- Hematophobia: fear of blood
- Microphobia: fear of germs
- Nyctophobia: fear of night or dark places
- Ophidiophobia: fear of snakes
- Phonophobia: fear of loud noises
- Photophobia: fear of light
- Pyrophobia: fear of fire
- Tropophobia: fear of a place, like a stage
- Xenophobia: fear of strangers
- Zoophobia: fear of animal or animals

Blood injection injury phobia merits special consideration because the phobia involves medical treatments. The physiologic processes that are exhibited during phobic exposure include a strong vasovagal response, which significantly increases blood pressure and pulse, followed by deceleration of the pulse and lowering of blood pressure in the patient. Monitor closely when giving required injections or medical treatments.

About 75% of patients with blood injection injury phobia report fainting on exposure (Mason et al., 2022). Factors that may predispose individuals to specific phobias may include traumatic events; unexpected panic attacks in the presence of the phobic object or situation; observation of others experiencing a trauma; or repeated exposure to information warning of dangers, such as parents/guardians repeatedly warning young children that dogs bite. Specific treatment for blood injection injury phobia is exposure therapy, CBT, and muscle-tension exercises where the patient contracts and releases muscle groups (Mason et al., 2022).

Phobic content must be evaluated from an ethnic or cultural background. In some cultures, fears of spirits or magic are common. They should be considered part of a disorder only if the fear is excessive in the context of the culture, causes the individual significant distress, or impairs the ability to function. Psychotropic drugs have not been effective in the treatment of specific phobia. Anxiolytics may give short-term relief of phobic anxiety, but no evidence confirms that they affect the course of the disorder. The treatment of choice for specific phobia is exposure therapy.

SOCIAL ANXIETY DISORDER (SOCIAL PHOBIA)

Social anxiety disorder, also called social phobia, involves a persistent fear of social or performance situations in which embarrassment may occur. Social anxiety is different than being shy, which is a personality trait that causes the individual to be reluctant to engage in social activities and interactions. In a social anxiety disorder, exposure to a feared social or performance situation nearly always provokes immediate anxiety and may trigger panic attacks. People with social anxiety disorder fear that others will scrutinize their behavior and judge them negatively. They often do not speak up in crowds out of fear of embarrassment. They go to great lengths to avoid feared situations. If avoidance is not possible, they suffer through the situation with visible anxiety (APA, 2022).

People with social anxiety disorder appear to be highly sensitive to disapproval or criticism, tend to evaluate themselves negatively, and have poor self-esteem and a distorted view of their personal strengths and weaknesses. They may magnify their personal flaws and underrate any talents. They often believe others would act with more assertiveness in a given social situation. Women are more likely to have social anxiety disorder, but people of all genders with this disorder tend to have difficulties with dating and with sexual relationships (Shechter Strulov & Akerka, 2024). Children tend to underachieve in school because of test-taking anxiety. This is an important area that should be assessed in all patients.

Generalized social anxiety disorder is diagnosed when the individual experiences fears related to most social situations, including public performances and social interactions. These individuals are likely to demonstrate deficiencies in social skills, and their phobias interfere with their ability to function (Rose & Tadi, 2022).

People with social anxiety disorder fear and avoid only one or two social situations. Classic examples of such situations are eating, writing, or speaking in public, or using public bathrooms. The most common fears for individuals with social anxiety disorder are public speaking, fear of meeting strangers, eating in public, writing in public, using public restrooms, and being stared at or being the center of attention.

Pharmacotherapy is a relatively new area of research in treating patients with social anxiety disorder. SSRIs are used to treat those with social anxiety disorder because they significantly reduce social anxiety and phobic avoidance. Benzodiazepines are also used to reduce anxiety caused by phobias. Providing referrals for appropriate psychiatric treatment is a critical nursing intervention.

SUMMARY OF KEY POINTS

- Anxiety is an unavoidable human condition. Anxiety becomes an anxiety disorder when anxiety and fear significantly interfere with social and occupational functioning.
- Anxiety-related disorders are the most common of all mental disorders and comprise several disorders, including panic disorder.
- The anxiety disorders share the common symptom of recurring anxiety but differ in symptom profiles. Panic attacks can occur in many different disorders. Physical symptoms can mimic a heart attack.
- Panic disorder can occur throughout the lifespan but is most common in adulthood. Those experiencing anxiety disorders have a high level of physical and emotional illness and often experience dual diagnoses with other anxiety disorders, substance use disorder, or depression. These disorders often render individuals unable to function effectively at home or at a job.
- There appears to be a familial predisposition to panic disorder. Serotonin, norepinephrine, and GABA are implicated in a panic disorder. The hypothalamic–pituitary–adrenal axis and activation of the stress hormones are also implicated in the expression of this disorder.
- Patients with panic disorder are often seen in various health care settings, frequently in hospital emergency departments or clinics, presenting with a confusing array of physical and emotional symptoms. Skillful assessment is required to eliminate possible life-threatening causes.
- Treatment approaches for all anxiety-related disorders are somewhat similar, including pharmacotherapy, psychological treatments, or often a combination of both.
- Antidepressants are the first-line medication treatment and are often included in psychosocial therapies such as cognitive-behavioral therapy, and exposure therapy. Virtual mental health strategies such as telehealth, mobile apps provide most of the same therapies as face-to-face therapies.
- Nursing interventions include helping patients manage a panic attack, promoting healthy diet, exercise, and sleep hygiene habits, medication administration and monitoring, psychoeducation, and cognitive interventions.
- Many people with a panic disorder have other health issues that are treated in primary care. Mental and physical health needs should be integrated with both primary and mental health services.

DEVELOPING CLINICAL JUDGMENT

1. A patient is unable to focus on your directions. They do not seem to notice others in the room; instead, they are intent on cutting their food into small pieces. Applying Peplau stages of anxiety, what level of anxiety is this patient experiencing?
2. Compare and contrast the following treatment modalities for anxiety disorders: exposure therapy, systematic desensitization, implosive therapy, and cognitive-behavioral therapy (CBT).
3. Identify the major nursing assessment areas for an individual experiencing a panic disorder.
4. A patient asks you how to prevent hyperventilation. How would you answer the question?
5. Delineate the differences in treatment effects of antidepressants versus antianxiety medication in the treatment of panic disorder.
6. Compare the various phobias that people experience. What interventions should a nurse use for an individual who has a blood injection injury phobia?
7. How might one differentiate shyness from social anxiety disorder?

MOVIES, TV, OR STREAMING PROGRAMS

***Woman in the Window:* 2021.** Anna Fox (Amy Adams), a child psychologist with agoraphobia, lives alone in Manhattan. Her daughter and husband are both deceased and she is unable to leave her house. She takes many medications and drinks alcohol regularly. She spends her days watching her neighbors, including the Russell family, from a second-story window. She meets Ethan Russell, the teenage son, and believes that he is being abused. The plot takes a dark turn when Anna observes the murder of Ethan's mother. The Russells deny that the mother was killed. The suspense thriller takes several twists and turns as Anna eventually becomes the target of a murder. Throughout the movie, Anna tries desperately to convince the police and others of the murder that she witnessed and her victimization.

The plot of this movie assumes that Anna Fox cannot be believed because of her mental disorder. The murder and Anna's victimization are thought by others to be symptoms of her mental disorder. The movie loosely linked Anna's agoraphobia with a trauma that she experienced when her husband and child were killed in an automobile accident when she was driving.

Viewing Points:

1. Are Anna's agoraphobia symptoms consistent with the *DMS-5-TR* diagnostic criteria?
2. Is it possible that the agoraphobia is related to the accident that killed her family?
3. What are examples of stigmatization in the movie?
4. Is it realistic that Anna would consider suicide?
5. Did Anna demonstrate countertransference as she interacted with Ethan and his family?
6. What similarities did Ethan see between his mother and Anna?

Unfolding Patient Stories: Linda Waterfall • Part 2

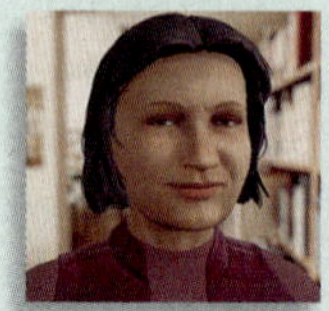

Recall from Chapter 6 Linda Waterfall, a 48-year-old recently diagnosed with an aggressive form of breast cancer. Linda's mother died when she was 10 years old, during surgery. While getting ready to go into surgery, Linda's initial anxiety about the recommended treatment (a mastectomy followed by chemotherapy) escalated when she realized she forgot her medicine bundle at home. How can an underlying diagnosis of anxiety contribute to Linda's physical decline from cancer? What psychosocial assessments and interventions should the nurse incorporate into the plan of care to manage her anxiety? How could the nurse use a trauma-informed approach in planning Linda's care?

REFERENCES

Alcan, E., Benke, C., & Melzig, C. A. (2024). A threat from within: Learning to fear by observing aversive bodily symptoms in others. *Behaviour Research and Therapy*, *178*, 104555. https://doi.org/10.1016/j.brat.2024.104555

American Psychiatric Association. (2022). *Diagnostic and statistical manual of mental disorders* (5th ed., text rev.). Author.

Amitani, H., Nishi, R., Sagiyama, K., Fukumoto, T., Funakoshi, K., Takayanagi, N., Watanabe, H., Hirose, M., Tagawa, K., Ota, K., Ito, Y. M., & Asakawa, A. (2023). The effect of lavender aroma for anxiety disorder: A study protocol for a multicenter, double-masked, randomized, placebo-controlled clinical trial. *BMC Complementary Medicine and Therapies*, *23*(1), 397. https://doi.org/10.1186/s12906-023-04231-1

Atchison, K., Wu, P., Samii, L., Walsh, M., Ismail, Z., Iaboni, A., & Goodarzi, Z. (2024). Detection of anxiety symptoms and disorders in older adults: A diagnostic accuracy systematic review. *Age and Ageing*, *53*(7), afae122. https://doi.org/10.1093/ageing/afae122

Baker, H. J., Hollywood, A., & Waite, P. (2022). Adolescents' lived experience of panic disorder: An interpretative phenomenological analysis. *BMC Psychology*, *10*(1), 143. https://doi.org/10.1186/s40359-022-00849-x

Bandelow, B., Allgulander, C., Baldwin, D. S., Costa, D. L. D. C., Denys, D., Dilbaz, N., Domschke, K., Eriksson, E., Fineberg, N. A., Hättenschwiler, J., Hollander, E., Kaiya, H., Karavaeva, T., Kasper, S., Katzman, M., Kim, Y. K., Inoue, T., Lim, L., Masdrakis, V., … Zohar, J. (2023). World Federation of Societies of Biological Psychiatry (WFSBP) guidelines for treatment of anxiety, obsessive-compulsive and posttraumatic stress disorders—Version 3. Part I: Anxiety disorders. *The World Journal of Biological Psychiatry*, *24*(2), 79–117. https://doi.org/10.1080/15622975.2022.2086295

Barbuti, M., Brancati, G. E., Calderone, A., Fierabracci, P., Salvetti, G., Weiss, F., Carignani, G., Santini, F., & Perugi, G. (2021). Prevalence of mood, panic and eating disorders in obese patients referred to bariatric surgery: Patterns of comorbidity and relationship with body mass index. *Eating and Weight Disorders*, *27*(3), 1021–1027. https://doi.org/10.1007/s40519-021-01236-y

Brunette, M. F., Erlich, M. D., Edwards, M. L., Adler, D. A., Berlant, J., Dixon, L., First, M. B., Oslin, D. W., Siris, S. G., & Talley, R. M. (2023). Addressing the increasing mental health distress and mental illness among young adults in the United States. *The Journal of Nervous and Mental Disease*, *211*(12), 961–967. https://doi.org/10.1097/NMD.0000000000001734

Cackovic, C., Nazir, S., & Marwaha, R. (2023). Panic disorder. In: *StatPearls [Internet]*. StatPearls Publishing. https://www.ncbi.nlm.nih.gov/books/NBK430973

Cho, Y., Kim, H., Seong, S., Park, K., Choi, J., Kim, M. J., Kim, D., & Jeon, H. J. (2024). Effect of virtual reality-based biofeedback for depressive and anxiety symptoms: Randomized controlled study. *Journal of Affective Disorders, 361*, 392–398. https://doi.org/10.1016/j.jad.2024.06.031

Crisp, Z. C., & Grant, J. E. (2024). Impulsivity across psychiatric disorders in young adults. *Comprehensive Psychiatry, 130*, 152449. https://doi.org/10.1016/j.comppsych.2023.152449

Docherty, C., McPeake, J., Quasim, T., MacTavish, P., Devine, H., O'Brien, P., Strachan, L., Lucie, P., Hogg, L., Sim, M., & Shaw, M. (2023). The relationship between pain, anxiety and depression in patients with post-intensive care syndrome. *Journal of Critical Care, 78*, 154359. https://doi.org/10.1016/j.jcrc.2023.154359

Forstner, A. J., Awasthi, S., Wolf, C., Maron, E., Erhardt, A., Czamara, D., Eriksson, E., Lavebratt, C., Allgulander, C., Friedrich, N., Becker, J., Hecker, J., Rambau, S., Conrad, R., Geiser, F., McMahon, F. J., Moebus, S., Hess, T., Buerfent, B. C., … Hoffmann, P. (2021). Genome-wide association study of panic disorder reveals genetic overlap with neuroticism and depression. *Molecular Psychiatry, 26*(8), 4179–4190. https://doi.org/10.1038/s41380-019-0590-2

Gonzales, G., & McKay, T. (2024). Negative LGBTQ+ news media means bad news for LGBTQ+ young adult mental health. *JAMA Pediatrics, 178*(11), 1101–1103. https://doi.org/10.1001/jamapediatrics.2024.3130

Gros, D. F., Pavlacic, J. M., Wray, J. M., & Szafranski, D. D. (2023). Investigating relations between the symptoms of panic, agoraphobia, and suicidal ideation: The Significance of comorbid depressive symptoms in veterans with panic disorder. *Journal of Psychopathology and Behavioral Assessment, 45*, 1154–1162. https://doi.org/10.1007/s10862-023-10082-4

Hamilton, M. (1959). The assessment of anxiety states by rating. *British Journal of Medical Psychology, 32*(1), 50–55.

Han, X., Shen, Q., Hou, C., Yang, H., Chen, W., Zeng, Y., Qu, Y., Suo, C., Ye, W., Fang, F., Valdimarsdóttir, U. A., & Song, H. (2024). Disease clusters subsequent to anxiety and stress-related disorders and their genetic determinants. *Nature Communications, 15*(1), 1209. https://doi.org/10.1038/s41467-024-45445-2

Holubova, M., Prasko, J., Vanek, J., Hodny, F., Nesnidal, V., Kasalova, P., Slepecky, M., & Kolek, A. (2021). Self-stigma, severity of psychopathology, dissociation, parental style and comorbid personality disorder in patient with neurotic spectrum disorders Part 1: Relationships between self-stigma and clinical, psychosocial and demograph. *Neuro Endocrinology Letters, 42*(2), 99–112.

Kempinski G. A. (2024). Creating LGBTQIA+-inclusive health care as a supportive care strategy. *Clinical Journal of Oncology Nursing, 28*(4), 342–349. https://doi.org/10.1188/24.CJON.342-349

Khazanov, G. K., Wolk, C. B., Lorenc, E., Candon, M., Pieri, M. F., Oslin, D. W., Press, M. J., Anderson, E., Famiglio, E., & Jager-Hyman, S. (2024). Change in suicidal ideation, depression, and anxiety following collaborative care in the community. *BMC Primary Care, 25*(1), 241. https://doi.org/10.1186/s12875-024-02494-2

Kim, H. J., Kim, J., Yook, K. H., Choi, T. K., & Lee, S. H. (2023). Early trauma subtypes are differentially related to anxiety symptomatology and suicidal ideation in panic disorder. *Psychiatry Investigation, 20*(12), 1211–1220. https://doi.org/10.30773/pi.2023.0371

López-Cepero, A. A., Spruill, T., Suglia, S. F., Lewis, T. T., Mazzitelli, N., Pérez, C. M., & Rosal, M. C. (2024). Shift-and-persist strategies as a potential protective factor against symptoms of psychological distress among young adults in Puerto Rico. *Social Psychiatry and Psychiatric Epidemiology, 59*(8), 1357–1365. https://doi.org/10.1007/s00127-023-02601-1

MacKay, M., Yang, B. H., Dursun, S. M., & Baker, G. B. (2024). The gut-brain axis and the microbiome in anxiety disorders, post-traumatic stress disorder and obsessive-compulsive disorder. *Current Neuropharmacology, 22*(5), 866–883. https://doi.org/10.2174/1570159X21666230222092029

Mason, E. C., Gaston, J. E., Pestell, C. F., & Page, A. C. (2022). A comprehensive group-based cognitive behavioural treatment for blood-injection-injury phobia. *The British Journal of Clinical Psychology, 61*(2), 494–509. https://doi.org/10.1111/bjc.12345

McEvoy, D., Brannigan, R., Cooke, L., Butler, E., Walsh, C., Arensman, E., & Clarke, M. (2023). Risk and protective factors for self-harm in adolescents and young adults: An umbrella review of systematic reviews. *Journal of Psychiatric Research, 168*, 353–380. https://doi.org/10.1016/j.jpsychires.2023.10.017

Moraes, A. C. N., Wijaya, C., Freire, R., Quagliato, L. A., Nardi, A. E., & Kyriakoulis, P. (2024). Neurochemical and genetic factors in panic disorder: A systematic review. *Translational Psychiatry, 14*(1), 294. https://doi.org/10.1038/s41398-024-02966-0

Nowak, J., Nikendei, C., Rollmann, I., Orth, M., Friederich, H.-C., & Kindermann, D. (2023). Characterization of different types of anxiety disorders in relation to structural integration of personality and adverse and protective childhood experiences in psychotherapy outpatients—a cross-sectional study. *BMC Psychiatry, 23*(1), 501. https://doi.org/10.1186/s12888-023-04988-2

Öğüt, Ç. (2024). Reflection impulsivity in patients with panic disorder. *Anxiety, Stress, and Coping, 38*(2), 234–246. https://doi.org/10.1080/10615806.2024.2393207

Oh, D. H., Park, D. H., Ryu, S. H., Ha, J. H., & Jeon, H. J. (2021). Psychological predictors of bipolarity in panic disorder. *World Journal of Psychiatry, 11*(6), 242–252. https://doi.org/10.5498/wjp.v11.i6.242

Pace, M., Heckendorn, M., Aouizerate, B., Hanon, C., Seigneurie, A. S., Lavaud, P., Hozer, F., Raykeer, R. P., Guerin-Langlois, C., Cormier, L., Raucourt, H. P., Limosin, F., & Hoertel, N. (2021). Management of panic disorder in the elderly. *Geriatrie et Psychologie Neuropsychiatrie du Vieillissement*. https://doi.org/10.1684/pnv.2021.0965

Peplau, H. (1989). Theoretic constructs: Anxiety, self, and hallucinations. In A. O'Toole & S. Welt (Eds.), *Interpersonal theory in nursing practice: Selected works of Hildegarde E. Peplau*. Springer.

Quagliato, L. A., & Nardi, A. E. (2023). The interplay between sexual abuse and inflammation, oxidative stress, and DNA damage in drug-naïve panic disorder patients. *Molecular Psychiatry, 28*(7), 2995–3001. https://doi.org/10.1038/s41380-023-02086-z

Remmerswaal, K. C. P., Ten Have, M., de Graaf, R., van Balkom, A. J. L. M., Penninx, B. W. J. H., & Batelaan, N. M. (2024). Risk factors of chronic course of anxiety and depressive disorders: a 3-year longitudinal study in the general population. *Social Psychiatry and Psychiatric Epidemiology, 59*(9), 1607–1615. https://doi.org/10.1007/s00127-023-02591-0

Rose, G. M., & Tadi, P. (2022). Social anxiety disorder. In *StatPearls*. StatPearls Publishing. www.ncbi.nlm.nih.gov/books/NBK555890

Roth-Rawald, J., Maaß, U., Mai, S., & Weck, F. (2023). Exposure therapy for health anxiety: Effectiveness and response rates in routine care of an outpatient clinic. *Journal of Clinical Psychology, 79*(12), 2884–2898. https://doi.org/10.1002/jclp.23587

Schröder, D., Wrona, K. J., Müller, F., Heinemann, S., Fischer, F., & Dockweiler, C. (2023). Impact of virtual reality applications in the treatment of anxiety disorders: A systematic review and meta-analysis of randomized-controlled trials. *Journal of Behavior Therapy and Experimental Psychiatry, 81*, 101893. https://doi.org/10.1016/j.jbtep.2023.101893

Seetharaman, R., Avhad, S., & Rane, J. (2024). Exploring the healing power of singing bowls: An overview of key findings and potential benefits. *Explore, 20*(1), 39–43. https://doi.org/10.1016/j.explore.2023.07.007

Shechter Strulov, T., & Aderka, I. M. (2024). Dating in social anxiety disorder: A daily diary study. *Journal of Anxiety Disorders, 107*, 102927. https://doi.org/10.1016/j.janxdis.2024.102927

Shi, K., Li, J., Zhang, H., Wang, K., Li, C., Xia, Y., Tian, T., Li, Y., Peng, X., & Yang, Y. (2024). The functional and structural alterations in brain regions related to the fear network model in panic disorder: A resting-state fMRI and T1-weighted imaging study. *Journal of Psychiatric Research, 177*, 59–65. https://doi.org/10.1016/j.jpsychires.2024.06.038

Smith, N. S., Bauer, B. W., & Capron, D. W. (2022). Comparing symptom networks of daytime and nocturnal panic attacks in a community-based sample. *Journal of Anxiety Disorders, 85*, 102514. https://doi.org/10.1016/j.janxdis.2021.102514

Surace, T., Buoli, M., Affaticati, L. M., Esposito, G., Capuzzi, E., Colzani, L., La Tegola, D., Biagi, E., Colmegna, F., Caldiroli, A., & Clerici, M. (2024). Which clinical factors delay proper treatment in panic disorder? A cross-sectional multicentric study. *Early Intervention in Psychiatry, 18*(8), 633–641. https://doi.org/10.1111/eip.13506

Tunnell, N. C., Corner, S. E., Roque, A. D., Kroll, J. L., Ritz, T., & Meuret, A. E. (2024). Biobehavioral approach to distinguishing panic symptoms from medical illness. *Frontiers in Psychiatry, 15*, 1296569. https://doi.org/10.3389/fpsyt.2024.1296569

Vickery, A. (2022). "It's made me feel less isolated because there are other people who are experiencing the same or very similar to you": Men's experiences of using mental health support groups. *Health & Social Care in the Community, 30*(6), 2383–2391. https://doi.org/10.1111/hsc.13788

Yadla, V. S., Nj, P., Kamarthy, P., & Matti, M. R. (2024). Effect of integrated yoga as an adjuvant to standard care for panic disorder: A randomized control trial study. *Cureus, 16*(1), e53286. https://doi.org/10.7759/cureus.53286

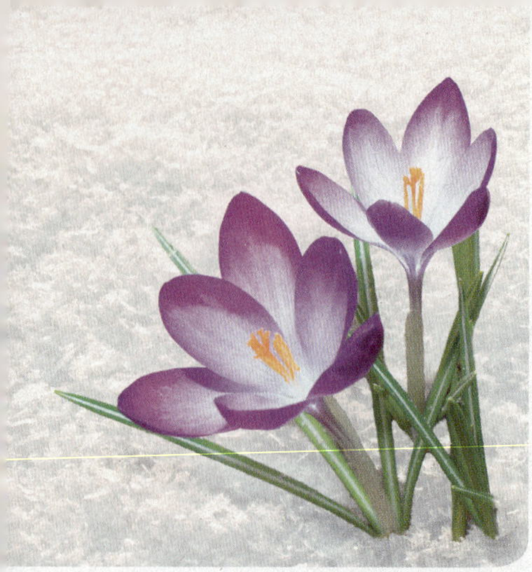

28 Obsessive-Compulsive and Related Disorders

Nursing Care of People With Obsessions and Compulsions

Patricia E. Freed

KEYCONCEPTS

- compulsions
- obsessions

LEARNING OBJECTIVES

After studying this chapter, you will be able to:

1. Explain the role of obsessions and compulsions in obsessive-compulsive disorder.
2. Relate the primary theories of obsessive-compulsive disorders to clinical symptoms and the course of the disorder.
3. Evaluate the significance of trauma in the appearance of obsessive-compulsive symptoms.
4. Examine the relationship between social determinants of health and obsessive-compulsive disorder.
5. Select strategies to establish a therapeutic relationship with people with obsessive-compulsive disorder.
6. Using a clinical judgment model, formulate a person-centered, recovery-oriented nursing care plan for people with obsessive-compulsive disorder.
7. Identify medications and therapies that are used to treat people with obsessive-compulsive disorder and evaluate their effectiveness.
8. Develop wellness strategies for people with obsessive-compulsive disorder.
9. Compare and contrast mental health care provided in emergency, inpatient, community, and virtual settings.
10. Support the integration of health and mental health care for people with obsessive-compulsive disorder
11. Compare and contrast other obsessive-compulsive and related disorders.

KEY TERMS

• acceptance and commitment therapy (ACT) • circumferential speech • cognitive-behavioral therapy • cyberchondria • dissociative absorption • ego-dystonic • ego-syntonic • excoriation • exposure and response prevention (ERP) • family accommodation • family map • isolation • mental contamination • mindfulness-based cognitive therapy • minority stress • OCD religious beliefs • pathologic doubt • reaction formation • religiosity • rituals • scrupulosity • subclinical symptoms • third-wave therapies • undoing

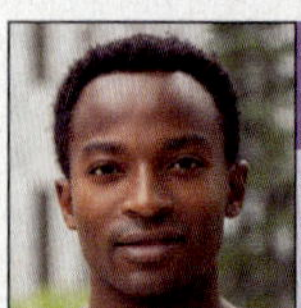

Case Study: Tim

Tim, a 32-year-old engineer, was diagnosed with OCD as a teenager when his obsession with cleanliness and compulsively washing his hands interfered with his friendships and school work.

INTRODUCTION

Most of us experience times when we are preoccupied with specific thoughts or ideas. Many also find that routines or *rituals* are important in organizing our work and home life. When these preoccupations and rituals interfere with daily life, they become atypical and may represent symptoms of a mental disorder. This chapter explains obsessions and compulsions and their role in obsessive-compulsive disorders (OCD). OCD is highlighted in this chapter.

OBSESSIONS AND COMPULSIONS

When thoughts become preoccupying, excessive, intrusive, or unwanted, and begin to interfere with daily functioning, such thoughts are considered to be obsessions.

> **KEYCONCEPT Obsessions** are excessive, unwanted, intrusive, and persistent thoughts, impulses, or images that cause anxiety and distress. Obsessions are not under the individual's control and are inconsistent with the individual's usual thought patterns.

Common obsessions include fears of contamination, fear of losing or misplacing something, the need for symmetry and completion, thoughts of hurting someone, and sexual-based thoughts or images.

Routines are a part of everyday life. Getting up in the morning at the same time and going to work or school structures our lives and helps us be productive. When routines become ritualistic and interfere with daily activities, they become compulsions.

> **KEYCONCEPT Compulsions** are repetitive behaviors and mental acts performed in a ritualistic fashion with the goal of preventing or relieving anxiety and distress caused by obsessions.

For example, making sure a stove is turned off before leaving the house can be a safety routine, but being late for work because of making several trips to the stove before leaving the house is a compulsion. Common compulsions include handwashing, excessive cleaning, checking, arranging things, counting, ordering, and hoarding. See Table 28.1.

OBSESSIVE-COMPULSIVE AND RELATED DISORDERS OVERVIEW

Obsessions and compulsions are characteristic of obsessive-compulsive and related disorders. These disorders include OCD, trichotillomania (i.e., compulsively pulling out one's hair), excoriation disorder (skin picking), body dysmorphic disorder (BDD; perceived flaws or defects in one's physical appearance), and hoarding disorder (excessive accumulation and/or difficulty discarding possessions). These disorders are closely related to anxiety disorders (American Psychiatric Association [APA], 2022).

OBSESSIVE-COMPULSIVE DISORDER

In OCD, affected people may have both obsessions and compulsions and believe that they have no control over them. Because of the nature of the disorder, nurses who work in settings other than psychiatric settings or in-home health care may be among the first to identify an individual's symptoms as OCD and make the appropriate referrals. Many individuals have good or fair insight regarding the accuracy of their beliefs. However, some show an absence of insight, similar to

TABLE 28.1 COMMON OBSESSIONS, COMPULSIONS, AND CONSEQUENCES

Obsession	Compulsion	Individual Consequences	Impact on Family Functioning
Fear of germs and contamination	Excessive cleaning or handwashing	Skin irritation, social isolation	Disrupts family routine
Fear of forgetting, losing, or misplacing something	Repeatedly checking things, such as that the door is locked, or the oven is off	Anxiety and worry. Unable to get to work, school on time.	Family frustration and disruption of routines
Fear of losing control over one's behavior	Focusing on maintaining safety, such as avoiding knives or sharp objects	Social isolation. Avoidance of activities related to objects triggering fear	Prevents family from participating in routine activities
Aggressive thoughts toward others or oneself	Avoiding others	Fear of hurting someone or self	Disrupts family social activities
Unwanted, forbidden, or taboo thoughts involving sex, religion, or harm	Praying, repeating words	Guilt, shame. Excessive religious behavior	Family members may distance themselves from individual
Desire to have things symmetrical or in perfect order	Ordering or arranging things in a particular, precise way	Anxiety and frustration	Irritation of family members

Source: National Institute of Mental Health. (2023). Obsessive-Compulsive Disorder: when unwanted thoughts or repetitive behaviors take over. NIH Publication No. 23-MH-4676. U.S. Department of Health and human Services. https://www.nimh.nih.gov/health/publications/obsessive-compulsive-disorder-when-unwanted-thoughts-or-repetitive-behaviors-take-over

delusional beliefs, which has been linked to worse long-term outcomes (APA, 2022). Though obsessive beliefs may be irrational, they are not as fixed and unyielding as delusions, and insight regarding these beliefs may change over the course of the disorder. Symptoms of OCD are often less severe than those in delusional disorder, and individuals with OCD generally have higher levels of educational attainment and experience higher quality of life (QoL) than those with delusional disorders.

Although it may seem that some symptoms of OCD overlap with obsessive-compulsive personality disorder (OCPD), they are separate disorders. OCPD is discussed in Chapter 30.

CLINICAL COURSE

OCD follows a chronic waxing and waning course. Symptoms of OCD often begin in childhood, but many receive treatment only after the disorder has significantly affected their lives. In preschool-age children, OCD is often misdiagnosed as separation anxiety disorder (Haque et al., 2023). Onset in early or middle childhood is associated with a better outcome than later onset (Schuyler & Geller, 2023).

Individuals with OCD may become incapacitated by their symptoms. They may even become unable to complete a task as simple as walking through a door without performing rituals. Interpersonal relationships suffer, and the individual may actively isolate and withdraw from contact with others. Individuals with OCD often engage in **dissociative absorption**, a tendency to become excessively absorbed in fantasy (movies, online gaming), leading to decreased self-awareness, and inattention to their surroundings.

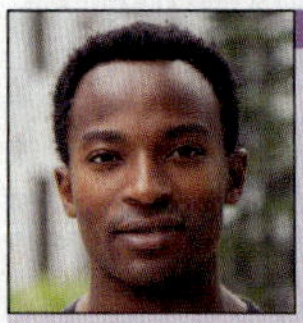

Remember Tim?

When Tim was in high school, he was unable to eat at the school cafeteria because he was afraid the other students' germs would contaminate his food. He avoided touching doorknobs and would wash his hands for 3 minutes if he inadvertently touched a doorknob.

DIAGNOSTIC CRITERIA

OCD is diagnosed when recurrent obsessions or compulsions (or both) take up more than 1 hour a day or cause considerable stress to the individual. These obsessions or compulsions are not caused by substance or medication use or other disorders. Some individuals recognize that these obsessions or compulsions are excessive and unrealistic; others have limited insight and are unsure whether the obsessive thoughts are true but continue to have the thoughts and feel compelled to perform the actions. Another group of individuals are convinced that their obsessive thoughts are true. These thoughts and compulsive behaviors are stressful and interfere with usual daily routines.

Obsessions

Mental contamination, an internal, diffuse feeling of dirtiness, infection, or impurity in the absence of contact with an external source (Millar et al., 2023) provides the bases for understanding many obsessional thoughts. Fear of contamination is the most common obsession, usually focuses on dirt or germs, but other materials may be feared as well, such as toxic chemicals, poisons, radiation, or exposures to heavy metals. Although most individuals experience their obsessive thoughts as **ego-dystonic** (unacceptable thoughts), there are varying degrees of insight involved. Poor insight is correlated with symptom severity and schizotypal personality traits (see Chapter 30) (Ottoni et al., 2023) and although still investigational, may be associated with different subtypes of OCD (de Avila et al., 2023). **Scrupulosity** is a specific OCD dimension in which obsessions center on religious or morally intrusive thoughts, followed by repetitive actions, such as going to confession or repeatedly asking for forgiveness or assurance. These types of obsessions clearly exceed cultural or religious norms, interfere with social obligations, and may appear at inappropriate times (Wetterneck et al., 2021).

Compulsions

Compulsions are performed to relieve the anxiety created by the obsession. Compulsions are repetitive, purposeful acts, or mental actions (such as counting), that the individual feels compelled to perform in accordance with an internal rule. Excessive washing, counting, checking, hoarding, asking for reassurance, and following strict inflexible routines may indicate the presence of a compulsion.

Rituals are common compulsions in which objects must be in a certain order, motor activities are performed in a rigid fashion, or things must be arranged in perfect symmetry. A ritualized behavior may be driven by obsessive thoughts or may be attributed to a distinctive urge that creates tension and pressure throughout the body. A ritual consumes a great deal of time to complete, interfering with even the simplest task.

Cyberchondria, characterized by excessive online searching for health information, is under investigation as another type of compulsive behavior. Excessive searching might provide some temporary reassurance while leading to ever-worsening anxiety and distress (Thomas, 2023).

Concept Mastery Alert

Although worries about contamination and germs or catching infectious diseases are common and took on new urgency during the COVID-19 pandemic, these actions undertaken with sensible guidance and restraint are not to be confused with pathologic compulsions.

OBSESSIVE-COMPULSIVE DISORDER ACROSS THE LIFESPAN

Although OCD is relatively common, it is still underrecognized and undertreated. OCD affects people of all ages. Identification, diagnosis, and treatment of OCD are necessary for recovery and optimal functioning.

Children and Adolescents

Obsessions and compulsions in children are more likely to change/evolve as well as to wax and wane, compared to the course of the disorder in adults. Typically, parents/caregivers notice that a child's grades begin to fall as a result of decreased concentration and a great amount of time spent performing rituals. Children often have at least one other mental disorder and are less likely than adults to recognize the irrationality of their symptoms.

Older Adults

Among older adults, OCD most likely began in childhood, but there are some older adults whose onset (beginning of individual distress and interference in work, family, and social activities associated with obsessions and compulsions) began later in life. In the older adult, continuing symptoms are linked to higher rates of depression and poorer mental and social functioning. Older adults who engage in checking compulsions and hoarding may have more thought disturbances and communication difficulties than those who engage in other types of compulsive behaviors (Nutley et al., 2024; Box 28.1).

BOX 28.1

Clinical Judgment Vignette: Obsessive-Compulsive Disorder in an Older Adult

Louise, a 76-year-old retired accountant, resides in an assisted living complex with her husband. Always very neat and organized, she recently began cleaning excessively, sometimes in the middle of the night. She developed a routine where she had to have everything cleaned before she could eat because of her fears of germs. Her husband expressed his concern to their primary care provider, who referred them to a geriatric psychiatrist. A diagnosis of OCD was made. Louise recognizes that her behavior has changed and is interfering with her life but says she gets too nervous if she does not conduct her routine.

Building Clinical Judgment

1. What are the behaviors that indicate that Louise has OCD symptoms?
   Answer: The behaviors that indicate that Louise has OCD symptoms are her cleaning in the middle of the night and needing to have everything cleaned before she eats.
2. What are the obsessive symptoms of OCD that Louise is experiencing?
   Answer: She experiences anxiety if she does not conduct her routine and she is fearful of germs.

EPIDEMIOLOGY AND RISK FACTORS

The lifetime prevalence of OCD among US adults over 18 was 2.3%, with slightly higher rates in people assigned female at birth during adolescence and adulthood (Brock et al., 2024). Identifying those at risk for more rapid symptom escalation may lessen the heavy public health burden of this chronic disorder for the more than 60 million people in the United States who experience OCD symptoms without meeting the formal criteria for diagnosis (Beyond OCD, 2023a). In most people, this chronic condition is associated with moderate to severe disability and carries a heavy health burden for the patient and family.

Age of Onset

The onset of the illness has a bimodal peak—in early adolescence and early adulthood (Vriend et al., 2024). Diagnosis over the age of 35 is unusual (APA, 2022), necessitating careful assessment for other serious causes. **Subclinical symptoms** (mental or emotional issues that are not severe enough to be considered diagnosable symptoms), are common in children and may not lead to a formal diagnosis of OCD, but they may still be troubling and may contribute to some level of impairment. In most cases, OCD develops gradually and an abrupt onset or overnight eruption of obsessive or compulsive symptoms following an infection in a toddler may herald an infection-triggered autoimmune encephalopathy.

Sex Assigned at Birth

Adults assigned male at birth (referred to as "male" hereafter in this section) have an earlier onset and greater symptom severity than adults assigned female at birth (referred to as "female" hereafter in this section), though OCD is slightly more common in adult females (APA, 2022; Benatti et al., 2022; Vellozo et al., 2021). Differences in age of onset may be associated with comorbid disorders, such that males are more strongly affected by comorbid developmental disorders like tic and autistic spectrum disorder, whereas OCD in females is influenced more by life events (marriage, pregnancy, and childbirth) and by comorbid mood or anxiety disorders (Vismara et al., 2024).

There are also considerable variations in symptom pattern presentation. For instance, more females have symptoms in the cleaning dimension and more males report symptoms in the symmetry and forbidden (taboo) thought dimension (APA, 2022). New guidelines compiled based on expert opinions and mothers' experience living with OCD, resulted in a novel presentation of best practices for OCD (Mulcahy et al., 2023). One notable highlight was agreement between mothers and the panel of experts on the importance of assessing whether infant-harming obsessions were experienced as **ego-syntonic** (agreeable to self) or ego-dystonic (unwanted, alien to self), because this would be essential information for treatment planning. Sex assigned at birth appears to be a fundamental contributor to OCD variation and severity, and a substantial number of females with OCD are at risk for OCD symptom exacerbation during pregnancy and should be closely monitored (Holingue et al., 2021).

LGBTQ+ Individuals and OCD

LGBTQ+ individuals with OCD face additional challenges and unique stressors when compared with their straight, cisgender peers. LGBTQ+ individuals are subjected to discrimination and violence that leads to vigilance, identity concealment, and discomfort. These experiences result in minority stress and are related to increased susceptibility to mental health issues (Pinciotti et al., 2022) and higher rates of mental health disorders than cisgender adults (Bedford et al., 2023). In fact, OCD may be more prevalent than other mental health disorders in this population because obsessions and compulsions around stigma and shame are perpetuated by the accumulation of identity-based stressors (Pinciotti & Orcutt, 2021). **Minority stress** takes many forms, including internalized stigma and self-hate, rejection and discrimination, microaggressions such as bullying and shaming, and keeping secrets and isolating—all of which make it difficult for the individual to seek help, despite the fact that early diagnosis and treatment minimizes severity and level of disability. See Box 28.2.

There may also be differences in symptom presentation, with LGBTQ+ individuals experiencing more severe obsessive-compulsive symptoms and troubling themes around violence, sex, or religion (Pinciotti & Orcutt, 2021). Taboo thoughts should be recognized as an independent risk for suicidality in those with OCD (Cervin et al., 2022). Although all types of obsessional thinking can be disabling, sexual obsessions threaten one's fundamental identity as a social–sexual being. For people questioning their emerging sexual identities, dysphoric thoughts about sexuality may be troubling enough to create doubt and confusion, for which the individual may want help. Being able to attain help from a reliable therapist or clinician who understands sexuality and gender issues is of the utmost importance. A gender-affirming health provider helps the individual sort through confusion about sexuality and helps the client manage troubling obsessional sexual thoughts in a safe, nonjudgmental environment. Finding both a gender-affirming therapist and a qualified, certified expert in OCD therapies is challenging.

Additional barriers to treatment within the LGBTQ+ community may arise because of an individual's youth, a person's inability to afford or access treatment, or because of fear of negative family or community reactions to disclosure (Trondsen, 2021).

BOX 28.2

Mental Health Inequities: Obsessive-Compulsive Disorder and Minority Stress

As a result of discrimination and violence, individuals with OCD and related disorders are subjected to minority stress, which may lead to vigilance, identity concealment, and discomfort. LGBTQ+ individuals may internalize self-stigma and low self-esteem. Historically, behavioral treatment of sexual orientation and gender-themed obsessive-compulsive behavior reinforced anti-LGBTQ+ stigma and contributed to minority stress. Contemporary treatment recommendations include eliminating exposures that reinforce negative stereotypes and replacing them with neutral and positive stimuli and exposures to uncertainty and core fears. Psychoeducation about LGBTQ+ identities is also an important recommended aspect of treatment.

Source: Pinciotti, C. M., Smith, Z., Singh, S., Wetterneck, C. T., & Williams, M. T. (2022). Call to Action: Recommendations for justice-based treatment of obsessive-compulsive disorder with sexual orientation and gender themes. *Behavior Therapy*, *53*(2), 153–169. https://doi.org/10.1016/j.beth.2021.11.001

Family, Ethnicity, and Culture

Culture, ethnic, and family beliefs shape the perception of OCD and influence the treatment of this disorder. Symptoms are interpreted and manifested within culturally accepted norms. At times, cultural or religious beliefs and practices may be misunderstood and mistaken for obsessions or compulsions. These beliefs and actions must be evaluated in the context of the individual's culture. If these beliefs are consistent with the patient's social, family, or cultural environment; are not harmful to the individual or others; and do not interfere with individual functioning in that environment, they should not be considered symptoms of OCD (Morris et al., 2024).

COMORBIDITY

High rates of comorbid conditions can be found in populations with OCD, most commonly, anxiety disorders, mood disorders, and other related OCDs (Singh et al., 2023). Having any comorbid condition is associated with a longer course of illness, and having two or more contributes to symptom severity and chronicity. Worsening levels of suicidality (thoughts) and suicide attempts are related to the severity of comorbid depression, anxiety and obsessive symptoms, feeling hopeless and to having a history of suicide attempts (Fernández de la Cruz et al., 2024).

OCD and eating disorders (EDs), such as anorexia and bulimia, are highly comorbid and share similarities such as obsessional thinking, ritualized behaviors, and perfectionism (Di Luzio et al., 2024). The presence of an ED complicates the treatment of OCD. In both disorders, individuals have difficulty controlling their thoughts. In OCD, there is difficulty controlling obsessional thoughts and in EDs, there is weight overvaluation, fear of loss of control, and concerns that others will see them eating (Di Luzio et al., 2024).

More than half of children with OCD have one or more comorbid conditions. Though understudied, Tics/Tourette syndrome, attention-deficit hyperactivity disorder (ADHD), and OCD frequently occur together. Symptom severity of each disorder decreases with age (Schuyler & Geller, 2023).

Obsessive-compulsive symptoms are common in people who have migraines and in individuals with schizophrenia, who are experiencing anxiety, mood symptoms, and psychosis. Although treatable, when obsessive-compulsive symptoms appear along with schizophrenia, they often go unrecognized and remain untreated (Singh et al., 2023).

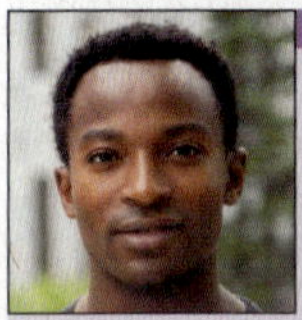

Consider This

As a child, Tim frequently went to the school nurse about multiple physical symptoms. Later, he was unable to engage in sexual relations with a long-time girlfriend because the thought of the sex act made him feel nauseous, and twice he experienced severe vomiting. At the time, he sought emergency treatment, but ultimately no physical reason was discovered.

ETIOLOGY

During the 1990s, research evidence from neuroimaging studies, neurochemical studies, and treatment advances substantiated a predominantly neurobiologic basis for OCD. The following sections provide a brief overview of these findings and evidence pointing to genetic vulnerability. Psychological factors are also discussed because of their contributions to the disorder. Because no single explanation accounts for all aspects of OCD, a combination of factors will probably be found to produce the disorder.

Biologic Theories

Genetic, neuropathologic, and biochemical research, reviewed in this section, suggests that OCD has a biologic basis involving several neuroanatomic structures.

Genetic Factors

Family and twin studies demonstrate that OCD is a multifactorial familial condition that involves multiple genes and environmental risk factors (Blanco-Vieira et al., 2023). OCD occurs more often in people who have first-degree relatives with OCD or with Tourette syndrome than it does in the general population. There appears to be an elevated risk of suicide attempts among the relatives of those with OCD, and the odds increase with closer relationships (Sidorchuk et al., 2021).

Neuropathologic Theories

Currently, OCD is conceptualized as a dysfunction of brain networks that manage fear-related information (Jalal et al., 2023). Individuals with OCD realize their behavior does not make sense but are unable to stop it. With increasing advances in studying the neurocircuitry of OCD, it is possible that future pharmacologic treatments can be designed to target involved brain circuits (Zrenner et al., 2023).

Biochemical Theories

Biochemical theories address imbalances of chemicals in the brain, but there is no persuasive evidence that any mental illness is caused by a single biochemical imbalance. There is strong evidence that drugs that increase the levels of serotonin in the brain have antiobsessional effects, and these studies have been used to support the role of serotonin dysregulation in OCD. However, other neurotransmitters (such as dopamine, glutamate, and GABA) imbalances have been identified (Jalal et al., 2023).

Psychological and Psychosocial Theories

Although psychological theories of OCD have not been scientifically tested, the rich literature describing clinical examples and case histories helps us understand the symptoms and behaviors related to OCD. In addition, behavioral treatment of individuals with severe compulsions improves symptoms. Cognitive-behavioral therapy (CBT), which should be considered in every treatment plan, is associated with lower relapse rates (Singh et al., 2023).

Psychosocial Theories

Psychosocial factors are known to have precipitating and maintaining effects on OCD (Hühne et al., 2024). Evidence-based treatments, particular for children and adolescents, within the context of family-focused or group formats are still offered, largely coupled with some variant of CBT. Although promising, more research is needed to establish the effectiveness of including interpersonal therapies or treatment programs designed to improve resilience, interpersonal relations, and coping (Di Salvo et al., 2024).

Psychodynamic Factors

The psychodynamic theory hypothesizes that OCD symptoms and character traits arise from three unconscious defense mechanisms: **isolation** (separation of affect from a thought or impulse), **undoing** (an act performed with the goal of preventing consequences of a thought or impulse), and **reaction formation** (behavior and consciously stated attitudes that oppose underlying impulses). Classic psychoanalytic theory describes OCD as regression from the oedipal phase to the anal phase of development, which includes preoccupations with anger and dirt (see Chapter 6). This regression occurs when the patient becomes anxious about retaliation or loss of love.

Behavioral Factors

Behavioral explanations for OCD stem from learning theory. From this viewpoint, obsessions are seen as conditioned stimuli. Compulsions develop as the individual discovers behaviors that successfully reduce the obsessional anxiety. The more the behaviors decrease the anxiety, the more likely the individual is to continue using them. Carefully interrupting this cycle is the focus of behavioral therapy in treating an individual with OCD. Nurses often use behavioral approaches to reinforce and encourage acceptable behaviors, to set limits, and to impose structure on the environment to make people feel safe, which can reduce anxiety and confusion.

FAMILY RESPONSE TO OBSESSIVE-COMPULSIVE DISORDER

OCD poses a considerable caregiving burden on families, which is heightened by severe symptoms, functional impairment, and comorbid psychopathologies in the patient or caregiver (Swisher et al., 2023). Caregivers are overwhelmed trying to find therapists, to book appointments and arrange schedules, and to pay for services, and their inability to find therapists and pay for services adds considerable guilt and stress for them (Frank et al., 2023). To maintain their own mental well-being, caregivers are likely to look to the nurse for resources for support and respite, as well as for knowledge of how to navigate the health care system.

Family assessment reveals the need for education and support and begins the partnership with the individual, family, and treatment team. The nurse can evaluate the family's understanding of the disorder and of proposed treatments with targeted questions. Is the family able and willing to help the patient practice cognitive and behavioral techniques? Is the family knowledgeable about prescribed medicines? These questions offer an opportunity for individual and family education.

Families often accommodate a family member's obsessive-compulsive symptoms in a variety of ways, such as taking part in rituals, contributing to ritual performance, contributing to avoidance, and/or by modifying their own daily routines around the compulsive behavior. **Family accommodation** is often done with good intentions, but high levels of accommodation are associated with negative effects for both family members and for the individual with OCD (Hermida-Barros et al., 2024). Standardized assessment tools such as the Family Accommodation Scale (FAS-SR) parental version, or the recently developed adult-patient rated questionnaire, the Family Accommodation Scale for OCD-Patient Version (FAS-PV), which examines family accommodation from the patient's perspective (La Buissonnière-Ariza et al., 2022), can be used to objectively assess the level of family accommodation.

Engaging with the family to build rapport, empathy, and respect coupled with a thorough investigation of family accommodation helps nurses plan care aimed at reducing the family's level of accommodation and replacing it with the promotion of autonomy and independence in the member with OCD. This can be achieved via family psychoeducation, helping the family offer emotional support to the member with OCD, and by encouraging the family to cooperate fully with the health care team. A helpful strategy for families trying to reduce their accommodating behavior is to help them develop a **family map**, which outlines specific behaviors family members can use to disengage from accommodation to specific compulsive behaviors. This plan can be developed mutually by the nurse and all family members and allows the individual with OCD to take on more responsibilities while reducing the caregiver's duties (Beyond OCD, 2023b).

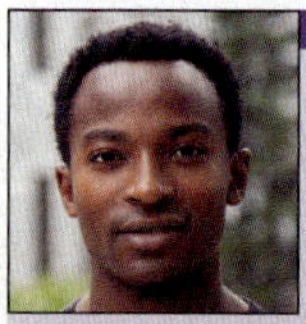

Tim's Family

Tim's parents recognized their son had unusual behaviors that interfered with his growth and development. When he was in high school, his parents took him to a psychiatrist who prescribed medication and offered brief counseling. Tim was able to successfully complete high school with honors and was accepted into a highly respected college. He was able to function when taking medications.

RECOVERY-ORIENTED CARE FOR PEOPLE WITH OBSESSIVE-COMPULSIVE DISORDER

Teamwork and Collaboration: Working Toward Recovery

OCD can be difficult to treat because obsessions and compulsions consistently interfere with recovery efforts. First-line treatments of OCD are **cognitive-behavioral**

therapy (see Chapter 13), exposure and response prevention therapy (ERP) (see discussion later in this chapter for more details), and medications (ADAA, 2021). Prolonged CBT or ERP treatment combined with selective serotonin reuptake inhibitors (SSRIs) is the most effective treatment (Brock et al., 2024). The overall goals for recovery are a decrease in symptoms, improvement of physical and mental health, and an improved QoL.

Staff may have differing opinions about the amount of control the individual has over the behavior, but these differences of opinion must be resolved. All staff must be consistent in their expectations and acceptance of the patient's behaviors to keep these patients from becoming frustrated or confused regarding expectations during treatment (see Box 28.3).

Electroconvulsive Therapy

The role of electroconvulsive therapy (ECT) in the treatment of OCD is unclear, and its effectiveness is limited (Li et al., 2022). ECT is used when there is limited or no response to other treatments and the patient is acutely symptomatic. Nursing's role in caring for the individual undergoing ECT is outlined in Chapter 11.

Transcranial Magnetic Stimulation

Transcranial magnetic stimulation (TMS), a noninvasive procedure that uses magnetic fields to stimulate brain cells, is a safe and effective treatment for OCD. Headache is the most commonly reported side effect of treatment, and other muscle discomforts or pain at the application site resolve shortly after treatment (Grassi et al., 2023).

Other Treatments

Psychosurgery is sometimes used to treat extremely severe OCD that has not responded to prolonged and intensive drug treatment, behavioral therapy, or a combination of the two. Modern stereotactic surgical techniques produce lesions that may bring about substantial clinical benefit without causing significant morbidity (Brock et al., 2024). Other treatment options include radiotherapy and deep brain stimulation, in which electrical current is applied through an electrode inserted into the brain (Brock et al., 2024).

BOX 28.3

Reflection of a Nurse: More Teamwork Needed

Incident

On an inpatient unit, a patient with obsessive-compulsive disorder (OCD) was engaging in compulsions that involved hoarding linens and monopolizing the shower. The staff, frustrated by this behavior, locked the shower door, which prevented the patient from engaging in their compulsions. The patient's nurse gave the patient a PRN medication for anxiety. Shortly afterward, the patient signed out of the unit against medical advice.

Reflection

Upon evaluation of the intervention, the nurse realizes that by preventing the compulsion and locking the door, the patient's anxiety increased.

1. What cues could help the nurse discern that the patient would leave the hospital?
2. If the medication had been effective in calming the patient, why would other interventions be necessary?

Safety Issues

Although individuals with OCD do not usually become suicidal as a direct result of anxiety, the disorder greatly distresses the individual who realizes the pointlessness and absurdity of the behaviors. The individual may feel a sense of hopelessness and helplessness and may contemplate suicide to end the suffering. An additional risk for suicide is created by the high probability of major depression and substance use, which often accompanies OCD. A suicide assessment must be completed. Some people have aggressive obsessions, so that if hospitalized, external limits may have to be imposed for the protection of others.

EVIDENCE-BASED NURSING CARE OF PEOPLE WITH OCD

People with OCD may be of any age; many have other disorders. Nursing care involves a careful assessment of the impact of the mental health disorder on an individual and a family. See Clinical Judgment Nursing Care Plan 28.1, which sets forth a plan of care for Tim, the patient in the case study in this chapter.

RECOGNIZING CUES: RELEVANT ASSESSMENT INFORMATION

The nurse should assess the type and severity of the individual's obsessions and compulsions. If the assessment occurs in a hospital, remember that some individuals with OCD experience a transient decrease in symptoms when admitted to a hospital; therefore, sufficient time must be allowed for an accurate assessment. If that time is unavailable, family members or significant others may provide an important source of information, with the individual's permission. Remember that individuals are often ashamed and embarrassed to reveal their obsessions and may have kept them secret for years. Because they are very worried about others' reactions, it is essential for the nurse to use an approach that is nonjudgmental, emotionally supportive, and patient.

Physical Health and Functioning

OCD has been associated with increased risk of premature death and increased morbidity. People with OCD have a higher prevalence of metabolic syndrome when

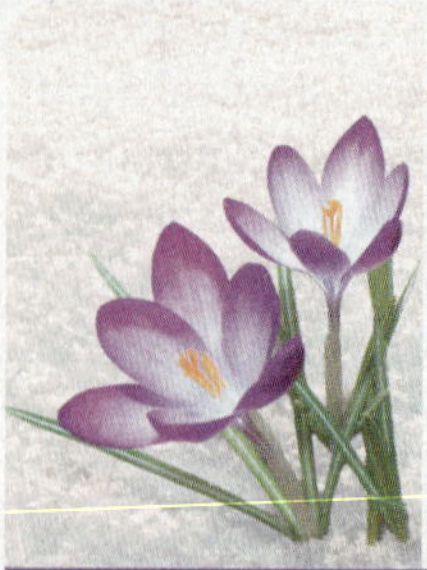

CLINICAL JUDGMENT NURSING CARE PLAN 28.1

The Person With Obsessive-Compulsive Disorder (OCD)

Tim, a 32-year-old engineer, is admitted to an inpatient unit for compulsively washing his hands and being unable to go to work. His wife is with him and is quite upset about his behavior. He was being successfully treated for OCD with clomipramine and sertraline but stopped taking his medications 3 months ago, shortly after his marriage. He denies suicidal ideation.

Setting: Acute Mental Health Unit

Assessment Cues: Tim is a casually dressed man, clean shaven. Hands are very red with small abrasions. He reports washing his hands several times a day to protect himself from germs. If he does not wash his hands, he gets very anxious. He has a specific routine for washing his hands that has interfered with his job. He stopped taking his medication and does not want to resume taking the same medications. He is concerned that his wife will leave him if he does not get better. He does understand that his behavior is unusual and is symptomatic of his disorder. He denies using alcohol or other substances. He works out regularly at a gym but has been unable to keep up with his routine because of his need to wash his hands. He is 6 ft 2 in, weighs 190, BMI 24.4; BP 135/70; P70, R 16. His goal is to manage his symptoms and resume his life.

Strengths: Wife wants him to get better and is supportive. He is motivated for change, does not use substances, and wants to return to exercise. Nutrition is excellent.

Associated Psychiatric Diagnosis	Medications
Obsessive-compulsive disorder	None

Priority Hypothesis Inability to Manage OCD Symptoms

Important Characteristics	Associated Considerations
Acceleration of symptoms of illness Lack of attention to illness Verbalizes desire to manage illness Verbalizes difficulty with prescribed regimen	Discontinuation of medication

Planning Recovery and Wellness Outcomes

Initial	Long Term
Recognize the need to treat symptoms	Reduce OCD symptoms
Identify acceptable strategies for managing symptoms	Return to work and resume usual lifestyle activities

Taking Action: Nursing Interventions

Interventions	Rationale	Ongoing Assessment
Initiate a nurse–patient relationship by using an accepting, nonjudgmental approach.	A therapeutic relationship will provide an opportunity for Tim to understand the reason for not discontinuing medication.	Determine the extent to which Tim is willing to trust and engage in a therapeutic relationship.
Encourage Tim to identify OCD symptoms.	By identifying symptoms, Tim will be able to discuss options for treatment.	Assess Tim's recognition of his symptoms and level of understanding of their relationship to his current distress.
Explore with Tim the reasons he discontinued taking his medications.	There are a variety reasons individuals stop taking medications. Understanding the reasons will help the nurse explore other alternatives.	Identify the reason(s) Tim discontinued taking his medication.
Discuss with Tim the evidence-based options for treating OCD including other medications, and cognitive-behavioral therapy (CBT).	Collaboration with patient is important in planning for successful outcomes.	Make sure that Tim takes his medication. Monitor for improvement in OCD symptoms and side effects (e.g., nervousness, nausea).

Clinical Judgment Nursing Care Plan 28.1 Continued

Priority Hypothesis Motivated to Learn New Coping Skills		
Defining Characteristics	**Related Factors**	
Aware of possible environmental changes Defines stressors as manageable Seeks knowledge of new strategies	Recognition that he needs symptom management	
Planning Recovery and Wellness Outcomes		
Initial	**Long Term**	
Commit to strategies to improve symptoms.	Implement strategies that control symptoms.	
Taking Action: Nursing Interventions		
Interventions	**Rationales**	**Ongoing Assessment**
Discuss evidence-based strategies for managing OCD including medications.	Evidence-based strategies include medication and psychotherapy.	Determine whether Tim discusses all possibilities.
Based on Tim's medication side effects, discuss other medication options.	Medications have helped Tim in the past and will probably work again.	Determine whether Tim is open to taking other medications and monitoring side effects.
Discuss psychotherapy opportunities including CBT, supportive therapy.	CBT can improve symptoms.	Determine if Tim has the time and commitment to CBT.

compared to the general population. They have an increased risk of cardiometabolic complications including obesity, dyslipidemia, and type 2 diabetes mellitus. Unhealthy lifestyle habits including physical inactivity, an unhealthy diet, smoking, and alcohol consumption contribute to their morbidity (Holmberg et al., 2024).

Skin

Each individual with OCD should be assessed for dermatologic lesions caused by repetitive handwashing, excessive cleaning with caustic agents, or bathing. Osteoarthritic joint damage secondary to cleaning rituals may also be observed. Undetected somatic compulsions, such as persistent nausea and vomiting, can contribute to diminished QoL and pose diagnostic challenges for clinicians.

Nutrition

A nutrition assessment should be included because of the increased risk of cardiometabolic complications. A nutrition assessment is especially important if OCD is accompanied by an ED or another comorbid disorder that interferes with eating or metabolism.

Sleep

Individuals with OCD often have insomnia because of the heightened anxiety levels they experience. Sleep issues are also common in youth with OCD. For youth, delayed bedtime and increased arousal decreases sleep duration, which contributes to symptom severity during the day and into the evening (Cox & Olatunji, 2022).

Physical Activity

Compulsive behaviors can become very time consuming with little time or energy left for exercise. The patient should be asked about regular exercise and current physical stamina for improving physical activity.

History of Trauma

The high prevalence of traumatic histories among those with OCD is not a recent discovery (Pinciotti et al., 2022). Traumatic life events occurring around the onset of their OCD symptoms are frequently recalled as stressful life events causing serious personal distress, often around some concern with contamination or an exposure to a toxin. Past traumas can complicate treatment, and some obsessive-compulsive symptoms may have developed as a way of coping with trauma. Trauma contributes to negative treatment outcomes in OCD (Hühne et al., 2024).

It is important that psychiatric nurses complete a trauma history, assess for comorbid conditions, and explore the time sequences of traumatic and stressful

BOX 28.4

Trauma-Informed Approaches: Obsessive-Compulsive Disorder After a Visit to Disneyland

Background

In the late 1990s, Disneyland was sued by the parents of children who were traumatized after seeing costumed Disney characters walking around with their costume heads removed. One child was reported to have become depressed and withdrawn afterward. At the time, response to reports of this incident was mixed with skepticism and sometimes amusement. Today we know that there is evidence that stressful life events can be shocking and distressing enough to constitute personal traumas and that individuals do associate these types of stressful events, which can cause depression and anxiety at the time of the event, with the onset of their OCD symptoms (Hühne et al., 2024).

Interventions

Remember that not all traumas are adverse childhood experiences (ACEs), so trauma interviewing should be broad. Understanding the trajectory of onset and exploring the meaning of the event to the individual are important considerations for treatment.

Source: Hühne, V., Dos Santos-Ribeiro, S., Moreira-de-Oliveira, M. E., de Menezes, G. B., & Fontenelle, L. F. (2024). Towards the correlates of stressful life events as precipitants of obsessive-compulsive disorder: A systematic review and metanalysis. *CNS Spectrums*, *29*(4), 252–260. https://doi.org/10.1017/S1092852924000269

life experiences (Wadsworth et al., 2023). When patients feel comfortable talking about the past, they should be encouraged to share previous stressful and traumatic experiences including their perceptions of how past experiences contributed to, and have meaning to, the symptoms they are currently experiencing. Perceptions of the significance of past traumatic experiences contribute to the severity of the symptoms (Pinciotti & Fisher, 2022). People with OCD often suffer from shame and embarrassment, and encouraging them to talk about why they have to behave the way they do and what it means can help them to relieve anxiety (Laving et al., 2023; Box 28.4).

Medication

A careful assessment of current and past medication helps in understanding and predicting the best medications. People with OCD are prescribed a variety of medications in addition to over-the-counter vitamins and herbal substances.

Substance Use

Many individuals self-medicate with substances including tobacco to relieve the anxiety produced by obsessive thoughts. About one third experience substance use disorder or dependence in their lifetime. In addition, some individuals may misuse benzodiazepines and other prescription medications. Since compulsivity plays a central role in both OCD and substance use disorder, there may be a common brain circuit dysfunction in these two disorders, which can help in identifying appropriate prevention and treatment targets (León et al., 2023). Social isolation can also lead to substance misuse, as individuals avoid being around others, and avoid social or family events. They are shamed and embarrassed by behaviors that they realize are irrational.

Psychosocial Cues

A psychosocial assessment involves gathering information by interviewing and talking with the patient and family, and by reviewing prior medical records.

Mental Status and Appearance

Most individuals appear neatly dressed and groomed, cooperative, and eager to answer questions. Most people with OCD recognize that their thoughts and behaviors are different than others. Speech is at an expected rate and volume, but often their thinking exhibits an obsessional, ruminative style with **circumferential speech** (i.e., speech that is loaded with irrelevant details); however, eventually they address the question. Listening may be frustrating and require considerable patience, but remember that such speech, which expresses the individual's thinking, is part of the disorder and may be beyond the individual's awareness. Continually interrupting and redirecting them can interfere with establishing a therapeutic relationship, especially in the initial assessment. Redirection should be done in a gentle and noncritical manner to allow the patient time to refocus.

Behavioral Responses

Observation of the patient's behavior during the assessment will give clues to the level of anxiety that is being experienced. Does the patient shift in the chair, seem restless, or are they unable to sit or stand still? Nonverbal behavior should be observed for an increase in anxiety or fear.

The nurse should ask about compulsive behaviors such as repeating, ordering, or counting actions such as opening and closing a door 3 or 4 times before leaving the house or washing hands several times a day. Some people with OCD are very inhibited and avoid touching others. Other people with OCD are impulsive. A nurse can determine if either behavior is typical by asking about interactions with others and their environment.

Self-Concept

Children and adults with OCD often have low self-concept. Their compulsive behaviors and obsessive thoughts are often internalized as personality quirks instead of understanding them as symptoms. They recognize that others do not have the same types of thoughts and behaviors and want to hide them. Their constant worrying and shame contributes to low self-esteem (Mavrogiorgou et al., 2024). The nurse should listen for negative self-statements or expressions of helplessness.

Stress and Coping Patterns

Assessment of stress and general mood states is essential. Information should be gathered about the stress of daily life and stress related to OCD symptoms to determine how the individual is coping. Levels of stress during crises, life transitions, or other events should be explored as these can exacerbate symptoms.

Social Network/Support Systems

Social networks and support systems are an important part of the assessment because low levels of social support are related to increased symptom severity. Although no studies show that lack of social support predicts relapse, empathy and positive interactions are associated with maintenance of gains, whereas negative family interactions (such as anger and criticism) can lead to poorer outcomes (Farrell et al., 2023; Palardy et al., 2018).

Functional Status

Functional status assessment focuses on the degree to which the OCD symptoms interfere with the patient's daily functioning. Several rating scales are available to identify symptoms and monitor improvement. Some of these scales are to be used by the nurse; others are self-rating scales for the patient, child, or family member. The Maudsley Obsessive-Compulsive Inventory is a 30-item, true–false, self-assessment tool that may help the individual recognize symptoms. See Table 28.2 for more information about psychometrically valid scales.

It is also important to assess for secondary complications related to compulsive behaviors (such as skin chafing, high use of soap and paper towels, unexplained high utility bills, frequent checking on family members that is excessive) as these factors need to be addressed in planning care. Also, be sure to explore the individual's insights, if any, about the accuracy of their obsessions and their ability to control them as this plays a role in treatment planning and outcomes.

TABLE 28.2 EVIDENCE-BASED ASSESSMENT TOOLS FOR OBSESSIVE-COMPULSIVE DISORDER

Rating Scale	Description
Yale-Brown Obsessive Compulsive Scale	A clinician-rated, 16-item scale with separate subtotals for the severity of obsessions and compulsions. Scoring changes after repeated measurement are used to identify response to treatment.
The Sheehan Disability Scale	Brief, self-rated, 3-item, visual analog scale to assess disability. A global measure of functioning can be determined. Recommended for tracking functional changes over time.
Family Accommodation Scale for Obsessive-Compulsive Disorder	This self-rated, 19-item rating scale can be used by the parent/caregiver, child, or others to track and monitor the family's response to symptoms during treatment.
The Brown Assessment of Beliefs Scale	A self-rated scale that scores on six dimensions: conviction, perception of other's views, explanation of differing views, idea fixity, attempts to reject beliefs, and insight. Helps rate the degree *of conviction and insight* patients have concerning their obsessions.

Spiritual Assessment

Using a nonjudgmental approach, the nurse should ask the patient about the importance of religion and the belief in a higher power. See Chapter 10. People with OCD often demonstrate **religiosity,** or strong religious beliefs that can provide comfort or can be distressing and contribute to their disorder. Because guilt and shame are common feelings for someone with OCD, the nurse should consider the relationship between guilt, the belief in a higher power, and OCD. **OCD religious beliefs** are symptoms of OCD that include **pathologic doubt** (negative belief about self, abilities, or future), religious themes, hypermorality, worry about sin, and excessive religious behavior within the context of their cultural group (Rakesh et al., 2021).

Quality of Life

Children with OCD have overall decreased QoL in social and school-related settings (Stiede et al., 2024). In adults, depressive symptoms are a strong predictor of poor QoL. Contamination fears and the need for things to be perfect, exact, or symmetrical contribute to lower satisfaction in social relationships. These fears can interfere with leisure activities and sexual functioning which in turn can negatively impact relational intimacy (Brock et al., 2024).

Strengths Assessment

The personal and social strengths of the individual should emerge during the assessment interview. Questions to ask could include: Does the child or adult enjoy good physical health? Is the individual motivated for treatment? Does the individual recognize that obsessions or compulsions are unusual? Are there social supports, and safe and stable housing? Does the individual have unique talents, interests, and character strengths? All this information will be useful in establishing a personalized recovery plan.

ANALYZING CUES AND DEVELOPING HYPOTHESES

Patients with OCD may present with various concerns and issues, depending on the particular obsessions and compulsions/rituals and on the presence of comorbid disorders. As a result, nursing hypotheses could run the gamut from safety concerns related to suicide and depression, psychological issues related to anxiety, poor self-concept, and loneliness to physical issues such as skin integrity. Medical treatment goals focus on reducing symptoms and improving functionality. Recovery outcomes, which are personalized, are determined collaboratively after the issues have been identified. The patient should be encouraged to commit to follow-up for long-term treatment and recovery.

PLANNING RECOVERY AND WELLNESS OUTCOMES: GENERATING SOLUTIONS

OCD can be persistent and disabling even when clinical symptoms are in remission. Good mental health encompasses more than a positive clinical response to treatment. When planning for recovery, the nurse should partner with the patient and family in identifying realistic treatment goals and mental health and wellness-promoting activities. Goals are collaboratively determined within the context of a therapeutic nurse–patient relationship. Ideally, the patient will want to reduce symptoms, learn about the disorder and treatment, manage health-related issues, and seek a higher level of wellness.

The planning process should also include steps to be taken during periods of stress that reduce anxiety and prevent an exacerbation of obsessions and compulsions. For example, the patient may learn to use mindfulness during stressful periods to reduce anxiety.

THERAPEUTIC RELATIONSHIP

Establishing a therapeutic relationship with an individual with OCD requires patience and active listening. The individual may go to great lengths to explain some minute aspect of their life. It is important not to interrupt or rush these explanations. Being unable to finish thoughts increases the patient's anxiety and frustration. For a therapeutic dialogue that involves Tim, the case study patient in this chapter, see Box 28.5.

The nurse's interpersonal skills are crucial to successful intervention with the patient who has OCD. Nurses must control their own anxiety. The nurse should interact with the individual in a calm, nonauthoritarian fashion without exhibiting any disapproval of the patient or the patient's behaviors while demonstrating empathy about the distress that the disorder has caused. This approach is one of the most effective means available for acknowledging the individual as separate from the illness.

TAKING ACTION: NURSING INTERVENTIONS

Nursing interventions for people with OCD should be individualized and holistic. Even though specialists implement CBT that address the obsessions and compulsions, nurses should reinforce the CBT interventions through their interactions and support. Patients also benefit from medications and other interventions such as addressing the physical and mental consequences of obsessive thinking and compulsive behaviors, supporting a healthy lifestyle, and managing medication side effects.

Priorities of Care

Safety is always the primary concern in caring for people with OCD. Suicide attempts and accidents are the primary concerns for life-threatening injuries (Fernández de la Cruz et al., 2024). Suicidal ideation should be closely monitored, especially if the patient is also depressed and hospitalized. The obsessions and compulsions can be so overwhelming that suicide seems to be the best option.

Incidents that appear to be accidents can be caused purposely in an attempt to end one's life or a result of being distracted with thoughts and behaviors. Nurses discuss with the patient the history of accidents or the extent of distraction that is experienced because of obsessions and compulsions.

Physical Care

Physical care is important because of the increased risk of morbidity and mortality for individuals with OCD. Inactivity and poor nutrition lead to cardiometabolic issues. Compulsions, such as excessive cleaning or exercise routines, can become habitual, repetitive behaviors that threaten physical health.

BOX 28.5

Therapeutic Dialogue: Obsessive-Compulsive Disorder

Tim is admitted to an inpatient unit; an initial assessment is currently being conducted.

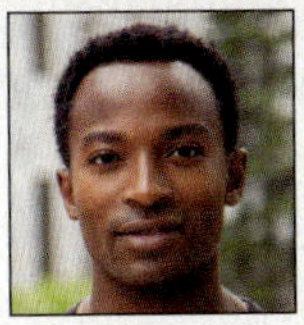

INEFFECTIVE APPROACH

Nurse: Could you tell me what brings you here?

Tim: What? Oh, sorry I get distracted easily. What did you say?

Nurse: I said, why are you here? What do you hope to accomplish while you are here?

Tim: Well, this is how I see it. We need to make sure everyone is healthy, and I want to make sure…

Nurse: (interrupts) No, you do not understand what I am asking. *Why* are you here?

Tim: Forget it. I want to see my wife.

EFFECTIVE APPROACH

Nurse: Tim, how can I help you?

Tim: Well, I am not sure. My wife thinks I am doing strange things. See, I want everyone to be protected, and it is important to stay healthy. There is an outbreak of staph infections, and I want to make sure that my family is safe, and I am just trying to figure things out.

Nurse: OK, it sounds like you are concerned about your family, and you are trying to protect them.

Tim: Yes, it is all of the germs. They are everywhere.

Nurse: And you are trying to get rid of them?

Tim: Yes, my wife thinks I am going overboard and wants me to take my medication.

Nurse: Your medication?

Tim: Yes, I used to take medication when I felt like this.

Nurse: You don't take your medication anymore?

Tim: No, I don't need it.

Nurse: I see. But your wife thinks you do?

Tim: Yes, but I don't like the side effects.

Nurse: Such as?

Tim: Well, to tell you the truth, I'd rather not talk about it.

Nurse: OK. While you are here, we can look at different options to help you feel more comfortable.

CRITICAL THINKING CHALLENGE

1. How did the first nurse's interaction block communication and increase Tim's frustration?
2. What effective communication techniques did the nurse use in the second scenario?

Maintaining Skin Integrity

For the patient with cleaning or handwashing compulsions, attention to skin condition is necessary. Encourage the individual to use tepid water when washing and hand cream after washing. Remove harsh abrasive soaps and replace them with moisturizing soaps. Attempt to decrease the frequency of washing by agreeing on a time schedule and time-limited washing (Box 28.6).

Wellness Challenges

Healthy living is a challenge for people who worry excessively, especially about health-related issues or who spend most of their waking hours cleaning. A wellness plan takes into account all of the dimensions of wellness: physical, mental, spiritual, emotional, intellectual, social, occupational, financial, and environmental. Helping the individual develop healthy eating habits and exercising regularly should be included in the recovery plan. Obsessional thinking can interfere with sleep and become a major issue for some with OCD. Sleep hygiene habits can help reduce some of the OCD symptoms as well as enhance overall well-being. Some specific challenges people with OCD face and some broad coping directions can be seen in Table 28.3.

Medication Interventions

SSRIs, including fluoxetine, fluvoxamine, paroxetine, and sertraline, are approved by the US Food and Drug Administration (FDA) for treatment of OCD. If there is no response to these medications, the tricyclic antidepressant clomipramine is recommended as the next medication to be prescribed. It is approved by the FDA for OCD treatment (ADAA, 2021). These medications are recommended along with concurrent CBT and ERP.

BOX 28.6

Building Clinical Judgment With SBAR: Nurse Communication With Provider Regarding a Patient With Obsessive-Compulsive Disorder

SBAR

S: Situation

John is a 33-year-old person assigned male at birth who is newly diagnosed with obsessive-compulsive disorder (OCD). He was admitted 2 days ago after an attempted suicide. At present he denies thoughts of suicide but says his handwashing is getting worse. The skin on his hands is splitting, and he is increasingly anxious and worried that he will get human immunodeficiency virus (HIV) by touching doorknobs, even though he knows that is irrational.

B: Background

John reports that he has had symptoms for as long as he can remember and that his symptoms got worse about 10 years ago following a few life stressors, but he felt he was able to manage the symptoms and never needed medical care. This was up until a few weeks ago, when everything worsened, and he became more fearful, would not leave the house, and eventually felt that he could not take it anymore. He planned a suicide that was interrupted by his wife, who brought him to the emergency department.

A: Assessment

Physical health: Ht. 5′11″, Wt. 185
Vital signs: BP 130/70, HR 88, R 10
Oriented X 4

Recommendation

Continue to monitor suicidal ideation.
Contact provider for medication evaluation.
Seek a dermatology referral.

Building Clinical Judgment

1. Why does the nurse recommend that the patient continue to be on suicide precautions?
2. Why does the nurse request a dermatology referral?

SSRIs or clomipramine lead to improvement in 40% to 60% of people who take them for OCD. Combining medications and using off-label medications such as other antidepressants, mood stabilizers, or antipsychotics is common in the treatment of OCD (Gautam, 2023). See Table 28.4.

Administering and Monitoring Medications

Antidepressants used to treat people with OCD are often given in higher doses than those usually used to treat patients with depression. The most common route of administration is oral. For refractory OCD, high-dose, intravenous treatment with antidepressant drugs may be indicated to bring the symptoms quickly under control. Medication effects must be closely monitored, including being alert to signs of toxicity, to provide safe and adequate care.

TABLE 28.3 WELLNESS CHALLENGES AND COPING STRATEGIES

Challenge	Coping Strategies
To cope effectively with daily obsessions/compulsions	Practice resisting urges to perform compulsive behaviors such as internet health searching; develop strategies to avoid obsessive thoughts, reframe thoughts
To seek environments that reduce the need for using compulsive behaviors	Seek safe living arrangement; maintain a structured living environment
To find satisfying and enriching work that can accommodate obsessive-compulsive behaviors	Satisfying and enriching work that can accommodate obsessive-compulsive behaviors
To recognize the need for physical activity, healthy foods, and sleep	Develop a plan for regular physical activity; discuss healthy diets; encourage establishing healthy sleep hygiene routines, including discussing benefits of going to bed at regular time; for those with OCD specifically: boosted mood, better judgment, heightened awareness, and better concentration
To develop a sense of connection, belonging, and a support system	Explore availability of support groups, family psychoeducation
To expand a sense of purpose and meaning in life	Focus on goals, values, and beliefs; read inspiring stories or essays

Because patients may become discouraged with a perceived lack of effect, they should be informed that these medications may take 10 to 12 weeks before their effects are realized. All patients should be warned not to stop taking prescribed antidepressant medications abruptly. See Chapter 11 for more information.

Monitoring for Drug Interactions

Because of the extensive list of drug–drug interactions associated with antidepressant medications, a prudent nurse will consult a drug reference or consult with a pharmacist before administering any other medications. As antidepressant treatment occurs over an extended period of time, the probability of a patient experiencing a drug interaction is high. Metabolic drug interactions can result in additive, synergistic, or antagonistic effects. For instance, fluoxetine can cause an increase in plasma concentrations of traditional antipsychotics and may interfere with the elimination of atypical antipsychotics and benzodiazepines. These patients must be monitored for the onset of akathisia or parkinsonian symptoms requiring

TABLE 28.4 ADMINISTRATION AND COURSE OF TREATMENT FOR OBSESSIVE-COMPULSIVE DISORDER

Medications	Suggested Therapeutic Dose Ranges
Selective Serotonin Reuptake Inhibitors	
Fluoxetine[a]	40–80 mg/day
Fluvoxamine[a]	200–300 mg/day
Paroxetine[a]	40–60 mg/day
Sertraline[a]	50–200 mg/day
Citalopram[b]	Up to 40 mg/day; (20 mg in those older than 60)
Escitalopram[b]	20–40 mg/day
Tricyclic Antidepressant	
Clomipramine[a]	100–250 mg/day
Serotonin-Norepinephrine Uptake Inhibitors	
Venlafaxine[b]	225–350 mg/day
SSRI's Administration and Safe Handling	

Start at a low dose to enhance tolerability, and the dose can be increased every week, or every other week as tolerated. Maintain at therapeutic level for at least 6 weeks before concluding the patient is nonresponsive to the drug.

SSRIs given in higher doses lead to greater response rates and/or greater mean rate of improvement compared with lower doses. However, higher doses are associated with higher dropouts due to side effects.

Patients who respond to an adequate trial of a serotonergic antidepressant should stay on that medication for at least 1–2 years.

To discontinue, slow taper at 10–25% every 1–2 months.

Refer to manufacturer's information. In general, tablets are kept dry and stored away from light.

[a]FDA approved for OCD.

[b]Used off-label for OCD.

Source: Drugs@FDA: FDA-Approved Drugs. Retrieved October 10, 2021, from https://www.accessdata.fda.gov/scripts/cder/daf/

anticholinergic medication. Quick recognition of signs and symptoms of interactions or toxic reactions is imperative for safe care. Allergic reactions are rare but can occur and can be fatal. Anaphylactic reactions (bronchospasm, angioedema) and/or the presence of urticaria (rash and intense itching) should alert the nurse to hold the next dose of medication and contact the primary care provider.

Management of Complications

Though all antidepressants have a boxed warning for suicidality in children, adolescents, and young adults, there is no current evidence to show that adults treated with SSRIs are at an increased risk of suicide (Lagerberg et al., 2022). Treatment with tricyclic antidepressants and the SSRIs citalopram and escitalopram can cause QTc prolongation (Bruggeman & O'Day, 2023). Symptoms include heart palpitations, rapid pulse, dizziness, chest pain, cold sweats, low blood pressure, and shortness of breath. Since other factors may contribute to this life-threatening cardiac condition known as *torsade de points*, a baseline ECG should be completed prior to initiating any type of antidepressant treatment. Sertraline and paroxetine are usually considered safest for breastfeeding because they have a low level of excretion in breast milk, but any antidepressant taken during pregnancy may endanger the fetus, or cause complications in the newborn, such that the benefits of treatment over the risks should always be carefully weighed. See Chapters 11 and 25.

Psychosocial Interventions

Psychosocial interventions are crucial to the successful treatment of OCD. Nurses can reinforce CBT strategies their patients are learning in therapy and help them practice and use them when anxiety is escalating. Nurses use basic behavioral interventions to reinforce change and avoid adding unnecessary stress to their patient's lives. Nurses can have a powerful impact on the successful use and acceptance of therapeutic techniques and practices including helping patients set realistic goals, adapt to the hospital milieu, discussing issues and concerns and by providing ongoing emotional support and encouragement.

Therapeutic Interactions

Interactions with people who are experiencing symptoms of OCD require a calm, nonjudgmental approach. It is important to validate the thoughts the individual is experiencing and be sensitive to their feelings. If they are experiencing anxiety, they may not be able to concentrate on verbal conversations or be able to sit still. The nurse can initiate a discussion about the triggers for the anxiety and the behaviors that the patient is using to control the anxiety. The nurse supports the patient as positive behaviors and thoughts replace the symptomatic obsessions and compulsions.

Enhancing Cognitive Functioning: Cognitive Restructuring

Cognitive restructuring based on CBT is a method of teaching the individual to restructure dysfunctional thought processes by defining and testing them. The goal of treatment is to alter the individual's immediate, dysfunctional appraisal of a situation and perception of long-term consequences. The individual is taught to monitor automatic thoughts and then to recognize the connection between thoughts, emotional response, and behaviors. The distorted thoughts are examined and tested by for-or-against evidence presented by the nurse, which helps the individual to realistically assess the likelihood that the feared event will happen if the compulsive behavior is not performed. The individual begins to analyze their thoughts as incongruent with reality.

Exposure and Response Prevention

For those who perform ritualized (time-consuming) compulsions, **exposure and response prevention (ERP)** is a very effective strategy. The individual is exposed to situations or objects that are known to trigger (induce) anxiety but is asked to refrain from performing the ritualized behavior. For example, people with contamination obsessions are asked to handle dirty objects without washing afterward. The goal is to help the individual understand that resisting the ritual is less anxiety producing and time consuming than performing rituals. Another goal is to confound the expectation of distressing outcomes, which eventually extinguish the compulsive behaviors. ERP has been shown to be as effective as medications and more effective than stress management therapy (Himle et al., 2024). Despite the success of ERP, barriers such as high cost, lack of access, and insufficient clinical expertise and training, still need to be addressed so that more individuals can benefit from evidence-based treatments.

Acceptance and Commitment Therapy

Nurses may have patients who are engaged in **acceptance and commitment therapy (ACT),** which is a form of CBT. ACT is, however, somewhat different than CBT or ERP in that it focuses more on altering obsessional thinking and the way it is experienced. Strategies here help the individual accept thoughts and anxiety without allowing them to interfere with life. Better functioning can be achieved without changing the frequency or severity of symptoms. ACT can be helpful for patients who relapsed after a course of ERP or CBT (Evey & Steinman, 2023).

Third-Wave Emerging Therapies

A number of other therapies for OCD are emerging. Referred to as **third-wave therapies**, these therapies give individuals with OCD more personalized choices and are specifically useful for those who do not respond or do not adequately respond to treatment (Castel et al., 2023). Though many remain investigational, evidence is increasing. Some are derivations of other successful therapies. For example, from trauma-focused therapy, there is eye movement desensitization (EMD) and imagery rescripting and narrative therapy (IRNT), which are being retooled for treatment of OCD. The Bergen Program is a concentrated version of ERP, which has shown promising results for OCD treatment (Skjold et al., 2024). Digital technologies (apps and websites) are playing a role in increasing OCD treatment access (Chaves et al., 2022). Although there is still a long way to go in terms of development, research, and dissemination of empirically supported treatments, they are gaining ground (Guzick et al., 2023; Hiranandani et al., 2023).

Behavioral Interventions

Although most patients with OCD are treated in outpatient settings, some are hospitalized with comorbidities and are unable to care for themselves or pose a substantial risk of harm to self or others. Some general behavioral-based strategies that can be used in any setting include the following:

- Unit routines must be carefully and clearly explained to decrease fear of the unknown.
- Assess and monitor the level of anxiety and disability.
- Monitor for psychiatric comorbidities and suicide risk.
- At least initially, do not prevent the individual from engaging in rituals because the individual's anxiety level will increase.
- Recognize the significance of the rituals to the individual and empathize with the individual's need to perform them.
- Make reasonable demands and set reasonable limits, avoid situations that provoke or increase frustration.
- Encourage discussions that identify disturbing topics that may relate to underlying anxiety or fear.
- Assist the individual in arranging a schedule of activities that not only incorporates some private time but also integrates the individual into unit activities.
- Help the individual recognize triggers to obsessive thoughts and ritualistic behaviors and the relationship between them.
- Give positive reinforcement for nonritualistic behavior and to acknowledge the individual's progress, strengths, and accomplishments.
- Reinforce the use of cognitive strategies, including constructive self-talk and cognitive restructuring.

Complementary Therapies

Clinical evidence supports the benefits of complementary therapies in the care of people with OCD. Some interventions directly impact OCD symptoms and others support overall mental health and well-being.

Mindfulness-based Cognitive Therapy

Studies show that adding the practice of mindfulness to CBT or ERP produces larger gains in QoL measures and in symptom improvement or reduction than use of CBT or ERP alone (Başkaya et al., 2021). **Mindfulness-based cognitive therapy** (MBCT) is an approach of focusing on the present moment and acceptance of psychological experiences such as anxiety. MCBT uses attention control, self-awareness, and emotion regulation. The goal of MBCT practice is to develop alternative approaches to deal with obsessions and a reduction in compulsions. For those with OCD, this might be difficult as they are struggling with painful, intrusive thoughts and sensations and making negative judgments about their unwanted thoughts. Still, increasing evidence suggests that MCBT is effective as an adjunctive therapy (De la Peña-Arteaga et al., 2024).

In mindfulness, no attempt is made to neutralize internal experiences with compulsions, and the nurse helps the patient accept and become aware that these are mental events, capable of being observed (perhaps reframing them as well intentioned, but "just a passing thought"). Exactly how mindfulness helps is unknown, but individuals with OCD recognize the transient nature of experience and begin to question the factual accuracy of their thoughts. Nurses can feel comfortable that mindfulness is an evidence-based intervention they can support and reinforce in their work with individuals with OCD.

Relaxation Techniques

Individuals with OCD experience insomnia because of heightened anxiety levels. Relaxation exercises may be helpful in improving sleep patterns. These exercises do not affect OCD symptoms but may be used to decrease anxiety and promote relaxation for sleep. The nurse may also teach and encourage the individual to use other relaxation measures, such as deep breathing, taking warm baths, going for a walk, enjoying music, or engaging in other quiet activities before bedtime.

Music Therapy

People with OCD appear to be more emotionally responsive to music than those who do not have OCD. Studies show that relaxing, sleep, or meditation music can be therapeutic and reduce OCD symptoms. Depending on the patient's interests, symptom reduction can occur with music that is either receptive (only listening to a track) or improvisational (involved in the creation or playing of the music) (Truong et al., 2021).

Exercise

Various forms of exercise (yoga, aerobic exercise) appear to be an effective intervention to improve the symptoms of OCD. Exercise also can reduce depression and anxiety symptoms (Bottoms et al., 2023). The nursing challenge is to help the individual commit to a safe exercise routine that is realistic. The discussion about exercise should be included in any wellness plan that is developed with the patient. See Box 28.7.

Vitamins

Vitamin D and folate play an important role in brain development. Research shows that OCD symptoms are negatively correlated with vitamin D and folic acid levels (Marazziti et al., 2024). People with OCD should be encouraged to consume adequate amounts of both vitamins. Whether the patient should try to obtain enough vitamins in their diet or take additional supplements needs to be determined on an individual basis with the provider.

Spiritual Interventions

Guilt and shame are OCD symptoms that often underlie strong religious beliefs. The nurse should separate the religious beliefs that are a part of the illness from the need to seek spiritual comfort and explore the patient's personal beliefs related to the meaning of life. If a patient is worrying excessively about sin and performing religious behaviors that are unusual for the individual, the nurse can assure the patient that the intensity of the feelings will decrease once symptoms are reduced. The nurse can make a referral to a chaplain for more in-depth spiritual counseling.

Psychoeducation

Psychoeducation is a crucial nursing intervention for the individual with OCD. Knowledge is power; the more the individual knows about their disorder, the more control

BOX 28.7

Research for Evidence-Based Practice: Long-term Exercise Engagement

Szuhany, K. L., Steinberg, M. H., McLaughlin, N. C. R., Mancebo, M. C., Brown, R. A., Greenberg, B. D., Simon, N. M., & Abrantes, A. M. (2023). Predictors of long-term exercise engagement in patients with obsessive-compulsive disorder: The role of physical activity enjoyment. Behavior Therapy, *54(4), 610–622. https://doi.org/10.1016/j.beth.2022.12.010*

THE QUESTION: What factors predict long-term behavioral change in exercise engagement for people with OCD?

METHODS: Fifty-six low-active patients with OCD were randomly assigned to aerobic exercise or health education program for 12 weeks. Participants completed measures of exercise engagement, physical activity enjoyment, behavioral activation, and positive and negative affect at baseline, postintervention, and 3-, 6-, and 12-month follow-up.

FINDINGS: Physical activity enjoyment was higher in the aerobic exercise group, but did not predict follow-up exercise engagement above and beyond baseline enjoyment.

IMPLICATIONS FOR NURSING: Exercise commitment is a complex process that requires additional research. Future research may link physical activity enjoyment to long-term commitment. Nurses should encourage patients to plan an exercise program that is realistic for them and that includes mechanisms for accountability.

BOX 28.8

Psychoeducation Checklist: Obsessive-Compulsive Disorder

When caring for a patient with OCD, be sure to include the family. If appropriate, address the following topic areas in the teaching plan.

- Explanation of mechanisms underlying OCD and selected therapies including length of treatment and expected outcomes
- Psychopharmacologic agents (SSRIs, MAOIs, lithium, anxiolytics, antipsychotics) as prescribed, including drug actions, dose, frequency, possible side effects, and common interactions with food or other drugs
- Skin care measures or issue resolution for other secondary consequences of OCD
- Alternatives to ritualistic behaviors
- Cognitive restructuring strategies
- Mindfulness and relaxation techniques
- Recovery strategies
- Community/internet resources and supports
- Addressing family factors (accommodation, family involvement)

SSRI, selective serotonin reuptake inhibitor; MAOI, monoamine oxidase inhibitor.

they will have over symptoms. The individual should be instructed not only about the biologic components of OCD but also about its treatments and disease course. Treatment is a shared responsibility between the individual and the health care provider; the individual should be included in the medication and treatment decision-making processes. If local support groups are available, the individual should be referred to reduce feelings of uniqueness and embarrassment about the disease. See Box 28.8 for components to include in psychoeducation for those with OCD.

Teaching Strategies

Educating children, youth, and adults who have OCD requires some special consideration. Modifying the environment can help the child manage anxiety, be less distracted, and ultimately prevent disruptions. In a school setting, teachers are encouraged to structure seating arrangements, provide private testing rooms, extend test times, have books on tape, provide access to laptops for writing, and break homework down into small chunks. Teachers should be aware of the child's triggering events, give advance notice of any change whenever possible, and have a plan that the child can use when things become too overwhelming (Child Mind Institute, 2024). These tips translate well to pediatric settings, where nurses frequently work with hospitalized children who have the triad of OCD–ADHD–Tics/Tourette syndrome.

Many of the same strategies can be used for adults. Adults often deal with intrusive thoughts, which make concentration difficult and frustrating. Avoid overloading them with too much information and keep things short, simple, and well organized.

Wellness Strategies

Wellness strategies for those with OCD are not too different than those for other people. Stress management, relaxation, and anxiety reduction strategies can best help the individual manage day-to-day stress. Structured QoL assessments can give the nurse a more accurate picture of mood states and information about other health domains. Self-help strategies can be introduced to help the individual manage symptoms and live with OCD, and these strategies are being identified as helpful in ways not previously known. For instance, running (predetermined bouts of running as exercise) reduced the frequency and intensity of OCD symptoms and improved mood (Bottoms et al., 2023).

Providing Family Education

The families of people with OCD need to be educated about the causes of the disorder and to learn about biologic and psychological treatment approaches. Understanding the biologic basis of the disorder should decrease some of the stigma and embarrassment they may feel about the bizarre nature of the patient's obsessions and compulsions. Families also need to learn how to be supportive and to avoid accommodating to a compulsion to the extent that their good intentions impede the individual's recovery. The International OCD Foundation offers families some excellent guidelines on what families can do to help them live with the individual who has OCD and to make life better for the whole family as well as how they can contribute to recovery and management of symptoms.

Family assistance in monitoring symptom remission and side effects of the medication is invaluable to mark progress, and the family can be enlisted (and taught how) to assist the individual with behavioral and cognitive interventions to manage symptoms.

Promoting Safety

Safety promotion should be highlighted in the care of every patient and family with OCD or related disorders. Suicide is a significant risk, with estimates of suicide attempts occurring in 1 out of 10 cases (Pellegrini et al., 2021). Assessment for suicidal ideations, for comorbid depression and traumatic histories, which increase risk, should always be conducted. Some individuals have specific suicide-related obsessions that are accompanied by compulsions such as reassurance seeking, avoidance, or comparing self to people who have died by suicide. Like others with OCD, these individuals can benefit from CBT or ERP therapy which can help them learn to resist the urges and recognize irrational thoughts. Nurses should also initiate suicide safety planning because it can be difficult for the individual to discriminate between a thought about an action and the intention to commit the action.

Safety issues for people with OCD, are compounded by the fact that neural processing differences make it difficult to make decisions about risks (Han et al., 2024). This means that the daily experience of making safe judgments about unclear situations is challenging for such individuals and may put them at risk. Knowing how neural processing is altered in individuals with OCD may lead to discoveries about how to better modify ERP to help those who do not respond to treatment (Apergis-Schoute et al., 2023).

Convening Support Groups

Patients with OCD are often members of support groups led by nurses. Group leaders should assess the ability of the individual with OCD to stay focused in the group. If a patient is having acute symptoms, the individual may not be able to sit through a group. A task-oriented group may allow the patient to be more active and thus reduce anxiety. The patient should be discouraged from compulsive behavior in a support group.

Developing Recovery Rehabilitation Strategies

OCD is a chronic condition requiring rehabilitation strategies that promote recovery. Strategies should be developed within the therapeutic relationship with the nurse guiding the decision-making process. Ideally, the patient should continue with the CBT and ERP therapies, adhere to the medication regimen, develop strategies to reduce stress, and develop plans for a healthy lifestyle.

Evaluation of Patient Outcomes

Several methods can be used to measure the response to treatment, including nursing observations, patient self-reports and changes in rating scales, remission of presenting symptoms, and the ability to complete activities of daily living. The individual should be able to participate in social or group activities, with a degree of comfort and without self-harm or aggressive intent. They should also be able to demonstrate common knowledge of OCD by describing its symptoms, biologic basis, and treatments. In addition to recognizing triggers, the patient should be able to summarize effective ways of interrupting thoughts and patterns of behavior that increase anxiety and should be able to explain what they are doing and why, to others, with less shame or embarrassment. The nurse could also assess for outcomes such as showing increased independence, paying more attention to self-care, demonstrating an increase in nonritualistic behaviors, and use of positive coping skills. Finally, the patient will have met outcomes by indicating that they have a plan in place to continue practicing what they are learning in therapy sessions at home.

Continuum of Care

The symptoms of OCD can become debilitating. The symptoms wax and wane throughout treatment. As the focus of treatment shifts from inpatient to outpatient environments, individuals must be assessed continually to ensure favorable outcomes through early intervention if symptoms resurface.

Emergency Care

Individuals with OCD frequently use medical services long before they seek specialized psychiatric treatment. Therefore, early recognition of symptoms and referral are important concerns for nurses working in primary care and other medical settings. After individuals are referred, most psychiatric treatment of OCD occurs on an outpatient basis. Individuals with severe OCD and/or self-harming thoughts and behaviors may be hospitalized for their own safety. In these settings, medications are the primary interventions.

Inpatient-Focused Care

In an inpatient setting, the presence of an individual with severe OCD may present a nursing management challenge. These individuals require a significant amount of staff time. They may monopolize bathrooms or showers or have disruptive rituals involving eating. The nurse should help the individual perform activities of daily living to ensure that they are completed. Monitoring medication effects, teaching psychoeducation groups, ensuring adequate caloric intake, and providing individual patient counseling are additional inpatient interventions.

Community Care

Partial hospitalization programs and day treatment programs help individuals in their quest for recovery. These programs can support independence while individuals begin medications and behavioral therapies. Some patients require outpatient treatment daily when symptoms increase. Maintenance outpatient therapy may be scheduled weekly or biweekly for several weeks until the symptoms are well controlled. Community agency visits are recommended to monitor medication.

Virtual Mental Health Care

Virtual approaches in the assessment and treatment of OCD and related disorders range from online individual and group psychotherapy (well established) to virtual assessment, online peer-support, and computerized programs designed to break neurocognitive habits (digital behavior change interventions). Virtual mental health care can help individuals cope with mental health issues while staying home. Communication with health professionals

TABLE 28.5 INTERNET RESOURCES FOR LIVING WITH OBSESSIVE-COMPULSIVE DISORDER

Website	URL
The TLC Foundation for Body-Focused Repetitive Behaviors	https://bfrb.org
International OCD Foundation	https://iocdf.org/
Body Dysmorphic Disorder Foundation	https://bddfoundation.org/
Peace of Mind Foundation	https://peaceofmind.com/
Psych Central-OCD and Mindfulness	https://psychcentral.com/lib/ocd-and-mindfulness/

via text, audio, or video messaging is available, and there are now easy-to-navigate mental health apps.

Several types of technology-enabled psychotherapy programs are available. With increasing demand and an expanding role, evidence about them has been accumulating. Technology programs vary by platform (internet, computerized), type of therapy, and the level of clinician involvement. Less-studied programs such as virtual reality exposure therapy and mobile therapy are also showing promise (Ferraioli et al., 2024). These programs also address cost, location, time, and access barriers (Feusner et al., 2022). Virtual access to therapy has obvious benefits for consumers and may help reduce stigma as some patients who cannot leave their homes can still get treatment. For those who are comfortable interacting via technology, online models may help normalize mental health care and make the process easier. See Table 28.5.

Integration With Primary Care

Effective treatment for those with OCD requires a continuum of preventive and restorative mental health and substance use disorder services, according to changing needs over time and across various levels of the health care system. A team-based approach for individuals and families with OCD and related disorders is best when mental health care and general medical care are offered in the same setting. Currently, there is little articulation between behavioral health and primary care systems. As virtual therapies and treatments become popular, it may be even more difficult to coordinate and integrate care. Policies to promote better integration and collaboration between behavioral health and primary care should be a priority for mental health advocates, such as nurses.

OTHER RELATED OBSESSIVE-COMPULSIVE DISORDERS

The other related OCDs are grouped together in the Diagnostic and Statistical Manual of Mental Disorders (DSM-5-TR) because evidence has accumulated to show a relationship, such as symptom similarity, presentation, frequent co-occurrence, genetic risks, and other common threads (APA, 2022). Grouping disorders together also allows for more discriminating research, which can improve screening, assessment, and earlier treatment. Trichotillomania, excoriation disorder, BDD, and hoarding disorder are briefly described here.

TRICHOTILLOMANIA DISORDER

Trichotillomania is chronic self-destructive hair pulling that results in noticeable hair loss, usually in the crown, occipital, or parietal areas of the head, although sometimes also involves the eyebrows and eyelashes. The individual has an increase in tension immediately before pulling out the hair or while attempting to resist the behavior. After the hair has been pulled, the individual feels a sense of relief. Hair ingestion may result in the development of a hair ball, which can lead to anorexia, stomach pain, anemia, intestinal obstruction, and peritonitis. Other medical complications include infection at the hair-pulling site. Hair pulling is usually done alone and people may deny it; for some there is little conscious awareness, and for others active pulling may regulate negative feelings (Pereyra & Saadabadi, 2023).

Clinical Course

The onset of trichotillomania occurs among children before the age of 5 years and in adolescents. For the young child, distraction or redirection may successfully eliminate the behavior. The behavior in adolescents may begin a chronic course that may last well into adulthood.

Diagnostic Criteria

Trichotillomania is diagnosed when recurrent pulling out of hair with hair loss occurs. The individual is unable to reduce or stop such hair pulling, which causes considerable distress (Torales et al., 2021).

Etiology and Treatment

This disorder is poorly understood. An etiologic relationship to OCD has not been established, but support is present for a familial connection. The prevalence of trichotillomania is estimated at 1% to 2% of the population (APA, 2022). No particular medication class demonstrates effectiveness in treatment. Studies of individual medications, including olanzapine (antipsychotic) and clomipramine (tricyclic antidepressant), show some treatment effectiveness. CBT and habit reversal training, a behavioral intervention, show more pronounced effect than medications (can improve the symptoms) (Pereyra & Saadabadi, 2023).

Evidence-Based Nursing Care of People With Trichotillomania

The assessment includes a review of current issues, developmental history (especially school conflicts and learning difficulties), family and social history, identification of support systems, previous psychiatric treatment, and general health history. The cultural context in which trichotillomania occurs must be taken into consideration because in some cultures, this behavior may be viewed as socially acceptable. The hair-pulling history and pattern are also used to determine the duration and severity of the disorder. Within the therapeutic relationship, a cognitive-behavioral approach can be used to help the individual identify when hair pulling occurs, the precipitating events, and the details of the episode.

EXCORIATION (SKIN-PICKING) DISORDER

Repetitive and compulsive picking of skin causing tissue damage characterizes **excoriation** or skin-picking disorder (Marazziti et al., 2024). Although face, arms, or hands are the most common sites for picking, it can occur at other body sites. Most affected people pick with their fingers, but tweezers or pins are also sometimes used. Similar to other disorders, skin picking causes significant distress to individuals. Prevalence is estimated at 3% of the population and occurs more frequently in people with OCD. Treatment data are limited but include behavioral and pharmacologic interventions. CBT and ACT are highly recommended. Nursing care is similar to caring for an individual with trichotillomania. Cold compresses or creams (antibiotics and corticosteroids) can also be applied. These disorders can carry a significant amount of shame and embarrassment, and individuals frequently try to camouflage skin lesions that could be detected. Possible medical sequelae, such as infections, lesions, scarring, and even severe physical disfigurement, can result (Mandarino et al., 2024).

BODY DYSMORPHIC DISORDER

Individuals with BDD focus on real (but slight) or imagined defects in appearance, such as a large nose, thinning hair, or small genitals. Preoccupation with the perceived defect causes significant distress and interferes with their ability to function socially. They feel so self-conscious that they avoid work or public situations. Some fear that their "ugly" body part will malfunction. Surgical correction of the issue by a plastic surgeon or a dermatologist does not correct their preoccupation and distress. BDD is an extremely debilitating disorder and can significantly impair an individual's QoL. BDD usually begins in adolescence and continues throughout adulthood. These individuals are not usually seen in psychiatric settings unless they have a coexisting psychiatric disorder, or a family member insists on psychiatric attention (see Box 28.9).

BOX 28.9

Clinical Judgment Vignette: Body Dysmorphic Disorder

K, age 16, for about 6 months has believed that her nose is becoming increasingly dislocated and prominent. She believes that everyone stares at it and talks about it. She does not remember a particular event related to the appearance of the symptom but is absolutely convinced that she can be helped only by a surgical correction of her nose.

She was treated recently for anorexia nervosa with marginal success. Although her weight is nearly back to how it was before her illness, she continues to be preoccupied with the looks of her body. She spends almost the entire day in her bedroom, refusing to leave the house and saying she wishes she would go to sleep and not wake up. Once or twice a day, she measures the length of her nose and is convinced that it is enlarging. She wears a nose guard to cover her nose. In desperation, her parents called the clinic for help.

The family was referred to a home health agency and a psychiatric home health nurse who arranged for an assessment visit.

Building Clinical Judgment

1. How should the nurse approach K? Should an assessment begin immediately?
2. From the vignette, prioritize areas of concern, outcomes, and interventions.

Source: Sobanski, E., & Schmidt, M. H. (2000). "Everybody looks at my pubic bone"—a case report of an adolescent patient with body dysmorphic disorder. *Acta Psychiatrica Scandinavica, 101*, 80–82.

This disorder occurs in adults with a prevalence of 1.7% to 1.8% in the United States (APA, 2022). The risk of depression, suicidal ideation, and suicide is high. The suicide risk in BDD is increased by the presence of other disorders such as substance use disorder, major depressive disorder, eating, and personality disorders. People with comorbid OCD–BDD have high morbidity, a decrease in insight, and poor psychosocial functions (Addison et al., 2024; Nicewicz et al., 2024). No single theory explains the cause of BDD. Unrealistic cultural expectations and genetic predisposition most likely underlie this disorder. There is emerging evidence that TMS may be effective in treatment-resistant cases of BDD (Wong et al., 2021).

HOARDING DISORDER

Difficulty parting with or discarding possessions, regardless of actual value, characterize hoarding disorder. Individuals with this disorder have a need to save items and experience distress if their items are discarded. Most affected individuals with hoarding disorder also exhibit excessive acquisition (excessive purchasing of items or collecting free items).

The prevalence of this disorder is estimated at 1.5% to 6% (APA, 2022). Hoarding may begin in childhood with an increase in severity throughout a lifespan. This disorder tends to be familial and present in different generations. Over 50% of the individuals have co-occurring depression or chronic anxiety. Treatment includes pharmacologic agents and CBT. There is some evidence that peer-led groups may be effective (Nutley et al., 2024).

Hoarding poses public health and safety risks for individuals, families, and communities. Excessive collection of items not only clutters living areas but can also lead to being trapped in an inaccessible environment and one that is at high risk for fire. Home health nurses are often the first health care providers that recognize the issue and so are a valuable resource in determining the safety hazards and helping the individual become aware of the issue and seek treatment. Currently, treatment includes CBT and medication for co-occurring mental disorders (Worden et al., 2024).

NCLEXNOTE Remember that NCLEX questions about OCD and related disorders are built on the nursing process and engage you in caring for a patient with a specific OCD or related disorder. NCLEX questions are NOT about what you would say or do personally in a similar situation. They are about applying evidence and/or theory to identify what is the BEST the nurse can say or do for the patient or family within the context and confines of the particular question.

SUMMARY OF KEY POINTS

- Obsessions are excessive, intrusive, or unwanted thoughts. Compulsions are repetitive behaviors performed in a ritualistic manner.
- The most common obsession is the fear of contamination.
- Compulsions relieve anxiety and should not be interrupted unless the behavior jeopardizes the safety of the individual or others. Interrupting compulsive behavior increases the individual's anxiety.
- OCD is characterized by obsessions, compulsion, or both. OCD can occur in children and adults.
- CBT, ERP, and medications can help affected individuals to get through episodes and reduce the compulsive behavior.
- Nursing care focuses on motivating the individual for change, administering and monitoring medication, providing psychoeducation, and supporting positive new behaviors.
- The primary characteristics of trichotillomania and excoriation disorders are compulsive behaviors that damage the hair or skin. Compulsive behaviors of both disorders cause significant distress to the individual who cannot stop or decrease the behaviors. Medications and psychotherapy can reduce these behaviors.
- BDD involves excessive focus on slight or imagined defects in appearance. The individual with these extremely distressing defects seeks treatment by plastic surgeons or dermatologists. Correction does not relieve the patient's preoccupation, which continues to interfere with their QoL. These individuals are at high risk for depression and suicide.
- Hoarding disorder can begin in childhood and last a lifetime. Individuals with this disorder need to save things and become very upset if items are removed. When excessive collection leads to extreme clutter, it becomes a safety issue.

DEVELOPING CLINICAL JUDGMENT

1. Differentiate an obsession from a compulsion.
2. List common obsession-compulsion dimensions and their consequences to the individual and family.
3. Describe the treatment priorities you would identify for a 35-year-old single parent who has been unable to work because they fear their apartment will burn down if they do not continually check the stove and furnace.
4. Develop a plan for a family who has been making many accommodations around the compulsions of a teenage family member with OCD.
5. Explain how nurses contribute to treatment using CBT and ERP behavioral strategies.
6. Identify patient teaching strategies for children and adults with OCD, including milieu modifications.
7. Describe the relationship between OCD and trauma.
8. Explain the behaviors associated with trichotillomania, excoriation disorder, body dysmorphic disorder, and hoarding disorder. What are the similarities and differences?

MOVIES, TV, OR STREAMING PROGRAMS

***Helen* (A Short Film on BDD): 2021.** This motion-capture short film conveys the themes underlying body dysmorphic disorder (BDD). We watch Helen, who has isolated herself in the bathroom (you can hear the muffled sounds of the party going on outside and see the shadows of others through the crack of the door). Helen engages in repetitious body checking, patting, and posturing. The viewer feels the tension and is acutely aware that something is wrong. When Helen finally gets a glimpse of herself in the mirror, the exaggerated perception of her body becomes apparent. But of course, the viewer does not really understand and feels confused—and Helen probably feels the same. At the end of the film, Helen falls and hits her head, and she does not get up. Now it is too late to find out more or to do anything about it (BDDF, 2021 https://youth.bddfoundation.org/helen-a-short-film/).

Viewing Points:

1. Does the short capture the emotional tone of what BDD must be like for people who have this disorder?
2. Can you recognize the pain of obsessing over bodily slights that may not even be present and, if present, others likely would not even notice?
3. What nursing interventions would you use to reach out to Helen to bring her out of the bathroom?
4. Did you sense the urgency of helping Helen (note that as many as 80% of those with BDD have suicidal ideations, and at least 24% have attempted suicide)?
5. Can you understand why the nurse would have needed to screen Helen for other symptoms and disorders such as depression, eating disorders, or anxiety disorders?
6. Would you have thought about completing a suicide assessment?

***Turtles All the Way Down:* 2024.** Aza Homles (Isabela Merced), a 16-year-old student who has obsessive-compulsive disorder, is negotiating high school and is getting ready for college. She is the only daughter of a single mother who is a high school teacher. Aza is seeing a therapist but refuses to take medication, and her symptoms prevent her from fully participating in social activities. She and her best friend, Daisy (Cree Cicchino), manage to connect with Aza's childhood crush. She struggles with her obsessive thoughts and compulsive behaviors as she tries to engage in a romantic relationship.

Viewing Points:

1. What obsessive-compulsive disorder symptoms does Aza have?
2. How do her symptoms interfere with her relationship with Daisy?
3. How do Aza's symptoms interfere with her relationship with Davis?
4. Does the protectiveness of Aza's mother, Gina, interfere with or support Aza's recovery?
5. How does Aza's obsession with germs relate to her sense of identity?
6. What will Aza have to do to recover from her disorder?

REFERENCES

Addison, M., James, A., Borschmann, R., Costa, M., Jassi, A., & Krebs, G. (2024). Suicidal thoughts and behaviours in body dysmorphic disorder: Prevalence and correlates in a sample of mental health service users in the UK. *Journal of Affective Disorders*, *361*, 515–521. https://doi.org/10.1016/j.jad.2024.05.145

American Psychiatric Association (APA). (2022). *Diagnostic and statistical manual of mental disorders (5th ed., text rev.)*. Author.

Anxiety & Depression Association of America (ADAA). (2021). *Clinical practice review for OCD*. https://adaa.org/resources-professionals/practice-guidelines-ocd

Apergis-Schoute, A. M., van der Flier, F. E., Ip, S. H. Y., Kanen, J. W., Vaghi, M. M., Fineberg, N. A., Sahakian, B. J., Cardinal, R. N., & Robbins, T. W. (2023). Perseveration and shifting in obsessive-compulsive disorder as a function of uncertainty, punishment, and serotonergic medication. *Biological Psychiatry Global Open Science*, *4*(1), 326–335. https://doi.org/10.1016/j.bpsgos.2023.06.004

Başkaya, E., Özgüç, S., & Tanrıverdi, D. (2021). Examination of the effectiveness of mindfulness-based cognitive therapy on patients with obsessive-compulsive disorder: Systematic review and meta-analysis. *Issues in Mental Health Nursing*, *42*(11), 998–1009. https://doi.org/10.1080/01612840.2021.1920652

Bedford, C. E., Trotter, A. M., Potter, M., & Schmidt, N. B. (2023). Minority stress and mental health in lesbian, gay, bisexual, transgender, and queer survivors of sexual assault. *Journal of Traumatic Stress*, *36*(6), 1031–1043. https://doi.org/10.1002/jts.22970

Benatti, B., Girone, N., Celebre, L., Vismara, M., Hollander, E., Fienberg, N. A., Stein, D. J., Nicolini, H., Lanzagorta, N. Marazziti, D., Pallanti, S, van Ameringen, M., Lochner, C., Karamustafalioglu O, Hranov, L., Eigee, M., Drummond, L. M., Grant, J. E., Denys, D., … Dell'Osso, B. (2022). The role of gender in a large international OCD sample: A report from the International College of Obsessive-Compulsive Spectrum Disorders (ICOCS) Network. *Comprehensive Psychiatry*, *116*, 152315. https://doi.org/10.1016/j.comppsych.2022.152315

Beyond OCD. (2023a). *Facts about obsessive compulsive disorder*. https://beyondocd.org/ocd-facts

Beyond OCD. (2023b). *Stop accommodating OCD*. https://beyondocd.org/information-for-friends-and-family/stop-accommodating-ocd

Blanco-Vieira, T., Radua, J., Marcelino, L., Bloch, M., Mataix-Cols, D., & do Rosário, M. C. (2023). The genetic epidemiology of obsessive-compulsive disorder: A systematic review and meta-analysis. *Translational Psychiatry*, *13*(1), 230. https://doi.org/10.1038/s41398-023-02433-2

Body Dysmorphic Disorders Foundation (BDDF). (2021). *"Helen" A short film (by L. Kenton & E. Prior)*. https://bddfoundation.org/helen-a-short-film

Bottoms, L., Prat Pons, M., Fineberg, N. A., Pellegrini, L., Fox, O., Wellsted, D., Drummond, L. M., Reid, J., Baldwin, D. S., Hou, R., Chamberlain, S., Sireau, N., Grohmann, D., & Laws, K. R. (2023). Effects of exercise on obsessive-compulsive disorder symptoms: A systematic review and meta-analysis. *International Journal of Psychiatry in Clinical Practice*, *27*(3), 232–242. https://doi.org/10.1080/13651501.2022.2151474

Brock, H., Rizvi, A., & Hany, M. (2024). *Obsessive-compulsive disorder*. In *StatPearls*. StatPearls Publishing. (nih.gov).

Bruggeman, C., & O'Day, C. S. (2023). *Selective serotonin reuptake inhibitor toxicity*. In *StatPearls*. StatPearls Publishing. (nih.gov).

Castle, D., Feusner, J., Laposa, J. M., Richter, P. M. A., Hossain, R., Lusicic, A., & Drummond, L. M. (2023). Psychotherapies and digital interventions for OCD in adults: What do we know, what do we need still to explore? *Comprehensive psychiatry*, *120*, 152357. https://doi.org/10.1016/j.comppsych.2022.152357

Cervin, M., do Rosário, M. C., Fontenelle, L. F., Ferrão, Y. A., Batistuzzo, M. C., Torres, A. R., Damiano, R. F., Fernández de la Cruz, L., Miguel, E. C., & Mataix-Cols, D. (2022). Taboo obsessions and their association with suicidality in obsessive-compulsive disorder. *Journal of Psychiatric Research*, *154*, 117–122. https://doi.org/10.1016/j.jpsychires.2022.07.044

Chaves, A., Arnáez, S., Castilla, D., Roncero, M., & García-Soriano, G. (2022). Enhancing mental health literacy in obsessive-compulsive disorder and reducing stigma via smartphone: A randomized controlled trial protocol. *Internet Interventions*, *29*, 100560. https://doi.org/10.1016/j.invent.2022.100560

Child Mind Institute. (2024). *Teacher's guide to OCD in the classroom*. https://childmind.org/guide/a-teachers-guide-to-ocd-in-the-classroom

Coles, M. E., Schubert, J., & Nota, J. A. (2021). Delayed sleep timing in obsessive-compulsive disorder is associated with diminished response to exposure and ritual prevention. *Behavior Therapy*, *52*(5), 1277–1285. https://doi.org/10.1016/j.beth.2021.02.006

Cox, R. C, & Olatunji, B. O. (2022). Delayed circadian rhythms and insomnia symptoms in obsessive-compulsive disorder. *Journal of Affective Disorders*, *18*, 94–102. https://doi.org/10.1016/j.jad.2022.08.118

de Avila, R. C. S., do Nascimento, L. G., Porto, R. L. M., Fontenelle, L., Filho, E. C. M., Brakoulias, V., & Ferrão, Y. A. (2023). Level of Insight in patients with obsessive-compulsive disorder: An exploratory comparative study between patients with "good insight" and "poor insight." *Frontiers of Psychiatry*, *3*(10), 413. https://doi.org/10.3389/fpsyt.2019.00413

De la Peña-Arteaga, V., Cano, M., Porta-Casteràs, D., Vicent-Gil, M., Miquel-Giner, N., Martínez-Zalacaín, I., Mar-Barrutia, L., López-Solà, M., Andrews-Hanna, J. R., Soriano-Mas, C., Alonso, P., Serra-Blasco, M., López-Solà, C., & Cardoner, N. (2024). Mindfulness-based cognitive therapy neurobiology in treatment-resistant obsessive-compulsive disorder: A domain-related resting-state networks approach. *European Neuropsychopharmacology*, *82*, 72–81. https://doi.org/10.1016/j.euroneuro.2024.02.011

Di Luzio, M., Bellantoni, D., Bellantoni, A. L., Villani, V., Di Vincenzo, C., Zanna, V., Vicari, S., & Pontillo, M. (2024). Similarities and differences between eating disorders and obsessive-compulsive disorder in childhood and adolescence: A systematic review. *Frontiers in Psychiatry, 15*, 1407872. https://doi.org/10.3389/fpsyt.2024.1407872

Di Salvo, G., Perotti, C., Ricci, V., Maina, G., & Rosso, G. (2024). Efficacy and suitability of adding short-term psychodynamic psychotherapy (STPP) to pharmacotherapy in patients with depressive disorders: A systematic review. *Trends in Psychiatry and Psychotherapy*. https://doi.org/10.47626/2237-6089-2023-0764

Evey, K. J., & Steinman, S. A. (2023). A systematic review of the use of acceptance and commitment therapy to treat adult obsessive-compulsive disorder. *Behavior Therapy, 54*(6), 1006–1019. https://doi.org/10.1016/j.beth.2022.02.009

Farrell, L. J., Waters, A. M., Storch, E. A., Simcock, G., Perkes, I. E., Grisham, J. R., Dyson, K. M., & Ollendick, T. H. (2023). Closing the gap for children with OCD: A staged-care model of cognitive behavioural therapy with exposure and response prevention. *Clinical Child and Family Psychology Review, 26*(3), 642–664. https://doi.org/10.1007/s10567-023-00439-2

Fernández de la Cruz, L., Isomura, K., Lichtenstein, P., Larsson, H., Kuja-Halkola, R., Chang, Z., D'Onofrio, B. M., Brikell, I., Rück, C., Sidorchuk, A., & Mataix-Cols, D. (2024). All cause and cause specific mortality in obsessive-compulsive disorder: Nationwide matched cohort and sibling cohort study. *British Medical Journal, 384*, e077564. https://doi.org/10.1136/bmj-2023-077564

Ferraioli, F., Culicetto, L., Cecchetti, L., Falzone, A., Tomaiuolo, F., Quartarone, A., & Vicario, C. M. (2024). Virtual reality exposure therapy for treating fear of contamination disorders: A systematic review of healthy and clinical populations. *Brain Sciences, 14*(5), 510. https://doi.org/10.3390/brainsci14050510

Feusner, J. D., Farrell, N. R., Kreyling, J., McGrath, P. B., Rhode, A., Faneuff, T., Lonsway, S., Mohideen, R., Jurich, J. E., Trusky, L., & Smith, M. (2022). Online video teletherapy treatment of obsessive-compulsive disorder using exposure and response prevention: Clinical outcomes from a retrospective longitudinal observational study. *Journal of Medical Internet Research, 24*(5), e36431. https://doi.org/10.2196/36431

Frank, H. E., Cain, G., Freeman, J., Benito, K. G., O'Connor, E., Kemp, J., & Kim, B. (2023). Parent-identified barriers to accessing exposure therapy: A qualitative study using process mapping. *Frontiers in psychiatry, 14*, 1068255. https://doi.org/10.3389/fpsyt.2023.1068255

Gautam, M. (2023). Clinical recommendations for augmentation agents in obsessive-compulsive disorder partially responsive to serotonin reuptake inhibitors. *Journal of Clinical Psychopharmacology, 43*(4), 369–377. https://doi.org/10.1097/JCP.0000000000001716

Grassi, G., Moradei, C., & Cecchelli, C. (2023). Will transcranial magnetic stimulation improve the treatment of obsessive-compulsive disorder? A systematic review and meta-analysis of current targets and clinical evidence. *Life (Basel), 13*(7), 1494. https://doi.org/10.3390/life13071494

Guzick, A. G., Schneider, S. C., Perozo Garcia, A.B., Kook, M., Greenberg, R. L., Riddle, D., McNeel, M., Rodriguez-Barajas, S., Yang, M., Upshaw, B., & Storch, E. A. (2023). Development and pilot testing of internet-delivered, family-based cognitive behavioral therapy for anxiety and obsessive-compulsive disorders in autistic youth. *Journal of Obsessive-Compulsive and Related Disorders, 37*, 100789. https://doi.org/10.1016/j.jocrd.2023.100789

Han, Y., Gao, F., Wang, X., Xia, J., Du, H., Liu, X., Cai, S., Tan, C., Fan, J., & Zhu, X. (2024). Neural correlates of risk taking in patients with obsessive-compulsive disorder during risky decision-making. *Journal of Affective Disorders, 345*, 192–199. https://doi.org/10.1016/j.jad.2023.10.099

Haque, U. M., Kabir, E., & Khanam, R. (2023). Early detection of paediatric and adolescent obsessive-compulsive, separation anxiety and attention deficit hyperactivity disorder using machine learning algorithms. *Health Information Science and Systems, 11*(1), 31. https://doi.org/10.1007/s13755-023-00232-z

Hermida-Barros, L., Primé-Tous, M., García-Delgar, B., Forcadell, E., Lera-Miguel, S., Fernández de la Cruz, L., Vieta, E., Radua, J., Lázaro, L., & Fullana, M. A. (2024). Family accommodation in obsessive-compulsive disorder: An updated systematic review and meta-analysis. *Neuroscience and Biobehavioral Reviews, 161*, 105678. https://doi.org/10.1016/j.neubiorev.2024.105678

Himle, J. A., Grogan-Kaylor, A., Hiller, M. A., Mannella, K. A., Norman, L. J., Abelson, J. L., Prout, A., Shunnarah, A. A., Becker, H. C., Russman Block, S. R., Taylor, S. F., & Fitzgerald, K. D. (2024). Exposure and response prevention versus stress management training for adults and adolescents with obsessive compulsive disorder: A randomized clinical trial. *Behaviour Research and Therapy, 172*, 104458. https://doi.org/10.1016/j.brat.2023.104458

Hiranandani, S., Ipek, S. I., Wilhelm, S., & Greenberg, J. L. (2023). Digital mental health interventions for obsessive compulsive and related disorders: a brief review of evidence-based interventions and future directions. *Journal of Obsessive-Compulsive and Related Disorders, 36*, 100765. https://www.sciencedirect.com/science/article/pii/S2211364922000586

Holingue, C., Samuels, J., Guglielmi, V., Ingram, W., Nestadt, G., & Nestadt, P. S. (2021). Peripartum complications associated with obsessive compulsive disorder exacerbation during pregnancy. *Journal of Obsessive Compulsive and Related Disorders*, 100641. https://doi.org/10.1016/j.jocrd.2021.100641

Holmberg, A., Martinsson, L., Lidin, M., Rück, C., Mataix-Cols, D., & Fernández de la Cruz, L. (2024). General somatic health and lifestyle habits in individuals with obsessive- compulsive disorder: An international survey. *BMC Psychiatry, 24*(1), 98. https://doi.org/10.1186/s12888-024-05566-w

Hühne, V., Dos Santos-Ribeiro, S., Moreira-de-Oliveira, M. E., de Menezes, G. B., & Fontenelle, L. F. (2024). Towards the correlates of stressful life events as precipitants of obsessive-compulsive disorder: A systematic review and metanalysis. *CNS Spectrums, 29*(4), 252–260. https://doi.org/10.1017/S1092852924000269

Jalal, B., Chamberlain, S. R., & Sahakian, B. J. (2023). Obsessive-compulsive disorder: Etiology, neuropathology, and cognitive dysfunction. *Brain and Behavior, 13*(6), e3000. https://doi.org/10.1002/brb3.3000

La Buissonnière-Ariza, V., Guzik, A. G., Schneider, S. C., Cepeda, S. L., Goodman, W. K., & Storch, E. A. (2022) Family accommodation of symptoms in adults with obsessive-compulsive disorder: Factor structure and usefulness of the Family Accommodation Scale for OCD-Patient Version. *Journal of Psychiatric Practice, 28*(1), 36–47. https://doi.org/10.1097/PRA.0000000000000597

Lagerberg, T., Fazel, S., Sjölander, A., Hellner, C., Lichtenstein, P., & Chang, Z. (2022). Selective serotonin reuptake inhibitors and suicidal behaviour: A population-based cohort study. *Neuropsychopharmacology, 47*(4), 817–823. https://doi.org/10.1038/s41386-021-01179-z

Laving, M., Foroni, F., Ferrari, M., Turner, C., & Yap, K. (2023). The association between OCD and shame: A systematic review and meta-analysis. *The British Journal of Clinical Psychology, 62*(1), 28–52. https://doi.org/10.1111/bjc.12392

León, J. J., Fernández-Martin, P., González-Rodríguez, A., Rodríguez-Herrera, R., García-Pinteño, J., Pérez-Fernández, C., Sánchez-Kuhn, A., Amaya-Pascasio, L., Soto-Ontoso, M., Martínez-Sánchez, P., Sánchez-Santed, F., & Flores, P. (2023). Decision-making and frontoparietal resting-state functional connectivity among impulsive-compulsive diagnoses. Insights from a Bayesian approach. *Addictive Behaviors, 143*, 107683. https://doi.org/10.1016/j.addbeh.2023.107683

Li, K., Long, J., Deng, W., Cheng, B., & Wang, J. (2022). Electroconvulsive therapy for obsessive-compulsive disorder: A retrospective study. *Frontiers in Psychiatry, 13*, 1040443. https://doi.org/10.3389/fpsyt.2022.1040443

Mandarino, M. J., Stummer, L., Trueba, A. F., Vahia, I., & Freedberg, A. (2024). Review of management considerations for excoriation disorder in older adults. *The American Journal of Geriatric Psychiatry, 32*(7), 879–894. https://doi.org/10.1016/j.jagp.2024.02.013

Marazziti, D., Massa, L., Carbone, M. G., Palermo, S., Arone, A., D'Angelo, G., Schulz Bizzozzero Crivelli, N., Gurrieri, R., Perrone, P., Palagini, L., & Dell'Osso, L. (2024). Silent infections are not so silent: The emerging role of combined infections, inflammation, and vitamin levels in OCD. *Clinical Neuropsychiatry, 21*(1), 7–21. https://doi.org/10.36131/cnfioritieditore20240101

Mavrogiorgou, P., Becker, S., & Juckel, G. (2024). Guilt and shame in patients with obsessive-compulsive disorders. *Psychopathology*, 1–11. https://doi.org/10.1159/000537996

Millar, J. F. A., Coughtrey, A. E., Healy, A., Whittal, M., & Shafran, R. (2023). The current status of mental contamination in obsessive compulsive disorder: A systematic review. *Journal of Behavior Therapy and Experimental Psychiatry, 80*, 101745. https://doi.org/10.1016/j.jbtep.2022.101745

Morris, O. J., Wiese, A. D., Pinciotti, C. M., Pacheco, R., Mallen, M. C. M., Schweissing, E. J., Soileau, K. J., Crowley, J. J., & Storch, E. A.; Latin American Trans-ancestry INitiative for OCD genomics (LATINO), Brazilian Obsessive-Compulsive Spectrum Work Group (GTTOC). (2024). Obsessive-compulsive disorder among individuals of Hispanic and Latin American ancestry: Cultural considerations for assessment and psychotherapy. *Bulletin of the Menninger Clinic, 88*(2), 148–170. https://doi.org/10.1521/bumc.2024.88.2.148

Mulcahy, M., Long, C., Morrow, T., Galbally, M., Rees, C., & Anderson, R. (2023). Consensus recommendations for the assessment and treatment of perinatal obsessive–compulsive disorder (OCD): A Delphi study. *Archives of Womens Mental Health, 26*, 389–399. https://doi.org/10.1007/s00737-023-01315-2

Nicewicz, H. R., Torrico, T. J., & Boutrouille, J. F. (2024). *Body dysmorphic disorder*. In *StatPearls*. StatPearls Publishing. https://www.ncbi.nlm.nih.gov/books/NBK555901

Nutley, S., Nguyen, B. K., Mackin, R. S., Insel, P. S., Tosun, D., Butters, M., Aisen, P., Raman, R., Saykin, A. J., Toga, A. W., Jack, C., Weiner, M. W., Nelson, C., Kassel, M., Kryza-Lacombe, M., Eichenbaum, J., Nosheny, R. L., & Mathews, C. A. (2024). Relationship of hoarding and depression symptoms in older adults. *The American Journal of Geriatric Psychiatry*, *32*(4), 497–508. https://doi.org/10.1016/j.jagp.2023.11.006

Ottoni, R., Pellegrini, C., Mora, L., Marchesit, C., & Tonna, M. (2023). Psychopathology of insight in obsessive-compulsive disorder. *Current Psychology*, *42*, 14760–14768. https://doi.org/10.1007/s12144-022-02806-8

Palardy, V., El-Baalbaki, G., Fredette, C., Rizkallah, E., & Guay, S. (2018). Social support and symptom severity among patients with obsessive-compulsive disorder or panic disorder with agoraphobia: A systematic review. *Europe's Journal of Psychology*, *14*(1), 254–286. https://doi.org/10.5964/ejop.v14i1.1252

Pellegrini, L., Maietti, E., Rucci, P., Burato, S., Menchetti, M., Berardi, D., Maina, G., Fineberg, N. A., & Albert, U. (2021). Suicidality in patients with obsessive-compulsive and related disorders (OCRDs): A meta-analysis. *Comprehensive Psychiatry*, *108*, 152246. https://doi.org/10.1016/j.comppsych.2021.152246

Pereyra, A. D., & Saadabadi, A. (2023). *Trichotillomania*. In *StatPearls*. StatPearls Publishing. (nih.gov)

Pinciotti, C. M., & Fisher, E. K. (2022). Perceived traumatic and stressful etiology obsessive-compulsive disorder. *Psychiatry Research Communications*, *2*(2), 1–8. https://doi.org/10.1016/j.psycom.2022.100044

Pinciotti, C. M., & Orcutt, H. K. (2021). Obsessive-compulsive symptoms in sexual minorities. *Psychology of Sexual Orientation and Gender Diversity*, *8*(4), 487–495. https://doi.org/10.1037/sgd0000437

Pinciotti, C. M., Smith, Z., Singh, S., Wetterneck, C. T., & Williams, M. T. (2022). Call to action: Recommendations for justice-based treatment of obsessive-compulsive disorder with sexual orientation and gender themes. *Behavior Therapy*, *53*(2), 153–169. https://doi.org/10.1016/j.beth.2021.11.001

Pinciotti, C. M, Wetterneck, C. T., & Riemann, B. (2022). Symptom severity and presentation in comorbid OCD and PTSD: A clinical replication. *Bulletin of the Menninger Clinic*, *86*(3), 183–203. https://doi.org/10.1521/bumc.2022.86.3.183

Rakesh, K., Arvind, S., Dutt, B. P., Mamta, B., Bhavneesh, S., Kavita, M., Navneet, K., Shrutika, G., Priyanka, B., Arun, K., Harkamal, K., & Jagdeep, K. (2021). The role of religiosity and guilt in symptomatology and outcome of obsessive compulsive disorder. *Psychopharmacology Bulletin*, *51*(3), 38–49.

Schuyler, M., & Geller, D. A. (2023). Childhood obsessive-compulsive disorder. *The Psychiatric Clinics of North America*, *46*(1), 89–106. https://doi.org/10.1016/j.psc.2022.10.002

Sidorchuk, A., Kuja-Halkola, R., Runeson, B., Lichtenstein, P., Larsson, H., Rück, C., D'Onofrio, B. M., Mataix-Cols, D., & Fernández de la Cruz, L. (2021). Genetic and environmental sources of familial coaggregation of obsessive-compulsive disorder and suicidal behavior: A population-based birth cohort and family study. *Molecular Psychiatry*, *26*(3), 974–985. https://doi.org/10.1038/s41380-019-0417-1

Singh, A., Anjankar, V. P., & Sapkale, B. (2023). Obsessive-compulsive disorder (OCD): A comprehensive review of diagnosis, comorbidities, and treatment approaches. *Cureus*, *15*(11), e48960. https://doi.org/10.7759/cureus.48960

Skjold, S. H., Hagen, K., Wheaton, M. G., Hjelle, K. M., Björgvinsson, T., & Hansen, B. (2024). The effectiveness and acceptability of the Bergen 4-day treatment for adolescents with OCD: A replication and extension. *BMC Psychiatry*, *24*(1), 148. https://doi.org/10.1186/s12888-024-05601-w

Stiede, J. T., Spencer, S. D., Onyeka, O., Mangen, K. H., Church, M. J., Goodman, W. K., & Storch, E. A. (2024). Obsessive-compulsive disorder in children and adolescents. *Annual Review of Clinical Psychology*, *20*(1), 355–380. https://doi.org/10.1146/annurev-clinpsy-080822-043910

Swisher, V. S., Ricketts, E. J., & Rogers, S. A. (2023). The impact of family functioning on help-seeking behavior and symptom severity in obsessive-compulsive disorder. *The Journal of Nervous and Mental Disease*, *211*(9), 670–678. https://doi.org/10.1097/NMD.0000000000001683

Thomas, S. P. (2023). Addressing gaps in knowledge about cyberchondria. *Issues in Mental Health Nursing*, *44*(7), 583–584. https://doi.org/10.1080/01612840.2023.2229718

Torales, J., Ruiz Díaz, N., Ventriglio, A., Castaldelli-Maia, J. M., Barrios, I., García, O., Navarro, R., González-Urbieta, I., O'Higgins, M., & Jafferany, M. (2021). Hair-pulling disorder (Trichotillomania): Etiopathogenesis, diagnosis and treatment in a nutshell. *Dermatologic Therapy*, *34*(1), e13466. https://doi.org/10.1111/dth.14366

Trondsen, C. (2021). *Barriers to OCD treatment for the LGBTQ community*. International OCD Foundation. https://iocdf.org/blog/2021/06/25/barriers-to-ocd-treatment-for-the-lgbtq-community/

Truong, T. P. A., Applewhite, B., Heiderscheit, A., & Himmerich, H. (2021). A systematic review of scientific studies and case reports on music and obsessive-compulsive disorder. *International Journal of Environmental Research and Public Health*, *18*(22), 11799. https://doi.org/10.3390/ijerph182211799

Vellozo, A. P., Fontenelle, L. F., Torresan, R. C., Shavitt, R. G., Farrao, Y. A., Rosario, M. C., Miguel, E. C., & Torres, A. R. (2021). Symmetry dimension in obsessive-compulsive disorder: Prevalence, severity and clinical correlates. *Journal of Clinical Medicine*, *10*(2), 274. https://doi.org/10.3390/jcm10020274

Vismara, M., Benatti, B., Fineberg, N. A., Hollander, E., Van Ameringen, M., Menchon, J. M., Zohar, J., & Dell'Osso, B. (2024). Lessons from a multicenter, international, large sample size analysis of patients with obsessive-compulsive disorders: An overview of the ICOCS Snapshot studies. *CNS Spectrums*, *29*(1), 40–48. https://doi.org/10.1017/S1092852923002432

Vriend, C., de Joode, N. T., Pouwels, P. J. W., Liu, F., Otaduy, M. C. G., Pastorello, B., Robertson, F. C., Ipser, J., Lee, S., Hezel, D. M., van Meter, P. E., Batistuzzo, M. C., Hoexter, M. Q., Sheshachala, K., Narayanaswamy, J. C., Venkatasubramanian, G., Lochner, C., Miguel, E. C., Reddy, Y. C. J., … van den Heuvel, O. A. (2024). Age of onset of obsessive-compulsive disorder differentially affects white matter microstructure. *Molecular Psychiatry*, *29*(4), 1033–1045. https://doi.org/10.1038/s41380-023-02390-8

Wadsworth, L.P., Van Kirk, N., August, M., Kelly, J. M., Jackson, F., Nelson, J., & Luehrs, R. (2023). Understanding the overlap between OCD and trauma: Development of the OCD trauma timeline interview (TTI) for clinical settings. *Current Psychology*, *42*(9), 6937–6947. https://doi.org/10.10.1007/s12144-021-02118-3

Wetterneck, C. T., Rouleau, T. M., Williams, M. T., Vallely, A., La Torre, J. T., & Björgvinsson, T. (2021). A new Scrupulosity Scale for the dimensional Obsessive-Compulsive Scale (DOCS): Validation with clinical and nonclinical samples. *Behavior Therapy*, *52*(6), 1449–1463. https://doi.org/10.1016/j.beth.2021.04.001

Wong, W. W., Rangaprakash, D., Larson, M. S., Diaz-Fong, J. P., Tadayonnejad, R., Leuchter, A. F., & Feusner, J. D. (2021). Can excitatory neuromodulation change distorted perception of one's appearance? *Brain Stimulation*, *14*(5), 1197–1200. https://doi.org/10.1016/j.brs.2021.07.010

Worden, B. L., Tolin, D. F., & Stevens, M. C. (2024). An exploration of neural predictors of treatment compliance in cognitive-behavioral group therapy for hoarding disorder. *Journal of Affective Disorders*, *345*, 410–418. https://doi.org/10.1016/j.jad.2023.10.148

Zrenner, B., Zrenner, C., Balderston, N., Blumberger, D. M., Kloiber, S., Laposa, J. M., Tadayonnejad, R., Trevizol, A. P., Zai, G., & Feusner, J. D. (2023). Toward personalized circuit-based closed-loop brain-interventions in psychiatry: Using symptom provocation to extract EEG-markers of brain circuit activity. *Frontiers in Neural Circuits*, *17*, 1208930. https://doi.org/10.3389/fncir.2023.1208930

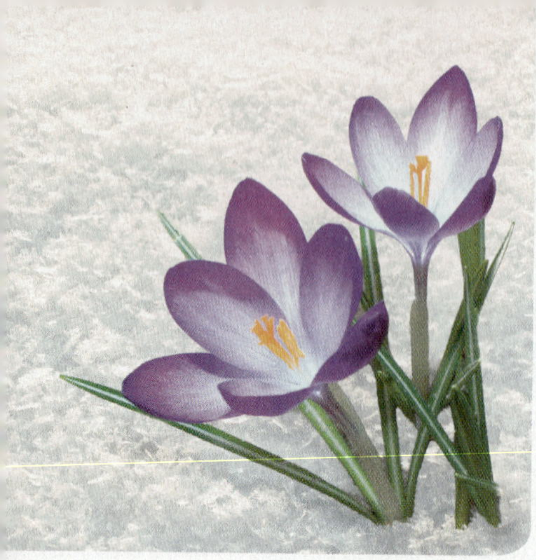

29 Trauma- and Stressor-Related Disorders

Nursing Care of People With Posttraumatic Stress and Related Disorders

Mary Ann Boyd

KEYCONCEPTS

- psychological trauma
- resilience
- traumatic events

LEARNING OBJECTIVES

After studying this chapter, you will be able to:

1. Examine the roles of psychological trauma and resilience with respect to mental disorders.
2. Relate the primary theories of posttraumatic stress disorder to clinical symptoms and the course of the disorder.
3. Evaluate the significance of trauma in the appearance of posttraumatic stress disorder.
4. Examine the relationship between social determinants of health and posttraumatic stress disorder.
5. Select strategies to establish a therapeutic relationship with people with posttraumatic stress disorder.
6. Using a clinical judgment model, formulate a person-centered, recovery-oriented nursing care plan for people with posttraumatic stress disorder.
7. Identify medications used to treat people with posttraumatic stress disorder and evaluate their effectiveness.
8. Develop wellness strategies for people with posttraumatic stress disorder.
9. Compare and contrast mental health care provided in emergency, inpatient, community, and virtual settings.
10. Support the integration of health care and mental health care for people with posttraumatic stress disorder.
11. Compare and contrast posttraumatic stress disorder and other trauma-related disorders.

KEY TERMS

• acute stress disorder • adjustment disorder • behavioral sensitization • cognitive-behavioral therapy • complex posttraumatic stress disorder (CPTSD) • depersonalization • depersonalization/derealization disorder • derealization • disengagement • disinhibited social engagement disorder • dissociation • dissociative amnesia • dissociative disorders • dissociative identity disorder • emotional numbing • emotional reaction • exaggerated negative beliefs • eye movement desensitization and reprocessing therapy • fear conditioning • flashbacks • hyperarousal • hypervigilant • intrusion • minority stress • positive emotions • posttraumatic stress disorder (PTSD) • psychodynamic psychotherapy • reactive attachment disorder • retraumatization • secondary trauma • sleep disturbance • social network • social support • survivor guilt • trauma-informed approach • virtual reality exposure therapy

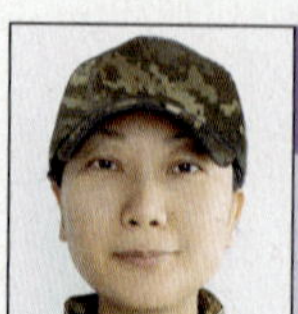

Case Study: Susan

Thirty-year-old Susan is admitted to an inpatient mental health unit following a suicide attempt. Her relationship with her husband has deteriorated since she returned from Iraq 6 months ago. She is overwhelmed by her responsibilities as a parent and wife. She has been diagnosed with posttraumatic stress disorder.

INTRODUCTION

All of us experience stress in our daily lives, but our responses vary from individual to individual. One individual may develop a severe **emotional reaction** (strong agitation of feelings), and another resilient individual is hardly aware of a traumatic event. Although most stressful events do not lead to mental disorders, sometimes, emotional issues and mental disorders develop as the response to trauma. This chapter explains the role of resilience in buffering the mental health consequences of psychological trauma and the nursing care for those who develop trauma- and stressor-related disorders. Posttraumatic stress disorder (PTSD) is highlighted in this chapter. Dissociative disorders are also discussed.

TRAUMA AND RESILIENCE

Trauma can be viewed from several different perspectives. Physical trauma may result from bodily injury resulting from an accident, self-inflicted damage, or violence perpetrated by others. Falls are a leading cause of accidents in the home. Automobile accidents are a major threat to adolescents. Self-inflicted physical trauma is often associated with mental disorders. Physical abuse of intimate partners and older person abuse are nationwide health issues. Rape and sexual abuse are physically traumatic and produce psychological trauma.

> **KEYCONCEPT Psychological trauma** is an emotional injury caused by an overwhelmingly stressful event that threatens one's survival and sense of security.

Harassment, embarrassment, child abuse, sexual abuse, employment discrimination, police brutality, bullying, and domestic violence are examples of events that can lead to psychological trauma. Family violence, loss of family members, acts of terrorism, and natural disasters are all traumatic events. Exposure to war, natural disasters, and witnessing catastrophic events may also cause psychological trauma.

Not everyone who experiences a traumatic event will be emotionally injured. One explanation for the variability in experiencing psychological trauma is resilience.

Resilience reduces the impact of risk factors and enhances the ability to "bounce back" and recover from stressful experiences. The stronger the resilience, the less likely the individual will experience reactions that lead to maladaptive behaviors and outcomes (Marazziti et al., 2024). An important mental health promotion nursing strategy is enhancing resilience, especially for people with mental and/or substance use disorders. See Box 29.1.

BOX 29.1

Clinical Judgment Vignette: Trauma and Resilience

Joe, a 22-year-old college student, experienced an armed robbery. His companion was shot and killed when Joe refused to give the robbers his money. After the incident, he was preoccupied with thoughts of the murder and felt personally responsible for his friend's death.

Joe sought psychological help from the college counseling center. During weekly counseling sessions, Joe was able to reframe his experience. Although he still has brief periods of sadness, he no longer blames himself for his friend's death. He is now resuming his usual activities and is no longer having intrusive thoughts.

Building Clinical Judgment

1. How would you document Joe's trauma?
2. How did Joe build resilience?

Resilience develops in association with a positive self-concept and self-worth, a feeling of being in control of one's life, and a feeling of power. Resilience is acquired over time, beginning in early childhood, as positive problem solving, communication, and coping skills are learned. Some children seem more resilient to trauma and are able to cope quite well with traumatic events. Family resilience and community support also play a role in developing resilience (McDorman et al., 2024).

> **KEYCONCEPT Resilience** is the capacity to withstand stress and catastrophe. It develops over time and is the culmination of multiple internal and external factors.

TRAUMA- AND STRESSOR-RELATED DISORDERS OVERVIEW

Exposure to a traumatic or otherwise stressful event can lead to a trauma- and stressor-related disorder such as reactive attachment disorder, disinhibited social engagement disorder, PTSD, acute stress disorder, and adjustment disorder.

Trauma- and Stressor-Related Disorders Across the Lifespan

Trauma- and stressor-related disorders can develop at any time throughout a lifespan. In children, exposure to trauma can cause enduring emotional issues that lead to any one of these disorders. One of the most traumatic losses for children is an unexpected death of a loved one, which can lead to multiple psychiatric disorders (Ennis et al., 2023).

Military violence is responsible for lifelong effects for deployed service members. There are reports of older adults who served in World War II developing symptoms of PTSD in later life (Bashian et al., 2024). There is a growing number of research studies that demonstrate the traumatic impact on children during military deployment and reintegration of their parents (Hébert et al., 2024). See Chapter 40.

Children

Childhood psychological and physical abuse including sexual abuse can lead to a lifelong struggle with a trauma- and stressor-related disorder. Adverse childhood events are categorized by the CDC-Kaiser Permanente Adverse Childhood Experiences (ACE) Study into three groups: abuse (emotional, physical, sexual); household challenges (birthing parent treated violently, household substance misuse, mental illness in household, parental separation or divorce, criminal household member); and neglect (emotional, physical). In this study of 8,667 adult members of a health maintenance organization, childhood physical and sexual abuse, as well as witnessing of maternal battering, was common. More than one-third of the members experienced more than one type of maltreatment. The more frequent and severe the abuse as a child, the greater the PTSD symptoms as an adult (da Silva et al., 2024).

Older Adults

When an older adult experiences trauma, memories of a lifetime of previous traumas and abuse influence the current experience. Loss of partners, friends, and family members through death, marriage, or relocation can add to the trauma. Elder abuse is discussed in Chapter 23.

POSTTRAUMATIC STRESS DISORDER

Posttraumatic stress disorder (PTSD) occurs following exposure to an actual or threatened traumatic event such as death, serious injury, or sexual violence (American Psychiatric Association [APA], 2022). Traumatic events include those that are directly experienced, witnessed, learned about from others, or repeated exposure to aversive events. Examples of traumatic events are violent personal assault, rape, military combat, natural disasters, terrorist attacks, being taken hostage, incarceration as a prisoner of war, torture, an automobile accident, or being diagnosed with a life-threatening illness.

KEYCONCEPT Traumatic events include those that are directly experienced, witnessed, learned about from others, or repeated exposure to adverse events.

CLINICAL COURSE

Most people who experience a traumatic event do not develop PTSD. However, for those who do, the symptoms often develop within several days of the event and must persist for a minimum of 30 days in order for the criteria of the diagnosis to be met. In some cases, the symptoms may initially occur substantially after the event, sometimes up to 6 months later. This is known as delayed-onset PTSD (Kang et al., 2024). About one third of the people diagnosed with PTSD develop chronic symptoms. For these individuals, symptoms fluctuate in intensity with time and usually are worse during periods of stress. Children with PTSD may react differently than adults. See Box 29.2.

BOX 29.2

Posttraumatic Stress Disorder Symptoms in Children and Adolescents

PTSD SYMPTOMS IN CHILDREN

- Bedwetting, after they had learned how to use a toilet
- Forgetting how or being unable to talk
- Acting out the scary event during playtime
- Being unusually clingy with a parent/caregiver or other adult

PTSD SYMPTOMS IN ADOLESCENTS

- May show symptoms similar to adult
- Develop disruptive, disrespectful, or destructive behaviors
- Feel guilty for not preventing injury or death
- Thoughts of revenge.

Source: U.S. Department of Health & Human Services. (2023). Post-Traumatic Stress Disorder. https://www.nimh.nih.gov/health/publications/post-traumatic-stress-disorder-ptsd

DIAGNOSTIC CRITERIA

PTSD is diagnosed following exposure to a traumatic event when symptoms in four general areas appear: (1) intrusive symptoms, avoidance of individual(s), places, or objects that are a reminder of the traumatic event; (2) negative mood and cognitions or negative thoughts associated with the event; (3) hyperarousal characterized by aggressive, reckless, or self-destructive behavior; and (4) sleep disturbances or hypervigilance for at least 1 month (National Institutes of Mental Health [NIMH], 2024).

Intrusion

In PTSD, **intrusion** is defined as the involuntary appearance of thoughts, memories, or dreams of traumatic events that cause psychological and sometimes physiologic distress. Often the intrusive thoughts are associated with cues that symbolize or resemble the original event. Sometimes, the traumatic images, thoughts, or perceptions are reexperienced, known as **flashbacks**. Nightmares are common. Intrusive symptoms also include dissociative reactions (i.e., feeling or acting as if the event is recurring). Sleeping is difficult. Terrifying flashbacks and nightmares often include fragments of traumatic events exactly as they happened. Many stimuli (e.g., loud noises, odors) associated with the trauma cause flashbacks and dreams. Consequently, affected individuals avoid such stimuli (Davis & Hamner, 2024).

In children, older than 6, repetitive play may occur that expresses the themes or aspects of the traumatic events.

They may reenact the specific trauma. Nightmares of these children may not have content (APA, 2022).

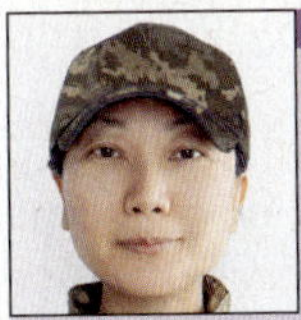

Remember Susan?

She suffers from flashbacks of exploding helicopters when she hears loud noises. Her husband tells her she screams while sleeping. She reports frightening nightmares.

Avoidance, Numbing, and Dissociation

Individuals with PTSD avoid reminders of the event including people, places, or activities associated with the event (e.g., fireworks may bring back memories of war). Many people suffering from this disorder escape situations by altering their state of consciousness or numbing by dissociating. **Dissociation** is a disruption in the linkages among subjective awareness, feelings, thoughts, behavior, and memories. An individual who dissociates is making themselves "disappear." That is, the individual has the feeling of leaving their body and observing what happens to them from a distance. During trauma, dissociation enables an individual to observe the event while experiencing no pain or only limited pain and to protect themselves from awareness of the full impact of the traumatic event. See Box 29.3. Examples of dissociation include (1) **derealization** (feelings of unreality) and **depersonalization** (the experience of self or the environment as strange or unreal); (2) periods of **disengagement** from the immediate environment during stress, such as "spacing out"; (3) alterations in bodily perceptions; (4) **emotional numbing**; (5) out-of-body experiences; and (6) amnesia about abuse-related memories.

Mood and Cognition

After a traumatic event, moods often become more irritable with episodes of explosive anger, fear, guilt, or shame. Individuals with PTSD often have difficulty experiencing **positive emotions** such as happiness or love. Consequently, they become estranged from loved ones who become frustrated with their family member's unpredictable moods and lack of emotional connection. In PTSD, the thought process becomes distorted with **exaggerated negative beliefs** or expectations about oneself, others, and the world. They may believe that no one can be trusted or that they are terrible people (Assmann et al., 2024).

BOX 29.3

Clinical Judgment Vignette: Dissociation

Carol, a 14-year-old high school student, was brutally raped by an older man in a park. When the accused person was arrested, Carol could not recall any part of the attack. Her last memory was walking home after school and seeing a man parked on the street.

Building Clinical Judgment

1. How would you document Carol's dissociative experience?
2. If Carol had experienced depersonalization, how would you expect her to describe the experience?

Hyperarousal and Hypervigilance

After a traumatic experience, the stress system seems to go on permanent alert, as if the danger might return at any time. In this state of physiologic **hyperarousal**, the traumatized individual is **hypervigilant** for signs of danger, startles easily, reacts irritably to small annoyances, and sleeps poorly. They are looking for physical danger, a repeat of a trauma, or something wrong in a relationship. The state of hyperarousal causes other issues for family members. The affected individual is irritable and overreacts to others, which causes others to avoid the individual who in turn maintains a state of continual arousal (Krupnik, 2021).

Sleep Disturbance

Sleep disturbance is one of the most commonly reported symptoms of PTSD. The disruptions fall into two categories—insomnia (persistent difficulty falling asleep or staying asleep) and nightmares. Many people with PTSD experience both. Sleep disturbances prior to the trauma are believed to be a risk factor for PTSD and insomnia immediately after the trauma is predictive of PTSD developing within 1 year. Improvement in sleep quality is associated with reduction of PTSD symptoms (Taylor et al., 2023).

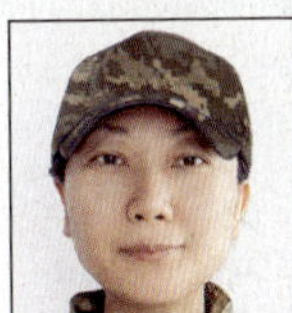

Susan and Her Family

Susan feels she does not fit into the family and no longer believes she has a role as a wife and mother. She is extremely irritable and argues with her husband constantly. She is suspicious of her neighbors and fearful that her children will be kidnapped.

COMPLEX POSTTRAUMATIC STRESS DISORDER

Complex posttraumatic stress disorder (CPTSD) is a subgroup of PTSD that occurs with severe chronic, repetitive trauma that continues for months or years. Whereas PTSD focuses on the threats and avoidance of harm, CPTSD is understood as a betrayal of trust and occurs in extreme childhood neglect, repeated sexual or physical abuse, domestic abuse, and human trafficking. These traumas result in fundamental damage to one's sense of self, personality changes, and significant impairment in personal, family, social, educational, and occupational functioning (Fung et al., 2024).

The CPTSD diagnosis is not specified in the *DSM-5-TR* but is accepted by several international organizations. For example, the World Health Organization's *International Classification of Diseases* (ICD-11) differentiates CPTSD from PTSD by symptoms. PTSD core symptoms are intrusion, avoidance, and hyperarousal. CPTSD symptoms include the core PTSD symptoms plus emphasis on symptoms of affective dysregulation, negative self-concept, and interpersonal issues (Kleva et al., 2024).

POSTTRAUMATIC STRESS DISORDER ACROSS THE LIFESPAN

Children

In children 6 years and younger, exposure to actual or threatened death, severe injury, or sexual violence may result in PTSD. The symptoms include recurrent, involuntary, and intrusive distressing memories of the events. These memories may not appear distressing and may be expressed as play. The child may not be able to explain or remember the content of the distressing dreams related to the event. Children with PTSD may avoid situations, thoughts, or moods that are associated with the traumatic event. They often become irritable and have angry outbursts with little or no provocation or distress. Although these behaviors seem illogical to adults, they represent the child's attempt to cope with the trauma (van Hemert et al., 2024).

Older Adults

PTSD in older adults can occur following a new trauma or to an event that happened several years earlier. Since there are multiple possible traumas that can precipitate PTSD, longevity increases the possibility of experiencing a traumatic event. There are many well-published accounts of Vietnam veterans who first experienced PTSD symptoms in later life (Kurth et al., 2024). Older adults are also exposed to other traumas associated with physical health issues such as cardiovascular and musculoskeletal conditions, pain (Wamser et al., 2023), and psychosocial issues such as loss of partners and changes in residences (Shakya et al., 2024).

EPIDEMIOLOGY AND RISK FACTORS

The lifetime prevalence of PTSD in the general population in the United States is 6%. The likelihood of developing PTSD varies and is often dependent on the type of traumatic event that was experienced (Schnurr, 2023; WHO, 2024). For example, violent and sexual trauma are associated with PTSD severity (Lathan et al., 2024).

For adults, the most impactful risk factor is a prior diagnosis of acute stress disorder (Haering et al., 2024). Other risk factors for PTSD include the extent, duration, and intensity of trauma involved and environmental factors (Chu et al., 2024). See Box 29.4. High levels of anxiety, low self-esteem, and existing personality difficulties

BOX 29.4

Research for Evidence-Based Practice: Gun Violence and Quality of Life

Paruk, J., & Semenza, D. (2024). Gun violence exposure and quality of life in nine US states. Journal of Urban Health, 101*(5), 942–950. https://doi.org/10.1007/s11524-024-00891-7*

THE QUESTION: Direct and indirect gun exposure is associated with a broad range of health effects including pain and PTSD. This study asks how four types of gun violence exposure (GVE) and cumulative GVE are associated with quality of life. Four types of gun violence exposure are: (1) being threatened with a firearm, (2) being shot with a firearm, (3) knowing a family member or friend has been shot on purpose, and (4) witnessing or hearing about someone being shot in your neighborhood.

METHODS: Data were collected through a survey distributed to noninstitutionalized adults living in nine states (CO, FL, MN, MS, NJ, OH, PA, TX, and WA). Gun violence exposure and quality of life (physical, psychological, social, environmental, and overall) were measured through an emailed survey. Surveys were distributed to 13,568 adults, and 7,785 agreed to participate. Participant demographics included 48% people assigned male at birth and 52% people assigned female at birth, ranging in age from 18 to 60+ years; race/ethnicity categories included White (61%), Black (11%), Hispanic (20%), and other (8%).

FINDINGS: Thirty-seven percent of the participants experienced at least one type of GVE and it was associated with decreases in all types of quality of life. Those with the highest exposure to gun violence reported the lowest quality of life. The most common type of GVE was witnessing or hearing about a shooting in the neighborhood, with decreases in all types of quality of life. The second most common GVE was knowing someone close to them (family or friend) who was shot.

IMPLICATIONS FOR NURSING: Gun violence is pervasive in US society and has a major impact on quality of life. Gun violence is a potential risk for PTSD because of its impact on quality of life. Nurses should routinely assess for gun violence and its impact on patients' lives. Gun violence prevention programs should be included in health education in all community settings.

may increase the likelihood that PTSD will develop (Bdier et al., 2023). Other risk factors include being a person assigned female at birth (hereinafter referred to as "female" in this section; the term "male" in this section refers to a person assigned male at birth), being a veteran, being a person in the LGBTQ+ community, being a member of an underrepresented group, and having family members with the disorder.

Sex Assigned at Birth

Females experience PTSD at two to three times the rate as males, with prevalence estimates at 9.7% for females and 3.6% for males (Vogt, 2023). Research differentiating PTSD risks between females and males is limited, but females consistently show higher psychological stress responses immediately after trauma leading to higher severity of PTSD symptoms. It is hypothesized that there may be several female-specific risk factors such as hormonal fluctuations or birth-related trauma that are not present in males and that are related to this heightened severity (Haering et al., 2024).

Females are more likely than males to experience sexual violence by their intimate partner leading to PTSD (White et al., 2024). The appearance of PTSD symptoms in females who are sexually assaulted depends on their age at the time of the first sexual assault. The younger the individual experiences their first assault, the more severe the symptoms (Weiss et al., 2023).

Veterans and PTSD

High rates of PTSD in veterans who returned from Iraq and Afghanistan are unprecedented in modern times. PTSD prevalence is estimated to be 15.7% of deployed veterans; female veterans have a higher rate than male veterans, with almost 20% prevalence (PTSD: National Center for PTSD, 2022). PTSD is more prevalent in the Army, among enlisted personnel when compared to officers, and more common among health care occupations, combat specialists, and service and supply personnel. PTSD in veterans is associated with postdeployment violence and alcohol misuse (Obuobi-Donkor et al., 2022). Suicide attempts are predicted by predeployment history of minor traumatic brain injury (TBI), frequent mental health treatment visits, young age, female sex assigned at birth, and relationship difficulties (Mash et al., 2023) (see Chapter 40).

LGBTQ+ Individuals and PTSD

Research data related to PTSD and people who identify as LGBTQ+ are limited, but evidence is emerging that rates of trauma exposure are elevated among lesbian, gay, bisexual, and transgender veterans compared to the general US population (Ellis et al., 2024). Minority stress in youth can be the cause or the result of PTSD (Thoma et al., 2024). For LGBTQ+ youths, **minority stress** not only includes discrimination and prejudice but also peer assault, family rejection, negative expectations for social rejection, negative disclosure experience, and internalized self-stigma.

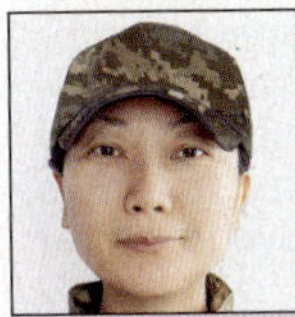

Consider This

Susan was exposed to exploding improvised explosive devices (IEDs) while serving in Iraq. Between the ages of 6 and 9 years, an uncle sexually abused her. She never told anyone.

Ethnicity and Culture

Discrimination is associated with higher rates of PTSD in underrepresented groups. PTSD symptoms are associated with Latinx immigrants' experiences of racial and ethnic discrimination (Estrada et al., 2021). African American individuals experience higher rates of PTSD than the general population and are more likely to develop PTSD following trauma exposure; discrimination contributes to the disparate rates of PTSD experienced by African American individuals (Torres et al., 2024). See Box 29.5. Asian American individuals experienced increased stress and PTSD during the COVID-19 pandemic because of heightened discrimination related to the initial source of the coronavirus (Nhan et al., 2024). Violent hate crime attacks on African American individuals contribute to an emerging increase in PTSD and comorbid psychiatric disorders (Hellyer & Gereke, 2024).

Familial Differences

There is evidence that PTSD has a heredity component, especially for females. In a large twin study, the heritability of PTSD was estimated at over 35% for females compared to 28% in males (Amstadter et al., 2024). This means that part of the etiology of PTSD can be attributed to heredity and the rest to the environment and that PTSD tends to run in families.

COMORBIDITY

Several medical and mental health conditions are associated with PTSD. Research shows that nearly 60% of individuals with PTSD also have an alcohol and/or a substance use disorder (Back et al., 2024). Depression, anxiety, suicidality, and insomnia are often present with PTSD (Kim et al., 2024). Medical illnesses associated with PTSD include cardiovascular disease, metabolic conditions, autoimmune diseases, neurocognitive disorders, and health complications such as preterm birth,

BOX 29.5

Mental Health Inequities: Racial Stress and PTSD in Pregnant Black Individuals

Black individuals are disproportionately affected by PTSD compared to other racial groups, and pregnant individuals in Black communities are at even higher risk for PTSD (lifetime rates as high as 56%) (Powers et al., 2020). One factor that could explain the disparity in rates of PTSD is racism, either individual racism (lack of respect, suspicion of committing a crime) or institutional racism (policies and procedures that deny underrepresented groups access to opportunities and resources). Because racism is traumatizing, it can lead to racial stress (psychological stress caused by racism).

In a study determining the existence of an indirect association between racial stress and PTSD symptoms through perceived barriers to psychological treatment, researchers found that experiencing racial stress predicted a negative evaluation of therapy, which in turn predicted higher PTSD symptoms. That is, experiencing individual and institutional racism can lead to mistrust of health care providers and mental health care systems, which can result in mental health needs being left untreated.

Source: Powers, A., Woods-Jaeger, B., Stevens, J. S., Bradley, B., Patel, M. B., Joyner, A., Smith, A. K., Jamieson, D. J., Kaslow, N., & Michopoulos, V. (2020). Trauma, psychiatric disorders, and treatment history among pregnant African American women. *Psychological Trauma: Theory, Research, Practice, and Policy, 12*(2), 138–146. https://doi.org/10.1037/tra0000507; Ravi, M., Lathan, E. C., Wallace, S., Hinojosa, C. A., Jones, D., Villalobos, J., Karra, S., Powers, A., & Michopoulos, V. (2024). Indirect effect of negative evaluations of therapy on the association between racial stress and posttraumatic stress disorder symptoms in pregnant Black persons. *Psychological Trauma: Theory, Research, Practice and Policy, 16*(3), 382–389. https://doi.org/10.1037/tra0001593

polycystic ovary syndrome, and endometriosis (Lawrence & Scofield, 2024).

ETIOLOGY

Biologic Theories

A growing body of research postulates that biologic factors, including neurobiology and genetics, interact with environmental factors, such as childhood experiences, and the severity and extent of the traumatic exposure, to affect susceptibility to PTSD. The amygdala and hippocampus appear to be important players in fear conditioning along with the thalamus, locus coeruleus, and sensory cortex. Interaction between the cortex and the amygdala may be necessary for specific stimuli to elicit traumatic memories (Traina & Tuszynski, 2023).

Fear conditioning occurs when a neutral stimuli, environment, situation, or action is associated with a negative event causing a fear response even when the negative event is not present. Several neurochemical systems are involved in regulating fear conditioning, including norepinephrine, dopamine, glutamate, and corticotropin-releasing systems. Hyperarousal symptoms such as anxiety and alertness with a sense of being threatened are characteristic of increased noradrenergic function, particularly in the locus coeruleus and in the limbic system (hypothalamus, hippocampus, and amygdala), and of increased dopamine activity, particularly in the prefrontal–cortical systems (Traina & Tuszynski, 2023).

Psychosocial Theories

Behavioral sensitization may be one mechanism underlying the hyperarousal seen in PTSD. The sensitized individual reacts with a magnified stress response to later, milder stressors. Research shows that traumatic exposure can alter neurotransmitter connectivity in the frontal areas resulting in severe reaction to a minor stressor. This finding would account for the fact that some individuals with PTSD experience intense fear, anxiety, and panic in response to minor stimuli. One example of behavioral sensitization is that PTSD after combat exposure is more likely to develop in veterans who experienced childhood abuse than in those who have not experienced prior trauma (Kerr et al., 2025).

FAMILY RESPONSE TO PTSD

A family member with PTSD can be difficult to live with. Startled responses, nightmares, and avoiding social situations frequently cause stress to family members who can feel hurt, angry, and discouraged. Initially, family members may be excessively sympathetic and overly protective, which can easily lead to resentment from the member with PTSD. Depression, caused by feelings of pain or loss, is common for family members. When one member has PTSD, other members are likely stressed (Larsen, 2024).

RECOVERY-ORIENTED CARE FOR PEOPLE WITH PTSD

Recovery from PTSD takes time and involves support and patience from family and friends, as well as a team of health care providers. A trauma-informed approach is important in supporting recovery and includes an understanding of trauma and an awareness of the impact it can have across settings, services, and populations. Early recognition of the symptoms and treatment lead to more successful outcomes with less likelihood of major complications. It is important to understand that there are several paths to recovery (see Chapters 2 and 8).

Teamwork and Collaboration: Working Toward Recovery

Major approaches to the treatment of PTSD include pharmacotherapy and psychotherapy. The selection of treatment is guided by practice guidelines that recommend various interventions based on medical and functional status, preexisting psychiatric and medical conditions, and current mental health assessment. The treatment guidelines, developed by the Department of Veterans Affairs and Department of Defense with the support of the Institute of Medicine, recommend education, brief psychotherapy sessions, and acute symptom management (sleep disturbance, hyperarousal, pain) for an acute reaction. For treatment of more chronic symptoms, trauma-focused therapy and stress management are recommended along with medication (Department of VA & DOD, 2023).

Psychotherapeutic approaches to the treatment of patients with PTSD include psychodynamic psychotherapy; **cognitive-behavioral therapy** (CBT); and eye movement desensitization and reprocessing. **Psychodynamic psychotherapy** focuses on different factors that may influence current PTSD symptoms such as early childhood experience and current relationships. There is emphasis on the unconscious mind. CBT focuses on the evaluation of situations, thoughts, feelings, and the problematic ways these events cause an individual to act (see Table 29.1).

Eye movement desensitization and reprocessing therapy is a process of reviewing and visualizing disturbing memories of traumatic or distressing experiences to reduce the long-term impact of the events. The patient is guided through images of the trauma, allowing for progressive desensitization. Under deep relaxation, the patient maintains an image of the traumatic event while focusing on the lateral movement of the clinician's finger. This recent approach has been successful in minimizing the fear response and avoidance pattern of those with PTSD (de Jongh et al., 2024).

Virtual Reality Exposure Therapy, the use of a virtual environment to facilitate emotional process of memories related to the trauma, is being used in some treatment settings. It can be used as a part of exposure therapy (Gausemel & Filkuková, 2024). See Chapter 28 for discussion of exposure therapy.

Group therapy and family therapy should also be considered in the treatment of those with PTSD. Sharing the traumatic experiences with family or with others who have experienced trauma can be both supportive and therapeutic. PTSD disrupts both the life of the patient and their significant others. **Social support** is a protective factor in the development of the disorder, and patients who have PTSD can benefit from the tangible social support they receive from spouses, family, and friends (Handelzalts et al., 2024).

TABLE 29.1 COGNITIVE-BEHAVIORAL THERAPIES

Therapy	Purpose
Exposure therapy	Helps people face and control their fear by exposing them to the trauma in a safe way. Strategies are mental imagery, writing, or visits to the place where the event happened.
Cognitive restructuring	Helps people make sense of the bad memories by reframing their experiences in a more realistic way. They may feel guilt or shame about what is not their fault.
Cognitive processing therapy	Helps people understand why recovery from traumatic events has been difficult and how symptoms of PTSD affect daily life. Focus is on identifying how traumatic experiences changed thoughts and beliefs and influenced current feelings and behaviors.
Stress inoculation training	Teaches an individual how to reduce anxiety. Like cognitive restructuring, this treatment helps people look at their memories in a healthy way.

Safety Issues

PTSD is associated with an increased risk of suicide, suicide attempts, aggression, and substance use disorder (Mann et al., 2024; Stanley et al., 2021; Zhan et al., 2024). The first contact the nurse often has with the patient is after a suicide attempt or an aggressive episode. A careful assessment should include determination of the risk for self-injury or aggression toward others. These individuals are at high risk for substance misuse and suicide, so a suicide risk assessment should be included in the nursing assessment. Safety measures such as suicide precautions may be needed, particularly if the individual is hospitalized.

EVIDENCE-BASED NURSING CARE FOR PEOPLE WITH POSTTRAUMATIC STRESS DISORDER

People with PTSD receive nursing services in a variety of settings throughout the continuum of care. Many will access care through a primary care setting, and others will seek out services in a mental health or primary health clinic. In many instances, the individual is reluctant to disclose information and has a tough time trusting others. Distrust is especially common in people whose trauma is associated with a violation of trust such as a rape. Gaining the individual's trust through a warm, empathic interaction, for example, offering the patient the opportunity to talk about the trauma without pressing them on the details, can lead to a meaningful therapeutic relationship.

RECOGNIZING CUES: RELEVANT ASSESSMENT INFORMATION

After the physical health needs are met and suicidal/aggressive safety measures are established, the mental health nursing assessment targets specific areas. These include the identification of the original trauma, specific physical symptoms, and the emotional and behavioral consequences of the patient's PTSD. The nursing assessment is best conducted through an interview to identify the impact of the trauma and the individual's physical and psychological strengths. The full assessment may need to take place over the course of one or more meetings, depending on the patient's capacity to discuss the traumatic events and sequelae without emotionally reexperiencing the trauma or **retraumatization**.

History of Trauma

Identifying the original trauma establishes the nature of the trauma and the length of time that the patient's PTSD has been present. However, if the individual does not want to talk about the details of the trauma, the nurse should not pursue the topic. The meaning of the trauma to the individual is much more important than what happened. The person who experienced trauma may be seeking help for the consequences of the trauma and is unable to discuss the original trauma. If the individual wants to share information related to the traumatic experience, the following questions can be used in the assessment:

- In what ways has your life been different since the trauma?
- What does the trauma mean to you?
- Do you feel that you are the same individual now as you were before the trauma? How are you the same? How are you different?
- Did anyone help you? Who are the supportive people in your life?
- Did you experience trauma or abuse prior to the trauma associated with PTSD?

Physical Health

The assessment should focus not only on the physical issues but also on healthy aspects. For example, nutrition, exercise, and self-care, such as hobbies and leisure activities, may be the individual's strengths. Information gathered from the physical health assessment can be used in developing wellness strategies. The assessment process should be similar to the one described in Chapter 10.

Nutrition

The nutritional status of an individual with PTSD can be severely compromised by a poor diet following a traumatic event. Over time, a poor diet can increase the risk of other chronic diseases. The unhealthy eating habits usually appear shortly after the trauma. The nurse should assess for changes in diet.

Sleep

In PTSD, sleep is often disrupted or practically nonexistent. Disturbing nightmares are common. The nurse should compare sleep patterns before and after the trauma. Insomnia is typically characterized by difficulty falling asleep, fragmented sleep, or panic-like awakenings. The nurse should also assess for nightmares including frequency and intensity. Family members may be able to provide detailed information that is out of the patient's awareness.

Pain

The original trauma may result in chronic pain. For example, physical abuse or wartime injury may result in long-term physical treatment and pain. Prescribed pain medication is often used for reasons other than those for which it was prescribed.

Other Somatic Responses

People with PTSD often have multiple unexplained physical issues (e.g., gastrointestinal, cardiovascular, neurologic, and musculoskeletal symptoms). Sometimes, the patient is reluctant to admit a trauma such as a rape or domestic assault and instead seeks out medical care for physical issues. Obtaining a trauma history becomes especially important when multiple physical symptoms are present.

Medication

Taking regularly prescribed medication is often difficult following a trauma. The nurse should determine the medications, vitamins, and herbal supplements the patient was taking prior to the trauma. If the individual has been unable to maintain a recommended medication regimen, medication adherence can be addressed when goals are established.

Substance Use

Commonly, individuals with PTSD self-medicate to relieve the discomfort, anxiety, or pain caused by the trauma. The use of alcohol or other drugs is common. Assessment of the use of substances and the frequency will give direction for interventions.

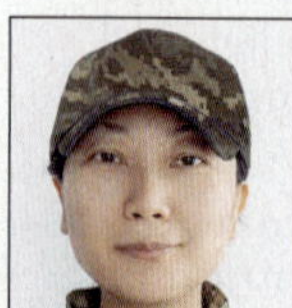

Consider This

Susan started drinking alcohol regularly in Iraq. After returning home, she continued to drink six to eight cans of beer every day.

Psychosocial Cues

The focus of the psychosocial assessment is identifying the severity of the PTSD symptoms, the disruptions that these symptoms cause the affected individual and family, and current coping approaches. The patient should be asked about the presence of intrusive thoughts, irritable moods, negative thoughts, avoidance behaviors, and arousal behaviors, and their impact on their daily lives.

Mental Status and Appearance

Behavioral Responses

Avoidance and isolation are common responses to trauma. The nurse should determine if the individual is avoiding others, situations, or environmental reminders of the trauma. Other responses associated with PTSD are agitation and aggression after the event or events. The nurse would want to determine if these behaviors are interfering with functioning and interpersonal relationships.

The nurse should assess for hyperarousal and hypervigilance such as checking surroundings and difficulty focusing on conversations. The individual may be easily startled or distracted and overreacts to environmental events.

Self-Concept

In PTSD, guilt, shame, and depression are often present. Guilt may relate to feeling responsible for the events that led up to the trauma. **Survivor guilt** occurs when one individual survives a traumatic event when others do not. Assessing self-esteem and self-concept will provide clues to the patient's resilience (see Chapter 10).

Stress and Coping Patterns

The amount of daily stress can impact the ability of the individual to manage PTSD symptoms. The individual may notice that the PTSD symptoms are worse on certain days or during certain circumstances. For example, one nurse noticed that hypervigilance was worse after working the night shift for several days. These stresses should be linked to the individual's current coping skills, which may be positive (meditation, relaxation) or negative (use of substances).

As the nurse and patient identify and evaluate the effectiveness of coping skills, the nurse should determine if the patient is resilient in dealing with stress. Some coping skills may be effective immediately but have negative consequences such as the use of substances. Developing new coping skills may be important in order to enhance resilience and positive consequences.

Social Network

By definition, a **social network** includes social interactions and personal relationships. When assessing the social network, the nurse should ask about the interactions with friends and family members and the significance of the interactions. Are the interactions with members of their social network important and frequent? Are the social network members supportive? The nurse should determine if there have been changes in the family dynamics since the trauma occurred. The nurse should also ask the individual about the use of internet social networks and how frequently they use social media in their daily living.

Functional Status

An important assessment component is determining the impact of PTSD symptoms on daily functioning. Is the individual able to maintain activities of daily living, shopping, and maintaining a household? Are there difficulties in school or work performance? If there are issues in these areas, the nurse will be able to address them during the recovery planning.

Social Determinants of Health

The impact of the social determinants of health (SDOH) should be considered when assessing an individual with PTSD because they can negatively affect symptoms. If individuals have high SDOH needs, they are more likely to experience psychological stress than those without such needs. For example, if an individual is experiencing food insecurity from lack of economic resources, they are likely to experience more psychological stress (Alegría et al., 2024).

Quality of Life

Quality of life is an overall measure of the culmination and impact of these previously discussed changes. The impact of the trauma and PTSD symptoms on overall quality of life should be examined. For example, a rape can leave an individual despondent and unable to function. Nightmares and flashbacks impede sleep and physical health.

Spiritual Assessment

Spirituality can be a source of coping and resilience for people experiencing traumas, especially those who experience multiple traumas such as firefighters and first responders. People who have PTSD and alcohol use disorder may be struggling with sobriety and no longer attend their self-help groups such as AA (Alcoholics Anonymous) (Kaufman & Rosmarin, 2024). Using the spiritual assessment questions in Chapter 10, the nurse should look for thoughts of abandonment such as "Why are you doing this terrible thing?" or loss of faith.

Strengths Assessment

Throughout the assessment, the nurse should be listening for evidence of individual physical and psychosocial strengths. Was the patient physically healthy before the traumatic event occurred? How does the patient cope with the stress of the trauma? Does the patient have family or friends who can support the individual? Is the patient motivated to deal with PTSD symptoms, develop new coping strategies, and engage in a collaborative, therapeutic relationship? Are there financial or social resources available? This information can be used in helping patients develop a safety and recovery plan.

ANALYZING CUES AND DEVELOPING HYPOTHESES

When analyzing assessment cues, safety information should be the first consideration. Is the individual suicidal or homicidal? If there is a risk for suicide, the nurse and patient should first begin to address ideations and behaviors. Other safety considerations include keeping the patient safe from acting on command hallucinations, delusional thinking, or poor judgment. Once safety needs are addressed, the nurse can examine the other cues such as the need for sleep, exercise, stress reduction, or anger management.

PLANNING RECOVERY AND WELLNESS OUTCOMES

For someone who has been traumatized and, as a result, developed PTSD, the nurse and patient can establish a recovery plan that addresses areas that interfere with coping and functioning such as feelings of anxiety, hopelessness, and powerlessness. For some individuals, a loss of impulse control results in angry outbursts or aggressive behavior that characterizes their difficulty with their quality of life and well-being.

The nurse needs to guide the patient in prioritizing goals. It is unrealistic to expect the patient to work on all goals at a time. Trauma can leave people feeling powerless. For example, one place to start is with reestablishing reasonable eating and sleeping patterns. By introducing small changes, the patient will be able to determine which interventions are likely to be effective.

THERAPEUTIC RELATIONSHIP

Establishing a trusting relationship with an individual with PTSD is the basis of nurse–patient collaboration. Needs and safety are defined by the person experiencing PTSD, who chooses the help that is wanted. Developing a relationship may take time because many people who have experienced PTSD have had their trust violated during the traumatic event. See Box 29.6. Trauma can have a lasting effect on the ability to trust others and form intimate relationships. Coping behaviors may be misinterpreted as being nonadherent and can lead to negative reactions by health care providers.

TAKING ACTION: NURSING INTERVENTIONS

Trauma-Informed Approaches

Trauma is linked to health challenges over the lifespan. A **trauma-informed approach** considers the events and circumstances causing the trauma, the individual's experience of these events, and the effects of the trauma (Substance Abuse and Mental Health Services Administration [SAMHSA], 2023). Adverse childhood events can lead to physiologic changes that lead to long-term health and social issues. When caring for an individual with PTSD, the impact of the trauma should be considered. People who have experienced trauma may respond to the present through the lenses of their past. See Box 29.7.

Physical Care

Many of the same nursing interventions discussed in Chapter 27 are used with the individual with PTSD. Proper nutrition and regular exercise can help fortify the resilience. See Box 29.8.

Sleep Enhancement

Sleep hygiene is also an important strategy because sleep disruption is common in PTSD. Early-life adversity and PTSD severity are associated with fewer hours of resting and sleeping when compared to those who had lower early-life adversity (Barone, 2024). Nurses should collaborate with the patient in finding a strategy that will help the individual sleep and manage nightmares. For example, the individual may want to sleep with the lights on because of the nightmares. However, light interferes with nighttime sleep for some people. It may be possible to go to sleep with the lights on but ask a family member to turn off the lights later. Some people with PTSD find that they cannot sleep in their bed but can sleep in a chair. Some of the following strategies may be helpful:

- Establish and maintain a regular bedtime and rising time.
- Avoid naps.
- Abstain from alcohol. Although alcohol may assist with sleep onset, an alerting effect occurs when it wears off.
- Refrain from caffeine after midafternoon. Avoid nicotine before bedtime and during the night. Caffeine and nicotine are strong stimulants and cause fragmented sleep.
- Avoid exercising 3 hours before bedtime.

BOX 29.6

Therapeutic Dialogue: Approaching Susan

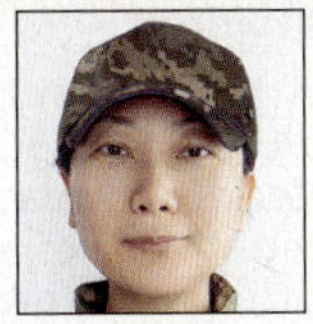

Susan did not want to be admitted to the inpatient unit and reported that she did not want to live. Her husband wants Susan to forget about Iraq and return to her former self. When she arrived on the unit, she was asked several assessment questions. She did not want to tell her story again to the nurse. The nurse needed to complete the admission assessment.

INEFFECTIVE APPROACH

Nurse: Susan, I need to ask you some questions.

Susan: Can't it wait?

Nurse: Oh—unfortunately, I have to ask questions.

Susan: I am tired of talking. Everyone is asking the same questions. For the record, I do not have a problem, I do not drink too much, and I wish my husband would go away.

Nurse: Your husband is a nice guy and is only trying to help.

Susan: You do not know what you are talking about. He wants to control me.

Nurse: If you just answer some questions, I can finish my assessment.

Susan: Not now. Go away.

EFFECTIVE APPROACH

Nurse: Hi Susan, my name is Jane, and I am your nurse today.

Susan: What do you want? I don't need a nurse.

Nurse: Well, we can just talk. What brought you here?

Susan: I am tired of talking. Everyone is asking the same questions. For the record, I do not have a problem, I do not drink too much, and I wish my husband would go away.

Nurse: Talking can be tiring. What questions have you been asked?

Susan: My whole life story—where I grew up, when I got married, how I get along with my husband and children, what happened in Iraq?

Nurse: You have had a lot of questions since you have been here. How were you able to answer all those questions?

Susan: The worst questions were about abuse and Iraq. I don't think I can talk about that yet.

Nurse: Why don't we stick to the easier ones for now?

Susan: OK, I can try.

CRITICAL THINKING CHALLENGE

1. What ineffective techniques did the nurse use in the first scenario? Whose needs was the nurse meeting?
2. What effective techniques did the nurse use in the second scenario?

BOX 29.7

Trauma-Informed Approaches: Understanding and Responding to Patient Trauma

Background

A trauma-informed approach provides a framework for understanding and responding to the effects of trauma. In this approach, the creation of a safe, supportive, and empowering environment is the priority of care. Trauma-informed approaches recognize that trauma can affect all aspects of an individual's life including interpersonal relationships, self-esteem, mood, interpretation of events, spirituality, and the environment.

Interventions

- An inpatient room for hospitalized patients should be selected that helps the patient feel safe from intruders, unnecessary sounds and lights, and other patients who may inadvertently wander into the patient's room.
- Outpatient offices should allow patients to feel there is an easily accessible exit.
- Nurses should respect patients' need for privacy and security.
- Nursing interventions should use a holistic approach and emphasize wellness strategies.

Source: Yadav, G., McNamara, S., & Gunturu, S. (2024). Trauma-Informed Therapy. In *StatPearls*. StatPearls Publishing. https://www.ncbi.nlm.nih.gov/books/NBK604200

BOX 29.8

Reflection of a Nurse: Changing Patient Behavior

Incident

A patient with PTSD states that they have been using alcohol to reduce anxiety and to improve sleep. The nurse decides to teach the patient about using alternative coping strategies and prepares a brief presentation outlining other strategies such as relaxation, sleep hygiene, and exercise. The patient listens quietly to the presentation and then agrees to change the questionable behavior. The nurse carefully documents the education session in the patient's chart.

Reflection

Upon evaluation of the intervention, the nurse realizes that even though the patient agreed to change their behavior, there was no discussion about whether the patient thought that it was likely the new behaviors would be realistic and doable.

1. What cues did the patient give that it would be unlikely there would be a behavior change?
2. What could the nurse have done differently during the education session?

Exercise

Severe PTSD symptoms are associated with poor physical performance and decreased physical functioning, and we know that exercise is associated with reduced PTSD symptoms (Kinsman et al., 2024). Nurses need to encourage patients with PTSD to engage in regular exercise, not only for health promotion but also to reduce symptoms.

Nutrition Interventions

PTSD and early-life adversity are associated with risk of obesity, diabetes, and cardiovascular disease. The greater the symptoms, the higher the body weight and blood pressure and lower the insulin sensitivity (Moriya et al., 2024). Poor diet quality including the consumption of *trans* fatty acids can be a major health issue with these individuals. Monitoring body weight and blood pressure should be included in the patient's plan of care. If these health issues are present, nurses should encourage patients to make different food choices and to choose healthy foods. Referral to a dietician may be necessary.

Smoking Cessation

Individuals with PTSD have higher smoking rates than others, and fewer have quit than the general population (Shevorykin et al., 2024). Smoking serves as a way of coping with the symptoms of PTSD. Smoking often co-occurs with alcohol use disorders and cannabis use. Nurses should discuss the health risks associated with these behaviors and encourage the patient to reduce their use. Smoking cessation programs are readily available in most communities

Medication Interventions

The selective serotonin reuptake inhibitors (SSRIs), serotonin-norepinephrine reuptake inhibitors, atypical antipsychotics, and mood stabilizers may be effective in reducing the symptoms of PTSD (see Chapters 11 and 25). Two SSRI antidepressants, sertraline and paroxetine, are approved for PTSD and are used to treat symptoms such as sadness, worry, anger, and feeling numb inside. See Box 29.9. Benzodiazepines are not recommended for people with PTSD (Bernardy et al., 2021). Recently, off-label use of prazosin, an alpha1 inhibitor, has been shown to be effective in treating nightmares and improving sleep in PTSD (Reist et al., 2021). When prescribed in conjunction with psychotherapy, pharmacotherapy can minimize the excessive fear and anxiety of PTSD (Burback et al., 2024).

Because the individual with PTSD may take many different types of medication, the nurse needs to monitor for any drug interactions and teach the individual about all the medications including expected therapeutic effect(s) and side effects. These individuals often take prescribed or over-the-counter pain medications that may interact with mood stabilizers, antidepressants, antianxiety agents, or antipsychotic agents.

Management of Complications

If the individual has been using substances to dull the feelings associated with the trauma, the nurse should educate the individual about the misuse of substances and refer them to a substance misuse treatment team. It is important for the nurse to use a nonjudgmental approach, recognizing the individual is suffering from the trauma and is trying to cope with intrusive thoughts and pain. The nurse should emphasize that there are more effective coping mechanisms and offer hope that the individual can find other means of alleviating the PTSD symptoms.

Psychosocial Interventions

Many of the same psychosocial interventions discussed in Chapter 27 can be used for people with PTSD. Relaxation strategies and stress-reduction techniques are particularly helpful for these individuals. Encouraging the individual to participate in a support group can decrease the isolation that may be present and learn how others deal with their symptoms. Service and companion dogs are also helpful in helping the individual address the stress of PTSD.

Therapeutic Interactions

One of the greatest treatment challenges is avoiding **secondary trauma** (distress or symptoms after being indirectly exposed to trauma). When caring for people

BOX 29.9

Medication Profile: Sertraline

DRUG CLASS: Antidepressant (SSRI)

RECEPTOR AFFINITY: Blocks the reuptake of serotonin

INDICATIONS: Major depressive disorder, obsessive-compulsive disorder, panic disorder, PTSD, premenstrual dysphoric disorder, social anxiety disorder

ROUTES AND DOSAGES: Available in 25-mg, 50-mg, 100-mg rts, 20 mg/mL

Adults: 50 to 200 mg PO once daily; start 50 mg PO once daily, may increase by 50 mg/day

HALF-LIFE (PEAK EFFECT): 62 to 104 hours

SELECTED ADVERSE REACTIONS: Nausea, headache, insomnia, diarrhea, dry mouth, ejaculatory dysfunction, somnolence, weakness, lack of energy, tremor, dyspepsia, anorexia, constipation, decrease in libido, nervousness, anxiety, rash, visual disturbance.

WARNINGS: Increase suicidality risk in children, adolescents, and young adults with major depressive or other psychiatric disorders. Contradicted in people being treated with monoamine oxidase inhibitors and pimozide, an antipsychotic. Risk for serotonin syndrome.

SPECIFIC PATIENT AND FAMILY EDUCATION

- Take exactly as prescribed.
- Can be taken with or without food.
- If a dose is missed, take missed dose as soon as the patient remembers unless time for next dose; then skip missed dose.
- Can cause sleepiness or may affect the ability to make decisions, think clearly or react quickly.
- Do not drive, operate heavy machinery until patient knows how medication will affect them.
- Do not drink alcohol while taking medication.
- Report any signs and symptoms of adverse reactions, suicidal thoughts, or actions.
- Notify your health care provider if severe agitation, hallucinations, coordination issues, muscle twitching, racing heartbeat, high or low blood pressure, muscle rigidity, sweating or fever, nausea, vomiting, diarrhea occur.

with PTSD, we should assume that they have a history of traumatic stress. Extreme stress occurs when shocking or unexpected events overwhelm an individual's ability to cope. The nurse should respect how and when an individual chooses to talk about the trauma. Healing from trauma requires finding and maintaining a sense of safety, gaining a sense of control over one's life and environment.

The focus of the interactions should be on understanding "what happened," not on what is wrong with the individual. The nurse seeks to understand the meaning of the experience to the individual. Similar events have different meanings to different people. When patients are describing traumatic events, it is important for the nurse to avoid responding in shock, dismay, or disgust. A welcoming approach creates a safe environment for the individual to discuss the trauma. Within a collaborative relationship, coping strategies, not symptoms, are the focus. In a safe environment, the individual can develop positive coping skills and make sense of who they are. See Box 29.10.

Enhancing Cognitive Functioning

There are several approaches to managing the intrusive thoughts, dissociative experiences, and hypervigilance that

BOX 29.10

Building Clinical Judgment With SBAR: Nurse Communication With Nursing Team

SBAR

S: Situation

Linda is a 54-year-old female assigned at birth who was admitted to a mental health unit for a suicide attempt. After the recent death of her daughter, she attempted suicide with an overdose.

B: Background

This is the second inpatient admission for Linda. According to her partner, she has a history of PTSD from witnessing a brutal murder of her parents but has been managing the symptoms without medication. She began drinking and using cannabis to deal with her irrational guilt about her daughter's death from cancer a month ago and intrusive thoughts about her parents' murder. She has not slept more than 3 hours at a time since her daughter's death.

A: Assessment

- Physical health: Ht. 5'2', Wt. 135
- Vital signs: BP 130/70, HR 85, R 12
- Oriented X 4;
- Depressed mood, denies suicidal thoughts
- No alcohol, cannabis for 72 hours

R: Recommendation

- Continue to assess for suicidal thoughts
- Establish a therapeutic relationship
- Request provider evaluate her for antidepressant
- Sleep enhancement interventions
- Consider referral for CBT

Building Clinical Judgment

1. Why did the nurse include "Continue to assess for suicidal thoughts" as the first recommendation?
2. Why did the nurse focus on sleep instead of intrusive thoughts?

the individual may be experiencing. The intrusive thoughts could be addressed through distraction, thought-stopping, meditation, or relaxation. Deep breathing or reframing the situation may reduce the hypervigilance and refocusing may reduce the dissociation. The specific approach will depend on the ability of the individual to use the techniques.

Complementary Therapies

Practicing yoga may motivate people with PTSD to increase physical activity along with enhancing self-efficacy. Simple stretching and breathing have shown to reduce unexpected cortisol levels and can be taught in many practice settings (Srour & Keyes, 2024).

Spiritual Interventions

Spirituality can support resilience in the face of trauma. Spiritual skills such as prayer, mindfulness, and meditation have been shown to help people having difficulty falling and staying asleep (Kaufman & Rosmarin, 2024).

Psychoeducation

Teaching About Symptoms

PTSD impacts every aspect of an individual's life. Trauma, genetic predisposition, brain changes, risk for multiple health issues, and risk for dependency are a part of PTSD. Education about the disorder, its consequences, health risks, and treatment become key topics for patient and family education. Psychoeducation should be customized to the individual's specific issues. There are general psychoeducation topics that should be considered for patient teaching. See Box 29.11.

Wellness Strategies

Many wellness strategies are used to treat the symptoms of PTSD. For example, sleep hygiene is important for those with sleeping issues. Managing stress is especially important for an individual with this disorder. Practicing healthy stress management techniques are critical for handling the events related to hyperarousal. A loud noise may be misinterpreted as a gunshot, causing an aggressive response. Exercise helps reduce stress and supports healthy functioning.

BOX 29.11

Psychoeducation Checklist: Posttraumatic Stress Disorder

When caring for an individual with PTSD, be sure to include the following topic areas in the teaching plan:

- Identification of individual triggers and cues that lead to reexperiencing trauma
- Safety plans for stressful periods
- Recovery plans that focus on personal strengths
- Risk factors for recurrence of symptoms
- Various treatment options: if one does not help, others exist
- Avoid substances such as alcohol and drugs
- Nutrition
- Exercise
- Sleep hygiene
- Follow-up appointments
- Community services

Providing Family Education

Families need support as they learn to cope with their family member with PTSD. Family members often feel hopeless in trying to understand the changes that their loved one is undergoing. In many instances, the member with PTSD is unable to share information about the trauma and the symptoms. If alcohol or other drugs are used to self-medicate, the family has additional challenges in dealing with the substance use. Support groups, education about PTSD, and family therapy are helpful.

Promoting Safety

Hospitalization provides a measure of safety for the patient. During hospitalization, the nurse should continue with suicide risk screening as needed and protection from triggering events such as loud noises or stimulating activities. A safety plan should be developed if the patient has had thoughts of dying by suicide (see Chapter 22).

Evaluation of Patient Outcomes

The treatment of PTSD may last several years with changing goals. Early in treatment, the goals may be to reduce intrusive thoughts and regulate sleep; later goals may include being able to establish a trusting relationship with a partner. The evaluation will be modified as the goals and interventions change.

Continuum of Care

The individual with PTSD is primarily treated in the community rather than a medical facility as an inpatient. Short-term hospitalization for safety may be needed if suicidal or homicidal thoughts are strong or for an adjustment of medication.

Emergency Care

When individuals with PTSD need emergency care, they are usually having suicidal ideation or thoughts to hurt others. Safety interventions should be implemented. It is important for the nurse to know the nature of the trauma to be able to approach the patient. For example, an individual previously exposed to combat may be sensitive to loud noises and is more likely to become aggressive when doors slam, whereas a person who has been raped may not tolerate anyone touching them.

Inpatient-Focused Care

Inpatient settings can provide a safe environment for the individual who is tormented with frequent flashbacks, has become depressed and potentially suicidal, or is harboring thoughts about hurting others. Medications may be initiated or adjusted. However, hospitalization and restrictive treatment can also retraumatize the patient. Being locked in a mental health unit or being restrained can be extremely traumatizing to the individual who has already been traumatized. See Clinical Judgment Nursing Care Plan 29.1, which sets forth a plan of care for Susan, the case study patient in this chapter.

Community Care

Treatment mostly occurs in the community with the individual attending group therapy, support groups, individual therapy, and medication management. Most appointments will occur after working hours. Nursing care can be delivered in all settings. The community setting is an excellent opportunity for patient and family education.

Virtual Mental Health Care

Virtual strategies are beneficial for the care of individuals with PTSD. Remote access to providers and treatment

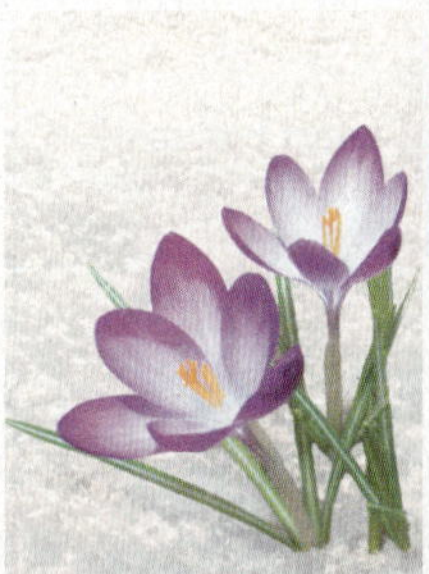

CLINICAL JUDGMENT NURSING CARE PLAN 29.1

The Person With Posttraumatic Stress Disorder

Susan, age 30, is admitted to an acute mental health unit after a suicide attempt with an overdose of benzodiazepines and alcohol. She was discharged from the Army 6 months ago and returned home to her husband and two children, ages 6 and 8. She was sexually assaulted by an uncle when she was 6 years old. While in Iraq, she was exposed to combat and was sexually assaulted by another soldier. She has been drinking alcohol heavily after her return home. She and her husband have been arguing since her return and are now discussing divorce. She decided to end it all.

Setting: Acute Mental Health Unit

Assessment Cues: Susan, assigned female at birth, is dressed in hospital scrubs following medical treatment of overdose. She is oriented X3. She is gazing downward, with flat affect, shoulders slightly hunched, soft voice. She reports she is no longer having suicidal thoughts but feels very depressed. "I don't know what to do. I don't feel close to my kids and my husband wants a divorce." She reports that she began taking her mother's benzodiazepines to help her sleep. She is having constant thoughts about the killings she saw in Iraq, cannot sleep, often has nightmares when she does sleep, does not want sexual relations with her husband, and sleeps on a couch close to the front door. She drinks six to eight beers a day. She has not worked since returning from Iraq. She is 5′5″ tall, weighs 140 lb (BMI 23.3), and has BP 120/70; P70, R16. Her goal is to have a typical life.

Strengths: Husband states he does not want a divorce and wants to stay married and is willing to engage in counseling. Mother is very supportive. She has work skills.

Associated Psychiatric Diagnosis

Posttraumatic Stress Disorder
Lorazepam 1 mg every 4 to 6 hours as needed
Zolpidem 5 mg PO HS as needed

Medications

Sertraline, 25 mg every morning for 1 week, then 50 mg PO every day.

Priority Hypothesis Post-Trauma Behaviors

Important Characteristics

Depression
Flashbacks
Intrusive thoughts

Associated Considerations

Abuse, witnessing violent death
Rape
Substance misuse

Planning Recovery and Wellness Outcomes

Initial

Motivate patient to reduce use of alcohol and misuse of benzodiazepines for stress reduction.
Discuss original trauma and the more recent trauma in Iraq.
Increase quality of sleep.
Practice stress reduction techniques.

Long Term

Engage in psychotherapy to reduce impact of trauma.
Develop positive healthy strategies for managing stress.

Continued

Clinical Judgment Nursing Care Plan 29.1 Continued

Taking Action: Nursing Interventions

Interventions	Rationale	Ongoing Assessment
Initiate a nurse–patient relationship by using an accepting, nonjudgmental approach.	A relationship with a therapist will provide an opportunity for Susan to discuss her trauma and strengths.	Determine the extent to which Susan is willing to trust and engage in a therapeutic relationship.
Encourage Susan to identify symptoms of PTSD.	By identifying symptoms, Susan will be able to recognize that the intrusive thoughts, insomnia, and other symptoms are related to her traumatic experience.	Assess Susan's recognition of her symptoms and her level of understanding of the symptoms' relationship to her current distress.
Help Susan develop a plan to address her current marital issues such as counseling or therapy after discharge.	Her marital issues may be related to her sexual assaults and exposure to combat.	Determine Susan's willingness to develop a plan.
Administer sertraline 50 mg as prescribed. Observe for target effects and side effects. Begin teaching about the medication and the importance of taking the medication as prescribed, avoiding consuming alcohol, and reporting any side effects.	Sertraline is an SSRI that blocks the reuptake of serotonin and is indicated for PTSD.	Make sure that Susan takes her medication. Monitor for improvement in PTSD symptoms and side effects such as nervousness, nausea, and any others.
Monitor sleep patterns and teach improved sleep hygiene. Administer zolpidem as prescribed.	Disturbed sleep is common in association with PTSD.	If Susan continues to have disturbed sleep or experience side effects from zolpidem therapy, notify the primary care prescriber.
Support development of resilience by examining Susan's strengths (e.g., social support, nutrition, exercise).	Resilience is important in reducing the impact of previous trauma. Positive social support, nutrition, and exercise help support resilience.	Determine Susan's social support, nutrition, and exercise regimen.

Priority Hypothesis Difficulty in Assuming Parenting Responsibilities

Important Characteristics	Associated Considerations
Decreased capacity to parent Inadequate coping with stresses of parenting	Substance use Stress Conflict with husband

Planning Recovery and Wellness Outcomes

Initial	Long Term
Resume parenting role. Decrease conflict with husband. Reduce use of substances.	Serve as role model to children. Develop positive relationship with husband. Eliminate the use of substances as a stress reliever.

Evaluation

Interventions	Rationales	Ongoing Assessment
Collaborate with Susan in identifying her current role perceptions.	Recovery-oriented nursing care engages the patient in decision-making.	Validate whether her current role perceptions accord with reality.
Identify the changes that she would like to make in her parenting role. Discuss her goals for her marriage.	Relationship rebuilding starts with self-awareness of personal goals.	Determine if she needs referral to community resources that can help her with her relationship and role issues.
Discuss strategies for reducing substance use for stress reduction. Offer relaxation, meditation, or imagery for stress reduction.	Substance use for stress reduction has negative outcomes with high risk of dependency.	Determine whether strategies are useful to Susan. May need referral to substance misuse counselor if necessary.

apps are readily available on cell phones and computers. More sophisticated virtual reality technology is also being used. For example, digital therapeutic tools and AI (artificial intelligence) assessment instruments make remote counseling therapy available to a wider geographical population (Wu et al., 2025).

Integration With Primary Care

People with PTSD may first seek help from a primary care provider. For example, sleeping issues in adults and behavior issues in children are often treated in a non–mental health environment. Conversely, when mental health clinicians care for people with PTSD, they must address the physical issues as well as their psychological issues. Because there is no one medication indicated for PTSD, there is a risk of multiple medications being prescribed to treat various physical and mental health issues. Ideally, individuals with PTSD should be treated in an integrated setting where close monitoring of all treatments is possible.

OTHER TRAUMA- AND STRESSOR-RELATED DISORDERS

ACUTE STRESS DISORDER

Acute stress disorder is similar to PTSD except that it is resolved within 1 month of the traumatic event. Acute stress disorder can develop into PTSD if the symptoms last longer than 1 month. Two trauma- and stressor-related disorders typically occurring in childhood are reactive attachment disorder and disinhibited social engagement disorder.

REACTIVE ATTACHMENT DISORDER

Reactive attachment disorder is characterized by inhibited, emotionally withdrawn behavior toward an adult caregiver. These children rarely seek or respond to comfort when distressed. This disorder usually occurs when the primary caregiver frequently changes.

DISINHIBITED SOCIAL ENGAGEMENT DISORDER

In **disinhibited social engagement disorder**, the child is overly familiar with others in ways uncharacteristic of cultural norms. For instance, the child does not hesitate to go somewhere with an unfamiliar adult.

ADJUSTMENT DISORDER

A common diagnosis for people who are hospitalized is **adjustment disorder**. This disorder occurs within 3 months of the stressor. Affected individuals experience distress that seems out of proportion to the severity of the stressor and may be unable to function socially. After the situation is resolved, the symptoms subside (APA, 2022).

DISSOCIATIVE DISORDERS

Dissociative disorders are thought to be responses to extreme external or internal events or stressors where dissociation, or a splitting from the self, occurs as a way of coping with severe anxiety. Prevalence is higher among people who experience childhood physical or sexual abuse than among others. The onset of these disorders may be sudden or may occur gradually; the course of each may be long term or transient. Dissociative disorders include **dissociative amnesia**, the inability to recall important yet stressful information; **depersonalization/derealization disorder**, the feeling of being detached from one's mental processes; and **dissociative identity disorder** (DID) (formerly called multiple personality disorder), the presence of at least two distinct personality or identity states.

The essential feature of these disorders involves a failure to integrate identity, memory, and consciousness. That is, unwanted intrusive thoughts disrupt one's contact with the here and now, or memories that are usually accessible are lost. These disorders are closely related to the trauma- and stressor-related disorders but are categorized separately. People with dissociative disorders may also have comorbid substance misuse, mood disorders, personality disorders, or PTSD (APA, 2022).

DID has long been a controversial diagnosis, with many skeptics challenging the legitimacy of this disorder. Recent empirical evidence supports DID as a complex, posttraumatic developmental disorder. Once believed to be relatively rare, prevalence rates are reported at approximately 1.1% to 1.5% of community samples. The highest prevalence is found in groups highly exposed to trauma or cultural oppression. There is also emerging evidence that there are structural brain changes in people with this disorder (Mitra & Jain, 2023).

Treatment options include the use of antidepressants to treat the patient's underlying mood and anxiety. Psychotherapy options include CBT and psychodynamic psychotherapy to determine the triggers that lead to heightened anxiety and dissociation.

SUMMARY OF KEY POINTS

- The development of psychological trauma depends on the meaning of the event and the resilience of the individual. The stronger the resilience, the more likely the individual will be able to withstand the negative impact of a potentially traumatic event.
- Resilience develops over time when there is a positive self-concept and measured self-worth, and when

problem-solving, communication, and coping skills have been learned.

- PTSD occurs after a traumatic event and is characterized by involuntary intrusive thoughts, avoidance and numbing, negative moods and thoughts, and hyperarousal. CPTSD develops when there is betrayal of trust and chronic repetitive trauma over months or years.
- People assigned female at birth are two to three times as likely as people assigned male at birth to experience PTSD. Service members who have returned from Iraq and Afghanistan have high rates of PTSD.
- There are several approaches to the treatment of PTSD including CBT, traditional psychotherapy, and medications.
- Nursing care focuses on assessing symptoms of PTSD, building strengths, enhancing resilience, and collaborating with the patient in counseling interventions, administration of medication, psychoeducation, and family support.

DEVELOPING CLINICAL JUDGMENT

1. What are the various traumatic events that can lead to PTSD? Why do some people develop PTSD and others, who have experienced the same trauma, do not?
2. Identify strategies the nurse can use to support the development of resilience.
3. Differentiate intrusive thoughts from dissociative symptoms.
4. Give examples of derealization and depersonalization.
5. Compare trauma- and stressor-related disorders with dissociative disorders. How are they similar? How are they different?
6. How should a nurse approach a military veteran who is having intrusive thoughts, is having nightmares, and is unable to sleep?

MOVIES, TV, OR STREAMING PROGRAMS

Scars: 2024. Eric (Allen Williamson) is a young adult who enlisted in the California National Guard as a medic and was quickly thrown into combat. Upon returning, he suffered severe symptoms of PTSD. When he was deployed to Afghanistan, he left his mother Roberta (Elizabeth Gast) to manage and save their family's wildfire-torn vineyard from bankruptcy. His girlfriend, Emilee (Cayla Black), worked at the vineyard and waited for Eric to return. He experienced the brutal deaths of friends and mentors killed in combat, and he also was injured. He recognizes that he was experiencing stress symptoms while being deployed but does not get the needed help. His transition to civilian life was not smooth, and he resisted accessing mental health care.

Viewing Points:

1. What made Eric at risk for PTSD even before he joined the National Guard?
2. What symptoms of PTSD did Eric demonstrate?
3. Did Eric demonstrate any characteristics of resilience?
4. What interventions would you recommend for Eric?

REFERENCES

Alegría, M., Cruz-Gonzalez, M., Markle, S. L., Falgas-Bague, I., Poindexter, C., Stein, G. L., Eddington, K., Martinez Vargas, A. E., Fuentes, L., Cheng, M., & Shrout, P. E. (2024). Referrals to community and state agencies to address social determinants of health for improving mental health, functioning, and quality of care outcomes for diverse adults. *American Journal of Public Health*, *114*(S3), S278–S288. https://doi.org/10.2105/AJPH.2023.307442

American Psychiatric Association. (2022). *Diagnostic and statistical manual of mental disorders* (5th ed., text rev.). Author.

Amstadter, A. B., Lönn, S. L., Cusack, S., Sundquist, J., Kendler, K. S., & Sundquist, K. (2024). Testing quantitative and qualitative sex effects in a national Swedish twin-sibling study of posttraumatic stress disorder. *The American Journal of Psychiatry*, *181*(8), 720–727. https://doi.org/10.1176/appi.ajp.20230104

Assmann, N., Rameckers, S. A., Schaich, A., Lee, C. W., Boterhoven de Haan, K., Rijkeboer, M. M., Arntz, A., & Fassbinder, E. (2024). Childhood-related PTSD: The role of cognitions in EMDR and imagery rescripting. *European Journal of Psychotraumatology*, *15*(1), 2397890. https://doi.org/10.1080/20008066.2024.2397890

Back, S. E., Jarnecke, A. M., Norman, S. B., Zaur, A. J., & Hien, D. A. (2024). State of the science: Treatment of comorbid posttraumatic stress disorder and substance use disorders. *Journal of Traumatic Stress*, *37*(6), 803–813. https://doi.org/10.1002/jts.23049

Barone, D. A. (2024). Trauma-associated sleep disorder. *Sleep Medicine Clinics*, *19*(1), 93–99. https://doi.org/10.1016/j.jsmc.2023.10.005

Bashian, H. M., Daks, J. S., Baird, L., Heintz, H., Moye, J., & Pless Kaiser, A. (2024). Home-based primary care providers' perspectives on the unique challenges of working with late life posttraumatic stress disorder within their population of veterans. *Psychological Services*, *21*(3), 613–620. https://doi.org/10.1037/ser0000872

Bdier, D., Mahamid, F., Fallon, V., & Amir, M. (2023). Posttraumatic stress symptoms and postpartum anxiety among Palestinian women: The mediating roles of self-esteem and social support. *BMC Women's Health*, *23*(1), 420. https://doi.org/10.1186/s12905-023-02567-x

Bernardy, N. C., Montano, M., Cuccurullo, L. A., Breen, K., & Cole, B. F. (2021). Taking the message to the rural patient: Evidence-based PTSD care. *Journal of Behavioral Medicine*, *44*(4), 519–526. https://doi.org/10.1007/s10865-020-00194-7

Burback, L., Brémault-Phillips, S., Nijdam, M. J., McFarlane, A., & Vermetten, E. (2024). Treatment of posttraumatic stress disorder: A state-of-the-art review. *Current Neuropharmacology*, *22*(4), 557–635. https://doi.org/10.2174/1570159X21666230428091433

Chu, B., Marwaha, K., Sanvictores, T., Awosika, A. O., & Ayers, D. (2024). Physiology, stress reaction. In *StatPearls*. StatPearls Publishing. https://www.ncbi.nlm.nih.gov/books/NBK541120

da Silva, H. C., Vilete, L., Coutinho, E. S. F., Luz, M. P., Mendlowicz, M., Portela, C. M., Figueira, I., Ventura, P., Mari, J. J., Quintana, M. I., Ribeiro, W. S., Andreoli, S. B., & Berger, W. (2024). The role of childhood cumulative trauma in the risk of lifetime PTSD: An epidemiological study. *Psychiatry Research*, *336*, 115887. https://doi.org/10.1016/j.psychres.2024.115887

Davis, L. L., & Hamner, M. B. (2024). Post-traumatic stress disorder: the role of the amygdala and potential therapeutic interventions—a review. *Frontiers in Psychiatry*, *15*, 1356563. https://doi.org/10.3389/fpsyt.2024.1356563

de Jongh, A., de Roos, C., & El-Leithy, S. (2024). State of the science: Eye movement desensitization and reprocessing (EMDR) therapy. *Journal of Traumatic Stress*, *37*(2), 205–216. https://doi.org/10.1002/jts.23012

Department of Veteran Affairs, & Department of Defense. (2023). VA/DoD clinical practice guideline for management of posttraumatic stress disorder and acute stress disorder. Version 4.0. Quality, Safety and Value, VA, & Office of Evidence Based Practice, U.S. Army Medical Command. https://www.healthquality.va.gov/guidelines/MH/ptsd/VA-DOD-CPG-PTSD-Full-CPGAug242023.pdf

Ellis, É., Wieling, E., & Tate, A. (2024). complex posttraumatic stress disorder links trauma exposure and suicidal behaviors among sexual minority populations: A new target in suicide prevention? *Journal of Homosexuality*, *71*(10), 2300–2318. https://doi.org/10.1080/00918369.2023.2233654

Ennis, N., Pastrana, F. A., Moreland, A. D., Davies, F., delMas, S., & Rheingold, A. (2023). Assessment tools for children who experience traumatic loss: A systematic review. *Trauma, Violence & Abuse*, *24*(5), 3205–3219. https://doi.org/10.1177/15248380221127256

Estrada, F., Cerezo, A., & Ramirez, A. (2021). An examination of posttraumatic stress disorder-related symptoms among a sample of Latinx sexual- and gender-minority immigrants. *Journal of Traumatic Stress*, *34*(5), 967–976. https://doi.org/10.1002/jts.22714

Fung, H. W., Yuan, G. F., Liu, C., Lin, E. S. S., Lam, S. K. K., & Wong, J. Y. (2024). Prevalence and clinical correlates of dissociative symptoms in people with complex PTSD: Is complex PTSD a dissociative disorder? *Psychiatry Research*, *339*, 116076. https://doi.org/10.1016/j.psychres.2024.116076

Gausemel, Å., & Filkuková, P. (2024). Virtual realities, real recoveries: exploring the efficacy of 3MDR therapy for treatment-resistant PTSD. *Frontiers in Psychology*, *15*, 1291961. https://doi.org/10.3389/fpsyg.2024.1291961

Haering, S., Seligowski, A. V., Linnstaedt, S. D., Michopoulos, V., House, S. L., Beaudoin, F. L., An, X., Neylan, T. C., Clifford, G. D., Germine, L. T., Rauch, S. L., Haran, J. P., Storrow, A. B., Lewandowski, C., Musey, P. I., Jr., Hendry, P. L., Sheikh, S., Jones, C. W., Punches, B. E., … Powers, A. (2024). Sex-dependent differences in vulnerability to early risk factors for posttraumatic stress disorder: results from the AURORA study. *Psychological Medicine*, *54*(11), 2876–2886. https://doi.org/10.1017/S0033291724000941

Handelzalts, J. E., Kalfon-Hakhmigari, M., Raichin, A., & Peled, Y. (2024). Postpartum acute stress disorder symptoms, social support, and quality of couple's relationship associations with childbirth PTSD. *Frontiers in Psychiatry*, *15*, 1310114. https://doi.org/10.3389/fpsyt.2024.1310114

Hébert, M. L., Tippe, J. M., Aquin, C., Maximos, M., Brémault-Phillips, S., & Sevigny, P. R. (2024). Military family-centred resilience-building programming across the deployment cycle: A scoping review. *International Journal of Environmental Research and Public Health*, *21*(10), 1378. https://doi.org/10.3390/ijerph21101378

Hellyer, J., & Gereke, J. (2024). The shadow of fear: Hate crime victimization and stress after Charlottesville. *Frontiers in Psychology*, *15*, 1384470. https://doi.org/10.3389/fpsyg.2024.1384470

Kang, S. G., Kim, J. W., Kang, H. J., Jang, H., Kim, J. C., Lee, J. Y., Kim, S. W., Shin, I. S., & Kim, J. M. (2024). Differential predictors of early- and delayed-onset post-traumatic stress disorder following physical injury: A two-year longitudinal study. *Frontiers in Psychiatry*, *15*, 1367661. https://doi.org/10.3389/fpsyt.2024.1367661

Kaufman, C. C., & Rosmarin, D. H. (2024). Spirituality in the line of duty: Perspectives from first responders with acute posttraumatic stress disorder and alcohol use disorder. *Psychological Services*. Advance online publication. https://doi.org/10.1037/ser0000856

Kerr, K., Mellor, R., Bennett, D., Wellauer, R., & McGaw, V. (2025). The impact of childhood abuse on future military sexual assault and PTSD symptomology in Australian veterans. *The Australian and New Zealand Journal of Psychiatry*, *59*(1), 40–47. https://doi.org/10.1177/00048674241289027

Kim, J. I., Min, B., Lee, J. H., Park, H., & Kim, J. H. (2024). Patterns of comorbid PTSD, depression, alcohol use disorder, and insomnia symptoms in firefighters: A latent profile analysis. *Journal of Affective Disorders*, *356*, 338–345. https://doi.org/10.1016/j.jad.2024.03.159

Kinsman, L. M., Norrie, H. J., Rachor, G. S., & Asmundson, G. J. G. (2024). Exercise and PTSD. *Current Topics in Behavioral Neurosciences*, *67*, 241–262. https://doi.org/10.1007/7854_2024_500

Kleva, C. S., Keeley, J. W., Evans, S. C., Maercker, A., Cloitre, M., Brewin, C. R., Roberts, M., & Reed, G. M. (2024). Examining accurate diagnosis of complex PTSD in ICD-11. *Journal of Affective Disorders*, *346*, 110–114. https://doi.org/10.1016/j.jad.2023.10.137

Krupnik, V. (2021). Tackling hyperarousal: An integrative multimodal approach. *Cognitive Neuropsychiatry*, *26*(3), 199–212. https://doi.org/10.1080/13546805.2021.1907177

Kurth, M. L., Witzel, D. D., Segerstrom, S. C., Choun, S., & Aldwin, C. M. (2024). Cohort differences in PTSD symptoms and military experiences: A life course perspective. *The Gerontologist*, *64*(2), gnad129. https://doi.org/10.1093/geront/gnad129

Larsen, S. E. (2024). PTSD and the family. PTSD: National Center for PTSD. Retrieved November 22, 2024, from https://www.ptsd.va.gov/professional/treat/specific/ptsd_family.asp

Lathan, E. C., McAfee, E. E., Spivey, B. N., Garcia, V., Kaslow, N., & Powers, A. (2024). Risk for posttraumatic stress disorder symptoms by trauma type: The role of self-compassion. *Psychological Trauma: Theory, Research, Practice and Policy*. https://doi.org/10.1037/tra0001707

Lawrence, S., & Scofield, R. H. (2024). Post traumatic stress disorder associated hypothalamic-pituitary-adrenal axis dysregulation and physical illness. *Brain, Behavior, & Immunity—Health*, *41*, 100849. https://doi.org/10.1016/j.bbih.2024.100849

Mann, S. K., Marwaha, R., & Torrico, T. J. (2024). Posttraumatic Stress Disorder. In *StatPearls*. StatPearls Publishing. https://www.ncbi.nlm.nih.gov/books/NBK559129

Marazziti, D., Fantasia, S., Palermo, S., Arone, A., Massa, L., Gambini, M., & Carmassi, C. (2024). Main biological models of resilience. *Clinical Neuropsychiatry*, *21*(2), 115–134. https://doi.org/10.36131/cnfioritieditore20240201

Mash, H. B. H., Ursano, R. J., Kessler, R. C., Naifeh, J. A., Fullerton, C. S., Aliaga, P. A., Dinh, H. M., Sampson, N. A., Kao, T. C., & Stein, M. B. (2023). Predictors of suicide attempt within 30 days of first medically documented major depression diagnosis in U.S. army soldiers with no prior suicidal ideation. *BMC psychiatry*, *23*(1), 392. https://doi.org/10.1186/s12888-023-04872-z

McDorman, S. A., Taylor-Robinette, E. K., & Romeo, R. R. (2024). Risk and resilience models in child development. *Advances in Child Development and Behavior*, *67*, 132–163. https://doi.org/10.1016/bs.acdb.2024.06.005

Mitra, P., & Jain, A. (2023). Dissociative identity disorder. In *StatPearls*. StatPearls Publishing. https://www.ncbi.nlm.nih.gov/books/NBK568768

Moriya, R. M., de Oliveira, C. E. C., Reiche, E. M. V., Passini, J. L. L., & Nunes, S. O. V. (2024). Association of adverse childhood experiences and overweight or obesity in adolescents: A systematic review and network analysis. *Obesity Reviews*, *25*(11), e13809. https://doi.org/10.1111/obr.13809

National Institutes of Mental Health [NIMH]. (2024). *Post-traumatic stress disorder*. Retrieved November 5, 2024, from https://www.nimh.nih.gov/health/topics/post-traumatic-stress-disorder-ptsd

Nhan, E. R., Williamson-Raun, A. R., Chan, R., & Yang, J. P. (2024). Ethnic identity protects and internalized racism harms health and coping in Asian Americans Following COVID-19 discrimination: A mixed-methods study. *Journal of Racial and Ethnic Health Disparities*. https://doi.org/10.1007/s40615-024-02000-5

Obuobi-Donkor, G., Oluwasina, F., Nkire, N., & Agyapong, V. I. O. (2022). A scoping review on the prevalence and determinants of post-traumatic stress disorder among military personnel and firefighters: Implications for public policy and practice. *International Journal of Environmental Research and Public Health*, *19*(3), 1565. https://doi.org/10.3390/ijerph19031565

PTSD: National Center for PTSD. (2022). Traumatic stress in women veterans. Retrieved November 7, 2024, from https://www.ptsd.va.gov/professional/treat/type/trauma_female_veterans.asp#:~:text=How%20Many%20Women%20Veterans%20Have,male%20Vietnam%20Veterans%20was%2031%25

Reist, C., Streja, E., Tang, C. C., Shapiro, B., Mintz, J., & Hollifield, M. (2021). Prazosin for treatment of post-traumatic stress disorder: A systematic review and meta-analysis. *CNS Spectrums*, *26*(4), 338–344. https://doi.org/10.1017/S1092852920001121

Schnurr, P. P. (2023). *Epidemiology and the Impact of PTSD*. PTSD: National Center for PTSD. Retrieved November 6, 2024, from https://www.ptsd.va.gov/professional/treat/essentials/epidemiology.asp

Shakya, S., Silva, S. G., McConnell, E. S., McLaughlin, S. J., & Cary, M. P. Jr. (2024). Psychosocial stressors associated with frailty in community-dwelling older adults in the United States. *Journal of the American Geriatrics Society*, *72*(4), 1088–1099. https://doi.org/10.1111/jgs.18821

Shevorykin, A., Hyland, B. M., Robles, D., Ji, M., Vantucci, D., Bensch, L., Thorner, H., Marion, M., Liskiewicz, A., Carl, E., Ostroff, J. S., & Sheffer, C. E. (2024). Tobacco use, trauma exposure and PTSD: a systematic review. *Health Psychology Review*, *18*(4), 649–680. https://doi.org/10.1080/17437199.2024.2330896

Srour, R. A., & Keyes, D. (2024). Lifestyle mindfulness in clinical practice. In *StatPearls*. StatPearls Publishing. https://www.ncbi.nlm.nih.gov/books/NBK599498

Stanley, I. H., Marx, B. P., Keane, T. M., & Vujanovic, A. A. (2021). PTSD symptoms among trauma-exposed adults admitted to inpatient psychiatry for suicide-related concerns. *Journal of Psychiatric Research*, *133*, 60–66. https://doi.org/10.1016/j.jpsychires.2020.12.001

Substance Abuse and Mental Health Services Administration [SAMHSA]. (2023). *Practical guide for implementing a trauma-informed approach*. SAMHSA Publication No. PEP23-06-05-005. National Mental Health and Substance Use Policy Laboratory. Substance Abuse and Mental Health Services Administration.

Taylor, D. J., Pruiksma, K. E., Mintz, J., Slavish, D. C., Wardle-Pinkston, S., Dietch, J. R., Dondanville, K. A., Young-McCaughan, S., Nicholson, K. L., Litz, B. T., Keane, T. M., Peterson, A. L., Resick, P. A., & Consortium to Alleviate PTSD. (2023). Treatment of comorbid sleep disorders and posttraumatic stress disorder in U.S. active duty military personnel: A pilot randomized clinical trial. *Journal of Traumatic Stress*, *36*(4), 712–726. https://doi.org/10.1002/jts.22939

Thoma, B. C., Biernesser, C. L., & Win, E. (2024). Gender nonconformity, minority stress, and psychological distress among sexual minority adolescents. *LGBT Health*. https://doi.org/10.1089/lgbt.2024.0059

Torres, L., Geier, T. J., Tomas, C. W., Bird, C. M., Timmer-Murillo, S., Larson, C. L., & deRoon-Cassini, T. A. (2024). Racial discrimination increases the risk for nonremitting posttraumatic stress disorder symptoms in traumatically injured Black individuals living in the United States. *Journal of Traumatic Stress*, *37*(4), 697–709. https://doi.org/10.1002/jts.23051

Traina, G., & Tuszynski, J. A. (2023). The neurotransmission basis of post-traumatic stress disorders by the fear conditioning paradigm. *International Journal of Molecular Sciences*, *24*(22), 16327. https://doi.org/10.3390/ijms242216327

van Hemert, M. T. C., de Jong, P. M., Vanaerschot, G., Brouwer, T. R., Zoon, J. S., & Gunst, E. (2024). Posttraumatic stress disorder following childhood sexual and physical abuse: a study protocol for an 11-week randomised controlled trial comparing imaginal exposure and imagery rescripting. *European Journal of Psychotraumatology*, *15*(1), 2358683. https://doi.org/10.1080/20008066.2024.2358683

Vogt, D. (2023). *Research on women, trauma and PTSD*. PTSD: National Center for PTSD. Retrieved November 6, 2024, from https://www.ptsd.va.gov/professional/treat/specific/ptsd_research_women.asp

Wamser, R. A., Walker, H. E., & Sager, J. (2023). Physical health outcomes of trauma exposure across the lifespan. *Journal of Interpersonal Violence*, *38*(23–24), 12025–12045. https://doi.org/10.1177/08862605231190670

Weiss, J., Steil, R., Priebe, K., Lindauer, P., Kleindienst, N., Fydrich, T., & Müller-Engelmann, M. (2023). Sexual dysfunctions in women with posttraumatic stress disorder following childhood sexual abuse: Prevalence rates according to DSM-5 and clinical correlates. *Archives of Sexual Behavior*, *52*(8), 3365–3378. https://doi.org/10.1007/s10508-023-02652-0

White, S. J., Sin, J., Sweeney, A., Salisbury, T., Wahlich, C., Montesinos Guevara, C. M., Gillard, S., Brett, E., Allwright, L., Iqbal, N., Khan, A., Perot, C., Marks, J., & Mantovani, N. (2024). Global prevalence and mental health outcomes of intimate partner violence among women: A systematic review and meta-analysis. *Trauma, Violence & Abuse*, *25*(1), 494–511. https://doi.org/10.1177/15248380231155529

World Health Organization (WHO). (2024). *Post-traumatic stress disorder*. Retrieved November 22, 2024, from https://www.who.int/news-room/fact-sheets/detail/post-traumatic-stress-disorder#:~:text=The%20likelihood%20of%20developing%20PTSD,following%20sexual%20violence%20(1)

Wu, J. Y., Tsai, Y. Y., Chen, Y. J., Hsiao, F. C., Hsu, C. H., Lin, Y. F., & Liao, L. D. (2025). Digital transformation of mental health therapy by integrating digitalized cognitive behavioral therapy and eye movement desensitization and reprocessing. *Medical & Biological Engineering & Computing*, *63*(2), 339–354. https://doi.org/10.1007/s11517-024-03209-6

Zhan, N., Zhang, L., Gong, M., & Geng, F. (2024). Clinical correlates of irritability, anger, hostility, and aggression in posttraumatic stress disorder. *Psychological Trauma: Theory, Research, Practice and Policy*, *16*(6), 1055–1062. https://doi.org/10.1037/tra0001498

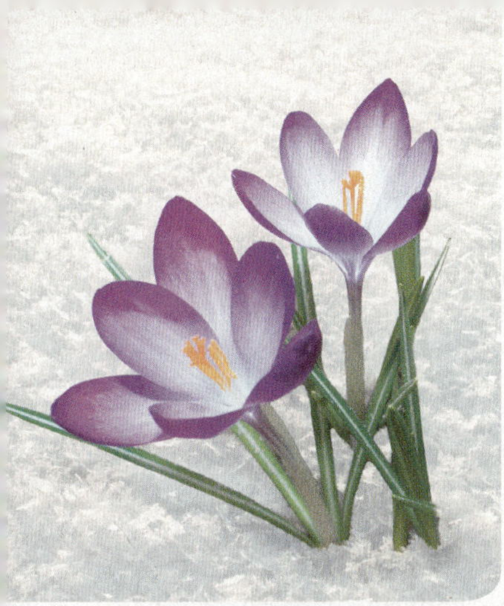

30 Personality Disorders

Nursing Care of People With Personality and Impulse-Control Disorders*

Rebecca Luebbert and Mary Ann Boyd

KEYCONCEPTS

- antisocial personality disorder (ASPD)
- borderline personality disorder (BPD)
- difficult temperament
- emotional dysregulation
- impulse-control disorders
- impulsivity
- personality
- personality disorder
- self-harm
- temperament

LEARNING OBJECTIVES

After studying this chapter, you will be able to:

1. Discuss the role of a personality in personality disorders.
2. Relate the primary theories of personality disorders to the clinical symptoms and the course of borderline and antisocial personality disorders, with emphasis on emotional dysregulation, self-harm, temperament, and impulsivity.
3. Evaluate the significance of trauma in the appearance of borderline and antisocial personality symptoms.
4. Examine the relationship between social determinants of health and borderline and antisocial personality disorders.
5. Select strategies to establish therapeutic relationships with people with borderline and antisocial personality disorders.
6. Using a clinical judgment model, formulate person-centered, recovery-oriented nursing care plans for people with borderline and antisocial personality disorders.
7. Identify medications that are used to treat people with borderline and antisocial personality disorders and evaluate their effectiveness.
8. Develop wellness strategies for people with borderline and antisocial personality disorders.
9. Compare and contrast mental health care provided in emergency, inpatient, community, and virtual settings.
10. Support the integration of health care and mental health care for people with borderline and antisocial personality disorders.
11. Compare and contrast other personality disorders.
12. Compare and contrast disruptive impulse-control disorders.

KEY TERMS

• affective instability • avoidant personality disorder • cognitive schemata • dependent personality disorder • dialectical behavior therapy (DBT) • dichotomous thinking • dissociation • histrionic personality disorder • identity diffusion • inhibited grieving • intermittent explosive disorder • invalidating environment • kleptomania • mentalization-based therapy (MBT) • mentalizing • narcissistic personality disorder • obsessive-compulsive personality disorder • paranoid personality disorder • parasuicidal behavior • personality traits • projective identification • pyromania • schizoid personality disorder • schizotypal personality disorder • schizotypy • separation-individuation • splitting

---

*In this chapter, "men," "women," "male," and "female" refer to people who identify as these genders.

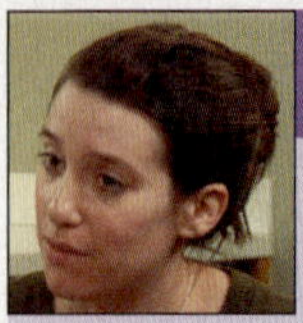

Case Study: Rebecca

Rebecca, age 23, lives alone. She has few friends but does attend regular psychotherapy sessions that help her understand her emotions and behaviors. She becomes very upset when her therapist leaves town for a planned vacation. Her family wants to help but is frustrated with Rebecca's inability to deal with everyday stresses.

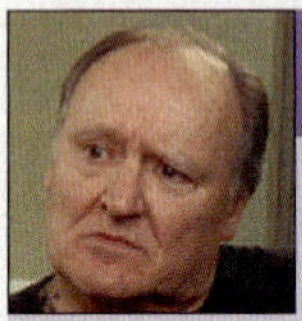

Case Study: Danny

Danny, age 55, was admitted to the inpatient mental health unit from the county jail after threatening suicide with a plan to hang himself. He was arrested after physically assaulting his girlfriend, with whom he lives.

INTRODUCTION

The concept of personality seems deceptively simple but instead is very complex. Historically, the term *personality* was derived from the Greek word *persona*, the theatrical mask used by dramatic players that had the connotation of a projected pretense or allusion. With time, the connotation changed from being an external surface representation to the internal traits of the individual.

KEYCONCEPT Personality is a complex pattern of characteristics, largely outside of the person's awareness, which comprise the individual's distinctive pattern of perceiving, feeling, thinking, coping, and behaving.

Personality traits are prominent aspects of personality that are exhibited in a wide range of social and personal contexts. Intrinsic and pervasive, personality traits emerge from a complicated interaction of biologic dispositions, psychological experiences, and environmental situations that ultimately comprise a distinctive personality.

No sharp division exists between typical and atypical personality functioning. Instead, personalities are viewed on a continuum from typical at one end to atypical at the other. Many of the same processes involved in the development of a "typical" personality are responsible for the development of a personality disorder.

This chapter provides an overview of personality disorders with borderline personality disorder (BPD) explained in detail and antisocial personality disorder (ASPD) emphasized. Disruptive impulse-control disorders, a closely related group of disorders, are also reviewed. Oppositional defiant disorder and conduct disorder, which are childhood diagnoses, are discussed in Chapter 37.

PERSONALITY DISORDERS OVERVIEW

A personality disorder is "an enduring pattern of inner experience and behavior that deviates markedly from the expectations of the individual's culture, is pervasive and inflexible, has an onset in adolescence or early adulthood, is stable over time, and leads to distress or impairment" (American Psychiatric Association [APA], 2022).

Historically there has always been the question of the cause of personality disorders. Is it "bad genes" and/or "bad environment"? There appears to be a general agreement that the main etiologic factors for personality disorder are heritably heightened affect states (excessive fear, anger, insecure attachments) and adverse environmental factors (ineffective parenting, childhood trauma), acting singly or in concert (Neves Horacio et al., 2023).

KEYCONCEPT A **personality disorder** diagnosis is based on pervasively inflexible behavior patterns of long duration—traced to adolescence or early adulthood—that deviates from acceptable cultural norms.

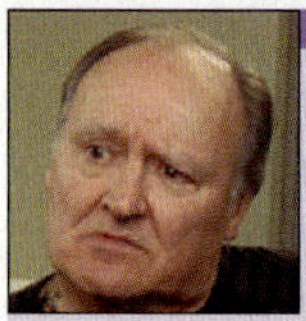

Consider Danny

Danny explains that rules are made to be broken.

The prevalence rate of any personality disorder in the adult population is estimated to be between 3% to 10% globally; prevalence is much higher in people affected by other psychiatric disorders (Solmi et al., 2021). These rates are of public health significance because of the extreme social dysfunction and high health care use of people with personality disorders. Many others do not seek treatment for the distress or impairment related to their personality disorder because they do not perceive themselves as having an issue. However, they frequently seek help for concurrent medical or mental health disorders.

At present, 10 personality disorders are recognized in the *DSM-5-TR* within three clusters. Cluster A disorders are characterized by odd or eccentric behavior, Cluster B disorders are characterized by dramatic, emotional, or erratic behavior, and in Cluster C disorders, individuals appear anxious or fearful (APA, 2022).

CLUSTER A DISORDERS: PARANOID, SCHIZOID, AND SCHIZOTYPAL PERSONALITY DISORDERS

PARANOID PERSONALITY DISORDER

Clinical Course and Diagnostic Criteria

Paranoid personality disorder is characterized by a long-standing suspiciousness and mistrust of people in general. Individuals with this disorder are distrustful and suspicious and assume that others may harm or deceive them. These individuals are suspicious, guarded, and hostile. They are consistently mistrustful of others' motives, even those of relatives and close friends. Actions of others are often misinterpreted as deception, deprecation, and betrayal, especially regarding loyalty or trustworthiness of friends and associates (Jain & Torrico, 2024).

People with paranoid personality disorder are unforgiving and hold grudges; their typical emotional responses are anger and hostility. They distance themselves from others and are outwardly argumentative and abrasive; internally, they feel powerless, fearful, and vulnerable. Other hallmark features of paranoid personality disorder are persistent ideas of self-importance and the tendency to be rigid and controlling. Blind to their own unattractive behaviors and characteristics, they often attribute these same traits to others. Their outward demeanor often seems cold, sullen, and humorless. They want to appear controlled and objective, yet often they react emotionally, displaying signs of nervousness, anger, envy, and jealousy. Orderly by nature, they are hypervigilant to any environmental changes that may loosen their control of the world. Occupational issues are common. In clinical populations, paranoid personality disorder is one of the strongest predictors of aggressive behavior, often associated with violence and stalking. People with this disorder do not seek mental health care until they have symptoms of comorbid disorders, such as a major depressive episode (Jain & Torrico, 2024).

Epidemiology and Risk Factors

The prevalence estimates for paranoid personality range from 0.5% to 4.4% in the general US population, up to 30% in inpatient psychiatric settings, and 23% in individuals who are incarcerated. Although prevalence rates for this disorder are higher in women, men seek clinical attention more frequently. Although studies have found a genetic relationship between paranoid personality and schizophrenia, there is an even stronger relationship between paranoid personality and delusion disorder and affective disorders (Jain & Torrico, 2024).

Etiology

The etiologic factors of paranoid personality remain unclear, but a genetic predisposition for an irregular maturation may be involved. Temperament is heritable and contributes to personality development. There is also a connection between social stress and childhood trauma and paranoid personality.

Evidence-Based Nursing Care of People With Paranoid Personality Disorder

Nurses most likely see these patients about other health issues but formulate nursing approaches based on the patient's underlying paranoia. Assessment of these individuals reveals disturbed or illogical thoughts that demonstrate misinterpretation of environmental stimuli. For example, a man was convinced that his wife was having an affair with the neighbor because his wife and the neighbor left their homes for work at the same time each morning. Although the man's beliefs were illogical, he never once considered that he was wrong. He frequently followed them but never caught them together. He continued to believe they were having an affair.

Because of their inability to develop relationships, these patients are often socially isolated and lack social support systems.

Mental health nursing interventions based on the establishment of a therapeutic relationship are difficult to implement because of the patient's mistrust. If a trusting relationship is established, the nurse helps the patient identify problematic areas, such as getting along with others or keeping a job. Through therapeutic techniques such as acceptance, confrontation, and reflection, the nurse and patient examine a problematic area to gain another view of the situation. Changing thought patterns takes time. Patient outcomes are evaluated in terms of small changes in thinking and behavior. There is evidence that change in interpersonal sensitivity, hostility, and paranoid ideation can occur (Cheli et al., 2021).

Continuum of Care

Individuals with paranoid personalities are unlikely to participate in treatment or recovery plans. If they have other comorbid disorders and are forced to seek treatment (through loss of their job or being ordered by a court in connection with an offense of a chargeable nature), they may seek help for depression or psychosis.

SCHIZOID PERSONALITY DISORDER

Clinical Course and Diagnostic Criteria

People with **schizoid personality disorder** are characterized as being seclusive and isolated, and having limited interest or involvement in everyday events. They have a diminished need for social connectedness and demonstrate little concern for others (Torrico & Madhanagopal, 2024). They tend to be unable to experience the joyful and pleasurable aspects of life, and rarely display strong emotions such as anger or joy. They are introverted, reclusive, and clinically seem distant, aloof, apathetic, and emotionally detached. Typically life-long loners, they have difficulty making friends, seem uninterested in social activities, and appear to gain little satisfaction in personal relationships. In fact, they appear to be incapable of forming social relationships. Their interests are directed at objects, things, and abstractions. They may do well at solitary jobs that other people might find difficult to tolerate. Often, people with schizoid personality disorders may daydream excessively and become attached to animals, and they frequently do not form long-lasting romantic relationships. As children, they engage primarily in solitary activities, such as stamp collecting, computer games, electronic equipment, or academic pursuits such as mathematics or engineering. In addition, they seem to have a cognitive deficit characterized by obscure thought processes, particularly about social matters. Communication with others is confused and lacks focus. These individuals reveal minimum introspection and self-awareness, and interpersonal experiences are described in a very mechanical way.

Epidemiology and Risk Factors

Schizoid personality disorder is rarely diagnosed in clinical settings. It is estimated that the US prevalence is 3.1% (APA, 2022).

Etiology

The etiologic processes are speculative. There may be neuroanatomical or neurotransmitter changes associated with schizoid disorder (Torrico & Madhanagopal, 2024). Schizoid pathology has also been hypothesized to be a reaction to trauma, particularly rejection experienced during childhood resulting in the person's inward retreat. Further research has found that traumatic events occurring in childhood, particularly physical and emotional abuse and neglect, are strong predictors of schizoid pathology. More recent research has examined the influence of interpersonal trauma that includes a high degree of betrayal (trauma perpetrated by someone that the person trusts or relies on for protection or support) on more severe pathology (Newcomb, 2024).

Evidence-Based Nursing Care of People With Schizoid Personality Disorder

Individuals with schizoid personality disorder have limited insight about their illness and consequently do not seek treatment on their own. It is usually only after their behaviors have resulted in significant distress to others that they present for treatment. Difficulty with social relations and low self-esteem are typical nursing priorities. The nurse should complete a thorough personal and social history to determine the disorder's impact on individuals' day-to-day living. Major treatment goals are to prevent social isolation, reduce interpersonal conflict, and increase emotional responsiveness to others. Because these individuals often lack customary social skills, social skills training is useful in enhancing their ability to relate in interpersonal situations. The primary focus is to increase the patient's ability to feel pleasure. The nurse balances interventions between encouraging enough social activity to prevent the individual from retreating into a fantasy world and too much social activity that becomes intolerable to the patient.

Establishing a therapeutic relationship with these individuals may be difficult due to their preference to shy away from interactions. They may not be motivated for treatment and may not reciprocate satisfaction or fulfillment in treatment interventions. The nurse should encourage the patient to engage in their available support networks. Evaluation of outcomes should be in terms of increasing the patient's feelings of satisfaction with solitary activities (Torrico & Madhanagopal, 2024).

Continuum of Care

People with schizoid personalities are rarely hospitalized unless they have a comorbid disorder. Family members may seek treatment for them in an outpatient setting.

SCHIZOTYPAL PERSONALITY DISORDER

Clinical Course and Diagnostic Criteria

Schizotypal personality disorder is characterized by a pattern of social and interpersonal deficits. The term **schizotypy** refers to traits that are similar to the symptoms of schizophrenia but are less severe. Cognitive perceptual symptoms are a primary characteristic and include magical beliefs (similar to delusions) and perceptual aberrations (similar to hallucinations). Other common symptoms include referential thinking (interpreting insignificant events as personally relevant) and paranoia (suspicion of others). Individuals with this disorder may express paranormal, supernatural, or astrologic preoccupations.

People with schizotypal personality disorder are more dramatically eccentric than those with schizoid personality disorder who are characteristically flat, neutral, and dull. These individuals are perceived as strikingly odd or strange in both appearance and behavior, even to laypersons. They may have unusual mannerisms, an unkempt manner of dress that does not quite "fit together," and inattention to usual social conventions (e.g., avoiding eye contact, wearing clothes that are stained or ill fitting, and being unable to join in the give-and-take banter of coworkers). Devoid of any close friends other than first-degree relatives, their mood is constricted or inappropriate, with excessive social anxieties. They usually exhibit an avoidant behavior pattern.

People with schizotypal personality disorder may respond to stress with transient psychotic episodes (lasting minutes to hours). Because of their short duration, the symptoms mirror but fall short of features that would justify the diagnosis of schizophrenia. Many individuals with schizotypal personality disorder also have a co-occurring major depressive disorder diagnosis when admitted to a hospital and are at greater risk for suicide (Sher et al., 2023). Schizotypal personality disorders may be slightly more common in males (APA, 2022; Francois & Torrico, 2024).

Epidemiology and Risk Factors

The lifetime prevalence of schizotypal personality disorder is 3.9%, with higher rates among men (4.2%) than women (3.7%). There are variations of traits across countries and cultures. People from some cultures express all of the symptoms of schizotypal personality disorder and others only one or two distinct symptoms (Francois & Torrico, 2024).

Etiology

Magnetic resonance imaging studies of individuals with schizotypal personality disorder show smaller gray matter volume, which is correlated with negative symptoms. Studies show dysfunction of brain circuits including striatal, frontal, temporal, limbic regions (and their networks), together with a dysregulation of the dopaminergic pathways (Attademo et al., 2021). There is also evidence that winter birth and prenatal exposure to influenza may be associated with schizotypy. Trauma-exposed individuals have a greater risk of developing schizotypal disorder (Dong et al., 2021).

Evidence-Based Nursing Care of People With Schizotypal Personality Disorder

Because some clinical features of schizotypal personality disorder mimic schizophrenia, a formal thought disorder should be first ruled out. Obtaining a detailed social history is also important to determine the disorder's impact on patients' daily functioning and relationships with others. Depending on the amount of decompensation (i.e., deterioration of functioning and exacerbation of symptoms), the assessment of a patient with a schizotypal personality disorder can generate a range of clinical priorities. If an individual has severe symptoms, such as delusional thinking or perceptual disturbances, the nursing priorities are similar to those for an individual with schizophrenia (see Chapter 24). Atypical antipsychotics may be beneficial in addressing paranoia. Assessment of depressive symptoms and suicidal ideation is also important. If symptoms are mild, social isolation, coping with stress and daily living, low self-esteem, and difficult social interactions are the focus of nursing care.

People with schizotypal personality disorder need help in developing recovery-oriented strategies to increase their sense of self-worth and recognize their positive attributes. They can benefit from social skills training and environmental management that increases their psychosocial functioning. Their eccentric thoughts and behaviors alienate them from others. Reinforcing socially appropriate dress and behavior can improve their overall appearance and ability to relate to the environment. Because they have a hard time generalizing from one situation to another, attention to cognitive skills is important.

Continuum of Care

Quality of life (QoL) for a patient with schizotypal personality disorder can be improved with supportive psychotherapy, but their suspiciousness, lack of trust, or impaired social interactions make it difficult to establish a therapeutic relationship. They are less likely to maintain long-term social relationships and are less likely to achieve stable employment. These individuals do not usually seek treatment unless more serious symptoms appear, such as depression or anxiety.

Nursing care is often provided in a home or clinic setting, with the personality disorder being secondary to the purpose of the care. This means that nurses focus on other aspects of patient care and may miss the underlying psychiatric disorder. A psychiatric nursing consultation may be needed for these patients to help identify the disorder (Francois & Torrico, 2024).

CLUSTER B DISORDERS: BORDERLINE, ANTISOCIAL, HISTRIONIC, AND NARCISSISTIC PERSONALITY DISORDERS

BORDERLINE PERSONALITY DISORDER

The term *borderline* was first coined by Adolph Stern in 1938 when he identified a "border line group of patients" who "fit frankly neither into the psychotic nor into the psychoneurotic group, and are extremely difficult to handle by any psychotherapeutic method" (Stern, 1938).

People with BPD have difficulty regulating their moods, developing a self-identity, maintaining interpersonal relationships, maintaining reality-based thinking, and avoiding impulsive or destructive behavior. The severity and difficulty in treating the disorder lead to enormous public health costs from health care utilization and functional disability (Hastrup et al., 2022).

> **KEYCONCEPT Borderline personality disorder (BPD)** is characterized by a disruptive pattern of instability related to self-identity, interpersonal relationships, and affect, combined with marked impulsivity and destructive behavior. BPD has historically been seen as a lifelong, highly disabling disorder; however, research over the past two decades has challenged that assumption. BPD can be accurately identified in adolescence, and the course of the disorder in adolescence and adulthood is generally similar, with reductions in symptoms over time (Liljedahl et al., 2023).

Clinical Course

Individuals with BPD appear more competent than they actually are and often set unrealistically high expectations for themselves. When these expectations are not met, they experience intense shame, self-hate, and self-directed anger. Their lives resemble never-ending drama—one crisis after another. Some of the crises are caused by the individual's dysfunctional lifestyle or inadequate social milieu, but many are caused by fate—the death of a spouse or a diagnosis of an illness. They react emotionally with minimal coping skills. The intensity of their emotions often frightens them and others. Friends, family members, and coworkers limit their contact with the person, which furthers the sense of aloneness, abandonment, and self-hatred. It also diminishes opportunities for learning self-corrective measures.

Remissions from the acute symptoms (e.g., self-injurious behaviors, suicide attempts, or threats about suicide) are fairly common, and the relapse rate is relatively low compared with other disorders. However, although clinical symptoms of BPD generally decrease over time, many individuals continue to present longer-lasting symptoms of low mood, feelings of emptiness, and poor psychosocial adjustment (Casellas-Pujol et al., 2024).

Diagnostic Criteria

BPD is a "pervasive pattern of instability of interpersonal relationships, self-image, and affects, and marked impulsivity beginning by early adulthood and present in a variety of contexts" (APA, 2022, p. 754). See Key Diagnostic Characteristics 30.1. Individuals with BPD also exhibit related cognitive and behavioral dysfunctions.

Unstable Interpersonal Relationships

People with BPD have an extreme fear of abandonment, as well as a history of unstable or insecure attachments. They suffer from difficulties in emotion regulation, which includes **affective instability**, impulsivity, fear of abandonment, eruptions of rage, feelings of emptiness, unstable interpersonal relationship, chronic dysphoria, or depression, as well as heightened risk-taking behaviors. Most have never experienced a consistently secure, nurturing relationship and are constantly seeking reassurance and validation. In an attempt to meet their interpersonal needs, they idealize others and establish intense relationships that violate others' interpersonal boundaries, which lead to rejection. The relationships of individuals with BPD may be chaotic, intense, and marked with difficulties (DiBenedetti et al., 2023). When these relationships do not live up to their expectations, they devalue the person. Continually disappointed in relationships, these individuals, who are already intensely emotional and have a poor sense of self, feel estranged from others and inadequate in the face of perceived social standards. Intense shame and self-hate follow. These feelings often result in self-injurious behaviors, such as wrist cutting, self-burning, or head banging. BPD is associated with high mortality by suicide. There is also a high risk to die prematurely because of impulsive risk-taking, as well as succumbing to violence from others. Even though the characteristics of BPD are easy to identify, the diagnosis is often overlooked. A key reason for this neglect is the perception that the overemotional,

KEY DIAGNOSTIC CHARACTERISTICS 30.1

***DSM-5-TR* DIAGNOSTIC CRITERIA: Borderline Personality Disorder**

A pervasive pattern of instability of interpersonal relationships, self-image, and diminished affect, and marked impulsivity, beginning by early adulthood and present in a variety of contexts, as indicated by five (or more) of the following:

1. Frantic efforts to avoid real or imagined abandonment. (**Note:** Do not include suicidal or self-mutilating behavior covered in Criterion 5.)
2. A pattern of unstable and intense interpersonal relationships characterized by alternating between extremes of idealization and devaluation.
3. Identity disturbance: markedly and persistently unstable self-image or sense of self.
4. Impulsivity in at least two areas that are potentially self-damaging (e.g., spending, sex, substance use, reckless driving, binge eating). (**Note:** Do not include suicidal or self-mutilating behavior covered in Criterion 5.)
5. Recurrent suicidal behavior, gestures, or threats, or self-mutilating behavior.
6. Affective instability due to a marked reactivity of mood (e.g., intense episodic dysphoria, irritability, or anxiety usually lasting a few hours and only rarely more than a few days).
7. Chronic feelings of emptiness.
8. Inappropriate intense anger or difficulty controlling anger (e.g., frequent displays of temper, constant anger, recurrent physical fights).
9. Transient stress-related paranoid ideation or severe dissociative symptoms.

sometimes theatrical, and self-injurious behaviors are signs of willfulness and manipulations rather than signs of an illness (Miller et al., 2023).

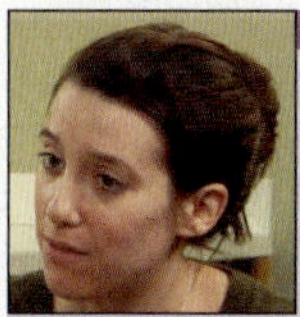

Consider Rebecca

Rebecca hates being alone, but her behaviors drive others away. When she feels rejected, anxious, or angry, she cuts her wrists, which decreases her anxiety.

Unstable Self-Image

Patients with BPD appear to have no sense of their own identity and direction. A typical expression of identity confusion is difficulty answering questions such as: Who am I? How can I be differentiated from anybody else? What do I want? It is not unusual for people with BPD to direct their actions in accord with the wishes of other people. For example, one person with BPD describes themselves as follows: "I am a singer because my mother wanted me to be. I live in the city because my manager thought that I should. I become whatever anyone tells me to be. Whenever someone recommends a song, I wonder why I didn't think of that. My boyfriend tells me what to wear." Individuals with BPD confuse their own attributes, feelings, and desires with those of another person, particularly in close relationships. This disturbance in identity contributes to people with BPD being more vulnerable in stressful situations (Ducasse, 2023).

Unstable Affect

Affective instability (i.e., rapid and extreme shift in mood) is a core characteristic of BPD and is evidenced by erratic emotional responses to situations and intense sensitivity to criticism or perceived slights. For example, an individual may greet a casual acquaintance with intense affection yet later be aloof with the same acquaintance. Friends describe individuals with BPD as moody, irresponsible, or intense. These individuals often fail to recognize their own emotional responses, thoughts, beliefs, and behaviors and have difficulty interpreting the facial effects of others. In this disorder, recognizing emotions in others is altered (Graumann et al., 2023).

Cognitive Dysfunctions

People with BPD often have **dichotomous thinking**. That is, they evaluate experiences, people, and objects in terms of mutually exclusive categories (e.g., good or bad, success or failure, trustworthy or deceitful). Their interpretation of normally occurring events is usually extremely positive or extremely negative. Sometimes their thinking becomes disorganized with irrelevant, bizarre notions, and vague or scattered thought connections, as well as delusions and hallucinations.

Another cognitive dysfunction common in BPD is **dissociation**, or times when thinking, feeling, or behaviors occur outside a person's awareness. It is a coping strategy for avoiding disturbing events. In dissociating, the person does not have to be aware of or remember traumatic events. There is evidence of functional changes in the frontolimbic regions (amygdala, anterior cingulate, inferior frontal gyrus, medial, and dorsolateral prefrontal cortices) and temporoparietal areas (Krause-Utz et al., 2021).

Impaired Problem Solving

In BPD, affected people often fail to engage in active problem solving. Instead, problem solving is attempted by soliciting help from others in a helplessly hopeless manner. Suggestions offered are rarely taken up.

Impulsivity

These individuals often have difficulty delaying gratification or thinking through the consequences before acting on their feelings; their actions are often unpredictable. Essentially, they act in the moment and clean up the mess afterward. Gambling, spending money irresponsibly, binge eating, engaging in unsafe sex, and abusing substances are typical of these individuals. They can also be physically or verbally aggressive. Job losses, interrupted education, and unsuccessful relationships are common.

Self-Harm Behaviors

The turmoil and unsuccessful interpersonal relationships and social experiences associated with BPD may lead the person to undermine themselves when a goal is about to be reached. The most serious consequences are suicide attempts or parasuicidal behavior (i.e., deliberate self-injury with intent to harm oneself).

KEYCONCEPT Self-harm is deliberate self-injurious behavior.

Self-harm behavior can be compulsive (e.g., hair pulling), episodic, or repetitive (e.g., cutting wrists, arms, other body parts) and is more likely to occur when the individual with BPD is depressed; has highly unstable interpersonal relationships, especially issues with intimacy and sociability; and is paranoid, hypervigilant (i.e., alert, watchful), and resentful. It is not unusual for people with this disorder to self-harm in unusual ways such as swallowing pens, staples, and even razor blades, or banging one's head against a brick wall. Individuals who have engaged in self-injurious behavior describe varied purposes for doing so, including to "feel something," "punish self," "escape feelings," "relieve anxiety," "stop feeling self-hatred," "stop feeling angry," "show how much they are hurting," and "create a hurt that can be soothed" (Sack et al., 2024). Regardless of intent, self-harm behaviors should be considered potentially life threatening and taken seriously.

Borderline Personality Disorder Across the Lifespan

Many children and adolescents show symptoms similar to those of BPD, such as moodiness, self-destruction, impulsiveness, lack of temper control, and rejection sensitivity. If a family member has BPD, the adolescent should be carefully assessed for this disorder. Because symptoms of BPD begin in adolescence, it makes sense that some children and adolescents would meet the criteria for BPD even though it is not diagnosed before young adulthood. More likely, some personality traits, such as impulsivity and mood instability, in many adolescents should be recognized and treated, whether or not BPD eventually develops.

Although BPD persists into later life, recognizing symptoms in older adults is difficult and subsequent treatment is understudied. Aging individuals present less overt manifestations of impulsivity. However, the basic patterns of instability, depressive symptoms, feelings of emptiness, anger, unstable interpersonal relationships, unpredictable responses, and somatic complaints are generally present (D'Agostino et al., 2022).

Epidemiology and Risk Factors

The estimated US prevalence of BPD is roughly 1.8% in community settings. In clinical settings, the prevalence of BPD is approximately 10% in outpatient mental health clinics and 15% to 20% in inpatient psychiatric settings. Rates of BPD among people who are incarcerated are reported to be as high as 30% (Bozzatello et al., 2024; Dahlenburg et al., 2024). Genetic, neurobiologic, psychological, and social factors have all been found to contribute to the risk for BPD. Brain imaging studies show that individuals with BPD experience disruption in the frontolimbic system, which is involved in emotional regulation, and the default-mode network, which is associated with self-regulation and self-related thinking (Ruocco & Marceau, 2024). BPD has a clear genetic predisposition, with studies showing over 45% heritability (Ansari et al., 2023). BPD has a heritability component on self-harm, with estimates ranging from 31% to 41%. Strong relationships demonstrated in twin studies demonstrated heritability of impulsive spending, risk of suicide and injury, and other risk-taking behaviors (Schermer et al., 2020). The association between familial adversities and the development of BPD has been studied, and findings show that maladaptive parenting, parental psychopathology, domestic violence, parental divorce, low socioeconomic status, parental hostility, overprotective and rejecting parenting styles, and attachment disorganization are all strong predictors. Childhood abuse is known to be a strong predictor of BPD development. Social factors contributing to BPD development include bullying, victimization, dating violence, and being a sexual underrepresented group (Gupta et al., 2023).

Age of Onset

BPD commonly starts and peaks in early to late adolescence and then largely declines over time. Because adolescence is a transition period with neurodevelopmental changes and is associated with mood swings, impulsivity, and emotional disturbances, many clinicians delay diagnosis even though symptoms of BPD are clearly present (Gupta et al., 2023). Unfortunately, delayed diagnosis contributes to delayed evidence-based treatment (Kingsley, 2022; Tedesco et al., 2023). Although uncommon, symptoms of BPD may present for the first time in middle adulthood. In these cases, presentation of symptoms tends to be more sudden in onset, with severe symptoms. Interpersonal issues, loss of employment, and reminders of past sexual trauma are key precipitators (Jo et al., 2022).

Gender Differences

In community settings, the US prevalence of BPD is believed to be comparable in women and men; in clinical populations, the diagnosis of BPD is three times higher in women. This increased rate in diagnosis may be due to bias and a labeling process. For example, "inappropriate and intense anger" may be considered to be more pathologic in women than in men. Another reason for increased rates in women is that childhood sexual abuse, which more commonly affects females, is one of the strongest risk factors for BPD. Still another explanation is that because eating disorders are more common in women with BPD, they have a greater likelihood of also having a mood, anxiety, or posttraumatic stress disorder. There are differences in the expression of symptoms; whereas women more often report affective instability, identity disturbance, chronic feelings of emptiness, and unstable relationships, men are more likely to be aggressive, impulsive and having substance use issues, and are less likely to be engaged in treatment (Bozzatello et al., 2024; Qian et al., 2022).

Rates of BPD in LGBTQ+ individuals are significantly higher than rates among their heterosexual peers (ranging from 14% to 57%), in both community and clinical settings. Whether these disparities are true differences or are due to measurement bias is unclear (Carsten et al., 2024). LGBTQ+ individuals experience social stressors related to being in an underrepresented group that inevitably increase their vulnerability to psychological symptoms. Environments that are invalidating, nonaccepting, and discriminatory contribute to the risk for developing borderline personality traits (Cano et al., 2024).

Ethnicity and Culture

The pattern of behavior seen in BPD has been identified in many settings around the world; however, research on diagnostic differences among racial and ethnic underrepresented groups is limited and inconsistent. Cultural differences in emotional expression, clinician biases, and diagnostic practices all contribute to variances (Becker et al., 2023).

Comorbidity

Comorbid psychiatric disorders are extremely common in patients with BPD. Mood disorders, particularly MDD and substance use disorder, anxiety disorder, and eating disorder are more frequently seen in patients with BPD, compared with patients with other personality disorders (Chapman et al., 2022). The coexistence of BPD with other disorders presents clinicians with the difficult choice of which disorder receives treatment priority. Symptoms associated with this disorder often provoke negative reactions on the part of clinicians, which interfere with clinicians' ability to provide effective care (Miller et al., 2023).

Etiology

Evidence supports a biopsychosocial etiology. Studies suggest that BPD traits are heritable, although the specific genetic factors remain unclear. There is clear evidence of differences in brain functioning between those with and without BPD. There is also clear evidence that psychological and social factors contribute to the development of the disorder (Yuan et al., 2023). The following discussion highlights the leading explanations for BPD.

Biologic Theories

Evidence of central nervous system dysfunction in BPD is now clear, including possible structural changes. Biologic anomalies are associated with three BPD characteristics: affective instability; transient psychotic episodes; and impulsive, aggressive, and suicidal behavior. Associated brain dysfunction occurs in the limbic system and frontal lobe and increases the behaviors of impulsiveness, parasuicide, and mood disturbance (Krause-Utz et al., 2021).

Psychosocial Theories

Psychoanalytic Theories

Using psychoanalytic methodology suggests people with BPD have not achieved the typical and healthy developmental stage of **separation-individuation**, during which a child develops a sense of self, a permanent sense of significant others (object constancy), and integration of seeing both bad and good components of oneself (Nitzan, 2024). Those with BPD lack the ability to separate from the primary caregiver and develop a separate and distinct personality or self-identity.

Projective identification, a defense mechanism by which people with BPD protect their fragile self-image, is believed to play an important role in the development of BPD. For example, when overwhelmed by anxiety or anger at being disregarded by another, they defend against the intensity of these feelings by unconsciously blaming others for what happens to them. They project their feelings onto a significant other with the unconscious hope that that person knows how to deal with it. Projective identification becomes a defensive way of interacting with the world, which leads to more rejection.

Maladaptive Cognitive Processes

Cognitive schemata are patterns of thought that determine how an individual interprets events. Each person's cognitive schemata screen, code, and evaluate incoming stimuli. In personality disorders, maladaptive cognitive schemata cause misinterpretation of other people's actions or reactions and of events that result in dysfunctional ways of responding. Cognitive schemata are important in understanding BPD (and ASPD as well).

Individuals with BPD develop dysfunctional beliefs and maladaptive schemata early in life, leading them to misinterpret environmental stimuli continuously, which, in turn, leads to rigid and inflexible behavior patterns in response to new situations and people (Thimm & Chang, 2022). Because those with BPD have been conditioned to anticipate rejection and disappointment in the past, they become entrenched in a pattern of fear and anxiety regarding encountering new people or situations. They have fears that disaster is going to strike at any minute. The work of cognitive therapists is to challenge distortions in thinking patterns and replace them with realistic ones.

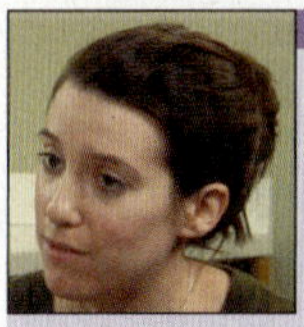

Remember Rebecca?

Rebecca does not see herself as contributing to her issue but believes her misfortunes are caused by others. For example, when she encounters new people, she shares too much personal information and is disappointed when they do not respond with the same intensity. She interprets their response as rejection.

Social Theories: Biosocial Theories

The biosocial viewpoint proposed by Marsha Linehan and colleagues sees BPD as a multifaceted issue, a combination of innate emotional vulnerability (sensitivity and reactivity to environmental stress), emotional dysregulation (inability to control emotions in social interactions), and the environment (Linehan, 1993) (Box 30.1).

BOX 30.1

Behavioral Patterns in Borderline Personality Disorder

1. Emotional vulnerability. Person experiences a pattern of pervasive difficulties in regulating negative emotions, including high sensitivity to negative emotional stimuli, high emotional intensity, and slow return to emotional baseline.
2. Self-invalidation. Person fails to recognize one's own emotional responses, thoughts, beliefs, and behaviors and sets unrealistically high standards and expectations for self. May include intense shame, self-hate, and self-directed anger. Person has no personal awareness and tends to blame social environment for unrealistic expectations and demands.
3. Unrelenting crises. Person experiences patterns of frequent, stressful, negative environmental events, disruptions, and roadblocks—some caused by the individual's dysfunctional lifestyle, others by an inadequate social milieu, and many by fate or chance.
4. Inhibited grieving. Person tries to inhibit and overcontrol negative emotional responses, especially those associated with grief and loss, including sadness, anger, guilt, shame, anxiety, and panic.
5. Active passivity. Person fails to engage actively in solving of own life problems but will actively seek problem solving from others in the environment, learned helplessness, hopelessness.
6. Apparent competence. Tendency for the individual to appear deceptively more competent than they actually are, usually because of failure of competencies to generalize across expected moods, situations, and time. Person fails to display adequate nonverbal cues of emotional distress.

Adapted from Linehan, M. (1993). *Cognitive-behavioral treatment of borderline personality disorder* (p. 10). Guilford Press.

KEYCONCEPT Emotional dysregulation is the inability to control emotions in social interactions and includes an instability of mood, marked shifts to or from depression, stress-related and transient mood crashes, rejection sensitivity, and inappropriate and intense outbursts of anger.

The emotional dysregulation and aggressive impulsivity entail both social learning and biologic regulation. Much of the neurobiologic research is directed at corticolimbic function and other cerebral functions (Krause-Utz et al., 2021). In fact, restoring balance in these systems permits more consistent neural firing between the limbic system and the frontal and prefrontal cortices. When these circuits are functional, the person has a greater capacity to think about their emotions and modulate behavior more responsibly.

The ability to control emotion is partly learned from private experiences and encounters with the social environment. BPD is believed to develop when emotionally vulnerable individuals interact with an **invalidating environment,** a social situation that negates private emotional responses and communication. When core emotional responses and communications are continuously dismissed, trivialized, devalued, punished, and discredited (invalidated) by respected or valued people, the vulnerable individual becomes unsure about their feelings. A minor example of an invalidating environment or response follows: The parents of Emily, a 4-year-old girl, tell her that the family is going to grandmother's house for a family meal. The child responds, "I am not going to Gramma's. I hate Stevie (her cousin)." The parents reply, "You don't hate Stevie. He is a wonderful child. He is your cousin, and only a spoiled and selfish little girl would say such a thing." The parents have devalued Emily's feelings and discredited her comments, thereby invalidating her feelings and sense of personal worth.

The most severe form of invalidation occurs in situations of child sexual abuse. Often, the abusing adult has told the child that this is a "special secret" between them. The child experiences feelings of fear, pain, and sadness, yet this trusted adult continuously dismisses the child's true feelings and tells the child what they should feel.

Family Response to Borderline Personality Disorder

Individuals with BPD are typically part of a chaotic family system, but their behavior adds to the chaos. Family members often feel captive to these patients. Family members are afraid to disagree with them or refuse to meet their multiple needs, fearing that self-destructive behavior will follow. During the course of the disorder, family members often get "burned out" and withdraw from the patient, only adding to the patient's fear of abandonment (Roca et al., 2024).

RECOVERY-ORIENTED CARE FOR PEOPLE WITH BORDERLINE PERSONALITY DISORDER

Teamwork and Collaboration: Working Toward Recovery

Treatment of BPD requires the collaboration of the entire mental health care team. Because people with BPD view the world in absolutes, nurses and other treatment team members are alternately categorized as all good or all bad. This defense is called **splitting** and presents clinicians with a challenge to work openly with each other as well as the patient until the issue can be resolved through team meetings and clinical supervision.

People with BPD are inadvertently highly stigmatized by many clinicians. Much of the stigma occurs when clinicians encounter these patients in crisis settings, such as the emergency department, crisis clinics, and general psychiatric inpatient wards. As these are not the settings in which treatment occurs, clinicians develop a biased perspective on these patients. Few clinicians have the opportunity to see these patients improve over time in specialized treatment clinics; nonetheless, these patients improve and are treatable. Staff often accuse these individuals of "manipulation" to get attention and say so in a very derogatory manner. In reality, all of us want attention from significant people in our lives. Most of us have the necessary skills to successfully meet our need for closeness and attention without alienating the very people who are important to us. People with BPD are unsuccessful in developing long-term meaningful relationships or getting what they want because their approach alienates others. Their need for attention and closeness to others is appropriate: It is how they seek attention that is problematic. See Box 30.2.

Psychotherapy is needed to help the individual with BPD manage their dysfunctional moods, impulsive behaviors, and self-injurious behaviors. Specially trained therapists who are comfortable with the many demands of these patients are needed. These therapists represent a variety of mental health disciplines, including psychology, social work, and advanced practice nursing. This disorder requires ongoing treatment as the individual copes with multiple interpersonal crises. Several types of medications are usually needed, including mood stabilizers, antidepressants, and anxiolytics. Careful medication monitoring is necessary.

Dialectical behavior therapy (DBT) combines cognitive and behavior therapy strategies with acceptance-based practice drawn from Zen and humanistic approaches. It was developed for people with BPD. Core interventions include problem-solving, exposure techniques (i.e., gradual exposure to cues that set off aversive emotions), skills training, contingency management (i.e., reinforcement of positive behavior), and cognitive modification. Skills groups are an integral part of DBT and are taught in group settings in which patients practice emotional regulation, interpersonal effectiveness, distress tolerance, core mindfulness, and self-management skills. Weekly individual therapy sessions focus on enhancing motivation and improving competence (Hernandez-Bustamante et al., 2024).

Mentalization-based therapy (MBT) is a psychodynamic psychotherapy that is used in both individual and group formats. In MBT, borderline personality symptoms are viewed as a result of distortion or reduction in **mentalizing,** which is the ability to understand the mental states of oneself and others, including thoughts and feelings, that lead to actions. The goal of MBT is to improve patients' capacity to accurately understand others' actions and develop self-awareness skills through a therapeutic relationship (Smits et al., 2022).

BOX 30.2

Mental Health Inequities: Experiences of Stigma and Discrimination in Borderline Personality Disorder: A Systematic Review and Qualitative Meta-Synthesis

Research shows that clinicians view BPD more negatively than other psychiatric conditions. Individuals with borderline personality disorder experience discrimination and stigma that directly impacts their care. A meta-synthesis of qualitative studies exploring stigma and discrimination among people with BPD discovered five themes:

1. Resistance from clinicians and withholding information
2. Othering from health care professionals and the public
3. Negative impact on self-image and self-esteem
4. Hopelessness surrounding the perceived permanency of BPD
5. Feeling like a burden

Specialized training for clinicians is needed to improve their understanding of BPD. Significant work is needed to reduce barriers and dispel myths around BPD and treatment.

Source: Stiles, C., Batchelor, R., Gumley, A., & Gajwani, R. (2023). Experiences of stigma and discrimination in borderline personality disorder: A systematic review and qualitative meta-synthesis. *Journal of Personality Disorders*, *37*(2), 177–194. https://doi.org/10.1521/pedi.2023.37.2.177.

Safety Issues

People with BPD can be extremely volatile emotionally. Because they experience emotions so intensely, they are at high risk for self-harm and suicide. Self-harm threats should be taken very seriously.

EVIDENCE-BASED NURSING CARE FOR PEOPLE WITH BORDERLINE PERSONALITY DISORDER

People with BPD may enter the mental health system early (during young adulthood or even before) because of their chaotic lifestyles. Behavior includes unstable moods, issues with interpersonal relationships, low self-esteem, and self-identity issues. Thinking and behavior are dysregulated (Box 30.3). They have issues in daily living, including maintaining intimate relationships, keeping a job, and living within the law (Box 30.4). See Clinical Judgment Nursing Care Plan 30.1, which sets forth a plan of care for Rebecca, one of the case study patients in this chapter.

RECOGNIZING CUES: RELEVANT ASSESSMENT INFORMATION

Physical Health

People with BPD are usually able to maintain personal hygiene and physical functioning. Because of the comorbidity of BPD and eating disorders and substance use, however, a nutritional assessment may be needed. The patient

BOX 30.3

Response Patterns of People With Borderline Personality Disorder

- Affective (mood) dysregulation
- Mood lability
- Issues with anger
- Interpersonal dysregulation
- Chaotic relationships
- Fears of abandonment
- Self-dysregulation
- Difficulties with sense of self
- Sense of emptiness
- Behavioral dysregulation
- Parasuicidal behavior or threats
- Impulsive behavior
- Cognitive dysregulation
- Dissociative responses
- Paranoid ideation

should be queried about physiologic responses of emotion. Sleep patterns also should be assessed because sleep alterations may suggest coexisting depression or mania.

Physical Indicators of Self-Injurious Behaviors

Patients with BPD should be assessed for self-injurious behavior or suicide attempts. It is important to ask the patient about specific self-abusive behaviors, such as cutting, scratching, or swallowing foreign objects. The patient may wear long sleeves to hide injury to the arms. Specifically, asking about thoughts of hurting oneself when experiencing a major upset provides an opportunity for prevention and for coaching the patient toward alternative self-soothing measures.

Nutrition

A nutritional assessment is important if the person is using food for self-soothing and anxiety control. In some instances, excessive food intake may indicate self-injury or impulse eating may occur. The assessment should also include the use of caffeinated beverages (e.g., coffee, tea, cola, energy drinks). Since there is often a comorbidity with anorexia nervosa and bulimia nervosa, an assessment focusing on eating patterns and food intake is important. In patients who engage in binging or purging, assessment should include examining the teeth for pitting and discoloration, as well as the hands and fingers for redness and calluses caused by inducing vomiting. See Chapter 32.

Sleep

Sleep disturbance is common in people with BPD. Impulsivity, emotion dysregulation, and aggressive behaviors contribute to increased vulnerability for poor sleep. Poor sleep quality is manifested through prolonged sleep onset, shorter sleep duration, more frequent awakenings, and lower sleep efficiency. Additionally, BPD is associated with disturbed sleep stages and wakefulness periods through the night. People with BPD report experiencing more nightmares and poorer sleep quality than those without BPD. Understanding and addressing sleep health in patients is critical because of the extensive negative repercussions of sleep disturbances. Sleep issues, particularly insomnia, can increase suicide and self-harm risk. The nurse should conduct a thorough sleep history by asking the patient about their sleep habits, including

BOX 30.4

Clinical Judgment Vignette: Borderline Personality Disorder

Joanne is a 22-year-old single woman who was recently fired from her job as a data entry clerk. She lives with her mother and stepfather, who brought her to the emergency department after finding her crouched in a fetal position in the bathroom, her wrists bleeding. She seemed to be in a daze. This is her first psychiatric admission although her mother and stepfather have suspected that she has "needed help" for a long time. In high school, she received brief treatment for a potential eating disorder. She remains very thin but is able to eat at least one meal per day. During periods of stress, she will go for days without eating. Joanne is the second of three children. Her parents divorced when she was 3 years old. She has not seen her father since he left. Although she has pleasant memories of her father, her mother has told her that he beat Joanne and her sisters when he was drinking. When Joanne was 6 years old, her older sister died as a result of an automobile accident. Joanne was in the car but was uninjured. As a child, Joanne was seen as a potential singing star. Her natural musical talent attracted her teachers' support, which encouraged her to develop her talent. She took singing lessons and entered statewide competitions in high school. Although she enjoyed the attention, she was never really comfortable in the limelight and felt "guilty" about having a talent that she sometimes resented. She was able to make friends but found that she was unable to keep them. They described her as "too intense" and emotional. She had one boyfriend in high school, but she was very uncomfortable with any physical closeness. After ending the relationship with the boyfriend, she concentrated on dieting to have a "perfect body." When her dieting attracted her parents' attention, she vowed to eat just enough to keep them "off her back about it." She spent much of her leisure time with her grandmother. She attended college briefly but was unable to concentrate. It was during college and after her grandmother's death that Joanne began cutting her wrists during periods of stress. It seemed to calm her.

After leaving college, Joanne returned home. She had several jobs and short-lived friendships. She was usually fired from her job because of "moodiness," and it took her several months before she would again find another. She spent days in her room listening to music. Her recent episode occurred after she was fired from work and spent 3 days in her bedroom.

Building Clinical Judgment

1. How would you describe Joanne's mood?
2. Are Joanne's losses of her father and sister really severe enough to affect her ability to relate to others now? Do the losses seem to relate to the self-injury?
3. What symptoms and behaviors indicating problems with self-esteem and self-identity are present?

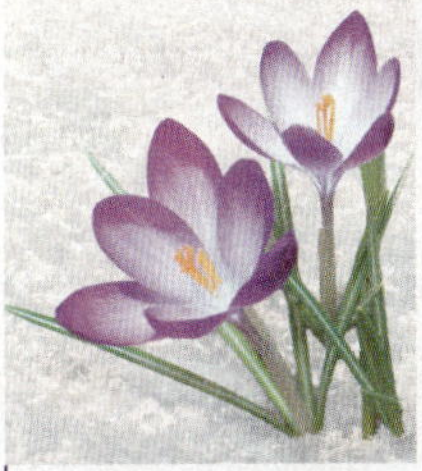

CLINICAL JUDGMENT NURSING CARE PLAN 30.1

The Patient With Borderline Personality Disorder

Rebecca, age 23, was admitted voluntarily to the inpatient mental health unit after cutting her wrists and arriving in the emergency department with blood-soaked towels wrapped around her wrists. She lives alone and has no close friends. Her relationships are intense, which drives people away. She often reveals too much personal information to strangers. Her therapist left town, and she fears that they will not return. This admission is one of multiple past admissions.

Setting: Inpatient Psychiatric Unit in a General Hospital

Assessment Cues: Rebecca's wrists have several fresh lacerations and many older cuts in various stages of healing. She also has several scars from self-harming incidents in the past. Before harming herself, Rebecca reports feeling angry, anxious, numb, empty, and feeling detached from her body. She states that after she cuts herself she feels a sense of relief. She has a poor self-concept and low self-esteem. She says she does not understand why everyone is so mean to her. She has a history of being sexually abused as a child by her uncle following the death of her mother at age 4. BP is 120/70, P 72, R 15, Ht. 5′4″, Wt. 130, BMI 22.3.

Associated Psychiatric Diagnosis

Borderline personality disorder

Medications

Sertraline (Zoloft) 150 mg daily for anxiety and depression

Priority Hypothesis: Self-Injury

Important Characteristics

Cuts and scratches on body
Self-inflicted wounds

Associated Considerations

Fears of abandonment secondary to therapist's vacation
Inability to handle stress

Planning Recovery and Wellness Outcomes

Initial

Remain safe and free of self-injury.
Identify feelings before and after cutting herself.
Identify ways of dealing with self-harming impulses if they return.

Discharge

Verbalize alternate thinking with more realistic expectations of others.
Identify community resources to provide structure and support while therapist is away.

Taking Action: Nursing Interventions

Interventions	Rationale	Ongoing Assessment
Monitor patient for changes in mood or behavior that might lead to self-injurious behavior.	Close observation establishes safety and protection of patient from self-harm and impulsive behaviors.	Document according to facility policy. Continue to observe for mood and behavior changes.
Discuss with patient need for close observation and rationale to keep her safe.	Explanation to patient for purpose of nursing interventions helps her cooperate with the nursing activity.	Assess her response to increasing level of observation. Observe for side effects.
Administer medication as prescribed and evaluate medication effectiveness in reducing depression, anxiety, and cognitive disorganization.	Allows for adjustment of medication dosage based on target behaviors and outcomes.	Observe for her willingness to agree to not harm herself.
After 6 to 8 hours, present written agreement to not harm herself.	Permits patient time to return to more thoughtful ways of responding rather than her previous reactive response. Avoids a power struggle if presented much earlier.	Review documentation of close observation for all shifts.
Communicate information about patient's risk to other nursing staff.	The close observation should be continued throughout all shifts until patient agrees to resist self-harm urges.	

Continued

Clinical Judgment Nursing Care Plan 30.1 Continued

Evaluation

Outcomes	Revised Outcomes	Interventions
Remained safe without further harming self. Identified fears of abandonment before cutting herself and relief of anxiety afterward. She identified friends to call when fears return and hotlines to use if necessary.	Use hotlines or call friends if fears to harm self-return.	Give patient hotline number and ask her to record friends' numbers in an accessible place.
Agreed to not harm herself over the next 3 days.	Does not harm self for 3 days.	Remind her to call someone if urges return.
Enrolled in a day hospital program for 4 weeks.	Attend day hospital program.	Follow-up on enrollment.

Priority Hypothesis: Feeling Abandoned

Important Characteristics	Associated Characteristics
Frequent feelings of abandonment	Therapist's absence

Planning Recovery and Wellness Outcomes

Initial	Discharge
Discuss being lonely. Identify previous ways of coping with loneliness.	Identify strategies to deal with loneliness while therapist is away.

Taking Action: Nursing Interventions

Interventions	Rationale	Ongoing Assessment
Develop a therapeutic relationship.	People with BPD are able to examine loneliness within the structure of a therapeutic relationship.	Assess her ability to relate and nurse's response to the relationship.
Discuss past experience with therapist being gone with emphasis on how she was able to survive it.	She has survived therapist's absences before. By identifying the strategies she used, she can build on those strengths.	Assess her ability to assume any responsibility for "living through it." This will become a strength.
Acknowledge that it may be expected to feel angry when the therapist is gone, but there are other strategies that may help the patient deal with the loneliness besides cutting.	Acknowledging feelings is important. Helping patient focus on the possibility of other strategies for dealing with the anger helps her regain a sense of control over her behavior.	Assess whether she is willing to acknowledge that there are other behavioral strategies to manage her anger.
Begin immediate discharge planning with focus on day hospitalization or day treatment for skills training and management of loneliness.	While patient is in the hospital, she is out of the stressful environment in which she can learn more effective behaviors and use the therapy. Moving out of the hospital and back into outpatient therapy decreases the possibility of regression and lost learning (Linehan, 1993).	Assess her willingness to learn new skills within a day treatment setting.
Teach her about stress management techniques. Assign her to anger management group while she is in the hospital.	Learning about ways of dealing with feelings and stressful situations helps the patient with BPD choose positive strategies rather than self-destructive ones.	Monitor whether she actually attends the groups. She should be encouraged to attend.

Clinical Judgment Nursing Care Plan 30.1 Continued

Evaluation

Outcomes	Revised Outcomes	Interventions
Rebecca was able to verbalize her anger about her therapist's absence and fears of abandonment. The last two times her therapist went on vacation, the patient became self-injurious and was hospitalized for 2 weeks.	None	
Rebecca was willing to be discharged the next day if she could attend day treatment while her therapist was gone.	Identify other strategies of dealing with her therapist's vacation besides cutting herself.	Attend stress management, communication, and self-comforting classes.

sleep duration and quality. Factors contributing to poor sleep, including psychosocial factors, physical health issues, and lifestyle habits should be explored. Physical indicators of sleep deprivation include yawning, irritability, difficulty sleeping, and daytime drowsiness. Formal sleep assessment tools may also be used.

History of Trauma

Childhood adversity and trauma play an important role in the development of BPD. Individuals with BPD are nearly 14 times more likely to disclose childhood adversity than the nonclinical population, and over three times more likely to report adversity than other psychiatric clinical groups. The experience of trauma, such as emotional abuse and neglect, physical or sexual abuse, and traumatic loss or separation from caregivers, contributes to a distorted sense of self and others. Emotional abuse and neglect result in emotional invalidation and rejection sensitivity (van Beeck, 2024). Routine assessment of abuse and neglect is important, as well as utilizing a trauma-informed approach to prevent further trauma (see Chapter 2). An individual with BPD will not just automatically trust the nurse simply because they are a member of their treatment team. Because of their innate fear of rejection and abandonment, establishing trust may take time. See Box 30.5.

Medication

Although there is no established pharmaceutical treatment for BPD, many patients with BPD receive psychotropic medication for comorbidities and other issues such as impulsivity, cognitive–perceptual issues, or anger. As mood dysregulation is a primary symptom, treatment with mood stabilizers (e.g., lithium, valproate, or lamotrigine) and/or a low-to-moderate dose of an atypical antipsychotic (e.g., aripiprazole or quetiapine) are common (Gartlehner et al., 2021). Depressive symptoms are frequently treated with selective serotonin reuptake inhibitors (SSRIs), serotonin and norepinephrine reuptake inhibitors (SNRIs), and tricyclic antidepressants (TCAs) and may be augmented with atypical antipsychotics and or lamotrigine. Benzodiazepines should be avoided for anxiety due to habituation and they are not meant for long-term use. Buspirone is considered a safer option for treating anxiety in patients with BPD. Initially, patients may be reluctant to disclose all the medications they are taking because, for many of them, trial and error has

BOX 30.5

Trauma-Informed Approaches: The Impact of a Trauma-Informed Approach on Social Climate in Forensic Inpatient settings

Background

People with BPD are overrepresented in forensic settings. The social climate of a forensic unit refers to the physical, social, and emotional conditions that impact how the environment is perceived and experienced. Conflicts between therapeutic and security needs can result in a social environment that presents challenges for mental health nurses and patients alike.

Interventions

Implementing a trauma-informed approach contributes to a therapeutic social climate, which in turn reduces the risk of retraumatization and leads to improved outcomes for both patients and staff. Principles of a trauma-informed approach include safety, trustworthiness and transparency, peer support, empowerment and choice, collaboration and mutuality, and cultural, historical, and gender sensitivity. Nurses must recognize the widespread impact of trauma and its potential impact on mental, physical, and emotional well-being.

Source: Rodwell, D., & Frith, H. (2024). Using a trauma-informed care framework to explore social climate and borderline personality disorder in forensic inpatient settings. *International Journal of Mental Health Nursing*, *33*(4), 1139–1150. https://doi.org/ 10.1111/inm.13300.

led to repeated prescriptions. They are fearful of having medication taken away from them. Development of rapport with special attention to a nonjudgmental approach is especially important when eliciting current medication practices. The effectiveness of the medication in relieving the target symptom needs to be determined.

Substance Use

Since nearly half of individuals with BPD have a co-occurring substance use disorder, use of alcohol, over-the-counter (OTC) medications, and street drugs should be carefully assessed (Waite et al., 2024). Use of benzodiazepines (i.e., alprazolam, lorazepam, or diazepam) is contraindicated due to the risk of dependence and misuse. Impulsiveness in patients with BPD must be considered. Alcohol can lower inhibition and lead to high-risk behaviors (e.g., suicide and parasuicide gestures or accidental overdosing).

Psychosocial Cues

People with BPD have usually experienced significant losses in their lives that shape their view of the world. They experience **inhibited grieving**, "a pattern of repetitive, significant trauma and loss, together with an inability to fully experience and personally integrate or resolve these events" (Linehan, 1993). They have unresolved grief that can last for years and will avoid situations that evoke those feelings of separation and loss. During the assessment, the nurse can identify the losses (real or perceived) and explore the patient's experience during these losses, paying particular attention to whether the patient has reached resolution. A history of physical or sexual abuse and early separation from significant caregivers may provide important clues to the severity of the disturbances.

Mood fluctuations are common and can be assessed by depression and anxiety screening scales or by asking the following questions:

- What things or events bother you and make you feel sad or angry?
- Do these things or events trouble you more than they trouble other people?
- Do friends and family tell you that you are moody?
- Do you get angry easily?
- Do you have trouble with your temper?
- Do you think you were born with these feelings, or did something happen to make you feel this way?

Mental Status and Appearance

Appearance and activity level generally reflect the person's mood and psychomotor activity. Many of those with BPD have been physically or sexually abused and thus should be assessed for depression. A disheveled appearance can reflect depression or an agitated state. When feeling good, these patients can be very engaging; they tend to be dramatic in their style of dress and attract attention, such as by wearing an unusual hairstyle or heavy makeup. Because physical appearance reflects identity, patients may experiment with their appearance and seek affirmation and acceptance from others. Body piercing, tattoos, and other perceived adornments provide a mechanism to define self.

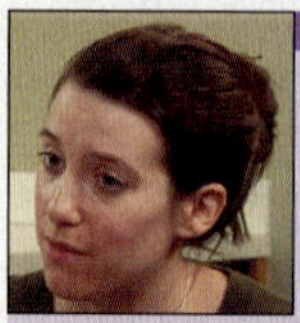

Rebecca's Assessment

Rebecca loves to project a dramatic appearance when she is feeling good. When she is in a good mood, she projects as an overly confident, engaging person. She has several body piercings. She refuses to discuss any childhood trauma or sexual abuse.

Cognitive Disturbances

The mental status examination of those with BPD usually reveals appropriate thought processes that are not disorganized or confused, except during periods of stress. Those with BPD usually exhibit dichotomous thinking, or a tendency to view things as absolute, either black or white, good or bad, with no perception of compromise. Dichotomous thinking can be assessed by asking patients how they view other people. Evidence of dichotomous thinking is indicated with responses of "good" or "bad," "wonderful" or "terrible."

Self-Concept and Identity Disturbance

Unstable self-image is often manifested as an identity disturbance or **identity diffusion**, a loss of the capacity for self-definition and commitment to values, goals, or relationships. There is not a consistent sense of self, and the process of identity formation is impaired. They have difficulties differentiating themselves from others and defining psychological boundaries. The nurse can recognize identity diffusion if the patient reports an ongoing "emptiness" or contradictory behavior. "I don't know if what I am saying is something I really mean; if what I feel is something I really feel." The person's thoughts and behavior will seem fragmented and superficial (Jorgensen & Boye, 2022).

Dissociation and Transient Psychotic Episodes

With BPD, periods of dissociation and transient psychotic episodes may occur. A history of trauma, especially childhood abuse and neglect, is a significant risk factor for dissociation (Schulze et al., 2024). Dissociation can be assessed by asking if there is ever a time when the patient does not remember events or has the feeling of being separate from their body. Some patients refer to this as "spacing out." By asking specific information about how often, how long, and when dissociation was first used, the nurse can get an idea of how important dissociation is as a coping skill. It is important to ask the person what happens in the environment when dissociation occurs. Frequent dissociation indicates a highly habitual coping mechanism that is difficult to change. Because transient psychotic states occur, it is also important to elicit data regarding the presence of hallucinations or delusions and their frequency and circumstances.

Impulsivity

Impulsivity can be identified by asking the patient whether they do things impulsively or at the spur of the moment. For example: "Have there been times when you were hurt by your actions or were sorry later that you acted in the way you did?" Direct questions about gambling, choices in sexual partners, sexual activities, fights, arguments, arrests, and habits related to the consumption of alcohol can also help in identifying areas of impulsive behavior.

From a neurophysiologic perspective, impulsively acting before thinking seems to be mediated by rapid nerve firing in the mesolimbic area. This activates psychomotor responses before pathways reach the prefrontal cortex (Krause-Utz et al., 2021). Teaching the patient strategies to slow down automatic responses (e.g., deep breathing, counting to 10) buys time to think before acting.

Interpersonal Skills

Assessment of the person's ability to relate to others is important because interpersonal issues are linked to dissociation and self-injurious behavior. Information about friendships, frequency of contact, and intimate relationships provide data about the person's ability to relate to others. Patients with BPD are often sexually active and may have numerous sexual partners. Their need for closeness clouds their judgment about sexual partners, so it is not unusual to find these patients in abusive, destructive relationships with people with ASPD.

Stress and Coping Skills

Coping with stressful situations is one of the major issues of people with BPD. Assessment of their coping skills and their ability to deal with stressful situations is important. Self-esteem is closely related to identifying with health care workers. Patients with BPD perceive their families and friends as being weary of their numerous crises and their seeming unwillingness to break the vicious self-destructive cycle. Feeling rejected by their natural support system, these individuals create one within the health system. During periods of crisis, especially during the late evening, early morning, or on weekends, they may call or visit various psychiatric units asking to speak to specific personnel who formerly cared for them. They even know different nurses' scheduled days off and make the rounds to several hospitals and clinics. Sometimes they bring gifts to nurses or call them at home. Because their newly created social support system cannot provide the support that is needed, the patient continues to feel rejected. One of the treatment goals is to help the individual establish a more natural support network.

Functional Status

Some individuals with BPD can function very well except during periods when symptoms erupt. They hold jobs, are active in communities, and can perform well. During periods of stress, symptoms often appear. Conversely, some individuals with severe BPD function poorly; they seem to be always in a crisis, which often they have created.

Social Support Systems

Identification of social supports (e.g., family, friends, religious organizations) is the purpose of assessing resources. Knowing how the patient obtains social support is important in understanding the quality of interpersonal relationships. For example, some patients consider as their "best friends" nurses, providers, and other health care personnel. Because these are not authentic friendships (i.e., not reciprocated), they inevitably lead to frustration and disappointment. However, helping the patient find ways to meet other people and encouraging the patient's efforts are more realistic.

Risk Assessment: Suicide or Self-Injury

It is critical that patients with BPD be assessed for suicidal and self-damaging behavior, including alcohol and substance use (see Chapter 22). The assessment should include direct questions, such as asking the patient whether they think about or engage in self-injurious behaviors. If so, the nurse should continue to explore the behaviors: what is done, how is it done, how frequently is it done, and what are the circumstances surrounding the self-injurious behavior. Changes in self-harming behavior, such as increased frequency or lethality, can be a sign of increased risk of suicidal ideation or attempts (Wheeler, 2024). It is helpful to explain briefly to the patient that sometimes people cut, scratch, or pick at themselves as a way of bringing some relief and comfort. Although the behavior brings temporary relief, it also places the person at risk for infection. Approaching the assessment in this way conveys a sense of understanding and is more likely to invite the patient to disclose honestly.

Quality of Life

BPD is associated with greater disability relative to other psychiatric disorders (Griffiths et al., 2024). People diagnosed with BPD are predisposed to have a substantial degree of functional impairment through a variety of social and occupational domains, including trouble with finding and maintaining adequate work, housing, or relationships. Patients with BPD have poor social functioning; they are often socially isolated and unemployed or on long-term sick leave. Many patients with BPD do not finish their education or complete it at a minimal level. Individuals with BPD often find themselves in problematic relationships and experience difficulties in parenting. Job environment can be one of the areas where patients with BPD struggle for maintaining their identity. Conflicts with boss and colleagues are frequent; individuals with BPD mostly fight against assumed injustice and nepotism and accuse others of incompetence, lack of diligence, and gaining benefits from their bosses. Occupational patterns are characterized by instability, intense preoccupation, the subsequent loss of interest in the job, lack of job satisfaction, and issues in relationships (Hastrup et al., 2022; Larcombe & Miller, 2022).

Strengths Assessment

The strengths assessment is important because these positive thoughts, skills, and behaviors can be supported as individuals replace self-defeating behaviors with positive ones. Many of these individuals are extremely resilient despite the trauma that they have often experienced. The person's strength will emerge in the assessment and increase as the nurse gets to know the patient better. Some key questions include the following:

- How do you make yourself feel better?
- How do you resist the urge to hurt yourself?
- How do you make friends?
- What is the most positive thought, skill, or behavior that you have?

ANALYZING CUES AND DEVELOPING HYPOTHESES

Maintaining patient safety is the priority. Self-injury and suicidal ideation should be considered when establishing recovery goals. If the patient is not experiencing suicidal or self-injurious thoughts or behavior, the patient's thought processes (dissociation) or ability to cope with everyday stress may emerge as priorities of care, especially if these interfere with daily living. If the individual copes with stressful situations by dissociating or hallucinating, the nurse should begin to help the patient identify other coping strategies. Patients who are very emotional sometimes find that they will be able to cope if they learn emotional regulation strategies. For other patients, identity issues, anxiety, or low self-esteem may become priorities of care.

Identified strengths should be included in the priorities. By including a person's strengths, such as being motivated to manage self-destructive thoughts, the nurse can channel these attributes to deal with specific issues.

PLANNING RECOVERY AND WELLNESS OUTCOMES: GENERATING SOLUTIONS

Changing or modifying personality traits is difficult. The person must want to change cognitive, emotional, and behavioral responses that were established in early childhood. Recovery goals should initially focus on the most problematic areas, and then shift as outcomes are achieved. The patient and nurse should establish specific wellness goals, such as reducing food intake or increasing exercise. There should be an agreed-upon plan between the patient and the nurse.

THERAPEUTIC RELATIONSHIP

Psychiatric–mental health (PMH) registered nurses do not function as the patient's primary therapists, but they do need to establish a therapeutic relationship that strengthens the patient's coping skills and self-esteem and also supports individual psychotherapy. The therapeutic relationship helps the patient to experience a model of healthy interaction with consistency, limit setting, caring, and respect (both self-respect and respect for the patient). Patients who have low self-esteem need help in recognizing genuine respect from others and reciprocating with respect for others. In the therapeutic relationship, the nurse models self-respect by observing personal limits, being assertive, and clearly communicating expectations (Box 30.6). The nurse should always avoid using stigmatizing language, such as describing the person's behavior as manipulating instead of reporting or documenting specific behaviors.

Nurses should use their own self-awareness skills to examine their personal response to the patient. How the nurse responds to the patient can often be a clue to how others perceive and respond to the person. For example, if the nurse feels irritated or impatient during the interview, that is a sign that others respond to this person in the same way; conversely, if the nurse feels empathy or closeness, chances are this patient can evoke these same feelings in others.

TAKING ACTION: NURSING INTERVENTIONS

Physical Care

Usually, the person can manage hydration and self-care fairly well. This section focuses on those areas that are more likely to be problematic.

Sleep Hygiene

Disturbed sleep patterns are common in BPD. The nurse can intervene by helping the person establish a regular bedtime routine by teaching sleep hygiene strategies such as avoiding foods and drinks that could interfere with sleep. If relaxation exercises are used, they should

BOX 30.6

Therapeutic Dialogue: Borderline Personality Disorder

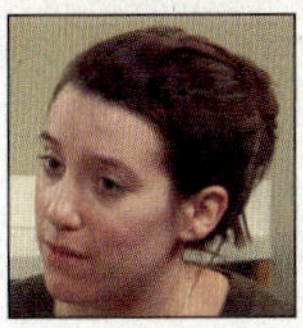

INEFFECTIVE APPROACH

Rebecca: Hey, you know what? You are my favorite nurse. That night nurse sure doesn't understand me the way you do.

Nurse: Oh, I'm glad you are comfortable with me. Which night nurse?

Rebecca: You know, Sue.

Nurse: Did you have problems with her?

Rebecca: She is terrible. She sleeps all night or she is on the telephone.

Nurse: Oh, that doesn't sound very professional to me. Anything else?

Rebecca: Yeah, she said that you didn't know what you were doing. She said that you couldn't nurse your way out of a paper bag (smiling).

Nurse: She did, did she? (Getting angry.) She should talk.

Rebecca: Well, I gotta go to group. Where will you be? I feel so much better if I know where you are. I don't know how I can possibly be discharged tomorrow.

EFFECTIVE APPROACH

Rebecca: Hey, you know what? You are my favorite nurse. That night nurse sure doesn't understand me the way you do.

Nurse: I really like you, Rebecca. Tomorrow you will be discharged, and I'm glad that you will be able to return home. (Nurse avoided responding to "favorite nurse" statement. Redirected interaction to impending discharge.)

Rebecca: That night nurse slept all night.

Nurse: What was your night like? (Redirecting the interaction to Sara's experience.)

Rebecca: It was terrible. Couldn't sleep all night. I'm not sure that I'm ready to go home.

Nurse: Oh, so you are not quite sure about discharge? (reflection)

Rebecca: I get so, so lonely. Then, I want to hurt myself.

Nurse: Lonely feelings have started that chain of events that led to cutting, haven't they? (validation)

Rebecca: Yes, I'm very scared. I haven't cut myself for 1 week now.

Nurse: Do you have a plan for dealing with your lonely feelings when they occur?

Rebecca: I'm supposed to start thinking about something that is pleasant—like spring flowers in the meadow.

Nurse: Does that work for you?

Rebecca: Yes, sometimes.

CRITICAL THINKING CHALLENGE

1. How did the nurse in the first scenario get sidetracked?
2. How was the nurse in the second scenario able to keep the patient focused on herself and her impending discharge?

be adapted to the tolerance of the individual. Special consideration must be made for people who have been physically and sexually abused and who may be unable to put themselves in a vulnerable position (e.g., lying down in a room with other people or closing their eyes). These patients may need additional safeguards to help them sleep, such as a night light or repositioning the furniture in the room to allow a quick exit.

Teaching Nutritional Balance

The nutritional status of the person with BPD can quickly become a priority, particularly if the patient has coexisting eating disorders, mood disorders, or substance dependence. Eating is often a response to stress, so patients can quickly become overweight. This is especially problematic when the patient has also been taking medications that promote weight gain, such as antipsychotics, antidepressants, or mood stabilizers. Helping the patient learn the basics of nutrition, make reasonable choices, and develop other coping strategies than eating are important interventions. If patients are engaging in purging or severe dieting practices, teaching the patient about the dangers of both practices is important (see Chapter 32). Referral to an eating disorders specialist may be needed.

Medication Interventions

Limiting medication is better for people with BPD. Patients should take medications only for target symptoms for a short time (e.g., an antidepressant for a period of depression) because they may be taking many medications, particularly if they have a comorbid disorder, such as a mood disorder or substance use. Medications are used to control emotional dysregulation, impulsive aggression, cognitive disturbances, and anxiety as an adjunct to psychotherapy.

Administering and Monitoring Medications

In inpatient settings, it is relatively easy to control medications; in other settings, however, patients must be aware that it is their responsibility to take their medication and monitor the number and type of drugs being taken. Patients who rely on medication to help them deal with stress and those who are periodically suicidal are at high risk for misuse of medications. Patients who experience unusual side effects are also at high risk for nonadherence. The nurse must determine whether the patient is actually taking medication, whether the medication is being taken as prescribed, its effect on target symptoms, and the use of any OTC drugs (e.g., antihistamines, sleeping pills, or herbal supplements with similar pharmacologic activity).

Monitoring Side Effects

Patients with BPD appear to be sensitive to many medications, so the dosage may need to be adjusted based on the side effects they experience. Listen carefully to the patient's description of the side effects. Any unusual side effects should be accurately documented and reported to the prescriber.

Teaching Points

Patients should be educated about the prescribed medications and their interactions with other drugs and substances, but they should be encouraged to avoid relying on medication alone. Interventions include teaching patients about the medication and how and where it acts in the brain and body, helping establish a routine for taking prescribed medication, reporting side effects, and facilitating the development of positive coping strategies to deal with daily stresses rather than relying on medications. Eliciting the patient's partnership in care improves adherence and thereby outcomes.

Psychosocial Interventions

Therapeutic Interactions

One key to helping patients with BPD is recognizing their fears of both abandonment and intimacy. Informing the patient of the length of the therapeutic relationship as much as possible allows the patient to engage in and prepare for termination with less sense of abandonment. If the patient's hospitalization is time limited, it is important to acknowledge the limit overtly and remind the patient with each contact how many sessions remain.

In day treatment and outpatient settings, the duration of treatment may be indeterminate, but the nurse may not be available that entire time. The termination process cannot be casual; this would stimulate abandonment fears. However, some patients end treatment prematurely when the nurse informs them of the impending end as a way to leave before being rejected. The best approach is to explore these anticipated feelings with the patient. After careful planning, the nurse and patient discuss how to cope with anticipated feelings, including the wish to run away, review the progress the patient has made, and summarize what the patient has learned from the relationship that can be generalized to future encounters.

Establishing Personal Boundaries and Limitations

Personal boundaries are highly context specific; for example, stroking the hair of a stranger on the bus would be inappropriate, but stroking the hair and face of one's intimate partner while sitting together would be appropriate. Clarifying limits requires making explicit what is usually implicit. This may mean having a standing time during each shift that the nurse will talk with the patient. The nurse should refrain from offering personal information, which is frequently confusing to the person with BPD. At times, the person may present in a somewhat arrogant and seemingly entitled way. It is important for the nurse to recognize such a presentation as reflective of internal confusion and dissonance. Responding in a very neutral manner avoids confrontation and a power struggle, which might also unwittingly reinforce the patient's internal sense of inferiority.

Some additional strategies for establishing the boundaries of the relationship include the following:

- Documenting in the patient's chart the agreed-on appointment expectations
- Sharing the treatment plan with the patient
- Confronting violations of the agreement in a nonpunitive way
- Discussing the purpose of limits in the therapeutic relationship and applicability to other relationships

When patients violate boundaries, it is important to respond right away but without taking the behavior personally. For example, if a patient is flirtatious, simply say something like, "Mr. J., I feel uncomfortable with your overly friendly behavior. It seems out of place because we have a professional relationship. That would be more fitting for an intimate relationship that we will never have."

Enhancing Cognitive Functioning

The nurse can often challenge the patient's dysfunctional ways of thinking and encourage the person to think about the event in a different way. When a patient engages in catastrophic thinking, the nurse can challenge by asking, "What is the worst that could happen?" and "How likely would that be to occur?" Or in dichotomous thinking, when the patient fixates on one extreme perception or alternates only between the extremes, the nurse should ask the patient to think about any examples of exceptions to the extreme. The point of the challenge is not to debate or argue with the patient but to provide different perspectives to consider. Encouraging patients to keep journals of real interactions to process with the nurse or therapist is another effective way of testing the reality of their thinking and anticipations, affording more choices and flexibility (Box 30.7).

In problem solving, the nurse might encourage the patient to debate both sides of the problem and then search for common ground. Practicing communication and negotiation skills through role playing helps the patient make mistakes and correct them without harm to their self-esteem. The nurse also encourages patients to use these skills in their everyday lives and report back on the results, asking patients how they feel applying the skills and how doing so affects their self-perceptions. Success, even partial success, builds a sense of competence and self-esteem (Table 30.1).

BOX 30.7

Clinical Judgment Vignette: Challenging Dysfunctional Thinking

Ms. S had worked for the same company for 20 years with a good job record. After an accident, she made some minor mistakes in her work that she quickly corrected. She informed her company nurse that her work was "really slipping" and that she was fearful of her coworkers' disapproval and of getting fired from her job. The nurse asked her to keep a journal of coworkers' comments for the next week. At the next visit, the following dialogue occurred:

Nurse: I noticed that you received several compliments on your work. Even a close friend of your boss expressed appreciation for your work.

Ms. S: It was a light week at work. I really don't believe they meant what they said.

Nurse: I can see how you can believe that one or two comments are not genuine, but how do you account for four and five good reports on your work?

Ms. S: Well, I don't know.

Nurse: It looks like your beliefs are not supported by your journal entries. Now, what makes you think that your boss wants to fire you after 20 years of service?

Building Clinical Judgment

1. What is behind Ms. S.'s inaccurate interpretation of the positive comments and compliments received by her coworkers?
2. Why does the nurse challenge Ms. S.'s dysfunctional thinking?

Behavioral Interventions

The goal of behavioral interventions is to replace dysfunctional behaviors with positive ones. The nurse has an important role in helping patients control emotions and behaviors by acknowledging and validating desired behaviors and ignoring or confronting undesired behaviors. Patients often test the nurse for a response, so nurses must decide how to respond to particular behaviors. This can be tricky because even negative responses can be viewed as positive reinforcement by the patient. In some instances, if the behavior is irritating but not harmful or demeaning, it is best to ignore, rather than focus, on it. However, grossly inappropriate and disrespectful behaviors require confrontation. If a patient throws a glass of water on an assistant because she is angry at the treatment team for refusing to increase her hospital privileges, an appropriate intervention would include confronting the patient with

TABLE 30.1 THOUGHT DISTORTIONS AND CORRECTIVE STATEMENTS

Thought Distortion	Corrective Statement
Catastrophizing	
"This is the most awful thing that has ever happened to me"	*"This is a sad thing but not the most awful."*
"If I fail this course, my life is over."	*"If you fail the course, you can take the course again. You can change your major."*
Dichotomizing	
"No one ever listens to me."	*"Your husband listened to you last night when you told him ..."*
"I never get what I want."	*"You didn't get the promotion this year, but you did get a merit raise."*
"I can't understand why everyone is so kind at first and then always dumps me when I need them the most."	*"It is hard to remember those kind things and times when your friends have stayed with you when you needed them."*
Self-Attribution Errors	
"If I had just found the right thing to say, she wouldn't have left me."	*"There is not a single right thing to say, and she left you because she chose to."*
"If I had not made him mad, he wouldn't have hit me."	*"He has a lot of choices in how to respond, and he chose hitting. You are responsible for your feelings and actions."*

her behavior and issuing the consequences, such as losing her privileges and apologizing to the assistant.

However, such an incident can be used to help the patient understand why such behavior is inappropriate and how it can be changed. The nurse should explore with the patient what happened, what events led up to the behavior, what the consequences were, and what feelings were aroused. Advanced practice nurses or other therapists explore the origins of the patient's behaviors and responses, but the generalist nurse needs to help the patient explore ways to change behaviors involved in the current situation. The laboriousness of this analytic process may be a sufficient incentive for the patient to abandon the dysfunctional behavior.

Complementary Therapies

Art therapy, facilitating the expression and sharing of a person's life story though words and images, is beneficial for people with BPD. Art therapy allows the person to explore and understand their previous traumatic experiences, fostering a sense of connection and recognition. In doing so, the person can see their history of resilience and personal accomplishments, ultimately leading to increased empowerment and hope (Haeyen et al., 2024).

Psychoeducation

Patient education within the context of a therapeutic relationship is one of the most important, empowering interventions for the generalist PMH nurse to use. Teaching patients skills to resist parasuicidal urges, improve emotional regulation, enhance interpersonal relationships, tolerate stress, and enhance overall QoL provides the foundation for long-term behavioral changes. These skills can be taught in any treatment setting as a part of the overall facility program (Box 30.8). If nurses are practicing in a facility where DBT is the treatment model, they can be trained in DBT and can serve as group skills leaders.

BOX 30.8

Psychoeducation Checklist: Borderline Personality Disorder

When caring for the patient with borderline personality disorder, be sure to include the following topic areas in the teaching plan:

- Management of medication, if used, including drug action, dosage, frequency, and possible adverse effects
- Regular sleep routines
- Nutrition
- Safety measures
- Functional versus dysfunctional behaviors
- Cognitive strategies (e.g., distraction, communication skills, thought stopping)
- Structure and limit setting
- Social relationships
- Recovery strategies
- Community resources

Teaching Emotional Regulation

A major goal of cognitive therapeutic interventions is emotional regulation—recognizing and controlling the expression of feelings. Patients often fail even to recognize their feelings; instead, they respond quickly without thinking about the consequences. Remember, the time needed for taking action is shorter than the time needed for thinking before acting. Pausing makes up for the momentary lag between the limbic and autonomic response and the prefrontal response.

Another element of emotional regulation is learning to delay gratification. When the patient wants something that is not immediately available, the nurse can teach patients to distract themselves, find alternate ways of meeting the need, and think about what would happen if they have to wait to meet the need.

Teaching Effective Ways to Communicate

Patients lack interpersonal skills in relating because they often had inadequate modeling and few opportunities to practice. The goals of relationship skill development are to identify problematic behaviors that interfere with relationships and to use appropriate behaviors in improving relationships. The starting point is with communication. The nurse teaches the patient basic communication approaches, such as making "I" statements, paraphrasing what the other party says before responding, checking the accuracy of perceptions with others, compromising and seeking common ground, listening actively, and offering and accepting reactions. Besides modeling the behaviors, the nurse guides patients in practicing a variety of communication approaches for common situations. When role playing, the nurse needs to discuss not only what the skills are and how to perform them but also the feelings patients have before, during, and after the role play.

In day treatment and outpatient settings, the nurse can give the patient homework, such as keeping a journal, applying role-playing skills to actual situations, and observing behaviors in others. In the hospital, the patient can experience the same process, where the nurse is available to offer immediate feedback. Whatever the setting or whatever the specific problems addressed, the nurse must keep in mind and remind the patient that change occurs slowly. Thus, working on the problems occurs gradually, with severity of symptoms as the guide to deciding how fast and how much change to expect.

Wellness Strategies

Whole Health is a cutting-edge approach to care that supports a person's health and well-being. This approach is currently being implemented throughout the US Department of Veterans Affairs. It is a nationally supported, grassroots movement that is bringing about system-wide transformation to health care in VA medical centers across the country. Whole Health centers around **what matters to you**, not what's the matter with you. The health care team gets to know you as an individual, and then works with you to develop an individual health plan that is based on your values, needs, and goals. Whole Health is wellness-oriented care. It has been found to be extremely effective for patients with all kinds of health care needs and is a great adjunctive care approach for people with psychiatric disorders. Whole Health programs such as meditation, yoga, acupuncture, Tai Chi, nutrition, and cooking classes serve as nonpharmaceutical approaches to health and wellness. Patients with BPD and depression especially, have reported enjoying and benefiting from Whole Health programs. Although some health care providers have implemented some type of wellness education and training in their practices for many years, the Whole Health approach to care is anticipated to be more formally included in all medical practices in the future.

Building Social Skills and Self-Esteem

In the hospital, the nurse can use group therapy to discuss feelings and ways to cope with their patients. Women with BPD benefit from assertiveness classes and women's health issues classes. Many of the women are involved in abusive relationships and lack the ability to resolve these relationships because of their extreme anxiety regarding separating from those they love and their extreme need to feel connected. These women verbalize desires to do it, but they do not have the strength and self-confidence needed to leave. Exposing them to a different style of interaction, as well as validation from other people, increases their self-esteem and ability to get away from negative influences.

Providing Family Education

Caring for or living with an individual with BPD is challenging. Families and friends experience high levels of anxiety, depression, and grief. They often feel that they are burdened with the person's problems and crises. These feelings are higher in families with a member with this disorder than in families of individuals with other severe mental disorders. Psychoeducation programs are currently being studied to support families and friends in their relationship with the affected person and reduce the feelings of grief, depression, anxiety, and burden (Benetti et al., 2024).

The awareness of these caregiver issues affords the nurse the opportunity to provide family educations in several areas:

- Educating the family about the diagnosis of BPD
- Educating the caregiver about mental health and support recourses for the person with BPD
- Educating the caregiver and normalizing their feelings that they too need support and care
- Educating the caregiver on access to mental health care for self-care and access to caregiver support resources (e.g., The National Alliance on Mental Illness.)

Promoting Safety

Patients with BPD are usually admitted to the inpatient setting because of threats of self-harm. Observing for antecedents of self-injurious behavior and intervening before an episode are important safety interventions. Patients can learn to identify situations leading to self-destructive behavior and develop preventive strategies (see Box 30.9).

Because patients with BPD are impulsive and may respond to stress by harming themselves, observation of the patient's interactions and assessment of mood, level of distress, and agitation are important indicators of impending self-injury. Remembering that self-harm is an effort to self-soothe by activating endogenous endorphins, the nurse can assist the patient to find more productive and enduring ways to find comfort. Linehan (1993) suggests using the Five Senses Exercise:

- Vision (e.g., go outside and look at the stars or flowers or autumn leaves)
- Hearing (e.g., listen to beautiful or invigorating music or the sounds of nature)
- Smell (e.g., light a scented candle, boil a cinnamon stick in water)
- Taste (e.g., drink a soothing, warm, nonalcoholic beverage)
- Touch (e.g., take a hot bubble bath, pet your dog or cat, get a massage)

Evaluation and Patient Outcomes

Evaluation and treatment outcomes vary depending on the severity of the disorder, the presence of comorbid disorders, and the availability of resources. For a patient with severe symptoms or continual self-injury, keeping the patient safe and alive may be a realistic outcome. Helping the patient resist parasuicidal urges may take years. In contrast, individuals who rarely need hospitalization and have adequate resources can expect to recover from the self-destructive impulses and learn positive interaction skills that promote a high-quality lifestyle. Most patients fall somewhere in between, with periods of symptom exacerbation and remission. In these patients, increasing the symptom-free time may be the best indicator of outcomes.

Continuum of Care

Treatment and recovery involve long-term therapy. Hospitalization is sometimes necessary during acute episodes involving **parasuicidal behavior**, but after

BOX 30.9

Building Clinical Judgment With SBAR: Managing Self-Injurious Behavior

SBAR

S: Situation

Samantha is a 26-year-old person assigned female at birth diagnosed with borderline personality disorder. She was admitted to the inpatient psychiatric unit due to affective instability, feelings of hopelessness, and self-injurious behavior which has increased in the past 24 hours.

B: Behavior

Samantha has a history of impulsivity and self-injury during periods of increased stress. She reports that her boyfriend broke up with her a few days ago after an argument. She has been relatively adherent to her current treatment regimen, which includes dialectical behavior therapy (DBT) and mood stabilizers.

A: Assessment

Samantha is visibly distraught. The nurse observes cuts on both forearms which appear to be recent. She is expressing feelings of hopelessness, worthlessness, and a desire to "make it all go away." She will not commit to a safety plan when one is presented by the nurse.

R: Recommendation

- Provide a safe environment.
- Monitor closely for further self-harm.
- Initiate 1:1 observation to promote safety and reduce opportunities for impulsive behaviors.
- Promote a consistent, structured environment.
- Contact health care provider for review of treatment plan to include more intensive therapeutic support.
- Provide Samantha with more structured coping strategies; provide ongoing support for managing distress, such as mindfulness practices or a Five Senses Exercise.

Building Clinical Judgment

1. How can the nurse foster a therapeutic relationship with Samantha?
2. What signs and behaviors might indicate that Samantha's condition is worsening?
3. What is the purpose of the Five Senses Exercise?

this behavior is controlled, patients are discharged. It is important for these individuals to continue with treatment in the outpatient or day treatment setting. Because these individuals often appear more competent and in control than they are, nurses must not be deceived by these outward appearances. These individuals need continued follow-up and long-term therapy, including individual therapy, psychoeducation, and positive role models (see Box 30.10). There is growing evidence that virtual psychosocial applications for people with BPD are clinically useful (Lindsay et al., 2024).

Integration With Primary Care

The mental health team should work closely with the primary care providers and explain the behaviors that interfere with receiving care. People with BPD often have multiple medical issues such as diabetes, obesity, and hyperlipidemia. The person may not show up for appointments yet expect the providers to call and remind them. Their interaction style and need for attention may quickly wear out a busy primary care staff, causing the staff to reject the person. Emotional dysfunction may erupt when the person is confronted with a stressful situation or diagnosis. The mental health team should be available to provide support to the primary care staff and help the patient negotiate the health care system.

ANTISOCIAL PERSONALITY DISORDER

ASPD is defined as "a pervasive pattern of disregard for, and violation of, the rights of others occurring since age 15 years" (APA, 2022, p. 749). This diagnosis is given to individuals 18 years of age or older who fail to follow society's rules—that is, they do not believe that society's rules are made for them and so are consistently irresponsible. ASPD has a long history in psychopathologic literature. A condition termed *moral insanity* was first described in the early 19th century. Since then the disorder has also been called psychopathy, and sociopathy. The term *psychopath*, or *sociopath*, an individual with a tendency toward antisocial and criminal behavior with little regard for others, is often used in describing the behaviors of people with ASPD.

KEYCONCEPT **Antisocial personality disorder** is characterized by a persistent pattern of disregarding and infringing upon the rights of others.

Clinical Course and Diagnostic Criteria

ASPD has a chronic course with antisocial behaviors tending to diminish later in life, particularly after the age of 40 years (APA, 2022). Individuals with ASPD are arrogant and self-centered and feel privileged and entitled. They are self-serving, and they exploit and seek power

BOX 30.10

Research for Evidence-Based Practice: Long-Lasting Symptoms in Borderline Personality Disorder: Defining an Emergent Population With Differential Clinical and Therapeutic Features

Casellas, P. E., Soler, J., Schmidt, C., Soriano, J., & Pascual, J. C. (2024). *Long-lasting symptoms in borderline personality disorder: Defining an emergent population with differential clinical and therapeutic features.* Personality & Mental Health, 18*(3), 248–258.*

THE QUESTION: What are sociodemographic, clinical, and therapeutic variables in individuals with BPD with and without long-lasting symptoms (LLS)?

METHODS: Patients who were admitted to a free outpatient clinic specializing in BPD during a 20-year period were included in this retrospective study. Patients were divided into two groups: those with LLS and those without. Only those over 18 years old, with a primary diagnosis of BPD, and with no comorbid psychotic or bipolar disorder or other severe physical conditions were included. Demographic and clinical data at baseline were described and compared between groups.

FINDINGS: There were 620 patients with a primary diagnosis of BPD included in the study. Of these, 71% were over the age of 40 with LLS. In this group, the average age of onset was 27 years old. Compared with non-LLS patients, the LLS group had less clinical severity, particularly related to impulsivity and issues with interpersonal relationships. The LLS group did have greater comorbidity with affective disorders and were more likely to be receiving disability payments. Despite lower overall severity of clinical symptoms, those with LLS had a higher use of medications. Of interest, individuals with LLS who completed dialectical behavior therapy (DBT) had a significant decrease in the use of benzodiazepines as well as the overall number of medications prescribed.

IMPLICATIONS FOR NURSING: Nurses should be aware of the specific features of LLS in BPD to best identify and address patient needs, as symptoms may vary according to age. DBT is found to be particularly effective for BPD and may also aid in reducing polypharmacy in older patients with LLS.

over others. They can be interpersonally engaging and charming, which is often mistaken for a genuine sense of concern for other people. In reality, they lack empathy; are unable to express human compassion; and tend to be insensitive, callous, and contemptuous of others. Deceit and manipulation for personal profit or pleasure are central features associated with this disorder. They are behaviorally impulsive and interpersonally irresponsible. Many with this disorder repeatedly perform acts that are grounds for arrest (whether they are arrested or not), such as destroying property, harassing others, stealing, or pursuing other illegal occupations. They act hastily and spontaneously, are temperamentally aggressive and shortsighted, and fail to plan ahead or consider alternatives. They fail to adapt to the ethical and social standards of the community. They lack a sense of personal obligation to fulfill social and financial responsibilities, including those involved with being a spouse, parent/caregiver, employee, friend, or member of the community. They lack remorse for their transgressions (APA, 2022).

Some of these individuals openly and flagrantly violate laws and end up in jail. But most people with ASPD never come in conflict with the law and instead find a niche in society, such as in business, the military, or politics, which rewards their competitively tough behavior. Although ASPD is characterized by continual antisocial acts, the disorder is not synonymous with criminality. See Key Diagnostic Characteristics 30.2.

Epidemiology and Risk Factors

Twelve-month US prevalence rates of ASPD are estimated between 0.6% and 3.6% (APA, 2022). The prevalence of ASPD increases through early adulthood, with a peak of 3.91% in younger adults and decline to 0.78% in adults ages over 65 years (Holzer et al., 2022). Males with alcohol use disorder and those released from substance misuse clinics, prisons, or other forensic settings have the highest rates. Adverse socioeconomic (i.e., poverty) or sociocultural (i.e., migration) factors also are associated with higher prevalence (APA, 2022). Gender differences also exist in how symptoms are manifested (Key Diagnostic Characteristics 30.2).

Age of Onset

To be diagnosed with ASPD, the individual must be at least 18 years old and must have exhibited one or more childhood behavioral characteristics of conduct disorder before the age of 15 years, such as aggression to people or animals, destruction of property, deceitfulness or theft, or serious violation of rules. The likelihood of developing adult ASPD is increased if onset of conduct disorder is seen before age 10 years as well as an accompanying childhood attention-deficit hyperactivity disorder diagnosis (APA, 2022).

Comorbidity

ASPD is associated with several other psychiatric disorders, including mood, anxiety, and other personality disorders. ASPD is strongly associated with alcohol and substance misuse (Low et al., 2024). However, a diagnosis of ASPD is not warranted if the antisocial behavior occurs only in the context of substance use. For example, some people who misuse substances sometimes engage in criminal behavior, such as stealing or prostitution, only

KEY DIAGNOSTIC CHARACTERISTICS 30.2

***DSM-5-TR* DIAGNOSTIC CRITERIA: Antisocial Personality Disorder**

A. A pervasive pattern of disregard for and violation of the rights of others, occurring since age 15 years, as indicated by three (or more) of the following:
   1. Failure to conform to social norms with respect to lawful behaviors, as indicated by repeatedly performing acts that are grounds for arrest.
   2. Deceitfulness, as indicated by repeated lying, use of aliases, or conning others for personal profit or pleasure.
   3. Impulsivity or failure to plan ahead.
   4. Irritability and aggressiveness, as indicated by repeated physical fights or assaults.
   5. Reckless disregard for safety of self or others.
   6. Consistent irresponsibility, as indicated by repeated failure to sustain consistent work behavior or honor financial obligations.
   7. Lack of remorse, as indicated by being indifferent to or rationalizing having hurt, mistreated, or stolen from another.

B. The individual is at least age 18 years.

C. There is evidence of conduct disorder with onset before age 15 years.

D. The occurrence of antisocial behavior is not exclusively during the course of schizophrenia or bipolar disorder.

when in pursuit of drugs. Therefore, it is crucial to assess whether the person with possible ASPD has engaged in illegal activities at times other than when pursuing or using substances.

Etiology

Biologic Theories

Perhaps more than any other personality disorder, an extensive number of biologically oriented studies explore the genetic bases, neuropsychological factors, and arousal levels among this group of pathologies. Many of these studies show neurobiologic changes associated with personality disorders or characteristics, but the evidence lacks that these changes caused the disorder (Deming et al., 2024). These studies often overlap with studies of aggression, temperament, and substance use (Dotterer et al., 2021; Kolla et al., 2021).

Psychosocial Theories

Temperament

Scientists believe temperament is neurobiologically determined, and many believe that it is central to understanding personality disorders. A temperament, the natural predisposition to express feelings and actions, is evident during the first few months of life and remains stable through development. For example, whereas some infants are more relaxed or calm and sleep a lot, others are extremely alert, startled by the slightest noise, cry more, and are sleepless.

Difficult temperaments are common in ASPD and are often on the basis of their aggression and impulsivity.

KEYCONCEPT Temperament is an innate attribute that defines the child's approach to the world and interaction with the environment across the following dimensions: *Easy or flexible* (friendly, easygoing, adheres to routines, adapts to changes, and calm disposition), *active or feisty* (fussy, does not follow routines, irregular feeding and sleeping schedules, apprehensive of a new environment and new people, intense reactions, and easily upset), and *slow to warm up or cautious* (less engaged or active than other children, shy disposition to a new situation and new people, withdraws or has a negative reaction to situations, becomes more comfortable and warms up with repeated exposure to a new environment or person) (Malik & Marwaha, 2022).

KEYCONCEPT A **difficult temperament** or negative emotionality is characterized by withdrawal from stimuli, low adaptability, and intense emotional reactions. Behaviors associated with a difficult temperament are aggression, inattention, hyperactivity, and impulsivity (Zhang et al., 2022). Individuals with a difficult temperament are more likely to experience mood disorders, major depression, disruptive behavior disorders, and drug misuse (Tharshini et al., 2021).

Attachment

One of the leading explanations of ASPD is that unsatisfactory attachments in early relationships lead to antisocial behavior in later life. Attachment, attaining, and retaining interpersonal connection to a significant person, begins at birth. In a secure attachment, a child feels safe, loved, and valued and develops the self-confidence to interact with the rest of the world. Experiences within the context of secure relationships enable the child to develop trust in others. Strong attachments between parents/caregivers and child may lower the risk of delinquency, assault, and other offenses that are characteristic of those who develop antisocial behavior (Bachmann et al., 2023).

In individuals with ASPD, a failure to make or sustain stable attachments in early childhood can lead to avoidance of future attachments. Risk factors for developing dysfunctional attachments include parental abandonment or neglect, loss of a parent or primary caregiver, and physical or sexual abuse. Parents/caregivers who lacked secure attachment relationships in their own childhoods may be unable to form secure attachment relationships with their own children.

Family Issues

In many cases, individuals with ASPD come from chaotic families in which alcohol use disorder and violence are the norm. Individuals who have been victims of abuse or neglect, live in a foster home, or have had several primary caregivers are more likely to be targeted by antisocial behaviors, especially aggression. Child abuse and growing up in a home with domestic violence increase the risk of antisocial behavior (Moreira et al., 2022). It is difficult to separate the influence of social factors on the development of the disorder because the symptoms of ASPD are expressed as social manifestations, including unemployment, multiple divorces and separations, and violence.

Family Response to Antisocial Personality Disorder

If family members are present in a patient's life, they have probably been abused, mistreated, or intimidated by these patients. For example, one patient sold their parents' possessions while they were at work. Another abused their spouse after drinking. However, family members may be fiercely loyal to the patient and blame themselves for their shortcomings.

RECOVERY-ORIENTED CARE FOR PEOPLE WITH ANTISOCIAL PERSONALITY DISORDER

See Clinical Judgment Nursing Care Plan 30.2, which sets forth a plan of care for Danny, one of the case study patients in this chapter.

Teamwork and Collaboration: Working Toward Recovery

People rarely seek mental health care for ASPD but rather for treatment of depression, substance use, uncontrolled anger, or forensic-related issues. Patients with psychiatric disorders who are admitted through the courts often have a comorbid diagnosis of ASPD. Patients with ASPD usually present for treatment as a result of an ultimatum. Treatment is often a choice between losing a job, being expelled from school, ending a marriage or relationship with children, or giving up on a chance at probation and psychological treatment. Under these circumstances, treatment is usually forced on them. Other times, people with ASPD who find themselves in trouble with the law will seek out psychiatric care on their own in an attempt

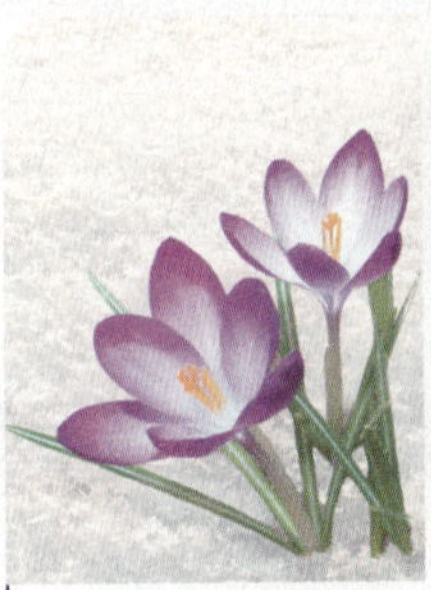

CLINICAL JUDGMENT NURSING CARE PLAN 30.2

The Patient With Antisocial Personality Disorder

Danny, age 55, was brought to the emergency department of the psychiatric hospital by the local police after threatening suicide. He was arrested and incarcerated after physically assaulting his girlfriend with whom he lives after she called the police. "I hit her because she nags me. I went to jail because my girlfriend called the police." Danny is now without stable housing after his girlfriend obtained a restraining order. Danny was diagnosed with conduct disorder at age 10 and has a history of being aggressive toward animals and people. He has not held a job more than a few months and has never been able to independently support himself. After he arrived on the unit, he told the staff that he really did not intend to kill himself. "The jail beds are uncomfortable, and the food is terrible."

Setting: Inpatient Psychiatric Unit in a General Hospital

Assessment Cues: Danny is highly interactive and engaging with others. He appears confident. After his arrest, he attempted suicide by hanging in his cell. He currently denies any suicidal ideation. His family reports that he has been in trouble all his life, most recently for selling drugs. Danny believes that he has to put his own needs above others and that he can exploit others because they will eventually take advantage of him. His father is currently in prison for murder.

Psychiatric Diagnosis	Medications
Antisocial personality disorder	None

Priority Hypothesis: Risk for Suicide

Important Characteristics	Associated Considerations
Threatened suicide	Has no real friends Arrested for assaulting girlfriend History of numerous arrests

Continued

Clinical Judgment Nursing Care Plan 30.2 Continued

Planning Recovery and Wellness Outcomes

Initial	Discharge
1. Remain safe and not harm himself. 2. Agree not to harm himself over the next 24 hours.	1. Identify ways of dealing with stress instead of suicide threats. 2. Verbalize alternate thinking with a more realistic base.

Taking Action: Nursing Interventions

Interventions	Rationale	Ongoing Assessment
Monitor the patient for changes in mood or behavior that might lead to self-injurious behavior.	Close observation establishes safety and protection of the patient from self-harm and impulsive behaviors.	Document according to facility policy. Continue to observe for mood and behavior changes.
Discuss with the patient the need for close observation and rationale to keep him safe.	Close observation should be continued throughout all shifts until the patient agrees to resist urge for self-harm.	Communicate information about the patient's risk to other nursing staff. Review documentation of close observation for all shifts.

Evaluation

Outcomes	Revised Outcomes	Interventions
Remained safe without further harming self	None	

Priority Hypothesis: Ineffective Role Performance

Important Characteristics	Associated Characteristics
Violence, harassment Inadequate coping Inadequate self-management System conflict	Inadequate role preparation Lack of education Unrealistic role expectations

Planning Recovery and Wellness Outcomes

Initial	Discharge
1. Identify need to learn new coping skills. 2. Begin to assume responsibility for actions. 3. Seek substance use treatment.	1. Develop a plan to finish high school. 2. Seek additional help in developing empathy for others.

Taking Action: Nursing Interventions

Interventions	Rationale	Ongoing Assessment
Discuss the importance of looking at lifestyle and relationship with others.	People with antisocial personality disorder often blame others for their misfortune. Focusing on lifestyle and relationships initiates a dialogue.	Observe the willingness of Danny to assume responsibility for own choices.

Evaluation

Outcomes	Revised Outcomes	Interventions
Expressed interest in changing lifestyle only if nurse agreed to maintain contact after discharge.	Continue to discuss lifestyle and developing positive relationships. None	Set boundary limits with Danny. Emphasize the importance of personal responsibility for behavior change.

to "prove" to the court they are seeking help for their offenses, when they are actually only manipulating the justice system through deception. Most prisons and other correctional facilities require inmates to attend psychotherapy sessions. In either case, working with people with ASPD is likely to be a frustrating and exasperating experience for the nurse due to the patient's clear lack of insight and/or motivation to change. Treatment is difficult and involves helping the patient alter their cognitive schemata.

Safety Issues

Although they can be interpersonally charming, these patients can become verbally and physically abusive if their expectations are not met. Protection of other patients and staff is a priority.

EVIDENCE-BASED NURSING CARE OF PEOPLE WITH ANTISOCIAL PERSONALITY DISORDER

People with ASPD usually enter the mental health system because of another disorder, such as a substance use disorder, or a court order. ASPD is rarely the primary diagnosis at admission. Nurses should maintain a professional relationship with patients who have this disorder, while remaining vigilant against manipulation by enforcing boundaries, avoiding unnecessary self-disclosure, and upholding unit rules.

RECOGNIZING CUES: RELEVANT ASSESSMENT INFORMATION

Physical Health and Functioning

ASPD does not significantly impair physical functioning except in the presence of coexisting substance use disorder or another psychiatric diagnosis involved. Because substance use is a major issue with this population, the physical effects of chronic use of addictive substances must be considered. If admitted inpatient, the nurse needs to keenly observe for possible withdrawal symptoms from substance use. Conversely, someone who has health issues secondary to chronic substance misuse should also be assessed for concurrent personality disorders. Substance use and ASPD are not mutually exclusive. Some people with substance use disorders are not antisocial but may commit crimes (e.g., selling drugs, robbery, theft) in the context of obtaining drugs for their personal use.

Psychosocial Cues

Eliciting psychosocial data from people with ASPD may be difficult because of their basic mistrust of authority figures. Many patients with ASPD are committed to mental health care by the court system. They may not give an accurate history or may embellish aspects to project themselves in a more positive light. They often deny any criminal activity, even if they are admitted to police custody.

Behavioral Responses

Key areas of assessment are determining the quality of relationships, impulsivity, and the extent of aggression. These individuals do not assume responsibility for their own actions and often blame others for their misfortune. Their disregard for others is manifested in their interactions. For example, one patient with human immunodeficiency virus was engaging in unprotected sex with several different people because he wanted to "have fun as long as I can." He was completely unconcerned about the possibility of transmitting the virus. These individuals often make good first impressions. Self-awareness is especially important for the nurse because of the initial charming quality of many of these individuals. When these patients realize that the nurse cannot be used or manipulated, they lose interest in the nurse and revert to their usual, egocentric behaviors.

Support Network

Social support for these individuals is often minimal, just as it is for individuals with BPD, but the reasons are different. These individuals have often taken advantage of friends and relatives who, in turn, no longer trust them. Helping the patient build a new support system after new skills are learned is usually the only option. For these individuals to develop friends and re-engage family members, they must learn to interact in new ways, develop empathy, and risk an attachment. For many, this never truly becomes a reality.

ANALYZING CUES AND DEVELOPING HYPOTHESES

People with ASPD are often admitted to psychiatric units following a violent incident, such as a physical confrontation or a suicide attempt. As with any patient, safety is a priority. One of the first priorities is to establish a safe environment for the patient and staff. After safety is established, other mutually agreed-upon priorities can be considered, such as improving interpersonal communication with family members or addressing anger issues.

PLANNING RECOVERY AND WELLNESS OUTCOMES

Recovery involves changing interpersonal and lifestyle behaviors. The overall treatment goals are to develop a nurturing sense of attachment and empathy for other people and situations and to live within the norms of society. Several current treatment modalities may be helpful in establishing these goals. Harm reduction is a pragmatic approach for managing high-risk behaviors, such as substance use or high-risk sexual behaviors, that are often characteristic of people with ASPD. For example, the harm reduction approach recognizes that reducing substance use from 7 to 3 days per week is progress. Reducing the harm of substance use is celebrated and built upon for further success. See Chapter 31. Motivational interviewing can help the person explore and resolve ambivalence to change. MBT, discussed earlier in this chapter, can also be for people with ASPD.

Outcomes should be short-term and relevant to a specific issue. For example, if a patient has been chronically unemployed, a reasonable short-term outcome is for the patient to set up job interviews rather than obtain a job.

THERAPEUTIC RELATIONSHIP

Therapeutic relationships are difficult to establish because these individuals do not attach themselves to others and are often unable to use a relationship to change behavior. The goal of the therapeutic relationship is to identify dysfunctional thinking patterns and develop new problem-solving behaviors. After the first few meetings with these patients, the nurse may believe that the relationship has a good start, but in reality, a superficial alliance is usually formed. Additional sessions reveal the lack of patient commitment to the relationship. These patients begin to revisit topics discussed in previous sessions or lose interest in trying to work on issues. Setting limits, providing clarity and structure to interactions, and being authentic, nonjudgmental, and genuinely involved are key elements in building a strong therapeutic alliance with the patient (Aerts et al., 2023). By using self-awareness skills and accessing supervision regularly, the nurse can identify blocks in the development of a therapeutic relationship (or lack of) and their response to the relationship.

TAKING ACTION: NURSING INTERVENTIONS

Physical Care

In instances in which there are comorbid disorders, the patient with ASPD may actually interfere with interventions aimed at improving physical functioning. For example, a patient with substance use disorder and ASPD may not develop enough trust within a relationship to examine their thoughts or other aspects of dysfunction, such as alcohol or substance misuse. A patient with ASPD who develops a case of pancreatitis may refuse to refrain from misusing alcohol. As a result, they may be hospitalized for multiple episodes of pancreatitis.

Medication Interventions

There are no medications to treat ASPD, only treatment for symptoms they may experience. For example, impulsive aggression may benefit from the use of atypical antipsychotics, lithium, anticonvulsants, and stimulants (Sesso & Masi, 2023).

Psychosocial Interventions

Facilitating self-responsibility (i.e., encouraging a patient to assume more responsibility for personal behavior) is an important intervention. The nursing activities that are particularly helpful include holding the patient responsible for the behavior, monitoring the extent that self-responsibility is assumed, and discussing the consequences of not dealing with responsibilities. The nurse needs to refrain from arguing or bargaining about the unit rules, such as time for meals, use of the television room, and smoking. Instead, positive feedback is given to the patient for accepting additional responsibility or changing behavior.

Psychoeducation

Patient education efforts must be creative and thought provoking. In teaching an individual with ASPD, a direct approach is best, but the nurse must avoid "lecturing," which the patient will resent. In teaching the patient about positive health care practices, impulse control, and anger management, the best approach is to engage the patient in a discussion about the issue and then direct the topic to the major teaching points. These patients often take great delight in arguing or showing how the rules of life do not apply to them. A sense of humor is important, as are clear teaching goals and avoiding being sidetracked (see Boxes 30.11 and 30.12).

Wellness Strategies

Enhancing self-awareness (i.e., exploring and understanding personal thoughts, feelings, motivation, and behaviors) is another nursing intervention that helps patients understand how to relate peacefully to the rest of the world. Encouraging patients to recognize and discuss their thoughts and feelings helps the nurse understand how the patient views the world. Psychotherapy may be effective in improving interpersonal relationships, reducing criminal behaviors, and managing anger in individuals with ASPD (Maden et al., 2023).

Providing Family Education

Family members of patients with ASPD usually need help in establishing boundaries. Because there is a long-term pattern of interaction in which family members feel responsible for the patient's antisocial behavior, these patterns need to be stopped. Families need help in recognizing the patient's responsibility for their own actions.

Promoting Safety

Aggressive behavior is often an issue for these individuals and their family members. Similar to patients with BPD, people with ASPD tend to be impulsive. Instead of self-injury, these individuals are more likely to strike out at

BOX 30.11

Therapeutic Dialogue: Antisocial Personality Disorder

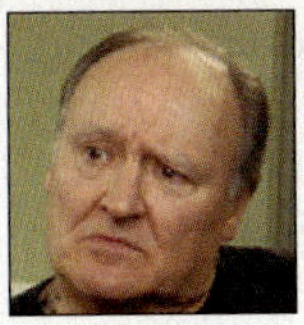

INEFFECTIVE APPROACH

Danny: Hey, I need a light for my cigarette.

Nurse: Really? You know the rules—no smoking on the unit.

Danny: I'm not going to smoke here. I just need a light so that I can have a cigarette when I leave here.

Nurse: I also need your cigarettes. Cigarettes are contraband.

Danny: You are terrible—just like the bitch who kicked me out. Who do you think you are anyway?

Nurse: You need to quiet down.

Danny: Yeah, says who?

Nurse: I will call security if you don't quiet down.

Danny: Call them, I don't care.

EFFECTIVE APPROACH

Danny: Hey, I need a light for my cigarette.

Nurse: A light? I don't have a light.

Danny: I need a light so that I can smoke later.

Nurse: Oh, I see. Did you have a lighter when you were admitted?

Danny: Yea, they took everything away including my belt and shoelaces.

Nurse: The reason for storing everything is for the safety of everyone. When you are discharged, you can retrieve everything. I also need to store any cigarettes you have.

Danny: What makes you think I have any cigarettes?

Nurse: Well, you asked for a light. Many patients manage to bring cigarettes into the unit. I need to put them with your things. You can retrieve them when you are discharged.

Danny: This place is something.

Nurse: I will put your cigarettes in a bag with your name on them.

Danny: This sucks. But here they are.

CRITICAL THINKING CHALLENGE

1. How did the nurse in the first scenario get sidetracked?
2. How was the nurse in the second scenario able to convince Danny to give up his cigarettes without escalating his anger?

those who are perceived to be interfering with their immediate gratification. Anger control assistance (helping to express anger in an adaptive, nonviolent manner) becomes a priority intervention. Because the expression of anger and aggression develops during a lifetime, these individuals can benefit from anger management techniques.

BOX 30.12

Psychoeducation Checklist: Antisocial Personality Disorder

When caring for the patient with ASPD, be sure to include the following topic areas in the teaching plan:

- Positive health care practices, including substance use control
- Effective communication and interaction skills
- Impulse control
- Anger management
- Group experience to help develop self-awareness and impact of behavior on others
- Analyzing an issue from the other person's viewpoint
- Maintenance of employment
- Interpersonal relationships and social interactions

Group Interventions

Group interventions are more effective than individual modalities because other patients and staff can validate or challenge the patient's view of a situation. Problem-solving groups that focus on identifying a problem and developing a variety of alternative solutions are particularly helpful because patient self-responsibility is reinforced when patients remind each other of better alternatives. Patients are likely to confront each other with dysfunctional schemata or thinking patterns. Teaching patients with ASPD the same communication techniques as those with BPD will also encourage self-responsibility. These patients often attend groups that focus on the development of empathy.

Implementing Milieu Therapy

Milieu interventions, such as providing a structured environment with rules that are consistently applied to patients who are responsible for their own behavior, are important. While living in close proximity to others, the individual with ASPD will demonstrate dysfunctional social patterns that can be identified and targeted for correction. For example, these patients often violate ward rules, such as no smoking or limitations on the number of visitors, and may bring contraband, such as illegal drugs, into the unit.

In an inpatient unit, interventions can be more intense and focus on helping the patient develop positive interaction skills and experience a consistent environment. For example, the focus of nursing interventions may be the patient's continual disregard of the rights of others. On one unit, a patient continually placed orders for pizzas in the name of another patient who had limited intelligence and was genuinely afraid of the person with ASPD. The victimized patient always paid for the pizza. When the nursing staff realized what was happening, they confronted the patient with ASPD about the behavior and revoked his unit privileges.

Evaluation and Patient Outcomes

The outcomes for patients with ASPD are evaluated in terms of managing specific issues, such as maintaining employment or developing a meaningful interpersonal relationship. The nurse will most likely see these patients for other health care issues, so adherence to treatment recommendations and development of health care practices (e.g., reducing smoking and alcohol consumption) can also be factored into the evaluation of outcomes.

Continuum of Care

People with ASPD rarely seek mental health care unless there is a comorbid condition, such as depression. Nurses are most likely to see these patients in medical–surgical settings for comorbid conditions. Consistency in interventions is necessary for treating the patient throughout the continuum of care.

HISTRIONIC PERSONALITY DISORDER

Clinical Course and Diagnostic Criteria

Attention seeking, *excitable*, and *emotional* are terms used to describe people with **histrionic personality disorder (HPD)**. HPD is one of the most ambiguous diagnostic categories in psychiatry. HPD made its first official appearance in the *Diagnostic and Statistical Manual of Mental Disorders II (DSM II)* and since its revisions through *DSM-5-TR*. HPD is the only modern category in diagnostic classifications that conserved a derivative of the old concept of Hysteria. Several psychiatric disorders are derived from the original term *hysteria* such as the *conversion disorder*, the *somatization disorder*, *somatoform disorders*, *phobic anxiety*, the term *mass hysteria*, and finally the *HPD*. The word *hysteria* is derived from the Greek term *hystera*, meaning the womb or uterus. It was believed that these behaviors were exclusive to people assigned female at birth and were caused by disturbances in the uterus. Freud proposed "hysteria" as being a psychological disorder primarily experienced by women and characterized by emotional excesses and attention seeking behavior. Although this theory is often criticized, it did lay the foundation for the exploration of histrionic symptoms and behaviors (Torrico et al., 2024).

Individuals with HPD are lively and dramatic and draw attention to themselves by their enthusiasm, dress, and apparent openness. They are the "life of the party" and, on the surface, seem interested in others. Their insatiable need for attention and approval quickly becomes obvious. Their need to be "center stage" arises in two ways: (1) their interests and topics of conversation focus on their own desires and activities and (2) their behavior, including their speech pattern, continually calls attention to themselves. These needs are inflexible and persistent even after others attempt to meet them. People with HPDs are quick to form new friendships and just as quick to become demanding. Because they are trusting and easily influenced by other opinions, their behavior often appears inconsistent. Their strong dependency need makes them overly trusting and gullible. They are moody and often experience a sense of helplessness when others are uninterested in them. They are sexually seductive in their attempts to gain attention and often are uncomfortable within a single relationship. Their appearance is provocative and their speech dramatic. They express strong opinions without supporting facts. Loyalty and fidelity are lacking (Babl et al., 2023; Yalch et al., 2023).

Gender influences the manifestations of this disorder. Women dress seductively, may express dependency on selected men, and may "play" a submissive role. Men may dress in a very masculine manner and seek attention by bragging about athletic skills or successes in their jobs. Men may also demonstrate more aggressive behaviors. Individuals with this disorder have difficulty achieving any true intimacy in interpersonal relationships. They seem to possess an innate sensitivity to the moods and thoughts of those they wish to please. This hyperalertness enables them to maneuver quickly to gain their attention. They then attempt to control relationships by their seductiveness at one level but become extremely dependent on their friends at another level. Their demand for constant attention quickly alienates their friends. They become depressed when they are not the center of attention.

Epidemiology and Risk Factors

The prevalence of HPD is estimated to affect up to 1.8% of the general population of the United States. Women are diagnosed four times as often as men. This may be due to societal norms where women are expected to be less sexually assertive. This disorder occurs concurrently with other mental disorders; anxiety disorder, obsessive-compulsive syndromes, somatic symptom disorder, substance use disorder, and mood disorders, in which they overplay their feelings of dysthymia by expressing them through dramatic and eye-catching gestures (Torrico et al., 2024).

Etiology

Research related to this personality disorder is minimal. Some speculate that there is a biologic component and that heredity may play a role but that the biologic influence is less than in some of the previously discussed personality issues. In infancy and early childhood, these individuals are extremely alert and emotionally responsive. The tendencies for sensory alertness may be traced to responses of the limbic and reticular systems. They demonstrate a high degree of dependence on others and a type of dissociation in which they have reduced awareness of their behavior in relation to others (Torrico et al., 2024).

It is believed that these highly alert and responsive infants seek more gratification from external stimulation during their first few months of life. Depending on the responsiveness of caregivers to them, they develop behavior patterns in response to their caregivers. It is believed that these children experience brief, highly charged, and irregular reinforcement from multiple caregivers (parents, siblings, grandparents, foster parents) who are unable to provide consistent experiences.

Parental behavior and role modeling are also believed to contribute to the development of HPD. Many of the women with this disorder reported that they are just like their mother, who is emotionally labile, bored with the routines of home life, flirtatious with men, and clever in dealing with people. It is believed that through role modeling, these children learn and mimic the behaviors observed in caregivers or adults (Torrico et al., 2024).

Childhood trauma, particularly sexual abuse, is another factor that may increase risk for HPD. Individuals demonstrating overly seductive and other sexualized behaviors may have learned such behaviors through experiencing childhood sexual abuse. A history of physical abuse and neglect are also noted in histories of people with severe HPD (Yalch et al., 2023).

Evidence-Based Nursing Care of People With Histrionic Personality Disorder

The ultimate treatment goal for patients with HPD is to correct the tendency to expect others to fulfill all of their needs. When these individuals seek mental health care, they have usually experienced a period of social disapproval or deprivation. Their hope is that the mental health providers will help fulfill their needs. Specific goals are needed to protect the person from becoming dependent on a mental health system. In the nursing assessment, the nurse focuses on the quality of the individual's interpersonal relationships. It is common that the person is dissatisfied with their partner, and sexual relations may be nonexistent.

During the assessment, the patient will make statements that indicate low self-esteem. Because these individuals believe that they are incapable of handling life's demands and have been waiting for a truly competent person to take care of them, they have not developed a positive self-concept or adequate problem-solving abilities.

Priority of care areas for people with this disorder include focusing on self-esteem and coping patterns. Outcomes focus on helping the patient develop autonomy, a positive self-concept, and mature problem-solving skills.

A variety of interventions support the outcomes. A nurse–patient relationship that allows the patient to explore positive personality characteristics and develop independent decision-making skills forms the basis of the interventions. Reinforcing personal strengths, conveying confidence in the patient's ability to handle situations, and examining the patient's negative perceptions of him- or herself can be done within the therapeutic relationship. Encouraging the patient to act autonomously can also improve the individual's sense of self-worth. Attending assertiveness groups can help increase the individual's self-confidence and improve self-esteem.

Continuum of Care

Patients with HPD do not seek mental health care unless they have a coexisting medical or mental disorder. They are likely to be treated within the community for most of their lives, with the exception of short hospitalizations for nonpsychiatric issues.

NARCISSISTIC PERSONALITY DISORDER

Clinical Course and Diagnostic Criteria

People with **narcissistic personality disorder** are grandiose, have an inexhaustible need for admiration, and lack empathy. Beginning in childhood, these individuals believe that they are superior, special, or unique and that others should recognize them in this way (Weinberg et al., 2024). They are often preoccupied with fantasies of unlimited success, power, beauty, or ideal love. They overvalue their personal worth, direct their affections toward themselves, and expect others to hold them in high esteem. They define the world through their own self-centered view. Their sense of entitlement is striking. People with narcissistic personality disorder are benignly arrogant and feel themselves above the conventions of their cultural group. They handle criticism poorly and may become enraged if someone dares to criticize them, or else they may appear totally indifferent to criticism. They believe they are entitled to be served and that it is their inalienable right to receive special considerations. People with this disorder want to have their own way and are frequently ambitious for fame and fortune. These individuals are often successful in their jobs but may alienate their significant others, who grow tired of their narcissism. They cannot show empathy, and they feign sympathy only for their own benefit to achieve their selfish ends. Clinically, those with narcissistic personality disorder show overlapping characteristics of BPD and ASPD (Mitra et al., 2024).

Epidemiology and Risk Factors

The prevalence of narcissistic personality disorder in community samples has been estimated as high as 7.7% for men and 4.8% for women. Narcissistic personality disorder can be found in professionals who are highly respected, such as those in law, medicine, and science and those associated with celebrity status. People with this disorder may impart an unrealistic sense of omnipotence, grandiosity, beauty, and talent to their children; therefore, children of parents with a narcissistic personality disorder have a higher than usual risk of developing the disorder themselves. It also commonly occurs in only children and among first-born boys in cultural groups in which males have special privileges (Mitra et al., 2024).

Etiology

Limited evidence suggests biologic factors contribute to the development of this disorder. One notion about its development is that it is the result of overvaluation and overindulgence of a child by parents/caregivers. These children are overly pampered and indulged, with every whim catered to. They learn to view themselves as special beings and to expect special treatment and subservience from others. They do not learn how to cooperate, share, or consider others' desires and interests. An alternate explanation is that the child never truly separated emotionally from their primary caregiver and therefore cannot envision functioning independently. According to another set of theories, these individuals try to avoid or reduce intense feelings of shame and engage in diverse strategies to gain attention for themselves (Koskinen et al., 2024; Ross et al., 2024).

Evidence-Based Nursing Care for People With Narcissistic Personality Disorder

The nurse usually encounters people with narcissism in medical settings and in psychiatric settings with a coexisting psychiatric disorder. They are difficult patients who often appear snobbish, condescending, and patronizing in their attitudes. It is unlikely that these individuals are motivated to develop sensitivity to others and socially cooperative attitudes and behaviors. Building a therapeutic relationship is a slow process because these patients avoid self-reflection and often reject the clinician's approaches. They may be dismissive and avoidant. They may consider contact with a clinician as being intrusive or demeaning, and suggestive that they are imperfect. It is important not to engage in power struggles with the patient. Nurses need to use their self-awareness skills in interacting with these patients and help the person identify concrete, realistic, and measurable treatment goals that the patient identifies as their own (Ronningstam & Weinberg, 2023; Weinberg, 2024).

Continuum of Care

Similar to patients with histrionic disorder, those with narcissistic personality disorder do not seek mental health care unless they have a coexisting medical or mental disorder. They are likely to be treated within the community for most of their lives, with the exception of short hospitalizations for nonpsychiatric issues.

CLUSTER C DISORDERS: AVOIDANT, DEPENDENT, AND OBSESSIVE-COMPULSIVE PERSONALITY DISORDERS

AVOIDANT PERSONALITY DISORDER

Clinical Course and Diagnostic Criteria

Avoidant personality disorder (AVPD) is characterized by extensive avoidance of social interaction driven by fears of rejection and feelings of personal inadequacy (Aghakishiyeva & Ozdel, 2023). Individuals with this disorder stay out of social situations in which interpersonal contact with others may be expected. Individuals appear timid, shy, and hesitant; they also fear criticism and feel inadequate. These individuals are extremely sensitive to negative comments and disapproval and appraise situations more negatively than others do. They perceive themselves as unwanted and isolated from others. This behavior becomes problematic when it restricts their social activities and work opportunities because of their extreme fear of rejection. In comparison to other personality disorders, AVPD is associated with a high level of impairment in daily functioning (Kealy et al., 2022). Comorbid anxiety and depressive disorders, some accompanied by suicidal ideation, contribute to functional impairment (Kealy et al., 2022; Kvarstein et al., 2021). Anxious and avoidant attachments with early caregivers have been shown to contribute to the development of AVPD. Fear, expectations of being shamed, and overuse of cognitive and behavioral avoidance contribute to the vicious cycles of maintenance in AVPD.

In childhood, people with AVPD are shy, but instead of growing out of the shyness, it becomes worse in adulthood. They perceive themselves as socially inept, inadequate, and inferior, which, in turn, justifies their isolation and rejection by others. Vocationally, people with AVPD often take jobs on the sidelines, rarely obtaining personal advancement or exercising much authority, but to employers, they seem shy and eager to please. They are reluctant to enter relationships unless they are given strong assurance of uncritical acceptances, so they consequently often have no close friends or confidants (Torrico & Sapra, 2024).

Epidemiology and Risk Factors

The prevalence of AVPD is 2.6% in the general US population (APA, 2022), but it has been reported in nearly 15% of outpatients in mental health clinics (Torrico & Sapra, 2024). The problem with examining the epidemiology of AVPD is its potential overlap with social anxiety disorder. Several studies found that a significant portion of the patients with diagnoses of social anxiety disorder also met criteria for AVPD. Emotional reactivity, introversion, passive behavior, and low self-worth are all predictive factors for AVPD (Wichstrom et al., 2024). More research is needed to clarify the relationship between avoidant personality and anxiety disorders. In light of prevalence rates, societal costs, and the current state of research, it needs to be stated that AVPD qualifies as a neglected disorder (Sveen et al., 2025).

Etiology

Several factors are hypothesized to contribute to the development of AVPD, including genetic predisposition, childhood experiences, and environmental factors. Medical conditions, particularly those that are known to damage neurons, such as head trauma, are associated with personality disorders (Torrico & Sapra, 2024).

Evidence-Based Nursing Care of People With Avoidant Personality Disorder

Assessment of these individuals reveals a lack of social contacts, a fear of being criticized, and evidence of chronic low self-esteem. The focus of nursing care is on increasing self-esteem and decreasing social isolation. The establishment of a therapeutic relationship is necessary to be able to help these individuals meet their treatment outcomes. The development of the nurse–patient relationship is a slow process and requires an extreme amount of patience on the part of the nurse. These individuals may not have had positive interpersonal relationships and need time to be able to be sure that the nurse will not criticize and demean them. Interventions should focus on refraining from any negative criticism, assisting the patient to identify positive responses from others, exploring previous achievements of success, and exploring reasons for self-criticism. The patient's social dimension should be examined for activities that increase self-esteem and interventions focused on increasing these self-esteem–enhancing activities (Dahl et al., 2024).

Continuum of Care

Long-term therapy is ideal for patients with AVPD because it takes time to make changes in one's behavior. Mental health nurses may initially see these individuals for other health issues. Encouraging the patient to continue with therapy and contacting the therapist when necessary are important in maintaining continuity of care. These patients are hospitalized only for a coexisting disorder.

DEPENDENT PERSONALITY DISORDER

Clinical Course and Diagnostic Criteria

People with **dependent personality disorder** cling to others in a desperate attempt to keep them close. Their need to be taken care of is so great that it leads to doing anything to maintain the closeness, including total submission and disregard for themselves.

Decision-making is difficult or nonexistent. They adapt their behavior to please those to whom they are attached. They lean on others to guide their lives. They ingratiate themselves with others and denigrate themselves and their accomplishments. Their self-esteem is determined by others. Behaviorally, they withdraw from adult responsibilities by acting helpless and seeking nurturance from others. In interpersonal relationships, they need excessive advice and reassurance. They are adherent, conciliatory, and placating. They rarely disagree with others and are easily persuaded. Friends describe them as gullible. They are warm, tender, and noncompetitive. They timidly avoid social tension and interpersonal conflicts (Hansen et al., 2024).

Epidemiology and Risk Factors

The US prevalence of dependent personality disorder is estimated at 0.6% (APA, 2022). The diagnosis is made more frequently in women than in men. This gender difference may represent a bias by clinicians because when standardized instruments are used, men and women receive diagnoses at equal rates. There is little difference among racial and ethnic groups, and it is more commonly diagnosed in young adults (Hansen et al., 2024). In older adults, dependent personality disorder is more common in older adults with depression when compared to other personality disorders (Heintz et al., 2021).

Etiology

Evidence-based studies on the etiology of depended personality disorder are limited. It is likely that a biologic predisposition exists to develop the dependency attachments of this disorder. However, no research studies support a biologic hypothesis. Dependent personality disorder is most often explained as a result of parents'/caregivers' genuine affection, extreme attachment, and overprotection. Children then learn to rely on others to meet their basic needs and do not learn the necessary skills for autonomous behavior. People with chronic physical illnesses or persistent separation anxiety in childhood may be prone to developing this disorder (Hansen et al., 2024).

Evidence-Based Nursing Care of People With Dependent Personality Disorder

Nurses can determine the extent of dependency by assessment of self-worth, interpersonal relationships, and social behavior. They should determine whether there is currently someone on whom the person relies (parent, spouse) or whether there has been a separation from a significant relationship by death or divorce.

Priorities of care that are usually identified include low self-esteem, difficulties in social situations, and coping with stresses of everyday life. Home management skills may be a priority if the patient does not have these skills and has to make decisions related to finances, shopping, cooking, and cleaning. The challenge of caring for these patients is to help them recognize their dependent patterns; motivate them to want to change; and teach them adult skills that have not been developed, such as balancing a checkbook, planning a weekly menu, and paying bills when they are due. Occasionally, if a patient is extremely fatigued, lethargic, or anxious, the disorder interferes with efforts at developing greater independence; antidepressants or antianxiety agents may be used in therapy.

These patients readily engage in a nurse–patient relationship and initially look to the nurse to make all decisions. The nurse can support patients to make their own decisions by resisting the urge to tell them what to do. Ideally, these patients are in individual psychotherapy and working toward long-term personality changes. The nurse can encourage patients to stay in therapy and to practice the new skills that are being learned. Assertiveness training is helpful.

Continuum of Care

Individuals with dependent personality disorder readily seek out therapy and are likely to spend years seeking therapy. Hospitalization occurs for comorbid conditions such as depression.

OBSESSIVE-COMPULSIVE PERSONALITY DISORDER

Clinical Course and Diagnostic Criteria

Obsessive-compulsive personality disorder (OCPD) stands out because it bears close resemblance to obsessive-compulsive disorder (OCD). Although these disorders have similar names, the clinical manifestations are quite different. A distinguishing difference is that those with OCD tend to use obsessive thoughts and compulsions when anxious but less so when anxiety decreases (Pozza et al., 2021). People with OCPD do not demonstrate obsessions and compulsions but rather a pervasive pattern of preoccupation with orderliness, perfectionism, and control. Individuals with this disorder attempt to maintain control by careful attention to rules, trivial details, procedures, and lists. They may be completely devoted to work, which typically has a rigid character, such as maintaining financial records or tracking inventory. They are uncomfortable with unstructured leisure time, especially vacations. Their leisure activities are likely to be formalized (e.g., season tickets to sports, organized tour groups). Hobbies are approached seriously (Pinto et al., 2022).

Behaviorally, individuals with OCPD are perfectionists, maintaining a regulated, highly structured, strictly organized life. A need to control others and situations is common in their personal and work lives. They are prone to repetition and have difficulty making decisions and completing tasks because they become so involved in the details. They can be overly conscientious about morality and ethics and value polite, formal, and correct interpersonal relationships. They also tend to be rigid, stubborn, and indecisive and are unable to accept new ideas and customs. Their mood is tense and joyless. Warm feelings are restrained, and they tightly control the expression of emotions (Pinto et al., 2022).

Epidemiology and Risk Factors

OCPD is one of the most prevalent personality disorders in the US general population, with estimated prevalence ranging from 2.1% to 7.9% (APA, 2022). This disorder is associated with higher education, employment, and marriage. Subjects with the disorder had a higher income than did those without the disorder.

Etiology

As with some other personality disorders, evidence for a biologic formulation is scant. The basis of the compulsive patterns that characterize OCPD is parental overcontrol and overprotection that is consistently restrictive and sets distinct limits on the child's behavior. Parents/caregivers teach these children a deep sense of responsibility to others and to feel guilty when these responsibilities are not met. Play is viewed as shameful, sinful, and irresponsible, leading to dire consequences. They are encouraged to resist the natural inclinations toward play and impulse gratification, and parents/caregivers try to impose guilt on the child to control behavior.

Evidence-Based Nursing Care of People With OCPD

These individuals seek mental health care when they have attacks of anxiety, spells of immobilization, sexual impotence, and excessive fatigue. The nursing assessment focuses on the patient's physical symptoms (sleep, eating, sexual), interpersonal relationships, and social issues. There may be multiple nursing care priorities such as anxiety, loneliness, decision-making, sexual issues, insomnia, and interpersonal relationships. People with OCPD realize that they can improve their QoL, but they find it extremely anxiety provoking to make the necessary changes. To change the compulsive pattern, psychotherapy is needed. Although no medications have Food and Drug Administration (FDA) approval for the treatment of OCPD, SSRIs are widely used to treat comorbid anxiety and mood symptoms (Pinto et al., 2022). A supportive nurse–patient relationship based on acceptance of the patient's need for order and rigidity will help the person have enough confidence to try new behaviors. Examining the patient's belief that underlies the dysfunctional behaviors can set the stage for challenging the childhood thinking. Because the compulsive pattern was established in childhood, it will take a long time to modify the behavior.

Continuum of Care

People with OCPD are treated primarily in the community. If there is a coexisting disorder or the person experiences periods of depression is present, hospitalization may be useful for a short period of time.

DISRUPTIVE, IMPULSE-CONTROL, AND CONDUCT DISORDERS

Disruptive, impulse-control, and conduct disorders are a group of psychiatric conditions that have the essential feature of irresistible impulsivity. Behaviors associated with these disorders violate the rights of others and/or are in conflict with societal norms (APA, 2022). Disorders discussed include intermittent explosive disorder (IED), kleptomania, and **pyromania**.

> **KEYCONCEPT Impulsivity,** acting without considering consequences or alternative actions, results when neurobiologic overactivity is stimulated by psychological, personality, or social factors related to personal needs of the individual.

> **KEYCONCEPT Impulse-control disorders** often coexist with other disorders and are characterized by an inability to resist an impulse or temptation to complete an activity that is considered harmful to oneself or others.

Tension increases before the individual commits the act and derives excitement or gratification when the act is committed. The release of tension is perceived as pleasurable, but remorse and regret usually follow the act. Disruptive behavior disorders, which include oppositional defiant disorder and conduct disorder, are a group of conditions marked by significant issues of conduct. See Chapter 37.

INTERMITTENT EXPLOSIVE DISORDER

Episodes of aggressiveness that result in assault or destruction of property characterize people with **intermittent explosive disorder**. The severity of aggressiveness is out of proportion to the provocation. The episodes can have serious psychosocial consequences, including job loss, interpersonal relationship issues, school expulsion, divorce, automobile accidents, or jail. This diagnosis is given only after all other disorders with aggressive components (e.g., delirium, dementia, head injury, BPD, ASPD, substance use) have been excluded. Little is known about this disorder, but it is a more common condition than previously thought.

Aggression is a destructive behavior that imposes a considerable burden on individuals and society. In clinical settings, recurrent problematic aggression is identified as IED. IED is associated with significantly more aggression than BPD or ASPD alone (Patoilo et al., 2021).

The prevalence of IED in the United States is about 2.7%. The onset is most common in childhood or adolescence and rarely begins for the first time after the age of 40 years. The mean age at onset is 14 years. It is more prevalent in individuals with a high school education or less (APA, 2022). The anger experience and expression of anger contribute to self-harm and suicidality (Ciesinski et al., 2024).

The treatment of this disorder is multifaceted. Psychopharmacological agents are sometimes used as an adjunct to psychotherapeutic, behavioral, and social interventions. Serotonergic antidepressants and gamma-aminobutyric acid-ergic mood stabilizers have been used. Anxiolytics are used to treat obsessive patients who experience tension states and explosive outbursts. Medication alone is insufficient, and anger management should be included in the treatment plan.

KLEPTOMANIA

In **kleptomania**, individuals cannot resist the urge to steal, so they independently steal items that they could easily afford. These items are not particularly useful or wanted. The underlying issue is the act of stealing. The term *kleptomania* was first used in 1838 to describe the behavior of several kings who stole worthless objects (Aboujaoude & Koran, 2010). These individuals experience an increase in tension and then pleasure and relief at the time of the theft. Kleptomania occurs in about 4% to 22% of individuals arrested for shoplifting. Its prevalence in the general population, however, is very rare, at approximately 0.3% to 0.6%. Kleptomania or compulsive stealing remains poorly understood with limited data regarding its underlying pathophysiology and appropriate treatment choices. Severity of kleptomania behaviors is associated with having more frequent urges to steal, feeling excited by stealing, having a current eating disorder, and having a current diagnosis of OCD. Furthermore, worse symptom severity was associated with a shorter transition time (between first stealing and developing kleptomania), as well as with more chance of stealing from relatives and seeking treatment at some point.

Females outnumber males at a ratio of 3:1 (APA, 2022). Because it is considered a "secret" disorder, little is known about it, but it is believed to last for years despite numerous convictions for shoplifting. It appears that kleptomania often has its onset during adolescence (Fariba & Gokarakonda, 2023).

Despite being described in medical literature for nearly 200 years, kleptomania still remains poorly understood with limited data regarding its underlying pathophysiology and appropriate treatment choices. It appears that behavior therapy is frequently used. Antidepressants, particularly SSRIs, have been successful in some cases. Mood stabilizers such as lithium, valproic acid, and topirate have been effective in dampening urges. Naltrexone is also promising in the treatment of kleptomania. More investigation is needed (Miyazaki & Uchiyama, 2023; Tahir et al., 2022).

PYROMANIA

Irresistible impulses to start fires characterize pyromania, repeated fire setting with tension or arousal before setting fires; fascination or attraction to the fires; and gratification when setting, witnessing, or participating in the aftermath of fire. These individuals often are regular "fire watchers" or even firefighters. They are not motivated by aggression, anger, suicidal ideation, or political ideology. Little is known about this disorder because only a small number of deliberate fire starters are apprehended, and of those individuals, only a few undergo psychiatric evaluation. The US prevalence of fire setting in the general population is about 1%, but most fire setting is not done by people with pyromania, which occurs infrequently, mostly in men. Prevalence rates are higher in those with mental health conditions, intellectual disabilities, autism, and criminal history (Kipoulas et al., 2024).

Early research demonstrated low serotonin and norepinephrine levels associated with arson. Little is known about treatment, and as with the other impulse-control disorders, no approach is uniformly effective. Historically, fire starters generally possess poor interpersonal skills, exhibit low self-esteem, battle depression, and have difficulty managing anger. Cognitive-behavioral therapy that includes education on fire setting, coping strategies, self-awareness and self-esteem, emotion management, communication skills, positive relationships, and relapse prevention may be used in the management of pyromania (Kipoulas et al., 2024; Winters et al., 2022).

CONTINUUM OF CARE FOR DISRUPTIVE, IMPULSE-CONTROL DISORDERS

Impulse-control disorders require long-term treatment, usually in an outpatient setting. Group therapy is often a facet of treatment because patients can talk in a community where people share common experiences. Hospitalization is rare except when patients have comorbid psychiatric or medical disorders.

SUMMARY OF KEY POINTS

- A personality is a complex pattern of characteristics, largely outside of the person's awareness, that comprise the individual's distinctive pattern of perceiving, feeling, thinking, coping, and behaving.
- A personality disorder is an enduring pattern of inner experience and behavior that deviates markedly from the expectations of the individual's culture, is pervasive and inflexible, has an onset in adolescence or early adulthood, is stable over time, and leads to distress or impairment.
- For many patients with personality disorders, maintaining a therapeutic nurse–patient relationship can be one of the most helpful interventions. Through this therapeutic relationship, the patient experiences a model of healthy interaction, establishing trust, consistency, caring, boundaries, and limitations that help to build the patient's self-esteem and respect for self and others. In some personality disorders, nurses will find it more difficult to engage the patient in a true therapeutic relationship because of the patient's avoidance of interpersonal and emotional attachment (i.e., ASPD or paranoid personality disorder).
- Patients with personality disorders are rarely treated in an inpatient facility except during periods of destructive behavior or self-injury. Treatment is delivered in the community and over time. Continuity of care is important in helping the individual change lifelong personality patterns.
- People with BPD have difficulties regulating emotion and have extreme fears of abandonment, leading to dysfunctional relationships; they often engage in self-injury.
- Medications, including mood stabilizers, antidepressants, and antipsychotics, are useful in regulating the symptoms. They should, however, only be taken for target symptoms for a short time because patients may

already be taking other medications, particularly for a comorbid disorder.

- During hospitalizations, keeping the patients safe by preventing self-harm is priority. Open communication and the use of DBT techniques are important interventions.
- Recovery-oriented approaches are grounded in cognitive-behavioral therapy. The interdisciplinary treatment or recovery team needs to maintain open communication to work effectively with an individual with BPD.
- ASPD, often synonymous with psychopathy, includes people who have no regard for and refuse to conform to social rules.
- The primary characteristic of disruptive, impulse-control disorders is impulsivity, which leads to inappropriate social behaviors that are considered harmful to oneself or others and that give the patient excitement or gratification at the time the act is committed.

DEVELOPING CLINICAL JUDGMENT

1. Define the concepts *personality* and *personality disorder*. When does a typical personality become a personality disorder?
2. Karen, a 36-year-old receiving inpatient care, was admitted for depression; she also has a diagnosis of BPD. After a telephone argument with her husband, she approaches the nurse's station with her wrist dripping with blood from cutting. What nursing approach best fits this behavior? What interventions should the nurse use with the patient after the self-injury is treated?
3. A 22-year-old man with BPD is being discharged from the mental health unit after a severe suicide attempt. As his primary psychiatric nurse, you have been able to establish a therapeutic relationship with him, but are now terminating the relationship. He asks you to meet with him "for just a few sessions" after his discharge because his therapist will be on vacation. What are the issues underlying this request? What should you do?
4. Compare the biologic theory with the psychoanalytic and Linehan's biosocial theory. What are the primary differences between these theories?
5. Compare the characteristics, epidemiology, and etiologic theories of ASPD and BPDs.
6. Compare and contrast ASPD with narcissistic personality trait.
7. Compare and contrast relationships in schizoid personality disorder and avoidant personality disorder.
8. Summarize the impulse-control disorders and identify key assessment data, nursing priorities, and outcomes.

MOVIES, TV, OR STREAMING PROGRAMS

***Fatal Attraction*: 1987.** This award-winning film portrays the relationship between a married attorney, Dan Gallagher (played by Michael Douglas), and Alex Forest, a single woman (played by Glenn Close). Their one-night affair turns into a nightmare for the attorney and his family as Alex becomes increasingly possessive and aggressive, demonstrating behaviors characteristic of borderline personality disorder, including anger, impulsivity, emotional lability, fear of rejection and abandonment, vacillation between adoration and disgust, and self-mutilation.

Viewing Points:

1. Identify the behaviors of Alex that are characteristic of borderline personality disorder.
2. Identify the feelings that are generated by the movie.
3. With which characters do you identify?
4. For which characters do you feel sympathy?
5. If Alex had lived and been admitted to your hospital, what would be your first priority?
6. How might this movie contribute to stigmatization of borderline personality disorder?

REFERENCES

Aboujaoude, E., & Koran, L. M. (2010). *Impulse control disorders*. Cambridge University Press.

Aerts, J. E. M., Rijckmans, M. J. N., Bogaerts, S., & van Dam, A. (2023). Establishing an optimal working relationship with patients with an antisocial personality disorder. Aspects and processes in the therapeutic alliance. *Psychology & Psychotherapy, 96*(4), 999–1014.

American Psychiatric Association. (2022). *Diagnostic and statistical manual of mental disorders* (5th ed., text rev.). Author.

Aghakishiyeva, T., & Özdel, K. (2023). Theory of mind in social anxiety disorder and avoidant personality disorder comorbidity. *Nöro Psikiyatri Arşivi, 60*(4), 316–321.

Ansari, D., Lakkimsetti, M., Olaleye, K. T., Bhullar, J. V. K., Shah, R. Z., Arisoyin, A. E., Nadeem, H., Sacal Slovik, S. C., Habib, F. Z., Abdin, Z. U., & Zia Ul Haq, M. (2023). Genetic influences on outcomes of psychotherapy in borderline personality disorder: A narrative review of implications for personalized treatment. *Cureus, 15*(8), e43702.

Attademo, L., Bernardini, F., & Verdolini, N. (2021). Neural correlates of schizotypal personality disorder: A systematic review of neuroimaging and EEG studies. *Current Medical Imaging, 17*(11), 1283–1298. https://doi.org/10.2174/1573405617666210114142206

Babl, A., Gómez Penedo, J. M., Berger, T., Schneider, N., Sachse, R., & Kramer, U. (2023). Change processes in psychotherapy for patients presenting with histrionic personality disorder. *Clinical Psychology & Psychotherapy, 30*(1), 64–72.

Bachmann, C. J., Humayun, S., Stevens, M., O'Connor, T. G., & Scott, S. (2023). Secure attachment predicts lower societal cost amongst severely antisocial adolescents. *Child and Adolescent Psychiatry and Mental Health, 17*(1), 1–9.

Becker, L. G., Asadi, S., Zimmerman, M., Morgan, T. A., & Rodriguez-Seijas, C. (2023). Is there a bias in the diagnosis of borderline personality disorder among racially minoritized patients? *Personality Disorders, 14*(3), 339–346.

Benetti, C., Whitehead, R., & Hopkins, L. (2024). "I feel like they understand me a bit more": The experiences of young people with borderline personality disorder following their parents taking part in a mentalisation-based intervention for parents and carers (MBT-FACTS). *Journal of Family Therapy, 46*(4), 406–422.

Bozzatello, P., Blua, C., Brandellero, D., Baldassarri, L., Brasso, C., Rocca, P., & Bellino, S. (2024). Gender differences in borderline personality disorder: A narrative review. *Frontiers in Psychiatry, 15*, 1320546.

Cano, S., Carreiras, D., Carvalho, S. A., & Cunha, M. (2024). To feel safe inside and out: The effect of self-compassion and social safeness underlie the relationship between parental invalidation and borderline features in sexual minority adults. *Psychology & Sexuality, 15*(1), 114–126.

Carsten, E. E., Bornovalova, M., & Rodriguez-Seijas, C. (2024). An evaluation of measurement invariance of Diagnostic and Statistical Manual of Mental Disorders, Fifth Edition borderline personality disorder criteria across heterosexual, lesbian, gay, and bisexual adults. *Personality Disorders, 15*(6), 436–445.

Casellas, P. E., Soler, J., Schmidt, C., Soriano, J., & Pascual, J. C. (2024). Long-lasting symptoms in borderline personality disorder: Defining an emergent population with differential clinical and therapeutic features. *Personality and Mental Health, 18*(3), 248–258.

Chapman, J., Jamil, R. T., Fleisher, C., & Torrico T. J. (2022). Borderline personality disorder. In *StatPearls*. StatPearls Publishing. https://www.ncbi.nlm.nih.gov/books/NBK430883/

Cheli, S., Cavalletti, V., Popolo, R., & Dimaggio, G. (2021). A case study on a severe paranoid personality disorder client treated with metacognitive interpersonal therapy. *Journal of Clinical Psychology*, 77(8), 1807–1820. https://doi.org/10.1002/jclp.23201

Ciesinski, N. K., McCloskey, M. S., & Coccaro, E. F. (2024). A latent class analysis of cognitive-affective heterogeneity in current intermittent explosive disorder. *Journal of Affective Disorders, 363*, 230–238.

D'Agostino, A., Pepi, R., & Starcevic, V. (2022). Borderline personality disorder and ageing: Myths and realities. *Current Opinion in Psychiatry 35*(1), 68–72.

Dahl, K., Bremer, K., & Wilberg, T. (2024). The significance of connectedness: Avoidant personality disorder patients' subjective experiences of change after attending a specialized treatment program. *Frontiers in Psychology, 15*, 1412665.

Dahlenburg, S. C., Bartsch, D. R., & Gilson, K. J. (2024). Global prevalence of borderline personality disorder and self-reported symptoms of adults in prison: A systematic review and meta-analysis. *International Journal of Law and Psychiatry*, 97, 102032.

DiBenedetti, D., Kosa, K., Waters, H. C., & Oberdhan, D. (2023). Understanding patients' experiences with borderline personality disorder: Qualitative interviews. *Neuropsychiatric Disease and Treatment, 19*, 2115–2125.

Deming, P., Griffiths, S., Jalava, J., Koenigs, M., & Larsen, R. R. (2024). Psychopathy and medial frontal cortex: A systematic review reveals predominantly null relationships. *Neuroscience and Biobehavioral Reviews, 167*, 105904.

Dong, F., Liu, J., Hodgson, N. A., & Medoff-Cooper, B. (2021). Early life factors of schizotypal personality disorder in adolescents: A systematic review. *Journal of Psychiatric and Mental Health Nursing, 28*(6), 1092–1112. https://doi.org/10.1111/jpm.12733

Dotterer, H. L., Tomlinson, R. C., Burt, S. A., Weigard, A. S., Klump, K. L., & Hyde, L. W. (2021). Neurocognitive abilities associated with antisocial behavior with and without callous-unemotional traits in a community sample. *Neuropsychology, 35*(4), 374–387. https://doi.org/10.1037/neu0000733

Ducasse, D. (2023). How to target disturbed identity in borderline patients? Self-identification program: A case study. *L'Encephale, 49*(6), 596–605.

Fariba, K., & Gokarakonda, S. B. (2023). Impulse control disorders. In *StatPearls*. StatPearls Publishing. https://www.ncbi.nlm.nih.gov/books/NBK562279/

Francois, Z., & Torrico, T. J. (2024). Schizotypal personality disorder. In *StatPearls*. StatPearls Publishing. https://www.ncbi.nlm.nih.gov/books/NBK603720/

Gartlehner, G., Crotty, K., Kennedy, S., Edlund, M. J., Ali, R., Siddiqui, M., Fortman, R., Wines, R., Persad, E., & Viswanathan, M. (2021). Pharmacological treatments for borderline personality disorder: A systematic review and meta-analysis. *CNS drugs, 35*(10), 1053–1067. https://doi.org/10.1007/s40263-021-00855-4

Graumann, L., Cho, A. B., Kulakova, E., Deuter, C. E., Wolf, O. T., Roepke, S., Hellmann-Regen J., Otte, C., & Wingenfeld, K. (2023). Impact of social exclusion on empathy in women with borderline personality disorder. *European Archives of Psychiatry and Clinical Neuroscience*, 273(4), 865–874.

Griffiths, K., Velichkova, N., Quadt, L., & Berni, J. (2024). Can atypical antipsychotics alleviate deficits in psychosocial impairments in patients with a diagnosis of borderline personality? A systematic review and meta-analysis. *Psychiatry Research Communications*, 4(3). https://doi.org/10.1016/j.psycom.2024.100187

Gupta, N., Gupta, M., Madabushi, J. S., & Zubiar, F. (2023). Integrating psychosocial risks with emerging evidence for borderline personality disorders in adolescence: An update for clinicians. *Cureus, 15*(6), e40295.

Hansen, B. J., Thomas, J., & Torrico, T. J. (2024). Dependent personality disorder. In *StatPearls*. StatPearls Publishing. https://www.ncbi.nlm.nih.gov/sites/books/NBK606086/

Hastrup, L. H., Jennum, P., Ibsen, R., Kjellberg, J., & Simonsen, E. (2022). Welfare consequences of early-onset borderline personality disorder: A nationwide register-based case-control study. *European Child and Adolescent Psychiatry, 31*(2), 253–260.

Haeyen, S., Heres, H., & Pol, S. (2024). Making meaning of one's own life story in words and images: A narrative case report of personal recovery from personality disorder through the interventions "An Empowering Story" and art therapy. *Journal of Clinical Psychology, 80*(8), 1736–1753.

Heintz, H. L., Freedberg, A. L., & Harper, D. G. (2021). Dependent personality in depressed older adults: A case report and systematic review. *Journal of Geriatric Psychiatry and Neurology, 34*(5), 445–453. https://doi.org/10.1177/0891988720933361

Hernandez-Bustamante, M., Cjuno, J., Hernandez, R. M., & Ponce-Meza, J. C. (2024). Efficacy of dialectical behavior therapy in the treatment of borderline personality disorder: A systematic review of randomized controlled trials. *Iranian Journal of Psychiatry, 19*(1), 119–129.

Holzer, K. J., Vaughn, M. G., Loux, T. M., Mancini, M. A., Fearn, N. E., & Wallace, C. L. (2022). Prevalence and correlates of antisocial personality disorder in older adults. *Aging & Mental Health, 26*(1), 169–178. https://doi.org/10.1080/13607863.2020.1839867

Jain, L. & Torrico, T. J. (2024). Paranoid personality disorder. In *Stat Pearls*. StatPearls Publishing. https://www.ncbi.nlm.nih.gov/books/NBK606107/

Jo, R., Broadbear, J. H., Hope, J., & Rao, S. (2023). Late manifestation of borderline personality disorder: Characterization of an under-recognized phenomenon. *Personality & Mental Health, 17*(2), 165–175.

Jørgensen, C. R., & Bøye, R. (2022). How does it feel to have a disturbed identity? The phenomenology of identity diffusion in patients with borderline personality disorder: A qualitative study. *Journal of Personality Disorders, 36*(1), 40–69.

Kealy, D., Ben, D. S., Spidel, A., Wadsley, R. S., & Kim, D. (2022). Self-reassurance moderated by identity dysfunction: Associations with distress and impairment. *Journal of Counseling & Development, 100*(2), 205–214.

Kingsley, D. (2022). Debate: Child and adolescent mental health professionals have a responsibility to diagnose personality disorder. *Child and Adolescent Mental Health, 27*(2), 196–198.

Kipoulas, E., Sideri, A., Driver, B., & Beazley, P. I. (2024). The effectiveness of psychological interventions for adults who set fires: A systematic review. *Aggression & Violent Behavior, 78*, 101945. https://doi.org/10.1016/j.avb.2024.101945

Kolla, N. J., Boileau, I., Karas, K., Watts, J. J., Rusjan, P., Houle, S., & Mizrahi, R. (2021). Lower amygdala fatty acid amide hydrolase in violent offenders with antisocial personality disorder: an [11C]CURB positron emission tomography study. *Translational Psychiatry, 11*(1), 57. https://doi.org/10.1038/s41398-020-01144-2

Koskinen, E., Henttonen, P., Kettunen, S. K., Pesonen, S., Piispanen, M., Voutilainen, L., Wuolio, M., & Peräkylä, A. (2024). Shame in social interaction: Descriptions of experiences of shame by participants with high or low levels of narcissistic traits. *British Journal of Social Psychology, 63*(3), 1429–1449.

Krause-Utz, A., Frost, R., Chatzaki, E., Winter, D., Schmahl, C., & Elzinga, B. M. (2021). Dissociation in borderline personality disorder: Recent experimental, neurobiological studies, and implications for future research and treatment. *Current Psychiatry Reports, 23*(6), 37. https://doi.org/10.1007/s11920-021-01246-8

Kvarstein, E. H., Antonsen, B. T., Klungsøyr, O., Pedersen, G., & Wilberg, T. (2021). Avoidant personality disorder and social functioning: A longitudinal, observational study investigating predictors of change in a clinical sample. *Personality Disorders, 12*(6), 594–605. https://doi.org/10.1037/per0000471

Larcombe, E., & Müller, A. (2022). The relationship between borderline personality disorder and occupational participation: An integrative review. *International Journal of Mental Health Nursing, 31*(5), 1141–1150.

Liljedahl, S. I., Mossberg, A., Grenner, H., & Waern, M. (2023). Life experienced as worth living and beyond: a qualitative study of the pathways to recovery and flourishing amongst individuals treated for borderline personality disorder. *BMC Psychiatry, 23*(1), 838.

Lindsay, J. A. B., McGowan, N. M., Henning, T., Harriss, E., & Saunders, K. E. A. (2024). Digital interventions for symptoms of borderline personality disorder: Systematic review and meta-analysis. *Journal of Medical Internet Research, 26*, e54941.

Linehan, M. (1993). *Cognitive-behavioral treatment of borderline personality disorder*. Guilford Press.

Low, A., Stiltner, B., Nunez, Y. Z., Adhikari, K., Deak, J. D., Pietrzak, R. H., Kranzler, H. R., Gelernter, J., & Polimanti, R. (2024). Association patterns of antisocial personality disorder across substance use disorders. *Translational Psychiatry*, *14*(1), 346.

Maden, Ö., Sinici, E., & Uzun, Ö. (2023). Primary and secondary capacities in the context of positive psychotherapy in individuals with antisocial personality disorder: The Relationship with Criminal Behaviors and Anger. *Turkish Journal of Psychiatry*, *34*(3), 191–201.

Malik, F., & Marwaha, R. (2022). Developmental stages of social emotional development in children. In *StatPearls*. StatPearls Publishing. https://www.ncbi.nlm.nih.gov/books/NBK534819/

Miller, J., Nguyen, E., Lam, A. Y. H., Brann, P., Innes, S., Buntine, P., Broadbear, J., & Hope, J. (2024). Experiences of consumers, carers and clinicians during borderline personality disorder presentations to the emergency department: An integrative review. *Journal of Psychiatric and Mental Health Nursing*, *31*(4), 572–582.

Mitra, P., Torrico, T. J., & Fluyau, D. (2024). Narcissistic personality disorder. In *StatPearls*. StatPearls Publishing. https://www.ncbi.nlm.nih.gov/books/NBK556001/

Miyazaki, K., & Uchiyama, M. (2023). An adolescent boy with kleptomania and attention-deficit hyperactivity disorder treated with methylphenidate and guanfacine: A case report. *Neuropsychopharmacology Reports*, *43*(4), 650–653.

Moreira, D., Moreira, D. S., Barbosa, F., Sousa-Gomes, V., & Fávero, M. (2022). Childhood traumatic experiences and psychopathy: A comprehensive review. *Psychological Trauma: Theory, Research, Practice, and Policy*, *14*(8), 1281–1287.

Neves Horácio, A., Bento, A., & Gama Marques, J. (2023). Personality and attachment in the homeless: A systematic review. *International Journal of Social Psychiatry*, *69*(6), 1312–1326.

Newcomb, K. M., Froehlich, M., & Yalch, M. M. (2024). Influence of betrayal trauma on schizoid personality pathology. *Journal of Trauma & Dissociation*, *25*(4), 456–466.

Nitzan U. (2024). Exploring Margaret Mahler's theory: Applications in borderline personality disorder treatment within psychiatric wards. *Psychodynamic Psychiatry*, *52*(3), 270–275.

Patoilo, M. S., Berman, M. E., & Coccaro, E. F. (2021). Emotion attribution in intermittent explosive disorder. *Comprehensive Psychiatry*, *106*, 152229. https://doi.org/10.1016/j.comppsych.2021.152229

Pinto, A., Teller, J., & Wheaton, M. G. (2022). Obsessive-compulsive personality disorder: A review of symptomatology, impact of functioning, and treatment. *Focus*, *20*(4), 389–396.

Pozza, A., Starcevic, V., Ferretti, F., Pedani, C., Crispino, R., Governi, G., Luchi, S., Gallorini, A., Lochner, C., & Coluccia, A. (2021). Obsessive-compulsive personality disorder co-occurring in individuals with obsessive-compulsive disorder: A systematic review and meta-analysis. *Harvard Review of Psychiatry*, *29*(2), 95–107. https://doi.org/10.1097/HRP.0000000000000287

Qian, X., Townsend, M. L., Tan, W. J., & Grenyer, B. F. S. (2022). Sex differences in borderline personality disorder: A scoping review. *PLoS One*, *17*(12), e0279015.

Roca, M., Vilaregut, A., Pretel-Luque, T., Calvo, N., Frías, Á., & Ferrer, M. (2024). Assessing family relations in borderline personality disorder: A relational approach. *Journal of Marital and Family Therapy*, *50*(2), 495–507.

Ronningstam, E., & Weinberg, I. (2023). Narcissistic personality disorder: Patterns, processes, and indicators of change in long-term psychotherapy. *Journal of Personality Disorders*, *37*(3), 337–357.

Ross, A. G., Giri, S., Anyasodor, A. E., Mahmood, S., Astawesegn, F. H., Huda, M. M., Ahmed, K. Y., Mondal, U. K., & Thapa, S. (2024). Adverse childhood experiences leading to narcissistic personality disorder: A case report. *BMC Psychiatry*, *24*(1), 842.

Ruocco, A. C., & Marceau, E. M. (2024). Update on the neurobiology of borderline personality disorder: A review of structural, resting-state and task-based brain imaging studies. *Current Psychiatry Reports*. https://doi.org/10.1007/s11920-024-01553-w

Sack, L., Seddon, J. A., Sosa-Hernandez, L., & Thomassin, K. (2024). Typologies of non-suicidal self-injury functions and clinical correlates among inpatient youth. *Child Psychiatry and Human Development*, *55*(4), 999–1009.

Schermer, J. A., Colodro-Conde, L., Grasby, K. L., Hickie, I. B., Burns, J., Ligthart, L., Willemsen, G., Trull, T. J., Martin, N. G., & Boomsma, D. I. (2020). Genetic and environmental causes of individual differences in borderline personality disorder features and loneliness are partially shared. *Twin Research and Human Genetics*, *23*(4), 214–220. https://doi.org/10.1017/thg.2020.62

Schulze, A., Hughes, N., Lis, S., & Krause-Utz, A. (2024). Dissociative experiences, borderline personality disorder features, and childhood trauma: Generating hypotheses from data-driven network analysis in an international sample. *Journal of Trauma & Dissociation*, *25*(4), 436–455.

Sesso, G., & Masi, G. (2023). Pharmacological strategies for the management of the antisocial personality disorder. *Expert Review of Clinical Pharmacology*, *16*(3), 181–194.

Sher, L., Challman, K. N., Smith, E. C., New, A. S., Perez-Rodriguez, M. M., McClure, M. M., Goodman, M., Kahn, R. S., & Hazlett, E. A. (2023). Clinical features of individuals with schizotypal personality disorder with and without suicidal ideation. *Psychiatry Research*, *322*, 115132.

Smits, M. L., Luyten, P., Feenstra, D. J., Bales, D. L., Kamphuis, J. H., Dekker, J. J. M., Verheul, R., & Busschbach, J. J. V. (2022). Trauma and outcomes of mentalization-based therapy for individuals with borderline personality disorder. *American Journal of Psychotherapy*, *75*(1), 12–20.

Solmi, M., Dragioti, E., Croatto, G., Radua, J., Borgwardt, S., Carvalho, A. F., Demurtas, J., Mosina, A., Kurotschka, P., Thompson, T., Cortese, S., Shin, J. I., & Fusar-Poli, P. (2021). Risk and protective factors for personality disorders: An umbrella review of published meta-analyses of case-control and cohort studies. *Frontiers in Psychiatry*, *12*, 679379.

Stern, A. (1938). Psychoanalytic investigation of and therapy in the border line group of neuroses. *The Psychoanalytic Quarterly*, 7, 467–489. https://doi.org/0.1080/21674086.1938.11925367

Sveen, C. A., Pedersen, G., Wilberg, T., & Kvarstein, E. H. (2025). The societal costs of avoidant personality disorder. *Personality and Mental Health*, *19*(1), e1644.

Tahir, T., Wong, M. M., Maaz, M., Naufal, R., Tahir, R., & Naidoo, Y. (2022). Pharmacotherapy of impulse control disorders: A systematic review. *Psychiatry Research*, *311*, 114499.

Tedesco, V., Day, N. J. S., Lucas, S., & Grenyer, B. F. S. (2024). Diagnosing borderline personality disorder: Reports and recommendations from people with lived experience. *Personality & Mental Health*, *18*(2), 107–121.

Tharshini, N. K., Ibrahim, F., Kamaluddin, M. R., Rathakrishnan, B., & Che Mohd Nasir, N. (2021). The link between individual personality traits and criminality: A systematic review. *International Journal of Environmental Research and Public Health*, *18*(16), 8663. https://doi.org/10.3390/ijerph18168663

Thimm, J. C., & Chang, M. (2022). Early maladaptive schemas and mental disorders in adulthood: A systematic review and meta-analysis. *International Journal of Cognitive Therapy*, *15*(4), 371–413.

Torrico, T. J., French, J. H., Aslam, S. P., & Shrestha, S. (2024). Histrionic personality disorder. In *StatPearls*. StatPearls Publishing. https://www.ncbi.nlm.nih.gov/books/NBK542325/

Torrico, T. J., & Madhanagopal, N. (2024). Schizoid personality disorder. In *StatPearls*. StatPearls Publishing. https://www.ncbi.nlm.nih.gov/books/NBK559234/

Torrico, T. J., & Sapra, A. (2024). Avoidant personality disorder. In *StatPearls*. StatPearls Publishing. https://www.ncbi.nlm.nih.gov/books/NBK559325/

Van Beeck, M. (2024). The relationship between experiencing childhood trauma and psychopathic personality traits: The mediating role of insecure attachment. *Journal of Aggression, Maltreatment, and Trauma*, *33*(9), 1055–1072.

Waite, E. E., Raudales, A. M., Newberger, N. G., Ferguson, J. J., Denning, D. M., Huffman, S., Weiss, N. H., & Dixon, G. K. L. (2024). Longitudinal examination of borderline personality disorder symptoms and drug use: The influence of negative and positive emotion dysregulation. *Personality & Mental Health*, *18*(2), 157–165.

Weinberg, I. (2024). Building hope for treatment of narcissistic personality disorder. *Journal of Clinical Psychology*, *80*(4), 721–732.

Weinberg, I., Ronningstam, E., Ravichandran, C., & Gunderson, J. G. (2024). Can patients with narcissistic personality disorder change? A case series. *The Journal of Nervous and Mental Disease*, *212*(7), 392–397.

Wheeler, J. (2024). Assessment of suicide risk in people with borderline personality disorder: A qualitative analysis of risk protocols. *Australian Psychologist*, *59*(5), 458–463.

Wichstrøm, L., Wilberg, T., Hartveit Kvarstein, E., & Steinsbekk, S. (2024). Childhood predictors of avoidant personality disorder traits in adolescence: A seven-wave birth cohort study. *Journal of Child Psychology and Psychiatry, and Allied Disciplines*. https://doi.org/10.1111/jcpp.14064

Winters, G. M., Brereton, A., & Zychlinski, N. (2022). Intervention for firesetting offenders: A case study. *Journal of Correctional Health Care*, *28*(6), 361–367.

Yalch, M. M., Ceroni, D. B., & Dehart, R. M. (2023). Influence of child abuse and neglect on histrionic personality pathology. *Journal of Trauma & Dissociation*, *24*(1), 111–124.

Yuan, Y., Lee, H., Eack, S. M., & Newhill, C. E. (2023). A systematic review of the association between early childhood trauma and borderline personality disorder. *Journal of Personality Disorders*, *37*(1), 16–35.

Zhang, X., Sayler, K., Hartman, S., & Belsky, J. (2022). Infant temperament, early-childhood parenting, and early-adolescent development: Testing alternative models of Parenting × Temperament interaction. *Development and Psychopathology*, *34*(3), 784–795. https://doi.org/10.1017/S0954579420002096

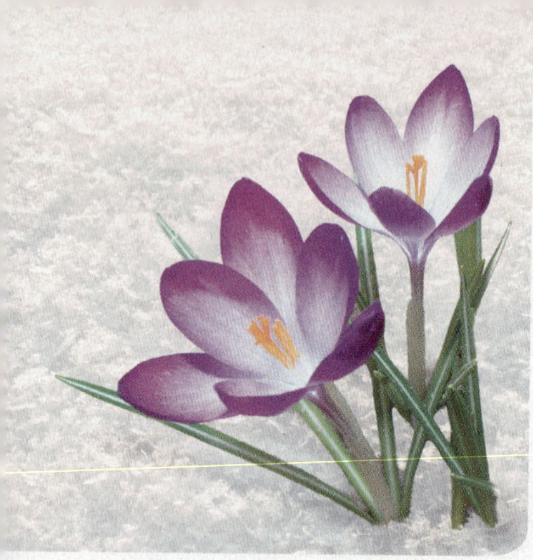

31 Substance-Related Disorders

Nursing Care of People With Substance Use and Other Compulsive Disorders

Susan Dawson and Patricia E. Freed

KEYCONCEPTS

- denial
- motivation
- substance dependence

LEARNING OBJECTIVES

After studying this chapter, you will be able to:

1. Discuss the diagnostic criteria for substance use disorders.
2. Relate the primary theories of substance use disorder to clinical symptoms and the course of the disorder.
3. Evaluate the significance of trauma in the development of a substance use disorder.
4. Examine the relationship between social determinants of health and substance use disorder.
5. Select strategies to establish a therapeutic relationship with people with a substance use disorder.
6. Using a clinical judgment model, formulate a person-centered, recovery-oriented nursing care plan for people with a substance use disorder.
7. Identify medications that are used to treat people with substance use disorders and evaluate their effectiveness.
8. Develop wellness strategies for people with substance use disorder.
9. Compare and contrast mental health care provided in emergency, inpatient, community, and virtual settings.
10. Support the integration of health care and mental health care for people with a substance use disorder.
11. Compare and contrast the actions, effects, and withdrawal symptoms of commonly used psychoactive substances.
12. Discuss impairment in nurses including recognizing possible cues, signs of diversion and the reporting obligations of nurses.

KEY TERMS

• acamprosate • addictive substance • adulterant • adverse childhood events • alcohol toxicity • alcohol withdrawal syndrome • alcoholics anonymous • amnestic disorders • anabolic steroid • anterograde amnesia • binge drinking • blood alcohol level • brief interventions • buprenorphine • codependence • comorbid disorders • confabulation • contingency management programs • co-occurring disorder • countertransference • cravings • delirium tremens • detoxification • dissociative drug • disulfiram • epigenetic • fentanyl • fetal alcohol syndrome • hallucinogen • harm reduction • inhalants • intoxication • Korsakoff syndrome • MDMA • methadone • misuse • motivational interviewing • naloxone • naltrexone • neonatal abstinence syndrome • opiate • opioid • opioid use disorder • physiologic dependence • recovery • relapse • rhabdomyolysis • screening • sobriety • substance use disorders • substance-induced disorders • subutex • therapeutic communities • tolerance • wernicke encephalopathy • Wernicke–Korsakoff syndrome • withdrawal • xylazine

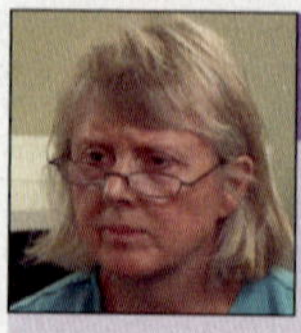

Case Study: Gladys

Gladys, a 68-year-old widow, lives by herself in a comfortable apartment. She spends her days with friends and visiting her grandchildren. At night, she frequently has an alcoholic drink to relax her and help her sleep. She denies that she is dependent on alcohol.

INTRODUCTION

The human use of alcohol and other drugs has been around since the beginning of history; so too have the subsequent social and emotional issues that accompany substance use. This chapter reviews substance use, types of substances used, biologic and psychological effects, current theories of substance-related disorders, and interventions. Gambling disorder is a non–substance-related compulsive behavioral disorder that is also discussed in this chapter.

SUBSTANCE USE DISORDERS OVERVIEW

Alcohol, tobacco, marijuana, and illegal prescription drug use has reached epidemic proportions in the United States, across all age groups (SAMSHA, 2024). One of the goals of *Healthy People 2030* is "to reduce substance misuse to protect the health, safety, and quality of life for all, especially children" (U.S. Department of Health and Human Services, 2020). A major challenge facing the United States is the opioid epidemic. The overriding concern about using mind-altering substances is that these substances compromise health, and their continued use can lead to dependence.

> **KEYCONCEPT Substance dependence** is a state of psychological and/or physical dependence on the use of alcohol or other addictive substances.

Many mind-altering (psychoactive) substances cause physiologic dependence and can easily lead to severe health and legal issues and exacerbate social and interpersonal issues. Use by ingestion, smoking, sniffing, or injection of some mind-altering substances such as alcohol, pain medications, tobacco, cannabis (in many states), or caffeine is legal for adults. Other substances such as cocaine and heroin are illegal in the United States, and marijuana use is still recognized as an illicit drug at the federal level. Synthetic drugs represent another group of illicit drugs that are produced to mimic the effects of existing illicit drugs. **Misuse** occurs when a person uses alcohol or substances for the purpose of **intoxication** or, in the case of prescription drugs, for purposes other than their intended use. Substance use disorders (SUDs) involve substances that are commonly misused (NIDA, 2023a). A chemical substance with significant potential for producing dependence is called an **addictive substance**.

Physiologic dependence can develop with many different types of medications such as beta-blockers, antidepressants, antipsychotics, opioids, antianxiety agents, and others. As long as medications are used for their intended purposes and under the supervision of qualified health care providers, physiologic dependence is an expectation of treatment. That is, dependence can be an expected response to some medications.

SUBSTANCE USE DISORDER

DIAGNOSTIC CRITERIA

The *Diagnostic and Statistical Manual of Mental Disorders, fifth edition, text revision* (*DSM-5-TR*) identifies 11 classes of substances including alcohol, caffeine, cannabis (marijuana), hallucinogens, inhalants, opioids, sedatives, hypnotics (anxiolytics), stimulants, tobacco, and others (APA, 2022). Gambling disorder is included within the SUD category because compulsive gambling behaviors can activate the brain's reward system similar to the SUDs.

There are two groups of substance-related disorders; the **substance-induced disorders** (SIDs) and the **substance use disorders** (SUDs). SIDs include intoxication, withdrawal, and other substance/medication induced mental disorders which are all caused by the effects of substances. SUDs occur when there is an underlying change in brain circuitry that may persist after **detoxification,** the process of safely and effectively withdrawing a person from an addictive substance, usually under medical supervision. These brain changes lead to repeated relapses and intense drug **cravings** when exposed to drug-related cues (e.g., a party, emotional experiences) (Day & Daly, 2022).

EPIDEMIOLOGY

Age of Onset

Use of drugs and/or alcohol may have an onset in early childhood, and some children are already abusing tobacco, alcohol, inhalants, marijuana, or prescription drugs by the time they are 12 or 13 years old. However, for most youths, early use does not progress to substance dependence. **Binge drinking,** a pattern of heavy alcohol consumption in a short period of time, continues to be problematic because it remains high in adolescents and is associated with many acute alcohol-related harms (such as alcohol poisoning, accidents, risky behaviors) that may persist into adulthood (Ranker et al., 2023). Although further study is needed, it is known that binge drinking contributes to neurobiologic changes in the brain (Lesnewich et al., 2022) that can lead to poor academic performance, as well as to alterations in memory and learning. Children and teens are attracted to illicit fentanyl, a synthetic opioid, because pills can look like candy or other medications; in addition, it is easier to access than some other drugs. These factors have led to increasing substance use and overdose among children and teens.

As with any high-risk behavior, prevention plays a more important role than intervention, and nurses are in a position to engage teens and their families in screening and preventive education.

LGBTQ+ Individuals and Substance Use

Individuals who identify as LGBTQ+ face social stigma and discrimination and greater risks of violence, and harassment than those who identify as cisgender. These and other stressors increase their risk for behavioral health issues. LGBTQ+ individuals who use opioids face additional discrimination because of the stigma associated with substance use. See Box 31.1. Substance use patterns in this population differ from those reported by cisgender people. For instance, LGBTQ+ individuals are at increased risk of cannabis and alcohol use when compared to cisgender women. This increased risk is thought to be related to the discrimination and stigma these individuals experience (Dyar et al., 2023). Transgender adults have a higher prevalence of nicotine, alcohol, and other SUDs than cisgender adults (Fahey et al., 2023). For some gay and bisexual men, alcohol and illegal drug use, especially methamphetamines (meth), amyl nitrates (poppers), and drugs used to treat erectile dysfunction, also contribute to a higher chance of getting human immunodeficiency virus (HIV) and other sexually transmitted infections (STIs) (Pepper et al., 2024). Using drugs or alcohol may also raise the chances of getting HIV or transmitting it to others because these people may engage in more risky sexual practices and behaviors or may be more likely to share needles or other injection equipment (SAMSHA, 2023a).

Youth identifying as LGBTQ+ have higher substance use, experience more violence, and are at a higher risk for suicide than other teens (Klein & Washington, 2023). These teens need access to crisis services, antibullying approaches, and screening for suicide prevention. Identifying differences and disparities among the diverse US population is essential to the design of programs, services, and policies that can effectively address specific population needs (Substance Abuse and Mental Health Services [SAMSHA], 2023a). The specific treatment needs of transgender and gender diverse groups require more research.

BOX 31.1

Mental Health Inequities: Opioid Use Disorder and Stigma

Narratives of people with opioid use disorder (OUD) were analyzed in this qualitative study to reveal patients' experiences of (1) social stigma (misconceptions of others, labeling, and enduring stigma in recovery), (2) self-stigma (internalized feelings, concealing while continuing use) and (3) structural stigma (resources and barriers, challenges to reintegration) around OUD. The authors concluded that the multifaceted impact of stigma poses continuing barriers to treatment and recovery that have not been adequately addressed. Recommendations for future research include studying stigma experiences from differing populations, discerning how stigma impacts decision-making and how that in turn impacts treatment seeking. Nurses who read this study should recognize that stigma around OUD is a continuing threat to the nation's health, and nurses must raise their voices to challenge stigma in all its forms (social, self, and structural).

Source: Judd, H., Yaugher, A. C., O'Shay, S., & Meier, C. L. (2023). Understanding stigma through the lived experiences of people with opioid use disorder. *Drug and Alcohol Dependence, 249*, 110873. https://doi.org/10.1016/j.drugalcdep.2023.110873

Sex Assigned at Birth

For most age groups, people assigned male at birth have higher rates of illicit drug and alcohol use than do people assigned female at birth. However, members of both groups are equally likely to develop an SUD (NIDA, 2022a). Differences around substance use depending on sex assigned at birth are well documented and show different patterns of use, prevalence rates, age-sex ratios, reporting rates, comorbidities, use, treatment, and response. People assigned female at birth often have comorbid mood disorders, anxiety disorders, eating disorders, and histories of trauma. They are less likely to seek or access substance use treatment unless it is for sedatives, sleep medication, or anxiety agents (NIDA, 2022a; Polak et al., 2023).

Neonatal abstinence syndrome (NAS) occurs when newborns go through opioid withdrawal after birth. NAS is caused by use of opioids during pregnancy. These infants are in crisis and must be medically managed for many days. **Fetal alcohol syndrome** (FAS) occurs when alcohol is consumed during pregnancy and leaves the infant with permanent disabilities. It is one of the leading causes of irreversible developmental delay. Cocaine, nicotine, and marijuana also affect the developing fetus, and the health consequences of these withdrawals are under investigation. It remains unclear if legalization of cannabis will increase use of this substance during pregnancy (Roberts et al., 2023). Effective prevention and treatment engagement programs must be developed to meet the needs of specific populations.

COMORBIDITY

Some **comorbid disorders**, chronic physical or neurologic conditions, are often a byproduct of long-term substance use; others predispose the individual to alcohol or drug dependence. Whatever the reason, nurses should be aware that patients who use substances often have comorbid disorders. People with SUDs experience comorbid, chronic physical health conditions, including chronic pain, cancer and heart diseases, diabetes mellitus (DM), gastrointestinal (GI) issues, hypertension, liver disease, and stroke (Lindenfeld et al., 2024; NIDA, 2021a).

The term **co-occurring disorder** is used when mental disorders such as depression or schizophrenia occur at the same time as an SUD. Nurses can expect that about half of patients with mental disorders experience an SUD. Higher prevalence of SUDs is associated with having a serious mental illness. Although there are fewer studies involving adolescents, research shows that adolescents with SUD also have higher rates of co-occurring mental disorders than their peers (Han et al., 2023).

Individuals who misuse substances are at high risk for death from drug overdoses and are at increased risk for death from other causes, including homicide, suicide, accidents, and opportunistic infections (such as HIV) (Swimmer & Sandelich, 2024).

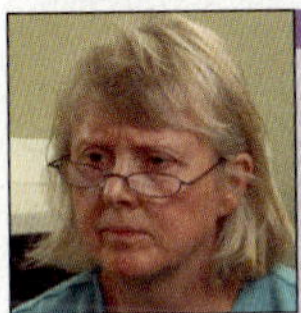

Consider Gladys

Gladys is depressed and spends many days in bed. During the last few months, her alcohol consumption has increased significantly.

ETIOLOGY

Recent findings show that a genetic vulnerability is highly prevalent in SUD, accounting for as much as 50% of the risk of dependence on nicotine, alcohol, marijuana, cocaine, heroin, fentanyl, or tobacco (Semaan & Khan, 2023). Human and animal studies confirm a genetic predisposition for behaviors involving drinking alcohol, misusing drugs, and self-administering mind-altering drugs. No precise genetic marker has been established yet, though clusters of genes are being identified that may play a role in substance dependence (Semaan & Khan, 2023).

Substance use can also cause **epigenetic** changes or modifications to DNA. Some epigenetic changes occur because of life experiences, including lifestyle, traumas, stress, and **adverse childhood events** (ACEs). Temperament, stress, self-concept, age, motivation for change, social consequences for problematic behaviors, relationships with parents/caregivers and other family members, and peer pressure all contribute to the expression of chronic and progressive SUDs.

FAMILY RESPONSES TO SUBSTANCE USE AND DEPENDENCE

The family (defined by the patient) continues to be the primary source of attachment, nurturing, and socialization. Family dynamics are dramatically affected when one member has a SUD that is associated with numerous medical, psychiatric, psychological, spiritual, economic, social, and legal issues. SUDs develop and persist within the family structure. The family can have a positive or negative influence on treatment (Lindeman et al., 2023).

Use of illegal substances can lead to arrest and imprisonment and heated disputes over child custody. Anticipation, concern, and dread can become a way of life for family members. Children may be at increased risk of substance misuse or neglect and the development of other physical or mental health issues. Birth parents with SUDs may be less sensitive to their infants' needs and may have difficulty establishing secure attachment bonds, engaging in nurturing, or promoting emotional regulation in the child (Hyysalo et al., 2022).

Poor family relationships and instability because of substance use cause higher rates of tension and conflict and can lead to family breakups. Family members may have different ideas about how to help the family member with the issue, which can lead to conflict and cause additional family burdens at a time when all resources are needed. Treating the individual without family involvement may limit the treatment's effectiveness because doing so ignores the devastating impact of SUDs on the family system, leaving family members unsupported (and/or untreated), and it does not recognize (nor facilitate) the family's potential for supporting change (Geijer-Simpson et al., 2023).

RECOVERY-ORIENTED CARE FOR PEOPLE WITH SUBSTANCE USE DISORDERS

For many individuals, a period of intense treatment is necessary to safely manage the physical and psychological **withdrawal** symptoms that occur when a substance is no longer used, or use was sharply cut back. Specific withdrawal symptoms depend on the substance and are explained in the following sections as the substances are discussed. The withdrawal process usually involves detoxification. After a person has safely withdrawn from the substance, the real work toward recovery can begin. Though periods of **relapse** often occur, prevention of relapse is desired because relapse compromises recovery. Recovery is a life-long journey.

Teamwork and Collaboration: Working Toward Recovery

A multidisciplinary approach provides individuals with the best chance of recovery. During periods of acute intoxication or overdose, medical teams treat the physical symptoms and give life-saving care. After the individual is medically stable and successfully withdrawn from the substance, care is provided by a team specializing in substance use. The team usually includes physicians, psychologists, social workers, nurses, chaplains, dependency specialists, and peer support specialists (PSS).

Recovery from SUDs is a process aimed at improving physical, psychological, and social well-being and health.

A recovery attitude in the patient indicates a dramatic shift in the individual's expectation of positive outcomes for the SUD and for any co-occurring disorders (SAMSHA, 2023b). The foundation of recovery is hope, and a belief that any individual can manage their own life successfully. Recovery is the lifelong pursuit of **sobriety**, which means working on the successful management of substance use, and regaining control of the rest of one's life.

Most SUD treatment occurs within a program setting, and the nurse is a member of a team. The team collaborates with the patient in setting recovery goals and wellness outcomes. It is important that the plan be individualized, holistic, and evidence based. A timeframe is agreed upon by the team and patient.

Discharge planning and relapse prevention are also essential components of successful treatment and so are incorporated into most programs. See Table 31.1 for an overview of the different treatment approaches used in drug and alcohol dependence. Several treatment modalities are used in most substance use programs including 12-step programs, cognitive-behavioral modalities, psychoeducation, group psychotherapy, and individual and family therapy.

Because patients with substance-related disorders differ greatly, no single type of treatment program will work for every individual. Often, several approaches can work together. Treatment programs usually combine many different interventions to provide a comprehensive approach based on the individual's needs. See Box 31.2.

BOX 31.2

Principles of Effective Treatment for SUD

1. Substance use disorder (SUD) is a complex but treatable disease that affects brain function and behavior.
2. No single treatment is appropriate for everyone.
3. Treatment needs to be readily accessible.
4. Effective treatment attends to multiple needs of the individual, not just their drug use.
5. Remaining in treatment for an adequate period of time is critical.
6. Behavioral therapies—including individual, family, or group counseling—are the most commonly used forms of drug use treatment.
7. Medications are an important element of treatment for many patients, especially when combined with counseling and other behavioral therapies.
8. An individual's treatment and service plan must be assessed continually and modified as necessary to ensure that it meets their changing needs.
9. Many individuals with SUDs also have concurrent mental disorders.
10. Medically assisted detoxification is only the first stage of treatment and by itself does little to change long-term drug misuse.
11. Treatment does not need to be voluntary to be effective.
12. Drug use during treatment must be monitored continuously because lapses during treatment do occur.
13. Use people-first language and do not reduce anyone's identity to a label.
14. Treatment programs should provide assessment for HIV/AIDS, hepatitis B and C, tuberculosis, and other infectious diseases, as well as provide targeted risk-reduction counseling, linking patients to treatment as necessary.

Source: National Institute on Drug Abuse. (2018). *Principles of drug addiction treatment: A research-based guide* (3rd ed., pp. 3–4). https://nida.nih.gov/sites/default/files/podat-3rdEd-508.pdf

Safety Issues

The primary concern for the individuals using substances is determining whether there is a danger of intoxication leading to a life-threatening condition such as opioid overdose or medical consequences of alcohol withdrawal. Patients are often admitted to inpatient settings with other medical conditions that are complicated by their substance use and may be in withdrawal. Staff and even the primary care provider may be unaware of the substance use. These topics will be discussed in later sections.

A priority is to determine substances that are being used or have been ingested, and if symptoms of poisoning (toxicity) are present. Nurses monitor for signs of respiratory depression and cardiac arrhythmias and begin rehydration with normal saline. As the patient may have been unconscious for some time before admission, creatine phosphokinase (CPK) should be drawn to rule out **rhabdomyolysis** (release of proteins from damaged muscle tissues which can permanently damage the heart and kidneys).

Equally important is the immediate threat of self-injury to self or others. Due to the psychosocial challenges (loss of job, loss of relationships, loss of custody) individuals may become despondent and feel that they are better off dead than to continue using. They believe that the world would be better off without them. They may have relapsed several times and do not trust themselves to try treatment again or they have just had a conflict or altercation. High risk for suicide is common. One-to-one for safety is instituted and the team may consider involuntary status for imminent threats to self and others.

Those with SUDs frequently go without food or usual sleep, often due to spending all their time and money on acquiring and using their drug(s) of choice. Medical issues are very common, including skin disorders, problematic pregnancies, seizures disorders, and GI disorders. For individuals with SUDs who are unhoused, immediate needs on admission might include hydration, nutrition, or thermal regulation due to heat or cold exposure. During the initial medical treatment, depending on the substance, there is always a risk for death and severe physical complications.

Once in recovery, relapse is a major threat to recovery. A safety plan should be developed to identify triggers for use and behaviors to counteract the urges to use substances.

TABLE 31.1 SUBSTANCE USE TREATMENT APPROACHES

Approach	Conception of Etiology	Conception of Patient	Conception of Treatment Outcome	Conception of Treatment Process	Advantages of Approach	Disadvantages of Approach
Psychiatric	Symptom of underlying emotional issue	Emotionally disturbed	Emotional conflicts are resolved; emotional health improves	Psychotherapy, medication to treat cause of substance dependence	Not punitive, treats comorbidity	Focus is only on treatment of mental disorder
Social	Society and environment cause dependence	Victim of circumstance	Improved social functioning or improved environment	Removal of environmental influences and increasing coping responses to it	Stresses social supports and coping skills	Blames "ills of society"—the person is not responsible for being dependent on substances
Learning	Misuse is a learned, reinforced behavior	Has distorted thinking, poor coping skills	Patient learns new ways of thinking and new coping skills	Cognitive therapy techniques and coping skills taught	Not punitive; teaches new coping skills	Places emphasis on control of use
Disease	Probably caused by genetic or biologic factors	Has a chronically progressive disease	Abstinence, arresting disease progression, and beginning of recovery process	Is treated as a primary disease, reinforces patient is sick	Not punitive, stresses support and education	Minimizes mental health disorders; discounts return to social use
12-Step	Combination of disease concept and "spiritual bankruptcy"	Misuses drugs or other substances and is powerless to resist temptation	Abstinence, ongoing spiritual recovery	Use 12 steps, seeking spiritual support, making amends, serving others in need	Widespread success, emphasis is on quality of life and spiritual growth	Self-help group, not a treatment program
Dual diagnosis	Both a primary substance dependency and a mental health disorder	Has both mental and substance use disorder	Improvement in both mental health and substance use disorders	Concurrent treatment of both disorders	Treats both mental health disorder and dependency, minimizing relapse potential	Not inclusive enough; does not include social or other issues
Biopsychosocial	Biologic basis, with social and psychological influences	Has deficiencies in all three interacting areas	Improvement in mental and physical health, utilization of social supports	Concurrent treatment of all issues	Uses different modalities; is more inclusive	Does not match patient and specific interventions
Multivariant	Many different causes; may be different for each individual	Has multiple issues to be assessed and addressed	Particular issues for individual addressed, so improvement occurs	Treatment strategies are matched with individual patient needs	Treatment matched to individual's needs	Logistical issues can occur during its implementation
Medication-Assisted Treatment	Primarily substance dependence is a brain-based disorder, involving the neurocircuitry in the brain associated with memory, reward and motivation and hijacking of mu receptors in the brain	Modification of behaviors related to alcohol or substance use and addictive behaviors	Use of medications to reestablish brain functions and support person through detoxification and recovery to prevent relapse	Controlled delivery of substance with no euphoria effects preventing further drug use	Improved quality of life, allows person to resume functioning and goal-oriented behavior unrelated to drug seeking.	Controversial Access issues for many; cost may not be covered. Patient continues to be dependent on substance
Complementary Therapies	Improves mood, coping, quality of life. Focuses on the interactions between mind, body, and behaviors.	Individual with talents and strengths capable of self-direction	Empowers person Improves self-efficacy and personal resources for recovery	Strengthens or augments traditional, neurobiologic, and psychological approaches	Wide variety of choices (e.g. yoga, tai chi, mindfulness, music and art therapy) may be cost effective or more easily accessed.	Research is limited for substance use disorders Not a replacement for traditional or standard medical support or treatment. Limited supply of providers with specialized training

Nurses can also be alert for those who try to cope by replacing the misuse of one psychoactive substance with another, or who substitute a compulsive behavior (such as compulsive gaming or compulsive eating) without recognizing that the replacement is harmful.

A careful suicide assessment and precautions are needed. There are frequent dangers involved in acquiring illicit (street) drugs, and some individuals may have a "kill or be killed" mentality just to survive and to maintain access to substances. Drug dealing and rivalry between gang members who may be involved in disputes might follow the patient to the hospital. Staff members need to be especially careful to maintain the safety of patients and other staff members when patients threaten homicide or express homicidal thoughts. Caution should be taken not to allow different gangs or their family members to access one another. When a threat is made, there is legal duty to warn and notify proper authorities. Gang violence protocols should be available in workplaces, and all staff members can request gang identification training. Escalated security protocols may need to be instituted, including locking down the emergency department (ED) and waiting areas.

EVIDENCE-BASED NURSING CARE FOR PEOPLE WITH SUBSTANCE USE DISORDERS

Because substance use and misuse are pervasive in Western society, all nurses will encounter people who are affected by substances. In most instances, substance use will be secondary to the health care issue, but the use of a substance can directly or indirectly affect the patient's goals, treatment, and outcome. Substance use needs to be considered for any patient who is seeking health care.

Assessment and interventions should include culturally relevant data, such as unique physiologic responses to substances, behavioral responses to dependence, and social expectations and sanctions. Nurses who are knowledgeable about cultural differences and issues are integral to successful treatment.

Recognizing Cues: Relevant Assessment Information

Screening for substances is the first step in identifying substance misuse. The purpose of screening for substance misuse is to identify people who are high risk for developing a substance use issue and who need further assessment for diagnosis and treatment (SAMHSA, 1997). In addition to previously discussed screening tools, there are a variety of tools available for screening. See Table 31.2.

When the results of a screening test are positive, a comprehensive SUD assessment is needed to determine the type and severity of substance use, diagnose the SUD or other comorbid and medical conditions, and explore the patient's perception of their condition and readiness to change including barriers and facilitators. Along with the psychiatric nursing interview (see Chapter 10), specific behavioral cues will help the nurse hypothesize about the substance use, misuse, or dependence. See Table 31.3. Patients often do not recognize the severity of the substance misuse and its consequences. It is important that the substance of misuse (including polysubstances) and the patterns of use (amount, route, first use, frequency, and length of use) are identified. See Clinical Judgment Nursing Care Plan 31.1, which sets forth a plan of care for Gladys, the case study patient in this chapter.

TABLE 31.2 SCREENING TOOLS FOR SUBSTANCE USE

	Substance Type		Patient Age		How Tool Is Administered	
Tool	Alcohol	Drugs	Adults	Adolescents	Self-Administered	Clinician-Administered
Screening to Brief Intervention (S2BI)	X	X		X	X	X
Brief Screener for Alcohol, Tobacco, and other Drugs (BSATD)	X	X		X	X	X
Tobacco, Alcohol, Prescription medication, and other Substance use (TAPS)	X	X	X		X	X
Alcohol Screening and Brief Intervention for Youth: A Practitioner's Guide (NIAAA)	X			X		X
Opioid Risk Tool – OUD (ORT-OUD) Chart		X	X		X	

Reprinted from National Institute on Drug Abuse. (2023). Screening and Assessment Tools Chart. https://nida.nih.gov/nidamed-medical-health-professionals/screening-tools-resources/chart-screening-tools

health issues (anemia, tooth decay, type 2 diabetes, malnutrition, etc.). It is important that a nutritional assessment be included.

Sleep

SUDs are associated with sleep disturbances such as insomnia and sleep fragmentation (Akinnusi et al., 2024). For many individuals, circadian rhythms are drastically disturbed as drug-seeking needs and the activities involved in using substances take priority over sleep. This misalignment between circadian rhythms and external cues worsens with the progression of the SUD (Tamura et al., 2021). Establishing healthy sleep hygiene and reestablishing circadian rhythms is necessary even if sleeping medications are needed.

Physical Signs of Substance Use

The nurse should document physical consequences of substance usage. There may be a "flushed face" from alcohol use, sores or abscesses from injecting drugs, or any of the many physical signs of substance withdrawal. Substance misuse often leads to lack of adherence to recommended treatment for physical and mental disorders. Unemployment and lack of medical and dental insurance are associated with physical deterioration. Substance misuse and dependence contributes to increased risk of mental illness (depression and anxiety) which in turn diminishes the ability to promote health and well-being (Keeney et al., 2025).

Physical Functioning

People with SUDs often experience comorbid chronic physical health conditions, including chronic pain, cancer, and heart disease. The use of the variety of psychoactive substances considered in this disorder has independent increased risks of cardiovascular and heart disease. Nurses include physical functioning in their assessment.

Smoking, which is five times more than the national average among people with SUDs (McCuistian et al., 2024), also contributes to age-related degeneration, manifesting in such disorders as diabetes, colorectal cancer, liver cancer, and respiratory disorders, chronic obstructive pulmonary disease (COPD), bronchitis (Rouland et al., 2024). For those with cancer, smoking contributes to adverse health outcomes such as tuberculosis, erectile dysfunction rheumatoid, arthritic inflammation, and impaired immune functioning, increasing their susceptibility to a variety of contagions and infections (Islami et al., 2024).

History of Trauma

The relationship between trauma and substance use is a two-way street. Substance use is a risk factor for trauma, and trauma is a risk for the use of substances. Studies show that 25% to 75% of teens who use substances began their use following trauma exposure or the onset of posttraumatic stress (PTS) symptoms. For teens, traumatic stress or the presence of PTS symptoms may make it more difficult to stop using substances (NCTSN, 2023). See Box 31.3.

Psychosocial Cues

Mental Status and Appearance

One of the first observations nurses make is the physical appearance of the patient. Nurses document evidence of poor hygiene, disheveled appearance, listlessness, sallow skin, and weight loss. If the patient is intoxicated or under the influence of a substance such as cocaine, their mental

BOX 31.3

Trauma-Informed Approaches: Adverse Childhood Experiences in Community Mental Health Settings

Background

Although many individuals in the United States experience trauma, little is known about the diverse populations being treated in community mental health settings. Hoping to shed more light on this topic, the Adverse Childhood Experience (ACE) questionnaire was used to survey 856 participants; 40% reported four or more ACEs. Emotional abuse, physical abuse, and emotional neglect were the most prevalent ACEs. Psychological symptoms, including posttraumatic stress disorder (PTSD), depression, impulse disorder, and substance use disorder were higher among those with high ACE scores, and higher scores were also associated with more comorbidities. Knowledge of an individual's ACEs can benefit therapeutic interventions, but more training is needed about the impact of ACEs on adults receiving mental health treatment.

Interventions

Nurses working in community mental health settings should expect a high prevalence of ACEs in those being treated and be prepared to engage in trauma screening and interviewing. Nurses can also endorse concepts of trauma-sensitive and trauma-informed approaches within these institutions.

Source: Sucich, J., Breitbart, V., Williams, S., Sanichar, N., Candelaria-Arce, E., Frankle, W. G., & Davison-Duffy, S. (2023). Prevalence of childhood trauma in a community-based mental health clinic. *Community Mental Health Journal*, *59*(6), 1136–1149. https://doi.org/10.1007/s10597-023-01094-1

status examination may show disorientation, confusion, speech changes, or hallucinations.

Behavioral Responses

Patients may be brought to the ED by police or by frightened, concerned family members following negative events that may have triggered the hospitalization or led to a suicide attempt (e.g., job loss, legal problems, assaults, theft, domestic disputes, custody battles). Substance misuse can lead to isolation, which in turn may increase substance use. In cases of long-term use of substances, in addition to establishing or reestablishing preventive care and physical health, the individual is likely to have other issues that will need attention and thoughtful problem solving as the person attempts to get on the road to recovery.

Stress and Coping Patterns

It is important to identify the stress and coping patterns of people who use substances. New coping skills to manage stress can be learned to replace long-entrenched, unhealthful coping patterns. The nurse can determine if the patient's social network is supportive of recovery. If the social network reinforces substance misuse, the development of new friendships and habits can be considered when setting goals and interventions. Functional status determines what the individual can do; some people manage to hold a job even with continued substance use, but missing days of work or causing accidents and errors can contribute to daily stress.

Interpersonal stresses are common among members of the patient's support system, who carry a heavy burden from worry. People who misuse substances often exhibit generally unpleasant behaviors; they may also direct harmful or dangerous behaviors (e.g., domestic or child abuse and neglect) at their family and friends. Relationships can pay a heavy toll; as many as 3% of marriages end in divorce due to SUD; substance use was reported as a motivating factor in 6% of divorces (BAART, 2023).

Denial

Denial is a coping mechanism that prevents people from recognizing or admitting their substance misuse. **Denial** is a complex emotional process that distorts an individual's perception of reality. It is not just a refusal to admit the truth. Denial can be expressed in diverse behaviors and attitudes and may not be expressed as an overt denial of the issue. For example, patients may admit to an issue and even thank the nurse for helping them to realize they have an issue but insist they can overcome the issue on their own and do not need outside help.

Denial is characterized by patient confusion, distorted comparisons with others' use of substances, difficulty reconciling past positive substance experiences with current issues, and misunderstandings about the diagnosis of substance use. Patients may also have a misguided belief that misuse can be overcome by sheer willpower and refuse to believe that drug or alcohol use has influenced thoughts, feelings, behaviors, or relationships with others.

Though further study is needed on the causes of denial is needed, a variety of neural networks may be involved in denial. Insight into misuse or dependence is thought to be impaired by neural deficits in monitoring and negative emotions. Because of the deficits, denial of substance use issues is perpetuated (Maracic & Moeller, 2021).

Usually, nurses encounter individuals during crises when they are seeking professional help. These situations offer an opportunity to explore the denial that keeps their substance use thriving. The nurse's approach should be caring, matter-of-fact, gentle, and direct. Approaches that are punitive or attempt to elicit feelings of guilt or shame are destructive to the therapeutic relationship.

Denial is often met with confrontation by nurses and other professionals, who argue with the patient and present evidence of dependence; however, this lecturing often fails to elicit in the patient admission of an issue or influence behavior change. Although we do not know how to target the specific areas of the brain involved in denial, nurses can continue to work with patients who use denial to cope with anxiety-provoking situations by offering their support, using active listening strategies, and by helping them solve issues in healthy ways.

KEYCONCEPT Denial is a coping mechanism that prevents people from recognizing or admitting their substance use issue. Denial is a complex emotional process that distorts an individual's perception of reality. It is not just a refusal to admit the truth.

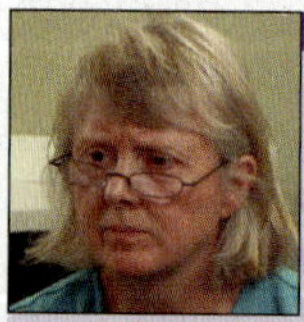

Gladys and Denial

Gladys continues to deny that she is dependent on alcohol. She is angry with her son for suggesting that she has a problem and refuses to sign a release of information for him.

Motivation for Change

Motivation is a key predictor of whether individuals will change their substance use behavior, but dependence is a chronic, relapsing biologic condition. The nurse can assess motivation by asking the patient about their intent to change behavior and lifestyle. **Motivational interviewing** is a method of therapeutic intervention that seeks to elicit self-motivational statements from patients, which creates a disconnect between the patient's goals and their continued alcohol and SUD. This communication skill can be used in other situations where healthy lifestyle changes will make a difference.

The nurse should explain that motivation alone may be insufficient without additional support and treatment. When an individual is dependent on substance, receptors in the brain can be hi-jacked by that substance. This means that in the absence of the substance, the individual does not experience pleasure and nothing besides the substance can take its place (not food, sex, or family). Urges to use can be so powerful that they overcome the best of motivations, even the desire to regain custody of one's children or to avoid going to jail. Although nurses can capitalize on the individual's motivation to change, they cannot be helpful unless they understand that recovery is a life-long process, requiring dramatic changes at the individual and family levels, which must indeed be dealt with, "one day at a time."

KEYCONCEPT Motivation is a goal-oriented attitude that propels action for change and can help sustain the development of new activities and behaviors when additional support and treatment are available

NCLEXNOTE Motivational approaches are priority interventions for patients with substance-related disorders. They help patients recognize an issue and begin to develop change strategies for continuing recovery and relapse prevention. Nurses at any level can be certified in motivational interviewing strategies.

Countertransference

Countertransference is the total emotional reaction of the treatment provider to the patient (see Chapter 9). Patients with substance-related disorders can generate strong feelings and reactions in nurses and other health care providers. These feelings can be triggered by overtly unpleasant patient behaviors such as lying, deceit, manipulation, or hostility, or these feelings may be more subconscious and stem from past experiences with relatives or others with substance dependence, or even from dealing with situations in the health care provider's own family. To be able to overcome countertransference feelings, nurses must recognize that the patient's behaviors are a part of the illness. Nurses should reflect on how their own behaviors toward patients who misuse substances can contribute or detract from the care they wish to provide. See Box 31.4.

BOX 31.4

Reflection of a Nurse: Avoiding Communication Blocks

Incident

Jessica is 48-year-old female assigned at birth on the medical surgical unit whose blood alcohol concentration (BAC) was 0.15% on admission 4 hours ago. The nurse begins the conversation by confronting Jessica about how much she was drinking. Jessica responds defensively, telling the nurse that she is not dependent on alcohol, but her father, who was a useless bum, was, and she is nothing like him. The nurse disagrees and Jessica says, "You're just like my son—you're just too young to appreciate all I've gone through."

Reflection

Upon evaluation of the interaction, the nurse realizes no rapport was developed with the patient and the interaction became a power struggle. On further reflection and discussion with a peer, the nurse considered how Jessica reminds the nurse of the nurse's own mother, who drinks heavily (unhelpful countertransference).

1. What priority assessments should the nurse have completed before beginning the conversation with Gladys about drinking?
2. What important cues can the nurse identify that will help in discussing alcohol use with the patient?
3. What can the nurse do to improve the nurse–patient relationship and be of assistance to the patient regarding alcohol use?

Codependence

The concept of **codependence** emerged out of studies of women's relationships with husbands who misused alcohol. Today, the scope of codependency includes people of all genders who grew up in any type of dysfunctional family system in which substance misuse may or may not have been an issue. Codependence has also been described as "enabling," in which an individual inadvertently reinforces the drinking behavior of the other person. The codependency label remains controversial and is viewed by some as an oversimplification of complex emotions and behaviors of family members. Nurses should be careful not to use it as a catch-all diagnosis and to take special care to assess and plan interventions that address each person's particular situation, issues, and needs (Mental Health America, 2024).

Spiritual Assessment

A spiritual assessment is an important part of any nursing assessment, but especially for patients with SUD. An effective recovery intervention for many people is a 12-step program grounded in the belief in a higher power. Using a spirituality scale, the nurse should ask the patient about the importance of religion to them and if they believe in a higher power. One validated scale is the adapted short-form Spirituality Scale that measures self-discovery (meaning in life, sense of purpose, happiness with self, and sacredness of everyday life) and transcendent connection (belief in and relationship to a higher power that helps in coping with challenges, use of prayer) (Britton et al., 2024).

Quality of Life (QoL)

It is well-documented that individuals with SUD experience a diminished quality of life. During the assessment, the nurse should consider how the substance usage impacts quality of life. Studies show that those who misuse cocaine or heroin have a lower quality of life than those who misuse alcohol and marijuana. A history of incarceration or those who have been injecting drugs for more than 10 years have lower QoL scores than others (Bratu et al., 2023).

The nurse should consider how the collected physical and psychological assessment data affects the patient's QoL. For example, how does the patient's poor health, pain, or discomfort impact the individual's quality of life? How does anxiety, depression, or lack of energy impact the patient?

Strength and Wellness Assessment

At the completion of the assessment, the nurse should be able to identify the patient's strengths such as positive support system, employment, and motivation to change. Based upon the assessment, the nurse can make a clinical judgment regarding the overall wellness of the patient.

ANALYZING CUES AND DEVELOPING HYPOTHESES

For a hospitalized patient, the priority is determining the type of substance(s) a person was using when admitted. With a brief assessment, the nurse should consider the patient's response to the substance—intoxication or withdrawal. If the individual is no longer in danger of toxicity or withdrawal, the nurse considers the possibility of suicide ideation (see chapter 10). If the patient is not at risk of self-harm, the nurse can initiate a discussion about the use of substances and their consequences. Denial of substance misuse is common. An essential first step toward recovery is for the patient to admit that there is an issue and that they want help. The nurse will guide the discussion according to the cues of the assessment.

Nurses are involved in the initial recovery process, including monitoring drug screens, administering medications, leading or assisting with recovery groups, and providing psychoeducation.

PLANNING RECOVERY AND WELLNESS OUTCOMES: GENERATING SOLUTIONS

The nurse and patient will establish outcomes based on the goals. Outcomes should include topics related to promotion of health and prevention of illnesses. For example, one patient might want to improve eating and sleeping, and another patient might want to develop strategies that improve medication adherence. The nurse is usually responsible for medication education (Fornili & Fogger, 2022).

THERAPEUTIC RELATIONSHIP

It is critical that the nurse establish a therapeutic relationship with patients and families. The following general guidelines can be used in establishing therapeutic interactions with patients with an SUD:

- Encourage honest expression of feelings.
- Listen to what the individual is really saying.
- Express caring for the individual.
- Hold the individual responsible for their behavior without being punitive
- Provide fair and consistent consequences for negative behaviors.
- Do not compromise your own values or nursing practice.
- Communicate the treatment plan to the patient and to others on the treatment team.
- Monitor your own reactions to the patient.
- Maintain healthy boundaries.

Confrontation can be very threatening to patients and should only occur within the context of a trusting relationship. Only by holding the patient in high regard and by separating the patient from the disorder can the nurse establish a trusting relationship that allows patient and nurse to fight substance misuse together. Box 31.5 provides an example of an SBAR that the nurse might use when calling the provider, as the therapeutic nurse–patient relationship begins.

TAKING ACTION: NURSING INTERVENTIONS

Nurses provide emotional support to families, establish a trusting alliance, engage patients in treatment, educate families about SUDs, and provide resources and information about the variety of treatment options available. Even though the nurse's role overlaps with the roles of other members of the interdisciplinary team, the nurse is still accountable to practice according to the *Psychiatric–Mental Health Nursing Scope and Standards of Practice* (ANA et al., 2022) and the *Addictions Nursing Scope and Standards of Practice* (Fornili & Fogger, 2022). Nursing care is based on the agreed-upon goals.

Nursing interventions vary depending on the nature of the current issues and their severity. For a patient who is undergoing detoxification, physical interventions (e.g., monitoring vital signs and neurologic functioning) are necessary. When the SUD is secondary to other physical or psychiatric issues, education of the patient and family may be a priority.

Priorities of Care

During detoxification, nurses are responsible for assessing progress and ensuring patient safety specific to the substance(s) the person had been using. The nurse also monitors IV fluids and administers medications as

BOX 31.5

Building Clinical Judgment With SBAR: Nurse Communication With Provider Regarding a Patient With Alcohol Use Disorder

SBAR

S: Situation

Stella, an 18-year-old college student, is adamant that her parents not be told about her alcohol use and states, "I don't drink any more than my friends do."

B: Background

Stella was brought to the emergency department (ED) after falling and hitting her head on the bathroom sink in her dorm. Her BAC was 0.17% on admission to the ED. The patient states, "my friends just left me there, and I don't even know who brought me to the hospital." A 3-inch laceration on the left side of her forehead has been treated, and stitches were required. Stella admits to drinking heavily at the party. She was given the AUDIT, and her score of 8 indicates a risk (moderate) for drinking.

A: Assessment

Stella is agitated about being in the hospital and was shocked when she saw the laceration on her forehead. No other injuries were noted, and concussion scans were negative. After explaining the results of the AUDIT, the patient consented to talking further with the nurse about her alcohol use.

- Vital signs: BP 122/80, P 76, R 18, T 36.8 °C
- Neuro checks: Stable, Oriented ×3
- Metabolic panel: WNL
- Computed tomography (CT) Scan: Negative
- Standardized assessment of concussion (SAC) Result: Mild
- Trauma screen: Denies trauma history

R: Recommendation

- Teach the patient how to change the dressing on the laceration and how to assess for infection.
- Provide postconcussion information and emergency precautions.
- Discuss the results of the AUDIT with patient and continue brief interventions/motivational interviewing.
- Provide instructions for self-help around similar upcoming social events, giving immediate personalized feedback, including advice and suggestions for protective behaviors and reminding Stella that underage alcohol use at any level is illegal.
- Engage in developing a safety plan including suggestions for protective behaviors (e.g., drinking water, eating, avoiding drinking games, planning how to get home, and how friends should stay together for safety).
- Engage patient in contracting for safety to convince her of the importance of informing family about the hospitalization for a medical emergency related to excessive alcohol consumption.
- Advise patient of possible resources in the community and suggest that she investigate services which may be available to her as a university student.
- Complete a follow-up contact 48 hours after discharge.

Building Clinical Judgment

1. Why did the nurse want to talk about developing a safety plan for continued drinking if underage drinking is illegal?
2. Why did the nurse request a 48-hour follow-up contact after discharge?

needed. After detoxification, the nurse provides supportive listening and referrals to recovery-oriented support groups that are online or in the community.

Patients who have SUDs are at high risk for suicide. Nurses should always be alert for changes in behavior that indicate an imminent suicide attempt.

In an inpatient or residential program, individuals sometimes bring prohibited or illegal items such as drugs or alcohol into the unit. The nurse and team should establish a process that prevents prohibited items from being brought to a unit; such strategies could include frequent room checks and a process of securing the items if found on the unit.

Physical Care

The nurse helps patients regain their physical health through education and referral to appropriate resources. Nurses working in recovery encourage patients to seek medical and dental exams on a regular basis.

Nutrition

Establishing a healthy diet is important in physical recovery. Reexamining the daily diet and investing in eating healthy food is a big step in recovering physically from abuse of the body. Vitamin and mineral replacement may be necessary. Nurses collaborate with the team and patient to make sure that there is a stable source of food. This is especially important for patients who are unhoused because they eat fewer meals each day and often lack food.

Exercise

Establishing an exercise routine can be the beginning of regenerating the patient's muscles and circulatory system. Physical inactivity and sedentary behavior are linked to an increased risk of alcohol consumption and cigarette smoking; physical exercise can contribute to abstinence and reduce cravings (Iob et al., 2023). Regular exercise is a way of reducing the risk of substance use and promoting a healthy lifestyle (Gústafsson et al., 2024).

Medication Interventions

People with SUDs may manifest behaviors characteristic of another mental disorder; for example, behaviors found in bipolar spectrum disorders (hyperthymic and cyclothymic temperament) can be caused by substance

TABLE 31.4 ANTIDEPRESSANTS AND THEIR ROLE IN SUBSTANCE USE DISORDER TREATMENT

Substance Misuse Issue	Antidepressant Effect
Nicotine Dependence	Bupropion used to reduce craving for tobacco and reduce nicotine dependence. Eases withdrawal symptoms and helps reduce the drive to acquire the drug.
Methamphetamine Dependence	Antidepressants may reduce cravings and reduce the efficacy of methamphetamine. Eases withdrawal symptoms, reduces psychological drive to get more of the drug. May reduce euphoria related to amphetamine use.
Pain, Headache, Insomnia	Antidepressants are a less addictive (habit-forming) method of treating these symptoms and are often used off-label. Those with substance use disorder (SUDs) may benefit from the mood-elevating effects of antidepressants as well as the relief of these symptoms which are common.
Negative moods and anxiety during detoxification	Antidepressants moderate and elevate mood which may help overcome the psychological effects of substance withdrawal.
Comorbid mental conditions	Antidepressants are used to treat underlying mental health conditions like anxiety and depression and are included in long-term SUD treatment along with psychotherapy.
Depression induced by long-term substance misuse	Long-term substance misuse leads to changes in brain chemistry which can induce anxiety or depression. A combination of antidepressants and psychotherapy during withdrawal could be effective in helping to taper the person off the misused substances.

Source: Laguna Treatment Hospital (2022). Can antidepressants prevent drug misuse, and what are the risks? American Addiction Centers. https://lagunatreatment.com/drug-abuse/antidepressants/

use—notably stimulants, alcohol, or cannabinoids. Mood stabilizers (carbamazepine, divalproex, and lamotrigine) may be prescribed for a short time to treat the symptoms. In some instances, benzodiazepines or antipsychotics may be given for acute mania.

SUD withdrawal symptoms may manifest as another mental disorder; for example, a person trying to overcome dependence on cocaine will experience depression as a withdrawal symptom, and antidepressants can relieve the intensity of the symptom (Gao et al., 2023), because during withdrawal, antidepressants can have mood-elevating effects and promote sleep. If the patient's symptoms persist after the intoxication or withdrawal has been treated, a co-occurring mental disorder most likely exists. In this situation, psychiatric medications will continue to be prescribed.

Antidepressants are not only helpful in treating SUDs; they are also used with other therapies to help the person overcome other conditions and gain relief from intolerable symptoms during detoxification and withdrawal. See Table 31.4. Antidepressants can ease withdrawal symptoms and may reduce cravings. They are also prescribed for insomnia, pain, and headaches. For those with an SUD, treating pain is an important consideration because antidepressants have less misuse potential than anxiolytics or opioid pain medications and are not as likely to lead to misuse and self-medicating The use of antidepressants in the treatment of gambling disorder is inconclusive, though some evidence suggests it may be promising (Farkouh et al., 2024).

Once the acute intoxication or withdrawal is treated, the patient and team may decide to administer medication for an SUD in combination with counseling and behavioral therapies. These medications help reduce urges and protect patients from relapse and include medications such as naltrexone, disulfiram. Medication programs for SUDs are carefully regulated because of their use of opioid agonists. These medications can be taken orally or as a long-acting injection. Nurses will be responsible for teaching patients about the action, side effects, and the importance of adherence. If injections are prescribed, the nurse will administer the medication.

When patients are treated for pain with opioids, there is always a risk of dependence. Nurses in EDs often encounter patients requesting pain medications from a lapsed prescription. See Box 31.6.

BOX 31.6

Clinical Judgment Vignette: Opioid Demands in the Emergency Department

Jabril is a 60-year-old who presents to the emergency department (ED) with chronic pain that remains following a work-related back injury that occurred over two years ago. The patient states that he took his last pain pill, but the pharmacy will not refill the prescription as his primary care provider is on vacation. He is anticipating that he will not be able to stand the pain until the doctor returns next week and is demanding a prescription for immediate-release oxycodone. He rates his pain as a 4 on a 10-point scale and says, "I really need the medicine." No changes were noted in his medical condition that could contribute to a change in symptoms. Jabril denies that he has an issue. Jabril has a history of running out of pills.

Building Clinical Judgment

1. How would the nurse approach this patient in the ED?
2. What other assessments should the nurse make?
3. What high-risk factors does Jabril have for opioid use disorder?
4. Prioritize Jabril's immediate needs.

Psychosocial Interventions

Screening, Brief Interventions, and Referral to Treatment (SBIRT)

Screening, brief intervention, and referral to treatment (SBIRT) is an approach to treating individuals with SUDs and those who are at risk of developing them. These services have been shown to be effective in helping individuals with high-risk alcohol use to seek help (Jones et al., 2024). Not everyone who is screened will need a brief intervention, and not everyone who needs a brief intervention will require treatment. In fact, the goals of screening and brief intervention are to reduce risky substance use before people become dependent.

The **brief intervention** (one to four sessions), focuses on increasing insight and awareness regarding substance use and motivation toward change. The acronym FRAMES (which is short form for feedback, responsibility, advice, menu of strategies, empathy, and self-efficacy) summarizes elements of brief interventions with patients. See Box 31.7. The nurse provides feedback about the screening results, impairment, and risks, informs the patient about safe consumption limits, and offers strategies for changing use behavior. The nurse determines the patient's readiness for change and negotiated goals and strategies. If substance use is moderate to severe, the patient is referred for a comprehensive assessment and treatment (SAMHSA, 2022).

Brief intervention is most successful when working with people who:

- Are experiencing few issues with their drug use
- Have low levels of dependence
- Have a short history of drug use
- Have stable backgrounds
- Are unsure or ambivalent about changing or ending their drug use

It is recommended that brief intervention at a minimum include:

- Advising how to reduce patient's drug use
- Providing harm-reduction information or self-help manuals relevant to the patient
- Giving the patient relevant information about the following:
  - The consequences of a drug conviction in terms of international travel and employment
  - Consequences of further or heavier drug charges

Discussing harm-reduction strategies, especially those relating to the following:

- Overdose
- Violence
- Driving under the influence
- Safe practices (e.g., safe injecting, safe sex)
- Offering and arranging a follow-up visit

> **BOX 31.7**
>
> **FRAMES—Effective Elements of Brief Intervention**
>
> **FEEDBACK**
>
> Provide patients with personal feedback regarding their individual status, such as personal alcohol and other drug consumption relative to norms, information about elevated liver enzyme values, and other factors. Invite them to review results of a standardized assessment. Remember to ask if they would like to hear or have more information if appropriate.
>
> **RESPONSIBILITY**
>
> Emphasize the individual's freedom of choice and personal responsibility for change. General themes are as follows:
> 1. It's up to you; you're free to decide to change or not.
> 2. No one else can decide for you or force you to change.
> 3. You're the one who has to do it if it's going to happen.
>
> **ADVICE**
>
> Include a clear recommendation or advice on the need for change, typically in a supportive and concerned, rather than in a judgmental, manner.
>
> **MENU**
>
> Offer a menu of options from which patients may pick those that seem more suitable, achievable, or appealing.
>
> **EMPATHIC SUPPORT**
>
> Show warmth, support, respect, and understanding in communication with patients.
>
> **SELF-EFFICACY**
>
> Reinforce self-efficacy or an optimistic feeling that they can change.

Cognitive Behavioral Interventions

Cognitive approaches to substance misuse hypothesize that if a patient can change the way they think about a situation, both the emotional reaction to it and the behavioral response will change. Cognitive-behavioral therapy (CBT) is a brief structured treatment that focuses on immediate issues. It enables patients to examine the thinking process that leads to decisions to use substances, analyze distortions in thinking, and develop rational responses to these distortions. Virtual treatment approaches, which became popular during the COVID-19 pandemic, were also used for SUD treatment, and some people have opted to continue their use. See Box 31.8.

Group Interventions

Isolation and alienation from friends and family are common themes in patients with substance-related disorders. In addition, thinking that has become distorted is left

BOX 31.8

Research for Evidence-Based Practice: Virtual Reality for SUD

Taubin, D., Berger, A., Greenwald, D., Greenwald, H., Burke, C., Gongora, D. S., & Wilens, T. (2023). A systematic review of virtual reality therapies for substance use disorders: Impact on secondary treatment outcomes. The American Journal on Addictions, 32*(1), 13–23. https://doi.org/10.1111/ajad.13342*

THE QUESTION: Is virtual reality (VR) therapy for SUD effective in treating urges and cravings and for mood, anxiety, and emotional regulation?

METHODS: A literature review of seven published research studies on the effectiveness of VR for secondary treatment outcomes was conducted.

FINDINGS: VR was effective in reducing cravings and urges but results were mixed for other secondary outcomes (symptoms of depression and anxiety). The authors conclude that more intentional targeting of other symptoms is necessary.

IMPLICATIONS FOR NURSING: This research should validate that virtual treatment can be effective against urges and cravings, and nurses know that these symptoms are often indicators of relapse and pose challenges for those striving toward recovery. As nurses engage in helping patients manage emotional regulation and use therapeutic strategies to help with dysregulated moods, they could offer some new and innovative ways of capturing their interventions in virtual reality. For instance, virtual care platforms that simplify the patient–clinician experience, innovate better care delivery, and are secure and reliable are being developed. These bring patients into closer collaboration with the health care team, inside or outside the facility. Nurses use their strengths and skills to be on the ground floor of the development of VR therapies.

unchallenged without contact with others; thus, change is difficult. When a patient enters a group that is working with the shared goal of continuing recovery, numerous healing advantages occur.

In treatment settings, groups focus on immediate goals of helping the individual enact a change in thinking and behavior patterns that support sobriety and abstinence. The emphasis is on using problem solving and other skills to deal with stressful events that threaten abstinence. This type of support group is also extremely effective in outpatient treatment settings. After a period of successful abstinence, group therapy can focus more on traditional psychotherapy work. Nurses may be involved in the facilitation of these groups and certainly encourage patients to attend and participate. Nurses may also help patients find support groups in the community and plan to attend meetings. Be ready to explain the benefits of support groups and of having networks of others to rely on, and offer continuing support as the patient strives for sobriety.

Individual Therapy

Often, individual therapy is helpful, particularly in conjunction with group therapy or family therapy. In substance use treatment settings, dependency therapists meet with individuals to maintain focus on the goals and objectives of their treatment, to review the fears and anxieties that often arise in early recovery, and to devise new and healthy responses and solutions to stressful and difficult situations. Psychiatric mental health advanced practice nurses (PMH-APRNs) who have specialized training and advanced education to provide group and individual psychotherapy may practice independently or in combination with medication management to provide services to those with SUDs.

Family Interventions

Family therapy, a vital part of substance use treatment, can be used in several beneficial ways to initiate change and help the family when the substance-abusing person is unwilling to seek treatment. Behavioral couples therapy for people who misuse alcohol and/or drugs can improve family functioning, reduce stressors, smooth marital adjustment, and lessen domestic violence and verbal conflict. When the person who misuses substances seeks help, family therapy can help stabilize abstinence and relationships. Often, inpatient substance use treatment programs have family education and group therapy components that help meet these goals. The nurse should explains how family therapy works and the benefits it offers and answers family members' questions.

Complementary Therapies

Substance use becomes a coping mechanism for physical and emotional issues and stress, leading to dependence on a substance and negative sequelae. Withdrawal symptoms can exacerbate other mental illness symptoms and there will be a struggle to maintain sobriety. The person in recovery needs healthy alternatives for coping. These could be anything from sports, exercising, and yoga to acupuncture, gardening, and joining a book club.

Person-centered care should guide nurses to help patients find activities that they will enjoy and that fit with their strengths and are realistic in face of the resources they still have or can gain access to. Many may need help with chronic illness management or adequate support to live with their disabilities. Access to recovery support services will help those in recovery achieve and sustain long-term wellness.

The most common complementary therapies associated with the treatment of SUD are acupuncture and integrative psychotherapies (such as mindfulness-based CBT) (Junyue et al., 2021). Research around complementary and integrative treatment has been increasing and shows promise for use with SUDs (Junyue et al., 2021).

Spiritual Interventions

Substance use treatment has a long tradition of advocating for a spiritual intervention. Several steps in 12-step programs (discussed later in chapter) refer to a power greater than self or God. There are also several other spiritual interventions that can be recommended such as readings from a religious book such as the Bible, Torah, or Quran, and reflexive readings (interpreting passages and finding personal meaning). Religiously integrated psychotherapy that includes meditating on religious meanings and cultivating forgiveness, hope gratitude, generosity, and motivation for community engagement is another approach (de Andrade et al., 2023). Referral to a chaplain should also be considered.

Psychoeducation

Psychoeducational materials, groups, and one-on-one interactions with nurses also impart information to reduce knowledge deficits related to alcohol and drug dependence. See Box 31.9.

Developing Recovery-Oriented Rehabilitation Strategies

Harm-Reduction Strategies

Harm reduction, a set of community health strategies designed to reduce the harm of substance use to the individual, the family, and society, has replaced a moral or criminal approach to drug use. It recognizes that the ideal is abstinence but works with the individual regardless of their commitment to reduce use. The goal is to reduce the potential harm and negative consequences associated with continued use of the alcohol or substance. Harm-reduction initiatives range from widely accepted designated driver campaigns to controversial initiatives, such as provision of condoms in schools, safe injection rooms, needle exchange programs, and heroin maintenance programs.

In 2023, the FDA approved over-the-counter naloxone to treat opioid overdose, and since then it has been a highly successful harm-reduction strategy used by first responders and family members to prevent fatal overdoses and save lives. Nurses offer patients who screen for moderate drinking a variety of harm-reduction strategies and include them in community education presentations. Remember that a main principle of harm reduction is that it includes a spectrum of strategies. What might be safe for one person, might not be safe for another. Harm reduction always depends on the individual's starting point (SAMHSA, 2024).

Several support groups include harm reduction philosophies and missions in their approach. See Table 31.5. Four such groups in the United States are Women for Sobriety, Moderation Management, Men for Sobriety, and Self-Management and Recovery Training (SMART) Recovery.

BOX 31.9

Psychoeducation Checklist: Substance Misuse

When caring for the patient with substance misuse and their family, be sure to include the following topic areas in the family's teaching plan:

- Psychopharmacologic agents, if used, including drug action, dosage, frequency, and possible side effects
- Manifestations of intoxication, overdose, and withdrawal
- Emergency medical system activation
- Nutrition
- Coping strategies
- Structured planning
- Safety measures
- Available treatment programs
- Family therapy referral
- Self-help groups and other community resources
- Follow-up laboratory testing, if indicated

Self-Help Group and 12-Step Program

Alcoholics Anonymous (AA) was the first 12-step, self-help program. See Box 31.10 for a list of these steps. AA is a worldwide fellowship of people with AUD, who provide support, individually and at meetings, to others who seek help. The program steps include spiritual, cognitive, and behavioral components. Many treatment programs discuss concepts from AA, hold meetings at the treatment facilities, and encourage patients to attend community meetings when appropriate. They also encourage continuing use of AA and other self-help groups as part of an ongoing plan for continued abstinence. Twelve-step programs do not solicit members; engage in political or religious activities; make medical or psychiatric diagnoses; engage in education about substance misuse to the general population; or provide mental health, vocational, or legal counseling (Alcoholics Anonymous, 2024). Using peer support and support groups is an accepted approach with many beneficial outcomes for participants, since nurses are often responsible for the selection and training of individuals who will serve as PSS. Much can be learned from studies that reveal member's ideas about what works best, and who they can best work with. Virtual support, prevention, and wellness programs may provide nurses a unique way of delivering care and empowering adolescents who are open to a variety of online health experiences.

Continuum of Care

Substance use treatment occurs primarily in an outpatient, residential, or community setting. Inpatient settings

TABLE 31.5 HARM REDUCTION STRATEGIES FOR ALCOHOL MISUSE

Strategy	Description
Sobriety homes	Group residences for people who are recovering from AUD maintain sobriety and live according to residential rules.
Managing alcohol consumption	Buy water or other nonalcohol beverages between alcoholic drinks. Avoid drinking in rounds with friends. Order smaller servings of beer, cider, and spirits, rather than pints or double servings. Do not let others top off glass if sharing a bottle of wine. Avoid high-alcohol content beverages, such as cocktails or spirits. Eat food before and while drinking. Occupy the time while drinking with other activities, such as playing pool. Do not leave drinks unattended.
Expectancy challenge alcohol literacy curriculum	Expectancy challenge interventions do not focus on abstinence or scare tactics but on an individual's perceptions of alcohol's effects and providing accurate information. Negative expectancies are associated with reducing alcohol consumption and other negative consequences of use. This intervention has been delivered in different ways, including experiential learning, informational campaigns, and peer-support sessions.
Resisting Negative Peer Pressure	Strategies to resist peer pressure for drinking are taught and practices. Strategies include what to say to peers, and what to do under continued pressure. Situations are rehearsed in anticipation of pressure, until the teen feels confident and comfortable using them.

Source: Alcohol and Drug Foundation. (n.d.). Retrieved January 5, 2024, from https://adf.org.au/reducing-risk/alcohol/; Dunn, M. E., Schreiner, A. M., Flori, J. N., Crisafulli, M. J., Willis, E. A., Lynch, G. T., Leary, A. V., & Dvorak, R. D. (2022). Effective prevention programming for reducing alcohol-related harms experienced by first year college students: Evaluation of the expectancy challenge alcohol literacy curriculum (ECALC). *Addictive Behaviors*, *131*, 107338. https://doi.org/10.1016/j.addbeh.2022.107338

are used for medical emergencies and detoxification. In the community, types of care include sober homes, long-term rehabilitation centers, private or federal clinics, and individual provider's offices. Integrating SUD services with primary care improves access to the millions of Americans who need SUD treatment and use psychoactive substances in risky ways, even without a diagnosis. Unfortunately, in 2021, 94% of people aged 12 or older with an SUD did not receive any treatment (USDHHS, 2023).

TYPES OF SUBSTANCE USE DISORDERS

This section provides an overview of the types of SUDs. Note that in an SUD diagnosis, the "S" of "SUD" is replaced with the substance being used—for example, "AUD" is "alcohol use disorder," "SUD" is "stimulant use disorder," and so on. Polysubstance use is common, and many patients may have a primary substance of misuse, such as alcohol, and also be dependent on another

BOX 31.10

The 12 Steps of Alcoholics Anonymous

1. We admitted we were powerless over alcohol—that our lives had become unmanageable.
2. Came to believe that a Power greater than ourselves could restore us to sanity.
3. Made a decision to turn our will and our lives over to the care of God as we understood Him.
4. Made a searching and fearless moral inventory of ourselves.
5. Admitted to God, to ourselves, and to another human being the exact nature of our wrongs.
6. We're entirely ready to have God remove all these defects of character.
7. Humbly asked Him to remove our shortcomings.
8. Made a list of all people we had harmed and became willing to make amends to them all.
9. Made direct amends to such people wherever possible, except when to do so would injure them or others.
10. Continued to take personal inventory and, when we were wrong, promptly admitted it.
11. Sought through prayer and meditation to improve our conscious contact with God, as we understood Him, praying only for knowledge of His will for us and the power to carry that out.
12. Having had a spiritual awakening as a result of these steps, we tried to carry this message to alcoholics and to practice these principles in all our affairs.

substance(s). A summary of effects of the classes of psychoactive substances can be seen in Table 31.6.

ALCOHOL USE DISORDER

Alcohol

Alcohol (ethanol, EtOH) is the most used substance in the United States and is consumed regularly throughout the world. An AUD is diagnosed when there is a problematic pattern of alcohol use with significant impairment or distress. There are often comorbid disorders (liver disease, pancreatitis, cancer of head, neck, liver, colon, or rectum), co-occurring disorders (depression, bipolar disorder) and psychosocial issues leading to injuries, aggression, violence, and suicide (Kranzler, 2023).

Etiology

Alcohol affects multiple neurotransmitters including dopamine, GABA, glutamate, norepinephrine, and serotonin. Initially, ingestion of alcohol is experienced as pleasurable and disinhibits social behavior. With continuing alcohol intake, the individual can become aggressive, angry, and assaultive and show signs of impaired judgment, motor functions, and speech. As **blood alcohol levels** (BAL) or blood alcohol concentration **(BAC)** rise further, severe intoxication becomes **alcohol toxicity** (poisoning), which can progress to coma, respiratory failure, and death (Semaan & Khan, 2023). **Intoxication** is determined by the BAC. See Table 31.7.

There are multiple etiologic risk factors associated with AUD. Twin heritability is 49% with the remainder attributed to other epigenetic factors such as verbal, physical and sexual abuse and household instability (Kranzler, 2023).

Effects of Long-Term Use

People who use alcohol regularly usually develop alcohol **tolerance**, the ability to ingest an increasing amount of alcohol before experiencing a "high" or a "buzz" and before showing cognitive and motor effects. Some individuals do not appear intoxicated but their BALs reflect the increased amount of alcohol, which affects their bodies, as described in Table 31.7. Excessive or long-term misuse of alcohol can adversely affect all body systems; the effects can be serious and permanent. Box 31.11 lists the major physical complications of alcohol misuse for the major organ systems.

Recognizing Cues: Relevant Assessment Information

The nurse's role and responsibilities vary according to the level of care and needs of the patient, but most often nurses assess for cues related to substance use and physical health needs, provide treatments and medications, assist with physical needs, and offer support for recovery.

In addition to the psychiatric nursing assessment, nurses expect to complete a routine screening for alcohol use, assessing for signs of risky drinking, and identifying drinking patterns such as social drinking, daily drinking, and binge drinking. Adolescents should be asked about risky behaviors, such as driving under the influence, or riding in a car with someone who has been drinking. Using standardized screening/assessment tools and asking permission to discuss the results provides the nurse with an opportunity to explore and discuss alcohol use and assess motivation for change or to give commendations to those who abstain or (if they are of age) to those who drink responsibly.

The CAGE Questionnaire is a common tool consisting of the four self-report responses to questions about the following aspects of alcohol use: (1) **C**utting back on alcohol, (2) feeling **A**nnoyed when others criticize your drinking, (3) feeling **G**uilty about drinking, and (4) needing an **E**ye-opener (a drink first thing in the morning).

Another early detection screening tool commonly used is the Alcohol Use Disorders Identification Test (AUDIT), a 10-item tool developed by the World Health Organization, which has been validated for use across genders and racial groups (Babor et al., 2001).

Taking Action: Nursing Interventions

Nurses are valued members of the interprofessional team that implement evidence-based practices for those with AUDs. Nurses have a role on the interdisciplinary team at all levels of care. In the management of alcohol withdrawal and detoxification, the nurse leads the team. The nurse is also the primary care provider for the care for the patient who is intoxicated, experiencing complications of alcohol consumption.

Alcohol Withdrawal and Detoxification

Withdrawal from alcohol can cause severe seizures and even death. For this reason, most alcohol detoxification takes place in a medically supervised setting. **Detoxification** is the gradual withdrawal of the misused substance, using medications to avoid dangerous withdrawal symptoms. Uncomplicated withdrawal from alcohol is usually completed within 48 to 96 hours.

Be aware that patients who are undergoing alcohol detoxification should not have access to hand sanitizers, mouthwash, cough medicines, and aftershave lotions because they contain high levels of alcohol. Remind family members to restrict access to these sources as well.

Withdrawal from alcohol presents many physiologic and psychological challenges. **Alcohol withdrawal syndrome** (AWS) is characterized by an increased heart rate and blood pressure, diaphoresis, mild anxiety, restlessness, and hand tremors. The most severe symptoms are **delirium tremens** (autonomic hyperarousal, disorientation, hallucinations), grand mal (tonic–clonic) seizures, and

TABLE 31.6 SUMMARY OF EFFECTS OF ADDICTIVE PSYCHOACTIVE SUBSTANCES, OVERDOSE, WITHDRAWAL SYNDROMES, AND PROLONGED USE

Substance	Route	Effects (E) and Overdose (O)	Withdrawal Syndrome	Prolonged Use
Alcohol	PO	E: Sedation, decreased inhibitions, relaxation, decreased coordination, slurred speech, nausea O: Respiratory depression, cardiac arrest	Tremors; seizures, elevated temperature, pulse, and blood pressure; delirium tremens	Affects all systems of the body. Can lead to other dependencies, and malnutrition
Stimulants (e.g., amphetamines, cocaine)	PO, IV, inhalation, smoking	E: Euphoria, initial CNS stimulation and then depression, wakefulness, decreased appetite, insomnia, paranoia, aggressiveness, dilated pupils, tremors O: Cardiac arrhythmias or arrest, increased or lowered blood pressure, respiratory depression, chest pain, vomiting, seizures, psychosis, confusion, seizures, dyskinesias, dystonia, coma	Depression: psychomotor retardation at first and then agitation; fatigue and then insomnia; severe dysphoria and anxiety; cravings, vivid, unpleasant dreams; increased appetite. Amphetamine withdrawal is not as pronounced as cocaine withdrawal.	Often alternates with use of depressants. Weight loss and resulting malnutrition and increased susceptibility to infectious diseases. May produce schizophrenia-like syndrome with paranoid ideation, thought disturbance, hallucinations, and stereotyped movements Deviated nasal septum, irreversible nasal damage
Cannabis (e.g., marijuana, hashish, THC)	Smoking, ingesting skin patches	E: Euphoria or dysphoria, relaxation and drowsiness, heightened perception of color and sound, poor physical coordination, spatial perception and time distortion, unusual body sensations (e.g., weightlessness, tingling), dry mouth, dysarthria, and cravings for particular foods O: Increased heart rate, reddened eyes, dysphoria, lability, disorientation		Can decrease motivation and cause cognitive deficits (e.g., inability to concentrate, impaired memory). Lung damage, may precipitate psychosis
Hallucinogens (e.g., LSD, MDMA)	PO	E: Euphoria or dysphoria, altered body image, distorted or sharpened visual and auditory perceptions, depersonalization, bizarre behavior, confusion, incoordination, impaired judgment and memory, signs of sympathetic and parasympathetic stimulation, palpitations (blurred vision, dilated pupils, sweating) O: Paranoia, ideas of reference, fear of losing one's mind, depersonalization, derealization, illusions, hallucinations, synesthesia, self-destructive or aggressive behaviors, tremors	"Flashbacks" or HPPD may occur after termination of use.	
PCP	PO, inhalation, smoking	E: Feeling superhuman, decreased awareness of and detachment from the environment, stimulation of the respiratory and cardiovascular systems, ataxia, dysarthria, decreased pain perception O: Hallucinations, paranoia, psychosis, aggression, adrenergic crisis (cardiac failure, cerebrovascular accident, malignant hyperthermia, status epilepticus, severe muscle contractions)		"Flashbacks," HPPD, organic brain syndromes with recurrent psychotic behavior, which can last up to 6 mo after not using the drug, numerous psychiatric hospitalizations and police arrests

Opioids (e.g., heroin, codeine)	PO, injection, smoking	E: Euphoria, sedation, reduced libido, memory and concentration difficulties, analgesia, constipation, constricted pupils O: Respiratory depression, stupor, coma	Abdominal cramps, rhinorrhea, watery eyes, dilated pupils, yawning, "goose flesh," diaphoresis, nausea, diarrhea, anorexia, insomnia, fever	Can lead to criminal behavior to get money for drugs, risk for infection related to needle use (e.g., HIV, endocarditis, hepatitis, abscesses)
Sedatives, hypnotics, anxiolytics	PO, injection	E: Euphoria, sedation, reduced libido, emotional lability, impaired judgment O: Respiratory depression, cardiac arrest	Anxiety rebound and agitation, hypertension, tachycardia, sweating, hyperpyrexia, sensory excitement, motor excitation, insomnia, possible tonic–clonic convulsions, nightmares, delirium, depersonalization, hallucinations	Often alternated with stimulants, use with alcohol enhances chance of overdose, risk for infection related to needle use
Inhalants (e.g., glue, lighter fluid, gasoline, screen-cleaners, hair spray, and other aerosol sprays)	Inhalation	E: Euphoria, giddiness, excitation O: CNS depression: ataxia, nystagmus, dysarthria, coma, and convulsions	Similar to findings with alcohol but milder, with anxiety, tremors, hallucinations, and sleep disturbance as the primary symptoms	Long-term use can lead to hepatic and renal failure, blood dyscrasias, damage to the lungs; CNS damage (e.g., OBS, peripheral neuropathies, cerebral and optic atrophy, parkinsonism)
Nicotine	Smoking	E: Stimulation, enhanced performance and alertness, and appetite suppression O: Anxiety	Mood changes (e.g., craving, anxiety) and physiologic changes (e.g., poor concentration, sleep disturbances, headaches, gastric distress, and increased appetite)	Increased chance for cardiac disease and lung disease (COPD, cancer)
Caffeine	PO	E: Stimulation, increased mental acuity, inexhaustibility O: Restlessness, nervousness, excitement, insomnia, flushing, diuresis, gastrointestinal distress, muscle twitching, rambling flow of thought and speech, tachycardia or cardiac arrhythmia, agitation	Headache, drowsiness, fatigue, craving, impaired psychomotor performance, difficulty concentrating, yawning, nausea	Physical consequences are under investigation, may have risks and benefits

CNS, central nervous system; HIV, human immunodeficiency virus; HPPD, hallucinogenic persisting perceptual disorder; LSD, d-lysergic acid diethylamide; MDMA, 3,4-methylenedioxymethamphetamine; OBS, organic brain syndrome; PO, oral; PCP, phencyclidine; THC, D-9-tetrahydrocannabinol.

TABLE 31.7 BLOOD ALCOHOL CONCENTRATIONS (BAC) AND BEHAVIOR

Number of Drinks	BAC (mg%)	Behavior
1–2	0.05	Impaired judgment, giddiness, mood changes
5–6	0.10	Difficulty driving and coordinating movements
10–12	0.20	Motor functions severely impaired, resulting in ataxia; emotional lability
15–20	0.30	Stupor, disorientation, and confusion
20–24	0.40	Coma
25	0.50	Respiratory failure, death

even status epilepticus (continuous seizures, lasting more than 30 minutes). These symptoms can be life-threatening and contribute to many bodily injuries and accidents. See Table 31.8.

Abrupt alcohol cessation increases the potential for serious withdrawal. In anticipation of withdrawal symptoms, nurses need to determine when the patient consumed the last alcoholic drink. AWS usually begins within 12 hours after abrupt discontinuation or attempt to decrease consumption. If seizures occur, they usually do so within the first 48 hours of withdrawal.

ED nurses play an important role in identifying those at risk for AWS. Assessing for vital sign changes, nausea, vomiting, tremors, perspiration, agitation, headache, and change in mental status are important nursing interventions. The *Clinical Institute Withdrawal Assessment for Alcohol Scale* (CIWA-Ar), a frequently used numerical rating tool for assessing the severity of withdrawal symptoms, is used to guide medical and nursing interventions. Close monitoring continues until there are no indications of withdrawal symptoms. See Box 31.12.

BOX 31.11

Medical Complications of Alcohol Misuse

- **Cardiovascular system:** Cardiomyopathy, congestive heart failure, hypertension
- **Digestive system and nutritional deficiencies:** Liver diseases (fatty liver, alcoholic hepatitis, cirrhosis), pancreatitis, ulcers, other inflammations of the GI tract, ulcers and GI bleeds, esophageal varices, cancers of the upper GI tract, pellagra, alcohol-amnestic disorder, dermatitis, stomatitis, cheilosis, scurvy
- **Endocrine and metabolic systems:** Increased incidence of diabetes mellitus, hyperlipidemia, hyperuricemia, and gout
- **Genitourinary system:** Hypogonadism, increased secondary female sexual characteristics in people assigned male at birth (hypoandrogenization and hyperestrogenization), erectile dysfunction, electrolyte imbalances due to excess urinary secretion of potassium and magnesium
- **Hematologic system:** Anemias, leukemia, hematomas
- **Immune system:** Impaired immune functioning, higher incidence of infectious diseases, including tuberculosis and other bacterial infections
- **Integumentary system:** Skin lesions, increased incidence of infection, burns, and other traumatic injury
- **Musculoskeletal system:** Increased incidence of traumatic injury, myopathy
- **Nervous system:** Withdrawal symptoms, irritability, depression, anxiety disorders, sleep disorders, phobias, paranoid feelings, diminished brain size and functioning, organic brain disorders, blackouts, cerebellar degeneration, neuropathies, palsies, gait disturbances, visual issues
- **Respiratory system:** Increased rate of pneumonia and other respiratory infections

TABLE 31.8 ALCOHOL WITHDRAWAL SYNDROME

	Stage I: Mild	Stage II: Moderate	Stage III: Severe
Vital signs	Heart rate elevated, temperature elevated, normal or slightly elevated systolic blood pressure	Heart rate, 100–120 bpm; elevated systolic blood pressure and temperature	Heart rate, 120–140 bpm; elevated systolic and diastolic blood pressures; elevated temperature
Diaphoresis	Slight	Usually obvious	Marked
Central nervous system	Oriented; no confusion; no hallucinations Mild anxiety and restlessness Restless sleep Hand tremors; "shakes"; no convulsions	Intermittent confusion; transient visual and auditory hallucinations and illusions (mostly at night) Painful anxiety and motor restlessness Insomnia and nightmares Visible tremulousness, rare convulsions	Marked disorientation, confusion, disturbing visual and auditory hallucinations, misidentification of objects, delusions related to the hallucinations, delirium tremens, disturbances in consciousness Agitation, extreme restlessness, and panic states Unable to sleep Gross uncontrollable tremors, convulsions common
Gastrointestinal system	Impaired appetite, nausea	Anorexia, nausea, and vomiting	Rejecting all fluid and food

BOX 31.12

Clinical Institute Withdrawal Assessment of Alcohol Scale, Revised (CIWA-Ar)

Patient: ______________ **Date:** ______________ **Time:** ______________ (24-h clock, midnight = 00:00)

Pulse or heart rate, taken for 1 min: ______________ **Blood pressure:** ______________

NAUSEA AND VOMITING—Ask, "Do you feel sick to your stomach? Have you vomited?" Observation.

0 no nausea and no vomiting
1 mild nausea with no vomiting
2
3
4 intermittent nausea with dry heaves
5
6
7 constant nausea, frequent dry heaves and vomiting

TACTILE DISTURBANCES—Ask, "Have you any itching, pins and needles sensations, any burning, any numbness, or do you feel bugs crawling on or under your skin?" Observation.

0 none
1 very mild itching, pins and needles, burning or numbness
2 mild itching, pins and needles, burning or numbness
3 moderate itching, pins and needles, burning or numbness
4 moderately severe hallucinations
5 severe hallucinations
6 extremely severe hallucinations
7 continuous hallucinations

TREMOR—Arms extended and fingers spread apart.

Observation.

0 no tremor
1 not visible but can be felt fingertip to fingertip
2
3
4 moderate, with patient's arms extended
5
6
7 severe, even with arms not extended

AUDITORY DISTURBANCES—Ask, "Are you more aware of sounds around you? Are they harsh? Do they frighten you? Are you hearing anything that is disturbing to you? Are you hearing things you know are not there?" Observation.

0 not present
1 very mild harshness or ability to frighten
2 mild harshness or ability to frighten
3 moderate harshness or ability to frighten
4 moderately severe hallucinations
5 severe hallucinations
6 extremely severe hallucinations
7 continuous hallucinations

PAROXYSMAL SWEATS—Observation.

0 no sweat visible
1 barely perceptible sweating, palms moist
2
3
4 beads of sweat obvious on forehead
5
6
7 drenching sweats

VISUAL DISTURBANCES—Ask, "Does the light appear to be too bright? Is its color different? Does it hurt your eyes? Are you seeing anything that is disturbing to you? Are you seeing things you know are not there?" Observation.

0 not present
1 very mild sensitivity
2 mild sensitivity
3 moderate sensitivity
4 moderately severe hallucinations
5 severe hallucinations
6 extremely severe hallucinations
7 continuous hallucinations

ANXIETY—Ask, "Do you feel nervous?" Observation.

0 no anxiety, at ease
1 mild anxious
2
3
4 moderately anxious, or guarded, so anxiety is inferred
5
6
7 equivalent to acute panic states as seen in severe delirium or acute schizophrenic reactions

HEADACHE, FULLNESS IN HEAD—Ask, "Does your head feel different? Does it feel like there is a band around your head?" Do not rate for dizziness or lightheadedness. Otherwise, rate severity.

0 not present
1 very mild
2 mild
3 moderate
4 moderately severe
5 severe
6 very severe
7 extremely severe

AGITATION—Observation.

0 normal activity
1 somewhat more than normal activity
2
3
4 moderately fidgety and restless
5
6
7 paces back and forth during most of the interview, or constantly thrashes about

ORIENTATION AND CLOUDING OF SENSORIUM—Ask, "What day is this? Where are you? Who am I?"

0 oriented and can do serial additions
1 cannot do serial additions or is uncertain about date
2 disoriented for date by no more than 2 calendar days
3 disoriented for date by more than 2 calendar days
4 disoriented for place/or person

Total **CIWA-Ar** Score ______
Rater's Initials ______
Maximum Possible Score 67

The ***CIWA-Ar*** is not copyrighted and may be reproduced freely. This assessment for monitoring withdrawal symptoms requires approximately 5 minutes to administer. The maximum score is 67 (see instrument). Patients scoring less than 10 do not usually need additional medication for withdrawal.

Sullivan, J. T., Sykora, K., Schneiderman, J., Naranjo, C. A., & Sellers, E. M. (1989). Assessment of alcohol withdrawal: The revised clinical institute withdrawal assessment for alcohol scale (**CIWA-Ar**). *British Journal of Addiction*, *84*, 1353–1357.

It can be challenging to recognize, prevent, and treat AWS. Astute assessment of withdrawal symptoms, use of appropriate screening tools, and closely following hospital protocols while simultaneous handling complex critically ill patients (who may be denying they need help) and the concerns of worried family members will test the knowledge and skills of the nurse.

Medications for Alcohol Withdrawal Syndrome

Several medications are used to prevent physiologic complications and provide a gradual withdrawal from alcohol. Antianxiety and sedating drugs, such as benzodiazepines, are titrated downwardly over several days as a substitution for alcohol. Chlordiazepoxide and diazepam have longer half-lives and smoother tapers. Lorazepam is better for older adults and people with liver impairment. Antidepressants, mood stabilizers, anticonvulsants, and antiemetics are all used as necessary. Sleep medications are used to promote a regular sleep pattern.

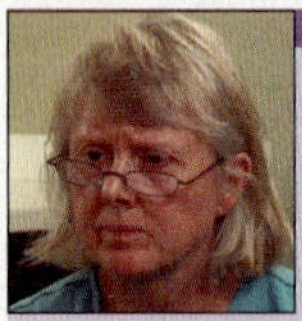

Remember Gladys?

Gladys abruptly stopped her alcohol intake when she was admitted to the hospital for depression and suicidal thoughts. She did not tell her primary care provider that her intake of alcohol was significant. She began to go through withdrawal.

Prevention of Relapse

Relapse prevention is important in the recovery of people with all substance-related disorders, including AUD.

Psychosocial Interventions

Prevention efforts include psychosocial interventions such as psychoeducation and self-help groups (e.g., **Alcoholics Anonymous** [AA], Alcoholics Anonymous Agnostics [AAA], and Smart Recovery). These interventions are discussed earlier in this chapter.

Medications

Medications are also used for recovery in AUD, include **disulfiram**, **acamprosate**, and naltrexone. Disulfiram is used to help deter some individuals from drinking. Disulfiram plus even small amounts of alcohol produces episodes of severe nausea and vomiting. These unpleasant reactions may deter drinking. Severe reactions may also occur, including respiratory depression, cardiovascular collapse, convulsions, and death. Those taking this drug must be informed about consuming or being in contact with unexpected sources of alcohol, such as food additives, aftershave, or hand sanitizers.

Acamprosate is used to decrease alcohol intake. Acamprosate is effective only if the individual is abstinent from alcohol prior to its initiation. The maintenance dose (333 to 666 mg orally) must be taken with meals three times daily, which can discourage adherence to treatment.

Naltrexone was originally used as a treatment for heroin misuse, but it is now also approved for the treatment of alcohol dependence. See Box 31.13. Naltrexone is formulated in a once-daily pill and a monthly injection (Vivitrol). It is given for alcohol and opioid dependence. Naltrexone does not treat withdrawal symptoms but totally blocks the effects of both alcohol and opioids. Warn patients not to use other drugs while on this medication. Those taking naltrexone should wear or carry an identification card in case of accidents, because no narcotic can be given for emergency use. Naltrexone has no misuse potential and does not result in the development of physical dependence. Naltrexone can: (1) reduce craving (the urge or desire to drink or use drugs despite negative consequences), (2) help maintain abstinence, and (3) interfere with the tendency to want to drink more if a recovering patient slips and has a drink. Patients have been known to stop using naltrexone if they plan to drink alcohol and restart it later, leaving them open to relapsing.

Naltrexone can also be administered via an intramuscular injection, which must be given after opioid detoxification and may cause injection site reactions, including intense hip pain, induration, swelling, bruising, and severe reactions such as open wounds or sterile abscesses. Patients must have adequate gluteal muscle mass to support a 4 mL injection, and nurses must carefully monitor and rotate injection sites. Adverse reactions and pain at the injection site can contribute to nonadherence with therapy.

Alcohol-Induced Amnestic Disorders

Patients with alcohol-induced **amnestic disorders** usually have a history of many years of heavy alcohol use. These individuals may experience **Wernicke encephalopathy** followed by **Korsakoff syndrome**, which are alcohol-induced amnesic disorders associated with deficiencies in dietary intake of folic acid and thiamine (and other B vitamins) (Canver et al., 2024). Wernicke encephalopathy is an acute neurologic condition characterized by ocular dysfunction, ataxia, and confusion. Wernicke encephalopathy causes brain damage in the thalamus and hypothalamus and is life-threatening. It is treated with thiamine. In a small number of cases, Korsakoff syndrome develops. These disorders are sometimes referred to as the **Wernicke–Korsakoff syndrome**.

The cardinal symptoms of Korsakoff syndrome are short-term memory disturbance and **confabulation** (i.e., telling a plausible but imagined scenario to compensate for memory impairment), ocular dysfunction, inability to speak coherently, and ataxia (Vasan & Kumar, 2023).

BOX 31.13

Medication Profile: Naltrexone

DRUG CLASS: Narcotic antagonist

RECEPTOR AFFINITY: Binds to opioid receptors in the CNS and competitively inhibits the action of opioid drugs, including those with mixed narcotic agonist–antagonist properties

INDICATIONS: Adjunctive treatment of alcohol or narcotic dependence as part of a comprehensive treatment program

DOSAGE AND ADMINISTRATION: Available in 50-mg tablets

Adults: For alcohol use disorder: 50 mg/day PO; for narcotic dependence: initial dose of 25 mg PO; if no signs or symptoms seen, complete dose with 25 mg. Usual maintenance dose is 50 mg/day PO.

Injectable intramuscular dose 380 mg/mo, rotate and inspect gluteal sites of injection.

Children: Safety has not been established for use in children younger than 18 yrs.

HALF-LIFE (PEAK EFFECT): 3.9 to 12.9 h (60 min)

SELECTED SIDE EFFECTS: Difficulty sleeping, anxiety, nervousness, headache, low energy, abdominal pain or cramps, nausea, vomiting, delayed ejaculations, decreased potency, rash, chills, increased thirst, joint and muscle pain

WARNINGS: Contraindicated in pregnancy and patients allergic to narcotic antagonists. Use cautiously in narcotic dependence because the drug may produce withdrawal symptoms. Do not administer unless patient has been opioid free for 7 to 10 days; verify with a negative urine screen. Also, use cautiously in patients with acute hepatitis, liver failure, depression, or suicidal tendencies and in those who are breastfeeding. Must make certain patient is opioid free before administering naltrexone.

SPECIFIC PATIENT AND FAMILY EDUCATION

- Understand that this drug will help facilitate abstinence from alcohol and block the effects of narcotics.
- Wear a medical identification tag to alert emergency personnel that you are taking this drug.
- Avoid the use of heroin or other opioid drugs; small doses may have no effect, but large doses can cause death, serious injury, or coma.
- Report any signs and symptoms of adverse effects.
- Notify other health care providers that you are taking this drug.
- Keep appointments for follow-up blood tests and treatment program.

CNS, central nervous system; PO, oral.

STIMULANT USE DISORDER

Amphetamines

Amphetamines, or stimulants, are known on the street as speed or uppers. They are used to treat attention-deficit hyperactivity disorder (ADHD) in adults and children, narcolepsy, depression, and obesity (on a short-term basis). Some people misuse these drugs to achieve the effects of alertness, increased concentration, a sense of increased energy, euphoria, and appetite suppression. The stimulation results in tachycardia, arrhythmias, increased systolic and diastolic blood pressures, and peripheral hyperthermia. The effects of amphetamine use, and the clinical course of an overdose, are like those of cocaine.

Methamphetamine

Methamphetamine, also known as meth, speed, ice, chalk, crank, and crystal, is an illegal potent CNS stimulant that releases excess dopamine responsible for the drug's toxic effects, including damage to nerve terminals. Highly addictive, it comes in many forms and can be smoked, snorted, orally ingested, or injected. This illegal substance is cheap, easy to make, and has devastating consequences. Methamphetamine has a much longer duration of action, and a larger percentage of the drug remains unchanged in the body.

High doses can elevate body temperature and stimulate seizures. Methamphetamine has a longer duration of action than cocaine and leads to prolonged stimulant effects. Long-term effects include dependence and psychosis (e.g., paranoia, hallucinations), mood disturbances, violent behavior, repetitive motor activity, stroke, intense itching leading to skin sores from scratching, weight loss, and extensive tooth decay

Long-term meth use, like cocaine use, can cause cardiac arrhythmias. Babies born to birth parents who used meth during pregnancy are highly irritable and frequently present with learning or other developmental delays. Parents/guardians dependent on methamphetamine often cannot meet parenting responsibilities even after abstaining. They often need continuing support to achieve the parenting role, including interdisciplinary support from child welfare and substance use treatment services (NIDA, 2022b).

See also the "MDMA and Other 'Club Drugs'" section in the "Other Types of Drugs That Can Be Misused" section later in this chapter.

Cocaine Use Disorder

Cocaine (also known as coke, crack, snow, nose candy, flake, blow, big c, lady, white, or snowbirds) is a white crystalline powder, commonly inhaled (or "snorted"), injected intravenously (with water), or smoked. Crack cocaine, often simply called "crack," is a form of free-base cocaine that gets its name from the crackling sound of the rock as it is heated. This extremely potent form produces a rapid high with intense euphoria and a dramatic crash. It is extremely addictive because of the intense and rapid onset of euphoric effects, which leave people who use it craving more. Enhanced sexual experiences and drive can get many started on regular use.

The cocaine high is followed by an intense let-down characterized by irritability, depression, fatigue, and intense drug cravings. As tolerance develops, and higher doses are needed to produce the high and prevent withdrawal, cocaine toxicity can increase the risk of overdose. Although people who use cocaine typically report that the drug enhances their feelings of well-being and reduces anxiety, cocaine is also known to bring on panic attacks. Behaviors around cocaine use can also contribute to STIs and to toxic, potentially catastrophic cardiovascular issues, which may become chronic even in those whose exposure to cocaine is limited to occasional, adult use (NIDA, 2024a).

Biologic Responses to Cocaine

Cocaine is absorbed rapidly through the blood–brain barrier and is also readily absorbed through skin and mucous membranes. Increased dopamine causes euphoria and psychotic symptoms. Cocaine also increases norepinephrine levels in the blood, causing tachycardia, hypertension, dilated pupils, and rising body temperatures. Serotonin excess contributes to sleep disturbances and anorexia. With prolonged cocaine use, these neurotransmitters are eventually depleted. Long-term cocaine misuse frequently leads to permanent cardiovascular damage and cardiovascular crisis (Cocaine Heart).

Cocaine Intoxication

Cocaine intoxication causes CNS stimulation, the length of which depends on the dosage and route of administration. With steadily increasing doses, restlessness proceeds to tremors and agitation followed by convulsions and CNS depression. In lethal overdose, death generally results from respiratory failure. Toxic psychosis is also possible; it may be accompanied by physical signs of CNS stimulation (e.g., tachycardia, hypertension, cardiac arrhythmias, sweating, hyperpyrexia, convulsions). Cocaine and alcohol taken together can cause drug-related death (van Amsterdam et al., 2024).

Cocaine Withdrawal

Cocaine withdrawal symptoms are not as life-threatening as in alcohol withdrawal. Withdrawal causes intense depression, craving (i.e., a strong desire to use cocaine despite negative consequences), and drug-seeking behavior that may last for weeks. Individuals who discontinue cocaine use often relapse because of the powerful effects it has on the brain's limbic system (reward center for pleasure and motivation) and the strong cravings that remain after withdrawal. Because cocaine has a short half-life, withdrawal symptoms can start within 90 minutes of the last dose.

> **NCLEXNOTE** In cocaine withdrawal, patients are excessively sleepy because of norepinephrine depletion. Recovery is difficult because of the intense cravings. Nursing interventions should focus on helping patients manage cravings because there is no medical detoxification.

Treatment

There are no medications approved to treat cocaine use disorder. Behavioral treatment programs that have shown to be effective include CBT and contingency management programs. **Contingency management programs** use motivational incentives such as a voucher or prize-based reward system to help patients abstain from cocaine and other drugs. **Therapeutic communities** are drug-free residences where residents can help each other understand and change their behaviors. These communities require a 6- to 12-month stay (NIDA, 2024a).

Nicotine Use Disorder (Tobacco Use Disorder; Nicotine Dependence)

Nicotine is the addictive chemical mainly responsible for the high prevalence of tobacco use. The use of e-cigarettes (vaping) has increased substantially over the last decade, especially among youth who have not been exposed to cigarettes (Lyzwinski et al., 2022). Additionally, smoking is two to three times more prevalent in people with mental illnesses than the general population and is two to three times higher among those with schizophrenia, bipolar disorder, posttraumatic stress disorder (PTSD), and alcohol/illicit drug use disorders (Sprenger & Anderson, 2024).

Biologic Response to Nicotine

Nicotine stimulates the central, peripheral, and autonomic nervous systems, causing increased alertness, concentration, attention, and appetite suppression. Nicotine activates dopamine, GABA, acetylcholine, and glutamatergic receptors. Readily absorbed, it is carried in the bloodstream to the liver, where it is partially metabolized. It is also metabolized by the kidneys and excreted in urine. There is emerging evidence that nicotine interacts with the epigenetic mechanism that enables nicotine-seeking behavior (Kim & Picciotto, 2023; Muenstermann & Clemens, 2024).

Smoking tobacco causes respiratory issues, lung cancer, emphysema, heart issues, and peripheral vascular disease. In fact, smoking is the largest preventable cause of premature death and disability.

Repeated use of nicotine produces both tolerance and dependence. Recent research has shown that nicotine use disorder is extremely powerful and is at least as strong as dependence on other drugs; 90% of the people who quit relapse within 1 year (NIDA, 2021; Truth Initiative, 2024).

Nicotine Withdrawal and Smoking Cessation

Nicotine withdrawal is marked by mood changes (e.g., craving, anxiety, irritability, depression) and physiologic changes (difficulty in concentrating, sleep disturbances, headaches, gastric distress, increased appetite). Nicotine replacements, such as nicotine transdermal patches, nicotine gum, nasal spray, and inhalers, have been used successfully to assist in withdrawal by reducing the craving for tobacco. The antidepressant bupropion is used to help people quit smoking. Many people who smoke purchase e-cigarettes (vaping) to attempt smoking cessation, and these products contain varying amounts of nicotine. The long-term health effects of e-cigarettes remain unknown, but cautions are increasing around possible lung damage (Gaba et al., 2023; Herzog et al., 2024); vaping cessation, which needs exploration, might be as difficult as stopping smoking. Individualized approaches that promote intentions, support attempts, and encourage cessation may be most effective (Amin et al., 2023). Youth are particularly drawn to vaping, and regulatory attempts to control vaping marketing to youth have not made much of an impact; according to the USFDA and the CDC, 1.61 million US middle and high school students reported e-cigarette use in the past 30 days in 2024 (U.S. FDA, 2024).

Caffeine Use Disorder

Caffeine is a stimulant found in many drinks (coffee, tea, cocoa, soft drinks), chocolate, and over-the-counter (OTC) medications, including analgesics, stimulants, appetite suppressants, and cold relief preparations. High-energy drinks, consisting of alcohol and caffeine, are being marketed to reduce the impairment caused by ingestion of alcohol. The reality is that these energy drinks give a false sense of physical and mental competence and decrease the awareness of impairment. Caffeine use disorder remains under investigation for inclusion in the DSM, but it is defined as a problematic pattern of caffeine consumption characterized by a persistent desire to cut down, or control use, along with unsuccessful efforts to do so, and issues caused by worsening use. Significant withdrawal symptoms or use of caffeine to avoid withdrawal symptoms are characteristic. This condition is still under study and attempts are being made to raise awareness of caffeine's potential to cause distress (Bodur et al., 2024).

Symptoms of caffeine intoxication can include the following: scattered thoughts, excessive talking, inability to focus on anything, irritability, elevated blood pressure, increased heart rate, nausea, anxiety, heart palpitations (arrhythmias), insomnia, sweating, dizziness, vomiting, cardiac arrest. These may also appear in people with no tolerance or high caffeine sensitivity (Brower & Swatek, 2024).

Caffeine withdrawal syndrome involves headache, drowsiness, and fatigue, sometimes with impaired psychomotor performance; difficulty concentrating; craving; and psychophysiological complaints, such as yawning or nausea.

CANNABIS (MARIJUANA) USE DISORDER

Marijuana

Marijuana is the common name for the plant *Cannabis sativa*, also known as hemp and many other names. Marijuana is fat soluble and is absorbed rapidly after being smoked or taken orally. After ingestion, the psychoactive substance THC can be stored for weeks in fat tissue and in the brain and is released extremely slowly. Urine drug screens will show positive for marijuana for 4 to 6 weeks after use. Marijuana use impairs the ability to form memories, recall events, and shift attention from one thing to another. It disrupts coordination of movement, balance, and reaction time. Contrary to popular belief, marijuana is an addictive substance, is an irritant to the lungs, and can produce the same respiratory issues experienced by people who use tobacco (i.e., daily cough, phlegm) (Gorelick, 2023). Emerging research suggests that frequent marijuana smoking contributes to the risk of breast and lung cancer (Niu et al., 2024).

It is a top research priority to understand how marijuana affects memory and learning in adolescents (APA, 2023), especially because use has increased among youth (Hughes et al., 2022). Smoking during pregnancy is extremely dangerous because cannabis exposure alters developmental regions in the fetal brain, with functional consequences associated with social behavior and executive functioning, lasting throughout life (Motamedi et al., 2023). See Box 31.14.

Marijuana causes relaxation, euphoria, at times dyscoria (i.e., unexpected pupillary reaction or shape), spatial misperception, time distortion, and food cravings. It also causes relaxation and drowsiness, unlike other hallucinogens, and is often associated with decreased motivation after long-term use The known safety issues related to marijuana use, especially in high doses, include impairment of short-term memory, altered judgment and decision-making, anxiety, and paranoia or psychosis (Gorelick, 2023).

The FDA has approved drugs containing marijuana, such as dronabinol and nabilone for therapeutic use, such as for anorexia associated with weight loss in acquired immunodeficiency syndrome (AIDS) and nausea and vomiting associated with cancer chemotherapy (NG & Keshock, 2023). Marijuana is legal for adult nonmedical use in some states in the United States.

"Spice" and "K2" are some of the trade names used for synthetic cannabinoid compounds found in various herbal mixtures that produce an experience like that of marijuana. The effects of synthetic cannabinoids can be

BOX 31.14

Research for Evidence-Based Practice: Prenatal Cannabis Use and Maternal Pregnancy Outcomes

Young-Wolff, K. C., Adams, S. R., Alexeeff, S. E., Zhu, Y., Chojolan, E., Slama, N. E., Does, M. B., Silver, L. D., Ansley, D., Castellanos, C. L., & Avalos, L. A. (2024). Prenatal cannabis use and maternal pregnancy outcomes. JAMA Internal Medicine, 184*(9), 1083–1093.* https://doi.org/10.1001/jamainternmed.2024.3270

THE QUESTION: Is prenatal cannabis use associated with maternal health outcomes?

METHODS: In a large retrospective cohort study of over 300,000 singleton pregnancies during 2011–2019 that lasted 20 weeks or longer, the exposure of cannabis was measured at the beginning of prenatal care via a self-administered questionnaire and urine toxicology test. Individuals were classified as having cannabis use since pregnancy if they self-reported cannabis use since pregnancy or had a positive confirmed toxicology test result.

FINDINGS: Over 20,000 screened positive for prenatal cannabis use. Prenatal cannabis use was associated with greater risk of gestational hypertension, preeclampsia, gestational weight gain outside of guidelines, and placenta abruption. Prenatal cannabis use was associated with a greater risk of eclampsia but did not reach level of significance. Prenatal cannabis use was also associated with a lower risk of gestational diabetes.

IMPLICATIONS FOR NURSING: These results suggest a complex relationship between prenatal cannabis use and neonatal outcomes. Nurses should educate patients about the association of prenatal cannabis use with negative neonatal outcomes in order for patients to make informed decisions about using cannabis during pregnancy.

unpredictable and severe or even life-threatening. Spice products are popular among young people, and they are legally sold in convenience stores, gas stations, drug paraphernalia shops, novelty stores, and online. Fatalities can occur, and there is no antidote available (de Oliveira et al., 2023). In recent years there has been significant growth in product manufacturing, sale, and use of synthetics. Although some states have passed legislation to prohibit use of specific synthetics, the volume and rapid emergence of new products has made it a challenge for regulatory control agencies to keep up.

OPIOID USE DISORDER

Opioids

The terms *opiates* and *opioids* are often used interchangeably, but they are different. The term **opiate** refers to a narcotic analgesic derived from an opium poppy and includes opium, morphine, and codeine. The term **opioid** refers to synthetic derivatives such as heroin, fentanyl, hydromorphone, methadone, buprenorphine. This text will use the term opioids to represent both opiates and synthetically derived opioids. **Opioid use disorder** (OUD) occurs when the chronic use of opioids causes significant distress or impairment (Dydyk et al., 2024).

Even centuries after their discovery, opioids are still the most effective pain relievers. Opioids also cause CNS depression, sleep, or stupor. Some opioids such as heroin have no medicinal use and are illegal in the United States, but others such as morphine and codeine are used to treat pain related to illnesses (e.g., cancer) and during medical and dental procedures. Still others such as methadone and buprenorphine are used in treatment of OUD. When used as directed by a clinician, opioids are safe and generally do not lead to OUD. However, opioids also possess very strong reinforcing properties and can quickly trigger dependence when used improperly. Even when pain is present, these medications should be used only as needed and never given on a schedule.

Two important effects produced by opioids are pleasure (or reward) and pain relief. Tolerance develops easily. When tolerance exists, a 100% increase in dose is often needed to achieve the same physical effects. Physical and psychological dependence develop rapidly. When the use of the drug is discontinued after a period of continuous use, withdrawal occurs. Table 31.9 describes the onset, duration, and symptoms of mild, moderate, and severe opioid withdrawal symptoms. See Table 31.9.

Epidemiology

Opioid use and misuse became a national public health issue in 2000, primarily in the United States. More recently, about one-fourth of the patients prescribed opioids for chronic pain misuse them, and between 8% and 12% develop OUD (Oelhaf et al., 2023). OUD occurs in individuals from all socioeconomic and educational backgrounds. Although people assigned female at birth are prescribed opioids for analgesia more often, people assigned male at birth account for the majority of opioid-related overdoses (Dydyk et al., 2024).

Heroin and Other Opioids

Heroin is the most misused and the most rapidly acting of the opioids. It can be sniffed, snorted, and smoked but is most frequently injected. Other opioids can have the same effect as heroin and pose risks for transmission of HIV, hepatitis C, and other diseases resulting from the sharing of needles or other injection equipment. Heroin produces profound degrees of tolerance and physical and psychological dependence, which are powerful motivating factors for compulsive misuse. People who use heroin

TABLE 31.9 SEVERITY OF OPIOID WITHDRAWAL SYNDROME

Initial Onset and Duration	Mild Withdrawal	Moderate Withdrawal	Severe Withdrawal
Onset: 8–12 h after last use of short-acting opioids. 1–3 days after the last use for longer-acting opioids, such as methadone	Physical: yawning, rhinorrhea, perspiration, restlessness, lacrimation, sleep disturbance	Physical: dilated pupils, bone and muscle aches, sensation of "goose flesh," hot and cold flashes	Nausea; vomiting; stomach cramps; diarrhea; weight loss; insomnia; twitching of muscles and kicking movements of legs; increased blood pressure, pulse, and respirations
Duration: Severe symptoms peak between 48 and 72 h. Symptoms abate in 7–10 days for short-acting opioids. Methadone withdrawal symptoms can last several weeks	Emotional: increased craving, anxiety, dysphoria	Emotional: irritability, increased anxiety, and craving	Emotional: depression, increased anxiety, dysphoria, subjective sense of feeling "wretched"

gradually spend more and more time and energy obtaining and using the drug until these activities become their primary purpose in life (Oelhaf & Azadfard, 2023).

Opioids act primarily on three receptors: mu, kappa, and delta. These are found in the central and peripheral nervous systems and in central respiratory centers. All opioids are selective for the mu receptor. The mu receptors are thought to be responsible for the analgesia, respiratory suppression, bradycardia, physical dependence, GI dysmotility, and euphoria. The kappa receptor is responsible for the hallucinations and dysphoria and the delta receptor for pain control and mood modulation effects (Oelhaf et al., 2023). Chronic use leads to physical dependence on an external source of opioids as the cells producing endogenous opioids cease to function and degenerate (Oelhaf & Azadfard, 2023).

Fentanyl

Between 2017 and 2023, there has been a sharp increase (67%) in opioid deaths attributed primarily to **fentanyl**, a powerful synthetic opioid that is 50 to 100 times more powerful than morphine and is available illegally and by prescription (Saunders et al., 2024). There are two types of fentanyl: pharmaceutical fentanyl and illegally made fentanyl. Although fentanyl prescription rates have remained relatively stable, there have been unprecedented increases in the global supply, processing, and distribution of illegally made fentanyl by criminal elements. See Figure 31.1. It is often added as an **adulterant** (contaminant) to other drugs because of its potency, which makes drugs cheaper, more powerful, and more dangerous (CDC, 2024).

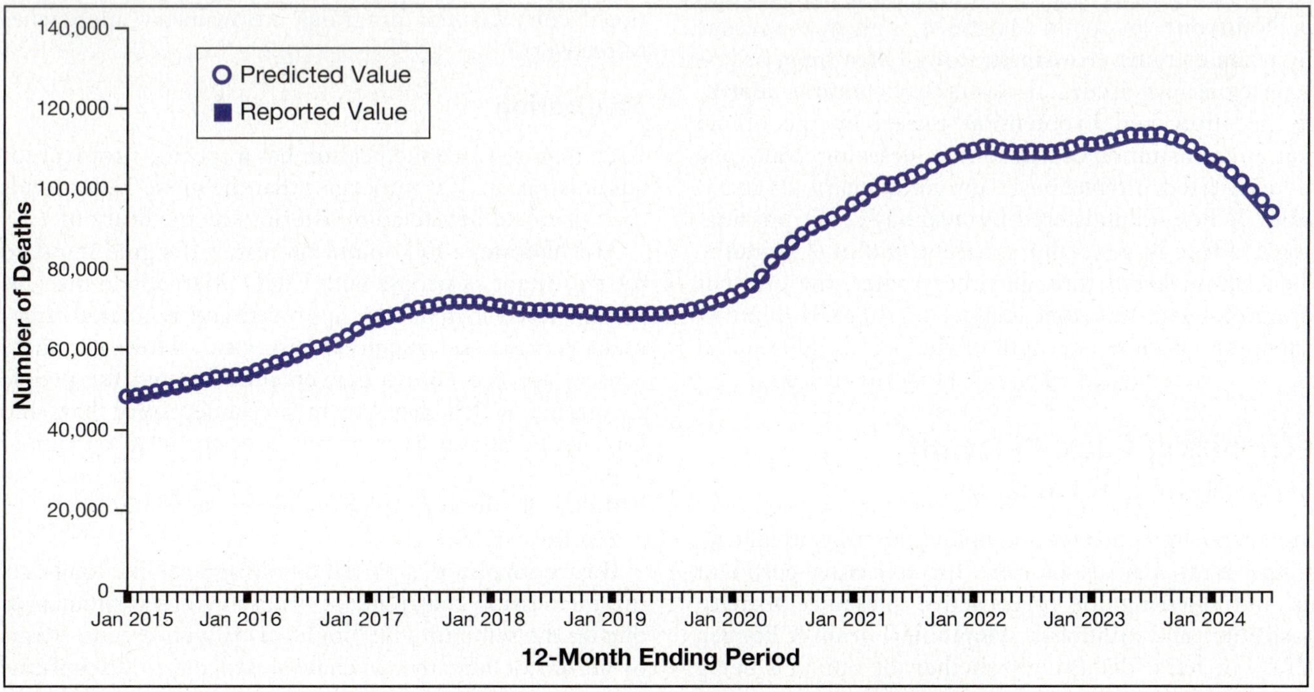

FIGURE 31.1 National provisional drug overdose death counts. (Reprinted from National Center for Health Statistics. VSRR Provisional Drug Overdose Death Counts. (2024). https://www.cdc.gov/nchs/nvss/vsrr/drug-overdose-data.htm)

Xylazine Adulterant

One of the deadliest drug threats the United States has ever faced is the introduction of **xylazine** as an adulterant into the supply of illicit drugs. This powerful, nonopioid, sedative, analgesic, and muscle relaxant is authorized only for veterinary use. Because of the stupor that it induces, it has been dubbed the "zombie drug" or "tranq" (short for tranquilizer). Xylazine and fentanyl drug mixtures place those who use these substances at a higher risk of suffering a fatal drug poisoning. Because xylazine is not an opioid, naloxone does not reverse its effects. Survival often depends on the availability of immediate respiratory support. However, experts always recommend administering naloxone if someone might be suffering from a drug overdose (Edinoff et al., 2024).

People who inject drug mixtures containing xylazine also can develop severe wounds, including necrosis that may lead to amputation (USDEA, 2023). Withdrawal is complicated by excruciating wounds, and the understanding of this drug's effects on humans is still in its infancy. As of the writing of this chapter, xylazine has not been added to the government's list of controlled substances, though the White House's Office of National Drug Control Policy has declared it an emerging threat.

Opioid Toxicity or Overdose

Emergency treatment of individuals with opioid intoxication is initiated with an assessment of CNS functioning, specifically arousal and respiratory functioning. Toxicity is primarily due to hypoxia from hypoventilation. **Naloxone**, an opioid antagonist, is given as a rescue drug when extreme drowsiness, slowed breathing, or loss of consciousness occurs. It reverses respiratory depression, sedation, and hypotension caused by the opioid agent. Administration of naloxone is lifesaving. Naloxone is administered intravenously, intramuscularly, or intranasally. When administered intravenously, the pharmacologic effect is generally apparent within 2 minutes. When administered through other routes, the effect is more prolonged. Naloxone is active for 30 to 81 minutes. Depending upon the strength of the opioid, subsequent doses are often needed when reversing the overdose.

Recognizing Cues: Relevant Assessment Information

People who are dependent on opioids are seen in all care settings. Nurses are responsible for collecting pertinent data and assessing for psychoactive substance toxicity, intoxication, and withdrawal symptoms (Fornili & Fogger, 2022). The nurse determines whether the opioid is being misused through a careful assessment of the amount, frequency, and pattern of use. Misuse occurs if the patient is not taking the opioid as prescribed or takes an opioid that is illegally obtained. The nurse also determines whether the patient is experiencing opioid toxicity with risk of overdose (medical emergency) or beginning to withdraw from opioids. The *Clinical Opiate Withdrawal Scale* (COWS) is a clinician-administered instrument that quantifies the degree of withdrawal on 11 physical findings and is used in many settings (Wesson & Ling, 2003).

Taking Action: Nursing Interventions

Opioid Detoxification

Opioid withdrawal is not life-threatening but is extremely uncomfortable and difficult. Ideally, opioid detoxification is achieved by gradually reducing an opioid dose over several days or weeks. Many treatment programs administer low doses of a substitute drug, such as buprenorphine or methadone, which can help satisfy the drug craving without providing the same subjective high. If opioids are abruptly withdrawn ("cold turkey") from someone who is physically dependent on them, severe physical symptoms occur, including body aches, diarrhea, tachycardia, fever, runny nose, sneezing, sweating, yawning, nausea or vomiting, nervousness, restlessness, or irritability, shivering or trembling, abdominal cramps, weakness, elevated blood pressure, and severe distress.

Maintenance Treatment

Psychosocial Approaches

Like other recovery approaches for SUD, OUD focuses on enhancing physical and psychological well-being and reducing the risk of relapse. CBT, self-help, and motivational enhancement programs are mainstay approaches to recovery.

Medication

Each maintenance medication has a specific protocol for administration. It is important that the nurse understands each protocol before administering the medication.

Methadone, a full opioid agonist, is the gold standard for treatment of people with OUD. Methadone must be administered in federally approved and regulated treatment centers and requires daily visits. However, these centers are not always conveniently located for people to attend, which can create an unnecessary hardship for anyone trying to maintain sobriety from an opioid dependence. Stopping methadone abruptly has the same withdrawal effects as stopping heroin suddenly.

See Box 31.15.

Buprenorphine, a partial opioid agonist, is a long-acting medication that relieves drug cravings without producing the same intense "high" or dangerous side effects of heroin or fentanyl. It enables patients to discontinue the misuse of opioids without experiencing withdrawal symptoms. Buprenorphine carries a lower risk of misuse and side effects, compared with full opioid agonists (methadone). See Box 31.16.

BOX 31.15

Medication Profile: Methadone

DRUG CLASS: Narcotic agonist, analgesic

RECEPTOR AFFINITY: Binds to opioid receptors in the CNS to produce analgesia, euphoria, sedation; the receptors mediating the effects of endogenous opioids, which are thought to be enkephalins or endorphins

INDICATIONS: Detoxification and temporary maintenance treatment of narcotic dependence; relief of severe pain

DOSAGE AND ADMINISTRATION: Available in 5-, 10-, and 40-mg tablets; oral concentrate

Adults: Detoxification: Initially 15 to 30 mg. Increase dosage to suppress withdrawal signs. 40 mg/day in single or divided dose is usually an adequate stabilizing dose; continue stabilizing dose for 2 to 3 days; then gradually decrease dosage. Usual maintenance dose is 20 to 120 mg/day in single dosing.

HALF-LIFE (PEAK EFFECT):

PO 90 to 120 min

IM 1 to 2 h

SC 1 to 2 h

SAFE HANDLING: Store in a safe, locked place, use a calibrated measuring device, supervised adherence may continue for at least 6 mo or longer. Dispense in a child-resistant container if home consumption is planned.

SELECTED SIDE EFFECTS: Lightheadedness, dizziness, sedation, nausea, vomiting, facial flushing, peripheral circulatory collapse, arrhythmia, palpitations, urethral spasm, urinary retention, respiratory depression, circulatory depression, respiratory arrest, shock, cardiac arrest

WARNINGS: Never administer in the presence of hypersensitivity to narcotics, diarrhea caused by poisoning (before toxins are eliminated), bronchial asthma, or chronic obstructive pulmonary disease. Use caution in the presence of acute abdominal conditions and cardiovascular disease. Increased effect and toxicity of methadone are observed if taken concurrently with cimetidine and/or ranitidine. Methadone hydrochloride tablets are for PO administration only and *must not* be used for injection. It is recommended that methadone hydrochloride tablets, if dispensed, be packaged in child-resistant containers and kept out of the reach of children to prevent accidental injection.

SPECIFIC PATIENT AND FAMILY EDUCATION

- Avoid use of alcohol in any form.
- Take the drug exactly as prescribed.
- Take the drug with food while lying quietly; this should minimize nausea.
- Eat small, frequent meals to treat nausea and loss of appetite.
- If experiencing dizziness and drowsiness, avoid driving a car or performing other tasks that require alertness.
- Administer mild laxative for constipation.
- Report severe nausea, vomiting, constipation, shortness of breath, or difficulty breathing. Methadone products, when used for treatment of narcotic dependence, shall be dispensed only by approved hospital and community pharmacies and maintenance programs approved by the FDA and designated state authorities.

CNS, central nervous system; IM, intramuscular; FDA, Food and Drug Administration; PO, oral; SC, subcutaneous.

BOX 31.16

Medication Profile: Buprenorphine

DRUG CLASS: Partial opioid agonist/antagonist

RECEPTOR AFFINITY: Partial agonist at the μ-opioid receptor and an antagonist at the kappa receptor. Will displace morphine, methadone, and other opioid full agonists from the receptor

INDICATIONS: For pain management and during detoxification and opioid dependence, and long-term maintenance treatment of opioid use disorder. May be initiated while the person is actively withdrawing from opioids.

DOSAGE AND ADMINISTRATION: Adults 4 mg to 36 mg/day in divided doses. Dosage level is related to the amount of narcotic and length of time patient has used opioids. The label indicates the dosage of buprenorphine and naloxone (4 mg/1 mg; 8 mg/2 mg, or 12 mg/3 mg).

Available as a sublingual film or sublingual tablet.

HALF-LIFE (PEAK EFFECT): Buprenorphine can take up to 37 (2 days to excrete 50% of the dose) naloxone has a shorter elimination half-life, 2 to 12 hours.

WARNING: Pregnant people should receive the buprenorphine-only sublingual tablet.

SAFE HANDLING: Pill counts may be useful to encourage treatment adherence. Because the injectable is a narcotic, arrangements should be made to have the injection delivered by the pharmacy to the office where it will be administered. Prescribing qualifications are required. Keep out of the reach of children. Store in a closed container at room temperature, away from heat, moisture, and direct light; keep from freezing. Dispose medications in Drug Enforcement Administration (DEA)-approved locations.

SELECTED SIDE EFFECTS: Lightheadedness, dizziness or fainting with position changes, cough, feeling of warmth or heat, flushing, headache, painful or difficult urination, slower back or side pain.

DRUG INTERACTIONS: Multiple drug interactions including antianxiety, antidepressant or antipsychotic medications, and many others can also cause serious allergic reactions and life-threatening anaphylaxis requiring immediate attention.

SPECIFIC PATIENT AND FAMILY EDUCATION

- Stopping this medication may cause withdrawal symptoms.
- Do not take other medications without first checking with your doctor.
- Tell your provider/dentist that you are using this medicine prior to any procedure.
- Notify your provider if you experience darkening or yellowing of the skin, diarrhea, tenderness in the upper stomach, pale stools, loss of appetite, nausea, or vomiting.
- Notify your provider should a rash, hives, hoarseness, trouble breathing or swallowing, swelling of hands, face, or mouth occur while you are using this medication.

Buprenorphine–naloxone, a sublingual film administered as a once-daily dose, is prescribed when there is a potential for relapse. The addition of naloxone prevents an overdose if the individual uses other opioids while taking buprenorphine.

Subutex, a buprenorphine-only preparation, is safe in pregnant people and provides consistent support. Fetal exposure to buprenorphine in utero is associated with significantly shorter hospitals stays, shorter length of NAS, and decreased duration and frequency of pharmacotherapy for NAS. Newborns should be assessed for NAS because the risks remain (Rana et al., 2023).

Naltrexone is similar to naloxone and has been used successfully to treat opioid dependence. Naltrexone blocks alcohol and opioid receptors and has long-acting coverage. If an individual who is opioid dependent takes naltrexone before they are fully detoxified from opioids, withdrawal symptoms may appear. See Table 31.9.

INHALANT USE DISORDER

Inhalants

Inhalants are organic solvents, which are carbon-based substances capable of dissolving or dispersing one or more other substance. Most inhalants other than nitrites depress the CNS in a manner like alcohol (e.g., slurred speech, lack of coordination, euphoria, dizziness). They may cause lightheadedness, hallucinations, and delusions. The nitrites enhance sexual pleasure by dilating and relaxing blood vessels. Although inhalant use disorder (IUD) is rare, it is important to remember that their use can be fatal and that inhalants can be a gateway to illegal, psychoactive drugs (NIDA, 2022c).

Inhalant Intoxication

Mild intoxication occurs within minutes. Often, the drugs are inhaled repeatedly to maintain an intoxicated state for hours. Initially, the person experiences a sense of euphoria, but as the dose increases, confusion, perceptual distortions, and severe CNS depression occur. People who use inhalants are also at risk for sudden sniffing death, which can occur when the inhaled fumes replace oxygen in the lungs and CNS, causing the person to suffocate. Inhalants can also cause death by disrupting the normal heart rhythm, which can lead to cardiac arrest (NIDA, 2024d).

Long-Term Complications

Chronic neurologic syndromes can result from long-term use, which is linked to widespread brain damage and atypical cognitive changes that can range from mild impairment to severe dementia. In recent studies, considerably more people who use inhalants than people who use cocaine had atypical brain results and their damage was more extensive. Magnetic resonance imaging scans of people who use inhalants demonstrate severe changes in cerebral white matter (NIDA, 2022c).

OTHER TYPES OF DRUGS THAT CAN BE MISUSED

ANABOLIC STEROIDS

Anabolic steroid is the name for synthetic substances related to the male sex hormones (androgens). Developed in the late 1930s to treat hypogonadism, they are also used to treat delayed puberty, some types of impotence, and wasting of the body caused by HIV infection or other diseases. They promote growth of skeletal muscle and the development of male sexual characteristics. More than 100 different types exist; to be used legally, all require a prescription. They can be taken orally or intramuscularly. Some are applied to the skin as a cream or gel. When misused, these preparations are taken at 10 to 100 times higher doses than are used for medical disorders. Although use among people assigned male at birth is higher, use among people assigned female at birth is growing (NIDA, 2024e).

Even though steroids do not produce euphoria or a "high" like typical addictive substances, the urge to continue use is related to the need to achieve a desired appearance and to continue feeling good about oneself, resulting in the compulsive need to seek out and use anabolic steroids. Cutting back or stopping use causes the appearance of withdrawal signs (low sex drive, loss of appetite, mood swings, fatigue, insomnia, and depression). Case reports and small studies indicate that in high doses, anabolic steroids increase irritability and aggression, often referred to as "roid rage." Some people who use steroids report that they have committed aggressive acts, such as physical fighting, armed robbery, using force to obtain something, committing property damage, domestic violence, stealing from stores, or breaking into a house or building. People who use steroids engage in these behaviors more often when they take steroids than when they are drug free. Other behavioral effects include euphoria, increased energy, sexual arousal, mood swings, distractibility, forgetfulness, and confusion (AlShareef et al., 2023).

With extended use, anabolic steroid use is associated with an increased risk for heart attacks and strokes, blood clotting, cholesterol changes, hypertension, depressed mood, fatigue, restlessness, loss of appetite, insomnia, reduced libido, muscle and joint pain, and severe liver issues. People assigned male at birth can have reduced sperm production, shrinking of the testes, and difficulty or pain in urinating. Other undesirable body changes in this population include breast enlargement; in people assigned female at birth, people's bodies can be masculinized.

People of all genders may experience hair loss and acne. Intravenous or intramuscular use of the drug and needle sharing put people who use steroids at risk for HIV, hepatitis B and C, and infective endocarditis, as well as bacterial infections at injection sites (NIDA, 2024e).

MDMA AND OTHER "CLUB DRUGS"

The drug 3,4-methylenedioxymethamphetamine (**MDMA**), also known as Ecstasy or Molly, is known as a "club drug" because it is used by teens and young adults as part of the nightclub, bar, and rave scenes. MDMA, chemically similar to both stimulants and hallucinogens, causes activity of dopamine, norepinephrine, and serotonin to increase. It produces feelings of increased energy, pleasure, emotional warmth, and distorted sensory and time perception. MDMA can cause hallucinations, confusion, depression, paranoia, sleep issues, drug craving, severe anxiety, nausea, muscle cramping, involuntary teeth clenching, blurred vision, chills, and sweating. In higher doses, MDMA can sharply increase body temperature (i.e., malignant hyperthermia), leading to muscle breakdown, kidney and cardiovascular failure, and death. MDMA effects last about 3 to 6 hours (NIDA, 2024b).

Other club drugs, such as flunitrazepam, gamma-hydroxybutyrate (GHB), and ketamine (discussed in the next section), are predominantly CNS depressants. Often colorless, tasteless, and odorless, the drugs can be ingested unknowingly. Known also as "date rape" drugs when mixed with alcohol, they can be incapacitating, causing a euphoric, sedative-like effect and producing an **anterograde amnesia**, which means that individuals may not remember events they experience while under the influence of these drugs.

HALLUCINOGENS AND DISSOCIATIVE DRUGS

A **hallucinogen** causes hallucinations and profound distortions in a person's perceptions of reality. When under the influence of hallucinogens, people report rapid, intense emotional swings and seeing images, hearing sounds, and feeling sensations that seem real but are not. Severe reactions may cause paranoia, fear of losing one's mind, depersonalization, illusions, delusions, and hallucinations. Intense mood and sexual behavior changes may occur; the person using the hallucinogen may feel unusually close to others or distant and isolated. Classic hallucinogens include LSD (D-lysergic acid diethylamide), psilocybin (4-phosphoryloxy-*N*, *N*-dimethyltryptamine), Peyote, and DMT (dimethyltryptamine). *Salvia divinorum* is an herb in the mint family that is used for its hallucinogenic effect. Many of the hallucinogenic drugs are being considered for use with psychotherapy and the United States is considering legalizing use for those purposes.

Dissociative drugs block the NMDA receptor, distort perception of sight and sound, and produce feelings of detachment from oneself or dissociation. PCP (phencyclidine) and ketamine are both manufactured illegally for recreational use. Ketamine is also manufactured legally and has FDA approval to be used as an anesthetic in humans and animals. Esketamine, a more potent form ketamine is used for treatment-resistant depression and only under the supervision of a physician. Ketamine is associated with an increased heart rate and blood pressure, impaired motor function, memory loss, numbness, and vomiting. At high doses, delirium, depression, respiratory depression, and cardiac arrest can occur (NIDA, 2024c).

Another dissociative drug, DXM (dextromethorphan), is a cough suppressant and expectorant ingredient in some OTC cold and cough medicines and is commonly misused by adolescents and young adults. DXM can cause a range of clinical effects from mild agitation to psychosis to seizures and coma (Journey et al., 2023).

PRESCRIPTION AND OVER-THE-COUNTER DRUGS

Misuse of prescription and OTC drugs occurs when one of the following criteria is met:

- Taking a medication that has been prescribed for someone else.
- Taking a drug in higher quantity or in another manner than prescribed.
- Taking a drug for another purpose than prescribed (NIDA, 2023).

The opioids (e.g., oxycodone, hydrocodone, morphine, fentanyl, codeine) prescribed for pain are some of the more commonly misused prescription medications. The most commonly misused CNS depressants are the benzodiazepines (diazepam, alprazolam, clonazepam, lorazepam), which are prescribed for anxiety and sleep. The *DSM-5-TR* diagnosis *sedative use disorder, hypnotic use disorder, or anxiolytic use disorder* would be given when these drugs are misused. Amphetamines and methylphenidate are stimulants prescribed for ADHD that are also frequently misused or diverted for illicit purposes. Nurses are well positioned to address the significant public health issue of drug diversion, through patient education and medication monitoring.

EMERGING DRUGS AND TRENDS

New drugs and drug-use trends rapidly enter our communities. NIDA continuously reports on these drugs. Some of the newer drugs include synthetic cathinones (bath salts, Flakka), nitazenes, and tianeptine.

Bath salts contain cathinone, an amphetamine-like stimulant naturally found in the Khat plant (*Catha edulis*). Severe intoxication and dangerous health effects are associated with these drugs. These drugs, which are chemically similar to methamphetamines and MDMA, produce euphoria, increased sociability, and increased sex drive, as well as paranoia, agitation, and hallucinatory delirium (NIDA, 2024f).

Nitazenes are synthetic opioids that may be as powerful or more powerful than fentanyl. They were developed in the 1950s but began to reemerge in 2019 after fentanyl-related substances were banned. Nitazenes have overdose potential, but research shows that naloxone may be effective (NIDA, 2024f).

Tianeptine is an antidepressant medication that is not approved by the FDA. It is marketed in dietary supplements as a cognitive enhancer. It may be combined with other cognitive enhancers but is also used with substances like kava and gabapentin (NIDA, 2024f).

CHEMICAL DEPENDENCY AND PROFESSIONAL NURSES

Although accurate epidemiologic data specific to nursing are scarce, evidence suggests that the prevalence of SUDs among nurses is similar to that of the general public.

RISK FACTORS

A nurse is just as susceptible to dependence as any other individual, but additional risk factors exist, such as access and availability of drugs, training in the administration and injection of drugs, and a familiarity with and a frequency of administering drugs. Nurses are most likely to misuse opioids rather than alcohol (Molloy, 2024).

Working conditions may be difficult and involve staffing shortages, acutely ill patients, inadequate patient-to-nurse ratios, shift rotations, shifts lasting longer than 8 hours, and increased overtime all add additional stress to the nurse, which increases the risk of substance misuse. Because of the risk of losing a license to practice, nurses are very reluctant to seek help.

INDICATIVE CUES

Ignoring, making excuses, or covering for an impaired colleague is not acceptable. Reporting can be a positive step toward protecting patients and supporting colleagues entering a treatment program.

Some cues to look for that might indicate a colleague is impaired or diverting drugs can be seen in Table 31.10. Legal requirements to report a nurse with an SUD vary among individual states, but nurses have an ethical and moral duty to patients, colleagues, the profession of nursing, and the community to act. Documents such as the American Nurses Association Code of Ethics for Nurses provide a framework for patient safety. Remember that SUDs are neurobiologic disorders; people do not consciously choose to misuse or become dependent on a substance. If you have suspicions about a colleague, talk with your manager, the human resources department, and/or substance use experts for advice.

TABLE 31.10 CUES A NURSING COLLEAGUE MIGHT HAVE AN SUD OR BE DIVERTING DRUGS

Type of Cue	Cues to Watch Out For
Behavioral and physical cues a colleague might have an SUD	• Severe mood swings, personality changes • Significant weight loss or gain • Nausea, vomiting, diarrhea • Refusing drug testing • Elaborate excuses • Frequent unexplained tardiness, work absences, illness and/or physical complaints • Deterioration in physical appearance
Cues a colleague might be diverting drugs	• Missing medications or prescription pads • Drugs and syringes carried in pockets. • Heavy drug wasting/miscounts • Inappropriate drug choices and doses for patients • Patients reporting lack of drug effect (pain relief) • Frequently volunteering to administer narcotics or relieve colleagues of casework where opioids are used.

Source: Healthy Nurse Healthy Nation. (2022). Warning signs of a substance use disorder in a nursing colleague. https://engage.healthynursehealthynation.org/blogs/10/3807.

NON–SUBSTANCE-RELATED COMPULSIVE DISORDERS

Certain compulsive behaviors characterized by risky use, urges, cravings, and "highs" make them similar to substance intoxication and dependence. At present, only compulsive gambling appears in the *DSM-5-TR*.

Compulsive sexual behavior disorder has been covered by the World Health Organization, making it billable for treatment with the International Classification of Disease (ICD-11) codes. This disorder is characterized by a persistent pattern of failure to control intense, repetitive sexual urges, resulting in repetitive sexual behavior that becomes a central focus of the person's life (Böthe et al., 2024).

Internet gaming disorder is under investigation for inclusion in this category of the *DSM*.

GAMBLING USE DISORDER (GUD)

Gambling use disorder (GUD) is characterized by compulsive and problematic gambling behavior that leads to significant impairments in functioning or distress. Individuals with gambling issues are more likely to die by suicide than those without such issues and are less likely to seek mental health treatment (Karlsson et al., 2023). Compulsive gamblers feel omnipotent in their ability to win back what was lost. This omnipotence serves as self-deception that leads to **denial**. Care of these patients involves confronting such omnipotent beliefs. Staff education about the disorder is important. Family involvement is also crucial. Families often have been dealing with the patient in a dysfunctional manner. Relapse prevention involves learning about specific cues that trigger the gambling behavior.

SUMMARY OF KEY POINTS

- Substance dependence is a condition of continued use of substances despite adverse consequences. Misuse occurs when a person uses alcohol or drugs for purposes for which they were not intended, to produce pleasurable feelings, or in excessive amounts.
- Accurate and comprehensive assessment is crucial in planning substance use treatment interventions. This assessment should consider all substances for pattern of use, including factors of tolerance; withdrawal symptoms; consequences of use; loss of control over amount, frequency, or duration of use; desire or efforts to cease or control use; and social, vocational, and recreational activities affected by use, history of previous substance use treatment, and family and social support systems.
- Denial of a substance use disorder is the individual's attempt to avoid accepting the diagnosis; it can be manifest in attempts to rationalize the substance use, minimize the harmful results, deflect attention from one's own issue to society's or someone else's, or blame childhood trauma.
- Nurses should use a nonconfrontational approach when dealing with patients in denial of their issues. Motivational interviewing approaches are most effective, using empathy and a nonjudgmental approach, to help the patient realize the discrepancy between life goals and engaging in substance use, thus motivating patients to change their self-destructive behaviors and make personal choices regarding treatment goals.
- Several effective modalities are used in substance use treatment, and many programs combine them, which may include 12-step programs, social skills groups, psychoeducational groups, group therapy, and individual and family therapies. No one best treatment method exists for all people.
- Substance use disorders have many social and political ramifications. No health profession is immune to having members who suffer with substance use disorders.
- Certain compulsive behaviors share characteristics with substance intoxication and dependence. Of these, only compulsive gambling appears in the *DSM-5-TR*.

DEVELOPING CLINICAL JUDGMENT

1. J. H., a 35-year-old patient who misuses cocaine, has entered a rehabilitation program. What goals would be realistic to achieve by the end of the projected 30-day inpatient stay?
2. M. L. has been admitted to an orthopedic unit for treatment for a fractured femur. The patient has been drinking recently and has a BAL of 0.08%. What further information in the following areas would the nurse need to plan nursing care?
   a. Medical
   b. Alcohol and drug use related
   c. Other psychosocial issues
3. Experimenting with alcohol or other substances during adolescence is common. How would you differentiate what is and what is not "risky" behavior?
4. J. M. is seeking treatment for depression and job stress. This individual came to your psychiatric assessment unit smelling of alcohol and claiming that the issue is not drinking but the job. What interventions would the nurse use to work with individuals who use denial to maintain substance use?
5. S. G. has been misusing heroin intravenously heavily for 2 years. The patient was admitted to the hospital with a leg abscess and a positive urine drug screen. What symptoms would you expect to observe during withdrawal? What medications would likely be used to ease these symptoms?
6. After S. G. is free from withdrawal symptoms, the patient expresses interest in obtaining medications for maintenance treatment. What are the options? How would you describe them?
7. R. L. has been treated for hypertension at your clinic. You notice that the patient complains of peripheral neuropathy and has an unsteady gait. What other medical signs would corroborate an alcohol use disorder? What experiences have you had with drug or alcohol misuse or dependence? What was your response? How do you think those experiences will affect you as you build your practice to help others who misuse alcohol and other substances?
8. Sending a family member to an often costly rehabilitation center for an extended in-patient stay is not always the best treatment option. What challenges around substance use disorders remain unaddressed by these centers?
9. Some states have enacted policies mandating point-of-sale warning signs with information on the harms of alcohol use during pregnancy, but these have not typically reduced use and are associated with increased support for punishment and other stigmatizing attitudes. What better methods should be used to

educate the public about the hazards of substance use during pregnancy?

10. If you could develop new harm-reduction strategies for commonly misused substances, what would they be? Often, good strategies (and even evidence-based harm-reduction strategies) are met with political resistance. Why do you think that happens and what could be done about it?

MOVIES, TV, AND STREAMING PROGRAMS

Dopesick: 2021. Dopesick is an American docudrama based on a nonfiction book by Beth Macy. The series focuses on opioid dependence across the United States, how individuals and families are affected, and the alleged conflicts of interest involving Purdue Pharma, the Food and Drug Administration, and the Department of Justice. There are eight episodes, available on streaming services. The legal case involving testing and marketing of the drug oxycodone is highlighted, and the Sackler family (owners of the pharmaceutical company) are portrayed. Viewers see dependence through the eyes of a distressed Virginia mining community as the filmmakers paint a disturbingly accurate portrayal of a major drug issue in America. Use of a legally manufactured drug for pain touted as a "miracle" increases after lies, despair, betrayal, greed, and aggressive marketing, which leads to the opioid epidemic in the United States and the high number of overdose deaths that we continue to experience to this day.

Nurses are on the front lines of caring for individuals and families experiencing the effects of opioid dependence. This documentary is an eye opener for those who consider drug misuse an individual or family issue that could be overcome by willpower or "just saying no." It reveals the broader picture of marketing influence and law enforcement and regulatory systems struggling to hold Purdue Pharma accountable, while being overwhelmed by the company's financial, legal, and lobbying resources.

Viewing Points:

1. After watching *Dopesick*, what views do you now have about dependence and who becomes dependent?
2. Consider the moral perspectives of all the major stakeholders.
3. What is it like to be a family in this Appalachian community who were already struggling, and to watch the progressive economic devastation that occurs as more community members and families succumb to dependence and overdose.

Uncut Gems: 2019. This film depicts the experience of a charismatic jeweler named Howard Ratner, who is involved in high-stakes betting scheme that could lead to a lifetime windfall or to the loss of everything he owns, including his family and even his life. The jeweler is entrenched in his gambling disorder, needing higher and higher stakes to sustain the pleasure, and ultimately rocketing out of control. Winning or losing doesn't really matter, as long as Howard gets an opportunity to make another bet and get on the roller coaster again. The film unfolds over a couple of days, but tension escalates at such a rapid, high-adrenaline pace that the viewer, for the space of this movie (only 135 minutes), is transported into the world of pathologic gambling. When the movie ends, there is an audible sigh of relief on the part of the audience.

Viewing Points:

1. Why is gambling, a non–substance-related activity, treated in a similar way to a substance use disorder?
2. What was Howard's level of self-deception, and how did he maintain it?
3. Notice how the dependency on gambling takes over Howard's life and the costs he is willing to pay to experience the high of gaming.
4. Notice his alertness and arousal as he is preoccupied with the bet and notice too, how short the pleasure lasts, before Howard must once again engage in another high-stakes game.
5. Look for Howard's lies, the level of his activity, the extent of measures he takes to hide his dependency.
6. See if you recognize other comorbidities in Howard's behavior. Were you concerned about his safety?
7. Could you identify the phases of compulsive gambling disorder: Winning, losing, desperation, and hopelessness?
8. How did you feel as you witnessed Howard self-destruct? What would it be like to be Howard's nurse?

Unfolding Patient Stories: Andrew Davis • Part 1

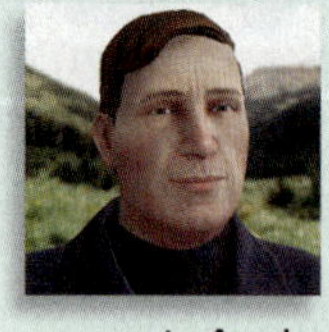

Andrew Davis, age 56, voluntarily admitted himself to an alcohol rehabilitation facility after his wife asked him to move out of their home due to his alcohol use. Although his son is still on speaking terms with him, his two daughters are not. Andrew refuses to attend group therapy or a self-help group meeting. How can the nurse establish a therapeutic relationship during the treatment stage of detoxification from alcohol and throughout recovery? What are the priority interventions during the initial phase of treatment for alcohol use disorder? Why is it important to cultivate trust between the nurse, Andrew, and his family? How can the nurse encourage him to attend group therapy and a self-help group meeting? (Andrew's story continues in Chapter 37.)

Care for Andrew Davis and other patients in a realistic virtual environment: ***vSim** for Nursing* (thepoint.lww.com/vSimMentalHealth). Practice documenting these patients' care in DocuCare (thepoint.lww.com/DocuCareEHR).

REFERENCES

Akinnusi, M., Martinson, A., & El-Solh, A. A. (2024). Treatment of insomnia associated with alcohol and opioid use: A narrative review. *Sleep and Biological Rhythms*, *22*(4), 429–445. https://doi.org/10.1007/s41105-024-00544-x

Alcoholics Anonymous. (2024). *Alcoholics anonymous information on AA [Online]*. http://www.aa.org

AlShareef, S., Gokarakonda, S. B., & Marwaha, R. (2023). Anabolic steroid use disorder. In *StatPearls*. StatPearls Publishing.

American Nurses Association [ANA], American Psychiatric Nurses Association, & International Society of Psychiatric-Mental Health Nurses. (2022). *Psychiatric-Mental Health Nursing: Scope and Standards of Practice* (3rd ed.). ANA.

American Psychiatric Association [APA]. (2022). *Diagnostic and statistical manual of mental disorders* (5th ed., text rev.). Author.

American Psychological Association [APA]. (2023). *How does marijuana affect the brain? Psychological researchers examine impact on different age groups over time*. https://www.apa.org/monitor/2023/06/marijuana-effects-brain

Amin, S., Pokhrel, P., Elwir, T., Mettias, H., & Kawamoto, C. T. (2023). A systematic review of experimental and longitudinal studies on e-cigarette use cessation. *Addictive Behaviors*, *146*, 107787. https://doi.org/10.1016/j.addbeh.2023.107787

BAART Programs. (2023). *Addiction, recovery and divorce*. https://baartprograms.com/addiction-recovery-and-divorce/#:~:text=Understanding%20the%20link%20between%20addiction,use%20as%20the%20motivating%20factor

Babor, T. F., Higgins-Biddle, J. C., Saunders, J. B., & Monteiro, M. B. (2001). *AUDIT: The alcohol use disorders identification test* (2nd ed.). World Health Organization.

Bodur, M., Kaya, S., Ilhan-Esgin, M., Çakiroğlu, F. P., & Özçelik, A. Ö. (2024). The caffeine dilemma: Unraveling the intricate relationship between caffeine use disorder, caffeine withdrawal symptoms and mental well-being in adults. *Public Health Nutrition*, *27*(1), e57. https://doi.org/10.1017/S1368980024000399

Böthe, B., Nagy, L., Koós, M., Demetrovics, Z., Potenza, M. N., International Sex Survey Consortium, & Kraus, S. W. (2024). Problematic pornography use across countries, genders, and sexual orientations: Insights from the International Sex Survey and comparison of different assessment tools. *Addiction*, *119*(5), 928–950. https://doi.org/10.1111/add.16431

Bratu, M. L., Sandesc, D., Anghel, T., Tudor, R., Shaaban, L., Ali, A., Toma, A. O., Bratosin, F., Turcu, I., Gantsa, A., Fericean, R. M., Bondrescu, M., & Barata, P. I. (2023). Evaluating the aspects of quality of life in individuals with substance use disorder: A systematic review based on the WHOQOL questionnaire. *Journal of Multidisciplinary Healthcare*, *16*, 4265–4278. https://doi.org/10.2147/JMDH.S440764

Britton, E. M., Taisir, R., Cooper, A., Remers, S., Chorny, Y., LaBelle, O., Rush, B., MacKillop, J., & Costello, M. J. (2024). Psychometric evaluation of an adapted short-form spirituality scale in a sample of predominantly white adults in an inpatient substance use disorder treatment program. *Assessment*, *31*(6), 1309–1323. https://doi.org/10.1177/10731911231217478

Brower, J. O., & Swatek, J. L. (2024). Beyond the buzz: The fatal consequences of caffeine overconsumption. *Journal of Analytical Toxicology*, *48*(8), 535–540. https://doi.org/10.1093/jat/bkae046

Canver, B. R., Newman, R. K., & Gomez, A. E. (2024). Alcohol withdrawal syndrome. In *StatPearls*. StatPearls Publishing. (nih.gov)

Centers for Disease Control and Prevention [CDC]. (2024). Fentanyl facts. Retrieved January 3, 2025, from https://www.cdc.gov/overdose-resources/pdf/CDC_Fentanyl-Fact-Sheet_General_508.pdf

Day, E., & Daly, C. (2022). Clinical management of the alcohol withdrawal syndrome. *Addiction*, *117*(3), 804–814. https://doi.org/10.1111/add.15647

Dyar, C., Lee, C. M., Rhew, I. C., & Kaysen, D. (2023). Sexual minority stress and substance use: An investigation of when and under what circumstances minority stress predicts alcohol and cannabis use at the event-level. *Journal of Psychopathology and Clinical Science*, *132*(4), 475–489. https://doi.org/10.1037/abn0000819

de Andrade, V. O., Monteiro, B. M. M., de Souza, V. C. R. P., & de Souza, J. C. R. P. (2023). A systematic review of interventions based on Judaeo-Christian principles for patients with substance dependence. *Journal of Religion and Health*, *62*(6), 4316–4333. https://doi.org/10.1007/s10943-023-01830-7

de Oliveira, M. C., Vides, M. C., Lassi, D. L. S., Torales, J., Ventriglio, A., Bombana, H. S., Leyton, V., Périco, C. A., Negrão, A. B., Malbergier, A., & Castaldelli-Maia, J. M. (2023). Toxicity of synthetic cannabinoids in K2/Spice: A systematic review. *Brain Sciences*, *13*(7), 990. https://doi.org/10.3390/brainsci13070990

Dydyk, A. M., Jain, N. K., & Gupta, M. (2024). Opioid use disorder. In *StatPearls*. StatPearls Publishing. https://www.ncbi.nlm.nih.gov/books/NBK553166/

Edinoff, A. N., Sall, S., Upshaw, W. C., Spillers, N. J., Vincik, L. Y., De Witt, A. S., Murnane, K. S., Kaye, A. M., & Kaye, A. D. (2024). Xylazine: A drug adulterant of clinical concern. *Current Pain and Headache Reports*, *28*(5), 417–426. https://doi.org/10.1007/s11916-024-01211-z

Fahey, K. M. L., Kovacek, K., Abramovich, A., & Dermody, S. S. (2023). Substance use prevalence, patterns, and correlates in transgender and gender diverse youth: A scoping review. *Drug and Alcohol Dependence*, *250*, 110880. https://doi.org/10.1016/j.drugalcdep.2023.110880

Farkouh, R., Audette-Chapdelaine, S., & Brodeur, M. (2024). Pharmacotherapy and gambling disorder: A narrative review. *Journal of Addictive Diseases*, *42*(4), 274–288. https://doi.org/10.1080/10550887.2023.2229725

Fornili, K. S., & Fogger, S. (Eds.). (2022). *Addictions nursing: Scope and standards of practice* (3rd ed.). American Nurses Association & International Nurses Society on Addictions.

Gaba, M., Kumar, N., Arumugam, P., & Dewan, A. (2023). Vape-associated lung injury in immediate postoperative period: An upcoming perioperative respiratory risk factor. *BMJ Case Reports*, *16*(7), e255250. https://doi.org/10.1136/bcr-2023-255250

Gao, Z., Winhusen, T. J., Gorenflo, M., Ghitza, U. E., Nunes, E., Saxon, A. J., Korthuis, T., Brady, K., Luo, S. X., Davis, P. B., Kaelber, D. C., & Xu, R. (2023). Potential effect of antidepressants on remission from cocaine use disorder—A nationwide matched retrospective cohort study. *Drug and Alcohol Dependence*, *251*, 110958. https://doi.org/10.1016/j.drugalcdep.2023.110958

Geijer-Simpson, E., Kaner, E., Lingam, R., McArdle, P., & McGovern, R. (2023). Effectiveness of family-involved interventions in reducing co-occurring alcohol use and mental health problems in young people aged 12–17: A systematic review and meta-analysis. *International Journal of Environmental Research and Public Health*, *20*(19), 6890. https://doi.org/10.3390/ijerph20196890

Gorelick D. A. (2023). Cannabis-related disorders and toxic effects. *The New England Journal of Medicine*, *389*(24), 2267–2275. https://doi.org/10.1056/NEJMra2212152

Gústafsson, B. J., Puljević, C., Davies, E. L., Barratt, M. J., Ferris, J., Winstock, A., & Piatkowski, T. (2024). Sweating for sobriety: Exploring the relationship between exercise engagement and substance use disorders. *Journal of Psychoactive Drugs*, 1–11. Advance online publication. https://doi.org/10.1080/02791072.2024.2311143

Han, B. H., Bronson, J., Washington, L., Yu, M., Kelton, K., Tsai, J., & Finlay, A. K. (2023). Co-occurring medical multimorbidity, mental illness, and substance use disorders among older criminal legal system-involved veterans. *Medical Care*, *61*(7), 477–483. https://doi.org/10.1097/MLR.0000000000001864

Healthy Nurse Healthy Nation. (2022). *Warning signs of a substance use disorder in a nursing colleague*. https://engage.healthynursehealthynation.org/blogs/10/3807

Herzog, C., Jones, A., Evans, I., Raut, J. R., Zikan, M., Cibula, D., Wong, A., Brenner, H., Richmond, R. C., & Widschwendter, M. (2024). Cigarette smoking and e-cigarette use induce shared DNA methylation changes linked to carcinogenesis. *Cancer Research*, *84*(11), 1898–1914. https://doi.org/10.1158/0008-5472.CAN-23-2957

Hughes, A. R., Grusing, S., Lin, A., Hendrickson, R. G., Sheridan, D. C., Marshall, R. C., & Horowitz, B. Z. (2023). Trends in intentional abuse and misuse ingestions in school-aged children and adolescents reported to US poison centers from 2000–2020. *Clinical Toxicology*, *61*(1), 64–71. https://doi.org/10.1080/15563650.2022.2120818

Hyysalo, N., Gastelle, M., & Flykt, M. (2022). Maternal pre- and postnatal substance use and attachment in young children: A systematic review and meta-analysis. *Development and Psychopathology*, *34*(4), 1231–1248. https://doi.org/10.1017/S0954579421000134

Iob, E., Pingault, J. B., Munafò, M. R., Stubbs, B., Gilthorpe, M. S., Maihofer, A. X., Psychiatric Genomics Consortium Posttraumatic Stress Disorder Working Group, & Danese, A. (2023). Testing the causal relationships of physical activity and sedentary behaviour with mental health and substance use disorders: a Mendelian randomisation study. *Molecular Psychiatry*, *28*(8), 3429–3443. https://doi.org/10.1038/s41380-023-02133-9

Islami, F., Marlow, E. C., Thomson, B., McCullough, M. L., Rumgay, H., Gapstur, S. M., Patel, A. V., Soerjomataram, I., & Jemal, A. (2024). Proportion and number of cancer cases and deaths attributable to potentially modifiable risk factors in the United States, 2019. *CA: A Cancer Journal for Clinicians*, *74*(5), 405–432. https://doi.org/10.3322/caac.21858

Jones, M., Seel, C. J., & Dymond, S. (2024). Electronic-screening, brief intervention and referral to treatment (e-SBIRT) for addictive disorders: Systematic review and meta-analysis. *Substance Use & Addiction Journal*, *45*(4), 736–752. https://doi.org/10.1177/29767342241248926

Journey, J. D., Agrawal, S., & Stern, E. (2023). Dextromethorphan toxicity. In *StatPearls*. StatPearls Publishing. (nih.gov)

Junyue, J., Siyu, C., Xindong, W., Qinge, X., Jingchun, Z., Liming, L., & Guohua, L. (2021). Complementary and alternative medicine for substance use disorders: A scientometric analysis and visualization of its use between 2001 and 2020. *Frontiers in Psychiatry*, *12*, 722240. https://doi.org/10.3389/fpsyt.2021.722240

Karlsson, A., Håkansson, A., & Hansson, H. (2023). Personal experiences of suicidality in women with gambling disorder—A qualitative interview study. *Journal of Behavioral Addictions*, *12*(2), 510–521. https://doi.org/10.1556/2006.2023.00024

Keeney, A. J., Ciro, D., Meng, Y., Coco, L., & Ekonomo, K. (2025). Depression, anxiety, and coping strategies among farmworkers exposed to substance use at work. *Journal of Agromedicine*, *30*(1), 105–113. https://doi.org/10.1080/1059924X.2024.2407384

Kim, K., & Picciotto, M. R. (2023). Nicotine addiction: More than just dopamine. *Current Opinion in Neurobiology*, *83*, 102797. https://doi.org/10.1016/j.conb.2023.102797

Klein, H., & Washington, T. A. (2023). The "triple whammy": Serious psychological distress, suicidal ideation, and substance misuse among transgender persons. *Acta Psychologica*, *241*, 104092. https://doi.org/10.1016/j.actpsy.2023.104092

Kranzler, H. R. (2023). Overview of alcohol use disorder. *The American Journal of Psychiatry*, *180*(8), 565–572. https://doi.org/10.1176/appi.ajp.20230488

Lesnewich, L. M., Pawlak, A. P., Gohel, S., & Bates, M. E. (2022). Functional connectivity in the central executive network predicts changes in binge drinking behavior during emerging adulthood: An observational prospective study. *Addiction*, *117*(7), 1899–1907. https://doi.org/10.1111/add.15828

Lindeman, S. K., Selseng, L. B., Lorås, L., & Løberg, A. H. (2023). Living with sibling' drug use. Bereaved siblings' family stories. *International Journal of Qualitative Studies on Health and Well-Being*, *18*(1), 2240576. https://doi.org/10.1080/17482631.2023.2240576

Lindenfeld, Z., Chen, K., Kapur, S., & Chang, J. E. (2024). Comparing rates of undiagnosed hypertension and diabetes in patients with and without substance use disorders. *Journal of General Internal Medicine*, *39*(9), 1632–1641. https://doi.org/10.1007/s11606-024-08718-6

Lyzwinski, L. N., Naslund, J. A., Miller, C. J., & Eisenberg, M. J. (2022). Global youth vaping and respiratory health: Epidemiology, interventions, and policies. *NPJ Primary Care Respiratory Medicine*, *32*(1), 14. https://doi.org/10.1038/s41533-022-00277-9

Maracic, C. E., & Moeller, S. J. (2021). Neural and behavioral correlates of impaired insight and self-awareness in substance use disorder. *Current Behavioral Neuroscience Reports*, *8*(4), 113–123. https://doi.org/10.1007/s40473-021-00240-x

McCuistian, C., Lisha, N. E., Campbell, B., Cheng, C., Le, J., & Guydish, J. (2024). Reducing tobacco use in substance use treatment: The California tobacco free initiative. *Addictive Behaviors*, *155*, 108025. https://doi.org/10.1016/j.addbeh.2024.108025

Mental Health America. (2024). *Co-dependency* [Online]. Retrieved June 26, 2024, from https://www.mhanational.org/issues/co-dependency

Molloy, P. A. (2024). Nurses and nursing students with substance use disorders. *Journal of Addictions Nursing*, *35*(1), 15–21. https://doi.org/10.1097/JAN.0000000000000562

Motamedi, S., Amleshi, R. S., Javar, B. A., Shams, P., Kohlmeier, K. A., & Shabani, M. (2023). Cannabis during pregnancy: A way to transfer an impairment to later life. *Birth Defects Research*, *115*(15), 1327–1344s. https://doi.org/10.1002/bdr2.2207

Muenstermann, C., & Clemens, K. J. (2024). Epigenetic mechanisms of nicotine dependence. *Neuroscience and Biobehavioral Reviews*, *156*, 105505. https://doi.org/10.1016/j.neubiorev.2023.105505

National Institute on Drug Abuse [NIDA]. (2021). *Introduction. Cigarettes and other tobacco products drug facts*. Retrieved June 22, 2024, from https://nida.nih.gov/publications/research-reports/tobacco-nicotine-e-cigarettes/introduction

National Institute on Drug Abuse [NIDA]. (2022a). *Sex differences in substance use*. https://nida.nih.gov/publications/research-reports/substance-use-in-women/sex-gender-differences-in-substance-use

National Institute on Drug Abuse [NIDA]. (2022b). *What is methamphetamine?* Retrieved June 21, 2024, from https://nida.nih.gov/research-topics/methamphetamine#what-is-methamphetamine

National Institute on Drug Abuse. [NIDA]. (2023). *What is the scope of prescription drug misuse in the United States?* Retrieved June 17, 2024, from https://nida.nih.gov/publications/research-reports/misuse-prescription-drugs/what-scope-prescription-drug-misuse

National Institute on Drug Abuse [NIDA]. (2024a). *Cocaine*. Retrieved June 21, 2024, from https://nida.nih.gov/research-topics/cocaine

National Institute on Drug Abuse [NIDA]. (2024b). *MDMA (Ecstasy/Molly)*. Retrieved June 21, 2024, from https://nida.nih.gov/research-topics/mdma-ecstasy-molly

National Institute on Drug Abuse [NIDA]. (2024c). *Ketamine*. Retrieved June 22, 2024, from https://nida.nih.gov/research-topics/ketamine

National Institute on Drug Abuse [NIDA]. (2024d). Inhalants. Retrieved April 9, 2025 from https://nida.nih.gov/research-topics/inhalants

National Institute on Drug Abuse [NIDA]. (2024e). *Anabolic steroids and other appearance and performance enhancing drugs (APEDs)*. Retrieved June 26, 2024, from https://nida.nih.gov/research-topics/anabolic-steroids

National Institute on Drug Abuse [NIDA]. (2024f). *Emerging drug trends*. Retrieved June 26, 2024, from https://nida.nih.gov/research-topics/emerging-drug-trends

Ng, T., & Keshock, M. C. (2023). Tetrahydrocannabinol (THC). In *StatPearls*. StatPearls Publishing. (nih.gov)

Niu, D., Li, C., Qu, H., & Zheng, Y. (2024). Does cannabis elevate cancer risk? Evidence from Mendelian randomization. *Wiener klinische Wochenschrift*, *136*(11–12), 311–318. https://doi.org/10.1007/s00508-023-02303-3

Oelhaf, R. C., & Azadfard, M. (2023). Heroin toxicity. In *StatPearls*. StatPearls Publishing. https://www.ncbi.nlm.nih.gov/books/NBK430736/

Oelhaf, R. C., Del Pozo, E., & Azadfard, M. (2023). Opioid toxicity. In *StatPearls*. StatPearls Publishing. https://www.ncbi.nlm.nih.gov/books/NBK431077/

Pepper, N., Zúñiga, M. L., & Corliss, H. L. (2024). Use of poppers (nitrite inhalants) among young men who have sex with men with HIV: A clinic-based qualitative study. *BMC Public Health*, *24*(1), 1741. https://doi.org/10.1186/s12889-024-19284-1

Polak, K., Haug, N. A., Dillon, P., & Svikis, D. S. (2023). Substance use disorders in women. *The Psychiatric Clinics of North America*, *46*(3), 487–503. https://doi.org/10.1016/j.psc.2023.04.006

Rana, D., McLeod, A. R., Gaston, P. K., Hill, D. M., & Pourcyrous, M. (2023). Assessing neonatal opioid withdrawal syndrome severity as a function of maternal buprenorphine dose and umbilical cord tissue concentrations. *The Annals of Pharmacotherapy*, *57*(8), 892–898. https://doi.org/10.1177/10600280221134643

Ranker, L. R., Ross, C. S., Rudolph, A. E., Weuve, J., & Xuan, Z. (2023). Identifying and describing trajectories of alcohol use frequency and binge drinking frequency among those aged 15–30 years in a national cohort of US adolescents: A group-based trajectory modeling approach. *Addiction*, *118*(9), 1739–1750. https://doi.org/10.1111/add.16216

Roberts, S. C. M., Zaugg, C., & Biggs, M. A. (2023). Association of mandatory warning signs for cannabis use during pregnancy with cannabis use beliefs and behaviors. *Journal of the American Medical Association Network Open*, *6*(6), e2317138. https://doi.org/10.1001/jamanetworkopen.2023.17138

Rouland, A., Thuillier, P., Al-Salameh, A., Benzerouk, F., Bahougne, T., Tramunt, B., Berlin, I., Clair, C., Thomas, D., Le Faou, A. L., Vergès, B., & Durlach, V. (2024). Smoking and diabetes. *Annales D'endocrinologie*, *85*(6), 614–622. https://doi.org/10.1016/j.ando.2024.08.001

Saunders, H., Panchal, N., & Zitter, S. (2024). Opioid deaths fell in mid-2023, but progress is uneven and future trends are uncertain. KFF. https://www.kff.org/mental-health/issue-brief/opioid-deaths-fell-in-mid-2023-but-progress-is-uneven-and-future-trends-are-uncertain/

Semaan, A., & Khan, M. K. (2023). Neurobiology of addiction. In *StatPearls*. StatPearls Publishing. (nih.gov)

Sprenger, S., & Anderson, J. S. (2024). Dying to quit: Understanding the burden of tobacco in psychiatric patients–A clinical review. *Journal of Psychiatric Practice*, *30*(1), 23–31. https://doi.org/10.1097/PRA.0000000000000764

Substance Abuse and Mental Health Services Administration [SAMSHA]. (1997). A guide to substance abuse services for primary care clinicians. Chapter 2—Screening for Substance Use Disorders. Available from: https://www.ncbi.nlm.nih.gov/books/NBK64820/

Substance Abuse and Mental Health Services Administration [SAMSHA]. (2022). *Screening, Brief intervention, and Referral to Treatment (SBIRT)*. Retrieved on July 3, 2024, from https://www.samhsa.gov/sbirt

Substance Abuse and Mental Health Services Administration [SAMSHA]. (2023a). *2020 National survey on drug use and health: Lesbian, gay and bisexual (LGB) adults. (NSDUH)*. https://www.samhsa.gov/data/data-we-collect/nsduh-national-survey-drug-use-and-health

Substance Abuse and Mental Health Services Administration [SAMSHA]. (2023b). Recovery and recovery support. https://www.samhsa.gov/find-help/recovery

Substance Abuse and Mental Health Services Administration [SAMSHA]. (2024). Results from the 2023 national survey of drug use and health (NSDUH): Key substance use and mental health indicators in the United States. Pub Id: PEP20-03-021. https://store.samhsa.gov/product/results-2023-nsduh/pep24-07-021

Swimmer, K. R., & Sandelich, S. (2024). Substance use disorder. *Emergency Medicine Clinics of North America*, *42*(1), 53–67. https://doi.org/10.1016/j.emc.2023.06.023

Tamura, E. K., Oliveira-Silva, K. S., Ferreira-Moraes, F. A., Marinho, E. A. V., & Guerrero-Vargas, N. N. (2021). Circadian rhythms and substance use disorders: A bidirectional relationship. *Pharmacology, Biochemistry, and Behavior*, *201*, 173105. https://doi.org/10.1016/j.pbb.2021.173105

The National Child Traumatic Stress Network [NCTSN]. (2023). Make the connections: Trauma and substance abuse. https://www.nctsn.org/sites/default/files/resources/making_the_connection_trauma_substance_abuse.pdf

Truth Initiative. (2024). Quitting tobacco. Quitting tobacco fact sheet. https://truthinitiative.org/sites/default/files/media/files/2024/04/Quitting%20Tobacco%20Fact%20Sheet%202024_approved.pdf

United States Drug Enforcement Administration [USDEA]. (2023). DEA reports widespread threat of fentanyl mixed with xylazine. https://www.dea.gov/alert/dea-reports-widespread-threat-fentanyl-mixed-xylazine

U.S. Department of Health and Human Services [USDHHS]. (2020). *Healthy People 2030*. U.S. Government Printing Office. https://health.gov/healthypeople/objectives-and-data/browse-objectives/addiction

U.S. Department of Health and Human Services [USDHHS]. (2023). SAMHSA announces national survey on drug use and health (NSDUH) results detailing mental illness and substance use levels in 2021. https://www.hhs.gov/about/news/2023/01/04/samhsa-announces-national-survey-drug-use-health-results-detailing-mental-illness-substance-use-levels-2021.html

U.S. Food & Drug Administration [FDA]. (2024). Results from the annual national youth tobacco survey. Retrieved January 3, 2025, from https://www.fda.gov/tobacco-products/youth-and-tobacco/results-annual-national-youth-tobacco-survey#2024%20Findings%20on%20Youth%20Use%20for%20E-Cigarette%20Products

van Amsterdam, J., Gresnigt, F., & van den Brink, W. (2024). Cardiovascular risks of simultaneous use of alcohol and cocaine-A systematic review. *Journal of Clinical Medicine*, *13*(5), 1475. https://doi.org/10.3390/jcm13051475

Vasan, S., & Kumar, A. (2023). Wernicke encephalopathy. In *StatPearls*. StatPearls Publishing. (nih.gov)

Wesson, D. R., & Ling, W. (2003). The Clinical Opiate Withdrawal Scale (COWS). *Journal of Psychoactive Drugs*, *35*(2), 253–259. https://doi.org/10.1080/02791072.2003.10400007

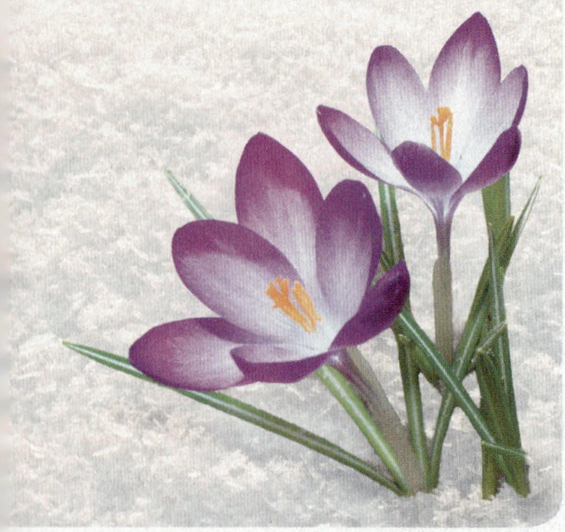

32 Eating Disorders

Nursing Care of People With Eating and Weight-Related Disorders

Jennifer Caires-Kennel and Mary Ann Boyd

KEYCONCEPTS

- binge eating
- body dissatisfaction
- body image distortion
- dietary restraint
- drive for thinness
- emotional dysregulation
- perfectionism
- purge
- shame

LEARNING OBJECTIVES

After studying this chapter, you will be able to:

1. Examine the roles of body image, body dissatisfaction, and gender differences in eating disorders.
2. Relate the primary theories of anorexia nervosa and bulimia nervosa to clinical symptoms and the course of the disorders.
3. Evaluate the significance of trauma in the appearance of anorexia nervosa and bulimia nervosa symptoms.
4. Examine the relationship between social determinants of health and anorexia nervosa and bulimia nervosa.
5. Select strategies to establish a therapeutic relationship with people with anorexia nervosa and bulimia nervosa.
6. Using a clinical judgment model, formulate a person-centered, recovery-oriented nursing care plan for people with anorexia nervosa.
7. Identify medications that are used to treat people with anorexia nervosa and bulimia nervosa and evaluate their effectiveness.
8. Develop wellness strategies for people with anorexia nervosa and bulimia nervosa.
9. Compare and contrast mental health care provided in emergency, inpatient, community, and virtual settings.
10. Support the integration of health care and mental health care for people with anorexia nervosa and bulimia nervosa.
11. Compare and contrast anorexia nervosa, bulimia nervosa, and related disorders.

KEY TERMS

• amenorrhea • anorexia nervosa (AN) • avoidant restrictive food intake disorder (ARFID) • binge-eating disorder (BED) • body image • body mass index (BMI) • body shame • bulimia nervosa (BN) • butyrate • diabulimia • disordered eating behaviors • dysphagia • eating disorders • enmeshment • faecalibacterium • food anxiety • guilt • high-caloric feeding protocols • hyperkinetic • lisdexamfetamine dimesylate • microbiota • orthorexia • other specified feeding or eating disorder (OSFED) • paraventricular thalamus (PVT) • pica • refeeding • refeeding syndrome • relapse prevention • rumination disorder • sarcopenia • self-monitoring • subclinical • superior mesenteric artery (SMA) syndrome

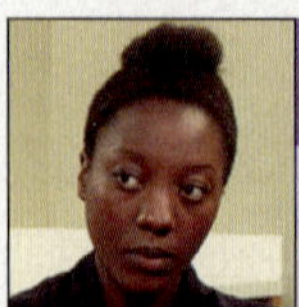

Case Study: Ellen

Ellen is a 20-year-old college sophomore admitted to an inpatient mental health unit after treatment in a medical unit, where she was admitted for dehydration and electrolyte imbalance. Ellen has been binging and purging while in school to maintain an optimal body weight.

INTRODUCTION

Since the 1970s, eating disorders have received national attention, primarily because several high-profile personalities and athletes with these disorders have received front-page news coverage. Since the 1960s, the increased incidence of anorexia nervosa (AN) and bulimia nervosa (BN) has prompted mental health professionals to address their causes and devise effective treatments.

Wellness depends on good nutritional status and healthy eating. Frequently, nurses and other health professionals recommend reduction or increase of body weight to maintain physical health and well-being. In some people, eating and body weight determine their behavior, self-esteem, and self-concept. They strive to reach an unrealistic and unhealthy body weight leading to the development of an eating disorder. Even though eating disorders are defined as mental disorders, the consequences of their disordered eating lead to serious impairment of physical health and sometimes death. All nurses should be able to recognize the symptoms of an eating disorder.

EATING DISORDERS OVERVIEW

Eating disorders are characterized by disturbed eating and eating-related behaviors. The *DSM-5-TR* classification of eating disorders includes anorexia nervosa (AN), bulimia nervosa (BN), binge-eating disorder (BED), pica, rumination disorder, avoidant restrictive food intake disorder (ARFID), and other specified feeding or eating disorders (OSFED) (APA, 2022). **Disordered eating behaviors** are often classified as **subclinical** or partial-syndrome cases of true eating disorders, such as AN and BN, which are psychiatric diagnoses. Individuals with disordered eating behaviors still need treatment despite not meeting the diagnostic criteria. Two other eating disorders—orthorexia and diabulimia—are not currently recognized in the *DSM-5-TR;* however they have gained attention from medical and psychiatric communities. **Orthorexia** is a fixation on eating only "healthy" foods. Although there may or may not be weight loss with orthorexia, the fixation on "healthy" eating can still cause great psychological distress to an individual. **Diabulimia** occurs when an individual with diabetes mellitus type 1 intentionally reduces insulin intake to lose weight. This can lead to diabetes ketoacidosis (DKA) and can be fatal (Poos et al., 2023).

Even though eating disorders differ in definition, clinical course, etiologies, and interventions, symptoms of these disorders, such as dietary restraint, binge eating, and preoccupation with weight and shape, overlap significantly. Viewing the symptoms along a continuum from less to more severe eating behaviors helps with this conceptualization, as shown in Figure 32.1. There are also common psychological characteristics of people with eating disorders (Box 32.1). This chapter highlights anorexia nervosa (AN), emphasizes bulimia nervosa (BN), and briefly discusses binge-eating disorder (BED) and other eating disorders.

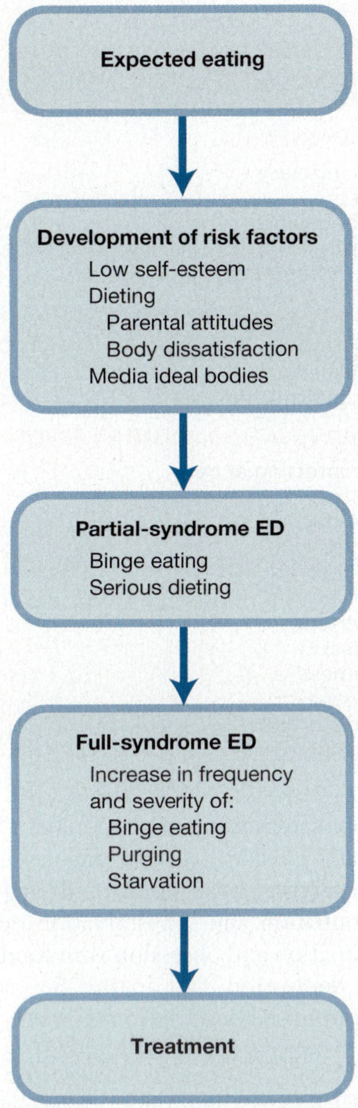

FIGURE 32.1 Progression of symptoms leading to an eating disorder.

KEYCONCEPT Dietary restraint is consciously restricting or controlling food intake. It is a common behavior in eating disorders.

ANOREXIA NERVOSA (AN)

Anorexia nervosa (AN) is a mixture of symptoms that include significantly low body weight, intense fear of gaining weight or becoming fat, and a disturbance in experiencing body weight or shape. People with AN are highly influenced by a distorted self-evaluation of weight or shape. Additionally, they lack recognition of the seriousness of low body weight.

BOX 32.1

Psychological Characteristics Related to Eating Disorders

ANOREXIA NERVOSA

- Issues with intimacy
- Maturity fears
- Ritualistic behaviors
- Perfectionism
- Emotional dysregulation

BULIMIA NERVOSA

- Impulsivity
- Boundary issues
- Limit-setting difficulties

ANOREXIA NERVOSA AND BULIMIA NERVOSA

- Difficulty expressing anger
- Low self-esteem
- Body dissatisfaction
- Powerlessness
- Ineffectiveness
- Perfectionism
- Dietary restraint
- Obsessiveness
- Compulsiveness
- Nonassertiveness
- Cognitive distortions

AN is further categorized into two major types: *restricting* (dieting and exercising with no binge eating or misuse of laxatives, diuretics, or enemas) and *binge eating and purging.* Malnutrition and semistarvation occur because of the preoccupation and obsession with food and weight, binge eating, depression, and apathy. Several body systems are compromised, leading to medical complications and, in some instances, death (APA, 2022).

> **KEYCONCEPT Binge eating** is rapid, episodic, impulsive, and uncontrollable ingestion of a large amount of food during a short period of time, usually for 2 hours. A **purge** is purposeful initiation of stomach or bowel evacuation through self-induced vomiting, misuse of laxatives, diuretics, or enemas.

CLINICAL COURSE

The onset of AN usually occurs in early adolescence. The onset can be slow, with serious dieting occurring before an emaciated body—the result of starvation—is noticed. This discovery often prompts diagnosis. Because the incidence of subclinical symptoms is higher than that of AN, many young people may not receive early treatment for their symptoms, or in some cases, they receive no treatment. Refusal to maintain an expected weight because of a distorted body image and an intense fear of becoming fat make people with this disorder difficult to identify and treat.

AN can be a chronic condition with relapses characterized by significant weight loss. Reporting conclusive outcomes for AN is difficult because of the variety of definitions used to determine recovery. Although patients considered to have recovered have restored expected weight, menses, and eating behaviors, some continue to have distorted body images and be preoccupied with weight and food; many develop BN, and many continue to have symptoms of other psychiatric illnesses, especially mood and anxiety disorders (Juli et al., 2023).

BODY DISTORTION

For most individuals, **body image** (a mental picture of one's own body) is consistent with how others view them. However, individuals with AN have a body image that is severely distorted from reality. Because of this distortion, they see themselves as obese and undesirable even when they are emaciated. They are unable to accept objective reality and the perceptions of the outside world.

> **KEYCONCEPT Body image distortion** occurs when the individual perceives their body disparately from how the world or society views it.

Concept Mastery Alert

People with anorexia nervosa have a distorted image of the appearance of their bodies. They can be very thin and still perceive that they are heavy and need to lose weight.

Drive for Thinness

Because of body distortion, individuals with AN have an intense drive for thinness. They see themselves as fat, fear becoming fatter, and are "driven" to work toward "undoing" this fear.

> **KEYCONCEPT Drive for thinness** is an intense physical and emotional process that overrides all physiologic body cues.

The individual with AN ignores body cues, such as hunger and weakness, and concentrates all efforts on controlling food intake. The entire mental focus of the young patient with AN narrows to only one goal: weight loss. Typical thought patterns are as follows: "If I gain a pound, I'll keep gaining." This all-or-nothing thinking keeps these patients on rigid regimens for weight loss.

The behaviors of patients with AN become organized around food-related activities, such as preparing food, counting calories, and reading cookbooks. Much behavior concerning what, when, and how they eat is ritualistic. Food combinations and the order in which foods may be eaten, and under which circumstances, can seem bizarre. One patient, for example, would eat only cantaloupe, carrying it with her to all meals outside of her home and consuming it only if it were cut in smaller than bite-sized pieces and only if she could use chopsticks, which she also carried with her. Because of the ritualistic behaviors, an all-encompassing focus on food and weight, and feelings of inadequacy, social contacts are gradually reduced, and the patient becomes isolated. More severe weight loss is associated with other symptoms, such as apathy, depression, and even mistrust of others (Tchanturia et al., 2023).

Emotional Dysregulation

KEYCONCEPT Emotional dysregulation is difficulty regulating and controlling feelings and emotions.

Emotions become dysregulated when feelings and their expressions cannot be controlled or regulated. In AN, emotional dysregulation is common. In particular, people with AN have difficulty recognizing, expressing, and understanding their emotions. They tend to avoid conflict and have difficulty expressing negative emotions, especially anger. They are less able to regulate emotions and have fewer strategies to use when upset when compared to people who do not have an eating disorder (Cogodi et al., 2024).

The relationship of emotional dysregulation to AN is unclear. One theory is that the maladaptive behaviors (i.e., binge eating, caloric restrictions) are an attempt to reduce and control negative emotions (Santos & Haynos, 2023). Another closely related theory is that emotional dysregulation is an adaptive response to emotional distress rather than an attempt to control emotions (Cogodi et al., 2024; Gratz & Roemer, 2004).

NCLEXNOTE When assessing patients with anorexia nervosa, the nurse should ask the patient to identify negative emotions that they experience and the strategies that are used to reduce the uncomfortable emotion. This information is critical in establishing goals and outcomes.

Perfectionism

Research findings demonstrate that **perfectionism** is a significant symptom of eating disorders (Robinson & Wade, 2021). Perfectionistic behaviors such as having high personal standards, excessive concern over mistakes, fear of negative evaluation, and self-criticism are typical significant symptoms of AN and BN. These perfectionistic behaviors occur long before the eating symptoms and remains present throughout the eating disorder and into the beginning of recovery. The more severe the disorder, the more perfectionistic the individual behaves. As symptoms are resolved, perfectionism may decrease (Longo et al., 2021).

KEYCONCEPT Perfectionism consists of personal standards (the extent to which the individual sets and tries to achieve high standards for oneself) and concern over mistakes and their consequences for their self-worth and others' opinions.

Shame and Guilt

Patients with AN experience both shame and guilt.

KEYCONCEPT Shame is conceptualized as a negative evaluation of self that leads to a sense of feeling small and worthless.

Shame negatively affects an individual's core identity and is associated with a desire to disappear. Shame is a central feature of AN (Panero et al., 2022). People with AN experience **body shame** (negative evaluation of body) and shame around eating (i.e., forbidden food) (Nechita et al., 2021). Body shame is related to the drive for thinness and body dissatisfaction and leads to pervasive feelings of worthlessness.

Shame can be devastating to people with AN. They report feeling lost in the world and want to disappear. Shame can lead to loss of identity, social isolation, and self-harm (Kiely et al., 2024). Shame also occurs in the parents/guardians of children with AN, making it difficult for them to help their children (Marchetti & Sawrikar, 2024).

Guilt occurs when a behavior such as eating a forbidden food is negatively evaluated and causes feelings of remorse and regret but does not affect the individual's identity. Guilt is associated with a desire to repair or undo (Panero et al., 2022). For someone with AN, guilt is associated with feeling fat and fear of weight gain. Feelings of having overeaten and feelings of fat are associated with fear of weight gain, which lead to dysfunctional behaviors such as diuretic/laxative use, self-weighing, binge eating, and diet restriction (Ralph-Nearman et al., 2024).

DIAGNOSTIC CRITERIA

The diagnosis of AN is made when there is a restriction of intake, leading to significantly low body weight. The **body mass index** (BMI) is used as a measure of severity. Other criteria include an intense fear of gaining weight or becoming fat, and body image issues including an undue influence of body weight on self-concept and lack of recognition of seriousness of low body weight (APA, 2022). See Key Diagnostic Characteristics 32.1 for an overview of diagnostic criteria and associated findings.

ANOREXIA NERVOSA ACROSS THE LIFESPAN

AN is primarily diagnosed in adolescence, with 90% of the cases in people assigned female at birth. The incidence in 10- to 14-year-olds in this population has increased from 8.6 to 38.6 per 100,000 (van Eeden et al., 2023). AN is also the most common eating disorder diagnosed in individuals over 50 years of age. Late-onset AN is mostly diagnosed in people assigned female at birth. AN in older adults is associated with significant psychiatric comorbidities and overall morbidity (Mulchandani et al., 2021).

KEY DIAGNOSTIC CHARACTERISTICS 32.1

***DSM-5-TR* DIAGNOSTIC CRITERIA: Anorexia Nervosa**

A. Restriction of energy intake relative to requirements, leading to a significantly low body weight in the context of age, sex, developmental trajectory, and physical health. *Significantly low weight* is defined as a weight that is less than minimally normal or, for children and adolescents, less than that minimally expected.
B. Intense fear of gaining weight or of becoming fat, or persistent behavior that interferes with weight gain, even though at a significantly low weight.
C. Disturbance in the way in which one's body weight or shape is experienced, undue influence of body weight or shape on self-evaluation, or persistent lack of recognition of the seriousness of the current low body weight.

***Specify* whether:**

- **Restricting type:** During the last 3 months, the individual has not engaged in recurrent episodes of binge-eating or purging behavior (i.e., self-induced vomiting or the misuse of laxatives, diuretics, or enemas). This subtype describes presentations in which weight loss is accomplished primarily through dieting, fasting, and/or excessive exercise.
- **Binge-eating/purging type:** During the last 3 months, the individual has engaged in recurrent episodes of binge-eating or purging behavior (i.e., self-induced vomiting or the misuse of laxatives, diuretics, or enemas).

***Specify* if:**

- **In partial remission:** After full criteria for anorexia nervosa were previously met, Criterion A (low body weight) has not been met for a sustained period, but either Criterion B (intense fear of gaining weight or becoming fat or behavior that interferes with weight gain) or Criterion C (disturbances in self-perception of weight and shape) is still met.
- **In full remission:** After full criteria for anorexia nervosa were previously met, none of the criteria have been met for a sustained period of time.

***Specify* current severity:**

The minimum level of severity is based, for adults, on current body mass index (BMI) (see below) or, for children and adolescents, on BMI percentile. The ranges below are derived from World Health Organization categories for thinness in adults; for children and adolescents, corresponding BMI percentiles should be used. The level of severity may be increased to reflect clinical symptoms, the degree of functional disability, and the need for supervision.

- **Mild:** BMI ≥17 kg/m^2
- **Moderate:** BMI 16 to 16.99 kg/m^2
- **Severe:** BMI 15 to 15.99 kg/m^2
- **Extreme:** BMI <15 kg/m^2

EPIDEMIOLOGY AND RISK FACTORS

The 12-month prevalence of AN among young people assigned female at birth is approximately 0.4%, but many researchers believe this figure does not reflect the true prevalence of this serious disorder (APA, 2022). The age of onset is typically between 14 and 16 years but can occur much earlier. Adolescents are vulnerable because of stressors associated with their development, especially concerns about body image, autonomy, peer pressure, and their susceptibility to such influences as the media, which extols an ideal body type (van Eeden et al., 2023).

Psychiatric disorders increase the risks of eating disorders. Low self-esteem, body dissatisfaction, and feelings of ineffectiveness also put individuals at risk. Bullying and weight teasing are other risk factors for the development of an eating disorder (Lie et al., 2021).

Elite athletes participating in lean sports (sports relying on a thin physique to maximize performance, for example, running, gymnastics, and wrestling) and nonelite athletes taking part in nonlean sports (e.g., soccer, powerlifting, and golf), experience a triad of symptoms (disordered eating, menstrual dysfunction, and osteoporosis). See Box 32.2. Athletes involved in lean sports are at higher risk of developing an eating disorder than other populations (Ghazzawi et al., 2024).

Eating disorders are not just about food but are associated with sexual interpersonal trauma, which can lead to psychological difficulties and emotional dysregulation. Individuals who have been sexually abused may restrict or binge and/or purge to cope with body dissatisfaction while hiding their emotions about the event from others (Convertino et al., 2022).

NCLEXNOTE A history of childhood trauma (bullying, neglect, physical or sexual abuse) is a risk factor for eating disorders. If sexually abused, individuals may intentionally lose or gain weight to be less attractive. However, if an individual has an eating disorder it does not necessarily mean they suffered from a traumatic event.

Sex Assigned at Birth

People assigned female at birth are 10 times more likely than people assigned male at birth to develop AN. (These populations are referred to hereafter in this section as "females" and "males," respectively.) This disparity has been attributed to society's pressure on females to internalize a thin body as ideal. Puberty is a risk period for the development of AN. Females often begin to diet at an early age because of body dissatisfaction, and the need for control of prepubertal weight increases. Restricting food can lead to starvation, binge eating, and purging. Males are more likely to engage in physical activity than dieting. Females demonstrate a drive for thinness; males have increased concern with muscularity and shape (Kadoura et al., 2024). See Box 32.3.

The LGBTQ+ population has risk factors that put them at increased risk for eating disorders. These risk factors include stigma related to their gender identity, low self-esteem, and mental health disorders (anxiety disorders, phobias, substance use disorders). Transgender

BOX 32.2

Research for Evidence-Based Practice: Eating Disorder Concerns in Elite Athletes

Fatt, S. J., George, E., Hay, P., Jeacocke, N., Gotkiewicz, E., & Mitchison, D. (2024). An umbrella review of body image concerns, disordered eating, and eating disorders in elite athletes. Journal of Clinical Medicine, 13*(14), 4171. https://doi.org/10.3390/jcm13144171*

THE QUESTION: What is the evidence regarding the prevalence and risk factors for disordered eating and body image concerns across various population of elite athletes?

METHODS: Five databases (Scopus, SPORTDiscus, MEDLINE, CINAHL, & PsycINFO) were reviewed and 1828 articles were screened for meeting the following inclusion criteria: peer-reviewed reviews or meta-analyses that reported on a sample of current or former elite athletes (national, international, professional, and NCAA D1), and synthesized findings on prevalence or risk factors for disordered eating or body image concerns. Twenty-four articles were included. Risk factors that were investigated included body dissatisfaction, sport type, pressures within sport, sport-specific psychological factors, and career changes.

FINDINGS: The prevalence for disordered eating ranged from 0% to 85.8%, and clinical eating disorders from 1.3% to 32.5%, with eating disorders not otherwise specified (EDNOS) the most common eating disorder diagnosis (up to 90%). For people assigned male at birth, 0% to 13.6% met the level of eating disorders in screening questions; for people assigned female at birth, 7.4% to 50% met the eating disorder level.

Disordered eating is significantly higher in elite athletes versus non-athletes. Athletes assigned female at birth typically reported higher disordered eating and body dissatisfaction than those assigned male at birth. Greater body dissatisfaction and negative affect were identified as risks for disordered eating and depression. Greater risk of disordered eating was found in people who played lean sports vs non-lean sports, high-energy expenditure sports (i.e., cyclists), wrestlers, and dancers. Pressure from coaches, internalization of sport-specific beliefs (i.e., ideal body for performance), and disruptions or changes in athletic career were identified as risks for disordered eating.

IMPLICATIONS FOR NURSING: Nurses should be aware that elite athletes have higher rates of disordered eating than the general population and should be assessed for eating disorders. Treatment should include a holistic approach that includes consideration of an individual's unique risk factors and also preventative measures. General and sport-specific pressures and mediating factors should be examined. Additional support may be needed for those involved in lean sports and high-energy expenditure sports.

BOX 32.3

Eating Disorders in People Assigned Male at Birth

Eating disorders in people assigned male at birth are becoming more prevalent. People in this population present with eating disorders between the ages of 16 and 24, with other specified eating disorders, night eating syndrome, and bulimia nervosa as the most prevalent disorders. Adolescents in this group are more likely to try to gain weight or bulk up and engage in muscle-enhancing behaviors, such as eating more or differently, using supplements, and taking androgenic-anabolic steroids. Overweight and obesity in people assigned male at birth may be associated with disordered eating behaviors including fasting, skipping meals, vomiting, using laxatives and diuretics, or binge eating. Identification of eating disorders in primary care settings may be difficult because the individual may be concealing their symptoms due to stigma associated with their perception that eating disorders are a disease of people assigned female at birth. In addition, because of the paucity of research related to eating disorders in people assigned male at birth, providers may not correctly diagnose this disorder. Because many of the assessment instruments and treatment protocols are geared toward people assigned female at birth, people assigned male at birth suffer from a lack of early identification of their disorders as well as a lack of early as well as successful treatment.

Source: Kadoura, B., Ganson, K. T., & Katzman, D. K. (2024). Anorexia nervosa in adolescent males. *CMAJ: Canadian Medical Association Journal 196*(6), E191. https://doi.org/10.1503/cmaj.230001

individuals are also at risk for eating-disordered behavior in efforts to prevent puberty onset or progression (Baker et al., 2024; Yesildemir & Akbulut, 2023).

Ethnicity and Culture

In the United States, recent studies show very few differences in prevalence of eating disorders in all racial, ethnic, and socioeconomic groups (Friedlich et al., 2024). Evidence shows that certain groups, such as Hispanic/Latino and African American adults, are at higher risk for eating disorders (Alexander et al., 2024). The diagnoses of AN and BN were developed based on research involving European and European American young adults assigned female at birth; these disorders were falsely believed to affect primarily people in this population who were White, young, thin, upper class, and cisgender (Alexander et al., 2024). It is important to recognize that eating disorders affect all individuals across ages, races, ethnicities, sexual orientations, gender identities, socioeconomic statuses, weight statuses, and their intersections.

COMORBIDITY

Depression is common in individuals with AN, and these individuals are at risk for suicide attempts (Amiri et al., 2023; Cadwallader et al., 2023). The most prevalent comorbid psychiatric disorders are mood disorders and substance use disorders. Anxiety disorders such as obsessive-compulsive disorder (OCD), phobias, and panic disorder are also associated with AN (Udo & Grilo, 2022). In fact, perfectionism is an aspect of both OCD and AN (Robinson & Wade, 2021). These comorbid conditions may often resolve when AN has been treated successfully. However, in many cases, an anxiety disorder may continue even following successful treatment of AN. AN is also associated with medical disorders such as fibromyalgia, cancer, anemia, and osteoporosis (Udo & Grilo, 2022).

COVID-19 Pandemic

People with eating disorders were negatively affected by the COVID-19 pandemic. Research suggests that individuals who were previously diagnosed with AN reported having worsening symptoms due to social isolation, increased anxiety, and reduced contact with their treatment team (J Devoe et al., 2023). Social isolation and feelings of uncertainty led to psychopathological changes, increased vulnerability, and treatment modifications. For some individuals, self-care and reduced social pressure were associated with resilience. Online treatment was an alternative to in-person treatment (Monteleone et al., 2021).

ETIOLOGY

The etiology of AN is multidimensional. Some of the risk factors (discussed earlier) and the etiologic factors overlap. For example, dieting is a risk factor for the development of AN, but it is also an etiologic factor, and in its most serious form—starving—it is also a symptom.

Biologic Theories

There is evidence that the volume of gray and white matter in the brains of people with AN is reduced but is normalized during weight restoration. These deficits may reflect malnourishment. Other studies suggest that there may structural alterations even after long-term recovery (Su et al., 2021). Research is ongoing.

Genetic Theories

Eating disorders are highly inheritable. First-degree relatives of people with AN have higher rates of this disorder. Rates of subthreshold cases among family members assigned female at birth of individuals with AN are even higher (Levine & Sadeh-Sharvit, 2023). Such relatives also have high rates of depression, leading researchers to hypothesize that a shared genetic factor may influence development of both disorders.

Genetic research indicates that a genetic vulnerability to AN exists, especially in people assigned female at birth. Genetic heritability is high among children of people with eating disorders; such children are 3 to 5 times more likely than the general population to develop an eating disorder. Separating genetic influences from environmental influences is difficult when twins share a similar family environment (Levine & Sadeh-Sharvit, 2023).

Neuroendocrine and Neurotransmitter Changes

Several neurobiologic changes occur in an eating disorder. The most common findings are increased activation of the amygdala and changes in the activation of the cingulate cortex (Wronski et al., 2023). An increase in endogenous opioids (through exercise) contributes to denial of hunger (Goldfarb et al., 2024). Malnutrition leads to a decrease in thyroid function (Haines, 2023). Serotonergic functioning is also blunted in low-weight patients (Alberts et al., 2023).

Gut Microbiome

The gut microbiome in AN shows depletion of faecalibacterium when compared to healthy-weight individuals. **Faecalibacterium** is an important group of gut bacteria that produce **butyrate** through fermentation of dietary fiber. Butyrate, a short-chain fatty acid, helps fight inflammation and repairs and enhances the barrier function of intestinal epithelial cells. In AN, reduced faecalibacterium in the gut microbiome leads to reduced anti-inflammatory effect at intestinal barrier cells (Zhao et al., 2024).

Psychological Theories

Historically, the most widely accepted explanation of AN was the psychoanalytic paradigm that focused on conflicts of separation–individuation and autonomy. Usually diagnosed between 14 and 18 years of age, AN was thought to occur as a result of a developmental arrest of typical adolescent struggles around identity and role, body image formation, and sexuality (Bruch, 1973). Dieting and weight control were viewed as a means to defend against these feelings of inadequacy and growing into adulthood.

The psychoanalytic paradigm explained the disparity in the prevalence of eating disorders between prepubescent individuals assigned female and male at birth as being related to the development of self-esteem in adolescents assigned female at birth. It was believed that the typical adolescent increase in self-doubt was linked to naturally occurring pubertal weight gain, which in turn resulted in confusion about one's identity. However, this view is only one of several possible explanations for the occurrence of AN in modern society (Jassogne et al., 2023).

Internalization of Peer Pressure

Some adolescents have reported that dieting, binge eating, and purging initially began as a result of peer pressure and a need to conform. Subsequently, many factors then converge that influence the initial behaviors to develop into a full syndrome eating disorder. Friends, as well as peers in the larger school system, influence unhealthy weight-control behaviors among preadolescents and adolescents assigned female at birth (Li & Li, 2022).

Body Dissatisfaction

Once the body is considered all-important, the individual begins to compare their body with others, such as those of celebrities. Images from social media are particularly powerful for preadolescents and adolescents assigned female at birth struggling with the tasks of identity and body image formation. Body dissatisfaction resulting from this comparison, in which one's own body is perceived to fall short of an ideal, may be dissatisfaction about one's weight, shape, size, or even a certain body part. Even in the absence of overweight, most adolescents surveyed in numerous studies were dissatisfied with their bodies (Vuong et al., 2021). Because this factor is so prevalent in people assigned female at birth and especially adolescents in this country, body dissatisfaction is considered less predictive for a diagnosis of AN. Yet it remains an important factor that follows the internalizing of an ideal body weight.

> **KEYCONCEPT Body dissatisfaction** occurs when the body is viewed negatively and becomes overvalued as a way of determining one's worth.

Many adolescents attempt to overcome this dissatisfaction through dieting and overexercising.

Social Theories

More than with any other psychiatric condition, society plays a significant role in the development of eating disorders with conflicting messages that young people assigned female at birth receive from society about their roles in life. Young prepubescent people assigned female at birth may interpret expectations about how they should look, what roles they should perform, and what they should achieve in society. Exposure to social media sites idealizing excessively thin bodies and glorifying extreme caloric restriction is associated with disordered eating behaviors (Jiotsa et al., 2021).

The media, the fashion industry, and peer pressure are significant social influences. Social media depicts preadolescents and adolescents assigned female at birth, with thin and often emaciated bodies, as glamorous, successful, popular, and powerful. People in this population diet because they want to be similar to these models both in character and appearance (Mushtaq et al., 2023).

Preadolescent children are extremely susceptible to the message to reduce intake and increase exercise as a way to lose weight and maintain health. Coupled with Internet videos that sanction self-starvation, emerging adolescents are already dissatisfied with their bodies and have the tools to lose weight through dieting and exercise.

Feminists have focused on the role of this pressure regarding the female body as one part of an explanation for the significant increase in eating disorders and for the greater prevalence in people assigned female at birth. Box 32.4 outlines some feminist assumptions regarding role, feminism, and the development of eating disorders.

> BOX 32.4
>
> **Feminist Ideology and Eating Disorders**
>
> Since the 1970s, proponents of the feminist cultural model of eating disorders have advanced a position to explain the higher prevalence of these disorders in people assigned female at birth (referred to hereafter in this box as "females"). Feminists believe females today are engaged in a struggle similar to the ones they believe females have had in history. They believe that during the Victorian era, "hysteria," a well-known emotional illness, developed as a result of oppression when females were not allowed to express their feelings and opinions and were "silenced" by a society dominated by people assigned male at birth. Feminist scholars today advance an explanation of the prevalence of eating disorders in females that suggests body dissatisfaction and eating dysfunction are associated with weight stigma and its internalization. Weight stigma—societal preference for thinner bodies and negative perceptions of higher-weight individuals—is internalized, leading to negative view of self. Weight stigma and societal weight bias lead to body image disturbance and disordered eating.
>
> Source: Martin-Wagar, C. A., Attaway, S. E., & Melcher, K. A. (2023). Differences among feminist and non-feminist women on weight bias internalization, body image, and disordered eating. *Journal of Eating Disorders, 11*, 129. https://doi.org/10.1186/s40337-023-00851-7

FAMILY RESPONSE TO DISORDER

Families of patients with anorexia are characterized as being enmeshed, overprotective, perfectionistic, rigid, and focused on success. Although an uninformed family can delay and complicate treatment, there is no evidence that family interactions are the cause of eating disorders, but their interactions can contribute to its development and delay in treatment (Mensi et al., 2021).

When conflict erupts and direct communication is blocked, family interaction can become dysfunctional. Since food is an integral part of family life, family conflict can easily occur around food choices and behaviors. In an enmeshed family, the individual gets lost in the family system. In **enmeshment**, boundaries that define individual autonomy are diffuse. Excessive togetherness intrudes on children's and adolescents' personal privacy that leads to difficulty differentiating and regulating emotions. When parents/guardians are overly protective

BOX 32.5

Research for Evidence-Based Practice: Parents' Weight Bias and Children's Eating Behaviors

Winograd, D., Goldschmidt, A. B., & Lydecker, J. (2024). Associations among parents' internalized weight bias, negative child-focused body talk, and feeding behaviors. Eating Behaviors, *52, 101848. https://doi.org/10.1016/j.eatbeh.2024.101848*

THE QUESTION: Does parental weight bias internalization and negative body talk relate to parents' feeding practices?

METHODS: Community-based adults (*n* = 242) over the age of 21 with at least one child (5 to 15 years old) were recruited to complete online assessments of parenting, bullying, eating, and weight. Parents were asked to have one child in mind when completing the surveys. The children's body mass index (BMI) was calculated based on parents' reports of their child's age, weight, and height. The BMI of the parents was also recorded. The parents completed (1) a self-report measure that evaluated how they speak to their child about their child's appearance and weight, (2) a weight-bias internalization scale, and (3) a child feeding questionnaire. Correlations among the scores were determined.

FINDINGS: Higher levels of parent weight-bias internalization and negative body talk were positively related to a child's weight and restrictive eating patterns. Parents may be acting on their concerns about their child's weight by trying to help their child lose weight.

IMPLICATIONS FOR NURSING: Nurses should assess the concerns of parents/guardians about their children's weight and restricting feeding practices. Nurses should educate parents/guardians about the link between restricting children's eating and the development of disordered eating and weight gain.

and parental control is exerted over the children and adolescents, difficulties in emotional regulation occur that contribute to dysfunctional eating behavior (Scotto Rosato et al., 2024).

The family, often unwittingly, can transmit unrealistic attitudes about weight, shape, and size. Adolescents are particularly sensitive to comments about their bodies because this is the stage for body image formation. Parental attitudes about weight have been found to influence body dissatisfaction and dieting; parental comments about weight or shape or even parents/guardians worrying about their own weight can influence adolescents in much the same way as the media does. See Box 32.5.

Hurtful weight-related comments by family members and significant others have been associated with disordered eating in people of all genders. Adolescents' perceived family functioning and the quality of their relationship with each parents/guardian have been shown to positively influence body image dissatisfaction and disordered eating. Therefore, healthy family relationships are believed to be a protective factor for developing an eating disorder and support research findings linking parental-focused treatment programs to positive outcomes for those with eating disorders (Chapman et al., 2021).

RECOVERY-ORIENTED CARE FOR PEOPLE WITH ANOREXIA NERVOSA

Teamwork and Collaboration: Working Toward Recovery

Treatment for the patient with AN focuses on initiating nutritional rehabilitation to restore the individual to a healthy weight, resolving psychological conflicts around body image disturbance, increasing effective coping skills, addressing the underlying conflicts related to maturity fears and role conflict, and assisting the family with healthy functioning and communication. Several strategies are used to accomplish these goals during the stages of illness and recovery.

The medical complications presented in Table 32.1 influence the decision to hospitalize an individual with an eating disorder. Suicidality is another reason for hospitalization. The criteria for hospital admission vary, and there is a lack of evidence-based studies determining when adolescents with AN should be hospitalized.

After an acceptable weight (at least 85% of ideal) is established, the patient is discharged to a partial hospitalization program or an intensive outpatient program. The intensive therapies needed to help patients with their underlying issues (e.g., body distortion and maturity fears) and to help families with communication and enmeshment usually begin after refeeding because concentration is usually impaired in severely undernourished patients with anorexia.

Family therapy typically begins while the patient is still hospitalized. Recently family-based therapies and caregiver-based approaches have shown promise in the treatment of eating disorders. These assist in improving overall communication within the family and helps members understand the disorder (Stewart & Baumann, 2024).

Interpersonal therapy (IPT) is a type of treatment that focuses on uncovering and resolving the developmental and psychological issues underlying the disorder. Role transitions and negative social evaluations typically are the focus (Russell et al., 2023). IPT and family-based therapies are sometimes combined.

Dialectic behavioral therapy (DBT) specifically designed for patients with AN has shown positive results. See Chapter 30. This skills training focuses on emotional dysregulation, viewed as a key symptom in AN (Cogodi et al., 2024).

TABLE 32.1 COMPLICATIONS OF EATING DISORDERS

Body System	Symptoms
From Starvation to Weight Loss	
Musculoskeletal	Loss of muscle mass, loss of fat (emaciation), osteoporosis
Metabolic	Hypothyroidism (symptoms include lack of energy, weakness, intolerance to cold, and bradycardia), hypoglycemia, decreased insulin sensitivity
Cardiac	Bradycardia; hypotension; loss of cardiac muscle; small heart; cardiac arrhythmias, including atrial and ventricular premature contractions, prolonged QT interval, ventricular tachycardia, sudden death
Gastrointestinal	Delayed gastric emptying, bloating, constipation, abdominal pain, gas, diarrhea
Reproductive	Amenorrhea, low levels of luteinizing hormone and follicle-stimulating hormone, irregular periods
Dermatologic	Dry, cracking skin and brittle nails caused by dehydration, lanugo (fine, baby-like hair over the body), edema, acrocyanosis (bluish hands and feet), thinning hair
Hematologic	Leukopenia, anemia, thrombocytopenia, hypercholesterolemia, hypercarotenemia
Neuropsychiatric	Unusual taste sensation (possible zinc deficiency) Apathetic depression, mild organic mental symptoms, sleep disturbances, fatigue
Related to Purging (Vomiting and Laxative Misuse)	
Metabolic	Electrolyte anomalies, particularly hypokalemia, hypochloremic alkalosis; hypomagnesemia; increased blood urea nitrogen
Gastrointestinal	Salivary gland and pancreatic inflammation and enlargement with increase in serum amylase, esophageal and gastric erosion (esophagitis) rupture, dysfunctional bowel with dilation, superior mesenteric artery syndrome
Dental	Erosion of dental enamel (perimylolysis), particularly of the frontal teeth, with decreased decay
Neuropsychiatric	Seizures (related to large fluid shifts and electrolyte disturbances), mild neuropathies, fatigue, weakness, mild organic mental symptoms
Cardiac	Ipecac cardiomyopathy arrhythmias

Safety Issues

Mortality is high among patients with AN, especially when compared with patients with other mental illnesses. Mortality is reported to be 3% to 7%, with a longer duration of the disorder predicting a higher range of the mortality rate. Suicide and cardiopulmonary arrest are the leading causes of death for individuals with AN (Akgül et al., 2024). These individuals tend to die by suicide with highly lethal means in which rescue is unlikely. Nurses need to pay special attention to the risk of suicide with these individuals (see Chapter 22). A significant number of individuals with eating disorders also self-injure without suicide attempts (Kirkpatrick et al., 2024).

EVIDENCE-BASED NURSING CARE FOR PEOPLE WITH ANOREXIA NERVOSA

Nurses must use a comprehensive and multidisciplinary approach when caring for an individual with AN. Physical health must be prioritized due to severe medical complications that may be present. Recovery also includes identifying and addressing any underlying psychosocial behaviors.

RECOGNIZING CUES: RELEVANT ASSESSMENT INFORMATION

Physical Health

Successful treatment of and recovery from AN depends upon early detection. The longer an individual suffers with AN, the higher the mortality risk. Therefore, nurses must understand the cues of AN. Common warning signs of AN in an individual include:

- Dramatic weight loss and low BMI
- Changes in eating patterns (such as not eating foods they once enjoyed)
- Excessive chewing or chewing and spitting
- Control of food
- Extreme dieting, restricting food groups, or engaging in food rituals
- Skipping meals
- Preoccupation with food, calories, and body weight. Possibly also frequent weighing or body-checking
- Body dissatisfaction
- Irregular or absent menstrual or delayed puberty in patients assigned female at birth

- Overexercising or visiting the bathroom immediately after meals
- Difficulty concentration
- Feeling cold all the time
- Cuts and calluses across the top of finger joints (Russell sign) from inducing vomiting
- Dental issues
- Lanugo (fine, soft hair that covers the body)

NCLEXNOTE Eating disorders are serious psychiatric disorders that threaten life. Careful assessment and referral for treatment are important nursing interventions.

Recognizing these warning signs, along with conducting a thorough evaluation of body systems, is important because many systems are compromised by starvation. The patient's current weight should be assessed and determined using the BMI and a scale. BMI, thought to reflect weight most accurately because exact height is used, is calculated by dividing weight in kilograms by height in meters squared. An acceptable BMI is between about 19 and 25. Currently, criteria for discharge require patients to be at least 85% of ideal weight according to height and weight tables.

Menses history also must be explored in that it provides information about possible estrogen depletion. However, it is often difficult to conclude that **amenorrhea** is present due to starvation because people in this age group may be prepubescent, have irregular periods, or may be on oral contraceptives. However, if menses was regular prior to AN, a return to regular menses after treatment can signify substantial body fat restoration. Fat and weight restoration have been hypothesized to aid in improving bone mineral density (Milano et al., 2022).

Medical Complications

While performing a head-to-toe assessment, nurses should document any findings of emaciation, hypotension, hypothermia, and bradycardia. Individuals who engage in purging behaviors may also exhibit dysfunctional bowels, inflammation of the salivary or parotid glands, erosion of enamel (specifically on front teeth), esophageal erosion, and Russell sign. Physical issues should be treated before the psychological issues can be meaningfully addressed.

Laboratory tests should also be examined for data. Electrolyte imbalances can be an indicator of AN due to dehydration or excess water consumption, starvation, or purging behaviors. One common electrolyte imbalance is hypokalemia. Laboratory tests that can help identify damage to the body include hemoglobin, hematocrit, hepatic enzymes, hormones (estrogen or testosterone), and BUN/creatinine. A complete metabolic panel (CMP) and complete blood count (CBC) are commonly completed since they check for all of these areas. Other tests such as an electrocardiogram (ECG), urinalysis, and bone densitometry should also be assessed. An ECG can assess if there is any damage to the heart from starvation. A urinalysis can detect dehydration by testing urine-specific gravity and presence of ketones. It is also important to do a bone densitometry because individuals with AN are at risk for bone density loss. Loss of bone density can be reversed if nutrition is introduced (osteopenia); however, in extreme cases bone density loss cannot be reversed (osteoporosis). Other tests usually included are stool examination for occult blood and an abdominal x-ray.

Psychosocial Assessment

Behavioral Responses

The psychological symptoms that patients with anorexia experience are listed in Box 32.1. The classic symptoms of body distortion—fear of weight gain, unrealistic expectations and thinking, and ritualistic behaviors—are easily noted during a clinical interview. Often, people with AN avoid conflict and have difficulty expressing negative emotions, such as anger. Other conflicts, such as issues with intimacy and feelings of ineffectiveness, may underlie this disorder. These symptoms may not be apparent during a clinical interview; however, instruments are available to determine their presence and severity. There is a high rate of nonsuicidal self-injury in patients with eating disorders, and the type and frequency of these behaviors should be assessed (Kirkpatrick et al., 2024).

The *Eating Attitudes Test* is frequently used in community samples (Garner et al., 1982). There is also a child version of this test, the CHEAT. The results of these paper-and-pencil tests can help identify the most significant symptoms for an individual patient and indicate a focus for interventions, especially therapy. In clinical settings, the *Eating Disorder Examination Questionnaire* (EDEQ) (Fairburn & Beglin, 1994) is frequently used.

Self-Concept

Individuals with eating disorders are usually struggling with their self-concept. It is important to determine their self-concept and self-esteem. In many instances, these individuals appear to be very competent, but when queried about their views, they often feel that they are not good enough and will describe their perceived faults in great detail.

Stress and Coping Patterns

Individuals with an eating disorder are often coping with stress and anxiety through controlling eating. In times of perceived stressful events, the dysfunctional eating pattern often becomes worse. An assessment of the stress the individual is experiencing and coping patterns is important because a part of successful treatment is developing healthy coping skills.

Social Network

Assessing social networks is important for individuals suffering from AN because they are at risk for social isolation. People with AN may struggle with eating with other people around them, including friends and family. Therefore, individuals with AN may avoid social settings that include food (i.e., weddings, family reunions, birthday parties, or even just a meal out with a friend). The assessment should also focus on family interaction, influence, and peer relationships. The role of the patient in the family and community should be considered, as well as the individual's ability to cope in social situations. For adolescents who are attending school, a conference with the teacher or counselor provides information regarding the amount and frequency of social contacts.

Spiritual Assessment

A spiritual assessment is important for people with AN because of the shame and guilt that is often present in these individuals. They can become isolated from others and their disorder becomes their identity (Cole, 2024). The nurse can determine the significance of religious beliefs and their impact on the patient's eating behavior. If individuals have been accessing pro-dieting sites on social media, discussions of bodily disgust and self-discipline can lead to calorie restriction and excessive exercise. These sites often use religious metaphors that suggest fasting is a purification ritual (Tragantzopoulou et al., 2024).

Quality of Life

People with AN have a lowered quality of life (QoL) than others with psychiatric disorders or those without psychiatric disorders. Behaviors that may lower the quality of life include low BMI, depression, anxiety, and purging. Individuals with AN often recall selective events and focus on negative aspect of the event, which, in turn, contributes to a low quality of life (Neipp et al., 2024).

Strengths Assessment

Strengths such as motivation to eat differently and have a more typical lifestyle may emerge during the interview. The following questions could be asked to elicit personal strengths:

- Do you remember a time when you did not have to worry about what you ate? If so, how old were you and what did you like to do?
- Have you found any strategy that prevented you from worrying about what you hate?
- Are you ready to change your eating patterns? What do you think will help you change your eating patterns?
- When you are successful in other areas (school, athletics), how do you reward yourself?

ANALYZING CUES AND DEVELOPING HYPOTHESES

Priorities of Care

Patients may complain of chest pain or heart palpitations, which can be signs of changes in heart structure and function. Arrhythmias are a result of electrolyte imbalances, specifically hypokalemia, hypomagnesemia, and hypocalcemia, and can be life threatening. Since the body has been starved of nutrients, it is unable to function properly and is forced to conserve energy. Therefore, the heart becomes weaker and cannot pump effectively. This in turn causes bradycardia and hypotension, which can lead to dizziness or syncope (Friars et al., 2023). Often a heart rate of less than 40 beats per minute and a blood pressure under 82/48 mmHg requires hospitalization. Bradycardia and hypotension can be reversed if weight is restored. It is important to note athletes with AN will have an even lower heart rate, which will become rapid with mild exertion.

Another symptom to consider is suicidality. Suicide risk is increased in those suffering with AN and is the second leading cause of death in these individuals (Akgül et al., 2024). Many individuals with AN have a depressed mood, past trauma, and become socially isolated due to their disordered eating and overexercise patterns. Therefore, suicidality and changes in mood are a high priority of nursing care and should be carefully assessed via the suicide risk assessment and the mental status exam. See Box 32.6.

Signs and symptoms of dehydration should also be taken seriously. Dehydration can be due to restricting or purging behaviors and can lead to electrolyte imbalances and kidney damage. Purging behaviors can also lead to hypovolemic shock, seizures, and kidney or heart failure. Blood in the vomit is a sign of an esophageal tear or rupture from repeated self-induced vomiting and can be fatal.

Refeeding syndrome is also of concern. Signs and symptoms are discussed later in this chapter.

Other Complications

Additional signs and symptoms that may occur with AN include the following:

- Anemia and lanugo are expected in a patient who is malnourished.
- Amenorrhea in patients assigned female at birth is not life threatening but can lead to long-term

BOX 32.6

Building Clinical Judgment With SBAR: Nurse Communication With Provider Regarding Patient With Anorexia Nervosa

SBAR

S: Situation

Lane is a 16-year-old individual assigned female at birth who is diagnosed with anorexia nervosa—restricting type. She was admitted 5 days ago to the eating disorder unit for severe weight loss, bradycardia, and hypotension. She is currently having suicidal thoughts but no plan; she denies homicidal thoughts and hallucinations. She has started olanzapine 2.5 mg once daily at bedtime.

B: Background

This is the first hospitalization for Lane. No previous suicide attempts were reported, but she reported seeing a therapist for self-harm behaviors and suicidal ideations that started 1 year ago.

A: Assessment

- Physical Health: Ht. 5′1″, Wt. 80 (BMI: 15.1 kg/m^2)
- Vital Signs: BP 90/60, HR 62, R 8
- Oriented X 4
- Mood: tearful; behavior: sleeps most of the day. Expresses feelings of hopelessness. Concerned about having to gain weight and not being able to exercise while in treatment
- Increased risk for suicide due to current suicidal ideations, mood, and history
- Increased risk for falls due to low BP, HR, and medication

R: Recommendation

- Institute suicide precautions.
- Staff check-in once per shift to assess mood and suicidal ideations.
- Conduct rounds every 15 minutes.
- Closely monitor patient for falls.

Building Clinical Judgment

1. Why did the nurse recommend checking on the patient every 15 minutes?
2. Why did the nurse associate fall risk with the medication?

complications due to decreased hormones (i.e., osteoporosis, cardiovascular disease, infertility, and reproductive cancers).

- **Dysphagia** (difficulty swallowing) may occur because of malnutrition and will require dietary modification. Low-fiber diets that are soft and easy to digest are recommended to reduce the feeding volume and the symptoms of early satiety. The patient may need tube feedings.
- **Superior mesenteric artery (SMA) syndrome** is a rare disorder in which acute angulation of the SMA causes compression of the third part of the duodenum between the SMA and the aorta. SMA syndrome can lead to obstruction of the duodenum, causing patients to have epigastric abdominal pain and a need for a liquid diet or tube feeding.
- **Sarcopenia** and other musculoskeletal complications can result in functional weakness and balance impairments, increasing fall risks and necessitating physical therapy evaluation and treatment.

PLANNING RECOVERY AND WELLNESS OUTCOMES: GENERATING SOLUTIONS

The mental health and wellness goals are very closely aligned for people with AN. Successful recovery involves establishing positive wellness habits of nutrition, physical activity, sleep, coping with stress, and developing a support system. The nurse and patient should prioritize long- and short-term goals. For example, a long-term goal is to maintain an optimal weight through healthy eating and exercise. A short-term goal is to increase food intake by 300 calories per day.

NCLEXNOTE One of the most helpful skills the nurse can teach patients with eating disorders is to set realistic goals around food and around other activities or tasks. Because of perfectionism, patients with anorexia nervosa often set unrealistic goals and end up frustrated. The nurse can help them establish smaller, more realistic, and attainable goals.

THERAPEUTIC RELATIONSHIP

Establishing a therapeutic relationship with individuals with AN may be difficult initially because they tend to be suspicious and mistrustful. These individuals believe authority figures and health personnel will intervene to disrupt their restricting and starvation behaviors, placing them in a position of extreme fear of becoming fat. At the time they are hospitalized, mistrust can almost reach a state of paranoia. Because of their low body weight and starvation, they are often impatient and irritable. A firm, accepting, and patient approach is important in working with these individuals. Providing a rationale for all interventions helps build trust, as does a consistent, nonreactive approach. Power struggles over eating are common, and remaining nonreactive is a challenge. During such power struggles, the nurse should always think about their own feelings of frustration and need for control.

TAKING ACTION: NURSING INTERVENTIONS

Physical Care

People with anorexia can usually perform self-care activities. They may actually be overly perfectionistic regarding daily self-care activities. If symptoms become severe, hospitalization may be necessary to re-establish a healthy body weight.

Nutritional Rehabilitation

Refeeding, the most important intervention during the hospital or initial stage of treatment, is also the most challenging. In AN, there is a shift from carbohydrate to fat and protein utilization, placing the body in a catabolic state. In this state, there is an altered insulin response and increased glucagon secretion. As nutritional balance is re-established, anabolic metabolism is restored and the body switches back to carbohydrate metabolism leading to lower levels of phosphate. During refeeding, patients typically gain a large proportion of their body weight within a few weeks (Lopes et al., 2023).

The traditional refeeding protocol typically starts with a low-calorie diet (i.e., 1,000 calories a day) and is increased slowly until the patient is consuming at least 3,500 calories a day in several meals. The aims of this diet are to develop somatic stability and to improve the mental state of the patient prior to psychotherapy.

Recently, **high-caloric feeding protocols** (i.e., starting with 1,500 calories a day) are being used that shorten hospital stays and increase initial weight gain (Haas et al., 2021). There is controversy regarding this type of aggressive refeeding. To prevent further weight loss, rapid increase of calories provides the best result. There is concern about the development of refeeding syndrome (discussed later in this section). Also, **food anxiety** (when thoughts about food become intrusive and distressing) is commonly experienced by people with AN. This is particularly true if there is a comorbid disorder such as depression, OCD, or PTSD. Increased anxiety can exacerbate the symptoms, making recovery more difficult. It is important that benefits of refeeding be weighed against the risk of increasing anxiety (Salter et al., 2024).

The nurse must monitor patients closely during meals and snacks for any eating-disordered behaviors. For example, the nurse must should ensure that all food is consumed and that the patient is not hiding food or participating in food rituals (e.g., cutting food into very small pieces, separating food on the plate, or excessively chewing before swallowing). All meal and snack portions have been decided by a dietician and are individualized for each patient in order for them to reach a healthy weight. Therefore, all of the portions must be consumed by the patient in a certain time frame. If the meal or snack is not consumed, oral liquid supplements such as Boost or Ensure are offered to the patient.

The individual will be fearful of weight gain or in denial about their illness and may refuse to eat. Commonly, staff on eating disorder units respond to multiple food refusals by placing a nasogastric tube (NG tube), and the patient will be given oral supplements through the NG tube.

Patients should be encouraged to use the bathroom before meals and snacks. Bathroom visits should be monitored to prevent purging behaviors or disposing of hidden food after meals and snacks. Bathrooms should be locked when they are not in use, and patients are not allowed to use the bathroom for at least 1 hour after meals and snacks.

Weight-increasing protocols usually include behavioral plans using positive reinforcements (i.e., excursion passes) and negative reinforcements (i.e., returning to bed rest) to encourage weight gain. The nurse should help patients to understand that these actions are not punitive. As patients begin gaining and maintaining weight, they are given more autonomy around nutrition. They can begin filling out their menus on the eating disorder units. They may also be able to attend cooking classes, practice portioning meals, and even choose from restaurant menus with the help of their dieticians.

Weights should also be closely monitored by the nurses. Patients should be weighed in a hospital gown every morning after they use the bathroom but before their first meal. Patients should not be allowed to see their weights, so they will need to step on the scale backwards. If there is any drastic change in weight, nurses should obtain a random weight. Patients may try to manipulate weight gain by hiding objects in their underwear or drinking excessive amounts of fluids before getting weighed. Often, patients do this to try and leave treatment early.

Electrolytes may be completely depleted in AN, so nursing care involves stabilizing electrolyte balance. Potassium depletion usually results from use of diuretics, diarrhea, and vomiting. Calcium depletion is related to large intake of dietary fiber, which decreases calcium absorption. Many individuals also need phosphorus replacement (Haas et al., 2021). During hospitalization, these electrolytes, if warranted, are replaced through oral or intravenous therapy.

A complication of refeeding is the development of **refeeding syndrome**, severe electrolyte disturbances leading to a decrease in serum phosphorus, and/or potassium, and/or magnesium levels, and/or organ dysfunction resulting from a decrease in any of these and/or due to thiamine deficiency, occurring within 5 days of reintroduction of calories (Brodie et al., 2024). This condition can develop during the refeeding process and include circulatory fluid overload, respiratory failure, and cardiac failure. Hypophosphatemia is a precursor to refeeding syndrome, which can result in sudden death. To decrease the risk of developing refeeding syndrome, calories should be increased slowly over time (Kells et al., 2023).

Emergency Care

Emergency care is not usually needed for individuals with AN. Family members and peers usually notice the weight loss and emaciation before patients' systems are compromised to the degree that they require emergency treatment. If systems are compromised enough to warrant emergency treatment, patients usually are admitted immediately for medical-surgical inpatient care.

Inpatient

Determining the level of care depends on the severity of the eating disorder. Hospitalization is typically required for AN and BN. For AN, typical indicators of hospitalization include severe weight loss (<75% ideal body weight), hypothermia, cardiac irregularities (bradycardia), hypotension, orthostatic changes in vital signs, dehydration, and electrolyte anomalies. If the BMI is severely low, there is a higher risk of mortality the first few days of hospitalization, thus it is crucial to begin treatment. Safety and mental status are thoroughly evaluated throughout the treatment process since there is an increased risk for self-harm and suicide. Some hospitals have specialized eating disorder units, which is more ideal than a mental health or medical surgical floor. Eating disorder units are staffed with teams of nurses, psychiatrists, medical doctors, dieticians, therapists, and social workers. Each patient's team will determine a dietary plan based on the individual's height, age, and developmental pattern. For children and adolescents, growth charts and BMI are referenced to determine healthy weights.

Promotion of Sleep

Sleep disturbance is also common, and these individuals are viewed as **hyperkinetic** (with restlessness or excessive movements). They sleep little, but they usually awaken in an energized state. A structured, healthy sleep routine must be established immediately to conserve energy and calorie expenditure because of low weight. To further conserve energy, patients are often relegated to bed rest until a certain amount of weight is regained. Exercise is generally not permitted during refeeding and only with caution after this phase. Inpatients must be closely supervised because they are often found exercising in their rooms, running in place, and doing calisthenics.

Medication Interventions

There are no medications approved by the Food and Drug Administration specifically for AN. However, certain medications are used to treat symptoms associated with AN. The atypical, second-generation antipsychotic, olanzapine, has shown to help patients gain weight and reduce anxiety and intensity of eating disordered thoughts. Selective serotonin reuptake inhibitors (SSRIs) have also been used in the treatment of AN and sometimes in combination with olanzapine, especially regarding comorbid influences and symptoms such as major depressive disorder and anxiety (Fornaro et al., 2023). SSRIs fluoxetine and sertraline are most commonly used. Because of the intense fear of weight gain, patients can experience panic attacks around meal and snack time and may require an anxiolytic. See Box 32.7.

BOX 32.7

Medication Profile: Fluoxetine Hydrochloride

DRUG CLASS: Selective serotonin reuptake inhibitor

RECEPTOR AFFINITY: Inhibits central nervous system neuronal uptake of serotonin with little effect on norepinephrine; thought to antagonize muscarinic, histaminergic, and α-adrenergic receptors.

INDICATIONS: Treatment of depressive disorders, obsessive-compulsive disorder, bulimia nervosa, and panic disorder.

ROUTES AND DOSAGE: Available in 10- and 20-mg capsules and 20-mg/5-mL oral solution.

Adults: 20 mg/d in the morning, not to exceed 80 mg/d. Full antidepressant effect may not be seen for up to 4 weeks. If no improvement, dosage is increased after several weeks. Dosages greater than 20 mg/d are administered twice daily. For eating disorders: typically, 60 mg/d is recommended.

Geriatric: Administer at lower or less frequent doses; monitor responses to guide dosage.

Children: Safety and efficacy have not been established.

HALF-LIFE (PEAK EFFECT): 2 to 3 days (6 to 8 hours)

SELECTED ADVERSE REACTIONS: Headache, nervousness, insomnia, drowsiness, anxiety, tremors, dizziness, light-headedness, nausea, vomiting, diarrhea, dry mouth, anorexia, dyspepsia, constipation, taste changes, upper respiratory infections, pharyngitis, painful menstruation, sexual dysfunction, urinary frequency, sweating, rash, pruritus, weight loss, asthenia, and fever.

BOXED WARNING: Increased risk of suicidal thoughts and behaviors in children, adolescents, and young adults.

WARNINGS: Avoid use in pregnancy and while breastfeeding. Use with caution in patients with impaired hepatic or renal function and diabetes mellitus. Possible risk for toxicity if taken with tricyclic antidepressants.

SPECIAL PATIENT AND FAMILY EDUCATION

- Be aware that the drug may take up to 4 weeks to get a full antidepressant effect.
- Take the drug in the morning or in divided doses, if necessary.
- Families and caregivers of pediatric patients being treated with antidepressants should monitor patients for agitation, irritation, and unusual changes in behavior.
- Report any adverse reactions.
- Avoid driving a car or performing hazardous activities because the drug may cause drowsiness or dizziness.
- Eat small, frequent meals to help with complaints of nausea and vomiting.

Psychosocial Interventions

Therapeutic Interactions

Identifying feelings, such as anxiety and fear, and especially negative emotions, such as anger, is the first step in helping patients decrease conflict avoidance and develop effective strategies for coping with these feelings.

Do not attempt to change distorted body image by merely pointing out that the patient is actually too thin. This symptom is often the last to resolve itself, and some individuals may take years to see their bodies realistically. However, although this symptom is difficult to abate, patients can continue to fear becoming fat but not be driven to act on the distortion by starving. The fear of becoming fat eventually lessens with time.

Enhancing Cognitive Functioning

The nurse can help individuals with cognitive distortions and unrealistic assumptions to restructure the way they view the world, especially relative to food, eating, weight, and shape. Faulty ways of viewing these situations result in ineffective coping. Table 32.2 lists some distortions commonly experienced by individuals with eating disorders and some typical restructuring responses or statements that challenge the distortion, which the nurse can present as more realistic ways of perceiving situations. Imagery and relaxation are often used to overcome distortions and to decrease anxiety stemming from a distorted body image.

TABLE 32.2 COGNITIVE DISTORTIONS TYPICAL OF PATIENTS WITH EATING DISORDERS, WITH RESTRUCTURING STATEMENTS BY THE NURSE

Distortion (Patient)	Clarification or Restructuring (Nurse)
Dichotomous or All-or-Nothing Thinking	
"I've gained 2 lb., so I'll be up to 100 lb. soon."	"You have never gained 100 lb., but I understand that gaining 2 lb. is scary."
Magnification	
"I binged last night, so I can't go out with anyone."	"Feeling bad and guilty about a binge are difficult feelings, but you are in treatment, and you have been monitoring and changing your eating."
Selective Abstraction	
"I can only be happy 10 lb. lighter."	"When you were 10 lb. lighter, you were hospitalized. You can choose to be happy about many things in your life."
Overgeneralization	
"I didn't eat anything yesterday and did okay, so I don't think not eating for a week or two will harm me."	"Any starvation harms the body, whether or not outward signs were apparent to you. The more you starve, the more issues your body will encounter."
Catastrophizing	
"I purged last night for the first time in 4 months—I'll never recover."	"Recovery includes ups and downs, and it is expected you will still have some mild but infrequent symptoms."

Using Behavioral Intervention

Many of the same behavioral interventions used in the care of people who are depressed or anxious are also implemented in the care of people with AN. See Chapter 6. Reinforcing and rewarding positive eating behaviors and avoiding reinforcement of perfectionistic and ritualistic behaviors can help the patient refocus on meaningful, healthy behaviors.

Complementary Therapies

Complementary therapies are often used as adjunctive treatments for symptoms of AN. Mindfulness and meditation can provide support (Owens et al., 2023). Yoga, virtual reality, eye movement desensitization and reprocessing, music therapy, and biofeedback are promising interventions (Zakers & Cimolai, 2023). Acupuncture is showing to be safe and effective in increasing food intake and body weight and shortening time to expected food intake (Chen et al., 2023).

Spiritual Interventions

Spiritual care can enhance treatment success by addressing feelings of shame and guilt. As individuals with AN struggle with hopelessness, religious/spiritual principles of hope, trust, acceptance, forgiveness, and power can help in healing. Helping patients connect or reconnect to a higher power can relieve feeling of isolation (Cole, 2024).

Psychoeducation

When weight is restored and concentration is improved, patients with AN can benefit from psychoeducation. Although these individuals have a wealth of knowledge about food and calories, they also have misinformation that needs clarifying. For example, they are often unclear about the role of "fats" in a healthy diet and try to be as "fat free" as possible. A thorough assessment of their knowledge is important because they seem to be "walking calorie books" with little information on the role of all of the nutrients and the importance of including them in a healthy diet. There are several topic areas that should be included in a teaching plan. See Box 32.8.

BOX 32.8

Psychoeducation Checklist: Anorexia Nervosa

When caring for a patient with anorexia nervosa, be sure to include the following topic areas in the teaching plan:

- Psychopharmacological agents, if used, including drug, action, dosage, frequency, and possible adverse effects
- Nutrition and eating patterns
- Effect of restrictive eating or dieting
- Weight monitoring
- Safety and comfort measures
- Avoidance of triggers
- Self-monitoring techniques
- Trust
- Realistic goal setting
- Resources

Teaching Strategies

Several factors influence the outcome of treatment for individuals with AN. Particularly long duration of symptoms and low weight when treatment begins predict poor outcomes, but family support and involvement generally improve outcomes. Comorbid conditions and their severity also influence recovery, especially anxiety disorders. Distorted thinking and eating patterns can set the stage for a relapse and later for the possible development of BN.

Wellness Strategies

Individuals with AN are very aware of wellness recommendations related to nutrition and exercise. Since they focus on nutrition, exercise, and weight control, their real challenge is to focus less on nutrition and exercise and more on developing positive self-concept and emotional wellness. They often ignore the other wellness dimensions, such as developing positive coping skills for stress management, developing a sense of connection with others, and searching for meaning or a purpose in life. See Table 32.3.

Providing Family Education

Denial, guilt, and subsequent greater overprotectiveness are common reactions of the family, especially when hospitalization has been necessary. In addition to family therapy with a skilled therapist, the nurse can help family members express their feelings, increase effective communication, decrease protectiveness, and resolve guilt. Often, siblings become resentful of the patient with an eating disorder because of the significant amount of attention they get from their parents/guardians. Having siblings discuss these feelings and the effect the illness has had on them is helpful. Families and friends are eager to help the patient with AN but often need direction. Box 32.9 provides a list of strategies that may assist them.

TABLE 32.3 WELLNESS CHALLENGES AND STRATEGIES

Challenge	Coping Strategy
To recognize the need for moderate physical activity, healthy foods, and sleep	• Limit physical activity to a reasonable schedule • Practice increasing amounts of healthy food • Track sleep and increase amount of sleep (if needed) and engage sleep hygiene techniques
To cope effectively with drive for thinness	• Identify times when the need to restrict diet occurs • Examine other strategies for dealing with the situation
To manage stress	• Practice meditation • Use cognitive strategies to examine beliefs and thoughts
Increase self-concept	• Keep a list of accomplishments • Help others • Keep busy • Participate in counseling or therapy
To develop a sense of connection, belonging, and a support system	• Develop a plan to increase social contact
To expand a sense of purpose and meaning in life	• Pray • Meditate • Help others • Volunteer

Developing Recovery-Oriented Rehabilitation Strategies

Recovery of people with AN focuses on physical, psychological, and social aspects. Maintaining an expected

BOX 32.9

What Family and Friends Can Do to Help Those With Eating Disorders

- Tell the individual you are concerned, you care, and you would like to help. Suggest that the individual seek professional help from a provider or therapist.
- If the individual refuses to seek professional help, encourage reaching out to an adult, such as a teacher, school nurse, or counselor.
- Do not discuss weight, the number of calories being consumed, or particular eating habits.
- Do try to talk about things other than food, weight, counting calories, and exercise.
- Avoid making comments about an individual's appearance. Concern about weight loss may be interpreted as a compliment; comments regarding weight gain may be felt as criticism.
- It will not help to become involved in a power struggle. You cannot force the individual to eat.
- You can offer support. Ultimately, however, the responsibility and the decision to accept help and to change rest with the individual.
- Read and educate yourself regarding these disorders.

weight and nutrition will require resisting urges to diet and overexercise. Motivation to continue to work toward recovery should be supported throughout recovery. Development of cognitive strategies to address these issues will need to be reinforced through attending support groups and maintaining a treatment alliance with a provider.

Relapse prevention plays a major role in recovery. The patient and family should work closely with a clinician to understand the patient's individual relapse process. Together, they identify the triggers and early warning signs of relapse and agree upon a relapse prevention plan that responds to the triggers. There is an increased risk of relapse in the first few months following discharge from acute care, indicating a need for frequent follow-up. After 2 months, the risk of relapse progressively decreases over time (Walsh et al., 2021).

Evaluation of Patient Outcomes

After implementing interventions, the nurse evaluates their effectiveness. Short-term outcomes for individuals with AN include becoming medically stable, stabilizing nutrition, restoring weight, and improving coping skills. Nurses can evaluate the extent these goals have been met. Long-term goals include improving body dissatisfaction, self-esteem, and social networks.

Continuum of Care

Community Care

Care does not end once an individual with AN is medically and nutritionally stable. Recovery from the psychological effects of the disorder can take years. Therefore, after being discharged from inpatient care, an individual may attend a partial hospitalization program to help them reintegrate back into their home life. They will start to eat meals at home and rely less on their team of dieticians, psychiatrists, and therapists. If their weight and nutrition is stable, they can begin outpatient treatment. An outpatient basis still includes individual and family therapy, nutrition counseling to reinforce healthy eating patterns and attitudes, and provider visits to monitor weight and evaluate somatic recovery. Support groups, which are often suggested, should not be substituted for therapy. Following an inpatient treatment program, many people with AN are referred for intensive outpatient therapy or day treatment programs prior to the usual outpatient therapy of 1 or 2 hourly sessions a week. In intensive outpatient therapy, patients may return to school but participate four to five evenings a week in a 4- to 5-hour structured program that includes group therapy, meeting with a dietician, and individual therapy. After full recovery, support groups are useful in maintaining recovery.

School Interventions

Younger patients with AN may have lost some school time because of hospitalization. Integrating back into a school and classroom setting is difficult for most. Shame and guilt about having an eating disorder and being hospitalized must be addressed. Because these patients typically have isolated themselves before hospitalization and treatment, renewing friendships and relationships with peers may provoke anxiety. Involving school nurses and teachers in the reentry process may help.

Prevention and early detection strategies for parents/guardians and schoolteachers are often the focus of school nurses and mental health nurses who work in the community. Some of these strategies appear in Box 32.10 and are based on the research on risk factors and protective factors.

National eating disorder awareness and advocacy groups work toward educating the general public, those at risk, and those who work with groups at risk, such as teachers and coaches. They also monitor the media and work to remove unhealthy advertisements and articles that appear in magazines appealing to preadolescents assigned female at birth. Policies, both health and social, can decrease the prevalence of eating disorders. Strategies include improving school-based curriculum to include content on prevention of eating disorders, implementing school-based antibullying policies that protect students from being bullied about their weight, and training educators including coaches and health providers on prevention and early identification.

BOX 32.10

Eating Disorder Prevention Strategies for Parents/Guardians and Children

EDUCATION FOR PARENTS/GUARDIANS

- Real versus ideal weight
- Influence of attitudes, behaviors, teasing
- Ways to increase self-esteem
- Role of media: TV, magazines, social media
- Signs and symptoms
- Interventions for obesity
- Boys at risk also
- Observe for rituals
- Supervision of eating and exercise

STRATEGIES FOR CHILDREN

Education:

- Peer pressure regarding eating, weight
- Menses, puberty, expected weight gain
- Strategies for obesity
- Ways to develop or improve self-esteem
- Body image traps: media, retail clothing
- Adapting and coping with issues
- Reporting friends with signs of eating disorders

Screening: Screen for risk factors
Assessment: Assess for treatment
Follow-up: Monitor for relapse

Virtual Mental Health Care

Virtual mental health care is available through electronic applications available for downloading on a cell phone from national helplines such as the National Eating Disorders Association and the National Association of Anorexia and Associated Disorders. Virtual applications are also being used in treatment of distorted body image to help people receive realistic representation of body size (Di Natale et al., 2024).

Integration With Primary Care

People with eating disorders are frequently treated in primary care for medical issues related to their eating disorder. Primary care services should coordinate with mental health services to treat mental health issues related to the individual's eating disorder. When there are few psychiatric services available, eating disorders are treated and monitored by the primary care provider. The patient should have access to a therapist and dietitian in any treatment setting. Due to the fast-paced nature of primary care, eating disorders are not as easily recognized in a general health care setting and are often missed.

BULIMIA NERVOSA

Bulimia nervosa (BN) was once thought to be a type of anorexia nervosa (AN). However, findings from extensive investigations have identified its characteristics as a separate entity. It is more prevalent than AN. Individuals with BN are usually older at onset than are those with AN. The disorder generally is not as life-threatening as AN. The usual treatment is outpatient therapy. Outcomes are better for BN than for AN, and mortality rates are lower (Jain & Yilanli, 2023).

CLINICAL COURSE

Few outward signs are associated with BN. Individuals binge and purge in secret and are typically of expected weight; therefore, it does not come to the attention of parents/guardians and peers as readily as does AN. Treatment consequently can be delayed for years as individuals attempt on their own to get their eating under control. Patients usually initiate their own treatment when control of their eating becomes impossible. When treatment is undertaken and completed, patients typically recover completely, except in cases in which personality disorders and comorbid serious depression are also present.

Patients with BN present as overwhelmed and overly committed individuals, "social butterflies" who have difficulty with setting limits and establishing appropriate boundaries. They have an enormous number of rules regarding food and food restriction, and they feel shame, guilt, and disgust about their binge eating and purging. They may also be impulsive in other areas of their lives, such as spending.

DIAGNOSTIC CRITERIA

BN involves eating a large amount of food within a discrete period of time (e.g., 2 hours) and engaging in recurrent episodes of binge eating and compensatory purging in various forms such as vomiting or using laxatives, diuretics, or emetics or in nonpurging compensatory behaviors, such as fasting or overexercising in order to avoid weight gain. These episodes must occur at least once a week for a period of at least 3 months to meet the *DSM-5-TR* criteria. Self-evaluation is excessively and inappropriately influenced by body weight and shape. Unlike AN, there is little or no weight loss. See Box 32.1 for psychological characteristics related to BN.

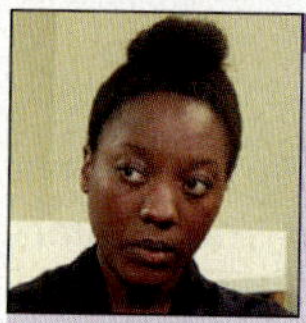

Remember Ellen?

Ellen is of expected weight but has been vomiting one to two times a week for several months after binging. She has calluses on her hands from her teeth when she gagged herself. She sees herself as very overweight.

Does Ellen have characteristics of bulimia nervosa? If she did not know that these behaviors were symptoms of bulimia, how would you explain to her what her symptoms might mean?

Binge eating is followed by feelings of guilt, remorse, and often self-contempt, leading to purging. To assuage the out-of-control feeling, dietary restraint is instituted and precipitates the next binge. The restrictions are viewed as "rules," such as no sweets, no fats, and so forth. The rules may be about what one can and cannot eat. Each binge sets up an out-of-control feeling, and thus the individual then sees the need for even stricter rules about what can and cannot be consumed, leading to more frequent binge eating. This cycle has prompted clinicians to focus treatment primarily on interventions related to dietary restraint. When dietary restraint is resolved, binge eating is decreased, and generally, the purging that follows binge eating also is decreased. Feeling out of control with food is often the major complaint when individuals seek treatment for BN.

Dieters' deprivation, or restraint, whether real or imagined, contributes to overeating and binging. Genetic predisposition for binge eating and deprivation may make dieters more prone to feel distressed over their dietary "failures," especially if dieting has become a way to overcome body dissatisfaction and to compensate for distress through dietary restraint that leads to overeating. Whether the eating is influenced by the attraction of forbidden foods or by internal needs to assuage failure, there is significant evidence that restraining one's intake can be related to bouts of overeating (Stewart et al., 2022).

BULIMIA NERVOSA ACROSS THE LIFESPAN

BN occurs in all age groups. It is not as common in children as in adolescents and adults; children appear more likely to have BED, discussed later. This finding has only recently been reported, and more data are needed to substantiate this finding (Matheson, 2024).

EPIDEMIOLOGY AND RISK FACTORS

The lifetime prevalence of BN is as high as 2.3% depending on whether clinical or community populations are sampled, with 1.3% of people assigned female at birth and 0.5% of assigned male at birth having BN. People assigned female at birth are five times more likely to develop bulimia than assigned male at birth (Jain & Yilanli, 2023).

There are numerous risk factors associated with BN, including genetic risk, being an individual assigned female at birth, obstetric complications and perinatal factors, higher BMI, frequent dieting, overexercising, and concern about body weight. Other risk factors include pressure to be thin, thin-ideal internalization, body dissatisfaction, negative emotionality, low parent/guardian support, and modeling of eating pathology (Yamamiya & Stice, 2024). Childhood sexual abuse and/or neglect has often been suggested as a risk factor for eating disorders (Hill et al., 2024). The beginning of puberty and the start of early adulthood are high-risk periods when adverse life events or peer teasing about appearance may trigger bulimic behavior, particularly if there is genetic susceptibility (Parsons & Clemens, 2023).

Age of Onset

Typically, the age of onset is between 15 and 24 years, which is later than the typical onset of AN. Some people assigned female at birth older than the typical age of onset have developed BN, and symptom cases have been identified as subsequent to life stressors such as a loss (Thompson et al., 2022).

Sex Assigned at Birth

As with AN, people assigned female at birth are more likely than people assigned male at birth to experience BN. Box 32.3 discusses people assigned male at birth who have eating disorders.

Ethnicity and Culture

BN is related to culture in the same way as AN. In Western cultures and those becoming Westernized in their norms, the focus on achieving a thin body ideal underlies the dieting and dietary restraint that set up the trajectory toward a diagnosable eating disorder. Any ethnic differences have to do with the degree to which individuals from specific cultural backgrounds internalize the thin ideal.

COMORBIDITY

The most common comorbid conditions are mood disorders, anxiety disorders, substance use disorders, and personality disorders (Juli et al., 2023; Matheson, 2024). If a comorbid condition occurs before the eating disorder develops, it may actually have a role in precipitating the disorder. The suicide rate for BN is around 17.5%%, with suicide attempts and ideation ranging from 15% to 40% (Akgül et al., 2024).

Several medical complications affect those with bulimia. Electrolyte imbalance can lead to cardiac arrhythmia, seizure, and death. Self-induced vomiting with loss of stomach acid can result in hyperchloremic alkalosis and hypokalemia. Chronic vomiting can result in subconjunctival hemorrhages, esophageal damage, acid reflux, and dental lesions (Nitsch et al., 2021).

ETIOLOGY

As with AN, theories do not individually explain the development of BN. Rather, the convergence of many of these factors at a vulnerable stage of individual development best explains causality.

Some of the predisposing or risk factors for AN and BN overlap with theories of causality. For example, dieting puts an individual at risk for the development of BN. The dieting can turn into dietary restraint, a symptom that leads to binge eating and purging. However, not all individuals who diet experience BN. The interplay of other risk factors (e.g., body dissatisfaction and separation–individuation issues) most likely explains the development of this disorder.

Biologic Theories

Some progress has been made in understanding the biologic changes in BN. Dieting, overeating, and stress cause changes in the intestinal **microbiota** and intestinal metabolism. These changes disinhibit the vagus nerve terminals in the gut leading to hyperactivation of the gut–brain axis, which in turn overstimulates the **paraventricular thalamus** (PVT). The PVT regulates seeking and consuming food and is involved in regulating ingestive behaviors under stress (Fan et al., 2023).

Genetic and Familial Predispositions

BN runs in families, with an increased risk for individuals if family members are diagnosed with this disorder.

Research shows that twins with gastrointestinal disease have more symptoms of eating disorders than twins without gastrointestinal disease. This overlap may be explained by genetic influences (Pascoe et al., 2024).

Psychosocial Theories

Symptoms of BN develop when psychological, sociocultural, or environmental events occur. Because the age of onset for BN is late adolescence—going away to college, for example—may represent the first physical separation for some adolescents, who are unprepared for the emotional separation. In addition, an inability to set limits and develop healthy boundaries leads to a sense of being overwhelmed and "drained." Overwhelming feelings often lead to binge eating, either to avoid or to distract oneself from feelings such as resentment, or binge eating can serve to assuage emptiness or to fill up a "drained" self with food (Adams & Hovel, 2024; Wetzel & Himmelstein, 2023).

Cognitive Theory

Many experts view BN as a disorder of thinking in that distortions are the basis for behaviors such as binge eating and purging. Psychological triggering mechanism models explain that cues such as stress, negative emotions, and even environmental cues (e.g., the presence of attractive food) play a role in etiology (Kwan & Dodd, 2024). These cognitive and triggering theories are viewed as an explanation for maintaining the binge eating after it has been established rather than an explanation of causality.

The same sociocultural factors that underlie AN play a significant role in the development of BN.

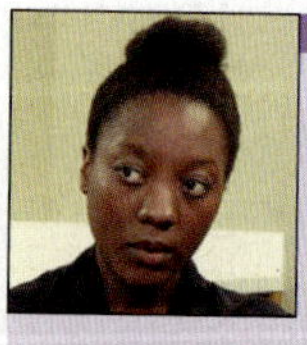

Ellen's Triggers

Some of Ellen's triggers are anxiety, boredom, alcohol use, exhaustion, anger, and social situations where food is readily available.

What are the theoretical explanations that relate her triggers to bulimia behavior? What interventions would you suggest for these triggers?

Family Factors

Dysfunctional family relationships of people with eating disorders have been implicated for years. Current research indicates that perceived lack of cohesion in a family relates to depressive and bulimic behaviors. That is, if an individual is depressed and views family members as less cohesive, close, or supportive, the individual would be more likely to have depression and/or bulimia (Laghi et al., 2021).

RECOVERY-ORIENTED CARE FOR PEOPLE WITH BULIMIA NERVOSA

Teamwork and Collaboration: Working Toward Recovery

Individuals with BN benefit from a comprehensive multimodal treatment approach. The goals for treatment for individuals with BN focus on stabilizing and then normalizing eating, which means stopping the binge–purge cycles; restructuring dysfunctional thought patterns and attitudes, especially about eating, weight, and shape; teaching healthy boundary setting; and resolving conflicts about separation–individuation. Treatment usually takes place in an outpatient setting except when the patient is suicidal or when past outpatient treatment has failed.

Pharmacologic interventions paired with cognitive-behavioral therapy (CBT) or interpersonal psychotherapy are also effective. Antidepressants demonstrate effectiveness in treating binge eating and purging even without comorbid depression. Nutrition counseling is an important part of outpatient treatment to stabilize eating. Some mental health professionals, psychologists, advanced practice psychiatric nurses, and social workers specialize in treating eating disorders, often working with nutritionists who also have expertise with this population. Group psychotherapy and support groups are also used. Family therapy is not usually a part of the treatment because many people with BN live on college campuses away from home or are older and live on their own. Usually, treatment becomes less intensive as symptoms remit. Therapy focuses on psychological issues, such as boundary setting and separation–individuation conflicts and on changing problematic behaviors and dysfunctional thinking using CBT.

Safety Issues

BN is associated with a high risk of suicide, independent of other comorbid disorders. Individuals with BN are also often at risk for self-harm. Because they display high levels of impulsivity, shoplifting, and overspending, financial and legal difficulties have been associated with this disorder (Akgül, 2024; Juli et al., 2023).

EVIDENCE-BASED NURSING CARE FOR PEOPLE WITH BULIMIA NERVOSA

Evidence-based nursing care for people with bulimia includes a comprehensive physical and psychological approach, including a thorough evaluation of eating behaviors and patterns. Establishing a therapeutic relationship will promote trust, safety, and collaboration with the patient, which will aid in their recovery.

RECOGNIZING CUES: RELEVANT ASSESSMENT INFORMATION

Although assessment of patients with BN involves many of the same cues as assessment of patients with AN, the following discussion highlights the unique cues of BN.

Physical Health and Functioning

Even though most individuals with BN maintain expected weights, the physical ramifications of this disorder may be similar to those of AN. The patient's height, weight, vital signs, and orthostatic hypotension should be assessed.

Warning signs of BN may include:

- Preoccupation with body weight and shape
- Visiting the bathroom right after meals
- Using laxatives, diuretics, enemas, or diet pills or self-induced vomiting
- Overexercising or fasting between binges
- Consuming a large quantity of food in a short period or hoarding food

Signs of purging behaviors include dysfunctional bowels, inflammation of the salivary or parotid glands, erosion of enamel (specifically on front teeth), esophageal erosion, and Russell sign. Russell sign or "bulimia knuckles" are abrasions, small lacerations, or calluses noted on the dorsal side of the hands. This is a positive sign of self-induced vomiting, as the incisor teeth scratch the knuckles. Neuropsychiatric disturbances, such as poor concentration and attention, and sleep disturbances, are common.

Laboratory results should be considered in the assessment. A comprehensive metabolic panel, complete blood count with differential, and urinalysis should be ordered by the provider. Vitamin B_{12}, serum magnesium, and phosphorous may also be ordered. An electrocardiogram will determine any unusual heart rhythms. Stool and urine test may be ordered for evidence of laxative use (Jain & Yilanli, 2023).

The nurse should assess current eating patterns, determine the number of times a day the individual binges and purges, and note dietary restraint practices. Sleep patterns and exercise habits are also important.

History of Trauma

Patients with BN have often experienced physical or sexual trauma during childhood. These traumatic experiences frequently underlie the eating dysregulation changes in the brain that patients experience (Cascino & Monteleone, 2024). Nurses should document cues relating to childhood trauma.

Substance Use

BN is associated with substance use, which should be assessed. BN is also highly associated with alcohol-related issues, including alcohol use disorder (Hirvelä et al., 2023) and cannabis use (Wilkinson et al., 2024). Because both alcohol and cannabis use are highly prevalent in society, careful assessment of these areas is important.

Psychosocial Assessment

Similar to AN, individuals with BN require a psychological assessment focusing on cognitive distortions. The psychological characteristics typical of patients with BN are presented in Box 32.1.

Individuals with BN display a significant number of cognitive distortions, examples of which are found in Table 32.2. These thought patterns form the basis for "rules" and lead the way to destructive eating patterns. During routine history taking, patients relate many of these erroneous assumptions. Situations that produce feelings of being overwhelmed and powerless need to be explored, as does the patient's ability to set boundaries, control impulsivity, and maintain quality relationships. These underlying issues precipitate binge eating. Body dissatisfaction should be openly explored. Mood is an important area for evaluation because many people with BN also have depression. Symptoms of depression should be thoroughly explored (see Chapter 25). Clinical Judgment Nursing Care Plan 32.1 sets forth a plan of care for Ellen, the case study patient in this chapter.

Quality of Life

Quality of life (QoL) is negatively impacted by BN as well as AN. In BN, binging and purging as well as dissatisfaction with perceived body shape and body image are related to poor quality of life; these behaviors and perceptions are also associated with alcohol binging (Mallaram et al., 2023; Wilkinson et al., 2024).

Strengths Assessment

People with bulimia can usually identify periods of time when they were able to resist binging and purging. They are usually motivated to reduce or eliminate the binging and purging. The following questions can be used if the strengths do not emerge during the assessment interview.

- How have you curtailed the binging and purging behavior in the past?
- What do you do to reduce your anxiety (instead of binging)?
- Is there anyone in your life that you feel understands your situation?
- How motivated are you to change your eating behaviors and work on body image issues?

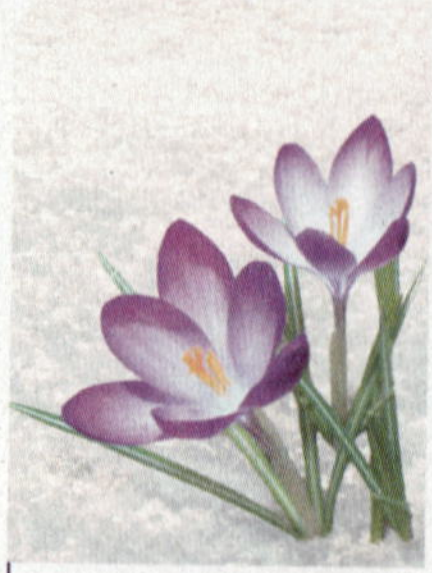

CLINICAL JUDGMENT NURSING CARE PLAN 32.1

The Patient With Bulimia Nervosa

Ellen, age 20, is admitted to the inpatient eating disorders unit for treatment of bulimia nervosa. She was discharged from a medical unit where she was treated for electrolyte imbalance and dehydration. She started binging and purging when she left home for college. She was introduced to ipecac but found that she could force herself to vomit by sticking her hand in her throat. She has agreed to admission in order to learn how to change her behavior.

Setting: Inpatient Psychiatric Unit

Assessment Cues: Ellen wants to maintain a typical weight but believes that she is overweight. She has been binging and purging for 2 years. When she is dieting, she becomes very hungry and binges on as many as 10,000 calories at once. She then becomes angry with herself and purges through vomiting. She feels better temporarily, but soon feels out of control, guilty, and remorseful. She does not use laxatives or diuretics to lose weight. She has dental issues, bilateral parotid enlargement, and tenderness. Her menstrual periods are irregular; cardiac arrhythmias related to electrolyte imbalance noted in chart. BP 110/60; P 70, R 16, Ht. 5 ft 3 in, Wt. 125, BMI 22.9.

Associated Psychiatric Diagnosis

Bulimia Nervosa

Medications

None

Priority Hypothesis: Body Image Disturbance

Important Characteristics

Considers herself too fat and unattractive despite contrary evidence

Associated Considerations

Inaccurate perceptions of body size

Believes that she is too fat despite evidence that she is typical weight.

Planning Recovery and Wellness Outcomes

Initial

Verbalizes feelings related to changing body shape and weight.

Identifies beliefs about controlling body size.

Long Term

Identifies positive aspects of her body and its ability to function.

Taking Action: Nursing Interventions

Interventions	Rationale	Ongoing Assessment
Explore Ellen's beliefs and feelings about body. Maintain a nonjudgmental approach.	To help patient gain a more positive body image, an understanding of her own views is important.	Monitor for statements that identify perceptions of her body. Is her view *distorted* or *dissatisfied*?
Assist patient in identifying positive physical characteristics.	In anorexia, the body is viewed negatively. By focusing on parts of the body that are positive, such as eyes or hands, the patient can begin to experience a positive image of her body.	Observe for patient's reaction to her body. Which areas are viewed positively? Observe for negative statements related to body size and self-esteem.
Clarify patient's views about an ideal body.	Many societal cues idealize an unrealistically thin female body.	Monitor for statements indicating external pressures to lose weight, experiences of teasing about body changes, or evidence of sexual abuse from others.
Provide education related to typical growth of women's bodies, role of fat in protection of body.	Providing education will help in reinforcing a broader view of the importance of a healthy body.	Assess patient's willingness to learn information.

Clinical Judgment Nursing Care Plan 32.1 Continued

Evaluation

Outcomes	Revised Outcomes	Interventions
Ellen revealed that she believes that she is too fat but does have positive physical traits—eyes. She believes that those who are overweight have lost control of their lives. She knows some models who are 6 ft and weigh barely 100 lb.	Accept alternative beliefs related to her own body.	Gradually, focus on other positive physical aspects of Ellen's body. Discuss grooming that encourages a more attractive look. Challenge her beliefs about body weights of models.
Willing to read information about typical body functioning.	Accept a new view of body functioning as a complex phenomenon.	Discuss the biologic aspect of the development of body weight. Emphasize multiple factors determine body weight.

Priority Hypothesis: Motivated for Change

Important Characteristics	Associated Considerations
Expresses willingness to change binging and purging behavior Choices of daily living are appropriate for meeting treatment goals.	History of dieting and purging. Wanting to resume usual eating patterns without purging.

Planning Recovery and Wellness Outcomes

Initial	Long Term
Desires to move to a higher level of wellness. Identify two new strategies to enhance management of bulimia nervosa.	Develop positive eating patterns.

Taking Action: Nursing Interventions

Interventions	Rationale	Ongoing Assessment
Encourage Ellen to discuss her strategies to meet higher wellness goals.	Patient needs to identify specific goals to meet wellness goals.	Determine if she is able to articulate realistic goals.
Help Ellen identify two new strategies to avoid dieting and purging.	Identification of specific, realistic plans to meet needs increases possibility of carrying out strategies.	Determine if goals are doable.

Evaluation

Evaluation	Revised Outcomes	Interventions
Met new wellness goals.	Completed	
Able to use new strategies to resist dieting and purging.	Completed	

ANALYZING CUES AND DEVELOPING HYPOTHESES

Priorities of Care

Mortality due to BN is often the result of medical complications and suicide. Medical complications are a result of binging and purging behaviors and their frequencies. Patients who purge, as well as misuse laxatives, risk fluid, and electrolyte anomalies that can further compromise cardiac status. Electrolyte anomalies are of most concern and should be monitored through frequent laboratory tests and cardiac monitoring. Hypokalemia can contribute to muscle weakness and fatigability, as well as to the development of cardiac arrhythmias, palpitations, and cardiac conduction defects.

PLANNING RECOVERY AND WELLNESS OUTCOMES: GENERATING SOLUTIONS

Important goals for people with bulimia are to establish an expected eating/elimination pattern and to develop positive self-esteem and positive body image. Since these individuals are not likely to be overexercising, helping them normalize physical activities and develop healthy sleep patterns are two possible wellness goals.

THERAPEUTIC RELATIONSHIP

Individuals with BN experience a great deal of shame and guilt (Nechita et al., 2021). They also often have an intense need to please and be liked and may approach the nurse–patient relationship in a superficial manner. They are too ashamed to discuss their symptoms but do not want to disappoint others, so they may discuss more social or unrelated issues in an attempt to engage the nurse. A nonjudgmental, accepting approach, stressing the importance of the relationship and outlining its purpose, is important at the outset (Box 32.11). Explaining the nature of the relationship and the goals of therapy will help clarify the boundaries.

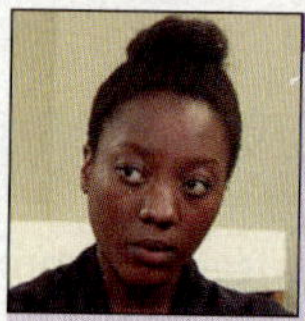

Consider This

Ellen feels shame and guilt over her binging and purging. She does not like to talk about it and is very reluctant to talk to the nurse about the behavior.

Which interventions would be helpful to help Ellen deal with her guilt? Would she be a candidate for a support group?

TAKING ACTION: NURSING INTERVENTIONS

Physical Care

If the patient is admitted to the hospital, meals and all food intakes are strictly monitored to normalize eating.

BOX 32.11

Therapeutic Dialogue: The Patient With an Eating Disorder

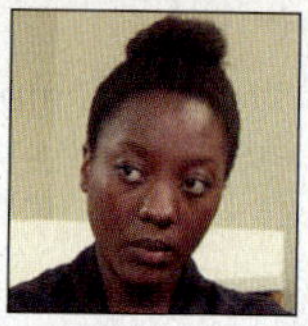

INEFFECTIVE APPROACH

Nurse: Ellen, I am glad to see that you ate your lunch.

Ellen: Thanks, I feel so fat after I eat.

Nurse: I will lock the bathroom so you are not tempted to purge.

Ellen: What, don't you trust me?

Nurse: It is not about trust, but I don't feel comfortable leaving you alone with bathroom access.

Ellen: Really? You have your nerve.

Nurse: We are just trying to help.

Ellen: Some help you are. I know you don't trust me.

Nurse: Ellen that is not what I said.

Ellen: No, but that is what you meant.

EFFECTIVE APPROACH

Nurse: Ellen, how was your lunch.

Ellen: I was ok. I always feel so fat after I eat.

Nurse: That is understandable. How long does that feeling last.

Ellen: Well, it depends on how much I have eaten. Since I didn't eat much, it will last for about an hour?

Nurse: Oh, I see. For many people with bulimia, the urges to purge are strongest after a meal. Is this a hard time for you?

Ellen: Sometimes it is.

Nurse: How can I help you resist the urges? Would you like me to stay with you until group time?

Ellen: That would be great.

CRITICAL THINKING CHALLENGE

- What effect did the first interaction have on Ellen's behavior? Why?
- In the second interaction, what theories and interventions regarding eating disorders did the nurse use in her approach to Ellen?

To prevent purging, bathroom visits may also be supervised (similar to treatment protocols used for patients with AN). Outpatients are asked to record their intake, binges, and purges. Because individuals with BN have chaotic lifestyles and are often overcommitted, sleep may be a low priority. Sleep-deprived individuals may assume that food would be helpful, and they begin to eat, triggering a binge. To encourage regular sleep patterns, sleep hygiene strategies are implemented.

Medication Interventions

Fluoxetine is approved by the FDA for treating BN. This SSRI has been shown to reduce vomiting and binging episodes (Lilly USA, 2023). Patients may be taking other medications for mood regulation or sleep.

Psychosocial Interventions

Using Cognitive and Behavioral Interventions

The behavioral techniques, such as cue elimination and response prevention, require self-monitoring to individualize the therapy. **Self-monitoring** is accomplished using a diary in which the patient records binges and purges and precipitating emotions and environmental cues. Emotional and environmental cues are identified, and alternative responses are suggested, tried, and reinforced. When a cue or stimulus leads to a dysfunctional or unhealthy response, the response can be eliminated or an alternate, healthier response to the cue can be substituted, tried, and then reinforced. Figure 32.2 gives two examples of behavioral interventions. In Example 1, for the patient with AN, the response is modified or altered to a healthier one; in Example 2, for the patient with BN, the cue is changed to produce a different, healthier response. Other techniques, such as postponing binges and purges through distraction, a technique to interrupt the cycle, are also effective.

> **NCLEXNOTE** Cognitive interventions within the context of a therapeutic relationship are a priority in the nursing care of patients with eating disorders.

Psychoeducation

Teaching Strategies

In addition to cognitive and behavioral techniques, educational strategies are also incorporated into treatment. For individuals with BN, psychoeducation focuses on setting boundaries and healthy limits, developing assertiveness, learning nutritional concepts related to healthy eating, and clarifying the many misconceptions they have about food and its influence on weight. Rules that result from dichotomous thinking must also be addressed because of their role in dietary restraint and resulting binge eating.

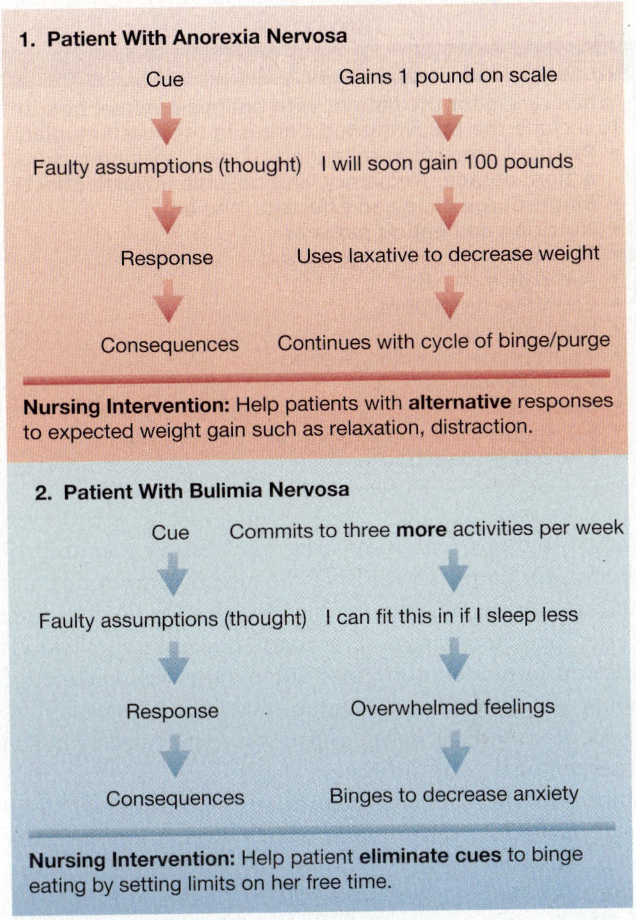

FIGURE 32.2 Examples of the relationship of cues, thoughts, responses, and behavioral interventions.

Teaching About Symptoms

The nurse can assist patients in understanding the binge–purge cycle and the role of rigid rules in contributing to this cycle. The value of eating meals regularly to ward off hunger and reduce the possibility of a binge is also important. Patients who misuse laxatives must be taught that although these drugs produce water-weight loss, they are ineffective for true, lasting weight loss because they work on the colon and not the small intestine or stomach where food is absorbed. Patients also need information about potassium depletion, electrolyte imbalances, dehydration, and the medical consequences of binge eating and purging. Other topics for psychoeducation are included in Box 32.12.

Convening Support Groups

Group interventions are cost-effective and increase learning more effectively than does individual treatment because patients learn from each other as well as from the nurse, therapist, or leader. Some experts have recommended 12-step programs for treating BN. However, many clinicians who work in this specialty have noted that

BOX 32.12

Psychoeducation Checklist: Bulimia Nervosa

When caring for the patient with bulimia nervosa, be sure to include the following topic areas in the teaching plan:

- Psychopharmacological agents, if used, including drug, action, dosage, frequency, and possible adverse effects
- Binge–purge cycle and effects on the body
- Nutrition and eating patterns
- Hydration
- Avoidance of cues
- Cognitive distortions
- Limit setting
- Appropriate boundary setting
- Assertiveness
- Resources
- Self-monitoring and behavioral interventions
- Realistic goal setting

these programs, with their strict rules, can be counterproductive for patients with BN, who already have rigid rules and are "abstinent" in many ways that lead to binge eating. Broad parameters regarding food choices (e.g., all foods allowed in moderation), in combination with knowledge about healthy eating, should be encouraged instead.

After symptoms subside, patients can concentrate on interpersonal issues in therapy, such as a fused relationship with their parents/guardians or feelings of inadequacy and low self-esteem, which often underlie their lack of assertiveness.

Developing Recovery-Oriented Rehabilitation Strategies

Strategies used for AN can also be applied to BN. There is emerging research that shows that physical exercise and dietary therapy may be a realistic approach that supports recovery (Mathisen et al., 2023).

Evaluation of Patient Outcomes

Over 50% of people with BN recover over time. Rates of recovery from bulimia peak within the first 10 years. Compared to other eating disorders, research indicates that BN has the highest rate of overall improvement but also the highest rate of relapse. Nutritional interventions, self-help, psychodynamic therapy, pharmacological treatment, and cognitive therapy are associated with the largest recovery rates (Solmi et al., 2024).

Continuum of Care

Emergency and Inpatient-Focused Care

Although patients with BN are less likely than those with AN to require hospitalization, those with extreme dehydration and electrolyte imbalance, depression and suicidality, or symptoms that have not remitted with outpatient treatment need hospitalization.

Inpatient admission to an eating disorder unit is usually required to avoid purging behaviors. Bathroom monitoring, nutrition rehabilitation, and positive reinforcement is part of treatment, similar to AN. Once purging behaviors and nutrition are addressed, patients can continue treatment in outpatient setting. Referrals to recovery groups and support groups are important to prevent relapse. Rarely do patients with BN require emergency care.

Community Care

As with AN, preventing BN requires effort on the part of teachers, school nurses, parents/guardians, and society as a whole. Because many of the risk factors are seen early in children attending elementary school, educating school nurses and teachers is an important focus for psychiatric–mental health nurses working in the community. Protective factors that mediate between risk factors and the development of an eating disorder must be emphasized and developed. Box 32.9 covers important prevention strategies for parents/guardians and their children or adolescents.

Society has begun to engage in an effort to help young preadolescents assigned female at birth. The federal government has developed a website called *girlshealth* that is devoted to areas such as body changes, body image, relationships, and self-confidence.

BINGE-EATING DISORDER

Binge-eating disorder (BED) is characterized by episodes of consuming large amounts of foods in a short period of time. These individuals binge in the same way as those with BN do, but they do not purge or compensate for binges through other behaviors. BED differs from other eating disorders in that there are few severe impairments. In the United States, the prevalence of BED is estimated to be 2.6% (Scrandis & Arnew, 2023).

RISK FACTORS

BED can result from psychological, social, and cultural factors. Some risk factors include childhood obesity, loss of controlled eating in childhood, intestinal microbiota alteration, distorted body image, perfectionism, conduct issues, and substance use.

DIAGNOSTIC CRITERIA

The diagnostic criteria for BED consist of binge eating, which includes both the ingestion of a large amount of food in a short period of time and a sense of loss of control during the binge, distress regarding the binge instead of eating until uncomfortably full, and feelings of guilt or depression after the binge. As mentioned, purging or other compensatory behavior does not follow the binge (Scrandis & Arnew, 2023).

MEDICATIONS

The first FDA-approved medication for BED is **lisdexamfetamine dimesylate,** a CNS stimulant that is also used to treat attention deficit hyperactivity disorder (ADHD). This drug is believed to increase dopamine, norepinephrine, and serotonin, which are the neurotransmitters that help regulate appetite and hunger thought to be low in people with BED (Gorgas, 2024). Lisdexamfetamine dimesylate is habit forming and may not be recommended for those with a comorbid condition of substance use disorder.

Weight loss medications such as orlistat have often been used by people with BED; however, these drugs have many negative side effects. Glucagon-like peptide-1 (GLP-1) receptor agonists such as tirzepatide and semaglutide have attracted interest, especially on social media, after several celebrities reported using a GLP-1 drug for weight loss (Wojtara et al., 2023). Although GLP-1 receptor agonists have shown promising results for weight loss, longer term studies have not yet been performed, nor is there any research on using these drugs for treatment of BED.

SYMPTOMS, ETIOLOGY, AND TREATMENT

Because this is a newly recognized disorder, additional research is needed to clarify its symptoms, etiology, and treatment. Symptoms of BED are discussed in the "Diagnostic Criteria section" earlier in this chapter. The etiology of BED is believed to be similar to that of BN. The treatment of individuals with BED includes psychotherapy, pharmacotherapy, and weight loss treatment.

OTHER EATING DISORDERS

A complete discussion of all the eating disorders is outside the scope of this text. Several additional eating disorders are briefly described below.

PICA

Pica is an eating disorder in which individuals consume nonnutritive, nonfood substances (e.g., dirt, starch, soap) over the course of 1 month. Pica involves eating substances that are inappropriate for the Individual's developmental stage (e.g., when a child over the age of 2 years repeatedly eats non-food substances) or that are not part of a culturally supported or accepted practice. Some psychiatric disorders (e.g., autism spectrum disorder, intellectual disabilities, and schizophrenia) may include symptoms of eating nonnutritive, nonfood substances; however, they may not meet the diagnostic criteria for a diagnosis of pica as listed above. About one third of pregnant patients have pica due to food insecurities and vitamin deficiencies (APA, 2022). The craving for ice is particularly common.

Depending on what the individual ingests, pica can result in intestinal obstructions, intestinal perforations, infections, and toxicity.

RUMINATION DISORDER

Rumination disorder occurs when an individual repeatedly regurgitates their food and such action is not associated with another medical condition or eating disorder. After food is regurgitated, it is either rechewed, reswallowed, or spit out, and this persists for at least 1 month (APA, 2022).

The onset of rumination disorder can occur in infancy (3 to 12 months), childhood, adolescence, or adulthood. If this disorder occurs in infancy, it can lead to severe malnutrition and can be fatal (APA, 2022).

AVOIDANT RESTRICTIVE FOOD INTAKE DISORDER

People with **avoidant restrictive food intake disorder** (ARFID) are perceived as "extreme picky eaters." Individuals with this disorder characterized by a lack interest in eating food, have sensory issues with food (i.e., textures, temperatures, odor, and color), and are concerned about adverse consequences of eating (i.e., choking, allergic reactions, fear of getting ill from food). Due to food avoidance and restrictiveness, individuals with ARFID experience significant weight loss, nutritional deficiencies, and poor psychosocial functioning. Although most children go through a picky phase of eating, those with ARFID do not consume enough calories to grow and develop properly (APA, 2022).

Risk factors for ARFID include autism spectrum disorder, ADHD, OCD, and anxiety disorders (APA 2022).

ARFID is similar to AN in that they both can involve restriction of food intake. However, unlike AN, people with ARFID do not present with issues of body shape or size, or fears of becoming overweight.

OTHER SPECIFIED FEEDING OR EATING DISORDERS

Other specified feeding or eating disorders (OSFED) include symptoms of feeding and eating disorders that cause significant distress or impairment in everyday functioning but do not meet the criteria to be diagnosed as any of the other eating disorders in the DSM-5-TR. Examples include the following:

- Atypical AN: All diagnostic criteria are met for AN, except significant weight loss. An individual's weight may be above or within expected range for age, height, sex assigned at birth, and developmental trajectory. Even though an individual's weight is above or within expected limits, they may still exhibit the complications associated with AN.

- Purging disorder: Individuals frequently purge but do not binge. Individuals with this disorder purge frequently and have an intense fear of gaining weight or becoming fat (Balasundaram & Santhanam, 2023). They restrict their dietary intake and purge after eating expected amounts of food due to the fear of eating, gaining weight, and/or appearing "fat."
- Night eating syndrome: An individual eats after awakening from sleep or consumes an excessive amount of food after the evening meal (Balasundaram & Santhanam, 2023). The individual is aware of overeating, which causes significant distress or impairment to the individual. There is a feeling of loss of control over consumption, sleep fragmentation, and morning anorexia. Night eating syndrome is conceptualized as a disorder of circadian modulation of food intake and sleep. It is mainly attributed to an endocrine, metabolic, or psychological trigger.
- Orthorexia: The individual obsessively focuses on healthy eating. Entire food groups may be eliminated because of fear that they are unhealthy.

SUMMARY OF KEY POINTS

- Although anorexia nervosa and bulimia nervosa have some common symptoms they are classified as discrete disorders.
- Eating disorders are best viewed along a continuum that includes subclinical or partial-syndrome disorders. Because these disorders occur more frequently than full syndromes, they are often overlooked but, after they are identified, they can be prevented from worsening.
- Similar factors predispose individuals to the development of anorexia nervosa and bulimia nervosa, and these factors represent a biopsychosocial model of risk. These disorders are preventable, and identifying risk factors assists with prevention strategies.
- Etiologic factors contribute in combination to the development of eating disorders; no one factor provides an explanation.
- Treatment of anorexia nervosa frequently includes hospitalization for refeeding; bulimia nervosa is treated primarily on an outpatient basis.
- Cognitive-behavioral therapy and medications improve the symptoms. Individual and group interpersonal psychotherapy are also effective in self-evaluation and communication.
- Research is ongoing related to bulimia nervosa treatment outcomes. The type and severity of comorbid conditions and the length of the illness influence outcomes.
- BED is characterized by periods of binge eating not followed by purging or any other compensating behaviors.

DEVELOPING CLINICAL JUDGMENT

1. Discuss the potential difficulties and risks in attempting to treat a patient with anorexia nervosa in an outpatient setting.
2. Parents/guardians are often in need of support and suggestions for how to help prevent eating disorders. Develop a teaching program and include the topics and rationale for suggestions chosen.
3. Identify the important nursing management components of a refeeding program for a patient who is hospitalized with anorexia nervosa.
4. Bulimia nervosa is often a concealed disorder with secretive binge eating and purging. Identify the signs and symptoms you may observe of someone with this disorder.
5. Positive outcomes for the recovery of bulimia nervosa and anorexia nervosa depend on many factors. Identify the factors that promote positive outcomes and those related to poorer outcomes and prognosis.

MOVIES, TV, OR STREAMING PROGRAMS

To the Bone: **2017.** This movie, written and directed by Marti Noxon, is based on her own experience with an eating disorder. The movie follows Ellen (played by Lily Collins), who is suffering from anorexia nervosa restricting type. Despite receiving treatment in several eating disorder treatment centers, Ellen (who later changes her name to Eli) found herself still struggling to recover. She enters a group home led by an unconventional doctor. The film shows the struggles of Ellen/Eli and her peers with eating as well as group therapy sessions. At first, Ellen/Eli is not willing to accept treatment, but later she accepts help.

Viewing Points:

1. Which eating disorders are depicted in this movie?
2. What are the behavioral and physical signs that Ellen/Eli had an eating disorder?
3. What were some risk factors that could have contributed to the development of an eating disorder for Ellen/Eli and Luke?
4. List three priority concerns to address in Ellen/Eli's care.
5. How did Ellen's/Eli's disorder affect her family?

REFERENCES

Adams, K. N., & Hovel, E. (2024). Eating Disorders: All that a pediatrician should know. *Advances in Pediatrics*, *71*(1), 69–86. https://doi.org/10.1016/j.yapd.2024.02.005

Alberts, C., Owe-Larsson, M., & Urbanska, E. M. (2023). New perspective on anorexia nervosa: tryptophan-kynurenine pathway hypothesis. *Nutrients*, *15*(4), 1030. https://doi.org/10.3390/nu15041030

Alexander, T., Burnette, C. B., Cory, H., McHale, S., & Simone, M. (2024). The need for more inclusive measurement to advance equity in eating disorders prevention. *Eating Disorders*, *32*(6), 798–816. https://doi.org/10.1080/10640266.2024.2328460

Akgül, S., Pehlivantürk Kızılkan, M., Yıldırım, A., & Derman, O. (2024). Prevalence of suicide attempt, suicide ideation and self-harm at diagnosis in adolescents with eating disorders. *International Journal of Psychiatry in Clinical Practice*, *28*(1), 63–67. https://doi.org/10.1080/13651501.2024.2337796

American Psychiatric Association. (2022). *Diagnostic and statistical manual of mental disorders, fifth edition, text revision*. Washington, DC, Author.

Amiri, S., & Khan, M. A. (2023). Prevalence of non-suicidal self-injury, suicidal ideation, suicide attempts, suicide mortality in eating disorders: a systematic review and meta-analysis. *Eating Disorders*, *31*(5), 487–525. https://doi.org/10.1080/10640266.2023.2196492

Baker, J. H., Freestone, D., Cai, K., Silverstein, S., Urban, B., & Steinberg, D. (2024). Eating disorder clinical presentation and treatment outcomes by gender identity among children, adolescents, and young adults. *The Journal of Adolescent Health*, *75*(2), 254–260. https://doi.org/10.1016/j.jadohealth.2023.11.015

Balasundaram, P., & Santhanam, P. (2023). Eating disorders. In *StatPearls*. StatPearls Publishing.

Brodie, E., van Veenendaal, N., Platz, E., Fleming, J., Gunn, H., Johnson, D., Griffin, H., & Wittholz, K. (2024). The incidence of refeeding syndrome and the nutrition management of severely malnourished inpatients with eating disorders: An observational study. *The International Journal of Eating Disorders*, *57*(3), 661–670. https://doi.org/10.1002/eat.24151

Bruch, H. (1973). *Eating disorders: Obesity, anorexia nervosa and the person within*. Basic Books.

Cadwallader, J. S., Orri, M., Barry, C., Falissard, B., Hassler, C., & Huas, C. (2023). Description of patients with eating disorders by general practitioners: a cohort study and focus on co-management with depression. *Journal of Eating Disorders*, *11*(1), 185. https://doi.org/10.1186/s40337-023-00901-0

Cascino, G., & Monteleone, A. M. (2024). Early traumatic experiences and the hypothalamus-pituitary-adrenal axis in people with eating disorders: A narrative review. *Psychoneuroendocrinology*, *159*, 106665. https://doi.org/10.1016/j.psyneuen.2023.106665

Chapman, L., Cartwright-Hatton, S., Thomson, A., & Lester, K. J. (2021). Parental eating disorders: A systematic review of parenting attitudes, behaviours, and parent-child interactions. *Clinical Psychology Review*, *88*, 102031. https://doi.org/10.1016/j.cpr.2021.102031

Chen, Y., Lun, T., Li, L., Yu, J., & Xiang, M. (2023). Acupuncture at Sifeng (EX-UE 10) for pediatric anorexia: A systematic review and meta-analysis. *Complementary Therapies in Medicine*, *78*, 102988. https://doi.org/10.1016/j.ctim.2023.102988

Cogodi, E., Ranieri, J., Martelli, A., & Di Giacomo, D. (2024). Emotional dysregulation in anorexia nervosa: Scoping review of psychological treatments. *Healthcare*, *12*(14), 1388. https://doi.org/10.3390/healthcare12141388

Cole, B. (2024). Understanding eating disorders and the nurse's role in diagnosis, treatment, and support. *Journal of Christian Nursing*, *41*(2), 80–87. https://doi.org/10.1097/CNJ.0000000000001147

Convertino, A. D., Morland, L. A., & Blashill, A. J. (2022). Trauma exposure and eating disorders: Results from a United States nationally representative sample. *The International Journal of Eating Disorders*, *55*(8), 1079–1089. https://doi.org/10.1002/eat.23757

Di Natale, A. F., Pizzoli, S. F. M., Brizzi, G., Di Lernia, D., Frisone, F., Gaggioli, A., Rabarbari, E., Oasi, O., Repetto, C., Rossi, C., Scerrati, E., Villani, D., & Riva, G. (2024). Harnessing immersive virtual reality: A comprehensive scoping review of its applications in assessing, understanding, and treating eating disorders. *Current Psychiatry Reports*, *26*, 470–486. https://doi.org/10.1007/s11920-024-01523-2

Eli Lilly and Co USA. (2023). Highlights of prescribing information. *Prozac*. Retrieved August 17, 2024, from https://www.accessdata.fda.gov/scripts/cder/daf/index.cfm?event=overview.process&ApplNo=018936

Fairburn, C. G., & Beglin, S. J. (1994). The assessment of eating disorders: Interview or self-report questionnaire? *International Journal of Eating Disorders*, *16*, 363–370.

Fan, S., Guo, W., Xiao, D., Guan, M., Liao, T., Peng, S., Feng, A., Wang, Z., Yin, H., Li, M., Chen, J., & Xiong, W. (2023). Microbiota-gut-brain axis drives overeating disorders. *Cell Metabolism*, *35*(11), 2011–2027.e7. https://doi.org/10.1016/j.cmet.2023.09.005

Fornaro, M., Mondin, A. M., Billeci, M., Fusco, A., De Prisco, M., Caiazza, C., Micanti, F., Calati, R., Carvalho, A. F., & de Bartolomeis, A. (2023). Psychopharmacology of eating disorders: Systematic review and meta-analysis of randomized controlled trials. *Journal of Affective Disorders*, *338*, 526–545. https://doi.org/10.1016/j.jad.2023.06.068

Friars, D., Walsh, O., & McNicholas, F. (2023). Assessment and management of cardiovascular complications in eating disorders. *Journal of eating disorders*, *11*(1), 13. https://doi.org/10.1186/s40337-022-00724-5

Friedlich, C. E., Park, H., Duval, C. J., Keshishian, T., & Murray, S. B. (2024). The prevalence of disordered eating in outpatient general psychiatry settings in publicly insured populations: a case series. *Eating Disorders*, *32*(2), 169–177. https://doi.org/10.1080/10640266.2023.2277055

Garner, D. M., Olmsted, M. P., Bohr, Y., & Garfinkel, P. E. (1982). The eating attitudes test: Psychometric features and clinical correlates. *Psychological Medicine*, *12*(4), 871–878. https://doi.org/10.1017/S0033291700049163

Ghazzawi, H. A., Nimer, L. S., Haddad, A. J., Alhaj, O. A., Amawi, A. T., Pandi-Perumal, S. R., Trabelsi, K., Seeman, M. V., & Jahrami, H. (2024). A systematic review, meta-analysis, and meta-regression of the prevalence of self-reported disordered eating and associated factors among athletes worldwide. *Journal of Eating Disorders*, *12*(1), 24. https://doi.org/10.1186/s40337-024-00982-5

Goldfarb, A. H., Kraemer, R. R., & Baiamonte, B. A. (2024). endogenous opioids and exercise-related hypoalgesia: modern models, measurement, and mechanisms of action. *Advances in Neurobiology*, *35*, 137–155. https://doi.org/10.1007/978-3-031-45493-6_8

Gorgas, D. L. (2024). Eating disorders. *Emergency Medicine Clinics of North America*, *42*(1), 163–179. https://doi.org/10.1016/j.emc.2023.06.024

Gratz, K. L., & Roemer, L. (2004). Multidimensional assessment of emotion regulation and dysregulation: development, factor structure, and initial validation of the difficulties in emotion regulation scale. *Journal of Psychopathology and Behavioral Assessment*, *26*(1), 41–54.

Haas, V., Kohn, M., Körner, T., Cuntz, U., Garber, A. K., Le Grange, D., Voderholzer, U., & Correll, C. U. (2021). Practice-based evidence and clinical guidance to support accelerated re-nutrition of patients with anorexia nervosa. *Journal of the American Academy of Child and Adolescent Psychiatry*, *60*(5), 555–561. https://doi.org/10.1016/j.jaac.2020.09.010

Haines, M. S. (2023). Endocrine complications of anorexia nervosa. *Journal of Eating Disorders*, *11*(1), 24. https://doi.org/10.1186/s40337-023-00744-9

Hill, N. G., Abber, S. R., & Keel, P. K. (2024). The role of sexual assault history and PTSD in responses to food intake among women with bulimic-spectrum eating disorders. *Eating Disorders*, *32*(3), 266–282. https://doi.org/10.1080/10640266.2023.2293597

Hirvelä, L., Keski-Rahkonen, A., & Sipilä, P. N. (2023). Associations of broad eating disorder symptoms with later alcohol problems in Finnish adult twins: A nationwide 10-year follow-up. *The International Journal of Eating Disorders*, *56*(10), 1854–1865. https://doi.org/10.1002/eat.24013

Jain, A., & Yilanli, M. (2023). Bulimia Nervosa. In *StatPearls*. StatPearls Publishing. (nih.gov)

Jassogne, C., Jacques, D., Dubois, T., & Zdanowicz, N. (2023). Is anorexia truly a contemporary disease? *Psychiatria Danubina*, *35*(Suppl 3), 24–28.

J Devoe, D., Han, A., Anderson, A., Katzman, D. K., Patten, S. B., Soumbasis, A., Flanagan, J., Paslakis, G., Vyver, E., Marcoux, G., & Dimitropoulos, G. (2023). The impact of the COVID-19 pandemic on eating disorders: A systematic review. *The International Journal of Eating Disorders*, *56*(1), 5–25. https://doi.org/10.1002/eat.23704

Jiotsa, B., Naccache, B., Duval, M., Rocher, B., & Grall-Bronnec, M. (2021). Social media use and body image disorders: Association between frequency of comparing one's own physical appearance to that of people being followed on social media and body dissatisfaction and drive for thinness. *International Journal of Environmental Research and Public Health*, *18*(6), 2880. https://doi.org/10.3390/ijerph18062880

Juli, R., Juli, M. R., Juli, G., & Juli, L. (2023). Eating disorders and psychiatric comorbidity. *Psychiatria Danubina*, *35*(Suppl 2), 217–220.

Kadoura, B., Ganson, K. T., & Katzman, D. K. (2024). Anorexia nervosa in adolescent males. *CMAJ: Canadian Medical Association Journal*, *196*(6), E191. https://doi.org/10.1503/cmaj.230001

Kells, M. R., Roske, C., Watters, A., Puckett, L., Wildes, J. E., Crow, S. J., & Mehler, P. S. (2023). Vitamin D and hypophosphatemia in patients with anorexia nervosa and avoidant/restrictive food intake disorder: a case control study. *Journal of Eating Disorders*, *11*(1), 195. https://doi.org/10.1186/s40337-023-00913-w

Kiely, L., Conti, J., & Hay, P. (2024). Anorexia nervosa through the lens of a severe and enduring experience: 'lost in a big world'. *Journal of Eating Disorders*, *12*(1), 12. https://doi.org/10.1186/s40337-023-00953-2

Kirkpatrick, R. H., Breton, E., Biorac, A., Munoz, D. P., & Booij, L. (2024). Non-suicidal self-injury among individuals with an eating disorder: A systematic review and prevalence meta-analysis. *The International Journal of Eating Disorders, 57*(2), 223–248. https://doi.org/10.1002/eat.24088

Kwan, M. Y., & Dodd, D. (2024). Social cognition and bulimic symptoms in male undergraduate students: The conditional effect of emotion dysregulation. *European Eating Disorders Review, 2*(6), 1220–1226. https://doi.org/10.1002/erv.3120

Laghi, F., Bianchi, D., Pompili, S., Lonigro, A., & Baiocco, R. (2021). Binge eating and binge drinking behaviors: The role of family functioning. *Psychology Health & Medicine, 26*(4), 408–420. https://doi.org/10.1080/13548506.2020.1742926

Levine, M. P., & Sadeh-Sharvit, S. (2023). Preventing eating disorders and disordered eating in genetically vulnerable, high-risk families. *The International Journal of Eating Disorders, 56*(3), 523–534. https://doi.org/10.1002/eat.23887

Li, Y., & Li, J. (2022). The boundary conditions by which body-esteem leads to eating disorders risk among adolescents. *The Journal of General Psychology, 149*(1), 97–115. https://doi.org/10.1080/00221309.2021.1915741

Lie, S. Ø., Bulik, C. M., Andreassen, O. A., Rø, Ø., & Bang, L. (2021). The association between bullying and eating disorders: a case-control study. *International Journal of Eating Disorders, 54*(8), 1405–1414. https://doi.org/10.1002/eat.23522

Longo, P., Aloi, M., Delsedime, N., Rania, M., Segura Garcia, C., Abbate-Daga, G., & Marzola, E. (2021). Different clusters of perfectionism in inpatients with anorexia nervosa and healthy controls. *Eating Disorders, 30*(5), 540–555. https://doi.org/10.1080/10640266.2021.1938937

Lopes, H. C. B., Mazzolani, B. C., Koritar, P., & Cordás, T. A. (2023). Characterization of refeeding protocols for under 18 years old hospitalized patients with anorexia nervosa: A systematic review. *General Hospital Psychiatry, 85*, 43–54. https://doi.org/10.1016/j.genhosppsych.2023.09.007

Mallaram, G. K., Sharma, P., Kattula, D., Singh, S., & Pavuluru, P. (2023). Body image perception, eating disorder behavior, self-esteem and quality of life: a cross-sectional study among female medical students. *Journal of Eating Disorders, 11*(1), 225. https://doi.org/10.1186/s40337-023-00945-2

Marchetti, D., & Sawrikar, V. (2024). Parents' illness representations of their child with anorexia nervosa: A systematic review of qualitative studies using the common-sense model. *The International Journal of Eating Disorders, 57*(5), 1049–1068. https://doi.org/10.1002/eat.24081

Matheson, B. E. (2024). Bulimia nervosa and binge-eating disorder across the lifespan. *Focus, 22*(3), 278–287. https://doi.org/10.1176/appi.focus.20240001

Mathisen, T. F., Pettersen, G., Rosenvinge, J. H., Schmidt, U., & Sundgot-Borgen, J. (2023). Effectiveness and acceptability of the physical exercise and dietary therapy in a healthy life center. *The International Journal of Eating Disorders, 56*(10), 1931–1940. https://doi.org/10.1002/eat.24020

Mensi, M. M., Orlandi, M., Rogantini, C., Provenzi, L., Chiappedi, M., Criscuolo, M., Castiglioni, M. C., Zanna, V., & Borgatti, R. (2021). Assessing family functioning before and after an integrated multidisciplinary family treatment for adolescents with restrictive eating disorders. *Frontiers in Psychiatry, 12*, 653047. https://doi.org/10.3389/fpsyt.2021.653047

Milano, W., Ambrosio, P., Carizzone, F., De Biasio, V., Foia, M. G., Saetta, B., Milano, M. F., & Capasso, A. (2022). Menstrual disorders related to eating disorders. *Endocrine, Metabolic & Immune Disorders Drug Targets, 22*(5), 471–480. https://doi.org/10.2174/1871530321666210625145345

Monteleone, A. M., Cascino, G., Barone, E., Carfagno, M., & Monteleone, P. (2021). COVID-19 pandemic and eating disorders: What can we learn about psychopathology and treatment? A systematic review. *Current Psychiatry Reports, 23*(12), 83. https://doi.org/10.1007/s11920-021-01294-0

Mulchandani, M., Shetty, N., Conrad, A., Muir, P., & Mah, B. (2021). Treatment of eating disorders in older people: A systematic review. *Systematic Reviews, 10*(1), 275. https://doi.org/10.1186/s13643-021-01823-1

Mushtaq, T., Ashraf, S., Hameed, H., Irfan, A., Shahid, M., Kanwal, R., Aslam, M. A., Shahid, H., Koh-E-Noor, Shazly, G. A., Khan, M. A., & Jardan, Y. A. B. (2023). Prevalence of eating disorders and their association with social media addiction among youths. *Nutrients, 15*(21), 4687. https://doi.org/10.3390/nu15214687

Nechita, D. M., Bud, S., & David, D. (2021). Shame and eating disorders symptoms: A meta-analysis. *The International Journal of Eating Disorders, 54*(11), 1899–1945. https://doi.org/10.1002/eat.23583

Neipp, M. C., Ruiz, Á., Manchón, J., León-Zarceño, E., Quiles, M. J., & Quiles, Y. (2024). Quality of life and clinical impairment in Spanish adolescent anorexia nervosa patients. *European Journal of Investigation in Health, Psychology and Education, 14*(5), 1425–1436. https://doi.org/10.3390/ejihpe14050094

Nitsch, A., Dlugosz, H., Gibson, D., & Mehler, P. S. (2021). Medical complications of bulimia nervosa. *Cleveland Clinic Journal of Medicine, 88*(6), 333–343. https://doi.org/10.3949/ccjm.88a.20168

Owens, R. A., Attia, E., Fitzpatrick, J. J., Phillips, K., & Nolan, S. (2023). Eating disorders: Identification and management in general medical and psychiatric settings. *Journal of the American Psychiatric Nurses Association, 29*(3), 241–251. https://doi.org/10.1177/1078390321999713

Panero, M., Longo, P., De Bacco, C., Abbate-Daga, G., & Martini, M. (2022). Shame, guilt, and self-consciousness in anorexia nervosa. *Journal of Clinical Medicine, 11*(22), 6683. https://doi.org/10.3390/jcm11226683

Parsons, M. A., & Clemens, J. P. (2023). Eating disorders among bariatric surgery patients: The chicken or the egg?. *JAAPA, 36*(11), 1–5. https://doi.org/10.1097/01.JAA.0000979532.00697.1a

Pascoe, L. A., Mikhail, M. E., Burt, S. A., Culbert, K. M., & Klump, K. L. (2024). Shared genetic influences between eating disorders and gastrointestinal disease in a large, population-based sample of adult women and men. *Psychological Medicine, 54*(6), 1184–1195. https://doi.org/10.1017/S003329172300301X

Poos, S., Faerovitch, M., Pinto, C., Jamalkhani, N., Chaudhri, F., Khan, S., Lo, D. F., McGowan, K., & Martin, A. (2023). The role of diabetes distress in Diabulimia. *Journal of Eating Disorders, 11*(1), 213. https://doi.org/10.1186/s40337-023-00924-7

Ralph-Nearman, C., Hooper, M. A., Hunt, R. A., & Levinson, C. A. (2024). Dynamic relationships among feeling fat, fear of weight gain, and eating disorder symptoms in an eating disorder sample. *Appetite, 195*, 107181. https://doi.org/10.1016/j.appet.2023.107181

Robinson, K., & Wade, T. D. (2021). Perfectionism interventions targeting disordered eating: A systematic review and meta-analysis. *The International Journal of Eating Disorders, 54*(4), 473–487. https://doi.org/10.1002/eat.23483

Russell, H., Aouad, P., Le, A., Marks, P., Maloney, D., National Eating Disorder Research Consortium, Touyz, S., & Maguire, S. (2023). Psychotherapies for eating disorders: findings from a rapid review. *Journal of Eating Disorders, 11*(1), 175. https://doi.org/10.1186/s40337-023-00886-w

Salter, F., Singh, U., Kerr, D., Zhao, Y., & Jeffery, E. (2024). A prospective observational study examining weight and psychosocial change in adolescent and adult eating disorder inpatients admitted for nutritional rehabilitation using a high-energy re-feeding protocol. *Journal of Eating Disorders, 12*(1), 58. https://doi.org/10.1186/s40337-024-01015-x

Santos, B. M., & Haynos, A. F. (2023). Difficulties with positive emotion regulation in anorexia nervosa. *European Eating Disorders Review, 31*(4), 520–528. https://doi.org/10.1002/erv.2973

Scotto Rosato, M., Cipriano, A., Napolano, R., & Cella, S. (2024). Maternal control and eating styles in children: The mediating role of emotion differentiation. *Clinical Child Psychology and Psychiatry, 29*(1), 76–89. https://doi.org/10.1177/13591045231199303

Scrandis, D. A., & Arnow, D. (2023). Binge-eating disorder. *The Nurse Practitioner, 48*(12), 22–28. https://doi.org/10.1097/01.NPR.0000000000000125

Solmi, M., Monaco, F., Højlund, M., Monteleone, A. M., Trott, M., Firth, J., Carfagno, M., Eaton, M., De Toffol, M., Vergine, M., Meneguzzo, P., Collantoni, E., Gallicchio, D., Stubbs, B., Girardi, A., Busetto, P., Favaro, A., Carvalho, A. F., Steinhausen, H. C., & Correll, C. U. (2024). Outcomes in people with eating disorders: a transdiagnostic and disorder-specific systematic review, meta-analysis and multivariable meta-regression analysis. *World Psychiatry, 23*(1), 124–138. https://doi.org/10.1002/wps.21182

Stewart, M. P., & Baumann, O. (2024). The effectiveness of adolescent-focused therapy and family-based therapy for anorexia nervosa. *Psychological Reports*, 332941241226687. https://doi.org/10.1177/00332941241226687

Stewart, T. M., Martin, C. K., & Williamson, D. A. (2022). The complicated relationship between dieting, dietary restraint, caloric restriction, and eating disorders: Is a shift in public health messaging warranted?. *International Journal of Environmental Research and Public Health, 19*(1), 491. https://doi.org/10.3390/ijerph19010491

Su, T., Gong, J., Tang, G., Qiu, S., Chen, P., Chen, G., Wang, J., Huang, L., & Wang, Y. (2021). Structural and functional brain alterations in anorexia nervosa: A multimodal meta-analysis of neuroimaging studies. *Human Brain Mapping, 42*(15), 5154–5169. https://doi.org/10.1002/hbm.25602

Tchanturia, K., Croft, P., Holetic, V., Webb, J., & Dapelo, M. M. (2023). Positive communication workshops: are they useful for treatment programmes for anorexia nervosa? *Frontiers in psychology, 14*, 1234928. https://doi.org/10.3389/fpsyg.2023.1234928

Thompson, K. A., DeVinney, A. A., Goy, C. N., Kuang, J., & Bardone-Cone, A. M. (2022). Subjective and objective binge episodes in relation to eating disorder and depressive symptoms among middle-aged women. *Eating and Weight Disorders: EWD, 27*(5), 1687–1694. https://doi.org/10.1007/s40519-021-01305-2

Tragantzopoulou, P., Fixsen, A., Ridge, D., & Cheshire, A. (2024). 'You are not alone, we've got you': Power plays, devotion, and punishment on healthy eating and pro-eating disorder websites. *Qualitative Health Research, 34*(12), 1216–1230. https://doi.org/10.1177/10497323241238628

Udo, T., & Grilo, C. M. (2022). Epidemiology of eating disorders among US adults. *Current Opinion in Psychiatry, 35*(6), 372–378. https://doi.org/10.1097/YCO.0000000000000814

van Eeden, A. E., van Hoeken, D., Hendriksen, J. M. T., & Hoek, H. W. (2023). Increase in incidence of anorexia nervosa among 10- to 14-year-old girls: A nationwide study in the Netherlands over four decades. *The International Journal of Eating Disorders, 56*(12), 2295–2303. https://doi.org/10.1002/eat.24064

Vuong, A. T., Jarman, H. K., Doley, J. R., & McLean, S. A. (2021). Social media use and body dissatisfaction in adolescents: The moderating role of thin- and muscular-ideal internalisation. *International Journal of Environmental Research and Public Health, 18*(24), 13222. https://doi.org/10.3390/ijerph182413222

Walsh, B. T., Xu, T., Wang, Y., Attia, E., & Kaplan, A. S. (2021). Time course of relapse following acute treatment for anorexia nervosa. *The American Journal of Psychiatry, 178*(9), 848–853. https://doi.org/10.1176/appi.ajp.2021.21010026

Wetzel, K. E., & Himmelstein, M. S. (2023). Constant vigilance: The impact of weight stigma, vigilance, and internalization on maladaptive eating behaviors. *Health Psychology, 42*(10), 712–722. https://doi.org/10.1037/hea0001324

Wilkinson, M. L., Trainor, C., Lampe, E., Presseller, E. K., & Juarascio, A. (2024). Cannabis use and binge eating: Examining the relationship between cannabis use and clinical severity among adults with binge eating. *Experimental and Clinical Psychopharmacology, 32*(4), 392–397. https://doi.org/10.1037/pha0000706

Wojtara, M., Mazumder, A., Syeda, Y., & Mozgała, N. (2023). Glucagon-like peptide-1 receptor agonists for chronic weight management. *Advances in Medicine, 2023*, 9946924. https://doi.org/10.1155/2023/9946924

Wronski, M. L., Geisler, D., Bernardoni, F., Seidel, M., Bahnsen, K., Doose, A., Steinhäuser, J. L., Gronow, F., Böldt, L. V., Plessow, F., Lawson, E. A., King, J. A., Roessner, V., & Ehrlich, S. (2023). Differential alterations of amygdala nuclei volumes in acutely ill patients with anorexia nervosa and their associations with leptin levels. *Psychological Medicine, 53*(13), 6288–6303. https://doi.org/10.1017/S0033291722003609

Yamamiya, Y., & Stice, E. (2024). Risk factors that predict future onset of anorexia nervosa, bulimia nervosa, binge eating disorder, and purging disorder in adolescent girls. *Behavior Therapy, 55*(4), 712–723. https://doi.org/10.1016/j.beth.2023.10.002

Yesildemir, O., & Akbulut, G. (2023). Gender-Affirming Nutrition: An overview of eating disorders in the transgender population. *Current nutrition reports, 12*(4), 877–892. https://doi.org/10.1007/s13668-023-00504-w

Zakers, A., & Cimolai, V. (2023). Complementary and integrative medicine and eating disorders in youth: Traditional yoga, virtual reality, light therapy, neurofeedback, acupuncture, energy psychology techniques, art therapies, and spirituality. *Child and Adolescent Psychiatric Clinics of North America, 32*(2), 421–450. https://doi.org/10.1016/j.chc.2022.08.014

Zhao, W., Kodancha, P., & Das, S. (2024). Gut microbiome changes in anorexia nervosa: A comprehensive review. *Pathophysiology, 31*(1), 68–88. https://doi.org/10.3390/pathophysiology31010006

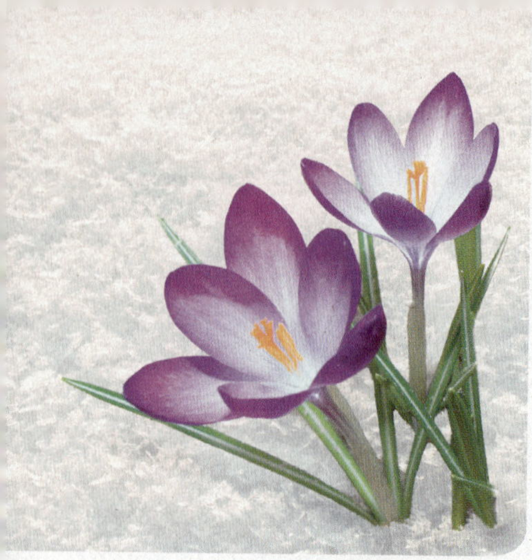

33 Somatic Symptom and Related Disorders

Nursing Care of People With Somatization

Patricia E. Freed

KEYCONCEPT

- health anxiety
- somatization

LEARNING OBJECTIVES

After studying this chapter, you will be able to:

1. Examine the role of somatization and health anxiety in somatic symptom disorders (SSD).
2. Relate the primary theories of somatization to clinical symptoms and the course of SSD.
3. Evaluate the significance of trauma in the appearance of SSD symptoms.
4. Examine the relationship between social determinants of health and SSD.
5. Select strategies to establish a therapeutic relationship with people with SSD.
6. Using a clinical judgment model, formulate a person-centered, recovery-oriented nursing care plan for people with SSD.
7. Identify medications that are used to treat people with SSD and evaluate their effectiveness.
8. Develop wellness strategies for people with SSD.
9. Compare and contrast mental health care provided in emergency, inpatient, community, and virtual settings.
10. Support the integration of health care and mental health care for people with SSD.
11. Compare and contrast somatic symptom disorder and related disorders.

KEY TERMS

• alexithymia • conversion • factitious disorder • factitious disorder imposed on another • functional cognitive disorder • functional neurologic symptom disorder • Hoover sign • hypochondriasis • illness anxiety disorder • malingering • nociceptors • pseudologia fantastica • psychogenic nonepileptic seizures • psychosomatic • somatic symptom disorder • symptom burden

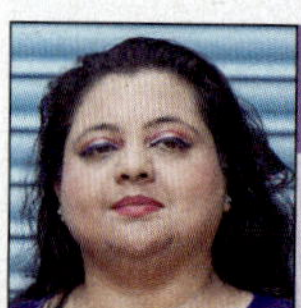

Case Study: Carol

Carol is a 48-year-old with obesity who is very angry at being forced to see a mental health care provider. She has had multiple surgeries, including hysterectomy, gastric bypass, and carpal tunnel release. She suffers from shoulder and neck pain and from vertigo. She takes multiple prescribed and over-the-counter medications.

INTRODUCTION

The connection between the "mind" and "body" has been hypothesized and described for centuries. The term **psychosomatic** has been traditionally used to describe, explain, and predict the psychological origins of illness and disease. Unfortunately, this notion perpetuates the stigma that certain disorders are purely "psychological" in nature and thus are not real or valid.

Somatization

The concept **somatization** acknowledges and respects that bodily sensations and functional changes are expressions of health and illness. Even though, in some instances they may be medically unexplained, they are not imaginary (van der Heijden et al., 2024).

> **KEYCONCEPT Somatization** (from *soma*, meaning body) is the manifestation of psychological distress as physical symptoms that may result in functional changes, somatic descriptions, or both.

Everyone experiences somatic symptoms at some point in their lives. Symptoms are usually associated with some stress, such as having a headache before an exam, or throwing up before an important performance. These common experiences are typically situational and temporary. These symptoms become an issue when somatization becomes a burden. A **symptom burden** occurs when the subjective symptoms become quantifiable, frequent, and severe, causing prolonged physical and emotional distress. As the somatic symptom burden increases, the emotional and behavioral manifestations often characterize the somatic symptom and related disorders (SSRD) presented in this chapter.

Somatic symptoms are not confined to the SSRDs. Other mental disorders may initially manifest with primarily somatic symptoms (i.e., depression, panic disorder) or occur comorbid to the SSRDs. Somatization crosses all cultures and is recognized in almost every society (Seiffge-Krenke et al., 2024). In many cultures, the expression of physical discomfort is more acceptable than acknowledging psychological distress. The disruption of routine body cycles, such as digestion, menstruation, or sleep, is more socially acceptable than having emotional responses related to interpersonal relationships, economic crises, adjustment to marriage, infertility, or the death of a spouse.

Health Anxiety

> **KEYCONCEPT Health anxiety** involves cycles of excessive worry about one's health fueled by misinterpretations of body sensations as indications of an undiagnosed disease or illness.

Worrying about one's health is likely a good motivation for engaging in self-care and seeking medical help when needed. But for some individuals, health and illness concerns become health anxiety. Different than somatization, the term **health anxiety** (also known as illness anxiety) is characterized by excessive worry about one's health fueled by misinterpretations of body sensations. In fact, worries become a pathologically anxious preoccupation with having or contracting a currently undiagnosed medical illness (Cassiday, 2022). Misinterpretation of bodily sensations and body distress fuels a vicious cycle of anxiety leading to psychological distress, functional impairment, excessive health care utilization, and relief-seeking.

Relief-seeking usually takes the form of excess primary care consultation, but other activities could be involved (overuse of over-the-counter [OTC] medications, seeking care from multiple providers, invalidism, etc.). There is a close relationship between health anxiety and somatic symptoms, which are more severe and distressing when they occur together (Sauer et al., 2023). Though they tend to cluster together, health anxiety and somatic symptom burden do not always occur together. For instance, an individual with health anxiety might not experience symptoms but still have an intense fear of developing a specific serious illness. Health anxiety has been identified as one of the factors that contribute to health disparities (see Box 33.1).

SOMATIC SYMPTOM AND RELATED DISORDERS OVERVIEW

This chapter explores the holistic evidence-based nursing care for people experiencing the *DSM-5-TR* group of disorders with prominent somatic symptoms and/or health anxiety. These symptoms are distressing to the person who has a negative and sometimes exaggerated interpretation of their seriousness, which leads to significant impairment (American Psychiatric Association

BOX 33.1

Mental Health Inequities: Health Anxiety and Socioeconomic Status (SES)

Persistent somatic symptoms (PSS) are more prevalent in those with low socioeconomic status (SES) and among migrants. A meta-analysis of 37 studies reported a significant association between SES and health anxiety, which was lower in those with higher SES. The presence of health anxiety in socially deprived individuals constitutes a health disadvantage that must be addressed in programs that aim to reduce health and social inequities (Barbek et al., 2022).

Source: Barbek, R. M. E., Makowski, A. C., & von dem Knesebeck, O. (2022). Social inequalities in health anxiety: A systematic review and meta-analysis. *Journal of Psychosomatic Research*, *153*, 110706. https://doi.org/10.1016/j.jpsychores.2021.110706

[APA], 2022). Somatic symptom disorder is highlighted and illness anxiety disorder, functional neurologic symptom disorder, and factitious disorders (FDs) are discussed.

SOMATIC SYMPTOM DISORDER

Nurses in primary care and medical-surgical settings are more likely than mental health nurses to encounter people with these issues.

CLINICAL COURSE

Somatic symptom disorder (SSD) is one of the most difficult disorders to manage because its symptoms tend to change and are diffuse and complex. They often vary and move from one body system to another. For example, initially gastrointestinal (e.g., nausea, vomiting, diarrhea) and neurologic (e.g., headache, backache) symptoms may be present that change to musculoskeletal (e.g., aching legs) and sexual issues (e.g., pain in the abdomen, pain during intercourse). Physical symptoms may last for more than 5 years (D'Souza & Hooten, 2023).

Individuals with SSD perceive themselves as being "sicker than the sick" and report all aspects of their health as poor. Many eventually believe that they are disabled and cannot work. They typically visit health care providers many times each month and quickly become frustrated because their primary health care providers do not understand their level of suffering and are unable to validate that a particular issue accounts for their extreme discomfort. Consequently, individuals with SSD tend to move from one provider to another until they find one who will give them new medication, hospitalize them, or perform surgery. Because the source of worrisome physical symptoms may not be confirmed through medical or laboratory tests, medical or psychiatric interviews, or medical imaging, they repeatedly seek a medical reason for their discomfort and ask for relief from suffering. Depending on the severity, these individuals undergo multiple surgeries and even develop iatrogenic illnesses. People with SSD often evoke negative subjective responses in health care providers because they overuse services and because they are dissatisfied with caregivers and with the results of their treatment.

The following are the most common characteristics:

- Somatic symptoms cause significant distress and anxiety that is persistent and excessive.
- Persistent attention to symptoms costs considerable time and energy and contributes to disruption in daily living.
- Receiving support from the environment that otherwise might not be forthcoming (e.g., gaining a spouse's attention because of severe back pain).
- Expressing concern about the physical issues inconsistent with the severity of the illness (being "sicker than the sick").

NCLEXNOTE Patients with SSD seek health care from multiple providers but often avoid mental health specialists.

DIAGNOSTIC CRITERIA

The diagnostic criteria of SSD include one or more symptoms that cause persistent distress or significant disruption in daily lives and excessive thoughts about the seriousness of the symptoms, feelings (such as anxiety about the symptoms or overall health), or behaviors related to the symptoms or health concerns (e.g., spending excessive time and energy focusing on these symptoms or health). These symptoms may or may not be explained by medical evidence. The course of SSD is chronic and fluctuating, influenced by the number of symptoms, the individual's age, level of impairment, and presence of any comorbidities.

SSD ACROSS THE LIFESPAN

SSD can occur in childhood, adolescence, or adulthood. SSD is found in all age groups though there are certain differences in symptom expression and number of comorbidities, and it is far higher in people assigned female at birth than those assigned male at birth, with a ratio of 10:1 in adult patients (D'Souza & Hooten, 2023).

Children and Adolescents

Although many children have somatic symptoms, SSD is not usually diagnosed until adolescence. However, when children have medical symptoms, further evaluation is needed so they are often referred to specialists to rule out physical, sexual, or emotional abuse or a comorbid psychiatric illness, such as depression or anxiety. In children, the most common symptoms are frequent abdominal pain, headache, fatigue, and nausea. Expression of somatic symptoms in children tends to be overlooked or minimized when it needs to be identified as a risk factor for follow-up (Barak et al., 2023). In adolescents, initial symptoms are typically menstrual difficulties, and pelvic or abdominal pain. Risk factors for both children and adolescents need to be taken seriously. Research has shown a link between childhood sexual abuse and somatization, substance use, and depression in adults (Landa-Blanco et al., 2024).

Older Adults

SSD can involve a lifelong pattern of symptoms that persists into old age. The symptoms of SSD, however, are often unrecognized by health care providers who tend to accept and minimize them as a part of the natural aging process after no medical cause is found. Somatic symptoms and concurrent medical illness are common and increase with age and comorbidities. When the diagnosis of SSD is made in older adults, it is critical to focus on assessing the thoughts, feelings, and behaviors related to the symptoms or health concerns and not merely the symptoms themselves. For most people diagnosed with SSD, the condition leads to chronic psychological disability, functional limitations, and a generally decreased quality of life (QoL) (D'Sousa & Hooten, 2023). As the world's population ages and longevity increases, more attention is needed to consider the heavy somatic symptom burden older adults carry from these disorders and comorbidities, and to improve their QoL (Wu et al., 2022).

EPIDEMIOLOGY AND RISK FACTORS

The estimated prevalence of SSD ranges from 4% to 6% (APA, 2022). Millions of dollars of lost revenue and the increased use of short- and long-term disability have prompted employers to study this unique population of employees. This disorder is believed to be higher than reported. In people with fibromyalgia syndrome, 13.3% to 40% meet the criteria for SSD (LoBrutto et al., 2024). Older age, female sex assigned at birth, and comorbid physical disease are predictive risk factors for SSD in older adults (Wu et al., 2022).

Age of Onset

SSD usually begins before the age of 30 years, with the first symptom often appearing during adolescence. It is rarely diagnosed until several years later; seeking help can last for many years, with the individual frequently going from one health care provider to another to no avail. The use of specific assessment instruments is increasing the likelihood of earlier diagnosis and treatment (APA, 2024).

Sex Assigned at Birth, Ethnic, and Cultural Differences

SSD has been reported globally even though its conceptualization is primarily Western. The symptoms may vary from culture to culture (Schrijvers et al., 2024). In some non-Western societies, where the mind–body distinction is not made and symptoms have different meanings and explanations, these physical manifestations are not labeled as a psychiatric disorder (Shu et al., 2023). In cultures that highly stigmatize mental illness, somatic symptoms are more likely to appear (Fox & Earnshaw, 2023). In Latin American and English-speaking Caribbean countries, depression is more likely described in somatic symptoms, such as headaches, gastrointestinal disturbances, or complaints of "nerves" rather than sadness or guilt (Gibson et al., 2024).

Epidemiologic studies show that SSD occurs more frequently in people assigned female at birth. People assigned male at birth are less likely to be diagnosed with SSD, partly because of stereotypic male traits, such as a disinclination to admit discomfort or seek help for their symptoms (APA, 2022).

LGBTQ+ Individuals and Somatization

People who identify as LGBTQ+ report higher levels of poor physical and mental health, including the expression of somatic symptoms. Pervasive trauma exposure, experiencing interpersonal violence, and minority stress are common (Nicholas & Bresin, 2024), and suicidality is higher among sexual underrepresented groups compared to their cisgender peers (Kingsbury et al., 2022).

Familial Differences

SSD tends to run in families, and children of parents/guardians with multiple unexplained somatic complaints are more likely to have somatic issues. Individuals with a tendency toward heightened physiologic arousal and a tendency to amplify somatosensory information have a greater risk of developing this disorder. Data have also confirmed a strong association between sexual trauma exposure and somatic symptoms, illness attitudes, and health care utilization in people assigned female at birth (Greenman et al., 2024).

COMORBIDITY

SSD frequently coexists with other psychiatric disorders, most commonly depression and anxiety. Others include posttraumatic stress disorder, panic disorder, social phobia, obsessive-compulsive disorder (OCD), psychotic disorders, and personality disorders (Sejdiu et al., 2023). Older adults are at particularly elevated risk for comorbid depression (Tu et al., 2024).

Ultimately, numerous unexplained medical issues also coexist with this disorder because many patients have received medical and surgical treatments, often unnecessarily, and are plagued with side effects. A disproportionately high number of people assigned female at birth who eventually receive diagnoses of SSD have been treated for irritable bowel syndrome (IBS), polycystic ovary disease, and chronic pain. Somatization may contribute to the suffering and symptom severity in both depression and functional bowel disorders even without a diagnosis of SSD or other mental disorder, such that psychological evaluation could lead to more effective management and treatment (Orzechowska et al., 2023; Prospero et al., 2021).

Etiology

Biologic Theories

The cause of SSD is unknown. General agreement exists that somatization has a biopsychosocial basis, with the possibility that the biologic dysfunction is common to other chronic disorders such as IBS, fibromyalgia, and chronic fatigue syndrome. There may be a triggering event such as an acute infection, injury, medical procedure, or stressful life events. Physical predisposing factors include previous or current medical conditions, high or low body mass index, genetic or epigenetic profiles, or endocrine, immunologic, or microbial predispositions. When predisposing factors such as dysregulation of the immune system persist, the somatic symptoms persist and become chronic (Löwe et al., 2024).

Emerging evidence suggests that psychological distress and somatic symptom severity are related to disorders of the gut–brain interaction (Trindade et al., 2024). The underlying theory is related to **nociceptors** (sensory fibers that respond to potentially damaging stimuli) in the gut that are involved in pain perception. These nociceptors detect noxious stimuli that initiate the sensation of pain in the brain; however, these nociceptors are activated below the expected threshold for pain detection.

Psychological Theories

Selective attention to and heightened perception of bodily sensations as well as health anxiety contribute to the persistence of SSD. People with this disorder often catastrophize and misinterpret these sensations. **Alexithymia**, difficulty identifying, expressing, and regulating emotions, is associated with SSD. There is a preoccupation with external events characterized by faulty emotional processing between the brain and the body, which results in alterations in the endocrine, immune, and pain-regulating systems (Berens et al., 2023).

Another explanation is that persistent physical symptoms are related to previously learned experiences or beliefs about the symptoms. That is, information from providers or previous experience with a disorder establishes beliefs and expectations about the severity of the current subjective symptom which is no longer severe (Löwe et al., 2024).

Cognitive behaviorists explain somatization symptoms as an interaction of negative views of the world with physical factors (e.g., pain, discomfort). In this model, individuals have a heightened response based on their experiences with a stressor, especially if the stressor is uncontrollable and unpredictable. Over time, their exaggerated responses become an automatic pattern, resulting in behavior that in turn provokes either a negative or positive response in others.

Family Response to Disorder

Family dynamics are shaped by all members, including the person with SSD. When one member has several ongoing chronic health issues, family members' activities and interactions are affected. See Box 33.2. The physical symptoms of the individual become the focus of family life, so activities are planned around that person. Because so much time and so many resources are used trying to discover an underlying illness, resources for other family members are reduced. Because the person is sick, expressing anger about the situation is difficult. The family members need support as they learn to understand the seriousness and difficulty of experiencing an SSD.

BOX 33.2

Research for Evidence-Based Practice: Parent Acceptance

Wiggins, A., Raniti, M., Gaafar, D., Court, A., & Sawyer, S. M. (2022). Pediatric somatic symptom and related disorders: Parent acceptance influences recovery. The Journal of Pediatrics, 241, *109–114. https://doi.org/10.1016/j.jpeds.2021.09.054*

THE QUESTION: The purpose of the study was to assess the influence of clinician's diagnostic-discussions on patient and parental acceptance of a diagnosis of SSRD, and to identify how the discussions relate to functional recovery.

METHODS: A cross-sectional design was used to analyze clinician/patient/parent diagnostic discussions over 18 months of pediatric medical records, and to determine the effect of influence the discussions had on diagnostic acceptance and recovery after 1 year.

FINDINGS: No significant findings were associated with the clinician's discussions and level of recovery even when no discussions were found. The authors concluded that recovery was not dependent on full parental acceptance. The authors emphasize the continuing importance of exploring the complexities around accepting a psychological rather than an organic reason for a child's illness. They conclude by suggesting for some families continuing resistance could contribute to further help seeking and unnecessary treatment, and even a differential diagnosis of factitious disorder imposed on another (FDIO) should be considered.

IMPLICATIONS FOR NURSING: This study supports the continuing importance of talking and teaching families and patients about mind–body connections (positive and negative), whether a diagnosis of SSRD has been made. Somatization can occur along with many other medical conditions, worsening distress even compromising expected treatment. Nurses are in trusted positions to explore diagnostic resistance and to provide education, as well as to introduce alternative strategies for anxiety, and coping which may well be more acceptable coming from a nurse who orients care holistically.

RECOVERY-ORIENTED CARE OF PEOPLE WITH SSD

Teamwork and Collaboration: Working Toward Recovery

The care of patients with SSD involves three approaches:

- Providing long-term supportive general management of the chronic condition.
- Treating symptoms of comorbid mental and physical issues.
- Providing care in special settings, including individual and group treatment and the use of complementary and alternative medicine (CAM).

The cornerstones of management are trust and belief. Ideally, the patient should see only one health care provider at regularly scheduled visits. During each primary care visit, the provider should conduct a holistic assessment, including a partial physical examination of the organ system, focusing on the areas where the patient has complaints. Physical symptoms are treated conservatively using the least intrusive approach. The provider should also assess for any stressors, life changes, and/or a history of trauma that has been linked to the excessive expression of somatic symptoms. In the mental health setting, the use of cognitive-behavioral therapy (CBT) can be effective (Sauer et al., 2023).

Safety Issues

SSD and related disorders are associated with a risk of suicide. If depression and anxiety are present, the risk is greater. Safety becomes even more of a concern because these individuals are not usually treated in a mental health setting where suicide assessments are routine (Torres et al., 2021).

EVIDENCE-BASED NURSING CARE OF PEOPLE WITH SSD

The nursing care for people with SSD requires patience, empathy, and a focus on using sound therapeutic communication techniques and the establishment of a trusting therapeutic relationship. Nurse self-awareness is critical when interacting with a patient with SSD.

RECOGNIZING CUES: RELEVANT ASSESSMENT INFORMATION

During the assessment interview, the nurse should allow enough time for the patient to explain all medical issues, discuss all symptoms, and describe what they do for relief. A hurried assessment interview blocks communication and may prevent full disclosure of past experiences and treatments which will have bearing on the current plan of care. See Clinical Judgment Nursing Care Plan 33.1, which sets forth a plan of care for Carol, the case study patient in this chapter.

NCLEXNOTE Encourage and allow patients with SSD to discuss their physical issues before focusing on psychosocial issues.

Physical Health

Psychiatric–mental health (PMH) nurses typically see these patients for issues related to coexisting psychiatric disorders, such as depression, not SSD. While taking the patient's history, the nurse may discover that the individual has had multiple surgeries or medical issues, making SSD a strong possibility. If the patient has not already received a diagnosis of SSD, the nurse should screen for it by determining the presence of the most reported issues associated with this disorder, which include dysmenorrhea, a lump in the throat, vomiting, shortness of breath, burning sensation in the sex organs, painful limbs, and amnesia. If the patient has these symptoms, they should be seen by a mental health provider qualified to make the diagnosis.

Somatization is common in the general population, among those with and without medical conditions. Older assessment tools focused on identifying somatic symptoms but did not screen effectively for SSD. A more recently developed instrument, the Somatic Symptom Disorder-B Criteria Scale (SSD-12), focuses less on symptom expression and more on excessive thoughts, behaviors, and feelings associated with the somatic symptoms (*DSM-5-TR* B criterion). The SSD-12 is more effective at recognizing those with SSD and identifying changes in severity of the disorder over the course of treatment (von Schrottenberg et al., 2024).

Review of Systems

Although these patients' symptoms have usually received considerable attention from the medical community, a careful review of systems is important because the appearance of physical issues is usually related to psychosocial issues. Even as the patient continues to be seen for mental health issues, an ongoing awareness of biologic symptoms is important, particularly because these symptoms are deemphasized in the overall case management.

Pain is the most common finding in people with this disorder. Because the pain is usually related to symptoms of all the major body systems, it is unlikely that a somatic intervention such as an analgesic will be effective on a long-term basis. Remember that although no medical explanation exists for the pain, the patient's pain is real and has serious psychosocial implications. A careful assessment should include the following questions:

- What is the pain like?
- What is the extent of the pain?

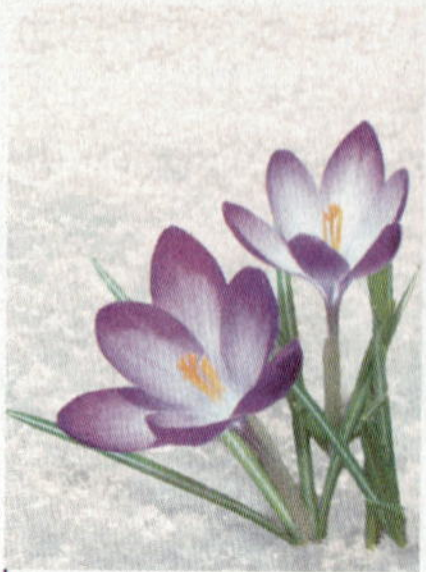

CLINICAL JUDGMENT NURSING CARE PLAN 33.1

The Patient With Somatic Symptom Disorder

Carol is, age 48, is making her weekly visit to her primary care provider for unexplained multiple somatic problems. This week, her concern is reoccurring abdominal pain that fits no symptom pattern. Upon physical examination, a cause for her abdominal pain could not be found. She is requesting a refill of alprazolam which is the only medication that relieves her pain. She is in the process of applying for disability income because of being completely disabled by neck and shoulder pain. The physician and office staff avoid her whenever possible. The physician will not refill the prescription until Carol is evaluated by the consulting mental health team that provides weekly evaluations and services.

Setting: Mental Health Clinic

Assessment Cues: Carol, age 48, has obesity and was referred by her primary care provider. She appears very angry, stating that she resents being forced to see a "shrink" for the only medication that works. She denies any psychiatric issues or emotional distress. Carol is wearing a short black top and snug slacks. Her hair is in curlers and she says that it is too much trouble to comb her hair.

Her mental status is within expected limits, but she admits to being slightly depressed and takes the alprazolam for her nerves. She says she has nothing to live for, but denies any thoughts of suicide. She depends on her children for everything and feels very guilty about doing so. She spends most of her waking hours going to various doctors and taking combinations of medications to relieve her pains. She has no friends or nonfamily social contacts. BP 144/80, P 80, R 18, Ht. 5′2″; Wt. 190; BMI 34.7.

Associated Psychiatric Diagnosis

R/O depression; SSD
S/P hysterectomy
S/P gastric bypass
S/P carpel tunnel release
Chronic shoulder, neck pain; vertigo

Medications

Premarin, 0.625 mg every day
Alprazolam, 25 mg tid
Ranitidine HCl, 150 mg with meals
Simethicone, 125 mg four times daily with meals
Calcium carbonate, 1,200 mg every day
Multiple vitamin, every day
Zolpidem tartrate, 10 mg at bedtime PRN
Ibuprofen, 600 mg q4h PRN pain
Simethicone 125 mg, PRN for indigestion
Phenylephrine topical suppositories PRN for hemorrhoid pain

Priority Hypothesis: Negative Self-Esteem

Important Characteristics

Slight depression
Dependency on others
Expresses guilt
Expresses feelings of helplessness

Associated Considerations

Feels she is a burden to family
Fleeting thoughts of suicide
Constant physical problems that interfere with usual social activities

Planning Recovery and Wellness Outcomes

Initial

Identify need to increase self-esteem

Long-Term

Participate in individual or group therapy for esteem building

Clinical Judgment Nursing Care Plan 33.1 Continued

Taking Action: Nursing Interventions

Interventions	Rationale	Ongoing Assessment
Establish rapport with patient.	Individuals with low self-esteem are reluctant to discuss true feelings.	Examine feelings that are provoked by patient (discuss with supervisor if interfering with care). Determine whether patient is beginning to engage in a relationship.
Encourage patient to spend time dressing and grooming appropriately.	Confidence and self-esteem improve when a person looks well-groomed.	Monitor response to suggestions.
Encourage patient to discuss various somatic problems but allow some time to discuss psychological and interpersonal issues.	Patients with SSD need time to express their physical problems. It helps them feel valued. The best way to build a relationship is to acknowledge physical symptoms.	Monitor time that patient spends explaining physical symptoms.
Explore opportunities for Carol to meet other people with similar, nonmedical interests.	Focusing Carol on meeting others will improve the possibilities of increasing contacts.	Observe willingness to identify other interests besides physical problems.

Evaluation

Outcomes	Revised Outcomes	Interventions
Carol admitted to having low self-esteem but was very reluctant to consider meeting new people.	Focus on building self-esteem.	Identify activities that will enhance personal self-esteem.

Priority Hypothesis: Using Medication Inappropriately

Important Characteristics	Associated Considerations
Lack of medication effectiveness. Verbalizes difficulty with prescribed regimens.	Uses medication for other conditions than prescribed.

Planning Recovery and Wellness Outcomes

Initial	Long-Term
Discuss the use of medications honestly.	Use nonpharmacologic means for stress reduction, especially avoiding continued use of antianxiety medications.

Taking Action: Nursing Interventions

Interventions	Rationale	Ongoing Assessment
Clarify the frequency and purpose of taking alprazolam.	Unsupervised polypharmacy is very common with these patients. Further clarification is usually needed.	Carefully track self-report of medication use; determine if patient is disclosing the use of all medications.
Educate patient about the effects of combining medications, emphasizing side effects.	Education about combining medication is the beginning of helping patient become effective in medication regimen.	Observe patient's ability and willingness to consider negative effects.
Recommend that patient gradually reduce number of medications and problem-solve other means of managing physical symptoms.	Giving patients clear directions about managing health care regimens needs to be followed up with specific strategies to change behavior.	Evaluate patient's ability to solve problems.

Evaluation

Outcomes	Revised Outcomes	Interventions
Carol disclosed use of medications but was unwilling to consider changing ineffective use of medication.	Identify next step if primary care physician does not refill prescription.	Discuss the possibility of not being able to obtain alprazolam.

- What helps the pain get better?
- When is the pain at its worst?
- What has worked in the past to relieve the pain?

Nutrition

Nutrition assessment is important because gastrointestinal disorders are highly comorbid with psychiatric disorders, especially SSD. Psychological distress and poorer psychosocial functioning associated with SSD contribute to the severity of IBS (Kleinstäuber et al., 2023). In IBS, there is a disordered communication between the gut and brain that results in motility disturbances, visceral hypersensitivity, and altered CNS processing. The primary treatment of IBS includes dietary changes, soluble fiber, and antispasmodic drugs (Patel & Shackelford, 2022).

Furthermore, the quality of the diet is associated with medically unexplained gastrointestinal symptoms. Diet patterns loaded with fruits, vegetables, low-fat dairy, dried fruits, and whole grains have fewer reported gastrointestinal disturbances than diets high in vegetable oil, meat, salt, hydrogenated oils, onions, egg, poultry, fish, and refined grains or diets loaded with processed meats, sweet desserts, and high-fat dairy (Pasta et al., 2024).

Sleep

Many sleep disturbances (insomnia, obstructive sleep apnea, restless leg syndrome) are common in people with SSD (Kundu et al., 2022). Somatic symptoms (aches, pains, fatigue) also contribute to poor-quality sleep. In all genders, trauma plays an aggravating role by increasing sleep disturbances and somatic symptoms (Challa et al., 2022). Among youth, increases in sleep disorders and somatic complaints may be a result of having had their daily routines disrupted during COVID-19, and this has not been resolved (Robert, & Kadhiravan, 2022). Sleep quality has major effects on multiple domains of functioning and mental/physical health; it should always be part of a comprehensive assessment that will help nurses formulate sleep interventions that target the specific needs of the individual.

Physical Functioning

The actual physical functioning of these individuals is often marginal. Fatigue is a constant issue for many people with SSD, and various physical issues interfere with usual activity. These patients report an overwhelming lack of energy, which makes maintaining usual routines or accomplishing daily tasks impossible. Fatigue is accompanied by the inability to concentrate on simple functions, leading to decreased performance and disinterest in surroundings. See Box 33.3.

BOX 33.3

Clinical Judgment Vignette: Somatic Symptom Disorder and Stress

Ms. J, age 42 years, has been coming to the mental health clinic for 2 years for her nerves. She has seen only the provider for medication but now has been referred to the nurse's new stress management group because she is experiencing side effects of all the medications that have been tried. The psychiatrist has diagnosed SSD and wants her to learn to manage her "nerves" without medication.

At the first meeting with the nurse, Ms. J was preoccupied with chest pain and bloating that had lasted for the past 6 months. Her chest pain is constant and sharp at times. The pain does not prevent her from going to her job as a restaurant server but does interfere with meal preparation at night for her family and her ability to have sexual intercourse. She has numerous other physical issues, including allergies to certain perfumes, dysmenorrhea, ovarian polycystic disease (ovarian cysts), chronic urinary tract infections, and rashes. She is constantly fatigued and has frequent leg cramps. She states that she is too tired to fix dinner for her family. On days off from work, she takes a nap in the afternoon, sleeping until evening. She is unable to fall asleep at night.

She believes that she will soon have to have her gallbladder removed because of occasional referred pain in her back and nausea that occurs a couple of hours after eating. She is not enthusiastic about a stress management group and does not believe it will help her issues. However, she has agreed to consider it.

Building Clinical Judgment

1. How should the nurse begin helping Ms. J. develop stress management strategies?
2. What are some possible interventions for Ms. J's fatigue?

Patients assigned female at birth with this disorder usually have had multiple gynecologic issues, so that the physical manifestations of SSD often lead to altered sexual behavior. Symptoms of dysmenorrhea and painful intercourse may indicate a history of sexual abuse and sexual trauma. Physiologic indicators, such as those produced by laboratory tests, are not available. However, a careful assessment of the patient's menstrual history, gynecologic issues, and sexual functioning is important. It is also important to assess whether abuse or trauma has occurred in the past or continues in the present, and whether such abuse is sexual, physical, or emotional.

NCLEXNOTE Focus on functions rather than symptoms—give acceptable explanations of symptoms, avoid unnecessary interventions, and arrange for more frequent (but brief) medical contacts.

History of Trauma

Credible evidence suggests a link between a history of childhood sexual abuse, rape, and domestic violence, and subsequent lifetime sequelae of somatic symptoms and somatic disorders (Greenman et al., 2024). The long-term trajectory of early trauma and future health impacts needs continuing study so that targeted interventions and policies for prevention and treatment can be developed.

Adverse childhood experiences (ACEs) increase the risk of developing ACE-related mental and somatic conditions in adulthood (Fernandez et al., 2024). In fact, emotional and sexual abuse during childhood predicts specific somatic symptoms in adolescents that are not explained by underlying pathology (Jacobsen et al., 2023) and physical health issues (cardiovascular disease, gastrointestinal disorders) in a strong and cumulative way (Eilers et al., 2023).

Cumulative adversities during adolescence may be more likely than single childhood events, and therefore are important to explore, since each will have strong, direct effects needing to be addressed via specific planning and intervention (Pinto et al., 2023). Although it is a tall order, and more research is needed to design and develop programs that will effectively reduce or prevent early adversities, nurses can help create conditions in which families and communities thrive, they can engage in community outreach programs, and they can advocate for policies that promote well-being for all. The Centers for Disease Control and Prevention (CDC) (2024) proposes five action strategies nurses could institute to help prevent ACEs (see Table 33.1).

Trauma Assessment

Because interpersonal trauma is so closely linked to somatic symptoms, a trauma assessment is essential. Not all people who experience trauma develop mental disorders, but higher levels of lifetime adversity and trauma are significantly associated with severe somatic symptoms (Greenman et al., 2024) and with high levels of health service utilization. Among underrepresented groups, cumulative histories of adverse/traumatic familial, community, and societal experiences (stigma and discrimination) carry disproportionate mental and physical health burdens (Snowden et al., 2023). As universal trauma screening becomes the norm rather than the exception, nurses should expect to conduct clinical interviews, use standardized trauma-screening measures, and make behavioral observations that provide an in-depth understanding of the severity and nature of the trauma, including the presence of additional trauma symptoms. Such wide-net screening can then drive treatment planning and referrals, and it can also be used to monitor progress over time.

TABLE 33.1 PREVENTING CHILD ABUSE AND NEGLECT: TIPS FROM THE CDC

Strategy	Approach
Strengthen economic supports to families	• Strengthening household financial security • Family-friendly work policies
Change social norms to support parents and positive parenting	• Public engagement and education campaigns • Legislative approaches to reduce corporal punishment
Provide quality care and education early in life	• Preschool enrichment with family engagement • Improved quality of child care through licensing and accreditation
Enhance parenting skills to promote healthy child development	• Early childhood home visitation • Parenting skill and family relationship approaches
Intervene to lessen harms and prevent future risk	• Enhanced primary care • Behavioral parent training programs • Treatment to lessen harms of abuse and neglect exposure • Treatment to prevent problem behavior and later involvement in violence

Reprinted from Centers for Disease Control and Prevention (CDC). (2024). Essentials for childhood: Creating safe, stable, nurturing relationships and environments for all children. https://www.cdc.gov/child-abuse-neglect/php/public-health-strategy/index.html

MEDICATION

A medication assessment of these patients can be challenging. Patients with SSD frequently seek help from numerous providers because they do not feel that they are believed, or they think that providers do not care about their suffering. Because they often receive medications from each provider, they usually take many drugs. A medication assessment is needed not only because of the number of medications but also because these individuals frequently experience unusual side effects, or they report that they are "sensitive" to medications. Because of their somatic sensitivity, they often overreact to medication. Research leaves many unanswered questions about dosing, drug-discontinuation, duration of treatment, long-term improvement, and differential responses to different drug classes which future studies may better address. As the mind-set around these disorders shifts away from overdependence on psychosocial explanations and the effectiveness of psychological treatments, complementary and integrative therapies may offer better options.

Substance Use

These patients spend much of their lives trying to find out what is wrong with them. When one health care provider after another can find little if any explanation for their symptoms, many patients become anxious and/or depressed. To alleviate their symptoms of anxiety, they sometimes self-medicate with OTC medications and/or substances of abuse (e.g., alcohol, marijuana), or they seek a health care provider who prescribes a benzodiazepine such as alprazolam. Because symptoms associated with their disorder cannot be treated within a few weeks with a benzodiazepine, they can become dependent on medication that should not have been prescribed in the first place.

Although benzodiazepines have a place in therapeutics, they are not recommended for long-term use and only complicate the treatment of individuals with SSD. These medications should also be avoided because of their dependent qualities, which place patients at risk of misuse. Unfortunately, by the time patients with SSD see a mental health provider, they often have already begun taking the medications for anxiety. Many times, they only agree to see a mental health provider because the last provider would no longer prescribe an anxiolytic without a psychiatric evaluation.

NURSES AND SOMATIZATION

The role of stress in the production of somatic symptoms should not be overlooked. A recent study of nurses found an association between concrete coping behaviors and distress and somatization. See Box 33.4. Nurses who identify with these experiences can recognize the role of stress in heightening emotional exhaustion and the production of somatic symptoms, and they may be better able to convey empathy and support those with somatic symptoms and related disorders to make connections between symptoms and stressors.

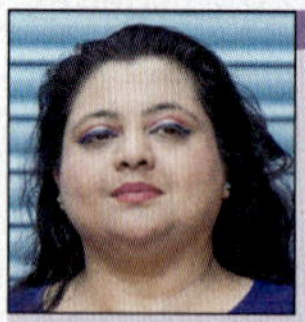

Remember Carol?

Carol has been taking alprazolam for stress for years. Her primary health care provider is refusing to prescribe it again until she has a complete mental health examination. No other health care providers will prescribe alprazolam for her.

PSYCHOSOCIAL CUES

The mental status of individuals with SSD can be within expected limits, although most patients report frustration, depression, and hopelessness about their situation. What is most noticeable is their intense focus on their bodies and the physical symptoms that are causing them distress and disability.

MENTAL STATUS AND APPEARANCE

Cognitive and Behavioral Responses

In general, cognition is not impaired in people with SSD, but it may be distorted, such as believing the pain means a life-threatening condition. These individuals seem preoccupied with the signs and symptoms of their illnesses and may even keep a record of their experiences. Living with illness, diseases, and suffering truly becomes a way of life.

Self-Concept

People with SSD usually have a negative self-concept of physical weakness and illness-related symptom evaluation. The self-concept can be determined by physical appearance, affect, and explanation of the current situation. Negative self-concept usually begins in childhood or adolescence when the child begins to see themselves as ill and cannot participate in usual school or recreational activities. Parents/guardians who focus on protecting children from illness can inadvertently reinforce the self-concept of being ill.

Stress and Coping Patterns

Some individuals with SSD have intense emotional reactions to life stressors and have led or are leading

BOX 33.4

Research for Evidence-Based Practice: Coping, Distress, and Somatization

Franck, E., Haegdorens, F., Goossens, E., van Gils, Y., Portzky, M., Somville, F., Abuaward, M., Slootmans, S., & Ban Bogaert, P. (2021). The role of coping behavior in healthcare workers' distress and somatization during the COVID-19 pandemic. Frontiers in Psychology, 12, 684618. *https://doi.org/10.3389/fpsyg.2021.684618*

THE QUESTION: How did the use of positive and negative stress-reducing activities affect health care workers' mental and physical well-being during the COVID-19 pandemic?

METHODS: A cross-sectional, online survey was sent to a network of health care workers. A total of 1,376 participants completed measures on demographics, coping behaviors, and showing signs of somatic symptoms and acute distress.

FINDINGS: Although use of coping strategies was related to demonstration of fewer somatic symptoms, health care workers who provided direct care to patients with COVID-19 were likely to decrease the use of positive coping strategies during the peak of the pandemic when they were highly stressed. Participants reported a variety of concrete coping mechanisms (watching TV, doing chores, playing cards, etc.) that effectively relieved their symptoms under ordinary circumstances.

IMPLICATIONS FOR NURSING: This study validates the link between the stressful work of caring during COVID-19 and the development of acute stress reactions and psychosomatic symptoms. It also emphasizes the importance of having a repertoire of concrete coping skills that work for the individual and committing to using them, especially during times of increased stress when their use might be compromised by competing demands on a nurse's time and energy. This study adds to the literature on the importance of self-care and universalizes the experience of somatizing, which might help nurses better understand and approach individuals with SSD or related disorders, without judging or stigmatizing them.

traumatic or chaotic lives. These patients usually have had a series of personal crises beginning at an early age. Examples include severe sexual and physical abuse and psychological trauma. Typically, a new symptom or medical issue develops during times of emotional stress, as well as during anniversaries of losses or traumas that have occurred in the patient's lifetime. It is critical that the link between the physical assessment data and the patient's psychological and social history are considered. A thorough history of major psychological events should be compared with the chronology of physical issues. Special attention should be paid to any history of sexual abuse or trauma in the patient's younger years. Early sexual abuse may also prevent the individual from being able to perform sexually or to endure chronic abdominal pain or discomfort during sexual relations.

The individual's mood is usually labile, often shifting from extremely excited or anxious to being depressed and hopeless. Response to physical symptoms is usually magnified, such as interpreting a simple cold as pneumonia or a brief chest pain as a heart attack. Family members may not believe the physical symptoms are real and may view them as attention-getting behavior because symptoms often improve when the patient receives attention. For example, a person who has been in bed for 3 weeks with severe back pain may suddenly feel much better when their children visit them.

Social Network

People with this disorder spend excessive time seeking medical care and treating their multiple illnesses. Because they believe themselves to be very sick, they also believe that they are disabled and cannot work. Many are unemployed, so frequently these individuals have changed jobs, had multiple positions over their lifetimes or careers, or have had absences or gaps in employment.

Because their symptoms are often inconsistent with any identifiable medical diagnosis, these individuals are rarely satisfied with their health care providers, who can find nothing wrong. However, their social network often consists of a series of health care providers, rather than peers or family members, who can also become weary of the individual's constant complaints of physical issues. Identifying a support network requires sorting out the health care providers from family and friends.

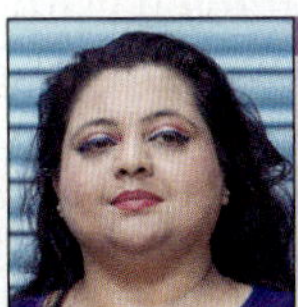

Consider Carol's Limited Social Network

Carol has no friends and spends her time going from provider to provider. Her anxiety about her symptoms has impacted her ability to maintain friendships and other close relationships.

Family Issues

Individuals with SSD sometimes live in chaotic families with multiple issues. In assessing the family structure, other members with psychiatric disorders must be identified. People may have abusive partners who have an antisocial personality disorder; substance use disorders are common. Identifying the positive and negative relationships within the family is important.

SSD is particularly problematic because it disrupts the family's social life. Changes in routine or major life events often precipitate the appearance of a symptom. For example, an individual may be planning a vacation with the family but at the last minute decides they cannot go because the back pain has returned, and they will be unable to sit in the car. These family disruptions are common. In addition, as already noted, employment history for the person with SSD may be erratic.

SPIRITUAL ASSESSMENT

A spiritual assessment should be conducted to determine the significance of spiritual beliefs impacting the perception of health. For example, does the patient believe the health issues are related to being punished for real or imagined transgressions? The spiritual assessment also provides information that can be used in planning care.

QUALITY OF LIFE

SSD has a negative impact on the QoL. Because many of the physical symptoms (25% to 50%) are unexplained, the person is continually told that there are no medical explanations, which leads to frustration and seeking out additional medical opinions. The pain or discomfort interferes with daily activities and prevents the person from participating fully with family and friends (Tu et al., 2024).

STRENGTHS ASSESSMENT

An individual with SSD may have difficulty identifying *any* personal strengths. The nurse should help the person focus on daily activities and suggest strengths that emerge. For example, some strengths might be that the person has a place to live, has a caring family, or some educational attainment. Recognizing a patient's strengths requires time and intentional effort. Nurses may be in the best position to develop system-level interventions that identify and build on a patient's strengths. For example, recognizing clever ideas and contributions the patient makes while collaborating in the development of the care plan is a great way to build strengths and self-esteem.

ANALYZING CUES AND DEVELOPING HYPOTHESES

Physical concerns and symptoms tend to dominate the individual's conversation and should not be dismissed. The patient may have several health issues to discuss, including fatigue, pain, and insomnia. Psychologically, depression and suicidal behavior should always be considered. Social isolation may be an outward expression of depression. Initially, hypothesizing about the meaning of somatic symptoms and the associated cognitive-affective disturbances (negative anticipation, attentional bias, pain catastrophizing, alexithymia, and negative emotions) may help the nurse and patient better understand the experience. Later, attempting to draw out the relationship between symptoms and the individual's life-stressors and their role in amplifying bodily distress is an effective nursing approach to begin the work of helping the patient regain a typical lifestyle.

PLANNING RECOVERY AND WELLNESS OUTCOMES: GENERATING SOLUTIONS

Establishing recovery and wellness goals, otherwise known as generating solutions, may seem to be out of the question with individuals who defines themselves as "ill," "sick," and/or in "chronic pain." However, helping such individuals define their symptoms and validate them is a start to recovery. Nurses are poised to educate individuals with multiple somatic issues to better understand their symptoms (e.g., what triggers them) and to define short-term goals for recovery.

The notion of recovery itself is patient centered and focused on what the patient believes is realistic and possible. For example, some patients with this disorder may choose to learn to live with their symptoms (e.g., pain) and find alternative ways of coping. Nursing interventions can help identify triggers that worsen symptoms and suggest coping strategies to address the symptoms. Even though a patient may suffer from multiple somatic symptoms and chronic health anxiety, together the nurse and the patient can work toward finding solutions that will promote health and well-being.

THERAPEUTIC RELATIONSHIP

The most difficult aspect of nursing care is developing a sound, positive, nonjudgmental nurse–patient relationship, yet this relationship is crucial. Without it, the nurse is just one more provider who fails to meet the patient's expectations. Developing this relationship requires time and patience. Therapeutic communication techniques should be used to refocus the patient on psychosocial issues related to the physical manifestations. During periods when symptoms of other psychiatric disorders surface, additional interventions are needed. For example, if depression occurs, additional supportive or cognitive approaches may be needed (see Box 33.5).

BOX 33.5

Reflection of a Nurse: The Importance of Empathy

Incident

On the inpatient unit, a patient with a diagnosis of somatic symptom disorder (SSD) begins demanding to leave the unit, refuses to eat, and complains of shooting leg pains. The nurse encourages the patient to eat before the tray is removed, but the patient pushes the tray away and says, "I don't belong here, this pain is real. No one believes me! How can I eat?" The nurse then begins explaining the reason the patient is in the hospital and about the diagnosis. After a few more exchanges the patient becomes even more angry and finally, they loudly tell the nurse, "Go away and leave me alone!"

Reflection

Upon evaluation of the interaction, the nurse realizes that by immediately trying to talk about the patient's diagnosis and not showing any empathy or acceptance that the patient was experiencing pain, the patient thought the nurse, just like everyone else, believed the symptoms were "all in their head," so the patient became angry and lashed out.

1. What interventions would have been more helpful initially to establish rapport with the patient?
2. What understandings about pain symptoms in SSD might help the nurse approach the patient differently?

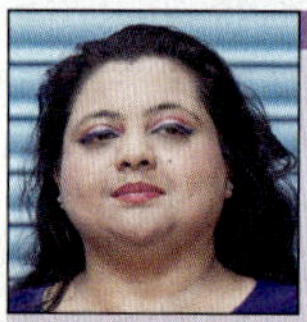

Carol's Behavior in the Mental Health Unit

Carol felt she was tricked into agreeing to be admitted to a mental health unit for medication evaluation. She believes she should be in a medical unit for her constant pain.

TAKING ACTION: NURSING INTERVENTIONS

Priorities of Care

Priorities of care are determined based on presenting issues. The risk of suicidal thoughts, attempts, past attempts, and even active plans are present in many with SSD (Torres et al., 2021). This risk calls for careful suicide screening and assuring that safety measures are in place, either via hospitalization or through negotiated suicide safety planning in outpatient or community settings. Although research is limited, a unique risk of all types of suicidal behavior—independent of other mental comorbidities—may be associated with anger, alexithymia, alcohol use, past hospitalizations, dissociation, and emotional abuse (Torres et al., 2021). Nurses should be alert to these additional risks for patients with SSDs.

Somatic symptoms are common expressions of distress in children and adolescents. The diagnosis of an SSD is often first made for severe somatic symptoms during an emergency department visit or in an inpatient setting (Roelf et al., 2025). Nurses who are aware of the link to trauma and the heightened risk of suicide in sexual underrepresented groups will follow suicide precautions and protocols closely.

Nurses should be able to provide emotional support, engage in reflective communication and problem-solving, and help individuals find appropriate resources including gender affirming therapists and providers to promote self-efficacy. As strong voices on the interprofessional health care team, nurses are not only a source of information about SSRDs but can help others understand how traumatic experiences, stigma, ACEs, and somatization cluster together. Nurses must also continue to serve as advocates who support policies and services that promote health equity and protect the rights of sexually underrepresented groups (see ANA, 2022).

Safety considerations also address the harmful effects of ordering unnecessary medical tests, especially those that are costly and carry potential dangers. So, the need to establish a trusting, therapeutic relationship is tantamount to protecting the patient from overzealous evaluations and ineffective treatment which may cause harm. A good therapeutic alliance can help minimize excessive and unnecessary evaluation and ineffective treatment, which improves patient satisfaction (Winograd et al., 2023). If the diagnosis has not been established, that should be the next priority. Although the primary care provider conducts the diagnostic discussion, nurses should follow up and be able to address the patient's questions. Accepting a functional diagnosis rather than receiving a typical medical diagnosis can be very challenging and frightening. Nurses must be careful not to strengthen a mind–body dichotomy or to create more defensiveness in patients who are already frustrated and confused about their experiences. Just telling a patient you believe them goes a long way in gaining their trust.

Symptom management follows as the next priority; the focus is on reducing the symptoms without reinforcing them while helping promote self-efficacy, improve healthy coping, and pursue health-related QoL. The nurse needs to have completed a thorough assessment to establish an individualized plan of care. Another priority is to focus on reducing the level of health anxiety. Helping the patient identify the relationship between stress and physical symptoms, facilitating emotional expression, and teaching emotion-focused strategies such as progressive relaxation, deep breathing, guided imagery, distraction via music, or other activities (Belleza, 2021) are some of the ways that nurses can intervene.

Physical Care

Nursing interventions that focus on physical health become especially important because medical treatment must be conservative; aggressive pharmacologic treatment must be avoided. Each time a nurse sees the patient, some of that time should be spent respectfully discussing physical complaints and validating the patient's distress. During the discussion, it is important that the nurse project the belief that the patient is truly experiencing the symptoms. Several physically focused interventions, including pain management, activity enhancement, nutrition regulation, relaxation, and pharmacologic interventions, may be useful in caring for patients with SSD.

Pain Management

In pain management, a single approach rarely works. Pain is a primary issue and was previously considered a separate disorder. Nursing care focuses on helping patients identify strategies to relieve pain and to examine stressors in their lives. After a careful assessment of the pain, nonpharmacologic strategies should be developed to reduce it. If gastrointestinal pain is frequent, eating and bowel habits should be explored and modified as needed. For back pain, exercises and consultation from a physical therapist may be useful. Headaches are a challenge. Self-monitoring and tracking them engages the patient in the therapeutic process and helps to identify psychosocial triggers. In addition, suggesting or referring the individual for complementary and alternative treatments may be useful. Relaxation techniques, identifying thoughts and feelings about pain or discomfort, and including family members in the intervention have also been shown to be useful.

Activity Enhancement

Helping the patient establish a daily routine may alleviate some of the difficulty with sleep but doing so may be difficult because most of these patients are not employed. Encouraging the patient to get up in the morning and go to bed at night at specific times can help the patient establish a routine. These patients should engage in regular exercise to improve their overall physical state, although they often have numerous reasons why they cannot. This is where the nurse's patience is tested; the nurse ultimately needs to remember that the patient's symptoms are an expression of suffering. Agreeing that daily exercise is difficult but continuing to emphasize the importance of exercise can counter some of the reluctance to exercise.

Nutrition Regulation

Patients with SSD often have gastrointestinal issues and may have special nutritional needs. The nurse should discuss the nutritional value of foods with the patient. Discussing the use of whole healthy food sources rather than processed or "junk" food is a strategy nurses can use to assist the patient with gastrointestinal distress to consider dietary changes. The act of talking with patients about ways that they can exert some control of their bodies can have a positive effect and assist them with managing some of their symptoms. If patients are being prescribed medications that promote weight gain, weight control strategies may be discussed, including exercise or increasing movement with physical therapy.

Relaxation

Patients taking anxiety-relieving medication can be taught relaxation techniques to alleviate stress. It is a challenge to help these patients really use these strategies. The nurse should consider various techniques, including simple relaxation techniques, distraction, and guided imagery. See Chapter 10.

Wellness Challenges

Individuals with SSD focus on signs of illness, not behaviors supporting wellness. Because these individuals have intense bodily sensations that are associated with illness, it is difficult to help them re-focus on wellness.

Medications Interventions

No medication is specifically recommended for patients with SSD; however, psychiatric symptoms of comorbid disorders, such as depression and anxiety, should be treated pharmacologically as appropriate. Usually, patients who are depressed or anxious take an antidepressant to treat their symptoms (see Chapter 25).

Multiple antidepressants have been shown to be effective for treating pain and the symptoms of depression. Duloxetine—a serotonin and norepinephrine reuptake inhibitor (SNRI) that is indicated for neuropathy, depression, and anxiety—is also used to manage pain (Jones et al., 2024). See Box 33.6.

Patients who report symptoms of anxiety are treated pharmacologically, like those with depression. The first line of treatment for all anxiety disorders is with an SSRI. Doses for SSD are generally higher than those prescribed for depression to relieve and manage the symptoms of anxiety disorders, including panic, social phobia, generalized anxiety, OCD, and posttraumatic stress disorder.

Nonpharmacologic approaches, such as biofeedback and relaxation, are also quite useful in conjunction with pharmacologic treatment. Benzodiazepines may be used initially in the treatment of those with anxiety but should

BOX 33.6

Medication Profile: Duloxetine

DRUG CLASS: Serotonin and norepinephrine reuptake inhibitor (SNRI)

RECEPTOR AFFINITY: Binds selectively and has a high affinity to both norepinephrine and serotonin (5-HT) transporters yet lacks affinity for monoamine receptors within the central nervous system.

INDICATIONS: Treatment of depression, generalized anxiety disorder, chronic musculoskeletal pain, diabetic peripheral neuropathic pain, fibromyalgia

ROUTE AND DOSAGE: Available as capsules: 30 mg, 60 mg

Adults: Initially, 60 mg daily and increasing to 90 mg/d consistent with patient tolerance. Therapy at 120 mg/d may be necessary before response occurs. Can be given in divided doses for individuals who are used to taking pain medication twice a day.

Geriatric: Adjust dosage as needed because older patients—particularly those on other medications—are more prone to develop side effects. May initiate dose of 30 mg daily for 2 weeks.

Pediatric: Not recommended for children younger than 18 years of age

HALF-LIFE (PEAK EFFECTS): Duloxetine has an elimination half-life of about 12 hours (the range is 8 to 17 hours). Steady state is usually achieved after 3 days.

SELECTED SIDE EFFECTS: Nausea, dry mouth, constipation, diarrhea, fatigue, difficulty sleeping, and dizziness. Increased blood pressure can occur and should be monitored. Seizures have been reported. Sexual dysfunction (decreased sex drive and delayed orgasm and ejaculation) has been associated with duloxetine.

BOXED WARNING: Suicidal thoughts and behaviors

WARNINGS: Screen for bipolar disorder, monitor for serotonin syndrome; monitor blood pressure before and after dosage is initiated (e.g., weekly for 1 month), screen for medication-to-medication interactions.

SPECIFIC PATIENT/FAMILY EDUCATION

- Take drug exactly as prescribed; do not stop taking it abruptly or without consulting your health care provider.
- If patients wish to stop the medication, they need to consult with their provider about tapering the dose due to discontinuation syndrome, a cluster of physical and emotional symptoms that are associated with decreasing SNRIs and selective serotonin reuptake inhibitors (SSRIs) too quickly. Symptoms of abrupt discontinuation can include the following: Symptoms of withdrawal include dizziness, anxiety, nausea, vomiting, nervousness, and diarrhea.
- Families and caregivers of patients should be advised to observe for the emergence of anxiety, agitation, panic attacks, insomnia, irritability, hostility, aggressiveness, impulsivity, hypomania, mania, other unusual changes in behavior, worsening of depression, and suicidal ideation. Such symptoms should be reported to the patient's prescriber or health professional, especially if side effects are severe, abrupt in onset, or were not part of the patient's presenting symptoms.
- Report any signs and symptoms of side effects.
- Combining duloxetine with aspirin, nonsteroidal anti-inflammatory drugs (NSAIDs), warfarin, or other drugs that are associated with bleeding may increase the risk of bleeding.

be slowly decreased and discontinued because of the psychological and physiologic dependence associated with these medications. Buspirone, a nonbenzodiazepine, does not lead to tolerance or withdrawal and may be useful for relief of acute anxiety. Buspirone should be used cautiously with other serotonin-related medications (such as SSRIs) because of its high affinity for serotonin receptors. If panic disorder is present, it should be treated aggressively with SSRIs and frequently at higher doses.

Pain medication should be prescribed conservatively. If mood disorders are also present, some mood stabilizers not only treat depression but also may treat the pain. An example is gabapentin, another frequently prescribed medication for neuropathic pain experienced during and after herpes zoster (also commonly known as shingles).

Administering and Monitoring Medications

In SSD, patients are usually treated in the community, where they commonly self-medicate. Carefully question patients about self-administered medicine and determine which medicines or substances they are currently using to relieve their pain and/or discomfort (including OTC, herbal supplements, and/or illicit substances). Also listen carefully to determine any side effects the patient attributes to the medication. This information should be documented and reported to the rest of the team. The patient should be encouraged to continue taking only prescribed medication and to seek approval before taking any additional OTC or other prescribed medications. SSD patients are at elevated risk for prescription drug misuse and abuse, as well as for purchasing substances illicitly. The current trends of prescription drug misuse have been linked to opioid use disorder and overdose.

Managing Side Effects

These individuals often have atypical reactions to their medications. Side effects should be assessed, but the patient should be encouraged to compare the benefits of the medication with any issues related to side effects. Patients should also be encouraged to give the medications enough time to be effective because many medications require up to 6 weeks before the patient has a response or experiences a relief of symptoms. This is especially true for patients who are prescribed some of the antidepressants that have been in use the longest, such as fluoxetine.

Management of Complications

In collaborating with patients with SSD, always be on the lookout for drug–drug interactions. Medications these patients take for physical issues could interact with psychiatric medications. Patients may be taking alternative medicines, such as herbal supplements, but they usually willingly disclose doing so. The patient should be encouraged to use the same pharmacy for filling all prescriptions so possible interactions can be checked and monitored.

Spiritual Interventions

For many patients, a discussion about their religious or spiritual beliefs can enhance the therapeutic relationship and support the patient's coping skills. Research shows that patients want to discuss their spiritual beliefs with their provider when patients believe they have a serious illness. Studies suggest that religious or spiritual interventions decrease depression and anxiety and increase spiritual well-being (Henry & Gilley, 2024). Nurses should consider referral to a chaplaincy service that can provide spiritual strategies for coping with health anxiety and somatic discomfort such as meditation, prayer, books, and audiovisual resources.

Psychosocial Interventions

The choice of psychosocial intervention depends on the specific issue the patient is experiencing. The most important and ongoing intervention is the maintenance of a therapeutic relationship.

Therapeutic Interactions

Nursing care should include listening to the patient's report of symptoms and fears, validating it by acknowledging that the fears may be real, asking the patient to monitor symptoms in a journal, and encouraging the patient to bring the journal to the next visit. By reviewing the symptom pattern, it is possible to continue to educate the patient and assess for significant symptoms. The outcome of this approach should be a decrease in fears and better control of the symptoms.

Enhancing Cognitive Functioning

Several interventions are effective in reducing patients' fears of experiencing serious illnesses. CBT, stress management, and group interventions can decrease the intensity and increase the control of symptoms (Sauer et al., 2023). Whether the positive outcomes result from the intervention itself or from the symptom validation and increased attention given to the patient remains unknown.

Counseling

Counseling with a focus on problem-solving is needed from time to time. These patients often have chaotic lives and need support through the multitude of crises. Although they may appear fascinating and at times self-assured, they can easily irritate others because of their constant complaints. The consequences of their impaired social interaction with others must be examined within a counseling framework. It will become evident that the patient's problem-solving and decision-making skills could be improved. Identifying stresses and strengthening positive coping responses help the patient deal with a chaotic lifestyle.

Complementary Therapies

Complementary therapies emphasize collaboration between the patient and the health care team and involve selecting different treatments from different orientations that are best suited for a particular patient. For example, in the treatment of SSD, studies on mindfulness-based cognitive therapy (MBCT) and mindfulness-based stress reduction support the effectiveness of these complementary treatments in reducing the severity and number of physical symptoms (Maas et al., 2023; Zargar et al., 2021) and improving health-related QoL (Wijnen et al., 2023).

CAM therapies include a broad range of techniques that are used alongside traditional treatments (e.g., yoga, relaxation techniques, deep breathing, acupuncture, and expressive therapies such as art, music, dance) that might seem to offer benefits for those with SSRDs. However, there is little if any research on these strategies with patients who have SSRDs and the quality of research on CAM in general is often low (Cutler et al., 2023). Interest in CAM for other somatic disorders and with conditions that have medically unexplained physical symptoms (depression, cancer pain, Parkinson disease, IBS, chronic fatigue syndrome) is increasing, and this may stimulate interest in complementary strategies for those with SSRDs.

Psychoeducation

Nurses provide psychoeducation to those with SSRD as they do those with other mental disorders. Sessions can be held for the individual, family, or community-based groups. For those experiencing medically unexplained symptoms and functional symptoms, utilization costs can be quite high on families and society (Christensen et al., 2023). Psychoeducation suggests a cost-effective option, but the willingness of those with SSRD to engage in group treatment remains to be shown.

Psychoeducation is effective and useful, especially in a busy primary care setting (Johnson et al., 2022). For those who typically refuse psychological services because they feel judged and shamed that no believes they are sick, psychoeducation promotes personal responsibility for health. See Box 33.7.

BOX 33.7

Psychoeducation Checklist: Somatic Symptom Disorder

When caring for a patient with SSD, be sure to include the following topic areas in the teaching plan:

- Psychopharmacologic agents (anxiolytics) if ordered, including drug, action, dosage, frequency, and possible side effects
- Nonpharmacologic pain relief measures
- Education about the physiology of stress and pain pathways in the brain
- Exercise
- Nutrition
- Sleep hygiene
- Social interaction and networking
- Appropriate health care practices
- Problem-solving
- Relaxation, mindfulness, and anxiety-reduction techniques
- Sexual functioning

Teaching About Symptoms

These patients have many questions about illnesses, symptoms, and treatments. Emphasize positive health care practices and minimize the effects of serious illness. Focus on helping the patient understand the relationship between stress and physical symptoms and establishing a daily routine that includes healthy behaviors around rest, nutrition, and activities. Since living with chronic diseases requires self-efficacy, a major barrier is low-health literacy in patients from diverse cultural and ethnic backgrounds. Nurses should demonstrate cultural humility as they include interventions to boost these patients' health literacy (Mariman et al., 2023). Simple strategies like using plain language, encouraging questions, providing access to patient portals, or suggesting mobile apps to collect health data, provide general health information, or assist with life-style change might be helpful and provide some assurance to health concerned individuals. Because of issues in managing medications and treatment, the therapeutic regimen needs monitoring, resulting in many opportunities for teaching.

A qualitative study queried nurses to see if they would accept the responsibility entailed in a "psychosomatic consultation," which basically charges the nurse with the responsibility of screening and educating patients about somatization and improving bodily awareness. The nurses in this qualitative study found such consultation to be acceptable and within the scope of their practice (Braunschneider et al., 2023). Although it would be helpful to have better resources and materials, training, and proper supervision, the idea of nurses engaging in screening and teaching about somatization is very much in keeping with the holistic framework espoused by all professional nurses.

Wellness Strategies

Wellness strategies should be included in the discussion of the interventions. The same interventions that were discussed in reducing the symptoms of SSD are also used as wellness strategies. Patients with SSD should focus on "staying healthy" instead of focusing on their illnesses. For these individuals, approaching the topic of health promotion usually must be within the context of preventing further issues. Setting aside time for themselves and identifying activities that meet their psychological and spiritual needs, such as going to church or synagogue, are important in maintaining a healthy balance.

Social Relationships

Patients with SSD are usually isolated from their families and communities. Strengthening social relationships and activities often becomes the focus of nursing care. The nurse should help the patient identify individuals with whom contact is desired, ask for a commitment to contact them, and encourage them to reinitiate the relationship. The nurse should counsel patients about talking too much about their symptoms with these individuals and emphasize that medical information should be shared with the nurse instead. The nurse must also ensure that patients know when their next appointments are scheduled.

Providing Family Education

The results of a family assessment often reveal that families of these individuals need education about the disorder, helpful strategies for dealing with the multiple complaints of the patient, and usually help in developing more effective communication patterns. Because of the chaotic nature of some of the families and the lack of healthy problem-solving, physical, sexual, and psychological abuse may be evident. It is important to be particularly sensitive to any evidence of current physical or sexual abuse because this may lead to a need for additional interventions.

Promoting Safety

Individuals with SSD can benefit from a crisis safety plan that could be used during times of stress or depression. The safety plan would list triggers for anxiety, suicidal ideation, and mood changes with specific behavioral strategies for each trigger. See Chapters 10 and 25.

Group Interventions

Although these patients may not be candidates for insight group psychotherapy, they do benefit from cognitive-behavioral groups that focus on developing coping skills for everyday life (Jongsma et al., 2023). Participation in groups that address feminist issues should be encouraged because such participation should strengthen patients' assertiveness skills and improve their generally low self-esteem.

When leading a group that has members with this disorder, redirection can keep the group from giving too much attention to an individual's illness. However, these individuals need reassurance and support while in a group. They may say that they do not fit in or belong in the group. In reality, they are feeling insecure and threatened by the situation. The group leader needs to show patience and understanding to engage the individual effectively in meaningful group interaction.

Evaluation of Patient Outcomes

Recovery outcomes for patients with SSD should be realistic. Because this is a lifelong disorder, small successes should be expected. Specific outcomes should be identified, such as gradually increasing social contact. Over time, a gradual reduction in the number of health care providers the individual contacts should occur and a slight improvement in the ability to cope with stresses should follow.

Continuum of Care

Emergency Care

The emergencies these individuals experience may be physical (e.g., chest pain, back pain, gastrointestinal symptoms) or stress responses related to a psychosocial crisis. Occasionally, these individuals become suicidal and require an intensive level of care. Generally speaking, nonpharmacologic interventions should be tried first, with very conservative use of antianxiety medications. All attempts should be made to retrieve records from other facilities.

Inpatient Care

Ideally, individuals with SSD spend minimal time in the hospital for treatment of their medical or comorbid mental disorders. While an inpatient, the patient should have consistency in providers who care or oversee all nursing care. Therapeutic interactions and relationships are especially important and can help move the individual toward recovery.

Community Care

Patients with SSD can spend a lifetime in the health care system and still have little continuity of care. Switching from one health care provider to others is detrimental to their long-term care. Most are outpatients. When they are hospitalized, it is usually for evaluation of medical issues or to receive care for comorbid disorders.

Virtual Mental Health Care

Digital applications provide immediate access to self-health programs such as relaxation, stress reduction, sleep, and imagery. Using these tools can reduce the intensity of distress and discomfort. Virtual primary care visits and health education sessions provide opportunities for patient–clinician interactions within a safe environment.

Integration With Primary Care

Primary care is the main treatment setting for people with SSD. Except in case of severe depression or comorbid mental health disorder, mental health specialists serve primarily as supportive consultants to primary care clinicians. The role of the mental health clinician is to validate the diagnosis to avoid unnecessary treatments. SSD will most likely be diagnosed if the primary care provider is aware of the patient medical and social history, recognizes a discrepancy between the symptoms presented by the patient and objective findings, and has concerns that the patient's thoughts or behaviors are hindering their recovery (Tuttle et al., 2024).

Health education in a familiar environment can help protect the patient from unnecessary procedures and use of resources. Education can improve perceptions of pain, views of health, and decrease feelings of loneliness (Johnson et al., 2022).

OTHER RELATED DISORDERS

ILLNESS ANXIETY DISORDER

Illness anxiety disorder (IAD) was a new classification in the *DSM-5*, a previous version of the *DSM-5-TR* (2022). Previously, the term **hypochondriasis** (or hypochondria) was used to designate this disorder. Most of the people with hypochondriasis were also diagnosed with SSD. However, there are some individuals who either do not have somatic symptoms or have only very mild symptoms, but who remain preoccupied with having or developing a medical illness (APA, 2022). These individuals would receive the diagnosis of IAD and would be encouraged to seek mental health treatment for their anxiety and preoccupation.

Individuals with IAD are fearful about developing a serious illness based on their misinterpretation of body sensations. The fear of having an illness continues despite medical reassurance and interferes with psychosocial functioning. They spend time and money on repeated examinations looking for feared illnesses. For example, an occasional cough or the appearance of a small sore results in the person making an appointment with an oncologist. They may repeatedly check their bodies for signs of illness or spend excessive time researching health information on the internet (French & Hameed, 2023). They are uncomfortable with their body sensations (interoceptive cues) and interpret them as pathologic. Over utilization of health services and help seeking is typical, but some with this disorder avoid contact with medical providers who may confirm their worst fears.

An IAD sometimes appears if the person has had a serious childhood illness or if a family member has a serious illness. Childhood or other traumas, extreme stress, presence of anxiety or depression, and a family history of anxiety disorders increase the risk of IAD. Incessant worrying about health concerns, avoiding situations or others they fear might jeopardize their health, and asking for reassurance causes considerable strain within the family (APA, 2022).

Evidence-Based Nursing Care for People With IAD

Nurses are most likely to care for people with IAD in medical settings. If a diagnosable medical condition is present, expect anxiety and preoccupation with the disorder to be disproportionate to the severity of the illness (APA, 2022). Nursing care for those with IAD is like those with SSD. The goal is to help them manage health anxiety and improve their ability to function and live a typical lifestyle.

FUNCTIONAL NEUROLOGIC SYMPTOM DISORDER (FNSD)

Functional neurologic symptom disorder (FNSD) (previously known as conversion disorder) is a complex condition characterized by sensory, neurologic, and motor symptoms. Typical sensory symptoms include loss of touch, vision difficulties, blindness, deafness, and hallucinations. Neurologic and motor symptoms often include impaired coordination or balance, paralysis, aphonia (i.e., inability to produce sound), difficulty swallowing or a sensation of a lump in the throat, and urinary retention (APA, 2022). In some instances, psychogenic nonepileptic seizures (PNES) occur (Peeling & Muzio, 2023).

Clinical Course

FNSD is usually a long-term disorder with symptoms that suggest an underlying recognizable condition, but laboratory, electroencephalographic, and neurologic test results do not fit standard diagnostic criteria. For example, if the arm is paralyzed and will not move, reflexes and muscle tone may still be present. FNSD symptoms do not follow an expected clinical course but rather change over time with one symptom suddenly appearing and increasing in intensity when attention is given to it. The symptoms interfere with how the person functions and copes in daily life (NINDS, 2024).

Symptoms of FNSD include limb weaknesses, jerks, spasms, speech and swallowing difficulties, dizziness, trouble walking, urinary bladder issues, memory impairment, and blurred vision. One of the most concerning symptoms is **psychogenic nonepileptic seizures** or dissociative seizures. These seizures may look like epileptic seizures but are caused by brain dysfunction (like dissociation) rather than unexpected electrical signaling in the brain (NINDS, 2024). There is typically a prodromal period with autonomic arousal and dissociation. These seizures tend to last longer than 5 minutes (longer than epileptic seizures) and include lateral limb flailing with side-to-side head shaking. Eyes close tightly and resist opening. Afterward the person can recall events during the seizure and may shake, cry, and be distressed by the experience (Stone, 2023). The person may also experience confusion, without shaking, and feel dissociated or somewhat disconnected from thoughts or feelings in the environment (NINDS, 2024).

People with FNSD become frustrated and worried when no one seems to know the diagnosis. If they have seizures, they begin to fear being injured during a seizure and embarrassed by having a seizure in public. They are highly stigmatized because they are often accused of feigning the illness (Stone, 2023).

Diagnostic Criteria

The diagnosis of FNSD remains difficult, costly, and lengthy, creating much frustration and in some cases, causing deterioration (detrimental waiting) as treatment is withheld. Although not clinically specific, some unexpected motor signs (Hoover sign), some sensory signs (pattern inconsistencies), and some unexpected gaits (walk-test) can give clues to the disorder and aid in the diagnosis.

Currently there are discussions over the benefit of using positive rule-in diagnosis (only a few selected, specific tests are administered) rather than traditional differential rule-out diagnosing requiring extensive, exhaustive, and costly testing (Perez et al., 2022). The clinical characteristic for diagnosing this disorder is **Hoover sign**—impairment of voluntary hip extension but expected automatic hip extension during contralateral hip flexion (flexing one hip while extending the hip on the opposite side). Ultimately, beginning rehabilitative treatment is essential to recovery. Although the "rule-in" approach is not universally accepted, the importance of early diagnosis, treatment, and especially education about the condition cannot be delayed.

Epidemiology

FNSD is a common condition that is diagnosed in 5% to 15% of patients seen by neurologists. The incidence is estimated at 4 to 12 per 100,00 per year. It occurs in all age groups but most commonly during puberty and adolescence. Twice as many people assigned female at birth as those assigned male at birth are diagnosed with FNSD. Patients from lower socioeconomic groups and with less education have a higher incidence of this disorder (Peeling & Muzio, 2023; Stone et al., 2024).

Comorbidities

There is evidence of several conditions that are comorbid with FNSD. Fatigue is highly prevalent and reported in 93% of patients with FNSD. **Functional cognitive disorder**, a disorder resulting in significant distress or impact on function that is not explained by another medical condition, is also highly comorbid with FNSD. Other common comorbidities are mental disorders such as mood, anxiety, dissociative, and psychotic disorders; neurodevelopmental disorders (autism spectrum disorder); and neurologic disorders (migraines, epilepsy, Parkinson disease, tics, restless leg syndrome, and traumatic brain injury) (Carle-Toulemonde et al., 2023).

Etiology

Biologic

The exact cause of FNSD is unknown. Some evidence suggests that neurobiologic changes in the brain may be responsible for the loss of sensation or control of movement (Sojka et al., 2022) or that brain circuity dysfunction may be involved in specific symptoms (Peeling & Muzio, 2023). Studies such as these, using advanced structural and functional brain magnetic resonance imaging techniques, are providing evidence that the symptoms are not feigned or made-up.

FNSD may be triggered by injury, pain, or infection. ACEs, stressful events, and psychiatric comorbidities also contribute to the development of this disorder (Stone et al., 2024). Though more study is needed, psychological processes following concussion, such as fear-avoidance, anxious arousal, and symptoms rumination, are involved (Picon, 2021).

Psychodynamic Model

A psychodynamic explanation for FNSD is that **conversion**, an underlying psychological process (defensive mechanism), is responsible for the development of somatic symptom (s) that help decrease anxiety around a repressed conflict. Conversion is no longer widely accepted as an explanation for most cases of FNSD, especially as emotional processing and related psychological constructs (alexithymia, dissociation, threat-avoidance) have become central to our understanding of this disorder.

Cognitive-Behavioral Model

A cognitive-behavioral explanation attributes symptom development to an automatic behavioral and perceptual processing error, in which symptoms stem from previously stored representational memories that are activated during intensive worrying and stress. These memories ultimately generate actual symptoms (Peeling & Muzio, 2023). It is helpful to explain this disorder as being due to an unintentional error in how the brain and nerves communicate with the body. It takes practice to relearn and retrain the connections as individuals get help in psychotherapy to deal with frustration, strong emotions, and issues that are delaying recovery (Nhan & Cheah, 2023).

Recovery-Oriented Care for People With Functional Neurologic Symptom Disorder

The treatment for FNSD is multidisciplinary, involving neurologists, psychiatrists, nurses, and others such as occupational, speech, and physical therapists. Psychotherapists also play a key role in treatment. Comorbidities such as migraines, insomnia, and depression will require medication management. An individualized, biopsychosocial-spiritual approach is needed based upon the patient's symptoms. Education is critical to help the patient understand the disorder and engage in their treatment (Finkelstein et al., 2023).

Evidence-Based Nursing Care for People With FNSD

The nurse can build a strong therapeutic relationship with the patient by acknowledging the symptoms are real and educating the patient about the complexity of the disorder. As trust develops within the nurse–patient relationship, the nurse can help the patient develop problem-solving approaches to everyday issues. See Boxes 33.8 and 33.9. Treatment depends on the type and extent of the functional changes and symptoms the person is experiencing. Promising evidence is accumulating

BOX 33.8

FNSD: Nurse–Patient Consultation Tips in FNSD

- Indicate that the patient's symptoms are real and that you understand how distressing they must be.
- Do **NOT** suggest the symptoms are only psychologically based.
- Give examples of medical diseases (CVA, Parkinson disease, IBS) that can be induced or worsened by stress, and highlight physical manifestations in other disorders (sweating, shaking, palpations) as examples of acute anxiety (mind–body connections).
- Explain how a diagnosis is made and point out differences in the physical exam and history that helped in the differentiation.
- Explain that their symptoms are potentially reversible because although they are not functioning properly, there is no underlying structural damage.
- Emphasize the fact that understanding and accepting the diagnosis of FNSD is essential for proper treatment and full engagement in treatment, and more helpful than focusing on finding out what is wrong.
- Emphasize the importance of continuing to collaborate with the therapist and completing rehabilitation tasks (empathize with their frustration, retraining is hard work!).
- Reach out to the interprofessional team to ensure that there is a cohesive approach in the presentation and treatment of the disorder.

Source: Nhan and Cheah (2023), Peeling and Muzio (2023).

BOX 33.9

Building Clinical Judgment With SBAR: Nurse Communication With Provider Regarding a Patient With FNSD

SBAR

S: Situation

Ruth, an 18-year-old college student, began experiencing cloudy thinking, along with coordination and walking difficulties. Ruth believes it started after experiencing a head injury during soccer practice last month. Ruth was admitted to the neuro-unit and was diagnosed with FNSD. Ruth's mother is upset and concerned today, saying she wants more tests run because "Ruth is stuttering now and she wasn't doing it yesterday."

B: Background

No past or family history of physical or mental or movement disorders. Psychiatric and psychosocial screening on intake were negative. Brain magnetic resonance imaging (MRI) and blood work (complete blood count, basic metabolic panel) were within expected limits. Ruth has met with the psychotherapist. The interprofessional team is being careful not to ascribe or reinforce any unconscious primary or secondary gain to Ruth's condition.

A: Assessment

Except for the onset of speech production difficulties, the patient is in no new distress and her neuro checks and vital signs are stable. The patient's mother is becoming more demanding and asking for more testing to make sure her daughter is "not just faking it." Ruth states she was beginning to accept the diagnosis of FNSD but now she is not so sure. Assurances that the provider would be notified of the new symptom helped relieve some of the mother's anxiety.

Recommendation

- Request consult with family therapist because there is an apparent tension between the mother and daughter that might affect recovery and discharge plans.
- Begin psychoeducation for FNSD, and help patient/family understand how the diagnosis was made.
- Continue offering emotional support and emphasizing our belief in the symptoms and the distress they are causing.
- Help Ruth with emotional regulation and to identify and connect with her feelings, and her physical symptoms, and reinforce any new skills she is learning in therapy or rehabilitation.
- Explore Ruth's interest in learning about mindfulness practice, yoga, or other somatic therapies to improve bodily awareness, and follow up with resources and teaching if Ruth is agreeable.
- Continue to work with the interprofessional treatment team regarding a consistent approach to treatment.

Building Clinical Judgment

1. What continues to make it so difficult for Ruth and her mother to accept a functional diagnosis?
2. What could be the onset of a new symptom (language difficulty) mean when it occurs within FNSD?

for treatments ranging from education and reassurance to extensive rehabilitation to combining approaches with other psychotherapies (Peeling & Muzio, 2023).

This disorder places heavy strains and financial costs on patients, families, and the health care system. Current research supports a biopsychosocial approach to address the needs of families (Vassilopoulos et al., 2022). A multidimensional, holistic approach to caring has prepared nurses to develop and deliver new ways of bridging the mind–body gap, promoting bodily awareness, and practicing somatic therapies (such as emotional self-regulation, mindfulness, and meditation) to promote mental health from their respected positions within the health care system.

FACTITIOUS DISORDERS

Factitious disorders are very different from other SSRDs. People with FDs intentionally cause an illness or injury to receive the attention of health care workers. These individuals are motivated solely by the desire to become a patient and develop a dependent relationship with a health care provider. There are two types of factitious disorders: factitious disorder (FD) and factitious disorder imposed on another (FDIA).

FACTITIOUS DISORDER

Although feigned illnesses have been described for centuries, it was not until 1951 that the term *Münchausen syndrome* was used to describe the most severe form of this disorder, which was characterized by fabricating a physical illness, having recurrent hospitalizations, and going from one health care provider to another. This disorder is now called **factitious disorder** and is differentiated from **malingering**, in which the individual who intentionally produces symptoms of illness and is motivated by another specific self-serving goal, such as being classified as disabled or avoiding work. Malingering is not classified as a mental disorder. There is no research evidence to support the effectiveness of any management strategy for factitious illness, but supported confrontation (involving at least two staff), and nonconfrontational approaches (nuanced, face-saving) are recommended (Carnahan & Jha, 2023).

Clinical Course and Diagnostic Criteria

Unlike people with borderline personality disorder, who typically injure themselves overtly and readily admit to self-harm, patients with FD injure themselves covertly. The illnesses are produced in such a manner that the health care provider is tricked into believing that a true physical or psychiatric disorder is present (Carnahan & Jha, 2023).

The self-produced physical symptoms appear as medical illnesses and involve all body systems. They include seizure disorders, wound-healing disorders, the abscess processes (i.e., introduction of infectious material below the skin surface), and feigned fever (rubbing the thermometer). These patients are extremely creative in simulating illnesses. They tell fascinating but false stories of personal triumph. These tales are referred to as pseudologia fantastica and are a core symptom of the disorder. **Pseudologia fantastica** are stories that are not entirely improbable and often contain a mixture of truth and falsehood. These patients falsify blood, urine, and other samples by contaminating them with protein or fecal matter. They self-inject anticoagulants to receive diagnoses of "bleeding of undetermined origin" or ingest thyroid hormones to produce thyrotoxicosis. They also inflict injury on themselves by inserting objects or feces into body orifices, such as the urinary tract, open wounds, or even intravenous tubing. They produce their own surgical scars, especially abdominal scars, and when treated surgically, they delay wound healing through scratching, rubbing, or manipulating the wound and introducing bacteria into the wound. These patients put themselves in life-threatening situations through actions such as ingesting allergens known to produce an anaphylactic reaction.

Patients who manifest primarily psychological symptoms produce psychotic symptoms such as hallucinations and delusions, cognitive deficits such as memory loss, dissociative symptoms such as amnesia, and conversion symptoms such as pseudoblindness or pseudoparalysis. These individuals often become psychotic, depressed, or suicidal after an unconfirmed tragedy. When questioned about details, they become defensive and uncooperative. Sometimes these individuals have a combination of both physical and psychiatric symptoms.

Epidemiology and Risk Factors

The prevalence of FD is unknown because diagnosing it and obtaining reliable data are difficult. The prevalence was reported to be high when researchers were looking for the disorder in specific populations. Within large general hospitals, FDs are diagnosed in about 1% of patients with whom mental health professionals consult. The age range of patients with the disorder is between 19 and 64 years. The median age of onset is the early 20s. Formerly thought to occur predominantly in people assigned male at birth, this disorder is now reported predominantly in people assigned female at birth. No genetic pattern has been identified, but it does seem to run in families. The presence of comorbid psychiatric disorders, such as mood disorders, personality disorders, and substance-related disorders, is common. Health care professionals, nurses, pharmacists, and physicians are overrepresented in the occurrence of this disorder (Carnahan & Jha, 2023).

Etiology

Many people with FD have experienced severe sexual abuse, trauma, and/or distress before the development of the disorder. The psychodynamic explanation is that these individuals, who were often abused as children, received nurturance only during times of illness; thus, they try to recreate illness or injury in a desperate attempt to receive love and attention. During the actual self-injury, the individual is reported to be in a trancelike, dissociative state. Many patients report having an intimate relationship with a health care provider, either as a child or as an adult, and then experiencing rejection when the relationship ended. The self-injury and subsequent attention are an attempt by the individual to reenact those experiences and gain control over the situation and the other person (Carnahan & Jha, 2023).

These patients are usually discovered in medical-surgical settings. They are hostile and distance themselves from others. Their network is void of friends and family and usually consists only of health care providers, who change at regular intervals. In FD, the patient fabricates a detailed and exaggerated medical history. When the interventions do not work and the fabrication is discovered, the health care team feels manipulated and angry. When the patient is confronted with the evidence, they become enraged and often leave that health care system, only to enter another. Eventually, the person is referred for mental health treatment. The course of the disorder usually consists of intermittent episodes.

EVIDENCE-BASED NURSING CARE FOR PEOPLE WITH FACTITIOUS DISORDER

The overall goal of treatment for a patient with FD is to replace the dysfunctional attention-seeking behaviors with positive behaviors. To begin treatment, the patient must acknowledge the deception. Because the pattern of self-injury is well established and meets overwhelming psychological needs, giving up the behaviors is difficult. The treatment is long-term psychotherapy. The PMH nurse will most likely care for the patient during or after periods of feigned illnesses.

Recognizing Cues: Relevant Assessment Information

A nursing assessment should focus on obtaining a history of medical and psychological illnesses. Physical disabilities should be identified. Early childhood experiences, particularly instances of abuse, neglect, or abandonment, should be identified to understand the underlying psychological dynamics of the individual and the role of self-injury. Family assessment is important because family relationships become strained as the members become aware of the self-inflicted nature of this disorder.

Analyzing Cues and Planning Recovery

The consequences of self-injury are the priority. Medical treatment may be needed. The patient is at elevated risk for self-abuse as discovery unfolds. Any nursing intervention must be implemented within the context of a strong nurse–patient relationship. A nonjudgmental attitude is imperative. Desired outcomes include decreased self-injurious behavior and increased positive coping behaviors.

Taking Action: Nursing Interventions

The fabrications and deceits of patients with FD provoke anger and a sense of betrayal in many nurses. To be effective with these patients, it is important to be aware of these feelings and resolve them by developing a better understanding of the underlying psychodynamic issues. Confronting the patient has been reported to be effective only if the patient feels supported and accepted and if there is clear communication among the patient, the mental health care team, and family members. All care should be centralized within one facility. The patient should see health care providers regularly even when not in active crisis. Offering the patient a tactful way of giving up the behaviors is often crucial. Behavioral techniques that shape new behaviors help the patient move forward toward a new life.

The health care team that knows the patient, agrees on a treatment approach, and follow-up is crucial to the patient's eventual recovery. For this to happen, the medical, psychiatric, inpatient, and outpatient teams need to communicate with each other on a regular basis. Family members must also be aware of the need for consistent treatment.

FACTITIOUS DISORDER IMPOSED ON ANOTHER

Factitious disorder imposed on another (FDIA) (previously *factitious disorder by proxy* or *Münchausen's by proxy*) is a rare disorder that involves an individual who inflicts injury on another person. It is commonly a birthing parent who inflicts injuries on their child to gain the attention of the health care provider through their child's injuries. These actions include inducing seizures, poisoning, or smothering. This most severe form of child abuse is usually identified in the emergency department. The person rarely admits injuring the child and thus is not amenable to treatment; the child is frequently removed from their care. This form of child abuse is distinguished from other forms by the routine unwitting involvement of health care workers, who subject the child to physical harm and emotional distress through tests, procedures, and medication trials. Some researchers suspect that children who are abused in this way may later experience FD themselves (Egge, 2023).

SUMMARY OF KEY POINTS

- Somatization is affected by sociocultural and gender factors. It occurs more frequently in people assigned female at birth than those assigned male at birth and in those who are less educated. It also has been strongly associated with individuals who have been sexually abused as children.
- SSD is a chronic relapsing condition characterized by multiple physical symptoms of unknown origin that develop during times of emotional distress.
- Identifying SSDs is complex because patients with these disorders reject any psychiatric basis to their health issues and often go for years moving from one health care provider to another to receive medical attention and avoid psychiatric assessment.
- Patients with SSD are often seen on the medical-surgical units of hospitals and go years without receiving a correct diagnosis. In most cases, they finally receive mental health treatment for comorbid conditions, such as depression, anxiety, and panic disorder.
- The development of the nurse–patient relationship is crucial to assessing these patients and identifying appropriate interventions. The nurse should use a flexible, relaxed, and nonjudgmental approach that acknowledges the symptoms, educates the patient about the disorder, and helps the patient learn new ways of coping with stress and avoiding recurrence of symptoms.
- Health teaching is important to help the individual develop positive lifestyle changes in place of somatization responses. Identifying personal strengths and supporting the development of positive skills improve self-esteem and personal confidence. Teaching the use of stress management provides the patient with positive coping skills.
- Nurses should be prepared to use complementary somatic therapies in their practices, to promote emotional regulation and increase awareness of body sensations. These strategies are employed to prevent or reduce somatization and to promote patient self-efficacy.
- IAD is characterized by excessive worry about having or developing a serious undiagnosed condition.
- FNSD is a condition of sensory, neurologic, and motor symptoms (e.g., impaired voluntary muscles or sensory stimulation) that are associated with severe emotional distress.
- Factitious disorders include two types, factitious disorder and factitious disorder imposed on another. In factitious disorder, physical or psychological symptoms (or both) are fabricated to assume the sick role. In factitious disorder imposed on another, the intentional production of symptoms is in others, usually children.

DEVELOPING CLINICAL JUDGMENT

1. A young adult who is depressed is admitted to a psychiatric unit in a state of agitation. They report extreme abdominal pain. Their admitting provider tells you that the patient has a classic case of SSD and to deemphasize their physical symptoms. The provider says that under no circumstances can the patient have any more pain medication. Conceptualize the assessment process and how you would approach this patient.
2. A nurse is developing a teaching plan for an individual who has a long history of somatization but who was recently diagnosed with breast cancer. How will the patient be able to differentiate the physical symptoms of somatization from those associated with the treatment of her breast cancer?
3. A patient was admitted for panic attacks and numerous somatic issues, ranging from dysmenorrhea to painful joints. The results of all medical examinations have been negative. They believe their panic attacks are caused by a weak heart. What approaches should the nurse use in providing culturally sensitive nursing care?
4. A nurse wants to take on more responsibilities in addressing somatization and health anxiety with patients/families and the health care team. What competencies would a nurse demonstrate in expanding services to manage and prevent somatization?
5. There may be a time in your nursing career when you suspect factitious disorder, although it is rare. What cues would be considered as evidence, and what action steps would a nurse need to take?

MOVIES, TV, OR STREAMING PROGRAMS

***Sharp Objects:* 2018.** This American psychological thriller is a miniseries based on Gillian Flynn's 2006 novel of the same name. Amy Adams plays the main character, Camille Preaker, a crime reporter who was recently discharged from an alcohol detoxification center and who has experienced years of self-mutilation. Camille returns home to investigate the murder of two young girls. The homecoming brings Camille back in contact with her family, under the cynical view of her mother, the laissez-faire attitude of her father, and her aloof younger sister. As the story unfolds, Camille becomes increasingly troubled as mysteries around the family's past and abuse begin to emerge, drawing everyone into the deceit, tension, and horrible family secrets.

Viewers could analyze many themes around mental disorders in this movie, including posttraumatic stress disorder, dissociative identity, substance use, and anxiety disorders. However, watch this film for evidence of factitious disorder imposed on another (FDIA), and see if you can recognize the mother's strong denial in the face of any accusation or evidence, the father's complicity and willingness to be uninvolved and separate from what is going on in the family, and the extent of both daughters' self-loathing.

Viewing Points:

1. What role does each character play in the dysfunctional family system?
2. How did the mother impose harm on Amma (the younger daughter)?
3. Did you believe that Camille might have been subjected to similar treatment?
4. What other errors or exaggerations can you detect?
5. Do you think the telling (airing) of this story has helped or hindered professionals who may ultimately collaborate with individuals with factitious disorder imposed on another (FDIA)?

REFERENCES

American Nurses Association [ANA]. (2022). The nurse's role and responsibility in unveiling and dismantling racism in nursing. *ANA Position Statement*, www.nursingworld.org

American Psychiatric Association [APA]. (2022). *Diagnostic and statistical manual of mental disorders, (5th ed., text rev.)*. Author.

American Psychiatric Association [APA]. (2024). *What is somatic symptom disorder?* https://www.psychiatry.org/patients-families/somatic-symptom-disorder/what-is-somatic-symptom-disorder

Barak, S., Landa, J., Gerner, M., Eisenstein, E., Bardach, A. C., & Silberg, T. (2023). A behavioral characteristics observational measure of youth with somatic symptom disorder during physical rehabilitation. *Life, 13*(10), 2078. https://doi.org/10.3390/life13102078

Barbek, R. M. E., Makowski, A. C., & von dem Knesebeck, O. (2022). Social inequalities in health anxiety: A systematic review and meta-analysis. *Journal of Psychosomatic Research, 153*, 110706. https://doi.org/10.1016/j.jpsychores.2021.110706

Belleza, M. (2021). Somatoform disorders Nursing care management. *Nurselabs*. https://nurseslabs.com/somatoform-disorders/

Berens, S., Ehrenthal, J. C., & Tesarz, J. (2023). Commentary: The framework for systematic reviews on psychological risk factors for persistent somatic symptoms and related syndromes and disorders (PSY-PSS). *Frontiers in Psychiatry, 14*, 1270497. https://doi.org/10.3389/fpsyt.2023.1270497

Braunschneider, L. E., Seiderer, J., Loeper, S., Löwe, B., & Kohlmann, S. (2023). Nurses' experiences of a screening and associated psychosomatic consultation service for mental comorbidities in somatic care inpatients—a qualitative study. *Frontiers in Psychiatry, 14*, 1148142. https://doi.org/10.3389/fpsyt.2023.1148142

Carle-Toulemonde, G., Goutte, J., Do-Quang-Cantagrel, N., Mouchabac, S., Joly, C., & Garcin, B. (2023). Overall comorbidities in functional neurological disorder: A narrative review. *L'Encephale, 49*(4S), S24–S32. https://doi.org/10.1016/j.encep.2023.06.004

Carnahan, K. T., & Jha, A. (2023). Factitious Disorder. In *StatPearls*. StatPearls Publishing. (nih.gov).

Cassiday, K. L. (2022). *Freedom from health anxiety: Understand and overcome obsessive worry about your health or someone else's and find peace of mind.* New Harbinger Publications, Inc.

Centers for Disease Control and Prevention (CDC). (2024). Essentials for childhood: Creating safe, stable, nurturing relationships and environments for all children. https://www.cdc.gov/child-abuse-neglect/php/public-health-strategy/index.html.

Challa, S. A., Graziano, R., Strasshofer, D. R., White, K. S., Sayuk, G. S., & Bruce, S. E. (2022). Perceived sleep quality mediates the relationship between posttraumatic stress and somatic symptoms. *Psychological Trauma: Theory, Research, Practice and Policy, 14*(7), 1080–1088. https://doi.org/10.1037/tra0000561

Christensen, O. R., Hedegaard, L., Rask, M. T., Clemensen, J., Frostholm, L., & Rosendal, M. (2023). Designing and developing an eHealth program for patients with persistent physical symptoms: Usability study. *JMIR Human Factors, 10*, e42572. https://doi.org/10.2196/42572

Cutler, J. B. R., Pane, O., Panesar, S. K., Updike, W., & Moore, T. R. (2023). Treatment of mood and depressive disorders with complementary and alternative medicine: Efficacy review. *Journal of Midwifery & Women's Health*, 68(4), 421–429. https://doi.org/10.1111/jmwh.13527

D'Souza, R. S., & Hooten, W. M. (2023). Somatic syndrome disorders. In *StatPearls*. StatPearls Publishing. https://www.ncbi.nlm.nih.gov/books/NBK532253/

Egge, M. K. (2023). Medical child abuse: A review by subspecialty. *Advances in Pediatrics, 70*(1), 59–80. https://doi.org/10.1016/j.yapd.2023.03.005

Eilers, H., Aan Het Rot, M., & Jeronimus, B. F. (2023). Childhood trauma and adult somatic symptoms. *Journal of Psychosomatic Medicine, 85*(5), 408–416. https://doi.org/10.1097/PSY.0000000000001208

Fernandez, A., Askenazy, F., Zeghari, R., Auby, P., Robert, P., Thümmler, S., & Gindt, M. (2024). Somatic and posttraumatic stress symptoms in children and adolescents in France. *JAMA Network Open, 7*(4), e247193. https://doi.org/10.1001/jamanetworkopen.2024.7193

Finkelstein, S. A., Carson, A., Edwards, M. J., Kozlowska, K., Lidstone, S. C., Perez, D. L., Polich, G., Stone, J., & Aybek, S. (2023). Setting up functional neurological disorder treatment services: Questions and answers. *Neurologic Clinics, 41*(4), 729–743. https://doi.org/10.1016/j.ncl.2023.04.002

Fox, A. B., & Earnshaw, V. A. (2023). The relationship between mental illness stigma and self-labeling. *Psychiatric Rehabilitation Journal, 46*(2), 127–136. https://doi.org/10.1037/prj0000552

French, J. H., & Hameed, S. (2023). Illness anxiety disorder. In *StatPearls*. (nih.gov).

Gibson, R. C., Lowe, G., Lipps, G., Jules, M. A., Romero-Acosta, K., & Daley, A. (2024). Somatic and depressive symptoms among children from Latin America and the English-speaking Caribbean. *Clinical Child Psychology and Psychiatry, 29*(2), 439–452. https://doi.org/10.1177/13591045231178890

Greenman, P. S., Renzi, A., Monaco, S., Luciani, F., & Di Trani, M. (2024). How does trauma make you sick? The role of attachment in explaining somatic symptoms of survivors of childhood trauma. *Healthcare, 12*(2), 203. https://doi.org/10.3390/healthcare12020203

Henry, N. L., & Gilley, N. (2024). Spiritual Assessment. In *StatPearls*. StatPearls Publishing. https://www.ncbi.nlm.nih.gov/books/NBK599554/

Jacobsen, S. A., Frostholm, L., Buhmann, C. B., Petersen, M. W., Ørnbøl, E., Dantoft, T. M., Bjerregaard, A. A., Eplov, L. F., & Carstensen, T. B. W. (2023). Are sexual assaults related to functional somatic disorders? A cross-sectional study. *International Journal of Environmental Research and Public Health, 20*(20), 6947. https://doi.org/10.3390/ijerph20206947

Johnson, K. K., Bennett, C., & Rochani, H. (2022). Significant improvement of somatic symptom disorder with brief psychoeducational intervention by PMHNP in primary care. *Journal of the American Psychiatric Nurses Association, 28*(2), 171–180. https://doi.org/10.1177/1078390320960524

Jones, E. A., Asaad, F., Patel, N., Jain, E., & Abd-Elsayed, A. (2024). Management of fibromyalgia: An update. *Biomedicines, 12*(6), 1266. https://doi.org/10.3390/biomedicines12061266

Jongsma, K., Darboh, B. S., Davis, S., & MacKillop, E. (2023). A cognitive behavioural group treatment for somatic symptom disorder: A pilot study. *BMC Psychiatry, 23*(1), 896. https://doi.org/10.1186/s12888-023-05141-9

Kingsbury, M., Hammond, N. G., Johnstone, F., & Colman, I. (2022). Suicidality among sexual minority and transgender adolescents: A nationally representative population-based study of youth in Canada. *CMAJ: Canadian Medical Association Journal. 194*(22), E767–E774. https://doi.org/10.1503/cmaj.212054

Kleinstäuber, M., Schröder, A., Daehler, S., Pallesen, K. J., Rask, C. U., Sanyer, M., Van den Bergh, O., Weinreich Petersen, M., & Rosmalen, J. G. M. (2023). Aetiological understanding of fibromyalgia, irritable bowel syndrome, chronic fatigue syndrome and classificatory analogues: A systematic umbrella review. *Clinical Psychology in Europe, 5*(3), e11179. https://doi.org/10.32872/cpe.11179

Kundu, K., Joshi, T., & Gupta, R. (2022). Somatic symptom disorder and sleep. In R. Gupta, D. N. Neubauer, & S. R. Pandi-Perumal (Eds.), *Sleep and neuropsychiatric disorders*. Springer. https://doi.org/10.1007/978-981-16-0123-1_23

Landa-Blanco, M., Vásquez, G., Portillo, G., Sproviero, F., & Echenique, Y. (2024). The impact of adverse childhood experiences on mental health, sexual risk behaviors, and alcohol consumption in adulthood. *Frontiers in Psychiatry, 15*, 1352824. https://doi.org/10.3389/fpsyt.2024.1352824

LoBrutto, L. R., Keeley, J. W., & Dautovich, N. D. (2024). Applying the somatic symptom disorder diagnosis to individuals with fibromyalgia: Strengths and limitations. *Journal of Clinical Psychology in Medical Settings, 31*(3), 607–613. https://doi.org/10.1007/s10880-024-10005-9

Löwe, B., Toussaint, A., Rosmalen, J. G. M., Huang, W. L., Burton, C., Weigel, A., Levenson, J. L., & Henningsen, P. (2024). Persistent physical symptoms: Definition, genesis, and management. *Lancet, 403*(10444), 2649–2662. https://doi.org/10.1016/S0140-6736(24)00623-8

Maas Genannt Bermpohl, F., Hülsmann, L., & Martin, A. (2023). Efficacy of mindfulness- and acceptance-based cognitive-behavioral therapies for bodily distress in adults: A meta-analysis. *Frontiers in Psychiatry*, *14*, 1160908. https://doi.org/10.3389/fpsyt.2023.1160908

Mariman, A., Vermeir, P., Csabai, M., Weiland, A., Stegers-Jager, K., Vermeir, R., & Vogelaers, D. (2023). Education on medically unexplained symptoms: A systematic review with a focus on cultural diversity and migrants. *European Journal of Medical Research*, *28*(1), 145. https://doi.org/10.1186/s40001-023-01105-7

National Institute of Neurological Disorders and Stroke [NINDS]. (2024). *Functional neurologic disorder*. https://www.ninds.nih.gov/health-information/disorders/functional-neurologic-disorder

Nhan, P., & Cheah, V. (2023). *Functional neurological disorder (FND) learning guide*. Mater Centre for Neurosciences. https://fndaustralia.com.au/resources/FND-Learning-guide-for-nurses.pdf

Nicholas, J., & Bresin, K. (2024). Everyday sexual and gender minority stress and health: A systematic review of experience sampling studies. *Archives of Sexual Behavior*, *53*(4), 1221–1243. https://doi.org/10.1007/s10508-023-02779-0

Orzechowska, A., Maruszewska, P., Gałecka, M., Hyland, P., Boduszek, D., Gałecki, P., & Bliźniewska-Kowalska, K. (2023). Emotional control in selected somatic and psychiatric diseases. *BMC Psychiatry*, *23*(1), 802. https://doi.org/10.1186/s12888-023-05321-7

Pasta, A., Formisano, E., Calabrese, F., Plaz Torres, M. C., Bodini, G., Marabotto, E., Pisciotta, L., Giannini, E. G., & Furnari, M. (2024). Food intolerances, food allergies and IBS: Lights and shadows. *Nutrients*, *16*(2), 265. https://doi.org/10.3390/nu16020265

Patel, N., & Shackelford, K. B. (2022). Irritable Bowel Syndrome. In *StatPearls*. StatPearls Publishing. (nih.gov).

Peeling, J. L., & Muzio, M. R. (2023). Functional Neurologic Disorder. In *StatPearls*. StatPearls Publishing. https://www.ncbi.nlm.nih.gov/books/NBK551567/?report=printable

Perez, D. L., Edwards, M. J., Nielsen, G., Kozlowska, K., Hallett, M., & LaFrance, W. C. (2022). A decade of progress in motor functional neurological disorder: Continuing the momentum *Journal of Neurology Neurosurgical Psychiatry*, *92*(6), 558–677. https://jnnp.bmj.com/content/92/6/668

Picon, E. L, Perez, D. L., Burke, M. J., Debert, C. T., Iverson, G. L., Panenka, W. J., & Silverberg, N. D. (2021). Unexpected symptoms after concussion: Potential links to functional neurological and somatic symptom disorders. *Journal of Psychosomatic Research*, *151*, 110661. https://www.sciencedirect.com/science/article/pii/S0022399921003068

Pinto, R. J., de Castro, M. V., Correia-Santos, P., Jongenelen, I., Maia, Â. C., & Levendosky, A. (2023). The mediating role of posttraumatic stress symptoms on somatization in adolescents: A two-wave longitudinal study. *Psychological Trauma: Theory, Research, Practice and Policy*, *15*(Suppl 1), S47–S54.

Prospero, L., Riezzo, G., Linsalata, M., Orglando, A., D'Attoma, B., Di Masi, M., Martulli, M., & Russo, F. (2021). Somatization in patients with predominant diarrhoea irritable bowel syndrome: The role of the intestinal barrier function and integrity. *BMC Gastroenterology*, *21*(1), 235. https://doi.org/10.1186/s12876-021-01820-7

Robert, S. J., & Kadhiravan, S. (2022). Prevalence of digital amnesia, somatic symptoms and sleep disorders among youth during COVID-19 pandemic. *Heliyon*, *8*(8), e10026. https://doi.org/10.1016/j.heliyon.2022.e10026

Roelf, K., Khare, M., Rungvivatjarus, T., Mannino Avila, E., Lenzen, C., Patel, A., Fisher, E. S., & Camera, M. (2025). Characteristics and resource utilization of hospitalized children with somatic symptoms. *Hospital Pediatrics*, *15*(1), 66–73. https://doi.org/10.1542/hpeds.2024-007847

Sauer, K. S., Witthöft, M., & Rief, W. (2023). Somatic symptom disorder and health anxiety: assessment and management. *Neurologic Clinics*, *41*(4), 745–758. https://doi.org/10.1016/j.ncl.2023.02.009

Schrijvers, K., Cosma, A., Potrebny, T., Thorsteinsson, E., Catunda, C., Reiss, F., Hulbert, S., Kostičová, M., Melkumova, M., Bersia, M., Klanšček, H. J., Gaspar, T., & Dierckens, M. (2024). Three decades of adolescent health: Unveiling global trends across 41 countries in psychological and somatic complaints (1994–2022). *International Journal of Public Health*, *69*, 1607774. https://doi.org/10.3389/ijph.2024.1607774

Seiffge-Krenke, I., & Sattel, H. (2024). How personality factors, coping with identity-stress, and parental rearing styles contribute to the expression of somatic complaints in emerging adults in seven countries. *Frontiers in Psychiatry*, *15*, 1257403. https://doi.org/10.3389/fpsyt.2024.1257403

Sejdiu, A., Jaka, S., Younis, H., Kidambi, N. S., Faruki, F., Patel, R. S., & Gunturu, S. (2023). Psychiatric comorbidities and risk of somatic symptom disorders in posttraumatic stress disorder: A cross-sectional inpatient study. *The Journal of Nervous and Mental Disease*, *211*(7), 510–513. https://doi.org/10.1097/NMD.0000000000001639

Shu, W., Ma, X., & Zhao, X. (2023). Changes in patient discourse: A qualitative study based on the treatment experience of Chinese patients with somatization symptoms. *Healthcare 11*(21), 2811. https://doi.org/10.3390/healthcare11212811

Snowden, L. R., Cordell, K., & Bui, J. (2023). Racial and ethnic disparities in health status and community functioning among persons with untreated mental illness. *Journal of Racial and Ethnic Health Disparities*, *10*(5), 2175–2184. https://doi.org/10.1007/s40615-022-01397-1

Sojka, P., Paredes-Echeverri, S., & Perez, D. L. (2022). Are functional (psychogenic nonepileptic) seizures the sole expression of psychological processes? *Current Topics in Behavioral Neurosciences*, *55*, 329–351. https://doi.org/10.1007/7854_2021_225

Stone, J. (2023). *Neurosymptoms FND Guide*. http://www.neurosymptoms.org/

Stone, J., Hoeritzauer, I., McWhirter, L., & Carson, A. (2024). Functional neurological disorder: Defying dualism. *World Psychiatry*, *23*(1), 53–54. https://doi.org/10.1002/wps.21151

Torres, M. E., Löwe, B., Schmitz, S., Pienta, J. N., Van Der Feltz-Cornelis, C., & Fiedorowicz, J. G. (2021). Suicide and suicidality in somatic symptom and related disorders: A systematic review. *Journal of Psychosomatic Research*, *140*, 110290. https://doi.org/10.1016/j.jpsychores.2020.110290

Trindade, I. A., Hreinsson, J. P., Melchior, C., Algera, J. P., Colomier, E., Törnblom, H., Drossman, D., Tack, J., Palsson, O. S., Bangdiwala, S. I., Sperber, A. D., & Simrén, M. (2024). Global prevalence of psychological distress and comorbidity with disorders of gut-brain interactions. *The American Journal of Gastroenterology*, *119*(1), 165–175. https://doi.org/10.14309/ajg.0000000000002500

Tu, C. Y., Liao, S. C., Wu, C. S., Chiu, Y. T., & Huang, W. L. (2024). Association of categorical diagnoses and psychopathologies with quality of life in patients with depression, anxiety, and somatic symptoms: A cross-sectional study. *Journal of Psychosomatic Research*, *182*, 111691. https://doi.org/10.1016/j.jpsychores.2024.111691

Tuttle, M. C., Ciampa, D. J., Godena, E., Kim, B. K., Sakmar, K. A., Vanwort-Meng, L., Verma, D., Stern, T. A., & Yeung, A. S. (2024). The evaluation and treatment of somatic symptom disorder in primary care practices. *The Primary Care Companion for CNS Disorders*, *26*(1), 23f03549. https://doi.org/10.4088/PCC.23f03549

van der Heijden, H., Goldman, M., Ray, A., Golden, E., Petty, C. R., Deaso, E., Hojlo, M., Sethna, N., Glahn, D. C., Gonzalez-Heydrich, J., & Upadhyay, J. (2024). Characterization of pain and somatization and its relationship with psychopathology in early onset psychosis. *Journal of Psychiatric Research*, *179*, 77–82. https://doi.org/10.1016/j.jpsychires.2024.09.006

Vassilopoulos, A., Mohammad, S., Dure, L., Kozlowska, K., & Fobian, A. D. (2022). Treatment approaches for functional neurological disorders in children. *Current Treatment Options in Neurology*, *24*(2), 77–97. https://doi.org/10.1007/s11940-022-00708-5

von Schrottenberg, V., Toussaint, A., Hapfelmeier, A., Teusen, C., Riedl, B., Henningsen, P., Gensichen, J., Schneider, A., & Linde, K. (2024). Lessons learned from applying established cut-off values of questionnaires to detect somatic symptom disorders in primary care: A cross-sectional study. *Frontiers in Psychiatry*, *14*, 1289186. https://doi.org/10.3389/fpsyt.2023.1289186

Wijnen, J., van't Hullenaar, G., Gordon, N. L., Pont, M. L., Geijselaers, M. W. H., Van Oosterwijck, J., & De Jong, J. (2023). An interdisciplinary multimodal integrative healthcare program for somatic symptom disorder, with predominant (spinal) pain. *Psychotherapy Research: Journal of the Society for Psychotherapy Research*, *33*(5), 581–594. https://doi.org/10.1080/10503307.2022.2144528

Winograd, D. M., Hyde, J. K., Bloeser, K., Santos, S. L., Anastasides, N., Petrakis, B. A., Pigeon, W. R., Litke, D. R., Helmer, D. A., & McAndrew, L. M. (2023). Exploring the acceptability of behavioral interventions for veterans with persistent "medically unexplained" physical symptoms. *Journal of Psychosomatic Research*, *167*, 111193. https://doi.org/10.1016/j.jpsychores.2023.111193

Wu, Y., Tao, Z., Qiao, Y., Chai, Y., Liu, Q., Lu, Q., Zhou, H., Li, S., Mao, J., Jiang, M., & Pu, J. (2022). Prevalence and characteristics of somatic symptom disorder in the elderly in a community-based population: a large-scale cross-sectional study in China. *BMC Psychiatry*, *22*(1), 257. https://doi.org/10.1186/s12888-022-03907-1

Zargar, F., Rahafrouz, L., & Tarrahi, M. J. (2021). Effect of mindfulness-based stress reduction program on psychological symptoms, quality of life, and symptom severity in patients with somatic symptom disorder. *Advanced Biomedical Research*, *10*, 9. https://doi.org/10.4103/abr.abr_111_19

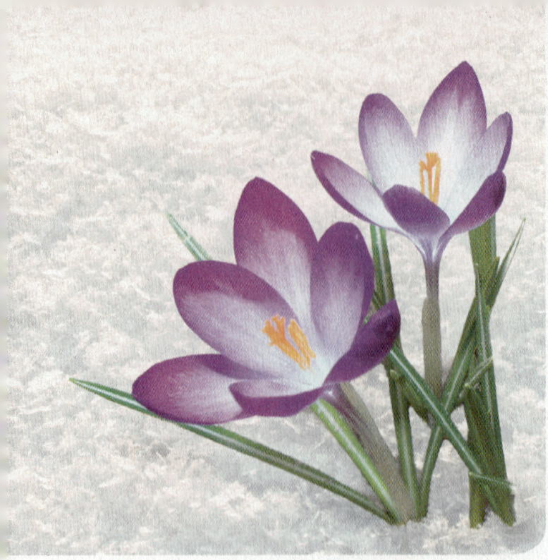

34
Sleep–Wake Disorders
Nursing Care of People With Insomnia and Sleep Disorders*

Sheri Compton-McBride

KEYCONCEPT

- insomnia
- rhythm
- sleep
- sleep–wake cycle

LEARNING OBJECTIVES

After studying this chapter, you will be able to:

1. Examine the role of the sleep–wake cycle in insomnia disorder.
2. Relate the primary theories of insomnia disorder to clinical symptoms and the course of the disorder.
3. Evaluate the significance of trauma in the appearance of insomnia disorder.
4. Examine the relationship between social determinants of health and insomnia disorder.
5. Select strategies to establish a therapeutic relationship with people with insomnia disorder.
6. Using a clinical judgment model, formulate a person-centered, recovery-oriented nursing plan for people with insomnia disorder.
7. Identify medications used to treat people with insomnia disorder and evaluate their effectiveness.
8. Develop wellness strategies for people with insomnia disorder.
9. Compare and contrast mental health care provided in emergency, inpatient, community, and virtual settings.
10. Support the integration of health care and mental health care for people with insomnia disorder.
11. Compare and contrast other sleep–wake-related disorders.

KEY TERMS

• benzodiazepine receptor agonists (BzRA) • benzodiazepines • cataplexy • chronic insomnia • chronotherapy • circadian rhythm • circadian rhythm sleep disorder • cognitive-behavioral therapy for insomnia (CBT-I) • continuous positive airway pressure (CPAP) • hypersomnolence disorder • hypocretins • hypnagogic hallucinations • imagery rehearsal therapy • insomnia disorder • luminotherapy • melatonin • multiple sleep latency test (MSLT) • narcolepsy • nightmare disorder • nonbenzodiazepines • non–rapid eye movement (NREM) • obstructive sleep apnea (OSA) syndrome • orexins • parasomnias • polysomnography • ramelteon • rapid eye movement (REM) sleep • relaxation training • restless legs syndrome (RLS) • short-term insomnia • sleep architecture • sleep debt • sleep diary • sleep efficiency • sleep health • sleep homeostasis • sleep hygiene • sleep latency • sleep paralysis • sleep restriction • sleep terrors • sleep–wake disorders • slow-wave sleep • somnambulism • stimulus control • suprachiasmatic nucleus • suvorexant • uvulopalatopharyngoplasty • valerian

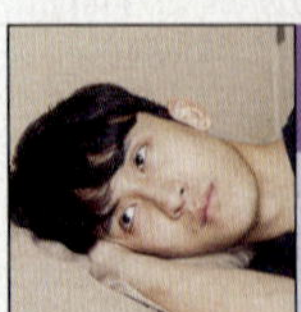

Case Study: Michael

Michael is a 20-year-old student who is majoring in nursing. He presents himself at Student Health Services with a complaint of insomnia. In assessing his issue, the nurse ascertains that he falls asleep 2 to 3 hours after turning the lights out.

**In this chapter, "male" refers to an individual assigned male at birth, and "female" refers to an individual assigned female at birth.*

INTRODUCTION

Sleep is a recurrent, altered state of consciousness that occupies nearly one third of our lives and occurs for sustained periods. Unlike a coma, sleep can be disrupted quite easily. Sleep is usually preceded by a period of sleepiness or the urge to fall asleep.

> **KEYCONCEPT Sleep,** which is necessary for human survival, is a state of decreased awareness of environmental stimuli and a relative state of unconsciousness with no memory of the state.

Sleep is important to our development, functioning, and health. Sleep has identifiable cycles and a variety of cognitive experiences, ranging from memory recall to feeling energetic. The consequences of disturbed sleep include impaired alertness and performance. Decades of research reveal sleep's critical role in optimizing biologic functions across the body, from genes to behavior. Biologic, environmental, and social factors collectively influence various dimensions of sleep, impacting health outcomes and functional aspects like alertness, satisfaction, and interpersonal relationships.

This chapter presents a discussion of typical sleep rhythms and patterns, sleep–wake disorders, and nursing care for people with sleep issues. Insomnia disorder is highlighted.

SLEEP AND WELLNESS

Adequate sleep is a critical aspect of wellness. **Sleep health** is a term that refers to the quality and quantity of sleep and includes the following concepts:

- adequate sleep duration (7 to 9 hours of sleep for adults)
- sleep continuity (easily falling asleep and staying asleep)
- sleep timing (getting enough sleep at the right time)
- alertness (feeling refreshed and alert during the day)
- sleep satisfaction (satisfied with overall sleep quality) (National Sleep Foundation [NSF], 2024a).

A closely related term is **sleep hygiene,** which describes healthy sleep habits and includes both the sleep environment and behavior. Good sleep hygiene includes setting a sleep schedule and sticking to it, following a bedtime routine, and optimizing the bedroom for sleep, such as darkening the bedroom, keeping the bedroom cool, and eliminating extraneous noise. Sleep hygiene also includes dietary modifications to reduce foods and nighttime behaviors that interfere with sleep and exercise (De Pasquale et al., 2024).

Sleeping less than the recommended 7 hours per night is associated with obesity, diabetes, high blood pressure, coronary heart disease, stroke, immune disorders, impaired reproductive health, and mental distress (Gale et al., 2024; Ma et al., 2024; Weng et al., 2024). More than one third of Americans report sleeping less than 7 hours per night (NSF, 2021), with the average sleep duration of US adults being between 6 and 6.5 hours, from a high of 8.5 hours in 1960. Sleepiness has been linked to catastrophic disasters, such as the Exxon Valdez oil spill, the nuclear meltdown at Chernobyl in Ukraine, the space shuttle *Challenger* accident, and the Three Mile Island disaster in the United States (Mitler et al., 1988; Rajaratnam & Arendt, 2001; Walsh et al., 2011).

Biologic Theories

The biology of sleep appears to involve dopamine, gamma-aminobutyric acid (GABA), adenosine, histamine, hypocretin, melatonin, and cortisol, which play roles in changing sleep states (Falup-Pecurariu et al., 2021; Meyer et al., 2024). Wakefulness is maintained by the reticular activating system in the brain. As the cycle of the reticular activating system dwindles, neurotransmitters that promote sleep take over (see Chapter 7).

Psychosocial Theories

Sleep is also related to psychosocial factors, such as lifestyle, stress, and work- and school-related factors. Underrepresented groups have short sleep duration. Short sleep duration is associated with lower socioeconomic groups and the unemployed. There is evidence that LGBTQ+ individuals experience more sleep issues than the general population and that family support can reduce the risk of sleep disturbances (Chum et al., 2021; Gueye-Ndiaye & Redline, 2024).

Pattern of Sleep

Sleep is a patterned activity and is one component of the biphasic 24-hour sleep–wake cycle.

> **KEYCONCEPT Sleep–wake cycle** is an endogenously generated rhythm close to 24 to 25 hours synchronized with the day–night cycle. The sleep–wake cycle is regulated by circadian rhythms and sleep homeostasis (Cable et al., 2021).

Sleep latency, the amount of time it takes to fall asleep, is measured from "lights out," or bedtime, to initiation of sleep. **Sleep architecture** is the pattern of **non–rapid eye movement** (NREM) and **rapid eye movement** (REM) that are in about a 90- to 110-minute cycle. Sleep occurs in stages, and the timing of sleep is regulated by circadian rhythms. **Sleep efficiency** is the ratio of total sleep time to time in bed.

Circadian Rhythms

> **KEYCONCEPT Rhythm** is movement with a cadence, a measured flow that occurs at regular intervals, with a cycle of coming and going, ebbing and rising, to return at the start point and begin again.

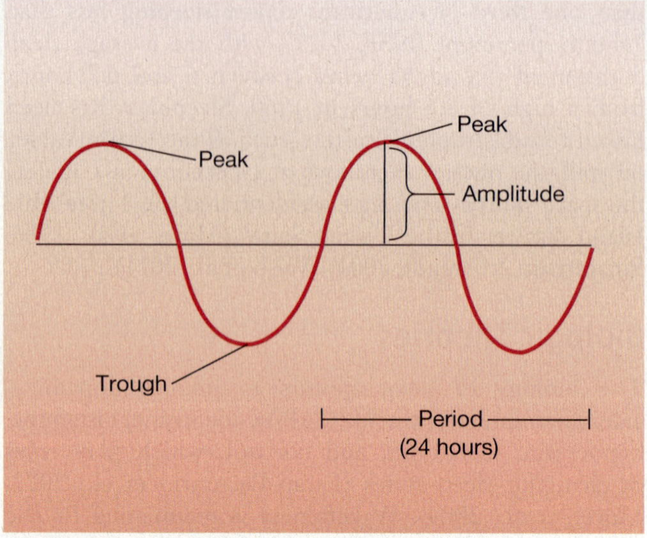

FIGURE 34.1 Circadian rhythms fluctuate in patterns. The peak is the point at which the rhythm reaches its maximum, and the trough is the point at which the rhythm reaches its minimum. The period is the time it takes to complete a cycle. The amplitude is the extent of the peak and is half the distance from peak to trough.

Nearly all physiologic and psychological functions fluctuate in a pattern that repeats itself in a 24-hour cycle, called **circadian rhythms** (Fig. 34.1). The biologic clock that regulates our circadian rhythms is located in the **suprachiasmatic nucleus**, an area of the hypothalamus that lies on top of the optic chiasm. However, it is now recognized that almost all cells and tissues in the body are circadian clocks (Koronowski & Sassone-Corsi, 2021). When two or more rhythms reach their peak at the same time, they are synchronized; if they reach their peak at different times, they are desynchronized.

Most physiologic functions reach their lowest levels during the middle of the sleep period. For example, body temperature follows a predictable pattern from lowest, in the early morning, to highest, in the mid-evening. Manual dexterity, reaction time, and simple recognition appear to coincide with the circadian rhythm of body temperature. Most circadian rhythms continue even when humans are unaware of the time of day. Natural age-related changes in circadian sleep rhythms generally regulate people as they get older, toward morning alertness and productivity and sleepiness at night (Sato et al., 2022).

Sleep Homeostasis

The circadian rhythms are not the only processes that regulate sleep. **Sleep homeostasis** is an internal biochemical system that operates as a timer or counter that generates pressure to sleep and regulates sleep intensity. This process reminds the body to sleep after a certain time. The longer we are awake, the stronger the desire and need for sleep becomes, and the likelihood of falling asleep increases. The longer we sleep, the pressure to sleep decreases and we are more likely to wake (Franken & Dijk, 2024).

Stages of Sleep

Sleep is biphasic, cycling between NREM and REM. During an 8-hour sleep period, the cycle of NREM and REM repeats itself. The duration of the cycles may change as the night progresses. In the first cycle, the amount of REM sleep is brief. With each succeeding cycle, the amount of time spent in REM lengthens. Conversely, NREM is most prominent during the initial cycle but declines as total sleep time progresses (Fig. 34.2).

Non–Rapid Eye Movement Sleep

NREM sleep occurs about 90 minutes after falling asleep and consists of four substages. Light sleep is characteristic of

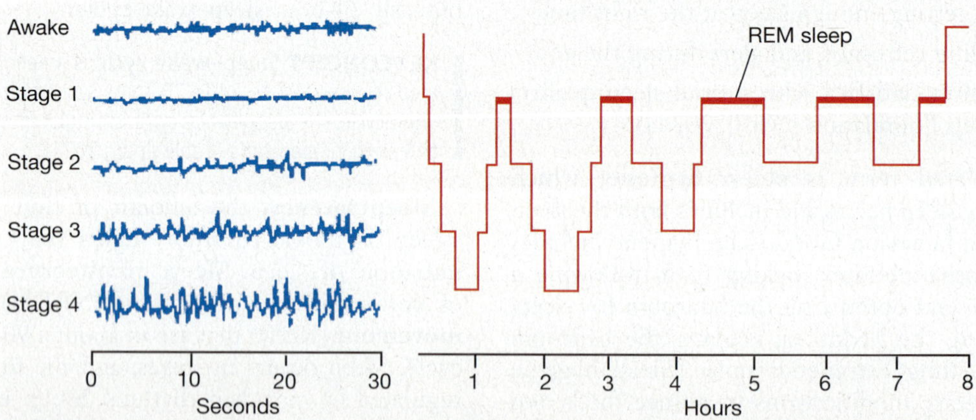

FIGURE 34.2 Brain waves during wakefulness and stages. Brain waves during wakefulness and stages 1, 2, 3, and 4 sleep on the *left* and duration of wakefulness, rapid eye movement (REM), and non–rapid eye movement (NREM) sleep on the *right.* In typical sleep architecture in young adults, NREM and REM sleep stages cycle every 90 to 110 minutes through the night. Wakefulness accounts for less than 5% of the night's sleep pattern. Slow-wave sleep dominates the first third of the night during NREM stages 3 and 4. REM sleep occurs in four to six separate episodes throughout the night (20% to 25% of sleep) and dominates the last third of the night's sleep. (Reprinted with permission from Norris, T. L. [2024]. *Porth's Pathophysiology: Concepts of altered health states* [11th ed.]. Wolters Kluwer.)

stages 1 and 2, in which the individual is easily aroused. An individual aroused from stage 1 sleep may even deny having been asleep, such as dozing while watching television and awakening minutes later during a loud commercial. Stage 1 accounts for only 2% to 5% of a night's sleep and is a transition between relaxed wakefulness and sleep. Stage 2 comprises about 45% to 55% of sleep. During phases 1 and 2, an electroencephalogram (EEG) shows an alpha rhythm gradually being replaced by a theta rhythm. Sleep spindles or "k complexes" occur in stage 2 (see Fig. 34.2).

Slow-wave sleep, or the deepest state of sleep, characterizes stages 3 and 4. Slow-wave sleep is believed to have a restorative function, although the exact mechanism for this is unclear. It may serve to conserve energy because metabolism and body temperature decrease during this part of sleep. These stages make up 10% to 23% of sleep. EEG findings show high-amplitude waves, slow waves, or delta waves. The difference between stages 3 and 4 is the amount of delta waves seen, with stage 3 demonstrating 20% to 50% of delta waves and stage 4 showing more than 50% of delta waves.

Rapid Eye Movement Sleep

REM sleep is a state characterized by bursts of REMs. REM sleep occurs in four to six separate episodes and makes up about 20% to 25% of a night's sleep. Although REM sleep is a deep sleep and muscles seem to be at rest, EEG findings demonstrate an active brain. Brain waves resemble a mixture of wakeful and drowsy patterns. Although vivid dreaming is the outstanding feature reported by adults when awakened out of REM sleep, people also report dreams when they awaken from NREM sleep.

During REM sleep, nerve impulses are blocked within the spinal cord. Muscle tone diminishes to the point of paralysis. Only stronger impulses are relayed, producing muscular twitches, eye movements, and impulses controlling heart rate and respiration. Breathing and heart rate may become irregular.

This type of sleep has a circadian rhythm that closely coincides with the body temperature rhythm. The greatest amount of REM sleep is seen when the body temperature cycle is at its lowest. People do not sweat or shiver during REM sleep because temperature regulation is impaired. Patterns of hormone release, kidney function, and reflexes change. Females have clitoral engorgement and an increase in blood flow to the vagina. Males have penile erections.

Factors Affecting Sleep Pattern and Quality

Sex Assigned at Birth

Sleep issues and poorer-quality sleep are reported more often by females than males. Disturbed sleep and daytime sleepiness have a cumulative effect on mental health (Harris et al., 2024). Females are at greater risk for insomnia and other sleep issues. Sleep in females is influenced by the sex hormones, which vary throughout the life cycle (Gadodia et al., 2023; Lin et al., 2024). Greater than 40% of pregnant people report experiencing insomnia during the third trimester (Salari et al., 2021). Socioeconomic factors contribute to poor sleep quality and daytime sleepiness in American females (Saini et al., 2021). Sleep deprivation and sleep quality in transgender and gender nonconforming adults (TGNC) have been reported and are compounded when TGNC individuals experience sexual victimization (Kolp et al., 2020). TGNC youth face a higher risk of experiencing depression, anxiety, and suicidal thoughts compared to cisgender individuals. This increased prevalence of mental health issues in TGNC youth has been linked to gender identity stigma and discrimination, further heightening their susceptibility to sleep disorders, as evidenced by recent studies involving college students (Gavidia et al., 2022; Leonard et al., 2024).

Age

Sleep patterns change dramatically over the course of the life span. Newborns need 17 to 18 hours of sleep each day, which occurs in 3- to 4-hour episodes throughout the day. By age 6 months, 12 hours of sleep at night and two 1- to 2-hour naps each day are needed. For toddlers (1 to 2 years old), 11 to 14 hours of sleep per 24 hours are recommended, with 1 to 2 hours of daily naps. For preschool (3 to 5 years old), 10 to 13 hours of sleep are recommended, with shortening of nap time. School-aged children (6 to 13 years old) should get 9 to 11 hours of sleep (Suni, 2022).

Preadolescents need about 10 hours of sleep each night, and napping is rare. A teenager's sleep need is only slightly less, at about 9 hours. During young adulthood, about 8 hours of sleep is needed. The amount of sleep required and sleep architecture typically remain unchanged during the middle-aged years. Poor sleep in females is associated with hormonal changes, such as during the menstrual cycle, pregnancy, and menopause.

The need for sleep does not decrease for older adults, but the ability to sustain sleep changes. Older people may spend more time in bed, sleep less, wake more often during the night, and take longer to fall asleep than younger adults. For some, sleep requirements are met by daytime napping. Furthermore, temperature rhythm in older people peaks earlier; early morning arousals may reflect an early rise in body temperature. Older people are at higher risk for sleep disorders (Winegar, 2024). Aging may include alterations in sleep-related hormone secretion, contributing to the multifactorial components that need to be considered when assessing for sleep disturbances (Li et al., 2022).

Environment

Sleep-related issues have multiple factors that make up the clinical picture. Whereas some are external, such as the noise and temperature, others are internal (e.g., stress and pain). An individual can be sleepy but may stay awake if in a stimulating environment with bright lights or a lot of activity. In contrast, a sleepy individual in a quiet place or engaged in sedentary activity cannot resist the urge to fall asleep. Sleepiness is a physiologic state, and although a stimulating environment can temporarily forestall it, when these stimuli are removed, the urge to sleep will persist. Even when someone who is chronically sleep deprived does not feel sleepy, the tendency to fall asleep is much greater and may manifest by causing the individual to doze off while sitting in lectures or during the monotonous operation of machinery or driving.

Lifestyles

Many factors can cause disrupted sleep patterns, such as travel across time zones, stress or anxiety, and changes in the sleep–wake pattern because of shift work. When traveling across time zones or working night shifts (and sleeping during the day), one's regular sleepiness–alertness rhythm may persist for several days (Leso et al., 2021). Even when daytime sleep is improved with a pharmacologic agent, sleepiness in the early morning hours usually continues for the first 2 to 3 nights. This extreme sleepiness often decreases after a 4- to 6-day reversal of the sleep–wake cycle (see Box 34.1).

Changes in Sleep

Sleep is sensitive to changes, and the body responds when deprived of certain phases of sleep, particularly REM sleep and slow-wave sleep. Certain activities, such as early rising, alcohol intake before bedtime, or consumption of certain medications, can suppress REM sleep. One example is the use of central nervous system (CNS)–acting medications. Fragmented sleep interrupts the restorative function of a good night's sleep. Not only does insufficient sleep cause daytime sleepiness, but disturbed sleep also affects daytime alertness and performance. A **sleep debt** occurs when there is recurrent long-term sleep deprivation.

When individuals are deprived of REM sleep, there is a subsequent "rebound effect," wherein the lost REM sleep is made up during the next sleep period. The body makes up for this lost REM sleep by earlier occurrence of REM sleep during the next night. The presence of REM at sleep onset implies REM deprivation.

Slow-wave sleep does not appear to have a circadian determinant, but it is more sensitive to the amount of previous sleep obtained. When one is deprived of both REM and slow-wave sleep, the body prefers to make up for the slow-wave before the REM sleep.

SLEEP–WAKE DISORDERS OVERVIEW

Sleep–wake disorders are diagnosed when an individual is dissatisfied with the quality, timing, and amount of their sleep, which is causing daytime distress and impairment. Sleep issues are more common in females, and prevalence increases with age in both males and females. Sleep–wake disorders occur independently of the diagnosis of other mental disorders, but they are also seen in people with mental disorders. For example, a core feature of posttraumatic stress disorder (PTSD) is sleep disturbance.

An occasional change in sleep pattern becomes a sleep disorder when mental and physical health is compromised as a result of issues in the sleep–wake cycle. Sleep–wake disorders include insomnia, hypersomnolence, and narcolepsy. Other disorders include breathing-related sleep disorders (such as obstructive sleep apnea [OSA]

BOX 34.1

Research for Evidence-Based Practice: Time Off Between Shifts

Holmelid, Ø., Harris, A., Pallesen, S., Bjorvatn, B., Vedaa, Ø., Waage, S., Nielsen, M. B., Djupedal, I. L. R., & Sunde, E. (2024). Acute effects of a simulated quick return on subjective sleepiness, mood, and cognitive performance: A laboratory crossover controlled trial. Chronobiology International, *41(8), 1116–1127. https://doi.org/10.1080/07420528.2024.2380736*

THE QUESTION: What are the acute effects of a quick return (8 hours off vs. 16 hours off) on sleepiness, mood, and cognitive performance in a simulated work day?

METHODS: The study followed a counterbalanced crossover design consisting of two simulated shift schedule conditions with 66 participants. The control condition was two simulated day shifts of 8 hours, 16 hours apart. The quick return condition was an 8-hour simulated evening shift followed by a day shift 8 hours later.

FINDINGS: Scores followed the circadian pattern in both groups with subjective sleepiness scores highest in the beginning of the day shifts and gradually lower as the shifts progressed. The differences between the groups were small, with the quick return group scoring higher sleepiness measures. No significant differences were found with mood and cognitive performance.

IMPLICATIONS FOR NURSING: Many nurses are shift workers, and the amount of rest time between shifts should be considered. Subjective sleepiness could be even higher in real-life context due to an accumulated effect of having multiple quick return shifts.

syndrome and circadian rhythm disorders) and parasomnias. This chapter will highlight insomnia disorder.

INSOMNIA DISORDER

KEYCONCEPT Insomnia, which is Latin for "no sleep," refers to difficulty falling asleep or maintaining sleep when opportunity and circumstances are adequate for sleep. Dissatisfaction with sleep quantity or quality may also be present (Sutton, 2021).

CLINICAL COURSE

Few studies describe the course of insomnia disorder, which can last for short periods in some patients and for decades in others. Since ancient times, providers have noted individuals having difficulty falling asleep, staying asleep, and early morning awakenings. **Short-term insomnia** is described as sleep disturbances present for more than 3 months. In **chronic insomnia**, sleep disturbances occur at least three times a week and have been present for the last 3 months (Kaur et al., 2023).

Individuals with mental illness are at a heightened risk of experiencing poor sleep quality compared to the general population. This subjective sleep impairment may serve as an early indicator of a potential sleep disorder and could signify a deterioration in the individual's overall psychological well-being. Importantly, the combination of poor mental health and poor sleep quality leads to a greater need for health care services, resulting in additional socioeconomic burdens (Corbo et al., 2023).

DIAGNOSTIC CRITERIA

Insomnia disorder is characterized by dissatisfaction with sleep quantity or quality and difficulty initiating or maintaining sleep, or in waking early in the morning, and being unable to return to sleep (Sutton, 2021).

INSOMNIA DISORDER ACROSS THE LIFE SPAN

Children and Adolescents

Sleep issues in children can occur in the presence of attention-deficit hyperactivity disorder (ADHD), epilepsy, and autism spectrum disorder or independently of a neurologic or psychiatric diagnosis (Ohi et al., 2021). Not unlike adults, cognition and emotional regulation are impacted when sleep quality and/or sleep quantity are impacted. Adolescence is a known time of change, and sleep is no exception.

Young adult students undergoing significant life changes associated with their studies—for example, relocation, increased independence, and higher consumption of stimulants—are at elevated risk of developing sleep disorders. Additionally, they often neglect basic sleep hygiene practices, further compromising sleep quality. The combination of late sleep phase preference, prolonged wakefulness, and early morning obligations results in insufficient sleep, particularly prevalent among college students. As concerns about mental health crises among teenagers persist, the 2024 Sleep in America Poll reveals a significant correlation between poor sleep health and depressive symptoms (NSF, 2024b). Insomnia and excessive daytime sleepiness are common conditions worldwide and are closely related, diminishing the quality of life of students (Babicki et al., 2023).

Older Adults

Cognitive impairment, depression, anxiety, and increased risk of falls are linked to insomnia in those 65 years and older. Increased rates of insomnia are seen in those residing in institutions versus those in a community setting. Older adults should be educated about the impact of poor quality sleep on daily functioning as well as vital organs, including cardiovascular, neurologic, and mental health implications (Lawson et al., 2024; Xu et al., 2023).

EPIDEMIOLOGY AND RISK FACTORS

Of all sleep-related issues, insomnia is the most prevalent. Thirty percent to 50% of the population experiences short-term, occasional insomnia. The prevalence of chronic or severe insomnia (occurring for at least 3 months and a minimum of three times per week) is estimated to range from 10% to 15% (Khachatryan, 2021). Insomnia is one of the most prevalent complaints in primary health care.

Insomnia has a greater prevalence among older people and among divorced, separated, and widowed adults. Increasing age, female sex, and comorbid disorders (e.g., medical, mental disorders, and substance use) are all risk factors for developing insomnia disorder (Khachatryan, 2021).

Age of Onset

Age of onset for insomnia varies and may be impacted by physical health issues and psychological and environmental experiences that impact sleep. Older adults and those with health issues are reportedly more likely to experience insomnia (Winegar, 2024).

Sex Assigned at Birth and Gender

Certain distinctions stem from biologic variances, whereas others arise from societal constructs such as roles, expectations, and cultural norms linked to gender. Females report a higher prevalence of insomnia compared to males within the United States and across countries in Europe and Asia (Polyné et al., 2021; Sato et al., 2021).

Hormone shifts contribute to sleep difficulties and occur most frequently during menstruation, pregnancy, and the transition to menopause (Haufe & Leeners, 2023).

Gender minority adolescents (GMA), whose gender identity differs from their sex assigned at birth, report poorer-quality sleep than non-GMAs (Levenson et al., 2021). LGBTQ+ adolescents commonly exhibit inadequate sleep duration, increased latency, and disturbances. These sleep issues are partially attributed to experiences of discrimination based on their sexuality (Bruzzese et al., 2023).

Disparities in sleep issues between the LGBTQ+ community and the general population exist with LGBTQ+ individuals more likely to experience short sleep duration, sleep latency, and low sleep quality. Population-based studies reveal that LGBTQ+ individuals are more prone to reporting less than 5 hours of sleep compared to cisgender individuals. In the United States, gay males exhibit a 32% higher prevalence of trouble falling asleep and a 22% higher prevalence of waking up unrested compared to cisgender males, whereas bisexual females have a 43% higher prevalence of trouble falling asleep compared to cisgender females (Chum et al., 2021).

Individuals who identify as LGBTQ+ present across all communities and often face negative health outcomes due to the intersection of their sex and gender minority (SGM) identities with other aspects of their identity. These communities include diverse members from various racial, ethnic, religious, physical ability/disability, mental capacity, age, and socioeconomic backgrounds. Healthy People 2020 and 2030 recognize the imperative of addressing health disparities for LGBTQ+ individuals compared to their cisgender counterparts, emphasizing the ongoing need for sustained efforts to achieve equity and inclusion goals (Ginaldi & DeMartinis, 2024).

Ethnicity and Culture

There is not an equal distribution of sleep disorders among ethnic and racial groups. It is crucial to address sleep disparities due to their connection to cardiometabolic diseases and the escalating health care expenses they entail. In the United States, individuals from underrepresented racial or ethnic backgrounds and low-income households bear a significantly heavier burden of sleep-related chronic illnesses compared. The elevated prevalence of metabolic diseases like obesity, hypertension, diabetes, and dyslipidemia in these communities is directly associated with the heightened prevalence of poor sleep (Jean-Louis et al., 2022).

People from racial and ethnic backgrounds that historically have been underrepresented, as well as those from underprivileged communities, do not experience the same advantages of getting enough sleep as others. See Box 34.2. This discrepancy leads to insufficient sleep and inequalities in sleep health. Studies investigating these gaps have identified various factors like social determinants of health, community violence, and structural challenges, all of which contribute to poor sleep. However, a strong body of evidence supports behavioral interventions that can be utilized to enhance sleep health among different racial and ethnic groups (Hughes et al., 2023).

BOX 34.2

Mental Health Disparities: Sleep Health and Social Determinants of Health

Poor sleep health factors such as insufficient sleep duration, sleep fragmentation, sleep irregularity, circadian misalignment, and sleep disordered breathing are associated with elevated rates of mortality, heart disease, diabetes, obesity, and cancer that are disproportionately prevalent in underrepresented groups.

Sleep health is influenced by the home, community, and work (including shift work) environments, economic status, discrimination, minority stress, and school conditions. Sleep health disparities occur because the opportunity to sleep is strongly patterned by social determinants of health. Reducing sleep health disparities requires an increased awareness of the root causes, recognition of vulnerable groups, and multilevel approaches for reducing adverse exposures and promoting healthy sleep. Risk reduction involves equitable screening, treatment, and disease management.

Source: Gueye-Ndiaye, S., & Redline, S. (2024). Sleep health disparities. *Annual Review of Medicine*, *76*, 403–415. https://doi.org/10.1146/annurev-med-070323-103130

Familial Differences

Fatal familial insomnia is a rare, fatal disease characterized not only by insomnia, but also by dysautonomia (malfunction of the autonomic nervous system), changes to motor function, rapidly progressive dementia, and myoclonic limb activity. Rarely does clinical onset occur before the age 32, with the average onset at 51 years of age, and with most cases reported from Europe and Asia. Genetically, the disorder is of an autosomal dominant pattern (Zhang et al., 2022).

The most widely regarded predictor of a familial risk for insomnia is a maternal history. It is challenging to distinguish differences among families and support systems due to the web of intricacies that can impact sleep, specifically insomnia. Known medical disorders and treatment regimens can impact sleep architecture, thereby making it challenging to determine if insomnia is idiopathic or a consequence of another component of overall health wellness management or treatment.

COMORBIDITY

Sleep disorders occur independently of the diagnosis of other mental disorders, but they often occur in people with mental disorders, such as PTSD and depression.

Insomnia often increases the risk of relapse of the mental disorder (Luik et al., 2024). Documented comorbid conditions include cardiovascular disorders, diabetes, musculoskeletal disorders (e.g., arthritis, chronic back/neck pain), respiratory disorders (e.g., chronic obstructive pulmonary disease [COPD], seasonal allergies, chronic bronchitis, emphysema), digestive disorders (e.g., gastroesophageal reflux disease, irritable bowel syndrome), pain conditions, and other sleep disorders such as sleep apnea, and restless legs syndrome (RLS) (Kaur et al., 2023).

Etiology

Many factors affect sleep, but one of the major reasons for insomnia is depression, which accounts for most cases. However, most people with insomnia do not have a psychiatric diagnosis (Hertenstein et al., 2023).

Family Response to Disorder

Living with a family member with insomnia disorder is challenging. Irritability, complaints of sleeplessness, and chronic fatigue interfere with the quality of interpersonal relationships. Family members become "exhausted" by living with someone who never sleeps.

RECOVERY-ORIENTED CARE FOR PEOPLE WITH INSOMNIA

Teamwork and Collaboration: Working Toward Recovery

Sleep disorders are best treated by clinicians specializing in this area, but primary and mental health care professionals should be able to identify sleep disturbances and provide education and interventions for improving sleep. However, because sleep disorders are common in individuals with mental health issues, psychiatric–mental health nurses should be prepared to provide care for those with sleep disorders. Optimal management and treatment of insomnia have been linked to improved outcomes in those with coexisting psychiatric disorders (Kraepelien et al., 2022).

Safety Issues

Safety is a priority for people with insomnia disorder. Sleep deprivation can lead to accidents, falls, and injuries, especially in older patients. Sedating medication could potentially increase falls (Cai et al., 2024).

EVIDENCE-BASED NURSING CARE FOR PEOPLE WITH INSOMNIA

Nursing assessment for the patient with insomnia focuses on difficulty falling asleep, staying asleep, and/or early morning awakenings. The following are examples of assessment questions.

- What time do you go to bed? In your estimation, how long does it take you to fall asleep?
- When did your symptoms begin? Did anything unusual or stressful precipitate the sleep disturbance pattern?

  Does anyone in your family experience the same symptoms?

  Do you find yourself awakening feeling sluggish or refreshed?
- Does your reported sleep issue impact your daily activities or ability to function?
- Do you nap? If so, what time and for how long?

Interventions stress the importance of sleep hygiene and helping the patient establish regular sleep patterns. If medications are given, the commonly prescribed over-the-counter (OTC) medications and supplements include diphenhydramine and melatonin. Prescription medications used for insomnia include benzodiazepine receptor agonists (BzRAs), melatonin receptor agonist, and orexin receptor antagonist.

RECOGNIZING CUES: RELEVANT ASSESSMENT INFORMATION

Assessment of a patient's sleep pattern is a part of every psychiatric nursing assessment (see Chapter 10). If a patient has a sleep disorder, a detailed sleep history should be included in the assessment process. See Clinical Judgment Nursing Care Plan 34.1, which sets forth a plan of care for Michael, the case study patient in this chapter.

Physical Health and Functioning

During the patient interview, the description, duration (when the issue began), stability (every night?), and intensity (how bad is it?) should be determined (Box 34.3). A sleep history includes current sleeping patterns, medical issues, current medications (including OTC and dietary supplements), current life events, use of alcohol and caffeine, and emotional and mental status that might be affecting sleep (see Boxes 34.4 and 34.5). A **sleep diary** is an individual's subjective written account of their sleep experience (Schyvens et al., 2024). The diary may cover a few days to several weeks. A simple diary is a record of the patient's daily, estimated bedtime, rise time, total sleep time, estimated time to fall asleep, number and length of awakenings, and naps. Electronic devices are also an option for monitoring sleep parameters. Complex sleep diaries involve recording the amount and time of alcohol and caffeine ingestion, activity level, ratings of fatigue, medication, and stressful events.

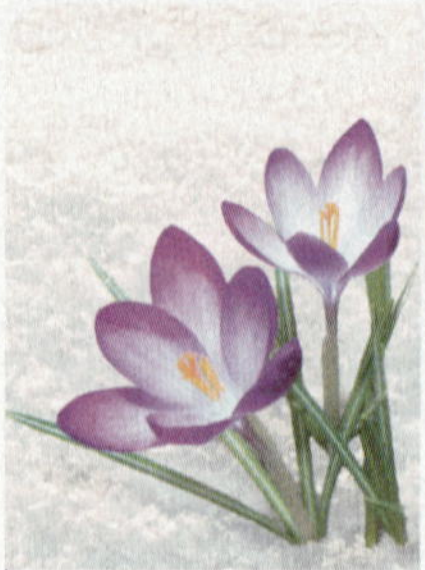

CLINICAL JUDGMENT NURSING CARE PLAN 34.1

Insomnia

Michael, age 20, is majoring in nursing. He presents himself at Student Health Services with issues sleeping. In assessing his issue, the nurse ascertains that Michael has insomnia because it takes 2 to 3 hours to fall asleep. During this interim of wakefulness, he lies in bed, calm but somewhat restless. He has had no prior difficulty with insomnia. His issue falling asleep occurs 3 nights a week—Monday, Wednesday, and Friday. He exercises vigorously during his physical education class (7–9 PM) on these three evenings. He denies any sleep issues during spring break, when he took a trip. The patient drinks 1 cup of coffee in the morning and denies the use of other stimulants. He reports that as a consequence he has had some irritability and difficulty concentrating on the days following a "bad night." He has tried an OTC sleep medication but does not remember the name of it. When he took these sleeping pills, he was able to fall asleep better, but found them to be costly. He would like a prescription for sleeping medication that would be covered by student health insurance.

Setting: Outpatient Student Health Service

Assessment Cues: A 20-year-old who presents with difficulty initiating sleep. After vigorous evening exercise, he takes 2–3 hours to fall asleep. Strengths: intelligence, motivated for treatment, adequate insurance coverage, good physical health.

Associated Psychiatric Diagnoses	Medications
Primary insomnia	None

Priority Hypothesis: Insomnia

Important Characteristics	Associated Considerations
Difficulty falling asleep, estimated sleep latency of 2–3 hours, three nights a week Changes in usual sleep environment Poor sleep hygiene	Mood alterations Poor concentration

Planning Recovery and Wellness Outcomes

Initial	Discharge
1. Describe factors that prevent or inhibit sleep. 2. Identify strategies to improve sleep hygiene.	1. Report an optimal balance of rest and activity.

Taking Action: Nursing Interventions

Interventions	Rationale	Ongoing Assessment
Teach patient good sleep hygiene habits.	Discussion of good sleep hygiene is the first treatment strategy.	Monitor Michael's reports of estimated sleep latency.
Instruct patient to keep a sleep diary for 1 week—including bedtime, sleep latency, rising time, naps, caffeine intake, time of exercise.	Keeping a sleep diary can give insight into insomnia issues by identifying alerting influences in relation to disturbed sleep. Exercise before sleep appears to be the primary factor that could be causing insomnia on Monday, Wednesday, and Friday.	Monitor other sleep hygiene issues.
Reassure patient that short-term insomnia will resolve when the factors that caused the issue are eliminated.	Anxiety about insomnia is a predisposing factor to the development of primary insomnia.	Determine Michael's level of anxiety about insomnia.
Determine whether it is possible to adjust the schedule so that vigorous exercise occurs several hours before sleep.	Physical exercise raises basal metabolism, which may interfere with sleep.	Determine whether it is possible to adjust the course schedule.
Problem solve with Michael how to adjust sleep schedule to avoid insomnia.	Problem-solving allows the patient to learn how to consider alternative strategies.	Evaluate whether strategies are reasonable.

Evaluation

Outcomes	Revised Outcomes	Interventions
After readjustment of exercise schedule, Matthew was able to resume typical sleep.	None	None

BOX 34.3

Therapeutic Dialogue: Sleep Assessment

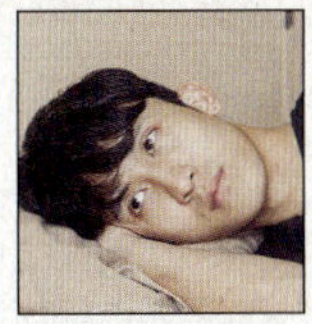

INEFFECTIVE APPROACH

Nurse: What time do you go to bed at night?

Michael: Oh, my bedtime varies between 10 PM and 2 AM.

Nurse: What time do you get up?

Michael: I get up anywhere between 6 AM and noon.

Nurse: How do you sleep during the night?

Michael: OK.

Nurse: OK?

Michael: Yeah, no problems sleeping.

EFFECTIVE APPROACH

Nurse: What time do you go to bed at night and what time do you get up?

Michael: Oh, my bedtime varies between 10 PM and 2 AM. I get up anywhere between 6 AM and noon.

Nurse: Let's be more specific. During a week's time, what time do you go to bed each night?

Michael: Well, this semester I have a morning clinical rotation Monday through Thursday. I'm usually up till 11 or midnight preparing for the next day. On Friday and Saturday nights, I typically go out with my friends and get to bed around 2 AM. On Sunday night, I get on to bed around 10 PM.

Nurse: What time do you get up each day of the week?

Michael: On the mornings that I have clinicals, I have to get up around 6 AM to be at the hospital by 6:45 AM. On Friday, I get up at 8 AM for a 9 o'clock class. Saturday morning, I get up around 8 AM so I can go to my part-time job. On Sunday, I get up by noon.

Nurse: How long do you take to fall asleep?

Michael: That's gotten much better. I fall asleep in 15 minutes or so.

Nurse: Do you take any naps?

Michael: Outside of class, I don't have time to nap. I'm just too busy with my classes, clinical, homework, job, and social life.

Nurse: Before this semester, how much sleep did you get?

Michael: That was last summer; I had a job that started at 1:30 PM, so I could sleep as late as I wanted. I bet I got 8 or even 9 hours of sleep every night. I don't remember being sleepy then.

CRITICAL THINKING CHALLENGE

1. Compare the quality and quantity of elicited data in the two scenarios.
2. What conclusions could be drawn from the first scenario?
3. Are the conclusions different for the second scenario? Explain.

BOX 34.4

Sleep History

- Perception of sleep issue
- Sleep schedule (bedtime and rise time)
- Difficulty falling asleep or maintaining sleep
- Quality of sleep
- Daytime sleepiness and impact of the sleep disorder on daytime functioning
- General emotional and physical issues (e.g., stress)
- Sleep hygiene (e.g., eating, drinking, or consuming caffeine immediately before bed)
- Use of OTC medications, herbal substances, prescription medication
- Use of substances such as alcohol, caffeine, tobacco, and illegal substances
- Sleep environment (e.g., room temperature, noise, light)

Adapted from Norris, T.L. (2024). Sleep and sleep-wake disorders. In T. L. Norris (Ed.), *Porth's pathophysiology: Concepts of altered health states* (11th ed., pp. 516–535). Wolters Kluwer.

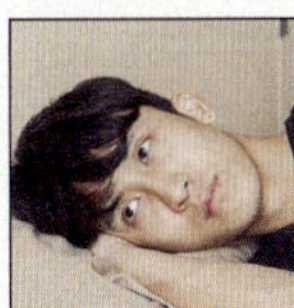

Consider Michael

His issue falling asleep occurs three nights a week—on Mondays, Wednesdays, and Fridays. He exercises vigorously during his physical education class (7 PM to 9 PM) on these three evenings. He denies any sleep issues during a spring break trip.

Should Michael keep a sleep diary? How would exercise impact his sleep? What does it mean that he has no issue sleeping during spring break?

History of Trauma

Experiencing traumatic stress during childhood can have profound effects on both neurologic and physiologic development. See Box 34.6. Epidemiologic research

BOX 34.5

Medications and Other Substances and Their Effects on Sleep

ALCOHOL

- Increases TST (total sleep time) during the first half of the night
- Decreases TST during the second half
- Decreases REM sleep during the first half of the night
- Withdrawal from long-term use of alcohol decreases TST, increased wakefulness after sleep onset, and REM rebound

AMPHETAMINES

- Disrupt sleep–wake cycle during acute use
- Decrease TST
- Decrease REM sleep
- Withdrawal may cause REM rebound

ANTIDEPRESSANTS (TRICYCLICS AND MAOIs)

- Sleep effects vary with sedative potential
- Increase slow-wave sleep (i.e., a recurrent period of very deep sleep, typically totaling 5 or 6 hours a night)
- Decrease REM sleep

BARBITURATES

- Increase TST
- Decrease WASO
- Decrease REM sleep
- Withdrawal may cause a decrease in TST and REM rebound

BENZODIAZEPINES

- Drugs vary in onset and duration of action
- Decrease SL
- Increase TST
- Decrease WASO
- Decrease REM sleep
- Daytime sedation may occur with long-acting drugs

BETA-ADRENERGIC BLOCKERS

- Decrease REM sleep
- Increase WASO, nightmares
- Daytime sedation may occur

CAFFEINE

- Increases SL
- Decreases TST
- Decreases REM sleep

L-DOPA

- Vivid dreams and nightmares

LITHIUM

- Increases slow-wave sleep
- Decreases REM sleep

OPIOIDS

- Effects vary with specific agents
- Increase WASO
- Decrease REM sleep
- Decrease slow-wave sleep

PHENOTHIAZINES

- Increase TST
- Increase slow-wave sleep

STEROIDS

- Increase WASO

MAOI, monoamine oxidase inhibitor; REM, rapid eye movement; SL, sleep latency; TST, total sleep time; WASO, wake after sleep onset.

indicates that adverse childhood experiences are linked to higher risks of various negative health outcomes throughout life, including premature morbidity, cardiovascular diseases, and psychiatric disorders. Sleep health, recognized as a crucial aspect of overall well-being, can be impaired in individuals who have experienced childhood adversity. Some studies suggest that sleep disturbances may act as a mediator, connecting childhood trauma to physical and mental health issues in adulthood (Ng & Chan, 2023).

Traumatic events can impact an individual's daily functioning, including sleep (Sanchez et al., 2022). Sleep disturbance is a common occurrence shortly after experiencing a traumatic event and is closely linked to emotional dysregulation, which is a significant risk factor for developing PTSD. PTSD is a prevalent and disabling psychiatric condition that can arise following exposure to trauma. It is characterized by intrusive thoughts about the traumatic event, avoidance of reminders, negative mood and thinking patterns, and heightened arousal. Sleep disturbance,

BOX 34.6

Trauma-Informed Approaches: Childhood Fears and Sleep Disturbances

Background

Children experiencing domestic violence often have sleep disturbances related to the fears associated with the trauma. They are unable to fall asleep because recurrent thoughts of the trauma are magnified, leading to poor sleep health. The amygdala is activated, resulting in automatic fear reactions and increased cortisol levels. Because these children do not get adequate sleep, they become tired and irritable during the day. A mental health evaluation should be trauma informed and include a specific assessment of sleep issues.

Interventions

Treatment that targets sleep-related symptoms can reduce daytime symptoms, increase well-being, and enhance readiness for treatment for psychotherapy.

Source: Fellman, V., Heppell, P. J., & Rao, S. (2024). Afraid and awake: The interaction between trauma and sleep in children and adolescents. *The Psychiatric Clinics of North America*, *47*(1), 229–253. https://doi.org/10.1016/j.psc.2023.06.015

particularly insomnia and nightmares, impacts 50% to 90% of individuals experiencing PTSD. Sleep issues can both contribute to and perpetuate PTSD symptoms, with evidence suggesting that early sleep disturbances following trauma can predict the development of PTSD months to years later in various populations, including accident victims, refugees, veterans, and people who have experienced natural disaster events (Zhou et al., 2023).

Substance Use and Medication

The bidirectionality of insomnia and substances must be acknowledged as substances impact the receptors and neurotransmitters directly involved with sleep–wake regulation. The development of sleep-related issues can be associated with the use of OTC products, such as nicotine and caffeine. Those who use products that are stimulating need to be informed about not only the effects on overall health but also the timing of consumption as it relates to initiating sleep and maintaining sleep and the impact on sleep quality. OTC and prescription medications that have a stimulating effect need to be avoided within 4 hours of sleep initiation. Though alcohol consumption may initially assist in helping individuals fall asleep, ultimately, alcohol use impacts sleep architecture and leads to disrupted, poor sleep quality; increases the likelihood of snoring or sleep apnea; and due to the diuretic effects, increases restroom visits (Zheng et al., 2021).

Psychosocial Cues

The assessment also includes evaluating the behavioral and social factors related to sleep issues. Though we each respond differently, stressful life events impact the quality and quantity of our sleep. Factors to consider include gender, coping skills, timing and perception of the stressor, and substance use or misuse. Recent changes in relationships, particularly a divorce or death of a loved one, can interfere with sleep significantly. A recent move, travel, and addition of a new family member can impact sleep.

Fatigue and stress increase when individuals assume the role of a caregiver in their personal lives and in those with occupations as professional health care providers. A rotating or variable work schedule compromises the circadian rhythm and contributes to insomnia (Cable et al., 2021).

Underrepresented groups, single parents/caregivers, employees in production-focused industries, and active-duty service members are more likely to report insufficient sleep.

Quality of Life

Health-related quality of life is decreased in adults who experience insomnia. There are numerous studies showing the quality of life is negatively impacted in people with insomnia. Although insomnia has a negative effect on quality of life in all genders, females with insomnia report a lower quality of life than males with insomnia (Kaur et al., 2023).

ANALYZING CUES AND DEVELOPING HYPOTHESES

The primary concern is sleep deprivation or insomnia, which can result in depression, cognitive dysfunction, and suicidal ideation. It is important to help the patient learn about sleep hygiene and the role that sleep plays in maintaining health and well-being.

PLANNING RECOVERY AND WELLNESS OUTCOMES: GENERATING SOLUTIONS

Sleep issues impact all aspects of health and wellness. Helping an individual examine current sleep patterns and their impact on any mental health issues is a beginning step in establishing wellness goals. Depending on the sleep issue, the nurse and patient should collaborate on establishing realistic goals. For example, going to bed at a regular hour each night or omitting caffeine after a set time of day could be a realistic goal. See Box 34.7.

TAKING ACTION: NURSING INTERVENTIONS

Priorities of Care

Safety is always a priority with sleep disorders. A patient should be protected from falls and in some severe cases, suicide which is associated with sleep deprivation (Wang et al., 2024a). Since depression is a risk for suicide, the patient who is depressed and sleep deprived should be carefully assessed for suicidal ideation.

Physical Care

With the emergence of smartphones and other portable devices, limiting screen time has been found to improve sleep quality and positively impact daytime vigilance (Brosnan et al., 2024). Night-time screen viewing not only contributes to inadequate sleep and poor diet, but ultimately to excess weight (Kracht et al., 2022). Exercise promotes sleep, but regular exercise should be planned to end 3 hours before bedtime. Routines are important, especially when preparing your body to sleep. Engaging in a quiet, relaxing activity, such as listening to soft music or reading nonstimulating material, is often suggested. Additional interventions include avoiding eating a heavy meal and avoiding drinking alcohol or caffeinated beverages. Patients should be encouraged to evaluate the temperature of the room. In general, a cooler environment enhances sleep.

BOX 34.7

Building Clinical Judgment With SBAR: Assessment and Recommendations for the Patient With Insomnia

SBAR

S: Situation

A 35-year-old presents to the outpatient clinic with complaints of severe insomnia and a recent onset of depression symptoms. She reports difficulty falling asleep, waking up frequently during the night, and feeling constantly fatigued during the day. Additionally, the patient admits to experiencing persistent feelings of sadness, hopelessness, and a loss of interest in activities she once enjoyed. She denies any recent significant life events or stressors.

B: Background

The patient has a past medical history of hypertension and panic attacks, for which she has been prescribed a selective serotonin reuptake inhibitor (SSRI) for the past 5 years. She has a history of intermittent adherence with medication, often discontinuing treatment when she starts feeling better. She is currently living alone, with limited family available for support. Her family history is significant for depression.

A: Assessment

Upon assessment, she appears disheveled and exhibits signs of fatigue and distress. She is tearful and expresses feelings of sadness, hopelessness, and worthlessness. The patient's vital signs are within expected limits, but she exhibits psychomotor agitation and poor concentration. The assessment reveals a high likelihood of depression exacerbating her insomnia symptoms.

R: Recommendation

1. **Medical Evaluation:**
   - Refer the patient for a comprehensive psychiatric evaluation to assess the severity of her symptoms and determine the appropriate treatment plan.
2. **Nonpharmacologic Interventions for Insomnia:**
   - Encourage sleep hygiene practices, such as maintaining a consistent sleep schedule, creating a comfortable sleep environment, and avoiding stimulating activities before bedtime.
   - Consider completion of sleep diary; customized preparation for sleep routine.
   - Suggest cognitive-behavioral therapy for insomnia (CBT-I), a nonpharmacologic treatment approach that addresses maladaptive thoughts and behaviors contributing to insomnia.
3. **Complementary Therapies:**
   - Recommend relaxation techniques, such as progressive muscle relaxation, deep breathing exercises, use of white noise machine, or guided imagery to promote relaxation and improve sleep quality.
   - Offer mindfulness-based interventions, such as meditation or yoga, to reduce stress and promote emotional regulation.
   - Explore the use of acupuncture or acupressure as adjunctive therapies for insomnia and anxiety management.
4. **Patient and Family Education:**
   - Educate patient and support people about the importance of incorporating nonpharmacologic interventions and complementary therapies into her routine as part of the treatment plan.
   - Provide psychoeducation about coping strategies for managing depression and insomnia, including mindfulness techniques and relaxation exercises.
5. **Follow-Up and Continuity of Care:**
   - Collaborate with her health care providers to ensure coordination of care and continuity of support, including assessment of the effectiveness of nonpharmacologic and complementary interventions.

Building Clinical Judgment

1. Why did the nurse refer the patient to a mental health provider?
2. Why did the nurse not recommend sleeping medications?

Wellness Challenges

Wellness activities are especially challenging because of the negative impact a lack of sleep has on daily life. Wellness can be severely compromised because the individual is tired and irritable from lack of sleep. The lack of energy can lead to poor nutrition and inadequate performance at work or school. Coping with everyday stress can be difficult (see Table 34.1).

Nonpharmacologic health-promoting interventions are the first choice before administering pharmacologic agents (Chun et al., 2021). Sleep hygiene strategies can be effective and should be encouraged. The goal is to adjust sleep patterns to improve well-being. The nurse can help the patient develop bedtime rituals and good sleep hygiene. Bedtime should be at a regular hour, and the bedroom environment should be conducive to sleep. Preferably, the bedroom should not be where the individual has access to technology or engages in work-related activities. The bedroom should be viewed as a room for either resting, sleeping, or sex (see Box 34.8).

Medication Interventions

Types of drugs used to treat symptoms of insomnia include BzRA, melatonin receptor agonists, sedating

TABLE 34.1 WELLNESS CHALLENGES AND COPING STRATEGIES RELATED TO SLEEP

Challenge	Coping Strategy
To cope effectively with daily stresses when not getting adequate sleep.	Reduce number of activities that require intense concentration
To seek pleasant environments that support well-being	Arrange for short periods of "quiet time" throughout the day
To recognize the need for physical activity, healthy foods, and sleep	Encourage regular physical activity, discuss healthy diets, encourage establishing healthy sleep hygiene routines
To develop a sense of connection, belonging, and a support system	Seek positive relationships and reduce number of unpleasant interactions.

antidepressants, and OTC medications and dietary supplements.

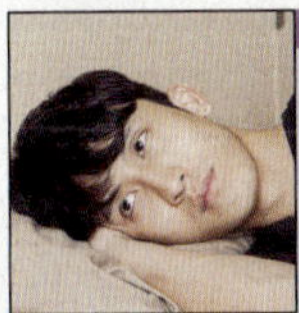

Consider Michael

Michael has tried OTC sleep medication, but does not remember the name of it. When he took these pills, he was able to fall asleep better, but found the pills to be costly. He wants a medication that will be covered by his student health insurance.

What nonpharmacologic interventions would you suggest before exploring less costly medications? Which sleeping medications requiring a prescription have the least side effects?

BOX 34.8

Teaching Tips for Sleep Hygiene Strategies

1. The most important healthy sleep habit is to *establish and maintain a regular bedtime and rising time.* Even if you awaken feeling unrefreshed, get up and out of bed at a regular, consistent time. "Sleeping in" can disturb sleep on the subsequent night. For most, time in bed should be limited to 8 hours.
2. Avoid naps.
3. Abstain from alcohol. Although alcohol may assist with sleep onset, there is an alerting effect when it wears off.
4. Refrain from caffeine after midafternoon. Avoid nicotine before bedtime and during the night. Caffeine and nicotine are strong stimulants and fragment sleep.
5. Exercise regularly, avoiding the 3 hours before bedtime. Exercising 6 hours before bedtime tends to strengthen the circadian rhythms of body temperature and sleepiness.
6. Use the bedroom only for sleep and sex. Promote the bedroom as a stimulus for sleep, not for studying, watching television, or socializing on the telephone.
7. Set a relaxing routine to prepare for sleep. Avoid frustrating or provoking activities before bedtime.
8. Provide for a comfortable environment. A cool room temperature, minimal light, and limiting noise are suggested.

Benzodiazepine Receptor Agonists

The **benzodiazepine receptor agonists (BzRAs)** hypnotics have US Food and Drug Administration (FDA) approval for insomnia. They include the **benzodiazepines** (e.g., triazolam, temazepam, estazolam, quazepam, and flurazepam) and the **nonbenzodiazepines** (e.g., zolpidem, zolpidem extended release, zaleplon, and eszopiclone) (Table 34.2). All these medications bind to benzodiazepine receptors and exert their effects by facilitating GABA effects. GABA, the most common inhibitory neurotransmitter, must be present at the benzodiazepine receptor for the BzRA to exert its effect. These medications are all absorbed rapidly and reduce sleep latency with medication at recommended doses (Cheung et al., 2024). Nonbenzodiazepine hypnotics, which provide immediate relief, are often used for short-term treatment of insomnia. The most common side effects are headache, dizziness, and residual sleepiness (Box 34.9).

The BzRAs are Schedule IV–controlled substances by federal regulation, have misuse and dependence potential, and produce withdrawal signs and symptoms after abrupt discontinuation. The risk for residual sedation on the day after using hypnotic medication is determined by the dose and rate of elimination (Cheung et al., 2024). The recommended therapeutic dose for using zolpidem (immediate release) is 5 mg and zolpidem CR is 6.25 mg.

TABLE 34.2 HYPNOTICS: BENZODIAZEPINE RECEPTOR

	Dosage (mg)	Half-life (h)
Estazolam	1–2	10–24
Flurazepam	15–30	48–120
Temazepam	15–30	8–20
Triazolam	0.125–0.25	2.4
Quazepam	7.5–15	48–120
Zolpidem	5–10	1.4–3.8
Zolpidem ER	6.25–12.5	2.8
Zaleplon	5–20	1
Eszopiclone	1–3	6

BOX 34.9

Medication Profile: Zaleplon

DRUG CLASS: Sedative-hypnotic (pyrazolopyrimidine nonbenzodiazepine hypnotic). It is readily absorbed and metabolized with only about 1% of zaleplon eliminated in urine.

RECEPTOR AFFINITY: Zaleplon acts at the GABA-benzodiazepine receptor complex.

INDICATION: Treatment of onset or maintenance insomnia

ROUTES AND DOSING: Zaleplon is available in 5- and 10-mg capsules. It should be taken at bedtime or after a nocturnal awakening with difficulty falling back to sleep (but at least 4 hours before the desired rise time).

Adults: The recommended starting dose is 10 mg with a maximum of 20 mg. An initial dose of 5 mg should be considered in adults with low body weight. Doses of over 20 mg have not been sufficiently studied.

Geriatric: Initially, 5 mg is recommended as a starting dose. Older adults should not exceed a 10-mg dose.

HALF-LIFE (PEAK PLASMA CONCENTRATION): 1 hour

SELECTED SIDE EFFECTS: Abdominal pain, headache, dizziness, depression, nervousness, difficulty concentrating, back pain, chest pain, migraine, conjunctivitis, bronchitis, pruritus, rash, arthritis, constipation, and dry mouth

WARNINGS: Zaleplon should not be administered to patients with severe hepatic impairment. Zaleplon potentiates the psychomotor impairments of ethanol consumption.

Melatonin Receptor Agonist

Melatonin is a hormone, released from the pineal gland that aids in the regulation of the sleep–wake cycle through activation of MT_1 and MT_2 receptors. Melatonin has been shown to shift circadian rhythm, decrease body temperature, alter reproductive rhythm, enhance immune function, and decrease alertness. Usually, levels of melatonin increase with decreasing exposure to light. **Ramelteon**, indicated for insomnia, is a melatonin receptor agonist with high affinity for melatonin receptors MT_1 and MT_2. This pharmacologic activity is believed to be related to its sleep-promoting properties (Box 34.10). Ramelteon has a low misuse potential and is not a controlled substance (Lou & Oks, 2021).

Orexin Receptor Antagonist

Orexins (also known as **hypocretins**) are neurotransmitters produced in the hypothalamus that trigger wakefulness, whereas low levels result in sleep. A deficiency is associated with narcolepsy. **Suvorexant** is an orexin receptor antagonist approved for the treatment of insomnia. Blocking the binding of orexins to receptors is thought to suppress the wake drive. This antagonism may also trigger signs of narcolepsy/cataplexy. There is emerging evidence that this group of medications is effective for other psychiatric disorders (Carpi et al., 2024).

Over-the-Counter Medications and Dietary Supplements

OTC sleeping pills are usually antihistamines. The most common agents are doxylamine and diphenhydramine. These histamine-1 antagonists have a CNS effect that includes sedation, diminished alertness, and slowing of reaction time. These drugs also produce anticholinergic side effects, such as dry mouth, accelerated heart rate, urinary retention, and dilated pupils. Drowsiness lasts from 3 to 6 hours after a single dose. Next-morning hangover can be an issue. Diphenhydramine decreases sleep latency and improves quality of sleep for those with occasional sleep issues but is not as effective as benzodiazepines for chronic sleep disturbances. It is not recommended for older adult patients (Lou & Oks, 2021).

BOX 34.10

Medication Profile: Ramelteon

DRUG CLASS: Sedative–hypnotic. It is readily absorbed and metabolized with median peak concentrations occurring 0.5 to 1.5 hours after fasted oral administration.

RECEPTOR AFFINITY: Ramelteon is a melatonin receptor agonist with high affinity for MT_1 and MT_2. No appreciable affinity for the GABA receptor complex.

INDICATION: Treatment of insomnia characterized by difficulty with sleep onset.

ROUTES AND DOSING: The recommended dose is 8 mg. It should be taken 30 minutes before bedtime.

It should not be taken with or immediately after a high-fat meal. Patients should be advised to use caution if they consume alcohol in combination with ramelteon.

Adolescents and Children: Ramelteon has been associated with an effect on reproductive hormones in adults, for example, decreased testosterone levels and increased prolactin levels.

Geriatric: No overall differences in safety or efficacy were observed between older and younger adult subjects.

HALF-LIFE (PEAK PLASMA CONCENTRATION): 1 to 2.6 hours

SELECTED ADVERSE REACTIONS: Somnolence, dizziness, nausea, fatigue, headache, and insomnia

WARNINGS: Ramelteon should not be used by patients with severe hepatic impairment. It should not be used in combination with fluvoxamine.

Melatonin has long been an available OTC and has been shown to have mild sleep-promoting properties when given outside the period of usual secretion. That is, melatonin can advance the sleep–wake cycle by making it easier to fall asleep earlier than usual. Some evidence suggests that in young and older individuals with insomnia, melatonin can be beneficial in ameliorating the symptoms (Savage et al., 2021).

Valerian, a dietary supplement, is used as a medicinal herb in many cultures. The mechanism of action is not fully understood and is believed to inhibit GABA reuptake. Valerian may be useful for sleeplessness, but not enough evidence from double-blind studies exists to confirm this. The American Academy of Sleep Medicine recommended against using valerian for chronic insomnia in adults. Mild side effects include headaches, dizziness, upset stomach, and tiredness the morning after its use (National Center for Complementary and Integrative Health, 2020).

Administering and Monitoring Medication

Sleeping medications are commonly used in all settings. They are usually given nightly for a short period of time to establish a wake–sleep pattern. Rebound insomnia can occur if a drug is abruptly discontinued. This side effect can be minimized or prevented by giving the lowest effective dose and tapering before discontinuing. Nurses should assess for confusion, memory issues, excessive sedation, and risk of falls.

Monitoring for Drug-to-Drug Interactions

Sleep medications generally have increased depressive effects when given with other CNS depressants. Sleep medications can interact with oral contraceptives, isoniazid (an antibiotic), fluvoxamine (a serotonin reuptake inhibitor [SSRI]), and verapamil (a calcium channel blocker) (see Chapter 11). Grapefruit juice should be avoided when taking these drugs. Ramelteon should not be given with fluvoxamine.

Teaching Points

Pharmacologic agents should complement sleep hygiene practices. These medications can be useful on a short-term basis. Alcohol use should be avoided when taking sleeping medications. Patients should use these medications when time for sleeping is adequate (at least 8 hours). Most sleep-related medications should be taken at bedtime. Patients should be instructed about the safe use of these medications and possible side effects.

Psychosocial Interventions

Enhancing Cognitive Functioning

Cognitive-behavioral therapy for insomnia (CBT-I) is useful in changing negative learned responses that perpetuate insomnia. This approach is especially helpful for those who also have comorbid depression or anxiety. This approach includes sleep hygiene, sleep restriction, stimulus control, cognitive therapy, and relaxation strategies, and it is recommended as first-line therapy (Cunnington, 2022). CBT-I aims to adjust daily habits, train the body to relax, and establish realistic and healthy associations to optimize sleep. There are a variety of CBT-I apps available as an online platform, where the content can be individualized to an individual's needs. Evidence indicates that these apps are helpful to use at home, with the sleep diary being the favorite feature (Erten Uyumaz et al., 2021).

Using Behavioral Interventions

Stimulus control is a technique used when the bedroom environment no longer provides cues for sleep but has become the cue for wakefulness. Patients are instructed to avoid behaviors in the bedroom incompatible with sleep, including watching television, doing homework, and eating. This allows the bedroom to be reestablished as a stimulus for sleep.

Another behavioral intervention is **sleep restriction**. Patients often increase their time in bed to provide more opportunity for sleep, resulting in fragmented sleep and irregular sleep schedules. Patients are instructed to spend less time in bed and avoid napping.

Relaxation training is used when patients complain of difficulty relaxing, especially if these patients are physically tense or emotionally distressed. Various procedures to reduce somatic arousal can be used, including progressive muscle relaxation, autogenic training, and biofeedback. Imagery training, meditation, and thought stopping are attention-focusing techniques that center on cognitive arousal.

Complementary Therapies

Insomnia ranks among the top five medical complaints for which complementary strategies are commonly sought. Analyses indicate that around 4.5% of adults with insomnia in the United States utilize complementary therapies to address their sleep issues, translating to over 1.6 million individuals, indicating a significant interest in nonconventional approaches to managing sleep issues (Zhao et al., 2023).

Meditative movements like tai chi and qi gong have been found to improve sleep quality across different populations. Yoga is associated with improvement in sleep quality (Cea et al., 2024). Other strategies include relaxation, massage therapy, and meditation (Tang et al., 2021). Aromatherapy, particularly with inhaled lavender oil, shows promise in improving sleep quality (Vora et al., 2024). Individuals in fragile health, such as older adults and patients receiving dialysis, may benefit from acupressure and acupuncture (Lu et al., 2024; Makhfudli et al., 2024).

Music therapy serves as a versatile instrument for enhancing sleep health and addressing sleep disorders in various populations. Its capacity to induce relaxation, alleviate stress, and regulate emotions provides a multifaceted strategy for enhancing sleep quality and overall well-being. Incorporating music therapy into current treatment modalities can provide individuals grappling with sleep disturbances with heightened therapeutic advantages and improved sleep results (Aasim, 2024). In addition to its broader applications, music therapy emerges as a valuable tool for addressing sleep disturbances in hospitalized patients. Factors like noise, pain, and unfamiliar environments often disrupt sleep in hospital settings, hindering patient recovery. Recognizing the importance of sleep in the healing process, nonpharmacologic and safe strategies to enhance sleep quality should be explored. Music interventions have demonstrated efficacy in improving sleep across various contexts, suggesting that music therapy could serve as a safe and cost-effective adjunctive intervention to promote better sleep outcomes for hospitalized patients (Jespersen et al., 2023).

Psychoeducation

Teaching Strategies

Education regarding interventions is crucial for patients with sleep disorders. An explanation of the sleep cycle and the factors that influence sleep are important for these patients. For those with insomnia, teaching about avoiding foods and beverages that might interfere with sleep should be highlighted (Box 34.11).

BOX 34.11

Psychoeducation Checklist: Sleep Disorders

When teaching patients with sleep disorders, be sure to include the following topics:

- Importance of developing a bedtime ritual and good sleep habits
- Allowing for 8 hours of sleep per night
- Maintenance of a regular sleep schedule, specifically a routine rise time
- Bedroom rituals
- Maintenance of a sleep log
- An occasional "bad night" happens to nearly everyone
- Foods to avoid before going to bed
- Avoidance of caffeine and rigorous exercise within the 6 hours before bedtime
- Avoidance of cigarette smoking 1 hour before bedtime and during nighttime awakenings
- Avoidance of alcohol. Alcohol disrupts sleep and is a poor hypnotic
- Use of sleep medications as prescribed
- Daytime sleepiness as a symptom of sleep disorders
- How to do relaxation exercises
- Appropriate family support

Wellness Strategies

There are sleep hygiene strategies that specifically promote sleep (Table 34.1), but there are many other activities associated with physical and psychological well-being that should also be considered. Eating a healthy diet, avoiding excessive weight gain, and identifying and managing psychological and physical stressors are examples of wellness strategies that promote sleep.

Providing Family Education

Family and friends should be encouraged to support the new habits the patient is trying to establish. Patients, spouses, and friends must understand that activities engaged in just before sleep can greatly affect sleep patterns and sleep difficulties, such as socializing, alcohol consumption, use of caffeine, and engaging in stimulating activities. Relaxing activities before bedtime are vital contributors to establishing a routine conducive to sleep. Family and friends can help create a positive environment with an emphasis on sleep as a priority.

Promoting Safety

Depending on the specific sleep disorder and associated risks, the nurse should implement safety measures during sleep, such as using bed rails or alarms for individuals at risk of falling out of bed, or ensuring a safe sleep environment for individuals prone to sleepwalking or night terrors. The nurse adjusts the sleep environment to optimize safety, such as removing tripping hazards, ensuring the bed is comfortable and supportive, and regulating the room temperature and lighting for better sleep quality.

Evaluation of Patient Outcomes

The primary treatment outcome is establishing an improved sleep cycle. Changes in diet and behavior (e.g., initiation of an exercise program) should be evaluated for their impact on the individual's sleep. Environmental modifications, such as a change in the level of lighting in the bedroom, decreased stimulation (e.g., turning off cell phone or moving the television out of the bedroom), or modification in room temperature, can be monitored for any changes affecting the sleep cycle.

Integration With Primary Care

Sleep issues are usually treated in the primary care setting. Cardiovascular and metabolic disorders are associated with sleep disturbances. Sleep deprivation is associated with obesity and hypertension (Hanson & Huecker, 2023). If a sleep disorder is being treated by a mental health specialist, it is important that the mental health specialist communicates with the primary care provider.

OTHER DISORDERS

HYPERSOMNOLENCE DISORDER

The essential characteristic of **hypersomnolence disorder** is excessive sleepiness at least three times a week for at least 3 months. Sleepiness occurs on an almost daily basis and causes significant impairment in social and occupational functioning. They have an excessive quantity of sleep, deteriorated quality of wakefulness, and sleep inertia (a period of impaired performance occurring during the sleep–wake transition characterized by confusion, ataxia, or combativeness) (Karna et al., 2023). This diagnosis is reserved for individuals who have no other causes of daytime sleepiness (e.g., narcolepsy, OSA syndrome).

Clinical Course

People with hypersomnolence typically sleep 8 to 12 hours per night. They fall asleep easily and sleep through the night, often having difficulty awakening in the morning. They often have difficulty meeting morning obligations. They exhibit poor concentration and memory. Excessive sleepiness may not be impacted by napping because they may awaken from a nap feeling unrefreshed. They may even describe dangerous situations, such as being sleepy while driving or operating heavy machinery.

Diagnosis

On the day after overnight **polysomnography** (a test that measures multiple body functions during sleep), a **multiple sleep latency test (MSLT)** may be used. The MSLT is a standardized procedure that measures sleep variables during a 20-minute period. The process is repeated every 2 hours, occurring approximately five times during the day (Iskander et al., 2023). The faster an individual falls asleep during testing, the greater the physiologic sleep tendency. The presence of sleep-onset REM (SOREM) during the MSLT and a report of cataplexy assist providers in determining a sleep diagnosis. Polysomnography shows short sleep latency, a typical-to-long sleep duration, and expected sleep architecture. Subjective symptoms of sleepiness are recognized as heavy eyelids, loss of initiative, reluctance to move, and yawning or slowed speech. Sleepiness is unique to the individual and situation, varying from mild to severe.

Evidence-Based Nursing Care of People With Hypersomnolence Disorder

Nursing assessment for the patient with hypersomnolence focuses on excessive sleepiness. The following are examples of assessment questions.

- Have you ever nodded off unintentionally?
- When did your sleepiness begin?
- Does anyone in your family experience the same sleepiness symptoms?
- Do you suddenly find yourself awakening feeling refreshed?

Interventions stress the importance of sleep hygiene and helping the patient establish regular sleep patterns. If medications are given, the most commonly prescribed stimulants for treating excessive daytime sleepiness are dextroamphetamine and amphetamine mixtures, modafinil, methylphenidate, and pemoline. These agents increase the patient's ability to stay awake and perform. Misuse of these medications should be assessed. In some cases, serotonin antagonists are used off-label.

People who are sleepy often self-medicate with caffeine. A cup of brewed coffee contains about 100 to 150 mg of caffeine. A 12-oz can of Mountain Dew contains 54 mg of caffeine. Caffeine contents of popular "energy" drinks range from 80 to 300 mg. Peak plasma concentration is reached 30 to 60 minutes after consumption, and the duration of effect is 3 to 5 hours in adults. Caffeine improves psychomotor performance, particularly tasks involving endurance, vigilance, and attention. High doses, especially in people who do not habitually use caffeine, may exhibit side effects such as irritability and anxiety.

NARCOLEPSY

The overwhelming urge to sleep is the primary symptom of **narcolepsy**. This irresistible urge to sleep occurs at any time of the day, regardless of the amount of sleep. Falling asleep often occurs in inappropriate situations, such as while driving a car or reading a newspaper. These sleep episodes are usually short, lasting 5 to 20 minutes, but may last up to an hour if sleep is not interrupted. Individuals with narcolepsy may experience sleep attacks and report frequent dreaming. They usually feel alert after a sleep attack, only to fall asleep unintentionally again several hours later.

Clinical Course

Narcolepsy is a chronic disorder that usually begins in young adulthood between the ages of 15 and 35 years. Excessive daytime sleepiness is the first symptom to appear. The severity of sleepiness may remain stable over the lifetime. Narcolepsy has no cure. Treatment is designed to control symptoms based on clinical presentation and severity. A secondary sleep disorder should be considered if the level of sleepiness changes (Anderson, 2021).

Narcolepsy is distinguished by a group of symptoms, including daytime sleepiness, cataplexy, hypnagogic hallucinations, and sleep paralysis. The symptom of daytime sleepiness is found in all individuals with narcolepsy, but existence of the other three symptoms varies.

- **Cataplexy** is the bilateral loss of muscle tone, triggered by a strong emotion, such as anger or laughter. This muscle atonia can range from subtle (drooping eyelids) to dramatic (buckling knees). Respiratory muscles are not affected. Cataplexy usually lasts for seconds. Individuals are fully conscious, oriented, and alert during the episode. Prolonged episodes of cataplexy may lead to unintentional sleep episodes. The frequency and severity of events generally increase when the individual is sleep deprived.
- **Hypnagogic hallucinations** are intense dream-like images that occur at sleep onset and usually involve the current environment. Hallucinations can be visual or auditory, such as hearing one's name called or a door slammed.
- **Sleep paralysis**, the inability to move or speak when falling asleep or waking up, is often described as terrifying and is accompanied by a sensation of struggling to move or speak. Although the diaphragm is not involved, patients may also complain of not being able to breathe or feeling suffocated. These episodes are typically brief and usually terminate spontaneously or when the individual is touched.

Diagnosis

Excessive daytime sleepiness and the presence of cataplexy are diagnostic of narcolepsy. It is possible to have narcolepsy without cataplexy. The diagnosis should be confirmed by an in-lab polysomnogram demonstrating at least 6 hours of sleep, followed by the MSLT showing a sleep latency of less than or equal to 8 minutes and two or more SOREM periods. The diagnosis can also be confirmed by a cerebrospinal fluid hypocretin-1 level less than or equal to 110 mg/mL (Anderson, 2021; Slowik et al., 2023).

Epidemiology and Etiology

The prevalence of narcolepsy is more than 65 per 100,000 people in the United States (Slowik et al., 2023). The etiology of most cases of narcolepsy is unknown, but it is thought that there are many triggers such as head trauma, viral illness, exposure to toxins, and development factors. In some patients, there is a deficiency of hypocretin, a hypothalamic peptide that may be linked to chromosome 6 in class II human leukocyte antigen. Hypocretin neurons are part of the neurologic system that wakes and maintains wakefulness (Slowik et al., 2023).

Evidence-Based Nursing Care of People With Narcolepsy

Nursing assessment is similar to that for insomnia. In general, sleepiness is treated with CNS stimulants. Methylphenidate, dextroamphetamine, modafinil, and pemoline are the most frequently prescribed stimulants. Cataplexy may be treated with tricyclic antidepressants because these drugs suppress REM. Sodium oxybate classified as a Schedule II drug, is indicated for excessive sleepiness and cataplexy. Because of its high misuse potential, patients who are prescribed this medication are closely monitored.

Patient education focuses on factors that can make symptoms worse, such as sleep deprivation. Patients need to develop strategies to manage symptoms. Naps can be integrated into their daily routines such as during work breaks or before engaging in activities that require sustaining alertness.

BREATHING-RELATED DISORDERS

Other breathing disorders include OSA–hypopnea, central sleep apnea, and sleep-related hypoventilation. This section will discuss OSA–hypopnea disorder (OSA syndrome). The term *obstructive sleep apnea syndrome* is more commonly used in nonpsychiatric areas and will be used in this section instead of the term *obstructive apnea–hypopnea disorder*. Central sleep apnea and sleep-related hypoventilation will not be discussed.

OBSTRUCTIVE SLEEP APNEA SYNDROME

Obstructive sleep apnea (OSA) syndrome, the most commonly diagnosed breathing-related sleep disorder, is characterized by snoring during sleep and episodes of sleep apnea (cessation of breathing) that fragments sleep and contribute to daytime sleepiness. The hallmark symptoms are snoring and daytime sleepiness. Often, snoring is so loud and disturbing that partners choose separate bedrooms for sleeping. A gasp, choke or pause in breathing during sleep or waking with a headache and dry mouth are signs of OSA. On physical examination, an enlarged, elongated uvula is associated with increased severity of snoring and apneic events (Olszewska et al., 2021). Snoring affects 57% of males, 40% of females, and 27% of children (NSF, 2022).

Clinical Course

Apneic episodes, which last from 10 seconds up to several minutes, cause disrupted sleep and abrupt awakenings with feelings of choking or falling out of bed; some people even leap out of bed to restore breathing. The individual may not later recall the awakening. These brief awakenings deprive essential sleep, resulting in excessive daytime sleepiness that may reach the same degree of pathologic sleepiness found in narcolepsy. Unlike narcolepsy, naps tend to be unrefreshing.

Esophageal reflux, or heartburn, is a common complaint. Genitourinary symptoms include nocturia (three to seven trips to the bathroom), nocturnal enuresis, and erectile dysfunction. Bradycardia, in association with tachycardia, is often seen with apneic events. Other cardiac arrhythmias are also seen, including sinus arrest. The onset of symptoms and sleepiness may coincide with weight gain. A 10% increase in weight may result in as much as a sixfold increase in developing moderate-to-severe sleep-disordered breathing. Obesity is a major risk factor for apnea and predictor across populations (Malhotra et al., 2021).

Diagnosis

Polysomnography, usually performed at night during sleep, monitors many body functions, including brain wave activity, eye movements, muscle activity, heart rhythm, breathing function, and respiratory effort. Polysomnography may show poor sleep continuity, increased stage 1 and decreased slow-wave and REM sleep, and an increased amount of EEG alpha wave activity while the individual is asleep. Clinical evaluation includes oral and nasal airflow, respiratory effort, oxyhemoglobin saturation, and electromyogram of limb muscle activity. Typically, patients with OSA demonstrate numerous respiratory events per night, resulting in intermittent hypoxemia and changes in intrathoracic pressure during polysomnographic measurement (Malhotra et al., 2021).

Epidemiology and Risk Factors

OSA occurs worldwide and is more common in males than females, but for all individuals, the prevalence increases as individuals age. It is thought that OSA is underdiagnosed in females. OSA is most common in males aged 45 to 65 years who are overweight. Males are more likely to report more frequent snoring than females, who tend to report nonspecific symptoms such as mood disturbances, lack of energy, daytime fatigue, morning headache, nightmares, and insomnia (Geer & Hilbert, 2021).

Research suggests that Black males have more severe OSA than White males, White females, and Black females; in addition, they are more likely to have a delayed diagnosis, resulting in greater severity of symptoms (Thornton et al., 2022). Lost workplace productivity, motor vehicle accidents, workplace injuries, and increased use of health care services are some of the societal consequences of untreated OSA (Tai et al., 2024). OSA is a risk factor for cardiac events and is commonly associated with metabolic syndrome disorders (Almendros et al., 2022; Yeghiazarians et al., 2021). OSA is more prevalent in people with mental health disorders than in the general population. Depression, anxiety, PTSD, and bipolar disorder are associated with OSA. The symptoms of depression, such as fatigue, irritability, depressed mood, and poor concentration, are similar to the symptoms of OSA. Evidence suggests that the successfully treated OSA may improve depressive symptoms (Gabryelska et al., 2024).

Etiology

An obstruction or collapse of the airway causes apnea, or cessation of breathing. In most cases, the site of obstruction is in the pharyngeal area. Vibrations of the soft, pliable tissues found in the pharyngeal airway cause the snoring sounds that occur during breathing.

Teamwork and Collaboration: Working Toward Recovery

There are nonsurgical and surgical options for the treatment of patients with OSA. Nonsurgical options vary based on the severity of the obstructive breathing. For patients with obesity who have less severe OSA, weight loss may help. For others, whose apnea is mild, changing sleeping position from supine to lateral can help control the severity of OSA. There has also been some effort in devising an oral appliance to reduce snoring and the occurrence of apnea. Currently, the most commonly used nonsurgical treatment is **continuous positive airway pressure (CPAP)** or bilevel positive airway pressure (BPAP). This treatment takes place during sleep and involves wearing a nose mask that is connected by a long tube to an air compressor. Airway patency is maintained with air pressure. Although this method of treatment is highly effective, adherence can be an issue. Individuals with severe OSA symptoms and daytime sleepiness are more adherent with CPAP treatment and report an improved quality of life (Anjan et al., 2024; Venkatnarayan et al., 2021).

Upper airway stimulation is FDA-approved for adults who have moderate-to-severe OSA, are unable to use or get consistent benefit from CPAP, and do not have significant obesity. A small impulse generator is implanted beneath the clavicle between the external and intercostal muscle. A tunneled stimulation lead is attached to the hypoglossal nerve, which produces tongue protrusion. When inspiration occurs, the impulse generator sends a signal via the stimulation lead to the hypoglossal nerve, which results in slight forward displacement of the stiffened tongue, resulting in fewer apnea episodes (Heiser et al., 2021).

The most commonly performed surgical procedure to treat patients with OSA is **uvulopalatopharyngoplasty**. This procedure involves the removal of redundant soft palate tissue, uvula, and tonsillar pillars. The surgery usually eliminates snoring and is judged to be about 50% effective in reducing the amount of sleep apnea. Severity of OSA, body mass index, and pharyngeal anatomic features are factors that impact surgical outcomes (Nomura et al., 2024).

CIRCADIAN RHYTHM SLEEP DISORDER

The chief feature of a **circadian rhythm sleep disorder** is the mismatch between the individual's internal sleep–wake circadian rhythm and the timing and duration of sleep (Basit et al., 2021). People with these disorders complain of insomnia at particular times during the day and excessive sleepiness at others. This diagnosis is reserved for those individuals with marked sleep disturbance or significant social or occupational impairment.

Diagnosis and Clinical Course

- *Delayed sleep phase type:* Individuals with delayed sleep phase type, or "night owls," tend to be unable to fall asleep before 2 AM to 6 AM; hence, their whole sleep patterns shift, and they have difficulty rising in the morning.
- *Advanced sleep phase type:* Opposite of the night owls, these individuals are "larks" or earlier risers. They are unable to stay awake in the evening and consistently wake up early.
- *Irregular sleep–wake type:* People with this type have a temporarily disorganized sleep pattern that varies in a 24-hour period.
- *Non–24-hour sleep–wake type:* Individuals with this type have an unexpected synchronization between the 24-hour light–dark cycle and their endogenous circadian rhythm, which leads to periods of insomnia, excessive sleepiness, or both. This type is most common among blind or visually impaired individuals.
- *Shift work type:* The endogenous sleep–wake cycle is typical but is mismatched to the imposed hours of shift work. Rotating shift schedules are disruptive because any consistent adjustment is prevented. Compared with day and evening shift workers, night and rotating shift workers have a shorter sleep duration and poorer quality of sleep. They may also be sleepier while performing their jobs. This disorder is further exacerbated by insufficient daytime sleep resulting from social and family demands and environmental disturbances (i.e., traffic noise, telephone). Because of the job requirements of the profession, nurses often experience this disorder. Furthermore, 20% of the US workforce is engaged in shift work and thereby at risk for circadian rhythm disorders.
- *Jet lag type:* This type of sleep disturbance occurs after traveling across time zones, particularly in coast-to-coast and international travel. The endogenous circadian sleep–wake cycle does not match the desired hours of sleep and wakefulness in a new time zone. Individuals traveling eastward are more prone to jet lag because it involves resetting one's circadian clock to an earlier time—it is easier to delay the endogenous clock to a later time period than adjust it to an earlier one.

Epidemiology and Etiology

There are no data regarding the prevalence of circadian rhythm disorders in the general population. The prevalence of circadian rhythm disorders among patients diagnosed at sleep disorder centers accounts for 2% or less of the total patients diagnosed. However, this is a gross underestimate, given that jet lag, a circadian rhythm disorder, affects nearly everyone traveling over three time zones.

Circadian rhythm disorders are caused by the dissociation of the internal circadian pacemaker and conventional time. The cause might be intrinsic, such as genetic factors called "clock genes" or extrinsic, as in jet lag and shift work. Each result is overwhelming daytime sleepiness and overflowing wakefulness at night.

Teamwork and Collaboration: Working Toward Recovery

The goals of treatment of circadian rhythm disorder are to strengthen timed clues (when to go to sleep), timed bright or blue light (stay awake during the day), and timed exogenous melatonin (initiate melatonin secretion at bedtime). Melatonin is often helpful in initiating sleep (Cruz-Sanabria, 2023).

Chronotherapy, timed interventions, manipulates the sleep schedule by progressively delaying bedtime until an acceptable bedtime is attained. Chronopharmacotherapy resets the biologic clock by using medications to induce sleep. Tasimelteon is a melatonin receptor agonist that is approved for the treatment of this disorder. Small amounts of hypnotics can also produce high-quality sleep in people who wish to reset their circadian schedules after long transmeridian flights. Conversely, for night shift workers, caffeine taken while working at night improves alertness and performance. However, caffeine should be used judiciously by night shift workers because they become quickly tolerant to the effects after a few nights (Palagini et al., 2021).

Luminotherapy (light therapy) is used to manipulate the circadian system. Timing, wavelength intensity, and prior light exposure are key factors when considering light therapy (Wang et al., 2024b). Exposure to moderate-intensity light and a shorter duration of light therapy is more effective in reducing sleepiness in shift workers compared with lower-intensity, higher-intensity, and longer-duration light therapy (Lam & Chung, 2021).

PARASOMNIAS

Parasomnias are sleep–wake disorders that occur in association with sleep, specific sleep stages, or sleep–wake transitions. The individual experiences unexpected behavioral, experiential, or physiologic events. Parasomnias are divided into two primary categories: NREM related and REM related. NREM sleep arousal disorders, including sleepwalking and sleep terror types, usually occur during the first third of the major sleep episode. REM sleep disorders consist of episodes of arousal during REM sleep. During REM sleep disorders, the individual appears to be awake acting out a dream which can be dangerous for the individual and their bed partners. Nightmare disorder is an REM disorder that generally occurs during the second half of the major sleep episode. RLS is considered a sleep disorder and is classified as a sleep-related movement disorder (Fariba & Tadi, 2023).

SLEEP TERRORS AND SLEEPWALKING

In **sleep terrors** (also called night terrors or pavor nocturnes), there are episodes of screaming, fear, and panic, causing clinical distress or impairing social, occupational, or other areas of functioning. Sleep terrors can last 45 to 90 minutes and can cause distress, panic, and a sense of helplessness. The individual may not remember the episode, but it is frightening to anyone witnessing it. Often, individuals abruptly sit up in bed screaming; others have been known to jump out of bed and run across the room. Other symptoms include a rapid heart rate and breathing, dilated pupils, and flushed skin. Usually, the individual having a sleep terror is inconsolable and difficult to awaken completely. Efforts to awaken the individual may prolong the episode. Once awake, most are unable to recall the dream or event that precipitated such a response. A few report a fragmentary image. Often, the individual does not fully awaken and cannot recall the episode the next morning (Van Horn & Street, 2023).

In sleepwalking or **somnambulism,** there are repeated episodes of complex motor behavior during sleep that may involve getting out of bed and walking around. While sleepwalking, people typically have a blank stare and are difficult to awaken. Often, they awaken to find themselves in a different place from where they went to sleep. If awakened during the episode, there is a brief period of confusion (Mundt et al., 2023; Zergham & Chauhan, 2021).

Clinical Course

Polysomnography shows that these disorders usually begin when slow-wave NREM sleep predominates during the first third of the night; they rarely occur during daytime naps. Telehealth consultation opportunities are a potential modality for the assessment of sleep-related issues (Rizzo et al., 2024). This delivery format may present some challenges because the polysomnography is usually followed with an immediate consultation, which may be difficult to schedule.

Epidemiology and Etiology

The prevalence of sleep terrors is estimated at 6.5% in children and 2.2% in adults. Males and females are affected equally. The prevalence of sleepwalking is 30% in children and 4% in adults. Sleepwalking peaks between 8 and 12 years of age; prevalence appears to be equal between male and female children (Van Horn & Street, 2023). Sleep terrors, confusional arousals, and sleepwalking are most common in childhood and typically lessen by adolescence (Mundt et al., 2023) Fever, stress, and sleep deprivation can increase the frequency of episodes. There appears to be some genetic predisposition for disorders of arousal, and they tend to run in families.

Teamwork and Collaboration: Working Toward Recovery

Learning about parasomnias and the need for safety precautions for patient and family should be the focus of the education. Hypnosis supplemented by psychotherapy may be considered. Treatment might also include medications, such as benzodiazepines.

Evidence-Based Nursing Practice for the People With Parasomnias

Although polysomnography may be used to diagnose or confirm a sleep disorder, the evaluation of a response to an NREM disorder involves a careful sleep history. Episodes of sleep terrors or sleepwalking are often unrealized by the patient but can be described in detail by the parent/caregiver or partner. Support people should be advised to avoid attempting to wake the individual/child and ensure a safe environment surrounds the individual. Safety features may include a sleep space absent of stairs, as well as securing windows and doors with locks. Sleep diaries should focus on the individual's bedtime activities, time of sleep onset and wake up, time to prepare for bed and fall asleep, use of medications, number of awakenings, subjective assessment of quality of sleep, and daytime naps. Sleep hygiene and a routine, to avoid insufficient sleep, should be promoted (Bruni et al., 2024).

Nursing interventions range from referring to sleep specialists to patient education about the disorder and strategies in dealing with the disorder. In some instances, nurses care for patients in the inpatient setting who have arousal disorders. In these instances, nurses should develop care plans that address the individual patient's needs. In instances of sleepwalking, staff should be alert to the safety issues and protect the patient from injury (see Box 34.12).

NIGHTMARE DISORDER

The repeated occurrence of frightening dreams that occur during REM sleep and often awaken an individual

BOX 34.12

General Safety Precautions for Sleepwalkers and Their Families

- Ensure adequate sleep. The occurrence of sleepwalking dramatically increases after sleep loss.
- Anticipate sleepwalking. Family members should be aware of the likelihood of sleepwalking for the first 2 to 3 hours after the sleepwalker goes to bed.
- Keep a sleep log to assist in identifying how much sleep is needed to prevent a sleepwalking event.
- Consider use of a noise device on the door of the sleepwalker's room to alert others that the sleepwalker is up.
- Deadbolt locks should be installed on doors leading outside. Windows should be secured to limit their opening.
- When the sleepwalker is spending the night away from home, alert appropriate individuals to the possibility that sleepwalking may occur. Ensure adequate sleep on the preceding nights.

is the essential characteristic of **nightmare disorder**. Typically, the individual can recall detailed dream content that involves physical danger (e.g., attack or pursuit) or perceived danger (e.g., embarrassment or failure). On awakening, the individual is fully alert and experiences a persisting sense of anxiety or fear. Many people have difficulty returning to sleep. Multiple same-night nightmares may be reported. Some people avoid sleep because of their fear of nightmares. Consequently, people may report that excessive sleepiness, poor concentration, and irritability disrupt their daytime activities. The occurrence of nightmares may be more serious than previously suspected. Nightmares are commonly experienced by military combat personnel who have PTSD (see Chapter 29).

Diagnosis and Clinical Course

Nightmares occur in REM sleep almost exclusively. They most often occur during the second half of the night when REM sleep dominates. Polysomnography demonstrates abrupt awakenings from REM sleep. In most cases, the REM sleep episode lasts for at least 10 minutes. Tachycardia and tachypnea may be evident.

Etiology and Epidemiology

The cause and prevalence of nightmares are unknown. Intriguing evidence provokes a debate as to whether nightmares are a symptom or an adaptive reaction to pathophysiologic factors. Negative emotions, primarily fear, are the most common dream emotions. Brain imaging demonstrates increased metabolic activity during REM sleep in the most primitive regions of the brain, the paralimbic and limbic regions. Many classes of drugs trigger nightmares, including catecholaminergic agents, beta-blockers, some antidepressants, barbiturates, and alcohol. In addition, withdrawal from barbiturates and alcohol causes REM rebound and more vivid dreaming.

Nightmares often begin in children between the ages of 3 and 6 years, and most children outgrow them. In adults, at least 50% of the population reports occasional nightmares. Females are more likely to report nightmares than males.

Teamwork and Collaboration: Working Toward Recovery

If the nightmares cause significant distress, an individual will be treated by multiple providers. Traditionally, psychotherapy aimed at conflict resolution has been the treatment of choice. Today, CBT is recommended, specifically **imagery rehearsal therapy**, a technique in which patients change the endings of their nightmares while they are awake. After rehearsing new, nonthreatening images and changing the content of the nightmare while awake, a reduction in the frequency of nightmares and associated distress has been shown (Isaac et al., 2023; Sahu et al., 2023; Vincent et al., 2023). Pharmacologically, the best-studied and most effective medication to treat nightmares with PTSD is prazosin, a centrally active alpha-1 adrenergic antagonist indicated for hypertension. The use of prazosin for PTSD-related nightmares is off-label. It does not have FDA approval for use with nightmares, but prazosin is recommended by the Standards of Practice Committee of the American Academy of Sleep Medicine for PTSD-associated nightmares (Morgenthaler et al., 2018).

Evidenced-Based Nursing Care

While caring for patients with other disorders, the nurse often is the first health professional to identify nightmares as an issue in a patient. Sleep assessment is vital in every nursing assessment. If nightmares are causing distress, a referral for a sleep evaluation should be made. Sleep hygiene techniques and education about the treatment of nightmares should be included in patient teaching. During hospitalization, the nurse should document that the patient has nightmares, and the nurses on the night shift should monitor for them.

RESTLESS LEGS SYNDROME

Restless legs syndrome (RLS) is a sleep–wake disorder characterized by an urge to move the legs, which begins or worsens at rest or periods of inactivity, typically in the evening or at night. The urge to move legs is reduced or relieved by movement.

Diagnostic Criteria and Clinical Course

RLS is a sensorimotor, neurologic disorder described as the intense desire to move legs accompanied by uncomfortable sensations such as creeping, crawling, tingling, burning, or itching. The diagnosis is made on the basis of self-report. These symptoms can interfere with sleep and cause considerable clinical distress or functional impairment. RLS is usually diagnosed in the second and third decades of life and can get progressively worse later in life.

Epidemiology and Etiology

RLS affects approximately 3% of adults in the United States. The prevalence is about twice higher in females than in males and increases with age in North America and Europe, but is not observed in Asian countries. RLS is consistently associated with comorbid conditions of insomnia, excessive sleepiness, and depressive and/or anxiety symptoms. RLS is the most common movement disorder occurring during pregnancy, usually developing in the third trimester (Brostrom et al., 2023; Lepuzanovic et al., 2024).

The etiology of RLS remains unclear, but genetic predisposition, dopaminergic dysfunction, and deficiencies in iron metabolism partially explain the underlying causes. RLS is linked to cardiovascular disease and metabolic syndrome (diabetes, obesity, hypertension, and dyslipidemia) (Hochstrasser et al., 2023; Mansur et al., 2023). There is emerging evidence that suggests inflammation and/or immunologic disorders have a role in RLS (Geng & Chen, 2024). Recent studies show an increase in prevalence of systemic lupus erythematosus and in cases of hepatitis C (Naqvi et al., 2021; Parperis et al., 2024).

Teamwork and Collaboration: Working Toward Recovery

The treatment of RLS involves a biopsychosocial approach using pharmacologic and nonpharmacologic treatment options. In cases of mild and intermittent RLS, behavioral therapy, sleep hygiene, and lifestyle interventions (avoiding caffeine, alcohol, and heavy meals) help reduce the likelihood of having an episode. If serum ferritin is <75 mcg/L, supplementation with ferrous sulfate is initiated (Silber et al., 2021). For moderate-to-severe RLS, there is strong evidence to support the use of pramipexole, rotigotine, cabergoline, and gabapentin enacarbil. There is moderate evidence to support the use of ropinirole, pregabalin, and IV ferric derisomaltose. Augmentation, also diagnosed as refectory RLS, can occur after multiple years of dopaminergic drugs. Assessment for augmentation, sleepiness, and compulsive behaviors are factors of focus for the health care team (Zhou et al., 2021).

Evidence-Based Nursing Practice for People With Restless Legs Syndrome

A thorough nursing assessment will provide direction for the nursing interventions for an individual with RLS. In many instances, there are underlying medical conditions such as diabetes or peripheral neuropathy, which contribute to the severity of RLS, particularly for the older adult. If the underlying medical condition is being treated adequately, the patient can be encouraged to engage in moderate regular physical activity 3 days a week or taking a hot bath before going to sleep. If medication is prescribed, the patient and family will benefit from medication education. If iron supplement is given, follow-up testing should be monitored to prevent overload. Sleep hygiene and encouragement to avoid exacerbating factors should be recommended.

SUMMARY OF KEY POINTS

- The sleep–wake cycle runs in a pattern called circadian rhythm. Most body systems follow a circadian rhythm and are often associated with the sleep–wake cycle. Hormones, such as melatonin and cortisol, help promote wakefulness during the day and sleepiness at night.
- Assessment is key. Information should focus on a comprehensive sleep history, including specific details of the sleep complaint, current sleep patterns, and sleep patterns before sleep difficulties, medical issues, current medications, current life events, and emotional and mental status.
- Nursing interventions for sleep disorders focus on nonpharmacologic approaches (e.g., exercise, nutrition, activity, thermoregulation) and pharmacologic interventions.
- Psychosocial nursing interventions for sleep disorders include educating patients about good sleep habits, instructing patients in relaxation exercises and sleep-promoting activities, providing patients with nutritional suggestions regarding foods and substances to avoid, and educating family members and friends regarding the importance of supporting the need for making high-quality sleep a priority.
- Insomnia disorder is characterized by difficulty falling asleep or difficulty maintaining sleep. Insomnia is often precipitated by feelings of stress or tension, with associations and behaviors persisting after the crisis or stressful situation has passed.
- OSA syndrome is a diagnosed breathing-related sleep disorder characterized by excessive snoring and episodes of apnea (i.e., cessation of breathing). These episodes disrupt sleep and may cause daytime sleepiness.
- In circadian rhythm sleep–wake disorders, a mismatch takes place between the individual's internal sleep–wake circadian rhythm and the timing and duration of sleep.
- Parasomnias occur in association with sleep, specific sleep stages, or sleep–wake transitions and include

sleepwalking, sleep terrors, nightmare disorders, and RLS. They are characterized by unexpected behavioral, experiential, or physiologic events. The etiology is unknown but appears to be of genetic predisposition. Unrestorative sleep, excessive sleepiness, poor concentration, and irritability are often the result.

DEVELOPING CLINICAL JUDGMENT

1. Describe the sleep hygiene interventions that would be useful for the individual with insomnia disorder.
2. Recognize the main issues and identify the primary issues related to sleep–wake disorders.
3. Construct a list of assessment questions for a 25-year-old who reports that she has not slept for 3 days.
4. A 55-year-old truck driver presents reporting unintentional episodes of excessive daytime sleepiness. Construct a list of assessment questions to explore the chief complaint of excessive daytime sleepiness.
5. Outline nursing interventions and educational highlights for the parents/caregivers of a 12-year-old child diagnosed with sleepwalking disorder.

MOVIES, TV, OR STREAMING PROGRAMS

Awake: **2021.** This apocalyptic thriller creates a scene of global disarray and fear as a mysterious event knocks out not only all electronics but also the ability to sleep for everyone around the world—except for one young girl (played by Ariana Greenblatt). Scientists race to find a cure for pervasive insomnia and its potentially fatal consequences. Produced by Mark Raso, the movie stars Gina Rodriguez as Jill, a US Army medic and widowed mother of two who is willing to do whatever it takes to protect her children.

Viewing Points:

1. How did the lack of sleep impact Jill's ability to make sound decisions?
2. What cues would you initially recognize that may lead you to assess sleep?
3. Is it realistic that insomnia can result in personality changes?

REFERENCES

Aasim, S. (2024). Harmonizing sleep: Exploring the multifaceted role of music therapy in sleep health. *International Journal of Science and Research, 13*(3), 662–663.

Almendros, I., Basoglu, Ö. K., Conde, S. V., Liguori, C., & Saaresranta, T. (2022). Metabolic dysfunction in OSA: Is there something new under the sun?. *Journal of Sleep Research, 31*(1), e13418. https://doi.org/10.1111/jsr.13418

Anderson, D. (2021). Narcolepsy: A clinical review. *JAAPA, 34*(6), 20–25. https://doi.org/10.1097/01.JAA.0000750944.46705.36

Anjan, T., Thakkar, S., Jahagirdar, A., Baddam, H., Pappulwar, S. M., Jha, K., & Prashant, M. C. (2024). Evaluation of treatment outcomes and quality of life in patients with obstructive sleep apnea receiving oral appliance therapy. *Journal of Pharmacy & Bioallied sciences, 16*(Suppl 3), S2634–S2636. https://doi.org/10.4103/jpbs.jpbs_375_24

Babicki, M., Piotrowski, P., & Mastalerz-Migas, A. (2023). Insomnia, daytime sleepiness, and quality of life among 20,139 College students in 60 countries around the world—A 2016–2021 study. *Journal of Clinical Medicine, 12*(2), 692.

Basit, H., Damhoff, T. C., & Huecker, M. R. (2021). Sleeplessness and circadian disorder. In *StatPearls*. StatPearls Publishing.

Brosnan, B., Haszard, J. J., Meredith-Jones, K. A., Wickham, S. R., Galland, B. C., & Taylor, R. W. (2024). Screen use at bedtime and sleep duration and quality among youths. *JAMA Pediatrics, 178*(11), 1147–1154. https://doi.org/10.1001/jamapediatrics.2024.2914

Broström, A., Alimoradi, Z., Lind, J., Ulander, M., Lundin, F., & Pakpour, A. (2023). Worldwide estimation of restless legs syndrome: A systematic review and meta-analysis of prevalence in the general adult population. *Journal of Sleep Research, 32*(3), e13783.

Bruni, O., DelRosso, L. M., Melegari, M. G., & Ferri, R. (2024). The parasomnias. *Psychiatric Clinics of North America, 47*(1), 135–146. https://doi.org/10.1016/j.psc.2023.06.009

Bruzzese, J. M., Leonard, S. I., Liu, J., Hughes, T. H., & Jackman, K. (2023). Sleep disparities among sexual minority early adolescents: The mediating role of sexual identity-based discrimination (abstract). *American Journal of Critical Care Medicine*. https://www.atsjournals.org/doi/abs/10.1164/ajrccm-conference.2023.207.1_MeetingAbstracts.A1103

Cable, J., Schernhammer, E., Hanlon, E. C., Vetter, C., Cedernaes, J., Makarem, N., Dashti, H. S., Shechter, A., Depner, C., Ingiosi, A., Blume, C., Tan, X., Gottlieb, E., Benedict, C., Van Cauter, E., & St-Onge, M. P. (2021). Sleep and circadian rhythms: Pillars of health—a Keystone Symposia report. *Annals of the New York Academy of Sciences, 1506*(1), 18–34. https://doi.org/10.1111/nyas.14661

Cai, A. W. T., Manousakis, J. E., Singh, B., Francis-Pester, E., Kuo, J., Jeppe, K. J., Rajaratnam, S. M. W., Lenné, M. G., Howard, M. E., & Anderson, C. (2024). Subjective awareness of sleepiness while driving in younger and older adults. *Journal of Sleep Research, 33*(1), e13933. https://doi.org/10.1111/jsr.13933

Carpi, M., Palagini, L., Fernandes, M., Calvello, C., Geoffroy, P. A., Miniati, M., Pini, S., Gemignani, A., Mercuri, N. B., & Liguori, C. (2024). Clinical usefulness of dual orexin receptor antagonism beyond insomnia: Neurological and psychiatric comorbidities. *Neuropharmacology, 245*, 109815. https://doi.org/10.1016/j.neuropharm.2023.109815

Cea, L. M., Brooks, C., Whipps, J., Wilkins, B., & Guseman, E. H. (2024). A routine within a routine: Can bedtime yoga improve sleep for the whole family? *Journal of Bodywork and Movement Therapies, 40*, 1724–1731. https://doi.org/10.1016/j.jbmt.2024.09.007

Cheung, J. M. Y., Scott, H., Muench, A., Grunstein, R. R., Krystal, A. D., Riemann, D., & Perlis, M. (2024). Comparative short-term safety and efficacy of hypnotics: A quantitative risk-benefit analysis. *Journal of Sleep Research, 33*(4), e14088. https://doi.org/10.1111/jsr.14088

Chum, A., Nielsen, A., & Teo, C. (2021). Sleep problems among sexual minorities: A longitudinal study on the influence of the family of origin and chosen family. *BMC Public Health, 21*(1), 2267. https://doi.org/10.1186/s12889-021-12308-0

Chun, W., Chao, D., Qi, H., Dongliang, Z., Zhenmei, L., & Jia, L. (2021). Pharmacological and non-pharmacological treatments for insomnia: A protocol for a systematic review and network meta-analysis. *Medicine (Baltimore), 100*(31), e26678. https://doi.org/10.1097/MD.0000000000026678

Corbo, I., Forte, G., Favieri, F., & Casagrande, M. (2023). Poor sleep quality in aging: The association with mental health. *International Journal of Environmental Research and Public Health, 20*(3), 1661.

Cruz-Sanabria, F., Carmassi, C., Bruno, S., Bazzani, A., Carli, M., Scarselli, M., & Faraguna, U. (2023). Melatonin as a chronobiotic with sleep-promoting properties. *Current Neuropharmacology, 21*(4), 951–987. https://doi.org/10.2174/1570159X20666220217152617

Cunnington, D. (2022). Cognitive behaviour therapy for insomnia works. It's time to make it accessible. *Sleep Medicine Reviews, 61*, 101586. https://doi.org/10.1016/j.smrv.2021.101586

De Pasquale, C., El Kazzi, M., Sutherland, K., Shriane, A. E., Vincent, G. E., Cistulli, P. A., & Bin, Y. S. (2024). Sleep hygiene—What do we mean? A bibliographic review. *Sleep Medicine Reviews, 75*, 101930. https://doi.org/10.1016/j.smrv.2024.101930

Erten Uyumaz, B., Feijs, L., & Hu, J. (2021). A review of digital cognitive behavioral therapy for insomnia (CBT-I Apps): Are they designed for engagement? *International Journal of Environmental Research and Public Health, 18*(6), 2929. https://doi.org/10.3390/ijerph18062929

Falup-Pecurariu, C., Diaconu, S', Tînt, D., & Falup-Pecurariu, O. (2021). Neurobiology of sleep (review). *Experimental and Therapeutic Medicine, 21*(3), 272. https://doi.org/10.3892/etm.2021.9703

Fariba, K. A., & Tadi, P. (2023). Parasomnias. In *StatPearls*. StatPearls Publishing. https://www.ncbi.nlm.nih.gov/books/NBK560524

Franken, P., & Dijk, D. J. (2024). Sleep and circadian rhythmicity as entangled processes serving homeostasis. *Nature reviews. Neuroscience*, *25*(1), 43–59. https://doi.org/10.1038/s41583-023-00764-z

Gabryelska, A., Turkiewicz, S., Białasiewicz, P., Grzybowski, F., Strzelecki, D., & Sochal, M. (2024). Evaluation of daytime sleepiness and insomnia symptoms in OSA patients with a characterization of symptom-defined phenotypes and their involvement in depression comorbidity-a cross-sectional clinical study. *Frontiers in Psychiatry*, *15*, 1303778. https://doi.org/10.3389/fpsyt.2024.1303778

Gadodia, R., Nandamuru, D., Akberzie, W., & Kataria, L. (2023). Sleep disorders and aging in women. *Sleep Medicine Clinics*, *18*(4), 545–557. https://doi.org/10.1016/j.jsmc.2023.06.017

Gale, E. L., James Williams, A., & Cecil, J. E. (2024). The relationship between multiple sleep dimensions and obesity in adolescents: A systematic review. *Sleep Medicine Reviews*, *73*, 101875. https://doi.org/10.1016/j.smrv.2023.101875

Gavidia, R., Whitney, D. G., Hershner, S., Selkie, E. M., Tauman, R., & Dunietz, G. L. (2022). Gender identity and transition: Relationships with sleep disorders in US youth. *Journal of Clinical Sleep Medicine*, *18*(11), 2553–2559.

Geer, J. H., & Hilbert, J. (2021). Gender issues in obstructive sleep apnea. *The Yale Journal of Biology and Medicine*, *94*(3), 487–496.

Geng, C., & Chen, C. (2024). Association between inflammatory cytokines and disease severity in restless legs syndrome. *Neurological Sciences*, *45*(12), 5765–5770. https://doi.org/10.1007/s10072-024-07736-w

Ginaldi, L., & De Martinis, M. (2024). Who needs education on LGBTQIA+ healthcare inclusion? *Medical Education Online*, *29*(1), 2329403.

Gueye-Ndiaye, S., & Redline, S. (2025). Sleep health disparities. *Annual Review of Medicine*, *76*(1), 403–415. https://doi.org/10.1146/annurev-med-070323-103130

Hanson, J. A., & Huecker, M. R. (2023). Sleep deprivation. In *StatPearls*. StatPearls Publishing. https://www.ncbi.nlm.nih.gov/books/NBK547676

Harris, R., Kavaliotis, E., Drummond, S. P. A., & Wolkow, A. P. (2024). Sleep, mental health and physical health in new shift workers transitioning to shift work: Systematic review and meta-analysis. *Sleep Medicine Reviews*, *75*, 101927. https://doi.org/10.1016/j.smrv.2024.101927

Haufe, A., & Leeners, B. (2023). Sleep disturbances across a woman's lifespan: What is the role of reproductive hormones? *Journal of the Endocrine Society*, 7(5), bvad036. https://doi.org/10.1210/jendso/bvad036

Heiser, C., Steffen, A., Hofauer, B., Mehra, R., Strollo, P. J. Jr., Vanderveken, O. M., & Maurer, J. T. (2021). Effect of upper airway stimulation in patients with Obstructive Sleep Apnea (EFFECT): A randomized controlled crossover trial. *Journal of Clinical Medicine*, *10*(13), 2880. https://doi.org/10.3390/jcm10132880

Hertenstein, E., Benz, F., Schneider, C. L., & Baglioni, C. (2023). Insomnia-A risk factor for mental disorders. *Journal of Sleep Research*, *32*(6), e13930. https://doi.org/10.1111/jsr.13930

Hochstrasser, K. J., Rogers, S. C., Quyyumi, A., Johnson, D., Pak, V., Shah, A. J., Rye, D. B., & Trotti, L. M. (2023). Restless legs syndrome, periodic limb movements of sleep, and subclinical cardiovascular disease. *Sleep and Biological Rhythms*, *22*(2), 259–267. https://doi.org/10.1007/s41105-023-00497-7

Hughes, A. J., Gunn, H., Siengsukon, C., Stearns, M. A., James, E., Donley, T., Grandner, M. A., Thomas, S. J., Hansen, K., & Williams, N. J. (2023). Eliminating sleep health disparities and achieving health equity: Seven areas for action in the behavioral sleep medicine community. *Behavioral sleep medicine*, *21*(5), 633–645.

Isaac, F., Toukhsati, S. R., DiBenedetto, M., & Kennedy, G. A. (2023). Cognitive behavioral therapy-based treatments for insomnia and nightmares in adults with trauma symptoms: A systematic review. *Current Psychology*, *42*(27), 23495–23505.

Iskander, A., Jairam, T., Wang, C., Murray, B. J., & Boulos, M. I. (2023). Normal multiple sleep latency test values in adults: A systematic review and meta-analysis. *Sleep Medicine*, *109*, 143–148. https://doi.org/10.1016/j.sleep.2023.06.019

Jean-Louis, G., Grandner, M. A., & Seixas, A. A. (2022). Social determinants and health disparities affecting sleep. *The Lancet Neurology*, *21*(10), 864–865.

Jespersen, K. V., Hansen, M. H., & Vuust, P. (2023). The effect of music on sleep in hospitalized patients: A systematic review and meta-analysis. *Sleep Health*, *9*(4), 441–448.

Karna, B., Sankari, A., & Tatikonda, G. (2023). Sleep disorder. In *StatPearls*. StatPearls Publishing. https://www.ncbi.nlm.nih.gov/books/NBK560720

Kaur, H., Spurling, B. C., & Bollu, P. C. (2023). Chronic Insomnia. In *StatPearls*. StatPearls Publishing. https://www.ncbi.nlm.nih.gov/books/NBK526136

Khachatryan, S. G. (2021). Insomnia burden and future perspectives. *Sleep Medicine Clinics*, *16*(3), 513–521. https://doi.org/10.1016/j.jsmc.2021.05.006

Kolp, H., Wilder, S., Andersen, C., Johnson, E., Horvath, S., Gidycz, C. A., & Shorey, R. (2020). Gender minority stress, sleep disturbance, and sexual victimization in transgender and gender nonconforming adults. *Journal of Clinical Psychology*, *76*(4), 688–698. https://doi.org/10.1002/jclp.22880

Koronowski, K. B., & Sassone-Corsi, P. (2021). Communicating clocks shape circadian homeostasis. *Science (New York, N.Y.)*, *371*(6530), eabd0951. https://doi.org/10.1126/science.abd0951

Kracht, C. L., Wilburn, J. G., Broyles, S. T., Katzmarzyk, P. T., & Staiano, A. E. (2022). Association of night-time screen-viewing with adolescents' diet, sleep, weight status, and adiposity. *International Journal of Environmental Research and Public Health*, *19*(2), 954. https://doi.org/10.3390/ijerph19020954

Kraepelien, M., Forsell, E., & Blom, K. (2022). Large-scale implementation of insomnia treatment in routine psychiatric care: Patient characteristics and insomnia-depression comorbidity. *Journal of Sleep Research*, *31*(1), e13448. https://doi.org/10.1111/jsr.13448

Lam, C., & Chung, M. H. (2021). Dose-response effects of light therapy on sleepiness and circadian phase shift in shift workers: A meta-analysis and moderator analysis. *Scientific Reports*, *11*(1), 11976. https://doi.org/10.1038/s41598-021-89321-1

Lawson, Y., Wilding, G. E., & El-Solh, A. A. (2024). Insomnia and risk of mortality in older adults. *Journal of Sleep Research*, *33*(6), e14229. https://doi.org/10.1111/jsr.14229

Leonard, S. I., Liu, J., Jackman, K. B., & Bruzzese, J. M. (2024). Sexual and gender minority sleep health disparities and minority stress in early adolescence. *The Journal of Adolescent Health*, *75*(3), 471–478. https://doi.org/10.1016/j.jadohealth.2024.05.022

Leso, V., Fontana, L., Caturano, A., Vetrani, I., Fedele, M., & Iavicoli, I. (2021). Impact of shift work and long working hours on worker cognitive functions: Current evidence and future research needs. *International Journal of Environmental Research and Public Health*, *18*(12), 6540. https://doi.org/10.3390/ijerph18126540

Lepuzanovic, M., Sinanovic, O., Aziraj-Smajic, V., Kapic, D., Basagic, E., & Muftic, M. (2024). Prevalence of restless legs syndrome during pregnancy and postpartum period. *Journal of Perinatal Medicine*, *52*(8), 852–857. https://doi.org/10.1515/jpm-2024-0208

Levenson, J. C., Thoma, B. C., Hamilton, J. L., Choukas-Bradley, S., & Salk, R. H. (2021). Sleep among gender minority adolescents. *Sleep*, *44*(3), zsaa185.

Li, J., Vitiello, M. V., & Gooneratne, N. S. (2022). Sleep in normal aging. *Sleep Medicine Clinics*, *17*(2), 161–171. https://doi.org/10.1016/j.jsmc.2022.02.007

Lin, Y., Chen, Y., Lin, Y., Xin, S., Ren, A., Zhou, X., Lin, X., & Li, X. (2024). Association between sleep quality and ovarian reserve in women of reproductive age: A cross-sectional study. *Fertility and Sterility*, *123*(3), 520–528. https://doi.org/10.1016/j.fertnstert.2024.09.018

Lou, B. X., & Oks, M. (2021). Insomnia: Pharmacologic treatment. *Clinics in Geriatric Medicine*, *37*(3), 401–415. https://doi.org/10.1016/j.cger.2021.04.003

Lu, G., Chen, F., Guo, C., & Wu, J. (2024). Acupuncture for senile insomnia: A systematic review of acupuncture point. *Archives of Gerontology and Geriatrics*, *127*, 105586. https://doi.org/10.1016/j.archger.2024.105586

Luik, A. I., van der Riet, J., Batelaan, N. M., & Ten Have, M. (2024). Insomnia and the incidence, recurrence and persistence of common mental disorders: Sex-differences in the general population. *Psychiatry Research*, *331*, 115658. https://doi.org/10.1016/j.psychres.2023.115658

Ma, Y., Yu, S., Li, Q., Zhang, H., Zeng, R., Luo, R., Lian, Q., Leung, F. W., Duan, C., Sha, W., & Chen, H. (2024). Sleep patterns, genetic susceptibility, and digestive diseases: a large-scale longitudinal cohort study. *International Journal of Surgery*, *110*(9), 5471–5482. https://doi.org/10.1097/JS9.0000000000001695

Malhotra, A., Ayappa, I., Ayas, N., Collop, N., Kirsch, D., Mcardle, N., Mehra, R., Pack, A. I., Punjabi, N., White, D. P., & Gottlieb, D. J. (2021). Metrics of sleep apnea severity: Beyond the apnea-hypopnea index. *Sleep*, *44*(7), zsab030. https://doi.org/10.1093/sleep/zsab030

Makhfudli, M., Tonapa, S. I., Has, E. M. M., Chong, M. C., & Efendi, F. (2024). Efficacy of mind-body exercise to reduce sleep disturbance and depression among older adults: A systematic review and meta-analysis. *Asian Nursing Research*, *18*(4), 408–419. https://doi.org/10.1016/j.anr.2024.08.002

Mansur, A., Castillo, P. R., Rocha Cabrero, F., & Bokhari, S. R. A. (2023). Restless legs syndrome. In *StatPearls*. StatPearls Publishing. https://www.ncbi.nlm.nih.gov/books/NBK430878

Meyer, N., Lok, R., Schmidt, C., Kyle, S. D., McClung, C. A., Cajochen, C., Scheer, F. A. J. L., Jones, M. W., & Chellappa, S. L. (2024). The sleep-circadian interface: A window into mental disorders. *Proceedings of the National Academy of Sciences of the United States of America, 121*(9), e2214756121. https://doi.org/10.1073/pnas.2214756121

Mitler, M. M., Carskadon, M. A., Czeisier, C. A., Dement, W. C., Dinges, D. F., & Graeber, R. C. (1988). Catastrophes, sleep, and public policy: Consensus report. *Sleep, 11*(1), 100–109.

Morgenthaler, T. I., Auerbach, S., Casey, K. R., Kristo, D., Maganti, R., Ramar, K., Zak, R., & Kartje, R. (2018). Position paper for the treatment of nightmare disorder in adults: An American Academy of Sleep Medicine position paper. *Journal of Clinical Sleep Medicine, 14*(6), 1041–1055.

Mundt, J. M., Schuiling, M. D., Warlick, C., Dietch, J. R., Wescott, A. B., Hagenaars, M., Furst, A., Khorramdel, K., & Baron, K. G. (2023). Behavioral and psychological treatments for NREM parasomnias: A systematic review. *Sleep Medicine, 111*, 36–53. https://doi.org/10.1016/j.sleep.2023.09.004

National Center for Complementary and Integrative Health. (2020). *Valerian*. National Institutes of Health, U.S. Department of Health and Human Services. https://www.nccih.nih.gov/health/valerian

National Sleep Foundation (NSF). (2021). *Sleep by the numbers*. https://www.thensf.org/sleep-facts-and-statistics/#:~:text=35%25%20of%20all%20adults%20in,to%20seven%20times%20a%20week

National Sleep Foundation (NSF). (2022). *Snoring and sleep*. [Online]. Retrieved February 17, 2022, from https://sleepfoundation.org/sleep-disorders-problems/other-sleep-disorders/snoring

National Sleep Foundation (NSF). (2024a). *Sleep health*. Retrieved December 3, 2024, from https://www.sleephealthjournal.org/content/professionalpracticegaps

National Sleep Foundation (NSF). (2024b). *Sleep in America poll: Teens' sleep and mental health are strongly connected*. Retrieved March 14, 2024, from https://www.thensf.org/wp-content/uploads/2024/03/NSF-Sleep-in-America-2024-Report_final.pdf

Naqvi, I. H., Ahmed, J., Salim, M., Ubaid, M., Malik, F., Afzal, R., Ashrafi, M. M., & Khan, M. A. A. (2021). Restless leg syndrome in patients with liver cirrhosis! its frequency, severity, and correlation. *CNS & Neurological Disorders Drug Targets, 20*(5), 465–472. https://doi.org/10.2174/1871527319666201208102104

Ng, A. S., & Chan, W. S. (2023). Sleep quality, sleep-related experiences, and dissociation in adult survivors of childhood trauma. *Behavioral Sleep Medicine, 21*(6), 659–670.

Nomura, T., Horikoshi, T., Kitano, Y., Yamada, M., Kondo, K., & Kikuchi, S. (2024). The morphometrical evaluation after uvulopalatopharyngoplasty. *Sleep & Breathing, 28*(2), 869–875. https://doi.org/10.1007/s11325-023-02926-w

Ohi, K., Ochi, R., Noda, Y., Wada, M., Sugiyama, S., Nishi, A., Shioiri, T., Mimura, M., & Nakajima, S. (2021). Polygenic risk scores for major psychiatric and neurodevelopmental disorders contribute to sleep disturbance in childhood: Adolescent Brain Cognitive Development (ABCD) Study. *Translational Psychiatry, 11*(1), 187. https://doi.org/10.1038/s41398-021-01308-8

Olszewska, E., Rogalska, J., & Brzóska, M. M. (2021). The association of oxidative stress in the uvular mucosa with obstructive sleep apnea syndrome: A clinical study. *Journal of Clinical Medicine, 10*(5), 1132. https://doi.org/10.3390/jcm10051132

Palagini, L., Manni, R., Aguglia, E., Amore, M., Brugnoli, R., Bioulac, S., Bourgin, P., Micoulaud Franchi, J. A., Girardi, P., Grassi, L., Lopez, R., Mencacci, C., Plazzi, G., Maruani, J., Minervino, A., Philip, P., Royant Parola, S., Poirot, I., Nobili, L., ... Geoffroy, P. A. (2021). International expert opinions and recommendations on the use of melatonin in the treatment of insomnia and circadian sleep disturbances in adult neuropsychiatric disorders. *Frontiers in Psychiatry, 12*, 688890. https://doi.org/10.3389/fpsyt.2021.688890

Parperis, K., Philippou, S., Christophi, C. A., Constantinou, A., Bargiotas, P., & Psarelis, S. (2024). Restless leg syndrome in systemic lupus erythematosus: Associations with disease activity, quality of life and depression. *Sleep Medicine, 121*, 111–116. https://doi.org/10.1016/j.sleep.2024.06.020

Polyné, N. C., Miller, K. E., Brownlow, J., & Gehrman, P. R. (2021). Insomnia: Sex differences and age of onset in active duty Army soldiers. *Sleep Health, 7*(4), 504–507. https://doi.org/10.1016/j.sleh.2021.03.003

Rajaratnam, S. M., & Arendt, J. (2001). Health in a 24-h society. *Lancet, 358*(9286), 999–1005. https://doi.org/10.1016/S0140-6736(01)06108-6

Rizzo, L., Barbetta, E., Ruberti, F., Petz, M., Tornesello, M., Deolmi, M., Fainardi, V., & Esposito, S. (2024). The role of telemedicine in children with obstructive sleep apnea syndrome (OSAS): A review of the literature. *Journal of Clinical Medicine, 13*(7), 2108. https://doi.org/10.3390/jcm13072108

Sahu, N., Patil, P. S. A., & Longkumer, I. (2024). Understanding and treating nightmares: A comprehensive review of psychosocial strategies for adults and children. *Cureus, 16*(9), e70044. https://doi.org/10.7759/cureus.70044

Saini, E. K., Keiley, M. K., Fuller-Rowell, T. E., Duke, A. M., & El-Sheikh, M. (2021). Socioeconomic status and sleep among couples. *Behavioral Sleep Medicine, 19*(2), 159–177. https://doi.org/10.1080/15402002.2020.1721501

Salari, N., Darvishi, N., Khaledi-Paveh, B., Vaisi-Raygani, A., Jalali, R., Daneshkhah, A., Bartina, Y., & Mohammadi, M. (2021). A systematic review and meta-analysis of prevalence of insomnia in the third trimester of pregnancy. *BMC Pregnancy and Childbirth, 21*(1), 284. https://doi.org/10.1186/s12884-021-03755-z

Sanchez, E., Blais, H., Duclos, C., Arbour, C., Van Der Maren, S., El-Khatib, H., Baril, A. A., Bernard, F., Carrier, J., & Gosselin, N. (2022). Sleep from acute to chronic traumatic brain injury and cognitive outcomes. *Sleep, 45*(8), zsac123. https://doi.org/10.1093/sleep/zsac123

Sato, S., Liu, Y., Ikeda, A., Filomeno, R., Suzuki, Y., Maruyama, K., Tomooka, K., Wada, H., Koyama, Y., & Tanigawa, T. (2021). Work-family conflict and insomnia symptoms among women working in aged care services in Japan. *Sleep Medicine, 82*, 155–158. https://doi.org/10.1016/j.sleep.2021.03.034

Sato, S., Solanas, G., Sassone-Corsi, P., & Benitah, S. A. (2022). Tuning up an aged clock: Circadian clock regulation in metabolism and aging. *Translational Medicine of Aging, 6*. 1–13. https://doi-org.libproxy.siue.edu/10.1016/j.tma.2021.11.003.

Savage, R. A., Zafar, N., Yohannan, S., & Miller, J. M. M. (2021). Melatonin. In *StatPearls*. StatPearls Publishing.

Schyvens, A. M., Van Oost, N. C., Aerts, J. M., Masci, F., Peters, B., Neven, A., Dirix, H., Wets, G., Ross, V., & Verbraecken, J. (2024). Accuracy of fitbit charge 4, garmin vivosmart 4, and whoop versus polysomnography: Systematic review. *JMIR mHealth and uHealth, 12*, e52192. https://doi.org/10.2196/52192

Silber, M. H., Buchfuhrer, M. J., Earley, C. J., Koo, B. B., Manconi, M., Winkelman, J. W., & Scientific and Medical Advisory Board of the Restless Legs Syndrome Foundation. (2021). The management of restless legs syndrome: An updated algorithm. *Mayo Clinic Proceedings, 96*(7), 1921–1937. https://doi.org/10.1016/j.mayocp.2020.12.026

Slowik, J. M., Collen, J. F., & Yow, A. G. (2023). Narcolepsy. In *StatPearls*. StatPearls Publishing. https://www.ncbi.nlm.nih.gov/books/NBK459236

Suni, E. (2024). How much sleep do babies and kids need? Sleep Foundation. Retrieved December 7, 2024, from https://www.sleepfoundation.org/children-and-sleep/how-much-sleep-do-kids-need

Sutton, E. L. (2021). Insomnia. *Annals of Internal Medicine, 174*(3), ITC33–ITC48. https://doi.org/10.7326/AITC202103160

Tai, J. E., Phillips, C. L., Yee, B. J., & Grunstein, R. R. (2024). Obstructive sleep apnoea in obesity: A review. *Clinical Obesity, 14*(3), e12651. https://doi.org/10.1111/cob.12651

Tang, Y., Gong, M., Qin, X., Su, H., Wang, Z., & Dong, H. (2021). The therapeutic effect of aromatherapy on insomnia: A meta-analysis. *Journal of Affective Disorders, 288*, 1–9. https://doi.org/10.1016/j.jad.2021.03.066

Thornton, J. D., Dudley, K. A., Saeed, G. J., Schuster, S. T., Schell, A., Spilsbury, J. C., & Patel, S. R. (2022). Differences in symptoms and severity of obstructive sleep apnea between Black and White patients. *Annals of the American Thoracic Society, 19*(2), 272–278. https://doi.org/10.1513/AnnalsATS.202012-1483OC

Van Horn, N. L., & Street, M. (2023). Night terrors. *In StatPearls*. StatPearls Publishing. https://www.ncbi.nlm.nih.gov/books/NBK493222

Venkatnarayan, K., Devaraj, U., Veluthat, C., Louis, V., Ramachandran, P., D'Souza, G., & Krishnaswamy, U. M. (2021). The effect of CPAP therapy on excessive daytime sleepiness and quality of life in subjects with obstructive sleep apnoea: An AB design study. *Sleep & Breathing, 25*(3), 1351–1357. https://doi.org/10.1007/s11325-020-02237-4

Vincent, N., Dirkse, D., Giannouli, E., & McQuarrie, A. (2023). Transdiagnostic cognitive behavioral therapy for nightmares and parasomnias. *Journal of Clinical Sleep Medicine, 19*(3), 499–509.

Vora, L. K., Gholap, A. D., Hatvate, N. T., Naren, P., Khan, S., Chavda, V. P., Balar, P. C., Gandhi, J., & Khatri, D. K. (2024). Essential oils for clinical aromatherapy: A comprehensive review. *Journal of Ethnopharmacology, 330*, 118180. https://doi.org/10.1016/j.jep.2024.118180

Walsh, J., Dement, W., & Dinges, D. (2011). Sleep medicine, public policy, and public health. In: M. H. Kryger, T. Roth, & W. C. Dement (eds.), *Principles and practice of sleep medicine* (5th ed., pp. 716–724). W.B. Saunders.

Wang, Z., Tang, Y., Wang, G., Deng, Y., Jiang, Y., Sun, W., Sun, X., Ip, P., Owens, J., Zhao, M., Xiao, Y., Jiang, F., & Wang, G. (2024a). Insufficient sleep is associated with increasing trends in adolescent suicidal behaviors. *The Journal of Adolescent Health, 74*(6), 1198–1207. https://doi.org/10.1016/j.jadohealth.2024.01.030

Wang, Q., Wu, S., Luo, Z., Pu, L., Wang, X., Guo, M., Zhang, M., Tang, H., Chen, M., Kong, L., Huang, P., Chen, L., Li, Z., Zhao, D., & Xiong, Z.

(2024b). Effects of light therapy on sleep and circadian rhythm in older type 2 diabetics living in long-term care facilities: A randomized controlled trial. *Frontiers in Endocrinology*, *15*, 1307537. https://doi.org/10.3389/fendo.2024.1307537

Weng, L., Hong, H., Zhang, Q., Xiao, C., Zhang, Q., Wang, Q., Huang, J., & Lai, D. (2024). Sleep deprivation triggers the excessive activation of ovarian primordial follicles via β2 adrenergic receptor signaling. *Advanced Science*, *11*(41), e2402393. https://doi.org/10.1002/advs.202402393

Winegar, R. (2024). Promoting healthy sleep among older adults. *Geriatric Nursing*, *58*, 298–303. https://doi.org/10.1016/j.gerinurse.2024.05.032

Xu, J., Zhang, L., Sun, H., Gao, Z., Wang, M., Hu, M., Ji, Q., & Guo, L. (2023). Psychological resilience and quality of life among middle-aged and older adults hospitalized with chronic diseases: Multiple mediating effects through sleep quality and depression. *BMC Geriatrics*, *23*(1), 752.

Yeghiazarians, Y., Jneid, H., Tietjens, J. R., Redline, S., Brown, D. L., El-Sherif, N., Mehra, R., Bozkurt, B., Ndumele, C. E., & Somers, V. K. (2021). Obstructive sleep apnea and cardiovascular disease: A scientific statement from the American Heart Association. *Circulation*, *144*(3), e56–e67. https://doi.org/10.1161/CIR.0000000000000988

Zergham, A. S., & Chauhan, Z. (2021). Somnambulism. In *StatPearls*. StatPearls Publishing.

Zhao, F. Y., Xu, P., Kennedy, G. A., Conduit, R., Zhang, W. J., Wang, Y. M., Fu, Q. Q., & Zheng, Z. (2023). Identifying complementary and alternative medicine recommendations for insomnia treatment and care: a systematic review and critical assessment of comprehensive clinical practice guidelines. *Frontiers in Public Health*, *11*, 1157419. https://doi.org/10.3389/fpubh.2023.1157419

Zhang, J., Chu, M., Tian, Z., Xie, K., Cui, Y., Liu, L., Meng, J., Yan, H., Ji, Y. M., Jiang, Z., Xia, T. X., Wang, D., Wang, X., Zhao, Y., Ye, H., Li, J., Wang, L., & Wu, L. (2022). Clinical profile of fatal familial insomnia: Phenotypic variation in 129 polymorphisms and geographical regions. *Journal of Neurology Neurosurgery and Psychiatry*, *93*(3), 291–297. https://doi.org/10.1136/jnnp-2021-327247

Zhou, A., McDaniel, M., Hong, X., Mattin, M., Wang, X., & Shih, C. H. (2023). Emotion dysregulation mediates the association between acute sleep disturbance and later posttraumatic stress symptoms in trauma exposed adults. *European Journal of Psychotraumatology*, *14*(2), 2202056.

Zheng, D., Yuan, X., Ma, C., Liu, Y., VanEvery, H., Sun, Y., Wu, S., & Gao, X. (2021). Alcohol consumption and sleep quality: A community-based study. *Public Health Nutrition*, *24*(15), 4851–4858. https://doi.org/10.1017/S1368980020004553

Zhou, X., Du, J., Liang, Y., Dai, C., Zhao, L., Liu, X., Tan, C., Mo, L., & Chen, L. (2021). The efficacy and safety of pharmacological treatments for restless legs syndrome: Systemic review and network meta-analysis. *Frontiers in Neuroscience*, *15*, 751643. https://doi.org/10.3389/fnins.2021.751643

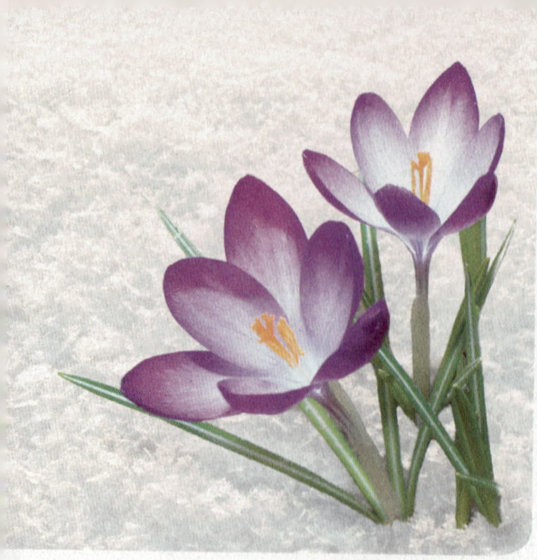

35 Sexual Disorders

Nursing Care of People With Sexual Dysfunction and Paraphilias*

Mary Ann Boyd

KEYCONCEPT

- sexual arousal
- sexual disorders
- sexual health
- sexuality

LEARNING OBJECTIVES

After studying this chapter, you will be able to:

1. Examine the role of sexuality and sexual response in sexual disorders.
2. Analyze primary theories of female orgasmic disorder and erectile dysfunction disorder and their relationships to comorbidities.
3. Evaluate the significance of trauma in the appearance of sexual disorders.
4. Select strategies to establish a therapeutic relationship with people with sexual disorders.
5. Using a clinical judgment model, formulate a person-centered, recovery-oriented nursing care plan for people with sexual disorders.
6. Identify medications used to treat people with sexual disorders and evaluate the effectiveness of the drugs.
7. Develop wellness strategies for people with sexual disorders.
8. Support the integration of health care and mental health care for people with sexual disorders.
9. Compare and contrast sexual disorders and related disorders.

KEY TERMS

• acquired premature ejaculation (PE) • ambiguous genitalia • anorgasmia • delayed ejaculation • disorders of sex development (DSDs) • dual-control model • dyspareunia • erectile disorder • excitement phase • female orgasmic disorder • female sexual interest/arousal disorder • flibanserin • human sexual response cycle • intracavernosal pharmacotherapy • lifelong premature ejaculation (PE) • male hypoactive sexual desire disorder • orgasmic phase • paraphilias • phosphodiesterase 5 (PDES5) inhibitors • plateau phase • premature ejaculation • resolution • sensate focus • sex determination • sex drive • sex therapist • sexual continuity • sexual differentiation • sexual desire • sexual dysfunctions • SRY gene • vaginismus

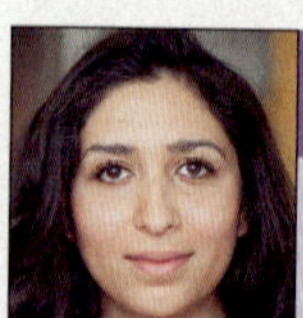

Case Study: Alice

Alice, age 35, was diagnosed with multiple sclerosis 3 years ago. She experiences transitory visual blurring, weakness of the lower limbs, and mood swings. She also has issues with urinary leakage and occasional bowel incontinence.

---

*In this chapter, "male" refers to a person assigned male at birth, and "female" refers to a person assigned female at birth.

INTRODUCTION

Sexuality is associated with sensuality, pleasure and pleasuring, intimacy, trust, communication, love and affection, attractiveness, and reverence for life. Sexuality influences how we view ourselves (self-concept) and, consequently, how we relate to others.

Sexuality is influenced by an individual's emotional and physiologic status, beliefs and values, and morals and laws of society. Barriers to sexual fulfillment can arise from medical issues (e.g., neurologic, musculoskeletal, cardiovascular, respiratory, renal, hepatic, and cognitive impairments); from pain, weakness, and fatigue; and from sequelae of surgical procedures and drugs. More often, sexual issues are a result of the interplay of multiple causes that can include intrapsychic, interpersonal, and sociocultural factors. This chapter focuses on sexuality and sexual functioning and discusses nursing care for people experiencing sexual dysfunction.

> **KEYCONCEPT Sexuality** is a life force that encompasses how we understand our bodies and relationships and how these characteristics relate to all that is human.

SEXUAL DEVELOPMENT

All of us are sexual beings. Sexuality is who we are, not what we do—the sum total of all our biologic and experiential influences. Sexuality encompasses all aspects of who we are—our values and beliefs, bodies, desires, relationships, and our thoughts and feelings about all of these. The innermost concept of self as male or female, neither, or both can be different from the physical state. Gender, gender identity, and sexual orientation are related concepts that are discussed in Chapter 3.

Sex Determination and Sexual Differentiation

Sexual development occurs in a precise sequence of two stages: sex determination and sexual differentiation. **Sex determination** is guided by the sex chromosomes inherited at conception and their effect on the undifferentiated gonad that has the potential to develop into either a testis (male) or ovary (female). At 6 weeks postfertilization there is no sexual difference. The **SRY gene** located on the inherited Y chromosome is responsible for the production of testosterone, which initiates the differentiation of the embryonic gonad resulting in male penis, prostate, and scrotum. After the male sex organs are formed, testosterone levels temporarily rise, causing a permanent sexual organization of the brain that is different from that of females. The absence of the Y chromosome results in the development of the female ovaries. The newly formed gonads secrete hormones to modulate the formation of internal and external genitalia (Mehmood & Rentea, 2023).

Sexual differentiation is the developmental process and pathway toward developing male or female phenotypes (observable traits). Sex differentiation typically follows a pathway consistent with the chromosomal sex of the embryo. Sex differentiation is complicated and involves multiple levels including chromosomal, gonadal, hormonal, phenotypic, and psychological factors (Aatsha et al., 2023). An in depth explanation of sexual differentiation is outside the scope of this text.

Disorders of sex development (DSDs) are congenital conditions associated with atypical development of gonads, internal genitalia, or external genitalia. In some people, there is a conflict between sex determination and sex differentiation of the gonads, external gonads, external genitalia, internal genitalia, or secondary sex characteristics. Any deviation from the usual pattern of differentiation can present as a DSD. People with these disorders are stigmatized, which negatively impacts their mental health and well-being (Aatsha et al., 2023).

For example, sex is often assigned at the time of birth based on the appearance of the external genitalia. The external genitalia are highly prone to variation from sexual differentiation and may present as **ambiguous genitalia;** that is, the genitalia are not clearly male or female. The genitals may either be incompletely developed, have characteristics of both sexes, or not match the infant's internal sex organs (Aatsha et al., 2023; Mehmood & Renea, 2023).

SEXUAL BEHAVIORS ACROSS THE LIFESPAN

Sexual Behaviors in Children and Adolescents

In infants, sexual behaviors are rare with the exception of hand-to-genital contact. As children become more aware of their body parts and the physical sensations deriving from their genitals, they become more interested in gender differences. For 2- to 5-year-old children, sexual behaviors are varied and more common than in older children, who are more aware of the social norms of concealing sexual behaviors. For example, young children observe and comment on body differences, demonstrate interest in bathroom habits and urination, and handle their genitals for pleasure and comfort. Their curiosity leads them to want to look at and touch adult bodies and breasts. Mutual genital exploration or urination among children may be seen at this time along with questions about where babies come from.

Age-appropriate solitary sexual behaviors (i.e., touching one's own genitals) are also common. At this early age, these behaviors do not have the sexualized meaning they do in adults. However, if young children are exposed to sexually explicit material (internet, movies, observation of parental sexual activities) or if their parents/caregivers overreact to age-appropriate behaviors, these activities can take on additional, more adult-like, meanings. If preoccupation with the sexual behaviors interferes with the child's ability to grow and function, then the behaviors are problematic. For example, an 8-year-old boy sneaking to the bathroom several times a day to touch his genitals needs help in addressing this behavior.

Sexual behaviors are common and occur in 42% to 73% of children by the time they reach 13 years of age. In general, the frequency of overt sexual behaviors decreases with age. These behaviors may not be as obvious because as children mature, they become increasingly more covert in their sexual behavior. For example, whereas 6- to 9-year-old children often touch their genitals at home, stand too close to others, and try to look at people when they are nude, 10- to 12-year-old children, who are actually more interested in and know more about sex, limit their behavior to looking at nudity in magazines, television, and the internet (American Academy of Pediatrics Council on Child Abuse and Neglect, 2023; Chouinard-Thivierge et al., 2021).

In the United States from 2015 to 2019, 40.5% of never-married female teenagers aged 15 to 19 and 38% of never-married male teenagers had had sexual intercourse (Abma & Martinez, 2023). A variety of circumstances lead to this sexual activity. Sex may be engaged in because of peer pressure or because friends or social groups condone sex. The need to be convinced of being in love, wanting to feel loved, and fear of rejection all precipitate risk-taking behavior. Depending on the family environment, stresses, and observation of adult sexual activities, children may exhibit more adult sexual behaviors, which may be considered typical for the environment in which they live. For children and adolescents, sexual behavior (usually involving other people) is considered atypical when it occurs at a greater frequency or at a much earlier age than would be developmentally or culturally expected.

Sexual Behaviors in Adulthood

Sexual activities occur throughout young adulthood and continue through middle and late adulthood. Although the frequency and types of sexual encounters may change, the quality need not change. During the fourth to fifth decades of life, physical changes become more obvious, and so various chronic illnesses, such as hypertension or arthritis, may also develop. As a result of decreased endocrine production, gradual changes to body tissues occur over a 15- to 20-year span.

In people assigned female at birth, estrogen deficiency during menopause affects the sexual system by causing a gradual thinning of the vaginal mucosa, decreasing the elasticity of muscles and orgasmic force, and increasing breast involution (sagging of breast tissue). Vaginal lubrication decreases, which may cause dyspareunia (i.e., pain during intercourse), often requiring the use of a water-soluble lubricant or saliva. Although many females experience little or no change in sexual function, both decreased and increased sexual activity and interest are possible. In some females, more time is required to lubricate the vulvovaginal areas and to strengthen clitoral response. Orgasmic capacity and breast response remain fairly constant in females who are appropriately stimulated. Most physical symptoms arise from vasomotor instability in females, which can include morning fatigue, vague pains, hot flashes, dizziness, chills, sweating, nervousness, crying spells, decreased sexual potency, and palpitations (Lugo & Tetrokalashvili, 2022).

In people assigned male at birth, decreasing testosterone production is responsible for sexual changes. The amount and viability of sperm decrease, erections become less firm, and more direct sexual stimulation is needed. The testicles begin to decrease in elasticity and size, ejaculation time increases, and the force of ejaculation decreases. Spermatogenesis decreases, although viable sperm, capable of impregnation, continue to be produced. Seminal fluid is less voluminous and viscous, and ejaculatory force is decreased (Mauvais-Jarvis & Lindsey, 2024). Older males, however, are capable of sustaining erection much longer with decreased ejaculatory demand, potentially benefiting older partners, who may require increased time to reach orgasm. Sexual activity is often perceived as more satisfactory than previously experienced (National Institute on Aging, 2022).

Sexual continuity (regularly engaging in sexual activity) depends to a great extent on good physical health, activity, and regular opportunities for sexual expression and sexual activity in all forms, including masturbation and same-gender behavior. An important influence on sexuality is the attitude of others, especially attitudes that define specific behaviors as acceptable or unacceptable. This is especially true in later life (Syme & Cohn, 2021). In healthy adults, sexual function, although modified by the aging process, should remain satisfying despite a differently timed sequence. Frequent sexual activity, whether by coitus, masturbation, or other practices, usually preserves sexual potency.

SEXUAL RESPONSES

Understanding typical sexual responses helps when discussing this very personal, but important, aspect of being human with patients. The following section provides an overview of major concepts and theories related to sexual responses.

Sexual Desire and Arousal

Sexual desire is the ability, interest, or willingness to receive or a motivational state to seek sexual activity. In healthy adults, the **sex drive** is the physical urge or motivation to engage in sexual activity. Sex drive is integrated through the central nervous system (CNS) with the autonomic nervous system governing extragenital changes (increased respiration and heart rate). The parasympathetic nervous system largely controls arousal, and the sympathetic nervous system largely controls orgasmic discharge (Waxenbaum et al., 2023). Sexual stimulation brings about a total-body response with dramatic changes seen in the genitals and breasts. Sex hormones, particularly androgen, influence desire in individuals, but less is known about hormonal influence in females. The higher centers of the brain apparently mediate the lower reflex response centers which supports the relationship between cognitive and affective states and sexual function (Pinto et al., 2024).

During sexual arousal, individuals experience an increased heart rate, blood pressure, respiration, and myotonia.

KEYCONCEPT Sexual arousal is the state of mounting sexual tension characterized by vasoconstriction and myotonia.

In males, visual stimulation (i.e., seeing a naked individual), fantasies, memories, or physical stimulation of the genitals or other regions (e.g., nipples) causes the parasympathetic system to involuntarily release chemicals that dilate penile arteries. A rapid inflow of arterial blood to the cavernous spaces of corpora cavernosa, facilitated by high levels of intrapenile nitric oxide, causes stiffening and elongation of the penis. With continued stimulation, an emission of semen and an ejaculation occurs. Subcortical structures (hypothalamus, brainstem, spinal cord) and cortical area regulate sexual response. Dopaminergic and serotonergic systems play an important role, along with other neurotransmitter systems such as the adrenergic and cholinergic systems. Testosterone is involved throughout the male sexual response (Bogacki-Rychlik et al., 2024).

Fantasies, visual stimuli, and physical stimulation are also important for sexual arousal in females, but physical stimulation seems more important for females and visual stimuli for males. The parasympathetic nervous system increases blood flow to the genitalia of the female, lubricating the vagina and enlarging the breast and clitoris. Estrogens and progestins are involved in female sexual functioning, but androgens are needed by both males and females to maintain arousal (Arias-Castillo et al., 2023).

Theoretical Models of Sexual Response

In 1966, Masters and Johnson described the classic **human sexual response cycle** as a linear model consisting of four phases: excitement, plateau, orgasm, and resolution. In the **excitement phase,** erotic feelings lead to a penile erection in males and vaginal lubrication in females. Heart rate and respirations also increase. The **plateau phase** is represented by sexual pleasure and increased muscle tension, heart rate, and blood flow to the genitals. For males, the **orgasmic phase** is ejaculation of semen, and for females it consists of rhythmic contractions of the vaginal muscles. Females also experience orgasm by clitoral stimulation as well as the vaginal–clitoral–urethral complex (part of the vulva or external genitalia). For most males, immediately after orgasm and before resolution, a refractory period occurs when no response is possible. In contrast to males, females do not have a refractory period and are capable of multiple orgasms (Arias-Castillo et al., 2023). **Resolution** is the gradual return of the organs and body systems to the nonaroused state. Muscle tension and vasocongestion subside. Breathing and heart rate gradually return to preexcitement rates. Usually, the individual feels a sense of relaxation, relief of tension, and satisfaction (Masters & Johnson, 1966, 1970). This model is considered relevant in 2024 and is used as a theoretical research model (Herder et al., 2023).

This linear approach is criticized as being primarily a biologic model and does not account for nonbiologic experiences such as pleasure, satisfaction, and the context of the relationship. To account for emotional and psychological aspects of sexual response, a circular model focusing on female sexual responses was developed by Basson (2001). This model proposes that nonsexual interpersonal factors, such as a desire for physical connection and intimacy needs, also motivate females to engage in sexual relations, not only sexual release. Arousal and desire appear to be interchangeable and inseparable from one another, with one reinforcing the other. Subjective feelings of interest may follow the sensation of arousal, and sexual satisfaction may be experienced without orgasm.

These two models—linear and circular—have been debated for years. Both models are supported empirically as being relevant to sexual responses in females, who report that sexual experiences are at times consistent with the linear and circular models at other times. There is also evidence that the circular model is relevant for males as well as the linear model (Balon, 2022; Parish et al., 2022).

Dual-Control Model

Another conceptualization, the **dual-control model,** focuses on individual variability and proposes that sexual responses involve an interaction between sexual excitement and sexual inhibition (Bancroft et al., 2009). This model assumes that (1) neurobiologic inhibition of sexual response is adaptive and occurs in situations when sexual activity would be a disadvantage, dangerous, or distracting; (2) individuals vary in their propensity for sexual excitation and inhibition; and (3) the context and cultural meaning attributed to the interaction of the individuals are important stimuli for both excitatory and inhibitory processes. Emerging research is showing that the dual-control model is an important framework in understanding how mood influences both subjective and genital sexuality in individuals (Granados et al., 2021; Janssen & Bancroft, 2023).

SEXUAL HEALTH AND WELLNESS

Sexual health is an important aspect of wellness. Sexual health is viewed holistically and positively and is relevant throughout the individual's lifespan. Influenced by gender norms, expectations, and power dynamics, sexual health is understood within specific social, economic, and political contexts (WHO, n.d.a). Major health threats related to sexuality are human immunodeficiency virus (HIV)/acquired immunodeficiency syndrome (AIDS), hepatitis, and sexually transmitted infections (STIs).

KEYCONCEPT According to the working definition of the World Health Organization (WHO), **sexual health** is "a state of physical, emotional, mental and social well-being in relation to sexuality; it is not merely the absence of disease, dysfunction or infirmity" (WHO, n.d.b). Sexuality and sexual relationships include the possibility of having pleasurable and safe sexual experiences that are "free of coercion, discrimination and violence"; in addition, sexual rights "must be respected, protected and fulfilled" for all people (WHO, n.d.b).

The mental health of the LGBTQ+ community is at risk due to discrimination in environments where they live, learn, and work (Shaikh et al., 2024). Sexual orientation discrimination is most prevalent in early young adulthood, but it occurs in all ages. Higher risks for alcohol, tobacco, and drug use disorders are associated with discrimination at older ages (Perez et al., 2024). One of the goals of *Healthy People 2030* is to improve the health, safety, and well-being of LGBTQ+ individuals (Healthy People 2030, 2021). Nurses are in a unique position to provide gender-affirming care in order to improve the safety and well-being of the LGBTQ+ communities. See Box 35.1.

BOX 35.1

Mental Health Inequities: Reducing LGBTQ+ Adolescent Mental Health Inequities

LGBTQ+ young people have elevated rates of mental health issues compared to their cisgender heterosexual peers. Systematic reviews and meta-analyses consistently report that LGBTQ+ students have a higher prevalence of depression, self-harm, suicidal ideation and attempts, and substance use compared to cisgender heterosexual youth. School environment is a leading predictor of emotional and behavioral outcomes of students. To improve the mental health of LGBTQ+ students, school-based interventions must address the silence, victimization, and misrecognition that these students experience. Research shows that developing a LGBTQ+ inclusive school environment needs policies that specifically address homophobic, biphobic, and transphobic bullying and discrimination by staff and students. A school program supporting the mental health of LGBTQ+ students includes staff training and support for implementing policies, an inclusive curriculum, school resources for LGBTQ+ support and activism, and ensuring that there are school staff available for LGBTQ+ students to talk to and trust.

Source: McDermott, E., Kaley, A., Kaner, E., Limmer, M., McGovern, R., McNulty, F., Nelson, R., Geijer-Simpson, E., & Spencer, L. (2024). Reducing LGBTQ+ adolescent mental health inequalities: A realist review of school-based interventions. *Journal of Mental Health*, *33*(6), 768–778. https://doi.org/10.1080/09638237.2023.2245894

SEXUAL DYSFUNCTIONS OVERVIEW

Sexual dysfunctions are a group of disorders that are characterized by clinically significant disturbances in the individual's ability to respond sexually or to experience sexual pleasure (American Psychiatric Association [APA], 2022). Unhealthy lifestyle and obesity contribute to the development of sexual dysfunctions, due to their negative impact on cardiovascular and metabolic functions. Tobacco smoking, alcohol use disorder, substance use disorder (SUD), and chronic stress lead to the development of sexual dysfunction (McCabe et al., 2024).

The *DSM-5-TR* identifies the following as sexual disorders: delayed ejaculation (DE), erectile disorder (ED), female orgasmic disorder, female sexual interest/arousal disorder, genitopelvic pain/penetration disorder, male hypoactive sexual desire disorder, and premature ejaculation (PE) and other specified and unspecified disorders. These dysfunctions can be lifelong or acquired and are categorized as mild, moderate, or severe. An occasional episode is not considered dysfunctional (APA, 2022).

In this chapter, female orgasmic disorder is highlighted because it is among the most commonly occurring sexual disorders in females, and **anorgasmia** (the inability to achieve an orgasm) is a frequent medication side effect. PE and ED are emphasized because they are among the most commonly occurring sexual disorders in people assigned male at birth. Paraphilias are also included in the discussion.

KEYCONCEPT **Sexual disorders** are clinical disturbances caused by the inability to respond sexually or to experience sexual pleasure.

FEMALE ORGASMIC DISORDER

A female orgasm is the least understood of all sexual responses; no universal definition exists (Basanta & Nuño de la Rosa, 2023). Descriptions of the orgasmic experience of females vary from altered consciousness to focused sensation. Many people require clitoral stimulation to reach orgasm, and only a small group of females report that they always experience orgasm during intercourse. An orgasmic disorder is the inability to reach orgasm by any means, either alone or with a partner, and/or markedly reduced intensity of orgasmic sensations for at least 6 months. The inability to experience an orgasm must cause clinically significant distress to be considered a disorder (Davis, 2024).

DIAGNOSTIC CRITERIA

Female orgasmic disorder is characterized by the inability of a female to experience orgasm or the intensity of the orgasm is markedly reduced at least 75% of the time. If other explanations for the anorgasmia exist, such as substance use, medications, or interpersonal issues, the diagnosis is not used (APA, 2022).

EPIDEMIOLOGY AND RISK FACTORS

Debate about the issue of female orgasms is considerable. Estimated prevalence of female's inability to reach orgasm ranges from 9% (in the United States) to 41.2% in Southeast Asia (Bancroft & Graham, 2011; Marchand, 2021).

Poor physical health, mental health, poor self-image, abuse, and relationship issues, especially partner difficulties, are the primary risk factors. Age, arousal difficulty, and lubrication difficulty are related to difficulty reaching orgasm (Davis, 2024).

ETIOLOGY

In general, any local genital or pelvic pathology, trauma, or surgery that causes pain on intercourse can produce impaired response to sexual stimulation. Spinal cord damage, endocrine disorders, systemic diseases, chronic pain, and general debility can interfere with sexual responses. CNS depressants (e.g., alcohol, barbiturates, narcotics), psychiatric disorders, infections, inflammatory disorders, and pregnancy have all been associated with female orgasmic disorder. Additionally, many medications such as antidepressants, contraceptives, antihypertensives, and substances (e.g., alcohol) can also affect the sexual response (Davis, 2024).

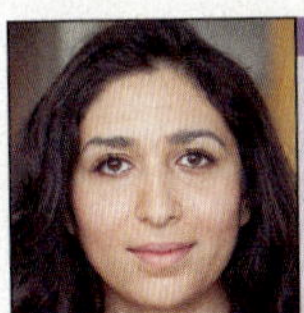

Consider Alice

Alice admits that her sexual activity is far less frequent than before her illness. She feels she is no longer attractive or interested in sexual activities.

How would you discuss her feelings? What information would you give her to help her look at her situation realistically?

Sexual responses can be inhibited by many different emotional and cognitions, including sexual anxiety and guilt, anger or hostility toward one's partner, indifference toward one's partner, depression, or excessive and intrusive thoughts. Misinformation or lack of information contributes to the inhibition. Cultural expectations also play an important role in the sexual experience; for example, religious prohibitions and cultural taboos may constrict an individual's sexuality.

RECOVERY-ORIENTED CARE FOR PEOPLE WITH FEMALE ORGASMIC DISORDER

Teamwork and Collaboration: Working Toward Recovery

Treatment of the individual with an orgasmic disorder is best left to clinicians who specialize in this area, but other health care providers can first treat underlying health, mental health, and relationship issues. If the orgasmic issue is not related to any of these areas, the patient should be referred to a qualified **sex therapist** who blends education and counseling with psychotherapy and specific sexual exercises. For example, **sensate focus** is a method for partners to learn what each finds arousing and to learn to communicate those preferences. It begins with nongenital contact and gradually includes genital touch and sexual intercourse (Huang et al., 2024).

Safety Issues

Low sexual functioning is linked to suicidal ideation in females who are service members and veterans. The low sexual functioning is associated with probable depression and posttraumatic stress disorder. It is important to include a suicide screening when caring for people with sexual dysfunction (Dargél et al., 2022).

EVIDENCE-BASED NURSING CARE FOR PEOPLE WITH FEMALE ORGASMIC DISORDER

Discussions of sexual issues or concerns are part of the psychiatric–mental health assessment. Developing implementation strategies depends on the reason the patient is seeking mental health service and the nurse's scope of practice. The nurse will most likely be seeing the patient for a different issue (e.g., psychiatric issue, acute

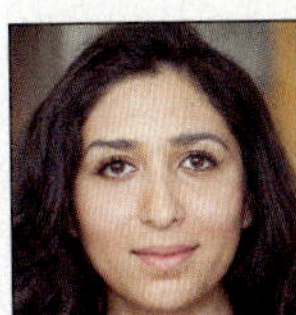

Remember Alice?

Alice believed that she could not have sexual relations with her husband because of her physical issues. Her nurse practitioner provided education and hope.

What information would you reinforce through discussion? What would you say to reinforce her self-esteem and hope for sexual relations?

If sexual dysfunction exists, one of the most important questions is: does the individual want to change sexual functioning? Many females may not see a need to pursue therapy even if a sexual issue exists. See Box 35.2.

BOX 35.2

Therapeutic Dialogue: Assessing Interest in Sexual Activity

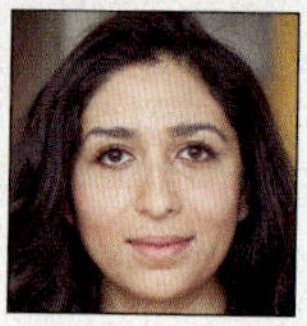

INEFFECTIVE APPROACH

Nurse: Alice, are you currently sexually active?

Alice: Once in a while.

Nurse: How would you describe your sexual activity?

Alice: How would you feel if you were in my condition?

Nurse: Well, you could still have sexual relations.

Alice: Sure thing. (Getting irritated)

Nurse: Is there a problem?

Alice: Look, I just don't want to talk about it.

EFFECTIVE APPROACH

Nurse: Alice, are you currently sexually active?

Alice: Once in a while.

Nurse: Once in a while?

Alice: Yeah, I really don't feel like it anymore.

Nurse: Oh (Silence)

Alice: My illness is messing up things in the bedroom.

Nurse: How so?

Alice: Well, I just feel so ugly—I have to urinate, my legs are weak.

Nurse: Are you feeling that you want to have sex?

Alice: Sometimes I think about it, but then I remember my illness. My poor husband. He should find someone else.

Nurse: Have you talked with him about your feelings?

Alice: Well, no. He is so patient.

Nurse: There are many people who have similar feelings but are able to begin to enjoy sex again. Is that something that you would like to consider?

Alice: Well, maybe.

Nurse: We can talk more about this. There are resources that can help you and your husband.

Alice: OK, sounds good.

CRITICAL THINKING CHALLENGE

1. Compare the course of the first dialogue with the second one. What did the second nurse do differently to elicit information about Alice's feelings and concerns?
2. What is problematic about the first dialogue?

or chronic physical health issue) and will discover sexual concerns during a health assessment. The nurse should document the concern and make a referral if agreeable to the patient.

Patients are sometimes reluctant to discuss sexual issues, especially those who may be socially stigmatized (e.g., same-sex couples, people with developmental issues, and older adults). Attention should be paid to special populations that are high risk for sexual concerns, such as those taking medications that impair sexual functioning and people with mental illnesses or chronic health issues. For older adults, poor physical health and lack of a partner are common barriers to sexual continuity. Other barriers include a lack of privacy or institutionalization. Sexual activity is also inhibited by lack of knowledge about the impact of aging or health conditions on sexuality, the normality of continued sexual desire and interest, and the alternatives for sexual gratification.

RECOGNIZING CUES: RELEVANT ASSESSMENT INFORMATION

Current sexual functioning, age, physical health, and the presence of any medical or psychiatric and substance use issues as well as factors that contribute to sexual functioning (e.g., rest, nutrition, personal hygiene) are considered in the sexual assessment (Box 35.3). The assessment should include a discussion about sexual trauma, especially if the individual is a veteran. A careful medication history is important because so many medications have a negative effect on sexual performance (see Chapter 11).

BOX 35.3

Medical Conditions and Substances Affecting Sexual Function

- Cardiovascular conditions and vascular conditions
- Endocrine conditions, particularly diabetes, which cause gradual erectile dysfunction in half of males and orgasmic dysfunction in one third of females
- Cancer or cancer treatments, such as radiation
- Surgery, particularly hysterectomy, mastectomy, prostatectomy, and bowel surgery
- Arthritis and neuromuscular disorders
- Spinal cord injury
- Head injury
- Cerebrovascular accident (stroke)
- Organic brain syndrome (senile dementia, Alzheimer disease)
- Cerebral palsy
- Asthma, emphysema, and chronic obstructive pulmonary disease
- Chronic renal failure
- Obesity
- Localized genital conditions, such as Sjögren syndrome, balanitis, vulvar ulcers, and psoriasis
- Prescription medications (e.g., antihypertensive drugs, anticholinergic drugs, some antidepressants)
- Chronic use of most recreational drugs
- Chronic alcohol misuse

Physical Health

Adults with chronic medical illnesses and disabilities who have issues with sensation, movement, body structure, fertility, or energy should be asked about the impact of the medical issues on their sexual function. Diabetes, heart disease, hormonal imbalances, menopause, and chronic illness such as kidney disease or liver failure are associated with sexual dysfunction in females (Sobel & David, 2024). Sexual activity often changes after a cardiac event because of fear about causing another attack (Ziapour et al., 2024). Obesity and pregnancy can both compromise sexual responses (Fernández-Carrasco et al., 2023; Saadedine et al., 2024).

The nurse should ensure that the individual understands the sexual responses, effects of medications, hormonal changes that occur during the life cycle of a female (e.g., adolescence, menstruation, pregnancy, menopause, aging), and the importance of adequate rest and nutrition.

Pain

Pain may be present and inhibiting the patient's ability to engage in sexual activity. The nurse should ask if there is pain present during intercourse and include pain descriptors such as the duration, location, intensity, and any psychological components (Tayyeb & Gupta, 2023).

History of Trauma

A history of trauma can significantly impact sexual function, and patients should be assessed for past and present traumas. Stress and trauma are highly prevalent among females and often contribute to sexual health concerns. Sexual function and satisfaction should be assessed in all females, but especially female veterans who have experienced sexual trauma and those who have experienced childhood sexual abuse. Research shows that these experiences significantly impact sexual health. A trauma-informed approach should be used when interviewing females who have experienced trauma (Lapping-Carr & Pappa, 2024). See Box 35.4.

BOX 35.4

Trauma-Informed Approaches: Childhood Maltreatment, Adult Sexual Functioning, and Self-Criticism

Background

Childhood maltreatment negatively affects sexual functioning in adulthood. Childhood maltreatment can disrupt the development of secure attachment, impair emotional regulation skills, and negatively shape an individual's self-perception. These factors can result in difficulties in forming and maintaining healthy intimate relationships, decreased sexual desire, sexual anxiety, and impaired sexual functioning.

When children are abused, they often internalize negative beliefs about themselves leading to a self-critical mindset that perpetuates negative self-perceptions and doubts about desirability, performance, and worthiness. Self-criticism is associated with childhood maltreatment and sexual functioning.

Interventions

- For individuals who experienced childhood maltreatment, sexual functioning and self-criticism should be routinely assessed.
- For individuals seeking counseling for sexual functioning, childhood maltreatment should be assessed.
- For individuals who are seeking help with improving sexual functioning and who experienced childhood maltreatment and are self-critical, interventions should focus on enhancing self-compassion and understanding one's own emotions, beliefs, and desires and the mental states of others.

Source: Lassri, D., & Gewirtz-Meydan, A. (2024). From trauma to intimacy: Examining the link between childhood maltreatment and adult sexual functioning—The mediating role of self-criticism. *Child Abuse & Neglect, 149*, 106663. https://doi.org/10.1016/j.chiabu.2024.106663

Mental Status and Appearance

A nurse conducts a mental status examination (as discussed in Chapter 10) if comorbid disorders with cognitive and mood disturbances are present. The following discussion focuses on specific assessment areas for people with orgasmic dysfunction.

Self-Concept

The nurse should assess the individual's self-concept, body image, and relationship with a partner. A poor self-concept can prevent a female from engaging in sexual relationships. Mood states, such as chronic depression and grief, can also affect the individual's ability to have an orgasm.

Stress and Coping

The nurse needs to assess the amount of stress the individual is experiencing and whether they have the ability to relax and focus on their sexuality. An unsatisfactory partner relationship may be at the core of the sexual issue. If the stress relates to earlier trauma, the nurse should consider a referral to a mental health provider.

Social Network and Support Systems

Cultural and family values play an important role in understanding a patient's response to orgasmic dysfunction and should be considered. Lifestyle disruptions, the birth of a child, a move to another city, or a change in financial or social status may coincide with sexual dysfunction. See Clinical Judgment Nursing Care Plan 35.1, which sets forth a plan of care for Alice, the case study patient in this chapter.

ANALYZING CUES AND DEVELOPING HYPOTHESES

Low self-esteem and depression are nursing care priorities for an individual with a sexual disorder. The nurse should determine the significance of this disorder to the individual. For some individuals, this issue may not be a major concern; for others, it may represent a loss of femininity.

PLANNING RECOVERY AND WELLNESS OUTCOMES: GENERATING SOLUTIONS

Sexual issues impact all aspects of health and wellness. The nurse should help the individual examine current sexual needs and identify ways to enhance sexual health. If there is a sexual issue, the nurse and patient can collaborate on establishing realistic goals. For example, encouraging the patient to discuss sexual needs with partner is a beginning step.

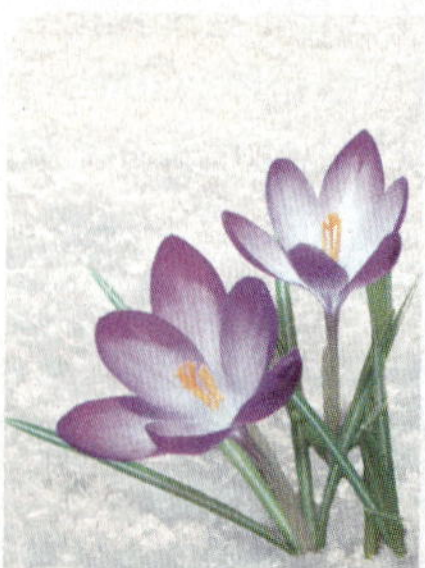

CLINICAL JUDGMENT NURSING CARE PLAN 35.1

The Person With Multiple Sclerosis and Sexual Dysfunction

Alice, a 35-year-old happily married for 11 years and the mother of two children, was diagnosed with multiple sclerosis 3 years ago. She is being seen for a periodic checkup by the nurse practitioner. Some of Alice's present symptoms include transitory visual blurring, weakness of the lower extremities, and mood swings. She also has had issues with urinary leakage and occasional bowel incontinence. She admits, with some obvious discomfort, that she is experiencing sexual difficulty and that her sexual activity is far less frequent than before her illness. Although Alice claims her husband has remained attentive and affectionate, she feels she is no longer attractive or comfortable with sexual activity. She says she wouldn't blame her husband if he found someone else.

Setting: Outpatient Clinic

Assessment Cues: The physical examination has demonstrated decreased sensation and reflexes in the lower extremities, decreased hand grasp, slight delayed blink response and nystagmus, clear speech pattern, nondistended bladder, typical bowel sounds, BP 124/76, P 76, and R 24. The patient wears an absorbent pad for urinary incontinence with a slight odor of urine. She is weepy and wrings her hands, and her eyes are downcast when discussing marital relationship. Alice's husband accompanied her to the appointment, holding her hand in the waiting room. He offered to be present during the examination or answer questions if desired. Alice has had difficulty experiencing orgasm for 2 years. She has difficulty communicating her needs.

Associated Diagnosis	Medications
Rule out: female orgasmic disorder multiple sclerosis	Interferon-beta-1b 22 mcg three times per week oxybutynin 5 mg three times a day

Clinical Judgment Nursing Care Plan 35.1 Continued

Priority Hypotheses: Low Self-esteem and Poor Body Image

Important Characteristics

Feels unattractive, uncomfortable with sexual activity, would understand husband finding another woman. "How would you feel if you had an 'accident' right before you were supposed to make love?" States husband has remained attentive and considerate but believes it's because he feels pity. States she has moods, "… really feeling sorry for myself. I suppose … I'm depressed … frustrated … MS affects you that way."

Associated Considerations

States she often feels tired and weak. Has some difficulty with mobility, requires assistance with bathing in tub and fastening back buttons and hooks. Frequently has urinary incontinence and occasional loss of bowel control. States she is usually unable to hold urine and sometimes bowels. Satisfactory sexual relationship before onset of illness, although had difficulty verbalizing sexual needs. Altered self-esteem Chronic illness

Planning Recovery and Wellness Outcomes

Initial

Alice and her husband will identify three barriers and three enhancers to effective communication regarding their sexual needs and issues.

Discharge

Alice will adapt to limitations and regain a positive body image. Alice and her husband will experience comfortable and satisfactory sexual expression.

Taking Action: Interventions

Interventions	Rationale	Ongoing Assessment
Lack of Knowledge		
Educate Alice and family; provide written materials; encourage questions.	Patients and families need factual information on the trajectory, treatment, and impact of multiple sclerosis.	Alice and her husband correctly explain the emotional aspects and pathophysiology of multiple sclerosis.
Communication		
Demonstrate empathy for Alice's difficulty in communicating sexual needs.	Talking about sex makes some people embarrassed.	Alice and her husband correctly identify factors that promote or impede their communication.
Explain common reasons for experiencing difficulty when discussing sexual issues.	Individuals may not know how to phrase what they mean. They may be afraid of insulting their partner or have a religious or cultural taboo.	The couple increases comfort in discussing sexual needs.
Emphasize the importance of being able to tell each other what is personally satisfying.	Clear communication is more successful than "telepathy."	Alice is able to identify her need for more time and foreplay.
Help Alice establish effective communication patterns by using role play or teaching assertive communication skills (e.g., beginning statements with "I really like it when you …").	Becoming assertive often requires changing male/aggressive and female/passive learned behavior patterns. Use of a fictional situation that can be role played and analyzed is an instructive nonthreatening model for learning new behaviors.	Alice and her husband report more open communication, which allows more sharing of true feelings and fears.
Encourage the establishment of a consistent, mutually agreeable, relaxed time to talk.	Communication is easier when it is planned and viewed as a value.	Alice and her husband report that communication is improved by allotting a half hour for "together time" each evening.
Encourage the use of support or self-help groups.	Communication can be enhanced through sharing thoughts, feelings, and experiences with others.	Has contacted Multiple Sclerosis Society.
Describe sexual concerns commonly identified by partners.	Partner may feel guilty about sexual desire when mate is ill; fear of harming, increasing discomfort, or overburdening mate; difficulty when mate assumes caretaking and lover role, often helped by use of a home health aide.	The couple is beginning to address their issues; express difficulty in adapting to the current and inevitable changes of the disease; express fear of complete loss of function in all aspects of function, not just sexuality.

Continued

Clinical Judgment Nursing Care Plan 35.1 Continued

Interventions	Rationale	Ongoing Assessment
Body Image Disturbance		
Related to illness and change in function	Common sequela of chronic illness.	Alice is able to express her thoughts and feelings about the effects of the disease.
Help Alice confront reality but identify positive aspects of her personality.	Allows Alice to focus on health function and inner being.	Sees herself as a good mother and wife.
Encourage Alice to maintain good hygiene, dress attractively, use grooming aids such as perfume, and treat herself to manicures.	Optimizing appearance is a mood enhancer.	Alice states she is having a friend take her to a hairdresser every other week; bought a new outfit through a catalogue.
Fatigue and Weakness		
Identify optimal time for sexual interaction.	Decreases stress; increases relaxation.	Reports using time when children are with grandparents for intimacy.
Do not eat or drink before activity.	Decreases expenditure of energy and potential for incontinence.	Able to cite correct rationale for food and fluid limitations.
Teach the use of side lying or rear entry position during intercourse.	Decreases energy expenditure of Alice.	Reports ability to use these positions.
Use pillows to support weakened limbs.	Assists positioning when there is muscle weakness.	Reports increased satisfaction in sexual activity when pillows are used for positioning.
Inform Alice of side effects of medications being taken.	Some drugs cause impaired sexual response and fatigue.	Not applicable at this time.
Impaired Mobility		
Teach active or passive range-of-motion exercises.	Helps to prevent contractures.	Has been evaluated by physical therapist; reports range of motion exercises done twice daily.
Consider use of a waterbed.	Assists with movement.	
Teach possibility and treatment of contractures or adductor spasms.	Antispasmodics may be needed and are effective when taken 10 to 15 minutes before sexual activity.	Not applicable at this time.
Bladder Incontinence		
For urinary leakage, teach Alice to empty her bladder in accordance with prescribed bladder training program.	To maximize urinary function, bladder training should be initiated as early as possible.	Reports following bladder training program.
Discuss decreasing fluids a few hours before sexual activity and having padding or towels on hand.	These techniques decrease urinary leakage or incontinence; protect bed linens if an accident occurs.	Alice empties her bladder and decreases fluid before attempting sexual intercourse; pads on bed. If using an indwelling catheter, tapes the catheter over her abdomen.
Before sexual activity, void on cue or via intermittent catheterization. If using an indwelling catheter, may advise temporary removal or moving the clamp and taping the catheter to one side.	Permits Alice to have coitus despite urinary retention or indwelling catheter.	
Bowel Incontinence		
Establish a regular bowel program.	Helps decrease the occurrence of accidental bowel elimination; may require preparatory use of a suppository or enema.	Reports following a regulated bowel training program.
Cover bed linens with towels.	Helps prepare for accidents.	

THERAPEUTIC RELATIONSHIP

Discussing sexual concerns can be anxiety provoking for the patient and requires the nurse to maintain a nonjudgmental, sex-positive approach that recognizes the importance of sexuality. A nurse should examine personal beliefs and implicit biases about sexuality and sexual functioning, and satisfaction. Patients will not feel comfortable disclosing personal information unless the patient trusts that the nurse is sensitive and concerned about the patient's sexual issues.

TAKING ACTION: NURSING INTERVENTIONS

Referral of the patient to a specialist in sexual disorders may be appropriate. The following interventions can be implemented with any patient who is experiencing sexual concerns, even if they are referred to a mental health provider.

Physical Care and Wellness Challenges

Wellness activities are especially important for sexual health and well-being. Co-occurring illnesses may interfere with sexual functioning. Feeling unattractive or stigmatized can compromise the willingness to discuss sexual needs. Wellness strategies are often needed to support sexual health (see Table 35.1).

Psychosocial Interventions

Nursing interventions include providing counseling, sex education, problem-solving opportunities, or referrals. Several health care practices are also known to promote sexual health, such as getting adequate rest, maintaining optimal nutrition, and exercising regularly. Explaining the dynamics of sexual responses is another important nursing action. Individuals who report difficulties with sexual response often benefit from factual information and helpful suggestions and do not need sex therapy. However, when long-standing or highly complex issues emerge in the assessment, it is better to refer the individual or couple to a formally trained, certified sex therapist. Nurses should be aware that certain processes, techniques, and adaptive devices can improve sexual functioning.

TABLE 35.1 WELLNESS CHALLENGES AND COPING STRATEGIES TO SUPPORT SEXUAL HEALTH

Challenge	Coping Strategy
To feel positive about sexuality and sexual health	Discuss the importance of sexual health to wellness
To seek pleasant environments that support sexual activities	Discuss realistic environmental changes that are conducive to sexual activity
To recognize the need for physical activity, healthy foods, and sleep	Encourage regular physical activity, discuss healthy diets, encourage establishing healthy sleep hygiene routines
To develop a sense of connection, belonging, and a support system	Seek positive relationships and reduce number of unpleasant interactions

Complementary Therapies

Few studies investigate the use of complementary therapies specifically for female orgasmic disorder. Yoga shows some improvement in female sexual function compared to a nonintervention control group (Rodrigues et al., 2024). The use of complementary therapies such as yoga, relaxation, and deep-breathing should improve well-being, which in turn supports sexual health.

Psychoeducation

Unless the nurse has had additional preparation in sexual counseling, the primary psychosocial interventions are providing information, helping patients identify issues related to sexual issues, and aiding them in developing problem-solving skills. Patients often benefit from learning how to communicate their sexual needs better in such areas as type of stimulation desired, positioning, and the amount of time required for maximum sexual pleasure. The nurse can recommend resource materials and referral sources. Box 35.5 outlines topics for patient education.

Support Groups

Individuals with orgasmic dysfunction can also benefit from a support group that includes people with similar issues. Group modalities are useful in helping patients decrease their embarrassment and uneasiness about sexual topics and increase their knowledge. Partner support is critical and should be encouraged throughout treatment.

Evaluation and Treatment Outcomes

Outcomes related to improved sexual functioning are developed with the patient and may vary from acquiring knowledge to increasing communication with their partner to deciding about a referral for specialized treatment.

BOX 35.5

Psychoeducation Checklist: Female Orgasmic Disorder

When caring for a patient with female orgasmic disorder, be sure to include the following topics in your teaching plan for the patient and partner:

- Possible etiologic factors
- Anxiety reduction techniques
- Communication skills
- Impact of medication on orgasm

Integration With Primary Care

Sexual disorders are treated by specialists, but often the patient's initial concern is shared with a nurse. It is important that mental and health issues are treated from a holistic perspective. Mental health and primary health clinicians should be monitoring the sexual health of the patient and provide appropriate, evidence-based interventions.

EJACULATORY DYSFUNCTIONS

Ejaculatory dysfunction is one of the most common sexual disorders of people assigned male at birth and ranges from **premature ejaculation** (PE) (inability to control ejaculation before or shortly after penetration) to **delayed ejaculation** (DE) (delay or absence of ejaculation). These dysfunctions cause negative personal consequences, clinical distress, frustration, and the avoidance of sexual intimacy (Allen et al., 2023). PE is subdivided into **lifelong PE**, present since first sexual experience, and **acquired PE,** which develops after a period of sexual function. A dysfunction needs to be present for approximately 6 months to be diagnosed as a sexual dysfunction and is not diagnosed in a male whose difficulty is caused by drug or alcohol misuse. In those cases, an SUD diagnosis is made, with the sexual disorder generally resolving when the SUD is treated (APA, 2022).

EPIDEMIOLOGY

Based on patient self-report, next to erectile dysfunction, PE is viewed as the most common sexual dysfunction of males, with prevalence rates of up to 30%. It is estimated that about 27% of males seeking treatment report PE as an issue. Most people with PE, however, do not seek treatment (Herkommer et al., 2024).

ETIOLOGY

The etiology of PE is unknown with few data to support suggested biologic or psychological theories such as anxiety, penile hypersensitivity, and serotonin receptor dysfunction. Lifelong PE is more likely related to an underlying neurobiologic functional disturbance, whereas acquired PE is more likely related to a medical, psychological, and interpersonal cause. Age does not seem to be an etiologic factor or a risk (van Raaij et al., 2024).

RECOVERY-ORIENTED CARE FOR PEOPLE WITH EJACULATORY DYSFUNCTIONS

Teamwork and Collaboration: Working Toward Recovery

The treatment of PE involves medication and behavioral strategies (Shechter & Gurenwald, 2024). People with PE are usually treated by specialists. Nurses are instrumental in teaching patients about the disorder and potential treatments and facilitating decision making about seeking treatment.

BOX 35.6

Psychoeducation Checklist: Premature Ejaculation

When caring for a patient with PE, be sure to include the following topics in your teaching plan for the patient and partner:

- Possible etiologic factors
- Pharmacologic agents, if indicated, including drug, dosage, action, frequency, and possible side effects
- Measures to decrease anxiety performance
- Communication skills
- Sexual counseling
- Sensate focus
- Sex therapy

EVIDENCE-BASED NURSING CARE FOR PEOPLE WITH EJACULATORY DYSFUNCTIONS

The issue of PE may become apparent during a health history that includes specific sexual data. Patients need assurance that many people have similar issues and that treatment is possible (Box 35.6). Patients can be referred to specialists for behavioral strategies. Younger people may find that masturbation before anticipation of sexual intercourse may help.

Integration With Primary Care

Treatment of PE should be coordinated within the context of primary care. Because medications and medical illness can impact sexual functioning, it is important for one provider to coordinate care. There is emerging evidence that alternative treatments, such as acupuncture, may be helpful (Wang et al., 2024).

ERECTILE DISORDER

Erectile disorder (ED) refers to the inability of a male to achieve or maintain an erection sufficient for satisfactory completion of the sexual activity. The term erectile dysfunction is often used interchangeably with the term ED. This text uses the term ED.

DIAGNOSTIC CRITERIA

Although most males experience an occasional lack of erection, intervention should be considered when there is consistent erectile inefficiency during masturbation, intercourse, or on awakening (Leslie & Sooriyamoorthy, 2024).

EPIDEMIOLOGY

ED may occur at any age, although incidence increases according to age. In the United States, 52% of males between 40 and 70 years of age have ED. After age 70, 70% will report having ED. Although less common in younger individuals, ED still affects 40% of males below age 40 (Leslie & Sooriyamoorthy, 2024).

People with diabetes, cardiovascular disease, or chronic renal failure also have a higher incidence of ED. For those undergoing treatment for prostate cancer, there is a high probability of ED. ED increases with age and with comorbidities such as diabetes, cardiovascular disease, depression, anxiety, obesity, metabolic syndrome, smoking, and substance use. Findings from these studies show that ED significantly impacts mood state, interpersonal functioning, and overall quality of life (Leslie & Sooriyamoorthy, 2024). Single people are more likely to experience ED than those with stable partners (Calzo et al., 2021).

ETIOLOGY

Biologic Theories

Common biologic causes of ED include genital trauma, vascular insufficiency, renal disease, hormonal deficiencies, Parkinson disease, diabetes, multiple sclerosis, surgical procedures, use of antihypertensive and antidepressant drugs, and heavy cigarette smoking. Long-term alcohol or cocaine consumption can affect the erectile response. It is also more common as an individual ages (Leslie & Sooriyamoorthy, 2024).

Many people with mental disorders attribute their ED to their psychiatric medication. If these individuals consequently stop taking their medications, they can have a psychiatric relapse within a few weeks to months.

Psychological Theories

ED may also have a psychological basis. Numerous psychosocial etiologies have been identified. Fear of failure, relationship stress, poor body image, fear of rejection, partner hostility, guilt, cultural taboos, religious proscriptions, lack of knowledge, and negative attitudes are some of the identified related factors (Leslie & Sooriyamoorthy, 2024).

RECOVERY-ORIENTED CARE FOR PEOPLE WITH ERECTILE DISORDER

Teamwork and Collaboration: Working Toward Recovery

The treatment of people with ED is usually managed in a primary care setting except for those with mental disorders, who may seek treatment within the mental health system. Since the introduction of the **phosphodiesterase 5 (PDE5) inhibitors**—pharmacologic agents such as sildenafil citrate, tadalafil, and vardenafil—many males choose the convenience of medication. For people with psychiatric disorders, monitoring medications and their potential interactions is important. However, behavioral interventions have also been shown to be useful.

EVIDENCE-BASED NURSING CARE FOR PEOPLE WITH ERECTILE DISORDER

ED is common in patients with mental health issues because of the side effects of many psychiatric medications. It is important to include interventions that address ED when implementing care because one of the major reasons people discontinue psychiatric medications is the sexual side effects. Care of patients with ED is within the scope of nursing practice.

RECOGNIZING CUES: RELEVANT ASSESSMENT INFORMATION

Some individuals are not comfortable discussing sexuality and sexual issues. The assessment should be conducted in an atmosphere of trust and understanding. In many cultures, self-esteem of males is related to the ability to perform sexually. When an individual has issues maintaining an erection, it is embarrassing and demeaning to that individual. Sensitivity to the patient's feelings should be reflected throughout the assessment.

Among the many medical issues that are reported to compromise male sexual activity and responses include obesity, smoking, diabetes, hypertension, hyperlipidemia, cardiovascular disease, and obstructive sleep disorder (Wang et al., 2023). ED is listed as a side effect in several medications such as antidepressants, cimetidine, ketoconazole, spironolactone, sympathetic blockers, thiazide diuretics, and other antihypertensive medications (Leslie & Sooriyamoorthy, 2024). In addition, low testosterone, chronic kidney disease, and some neurologic disorders are also associated with male sexual dysfunction (Fu et al., 2024; Lee et al., 2024).

Assessment should include a discussion about the impact of sexual dysfunction on the quality of the relationship with the partner. If a mental disorder, such as depression or posttraumatic stress disorder, is present, comparing the timing of the dysfunction with the onset of symptoms and prescribed medication can determine whether the ED is related to the disorder and medication. See Box 35.7.

ANALYZING CUES AND DEVELOPING HYPOTHESES

ED affects people differently, and the priorities of care will depend on its meaning to the patient. Low self-esteem and self-identity are two priorities that should be

BOX 35.7

Building Clinical Judgment With SBAR: Nurse Assessment of Medication History

SBAR

S: Situation

Steven, age 24, has a diagnosis of bipolar I disorder. He was admitted for impersonating a law officer and arresting people who did not obey his commands. He admitted that he was given a prescription for mood stabilization (valproic acid 250 mg twice a day) and an antipsychotic (risperidone 2 mg daily) to manage his hallucinations and racing thoughts 6 months ago and took the medication for 3 months.

B: Background

Steven was diagnosed with bipolar I disorder a year ago after he had a manic episode at work. He stopped taking his medication 3 months ago and his bipolar symptoms reappeared 4 weeks ago. Three months ago, he started dating a new person and recently asked her to move in with him.

A: Assessment

- Physical health: Ht. 5′10′, Wt. 160
- Vital signs: BP 130/70, HR 85, R 12
- Oriented × 3
- Mental Status: Mood labile, believes that he is a law officer, denies suicidal ideation
- Medication status: Discontinued medication 3 months ago because it interfered with his sexual performance
- Psychosocial: Has a new partner and is concerned that she will now move out.

R: Recommendation

- Consider medication that has less impact sexual functioning
- Consider medication to enhance sexual performance (PDE5 inhibitor)
- Sexual health psychoeducation

Building Clinical Judgment

1. Why did the nurse associate the patient's discontinuation of medication with sexual functioning?
2. Why did the nurse recommend changing medications rather than discontinuing the antipsychotics?

considered. ED may indicate an undiagnosed medical disorder such as diabetes or a medication side effect. Wellness priorities such as diet and exercise modifications may emerge. If ED is a side effect of medications such as antidepressants or antipsychotics, it is important to communicate with the prescriber who can consider a medication adjustment.

PLANNING RECOVERY AND WELLNESS OUTCOMES: GENERATING SOLUTIONS

There are various approaches with multiple potential outcomes for individuals with ED, depending on the underlying cause. Recovery approaches should be planned with the patient. If the ED is related to lifestyle issues such as diet, exercise, or smoking, encouraging a realistic plan to address these factors should be developed. If the ED is related to trauma or psychological issues, referral to mental health specialists should be considered. For a patient whose ED is related to medical disorders or medication side effects, the patient should seek help from the medical provider.

THERAPEUTIC RELATIONSHIP

As with patients with female orgasmic disorder, a trusting therapeutic relationship is necessary for patients to feel comfortable discussing personal information. A matter-of-fact, nonjudgmental approach works best.

TAKING ACTION: NURSING INTERVENTIONS

Wellness Strategies

Promotion of positive health practices that focus on adequate nutrition, rest, and exercise is important in promoting erectile functioning. Weight loss may improve overall health and enhance the strength of the erection. Regular exercise is also related to sexual health. Helping the patient develop a better lifestyle is important in promoting sexual functioning. Reducing alcohol consumption can also improve sexual performance.

Medication Interventions

PDE5 inhibitors are the treatment of choice. With sexual stimulation, nitric oxide is released into the nerve terminations and endothelial cell, stimulating the production of cyclic guanosine monophosphate (cGMP), a substance that enables the smooth muscle cells of the corpora cavernosa to relax. The PDE enzymes are involved in the breakdown of cGMP. The PDE inhibitors inactivate PDE5, thereby enabling the buildup of cGMP, sustaining relaxation of the corpora cavernosa (Dhaliwal & Gupta, 2023).

Approved PDE5 inhibitors include sildenafil citrate, vardenafil HCl, tadalafil, and avanafil. These medications enhance the effect of nitric oxide, which is released in the corpora cavernosa during sexual stimulation. These medications are rapidly absorbed, with maximum observed plasma concentrations reached within 30 to 120 minutes of oral dosing in the fasted state. Tadalafil acts for up to 36 hours (Dhaliwal & Gupta, 2023).

Although these medications are approved for the treatment of ED, they generally have not been shown to be efficacious in sexual arousal disorders in females. There is evidence of preliminary efficacy of topical sildenafil cream for treatment of female sexual arousal disorder (Johnson et al., 2024).

Before the introduction of PDE5 inhibitors, **intracavernosal pharmacotherapy** was the treatment of choice for ED. A vascular smooth muscle relaxant such as papaverine hydrochloride, phentolamine mesylate, or prostaglandin is directly injected into the corpora cavernosa by the patient or partner. This increases arterial flow of blood into the corpora cavernosa and decreases venous outflow. Neurogenic, rather than vascular, ED appears to respond better. Complications can include excessive bleeding, scarring and priapism, and potential hepatic involvement. Counseling, strict monitoring, and specific teaching are required (Furtado et al., 2024).

Another treatment is the use of alprostadil (prostaglandin) in microsuppository form inserted into the urethra using a special applicator. The intracavernous injection causes a rapid absorption of the medication through the urethral mucosa into the corpus spongiosum. It is particularly useful for males who are unable to inject themselves (Jain & Iqbal, 2023).

Other Interventions

When erection is determined to be permanently impaired, several options may be considered to facilitate intercourse. An external penile prosthesis can be placed over the flaccid penis, although some find this esthetically displeasing. A pumping device that creates a vacuum can be used for blood entrapment followed by placement of a rubber band at the base of the penis. Surgical techniques for improving vascular sufficiency are also showing promising results.

Psychoeducation

Education is important for a patient with ED. Teaching the patient about positive health practices and treatment options (i.e., mechanical devices, medications, surgical procedures) is usually needed (Box 35.8). The patient's concern about their partner's satisfaction needs to be explored. Many times, males believe that partner satisfaction is related only to penile penetration and their ability to sustain an erection. Encouraging the patient to talk with their partner about their partner's sexual needs and other aspects of their sexual experience (physical closeness, kissing, hugging, mutual exploration of their bodies) helps the patient broaden understanding of the sexual experience.

BOX 35.8

Psychoeducation Checklist: Erectile Disorder

When caring for a patient with male erectile disorder, be sure to include the following topics in your teaching plan for the patient and partner:

- Possible etiologic factors
- Psychopharmacologic agents (e.g., intracavernosal therapy, yohimbine), including drug, action, frequency, administration technique, and possible side effects
- Alternative methods of sexual expression
- Prosthesis use
- Sexual education and counseling
- Communication skills
- Sex therapy

Evaluation and Treatment Outcomes

The primary outcome for ED is improved sexual functioning. Acceptance of change of physical status is an outcome that is difficult to obtain. Improvement in sexual satisfaction may include increasing the ability for erectile functioning. If ED is permanent, exploration of other avenues of sexual expression may indicate a successful outcome. In this disorder, partner satisfaction is usually of prime concern. Improved communication with the partner may also be a positive outcome.

OTHER SEXUAL DISORDERS

FEMALE SEXUAL INTEREST/AROUSAL DISORDER

A **female sexual interest/arousal disorder** may occur at any age and may cause relationship difficulties and personal stress along with avoidance of sexual activity and impaired communication. Other etiologic factors, such as anxiety, guilt, and history of sexual abuse, and changes in androgen levels during the menstrual cycle have been shown to affect arousal. Aging also affects sexual arousal because vasocongestion develops more slowly in older females, so vaginal lubrication decreases after menopause; lower estrogen levels at this life stage may affect sexual arousal.

Interventions include psychosocial therapies such as counseling, mindfulness meditation therapy, body awareness education, and relationship counseling and medications. CBT is effective is exploring thoughts and behaviors related to sexuality and sexual functioning (Adebisi & Carlson, 2024). See Box 35.9.

Flibanserin, a medication formulated for premenopausal females, is approved by the US Food and Drug Administration (FDA) for generalized hypoactive

BOX 35.9

Research for Evidence-Based Practice: Motivational Interviewing on Sexual Health

Kamalak, H., & Aksoy Derya, Y. (2024). The effects of motivational interviewing on sexual quality of life and sexual self-efficacy in postmenopausal women with sexual dysfunction. Menopause, *31(10), 862–870. https://doi.org/10.1097/GME.0000000000002418*

THE QUESTION: What are the effects of motivational interviewing on sexual quality of life and sexual self-efficacy in postmenopausal females with sexual dysfunction?

METHODS: A randomized controlled study was conducted with 164 (82 = experimental, 82 = control) postmenopausal females with sexual dysfunction who presented to the gynecology outpatient clinic. The data were collected using a personal information form, the Arizona Sexual Experiences Scale-Female Version Questionnaire, the Sexual Quality of Life-Female Questionnaire, and the Sexual Self-Efficacy Scale. Four motivational interview sessions were conducted with the postmenopausal females in the experimental group at 1-week intervals, and those in the control group did not receive any intervention. The data were analyzed using descriptive statistics.

FINDINGS: Sexual quality of life and self-efficacy levels of the two groups were similar in the pretest stage ($P > .05$). After the motivational interviews, sexual dysfunction in the experimental group was determined as 82.9% and 98.8% in the control group. Additionally, after the motivational interviews, the sexual quality of life and sexual self-efficacy levels in the experimental group increased significantly compared to those in the control group ($P < .001$).

IMPLICATIONS FOR NURSING: Motivational interviewing is an option for females experiencing sexual dysfunction. This study showed that sexual dysfunction decreased for some participants.

sexual desire disorder. The primary side effects of the daily pill are dizziness, sleepiness, and fatigue (Sprout Pharmaceuticals, 2024). Bremelanotide, a melanocortin agonist, is administered subcutaneously as needed once daily, approximately 45 minutes before sexual activity (Cosette Pharmaceuticals, Inc, 2024).

MALE HYPOACTIVE SEXUAL DESIRE DISORDER

Male hypoactive sexual desire disorder is a recurrent deficiency or absence of sexual fantasies and desire for sexual activity. Individuals with this disorder are not interested in sex, do not or cannot get "turned on," and require no sexual gratification. Active avoidance of potential sexual relationships may exist. The prevalence is unknown, but it is believed to affect only a small proportion of males. Often, the disorder develops in adulthood after a period of adequate sexual interest and is associated with psychological distress, stressful life events (e.g., childbirth), or relationship difficulties (McClung et al., 2024).

Therapy for psychological issues related to hypoactive sexual desire aims at helping the patient understand the issue and develop strategies to enhance sexual arousal. Treatment approaches may include individual and couples therapy, sex-therapy techniques, clinical hypnosis, cognitive behavioral therapy, guided fantasy exercises, and sexual assertiveness training. If the issue is related to medication, changing to another class of medication, giving drug holidays, or lowering the dose may help.

GENITOPELVIC PAIN/PENETRATION DISORDER

Genitopelvic pain/penetration disorder is characterized by genital pain associated with sexual intercourse (dyspareunia) and involuntary spasm/tension of perineal and levator muscles, making penetration difficult or not possible (vaginismus). There is intense fear of pain. Chronic neuropathic-like pain in the vulvar area can persist independent of physical contact (Brown, 2024).

Dyspareunia is a term used to describe the genital pain associated with sexual intercourse that may be caused by **vaginismus,** which is spastic involuntary constriction of the perineal and outer vaginal muscles fostered by imagined, anticipated, or real attempts at vaginal penetration. This disorder may be related to interpersonal or emotional factors such as sexual dissatisfaction or poor technique leading to inadequate relaxation and lubrication. Biologic etiologies include intact or biperforate hymen, postmenopausal atrophic changes, trauma, malignancy, intestinal disease, or other pelvic disorders (Brown, 2024).

PARAPHILIAS

Paraphilias are characterized by recurrent, intense sexual urges, fantasies, or behaviors involving unusual objects, activities, or situations. These interests cause significant distress to the individual or impair social or occupational functioning. Paraphilias include voyeurism, exhibitionism, frotteurism, sexual masochism, sexual sadism, pedophilia, and fetishism disorders (APA, 2022).

Paraphilias are rarely diagnosed; the situation is complicated across cultures because acceptability of sexual practices varies across cultures. The exact etiology of paraphilias is unknown but is thought to be a combination of neurobiologic, interpersonal, and cognitive processes. Evidence suggests dopamine, serotonin, and norepinephrine are involved in the pathogenesis of these disorders and in the disturbance of conscious regulation of behavior. A history of childhood sexual abuse is common.

TABLE 35.2 PARAPHILIAS

Paraphilia	Description
Exhibitionism	The behavior involves exposing one's genitals to strangers, with occasional masturbation. There may be an awareness of the desire to shock an individual or the fantasy that the individual will become sexually aroused on observation of the exposure.
Fetishism	An object such as a female undergarment or foot apparel is used for sexual arousal. The individual usually masturbates while holding, rubbing, or smelling the item, or it is worn by a partner during sexual activity. Fetishism usually begins in adolescence and continues throughout life.
Frotteurism	Sexually arousing urges, fantasies, and behaviors occur when touching or rubbing one's genitals against the breasts, genitals, or thighs of a nonconsenting individual. This paraphilia usually begins in early adolescence or young adulthood and diminishes with age.
Pedophilia	Sexual activity occurs with a child usually 13 years of age or younger by an individual at least 16 years of age or 5 years older than the child. Pedophilic acts include fondling, oral sex, and anal or vaginal intercourse with the penis, fingers, or objects, with varying amounts of force.
Sexual masochism	This behavior involves the act of being humiliated, beaten, bound, or made to suffer. Self-induced masochistic acts include use of electric shock, pin sticking, restraints, and mutilation; partner-induced acts may include bondage, whipping, being urinated or defecated on; and being forced to crawl, bark, or wear diapers. One dangerous form of sexual masochism that may be practiced alone or with a partner is "hypoxyphilia." Oxygen deprivation by means of a noose, plastic bag, chest compression, or drug effect is used during sexual activity to heighten orgasmic sensation. Deaths have occurred as a result of these techniques.
Sexual sadism	Sexual excitement occurs when causing physical or psychological suffering to another individual. Commonly, the individual with sadistic behavior interacts with a masochistic partner. Sadistic behavior includes various forms of physical punishment, use of restraints, rape, burning, stabbing, strangulation, torture, and murder. This is usually a chronic paraphilia that begins as early sexual fantasies and increases in severity over time.
Voyeurism	This behavior involves "peeping," for the purpose of sexual excitement, at unsuspecting people who are nude, undressing, or engaged in sexual activity.
Other paraphilias	Sexual fantasies, urges, and activities involving animals (zoophilia), corpses (necrophilia), feces (coprophilia), urine (urophilia), body parts (partialism), and obscene telephone calls (telephone scatalogia).

Treatment for paraphilias is rarely sought by an individual; rather, treatment occurs as a result of psychosocial or legal ramifications. People with these disorders are highly stigmatized by society. A nonjudgmental approach helps build a therapeutic relationship. Treatment incorporates both psychological and biologic approaches. Cognitive-behavioral therapy has overall positive outcomes. Medications used in managing paraphilic behaviors include SSRIs, synthetic steroids, and antiandrogens (Fisher & Marwaha, 2023).

Certain behaviors and fantasies associated with paraphilias are said to begin in childhood and become more elaborate and better defined during adolescence and early adulthood. The disorders are often found to be chronic and lifelong, with the fantasies and behaviors finally diminishing with aging. Table 35.2 includes the different categories of paraphilias along with their descriptions (Fisher & Marwaha, 2023).

SUMMARY OF KEY POINTS

- Female orgasmic disorder is a common disorder affecting females; ED and PE are the most common disorders affecting males.
- Nursing interventions for people experiencing sexual dysfunction include (but are not limited to) counseling, education, and referral to sex therapists.
- Various medical conditions, psychological states, and medications negatively affect the sexual response cycle. Education about medication side effects and sexual experiences is important in maintaining health.
- Paraphilias are rarely diagnosed, and treatment is rarely sought.

DEVELOPING CLINICAL JUDGMENT

1. A 36-year-old female was recently diagnosed with depression and treated with a selective serotonin reuptake inhibitor (an antidepressant). Her depression is improving, but she has not been interested in sexual relations with her partner. Her lack of sexual interest is beginning to cause issues in her relationship. What could account for the changes in sexual interest?
2. A 52-year-old being successfully treated with lithium carbonate for his bipolar disorder was recently diagnosed with diabetes. He was told that his diabetes could be controlled by weight loss and diet. His major worry is that

the disease and lithium are causing his erectile dysfunction. He casually mentions that he is considering stopping the lithium. What issues should the nurse explore with the patient? What actions could the patient begin that would improve his sexual health?

MOVIES, TV, AND STREAMING PROGRAMS

***Men Up:* 2023.** This movie depicts the story of five Welshmen with diabetes who were dealing with erectile dysfunction as a result of the disease. They all participated in the first clinical trial for sildenafil in 1994 at Morriston Hospital in the United Kingdom. Each man had his own interpersonal relations that were impacted because of their erectile dysfunction. As the story unfolds, the men become supportive friends who recognize that the pill did not fix their relationship issues.

Viewing Points:

1. Why was it so difficult for Meurig (Iwan Rheon) to explain his erectile dysfunction to his wife?
2. Eddie (Mark Lewis Jones) was unable to admit that the pill was not working for him. How did the audience know that he associated his happiness with his ability to get an erection?
3. How did the clinical protocol discriminate against LGBTQ+ people?
4. How did the men's friendship help Peetham (Phaldut) and Eddie develop a different perspective on their relationships?
5. What was the main lesson that the men learned as a result of participating in the clinical trial?

REFERENCES

Aatsha, P. A., Arbor, T. C., & Krishan, K. (2023). Embryology, sexual development. In *StatPearls*. StatPearls Publishing. https://www.ncbi.nlm.nih.gov/books/NBK557601

Abma, J. C., & Martinez, G. M. (2023). Teenagers in the United States: Sexual activity, contraceptive use, and childbearing, 2015–2019. *National health Statistics Reports*, (196), 1–23.

Adebisi, O. Y., & Carlson, K. (2024). Female sexual interest and arousal disorder. In *StatPearls*. StatPearls Publishing. https://www.ncbi.nlm.nih.gov/books/NBK603746

Allen, M. S., Wood, A. M., & Sheffield, D. (2023). The psychology of erectile dysfunction. *Current Directions in Psychological Science*, *32*(6), 487–493.

American Academy of Pediatrics Council on Child Abuse and Neglect. (2023). *Sexual behaviors in young children: What's normal, what's not*. https://www.healthychildren.org/English/ages-stages/preschool/Pages/Sexual-Behaviors-Young-Children.aspx

American Psychiatric Association. (2022). *Diagnostic and statistical manual of mental disorders* (5th ed., text rev.). Author.

Arias-Castillo, L., García, L., & García-Perdomo, H. A. (2023). The complexity of female orgasm and ejaculation. *Archives of Gynecology and Obstetrics*, *308*(2), 427–434. https://doi.org/10.1007/s00404-022-06810-y

Balon, R. (2022). Is Basson's model of sexual response relevant? A commentary. *Journal of Sex & Marital Therapy*, *48*(1), 1–4. https://doi.org/10.1080/0092623X.2021.1887986

Bancroft, J., Graham, C. A., Janssen, E., & Sanders, S. A. (2009). The dual control model: Current status and future directions. *Journal of Sex Research*, *46*(2–3), 121–142.

Bancroft, J., & Graham, C. A. (2011). The varied nature of women's sexuality: Unresolved issues and a theoretical approach. *Hormones and Behavior*, *59*(5), 717–729.

Basanta, S., & Nuño de la Rosa, L. (2023). The female orgasm and the homology concept in evolutionary biology. *Journal of Morphology*, *284*(1), e21544. https://doi.org/10.1002/jmor.21544

Basson, R. (2001). Female sexual response: The role of drugs in the management of sexual dysfunction. *Obstetrics & Gynecology*, *98*(2), 350–353.

Bogacki-Rychlik, W., Gawęda, K., & Bialy, M. (2024). Neurophysiology of male sexual arousal-Behavioral perspective. *Frontiers in Behavioral Neuroscience*, *17*, 1330460. https://doi.org/10.3389/fnbeh.2023.1330460

Brown, B. (2024). Female pelvic conditions: Dyspareunia and vulvodynia. *FP essentials*, *547*, 8–15.

Calzo, J. P., Austin, S. B., Charlton, B. M., Missmer, S. A., Kathrins, M., Gaskins, A. J., & Chavarro, J. E. (2021). Erectile dysfunction in a sample of sexually active young adult men from a U.S. cohort: Demographic, metabolic and mental health correlates. *The Journal of Urology*, *205*(2), 539–544. https://doi.org/10.1097/JU.0000000000001367

Chouinard-Thivierge, S., Lussier, P., & Daignault, I. V. (2021). A longitudinal examination of developmental covariates of sexual behavior problems among youth referred to child protection services. *Sexual Abuse*, *34*(5), 537–567. https://doi.org/10.1177/10790632211047184

Cosette Pharmaceuticals, Inc. (2024). Vyleesi. Retrieved December 20, 2024 https://vyleesi.com/

Dargél, A. A., Mosconi, E., Volant, S., Taieb, D., & Brenot, P. (2022). Sexual dysfunction among males and females with bipolar disorder and healthy subjects: The burden of illness severity. *Bipolar Disorders*, *24*(6), 637–646. https://doi.org/10.1111/bdi.13249

Davis S. R. (2024). Sexual dysfunction in women. *The New England Journal of Medicine*, *391*(8), 736–745. https://doi.org/10.1056/NEJMcp2313307

Dhaliwal, A., & Gupta, M. (2023). PDE5 inhibitors. In *StatPearls*. StatPearls Publishing. https://www.ncbi.nlm.nih.gov/books/NBK549843

Fernández-Carrasco, F. J., Batugg-Chaves, C., Ruger-Navarrete, A., Riesco-González, F. J., Palomo-Gómez, R., Gómez-Salgado, J., Rodriguez Diaz, L., Vázquez-Lara, M. D., Fagundo-Rivera, J., & Vázquez-Lara, J. M. (2024). Influence of pregnancy on sexual desire in pregnant women and their partners: Systematic review. *Public Health Reviews*, *44*, 1606308. https://doi.org/10.3389/phrs.2023.1606308

Fisher, K. A., & Marwaha, R. (2023). Paraphilia. In *StatPearls*. StatPearls Publishing. https://www.ncbi.nlm.nih.gov/books/NBK554425

Fu, R., He, P., Hong, W., Liang, Y., Wang, W., Yuan, S., & Liu, L. (2024). Male sexual dysfunction in patients with chronic kidney disease: a cross-sectional study. *Scientific Reports*, *14*(1), 9207. https://doi.org/10.1038/s41598-024-59844-4

Furtado, T. P., Teloken, P. E., Ortega, Y., Narus, J., Wolchasty, N. P., & Mulhall, J. P. (2024). Delineating patient errors in an intracavernosal injection program. *The Journal of Sexual Medicine*, *21*(6), 529–532. https://doi.org/10.1093/jsxmed/qdae031

Granados, R., Carvalho, J., & Sierra, J. C. (2021). Preliminary evidence on how the dual control model predicts female sexual response to a bogus negative feedback. *Psychological Reports*, *124*(2), 502–520. https://doi.org/10.1177/0033294120907310

Healthy People 2030. (2021). *LGBT*. https://health.gov/healthypeople/objectives-and-data/browse-objectives/lgbt

Herder, T., Spoelstra, S. K., Peters, A. W. M., & Knegtering, H. (2023). Sexual dysfunction related to psychiatric disorders: a systematic review. *The Journal of Sexual Medicine*, *20*(7), 965–976. https://doi.org/10.1093/jsxmed/qdad074

Herkommer, K., Meissner, V. H., Dinkel, A., Jahnen, M., Schiele, S., Kron, M., Ankerst, D. P., & Gschwend, J. E. (2024). Prevalence, lifestyle, and risk factors of erectile dysfunction, premature ejaculation, and low libido in middle-aged men: First results of the Bavarian Men's Health-Study. *Andrology*, *12*(4), 801–808. https://doi.org/10.1111/andr.13524

Huang, S., Li, Z., & Santtila, P. (2024). The effectiveness of online sensate focus exercises in enhancing sexual function and intimacy among Chinese heterosexual couples: A randomized controlled trial. *Journal of Sex & Marital Therapy*, *50*(6), 707–724. https://doi.org/10.1080/0092623X.2024.2355229

Jain, A., & Iqbal, O. A. (2023). Alprostadil. In *StatPearls*. StatPearls Publishing. https://www.ncbi.nlm.nih.gov/books/NBK542217

Janssen, E., & Bancroft, J. (2023). The dual control model of sexual response: A scoping review, 2009–2022. *Journal of Sex Research*, *60*(7), 948–968. https://doi.org/10.1080/00224499.2023.2219247

Johnson, I., Thurman, A. R., Cornell, K. A., Hatheway, J., Dart, C., Brainard, C. P., Friend, D. R., & Goldstein, A. (2024). Preliminary efficacy of topical sildenafil cream for the treatment of female sexual arousal disorder: A randomized controlled trial. *Obstetrics and Gynecology*, *144*(2), 144–152. https://doi.org/10.1097/AOG.0000000000005648

Lapping-Carr, L., & Pappa, M. L. (2024). Evidence for the impact of stress and trauma on sexual function in women: Review and clinical recommendations. *Obstetrics and Gynecology Clinics of North America*, *51*(2), 285–298. https://doi.org/10.1016/j.ogc.2024.02.003

Lee, H., Hwang, E. C., Oh, C. K., Lee, S., Yu, H. S., Lim, J. S., Kim, H. W., Walsh, T., Kim, M. H., Jung, J. H., & Dahm, P. (2024). Testosterone replacement in men with sexual dysfunction. *The Cochrane Database of Systematic Reviews*, *1*(1), CD013071. https://doi.org/10.1002/14651858.CD013071.pub2

Leslie, S. W., & Sooriyamoorthy, T. (2024). Erectile dysfunction. In *StatPearls*. StatPearls Publishing. https://www.ncbi.nlm.nih.gov/books/NBK562253

Lugo, T., & Tetrokalashvili, M. (2022). Hot flashes. In *StatPearls*. StatPearls Publishing. https://www.ncbi.nlm.nih.gov/books/NBK539827

Marchand, E. (2021). Psychological and behavioral treatment of female orgasmic disorder. *Sexual Medicine Reviews*, *9*(2), 194–211. https://doi.org/10.1016/j.sxmr.2020.07.007

Masters, W. H., & Johnson, V. E. (1966). *Human sexual response*. Little, Brown.

Masters, W. H., & Johnson, V. E. (1970). *Human sexual inadequacy*. Little, Brown.

Mauvais-Jarvis, F., & Lindsey, S. H. (2024). Metabolic benefits afforded by estradiol and testosterone in both sexes: clinical considerations. *The Journal of Clinical Investigation*, *134*(17), e180073. https://doi.org/10.1172/JCI180073

McCabe, S. E., Dickinson, K., Engstrom, C. W., Kcomt, L., Veliz, P. T., Boyd, C. J., Parra, L. A., & Evans-Polce, R. (2024). A national longitudinal study of sexual orientation discordance, sexual identity fluidity, and alcohol and other drug use disorder symptoms. *The American Journal of Drug and Alcohol Abuse*, *50*(4), 481–491. https://doi.org/10.1080/00952990.2024.2378837

McClung, E., Rosen, N. O., Dubé, J. P., Wang, G. A., & Corsini-Munt, S. (2024). Motivation when desire is low: Associations between sexual motivation and sexual intimacy, sexual satisfaction, and sexual distress for men with hypoactive sexual desire disorder and their partners. *Archives of Sexual Behavior*, *53*(3), 1075–1089. https://doi.org/10.1007/s10508-023-02752-x

Mehmood, K. T., & Rentea, R. M. (2023). Ambiguous genitalia and disorders of sexual differentiation. In *StatPearls*. StatPearls Publishing. https://www.ncbi.nlm.nih.gov/books/NBK557435

National Institute on Aging. (2022). Sexuality and intimacy in older adults. National Institutes of Health. https://www.nia.nih.gov/health/sexuality/sexuality-and-intimacy-older-adults

Parish, S. J., Clayton, A. H., & Kingsberg, S. A. (2022). Response to Balon's commentary: Is Basson's model of sexual response relevant? *Journal of Sex & Marital Therapy*, *48*(1), 17–19. https://doi.org/10.1080/0092623X.2021.1995092

Perez, L. G., Troxel, W. M., Tucker, J. S., Dunbar, M. S., Rodriguez, A., Klein, D. J., & D'Amico, E. J. (2024). Discrimination experiences and problematic alcohol and cannabis use in young adulthood. *The American Journal on Addictions*, *34*(1), 30–39. https://doi.org/10.1111/ajad.13632

Pinto, J., Comprido, C., Moreira, V., Maccarone, M. T., Cogoni, C., Faustino, R., Pignatelli, D., & Cera, N. (2024). The complex role played by the default mode network during sexual stimulation: A cluster-based fMRI meta-analysis. *Behavioral Sciences*, *14*(7), 570. https://doi.org/10.3390/bs14070570

Rodrigues, A. M. B. P., Neto, O. B., Seguro, C. S., da Silva, W. F., Gonzalez, R. H., Santos, D. A. T., de Lira, C. A. B., & Viana, R. B. (2024). Does yoga improve sexual function? A systematic review and meta-analysis of randomized clinical trials. *Complementary Therapies in Clinical Practice*, *56*, 101864. https://doi.org/10.1016/j.ctcp.2024.101864

Saadedine, M., Faubion, S. S., Grach, S. L., Nordhues, H. C., & Kapoor, E. (2024). Association between obesity and female sexual dysfunction: a review. *Sexual Medicine Reviews*, *12*(2), 154–163. https://doi.org/10.1093/sxmrev/qead047

Shaikh, A., Kamble, P., Daulatabad, V., Singhal, A., Madhusudhan, U., & John, N. A. (2024). Mental health challenges within the LGBTQ community: A societal imperative. *Journal of Family Medicine and Primary Care*, *13*(9), 3529–3535. https://doi.org/10.4103/jfmpc.jfmpc_321_24

Shechter, A., & Gruenwald, I. (2024). New technologies developed for treatment of premature ejaculation. *International Journal of Impotence Research*, *36*(7), 700–705. https://doi.org/10.1038/s41443-024-00875-w

Sobel, T., & David, P. (2024). Impact of chronic medical disease on sexual function and other conditions. *Obstetrics and Gynecology Clinics of North America*, *51*(2), 323–340. https://doi.org/10.1016/j.ogc.2024.02.006

Sprout Pharmaceuticals. (2024). Prescribing Information ADDYI (flibanserin) tablets. Retrieved December 20, 2024, from https://addyi.com/

Syme, M. L., & Cohn, T. J. (2021). Aging sexual stereotypes and sexual expression in mid- and later life: Examining the stereotype matching effect. *Aging & Mental Health*, *25*(8), 1507–1514. https://doi.org/10.1080/13607863.2020.1758909

Tayyeb, M., & Gupta, V. (2023). Dyspareunia. In *StatPearls*. StatPearls Publishing. https://www.ncbi.nlm.nih.gov/books/NBK562159

van Raaij, J. J., Serefoglu, E. C., van Amelsvoort, T. A. M. J., & Janssen, P. K. C. (2024). Possible pathophysiologic roles of neurotransmitter systems in men with lifelong premature ejaculation: a scoping review. *Sexual Medicine Reviews*, *12*(4), 638–651. https://doi.org/10.1093/sxmrev/qeae048

Wang, A., Wang, H., Ma, D., Chang, H., Zhao, Z., Luo, D., & Wang, F. (2024). The role of acupuncture in treating premature ejaculation and its probable neurobiological mechanism. *Basic and Clinical Andrology*, *34*(1), 20. https://doi.org/10.1186/s12610-024-00239-w

Wang, C. M., Wu, B. R., Xiang, P., Xiao, J., & Hu, X. C. (2023). Management of male erectile dysfunction: From the past to the future. *Frontiers in Endocrinology*, *14*, 1148834. https://doi.org/10.3389/fendo.2023.1148834

Waxenbaum, J. A., Reddy, V., & Varacallo, M. (2023). Anatomy, autonomic nervous system. In *StatPearls*. StatPearls Publishing. https://www.ncbi.nlm.nih.gov/books/NBK539845

World Health Organization (WHO). (n.d.a). *Sexual health*. Retrieved December 12, 2024, from https://www.who.int/health-topics/sexual-health#tab=tab_1

World Health Organization (WHO). (n.d.b). *Sexual and reproductive health and research (SRH)*. Retrieved December 12, 2024, from http://www.who.int/reproductivehealth/topics/sexual_health/sh_definitions/en/

Ziapour, A., Kazeminia, M., Rouzbahani, M., Bakhshi, S., Montazeri, N., Yıldırım, M., Tadbiri, H., Moradi, F., & Janjani, P. (2024). Global prevalence of sexual dysfunction in cardiovascular patients: A systematic review and meta-analysis. *Systematic Reviews*, *13*(1), 136. https://doi.org/10.1186/s13643-024-02525-0

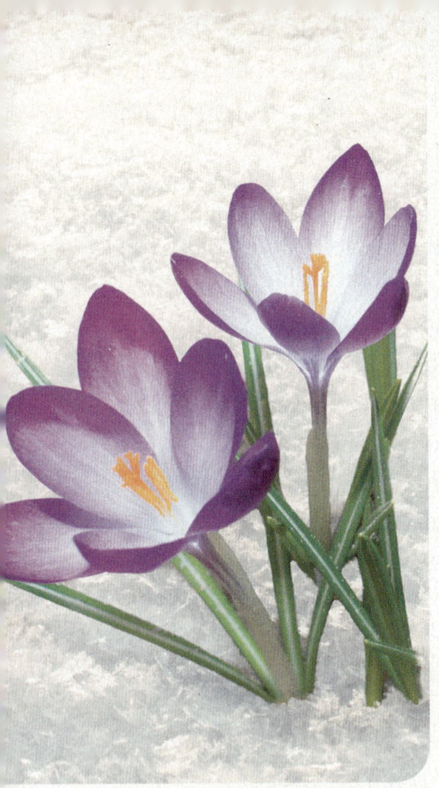

UNIT VII

Care of Children and Adolescents

36

Mental Health Assessment of Children and Adolescents*

Valerie Griffin and Rebecca Luebbert

KEYCONCEPTS

- assortative mating
- comprehensive assessment

LEARNING OBJECTIVES

After studying this chapter, you will be able to:

1. Define the assessment process for children and adolescents.
2. Discuss techniques of data collection used with children and adolescents.
3. Delineate important areas of assessment for children and adolescents, including evaluation of social determinants of health and presence of adverse childhood experiences.

KEY TERMS

• attachment • attachment disorganization • developmental delays • egocentrism • maturation • temperament

INTRODUCTION

The mental health assessment of children and adolescents is a specialized process that considers their unique issues and responses within the context of their development. Any nurse who cares for a child should be comfortable with conducting a mental health nursing assessment because the emotional and psychological aspects are central to understanding health needs and behaviors.

The assessment of children and adolescents generally follows the same format as for adults (see Chapter 10), but there are significant differences. Children think in more concrete terms; thus, the nurse needs to ask more specific and fewer open-ended questions than would typically be asked of adults. The nurse should use simple phrasing because children have a narrower vocabulary than do adults. Examples include saying "sad" instead of "depressed" or "nervous" instead of "anxious." The nurse needs to corroborate information that children offer with more sources (e.g., parents, caregivers, teachers) than they would for adults. The nurse may want to use artistic and play media (e.g., puppets, family drawings) to engage children and evaluate their perceptions, inner worlds, fine motor skills, and intellectual functions. Children have a less specific sense of time and a less developed memory than do adults. When children are asked about a sequence of events or specific times when events occurred, they may not be able to provide accurate information.

**In this chapter, "parent" refers to the primary caregiver of a child.*

A comprehensive evaluation includes a history, mental status examination, additional testing (e.g., cognitive or neuropsychological), if necessary, records of the child's school performance and medical–physical history, and information from other agencies that may be providing services (e.g., Department of Child and Family Services [DCFS], juvenile court, specialists). The nurse may use various assessment tools including, but not limited to, the Behavior Assessment System for Children (BASC), Child Behavior Checklist (CBCL), ADHD-specific rating scales, Patient Health Questionnaire (PHQ), General Anxiety Disorder-7 (GAD-7), Screen for Child Anxiety-Related Disorders (SCARED), Pediatric Symptom Checklist (PSC), Survey of Well-Being of Young Children (SWYC), or the Pediatric ACEs and Related Life-events Screener (PEARLS).

NCLEXNOTE Whenever assessing children or adolescents, developmental level will frame the assessment and implementation of the management plan.

THE CLINICAL INTERVIEW

The clinical interview is the primary assessment tool used in child and adolescent psychiatry. A unique set of skills is necessary for interviewing children and adolescents. How the nurse obtains mental health information depends on the developmental level of each child, specifically considering the child's language, cognitive, social, and emotional skills. For example, the nurse should simplify questions for young children or children with developmental delays so they can understand and respond appropriately.

The assessment interview may be the initial contact between the child and parent or guardian and the nurse. The first step is to establish a therapeutic alliance with both the child and parent, and the second is to assess the interactions between the child and parent.

Establishment of a Therapeutic Alliance

The nurse can establish rapport by greeting the child or adolescent in a friendly, polite, open manner, and putting them at ease. Speaking clearly and at a typical volume and using friendly, reassuring tones are essential measures. The nurse can establish a treatment alliance by recognizing the child's individuality and showing respect and concern for them. The nurse should demonstrate sensitivity, objectivity, and confidentiality. The child will be more forthcoming if they feel that the nurse is listening carefully and is interested in what they have to say.

Child and Parent Observation

Because the child's primary environment is with the parent or guardian, child–parent interactions provide important data about the child–parent attachment and parenting practices. The nurse's observations focus on both the child alone and the child within the family. The nurse can actually make some of these observations while the family is in the waiting area, including:

- How the child and parent talk to each other, including how frequently each initiates conversation
- How the parent disciplines the child
- How attached the parent and child appear
- How the child and parent separate
- If the parent and child play together
- How the child gets the parent's attention and how responsive the parent is to the child's attention-seeking behaviors
- How the parent and child show affection to each other

Separate Child and Parent Interviews

To get an accurate picture of the child, the nurse should interview the child and parent individually because each can provide unique meaningful information. Research has shown that when parent and child are interviewed separately in a structured interview about the child's psychopathology, they rarely agree on the presence of diagnostic criteria, particularly regarding depression and anxiety (De Los Reyes & Epkins, 2023; Lochner et al., 2023). Generally, there is greater child–parent agreement on external symptoms and behaviors than on nonobservable symptoms, such as mood, feelings, and emotions (Hu & Zhou, 2024; Nelemans et al., 2022).

Discussion With the Child

After talking with the parent and child together, the nurse should ask to speak with the child alone for a while. Young children may fear separating from their parents. The nurse can reassure children by showing them where the waiting area is and telling them that if they get scared, the nurse will accompany them to check on their parents. Introducing a toy or game or allowing the child to hold a transitional object may help. Remember that observing how the child separates from the parent is part of the data needed to complete the assessment.

Adolescents may act indifferent or even hostile when the nurse asks to speak with them alone. Teens tend to be skeptical that adults can really understand their experience, suspicious that they will be blamed for their issues, and fearful that their thoughts and feelings are unusual. The nurse should convey their genuine interest in wanting to hear the adolescent's perspective. The nurse should be patient with adolescents and say something like, "I can see you're pretty angry about being here. What are you particularly angry about? Perhaps there is some way I can help you." Another useful and reassuring question is, "During the last few minutes, you've been quiet. I'm wondering what you are feeling." Or the nurse may ask, "It can be uncomfortable to tell personal information to someone you don't know. Do you feel this way?" (Frick et al., 2020).

To begin the initial assessment of a child, the nurse introduces themself and explains briefly what they will be doing. For children younger than 11 years of age, the nurse should explain that they help worried or upset children by talking, playing, and giving advice to them and their parents. The nurse should then ask about the child's understanding of why they are there. This question often helps to identify children's misperceptions (e.g., believing the nurse is going to give them an injection, thinking they have done something bad) that could create barriers to working with them. When conducting the child interview, the nurse needs to get several releases of information from the child's guardian to obtain the corroborating reports, such as the child's physical assessment from the primary care provider; the school's report about the child's academic and behavioral performance, including the child's report card, behavior at school, peer interactions, and adult interactions; and records of diagnosis and treatment from any previous psychiatric provider.

The nurse must adapt communication to the child's age level (Box 36.1). The challenge is to avoid using overly complex vocabulary or talking down to children. Young children often express themselves more easily in the context of play than through adult like conversation. For example, a child may reenact a conversation that they had with a sibling or parent using puppets. Children respond well to third-person conversation prompts, such as "Some kids don't like being compared with their brothers and sisters," or "I know a kid who was so sad when their dog got lost that they thought they'd never be happy again."

Early in the interview, the goal is to explain the nurse's purpose, elicit any concerns the child may have about what is happening, and establish rapport with the child by engaging in unthreatening discussion. Many adults rarely ask children about things that truly interest them but expect children to respond readily to adult conversation. The nurse can establish a high degree of credibility simply by taking note of and asking about things that are obviously important to children (e.g., a sport the child participates in, a rock group displayed on a shirt, a toy a child has brought with them). However, children have an uncanny natural "radar" for phony adult behavior. Attempts to establish rapport work only when the nurse is genuinely interested in the child's life.

BOX 36.1

Strategies for Interviewing Children

- Use a simple vocabulary and short sentences tailored to the child's developmental and cognitive levels.
- Be sure that the child understands the questions and that you do not lead the child to give a particular response. Phrase your questions so the child does not receive any hint that one response is more acceptable than another.
- Select the questions for your interview on an individual basis using judgment and discretion and considering the child's age and developmental level.
- Be sure that the manner and tone of your voice do not reveal any personal biases.
- Speak slowly and quietly and try to allow the interview to unfold, using the child's verbalizations and behavior as guides.
- Use simple terms (e.g., "sad" for "depressed") in exploring affective reactions and ask the child to give examples of how they behave or how other people behave when emotionally aroused.
- Assume an accepting and neutral attitude toward the child's communications.
- Learn about children's current interests by looking at children's television programs, talking with parents, visiting toy stores, looking at children's books, and visiting day care centers and schools to observe children in their natural habitats.

Discussion With the Parents

After meeting alone with the child, the nurse should spend some time alone with the parents and ask for a detailed description of their view of the issue. When alone, parents may feel comfortable discussing their children in depth and sharing concerns with their behavior. Parents need this opportunity to speak freely without being constrained by concern for the child's feelings. In some cases, it would be detrimental for the child to hear the full impact of the parents' complaints and feelings, such as helplessness, anger, or disappointment. Parents need the nurse to allow them to express their feelings without passing judgment. This is the nurse's opportunity to enlist the help of parents as partners in the child's evaluation and treatment. This time is also good for filling in any gaps in the history and clarifying the data obtained from the interview with the child.

Parents need the chance to describe the presenting issue in their own words. The nurse can encourage them by asking general questions, such as, "What brings you here today?" or "How have things been in your family?" The nurse should then reflect their understanding of the issue, showing empathy and respect for both the parent and child. Asking any other family members about their view of the issue is always a good idea to clarify discrepant points of view, obtain additional data, and communicate awareness that different family members experience the same concern in different ways.

DEVELOPMENT OF RAPPORT

To reduce anxiety about the evaluation, the nurse must develop a rapport with the family. Establishing rapport can be facilitated by maintaining appropriate eye contact;

speaking slowly, clearly, and calmly with friendliness and acceptance; using a warm and expressive tone; reacting to communications from interviewees objectively; showing interest in what the interviewees are saying; and making the interview a joint undertaking (see Chapter 10). Suggestions for building rapport with children and adolescents are also addressed in each of the developmental sections that follow. The information in Box 36.2 can serve as a guide to asking specific questions during a comprehensive assessment.

KEYCONCEPT A **comprehensive assessment** includes a very detailed, focused interview that elicits all aspects of the responses and health promotion information that provides direction for care.

BOX 36.2

Semi-Structured Interview With School-Aged Children

Precede the following questions with a preliminary greeting, such as the following: "Hi, I am (your name and title). You must be (child's name). Come in."

FOR ALL SCHOOL-AGED CHILDREN

1. Has anyone told you about why you are here today?
2. (If yes) Who?
3. (If yes) What did they tell you?
4. Tell me why *you* think you are here. (If child mentions an issue, explore it in detail.)
5. How old are you?
6. When is your birthday?
7. What is your address?
8. What is your telephone number?

School

9. Let's talk about school. What grade are you in?
10. What is your teacher's name?
11. What grades are you getting?
12. What subjects do you like the best?
13. And what subjects do you like least?
14. What subjects give you the most trouble?
15. And what subjects give you the least trouble?
16. What activities are you in at school?
17. How do you get along with your classmates?
18. How do you get along with your teachers?
19. Tell me how you spend a usual day at school.

Home

20. Now let's talk about your home. Who lives with you at home?
21. Tell me a little about each of them.
22. What does one of your parents do for work?
23. What does your other parent do for work?
24. Tell me what your home is like.
25. Tell me about your room at home.
26. What chores do you do at home?
27. How do you get along with one of your parents?
28. What do they do that you like?
29. What does they do that you don't like?
30. How do you get along with your other parent?
31. What do they do that you like?
32. What do they do that you don't like?
33. (When relevant) How do you get along with your siblings?
34. What do they do that you like?
35. What do they do that you don't like?
36. Who handles the discipline at home?
37. Tell me about how they handle it.

Interests

38. Now let's talk about you. What hobbies and interests do you have?
39. What do you do in the afternoons after school?
40. Tell me what you usually do on Saturdays and Sundays.

Friends

41. Tell me about your friends.
42. What do you like to do with your friends?

Moods and Feelings

43. Everybody feels happy at times. What things make you feel happiest?
44. What are you most likely to get sad about?
45. What do you do when you are sad?
46. Everybody gets angry at times. What things make you angriest?
47. What do you do when you are angry?

Fears and Worries

48. All children get scared sometimes about some things. What things make you feel scared?
49. What do you do when you are scared?
50. Tell me what you worry about.
51. Any other things?

Self-Concerns

52. What do you like best about yourself?
53. Anything else?
54. What do you like least about yourself?
55. Anything else?
56. Tell me about the best thing that ever happened to you.
57. Tell me about the worst thing that ever happened to you.

Somatic Concerns

58. Do you ever get headaches?
59. (If yes) Tell me about them. (How often? What do you usually do?)
60. Do you get stomach aches?
61. (If yes) Tell me about them. (How often? What do you usually do?)
62. Do you get any other kinds of body pains?
63. (If yes) Tell me about them.

Thought Disorder

64. Do you ever hear things that seem funny or usual?
65. (If yes) Tell me about them. (How often? How do you feel about them? What do you usually do?)
66. Do you ever see things that seem funny or unreal?
67. (If yes) Tell me about them. (How often? How do you feel about them? What do you usually do?)

Memories and Fantasy

68. What is the first thing you can remember from the time you were a very little baby?
69. Tell me about your dreams.
70. Which dreams come back again?
71. Who are your favorite television characters?
72. Tell me about them.

BOX 36.2 (*Continued*)

73. What animals do you like best?
74. Tell me about these animals.
75. What animals do you like least?
76. Tell me about these animals.
77. What is your happiest memory?
78. What is your saddest memory?
79. If you could change places with anyone in the whole world, who would it be?
80. Tell me about that.
81. If you could go anywhere you wanted to right now, where would you go?
82. Tell me about that.
83. If you could have three wishes, what would they be?
84. What things do you think you might need to take with you if you were to go to the moon and stay there for 6 months?

Aspirations

85. What do you plan on doing when you become an adult?
86. Do you think you will have any problem doing that?
87. If you could do anything you wanted when you become an adult, what would it be?

Concluding Questions

88. Do you have anything else that you would like to tell me about yourself?
89. Do you have any questions that you would like to ask me?

FOR ADOLESCENTS

These questions can be inserted after number 67.

Sexual Relations

1. Do you have any special romantic partner?
2. (If yes) Tell me about that person.
3. What kind of sexual concerns do you have?
4. (If present) Tell me about them.

Drug and Alcohol Use

5. Do your parents/caregivers drink alcohol?
6. (If yes) Tell me about their drinking. (How much, how frequently, and where?)
7. Do your friends drink alcohol?
8. (If yes) Tell me about their drinking.
9. Do you drink alcohol?
10. (If yes) Tell me about your drinking.
11. Do your parents use drugs?
12. (If yes) Tell me about the drugs they use. (How much, how frequently, and for what reasons?)
13. Do your friends use drugs?
14. (If yes) Tell me about the drugs they use.
15. Do you use drugs?
16. (If yes) Tell me about the drugs you use.

Preschool-Aged Children

When interviewing preschool-aged children, the nurse should understand that they may have difficulty putting their feelings into words and that their thinking is very concrete. For example, a preschool-aged child might assume that a tall container holds more water than a wide container even if both containers hold the same amount of fluid.

The nurse can achieve rapport with preschool-aged children by joining their world of play. Play is a pleasurable physical or mental activity by which children transform an experience from real life into a symbolic, nonliteral representation. Play impacts all brain areas, structures, and functions. As a natural form of expression, play encourages verbalizations and socializing with others, promotes manual strength, teaches rules and problem solving, and helps children master control over their environment (Burgin & Ray, 2022; Elbeltagi et al., 2023; Hartwig & Taylor, 2022). With children younger than 5 years of age, the nurse may conduct the assessment in a playroom. Useful materials are paper, pencils, crayons, paints, paintbrushes, easels, clay, blocks, balls, dolls, doll houses, puppets, animals, dress-up clothes, and a water supply. The nurse must inform preschool-aged children about any rules for the play. For example, the nurse must tell the child that the nurse must ensure safety, so there will be no hitting in the playroom.

When observing the child in a free play setting, the nurse should pay attention to initiation of play, energy level, manipulative actions, tempo, body movements, tone, integration, creativity, products, age appropriateness, and attitudes toward adults. In addition, themes of play, expression of emotions, and temperament are important to observe. The nurse must allow children to direct and initiate these themes. When evaluating a young child's peer relationships through play therapy in a playgroup or school setting, observe play settings and themes, initiation of play, response to peer initiations of play, integration of affect and action during play, resolution of conflicts, responses to suggestions of others during play, and the ability to engage in role taking and role reversals.

The nurse's roles include being a good listener; using appropriate vocabulary; tolerating a child's anxious, angry, or sad behavior; and using reflective comments about the child's play. Through play, the nurse can assess the child's sensorimotor skills, cognitive style, adaptability, language functioning, emotional and behavioral responsiveness, social level, moral development, coping styles, problem-solving techniques, and approaches to perceiving and interpreting the surrounding world. Lidz (2003) developed a tool that clinicians can use to assess preschoolers' play (Box 36.3). Analyzing children's perceptions of fairy tales can provide clinicians with clues to culture, issues, solutions, and elements of mental functioning (Masri et al., 2025).

Drawings may be used in conjunction with other assessment strategies and are especially useful when assessing children who are less able to articulate their

BOX 36.3

LIDZ Assessment Tool

Child's Name: ________ Birth Date: ________ Age: _____
Assessor: ____________ Date of Assessment: __________

Describe typical play style/sequence.
Describe range of levels of play from lowest to highest level with age estimates and within contexts of independent/facilitated, familiar/unfamiliar, single/multiple toys.
Describe language and evidence of self-talk and internalized speech.
Describe interpersonal interactions with assessor and facilitator (if not assessor).
Describe content of any play themes.
What held the child's attention the longest? (For how long?) And what were the child's toy/play preferences?
Describe the child's affective state during play.
Implications of aforementioned for intervention.

thoughts and emotions verbally. Drawing can also be useful when communication is affected due to language and cultural differences (Efe et al., 2023). Through drawings, children can depict basic emotions such as happiness, sadness, fear, and anger. Social emotions, such as pride, shame, and jealousy, can also be conveyed through drawings (Fig. 36.1). Clinicians including child drawings in their assessments should note verbal, paraverbal, and nonverbal observations during the drawing activity. Assessment of human figure drawings generally include shapes and colors, facial expressions, posture, proximity to others, and context included in the drawing (Shinohara et al., 2022; Vettori et al., 2022).

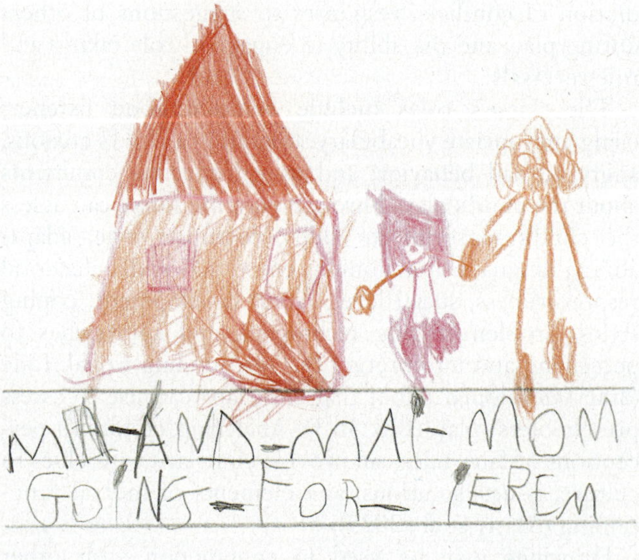

FIGURE 36.1 Drawing and writing by a 5-year-old child.

School-Aged Children

Unlike preschool-aged children, school-aged (5 to 12 years) children can use more constructs, provide longer descriptions and make better inferences of others, and acquire more complete conceptions of various social roles. Children in middle school are more capable of verbal exchange and can tolerate limited periods of direct questioning (Box 36.4). The nurse can establish rapport with school-aged children by using competitive board games, such as checkers and playing cards. A therapeutic game helpful in assessing the child's perceptions, cognition, and emotions and in establishing rapport between a clinician and child is the thinking–feeling–doing game. In this game, the clinician and child take turns drawing cards that pose hypothetical situations and ask what an individual might think, feel, or do in such scenarios. For example, one card might say, "A child has something on their mind that they are afraid to tell their parent. What are they scared to talk about?" Another might read, "A child heard their parents fighting. What were they fighting about? What was the child thinking while listening to their parents?"

Adolescents

Adolescents have an increased command of language concepts and have developed the capacity for abstract and formal operations thinking. Their social world is also more complex. Some early adolescents tend to assume that their subjective experiences are real and congruent with objective reality, which can lead to **egocentrism**. Egocentrism includes the concepts of the imaginary audience (others are watching them) and the personal fable (they are special and unique and omnipotent) (Rycek et al., 1998). Egocentrism is a preoccupation with one's own appearance, behavior, thoughts, and feelings. For example, a preteen may think they caused their parents to divorce because of a fight with one of their parents the day before the parents announced their decision to separate. Egocentrism is increased when emotions associated with uncertainty increase (Weidema et al., 2023). Because teenagers have a heightened sense of self-consciousness, they may be preoccupied during the interview with applying makeup or other self-grooming tasks.

During early adolescence, cognitive changes include increased self-consciousness, fear of being shamed, and demands for privacy and secrecy. An adolescent's willingness to talk to a nurse will depend partly on their perception of the degree of rapport between them. The nurse's ability to communicate, respect, cooperation, honesty, and genuineness is important. Rejection by the adolescent, even outright hostility, during the first few interactions is common, especially if the teen is having behavioral issues at home, at school, or in the community.

BOX 36.4

Psychiatric–Mental Health Nursing Assessment of Children and Adolescents

IDENTIFYING INFORMATION

Name
Gender/gender identity
Date of birth
Age
Birth order
Grade
Ethnic background
Religious preference
List of others living in household

MAJOR REASON FOR SEEKING HELP

Description of presenting issues or symptoms
When did the issues (symptoms) start?
Describe both the child's and the parent's perspective.

PSYCHIATRIC HISTORY

Previous mental health contacts (inpatient and outpatient)
Other mental health issues or psychiatric diagnosis (besides those described currently)
Previous medications and adherence
Family history of depression, substance misuse, psychosis, etc., and treatment

CURRENT AND PAST HEALTH STATUS

Medical issues
Current medications
Surgery and hospitalizations
Allergies
Diet and eating habits
Sleeping habits
Height and weight
Hearing and vision
Menstrual history (if relevant)
Immunizations
If sexually active, if birth control is being used, method used
Date of last physical examination
Primary care provider's name and telephone number

MEDICATIONS

Prescription (dosage, side effects)
Over-the-counter drugs

NEUROLOGIC HISTORY

Right handed, left handed, or ambidextrous
Headaches, dizziness, fainting
Seizures
Unusual movement (tics, tremors)
Hyperactivity
Episodes of weakness or paralysis
Slurred speech, pronunciation issues
Fine motor skills (eating with utensils, using crayon or pencil, fastening buttons and zippers, tying shoes)
Gross motor skills and coordination (walking, running, hopping)

RESPONSES TO MENTAL HEALTH ISSUES

What makes issues (symptoms) worse or better?
Feelings about those experiences (what helped and did not help)
What interventions have been tried so far?
Major loss or changes in past year
Fears, including punishment

MENTAL STATUS EXAMINATION

See Box 36.6.

DEVELOPMENTAL ASSESSMENT

Biological mother's pregnancy, delivery
Child's Apgar score
Physical maturation
Psychosocial
Language
Developmental milestones: walking, talking, toileting

ATTACHMENT, TEMPERAMENT OR SIGNIFICANT BEHAVIOR PATTERNS

Attachment
Concentration, distractibility
Eating and sleeping patterns
Ability to adjust to new situations and changes in routine
Usual mood and fluctuations
Excitability
Ability to wait, tendency to interrupt
Responses to discipline
Lying, stealing, fighting, cruelty to animals, fire setting

SELF-CONCEPT

Beliefs about self
Body image
Self-esteem
Personal identity

RISK ASSESSMENT

History of suicidal thoughts, previous attempts
Suicidal ideation, plan, lethality of plan, accessibility of plan
History of violent, aggressive behavior
Homicidal ideation

FAMILY RELATIONSHIPS

Relationship with parents
Deaths or losses
Family conflicts (nature and content)
Disciplinary methods
Quality of sibling relationship
Sleeping arrangements
Who does the child relate to or trust in the family?
Relationships with extended family

SCHOOL AND PEER ADJUSTMENT

Learning difficulties
Behavior issues at school
School attendance
Relationship with teachers
Special classes
Best friend
Relationships with peers
Dating, drug, and alcohol use
Participation in sports, clubs, other activities
After-school routine

COMMUNITY RESOURCES

Professionals or agencies working with child or family
Day care resources

FUNCTIONAL STATUS

Global Assessment of Functioning Scale (GAF)

STRESSES AND COPING BEHAVIORS

Psychosocial stresses
Coping behaviors (strengths)

SUMMARY OF SIGNIFICANT DATA

The nurse should be patient and avoid jumping to conclusions. Hostility or defiance may be a test of how much the teen can trust the nurse, a defense against anxiety, or a transference phenomenon (see Chapter 9).

Adolescents are likely to be defensive in front of their parents and concerned with confidentiality. At the start of the interview, the nurse should clearly convey to the adolescent what information will and will not be shared with parents. Adolescents generally prefer a straightforward, candid approach to the interview because they often distrust those in authority. Mentioning to adolescents that they do not have to discuss anything that they are not ready to reveal is also a good idea, so they will feel in control while they gradually build trust.

MENTAL HEALTH NURSING ASSESSMENT OF CHILDREN AND ADOLESCENTS

As discussed, the comprehensive assessment of the child or adolescent includes interviews with the child and parents, child alone, and parents alone. After completing these components, the nurse should bring the child and parents back together to summarize their view of their concerns and to ask for feedback regarding whether these perceptions agree with theirs. The nurse must give the family a chance to share additional information and ask questions. Then the nurse should thank them for their willingness to talk and give them some idea of the next steps. The use of an assessment tool is helpful in organizing data for mental health planning and intervention.

When interviewing both a child and parents, directly asking the child as many questions as possible is generally the best way to get accurate, firsthand information and to reinforce interest in the child's viewpoint. Asking the child questions about the history of the current issue, previous psychiatric experiences (both good and bad), family psychiatric history, medical issues, developmental history (to get an idea of what the child has been told), school adjustment, peer relationships, and family functioning is particularly important. If necessary, the nurse can ask some or all of these same questions of the parents to verify the accuracy of the data, attain supplemental information, or both. Keep in mind that developmental research shows moderate to low correlation between parent and child reports of family behavior.

Children's Rating Scales for Psychiatric Disorders

A number of children's rating scales can assist in the assessment of various psychiatric disorders (Table 36.1). The BASC, developed by Reynolds and Kamphouse (1998), is a tool used to measure behaviors and emotions in children aged 2 to 21 years. The scales include a teacher rating scale, a parent rating scale, and a self-report of personality. The scale evaluates several dimensions, including attitude to school, attitude toward teachers, sensation seeking, atypicality, locus of control, somatization, social stress, anxiety, depression, sense of inadequacy, relations with parents, interpersonal relations, self-esteem, and self-reliance. The CBCL, developed by Achenbach and Edelbrock (1983), is a 113-item self-report tool used to identify forms of psychopathology and competencies that occur in children aged 6 to 18 years. This instrument provides scores on internalizing and externalizing behaviors.

The PSC is a 35-item psychosocial screen to help identify cognitive, emotional, and behavioral issues in children aged 4 to 11 years (Jellinek et al., 1988). The Strengths and Difficulties Questionnaire (SDQ) screens for developmental milestones, behavioral/emotional development, family risk factors, and social determinants of health in children aged 4 to 17 years (Goodman, 1997). The SWYC assesses risk for developmental and behavioral concerns, including autism, parental depression, and family risk factors in young children (Sheldrick & Perrin, 2013). The PHQ was created in 1999 and is considered a valid, reliable tool used to measure depression severity (Kroenke et al., 1999).

The Vanderbilt Assessment Scales are used to assess children aged 6 to 12 years for attention-deficit hyperactivity disorder (ADHD) (Wolraich et al., 2003). The Children's Yale-Brown Obsessive Compulsive Scale, developed by Goodman et al. (1989), is a 19-item scale that can help diagnose childhood obsessive–compulsive disorder in children 6 to 17 years of age.

Spitzer et al. (2006) developed the GAD-7 as a screening tool and severity indicator for generalized anxiety disorder. The SCARED tool was developed in 1997 to screen for specific anxiety disorders such as GAD, separation anxiety disorder, panic disorder, and symptoms related to social phobia (Birmaher et al., 1997).

Safety Issues

The nurse must ask the child about any suicidal or violent thoughts. The best way to assess these areas is to ask straightforward questions, such as, "Have you ever thought about hurting yourself? Have you ever thought about hurting someone else? Have you ever acted on these thoughts? Have you thought about how you would do it? What did you think would happen if you hurt yourself? Have you ever done anything to hurt yourself before?" Contrary to popular belief, even young children attempt suicide, and they are capable of violent acts toward other children, adults, and animals. When a child shares the intent to commit a suicidal or violent act, the nurse must remind them that they will have to discuss this concern with the parent to keep the child and others safe.

TABLE 36.1 CHILDREN'S RATING SCALES FOR PSYCHIATRIC DISORDERS

Instrument	Use
Behavior Assessment System for Children (BASC)	• Assesses for behavioral and emotional issues • Age range: 2–21 years • 105–165 items • Estimated time to complete: 10–20 minutes
Child Behavior Checklist (CBCL)	• Screens for emotional, behavioral, and social issues • Age range: 6–18 years • 113 items • Estimated time to complete: 10 minutes
Children's Yale-Brown Obsessive Compulsive Scale (CY-BOCS)	• Rates the severity of obsessive and compulsive symptoms • Age range: 6–17 years • 19 items • Estimated time to complete: 30–45 minutes
General Anxiety Disorder (GAD-7)	• Screening for diagnosis and severity assessment of anxiety disorder • Age range: 11 years and older • 7 items • Estimated time to complete: 1–2 minutes
Patient Health Questionnaire (PHQ)	• Screens for depression • Age range: 12 years and older • 10 items • Estimated time to complete: 10 minutes
Pediatric Symptom Checklist (PSC)	• Psychosocial screen designed to recognize cognitive, emotional, and behavioral issues • Age range: 4–11 years • 35 items • Estimated time to complete: 5–10 minutes
Screening for Child Anxiety Related Disorders (SCARED)	• Screens for childhood anxiety disorders, including general anxiety, separation anxiety, panic disorder, and symptoms related to school phobias • Age range: 8–18 years • 41 items • Estimated time to complete: 10 minutes
Strengths and Difficulties Questionnaire (SDQ)	• Screens behaviors, emotions, and relationships • Age range: 4–17 years • 25 items • Estimated time to complete: 5 minutes
The Survey of Wellbeing of Young Children (SWYC)	• Screens for developmental milestones, behavioral/emotional development, family risk factors, and social determinants of health • Age range: 2–60 months • 12 items • Estimated time to complete: 5–10 minutes
NICHQ Vanderbilt Assessment Scales	• Screens for ADHD • Age range: 6–12 years • 55-item parent scale; 43-item teacher scale • Estimated time to complete: 10 minutes

Physical Health and Functioning

Nurses should include a thorough history of psychiatric and medical conditions in any comprehensive assessment. A physical assessment is necessary to rule out any medical issues that could be mistaken for psychiatric symptoms (e.g., weight loss resulting from diabetes, not depression; substance-induced psychosis).

Genetic Vulnerability

The line between nature and nurture is not always clear. Characteristics that appear to be inborn may influence parents and teachers to respond differently toward different children, thus creating issues in the family environment. A phenomenon called **assortative mating** may contribute to the genetic transmission of psychiatric disorders (Torvik et al., 2022).

Research increasingly shows that major psychiatric disorders (e.g., depression, anxiety disorder, schizophrenia, bipolar disorder, substance misuse) run in families. Thus, having a parent or sibling with a psychiatric disorder usually indicates an increased risk for the same or another closely related disorder in a child or adolescent. In addition, many childhood psychiatric disorders, such as autism spectrum disorder, intellectual disability, developmental learning disorders, some language disorders (e.g., dyslexia), ADHD, and Tourette syndrome, appear to be genetically transmitted (Johnson et al., 2023; Yasuda et al., 2023).

KEYCONCEPT Assortative mating is the tendency of individuals to select mates who are similar in genetically linked traits such as intelligence and personality style.

Neurologic Examination

A full neurologic evaluation is beyond the scope of practice for a baccalaureate-level or master's-level nurse without specific neuropsychiatric training. However, a screening of neurologic soft signs can help establish a database that will clarify the need for further neurologic consultation. The nurse should assess the neurologic screening items suggested in Box 36.4 of the child and should also note any soft signs of neurologic dysfunction, such as slurred speech, unusual movements (e.g., tics, tremors), hyperactivity, and coordination issues. The nurse can ask young children to hop on one foot, skip, or walk from toe to heel to assess their gross motor coordination and to draw with a crayon or pencil or play pickup sticks or jacks to assess their fine motor coordination.

Medication

Pharmacologic assessment should include prescription and over-the-counter medications. Nurses should ask about any allergies to food, medications, or environmental triggers. Adherence to the prescribed regimen should be assessed. Specifically, the nurse should assess whether the medication is producing the desired effect, the presence of adverse effects, and logistical barriers associated with obtaining or administering the medication. Individuals taking medications requiring dosing during school hours may find administration to be disruptive to their day, thus individualized treatment options should be considered (Soutullo et al., 2023; Titheradge et al., 2022).

Substance Use

Substance use disorders across the lifespan account for more deaths, illness, and disabilities than any other preventable health condition. Screening for potential use and misuse of substances is a priority in mental health assessment of adolescents. House (2002) developed an interview protocol that can be useful in identifying substance misuse issues in youth (Box 36.5). It is important to determine the use of substances, including prescription drugs and polysubstance use. The child and family should be referred to community resources. *The Adolescent Screening, Brief Intervention and Referral for Treatment for Alcohol and other Drug Use (SBIRT) Toolkit for Providers* is a useful resource (Levy & Shrier, 2015).

Psychological Assessment

Children can usually identify and discuss what improves or worsens their issues. The assessment may be the first time that someone has asked the child to explain their view of the issue. It is also a perfect opportunity to discuss any life changes or losses (e.g., death of grandparents or pets, parental divorce) and fears, especially of punishment.

Mental Status Examination

As discussed in Chapter 10, the mental status examination is an organized systematic approach to assessment of an individual's current psychiatric condition. It is essential in formulating a diagnosis. It can provide initial data that alert the clinician to obtain further cognitive, neurologic, or psychological testing. The mental status examination of children combines observation and direct questioning (Box 36.6). The nurse should note any areas where the child or adolescent is symptomatic or has difficulty with the task. A mental status examination should be obtained on subsequent visits so improvements or changes in the patient's functioning can be noted.

The nurse should note the child's general appearance, including the level of attractiveness. Although it should not be so, social–psychological research shows that the appearance and attractiveness of both children and adults strongly influence their social relationships (Jacobson et al., 2020). The nurse also should note the following:

- Do they seem to have difficulty focusing on the interview, sitting still, refraining from impulsive behavior, and listening without interrupting? (possible signs of ADHD)
- Does the child seem underactive, lethargic, distant, or hopeless? (possible signs of depression)
- Are there issues with speech patterns, such as rate (overly fast or slow), clarity, and volume, or any speech dysfluencies (e.g., stuttering, halting)?
- Are there possible mood disorders (e.g., depression, mania), language disorders, or psychotic processes?

When assessing thought processes, keep in mind that whereas young children are in the concrete operations stage, middle schoolers can begin to use logic and understand conversations. Adolescents should be able to demonstrate abstract thinking and think hypothetically, although they may appear to be self-conscious and introspective. Assessment of preteens and adolescents should address substance use and sexual activity because responses may provide useful information about high-risk behavior. In addition, the nurse should inquire about

BOX 36.5

Practice Note: An Interview Protocol for Reviewing Chemical Use in Youths

As with other topics, questions about substance use are interactive—the answers given determine to some extent the subsequent questions. However, certain topics and areas should be addressed irrespective of the previous responses.

- Now I'd like to ask you about your experience with cigarettes, alcohol, and other drugs.
- When was the last time you smoked tobacco?
- Have you ever smoked? Tell me about that.
- How old were you when you first smoked a cigarette?
- How many cigarettes do you smoke a day now?
- How long have you smoked this much?
- Where do you usually smoke?
- Where do you usually get your cigarettes?
- What kind of issues has smoking caused for you?
- How do your parents feel about your smoking?
- Have you gotten into trouble at school for smoking?
- Have you lost any friends or had issues with friends over smoking?
- What other tobacco products have you used?
- When was the last time you drank any alcohol?
- How much alcohol did you drink? What kinds of alcohol were you drinking? What happened afterward?
- Who was with you the last time you were drinking? What happened?
- How about the time before that? Tell me about that.
- What is the most alcohol you have ever drunk? What happened?
- How do you get alcohol?
- What kinds of issues have drinking caused for you?
- How do your parents feel about your drinking?
- Have you ever had issues at school because of drinking?
- Have you ever gotten into legal issues because of drinking?
- Have you had issues with your friends because of drinking?
- What is the worst thing that has happened while you were drinking?
- How old were you the first time you drank alcohol? When did most of your friends start drinking? How does your drinking compare with other kids in your classes at school or other kids your age?
- How has your drinking changed over the past year?
- When was the last time you used any marijuana?
- How old were you when you first tried marijuana?
- How often have you used marijuana in the past month?
- What is usually going on when you use marijuana?
- What other drugs have you used?
- When was the first time you used _____?
- When was the last time you used _____?
- How many times have you used _____?
- Where did you get the _____? How did you know that's what it was?
- How did _____ affect you?
- What has been the biggest effect you have obtained using _____?
- What has been the worst thing about using _____?
- Have you ever "huffed" or inhaled something to get high? Tell me about that.
- Have you ever used another individual's prescription medications? Tell me about that.
- How many people do you regularly do things with—hang out, party with, talk to?
- How many of your friends smoke tobacco occasionally?
- How many of your friends smoke tobacco regularly?
- How many of your friends drink alcohol occasionally?
- How many of your friends drink alcohol regularly?
- How many of your friends smoke marijuana occasionally?
- How many of your friends smoke marijuana regularly?
- What other drugs do your friends use?
- How has drug use affected your friends?

The first session with children and adolescents: conducting a comprehensive mental health evaluation by House, Alvin E. Adapted with permission of Guilford via Copyright Clearance Center.

any obsessions or compulsions (e.g., worries about germs, severe handwashing).

Temperament and Behavior

Temperament is an individual's characteristic intensity, activity level, threshold of responsiveness, rhythmicity, adaptability, energy expenditure, and mood. According to research findings, temperamental differences can be observed early in life, suggesting that they are at least partly biologically determined, and patterns of temperament can be correlated with emotional and behavioral issues (Liu et al., 2023). When looking at the cerebral activity in 9-month-old infants, consistent with early development of externalizing behaviors, electroencephalographic activity increased in response to fear rather than love and comfort (Santesso et al., 2007).

The classic *New York Longitudinal Study* (Thomas et al., 1968) identified three main patterns of temperament seen in infancy that often extend into childhood and later life:

- *Easy temperament* characterized by a positive mood, regular patterns of eating and sleeping, positive approach to new situations, and low emotional intensity
- *Difficult temperament* characterized by irregular sleep and eating patterns, negative response to new stimuli, slow adaptation, negative mood, and high emotional intensity
- *Slow-to-warm-up temperament* characterized by a negative, mildly emotional response to new situations that is expressed with intensity and initially slow adaptation but evolves into a positive response

On the positive side, an easy temperament can serve as a protective factor against the development of psychopathology. Children with easy temperaments can adapt to change without intense emotional reactions. Difficult temperament places children at high risk for adjustment issues, such as with adjustment to school or bonding with parents.

BOX 36.6

Mental Status Examination

APPEARANCE

Provide a head-to-toe assessment: Describe head shape and size (Down syndrome, fragile X syndrome, Turner syndrome, fetal alcohol syndrome), eyes (clarity, gaze, glasses, eye contact), height, weight, cleanliness, facial expressions, mannerisms, ears, hearing, skin (bruising could indicate physical abuse), gait, posture, nutritional status (possible eating disorder).

Evaluate dress: Is it appropriate for the weather? Does the child wear shirts with logos or groups? Does the child appear older or younger looking? Inquire about symptoms of physical illness.

MOTOR ACTIVITY

Use the following descriptors to assess motor activity: calm, psychomotor impairment, akathisia, agitated, hyperalertness, tics, muscle spasms, nail biting, hyperactivity, anxiety, restlessness, or compulsions.

SELF-CONCEPT

Ask about play, favorite stories, and three wishes. Ask the child to draw a self-portrait, describe best-liked and least-liked qualities. Ask what they imagine doing for an occupation when grown up. Also evaluate planning ability and sense of a future.

BEHAVIOR

Observe for temper tantrums, attention span, separation from family member, self-care activities, dressing, toileting, feeding, oppositionality, adherence, and so on.

SOCIAL INTERACTION

How does the child relate to the examiner? Is the child wary, submissive, attentive, friendly, manipulative, approval seeking, conforming, hostile, or guarded? Assess the child's relationships with the child's parent or guardian, siblings, and friends.

GENERAL INTELLIGENCE

Assess the child's general vocabulary, fund of knowledge, alertness, orientation, concentration, memory, calculations, organization, abstract reasoning creativity, spontaneity, and frustration tolerance. Ask about school, including regular or special education, grades, and grade retention.

FUND OF KNOWLEDGE

Ask child the following: How many legs does a dog have? How many pennies in a nickel? Have child identify body parts, draw a person, name colors, count as high as possible, and inquire about letter identification (younger children).

Inquire about the time. How many states are in the United States? Who was George Washington? How many days are in a week? What are the seasons of the year? (middle schoolers) What does the stomach do? Who is Charles Darwin? (teenagers)

ORIENTATION

Ask questions such as the following: How old are you?
Who is the current president of the United States?
Do you know who was the president before our current president?
What are two major news events in the past month? (older children)
What are the year, seasons, date, day, and month?
Where are we? (country, state, city, clinic)

RECENT MEMORY

Ask the child to repeat a memory phrase; remember three to five objects that you say or show and then recall them in a few minutes. Ask the following: What school do you currently attend? What did you have for breakfast or lunch today?

REMOTE MEMORY

Ask questions such as the following: What did you do last weekend? What was your last birthday like? What is your address and telephone number? Who is your first best friend? How old were you when you learned to ride a bike? What was the name of your kindergarten teacher?

ABSTRACT REASONING AND ANALOGIES

Ask what is meant by a stitch in time saves nine; a rolling stone gathers no moss; a bird in the hand is worth two birds in a tree; too many cooks spoil the broth.

Which object does not belong in this group: fish, tree, rock? Why?

Assess the similarity about objects such as peaches and lemons, oceans and lakes, a pencil and typewriter, a bicycle and a bus.

To evaluate comparative ability, complete this sentence: An engine is to an airplane as an oar is to a _______.

ARITHMETIC CALCULATIONS

Provide simple addition and subtraction questions based on the child's age. Ask older children multiplication and division problems. Count backward 20 to 1 for younger children. Ask how many quarters are in $3.50 or if you buy something that cost $2.50 and you have $5, how much change you will receive.

WRITING AND SPELLING ABILITY

Ask a first or second grader to spell *cat, hat, bad, old, dog*. Ask a third or fourth grader to spell words such as *clock, face, house*, or *flower*. Ask older children to write a sentence such as: "The grass is greener on the mountains."

READING

Have the child read a paragraph from an age-appropriate book. Reading begins in first grade. Children should demonstrate basic reading skills by the end of second grade.

GROSS MOTOR SKILLS

Assess level of activity, type of activity, and any unusual gestures or mannerisms and compulsions.
Have the patient walk, jump, hop on one foot, and walk heel to toe, throw a ball, balance and climb stairs.
By age 3 years, a child should walk up stairs with alternating feet, pedal a tricycle, jump in one place, and broad jump.
By age 4 years, a child can balance on one foot for 5 seconds and catch a bounced ball two of three times.
By age 5 years, a child can do heel-to-toe walking.
By age 6 years, a child should jump, tumble, skip, hop, walk a straight line, skip rope with practice, and ride a bicycle.
By age 7 years, a child should skip and play hopscotch, and run and climb with coordination.
By age 9 years, a child should have highly developed eye–hand coordination.

BOX 36.6 (*Continued*)

FINE MOTOR SKILLS

Have the child draw a picture or self-portrait as well as pickup sticks.

Have the child copy a design that you have drawn. Ask the child to draw a circle (age 3 years), an X (ages 3 to 4 years), a square (age 5 years), a triangle (age 6 years), a diamond (age 7 years), and connecting diamonds (age 8 years).

At age 3 years, a child should unbutton front buttons, copy a vertical line, copy a circle, and build an eight-block tower.

By age 4 years, a child should copy a cross and button large buttons.

By age 5 years, a child should dress themselves with minimal assistance, color within lines, and draw a three-part human.

By age 6 years, a child should be able to draw a six-part human.

By age 7 years, a child should print well and begin to write script.

By age 8 years, a child should demonstrate mature handwriting skills.

ATTENTION SPAN

Ask the patient to follow a series of short commands. Observe motor activity, attention, concentration, impulsivity, hyperactivity, outbursts, and organization.

Observe the child's ability to stay on task and focus during the course of the interview. Tasks include counting backward by seven, spelling the word "world" backward, and saying the letters of the alphabet backward.

INSIGHT AND JUDGMENT

Ask the child to provide a solution to a hypothetical situation such as what would you do if you found a stamped envelope lying on the ground? What would you do if a police officer stopped you for driving your bike through a red light? What would you do if you saw two children fighting on the school grounds? Assess the child's ideas about the current issue and the solutions tried so far. Assess if child can make use of assistance. Evaluate how impaired child is in activities of daily living, including attending school, attending recreational activities, making friends, self-care activities, and so on.

COMPREHENSION

Read a few pages or paragraphs from a short book or news article and ask the child to relate what happened in the story.

MOOD AND FEELINGS

Affect is the child's emotional tone. Evaluate the child's range of emotions, intensity, and appropriateness.

Assess for any mood swings, crying, anxiety, depression, anger, hostility, hyperalertness, lability, or pressured speech. Assess mood by asking how many times a week do you feel sad and how often do you cry? What makes you sad, angry, anxious, and so on? Risk assessment questions include the following: Have you ever wanted to hurt yourself or someone else? Do you have a plan to hurt yourself? Have you ever done anything to hurt yourself in the past?

THOUGHT PROCESS AND CONTENT

Were there any recurrent themes?

Observe the child's patterns of thinking for appropriateness of sequence, logic, coherence, and relevance to the topics discussed. Does the child talk about age-appropriate topics; is there any thought blocking, or disturbance in the stream of thinking, repetition of words, circumstantial or tangential thinking, perseverations, preoccupations, obsessive thoughts, actions, or compulsive behaviors, any grandiose reasoning, ideas of reference, or paranoia (feelings of being watched or followed, controlled, manipulated, and ritual or checking routines)?

Evaluate the child's perceptions for hallucinations (false perceptions or false impressions or experiences) and delusions (false beliefs that contradict social reality, such as hears voices, sees images or shadowy figures, smells offensive odors, tastes offensive flavors, feels worms crawling on skin). Assess hallucinations in all five senses: auditory, visual, tactile, gustatory, and olfactory. Assess for command hallucinations, which tell the patient to do something.

SPEECH AND LANGUAGE

Note any speech impediments and incongruence between verbal and nonverbal communication. Show a pencil and a watch and ask the patient to name them. Have the patient repeat "no ifs, ands, or buts."

Assess communication skills, including expressive language, vocabulary, and the ability to understand what you are saying (receptive language). Check voice quality, articulation, pronunciation, fluency, rhythm, rate, and ease of expression and volume.

Assess comprehension by giving the child a task. Assess coherence for flight of ideas, loose associations, word salad (meaningless, disconnected word choices), neologisms, clang associations (words that rhyme in a nonsensical way), echolalia (repetition of another individual's words), thought blocking, perseveration, irrelevance, and vagueness. Check for aphasia by listening for an omission or addition of letters, syllables, and made-up words or misuse or transposition of words.

Temperament has a major influence on the chances that a child may experience psychological issues; however, temperament is not unchangeable, and environmental influences can change or modify a child's emotional style (Miller et al., 2020). Children who respond positively to the environment continue in this pattern. Children who have other temperaments may develop positive temperaments at a later time.

The concept of temperament provides an excellent example of the interaction between biologic–genetic and environmental factors in producing child psychopathology. Although a child may be born with a particular temperament, longitudinal studies show that the temperament can be influenced by other factors such as parental control (Perlstein et al., 2022; Smith et al., 2022). However, difficult children, in particular, may evoke negative reactions in parents and teachers, thereby creating environments that exacerbate their biologically based behavior issues, initiating a vicious cycle. Difficult temperament that persists beyond 3 years of age is correlated with the development of child psychopathology (Wu et al., 2022). The nurse can help parents accept biologically based differences in their children and learn to adapt their behavior to each child's needs.

Developmental Assessment

Children respond to life's stresses in different ways and in accord with their developmental level. Knowing the difference between typical child development and psychopathology is crucial in helping parents view their children's behavior realistically and respond appropriately. The key areas for assessment include maturation, psychosocial development, and language.

Maturation

Healthy development of the brain and nervous system during childhood and adolescence provides the foundation for successful functioning throughout life. Such development, called **maturation**, unfolds through sequential and orderly growth processes. These processes are biologically and genetically based but depend on constant interactions with a stimulating and nurturing environment. If trauma or neglect impairs the process of typical biologic maturation, **developmental delays** and disorders that may not be fully reversible can result. For example, babies born with fetal alcohol syndrome experience permanent brain damage, often resulting in intellectual disability, learning disabilities, behavior disorders, and delays in language (Popova et al., 2023). A pregnant patient's use of crack cocaine deprives the fetus of nutrients and oxygen, leading to developmental delays, speech and language issues, deformities, and behavior disorders (e.g., impulsivity, withdrawal, hyperactivity). The nurse can assess for developmental delays by asking questions from specific sections of the mental status examination:

- *Intellectual functioning:* Evaluate the child's creativity, spontaneity, ability to count money and tell time, academic performance, memory, attention, frustration tolerance, and organization.
- *Gross motor functioning:* Ask the child to hop on one foot, throw a ball, walk up and down the hall, and run.
- *Fine motor functioning:* Ask the child to draw a picture or pickup sticks.
- *Cognition:* The nurse can evaluate the child's general level of cognition by assessing the child's vocabulary, level of comprehension, drawing ability, and responsiveness to questions. Testing, such as the Wechsler Intelligence Scale for Children (WISC-V), provides measures of intelligence quotient (IQ). A psychologist usually performs such tests. The nurse can request cognitive testing if they have concerns about a child's developmental delays or learning disabilities.
- *Thinking and perception:* Evaluate level of consciousness; orientation to date, time, and person; thought content; thought process; and judgment.
- *Social interactions and play:* Assess the child's organization, creativity, drawing capacity, and ability to follow rules. Children experiencing developmental delays may remain engaged solely in parallel play instead of moving to reciprocal play. They may consistently play with toys designed for younger children, draw crude body pictures, or display receptive or expressive language issues.

Psychosocial Development

Assessment of psychosocial development is very important for children with mental health issues. Various theoretical models are available from which to choose; the most commonly used model is Erikson stages of development. When considering this model, the nurse should examine the child's gender and cultural background for appropriateness.

Language

At birth, infants can emit sounds of all languages. Maturation of language skills begins with babbling, or the utterance of simple, spontaneous sounds. By the end of the first year, children can make one-word statements, usually naming objects or people in the environment. By age 2 years, they should speak in short, telegraphic sentences consisting of a verb and noun (e.g., "want cookie"). Between ages 2 and 4 years, vocabulary and sentence structure develop rapidly. In fact, a preschooler's ability to produce language often surpasses motor development, sometimes causing temporary stuttering when the child's mind literally works faster than their mouth.

Language development depends on the complex interaction of physical maturation of the nerves, development of head and neck musculature, hearing abilities, cognitive abilities, exposure to language, educational stimulation, and emotional well-being. Social needs create a natural inclination toward communication, but children need reinforcement to develop correct pronunciation, vocabulary, and grammar.

Before a diagnosis of a communication disorder (i.e., impairment in language expression, comprehension, or both) can be made, the child must be tested to rule out hearing, visual, or other neurologic issues. Brain damage, especially to the left hemisphere (dominant for language in most individuals), can seriously impair the development of communication abilities in children. Any child who has experienced brain damage from anoxia at birth, congenital trauma, head injury, infection, tumor, or drug exposure should be closely monitored for signs of a communication disorder. Before the age of 5 years, the brain has amazing plasticity, and sometimes other intact areas of the brain can take over functions of damaged areas, especially with immediate speech therapy. Genetically based disorders such as autism spectrum disorder cause language delays that are sometimes permanent and severe.

The nurse must recognize expected variations in child development and assess lags in the development of vocabulary and sentence structure during the critical preschool years. Delays in this area can seriously affect other areas, such as cognitive, educational, and social development. Many children who receive psychiatric treatment have speech and language disorders that are sometimes undetected, either leading to or compounding their emotional issues (Hancock et al., 2023).

Self-Concept

For young children, eliciting their view of themselves and the world is helpful. One technique is asking them what they would wish for if they had three wishes. Answers can be revealing. Whereas an inability to wish for anything beyond a nice meal or place to live may reflect hopelessness, wishes to conquer the world or put one's teacher in jail may indicate feelings of grandiosity. Another technique is to tell a story and ask the child to make up an ending for it. For example, a baby bird fell out of a nest—what happened to it? The nurse may design stories to elicit particular fears or concerns that may be relevant for the individual child.

Drawings also provide an excellent window into the child's internal world (Fig. 36.2). Asking the child to draw a picture of a person can provide data about the child's self-concept, sexual identity, body image, and developmental level. By age 3 years, children should be able to draw some facial features and limbs, but their drawings may have an "X-ray" quality, in which clothing is transparent and the body can be seen underneath. Older children should produce more sophisticated drawings unless they are resistant to the task. After the child has finished the drawing, the nurse can ask what the person in the drawing is thinking and feeling, using this device to assess the child's mental processes. For example, one adolescent with school phobia drew an individual fully dressed, in great detail, but with no feet. When asked about the drawing, he said that the child could not go anywhere because their parent was afraid to let them leave home.

Other ways to assess children's self-concepts include asking them what they want to do when they grow up, what their best subjects are in school, what things they are really good at, and how well-liked they are at school. Before concluding the individual interview with a child, the nurse should always ask if the child has any other information to share and whether they have any questions.

Stress and Coping Behaviors

Physical, behavioral, and personality predispositions; family; and community environment may affect a child's

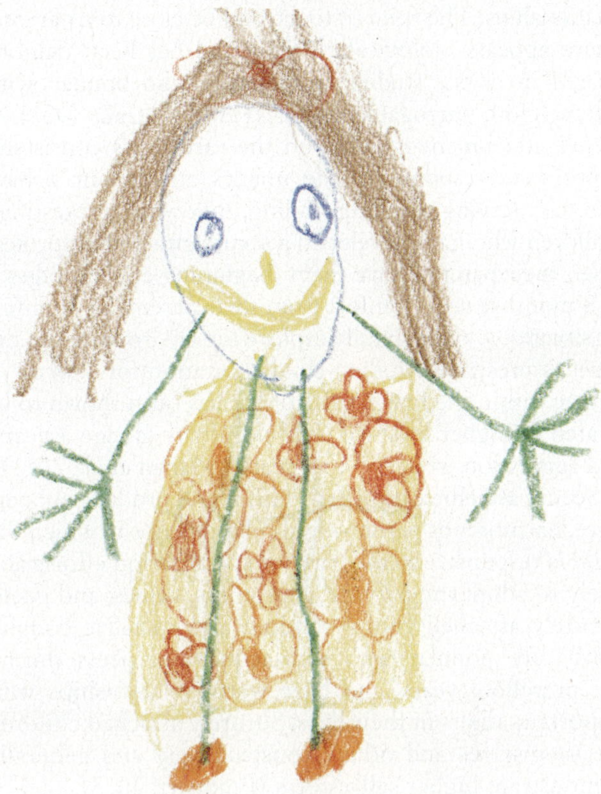

FIGURE 36.2 Self portrait of a child, age 5 years.

ability to cope with stressful life events. Stressful experiences for children include the death of a loved person or pet, parental divorce, violence, physical illness (especially chronic illness), mental illness, social isolation, racial discrimination, neglect, and physical and sexual abuse.

The number of stressful events that a child experiences (including trauma), the supports that the child has in place, and the child's developmental stage may also influence their ability to cope with stressors. Children who appear to have experienced early life stress may manifest posttraumatic stress symptoms (Hales et al., 2023). It is important to consider a stressful situation within the context of each child's support system and developmental stage.

As we learn more about trauma-informed approaches, it is important for nurses to screen patients for adverse childhood experiences (ACEs). ACEs can include abuse (emotional, sexual, and physical), neglect, substance use, violence, parental abandonment, and incarceration. These experiences put a child at risk for developing chronic conditions and understanding a child's ACEs can help the nurse to identify appropriate resources. One tool used to identify ACEs is the PEARLS (Thakur et al., 2020).

Attachment

Attachment is the emotional bond between an infant and their parental figure. Studies of attachment show that the quality of the emotional bond between the infant and parental figures provides the groundwork for future relationships. The need to touch and be close to a parental figure appears biologically driven and has been demonstrated in classic studies of monkeys who bonded with a terry-cloth surrogate mother (Harlow et al., 1971). A secure attachment is based on the caretaker's consistent, appropriate response to the infant's attachment behaviors (e.g., crying, clinging, calling, following, protesting). Children who have developed a secure attachment protest when their parents leave them (beginning at about ages 6 to 8 months), seek comfort from their parents in unfamiliar situations, and playfully explore the environment in the parent's presence. Mother–child separation for 1 week or longer within the first 2 years of life has been shown to be related to higher levels of child negativity (at age 3 years) and aggression (at ages 3 to 5 years) (Martin et al., 2011).

Secure attachments in early childhood produce cooperative, harmonious parent–child relationships in which the child is responsive to the parents' socialization efforts and likely to adopt the parents' viewpoints, values, and goals. Securely attached young children also socialize competently, are popular with well-acquainted peers during the preschool years, and have warm relationships with important adults in their lives. Securely attached children see themselves and others constructively and generally demonstrate higher self-esteem (Pinquart, 2023).

Although the importance of the parent's responsiveness is unquestionable in determining the development of a secure attachment, the process works both ways. Some babies seem to encourage attachment naturally with their parents by responding positively to holding, cuddling, and comforting behaviors. Others, such as those with developmental delays or autistic disorders, may respond less readily and even reject parental attempts at bonding.

Attachment Theories

Bowlby's early studies (1969) of maternal deprivation formed the initial framework for attachment theory based on the notion that the infant tends to bond to one primary parental figure, usually the birthing parent. Although this pattern is common, recent studies show that children make multiple attachments to parents and other caregivers, but high-quality, intense bonds remain essential for healthy development. Contemporary nursing theories, such as Barnard parent–child interaction model, have stressed the importance of the interaction between the child's spontaneous behavior and biologic rhythms and the birthing parent's ability to respond to cues that signal distress (Barnard & Brazelton, 1990). Whereas a positive attachment is likely to result in a happy child with a sense of self-worth, insecure attachment is associated with depressive symptoms (Kohler-Dauner et al., 2022; Spruit et al., 2020). Although most attachment research has been done with birthing parents, their partner's role in child development has become better understood through research done during the past 2 decades. Partners' emotional support tends to enhance the quality of the child's relationship with the birthing parent and facilitates positive adjustment by children. When partners are unsupportive and marital conflict is high, children suffer (Islamiah et al., 2023).

Partners of birthing parents play an important role in children's play, which affects the quality of the child's attachment. Playful interactions involving emotional arousal provide an especially good opportunity to learn how to get along with peers by reinforcing turn taking, affect regulation, and acceptable ways of competing. Evidence supports the importance of including the partner in the mental health care of their child (Gonzalez et al., 2023; Verschueren, 2020).

Disrupted Attachments

Disrupted attachments may result from deficits in infant attachment behaviors, lack of responsiveness by caregivers to the child's cues, or both and may lead to reactive attachment disorder, feeding disorder, failure to thrive, or anxiety disorder. A reactive attachment disorder is a state in which a child younger than 5 years of age fails to initiate or respond appropriately to social interaction and the caregiver subsequently disregards the child's physical and emotional needs. Attachment disorder behaviors are related to attention and behavior issues (Wylock et al., 2023).

Attachment disorganization is a consequence of extreme insecurity that results from feared or actual separation from the attached figure. Disorganized infants appear to be unable to maintain the strategic adjustments in attachment behavior represented by organized avoidant or ambivalent attachment strategies, with the result that both behavioral and physiologic dysregulation occurs. Preschoolers with disorganized attachment manifest behaviors of fear, contradictory behavior, or disorientation or disassociation in the caregivers' presence. Attachment disorganization appears moderately stable over time and has been associated with distinct, apparently genetically based, physiologic profiles (Zdebik et al., 2022).

Social Network

Family Relationship

Children depend on adults to create a safe, nurturing, and appropriate environment to support their development. The nurse should assess the quality of the home, including living space, sleeping arrangements, safety, cleanliness, and childcare arrangements, either through a home visit or by discussing these issues with the family. When gathering a family history, a genogram and timeline are useful tools to map family members' birth order and medical and psychiatric histories; family roles, norms, boundaries, strengths, and family subgroups; birth dates, deaths, and relationships; stage in the family cycle; and critical events. To understand fully the family's values,

BOX 36.7

Research for Evidence-Based Practice: Person-Centered Culture Assessment

Sanchez, A. L., Jent, J., Aggarwal, N. K., Chavira, D., Coxe, S., Garcia, D., La Roche, M., & Comer, J. S. (2022). Person-centred cultural assessment can improve child mental health service engagement and outcomes. Journal of Clinical Child & Adolescent Psychiatry, 51*(1), 1–22.*

THE QUESTION: Does including a brief caregiver assessment of cultural factors impact mental health service engagement and outcomes?

METHODS: Eighty-nine families receiving services for child externalizing problems were randomized to receive either Assessment as Usual (AAU) or AAU augmented with the Cultural Formulation Interview (CFI + AAU).

FINDINGS: Caregivers in the CFI + AAU group reported feeling better understood by their provider. Providers were more satisfied with their assessment when it included the CFI and reported having a better understanding of family values. Families in the CFI + AAU group were better engaged in treatment and were more likely to complete the first phase of treatment than families who received AAU.

IMPLICATIONS FOR NURSING: Evidence-based practice includes integrating the best available evidence with provider expertise and client preferences. Including a cultural assessment is a valuable person-centered approach to facilitate provider understanding of the child's/family's culture, beliefs, and values.

goals, and beliefs, the nurse must consider the family's ethnic, cultural, educational, and economic background throughout the assessment. Inclusion of these components facilitates engagement and adherence to treatment, ultimately contributing to improved outcomes (see Box 36.7). A comprehensive family assessment should be considered (see Chapter 15).

School and Peer Adjustment

The child's adjustment to school is also significant. Often, children are referred for a mental health assessment as a result of changes in behavior at school. Falling grades, loss of interest in usual activities, decreased concentration, or withdrawal from or aggression toward peers may indicate that the child is experiencing emotional issues. It is very important that the nurse obtain signed permission from the parents to talk to the child's teacher for their observations of the child. The nurse may want to observe the child in school, if feasible, to see how the child functions there. The parent can request a treatment planning conference in which the teacher, parent, and nurse discuss the child's school performance and plan ways to promote the child's emotional, cognitive, and social functioning in school. Suggestions may range from having the child tested for learning disabilities to designing behavior plans that include rewards for improved functioning, such as computer time at the end of the day.

Peers are an important aspect of child and adolescent social development. Assessment of peer relationships and activities with friends provides a rich source of information about the adolescent. Assessment of victimization by peers in the form of bullying is important because it can have a negative impact on social development and self-esteem.

Children and Adolescents Who Identify as LGBTQ+

Children and adolescents who identify as lesbian, gay, bisexual, transgender, questioning/queer (LGBTQ+) are highly stigmatized and often face discrimination and victimization because they do not adhere to conventional gender expectations. Transgender children and youth are especially affected by lack of understanding and social support. The health and mental health care needs of these children and adolescents are unique, and they often have difficulty accessing health care services (Holt et al., 2023).

Mental health issues are the leading causes of morbidity and mortality in this population. LGBTQ+ youth have a higher risk for depression, suicide, and substance use than other adolescents. They are also at increased risk for violence, including being targeted with bullying, teasing, harassment, and physical assault (Centers for Disease Control and Prevention [CDC], 2022). Social prejudice, family rejection, and self-nonacceptance are major risk factors. Protective factors include self-esteem, social support at home, positive relationships with peers, and positive school climates. It is important that the nurse inquire about anti-LGBTQ+ experiences that could lead to increased mental health issues. For children and adolescents to thrive, it is essential that they feel socially, emotionally, and physically safe and supported. Nurses can contribute to creating safe spaces by helping to create policies that support LGBTQ+ youth, participating in LGBTQ+-related trainings, incorporating inclusive language in their communication, normalizing the use of pronouns, and providing an environment (physical or digital) where the individual can freely seek care without stigma (Advocates for Youth, 2021).

Social Determinants of Health and Social Systems

Exposure to poverty, financial and food insecurity, and poor housing quality can negatively impact the overall health of a child. Children living in poverty and children from underrepresented groups have been found to have increased risk factors and prevalence of certain mental health conditions, all while having less access to care. It is critical that child assessment includes routine assessment of social determinants in order to provide necessary resources and interventions designed to protect children from further harm. ACEs, when layered with the effects of social determinants of health, further exacerbate negative mental health outcomes (Shim et al., 2022; Yaun et al., 2022).

Youth in healthy communities have been shown to be more likely to attend religious services, to believe their schools are places of caring and encouragement, to be involved in structured activities, and to remain committed to their own learning. Assessing the child's economic status, access to medical care, adequate home environment, exposure to environmental toxins (e.g., lead), neighborhood safety, and exposure to violence is important because these community factors place the child at risk (Yang et al., 2023).

Children and adolescents function better if they are linked to community supports, such as churches, recreational programs, park district programming, and after-school programming. The Big Brother/Big Sister program fosters mentoring relationships for children. A parent or child may call the local Big Brother/Big Sister organization to request a mentor for the child. The mentor may perform a wide range of services, from taking a child to community events, helping with homework, or talking about how the child can achieve their dreams and goals. Some towns offer community-based juvenile justice programs to rehabilitate children who have had altercations with the legal system. Juvenile justice programs provide support, such as individual and family counseling and prosocial recreational activities; teach children how to make positive choices about spending free time; and closely monitor their behaviors.

Religious and Spiritual Assessment

Spiritual assessment is an integral part of mental health assessment. There is a growing body of research suggesting that religious and spiritual practices may promote both physical and mental health (Aggarwal et al., 2023). The Joint Commission requires that each psychiatric evaluation include spiritual assessment questions.

Questioning about a patient's spiritual life should include interviewing strategies that are unbiased and facilitate understanding of the client's spiritual values. Questions can include but are not limited to the child's and family's specific faith background, level of activity with that group, support received from spiritual practices, religious rituals of importance, and religious influences on lifestyle and health choices. During a child interview, appropriate questions include, "Where is God?" or asking if the child could talk to God.

Childhood Sexual Abuse

There are several special considerations in interviewing an abused child. First, the nurse must establish a safe and supportive environment in which to conduct the evaluation. Second, the nurse needs to understand the forensic implications of assessment so that the interview format will be acceptable for disclosure in a court hearing. The American Academy of Pediatrics offers practice guidelines for evaluating children who may have been abused (Adams et al., 2016). If the child reports abuse, the nurse has a legal responsibility to report the abuse to child protection agencies. The nurse must use the same language and vocabulary that the child uses to describe the abuse or anatomical terms and ask nonleading questions. Nursing professionals who regularly interview children who have been abused may have special training in the use of anatomically correct dolls to obtain information about the abuse.

SUMMARY OF KEY POINTS

- Mental health assessment of children and adolescents includes evaluating the child's biologic, psychological, and social factors, primarily through interviewing and observation.
- Assessment of children and adolescents differs from assessment of adults in that the nurse must consider the child's developmental level, specifically addressing the child's language, cognitive, social, and emotional skills. Establishing a treatment alliance and building rapport are essential to obtaining a good mental health history.
- The mental status examination includes observations and questions about the child's appearance, motor activity, self-concept, behavior, social interaction, general intelligence, fund of knowledge, attention span, insight and judgment, comprehension, mood and feelings, thought process and content, speech and language, orientation, memory, reasoning, writing and spelling, reading, and motor skills. Assessment of the child and caregiver together provides important information regarding child–parent attachment and parenting practices.
- The three main types of temperament include the easy temperament, difficult temperament, and slow-to-warm-up temperament. Temperament can be evaluated by assessing the child's sleep and eating habits, mood, emotional intensity, and responses to new stimuli.
- A child's self-concept can be evaluated using tools such as play, stories, asking three wishes, and asking the child to draw a picture of themselves.
- If a child reveals suicidal ideation in the interview, the nurse must determine whether the child has a plan; let the parent know the child is suicidal; and make a plan to keep the child safe, such as inpatient hospitalization.

- If a child reports to the nurse neglect or physical or sexual abuse, the nurse must by law report the child's disclosure to the state's DCFS.

DEVELOPING CLINICAL JUDGMENT

1. What are some strategies for building rapport with children?
2. A child reports that they are suicidal. What would be your next question? What measures would you take next?
3. What are some techniques and media for obtaining information about a child's inner world, such as self-concept, sexual identity, body image, and developmental level?
4. Explain why it may be detrimental to interview a child in front of their parent. Why may it be detrimental to interview a parent in front of their child?
5. Why is obtaining the mental health histories of parents relevant to the child's mental health assessment?
6. What assessment questions would be important for a child who is transgender?
7. What are useful tools in obtaining a family history from the child and parent?
8. What types of questions would you ask to inquire about a child's spiritual life?

MOVIES, TV, OR STREAMING PROGRAMS

***The Perks of Being a Wallflower*: 2012.** Charlie is a lonely freshman in high school, a *wallflower*, who befriends two seniors who bring him into their friend group of misfits. This film highlights many societal issues, including mental illness, sexual abuse, intimate partner violence, bullying, substance use, suicidality, LGBTQ+ issues and lack of acceptance, and loneliness.

Viewing Points:

1. What are signs that Charlie was in a mental health crisis?
2. When Charlie is intimate with Sam, he has a sudden flashback of being sexually abused by his aunt when he was a child. Why hadn't he remembered this before?
3. Aunt Helen tells Charlie not to tell anyone about their sexual encounters, saying "It is our secret." Why do people who abuse others often instruct the people they abuse to do this?
4. Why did Charlie black out and not remember anything that happened during the fight in the school cafeteria?
5. Throughout the film, Charlie writes letters to a "friend." The friend is never specifically identified. What is the purpose of these letters?

REFERENCES

Achenbach, T. M., & Edelbrock, C. (1983). *The child behavior checklist: Manual for the child behavior checklist and revised child behavior profile*. Queen City Printers.

Adams, J. A., Kellogg, N. D., Farst, K. J., Harper, N. S., Palusci, V. J., Frasier, L. D., Levitt, C. J., Shapiro, R. A., Moles, R. L., & Starling, S. P. (2016). Updated guidelines for the medical assessment and care of children who may have been sexually abused. *North American Society for Pediatric and Adolescent Gynecology*, *29*(2), 81–87.

Advocates for Youth. (2021). Creating safer spaces for LGBTQ youth: A toolkit for education, healthcare, and community-based organizations. Creating-Safer-Spaces-Toolkit-Nov-13.pdf (advocatesforyouth.org).

Aggarwal, S., Wright, J., Morgan, A., Patton, G., & Reavley, N. (2023). Religiosity and spirituality in the prevention and management of depression and anxiety in young people: A systematic review and meta-analysis. *BMC Psychiatry*, *23*(1), 729.

Barnard, K. E., & Brazelton, T. B. (1990). *Touch: The foundation of experience*. International Universities Press.

Birmaher, B., Khetarpal, S., Brent, D., Cully, M., Balach, L., Kaufman, J., & Neer, S. M. (1997). The Screen for Child Anxiety Related Emotional Disorders (SCARED): Scale construction and psychometric characteristics. *Journal of the American Academy of Child and Adolescent Psychiatry*, *36*(4), 545–453. https://doi.org/10.1097/00004583-199704000-00018

Bowlby, J. (1969). *Attachment (Vol. 1 of Attachment and loss)*. Basic Books.

Burgin, E. E., & Ray, D. C. (2022). Child-centered play therapy and childhood depression: An effectiveness study in schools. *Journal of Child & Family Studies*, *31*(1), 293–307.

Centers for Disease Control and Prevention. (2022). Lesbian, Gay, Bisexual, and Transgender Health. https://www.cdc.gov/lgbthealth/index.htm

De Los Reyes, A., & Epkins, C. C. (2023). Introduction to the special issue: A dozen years demonstrating that informant discrepancies are more than measurement error: Toward guidelines for integrating data from multi-informant assessments of youth mental health. *Journal of Clinical Child & Adolescent Psychology*, *52*(1), 1–18.

Efe, Y. S., Soyunmez, S., Zuikar, Y., & Basdas, O. (2023). Determining family relations through drawing: Family relations in images drawn by immigrant children. *Journal of Pediatric Nursing*, *72*, e105–e113.

Elbeltagi, R., Al-Beltagi, M., Saeed, N. K., & Alhawamdeh, R. (2023). Play therapy in children with autism: Its role, implications, and limitations. *World Journal of Clinical Pediatrics*, *12*(1), 1–22.

Frick, P. J., Barry, C. T., & Kamphaus, R. W. (2020). *Clinical assessment of child and adolescent personality and behavior* (4th ed.). Springer.

Gonzalez, J. C., Klein, C. C., Barnett, M. L., Schatz, N. K., Garoosi, T., Chacko, A., & Fabiano, G. A. (2023). Intervention and implementation characteristics to enhance father engagement: A systematic review of parenting interventions. *Clinical Child and Family Psychology Review*, *26*(2), 445–458.

Goodman, R. (1997). The strengths and difficulties questionnaire: A research note. *Child Psychology & Psychiatry & Allied Disciplines*, *38*(5), 581–586. https://doi.org/10.1111/j.1469-7610.1997.tb01545.x

Goodman, W. K., Price, L. H., Rasmussen, S. A., Mazure, C., Fleischmann, R. L., Hill, C. L., Heninger, G. R., & Charney, D. S. (1989). The Children's Yale-Brown Obsessive Compulsive Scale (CYBOCS) I. Development, use, and reliability. *Archives of General Psychiatry*, *46*(11), 1006–1011.

Hales, G. K., Saribaz, Z. E., Debowska, A., & Rowe, R. (2023). Links of adversity in childhood with mental and physical health outcomes: A systematic review of longitudinal mediating and moderating mechanisms. *Trauma, Violence, & Abuse*, *24*(3), 1465–1482.

Hancock, A., Northcott, S., Hobson, H., & Clark, M. (2023). Speech, language and communication needs and mental health: The experiences of speech and language therapists and mental health professionals. *International Journal of Language & Communication Disorders*, *58*(1), 52–66.

Harlow, H. F., Harlow, M. K., & Suomi, S. J. (1971). From thought to therapy: Lessons from a private laboratory. *American Scientist*, *59*(5), 538–549.

Hartwig, E. K., & Taylor, E. R. (2022). Small steps can lead to big changes: Goal setting in schools using solution-focused play therapy. *International Journal of Play Therapy*, *31*(3), 131–142.

Holt, N. R., Obasi, S. N., Nisley, C., LeBlanc-Ralston, A. L., Lash, B., Huit, T. Z., Hope, D. A., Woodruff, N., & Mocarski, R. (2023). Transgender and gender diverse community perspectives on barriers and benefits of the psychosocial assessment for gender-affirming medical care. *Journal of Health Care for the Poor & Underserved*, *34*(2), 569–584.

House, A. (2002). *The first session with children and adolescents: Conducting a comprehensive mental health evaluation*. Guilford Press.

Hu, J., & Zhou, T. (2024). Parent-adolescent congruence and discrepancy in perceived parental emotion socialization to anger and sadness: Using response surface analysis to examine the links with adolescent depressive symptoms. *Journal of Youth & Adolescence*, *53*(1), 67–78.

Islamiah, N., Breinholst, S., Walczak, M. A., & Esbjorn, B. H. (2023). The role of fathers in children's emotion regulation development: A systematic review. *Infant & Child Development*, *32*(2), 1–43.

Jacobson, A. S., Trivers, R., & Palestis, B. G. (2020). Number of friends and self-perception among Jamaican children: The role of attractiveness and fluctuating asymmetry. *Journal of Biosocial Science*, *52*(2), 184–197.

Jellinek, M., Murphy, J., Robinson, J., Feins, A., Lamb, S., & Fenton, T. (1988). Pediatric symptom checklist: Screening school-age children for psychosocial dysfunction. *Journal of Pediatrics*, *112*(2), 201–209. https://doi.org/10.1016/s0022-3476(88)80056-8

Johnson, K. A., Worbe, Y., Foote, K. D., Butson, C. R., Gunduz, A., & Okun, M. S. (2023). Tourette syndrome: Clinical features, pathophysiology, and treatment. *Lancet Neurology*, *22*(2), 147–158. https://doi.org/10.1016/S1474-4422(22)00303-9

Kohler-Dauner, F., Buchheim, A., Hildebrand, K., Mayer, I., Clemens, V., Ziegenhain, U., & Feger, J. M. (2022). Maternal attachment representation, the risk of increased depressive symptoms and the influence on children's mental health during the SARS-CoV-2-pandemic. *Journal of Child & Family Studies*, *31*(2), 392–408.

Kroenke, K., Spitzer, R. L., & Williams, J. B. W. (1999). Patient Health Questionnaire-9 (PHQ-9) [Database record]. APA PsycTests. https://doi.org/10.1037/t06165-000

Levy, S., & Shrier, L. (2015). Adolescent SBIRT toolkit for providers. Massachusetts Department of Mental Health, Boston Children's Hospital, Massachusetts Department of Public Health, Massachusetts Child Psychiatry Access Project, SA3541. https://massclearinghouse.ehs.state.ma.us/PROG-BSAS-SBIRT/SA1099.html

Lidz, C. S. (2003). *Early childhood assessment*. John Wiley & Sons, Ltd.

Liu, C., Zheng, Y., Ganiban, J. M., & Saudino, K. J. (2023). Genetic and environmental influences on temperament development across the preschool period. *Journal of Child Psychology and Psychiatry*, *64*(1), 59–70.

Lochner, J., Hammerle, S., Ghezih, S., Starman-Wohrle, K., Schulte-Kome, G., & Platt, B. (2023). Parent-child agreement on children's psychopathology and the impact of parental depression. *International Journal of Methods in Psychiatric Research*, *33*(1), e1993. https://doi.org/10.1002/mpr.1993

Martin, H. K., Martin, A., Berlin, L. J., & Brooks-Gunn, J. (2011). Early mother-child separation, parenting, and child well-being in early head start families. *Attachment & Human Development*, *13*(1), 5–26.

Masri, A. S., Nuryatin, A., Subyantoro, S., Doyin, M., & Prusdianto, P. (2025). Therapeutic fairytales for holistic child development: A systematic literature review of clinical, educational, and family-based practices. *Journal of Mother and Child*, *28*(1), 136–145.

Miller, J. R., Cheung, A., Novilla, L. K., & Crandall, A. (2020). Childhood experiences and adult health: The moderating effects of temperament. *Heliyon*, *6*(5), e03927.

Nelemans, S. A., Mastrotheodoros, S., Ciftci, L., Meeus, W., & Branje, S. (2022). Do you see what I see? Longitudinal associations between mothers and adolescents' perceptions of their relationship and adolescent internalizing symptoms. *Research on Child and Adolescent Psychopathology*, *51*(2), 177–192.

Perlstein, S., Hawes, S., Vazquez, A. Y., Pacheco-Colon, I., Lehman, S., Parent, J., Byrd, A., & Waller, R. (2022). Genetic versus environmental influences on callous-unemotional traits in preadolescence: The role of parenting and parental psychopathology. *Development and Psychopathology*, *34*(5), 1686–1701. https://doi.org/10.1017/S0954579422000888

Pinquart, M. (2023). Associations of self esteem with attachment to parents: A meta-analysis. *Psychological Reports*, *126*(5), 2101–2118.

Popova, S., Charness, M. E., Burd, L., Crawford, A., Hoyme, H. E., Mukherjee, R. A. S., Riley, E. P., & Elliott, E. J. (2023). Fetal alcohol spectrum disorders. *Nature Reviews. Disease Primers*, *9*(1), 11. https://doi.org/10.1038/s41572-023-00420-x

Reynolds, C. R., & Kamphouse, R. W. (1998). *Behavior assessment system for children (BASC)*. American Guidance Service.

Rycek, R., Stuhr, S. L., McDermott, J., Benker, J., & Swartz, M. D. (1998). Adolescent egocentrism and cognitive functioning during late adolescence. *Adolescence*, *33*(132), 745–749.

Santesso, D. L., Schmidt, L. A., & Trainor, L. J. (2007). Frontal brain electrical activity (EEG) and heart rate in response to affective infant-directed (ID) speech in 9-month-old infants. *Brain & Cognition*, *65*(1), 14–21.

Sheldrick, R. C., & Perrin, E. C. (2013). Evidence-based milestones for surveillance of cognitive, language, and motor development. *Academic Pediatrics*, *13*(6), 577–586.

Shim, R., Szilagyi, M., & Perrin, J. M. (2022). Epidemic rates of child and adolescent mental health disorders require an urgent response. *Pediatrics*, *149*(5). https://doi.org/10.1542/peds.2022-056611

Shinohara, A., Narazaki, M., & Kobayashi, T. (2022). Children's affiliation toward peers reflected in their picture drawings. *Behavior Research Methods*, *55*(5), 2733–2742.

Smith, M. R., Parrish, K. H., Shimomaeda, L., Zalewski, M., Rosen, M. L., Rodman, A., Kasparek, S., Mayes, M., Meltzoff, A. N., McLaughlin, K. H., & Lengua, L. J. (2022). Early-childhood temperament moderates the prospective associations of coping with adolescent internalizing and externalizing symptoms. *Frontiers in Psychology*, *13*, 1011095.

Soutullo, C. A., Are, F., & Schield-Grant, S. (2023). Factors associated with adherence to pharmacological treatment of attention deficit hyperactivity disorder (ADHD): Preliminary review. *Medicana*, *83*(2), 27–31.

Spitzer, R. L., Kroenke, K., Williams, J. B., & Löwe, B. (2006). A brief measure for assessing generalized anxiety disorder: the GAD-7. *Arch Intern Med*. *166*(10), 1092–1097. https://doi.org10.1001/archinte.166.10.1092

Spruit, A., Goos, L., Weenink, N., Rodenburg, R., Niemeyer, H., Stams, G. J., & Colonnes, C. (2020). A relation between attachment and depression in children and adolescents: A multilevel meta-analysis. *Clinical Child and Family Psychology Review*, *23*(1), 54–69.

Thakur, N., Hessler, D., Koita, K., Ye, M., Benson, M., Gilgoff, R., Bucci, M., Long, D., & Harris, N. B. (2020). Pediatrics Adverse Childhood Experiences and Related Life Events Screener (PEARLS) and health in a safety-net practice. *Child Abuse & Neglect*, *108*, 104685. https://doi.org/10.1016/j.chiabu.2020.104685

Thomas, A., Chess, S., & Birch, H. G. (1968). *Temperament and behavior disorders in childhood*. University Press.

Titheradge, D., Godfrey, J., Eke, H., Price, A., Ford, T., & Janssens, A. (2022). Why young people stop taking their attention deficit hyperactivity disorder medication: A thematic analysis of interviews with young people. *Child: Care, Health and Development*, *48*(5), 724–735. https://doi.org/10.1111/cch.12978

Torvik, F. A., Eilertsen, E. M., Hannigan, L. J., Cheesman, R., Howe, L. J., Magnus, P., Reichborn-Kjennerud, T., Andreassen, O. A., Njolstad, P. R., Havdahl, A., & Ystrom, E. (2022). Modeling assortative mating and genetic similarities between partners, siblings, and in-laws. *Nature Communications*, *13*(1), 1108.

Verschueren, K. (2020). Attachment, self-esteem, and socio-emotional adjustment: There is more than just the mother. *Attachment and Human Development*, *22*(1), 105–109.

Vettori, G., Ruffini, C., Andreini, M., Megli, G., Fabbri, E., Labate, I., Bianchi, S., & Pecini, C. (2022). Investigating children's ability to express internal states through narratives and drawings: Two longitudinal studies during pandemic. *Children*, *9*(8), 1165.

Weidema, A., Hollarek, M., Sijtsma, H., Lee, N. C., Walsh, R. J., van Buuren, M., & Krabbendam, L. (2023). Increased interference from conflicting perspectives and gender differences: A longitudinal study during adolescence. *Journal of Experimental Child Psychology*, *235*, 105717.

Wolraich, M., Lambert, W., Doffing, M., Bickman, L., Simmons, T., & Worley, K. (2003). Psychometric properties of the Vanderbilt ADHD diagnostic parent rating scale in a referred population. *Journal of Pediatric Psychology*, *28*(8), 559–567. https://doi.org10.1093/jpepsy/jsg046

Wu, T. C. H., Meehan, A. J., Rijlaarsdam, J., Maughan, B., Fearon, P., & Barker, E. D. (2022). Developmental pathways from toddler difficult temperament to child generalized psychopathology and adult functioning. *Journal of Affective Disorders*, *301*, 14–22.

Wylock, J. F., Borghini, A., Slama, H., & Delvenne, V. (2023). Child attachment and ADHD: A systematic review. *European Child & Adolescent Psychiatry*, *32*(1), 5–16.

Yang, P., Hernandez, B. S., & Plastino, K. A. (2023). Social determinants of mental health and adolescent anxiety and depression: Findings from the 2018 to 2019 national survey of children's health. *International Journal of Social Psychiatry*, *69*(3), 795–798.

Yasuda, Y., Matsumoto, J., Miura, K., Hasegawa, N., & Hashimoto, R. (2023). Genetics of autism spectrum disorders and future direction. *Journal of Human Genetics*, *68*(3), 193–197. https://doi.org10.1038/s10038-022-01076-3

Yaun, J. A., Rogers, L. W., Marshall, A., McCullers, J. A., & Madubuonwu, S. (2022). Whole child well-child visits: Implementing ACEs and SDOH screenings in primary care. *Clinical Pediatrics*, *61*(8), 542–550.

Zdebik, M. A., Pascuzzo, K., Bureau, J. F., & Moss, E. (2022). Childhood behavioral inhibition and attachment: Links to generalized anxiety disorder in young adulthood. *Frontiers in Psychology*, *13*, 933213. https://doi.org/10.3389/fpsyg.2022.933213

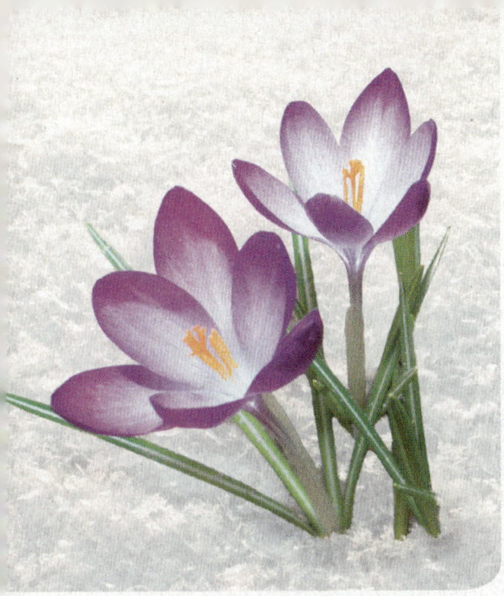

37 Mental Disorders of Childhood and Adolescence*

Valerie Griffin and Rebecca Luebbert

KEYCONCEPTS

- Attention
- Hyperactivity
- Impulsiveness
- Neurodevelopmental delay
- Tics

LEARNING OBJECTIVES

After studying this chapter, you will be able to:

1. Describe mental disorders usually diagnosed in childhood or adolescence.
2. Discuss prevailing theories relevant to mental disorders in childhood and adolescence.
3. Examine the relationship between social determinants of health and mental disorders of childhood and adolescence.
4. Using a clinical judgment model, discuss the nursing care of children with neurodevelopmental disorders.
5. Using a clinical judgment model, formulate a person-centered, recovery-oriented nursing plan for children with attention-deficit hyperactivity disorder.
6. Discuss the priority hypotheses for nursing care of children and adolescents with disruptive behavior disorders.
7. Discuss epidemiology, etiology, medications, and nursing care of children with tic disorders.
8. Using a clinical judgment model, discuss the nursing care of children and adolescents with separation anxiety and obsessive-compulsive disorders.
9. Differentiate the nursing care of children and adolescents with mood disorders and schizophrenia with that of adults with similar disorders.
10. Discuss the significance of behavioral intervention strategies for children who have elimination disorders.

KEY TERMS

• adaptive behavior • attention-deficit hyperactivity disorder (ADHD) • autism spectrum disorder (ASD) • communication disorders • conduct disorder • disruptive behavior disorders • dyslexia • encopresis • enuresis • intellectual developmental disorder • learning disorder • motor tics • oppositional defiant disorder • phonologic processing • separation anxiety disorder • Tourette syndrome • vocal tics

INTRODUCTION

Psychiatric issues are less easily recognized in children than in adults. Typical growth and development behaviors of one age group may be a symptom of a disorder in another age group. For example, an imaginary friend is age appropriate for a 4-year-old child but not for an adolescent. Despite the difficulty in diagnosis, an estimated one in six youths in the United States experiences a mental disorder in a given year, with three million having serious thoughts of suicide (National Alliance on Mental Illness [NAMI], 2024). Among the most commonly diagnosed disorders in children and adolescents are **attention-deficit hyperactivity disorder (ADHD)**

**In this chapter, "male" refers to an individual assigned male at birth, and "female" refers to an individual assigned female at birth. Also, "parent" refers to the primary caregiver of a child.*

(11.4%), behavior issues (7.4%), anxiety (10%), and depression (4%) (Centers for Disease Control and Prevention [CDC], 2024a). One in five children and adolescents reports the pandemic having a significant negative impact on their mental health (NAMI, 2024). Unfortunately, despite this prevalence, significant gaps in treatment exist, particularly for children in low-income, underrepresented, and underserved communities (Chang & Slopen, 2024; Ilori et al., 2024).

This chapter presents an overview of selected childhood disorders and discusses nursing care for children and their families with these issues. Because it is beyond the scope of this text to present all child psychiatric disorders, this chapter discusses selected ones, including neurodevelopmental disorders (**intellectual developmental disorder, autism spectrum disorder [ASD]**, and ADHD), disruptive behavior disorders (oppositional defiant and conduct disorders), tic disorders, **separation anxiety disorder,** and obsessive-compulsive disorder (OCD), mood disorders, childhood schizophrenia, and elimination disorders (**enuresis** and **encopresis**).

NCLEXNOTE All psychiatric disorders of childhood and adolescence should be viewed within the context of growth and development models. Safety and self-esteem are priority considerations.

NEURODEVELOPMENTAL DISORDERS OF CHILDHOOD THAT CAUSE SIGNIFICANT DELAY IN DEVELOPMENT

Neurodevelopmental disorders occur early in a child's development, often before beginning grade school. These disorders affect cognitive and developmental functioning resulting in deficits that range from very specific limitations of learning to global impairments of social skills. They impact personal, social, academic, or behavioral functioning. Under the primary influences of genes and environment, neurodevelopment of attention, cognition, language, affect, and social and moral behavior proceeds along several pathways. Developmental pathways and developmental delays are closely interwoven. For example, a language delay can interfere with a child's social development and contribute to difficulties in behavior and emotions (Abin et al., 2024; Tamayo et al., 2024). This section reviews neurodevelopmental disorders of childhood that include several conditions that are etiologically unrelated; however, their common feature is a significant delay in one or more lines of development.

KEYCONCEPT Neurodevelopmental delay means that the child's development in attention, cognition, language, affect, and social or moral behavior is outside the norm and is manifested by delayed socialization, communication, peculiar mannerisms, and idiosyncratic interests.

INTELLECTUAL DEVELOPMENTAL DISORDER

Intellectual developmental disorder, also known as intellectual disability, is a condition characterized by significant limitations in both intellectual function and in **adaptive behavior** that originates during the developmental period before the age of 22 (American Association on Intellectual and Developmental Disabilities [AAIDD], 2024).

Diagnostic Criteria and Clinical Course

The diagnosis of intellectual developmental disorder involves an assessment of intellectual function such as reasoning, problem-solving, and adaptive function in personal independence and social responsibility (AAIDD, 2024). A diagnosis is made through clinical assessment of behavioral features; historical accounts from parents and teachers; and performance on standardized tests such as the Stanford–Binet or the Wechsler Intelligence Scales for Children. The usual threshold for intellectual developmental disorder is an intelligence quotient (IQ) of 70 or less (i.e., two standard deviations below the population mean).

Adaptive behavior is composed of three skill types: conceptual skills (e.g., language and literacy, money, time, number concepts, and self-direction); social skills (e.g., interpersonal skills, social responsibility, self-esteem, gullibility, social problem-solving, and the ability to follow rules and obey laws and to avoid being victimized); and practical skills (e.g., activities of daily living [ADLs], occupational skills, health care, travel and transportation, schedules and routines, safety, use of money, and use of telephone). Although standardized tests may help to determine impaired adaptive functioning, this determination is primarily a clinical judgment based on the child's capacity to manage age-appropriate ADLs (AAIDD, 2024).

An intellectual developmental disorder is not necessarily lifelong. Some children may be diagnosed at school age as having an intellectual disability, but their level of life functioning may improve with sustained individualized support.

Epidemiology and Etiology

The prevalence of intellectual disabilities to be about 3% in the United States and worldwide. A considerable variability exists worldwide, with low- and middle-income countries reporting significantly higher rates of disability than high-income countries (Olusanya et al., 2023). Children and adolescents with intellectual developmental disorder are at higher risk for developing co-occurring mental health conditions, including major depression, bipolar disorder, anxiety disorders, psychotic illnesses, impulse control disorders, and others. ADHD is present in approximately 39% of children with intellectual disability. Such children are also more likely to have medical conditions that are overlooked because they are less able to localize pain, describe symptoms, or provide other assessment data (Pinals et al., 2022; Totsika et al., 2022).

Intellectual disabilities result from a variety of causes with the most common etiology related to genetic syndromes. Chromosomal changes or defects (e.g., Down syndrome) and exposure to toxins during prenatal development (e.g., fetal alcohol syndrome), heredity, pregnancy and perinatal complications, medication conditions, and environmental influences are all associated with intellectual disabilities (Shaffer et al., 2023; Tartaglione et al., 2024; van Wijngaarden et al., 2024).

EVIDENCE-BASED NURSING CARE OF CHILDREN WITH INTELLECTUAL DEVELOPMENTAL DISORDER

Person-centered care of a child with intellectual developmental disorder focuses on their strengths, capability, and ability to contribute to their community instead of their deficits. Nursing assessment focuses on current adaptive skills, intellectual status, and social functioning. A developmental history is a useful way to gather information about past and current capacities (Box 37.1). The nurse compares these data with typical growth and development. Developmentally delayed children who have not had a psychological evaluation should be considered for referral. Children with intellectual developmental disorder also require evaluation for other comorbid psychiatric disorders, which may be a challenge because of the child's cognitive limitations. Discussions about feelings and behavior may be too complex for these children. If children or adolescents with intellectual disabilities have a comorbid psychiatric disorder or serious behavioral issues, a carefully constructed interdisciplinary behavioral plan will guide care and treatment.

BOX 37.1

History and Hallmarks of Childhood and Adolescent Disorders

- Maternal age and health status during pregnancy
- Exposure to medication, alcohol, or other substances during pregnancy
- Course of pregnancy, labor, and delivery
- Infant's health at birth
- Eating, sleeping, and growth in first year
- Health status in first year
- Interest in others in first 2 years
- Motor development
- Mastery of bowel and bladder control
- Speech and language development
- Activity level
- Response to separation (e.g., school entry)
- Regulation of mood and anxiety
- Medical history in early childhood
- Social development
- Interests

The nurse also assesses the child's support systems (family, school, rehabilitative, and psychiatric) to ensure that the child's special needs have been identified and are being addressed. For example, occupational therapy may be recommended to improve motor coordination, but the family may not have transportation to these services available, so availability of alternative services should be explored.

The child and family's response to intellectual disability and other comorbid conditions will determine the nursing interventions. Interventions most often include promoting coping skills (i.e., interventions directed at building strengths, adapting to change, and maintaining or achieving a higher level of functioning), patient education, and parent education.

The overall goals of treatment and nursing care are an optimal level of functioning for the family and eventual independent functioning within an expected social environment for the child. For many children with intellectual disability, achieving independence in adulthood will be delayed but possible.

Continuum of Care

Children and families require varying levels of interventions at different times throughout the life cycle, with an ultimate goal to increase self-direction and promote full community inclusion. When a child is young, the family requires special educational support and, for some, residential services. The need for psychiatric intervention varies according to the severity of disability, family functioning, and the coexistence of other disorders. Feelings of grief and uncertainty in family members (especially parents) related to having a child with a disability may be relieved through family therapy. More specific parent training may be needed to deal with emerging maladaptive behaviors. See Clinical Judgment Nursing Care Plan 37.1.

AUTISM SPECTRUM DISORDER

ASD is characterized by persistent impairment in social communication and social interaction with others, and restricted and repetitive behaviors (APA, 2022). Children with ASD may or may not have an intellectual disability, but they commonly show an uneven pattern of intellectual strengths and limitations. This condition may be a lifelong pattern of being rigid in manner, intolerant of change, and prone to behavioral outbursts in response to environmental demands or changes in routine. Two conditions, autism disorder and Asperger syndrome, were previously diagnosed as separate disorders. However, because they have many overlapping symptoms and are difficult to differentiate from each other. The DSM-5-*TR* no longer considers autism and Asperger syndrome as separate disorders but considers both as an ASD differentiated by language or intellectual impairment (APA, 2022).

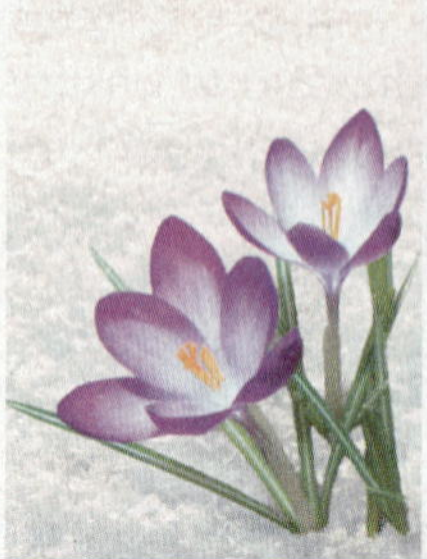

CLINICAL JUDGMENT NURSING CARE PLAN 37.1

The Child With ADHD

Jamie was referred to a home health agency for evaluation by the school counselor who was alerted by the teacher of impulsive and disruptive behavior in class. His mother Lillian had not realized that Jamie's behavior as unusual but willingly followed up with an appointment.

Setting: Psychiatric Home Care Agency

Assessment Cues: Jamie is a 6-year-old with prominent hyperactivity and disruptive behavior. He lives with Lillian, his single mother. These issues interfere with his interpersonal relationships and academic progress. Lillian is discouraged and feels unable to manage Jamie's behavior.

Associated Psychiatric Diagnosis

Attention-deficit hyperactivity disorder (ADHD)

Medications

Methylphenidate 7.5 mg at breakfast and lunch (i.e., at 8 AM and 12 noon) and then adding 5 mg at 7 PM

Priority Hypothesis: Difficulty in Social Relationships

Important Characteristics

Cannot establish and maintain developmentally appropriate social relationships
Has interpersonal difficulties at school
Is not well accepted by peers
Is easily distracted
Interrupts others
Cannot wait his turn in games
Speaks out of turn in the classroom

Associated Considerations

Impulsive behavior
Overactive
Inattentive
Risk-taking behavior (tried to climb out the window to get away from his mother)
Failure to recognize effects of his behavior on others

Planning Recovery and Wellness Outcomes

Initial

Decrease hyperactivity and disruptive behavior.
Improve attention and decrease distractibility.
Decrease frequency of acting without forethought.

Discharge

Improve capacity to identify alternative responses in conflicts with peers.
Improve capacity to interpret behavior of age mates.

Taking Action: Nursing Interventions

Intervention	Rationale	Ongoing Assessment
Educate mother and teach about ADHD and use of stimulant medication.	Better understanding helps to ensure adherence; also, parents and teachers often miscast children with ADHD as "troublemakers."	Determine the extent to which parent or teacher "blames" Jamie for his issues.
Monitor adherence to medication schedule.	Uneven adherence may contribute to failed trial of medication.	Administer parent and teacher questionnaires; inquire about behavior across entire day.
Ensure that medication is both effective and well tolerated.	Stimulants can affect appetite and sleep.	Administer parent and teacher questionnaires; check height and weight; ask about sleep and appetite.

Evaluation

Outcomes	Revised Outcomes	Interventions
Jamie shows decreased hyperactivity and less disruption in the classroom.	Improve ability to identify disruptive classroom behavior.	Initiate point system to reward appropriate behavior.

Clinical Judgment Nursing Care Plan 37.1 Continued

Jamie shows improved attention and decreased distractibility.	Improve school performance.	Move to front of classroom as an aid to attention.
Mother and teacher attest to Jamie's decreased impulsive behavior.	Increase Jamie's capacity to recognize the effects of his behavior on others.	Encourage participation in structured activities.
Jamie identifies alternative responses such as walking away until it is his turn.	Increase frequency of acting on these alternative approaches.	Inquire about social skills group at school, if available.
Jamie demonstrates more understanding of motives and behaviors of others.	Improve acceptance by peers.	Encourage participation in community activities.

Priority Hypothesis: Difficulty Parenting

Important Characteristics	Associated Considerations
Verbalizes discouragement and inability to handle situation with Jamie	Chronicity of ADHD More-than-average childrearing issues

Planning Recovery and Wellness Outcomes

Initial	Discharge
Verbalize frustration at trying to raise a child with ADHD alone.	Identify coping patterns that decrease the sense of frustration and increase parental competence.
Identify positive methods of interacting with and disciplining Jamie that will support the parent–child relationship as well as meet Jamie's development needs.	Initiate a collaborative relationship with the schoolteacher. Identify sources of support in the community and begin to access these resources.

Taking Action: Nursing Interventions

Intervention	Rationale	Ongoing Assessment
Assess mother's discouragement and feelings about parenting, identifying specific problem areas.	Helping the mother verbalize her feelings and identify problem areas helps in formulating problem-solving strategies.	Assess the severity of the issues with which she is living.
Refer mother to Community Mental Health Center for free parenting class.	Parent training based on clear directives and rewards can be effective for decreasing impulsive and disruptive behavior.	Monitor mother's level of confidence and perceived change in Jamie's behavior.
Refer mother to self-help organization.	Parent groups such as Children and Adults with Attention-deficit Disorder (CHADD) can be sources of support and information.	Determine whether contact was made and whether it was helpful.
Make contact with school to enhance collaboration with mother.	Assess effectiveness of medication and other interventions; need feedback from teachers.	Determine whether mother has been able to contact teacher.

Evaluation

Outcomes	Revised Outcomes	Interventions
After four sessions, Lillian expresses her frustrations, but she has begun to identify different ways of relating to Jamie and his developmental needs.	None	None
Through attending the parenting class and joining a support group, Lillian begins to change her coping patterns, decrease her frustrations, and increase her parental competence.	Complete parenting class; attend at least two support group meetings each month.	If necessary, refer for additional parent counseling.
Lillian initiates a collaborative relationship with Jamie's teacher.	Lillian and teacher mutually develop and implement behavior plans for home and school.	Have mother observe in the classroom; have mother visit highly structured classroom.

ASD with restricted repetitive patterns of behavior such as stereotypic or repetitive motor movement, use of objects, inflexible adherence to routine or ritualized patterns, and fascination with lights or movement has been a subject of considerable interest and research effort since its original description more than 70 years ago. Kanner (1943) described the profound isolation of these children and their extreme desire for sameness. These children appear aloof and indifferent to others and often seem to prefer inanimate objects.

Impairment in communication is severe and affects both verbal and nonverbal communication. Children with ASD may manifest delayed and deviant language development, as evidenced by echolalia (repetition of words or phrases spoken by others) and a tendency to be extremely literal in interpretation of language. Pronoun reversals and atypical intonation are also common. Other common features of ASD are stereotypic behavior, self-stimulating, nonfunctional repetitive behaviors, such as repetitive rocking, hand flapping, and an extraordinary insistence on sameness. These children may also engage in self-injurious behavior, such as hitting, head banging, or biting. In some children, their unusual interests may evolve into fascination with specific objects, such as fans or air conditioners, or a particular topic, such as transportation schedules.

A child with ASD may have age-appropriate language and intelligence but also have severe and sustained impairment in social interaction and restricted, repetitive patterns of behavior, interests, and activities. This type of ASD was previously known as Asperger syndrome and appears to be a milder form of ASD. These children have social deficits marked by inappropriate initiation of social interactions, an inability to respond to typical social cues, and a tendency to be literal in their interpretation of language (CDC, 2024c). They may also display stereotypic behaviors, such as rocking and hand flapping, and have highly restricted areas of interest, such as train schedules, fans, air conditioners, or dogs. Signs of developmental delay may not be apparent until preschool or school age, when social deficits become evident (Box 37.2).

BOX 37.2

Clinical Judgment Vignette: Autism Spectrum Disorder

A pediatrician refers Frank, age 5 years, 6 months, for an evaluation because of Frank's unusual preoccupation with ceiling fans and lawn sprinklers. According to his mother, Frank became interested in ceiling fans at age 3 years when he began drawing them, tearing pictures of them out of magazines, and engaging others in discussions about them. In the months before the evaluation, Frank also became fascinated by lawn sprinklers. These preoccupations dominated Frank's interactions with others so much that he was practically incapable of discussing any other topics. He remained on the periphery of his kindergarten class and had few friends. Although he tried to make friends, his approaches were not successful and he had trouble reading others.

Frank was the product of a full-term uncomplicated pregnancy, labor, and delivery to his then 25-year-old mother. It was her first pregnancy, and both parents eagerly anticipated Frank's birth. As an infant, Frank was healthy but seemed to cry a lot and it was difficult to comfort him, causing his mother to feel inadequate and depleted. His motor development was also delayed, and at age 3 years, nonfamily members had difficulty understanding his speech. His articulation, however, was within expected limits at the time of consultation. Frank received regular pediatric care and had no history of serious illness or injury. There was no family history of intellectual disability or psychiatric illness; results of genetic testing for chromosomal anomaly were negative.

In addition to his unusual preoccupations and social deficits, Frank resisted any change in his routine, was easily frustrated, and was prone to temper tantrums. His parents sharply disagreed about the nature of and appropriate response to his issues.

Building Clinical Judgment

1. What effect do you think Frank's preoccupation may have on his family and their relationships?
2. What kind of teaching program would you develop if you were the nurse assigned to this family?

Epidemiology and Etiology

Recent studies by the CDC find that approximately 1 in 36 children has been identified with ASD. It is nearly four times as prevalent among male children as among female children, and is found in all racial, ethnic, and socioeconomic groups (Maenner et al., 2023). Intellectual disability and epilepsy often occur in ASD (Assuah et al., 2023; Pinals et al., 2022). Although the annual prevalence of ASD is increasing, a broader definition and change in diagnostic criteria, changes in screening methods, and increased awareness of the disorder contribute to this increase (Talantseva et al., 2023). Additionally, racial disparities among youth with ASD related to diagnostic processes and access to services have been found (see Box 37.3).

Although research has not identified an exclusive cause for ASD, evidence has identified many likely contributing factors, including environmental, biologic, and genetic factors. There is strong evidence supporting the majority of risk for ASD is from genetic factors. In a multinational cohort study of over 2 million individuals, of whom 22,000 were diagnosed with ASD, the heritability rate was estimated to be approximately 80% (Bai et al., 2020). Other risk factors identified as possible contributors to ASD include having a sibling with ASD, being born to older parents and preterm birth, individuals with certain genetic or chromosomal conditions, such as fragile X syndrome or tuberous sclerosis, and experiencing complications at birth. Studies have shown that vaccines and maternal smoking and alcohol consumption are not linked to increased risk of ASD (CDC, 2024c; Yenkoyan et al., 2024).

BOX 37.3

Mental Health Inequities: Experiences of Racism and Racial Disparities in Health Care Among Youth With Autism Spectrum Disorder (ASD) and Their Caregivers

A systematic review of six databases included 37 studies of experiences of racism and racial disparities. The studies included over 733,000 children and youth with autism spectrum disorder (ASD) and 533 caregivers. A narrative synthesis revealed four themes:

1. Experiences and aspects of racism and disparities, including language and cultural barriers, poor-quality health care interactions, stereotypes and discrimination, family and community stigma, and indirect barriers.
2. Racial disparities in health care, including screening and referral, diagnosis, health care services, and care coordination.
3. Facilitators to accessing services, including advocating and taking action, building community networks, and strong provider-caregiver relationships.
4. Recommendations from caregivers, including cultivating a trusted relationship between caregivers and care providers, increasing training and education, and improved care coordination for different systems of care.

Source: Lindsay, S., Li, Y., Joneja, S., & Hsu, S. (2024). Experiences of racism and racial disparities in health care among children and youth with autism and their caregivers: A systematic review. *Disability and Rehabilitation, 12*, 1061–1080. https://doi.org/10.1080/09638288.2024.2364823

Teamwork and Collaboration: Working Toward Recovery

Patients with ASD require long-term care at various levels of intensity. The total costs per year for children living with ASD in the United States is estimated to be between $11 billion and $61 billion due to a culmination of direct and indirect costs, exceeding the costs associated with stroke and hypertension. Medical costs for children and adolescents with ASD to address impairments and comorbidities are 4.1 to 6.2 times higher than those without ASD (Yenkovan et al., 2024; Zuvekas et al., 2021). Treatment consists of designing academic, interpersonal, and social experiences that support the child's development. Children with autism, even those who are severely affected, may be able to live at home and attend special schools that use behavioral techniques. Other outpatient services may include family counseling, home care, and medication. As the child moves toward adulthood, living at home may become more difficult given the appropriate need for greater independence. The level of structure required depends primarily on IQ and adaptive functioning.

EVIDENCE-BASED NURSING CARE FOR CHILDREN WITH ASD

As the nurse begins caring for a child with ASD, it is important to remember that the symptoms and care are on a spectrum and vary from very little needs to major care needs. Each child and family is unique with their own level of symptoms and needs.

RECOGNIZING CUES: RELEVANT ASSESSMENT INFORMATION

A comprehensive nursing assessment of a child with ASD includes evaluation of developmental history, communication abilities, social interactions, behavior patterns, and sensory sensitivities. It is important for the nurse to also review relevant medical history and co-occurring disorders and medications.

Physical Health

Physical symptoms may result from ASD-associated disorders as well as from adverse effects of frequently prescribed medications. Individuals with ASD are at an increased risk for concurrent neurologic disorders such as cerebral palsy, macrocephaly, and epilepsy. They are also at greater risk for psychiatric disorders, including ADHD (28%), anxiety (20%), sleep disorders (13%), and depression (11%). Individuals with ASD are three times more likely to develop gastrointestinal (GI) symptoms such as chronic constipation, diarrhea, gastroesophageal reflux, and inflammatory bowel disease than their peers without ASD. Physical health assessment should include a review of physical health and neurologic status, giving particular attention to coordination, childhood illnesses, hospitalizations, and injuries. Self-injurious behavior may result in bruising to the forehead or nasal bridge (from head banging); marks from biting, scratching, slapping, or pinching; or injury to eyes (from eye poking). The nurse should assess sleep, appetite, and activity patterns because they may be disturbed in affected children. Lack of adequate sleep can increase irritability and contribute to poorer outcomes with therapy. Children with comorbid disorders may require the care of several providers and may be receiving multiple medications. Assessment should include a careful review of current medications and complementary therapies, paying special attention to potential interactions (Kaye et al., 2024).

Psychosocial Cues

Communication, behaviors, and flexibility are critical assessment areas. Direct behavioral observation is important to evaluate the child's ability to relate to others, to verify the selection of age-appropriate activities, and to watch for stereotypic behaviors. Assessment of the child with ASD can be based on the following categories:

- Communication
    - Verbal and nonverbal
    - Use of picture cards, writing, or drawing

  - Use of eye contact
  - Understanding of emotional cues
  - Presence of pain
  - Preoccupation with restricted interests
- Behaviors
  - Items of fixation (how does family manage?)
  - Triggers for agitation
  - Early signs that indicate beginning of agitation
  - Interventions that work when child is overstimulated or agitated
  - Repetitive behaviors
- Flexibility or adherence to routine
  - Home schedule
  - What aggravates or irritates the child
  - Early warning signs of agitation
  - When overagitated, what interventions work best

The child's behavior, need for structure, and communication style may affect the functioning of the whole family unit. Social and communication deficits are bound to influence family interaction which may adversely affect family functioning and result in increased stress among the family. For example, the ability for a parent to respond to the needs of other children within the family may be limited.

ANALYZING CUES AND DEVELOPING HYPOTHESES

Ensuring physical safety is a priority for the nurse. The nurse will need to develop a plan of care that takes into consideration the child's ability to communicate effectively with others. The child may also have difficulty completing ADLs and may demonstrate poor coping and impaired skills. Determining the need for predictability and stability in routine for the child is also important.

PLANNING RECOVERY AND WELLNESS OUTCOMES: GENERATING SOLUTIONS

Treatment outcomes need to be individualized to the child, family, and social environment and may change with time. Planning interventions for children with an ASD consider the child, family, and community supports, such as schools, rehabilitation centers, or group homes. First and foremost, the clinicians involved in the child's treatment should collaborate with the family toward the same general goals. As the number of clinicians and educators involved increases, the chance of fragmentation in treatment planning also increases. The nurse can serve as a case coordinator.

Residential care may be necessary in some cases. After making the decision to place a child into a residential facility, family members may experience guilt, loss, and a sense of failure concerning their inability to care for the child at home.

TAKING ACTION: NURSING INTERVENTIONS

Physical Health Interventions

In teaching self-care skills, the nurse needs to consider the child's current adaptive skills and language limitations. Developing a list of activities for the child to post in their bedroom may be effective for some children. Drawings or symbols may be useful for nonverbal children. Physical safety is an important concern for children who are cognitively delayed and may have impaired judgment.

Medication Interventions

No medication has proved effective at changing the core social and language deficits of autism. However, some atypical antipsychotics (i.e., risperidone, aripiprazole) are beneficial for the management of hyperactivity, impulsivity, agitation, temper outbursts, self-injury, or aggression associated with autism. Weight gain and metabolic syndrome are concerns with these agents (Iffland et al., 2023; Salazar de Pablo et al., 2023). Medications used for ADHD, both stimulants and nonstimulants, may be effective for symptoms of hyperactivity, irritability, and inattention (Martins et al., 2024). Antidepressants may be effective in treating restricted and repetitive behaviors associated with ASD (Liang et al., 2022; Maneeton et al., 2024). Evidence is unclear that anticonvulsants and traditional mood stabilizers are useful in managing mood lability and aggression (Sesso et al., 2023).

Psychosocial Interventions

When working with children with neurodevelopmental disorders, building on their strengths and using positive reinforcement are very important. If these children feel that they are constantly criticized or need "fixing," their self-esteem may be diminished and they may be less engaged in their treatment. Developmental approaches for children with ASD often focus on improving language and physical skills. Speech and language therapy will help the child improve their understanding and use of speech and language. Occupational therapy is beneficial in promoting independence, and may include building skills with eating, grooming, and bathing. Sensory integration therapy may be useful for individuals who struggle with sensory input (CDC, 2024c). Cognitive-behavioral therapy (CBT) and mindfulness therapy may be helpful in reducing anxiety and depression (Linden et al., 2023).

Promoting Interaction

Structuring interventions for social isolation should fit the child's cognitive, linguistic, and developmental levels. Interventions fostering nonverbal social interactions may be more useful than those based on speech. For higher-functioning children, activities such as getting the mail, passing out snacks, or taking turns in the context of simple games can engage them in social activities without requiring the use of their limited language skills. Structuring social interactions so that the child shares a task with another, such as carrying a load of books, may help boost confidence in relating to others.

ASD calls for extraordinary patience and determination. With help, these children can learn social and communication skills, such as taking turns in conversation and warning the listener before changing the subject in the context of milieu.

Ensuring Predictability and Safety

When children with ASD are hospitalized, milieu management—a consistent, structured environment with predictable routines for activities, mealtimes, and bedtimes—is necessary for successful treatment. Changes in routine may provoke disorganization in the child, leading to emotional disequilibrium and explosive behavior. The safety of the inpatient unit offers an opportunity to try behavioral strategies, such as rewards for managing transitions. Health care professionals can pass on successful strategies to parents or primary caretakers (Carruthers et al., 2023).

A structured physical environment will most likely be important to a child with a development disorder. Keeping furniture, dishes, and toys in the same place helps ease anxiety and fosters secure feelings. The nurse should identify the child's individual specific needs for structure.

Behavioral Interventions

Children with ASD often need specific behavioral interventions to reduce the frequency of inappropriate or aggressive behavior (Nuske et al., 2024). For example, a child may have angry outbursts in response to routine transitions. If the tantrum is dramatic, the consequence may be that the transition does not take place. By structuring the environment and using visual cues to signal the end of one activity and the start of another, it may be possible to reduce the number and intensity of responses to transitions. Safety is always a concern. Self-injury and aggression are sometimes present, so children may need to be protected from hurting themselves and others. If aggressive or assaultive behavior is an issue, a brief "time out" followed by prompt reentry into activities is usually effective.

Managing the repetitive behaviors of these children depends on the specific behavior and its effects on others or the environment. If the behavior, such as rocking, has no negative effects, ignoring it may be the best approach. If the behavior, such as head banging, however, is unacceptable, redirecting the child and using positive reinforcement are recommended. In some cases, especially in severely delayed children, these strategies may not work, and environmental alterations and perhaps protective headgear will be needed (see Box 37.4).

BOX 37.4

Building Clinical Judgment With SBAR: Managing Stereotypic Behavior of a Patient With Autism

SBAR

S: Situation

Ben, age 9, has been diagnosed with autism spectrum disorder (ASD). He was admitted to the inpatient child psychiatric unit due to aggressive outbursts and episodes of self-harm.

B: Background

Ben's parents report that he has been increasingly "unpredictable" and has had more frequent outbursts since his teacher was reassigned to a different classroom a week ago. They have noticed an increase in pacing, hand flapping, and vocal stimming. Yesterday in school, Ben was found repeatedly banging his head on his desk, prompting a referral to his health care provider. Ben is nonverbal, but able to communicate somewhat using picture cards.

A: Assessment

The nurse finds Ben pacing in the day room during a group therapy session. His body language is tense and he is avoiding eye contact. He is covering his ears with his hands and shaking his head back and forth.

R: Recommendation

- Reduce environmental stimuli. Accompany Ben to a quieter location, away from day room and other patients.
- Provide a safe environment. Assess for evidence of self-injurious behaviors. Consider providing helmet if head banging behavior returns.
- Monitor and manage sensory sensitivities.
- Promote a consistent, structured environment.
- Contact health care provider for medication evaluation.
- Explore referral to speech language specialist.

Family Interventions

Unfortunately, lack of integration of medical, psychiatric, social, and educational services can add to the family's burden. Parents may manifest denial, grief, guilt, and anger at various points as they adjust to their child's disability. The nurse can offer parents the opportunity to express their frustrations and disappointments and can be alert for indications that parents need additional assistance, such as parent support groups or respite care.

Family interventions include support, education, counseling, and referral to self-help groups. Whenever possible, the nurse provides education to help parents determine appropriate expectations for their child and to meet the child's special needs. The following are examples of potentially useful nursing interventions focusing on the family:

- Interpreting the treatment plan for parents and child
- Modeling appropriate behavior modification techniques
- Including the parents as co-therapists for the implementation of the care plan
- Assisting the family in identifying and resolving their sense of loss related to the diagnosis
- Coordinating support systems for parents, siblings, and family members
- Maintaining interdisciplinary collaboration

Evaluation of Patient Outcomes

Evaluation of patient and family outcomes is an ongoing process. Short-term outcomes might consist of discrete behavioral improvements, such as reducing self-injurious behavior by 50%. The long-term goal is for the patient to achieve the highest level of functioning.

ATTENTION-DEFICIT HYPERACTIVITY DISORDER

ADHD is one of the most commonly diagnosed disorders in school-aged children (CDC, 2024b). It is almost certainly a heterogeneous disorder with multiple etiologies. The relatively high frequency of ADHD and associated behavior issues virtually guarantees that nurses will meet affected children in all pediatric treatment settings. ADHD is also diagnosed in adults, but it is less common than in children (Popit et al., 2024).

Diagnostic Criteria and Clinical Course

A persistent pattern of inattention, hyperactivity, and impulsiveness that interferes with functioning characterizes ADHD (APA, 2022). A diagnosis is made based on school behavior, parents' reports, and direct observation of inattention and hyperactivity–impulsivity that are inconsistent with developmental level. Parents and teachers describe children with ADHD as restless, always on the go, highly distractible, unable to wait their turn, heedless, and frequently disruptive. It is often disruptive behavior that brings these children in for treatment.

> **KEYCONCEPT Attention** involves concentrating on one activity to the exclusion of others, as well as the ability to sustain focus.

In ADHD, the individual finds it difficult to attend to one task at a time and is easily distracted. For some, the lack of attention is related to being unable to filter incoming information, which leads to being unable to screen and select the important information. That is, all incoming stimuli are treated the same (e.g., directions from a teacher elicit the same importance as noise in the hallway). For others, the distractibility may be related to stimuli-seeking behavior. Given the heterogeneity of ADHD, either of these models may explain issues of attention for subgroups of affected children.

Children with ADHD are prone to impulsive, risk-taking behavior and often fail to consider the consequences of their actions (CDC, 2024b). They tend to demonstrate poor judgment and seem to have more accidental injuries due to their risk-taking behavior. They often require a high degree of structure and supervision (Lillvis et al., 2024).

> **KEYCONCEPT Impulsiveness** is the tendency to act on urges, notions, or desires without adequately considering the consequences.

Although hyperactivity is a characteristic often associated with ADHD, controversy is long-standing about whether attention-deficit disorder can occur without overactivity. In many cases, it is the hyperactivity that prompts the search for treatment. Parents typically report that a child's hyperactivity was manifested early in life and is evident in most situations (APA, 2022). Hyperactivity and impulsivity in childhood are associated with increased risk of being involved in cases of violence, particularly intimate partner violence and sexual violence, either as victims or perpetrators (Arrondo et al., 2023).

> **KEYCONCEPT Hyperactivity** is excessive motor activity, as evidenced by restlessness, an inability to remain seated, and high levels of physical motion and verbal output.

ADHD Across the Lifespan

ADHD is usually diagnosed in childhood and was traditionally viewed as an issue of children. We now understand that ADHD persists into adulthood, and it is sometimes first diagnosed later than in childhood. In adults, symptoms of hyperactivity and impulsivity tend to decline with age and deficit of attention persist and become more varied. However, most adults with ADHD are undiagnosed and untreated (Plowden et al., 2022).

Epidemiology and Risk Factors

Although prevalence estimates vary depending on the diagnostic criteria used, the sources of data, and the sampling procedure, ADHD has been diagnosed in as many as 9.8% of children aged 3 to 17 years, an estimated 7 million of children in the United States. Male children are more likely to be diagnosed than female children (15% compared to 8%) (CDC, 2024b). Researchers believe that several risk factors may contribute to the development of ADHD, including a family history of ADHD, environmental factors (such as brain injuries, nutrition, and social environments), substance use during pregnancy, exposures to environmental toxins (such as lead) during pregnancy and/or at a young age, and low birth weight (National Institute of Mental Health [NIMH], 2024a; Sears et al., 2022).

Etiology

No single explanation for the occurrence of ADHD exists; instead, this disorder is viewed as having multiple causes. Genetic factors are implicated in the etiology of ADHD. They clearly play a fundamental role in the manifestation of ADHD behavior (Kleppesto et al., 2024; Lopez-Martin et al., 2024). In some children, dietary patterns have been investigated as a potential contributing factor to the development of ADHD, specifically those characterized by high consumption of refined grains, processed meats, soft drinks, and saturated fat (Pinto et al., 2022).

Biologic Theories

Although the etiology of ADHD is uncertain, evidence about neurobiologic dysfunction is pervasive. Research has shown that the frontal lobe and functional connections impacted with specific subcortical structures also are dysregulated. One clearly dysfunctional area is the dorsolateral prefrontal cortex, the center of directed attention and the ability to manage emotions or delay emotional reactions. Several neurotransmitters (e.g., dopamine, serotonin, and norepinephrine) are dysregulated (Chepke et al., 2024; Lin et al., 2023; Predescu et al., 2024). Clinically, the hyperactive-impulsive behavior characteristic of ADHD has been shown to be predominantly related to biologic factors, not psychosocial factors.

Psychosocial Theories

Although genetic endowment is clearly a fundamental element in the etiology of ADHD, psychosocial factors are also important risk factors. Critical life events, family stress, marital discord, and parental substance use are also associated with exacerbation of ADHD behaviors. Other implicated psychosocial factors are poverty, overcrowded living conditions, and family dysfunction (Jendreizik et al., 2023; Spencer et al., 2022).

Family Response to ADHD

Living with a child who has ADHD is a challenge for all family members, particularly those members who also have issues similar to those of the affected child. The family will raise a child who needs a structured environment that helps support focus and attention, and the parents must partner with their children's school system. For some families, the relationship with the school is positive and supportive. For others, the relationship with the school can be strained and lead to additional stress. It is important that the teachers and parents work together and provide consistent directions to the child.

If parents also have issues related to attention, impulse, and hyperactivity, home chaos and ineffective parenting practices can occur. If the parents also have ADHD, they might not be able to provide a calm structured environment for the child. Effective parenting requires resisting overreacting emotionally, focusing on the child, keeping track of activities, and providing consistency in discipline (Morgan & O'Keefe, 2022).

RECOVERY-ORIENTED CARE FOR CHILDREN WITH ADHD

Teamwork and Collaboration: Working Toward Recovery

Children with ADHD and their families benefit from symptom management, education, and support from various disciplines to have a high-quality life. Successful recovery efforts involve early recognition and treatment. By recognizing the issue early, family members and teachers can structure the child's interactions, develop meaningful discipline strategies, and modify the physical environment so the child can learn coping skills to deal with impulsivity, distractibility, and hyperactivity. Evidence has accumulated over the years that medication is helpful, especially in the early years, but for long-term effects, a combination of medication management and behavioral approaches results in the best outcomes for the children and their families (Peterson et al., 2024; Rios-Davis et al., 2023).

ADHD is not an easy disorder to treat or manage. Comorbidity complicates successful recovery. Children with ADHD have more behavior or conduct issues (e.g., run-ins with police), learning disorders, anxiety, and depression (CDC, 2024b). Many other issues interfere with recovery efforts, such as family disruptions and economic issues, as well as naturally occurring changes such as maturational issues during their adolescent years. In addition, children from disadvantaged backgrounds fare worse than those children who have socioeconomic and educational support (Habdank-Kolaczkowski et al., 2023; Hall et al., 2023).

Safety Issues

Due to increased impulsivity and inattention, children and adolescents with ADHD are at greater risk for injury than those without ADHD. Research finds that children with ADHD are significantly more likely to experience injury when riding a bike, have more head injuries and injuries to multiple body parts, and are more likely to be hospitalized for unintentional poisoning. Teenagers with ADHD are more likely to break traffic rules and are more likely to be involved in a car accident than those without ADHD (CDC, 2024b).

Individuals of all ages with ADHD are at high risk for mood changes that could lead to risk-taking behavior and suicidal ideation or attempts. Mood lability, the presence of depression, and potential for self-harm should be carefully assessed in these individuals. The risk of suicide attempts in children and adolescents with ADHD may be increased due to possible exposure to certain environmental risk factors, such as poor performance in school, impaired interpersonal relationships, socioeconomic hardship, depression, and substance use (Lin et al., 2023; Todzia-Kornas et al., 2024). Studies find that hospitalized patients with ADHD are twice as likely to have suicidal ideation/attempts than those without ADHD (Trivedi et al., 2023).

EVIDENCE-BASED NURSING CARE FOR CHILDREN WITH ATTENTION-DEFICIT HYPERACTIVITY DISORDER

The planning of nursing interventions must be done within the context of the family, treatment setting, and school environment. With the parents, clinical team members, and school personnel, the nurse participates in designing a plan of care that fits the child's and family's needs. Individuals with ADHD and their families will benefit from nursing care at many different times in the course of the disorder. Unless hospitalized for a comorbid mental health issue, most treatment will occur outside the mental health system. School nurses often provide most of the nursing care and family education.

RECOGNIZING CUES: RELEVANT ASSESSMENT INFORMATION

In the school setting, the primary focus of the assessment is the impact of ADHD on classroom behavior and school performance. In the hospital, the nurse tries to determine the contribution of ADHD to the acute psychiatric issue. In both cases, the nurse collects assessment data through direct interview, observation of the child and parent, and teacher ratings. Because children with ADHD may have difficulty sitting through long sessions, interviews are typically brief. Parents and teachers are extremely important sources for assessment data (Box 37.5). To this end, the nurse can make use of several standardized instruments (Box 37.6).

Physical Health

As with other psychiatric disorders with onset in childhood, the nursing assessment of children with ADHD begins with identification and exploration of the presenting issues, usually hyperactivity, impulsivity, and inattention. This typically entails a review of the child's developmental course, the onset and pattern of the current symptoms, factors that have worsened or improved the child's issues, and prior treatment or self-initiated efforts to remedy the situation. Medical history is also essential, consisting of perinatal course, childhood illnesses, hospital admissions, injuries, seizures, tics, physical growth, general health status, and date of the child's last physical examination.

The behavior of these children is characteristically very active and can often be observed in the office. They cannot sit still. They fidget. Even in sleep, they may be more active than other children. Thus, a careful assessment of eating, sleeping, and activity patterns is essential. Assessing daily food intake, typical diet, and frequency of eating will help identify any nutritional issues.

BOX 37.5

Research for Evidence-Based Practice: Evidence-Based Assessment for ADHD

Eng, A. G., Bansal, P. S., Goh, P. K., Nirjar, U., Petersen, M. K., & Martel, M. M. (2024). Evidence-based assessment for attention-deficit/hyperactivity disorder. Assessment, *31(1), 42–52.*

PURPOSE: Review best-practice evidence-based assessment of ADHD.

FINDINGS: Assessment of ADHD should include both ADHD-specific and broadband rating scales from multiple informants. IQ, academic achievement, and executive functioning should be evaluated when there are concerns about learning. For children under the age of 12, parent and teacher ratings should be averaged. For those over 12 years old, when self and other reports are inconsistent, the informant reports should be prioritized.

IMPLICATIONS FOR NURSING: Inaccurate assessment leads to undiagnosed and untreated ADHD. Evidence-based assessment is essential for accurate assessment and early intervention. Although much is known about evidence-based assessment, more research is needed about assessment among varied populations. Females with ADHD are underidentified, and this may be due to lack of comprehensive assessment. Another heavily understudied area of ADHD assessment is the impact of race and ethnicity. A multipronged assessment approach is needed.

BOX 37.6

Standardized Tools for Attention-Deficit Hyperactivity Disorder Diagnosis[a]

CONNERS QUESTIONNAIRES

The Conners Parent Questionnaire is a 48-item scale that a parent completes about their child. Each item is a statement that the parent rates on a 4-point scale from 0 (not at all) to 3 (very much). The Conners Teacher Questionnaire is a 28-item questionnaire that the child's teacher completes according to the same 4-point scale as the Parent Questionnaire. Both questionnaires have been standardized by age and gender for a mean of 50 and a standard deviation of 10 (Conners, 1997; Goyette et al., 1978).

CHILD BEHAVIOR CHECKLIST

The Child Behavior Checklist (CBCL) is a 118-item questionnaire that a parent completes. In addition to the 118 questions about specific behaviors and psychiatric symptoms, the CBCL also includes questions concerning the child's competence in social and academic spheres as well as age-appropriate activities. Normative data are available, allowing the conversion of raw scores to standard scores for age and gender. A teacher version of this scale is also available.

[a]Note that the diagnosis of ADHD is not made on the basis of questionnaires alone. Data from these rating scales augment the information gathered through interview and observation. These questionnaires can be especially useful before and after initiating a treatment plan to measure change.

Caffeinated products can contribute to hyperactivity in some children. Sleep is often disturbed for children with ADHD and consequently also the family. A detailed sleep assessment can provide points for interventions and help the interpretation of drug effects.

Psychosocial Cues

Data regarding school performance, behavior at home, and comorbid psychiatric disorders are essential for developing school interventions and behavior plans and establishing the baseline severity for medication. Children with ADHD are more likely to have issues with their cognitive process during changing demands of teachers and parents (cognitive processing, attention, language, and memory) (Sadozai et al., 2024). Consequently, they may have more difficulty in school with decision-making. These children are often behind in their work at school because of poor organization, off-task behavior, and impulsive responses (Shroff et al., 2024).

Dysfunctional interactions can develop within the family. Discipline is frequently an issue because parents may have difficulty controlling their child's behavior, which is disruptive and occasionally destructive. They can exhaust their parents, aggravate teachers, and annoy siblings with their intrusive and disruptive actions. Reviewing the problematic behaviors and the situations in which they occur is a way to identify negative interaction patterns.

Because ADHD often occurs in the context of psychosocial adversity, it is important to review the family situation, including parenting style, stability of household membership, consistency of rules and routines, and life events (e.g., divorce, moves, deaths, job loss). Identification of these factors can be useful in shaping a care plan that builds on potential strengths and mitigates the effects of environmental factors that may perpetuate the child's disruptive behavior.

ANALYZING CUES AND DEVELOPING HYPOTHESES

Priorities of nursing care will depend on the severity of the responses, family situation, and school environment. Increased impulsivity and inattention put the child or adolescent at greater risk for injury. Comorbid disorders, such as mood or conduct disorders, may also be present. Sleep deprivation, inadequate nutrition, and the inability to carry out daily routines may require intervention. The child may demonstrate poor coping skills and may not function well in social settings or in structured activities (such as in the school environment).

PLANNING RECOVERY AND WELLNESS OUTCOMES

Outcomes should be individualized to the child. Short-term outcomes, such as decreasing the number of classroom ejections within a 2-week period, may be useful for one child, but reducing the frequency and amplitude of angry outbursts at home may be relevant to another child.

TAKING ACTION: NURSING INTERVENTIONS

Physical and psychosocial development must be considered when developing interventions for children and adolescents. Just as family relationships change during growth development, ADHD symptoms also change and influence the child and family's abilities to cope with these changes.

Physical Care

The following discussion of physical is applicable to children and adolescents. As a child transitions to adolescence, the personal responsibility for these interventions shift for the parent to the adolescent.

Modifying Nutrition

A link between adverse reactions to food (e.g., dietary salicylates and artificially added food colors, flavors, preservatives) and ADHD was suggested many years ago when the Feingold diet was introduced (Feingold, 1975). Over the years, interest in the link between food and behavior continues to spark interest in ADHD as an issue related to food. Agreement exists that in some children the behaviors associated with ADHD can be decreased with diet changes (Chatfield, 2023). The free foods diet may be an option in ADHD treatment. The few foods diet includes basic foods that are not likely to produce adverse effects such as lamb, chicken, potatoes, bananas, and apples. Grains, dairy products, and processed foods are avoided in the few foods diet. The restricted elimination diet includes all-natural, chemical-free foods. Fruits, vegetables, nuts, nut butters, beans, seeds, gluten-free grains such as rice and quinoa, fish, lamb, wild game meats, organic turkey, and large amounts of water are consumed. This diet is very restricted and consequently difficult to follow all of the time. The polyunsaturated diet suggests that children with ADHD have low levels of omega-3 polyunsaturated fatty acids. Supplements are encouraged for these individuals (Lange et al., 2023; Liu et al., 2023).

Supplementation with free fatty acids has been shown to be helpful for children who have deficiencies in free fatty acid such as omega-3 free fatty acid, omega-6 free fatty acid, and linolenic acid. This supplementation is usually achieved with capsule-containing oils or diets rich in fish products (Chatfield, 2023).

If patients adhere to any of these diets, the nurse should support the patient and family in providing the nutritional information needed for the diet. In addition, the patient and family will need education regarding those foods that are chemical free. A referral to a dietitian will benefit both patient and family.

Children with ADHD seem to be more susceptible to being overweight and developing obesity, with over half of children with ADHD demonstrating atypical eating behaviors. Factors contributing to the relationship between ADHD and being overweight may include the child's environment, genetics, atypical eating patterns, executive dysfunction, low physical activity, and sleep disturbances (Zhu et al., 2024). Because of the impulsivity and inattention characteristic of ADHD, children with ADHD may be unable to self-regulate and engage in healthy eating behaviors. They are more likely to consume sweetened beverages, sweets, candies, and other types of junk foods (Khazdouz et al., 2024). The nurse can help the family and patient structure the external environment, so the child has healthy choices available.

Promoting Sleep

Up to 70% of children with ADHD experience difficulty with sleep. Issues include bedtime resistance, sleep onset difficulties, lighter sleep, poor-quality sleep, fragmented sleep due to restlessness, and shorter sleep duration. Sleep disturbance contributes to poorer academic performance, higher parental stress, and poorer parental health (Larsson et al., 2022). There are many things contributing to sleep disturbance, including the overactivity of the disorder itself and the side effects of the psychostimulants. A sleep history should be taken before medications are prescribed. If issues exist, atomoxetine should be considered before the psychostimulants (see next section). If sleep issues arise while taking medications, sleep diaries should be kept. Sleep hygiene and behavior therapy techniques, including emphasis on a bedtime routine, electronic media restriction, caffeine restriction, exposure to morning light, scheduling physical activity during the day and optimization of the sleep environment should be implemented (Russell & Arnold, 2023). See Chapter 34.

Medication Interventions

Approved medications for ADHD in children as young as 6 years include stimulants and nonstimulants. Psychostimulants, including methylphenidate, dextroamphetamine, and mixed amphetamine salts (see Chapter 11), are by far the most commonly used medications for the treatment of ADHD and are found to effective in reducing ADHD symptoms in 70% to 80% of children. These medications enhance dopamine and norepinephrine activity, which thereby improves attention and focus, decreases hyperactivity and impulsivity, and decreases disruptive behaviors (CDC, 2024b; Cortese, 2023; NIMH, 2024a; Peterson et al., 2024).

Methylphenidate has a total duration of action of about 4 hours (Box 37.7). Thus, parents or teachers often describe a return of overactivity and distractibility as the first dose of medication wears off. This "rebound effect" can often be managed by moving the second dose of the day slightly closer to the first dose. Longer-acting preparations of methylphenidate or amphetamine–dextroamphetamine do not require such frequent dosing and may be a better fit with a school day schedule. The most common side effects associated with stimulants for ADHD include appetite suppression, insomnia, dry mouth, and nausea. Drug holidays are sometimes implemented to determine the need for continued medication and to manage side effects.

One major concern with psychostimulants is the potential for misuse. With the increase in recognition of ADHD, psychostimulant prescriptions have increased, as well as an increase in diversion for cognitive enhancement or appetite suppression. These misused prescription medications are most often acquired from peers who share, sell, or trade their medication. Nurses should caution parents about the potential for misuse and prevent their child's medication from being a source of recreational use (Cortese, 2023).

Nonstimulant medications do not work as quickly as stimulants, though they are an alternative for those who do not tolerate stimulants well, when a stimulant is

BOX 37.7

Medication Profile: Methylphenidate

DRUG CLASS: Central nervous system stimulant

RECEPTOR AFFINITY: The mechanisms of pharmacologic effect are not completely clear. At low doses, it provides mild cortical stimulation similar to that of amphetamines. This stimulation results from methylphenidate's ability to promote release and interfere with the reuptake of dopamine in the synaptic cleft. Main sites appear to be the brain stem arousal system and cortex to produce its stimulant effect.

INDICATIONS: Treatment of narcolepsy, attention-deficit disorders, and hyperkinetic syndrome.

ROUTES AND DOSAGE: Available in 5- to 10-mg immediate-release tablets and 20-mg sustained-release tablets. Long-acting preparations in various dose strengths are also available.

Adult Dosage: Must be individualized; range from 10 to 60 mg/day orally in divided doses bid (twice a day) to tid (three times a day), preferably 15 to 30 minutes before meals. If insomnia is an issue, drug should be administered before 6 pm.

Child Dosage: The immediate-release formulation can be started at 5 mg twice or three times daily on a 4-hour schedule with weekly increases depending on response. Starting doses of the long-acting preparations are equivalent to the total tid dose (e.g., 5 tid of short acting would translate into 18 mg of the long-acting preparation). Usually given on a tid schedule, with the last dose being roughly half that of the first and second doses. Daily dosage of more than 60 mg is not recommended. Discontinue after 1 month if no improvement is seen.

PEAK EFFECT: 1 hour; half-life: 3 to 4 hours for the immediate-release preparations

SELECT SIDE EFFECTS: Nervousness, insomnia, dizziness, headache, dyskinesias (including tics), toxic psychosis, anorexia, nausea, abdominal pain, increased pulse and blood pressure, palpitations, tolerance, psychological dependence.

WARNING: The drug is discontinued periodically to assess the patient's condition. Contraindications include marked anxiety, tension and agitation, glaucoma, severe depression, and obsessive-compulsive symptoms. Use cautiously in patients with a personal or family history of tic disorders, seizure disorders, hypertension, drug dependence, alcohol use disorder, or emotional instability.

SPECIFIC PATIENT AND FAMILY EDUCATION

- Do not chew or crush sustained-release tablets; they must be swallowed whole.
- Take the drug exactly as prescribed; if insomnia is an issue, the time and dose may need adjustment. The drug is rarely taken after 5 pm.
- Avoid alcohol and over-the-counter products, including decongestants, cold remedies, and cough syrups; these could accentuate side effects of the stimulant.
- Keep appointments for follow-up, including evaluations for monitoring the child's growth and use of parent and teacher ratings to monitor benefit.
- Note that the prescriber may discontinue the drug periodically to confirm effectiveness of therapy.

ineffective, or in combination with a stimulant to increase effectiveness. The four Food and Drug Administration (FDA)-approved nonstimulants for ADHD are a norepinephrine update inhibitor (atomoxetine), a norepinephrine reuptake inhibitor (viloxazine), and alpha-2 receptor agonists (guanfacine and clonidine) (CDC, 2024b; NIMH, 2024a; Peterson et al., 2024). Nonstimulants are less likely to be misused than stimulant medications due to a lack of immediacy of effect (a lower speed of action and feeling stimulated) and therefore are often used for those who are more likely to be substance dependent. These medications are generally well tolerated in children and adults.

Common side effects associated with atomoxetine and viloxazine include GI symptoms, somnolence, headaches, moodiness, and irritability. The more common adverse effects experienced by individuals taking the alpha-2 receptor agonists include fatigue, sedation, and somnolence (Peterson, 2024).

Teaching Points

Medication can help the child's hyperactivity, impulsiveness, and inattention; therefore, teaching the parent, child, and school personnel about the importance of the medication in ADHD and the potential side effects is a place to begin. Explaining to the child that the medication improves concentration and the ability to sit still can help strengthen patient motivation.

Often, parents are reluctant to initiate treatment with psychostimulants because of the fear that their use in childhood will increase the risk of using substances in adulthood. Studies show that children and adolescents who have taken simulants medications for ADHD are no more likely to develop later substance use than those who did not take stimulant medications (Molina et al., 2023). Teaching patients and families about the biologic basis of ADHD helps parents understand that these children are not "bad" kids but that they have issues with impulse control and attention. It may be helpful to review the purposes of the medications and assure parents that evidence shows that medications help most affected children.

Psychosocial Interventions

Behavioral programs based on rewards for positive behavior, such as waiting turns and following directions, can foster new social skills. Behavioral parent training, behavioral classroom management, and behavioral peer interventions are well-established treatments. Specific cognitive-behavioral techniques are helpful in which the child learns to "stop, look, and listen" before doing. These approaches have been refined and several useful recommendations are available (Dentz et al., 2024;

Rios-Davis et al., 2023). In general, interactions with children can be guided by the following:

- Set clear limits with clear consequences. Use few words and simplify instructions.
- Establish and maintain a predictable environment with clear rules and regular routines for eating, sleeping, and playing.
- Promote attention by maintaining a calm environment with few stimuli. These children cannot filter out extraneous stimuli and react to all stimuli equally.
- Establish eye contact before giving directions; ask the child to repeat what was heard.
- Encourage the child to do homework in a quiet place.
- Help the child work on one assignment at a time (reward with a break after each completion).

Family treatment is nearly always a component of cognitive behavioral treatment approaches with the child. This may involve parent training that focuses on principles of behavior management, such as appropriate limit setting and use of reward systems, as well as revising expectations about the child's behavior. School programming often involves increasing structure in the child's school day to offset the child's tendency to act without forethought and to be easily distracted by extraneous stimuli. Specific remediation is required for the child with comorbid deficits in learning or language. Some children may require small self-contained classrooms.

Complementary Therapies

Although not found to be as effective as conventional treatment, yoga and meditation have shown small to moderate beneficial effects on the core symptoms of ADHD of attention, hyperactivity, and impulsivity. There is insufficient evidence to support use of acupuncture in children with ADHD. Evidence of the effectiveness of neurofeedback is mixed, with studies showing benefit pointing to "nonspecific" psychological and behavioral effects versus impact of brain waves training. Newer emerging therapies under study include game-based digital therapeutics and trigeminal nerve stimulation (Caterfino et al., 2024; National Institutes of Health, National Center for Complementary and Integrative Health [NCCIH NIH], 2023; Russell & Arnold, 2023).

Evaluation of Patient Outcomes

Children may not notice any effects after taking medication, but people in their environment do. Often, within 1 to 2 weeks of initiating therapy, children with ADHD become more attentive, less impulsive, and less active. Parents and teachers are often the first to notice improvement. With time, academic achievement also may improve (Fig. 37.1).

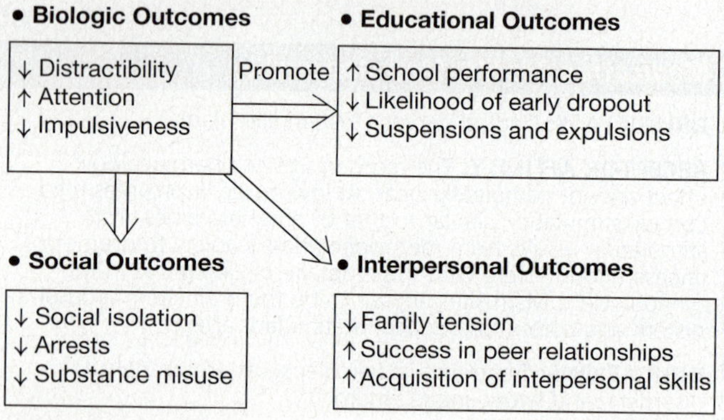

FIGURE 37.1 Long-term outcomes of optimal treatment for patients with attention-deficit hyperactivity disorder.

Continuum of Care

Treatment of ADHD typically is conducted in outpatient settings. Optimal treatment is multimodal (i.e., includes several types of interventions), encompassing four main areas: individual treatment for the child, family treatment, school accommodations, and medication. Parent training and social skills training also help diminish disruptive and defiant behavior.

OTHER NEURODEVELOPMENTAL DISORDERS

Other neurodevelopmental disorders are characterized by a narrower range of deficits. These include specific neurodevelopmental disorders generally classified as learning, communication, and motor skills disorders. This section focuses primarily on learning and communication disorders.

In general, a **learning disorder** (a diagnostic term) or learning disability (a legal term) is defined as a discrepancy between actual achievement and expected achievement based on the individual's age and intellectual ability. The definition varies depending on the source and state statute. Learning disorders are typically classified as verbal (e.g., reading, spelling) or nonverbal (e.g., mathematics).

Reading disability, also called **dyslexia**, has been recognized for more than 100 years. It is defined as a significantly lower score for mental age on standardized tests in reading that is not the result of low intelligence or inadequate schooling. This relatively common issue affects about 5% of school-aged children, with some studies reporting higher prevalence. In clinical samples, dyslexia affects male children more often than female children. This discrepancy can be explained by slower and variable processing speed and less inhibitory control in males than females. Approximately 40% of children with dyslexia have another comorbid neurodevelopmental disorder (Bozatli et al., 2024).

Although it is clear that no single cause will provide a sufficient explanation for reading disability, the underlying issue appears to be a deficit in **phonologic processing**, which involves the discrimination and interpretation of speech sounds. A disturbance in the development of the left hemisphere is believed to cause this deficit. Both genetic and environmental factors have been implicated in the etiology of reading disability. Data from family studies show that reading disability is familial and that shared environmental factors alone cannot explain the high rate of recurrence in affected families (Gialluisi et al., 2021).

Another learning disorder that is frequently comorbid with dyslexia is mathematics disorder, or dyscalculia. Dyscalculia affects approximately 5% to 7% of children worldwide (Li et al., 2023). Children with mathematics disorder struggle in comprehending even basic numeric and arithmetic concepts, despite average intelligence. This poses significant challenges due to the predominant use of numbers in everyday life that may also impact an individual's job opportunities and learning potential as an adult. An estimated 30% to 70% of children with mathematics disorder also have dyslexia, and 11% have comorbid ADHD (Hussain & Soares, 2022).

COMMUNICATION DISORDERS

Communication disorders involve speech or language impairments. Speech refers to the motor aspects of speaking; language consists of higher-order aspects of formulating and comprehending verbal communication. Communication disorders can affect the individual's ability to speak, listen, read, and write. Communication disorders are fairly common, occurring in approximately 1 in 14 children in kindergarten, with the impact generally persisting into adulthood. Although the exact cause of communication disorders is unknown, evidence points to a strong genetic link, with 50% to 70% of children affected having at least one family member with the disorder (National Institute of Health, National Institute on Deafness and Other Communication Disorders [NIH, NIDOCD], 2023). Language difficulties are an associated risk factor for reading and mathematics disorders (Duff et al., 2023).

A delay in speech or language development can adversely affect the child's socialization and education. For example, peers may rebuff or tease a child with an articulation defect or stutter, contributing to withdrawal and a negative self-image. The resulting isolation could limit opportunities to negotiate rules, take turns, and learn cooperation. These same tasks could also be difficult for children with language delay. For school-aged children, interventions may focus on helping the child follow directions, understand the meaning of words being used in class, organize information, and improve speaking, reading, and writing skills (NIH, NIDOCD, 2023).

EVIDENCE-BASED NURSING CARE FOR CHILDREN WITH COMMUNICATION DISORDERS

Nursing assessment of children with a known specific developmental disorder includes (1) evidence of interference in daily life, (2) determination of the child's ability (and limitations) to communicate during the interview, (3) assessment of the child's perception about their disability, (4) observation for impaired learning and communication, and (5) past and current interventions for the learning or communication deficit with data gathered through direct interview of the child and significant others such as parents. Several nursing diagnoses can be generated from these data, such as impaired verbal communication and social isolation.

For the child with learning disabilities, nurses can focus on building self-confidence and helping the family connect with guidance and educational resources that support the child's development into adulthood. For the child with communication disorders, the interventions focus on fostering social and communication skills and making referrals for specific speech or language therapy. Modeling appropriate communication in spontaneous situations with the child can be a useful intervention for some children. The following is an overview of nursing interventions for the child with specific developmental difficulties:

- Introduce strategies for increasing communication skills (e.g., initiating conversation, taking turns in conversation, facing the listener).
- Identify and develop specific intervention strategies for issues secondary to learning communication disorders, such as low self-esteem.
- Provide parental support for coping with the disorder.
- Maintain interdisciplinary medical, dental, and speech therapy, and also educational collaboration.
- Refer to learning or speech specialist for evaluation and assistance.

Continuum of Care

Children with learning disabilities obviously require careful psychoeducational and cognitive testing to identify their strengths and deficits. School or clinical psychologists usually perform this type of specialized testing. When a learning disability has been identified, the U.S. Education for All Handicapped Children Act (Public Law 94–142) mandates that public school systems provide remedial services in the least restrictive educational setting. Families occasionally need help in advocating for these services.

The same is true for children with communication disorders, although the services requested may be different. Speech pathologists conduct the diagnostic assessment of speech and language disorders. Nurses may be involved with formal screening for communication disorders. Services such as speech therapy (directed at the motor aspects of speaking) or social skills groups (directed at the social and interpersonal aspects of language) are often available in school districts and can be obtained if a speech or language disorder has been identified. For some children with communication disorders, the services offered by the school may be insufficient. In such cases, the nurse can help the family locate a facility that can provide these needed services.

DISRUPTIVE BEHAVIOR DISORDERS

Disruptive behavior disorders, which include oppositional defiant disorder and conduct disorder, are conditions marked by significant issues of conduct. Behaviors associated with these disorders violate the rights of others and/or are in conflict with societal norms (APA, 2022).

OPPOSITIONAL DEFIANT DISORDER AND CONDUCT DISORDER

Oppositional defiant disorder (ODD) is characterized by a persistent pattern of disobedience, argumentativeness, angry outbursts, low tolerance for frustration, and tendency to blame others for misfortunes, large and small. Children with oppositional defiant disorder are more likely to demonstrate oppositional behavior with people they know, such as family members or school teachers. Although it is not uncommon for all children to test limits at times, children with ODD do this more often than others their age. Their behaviors lead to issues with making friends with their peers, and they often find themselves in conflict with adults. ODD typically begins before the age of 8, and generally no later than 12 years old. Some children with ODD will develop conduct disorder (CDC, 2024e).

Conduct disorder (CD) is characterized by more serious violations of social norms, including aggressive behavior (such as bullying and fighting), destruction of property, and cruelty to animals. Conduct disorder generally occurs later than ODD, most often in adolescence. Children and adolescents with conduct disorder often lie to achieve short-term ends, may be truant from school, may run away from home, and may engage in breaking the law, resulting in arrest (CDC, 2024e). See Box 37.8.

BOX 37.8

Clinical Judgment Vignette: Conduct Disorder

Leon, age 14, was admitted to the child psychiatric inpatient service from the emergency department (ED) after a fight with his mother. His mother reported that she and Leon had argued earlier in the evening and that he stormed out of the house screaming and vowing he would never return. Several hours later, Leon came back, yelling, and demanding entry into the apartment. Leon's father was working. While his mother was getting up to open the door, Leon continued to yell and scream, waking the neighbors. This led to further arguments between Leon and his mother. Before long, the police were called, and Leon was taken to the ED.

The admission interview revealed that Leon had run away on several occasions and had even stayed away overnight. Although he strongly denied drug use, he had gotten drunk on several occasions. He had also been in several fights, the latest of which resulted in an expulsion from school. Three months before admission, he was caught trying to steal a video game from an electronics store. More recently, he boasted that he and his friends had snatched a purse at an outdoor concert and had broken into a car to steal its contents. Leon's school performance has been declining; he was truant on several occasions and will probably have to repeat ninth grade.

Leon was born in Puerto Rico and is the oldest of three children. His family moved to the mainland shortly after his birth, and the primary language at home is Spanish. His father is employed as a janitor and speaks very little English. His mother works as a secretary and has achieved fairly good command of English. He has received no treatment except for consultation with the school social worker.

Building Clinical Judgment

1. When conducting a nursing assessment, what would you want to learn about Leon's school performance?
2. What information could you provide Leon's parents about pharmacotherapy? About behavior management?

Epidemiology

Children and adolescents with disruptive behavior disorders frequently present to psychiatric treatment settings. The estimated global prevalence rate of conduct disorder in children and adolescents is 3%, with a rate 2.6 times higher in males than females. The disorder appears to be fairly consistent across various countries that differ in race and ethnicity (Ayano et al., 2024). Males with conduct disorder frequently are involved in fighting, stealing, vandalism, and school disciplinary issues. Females with the diagnosis are more likely to practice lying, truancy, running away, substance use, and prostitution. Whereas males tend to exhibit both physical aggression and relational aggression (i.e., behaviors that harm social relations of others), females tend to exhibit relatively more relational aggression (APA, 2022). Conduct disorder is a frequently diagnosed disorder in children in mental health facilities. Individuals with conduct disorder are at risk for comorbid substance use disorders, anxiety, and depressive disorders (Jandac & Lenka, 2024).

BOX 37.9

Trauma-Informed Approaches: Childhood Adversity in Youth Entering Residential Care

Background

Records of over 2,000 youth entering a family-style residential program were reviewed to examine profiles of patterns of childhood adversity. Five profiles were found: (1) Low Exposure, (2) Familial Dysfunction, (3) Neglect/Emotional Abuse, (4) High Exposure without Sexual Abuse, (5) High Exposure with Sexual Abuse. Overall, female children were more likely than male children to have profiles of Neglect/Emotional Abuse and High Exposure with Sexual Abuse. Each of the five profile patterns were associated with different clinical outcomes.

Interventions

The nurse must consider patterns of childhood adversity when working with children and adolescents with behavioral issues. This screening information can better inform interventions for children and their families.

Source: Gordon, C. T., Nguyen, P. T., Mitchell, A. K., & Tyler, P. M. (2023). Profiles of childhood adversity and associated psychopathology in youth entering residential care. *Psychological Trauma: Theory, Research, Practice & Policy, 15*, S82–S91.

Etiology

The etiologies of oppositional defiant disorder and conduct disorder are complex. More attention has been paid to conduct disorder, probably because it is the more serious of the two. Models used to understand aggressiveness (see Chapter 20) are useful in examining these childhood disorders, which appear to have both genetic and environmental components (Tesli et al., 2024). Exposure to childhood adversity is known to increase a child's risk for internalizing and externalizing issues (Gordon et al., 2023). See Box 37.9.

EVIDENCE-BASED NURSING CARE FOR CHILDREN WITH DISRUPTIVE BEHAVIOR DISORDERS

Recognizing Cues: Relevant Assessment Information

The nurse gathers data from multiple sources. Adolescents with disruptive behavior disorders are at high risk for physical injury as a result of fighting and impulsive behavior. Sexual promiscuity is common in conduct disorder, resulting in an increased frequency of pregnancy and sexually transmitted infections.

An important aspect of assessment is to rule out comorbid conditions that may partially explain or complicate the individual's lack of behavioral control. These conditions include ADHD, learning disabilities, chemical dependency, depression, bipolar disorder, or anxiety disorders. Children and adolescents who are chronically depressed may be irritable and easily frustrated. Given the tendency of adolescents to act out their frustration, chronic depression may exacerbate their behavior. Conduct issues can also elevate the risk for depression because young people who regularly elicit negative attention from parents and teachers and are constantly at odds with their environment may become despondent.

Adolescents with conduct issues are usually brought or forced into the mental health system by family, school, or the court system because of fighting, truancy, speeding tickets, car accidents, petty crimes, substance misuse, or suicide attempts. They may be hostile, sarcastic, defensive, and provocative. At the same time, they may appear calm, outgoing, and engaging. Inconsistencies, distortions, and misrepresentations of the truth are common when interviewing these children and adolescents, so obtaining a clear history may be difficult. Therefore, instead of asking whether an event or behavior occurred, it may be better to ask when it occurred. These adolescents are adept at changing the subject and diverting discussions from sensitive issues. They often use denial, projection, and externalization of anger as defense mechanisms when asked for self-disclosure. The assessment, which may take several sessions, should be conducted in a nonjudgmental fashion. High levels of marital conflict, parental substance misuse, and parental antisocial behavior often mark family history.

Planning Recovery and Wellness Outcomes: Generating Solutions

After patient and staff safety are established, improving communication and coping skills should be the patient's priorities. The nurse can help the patient develop insight into the need for enhanced communication and positive coping.

Taking Action: Nursing Interventions

Children with oppositional defiant disorder or conduct disorder who also have specific neurodevelopmental disorders should be placed in appropriate programs for remediation. If a diagnosis of ADHD or depression emerges from the evaluation, appropriate pharmacotherapy should be considered (see previous discussion of ADHD and later discussion regarding depression). In planning interventions for patients with oppositional defiant disorder or conduct disorder, the focus is on problematic behaviors. Therapeutic progress may be slow, at least partly because these patients often lack trust in authority figures.

Social Skills Training

The nurse should communicate behavioral expectations clearly and enforce them consistently. Consequences of appropriate and inappropriate actions should also be clear. Specific approaches for improving social and problem-solving skills are fundamental features for school-aged children and adolescents. As far as children and adolescents with disruptive behavior issues fail to recognize the adverse effects of their verbal and nonverbal behavior, their deficit can be formulated as an interpersonal issue. Social skills training teaches adolescents with these behavior disorders to recognize the ways in which their actions affect others. Training involves techniques such as role-playing, modeling by the therapist, and giving positive reinforcement to improve interpersonal relationships and enhance social outcomes.

Problem-Solving Therapy

In contrast to social skills training, which proposes that issues of conduct are the result of poor interpersonal skills, problem-solving therapy conceptualizes conduct issues as the result of deficiencies in cognitive processes. These processes include assessment of situations, interpretation of events, and expectations of others that are congruent with behavior. These children often misinterpret the intentions of others and may perceive hostility with little or no cause. Problem-solving skills training teaches these children to generate alternative solutions to social situations, sharpen thinking concerning the consequences of those choices, and evaluate responses after interpersonal conflicts.

Parent Training and Education

Parent training begins with educating parents about disruptive behavior disorders, focusing particularly on impulsiveness, impaired judgment, and self-control. Children and adolescents with long-standing issues in these areas often elicit punitive responses and negative attributions about their behavior from their parents. Ironically, because these parental responses focus on the child's failure, they may contribute to the child's behavior issues. An important second step is to clarify parental expectations and interpretation of the child's behavior. Parent training may be offered to a group of parents or to individuals.

The aims of education are to provide parents with new ways of understanding their child's behavior and to promote improved interactions between parent and child. The most commonly presented techniques include the importance of positive reinforcement (praise and tangible rewards) for adaptive behavior, clear limits for unacceptable behavior, and use of mild punishment (e.g., a time out) (Box 37.10).

BOX 37.10

Time-Out Procedure

Labeling behavior: Identify the behavior that the child is expected to perform or cease. The aim of this statement is to make clear what is required of the child. It typically takes the form of a simple declarative sentence: "Threatening is not acceptable."

Warning: In this step, the child is informed that if they do not perform the expected behavior or stop the unacceptable behavior, they will be given a "time out." "This is a warning: if you continue threatening to hit people, you'll have a time out."

Time out: If the child does not heed the warning, they are told to take a time out in simple straightforward terms: "Take a time out."

Duration: The usual duration for a time out is 5 minutes for children 5 years of age or older.

Location: The child sits in a designated time-out chair without toys and without talking. The chair should be located away from general activity but within view. A kitchen timer can be used to mark the time, but the clock does not start until the child sits quietly in the designated spot.

Follow-up: The child is asked to recount why they were given the time out. The explanation need not be detailed, and no further discussion of the matter is required. Indeed, long discourse about the child's behavior is not helpful and should be avoided.

Referral to Family Therapy

Family therapy is directed at assisting the family with altering maladaptive patterns of interaction or improving adjustment to stressors, such as changes or loss in family membership (Nuntavisit & Porter, 2022). Multisystem family therapy, which considers the child in the context of multiple family and community systems, has shown promise in the treatment of adolescents with conduct disorder (Lee et al., 2024).

Evaluation of Patient Outcomes

The nurse can review treatment goals and objectives to assess the child's progress with respect to verbal and physical aggression, socially appropriate resolution of conflicts, adherence with rules and expectations, and better management of frustration. As is true for the initial assessment, evaluation of treatment outcomes relies on input from parents, teachers, and other health care team members.

Continuum of Care

Children and adolescents with conduct disorders may be involved with many different agencies in the community, such as child welfare services, school authorities, and the legal system. Mental health services are requested when a child or adolescent's behavior is out of control or when a comorbid disorder is suspected. Helping the patient and family negotiate their way through this maze of services may be an essential part of the treatment plan.

TIC DISORDERS AND TOURETTE SYNDROME

Tics are sudden twitches, movements, or sounds that individuals do repeatedly without their control. Tics can be transient or chronic. **Motor tics** are generally quick jerky movements of the eyes, face, neck, and shoulders, although they may involve other muscle groups as well. Occasionally, tics involve slower, more purposeful, or dystonic movements. Vocal tics typically include repetitive throat clearing, grunting, or other noises but may also include more complex sounds, such as words; parts of words; and in a small percentage of patients, obscenities. Transient tics by definition do not endure over time and appear to be fairly common in school-aged children. Tic disorder is a general term encompassing several syndromes that are chiefly characterized by motor tics, vocal tics, or both.

KEYCONCEPT Tics are sudden, rapid, repetitive, stereotyped motor movements or vocalizations.

TOURETTE SYNDROME

Tourette syndrome, the most severe tic disorder, is defined by multiple motor and **vocal tics** for at least 1 year. Because no diagnostic tests are used to confirm this disorder, the diagnosis is based on the type and duration of tics present. Early symptoms of Tourette syndrome (generally in the head and neck area) typically occur in early childhood, with an average onset between the ages of 5 and 10 years. Most individuals with Tourette syndrome experience their most severe tics in their early teens, with tics typically lessening and becoming more controllable by late teens to early 20s (National Institute of Health, National Institute of Neurologic Disorders and Stroke [NIH NINDS], 2024). Motor tics generally precede vocal tics, and parents often describe the seeming replacement of one tic with another. In addition to this changing repertoire of motor and vocal tics, Tourette syndrome exhibits a waxing and waning course. The child can suppress the tics for brief periods. Thus, it is common to hear from parents that their child has more frequent tics at home than at school. Older children and adults may describe an urge or a physical sensation before having a tic.

Epidemiology and Etiology

Studies estimate that 1 out of every 162 children (0.6%) has Tourette syndrome, of which only half are diagnosed. Among those diagnosed, 44% report moderate to severe symptoms. Symptoms generally occur for around 2 years before receiving a formal diagnosis. Male children are three times more likely to have Tourette syndrome than female children, and rates are similar among children from all racial and ethnic groups or socioeconomic backgrounds. Over 80% of children diagnosed with Tourette syndrome to have a comorbid mental, behavioral, or developmental disorder. More than a third of individuals with Tourette syndrome have OCD. Other comorbid diagnoses include anxiety (61%), ADHD (52%), behavioral issues (34%), learning disabilities (34%), developmental delays (26%), autism spectrum disorder (21%), and depression (20%). In addition, over 40% of children with Tourette syndrome have a co-occurring chronic health condition (CDC, 2024d).

The precise nature of the underlying pathophysiology in this primarily inherited disorder is unclear, but the basal ganglia and functionally related cortical areas are presumed to play a central role. Findings from neuroimaging studies are consistent with the presumption that a dysregulation of the corticostriatal–thalamic circuitry of the brain underlies Tourette syndrome. In addition, multiple genes on different chromosomes interacting with environmental factors are involved. Several neurotransmitters (dopamine, serotonin, and norepinephrine) have been implicated in the etiology of Tourette syndrome (NIH NINDS, 2024).

Family Response to Disorder

Before evaluation and diagnosis of Tourette disorder, most families struggle with various explanations for the child's tics. Because tics fluctuate in severity with time and may be more prominent in some settings than in others, family members may have difficulty understanding their involuntary nature. Some parents may be convinced that the tics are deliberate and done to secure attention; others may judge that the tics are "nervous habits" indicative of underlying trouble. Such views require reconciliation with the currently accepted view that tics are involuntary. Some parents may conclude that the child is incapable of controlling any behavior because of Tourette disorder. They may subsequently feel uncertain about setting limits. In these families, delineating the boundaries of Tourette syndrome can be helpful (CDC, 2024d).

On learning that this disorder is probably genetic, some parents may harbor guilt for having passed it on to their child. The nurse can assist such families by listening to these concerns and providing information about the natural history of Tourette disorder—it is not a progressive condition, tics often diminish in adulthood, and it need not restrict what the child can achieve in life.

EVIDENCE-BASED NURSING CARE FOR CHILDREN WITH TOURETTE SYNDROME

Recognizing Cues: Relevant Assessment Information

Nursing assessment of a child with tics includes a review of the onset, course, and current level of the symptoms. Goals of the assessment are to identify the frequency, intensity, complexity, and interference of the tics and their effects on functioning; determine the child's level of adaptive functioning; identify the child's areas of strength and weakness in general and in school; and identify social supports for the child and family.

Another important aspect of the assessment is to determine the effects of the tic symptoms on the child and family. Some children and families adjust well; however, others are embarrassed or devastated and tend to withdraw socially. Because of the likelihood of comorbid mental, behavioral, or developmental disorders, in addition to inquiring about tics, the nurse should assess the child's overall development, activity level, and capacity to concentrate and persist with a single task, as well as explore repetitive habits and recurring worries.

Analyzing Cues and Developing Hypotheses

Children with Tourette syndrome generally have typical intellectual ability, but their tics can interfere with their ability to relate to others and perform well in school. The nurse should determine the degree of anxiety experienced by the child, the impact of the tics on the child's ability to cope, and whether the tics contribute to interference with social relationships and interactions.

Taking Action: Nursing Interventions

The approach to planning nursing interventions depends on the primary source of impairment: tics themselves; OCD symptoms; or the triad of hyperactivity, inattention, and poor impulse control. The nurse can provide counseling and education for the patient, education for the parents, and consultation for the school. Most children and their families need some education about Tourette syndrome. Individual psychotherapy with a mental health specialist (e.g., a psychologist or an advanced practice nurse) may be indicated for some children and adolescents with Tourette syndrome to deal with maladaptive responses to the chronic condition. There is evidence that comprehensive behavior therapy is effective in reducing the tics (Kohler et al., 2024).

Medications

Although there is no cure for Tourette syndrome, medications can be prescribed to help control tics that interfere with daily activities. Two classes of drugs are commonly used in the treatment of tics: antipsychotics and alpha-adrenergic receptor agonists. Aripiprazole is replacing the use of older antipsychotics, such as haloperidol and pimozide (He et al., 2024). These potent dopamine blockers are often effective at low doses. Attempts to eradicate all tics by increasing the dosages of these antipsychotics almost certainly will result in diminishing therapeutic returns and additional side effects. The most frequently encountered side effects include drowsiness, dulled thinking, muscle stiffness, akathisia, increased appetite and weight gain, and acute dystonic reactions. Long-term use carries a small risk for tardive dyskinesia. Stimulant medications, such as methylphenidate and dextroamphetamine, can reduce symptoms of ADHD in individuals with Tourette syndrome without increasing tic severity (Farhat et al., 2023; NIH NINDS, 2024).

Psychoeducation

Teachers, guidance counselors, and school nurses may need current information about Tourette syndrome and its related issues. Discussions with school personnel often include issues such as how to deal with tic behaviors that are disruptive in the classroom, how to manage teasing from other children, and how to handle medication side effects. A careful discussion of the boundaries of Tourette syndrome and tic symptomatology can usually resolve these matters. Teachers who understand the involuntary nature of tics can often generate creative solutions, such as excusing the child to do errands. This strategy allows the child to step out of the classroom briefly to release a bout of tics, thereby reducing stress. In some situations, a brief presentation about Tourette syndrome to the class will reduce teasing and help both teachers and classmates tolerate the tic symptoms (Box 37.11).

Before initiating these interventions with the school personnel, it is essential to identify the child's needs and to pursue these strategies in collaboration with the family and other clinical team members. The Education for the Handicapped Act (Public Law 94–142) ensures that children with conditions such as Tourette syndrome are eligible for special education services even if they do not meet full criteria for having a learning disability. Thus, if evidence shows that Tourette disorder is hindering academic progress, parents can demand special education services for their child. Nurses can help families negotiate with the school to obtain appropriate services.

Evaluation of Patient Outcomes

Treatment outcomes will vary over the years and will be influenced by growth and development changes, family interaction and understanding of the disorder, and reduction or elimination of the frequency of the tics. Outcomes should include improvement of the child's quality of life and ability to learn to manage the symptoms of the disorder.

OTHER MENTAL DISORDERS

SEPARATION ANXIETY DISORDER

Separation anxiety is not unusual for very young children but typically declines between the ages of 3 and 5 years.

BOX 37.11

Therapeutic Dialogue: Tics and Disruptive Behaviors

INEFFECTIVE APPROACH

Teacher: I see the tics. He jerks his head, makes faces, and flicks his hands.

Nurse: What do you do about them?

Teacher: What can I do? If he isn't disrupting the class, I leave him alone. Even when he is throwing spitballs.

Nurse: Spitballs! He shouldn't be allowed to throw spitballs.

Teacher: Oh, I thought that was a part of his problem.

Nurse: Well, throwing spitballs has nothing to do with tics.

EFFECTIVE APPROACH

Teacher: I see the tics. He jerks his head, makes faces, and flicks his hands.

Nurse: He cannot help the tics that you are seeing. Tic disorders can exhibit a wide range of severity, from mild to severe and from simple to complex. Some complex tics may be difficult to distinguish from habits or rituals.

Teacher: What about things like throwing spitballs? When he does things like that, I try to ignore that behavior.

Nurse: Sounds like you give him the benefit of the doubt. (Validation) However, throwing a spitball is not a tic behavior.

Teacher: What should I do?

Nurse: How do you usually handle that type of behavior? (A modification of reflection)

Teacher: I'd ask him to stop and sometimes go into the hall.

Nurse: Disruptive behavior that is voluntary in a student with a tic disorder should be handled as you would handle any other child.

CRITICAL THINKING CHALLENGE

1. Compare the responses of the nurse in these scenarios. What made the difference in the teacher's responsiveness to the nurse?

When the child's fear and anxiety around separation become developmentally inappropriate, separation anxiety disorder is diagnosed. Separation anxiety disorder is the most common childhood anxiety disorder (Patel & Bryant, 2021). Although many children experience some discomfort on separation from their attachment figures, children with separation anxiety disorder suffer great worry or fear when faced with ordinary separations or being away from home, such as when going to school. When separation is about to occur, children often resist by crying or hiding from their parents. When asked, most children with separation anxiety disorder will express worry about harm to or permanent loss of their major attachment figure. Other children may express worry about their own safety. For a discussion of other anxiety disorders, see Chapter 27.

A common manifestation of anxiety is school phobia, in which the child refuses to attend school, preferring to stay at home with the primary attachment figure. The term school phobia was coined to distinguish it from truancy; whether it is a phobia in the usual sense is a matter of some debate. However, school phobia is a common comorbidity with other disorders such as general anxiety disorder, social phobia, OCD, depression, and conduct disorder. When a comorbid disorder such as depression is identified, it becomes the focus of treatment. In some cases, school phobia may resolve when the primary disorder is successfully treated (Tekin & Aydin, 2022).

Epidemiology and Etiology

Separation anxiety disorder is estimated at 1% to 6% of school-aged children, with symptoms usually emerging before age 10. Insecure attachment, difficult temperaments, and genetic factors contribute to the development of separation anxiety disorder. Anxiety disorders are often familial, so it appears that both environmental and genetic factors affect the risk for separation anxiety disorder. Risk factors for separation anxiety disorder include family history of anxiety disorders, loss or trauma to an attachment figure, life stresses (e.g., parental divorce), or changes in the child's environment (e.g., relocation to a new home or school) (Rapee et al., 2023).

Family Response to Disorder

There is no single family response to a child who is experiencing separation anxiety. Parenting style, life events, and environmental factors vary from family to family. The family dynamics related to the child's behavior have to be carefully assessed. In some instances, the family may be undergoing a separation of a significant family member through death, divorce, or military deployment. In other situations, the arrival of a new family member may precede the child's separation anxiety. A family assessment is important in determining the relationship of the child's fears and anxiety and the family dynamics.

Teamwork and Collaboration: Working Toward Recovery

An interdisciplinary approach is needed for the treatment of separation anxiety disorder. Effective treatment includes child and parent psychoeducation, school consultation, CBT, and if severe, selective serotonin reuptake inhibitors (SSRIs) (Giani et al., 2022; Tekin & Aydin, 2022).

EVIDENCE-BASED NURSING CARE FOR CHILDREN WITH SEPARATION ANXIETY DISORDER

School refusal is often what prompts the family to seek consultation for the child. Because school refusal can be a behavioral manifestation of several different child psychiatric disorders, it requires careful assessment. Issues to consider are whether the parents have been aware that the child is avoiding school (separation anxiety vs. truancy); what efforts the family has used to return the child to school; the presence of significant subjective distress in the child with anticipation of going to school; and whether the school refusal occurs in the context of other behavioral, social, or emotional issues. The nurse should also review the purpose and dose of current medications.

The child's developmental history and response to new situations and prior separations provide essential background information for understanding the child's current separation anxiety. The assessment should also include a review of recent life events and the methods the family has used to promote the child's return to school. Finally, the family history with respect to anxiety, panic attacks, or phobias is also informative.

Nursing priorities will depend on the role of the nurse (school nurse, acute care, or community practice) and the relationship with the child and family. In some instances, the nurse will be responsible for education of the child and family. If the child is receiving medication, nursing care related to administration of medications and education should be implemented. Nurses will also be involved in educating teachers and serving as a liaison between treating providers, family and child, and school.

OBSESSIVE-COMPULSIVE DISORDER

OCD is characterized by intrusive thoughts that are difficult to dislodge (i.e., obsessions) or ritualized behaviors that the child feels driven to perform (i.e., compulsions) (see Chapter 28). Children tend to exhibit both multiple obsessions and compulsions that relate to fear of catastrophic family event, contamination, sexual or somatic obsessions, and overly moralistic thoughts. Washing, checking, repeating, and ordering are the most commonly reported compulsions (Geller, 2022; Schuyler & Geller, 2023).

Epidemiology and Etiology

The prevalence rate of OCD is estimated at 1% to 2% with two peaks of incidence across the lifespan, one occurring in preadolescent children and later a peak in early adult life. More than half of the cases of OCD in youth involve a comorbid psychiatric disorder, with ADHD, conduct disorders, autism spectrum disorder, and Tourette syndrome being most frequent, particularly in males. The etiology of OCD in children is thought to be similar to that of adults (see Chapter 28). However, there is a subset of children whose OCD behavior may be related to an immune response to group A beta-hemolytic streptococcal infections that led to inflammation of the basal ganglia (Schuyler & Geller, 2023; Vreeland et al., 2023).

Family Response to Disorder

Pediatric OCD often impacts a child's entire family unit. Family plays an important role in the maintenance of OCD, and parents' responses to their child's obsessions and compulsions depend on their understanding of the thoughts and behaviors. Family accommodation—that is, when family members participate in the child's OCD-related symptoms and behaviors—is intended to be helpful but is ultimately counterproductive. For example, when a family member gives frequent reassurance, facilitates the child's rituals, assists with avoidance, and modifies routines around symptoms, they unintentionally reinforce reliance on the obsessive-compulsive behaviors and family help. Parents need education and support to help their child (Chessell et al., 2023; Schuyler & Geller, 2023).

Teamwork and Collaboration: Working Toward Recovery

Interdisciplinary treatment including school personnel is important for the child and family with OCD. SSRIs and CBT, including psychoeducation, cognitive training, exposure and response preventions, and relapse prevention, are the treatment of choice (Schuyler & Geller, 2023).

EVIDENCE-BASED NURSING CARE FOR CHILDREN WITH OCD

Recurrent worries and ritualistic behavior can occur in children at particular stages of development. The first step in the assessment of OCD in children is to

BOX 37.12

Clinical Judgment Vignette: Obsessive-Compulsive Disorder

Kim, an 11-year-old fifth grader, comes for evaluation because her mother and teacher have become increasingly concerned about her repetitive behaviors. In retrospect, Kim's mother recalls first noticing repetitive rituals about 2 years before, but she did not become alarmed about these behaviors until recently when they began to interfere with daily living. At the time of referral, Kim exhibits complicated jumping rituals that involve a specific number of jumps and a particular manner of jumping. She also turns light switches off and on and performs complex movements, such as blinking in patterns and thrusting her arms back and forth a certain number of times. Her mother also reports Kim's near-constant request for reassurance about her own safety. In recent months, her incessant demands for reassurance have been more frequent and elaborate. For example, Kim's mother has to answer three times that everything is all right and then say, "I swear to it."

At the evaluation, Kim expresses fears that some ill fate, such as catastrophic illness or injury, will befall her. This fear is triggered by contact with any individual who seems sick, chance exposures to foul smells or dirt, and minor scrapes or bumps. When the fear is triggered, she becomes increasingly anxious and consumed with the fear that she will develop an illness and die. Sometimes her fears are specific, such as cancer or AIDS. Other times her fears are more ambiguous, as evidenced by statements such as "Something bad will happen" if she doesn't complete the ritual. Kim acknowledges that the ritual is probably not related to the feared event, but she is reluctant to take a chance. If the ritual does not reduce her anxiety, she seeks reassurance from her mother.

Kim's medical history was negative for serious illness or injury. She was born after an uncomplicated pregnancy, labor, and delivery and achieved developmental milestones at appropriate times. Indeed, her mother could recall no unusual issues in the first few years of life except that Kim was typically anxious in unfamiliar situations. Kim's mother reports a prior history of panic attacks, but the family history is otherwise negative for anxiety disorders, including OCD.

Building Clinical Judgment

1. What assessment information would you want to elicit from Kim?
2. What additional information should be considered from Kim's mother about her history of panic attacks?
3. What nursing interventions should be considered if Kim were your patient?

distinguish between typical childhood rituals and worries and pathologic rituals and obsessional thoughts. Obsessional thoughts are recurrent, nagging, and bothersome. Although children may describe obsessions as occurring "out of the blue," external events may trigger obsessions. For example, a child may fear contamination whenever they are in contact with a certain individual or object. Likewise, compulsions waste time, cause distress, and interfere with daily life (Box 37.12).

The severity of the child's and family's response to OCD will determine the appropriate interventions. When the obsessions and compulsions emerge, these children or adolescents are in distress because of the disturbing and relentless nature of the symptoms.

The needs of the family and the developmental needs of the child or adolescent will guide nursing interventions. If medication is prescribed, it is important to emphasize safe management of medications. Because the antidepressants have a boxed warning regarding suicide risk in adolescents, the nurse must discuss with the parents and child the importance of monitoring moods and keeping regularly scheduled mental health appointments.

MOOD DISORDERS

Mood disorders in children and adolescents are a major public health concern. The prevalence of depression is estimated to be 21% (5 million) of the U.S. population. Rates of depressive episodes are higher in females (29.2%) as compared to males (11.5%). Nearly 55% of adolescents with depression report that they are not receiving treatment for their illness (NIMH, 2023). Lifetime prevalence of bipolar disorder among adolescents aged 13 to 18 years is estimated to be 2.9%, of which 2.6% have severe impairment. Bipolar disorder in adolescents is found to be higher in females (3.3%) than in males (2.6%) (NIMH, 2024b). (See Chapters 25 and 26 for a complete discussion of these disorders.)

Recognizing Cues: Relevant Assessment Information

Children with mood disorders may not spontaneously express feelings (e.g., sadness, irritability) and are more likely to show their suffering through their behavior. These children may act out their feelings rather than discuss them. Thus, behavior issues may accompany depression. Reports from parents are important sources of information about changes in sleep patterns, appetite, activity level and interests, and emotional stability.

Spirituality Assessment

For many people, religious practices and spirituality shape their values, belief systems and traditions, and provide a sense of meaning and belonging (Camino-Gaztambide et al., 2022). Religion and spirituality have distinct effects on both physical and mental health (Hochstetler & Hill, 2024). Spiritual well-being can be a protective factor against depression (Aggarwal et al., 2023). Spiritual health also has a role in suicide prevention in that it has been found to give meaning to life and create hope and motivation (Atoofi et al., 2024; van den Brink et al., 2023). Negative religious coping (e.g., religious guilt or feeling abandoned by or blaming God), however, has been associated with increased depressive symptoms (Aggarwal et al., 2023; Leavitt-Alcantara et al., 2023).

Taking Action: Nursing Interventions

Priorities of nursing care for children or adolescents who are depressed are similar to those for adults. Treatment goals include improving the mood and restoring sleep, appetite, and self-care. Interventions for responses to mood disorders in children and adolescents are also similar to those for adults. The psychiatric nurse develops a therapeutic relationship with the child and provides parent education and support. Developing sensitivity to the influence of environmental events on the child is important for the nurse, parents, and teachers (Box 37.13).

Medication Interventions

Children and adolescents may be treated with medication. Antidepressant medications are used for depression and mood antipsychotics for bipolar disorder. The controversy surrounding the use of SSRIs in children reminds us that all treatments involve a risk–benefit equation. Given the modest benefit of the SSRIs and the potential for side effects, these medications merit careful monitoring in children and adolescents. Patient monitoring should focus on evidence of benefit and side effects, including sleep issues, hyperactivity, sudden changes in mood or behavior, suicidal ideation, or self-injurious behavior.

> **BOX 37.13**
>
> **Questions, Choices, and Outcomes**
>
> Mrs. S has just returned with her son Jared to the child psychiatric inpatient services facility after an overnight pass. She reports that the visit did not go well because of Jared's anger and defiance. She remarked that this behavior was distressingly similar to his behavior before the hospitalization. She expressed additional concern because of the upcoming discharge from the hospital. After saying goodbye to Jared, she pulled the nurse aside and stated that she had decided to file for divorce.
>
> Mrs. S indicated that she had not told her husband or the family therapist. When asked whether Jared knew about her decision, Mrs. S suddenly realized that he may have overheard her discussing the matter with her sister on the telephone during this home visit.
>
> How should the nurse approach this situation?
>
> **CHOICE**
>
> **Possible Outcomes**
>
> Discuss her hypothesis about Jared's behavior and his uncertainty
>
> Mother can see relationship between Jared's behavior and her plan for divorce. Mother ignores the nurse. Mother is interested but does not see the connection.
>
> Ignore the statement
>
> Child and family did not learn about the connection between Jared's behavior and the events at home.
>
> Encourage Jared's mother to sort out her issues.
>
> The focus is then on mother's issues.
>
> **Analysis**
>
> The best response is focusing on the possible relationship between Jared's recent behavioral deterioration and his uncertainty about his family's future. If the nurse ignores the statement or focuses on the mother's interpretation of Jared's behavior, the mother is less likely to appreciate the connection between her pending divorce and Jared's behavior. The nurse should also emphasize the importance of discussing the matter in family therapy.

Spiritual Interventions

Nurses should keep in mind the role of religion and spirituality in their patients' lives. Integrating religious and spiritual practices—for example, forgiveness, gratitude, compassion, and acceptance—into a plan of care may be effective in adolescents with depression and anxiety. These practices may also contribute to the development of positive identity; provide opportunities for strength, support, and social connectedness; and facilitate positive coping mechanisms. Additionally, religious beliefs and spiritual practices can strengthen family bonds and serve as inspiration and comfort in times of difficulty, trauma, or loss (Aggarwal et al., 2023; Camino-Gaztambide et al., 2022).

CHILDHOOD SCHIZOPHRENIA

Childhood (early-onset) schizophrenia is diagnosed by the same criteria as those used in adults (see Chapter 24). Difficulty in diagnosing a psychiatric disorder in children has led to years of debate and controversy regarding whether childhood schizophrenia differs from the adult type or is merely an early manifestation of the same disorder. For many years, it was believed that autism represented the childhood form of schizophrenia. However, today autism and childhood schizophrenia are differentiated. As currently defined, childhood schizophrenia (onset before the age of 13 years) is very rare, but prevalence increases sharply during adolescence, especially in young males (Sunshine & McClellan, 2022).

Childhood schizophrenia is usually characterized by poorer premorbid functioning than late-onset schizophrenia. Common premorbid difficulties include social, cognitive, linguistic, attentional, motor, and perceptual delays. Taken together, these findings suggest that early-onset schizophrenia is a more severe form of the disorder.

Nursing care for children with schizophrenia follows an approach similar to that for ASD. Antipsychotic medications are not generally approved for use in children, although the newer atypical antipsychotic medications appear to have a lower risk for neurologic effects; other side effects such as weight gain also warrant careful monitoring.

Development of an individualized care plan for children with schizophrenia begins with a nursing assessment to identify functional issues specific to the child. Similarly, the recognition that childhood schizophrenia is a chronic and severe condition should guide the identification of outcomes. Goals should be realistic; the nurse should pay special attention to the child's support systems. Parent education about the disorder, medications, and long-term management (including use of community resources) is an essential part of the treatment plan. Long-term management also requires monitoring of chronic antipsychotic therapy.

ELIMINATION DISORDERS

ENURESIS

Enuresis is the involuntary excretion of urine after the age at which the child should have attained bladder control. It usually involves involuntary bedwetting at night, but repeated urination on clothing during waking hours can occur (diurnal enuresis). Enuresis is a self-limiting disorder, with most children experiencing a spontaneous remission.

Epidemiology and Etiology

The prevalence of nocturnal enuresis varies with age and sex assigned at birth, being most common in young male children—an estimated 20% of 5-year-old and 10% of 7-year-old children have nocturnal enuresis (AACAP, 2023). The frequency in female children is about half that of male children in each age group. The etiology of enuresis is unknown, with probably no single cause. Most children with nocturnal enuresis have no urologic anomalies. Causes of bedwetting might include the inability of the child's bladder to hold urine overnight, constipation that is placing pressure on the bladder, and deep sleep resulting in the inability of the child to wake up. Bedwetting may also be a result of stress and emotions. For example, a child may begin bedwetting following a significant life change such as moving to a new home, parental divorce, loss of a loved one, or trauma (AACAP, 2023).

EVIDENCE-BASED NURSING CARE OF CHILDREN WITH ENURESIS

Nursing assessment should include the child's developmental history, the onset and course of enuresis, prior treatment, presence of emotional issues, and medical history. Routine laboratory tests such as urinalysis and a urine culture are used to identify the presence of infection. The nurse should obtain baseline data regarding toileting habits, including daytime incontinence, urinary frequency, and constipation. They should refer children with persistent daytime enuresis for consultation with a urologist. The nurse should also explore the family's home environment, family attitudes about the child's enuresis, and the family's medical history. Parents should be educated that children rarely wet the bed intentionally, and that children generally feel ashamed. Parents should provide encouragement to their child.

In many cases, limiting fluid intake in the evening and treating constipation (if present) is sufficient to decrease the frequency of bedwetting. One of the most effective methods is the bell and pad. In this approach, the child sleeps on a pad that has wires on it, and when the child voids, a bell sounds, waking up the child. With use, the child either wakes up to urinate or learns to sleep through the night without voiding. A more temporary solution is the use of desmopressin (DDAVP), a synthetic antidiuretic hormone that actually inhibits production of urine. After medication is withdrawn, the enuresis frequently returns (Tsuji & Kaneko, 2023).

ENCOPRESIS

Encopresis involves soiling clothing with feces or depositing feces in inappropriate places. Additional diagnostic criteria include that the child is older than 4 years; that the soiling occurs at least once per month; and that the soiling is not the result of a medical disorder, such as congenital aganglionic megacolon (Hirschsprung disease). The most common form of encopresis is fecal impaction accompanied by leakage around the hardened mass of stool. Because of the loss of muscle tone in the lower bowel, the child loses the usual urge to defecate and may not feel the leakage. Surprisingly, the child may not detect the smell of the stool because the olfactory apparatus becomes accustomed to the odor. If left untreated, this issue generally resolves independently by middle adolescence. Nonetheless, the social consequences may be substantial (DeLeon et al., 2022).

Epidemiology and Etiology

As with enuresis, encopresis is more common in male children, and the frequency of the condition declines with age. The current estimate of prevalence is 1% to 4% of school-aged children, with a three to six times greater prevalence in male children. Approximately 20% to 30% of children with encopresis also have enuresis (DeLeon et al., 2022).

The reasons for withholding stool and starting the cycle of fecal impaction are unclear but are not usually the result of physical causes. However, as noted, when fecal impaction occurs, there is an accompanying loss of tone in the bowel and subsequent leakage.

EVIDENCE-BASED NURSING CARE OF CHILDREN WITH ENCOPRESIS

Assessment includes a detailed interview with the child and parent regarding the pattern of the encopresis. A calm matter-of-fact approach can help to reduce the child's embarrassment. Physical examination is also necessary; thus, collaboration with the child's primary care provider or consulting pediatric specialist is essential. Diagnosis of encopresis is presumed, given a history of intermittent constipation and soiling. Collaboration with primary care consultants is often helpful to rule out rare medical conditions, such as Hirschsprung disease. The presence of encopresis does not necessarily signal severe emotional or behavioral disturbances, but the nurse should inquire about other psychiatric disorders. Psychiatric comorbidities, including attention difficulties, anxiety, and behavioral issues may make encopresis more challenging to treat (Baroud et al., 2022).

Effective intervention begins with educating the parents and the child about expected bowel function and the self-perpetuating cycle of fecal impaction and leakage of stool around the hardened mass of feces. The short-term goal of this educational effort is to decrease the anger and recrimination that often complicate the picture in these families. Because encopresis often results in a loss of bowel tone, it may help to motivate children by emphasizing the need to strengthen their anal muscles.

In many cases, cleaning out the bowel is necessary before initiating behavioral treatment through administration of laxatives, rectal suppositories, or enemas. A high-fiber diet and behavior modification is often recommended.

The behavioral treatment program involves daily sitting on the toilet after each meal for a predetermined period (e.g., 10 minutes). The child and parents can measure the time with an ordinary kitchen timer. The parents can encourage the child to read or look at picture books while sitting. They can give the child rewards in the form of stars, stickers, or points for adhering to the retraining program and add bonuses for successful defecation. The family can tally stickers or points on a calendar, and the child can "cash in" collected points for small prizes.

Caring for children with encopresis on an inpatient unit is a challenge, because very little research provides direction for positive outcomes. Staff can become frustrated with the child's seemingly unwillingness to cooperate. Possible interventions include maintaining discretion, assisting children with the development of age-appropriate social skills and empathy, and small rewards for treatment adherence (Baroud et al., 2022).

SUMMARY OF KEY POINTS

- A one in six American youths is affected by a mental disorder that impairs their ability to function.
- In addressing intellectual developmental disorder, the emphasis is on determining adaptive behaviors (e.g., conceptual skills, concepts, self-direction), social skills, and practical skills. With guidance and education, many children will no longer have a disability as adults.
- Children with ASD benefit from structure and specific behavioral interventions.
- ADHD is defined by the presence of inattention; impulsiveness; and in most cases, hyperactivity. As currently defined, ADHD is the most common disorder of childhood. This heterogeneous disorder affects male children more often than female children. Nursing interventions involve family and child education and support. The family must partner with the school system to help the child receive the best educational experience. Effective treatment of ADHD often involves multiple approaches, including medication and parental education and support.
- Tourette syndrome is a tic disorder characterized by motor and vocal tics. It is a frustrating disorder that requires patience and understanding. About half of the children with this disorder also have ADHD.
- Separation anxiety is relatively common in school-aged children. OCD becomes more common in adolescents. Treatment of separation anxiety and OCD may include medication, behavioral therapy, or a combination of these treatments.
- Elimination disorders include encopresis and enuresis. Behavioral therapy approaches are the most effective treatment for these disorders. Medication may also be used.
- Major depression in children is believed to be similar to major depression in adults.
- Childhood schizophrenia is a rare disorder, so other diagnoses should be carefully considered. Nursing care is similar to care of children with ASD.

DEVELOPING CLINICAL JUDGMENT

1. What are some approaches to obtaining assessment data about a child with a mental disorder?
2. When interviewing parents of a child with an intellectual developmental disorder, what questions might you ask?
3. Examine the differences and similarities between ASD with and without intellectual and language impairment.
4. Compare and contrast nursing approaches for a child with ADHD with those used for a child with ASD. How are they different? How are they similar?
5. Learning disabilities and communication disorders are more common in children with psychiatric disorders than in the general population. How might a learning disability or a communication disorder complicate a psychiatric illness in a school-aged child?
6. How would you answer these questions from a parent: "What causes ADHD? Is it my fault"?

MOVIES, TV, OR STREAMING PROGRAMS

Tyson's Run: **2022.** This inspirational drama follows the story of Tyson, a 15-year-old male with autism spectrum disorder who faces significant challenges in his everyday life, particularly in the areas of social interaction. Tyson forms a friendship with a marathon runner and decides he wants to run in his first marathon. Through determination and support from his family and his new friend, he starts to overcome his fears and doubts. As he trains and becomes more confident, Tyson learns not only to run but also to confront his personal obstacles and discover his own potential.

The film explores themes of perseverance, acceptance, and the power of community, showing Tyson's journey of self-discovery and growth as he pushes past barriers and achieves success in ways he never imagined. Ultimately, it's a heartwarming story about finding strength within oneself and embracing differences.

Viewing Points:

1. How does Tyson's perseverance help him?
2. What characteristics indicate that Tyson is on the autism spectrum?
3. What traits might make Tyson's life more difficult?

Unfolding Patient Stories: Andrew Davis • Part 2

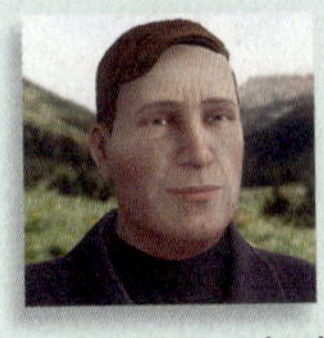

Recall from Chapter 31 **Andrew Davis**, who admitted himself to an alcohol rehabilitation facility. His alcohol misuse began in early adolescence. What factors can increase the risk for substance use disorder in an adolescent? What assessments can help the nurse identify the signs of alcohol use disorder? What assessment tools might the nurse use to ensure Andrew is safe during the withdrawal phase of his treatment? What are the implications to the family when a member has substance use disorder?

Care for Andrew Davis and other patients in a realistic virtual environment: ***vSim** for Nursing* (thepoint.lww.com/vSimMentalHealth). Practice documenting these patients' care in DocuCare (thepoint.lww.com/DocuCareEHR).

REFERENCES

Abín, A., Pasarín-Lavín, T., Areces, D., Rodríguez, C., & Núñez, J. C. (2024). The emotional impact of family involvement during homework in children with neurodevelopmental disorders: A systematic review. *Children, 11*(6), 713.

Aggarwal, S., Wright, J., Morgan, A., Patton, G., & Reavley, N. (2023). Religiosity and spirituality in the prevention and management of depression and anxiety in young people: A systematic review and meta-analysis. *BMC Psychiatry, 23*, 729.

American Academy of Child & Adolescent Psychiatry. (2023). *Bedwetting.* https://www.aacap.org/AACAP/Families_and_Youth/Facts_for_Families/FFF-Guide/Bedwetting-018.aspx

American Association on Intellectual and Developmental Disabilities. (2024). *Definition of intellectual disability.* https://www.aaidd.org/intellectual-disability/definition

American Psychiatric Association. (2022). *Diagnostic and statistical manual of mental disorders* (5th ed., text rev.). Author.

Arrondo, G., Osorio, A., Magallón, S., Lopez-del Burgo, C., & Cortese, S. (2023). Attention-deficit/hyperactivity disorder as a risk factor for being involved in intimate partner violence and sexual violence: A systematic review and meta-analysis. *Psychological Medicine, 53*(16), 7883–7892.

Assuah, F. B., Emanuel, B., Lacasse, B. M., Beggs, J., Lou, J., Motta, F. C., Nemzer, L. R., Worth, R., & Cravens, G. D. (2023). A literature review of similarities between and among patients with autism spectrum disorder and epilepsy. *Cureus, 15*(1), e33946.

Atoofi, M. K., Khodadadi, F. R., & Djalalinia, S. (2024). A comprehensive analysis of spiritual interventions in the prevention and management of student suicide: A three stage study. *International Journal of High Risk Behavior and Addiction, 13*(2), e143429.

Ayano, G., Abraha, M., Tsegay, L., & Gizachew, Y. (2024). Umbrella review of the global prevalence of conduct disorder in children and adolescents. *The Psychiatric Quarterly, 95*(1), 173–183.

Bai, D., Marrus, N., Yip, B. H. K., Reichenberg, A., Constantino, J. N., & Sandin, S. (2020). Inherited risk for autism through maternal and paternal lineage. *Biological Psychiatry, 88*(6), 480–487.

Baroud, E., Zar-Kessler, C., & Bender, S. (2022). A child psychiatry perspective on encopresis. *Journal of the American Academy of Child and Adolescent Psychiatry, 61*(7), 851–853.

Bozatlı, L., Aykutlu, H. C., Sivrikaya Giray, A., Ataş, T., Özkan, Ç., Güneydaş Yıldırım, B., & Görker, I. (2024). Children at risk of specific learning disorder: A study on prevalence and risk factors. *Children, 11*(7), 759.

Camino-Gaztambide, R. F., Fortuna, L. R., & Stuber, M. L. (2022). Religion and spirituality: Why and how to address it in clinical practice. *Child and Adolescent Psychiatric Clinics of North America, 31*, 615–630.

Carruthers, S., Mleczko, N., Page, S., Ahuja, S., Ellis, C., Howlin, P., Leadbitter, K., Taylor, L., Slonims, V., & Charman, T. (2023). Using implementation science frameworks to explore barriers and facilitators for parents' use of therapeutic strategies following a parent-mediated autism intervention. *Autism: The International Journal of Research and Practice, 27*(4), 1011–1025.

Caterfino, A., Krishna, S., & Chen, V. (2024). Novel and complementary treatment approaches in attention-deficit/hyperactivity disorder. *Current Opinion in Pediatrics, 36*(5), 562–569.

Centers for Disease Control and Prevention (CDC). (2024a). *Data and statistics on children's mental health.* https://www.cdc.gov/childrensmental-health/data.html

Centers for Disease Control and Prevention (CDC). (2024b). *About attention-deficit/hyperactivity disorder (ADHD).* https://www.cdc.gov/adhd/about/index.html

Centers for Disease Control and Prevention (CDC). (2024c). *About autism spectrum disorder.* https://www.cdc.gov/autism/about/index.html

Centers for Disease Control and Prevention (CDC). (2024d). *What is Tourette syndrome?* https://www.cdc.gov/ncbddd/tourette/facts.html

Centers for Disease Control and Prevention (CDC). (2024e). *Behavior or conduct problems in children.* https://www.cdc.gov/children-mental-health/about/about-behavior-or-conduct-problems-in-children.html#:~:text=A%20behavior%20disorder%20may%20be%20diagnosed%20when%20these,the%20needs%20of%20the%20specific%20child%20and%20family.

Chang, A. R., & Slopen, N. (2024). Racial and ethnic disparities for unmet needs by mental health condition: 2016 to 2021. *Pediatrics, 153*(1), 1–8.

Chatfield, S. (2023). The role of nutrition in ADHD. *Today's Dietician, 25*(3), 44–49.

Chepke, C., Brunner, E., & Cutler, A. J. (2024). Serotonergic drugs for the treatment of attention-deficit/hyperactivity disorder: A review of past development, pitfalls and failures, and a look to the future. *Psychopharmacology Bulletin, 54*(4), 45–80.

Chessell, C., Harvey, K., Halldorsson, B., Farrington, A., & Creswell, C. (2023). Parents' experiences of parenting a preadolescent child with OCD: A qualitative study. *Emotional & Behavioural Difficulties, 28*(1), 68–85.

Conners, C. K. (1997). *Conners' rating scales-revised: User's manual.* Multi-Health Systems, Inc.

Cortese, S. (2023). Evidence-based prescribing of medications for ADHD: Where are we in 2023? *Expert Opinion on Pharmacotherapy, 24*(4), 425–434.

DeLeon, J., Shrestha, M., Mahmood, Z., & Patel, D. R. (2022). Encopresis. *Journal of Alternative Medicine Research, 14*(3), 341–349.

Dentz, A., Soelch, C. M., Fahim, C., Torsello, A., Parent, V., Ponsioen, A., Guay, M. C., Bioulac-Rogier, S., Clément, C., Bader, M., & Romo, L. (2024). Non-pharmacological treatment of attention deficit disorder with or without hyperactivity (ADHD). Overview and report of the first international symposium on the non-pharmacological management of ADHD. *L'Encephale, 50*(3), 309–328.

Duff, D. M., Hendricks, A. E., Fitton, L., & Adlof, S. M. (2023). Reading and math achievement in children with dyslexia, developmental language disorder, or typical development: Achievement gaps persist from second through fourth grades. *Journal of Learning Disabilities, 56*(5), 371–391.

Farhat, L. C., Behling, E., Landeros-Weisenberger, A., Levine, J. L. S., Macul Ferreira de Barros, P., Wang, Z., & Bloch, M. H. (2023). Comparative efficacy, tolerability, and acceptability of pharmacological interventions for the treatment of children, adolescents, and young adults with Tourette's syndrome: A systematic review and network meta-analysis. *The Lancet. Child & Adolescent Health*, 7(2), 112–126.

Feingold, B. F. (1975). Hyperkinesis and learning disabilities linked to artificial food flavors and colors. *American Journal of Nursing, 75*(5), 797–803.

Geller, D. (2022). Obsessive-compulsive disorder. In M. K. Dulcan (Ed.), *Dulcan's textbook of child and adolescent psychiatry* (3rd ed.). American Psychiatric Publishing.

Gialluisi, A., Andlauer, T. F. M., Mirza-Schreiber, N., Moll, K., Becker, J., Hoffmann, P., Ludwig, K. U., Czamara, D., Pourcain, B. S., Honbolygó, F., Tóth, D., Csépe, V., Huguet, G., Chaix, Y., Iannuzzi, S., Demonet, J. F., Morris, A. P., Hulslander, J., Willcutt, E. G., ... Schulte-Körne, G. (2021). Genome-wide association study reveals new insights into the heritability and genetic correlates of developmental dyslexia. *Molecular Psychiatry, 26*(7), 3004–3017.

Giani, L., Caputi, M., Forresi, B., Michelini, G., & Scaini, S. (2022). Evaluation of cognitive-behavioral therapy efficacy in the treatment of separation anxiety disorder in childhood and adolescence: A systematic review of randomized controlled trials. *International Journal of Cognitive Therapy, 15*(1), 57–80.

Gordon, C. T., Nguyen, P. T., Mitchell, A. K., & Tyler, P. M. (2023). Profiles of childhood adversity and associated psychopathology in youth entering residential care. *Psychological Trauma: Theory, Research, Practice & Policy, 15*, S82–S91.

Goyette, C. H., Conners, C. K., & Ulrich, R. F. (1978). Normative data on the Conners parent and teachers rating scales. *Journal of Abnormal Child Psychology, 6*(2), 221–236.

Habdank-Kolaczkowski, J. S., Akahara, P. C., Ishola, F., Salawu, M. A., Augustine, S. W., Ezeamii, V. C., David, A. B., Okobi, E., & Okobi, O. E. (2023). Attention-deficit hyperactivity disorder among American youth: A comprehensive 20-year analysis of National Center for Health Statistics (NCHS) Data. *Cureus, 15*(11), e48781.

Hall, J. M., Chakrabarti, C., Mkuu, R., Thompson, L. A., Shenkman, E. A., & Theis, R. P. (2023). The association of socioeconomic vulnerability and race and ethnicity with disease burden among children in a statewide Medicaid population. *Academic Pediatrics, 23*(2), 372–380.

He, F., Luo, J., Huang, Y., Hao, Y., Sun, L., Ke, X., Wu, B., Chen, Y., Han, Y., Zhang, Y., Liu, J., Han, H., Xian, M., Uki, M., & Zheng, Y. (2024). Randomized, double-blind, placebo-controlled trial of aripiprazole oral solution in children and adolescents with Tourette's disorder. *Child & Adolescent Psychiatry & Mental Health, 18*(1), 1–10.

Hochstetler, E., & Hill, H. (2024). Mobilizing meaning: Religion and spirituality among future generations. *Child and Adolescent Psychiatric Clinics of North America, 33*, 411–421.

Hussain, K., & Soares, N. (2022). Dyscalculia. *International Journal of Child Health & Human Development, 15*(3), 249–262.

Iffland, M., Livingstone, N., Jorgensen, M., Hazell, P., & Gillies, D. (2023). Pharmacological intervention for irritability, aggression, and self-injury in autism spectrum disorder (ASD). *The Cochrane Database of Systematic Reviews, 10*(10), CD011769.

Ilori, E. O., Eziechi, N. M., Erechukwu, C., Obijiofor, N. B., Agazie, O., Obitulata-Ugwu, V. O., Okobi, O. E., Aderemi, L., Salawu, M. A., Ewuzie, Z. D., Anamazobi, E. G., & Alozie, A. S. (2024). Analyzing trends in mental and behavioral health support for children: A comprehensive study using national survey of children's health database. *Cureus, 16*(5), e59499.

Jandac, T., & Stastna, L. (2024). The prevalence of dual diagnoses in children and adolescents with substance use disorders, systematic review. *Journal of Substance Use, 29*(3), 393–398.

Jendreizik, L. T., von Wirth, E., & Döpfner, M. (2023). Familial factors associated with symptom severity in children and adolescents with ADHD: A meta-analysis and supplemental review. *Journal of Attention Disorders, 27*(2), 124–144.

Kanner, L. (1943). Autistic disturbances of affective contact. *Nervous Child, 2*, 217–250.

Kaye, A. D., Allen, K. E., Smith Iii, V. S., Tong, V. T., Mire, V. E., Nguyen, H., Lee, Z., Kouri, M., Jean Baptiste, C., Mosieri, C. N., Kaye, A. M., Varrassi, G., & Shekoohi, S. (2024). Emerging treatments and therapies for autism spectrum disorder: A narrative review. *Cureus, 16*(7), e63671.

Khazdouz, M., Safarzadeh, R., Hejrani, B., Hasani, M., Mahdavi, F. S., Ejtahed, H. S., & Qorbani, M. (2024). The association between junk foods consumption and attention deficit hyperactivity disorder in children and adolescents: A systematic review and meta-analysis of observational studies. *European Child & Adolescent Psychiatry, 34*(3), 825–834. https://doi.org/10.1007/s00787-024-02521-8

Kleppesto, T. H., Eilertsen, E. M., van Bergen, E., Sunde, H. F., Zietsch, B., Nordmo, M., Eftedal, N. H., Havdahl, A., Ystrom, E., & Torvik, F. A. (2024). Intergenerational transmission of ADHD behaviors: Genetic and environmental pathways. *Psychological Medicine, 54*(7), 1309–1317.

Kohler, K., Rosen, N., & Piacentini, J. (2024). Description, implementation, and efficacy of the comprehensive behavioral intervention for tics as first-line treatment for Tourette and other tic disorders. *Journal of Child and Adolescent Psychopharmacology, 35*(3), 126-134. https://doi.org/10.1089/cap.2024.0023

Lange, K. W., Lange, K. M., Nakamura, Y., & Reissmann, A. (2023). Nutrition in the management of ADHD: A review of recent research. *Current Nutrition Reports, 12*(3), 383–394.

Larsson, I., Aili, K., Lönn, M., Svedberg, P., Nygren, J. M., Ivarsson, A., & Johansson, P. (2023). Sleep interventions for children with attention deficit hyperactivity disorder (ADHD): A systematic literature review. *Sleep Medicine, 102*, 64–75.

Leavitt-Alcantara, S., Betz, J., Almeida, D. M., Ferrara, B., Xu, Y., Diop, E., Hamilton, O., Young, C., & Ragsdale, J. R. (2023). Religiosity and religious and spiritual struggle and their association to depression and anxiety among adolescents admitted to inpatient psychiatric units. *Journal of Health Care Chaplaincy, 29*(1), 1–13.

Lee, V., Watson, S., Shlonksy, A., & Tarren-Sweeney, M. (2024). A scoping review of randomized controlled trials of parenting and family-based interventions for 10- 17 year olds with severe and persistent conduct problems. *Journal of Evidence-Based Social Work, 21*(6), 720–748.

Li, D., Zhang, X., & Zhang, L. (2023). What skills could distinguish developmental dyscalculia and typically developing children: Evidence from a 2-year longitudinal screening. *Journal of Learning Disabilities, 56*(4), 257–277.

Liang, S. C., Sun, C. K., Fan, H. Y., Chung, W., Tzang, R. F., Hung, K. C., Chiu, H. J., Cheng, Y. S., & Yeh, P. Y. (2022). Therapeutic effects of antidepressants for global improvement and subdomain symptoms of autism spectrum disorder: a systematic review and meta-analysis. *Journal of Psychiatry & Neuroscience : JPN, 47*(4), E299–E310.

Lillvis, D. F., Harmon, B., Osei, H., Ribeiro, S., Zrik, A., Janjua, V., Assioun, J., Aronoff, N., & Kuo, D. Z. (2024). Accidental physical trauma in children and youth with special health care needs: A scoping review. *Academic Pediatrics, 25*(2), 102590.

Lin, H., Haider, S. P., Kaltenhauser, S., Mozayan, A., Malhotra, A., Constable, R. T., Scheinost, D., Ment, L. R., Konrad, K., & Payabvash, S. (2023). Population level multimodal neuroimaging correlates of attention-deficit hyperactivity disorder among children. *Frontiers in Neuroscience, 17*, 1138670.

Linden, A., Best, L., Elise, F., Roberts, D., Branagan, A., Tay, Y. B. E., Crane, L., Cusack, J., Davidson, B., Davidson, I., Hearst, C., Mandy, W., Rai, D., Smith, E., & Gurusamy, K. (2023). Benefits and harms of interventions to improve anxiety, depression, and other mental health outcomes for autistic people: A systematic review and network meta-analysis of randomised controlled trials. *Autism: The International Journal of Research & Practice, 27*(1), 7–30.

Liu, T. H., Wu, J. Y., Huang, P. Y., Lai, C. C., Chang, J. P. C., Lin, C. H., & Su, K. P. (2023). Omega-3 polyunsaturated fatty acids for core symptoms of attention-deficit/hyperactivity disorder: A meta-analysis of randomized controlled trials. *The Journal of Clinical Psychiatry, 84*(5), 22r14772.

López-Martín, S., Albert, J., Calleja-Pérez, B., Fernández-Mayoralas, D. M., Fernández-Perrone, A. L., Jiménez De Domingo, A., & Fernández-Jaén, A. (2024). Genetics of ADHD in clinical practice. *Medicina, 84*(Suppl 1), 26–30.

Maenner, M. J., Warren, Z., Robinson Williams, A., Amoakohene, E., Bakian, A. V., Bilder, D. A., Durkin, M. S., Fitzgerald, R. T., Furnier, S. M., Hughes, M. M., Ladd-Acosta, C. M., McArthur, D., Pas, E. T., Salinas, A., Vehorn, A., Williams, S., Esler, A., Grzybowski, A., Hall-Lande, J., & Nguyen, R. H. N. (2023). Prevalence and characteristics of autism spectrum disorder among children aged 8 years—Autism and developmental disabilities monitoring network, 11 sites, United States, 2020. *MMWR Surveillance Summaries, 72*(1/2), 1–14.

Maneeton, P., Maneeton, B., Winichaikul, Y., Kawilapat, S., Kienngam, N., & Maneeton, N. (2024). Updated systematic review and meta-analysis of randomized controlled trials: Antidepressants for restricted and repetitive behaviors in autism spectrum disorder. *Neuropsychiatric Disease and Treatment, 20*, 1711–1723.

Martins, P. L. B., Torquato, G. C. P., Dias, G. A. P. F., Leite, I. B., Gaspar, T. M., Pinto, J. P., & Macedo, D. S. (2024). Effectiveness of pharmacological interventions for managing ADHD symptoms in individuals with autism

spectrum disorder: A systematic review and meta-analysis. *Progress in Neuro-Psychopharmacology & Biological Psychiatry, 134*, 111089.
Molina, B. S. G., Kennedy, T. M., Howard, A. L., Swanson, J. M., Arnold, L. E., Mitchell, J. T., Stehli, A., Kennedy, E. H., Epstein, J. N., Hechtman, L. T., Hinshaw, S. P., & Vitiello, B. (2023). Association between stimulant treatment and substance use through adolescence into early adulthood. *JAMA Psychiatry, 80*(9), 933–941.
Morgan, T. C., & O'Keefe, L. C. (2022). Does a behavioral parent training program for parents of ADHD children improve outcomes? A pilot project. *Comprehensive Child & Adolescent Nursing, 45*(3), 264–274.
National Alliance on Mental Illness (NAMI). (2024). *Mental health conditions*. https://www.nami.org/about-mental-illness/mental-health-conditions/
National Institutes of Health, National Center for Complementary and Integrative Health (NCCIH NIH). (2023). *ADHD and complementary health approaches: What the science says*. https://www.nccih.nih.gov/health/providers/digest/adhd-and-complementary-health-approaches-science#meditation-therapies-and-yoga
National Institute of Health, National Institute of Neurologic Disorders and Stroke (NIH NINDS). (2024). *Tourette syndrome*. https://www.ninds.nih.gov/health-information/disorders/tourette-syndrome
National Institute of Health, National Institute on Deafness and Other Communication Disorders (NIH, NIDOCD). (2023). *Developmental language disorder*. https://www.nidcd.nih.gov/health/developmental-language-disorder
National Institute of Mental Health (NIMH). (2023). *Major depression*. https://www.nimh.nih.gov/health/statistics/major-depression.shtml#part_155031
National Institute of Mental Health (NIMH). (2024a). *Attention-deficit/hyperactivity disorder*. https://www.nimh.nih.gov/health/topics/attention-deficit-hyperactivity-disorder-adhd#part_2288
National Institute of Mental Health (NIMH). (2024b). *Bipolar disorder*. https://www.nimh.nih.gov/health/statistics/bipolar-disorder
Nuntavisit, L., & Porter, M. (2022). Mediating effects of discipline approaches on the relationship between parental mental health and adolescent antisocial behaviours: Retrospective study of a multisystemic therapy intervention. *International Journal of Environmental Research and Public Health, 19*(20), 13418.
Nuske, H. J., Young, A. V., Khan, F. Y., Palermo, E. H., Ajanaku, B., Pellecchia, M., Vivanti, G., Mazefsky, C. A., Brookman-Frazee, L., McPartland, J. C., Goodwin, M. S., & Mandell, D. S. (2024). Systematic review: emotion dysregulation and challenging behavior interventions for children and adolescents on the autism spectrum with graded key evidence-based strategy recommendations. *European Child & Adolescent Psychiatry, 33*(6), 1963–1976.
Olusanya, B. O., Smythe, T., Ogbo, F. A., Nair, M. K. C., Scher, M., & Davis, A. C. (2023). Global prevalence of developmental disabilities in children and adolescents: A systematic umbrella review. *Frontiers in Public Health, 11*, 1122009.
Patel, A. K., & Bryant, B. (2021). Separation anxiety disorder. *JAMA, 326*(18), 1880.
Peterson, B. S., Trampush, J., Maglione, M., Bolshakova, M., Rozelle, M., Miles, J., Pakdaman, S., Brown, M., Yagyu, S., Motala, A., & Hempel, S. (2024). Treatments for ADHD in children and adolescents: A systematic review. *Pediatrics, 153*(4), 1–11.
Pinals, D. A., Hovermale, L., Mauch, D., & Anacker, L. (2022). Persons with intellectual and developmental disabilities in the mental health system: Part 1. Clinical considerations. *Psychiatric Services (Washington, D.C.), 73*(3), 313–320.
Pinto, S., Correia-de-Sá, T., Sampaio-Maia, B., Vasconcelos, C., Moreira, P., & Ferreira-Gomes, J. (2022). Eating patterns and dietary interventions in ADHD: A narrative review. *Nutrients, 14*(20), 4332.
Plowden, K. O., Legg, T., & Wiley, D. (2022). Attention deficit/hyperactivity disorder in adults: A case study. *Archives of Psychiatric Nursing, 38*, 29–35.
Popit, S., Serod, K., Locatelli, I., & Stuhec, M. (2024). Prevalence of attention-deficit hyperactivity disorder (ADHD): Systematic review and meta-analysis. *European Psychiatry : The Journal of the Association of European Psychiatrists, 67*(1), e68.
Predescu, E., Vaidean, T., Rapciuc, A. M., & Sipos, R. (2024). Metabolomic markers in attention-deficit/hyperactivity disorder (ADHD) among children and adolescents: A systematic review. *International Journal of Molecular Sciences, 25*(8), 4385.
Rapee, R. M., Creswell, C., Kendall, P. C., Pine, D. S., & Waters, A. M. (2023). Anxiety disorders in children and adolescents: A summary and overview of the literature. *Behaviour Research and Therapy, 168*, 104376.
Rios-Davis, A., Sibley, M. H., Delgado, A., & Zulauf-McCurdy, C. (2023). Identifying common and unique elements of evidence-based treatments for adolescent ADHD. *Journal of Child & Family Studies, 32*(2), 466–480.
Russell, D., & Arnold, L. E. (2023). Complementary and integrative treatments for attention-deficit/hyperactivity disorder in youth. *Child and Adolescent Psychiatric Clinics of North America, 32*(2), 173–192.
Sadozai, A. K., Sun, C., Demetriou, E. A., Lampit, A., Munro, M., Perry, N., Boulton, K. A., & Guastella, A. J. (2024). Executive function in children with neurodevelopmental conditions: A systematic review and meta-analysis. *Nature Human Behaviour, 8*, 2357–2366. https://doi.org/10.1038/s41562-024-02000-9
Salazar de Pablo, G., Pastor Jordá, C., Vaquerizo-Serrano, J., Moreno, C., Cabras, A., Arango, C., Hernández, P., Veenstra-VanderWeele, J., Simonoff, E., Fusar-Poli, P., Santosh, P., Cortese, S., & Parellada, M. (2023). Systematic review and meta-analysis: Efficacy of pharmacological interventions for irritability and emotional dysregulation in autism spectrum disorder and predictors of response. *Journal of the American Academy of Child and Adolescent Psychiatry, 62*(2), 151–168.
Schuyler, M., & Geller, D. (2023). Childhood obsessive-compulsive disorder. *Psychiatric Clinics of North America, 46*(1), 89–106.
Sears, C. G., Lanphear, C. P., Xu, Y., Chen, A., Yolton, K., & Braun, J. M. (2022). Identifying periods of heightened susceptibility to lead exposure in relation to behavioral problems. *Journal of Exposure Science & Environmental Epidemiology, 32*(1), 1–9. https://doi.org/10.1038/s41370-021-00389-3.
Sesso, G., Brancati, G. E., & Masi, G. (2023). Comorbidities in youth with bipolar disorder: Clinical features and pharmacological management. *Current Neuropharmacology, 21*(4), 911–934.
Shaffer, R. C., Reisinger, D. L., Schmitt, L. M., Lamy, M., Dominick, K. C., Smith, E. G., Coffman, M. C., & Esbensen, A. J. (2023). Systematic review: Emotion dysregulation in syndromic causes of intellectual and developmental disabilities. *Journal of the American Academy of Child & Adolescent Psychiatry, 62*(5), 518–557.
Shroff, D. M., Dunn, N. C., Green, C. D., Breaux, R., Becker, S. P., & Langberg, J. M. (2024). Predictors of executive function trajectories in adolescents with and without ADHD: Links with academic outcomes. *Development and Psychopathology, 36*(3), 1489–1502.
Spencer, A. E., Oblath, R., Sheldrick, R. C., Ng, L. C., Silverstein, M., & Garg, A. (2022). Social determinants of health and ADHD symptoms in preschool-age children. *Journal of Attention Disorders, 26*(3), 447–455.
Sunshine, A., & McClellan, J. M. (2022). Early-onset schizophrenia. In M. K. Dulcan (Ed.), *Dulcan's textbook of child and adolescent psychiatry* (3rd ed.). American Psychiatric Publishing.
Talantseva, O. I., Romanova, R. S., Shurdova, E. M., Dolgorukova, T. A., Sologub, P. S., Titova, O. S., Kleeva, D. F., & Grigorenko, E. L. (2023). The global prevalence of autism spectrum disorder: A three-level meta-analysis. *Frontiers in Psychiatry, 14*, 1071181.
Tamayo, N., Wareham, H., Franken, M. C., McKean, C., Tiemeier, H., & Jansen, P. W. (2024). Bidirectional associations between mental health problems and language ability across 8 years of childhood. *European Child & Adolescent Psychiatry, 33*(3), 787–797.
Tartaglione, A. M., Camoni, L., Calamandrei, G., Chiarotti, F., & Venerosi, A. (2024). The contribution of environmental pollutants to the risk of autism and other neurodevelopmental disorders: A systematic review of case-control studies. *Neuroscience and Biobehavioral Reviews, 164*, 105815.
Tekin, I., & Aydin, S. (2022). School refusal and anxiety among children and adolescents: A systematic scoping review. *New Directions for Child and Adolescent Development, 185–186*, 43–65.
Tesli, N., Jaholkowski, P., Haukvik, U. K., Jangmo, A., Haram, M., Rokicki, J., Friestad, C., Tielbeek, J. J., Næss, Ø., Skardhamar, T., Gustavson, K., Ask, H., Fazel, S., Tesli, M., & Andreassen, O. A. (2024). Conduct disorder: A comprehensive exploration of comorbidity patterns, genetic and environmental risk factors. *Psychiatry Research, 331*, 115628.
Todzia-Kornaś, A., Szczegielniak, A., & Gondek, T. M. (2024). Suicidality and nonsuicidal self-injury in females diagnosed with attention-deficit hyperactivity disorder: A narrative review. *Current Opinion in Psychiatry, 37*(1), 38–42.
Totsika, V., Liew, A., Absoud, M., Adnams, C., & Emerson, E. (2022). Mental health problems in children with intellectual disability. The Lancet. *Child & Adolescent Health, 6*(6), 432–444.
Trivedi, C., Nandakumar, A. L., Yousefzadehfard, Y., Goriparthi, T. S. K., Chaudhari, G., Vora, D., Mansuri, Z., & Jain, S. (2023). Suicide risk among adolescents with ADHD: An overview from the National Inpatient Sample Data Set. *The Journal of Nervous and Mental Disease, 211*(3), 216–220.
Tsuji, S., & Kaneko, K. (2023). Management of treatment-resistant nocturnal enuresis. *Pediatrics International: Official Journal of the Japan Pediatric Society, 65*(1), e15573.
Van den Brink, B., Roodnat, R., Rippe, R. C. A., Cherniak, A. D., van Lieshout, K., Helder, S. G., Braam, A. W., & Schaap-Jonker, S. (2024). Religiosity, spirituality, meaning-making, and suicidality in psychiatric

patients and suicide attempters: A systematic review and meta-analysis. *Harvard Review of Psychiatry, 32*(6), 195–206.

van Wijngaarden, V., de Wilde, H., Mink van der Molen, D., Petter, J., Stegeman, I., Gerrits, E., Smit, A. L., & van den Boogaard, M. J. (2024). Genetic outcomes in children with developmental language disorder: a systematic review. *Frontiers in Pediatrics, 12*, 1315229.

Vreeland, A., Thienemann, M., Cunningham, M., Muscal, E., Pittenger, C., & Frankovich, J. (2023). Neuroinflammation in obsessive-compulsive disorder: Sydenham chorea, pediatric autoimmune neuropsychiatric disorders associated with streptococcal infections, and pediatric acute onset neuropsychiatric syndrome. *The Psychiatric Clinics of North America, 46*(1), 69–88.

Yenkoyan, K., Mkhitaryan, M., & Bjørklund, G. (2024). Environmental risk factors in autism spectrum disorder: A narrative review. *Current Medicinal Chemistry, 31*(17), 2345–2360.

Zhu, Y., Wang, N. N., Pan, D., & Wang, S. (2024). Risk of overweight and obesity in children and adolescents with attention-deficit/hyperactivity disorder: A systematic review and meta-analysis. *Childhood Obesity (Print), 20*(2), 119–127.

Zuvekas, S. H., Grosse, H. D., Lavelle, T. A., Maenner, M. J., Dietz, P., & Ji, X. (2023). Healthcare costs of pediatric autism spectrum disorder in the United States, 2003–2015. *Journal of Autism and Developmental Disorders, 51*(8), 2950–2958.

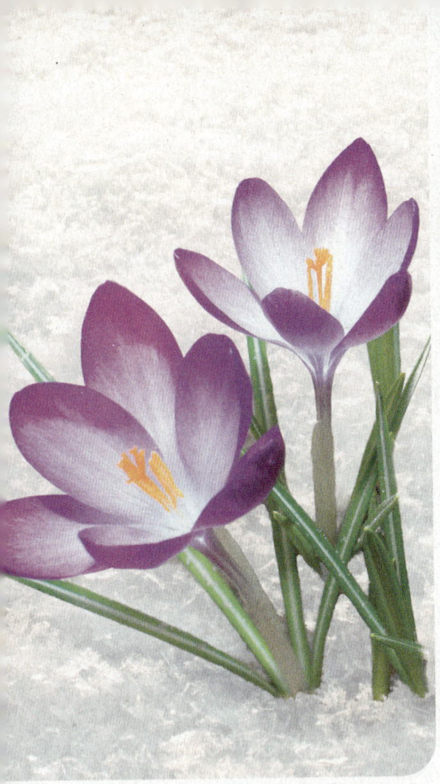

UNIT VIII
Care of Older Adults

38 Mental Health Assessment of Older Adults

Mary Ann Boyd and Rebecca Luebbert

KEYCONCEPTS

- psychiatric–mental health nursing assessment for the older adult
- typical aging

LEARNING OBJECTIVES

After studying this chapter, you will be able to:

1. Compare changes in typical aging with those associated with mental health issues in older adults.
2. Select various techniques in assessing older adults who have mental health issues.
3. Delineate important areas of assessment in the geropsychiatric nursing assessment, including evaluation of social determinants of health.

KEY TERMS

• dysphagia • financial exploitation • functional activities • instrumental activities of daily living • polypharmacy • xerostomia

INTRODUCTION

The average life span in the United States has increased from 47 years in 1900 to 79.9 years in 2021 (Arias et al., 2024). Health care providers have been facing increased challenges as the Baby Boomers (those born between 1946 and 1964) have moved into the ranks of the older adult population. Over the next 30 years, the number of adults over the age of 65 is expected to increase from 48 million to 88 million, with life expectancy increasing by 8 years (Davies, 2023).

KEYCONCEPT Typical aging is associated with some physical decline, such as decreased sensory abilities and decreased pulmonary and immune function, but many important functions do not change.

Intellectual function, capacity for change, and productive engagement with life remain stable with typical aging. Many myths exist about aging. Some people believe that "senility" is usual or that depression or hopelessness is natural for older adults. Ageist views, or discriminatory attitudes or beliefs based on a person's age, include that older adults are disabled, sick, frail, and tired. Individuals may be less likely to adopt healthy lifestyle habits and pursue needed medical treatment if their symptoms are believed to be natural processes of aging (Coelho-Junior et al., 2024). For example, a person with depressive symptoms might be experiencing early manifestations of dementia; however, this potential diagnosis may be overlooked if the individual or family members believe that the depressive symptoms are simply typical factors of aging (Elefante et al., 2023).

The most common mental health issues in older people are depression, anxiety disorders, and dementia which commonly occur with somatic conditions (Liu et al., 2023; Yang et al., 2022). Older adults with mental health issues comprise different population groups. One group consists of those with long-term mental illnesses who have reached the ranks of the older adult population. These individuals usually understand their disorders and treatments. Unfortunately, the changes associated with aging can affect a person's control of their chronic mental illness. Symptoms may reappear, and medications may need to be adjusted. Another group comprises individuals who are relatively free of mental health issues until their older adult years. These individuals, who may already have other health issues, develop late-onset mental disorders, such as depression, schizophrenia, or dementia. For these individuals and their family members, the development of a mental disorder can be very traumatic.

Mental health issues in older adults can be especially complex because of coexisting medical issues and treatments. Many symptoms of somatic disorders mimic or mask psychiatric disorders. For example, fatigue may be related to anemia, but it also may be symptomatic of depression. In addition, older people are more likely to report somatic symptoms, such as pain, gastrointestinal (GI) distress, or difficulty sleeping, rather than psychological ones, making identification of a mental disorder even more difficult (Davies, 2023).

The purpose of this chapter is to present a comprehensive geropsychiatric–mental health nursing assessment process that serves as the basis of care for older adults. A mental health assessment is necessary when psychiatric or mental health concerns are identified or when patients with mental illnesses reach their later years (usually about age 65 years). The assessment generally follows the same format as described in Chapter 10. However, the overall health care issues for older adults can be very complex, so it follows that certain components of the geropsychiatric nursing assessment are unique. Thus, the geriatric assessment emphasizes some areas that are less critical to the standard adult assessment.

TECHNIQUES FOR DATA COLLECTION

The nurse assesses the patient using an interview format that may take a few sessions to complete. Assessment may also include self-report standardized tests, such as depression and cognitive functioning tools. A wide variety of physiologic disorders may cause changes in mental status for older adults; thus, results of laboratory tests often are significant. For example, urinalysis can detect a urinary tract infection that has affected a patient's cognitive status. Box 38.1 contains a representative listing of common physiologic causes of changes in mental status. In addition, medical records from other health care providers are useful in developing a complete picture of the patient's health status.

BOX 38.1

Changes That Affect Mental Status in Older Adults

- Acid–base imbalance
- Dehydration
- Drugs (prescribed and OTC)
- Electrolyte changes
- Hypothyroidism
- Hypothermia and hyperthermia
- Hypoxia
- Infection and sepsis

An important source of patient data is family members, who often notice changes that the patient overlooks or fails to recognize. A patient with memory impairment may be unable to give an accurate history. By interviewing family members, the nurse expands the scope of the patient assessment. Moreover, the nurse has an opportunity to evaluate the caregivers themselves to determine whether they can care for the patient adequately and how they are coping with the situation. For example, a person may be unable to care for their partner but is unwilling to admit it. If the nurse can establish rapport with the person, the assessment interview may be used as an opportunity to help them examine their partner's care requirements realistically.

PSYCHIATRIC–MENTAL HEALTH NURSING ASSESSMENT OF THE OLDER ADULT

KEYCONCEPT A psychiatric–mental health nursing assessment for the older adult is the comprehensive, deliberate, and systematic collection and interpretation of data based on the special needs and concerns of the older adult. The purpose is to determine the current and past health, functional status, and human responses to mental health issues, both actual and potential (Box 38.2). As a person's lifespan increases, the likelihood of exposure to various levels of trauma also increases. Approximately 70% to 90% of adults 65 years and older have experienced at least one traumatic event in their lifetime. Using a trauma-informed approach creates a safe space for a more comprehensive nursing assessment. The nurse should recognize the cumulative effects of trauma as underlying factors in the development and severity of mental health issues (Davies, 2023).

At the beginning of the assessment, the nurse should determine the patient's ability to participate. A key component in a successful interview with an older adult is the formation of an atmosphere of respect for the person. Use of childlike language with the older adult signifies an ageist attitude and often results in poor communication. For example, if a patient is using a wheelchair, they may

BOX 38.2

Psychiatric–Mental Health Nursing Assessment for the Older Adult

I. Major reason for seeking help ____________

II. Initial information

Name ____________

Age ____________ Current marital status ____________

Gender ____________ Caregiver's name ____________

Living arrangements ____________

III. Level of independence:

High (needs no help) ____________

Moderate (lives independently, but needs some help with instrumental activities) ____________

Low (relies on others for help in meeting functional and instrumental activities) ____________

Physical limitations ____________

Level of education completed ____________

	As Expected	Treated	Untreated
Physical functions: system review	☐	☐	☐
Activity/exercise	☐	☐	☐
Sleep patterns	☐	☐	☐
Appetite and nutrition	☐	☐	☐
Hydration	☐	☐	☐
Sexuality	☐	☐	☐
Existing physical illnesses	☐	☐	☐

List any chronic illnesses ____________

Presence of pain (use standardized instrument if pain is present.) No ____________ Yes ____________

Score ____________ Treatment of pain ____________

IV. Responses to mental health issues

Major concerns regarding mental health issue

Major loss/change in past year: No ______ Yes ______

Fear of violence: No ____________ Yes ____________

Strategies for managing issues/disorder ____________

V. Mental status examination

General observation (appearance, psychomotor activity, attitude) ____________

Orientation (time, place, person) ____________

Mood, affect, emotions (GDS should be used if evidence of depression) Speech (verbal ability, speed, use of words correctly)

Thought processes (hallucinations, delusions, tangential, logic, repetition, rhyming of words, loose connections, disorganized) *(Describe the content of hallucinations, delusions.)*

Cognition and intellectual performance *(Use standardized test scores as well as observations.)*

Attention and concentration ____________

Abstract reasoning and concentration ____________

Memory (recall, short-term, long-term) ____________

Judgment and insight ____________

VI. Significant behaviors (psychomotor, agitation, aggression, withdrawn) *(use standardized test if behaviors are problematic.)*

When did problem behavior begin? Has it gotten worse?

VII. Self-concept (beliefs about self-body image, self-esteem, personal identity) ____________

VIII. Risk assessment

Suicide: High ____________ Low ____________

Assault/homicide: High ____________ Low ____________

Suicide thoughts or ideation: No ______ Yes ______

Current thoughts or harming self ____________

Plan ____________

Means ____________

Means available

Assault/homicide thoughts: No ______ Yes ______

What do you do when angry with a stranger? ____________

What do you do when angry with family or partner? ____________

Have you ever hit or pushed anyone? No ___ Yes ___

Have you ever been arrested for assault? No ___ Yes ___

Current thoughts of harming others ____________

IX. Functional status (*use standardized test such as FAQ*) ____________

X. Cultural assessment

Cultural group ____________

Cultural group's view of health and mental illness ____________

By what cultural rules do you try to live? ____________

Special, cultural foods that are important to you ____________

XI. Stresses and coping behaviors

Social support ____________

Family members ____________

Which members are important to you? ____________

On whom can you rely? ____________

Community resources ____________

XII. Spiritual assessment ____________

XIII. Economic status ____________

XIV. Legal status ____________

XV. Quality of life ____________

XVI. Summary of significant data that can be used in formulating clinical judgment.

SIGNATURE/TITLE ____________ Date ____________

have physical limitations that prevent full participation in the assessment. However, physical limitations should not be assumed to indicate decreased mental capacity. The patient must be able to hear the nurse. For a patient with compromised hearing, the nurse must attend to voice projection and volume. Shouting at the older patient is unnecessary. The nurse should remember to lower the pitch of their voice because higher-pitched sounds are often lost with presbycusis (loss of hearing sensitivity associated with aging). The nurse should eliminate distracting noises, such as from a television or radio, and ensure that required assistive medical devices or technologies, such as hearing aids, are available. Facing the patient and using distinct enunciation will help lip-reading patients understand what is being said. Sometimes deafness is mistaken for cognitive dysfunction. If a patient's hearing is questionable, the nurse should enlist the help of a speech and language specialist. Generally, the pace of the interview should mirror the patient's ability to move through the assessment. The pace of the interview may be slower than that used with a younger population.

Physical Assessment

Collecting and analyzing data for the physical assessment include areas similar to those discussed in Chapter 10. The assessment components include present and past health status, physical examination results, physical functioning, and pharmacology review. When focusing on physical health, the nurse pays special attention to the patient's general physical appearance as well as any observable manifestations of illness. The nurse should assess how all physical issues affect the patient's mental well-being. For example, pain and immobility are physical issues that can negatively affect mental health. A low-energy level may be immediately apparent. People with obvious osteoporosis may be experiencing frequent pain. Patients undergoing radiation for prostate cancer may worry about sexual functioning and urinary incontinence.

Present and Past Health Status

A review of the patient's current health status includes examining health records and collecting information from the patient and family members. The nurse must identify chronic health issues that could affect mental health care. For example, the patient's management of diabetes mellitus could provide clues to the likelihood of complications such as retinopathy or neuropathy, which in turn will affect the patient's ability to follow a mental health treatment regimen. The nurse must document any history of psychiatric treatment.

Physical Examination

The psychiatric nurse reviews the physical examination findings, paying special attention to recent laboratory values, such as urinalysis, white and red blood cell counts, thyroid studies, and fasting blood glucose data (see Chapter 10). Results of neurologic tests could indicate compromise of the neuromuscular systems. Many psychiatric medications lower the seizure threshold, making a history of seizures, which can cause behavior changes, an important assessment component. The nurse should note any evidence of movement disorders, such as tremors, unusual movements, or shuffling. If a patient has been taking antipsychotics, the nurse should consider assessment for symptoms of tardive dyskinesia using one of the appropriate assessment tools (see Chapter 24 for an additional discussion of tardive dyskinesia).

The nurse should take routine vital signs during the assessment. They should note any unusual readings in blood pressure (i.e., hypertension or hypotension) because many psychiatric medications affect blood pressure. Generally, these medications may cause orthostatic hypotension, which can lead to dizziness, an unsteady gait, and falls. A baseline blood pressure is needed for future monitoring of medication side effects. Lying, sitting, and standing blood pressures are especially useful in assessing for orthostatic hypotension.

Physical Functions

The nurse must consider the patient's physical functioning within the context of the expected changes that accompany aging and the presence of any chronic disorders. The nurse should note the patient's use of any personal assistive devices, such as canes, walkers, or wheelchairs; oxygen; or environmental devices, such as grab bars, shower benches, or hospital beds. Specific areas to consider are nutrition and eating, elimination, and sleep patterns.

Nutrition and Eating

Assessment of the type, amount, and frequency of food eaten is standard in any geriatric assessment. Weight loss of more than 10 pounds should be noted. The nurse must consider such nutrition changes in light of mental health issues. For example, is a patient's weight loss related to an underlying physical issue or to the patient's belief that she is being poisoned, which makes her afraid to eat?

Eating is often difficult for older patients, who may experience a lack of appetite. The nurse must assess eating and appetite patterns because many psychiatric medications can affect digestion and may impair an already compromised GI tract. A common issue of older adults who live in nursing homes is dysphagia, or difficulty swallowing. **Dysphagia** can lead to dehydration, malnutrition, pneumonia, or asphyxiation. People who have been exposed to conventional antipsychotics (e.g., haloperidol, chlorpromazine) may have symptoms of tardive dyskinesia, which can make swallowing difficult. Thus, the nurse should evaluate any patient who has been exposed to older psychiatric medications for symptoms of tardive dyskinesia.

Xerostomia, or dry mouth, which is common in older adults, also may impair eating. The nurse should pay particular attention to those who are currently receiving treatment for mental illnesses, particularly with medications that have anticholinergic properties. Dry mouth is also a side effect of many other anticholinergic medications, such as cimetidine, digoxin, and furosemide. Frequent rinsing with a nonalcohol-based mouthwash will help to correct the dry condition. The nurse should observe for the frequent use of candy or sugar-based gum for patients because dental caries and gum disease provide a portal of entry for sepsis in older adults. Decreased taste or smell is common among older adults and may reduce the pleasure of eating resulting in the patient eating less. Making meal times social and relaxing experiences can help the patient compensate for some of the loss of pleasure associated with decreased taste or smell. Preparing favorite foods will also enhance the quality of meals and meal times.

Substance Use

Substance use in older adults is increasing, though it is often overlooked by health care providers. The number of adults over the age of 65 needing treatment for substance use increased from 1.7 million in 2001 to 4.4 million in 2020. Approximately two-thirds of older adults with substance use disorder began using substances in early adulthood; consequently, these individuals are at greater risk for chronic health conditions because of such long-term use. The remaining one third of adults began using substances in middle adulthood, typically in response to a stressful life event. Substance misuse in older adults is expected to increase as the Baby Boomer generation ages, with its higher rates of substance use compared to preceding generations. Social isolation, lack of social support, and bereavement increase the risk for substance use, particularly among people assigned female at birth (Stewart et al., 2023). Misuse of alcohol, prescription benzodiazepines, and opioids are among the most significant sources of concern (Arcadepani & Fidalgo, 2023).

Nearly 7% of older adults are considered heavy drinkers or binge drinkers (Arcadepani & Fidalgo, 2023). Older adults are more vulnerable to the effects of alcohol because of the physiologic changes associated with aging, increases in chronic diseases, and medication use (Stewart et al., 2023). Alcohol use in older adults has been associated with functional impairments, falls, delirium, and increased mortality. Indications of alcohol use include observable changes in sleep patterns and unusual fatigue, changes in mood, jerky eye movement, seizures, unexplained complaints about chronic pain or vision issues, poor hygiene and self-neglect, unexplained nausea or vomiting, and slurred speech. Use of an assessment tool such as the CAGE questionnaire (discussed in Chapter 31) may be helpful.

BOX 38.3

Research for Evidence-Based Practice: Comorbidities With Opioid Use Disorders

Baumann, S. L., & Samuels, W. E. (2022). Comorbidities in older adults with opioid use disorders. Journal of the American Association of Nurse Practitioners, *34(12), 1280–1288.*

THE QUESTION: What medical and psychiatric conditions are found in older adults with opioid use disorders (OUDs)?

METHODS: Demographic and medical history data of adults over age 55 with an active diagnosis of OUD were analyzed. Researchers identified 644 patients, with a mean age of 60 years; 47% of the patients were between 50 and 59 years of age.

FINDINGS: Patients with OUD were two to three times more likely than a national sample of older adults without OUD to have medical and psychiatric co-occurring disorders. The most frequently co-occurring medical conditions included heart/circulatory, movement, respiratory, pain, nutritional, and metabolic disorders. Chronic pain conditions were found in 44% of the patients. Co-occurring psychiatric disorders included anxiety, depression, posttraumatic stress disorder (PTSD), and bipolar disorder.

IMPLICATIONS FOR NURSING: Treatment of older adults with OUD is complex as they often have one or more comorbid medical and psychiatric conditions. Nurses should provide comprehensive, holistic care. Care should be compassionate and trauma-informed; nurses should avoid overgeneralizations and be aware of their own implicit biases.

Prescription opioids and benzodiazepines are more likely to be given to older adults due to a high number of medical comorbidities, particularly chronic pain (Box 38.3). An estimated 25% of older adults have access to prescription medications with misuse potential. Older adults are more sensitive to prescription medication and prone to side effects due to changes in metabolism of medication as they age. They may be more vulnerable to developing tolerance and dependence due to a longer duration of metabolization. Prescription misuse in older adults is associated with a worsening of cognition and changes in mood, particularly depression. Older adults are also at greater risk for confusion and falls (Arcadepani & Fidalgo, 2023; Stewart et al., 2023).

Recent data suggest that 6% to 7% of older adults use cannabis, with 75% of them using it for medical reasons (e.g., chronic pain, insomnia). Cannabis use has been found to increase symptoms of depression, anxiety, cognitive impairment, accidents/injuries, and substance use. Evidence is limited regarding whether the benefits of cannabis use outweigh the harm (Wolfe et al., 2023).

Elimination

The nurse must assess the patient's urinary and bowel functions. Older adults are more likely to experience constipation caused by a change in eating or activity patterns or intentional reduction in fluid intake. Medications with anticholinergic properties can cause constipation, leading to fecal impaction. Misuse of laxatives is common among older adults and requires evaluation. Although the addition of fiber is recommended for constipation, such measures may cause bloating and excessive gas production. Older patients are also more likely to experience urinary frequency because the strength of the sphincter muscles decreases. Because many older adults drink fewer fluids to manage urinary incontinence, fluid intake also becomes an important factor in assessing urinary functioning and constipation. The nurse should remember that urinary incontinence is not an expected age-related finding but a symptom of a disorder that requires follow-up and treatment.

Sleep

During the expected aging process, sleep patterns change, and patients may sleep more or less than they did when younger. The nurse must assess any recent changes in sleep patterns and evaluate whether they are related to expected aging or are symptomatic of an underlying disorder. Insomnia, the inability to fall or remain asleep throughout the night, may be the result of depression or can lead to an increased risk for depression and regular use of sleep medications (Kristiansen et al., 2024). Sleep disturbances, such as waking after onset of sleep and spending time in bed, are one of the early signs of Alzheimer dementia (He et al., 2023). Disturbed sleep patterns are also associated with loneliness and social isolation (McLay et al., 2021). If a patient reports sleep issues, the nurse should ask about the patient's use of alcohol, over-the-counter (OTC) medications, and prescription drugs, which can interfere with sleep.

Pain

Older adults are more likely to experience persistent pain than younger adults because they are at increased risk for chronic illness and may be experiencing the consequences of a lifetime of injuries. For many older adults, chronic pain is a constant companion and contributes to unexplained behavior and personality changes. Chronic pain assessment is more difficult because of the person's perception of pain or cognitive impairment, which interferes with communication. Older people are often reluctant to report pain or believe that they have to be stoic about pain and "not make a big deal" about it.

Although an in-depth discussion of pain assessment is beyond the scope of this text, it is important for the mental health nurse to understand the pain assessment approaches. A common practice of asking a patient if they are experiencing pain on a scale of 1 to 10 is being replaced with a more meaningful assessment of the impact of the pain on the person. The emerging trend in pain assessment is to determine the intensity of the pain and the extent to which the pain interferes with movement (physical activity) and function (performance of daily or overall function). It is important to understand how pain limits their functional ability and mobility. A movement-based pain assessment involves assessing the pain intensity and interference on function during movement or physical activities (Fullen et al., 2023).

Pharmacologic Assessment

One of the most important aspects is the pharmacologic assessment. **Polypharmacy**, the use of duplicate medications, interacting medications, or drugs used to treat adverse drug interactions, is common in older adults. The nurse must ask the patient and collateral sources to list all medications and times that the patient takes them. Asking the patient's support people to bring in all the medications the patient is taking, including OTC medications, vitamins, and herbal supplements, allows for a careful assessment of polypharmacy. Because older adults are more sensitive than younger people to medications, the possibility of drug-to-drug interactions is greater. When considering potential drug interactions, the nurse should ask the patient about their consumption of grapefruit juice, which contains naringin, a compound that inhibits the CYP3A4 enzyme involved in the metabolism of many medications (e.g., antidepressants, antiarrhythmics, erythromycin, and several statins).

Risk for Falls

Falls are a significant concern in older adults, with an estimated prevalence rate of 30%. Falls are a leading cause of injury and injury-related death among older adults. People who experience falls are often left with physical limitations and frailty. Screening for fall risk is important and can be completed using a structured evaluation tool (Beauchet et al., 2025; Lafontant et al., 2024). In a national survey of falls resulting in emergency room treatment, nearly 80% of falls occurred within the home, most commonly in the bedroom, bathroom, or on stairs. Nearly 70% of older adults report a fear of falling. A decline in sensory perception, cognitive processing, and motor abilities contribute to fall risk. Medical comorbidities, including Parkinson disease, stroke, and arthritis contribute to risk. Additionally, medications affecting balance and coordination (e.g., medications causing orthostatic hypotension, drowsiness, dizziness, or blurry vision) increase a person's likelihood of falling. Functional exercises that improve balance and strength are recommended for fall prevention (Colón-Emeric et al., 2024).

Psychological Assessment

The psychological assessment provides the nurse with the opportunity to identify limitations, behavior symptoms, and reactions to illness. The nurse assesses many of the same areas as in other adult assessments, but again, the emphasis may be different. The following discussion focuses on the responses of older patients to mental health issues, mental status examination, behavior changes, stress and coping patterns, and risk assessments.

Responses to Mental Health Issues

Many older patients are reluctant to admit that they have psychiatric symptoms, particularly if their culture stigmatizes mental illness, and may deny having mental or emotional issues. They may also fear that if they admit to any symptoms, they may be placed outside their home or have certain freedoms taken away. If patients do not recognize or admit to having psychiatric symptoms, their vulnerability to being taken advantage of or injured increases.

Throughout the assessment, the nurse evaluates the patient's verbal reports, notable symptoms, and reports from collateral sources. If a patient flatly denies any psychiatric symptoms (e.g., depression, mood swings, outbursts of anger, memory issues), the nurse should respectfully accept the patient's answer and avoid arguments or confrontation (Box 38.4). If the patient's support network contradicts

BOX 38.4

Therapeutic Dialogue: Assessment Interview

Tom, age 79, is being seen for the first time in a geropsychiatric clinic because of recent changes in his behavior and his accusations that family members are trying to steal his house and car. He locked his wife out of the house, accusing her of being unfaithful. When Susan, the psychiatric nurse assigned to his case, is conducting the assessment interview, Tom cooperates and is very pleasant until the nurse begins the psychological assessment.

INEFFECTIVE APPROACH

Nurse: Have there been times when you have had problems with any members of your family?

Patient: No. (Silence)

Nurse: Have you noticed that lately you have been getting more upset than usual?

Patient: No. Who has been talking to you?

Nurse: Your wife seems to think that you may be getting a little more upset than usual.

Patient: You are just like her. She keeps telling me something is wrong with me. (Getting very agitated)

Nurse: Please, I'm trying to help you. I understand that you locked your wife out of the house last week.

Patient: Leave me alone. (Gets up and leaves)

EFFECTIVE APPROACH

Nurse: How have things been going at home?

Patient: All right.

Nurse: (Silence)

Patient: Well, my wife and I sometimes argue.

Nurse: Oh. Most husbands and wives argue. Any special arguments?

Patient: No. Just the usual. I don't pick up after myself enough. I don't dress right to suit her. But, lately, she's gone a lot.

Nurse: She is gone a lot?

Patient: Yeah! A lot.

Nurse: The way you say that, it sounds like you have some feelings about her being gone.

Patient: You're damned right I do—and you would, too.

Nurse: I'm missing something.

Patient: Well, if you must know, I think she's having an affair with the man next door.

Nurse: Really? That must upset you to think your wife is having an affair.

Patient: I am devastated. I feel so bad.

Nurse: Would you say that you are depressed?

Patient: Well, wouldn't you be? Yes, I'm feeling pretty low.

CRITICAL THINKING CHALLENGE

- How do the very first questions differ in the two interviews?
- What therapeutic techniques did the nurse use in the second interview to avoid the pitfalls the nurse encountered in the first scenario?
- How did the nurse in the second scenario elicit the patient's delusion about his wife's affair?
- From the data that the second nurse gathered, how many patient issues can be identified?

the patient's report or if symptoms are obvious during the interview, the nurse can approach the issue while planning care. Nurses may need to use conflict resolution strategies in helping families and patients arrive at mutually agreed on reports.

Mental Status Examination

The areas of special interest in the mental status examination are mood and affect, thought processes, and cognitive functioning. The nurse should interpret the results in light of any accompanying physical issues, such as chronic pain, or life changes, such as loss of a partner.

Mood and Affect

Depression in older adults is common and associated with the following risk factors: loss of a partner, physical illness, low socioeconomic status, impaired functional status, and heavy alcohol consumption. In older people, other disorders may mask depression. When symptoms are present, they may be attributed to expected aging or other age-related issues. Older patients are less likely to report feeling sad or worthless than younger patients. As a result, family members and primary care providers often overlook depression in older patients.

The term *late-onset depression* refers to the development of depression or depressive symptoms that impair functioning after 60 years of age. In late-onset depression, the risk for recurrence is relatively high. Emerging evidence suggests that late-life depression is associated with changes in the cortical network (Ribeiz et al., 2023; Tan et al., 2023).

The Geriatric Depression Scale (GDS) is a useful screening tool with demonstrated validity and reliability (Hyer & Blount, 1984). The GDS was designed as a self-administered test, although it also has been used in observer-administered formats. One advantage of the test is its "yes/no" format, which may be easier for older adults than the Hamilton Rating Scale for Depression (HAM-D), which uses a scale from 0 to 4 (see Chapter 25). This tool is easy to administer and provides valuable information about the possibility of depression (Box 38.5). If the results are positive, the nurse should refer the patient to a psychiatrist or advanced practice nurse for further evaluation. Among nursing home residents, the usefulness of the GDS depends on the degree of cognitive impairment. Residents who are mildly impaired may be able to answer the yes/no questions; however, moderate to severely impaired patients will be unable to do the same. The best validated scale for patients with dementia is the Cornell Scale for Depression in Dementia (CSDD) (Alexopoulos et al., 1998). The CSDD is an interview-administered scale that uses information both from the patient and an outside informant.

Anxiety is another important mood for nurses to assess in older adults because it can interfere with usual functioning. In dementia, anxiety is common (Brieler et al., 2023). The Rating Anxiety in Dementia (RAID) scale was developed as a global scale to assess anxiety in patients with dementia (Shankar et al., 1999). The domains that the RAID scale assesses include worry, apprehension and vigilance, motor tension, autonomic hyperactivity, and phobias and panic attacks.

BOX 38.5

Geriatric Depression Scale (Short Form)

1. Are you basically satisfied with your life?	Yes	No
2. Have you dropped many of your activities and interests?	Yes	No
3. Do you feel that your life is empty?	Yes	No
4. Do you often get bored?	Yes	No
5. Are you in good spirits most of the time?	Yes	No
6. Are you afraid that something bad is going to happen to you?	Yes	No
7. Do you feel happy most of the time?	Yes	No
8. Do you often feel helpless?	Yes	No
9. Do you prefer to stay at home rather than go out and do new things?	Yes	No
10. Do you feel you have more problems with memory than most?	Yes	No
11. Do you think it is wonderful to be alive now?	Yes	No
12. Do you feel pretty worthless the way you are now?	Yes	No
13. Do you feel full of energy?	Yes	No
14. Do you feel that your situation is hopeless?	Yes	No
15. Do you think that most people are better off than you are?	Yes	No

Score: __/15. One point for "No" to questions 1, 5, 7, 11, 13; one point for "Yes" to other questions.

Normal	3 ± 2
Mildly depressed	7 ± 3
Very depressed	12 ± 2

From Sheikh, J. I., & Yesavage, J. A. (1986). Geriatric Depression Scale (GDS): recent evidence and development of a shorter version. *Clinical Gerontologist, 5*(1–2), 165–173. Reprinted by permission of Taylor & Francis Ltd, https://www.tandfonline.com.

Thought Processes

Thought processes and content are critical in the assessment of older patients. Can the patient express ideas and thoughts logically? Can the patient understand questions and follow the conversation of others? If the patient shows any indication of hallucinations or delusions, the nurse should explore the content of the hallucination or delusion. If the patient has a history of mental illness, such as schizophrenia, these symptoms may be familiar to family members, who can validate whether they are old or new issues. If this is the first time the patient has experienced these atypical thought processes, the nurse should further evaluate the content. Suspicious and delusional thoughts that characterize dementia often include some of the following beliefs:

- People are stealing my things.
- The house is not my house.
- My relative is an impostor.

Cognition and Intellectual Performance

Cognitive functioning includes parameters such as orientation, attention, short- and long-term memory, consciousness, and executive functioning. Intellectual functioning, also considered a cognitive measure, is rarely formally assessed with a standardized intelligence test in older adults. Considerable variability among individuals depends on lifestyle and psychosocial factors. Some changes in cognitive capacity may accompany aging, but important functions are spared. Typical cognitive changes during aging include a slowing of information processing and memory retrieval. Changes in consciousness, orientation, judgment, speech, or language are not related to age but to underlying neuropathologic changes. Cognitive changes in older adults are associated with delirium or dementia (see Chapter 39) or with schizophrenia (see Chapter 24).

The assessment includes the number of years of education. An inverse relationship between Alzheimer disease and the number of years of education exists. Evidence suggests that severe cognitive deterioration may occur in older adults with schizophrenia. An easy-to-administer and easily accessible screening tool is the SLUMS (Saint Louis University Mental Status Examination) (see Chapter 39).

Behavior Changes

Behavior changes in older adults can indicate neuropathologic processes and thus require nursing assessment. If such changes occur, it is most likely that family members will notice them before the patient does. Apraxia (an inability to execute a voluntary movement despite expected muscle function) is not attributed to age but indicates an underlying disease process, such as Alzheimer disease, Parkinson disease, or other disorders. Various other behavior issues s are associated with psychiatric disorders in older adults, including irritability, agitation, apathy, and euphoria. Other behaviors in older adults who are experiencing psychiatric issues s include wandering and aggressive behaviors.

The Neuropsychiatric Inventory (NPI) was developed in 1994 to assess behavior issues associated with dementia. The scale assesses 10 behavior issues: delusions, hallucinations, dysphoria, anxiety, agitation or aggression, euphoria, inhibition, irritability or lability, apathy, and aberrant motor behavior (Cummings et al., 1994). This very popular tool is used in many medication clinical trials. There are two versions. The standard version is used when the patient is still at home; the second version (NPI-NH) is used when the patient is in a nursing home.

Stress and Coping Patterns

Identifying stresses and coping patterns is just as important for older patients as it is for younger adults. Unique stresses for older patients include living on a fixed income, handling declining health, losing partners and friends, and ultimately confronting death. Coping ability varies, depending on patients' unique circumstances. For example, some patients respond to stressful events with amazing adaptability, but others become depressed and suicidal.

Bereavement, a natural response to the death of a loved one, includes crying and sorrow, anxiety and agitation, insomnia, and a loss of appetite. These symptoms, although overlapping with those of major depression, do not constitute a mental disorder. Although bereavement is a natural response, the nurse must identify it and develop interventions to help the individual successfully resolve the loss. Bereavement is an important and well-established risk factor for depression (see Chapter 21).

Risk Assessment

Suicide is a major mental health risk for older adults. In 2022, people over the age of 85 had the highest rates of suicide, with the next highest rates among individuals between the ages of 75 and 84 (CDC, 2024). Depression is the greatest risk factor for suicide and contributes to the desire to die. Hopelessness is also a strong factor related to death by suicide. Hopelessness is driven by a low mood, perceptions of poor physical health, and social isolation (Chan et al., 2024). Social disconnectedness, characterized by social isolation and a lack of social support, increases with age and increases the risk of suicidal behavior (Solomonov et al., 2023). Individuals who are suicidal often believe that they are a burden to their families who would be better off without them (see Chapter 22). In assessing an older patient, the nurse should consider the following characteristics as indications of high risk for suicide:

- Depression
- Attempted suicide in the past
- Family history of suicide
- Firearms in the home
- Misuse of alcohol or other substances

- Unusual stress
- Burden to family
- Chronic medical condition (e.g., cancer, neuromuscular disorders)
- Social isolation

NCLEXNOTE Suicide assessment is a priority for the older adults experiencing mental health issues. It is important to carefully assess recent behavior changes and loss of support.

Social Assessment

The social assessment includes determining the patient's interactions with others in their family and community. The nurse targets social support because it is so important to the well-being of the older adult's functional status and because of the potential physical changes that can affect this area and social systems, which encompasses all community resources.

Social Support

Remaining active throughout one's life is one of the best predictors of mental health and wellness in an older patient. People obtain their sense of self-worth through their interactions with others in their environment. A sense of "who one is" is closely tied to the roles that a person assumes in life. When older adults relinquish such roles because of physical disabilities, become isolated from friends and family, or begin to sense that they are a burden to those around them rather than contributing members of society, a sense of hopelessness and helplessness often follows.

The role of social support is critical to assess in this age group. Social support is a reciprocal concept, meaning that simply receiving assistance increases the person's sense of being a burden. Those older adults who believe that they contribute to the welfare of others are most likely to remain mentally healthy. For this reason, pets are often "life savers" for older adults who live alone. Nothing can be more understanding and accepting of an older adult's behavior or disabilities than a beloved pet.

The nurse should assess the patient's number of formal and informal social contacts. The nurse should ask about the frequency of contact with others (in person and through telephone calls, letters, and cards). Determining whether these contacts are satisfying and supporting to the patient is essential. If family members are important to the patient's well-being, the nurse should complete a more in-depth family assessment (see Chapter 15).

The nurse can use the following questions to focus on social support:

- In the past 2 weeks, how often would you say that family members or friends let you know that they care about you?
- In the past 2 weeks, how often has someone provided you with help, such as giving you a ride somewhere or helping around the house?
- Do you have a family member or a special person you could call or contact if you need help? Who?
- In general, other than your children, who do you consider a close friend or companion?

For patients who are isolated with few social contacts, the nurse can develop interventions to improve social support.

Functional Status

As part of a complete assessment, the nurse will need to assess the older adult's functional status. **Functional activities** or activities of daily living (ADLs) are the activities necessary for self-care (i.e., bathing, toileting, dressing, and transferring). **Instrumental activities of daily living (IADLs)** include those that facilitate or enhance the performance of ADLs (i.e., shopping, using the telephone, using transportation). These aspects are critical to consider for any older adult living alone. The most common tools used to assess functional status are the Index of Independence in the ADLs and the IADLs (Katz & Akpom, 1976).

Older Adults Who Identify as LGBTQ+

Approximately 2.7 million (2.4%) of adults over age 50 identify as LGBTQ+. This number is expected to increase to 5 million by 2060. People who identify as LGBTQ+ experience greater health disparities, including poorer physical and mental health outcomes, than their heterosexual peers (Srithumsuk et al., 2024). Individuals requiring long-term support services are at greater risk due to experiences of rejection and discrimination, particularly when facilities lack inclusive policies (Shippee et al., 2024). LGBTQ+ individuals report higher levels of loneliness and lower mood compared to heterosexual individuals. For older adults in this population, living with someone else and having meaningful contact with family or friends are protective factors against loneliness. Older adults who identify as LGBTQ+ may experience less sense of belonging if they are not closely connected to younger generations of individuals who identify as LGBTQ+, which may also contribute to loneliness (Buczak-Stec et al., 2023). Because LGBTQ+ individuals may have experienced negative encounters in prior health care settings, coupled with potentially hostile and social climates in their earlier years, they may demonstrate lower levels of confidence and trust in the health care system and with their providers (Moriarty & Willis, 2024). Unfortunately, sexual health is often overlooked in assessment. Barriers to rapport, patient embarrassment, uncertainty about finding solutions, ageism, and other structural barriers contribute to this lack of assessment. Establishing therapeutic rapport and providing a safe environment with sufficient time to discuss concerns is important. Opportunities to discuss sexual health may present when reviewing adjacent concerns, such as incontinence, menopause, and prostate health (Bourchier et al., 2024).

Social Determinants of Health and Social Systems

Many socioeconomic factors—poverty, inequality, educational level, occupation, income, housing, and lifestyle—impact mental health. Further, although poor socioeconomic conditions contribute to mental disorders, the mental disorder may, in turn, exacerbate socioeconomic difficulties (Ilgun, 2022). Community resources are essential to an older adult's ability to maintain mental health and wellness, as well as to their ability to remain at home throughout the later years. Senior centers are federally funded community resources that provide a wide array of services to the nation's older population. They provide daily balanced meals at a nominal cost. In addition, they provide opportunities for socialization, which is a key to combating loneliness and social isolation. Many senior centers provide annual vaccination clinics and education on such topics as fall prevention and recognition and prevention of elder abuse. Additional community resources that are specific to older adults include geriatric assessment clinics and adult day care centers.

During the assessment, the nurse must determine which community resources are available and if the patient uses them. Lack of transportation to and from these community resources may be a barrier to use. Most communities have buses available for older people or those with disabilities. The nurse may need to assist the older adult in accessing this important resource.

Many older citizens rely on the Social Security Administration for their monthly income. For many, this financial support, although less than adequate in most instances, is their only source of income. In addition to Social Security, the federal government provides basic health care coverage in the form of the state-administered Medicare program. Together, these programs contribute to the patient's ability to live independently and receive health care. The nurse should assess a patient's sources of financial support. Sometimes nurses are uncomfortable asking for financial information, fearing that they are invading the patient's privacy. However, such data are important for the nurse to determine whether a patient's resources adequately meet their needs. The source of financial support is also important. For example, a patient whose income is adequate and from personal resources is more likely to be independent than the patient who depends on family members for income.

The nurse should ask the patient about accessible clinics, support groups, and pharmaceutical services. Information about available health care resources can provide useful data regarding the patient's ability to access services and can also provide potential referral sources. In urban areas that are likely to have adequate health care resources, cultural and language barriers may prohibit access. People who live in rural areas where health care resources are limited are less likely to utilize the full range of health care resources than are those in urban areas. Overall, the use of mental health services by older adults with mental illnesses is low (Gao et al., 2024). If older adults are married and have insurance, they are more likely to seek mental health services.

Spiritual Assessment

Spiritual needs are basic for all age groups and are requirements for establishing meaning and purpose, love and relatedness, and forgiveness. With advanced age, many people begin to reflect on their successes and failures. During such reflection, many seek out God or a higher power to make sense of the past and establish hope for the future.

The process of spiritual assessment involves active listening, thoughtful observation, and sensitive questioning. The nurse may simply ask if the person would find comfort from a visit from a spiritual leader. Many forms of religion use various rituals that are important to the person's daily routine. The nurse should explore and honor these aspects to the extent possible.

Legal Status and Risk for Exploitation

A growing trend in the United States is to view older adults as a special population whose rights deserve increased attention. Instances involving violation of the rights of older adults are far too common, with one in six people over age 60 experiencing abuse (Mosafer et al., 2025). Every nurse must consider themselves a patient advocate and be vigilant in recognizing the signs of neglect or abuse, such as unexplained injuries. At times, abuse can take the form of another individual usurping the rights of the older individual. Unless the older individual is determined to be incompetent, they have the same rights to personal decision making as any other adult, including the right to refuse treatment.

Among all types of abuse, the most common form experienced by older adults is **financial exploitation**. This involves the illegal taking, misuse, or concealment of funds, property, or assets. The prevalence of financial exploitation is alarming; over 25% of older people experience such abuse, with an estimated loss of approximately 36 billion dollars annually. Because the financial exploiter is most often a person close to them, such as a relative, caregiver, or friend, the older adult is less likely to report the exploitation. Financial exploitation results in detrimental effects beyond the loss of financial resources. The older adult's independence and security are at risk, and research finds that people who experience exploitation are exposed to a 300% increase in mortality. Older adults with cognitive decline are more susceptible to being victims of financial exploitation, as are individuals with depression or emotional distress. Social isolation and lack of support networks also increase risk. Racial underrepresented groups, particularly African Americans, have higher prevalence rates of exploitation. Systemic inequalities, including socioeconomic disparities, limited access to financial education, and historical patterns of exploitation contribute to this increased prevalence. The nurse should screen for financial exploitation, for early identification and intervention (Mosafer et al., 2025).

Quality of Life

A sense of quality of life is closely tied to values and beliefs. For many older adults, quality of life is not reflected in material possessions or physical health. At this stage, quality of life is connected more with contentment over how the person has lived life and the extent to which their life has had meaning and purpose. Keeping close personal contact with friends and family and having the opportunity to share stories of lifetime experiences are essential to maintaining mental health and wellness for older adults. For older adults, physical illnesses may affect the quality of life more than psychiatric disorders. The assessment of quality of life becomes especially important when assessing a patient living in a nursing home or isolated in their own home. The assessment of quality of life of older adults is similar to that of younger adults (see Chapter 10).

SUMMARY OF KEY POINTS

- Typical aging is associated with some physical decline, but most functions do not change. Intellectual functioning, capacity for change, and productive engagement with life remain stable.
- Mental health assessments are necessary when older patients face psychiatric or mental health issues. The biopsychosocial geropsychiatric nursing assessment examines many sources of data, including self-reports, laboratory test results, and reports from collateral sources.
- The psychiatric–mental health nursing assessment for the older adult is based on the special needs and concerns of the older adult. This assessment examines current and past health, functional status, and human responses to mental health issues.
- The physical assessment involves collecting data about past and present health status, physical examination findings, physical functions (i.e., nutrition and eating, elimination patterns, sleep), pain, fall risk, and pharmacologic information.
- The psychological assessment includes the patient's responses to mental health issues, mental status examination, behavioral changes, stress and coping patterns, and risk assessment.
- The social assessment includes social systems, spiritual assessment, legal information and risk for exploitation, and quality of life.
- When conducting an assessment, the nurse may find several tools useful. For patients with possible depression, the GDS may be helpful. For patients with anxiety, nurses can use the RAID scale.
- Coping with the stress of aging varies among patients. Determining stressors and coping skills for dealing with stress is important.
- Social support is critical to patients in this age group and requires assessment.
- Determination of the patient's ability to perform functional and instrumental ADLs is critical in the assessment of the older adult.

DEVELOPING CLINICAL JUDGMENT

1. The director of your community's senior center has asked you to be the guest speaker at the monthly meeting of the Retired Active Citizens group. The subject is to be “Maintaining Your Mental Health After Retirement.” What key points will you touch on in your presentation? What activities or handouts will you use to highlight your talk?
2. When asking about current illnesses, a patient begins telling you their whole life story. What approach would you take to elicit the most important needed to develop an individualized plan of care for your older patient?
3. A caregiver tells you that their mother has become suspicious of the neighbors and other family members. How would you assess this perceptual experience? What other data should you gather from this patient?
4. A caregiver brings a sack of medications to the patient's assessment interview. What information should you obtain from the caregiver regarding the patient's use of these medications?
5. An individual brings their parent, who has a long history of frequent psychiatric hospitalizations for depression, to the clinic. The patient's partner recently died, and the adult child fears that their parent is becoming depressed again. What approach would you use in assessing for changes in mood?

6. Obtain a listing of the social services available in your community. Examine the list for areas of duplication and omission of services needed by an older adult living alone in their own home.

MOVIE, TV, OR STREAMING PROGRAMS

Still Alice: **2014.** This drama follows the life of Alice Howland, a renowned linguistics professor who develops early-onset dementia in her early 50s. The film follows Alice's cognitive and emotional struggles as her illness progresses. Challenged by the loss of her independence and intellectual abilities, Alice her husband and her children are faced with accepting the diagnosis while trying to maintain a sense of normalcy in their personal and professional lives.

Viewing Points:

1. What are some of the symptoms Alice noted in herself that resulted in her consulting with the neurologist?
2. Why did the neurologist ask Alice to bring her husband to the next visit? Why do you believe she did not do so initially?
3. How does Alice's family react to her diagnosis?
4. When completing the nursing assessment, what does the nurse note about Alice's ability to perform activities of daily living (ADLs) as her condition progresses?
5. Why does Alice make plans for suicide when she reached the point that her symptoms progressed too much? What risk factors for suicide does Alice have?
6. How can the nurse help manage the emotional effects of Alzheimer disease for both Alice and her family?

Unfolding Patient Stories: George Palo • Part 2

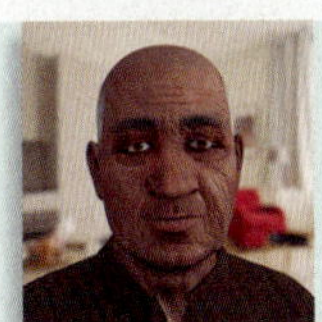

Recall from Chapter 21 George Palo, a 90-year-old who is diagnosed with minor neurocognitive impairment, Alzheimer's type, and who has been living independently in a retirement community since his wife died 3 years ago. His daughter has noticed some cognitive decline and social isolation after the recent loss of his dog. What assessments should the nurse perform during a home visit? How can the nurse develop a therapeutic relationship with George to determine if he is receptive to community resources for supporting his independent living? Considering his neurocognitive impairment, what are the factors the nurse would consider when assessing George's ability to continue to live independently? What factors may indicate the need to transfer to a higher level of care?

Care for George Palo and other patients in a realistic virtual environment: ***vSim** for Nursing* (thepoint.lww.com/vSimMentalHealth). Practice documenting these patients' care in DocuCare (thepoint.lww.com/DocuCareEHR).

REFERENCES

Alexopoulos, G. S., Abrams, R. C., Young, R. C., & Shamoian, C. A. (1998). Cornell scale for depression in dementia. *Biological Psychiatry, 23*(3), 271–284.

Arcadepani, F. B., & Fidalgo, T. M. (2023). Substance use among older adults: A review of the literature. *Journal of Addictive Diseases, 41*(4), 289–299.

Arias, E., Xu, J., Tejada-Vera, B., & Bastian, B. (2024). U.S. state life tables, 2021. *National Vital Statistics Reports*, 73(7). https://doi.org/10.15620/cdc/157499

Beauchet, O., Matskiv, J., Gaudreau, P., Allali, G., Vaillant-Ciszewicz, A. J., Guerin, O., & Gros, A. (2025). Fall risk screening in older adults using the "CARE" frailty scale: The NuAge cohort results. *Maturitas, 191*, 108134.

Bourchier, L., Temple-Smith, M., Hocking, J. S., & Malta, S. (2024). Older patients want to talk about sexual health in Australian primary care. *Australian Journal of Primary Health, 30*(4), 1–8.

Brieler, J. A., Salas, J., Amick, M. E., Sheth, P., Keegan-Garrett, E. A., Morley, J. E., & Scherrer, J. F. (2023). Anxiety disorders, benzodiazepine prescription, and incident dementia. *Journal of the American Geriatrics Society, 71*(11), 3376–3389.

Buczak-Stec, E., König, H. H., & Hajek, A. (2023). Sexual orientation and psychosocial factors in terms of loneliness and subjective well-being in later life. *Gerontologist, 63*(2), 338–349.

Centers for Disease Control and Prevention (CDC). (2024). *Suicide prevention.* https://www.cdc.gov/suicide/facts/data.html

Chan, E. C., Conlon, K., & Gagnon, L. (2024). Risk factors and methods in suicides of elderly patients connected to mental health services from 1999–2024. *Frontiers in Psychiatry, 15*, 1425371.

Coelho-Junior, H. J., Calvani, R., Picca, A., Landi, F., & Marzetti, E. (2024). The influence of ageism on the hallmarks of aging: Where age stigma and biology collide. *Experimental Gerontology, 196*, 112575.

Colón-Emeric, C. S., McDermott, C. L., Lee, D. S., & Berry, S. D. (2024). Risk assessment and prevention of falls in older community-dwelling adults: A review. *JAMA, 331*(16), 1397–1406.

Cummings, J. L., Mega, M., Gray, K., Rosenberg-Thompson, S., Carusi, D. A., & Gornbein, J. (1994). The neuropsychiatric inventory: Comprehensive assessment of psychopathology in dementia. *Neurology, 44*(12), 2308–2314.

Davies, T. L. (2023). Tailoring the mental health assessment to older adults. *Nurse Practitioner, 48*(1), 10–18.

Elefante, C., Brancati, G. E., Ismail, Z., Ricciardulli, S., Beatino, M. F., Lepri, V., Famà, A., Ferrari, E., Giampietri, L., Baldacci, F., Ceravolo, R., Maremmani, I., Lattanzi, L., & Perugi, G. (2023). Mild behavioral impairment in psychogeriatric patients: Clinical features and psychopathology severity. *Journal of Clinical Medicine, 12*(16), 5423.

Fullen, B. M., Wittink, H., De Groef, A., Hoegh, M., McVeigh, J. G., Martin, D., & Smart, K. (2023). Musculoskeletal pain: Current and future directions of physical therapy practice. *Archives of Rehabilitation Research and Clinical Translation, 5*(1), 100258.

Gao, Y., Burns, R., Leach, L., Chilver, M. R., & Butterworth, P. (2024). Examining the mental health services among people with mental disorders: A literature review. *BMC Psychiatry, 24*(568). https://doi.org/10.1186/s12888-024-05965-z

He, X., Hao, J., Song, Y., Cao, H., Chen, Y., & Yang, H. (2023). Effectiveness of non-pharmacological interventions for sleep disturbances in people living with dementia: A systematic review and meta-analysis. *Geriatric Nursing, 51*, 76–83.

Hyer, L., & Blount, J. (1984). Concurrent and discriminant validities of the geriatric depression scale with older psychiatric inpatients. *Psychological Reports, 54*(2), 611–616.

Ilgun, G. (2022). What are the socioeconomic determinants of mental disorders? *Perspectives of Psychiatric Care, 58*, 2881–2887.

Katz, S., & Akpom, C. A. (1976). A measure of primary sociobiological functions. *International Journal of Health Science, 6*(3), 493–508.

Kristiansen, S., Lyhne, C., Kragh, M., Sigaard, K., Videbech, P., Larsen, E., & Bjerrum, M. (2024). Experiences of adult patients living with depression-related insomnia: A qualitative systematic review. *JBI Evidence Synthesis, 22*(12), 2447–2517.

Lafontant, K., Blount, A., Suarez, J. R. M., Fukuda, D. H., Stout, J. R., Trahan, E. M., Lighthall, N. R., Park, J. H., Xie, R., & Thiamwong, L. (2024). Comparing sensitivity, specificity, and accuracy of fall risk assessments in community-dwelling older adults. *Clinical Interventions in Aging, 19*, 581–588.

Liu, Y., Xu, Y., Yang, X., Miao, G., Wu, Y., & Yang, S. (2023). The prevalence of anxiety and its key influencing factors among the elderly in China. *Frontiers in Psychiatry, 14*, 1038049.

McLay, L., Jamieson, H. A., France, K. G., & Schluter, P. J. (2021). Loneliness and social isolation is associated with sleep problems among older community dwelling women and men with complex needs. *Scientific Reports, 11*(1), 4877.

Moriarty, Y., & Willis, P. (2024). Interventions addressing care staff views of older LGBTQ+ people in residentials and homecare settings: A scoping review protocol. *BMJ Open, 14*, e086497.

Mosafer, H., Soltani, S., Rostami, Z., Sharifi, S., & Mohammadi, M. (2025). Factors associated with financial exploitation in older adults: A systematic review. *Geriatric Nursing (New York, N.Y.), 61*, 662–671. https://doi.org/10.1016/j.gerinurse.2024.10.028

Ribeiz, S. R. I., Duran, F. L. S., da Costa, D. L., Alves, T. C. de T. F., & Filho, G. B. (2023). Structural brain changes in late onset depression. *Alzheimer's & Dementia: The Journal of the Alzheimer's Association, 19*, e076561.

Shankar, K. K., Walker, M., Frost, D., & Orrell, M. W. (1999). The development of a valid and reliable scale for rating anxiety in dementia (RAID). *Aging & Mental Health, 3*(1), 39–49.

Shippee, T., Rosser, B. R. S., Wright, M. M., Aumock, C., Moone, R., Talley, K. M. C., Duran, P., Henning-Smith, C., Cahill, S., Flatt, J. D., Slaughter-Acey, J., Greenwald, S., McCarthy, T., & Ross, M. W. (2024). Scoping literature review: Experiences of sexual and gender minority older adults, with diagnoses of dementia, who use residential long-term services and supports. *Journal of Applied Gerontology, 43*(5), 562–576.

Solomonov, N., Green, J., Quintana, A., Lin, J., Ognyanova, K., Santillana, M., Druckman, J. N., Baum, M. A., Lazer, D., Gunning, F. M., & Perlis, R. H. (2023). A 50-state survey study of thoughts of suicide and social isolation among older adults in the United States. *Journal of Affective Disorders, 334*, 43–49.

Srithumsuk, W., Thummapol, O., & Bhatarasakoon, P. (2024). Social determinants of health inequities for older LGBT adults: A scoping review. *Journal of Transcultural Nursing, 35*(5), 368–380.

Stewart, S. A., Copeland, A. L., & Cherry, K. E. (2023). Risk factors for substance use across the lifespan. *The Journal of Genetic Psychology, 184*(2), 145–162.

Tan, W., Ouyang, X., Huang, D., Wu, Z., Liu, Z., He, Z., & Long, Y. (2023). Disrupted intrinsic functional brain network in patients with late-life depression: Evidence from a multi-site dataset. *Journal of Affective Disorders, 323*, 631–639.

Wolfe, D., Corace, K., Butler, C., Rice, D., Skidmore, B., Patel, Y., Thayaparan, P., Michaud, A., Hamel, C., Smith, A., Garber, G., Porath, A., Conn, D., Willows, M., Abramovici, H., Thavorn, K., Kanji, S., & Hutton, B. (2023). Impacts of medical and non-medical cannabis on the health of older adults: Findings from a scoping review of the literature. *PloS One, 18*(2), e0281826.

Yang, S. N., Chueh, C. H., Peng, L. N., & Tsai, Y. W. (2022). Impacts of intervals between sequential development of depression and dementia in older adults: A nationwide population-based study. *Archives of Gerontology & Geriatrics, 101*, 104693. https://doi.org/10.1016/j.archger.2022.104693

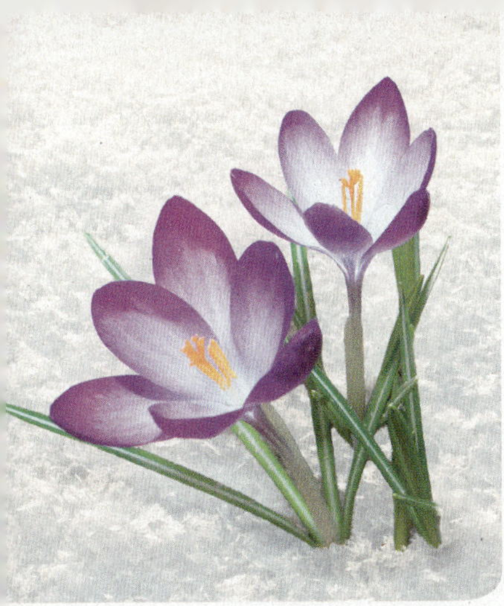

39 Neurocognitive Disorders

Nursing Care of Older Adults With Delirium and Dementia

Mary Ann Boyd and Rebecca Luebbert

KEYCONCEPTS

- cognition
- delirium
- dementia
- memory

LEARNING OBJECTIVES

After studying this chapter, you will be able to:

1. Examine the role of cognition and memory in neurocognitive disorders.
2. Relate the primary theories of Alzheimer disease to clinical symptoms and the course of the disorder.
3. Develop strategies to establish a person-centered therapeutic relationship with an individual with Alzheimer disease.
4. Using a clinical judgment model, formulate a person-centered, recovery-oriented nursing process for an individual with delirium and an individual with Alzheimer disease.
5. Differentiate medications used to treat people with Alzheimer disease and evaluate their effectiveness.
6. Develop wellness strategies for people with Alzheimer disease.
7. Contrast the mental health care provided for people with Alzheimer disease in inpatient-focused care and in community mental health care.
8. Support the integration of health and mental health care for people with Alzheimer disease.
9. Describe other types of neurocognitive disorders.

KEY TERMS

• acetylcholine (ACh) • acetylcholinesterase (AChE) • acetylcholinesterase inhibitors (AChEIs) • agnosia • amnestic MCI • amyloid precursor protein (APP) • antiamyloid immunotherapy • apathy • aphasia • APOE gene • apraxia • beta-amyloid plaques • catastrophic reactions • chronic traumatic encephalopathy (CTE) • confabulate • cortical dementia • disinhibition • disturbance of executive functioning • early-onset AD • free radicals • hypersexuality • hypervocalizations • illusions • impaired consciousness • late-onset AD • metabolic syndrome • mild cognitive impairment (MCI) • neurocognitive disorders • neurofibrillary tangles • nonamnestic MCI • oxidative stress • subcortical dementia • traumatic brain injury (TBI) • vascular neurocognitive disorder • visuospatial impairment • Alzheimer disease (AD)

INTRODUCTION

This chapter focuses on changes in cognitive functioning and neurocognitive disorders that are associated with the older adult. Although the first disorder discussed in this chapter, delirium, can occur at any time in an individual's life, it frequently occurs in the older adult. The other disorders discussed in this chapter are generally unique to the older adult.

Cognition is an intellectual process of acquiring, using, or manipulating perceptions and information. It involves the perception of reality and an understanding of its representations. Cognitive functions to be noted include the acquisition and use of language, the orientation of time and space, and the ability to learn and solve problems. Cognition also is the basis of judgment, reasoning, attention, comprehension, concept formation, planning, and the use of symbols (e.g., numbers and letters used in mathematics and writing).

KEYCONCEPT Cognition is based on a system of interrelated abilities, such as perception, reasoning, judgment, intuition, and memory, that allow one to be aware of oneself and one's surroundings. Individuals with impaired cognition may be unable to recognize that they are ill and in need of treatment.

Memory, a facet of cognition, refers to the ability to recall or reproduce what has been learned or experienced. It is more than simple storage and retrieval; it is a complex cognitive mental function that includes most areas of the brain, especially the hippocampus, which is believed to be essential to the transfer of some memories from short- to long-term storage. Defects of memory are an essential feature of many cognitive disorders, particularly dementia.

KEYCONCEPT Memory is a facet of cognition concerned with retaining and recalling past experiences, whether they occurred in the physical environment or internally as cognitive events.

Neurocognitive disorders are characterized by a decline in cognitive function from a previous level of functioning. These disorders are acquired and have not been present since early life. The diagnosis of a neurocognitive disorder is based on deficits in the following cognitive domains: *attention* (distractibility with multiple stimuli), *executive function* (planning, decision-making, working memory), *learning and memory* (recall and recognition), *language* (expressive including naming, work finding, fluency, grammatical syntax, and receptive language), *perceptual-motor* (visual perception, visuoconstructional, perceptual-motor), and *social cognition deficits* (recognition of emotions, ability to consider another's mental state) (American Psychiatric Association [APA], 2022).

The neurocognitive disorders discussed in this chapter include delirium, a disorder of acute cognitive impairment usually caused by a medical condition (e.g., infection), and dementia, characterized by chronic cognitive impairment. Dementia is differentiated from delirium by underlying cause, not by symptom patterns, which are often similar.

KEYCONCEPT Delirium is a disorder of acute cognitive impairment that is caused by a medical condition (e.g., infection), substance misuse, or multiple etiologies.

KEYCONCEPT Dementia is an umbrella term used to describe a decline in mental abilities that affects thinking, memory, reasoning, and behavior. Dementia impacts daily life and activities. It can be caused by certain neurologic conditions that affect the brain, and it worsens over time (NIA, 2024a).

Dementia can be further classified as cortical or subcortical to denote the location of the underlying pathology. **Cortical dementia** results from a disease process that globally afflicts the cortex. **Subcortical dementia** is caused by dysfunction or deterioration of deep gray- or white-matter structures inside the brain and brain stem. Symptoms of subcortical dementia may be more localized and tend to disrupt arousal, attention, and motivation, but they can produce a variety of clinical behavioral manifestations. In this chapter, one type of cortical dementia, Alzheimer disease (AD), is highlighted because it is the most prevalent form of dementia.

DELIRIUM

CLINICAL COURSE

Delirium is a disturbance in consciousness and an acute change in cognition and mental status that develops over a short time. It is usually reversible if the underlying cause is identified and treated quickly. It is a serious disorder and should always be treated as a medical emergency.

EMERGENCY CARE ALERT Individuals with delirium are in a state of confusion and disorientation that develops during a period of a few hours or days. If delirium is not treated in a timely manner, irreversible neurologic damage can occur. Delirium is a common complication in patients admitted to intensive care units and inpatient psychiatric units (Sakusic & Rabinstein, 2025).

DIAGNOSTIC CRITERIA

Impaired consciousness is the key diagnostic criterion for delirium. The patient becomes less aware of their environment and loses the ability to focus, sustain, and shift attention. Cognitive changes include issues with memory, orientation, and language. The patient may not know where they are, may not recognize familiar objects, or may be unable to carry on a conversation.

Delirium develops during a short period (compared with dementia, which develops gradually) (Patti & Gupta, 2023). Impaired alertness, apathy, anxiety, disorientation, and hallucinations commonly occur. Patients with delirium have a reduced ability to focus, difficulty in sustaining or shifting attention, changes in cognition, or perceptual disturbances. Although delirium may occur in any age group, it is most common among older adults. In this age group, delirium is often mistaken for dementia, which in turn leads to inappropriate treatment (Ramírez Echeverría et al., 2022).

Delirium can be categorized as *hyperactive* with agitation, increased psychomotor activity, and heightened level of arousal; *hypoactive* with somnolence and psychomotor retardation; or *mixed* with alternating hypoactive and hyperactive states. Hyperactive delirium is easily recognized, but hypoactive delirium is most common (Ramírez Echeverría et al., 2022). Delirium is different than dementia, although the presenting symptoms are often similar. Table 39.1 highlights the differences between delirium and dementia.

NCLEXNOTE Delirium and dementia have similar presentations. Because delirium can be life-threatening, identifying the potential underlying cause for the symptoms is a priority.

TABLE 39.1 DIFFERENTIATING DELIRIUM FROM DEMENTIA

Characteristics	Delirium	Dementia
Onset	Sudden	Slow development
24-hr course	Fluctuating	Stable
Consciousness	Reduced	Clear
Attention	Globally disoriented	Usually as expected
Cognition	Globally disoriented	Globally impaired
Hallucinations	Visual auditory	Possible
Orientation	Usually impaired	Often impaired
Psychomotor activity	Increased, reduced, or shifting	Often as expected
Speech	Often incoherent; slow or rapid	Often as expected
Involuntary movement	Often asterixis or coarse tremor	Rare
Physical illness or drug toxicity	One or both	Rare

Source: Alzheimer's Society. (2025). Delirium—symptoms, diagnosis and treatment. https://www.alzheimers.org.uk/get-support/daily-living/delirium

EPIDEMIOLOGY AND RISK FACTORS

Statistics concerning prevalence are based primarily on older adults in acute care settings. Estimated prevalence rates among patients in inpatient units worldwide are 17.7%. Among hospitalized older adults, the worldwide incidence of delirium ranges from 29% to 80% (Taylor et al., 2024). Delirium is particularly common in older postoperative patients. In some groups, such as those with dementia, the prevalence may be higher. Preexisting cognitive impairment is one of the greatest risk factors for delirium (Lindroth et al., 2024; see Boxes 39.1 and 39.2).

BOX 39.1

Risk Factors for Delirium

- AIDS
- Acute or chronic stress
- Admission to a long-term care institution
- Advanced age
- Bone fracture
- Changes in vital signs (including hypotension and hyper- or hypothermia)
- Electrolyte or metabolic imbalance (dehydration, renal failure, hyponatremia)
- Endocrine and metabolic disorders
- Functional dependence
- Infection (pneumonia, urinary tract)
- Medications (anticholinergic side effects)
- Pain
- Postcardiotomy
- Preexisting dementia
- Substance use and alcohol withdrawal

BOX 39.2

Clinical Judgment Vignette: Delirium

Margaret, a widowed 72-year-old living in her own home, has been having trouble sleeping. Her daughter visits her and suggests that she try an over-the-counter (OTC) sleeping medication. Margaret also takes antihistamines for allergies and the antidepressant amitriptyline. Three nights later, a neighbor calls the daughter, concerned because Margaret is wandering the streets, unable to find her home. When the neighbor approached Margaret to help her home, she began to scream and strike out at the neighbor.

The daughter visits immediately and discovers that her mother does not know who she is, does not know what time it is, appears disheveled, and is suspicious that people have been in her home stealing the things she cannot find. Margaret does not recall taking any medication, but when her daughter investigates, she finds that 10 pills of the new sleeping aid have already been used.

Building Clinical Judgment

1. Identify risk factors that may have contributed to Margaret's experiencing delirium.
2. How could the addition of an OTC sleeping medication interact with the antihistamine and antidepressant to be responsible for Margaret's delirium?

ETIOLOGY

Delirium in the older adult is associated with medications, infections, fluid and electrolyte imbalances, metabolic disturbances, hypoxia, or ischemia. The probability of the syndrome developing increases if some predisposing factors, such as advanced age, brain damage, or dementia, are also present. Sensory overload or underload, immobilization, sleep deprivation, infection, and psychosocial stress also contribute to delirium (Gogia & Fang, 2023).

RECOVERY-ORIENTED CARE FOR PEOPLE WITH DELIRIUM

Delirium is a medical emergency that is easily misdiagnosed as a dementia. Prompt treatment leads to recovery.

Teamwork and Collaboration: Working Toward Recovery

Although delirium may be recognized and diagnosed in any health care setting, appropriate intervention usually requires that the patient be admitted to an acute care setting for rigorous assessment and rapid treatment. Priority in care is identifying the underlying cause of the delirium. Interdisciplinary management of delirium includes two primary aspects: (1) elimination or correction of the underlying cause and (2) symptomatic and supportive measures (e.g., adequate rest, comfort, maintenance of fluid and electrolyte balance, and protection from injury).

Safety Issues

If possible, the use of all suspected medications should be stopped and vital signs should be monitored at least every 2 hours. Close observation of the patient with particular regard to changes in vital signs, behavior, and mental status is required. Patients are monitored until the delirium subsides or until discharge. If the delirium still exists at discharge, it is critical that referrals for postdischarge follow-up assessment and care be implemented.

EVIDENCE-BASED NURSING CARE FOR PEOPLE WITH DELIRIUM

The best management is prevention or early recognition of delirium. Special efforts should be made to include family members in the nursing process.

RECOGNIZING CUES: RELEVANT ASSESSMENT INFORMATION

The onset of symptoms is typically signaled by a rapid or acute change in behavior. Delirium is underdiagnosed, and symptoms are easily missed in people with mental disorders when it is assumed that the cognitive and behavioral changes are related to the mental disorder. An underlying medical cause should always be the first consideration.

Assessing the symptoms requires knowing what is expected for the individual. Caregivers, family members, or significant others should be interviewed because they can often provide valuable information. Family members may be the only resource for accurate information.

Physical Health Assessment

History should include a description of the onset, duration, range, and intensity of associated symptoms. Recent physical illness, dementia, depression, or other psychiatric illnesses should be identified. A physical examination should be conducted. Vital signs are crucial. Changes in activities of daily living (ADLs), use of sensory aids (eyeglasses and hearing aids), pain, and sleep should be documented. Recent laboratory results that might indicate hypoxia, hypoglycemia, and ST-segment elevation myocardial infarction (STEMI) should be considered. Assessment for infections that commonly underlie delirium, such as urinary tract infection, pneumonia, and sepsis from other sources, should be included. An unexpected neurologic assessment would suggest a transient ischemic attack (TIA), stroke, intracranial hemorrhage, or mass.

Medication

Many medications are associated with delirium (see Table 39.2). Medications and recent changes in the type and number, including over-the-counter (OTC)

TABLE 39.2 EXAMPLES OF MEDICATIONS THAT CAN CAUSE DELIRIUM

Class	Specific Medications
Anticholinergic	Antihistamines Chlorpheniramine Antiparkinsonian drugs (e.g., benztropine biperiden, or trihexyphenidyl) Atropine Belladonna alkaloids Diphenhydramine Phenothiazines Scopolamine Tricyclic antidepressants
Anticonvulsant	Phenobarbital Phenytoin Sodium valproate
Anti-inflammatory	Corticosteroids Ibuprofen Indomethacin Naproxen
Antiparkinsonian	Amantadine Carbidopa Levodopa
Antibiotics	Isoniazid Rifampin
Analgesic	Opioids Salicylates Synthetic narcotics
Cardiac	Beta-blockers Propranolol Clonidine Digitalis Lidocaine Methyldopa Quinidine Procainamide
Sedative—hypnotic	Barbiturates Benzodiazepines
Sympathomimetic	Amphetamines Phenylephrine Phenylpropanolamine
Over-the-counter medications	Compoz Excedrin PM Sleep-Eze Sominex
Miscellaneous	Acyclovir (antiviral) Aminophylline Amphotericin (antifungal) Bromides Cephalexin Chlorpropamide Cimetidine Disulfiram Lithium Metronidazole Theophylline Timolol ophthalmic

Source: Vanderbilt University Medical Center. (n.d.). Drugs that may cause delirium or problem behaviors. Retrieved January 15, 2025, https://www.caltcm.org/assets/HSAG/tab%2016-c_drugs%20that%20cause%20delirium%20or%20problem%20behaviors.pdf

medications, should be documented. Combinations of medications can interact and cause delirium. Cold medications, taken in sufficient quantities, may cause confusion, especially in older adults. A substance use history (including alcohol intake and smoking history) should be taken.

Psychosocial Cues

The following discussion highlights important psychosocial cues.

Mental Status

Rapid onset of global cognitive impairment that affects multiple aspects of intellectual functioning is the hallmark of delirium. Mental status evaluation reveals several changes:

- Fluctuations in level of consciousness with reduced awareness of the environment
- Difficulty focusing and sustaining or shifting attention
- Severely impaired memory, especially immediate and recent memory

Patients may be disoriented to time and place but rarely to person. Environmental perceptions are often disturbed. The patient may believe shadows in the room are really people. Thought content is often illogic, speech may be incoherent or inappropriate to the context. Mental status tends to fluctuate over the course of the day.

Behavior

People with delirium exhibit a wide range of behaviors, complicating the process of making a diagnosis and planning interventions. At times, the individual may be restless or agitated and at other times lethargic and slow to respond.

Family Environment

An assessment of living arrangements may provide information about sensory stimulation or social isolation. Assessing family interactions, support for the patient, and family members' ability to understand delirium is also important. The behaviors exhibited by the individual experiencing delirium may be frightening or at least confusing for family members. Some family members may actually contribute to the patient's increased agitation. At the same time, however, the family's presence may help to calm and reassure the patient.

ANALYZING CUES AND DEVELOPING HYPOTHESES

If delirium is established as the medical diagnosis, the nurse must address any life-threatening issues related to respiration and cardiovascular impairment. If the patient is combative, de-escalation becomes a priority. Because there are many potential issues that could be underlying delirium, other priorities will be based on the identified causes.

PLANNING RECOVERY AND WELLNESS OUTCOMES: GENERATING SOLUTIONS

The primary treatment goal is resolution of the delirious episode with return to the previous cognitive status and identification of the underlying causes of this disorder. Outcomes include the following:

- Correction of the underlying physiologic alteration
- Resolution of confusion
- Family member verbalization of understanding of confusion
- Prevention of injury

The planning should also include steps to prevent the reoccurrence of the delirium.

TAKING ACTION: NURSING INTERVENTIONS

Important interventions include providing a safe and therapeutic environment, maintaining fluid and electrolyte balance and adequate nutrition, and preventing aspiration and decubitus ulcers, which are common complications. Other interventions relate to individual symptoms and underlying causes.

Complementary Therapies

There is strong evidence that complementary interventions are effective in reducing agitation and delirium in older adults. Aromatherapy, massage, acupuncture, and therapeutic touch have been used successfully in reducing agitation and aggressive behavior (Devlin, 2024).

Medications

There is no medication for delirium, but as the underlying medical issue is treated, the individual may be given medication to treat the symptoms associated with delirium, such as agitation, inattention, combativeness, insomnia, and psychosis. Dosages are usually kept very low, especially with older adults, and the medication is selected in light of the potential side effects (particularly anticholinergic effects, hypotension, and respiratory suppression).

Research suggests that supportive measures and treatment of precipitating factors are more effective than antipsychotics (Torbic et al., 2024). Benzodiazepines are also used when the delirium is related to alcohol withdrawal. In some patients, benzodiazepines may further impair cognition because of the sedation.

Patients should be monitored for sedation, hypotension, or extrapyramidal symptoms. Although mental status often fluctuates during delirium, it may also be influenced by these medications, so any changes or worsening of mental status after administration of the medication should be reported immediately to the prescriber. Some side effects may also be confused with the symptoms of delirium. For example, akathisia (see Chapter 11), a side effect of antipsychotics, may appear as agitation or restlessness. Medications for treating symptoms related to delirium should be discontinued as soon as possible.

Psychosocial Interventions

Patients with delirium need frequent interaction and support if they are confused or hallucinating. Patients should be encouraged to express their fears and discomforts that result from frightening or disconcerting psychotic experiences. Adequate lighting, easy-to-read calendars and clocks, a reasonable noise level, and frequent verbal orientation may reduce this frightening experience. If the patient wears eyeglasses or uses hearing aids, these devices should be used. Including familiar personal possessions in the environment may also help. These interventions have been shown to reduce the need for antipsychotic medication and reduced length of hospitalization (Ryan, 2024).

A safe environment is important to protect the patient from injury. A predictable, orienting environment will help to reestablish order to the patient's life. That is, a calendar, clocks, and other items may be provided to help orient the patient to time, place, and person. If the patient is agitated, de-escalation techniques should be used (see Chapter 20). Physical restraint should be avoided.

Families can also be encouraged to work with staff to reorient the patient and provide a supportive environment. Families need to understand that important decisions requiring the patient's input should be delayed if possible until the patient has recovered. Although patients may be able to participate in decision-making, they may not remember the decision later.

Psychoeducation

To prevent future occurrences, provide education to the patient and family about the underlying cause of the delirium. If the delirium is not resolved before discharge, family members need to know how to care for the patient at home.

Promoting Safety

Behaviors exhibited by the individual with delirium, such as hallucinations, delusions, illusions, aggression, or agitation (restlessness or excitability), may pose safety issues. Because individuals with delirium are more likely to fall or injure themselves during a confused state, special precautions and safety measures should be considered. The patient must be protected from physical harm by using low beds, guardrails, and careful supervision. Delirium management and fall prevention may be implemented for any patient at risk for falls.

BOX 39.3

Psychoeducation Checklist: Delirium

When caring for the patient with delirium, be sure to include the caregivers, as appropriate, and address the following topic areas in the teaching plan:

- Psychopharmacologic agents, if used, including drug action, dosage, frequency, and possible adverse effects
- Underlying cause of delirium
- Mental status changes
- Safety measures
- Hydration and nutrition
- Avoidance of restraints
- Decision-making guidelines

Evaluation

Resolution of confusion is the primary goal. The end result of delirium may be full recovery, incomplete recovery, incomplete recovery with some residual cognitive impairment, or a downward course leading to death.

Continuum of Care

Patients with delirium may present in a number of treatment settings (e.g., home, nursing home, ambulatory care, day treatment, outpatient setting, hospital). Patients usually are admitted to an acute care setting for rapid evaluation and treatment of the underlying etiology. For more information on caring for patients with delirium, see Box 39.3.

ALZHEIMER DISEASE

One of the most challenging disorders is **Alzheimer disease (AD)**—a progressive dementia that impacts most families either directly or indirectly. Nurses in all areas of practice may encounter patients—or patients' family members—with this disorder.

CLINICAL COURSE

AD is a degenerative, progressive, neuropsychiatric disorder that results in cognitive impairment, emotional and behavioral changes, physical and functional decline, and ultimately death. Gradually, the patient's ability to carry out ADLs declines, although physical status often remains intact until late in the disease. Although primarily a disorder of older adults, AD has been diagnosed in patients as young as 35 years.

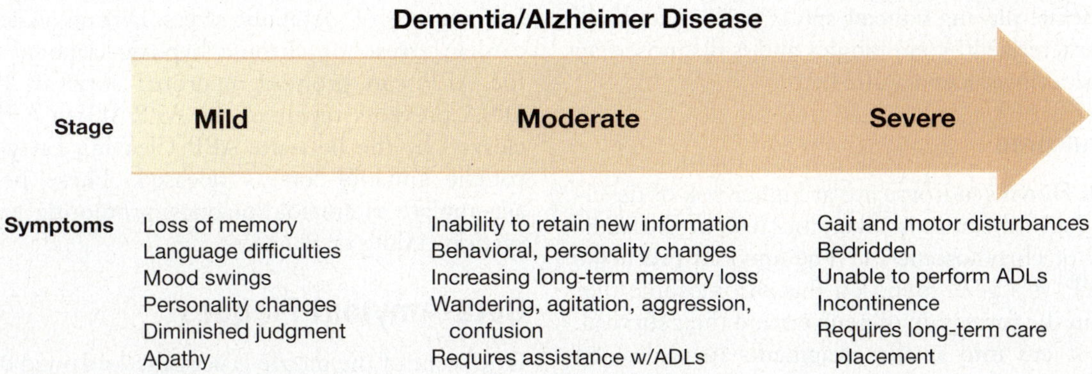

FIGURE 39.1 Alzheimer disease progression. ADLs, activities of daily living.

Two subtypes have been identified: **early-onset AD** (age 65 years and younger) and late-onset AD (age older than 65 years). **Late-onset AD** is much more common than early-onset AD, but early-onset AD has a more rapid progression. AD is also routinely conceptualized in terms of three stages: mild, moderate, and severe. Signs and symptoms of AD change as the patient passes from one phase of the illness to another (Fig. 39.1).

DIAGNOSTIC CRITERIA

The diagnosis of AD is made on clinical grounds, but verification is only confirmed during autopsy. The essential feature of AD is cognitive decline from a previous level of functioning in one or more cognitive domains (attention, executive function, learning and memory, language, perceptual-motor, or social cognition) (National Institute on Aging [NIA], 2024b). These deficits interfere with independence in ADLs. Typical deficits include **aphasia** (i.e., alterations in language ability), **apraxia** (i.e., impaired ability to execute motor activities despite intact motor functioning), **agnosia** (i.e., failure to recognize or identify objects despite intact sensory function), or a **disturbance of executive functioning** (i.e., ability to think abstractly, plan, initiate, sequence, monitor, and stop complex behavior).

Alzheimer Disease Across the Life Span

AD is diagnosed when clinical symptoms first appear. Although the disease process begins prior to clinical symptoms, neuropathologic changes occur asymptomatically. The disease is first evident with the appearance of biomarkers involving the processing and clearance of protein fragments. Research is ongoing to determine when the neuropathologic changes first appear (Jack et al., 2024).

EPIDEMIOLOGY AND RISK FACTORS

In 2024, an estimated 6.9 million Americans had AD. One in 9 (11.3%) Americans older than 65 years had AD, and approximately 200,00 Americans younger than 65 years had early onset (2024 Alzheimer's disease facts and figures, 2024). By 2050, the population of Americans over the age of 65 is projected to grow from 56 million in 2022 to 82 million (Mather & Scommegna, 2024). With this increase in the older-adult population, the number of those with AD will also grow. Almost two-thirds of Americans with AD are people assigned female at birth (Alzheimer's Association, 2025b).

Dementia appears to affect all groups, but studies in the United States reveal a higher incidence in Black individuals (twice as likely; Alzheimer's Association, 2025c) and Latinx individuals (1.5 times as likely) than in White individuals (2024 Alzheimer's disease facts and figures, 2024; American Brain Foundation, 2024). AD is the fifth leading cause of death among older adults in the United States (2024 Alzheimer's disease facts and figures, 2024).

General Risk Factors

The greatest risk factors for late onset are older age, genetics, family history of AD, and traumatic brain injury (TBI). After age 65, the risk of AD doubles every five years. Researchers have found several genes that increase the risk of AD (discussed later in this chapter). Compared with the general population, first-degree biologic relatives of individuals with early-onset AD are more likely to experience the disorder. The risk of developing AD is increased in medical conditions such as hypertension and diabetes. Studies show that those with fewer years of education or those who have had a prior head injury are at higher risk of developing AD (Alzheimer's Association, 2025d).

Traumatic Brain Injury (TBI)

Traumatic brain injury (TBI), disruption of expected brain function caused by a blow to the head or penetration of the skull, is associated with dementia. The greater the number of TBIs, the greater the risk of developing AD. **Chronic traumatic encephalopathy (CTE)** is caused by repeated blows to the head, such as those that occur while playing contact sports such as football. CTE is characterized by tau tangles and is diagnosed by autopsy (Pszczołowska et al., 2024).

Down Syndrome

People with Down syndrome are at higher risk of developing AD than others, most likely because of the additional copy of chromosome 21. The amyloid precursor protein (APP) is a gene found on this chromosome that is involved in the formation of neurons and their survival. This gene is cut into smaller fragments (peptides) by enzymes. The extra copy of chromosome 21 increases the amount of amyloid beta (A-beta) fragments in the brain, which in turn increases the possibility of formation of **beta-amyloid plaques**. By the age of 50 years, most people with Down syndrome have increased levels of beta-amyloid plaques and tau tangles in their brain (Alzheimer's Association, 2025e).

Metabolic Syndrome

Metabolic syndrome is associated with the development of AD. **Metabolic syndrome**, a cluster of conditions (hypertension, hyperglycemia, abdominal obesity, and hyperlipidemia) that occur together, increases the risk of heart disease, stroke, and diabetes. Metabolic syndrome is associated with microvascular changes in the brain, which in turn appear to cause mitochondrial dysfunction. Insulin resistance is thought to play a key role in the neuroinflammation and loss of synapses (Azizan et al., 2024).

Other Risk Factors

Other general risks factors associated with AD include smoking, physical inactivity, elevated body mass index (BMI), and diet, Emerging evidence suggests that diets rich in antioxidants and omega-3 fatty acids may have a protective effect against AD.

ETIOLOGY

Researchers have yet to identify a definitive cause of AD, but a combination of genetic, environmental, and lifestyle factors influences an individual's risk for developing the disease. Changes in the brain may begin decades before symptoms appear. During the very early stage of AD, changes are occurring in the brain including unexpected buildup of proteins that form the amyloid plaques and tau tangles. Healthy neurons stop functioning (National Institute on Aging [NIH], 2023).

Amyloid Precursor Protein (APP)

The **amyloid precursor protein (APP)** located on the cell membrane appears to have a neuroprotective role in situations of metabolic stress. During an acute stroke, cardiac arrest, or chronic hypoxic–ischemic condition, the APP can promote neuronal survival. Damage to DNA prevents repair of the APP. When APP is cut or cleaved by the beta-site APP Cleaving Enzyme 1, neurotoxic amyloid-beta is released. These peptides can accumulate as amyloid plaques, promoting neurodegeneration (Wang et al., 2024).

Beta-Amyloid Plaques

One piece of the puzzle is partially explained by a leading theory that **beta-amyloid plaques**, made up of proteins, clump together in the brain and destroy cholinergic neurons. Research suggests that beta-amyloid deposits impair the expected function of pericytes, which are cells important for controlling the removal of protein from the brain. This leads to further accumulation of the protein. Beta-amyloid is hypothesized to interfere with the process of storing memories through interrupting synaptic connection. Symptoms such as aphasia and visuospatial anomalies are attributable to plaque formation (Azargoonjahromi, 2024).

Neurofibrillary Tangles

Neurofibrillary tangles are made of unexpectedly twisted protein threads found inside the brain cells. The main component of the tangles is *tau*, a protein that stabilizes the microtubules of transport cells. In AD, tau separates from the microtubules. Loose tau proteins tangle with each other, causing the characteristic neurofibrillary tangles. When microtubules disintegrate, the neuron's transport system collapses, resulting in cell death (Liu et al., 2024).

Synaptic Micron RNA and Neurotransmission

In patients with AD, neurotransmission is reduced, neurons are lost, and the hippocampal neurons degenerate. Several major neurotransmitters are affected, such as **acetylcholine** (ACh), norepinephrine, and serotonin important, in cognitive functioning and memory. Researchers hypothesize that alterations in microRNA (molecules involved in gene expression) occur impacting synaptic transmission (see Chapter 7) (Dalal et al., 2024).

One of the early hypotheses was that cholinergic dysfunction contributed to cognitive deficits associated with aging and AD. This hypothesis was based on evidence that alterations in the cholinergic systems induced cognitive deficits similar to those in AD and aging. When cholinergic functioning was increased, there were beneficial effects. We now understand that the pathogenesis of AD is much more complicated than a single cause, even though the primary medications for AD target the cholinergic system (Dalal et al., 2024).

Genetic Factors

Mutations on three genes are identified as causing AD through altering amyloid-beta processing and are transmitted through genetic inheritance—*APP*, *PSEN1*, and *PSEN2*. These mutations are associated with early-onset AD and explain 5% to 10% of the occurrence of early-onset AD. Most early-onset AD cases do not have a clear genetic pattern of inheritance (Krishnamurthy et al., 2024).

Late-onset AD is associated with the **APOE gene** which transports cholesterol in the bloodstream. Three forms of the *APOE* gene (e2, e3, and e4) are inherited from each biologic parent. The e3 form is the most common and is believed to neither increase nor decrease the risk of AD. The e4 form is the next most common and is found to increase the risk of developing AD. People with one copy of the e4 form are three times as likely to develop AD compared with those who have the e3 form, and those with two copies of the e4 form have an 8 to 12 times greater risk. The least common *APOE* gene, e2, is relatively rare and may decrease one's risk of AD (Jackson et al., 2024).

Oxidative Stress, Free Radicals, and Mitochondrial Dysfunction

It is hypothesized that in AD-affected brains, there is a rapid increase in the formation of **free radicals** (i.e., highly reactive molecules), which can lead to **oxidative stress** that damages other cellular molecules such as proteins, lipids, and nucleic acids. Studies suggest that oxidative stress may result in changes in mitochondria which may lead to dysfunctional gene expression (Ekundayo et al., 2024).

Inflammation

Inflammation is now considered as one of the many factors that contribute to the development of AD. The hypothesis is that inflammation may damage small blood vessels and brain cells, initiating a cascade of pathologic events related to oxidative damage and dysregulated amyloid metabolism (Seddon et al., 2024).

Gut–Brain Axis Alteration

The gut microbial composition is thought to influence several age-related neurologic disorders including AD. It is proposed that alterations in gut microbial composition contribute to the pathogenesis of AD. Typically, the gastrointestinal (GI) tract epithelium and the blood–brain barrier are protective physiologic barriers. After aging, these protective barriers become more permeable. If repeated chronic infection occurs, exposure to exotoxins such as lipopolysaccharides (LPS) and bacterial amyloids occurs because they pass more easily through the compromised GI tract and blood–brain barrier. Evidence reveals that aging together with repeated chronic infections lead to altered activation of microglial cells that aggravates inflammatory responses, A-beta fibrillation, and the aggregation of amyloid-beta in the brain (Qu et al., 2024).

Family Response to Disorder

Families are the first to be aware of the cognitive issue, often before the patient, who can be unaware of the extent of memory impairment. When finally confirmed, the actual diagnosis can be devastating to the family. Unlike delirium, a diagnosis of AD means long-term care responsibilities, while the essence of a family member diminishes day by day. Most families keep their relative at home as long as possible to maintain contact and to avoid costly nursing home placement. The two symptoms that often result in nursing home placement are incontinence that cannot be managed and behavioral issues, such as wandering and aggression.

RECOVERY-ORIENTED CARE FOR PEOPLE WITH ALZHEIMER DISEASE

AD has a long clinical course—at least 20 years. AD research is quickly advancing, and it is likely that treatment will provide more options to reduce or reverse the illness trajectory. Hope for the future should be instilled in patients and families. Recovery is an important focus for people with AD, reminding families that wellness is possible despite the presence of a chronic disease.

Teamwork and Collaboration: Working Toward Recovery

The nature and range of services needed by patients and families throughout the illness can vary dramatically at different stages. As with any other patient, the individual with AD should be the center of the decision-making process. The plan should include educational and supportive programs individualized for the patient's self-identified needs. Ideally, plans should be designed to support self-awareness, self-esteem, maintenance of abilities, and management of behavioral symptoms and health promotion.

Treatment efforts currently focus on managing cognitive symptoms, delaying cognitive decline (e.g., memory loss; confusion; and issues with learning, speech, reasoning), treating the noncognitive symptoms (e.g., psychosis, mood symptoms, agitation), and supporting the caregivers to improve the quality of life for both patients and their caregivers.

Safety Issues

The priority of care changes throughout the course of AD. Initially, the priority is delaying cognitive decline and supporting family members. Later, the priority is protecting the patient from injury because of the patient's lack of judgment. Near the end, the physical needs of the patient are the focus of care.

EVIDENCE-BASED NURSING CARE FOR PEOPLE WITH ALZHEIMER DISEASE

Development and implementation of appropriate, effective, and safe nursing services for the care and support of patients with AD and their families is a particular challenge because of the complex nature of the illness. See Nursing Care Plan 39.1.

> **NCLEXNOTE** Needs and problematic behaviors of patients with AD vary throughout the course of the disorder. Early in the disorder, the nurse focuses on support, education, and cognitive interventions for depression. As AD progresses, priority care becomes safety interventions.

RECOGNIZING CUES: RELEVANT ASSESSMENT INFORMATION

The assessment begins with the physical health of the individual because the nurse will make a recommendation regarding the extent of physical care that is needed. The nurse should be alert to medical issues that contribute to dementia such as hypertension and diabetes.

Physical Health

A review of body systems must be conducted on each patient suspected of having AD. The neurologic function of the patient with AD is usually preserved through the early and middle stages of the disease, although seizures, gait disturbances, and tremors may occur at any time. In the later stages of the disease, neurologic signs, such as flexion contractures and primitive reflexes, are prominent features.

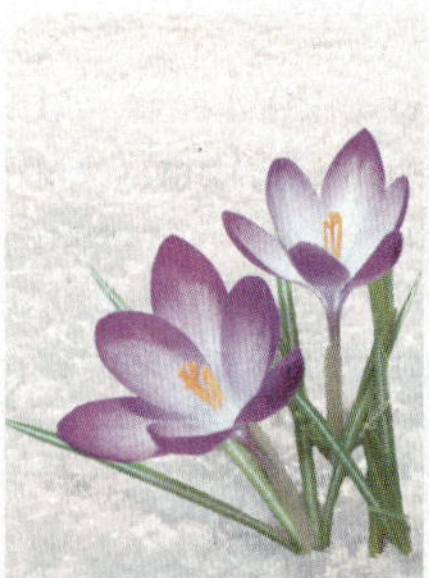

CLINICAL JUDGMENT NURSING CARE PLAN 39.1

The Patient With Dementia

Lorine is an 86-year-old widow who lives independently. Recently, her children have noticed that she is becoming more forgetful and seems to have periods of confusion. She has agreed to have someone help her during the day. Her oldest son lives with her and is with her during the evening and night. Lorine refuses to see a health care provider but did agree to go in for a routine checkup. Her daughter helped her get dressed and took her to the primary care office.

Setting: Primary Care Office

Assessment Cues: Lorine, well-groomed and accompanied by her daughter, says there is nothing wrong, but her daughter disagrees. A review of body systems reveals poor hearing and vision but is otherwise unremarkable. Her daughter reports that Lorine has become very suspicious of her neighbors and has changed her locks several times.

Associated Psychiatric Diagnosis	Medications
Probable Alzheimer disease	Galantamine 4 mg twice a day (BID); titrate to 8 mg BID over 4 weeks.

Priority Hypothesis: Changes in Memory

Important Characteristics	Associated Considerations
Inability to recall information Inability to recall past events Observed instances of forgetfulness Forgets to perform daily activities (e.g., grooming)	Neurocognitive changes associated with dementia

Planning Recovery and Wellness Outcomes

Initial	Long Term
Maintain or improve current memory	Delay cognitive decline associated with dementia

Clinical Judgment Nursing Care Plan 39.1 Continued

Taking Action: Nursing Interventions

Interventions	Rationale	Ongoing Assessment
Develop memory cues in home. Have clocks and calendars clearly displayed. Make lists for the patients.	Maintaining current level of memory involves providing cues that will help the patient recall information.	Contact family members for the patient's ability to use memory cues.
Teach the patient and family about taking an acetylcholinesterase inhibitor. Review expected effects and side effects. Develop a titration schedule with the family to decrease the appearance of side effects.	Confidence and self-esteem improve when a person looks well groomed.	Monitor response to suggestions.
Observe patient for visuospatial impairment. If present, sequence habitual activities such as eating, dressing, and bathing.	Visuospatial impairment is one of the symptoms of dementia.	Observe for appropriate dress, bathing, eating, and so on.

Evaluation

Outcomes	Revised Outcomes	Interventions
Lorine did have some improvement in memory. Suspiciousness and behavioral symptoms improved.	Continue maintaining memory.	Continue with memory cues and galantamine.

Physical Functions

Assessment of physical functions includes ADLs, recent changes in functional abilities, use of sensory aids (e.g., eyeglasses, hearing aids), activity level, and assessment of pain. Eyeglasses and hearing aids may need to be in place before other assessments can be made.

At first, limitations may primarily involve instrumental activities of daily living (IADLs) (e.g., shopping, preparing meals, performing other household chores). Later in the disease process, basic physical dysfunctions occur, such as incontinence, ataxia, dysphagia, and contractures. Incontinence can be a major source of stress and a considerable burden to family caregivers. Evaluation of the patient's functional abilities includes bathing, dressing, toileting, feeding, nutritional status, physical mobility, sleep patterns, and pain.

Self-Care

Alterations in the central nervous system (CNS) associated with AD impair the patient's ability to collect information from the environment, retrieve memories, retain new information, and give meaning to current situations. Therefore, patients with AD often neglect self-care activities. Periodically, assessment parameters need to be reevaluated because patients with AD may neglect activities such as bathing, eating, or skin care.

Sleep–Wake Disturbances

Patients with AD have frequent daytime napping and nighttime periods of wakefulness, with little rapid eye movement (REM) sleep. Circadian rhythms are disrupted as the amyloid beta (A-beta) increases. Tau pathology and increases in beta-amyloid plaques are associated with restlessness, irritability, and general sleep impairment (Chen et al., 2024a; Gonzales et al., 2024).

Activity and Exercise

One of the earliest symptoms of AD is withdrawal from expected activities. Motor activity is affected in the mild stages of AD and can lead to early issues in functional performance (Chen et al., 2024b). As the disease progresses, the patient may just sit staring at a blank wall.

Nutrition

Malnutrition is the most common nutritional issue in patients with AD (He et al., 2024). Nutritional assessment is very important in light of the recent understanding that changes in gut microbiota affect the brain's physiologic, behavioral, and cognitive functions (Samuelsson et al., 2021). Foods high in fat content and foods highly processed are detrimental to the support of a healthy gut microbiome.

Eating can become an issue for a patient with AD and is associated with rapid cognitive decline. As the disease progresses, patients may lose the ability to feed themselves or recognize that what is being offered is food. Some patients with AD are bulimic or hyperoral (eating or chewing almost everything possible and sometimes with an insatiable appetite). Other patients with AD experience anorexia and have no appetite.

Pain

Although AD is not usually considered a physically painful disorder, patients often have other comorbid physical diseases that may be painful. In the early stages of AD, the patient can usually respond to verbal questions regarding pain. Later, it may be difficult to assess the comfort level objectively, especially if the patient cannot communicate. Some patients in the end stage of AD become hypersensitive to touch.

Subtle behavioral changes, such as lethargy, anxiety, or restlessness, or more obvious physical signs, such as pyrexia, tachypnea, or tachycardia, may be the only indications of actual or impending illness. Observing for changes in patterns of nonverbal communication, such as facial expressions, may help in identifying indicators of pain. **Hypervocalizations** (disturbed vocalizations such as screams, curses, moans, groans, and verbal repetitiveness), restlessness, and agitation are other possible signs of pain.

Psychosocial Cues

Personality changes almost always accompany AD. Researchers have identified two contrasting patterns. One is marked by apathy, lack of spontaneity, and passivity. The other involves growing irritability, sarcasm, self-preoccupation, and intolerance of and lack of concern for others.

Mental Status and Appearance

The mental status assessment can be difficult for the patient with AD because cognitive disturbance is the clinical hallmark of AD. However, family members should also be a part of any assessment, especially early in the disease process. There are several screening instruments that can be used in detecting symptoms of dementia. The Mini-Cog is used by clinicians in assessing whether an individual has symptoms of AD (Borson et al., 2003). The AD8 Dementia Screening Interview, which is given to a family member, is a brief, sensitive measure that differentiates between those with and without dementia (Galvin et al., 2005, 2006). The AD8 contains eight questions asking the family member to rate any change ("yes" or "no") in memory, problem-solving abilities, orientation, and ADLs. The higher the number of changes, the more likely dementia is present. The nurse should suspect delirium in instances where cognitive deterioration occurs rapidly.

Memory

The most dramatic and consistent cognitive impairment is in memory. Patients with dementia appear mildly forgetful and repetitive in conversation. They misplace objects, miss appointments, and forget what they were just doing. They may lose track of a conversation or television show. Initially, they may complain of memory issues, but rapidly in the course of the illness, insight is lost, and they become unaware of what is lost. Sometimes, they may **confabulate**, making what appears to be an appropriate explanation of why the information or object is missing. Eventually, all aspects of memory are impaired and even long-term memories are affected. During the interview, short-term memory loss is usually readily evident by the patient's inability to recall three or four words given to them at the beginning of the assessment. Often, the earliest symptom of AD is the inability to retain new information.

Language

Language is also progressively impaired. Individuals with AD may initially have agnosia (difficulty finding a word in a sentence or in naming an object). They may be able to talk around a topic in an attempt to answer a question, but the loss is noticeable. Later, fluent aphasia develops; comprehension diminishes; and, finally, they become mute and unresponsive to directions or information.

Visuospatial Impairment

Visuospatial impairment, a deficit in the ability to perform tasks that require sensory and motor coordination (e.g., drawing and writing), develops early in AD. An inaccurate clock drawing is diagnostic of impairment in this area (Fig. 39.2). Sequencing tasks, such as cooking or other self-care skills, become impaired. The individual becomes unable to complete complex tasks that require calculations, such as balancing a check book.

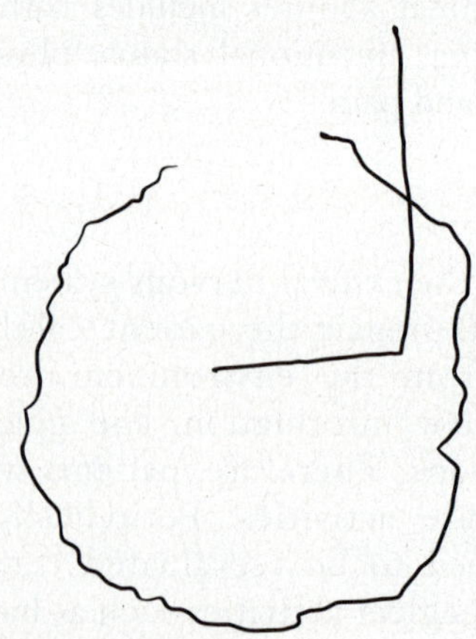

FIGURE 39.2 Clock drawing by a patient with moderate Alzheimer disease. The patient was asked to draw a clock at 3:00 PM.

Executive Functioning

Judgment, reasoning, and the ability to problem solve or make decisions are also impaired later in the disorder, closer to the time of nursing home placement. It is hypothesized that as the disease progresses, the degeneration of neurons is spread diffusely throughout the neocortex.

Psychotic Symptoms

Delusional thought content and hallucinations are common in people with AD. These psychotic symptoms differ from those of schizophrenia.

Suspiciousness, Delusions, and Illusions

Illusions, or mistaken perceptions, are also common in patients with AD. For example, an individual with AD mistakes their spouse for their parent. The spouse resembles the parent in that the spouse is roughly the age the parent was when they died. If an illusion becomes a false fixed belief, it is a delusion.

As the disease progresses, delusions often develop in people with AD (Cloak et al., 2024). These characteristic delusions are different from those discussed in the psychotic disorders. Common delusional beliefs include the following:

- Belief that their partner is engaging in marital infidelity
- Belief that other patients or staff are trying to hurt them
- Belief that staff or family members are impersonators
- Belief that people are stealing their belongings
- Belief that strangers are living in their home
- Belief that people on television are real and not actors

Hallucinations

Visual, rather than auditory, hallucinations are the most common in AD (Alzheimer's Society, 2021). A frequent complaint is that children, adults, or strange creatures are entering the house or the patient's room. These hallucinations may not seem unusual to the patient. If possible, the content and form of hallucination should be ascertained and documented because this information may suggest a treatable symptom or another disorder. For example, an auditory hallucination commanding the patient to kill themselves may be caused by a treatable depression, not AD. In some cases, hallucinations may be pleasant, such as children being in the room, or the hallucinations may be frightening and uncomfortable.

Mood Changes

A depressed mood is common, but major depression and AD appear to be separate disorders. Many people with AD experience one or more depressive episodes with symptoms such as psychomotor retardation, anxiety, feelings of guilt and worthlessness, sadness, frequent crying, insomnia, loss of appetite, weight loss, and suicidal rumination. Depressive symptoms are most prevalent in the early stages of AD, which may be attributed to the patient's awareness of cognitive changes, memory loss, and functional decline (Huang et al., 2024).

Anxiety

Moderate anxiety is a natural reaction to the fear engendered by gradual deterioration of intellectual function and the realization of impending loss of control over one's life. Failure to complete a task formerly regarded as simple creates a source of anxiety in patient with AD. As patients with AD become unsure of their surroundings and the expectations of others, they frequently react with fear and distress. Anxious behavior occurs when the patient is pressed to perform beyond their ability.

Catastrophic Reactions

Catastrophic reactions are overreactions or extreme anxiety reactions to everyday situations. Catastrophic responses occur when environmental stressors are allowed to continue or increase beyond the patient's threshold of stress tolerance. Behaviors indicative of catastrophic reactions typically include verbal or physical aggression, violence, agitated or anxious behavior, emotional outbursts, noisy behavior, compulsive or repetitive behavior, agitated night awakening, and other behaviors in which the patient is cognitively or socially inaccessible. Factors that contribute to catastrophic responses in patients with progressive cognitive decline include fatigue, a change in routine (e.g., faster pace, caregiver), demands beyond the patient's ability, overwhelming sensory stimuli, and physical stressors (e.g., pain, hunger).

Behavioral Responses

Characteristic behaviors are associated with AD. The following discussion summarizes the most common ones.

Apathy and Withdrawal

Apathy, the inability or unwillingness to become involved with one's environment, is common in AD, especially in the moderate to late stages. Apathy leads to withdrawal from the environment and a gradual loss of empathy for others. This lack of empathy is very difficult for families and friends to understand.

Restlessness, Agitation, and Aggression

Restlessness, agitation, and aggression are relatively common in the moderate to late stages of AD. Restlessness should be further evaluated to determine its underlying cause. If the restlessness occurs during medication change or adjustment, side effects should be suspected.

Aberrant Motor Behavior

Symptoms such as fidgeting, picking at clothing, wringing hands, loud vocalizations, and wandering may all be signs of such underlying conditions as dehydration, medication reaction, pain, or infection (suggesting delirium). One of the most difficult behaviors for which to determine an underlying cause is hypervocalization, common in the later stages of AD. Hypervocalizations often occur during a hospitalization or nursing home placement. In the assessment of hypervocalizations, it is important to identify when the behavior is occurring; antecedents of the behavior; and any related events, such as a family member leaving or a change in stimulation.

Disinhibition

One of the most frustrating symptoms of AD is **disinhibition,** acting on thoughts and feelings without exercising appropriate social judgment. In AD, the patient may decide that they are more comfortable naked than with clothes. Or the patient may not be able to find their clothes and may walk into a room of people without any clothes on. This behavior is extremely disconcerting to family members and can also lead to nursing home placement.

Hypersexuality

A closely related symptom is **hypersexuality,** which is inappropriate and socially unacceptable sexual behavior. The patient begins talking and behaving in ways that are uncharacteristic of premorbid behavior. This behavior is very difficult for family members and nursing home staff.

Stress and Coping Skills

Patients with AD seem extremely sensitive to stressful situations and often do not have the coping abilities to deal with such situations. A careful assessment of the triggers that precede stressful situations will help in understanding a provoking event.

Social Network and Support System

AD interferes with an individual's ability to interact socially as much as it disrupts intellectual functioning. The patient's whole social network is affected by AD, and the primary caregiver of an individual with AD (usually the partner or offspring in a community setting) is often considered a copatient. It is important to assess the family caregiver's ability to use supportive mechanisms to maintain their own integrity and mental health throughout the disease process.

If the patient still resides in the community, a home visit will prove useful because it provides information about the patient in the natural environment. From this assessment, the situational and psychosocial stressors that affect the family and patient can be identified, so interventions to strengthen coping strategies, including the ability to seek help from appropriate community resources, can be developed.

Spiritual Assessment

The diagnosis of AD can be a devastating moment for the patient and family. For individuals who practice a faith or religion, they most likely will want to reach out to their religious/spiritual community for support. Using the religious assessment section in Chapter 10 can help the patient and family identify religious or spiritual resources. Establishing a religious/spiritual connection early in the disease process is important not only for the patient, but especially for the caregiver and family. For patients and families who do not identify with any faith or spiritual family, they may be interested in establishing a relationship within a spiritual or religious group.

Quality of Life

Quality of life is always a concern for someone with a progressive dementia. Care arrangements will ultimately impact the individual's quality of life. That is, as the dementia progresses, the individual will require more care that leads to a loss of independence. Eliciting the patient's perspective of their quality of life can provide direction for nursing interventions to help improve and maintain their quality of life.

Strength and Wellness Assessment

Determining a baseline of strengths and personal wellness practices can provide cues about future interventions. For example, if an individual is an avid reader or card player, that activity can be encouraged. If a patient does not engage in any wellness activities such as walking or yoga, this is an opportunity to enhance wellness by providing opportunities for the patient to engage in these activities.

ANALYZING CUES AND DEVELOPING HYPOTHESES

The unique and changing needs of these patients present a challenge for nurses in all settings. Priorities of care vary according to the stage of the disease. Early on, memory impairment and confusion may be present. An individual may begin to feel less connected and engaged in usual activities. As the disease progresses, the patient may have difficulty with their ADLs. Safety concerns may be present, especially if the patient is agitated, aggressive, or prone to wondering. In late stages of AD, the patient may be completely reliant on others in meeting basic health care needs.

PLANNING FOR RECOVERY AND WELLNESS OUTCOMES: GENERATING SOLUTIONS

Planning for outcomes involves both the patient and caregiver. For the patient with dementia, recovery means short-term goals that are meaningful within the patient's ability. In the beginning of the disease process, the goals may focus on memory enhancement, maintaining physical functioning, and supporting independence. As the disease progresses, new goals may include safety issues, nutrition, and medication adherence.

THERAPEUTIC RELATIONSHIP

The therapeutic relationship is the basis for interventions for the patient with dementia and their family. Care of the patient entails a long-term relationship needing much support and expert nursing care. Interventions should be delivered within the relationship context.

TAKING ACTIONS: NURSING INTERVENTIONS

The nursing interventions should be modified throughout the course of the disorder. The following discussion includes interventions that are used throughout the progression of the dementia.

Self-Care Interventions

Patients should be encouraged to maintain as much self-care as possible. If eyeglasses and hearing aids are needed but not used, patients are more likely to have false perceptual experiences (hallucinations).

Oral hygiene can be an issue and requires excellent basic nursing care. Aging and many medications reduce salivary flow, which can lead to a painfully dry and cracking oral mucosa. Periodontal disease (a persistent low-grade inflammatory condition caused by pathogenic microorganisms) has been linked to increase in the amyloid beta (A-beta) load (Liao et al., 2025). For patients with xerostomia (dry mouth), hard candy or chewing gum may stimulate salivary flow or modification of the drug regimen may be necessary. Glycerol mouthwash can provide as much relief from xerostomia as artificial saliva.

During later stages of AD, bathing can be problematic for the patient and nursing staff. Bath time is a high-risk time for agitation and aggression. The person-centered approach focuses on personalizing care to meet patients' needs, accommodating to individual preferences, attending to the relationship and interaction with the patient, using effective communication and interpersonal skills, and adapting the physical environment and bathing procedures to decrease stress and discomfort.

Physical Health Interventions

Aging, dementia progression, treatment, and other age-related medical conditions impact the physical health of individuals with AD. The astute nurse will make connections among these factors when caring for people with AD.

Supporting Bowel and Bladder Function

Urinary or bowel incontinence affects many patients with AD. During the middle phases of the disease, incontinence may be caused by the patient's inability to communicate the need to use the toilet or locate a toilet quickly, undress appropriately to use the toilet, recognize the sensation of fullness, signaling the need to urinate or defecate, or apathy with lack of motivation to remain continent.

For the patient who is incontinent because of an inability to locate the toilet, orientation may be helpful. Signs and active training should help to modify disorientation. Displaying pictures or signs on bathroom doors provides visual cues; words should use appropriate terminology. For the individual who has lost motivation to remain continent, frequent reminders and urinary shields are helpful.

Sleep Interventions

Sedative–hypnotic agents may be prescribed for a short time for restlessness or insomnia, but they may also cause a paradoxical reaction of agitation and insomnia (especially in older adults). Sleep hygiene interventions are appropriate for patients with AD, although morning and afternoon naps (or rest periods for patients who do not nap) may be the most effective intervention for a patient with altered diurnal rhythms.

Activity and Exercise Interventions

Activity and exercise are important nursing interventions for patients with AD. To promote a feeling of success, any activity or exercise plan must be culturally sensitive and adapted to the patient's functional ability and interests. The activity or exercise must be designed to prevent excess stress (both physical and psychological), which means that it must be individualized for each patient with AD based on their relative strengths and deficits.

Nutritional Interventions

Maintenance of nutrition and hydration are essential nursing interventions. The patient's weight, oral intake, and hydration status should be monitored carefully. Patients with AD should eat well-balanced meals appropriate to their activity level and eating abilities, with special attention given to electrolyte balance and fluid intake. A Mediterranean diet (vegetables, whole grains and olive oil, fermented dairy products, nuts, seeds and herbs/spices, plant protein and seafood) supports a healthy gut and brain (Dominguez et al., 2024).

Watch for swallowing difficulties that may put the patient at risk for aspiration and asphyxiation. Swallowing difficulties may result from changes in esophageal motility and decreased secretion of saliva.

Pain and Comfort Management

Nursing care of noncommunicative patients who have AD and who also have pain can be challenging. Because of the difficulty in identifying and monitoring the pain, the patients are often undertreated. However, several measures may be used to assess the efficacy of pharmacologic interventions, such as decreased restlessness and agitation. Small doses of oral morphine solution appear to reduce discomfort during routine nursing procedures. The main side effect of morphine is constipation.

Relaxation

Approaching patients in a calm, confident, unhurried manner; maintaining a soothing, quiet environment; avoiding unnecessary noise or chatter around patients and lowering vocal tone and rate when addressing them; maintaining eye contact; and using touch judiciously are likely to promote a sense of security conducive to patient relaxation and comfort. Simple relaxation exercises can be used to reduce stress and should be performed by the patient.

Medication Interventions

Medications have two goals: restoration or maintenance of cognitive function and treatment of related psychiatric and behavioral disturbances that cause discomfort for the patient, interfere with treatment, or worsen the individual's cognitive status. Doses must be kept extremely low, and patients should be monitored closely for any side effects or worsening of cognitive status. "Start low and go slow" is the principle guiding the administration of psychopharmacologic agents in older patients.

Cholinesterase Inhibitors

Acetylcholinesterase inhibitors (AChEIs) are the mainstay of pharmacologic treatment of AD because they inhibit **acetylcholinesterase (AChE)**, an enzyme necessary for the breakdown of ACh. Inhibition of AChE results in an increase in cholinergic activity. Because these medications have been shown to delay the decline in cognitive functioning but generally do not improve cognitive function after it has declined, it is important that this medication be started as soon as the diagnosis is made. The primary side effect of these medications is GI distress, including nausea, vomiting, and diarrhea.

Cholinesterase inhibitors are indicated for the treatment of AD. These drugs may help to delay or prevent symptoms from becoming worse (see Table 39.3). Cholinesterase inhibitors are oral medications usually taken once or twice a day. The earlier in the disease process these medications are initiated, the more likely they will delay cognitive decline. Although there are no special monitors for the cholinesterase inhibitors, the prolonged concurrent use of nonsteroidal anti-inflammatory drugs (NSAIDs) with them can increase the risk of stomach ulcers.

N-Methyl-D-Aspartic Acid Antagonists

In AD, it is hypothesized that the chronic release of glutamate leads to neuronal degeneration. Memantine is an *N*-methyl-D-aspartic acid (NMDA) receptor antagonist that has been shown to improve cognition and ADLs in patients with moderate to severe symptoms of AD (Ning et al., 2024).

Memantine and Donepezil Combination

Patients stabilized on daily donepezil may be prescribed a combination of memantine and donepezil in one capsule (Box 39.4). This medication is formulated in various strengths of memantine (7, 14, 21, and 28 mg) combined with 10-mg donepezil.

Amyloid Beta-Directed Antibody

In AD, there is a build-up of the amyloid-beta plaque which interferes with neurotransmission. Another approach, **antiamyloid immunotherapy**, is viewed as the first disease-modifying therapy for the treatment of AD (Perneczky et al., 2024). Three medications are approved for the treatment of AD and target different stages of amyloid protein in the brain. *Aducanumab-avwa* was approved for the treatment of AD in 2021. This medication is a human, immunoglobulin gamma-1 (IgG1) monoclonal antibody that reduces the amyloid-beta plaques (Biogen, 2023). *Lecancemab-irmb* was approved in 2023 (Eisai Inc. & Biogen, 2024) and *donanemab-azbt* in 2024 (Eli Lilly and Company, 2024). All are intravenous injections and are amyloid beta-directed–antibodies that are initiated in patients with mild stages of AD or mild cognitive impairment.

Other Medications

Even though antipsychotics are not approved for use in dementia-related psychosis and most have a boxed warning for this population, off-label use of antipsychotics for psychosis is common. There is evidence for the use of antidepressants for treating symptoms of depression and in reducing agitation (Huang et al., 2024). Benzodiazepines should be used with caution and only on a short-term basis to treat anxiety in older adults.

TABLE 39.3 MEDICATIONS TO TREAT ALZHEIMER DISEASE (AD)

Drug	Drug Type and Use	Dose	Common Side Effects	Drug–Drug Interactions
Cholinesterase Inhibitors				
Donepezil				
Prevents the breakdown of acetylcholine in the brain	Cholinesterase inhibitor treats symptoms of mild, moderate, and severe AD	5 mg once a day. Increase after 4–6 wk to 10 mg/day	Nausea, diarrhea, vomiting	None observed in laboratory studies. NSAIDs should be used with caution in combination with this medication
Galantamine				
Prevents breakdown of acetylcholine and modulates nicotinic receptors that release acetylcholine in the brain	Cholinesterase inhibitor treats symptoms of mild and moderate AD	4 mg BID Titrate to 16–24 mg/day over 8 wk	Nausea, vomiting, diarrhea, weight loss	Some antidepressants, such as paroxetine, amitriptyline line, fluoxetine, fluvoxamine, and other drugs with anticholinergic action, may cause retention of excess galantamine in the body. NSAIDs should be used with caution in combination with this medication
Benzgalantamine				
Prevents breakdown of acetylcholine and modulates nicotinic receptors that release acetylcholine in the brain	Cholinesterase inhibitor treats symptoms of mild and moderate AD. Developed for less digestive upset than galantamine	5 mg BID by mouth	Nausea, vomiting, diarrhea, weight loss	No known serious interactions with any other drugs. Can interact with donepezil, escitalopram, metoprolol succinate ER, mirabegron, seroquel, and sertraline
Rivastigmine				
Prevents the breakdown of acetylcholine and butyrylcholine in the brain.	Cholinesterase inhibitor treats symptoms of mild and moderate AD (patch is also for severe AD)	1.5 mg BID Titrate to 24 mg/day by increasing 3 mg/day every 2 wk	Nausea, vomiting, weight loss, upset stomach, muscle weakness	None observed in laboratory studies. NSAIDs should be used with caution in combination with this medicine
NMDA Antagonist				
Memantine				
Blocks toxic effects of excess glutamate and regulates glutamate activation	NMDA antagonist to treat moderate to severe symptoms of Alzheimer	Initial dose 5 mg once a day; may increase to 10 mg/day, 15 mg/day, 20 mg/day at weekly intervals	Dizziness, headache, diarrhea, constipation, confusion	A total of 174 drugs (1,401 brand and generic names) are known to interact with memantine. Other prescribed medications and substances should be checked for interactions
NMDA Antagonist and Cholinesterase Inhibitor				
Memantine Extended-Release and Donepezil				
Blocks the toxic effects associated with excess glutamate and prevents the breakdown of acetylcholine in the brain	NMDA antagonist and Cholinesterase inhibitor to treat symptoms of moderate to severe AD	Recommended dose is 28 mg/10 mg once daily	Headache, nausea, vomiting, diarrhea, dizziness	Combined use with NMDA antagonists, anticholinergic medications, succinylcholine, similar neuromuscular blocking agents, or cholinergic agonists
Amyloid Beta-directed Antibody				
Lecanemab				
A humanized immunoglobulin gamma 1 (IgG1) monoclonal antibody directed against amyloid beta	Treats early-stage AD by targeting the protein beta-amyloid to help reduce amyloid plaques	10 mg/kg diluted then administered as an IV infusion over 1 hour, once 2 wk	Amyloid-related imaging abnormality (ARIA) with edema. Symptoms are headache, nausea, aphasia, weakness, or seizure	44 drugs interact with lecanemab. Major interactions occur with aspirin, ticagrelor, warfarin, apixaban, clopidogrel, dabigatran

(*continued*)

TABLE 39.3 MEDICATIONS TO TREAT ALZHEIMER DISEASE (AD) (*Continued*)

Drug	Drug Type and Use	Dose	Common Side Effects	Drug–Drug Interactions
Donanemab				
A humanized IgG1 monoclonal antibody directed against amyloid beta	Treats early-stage AD by targeting the protein beta-amyloid to reduce amyloid plaques	Recommended dosage is 700 ng every 4 weeks for 3 doses, then 1,400 mg every 4 wk. It is administered through IV infusion over 30 minutes	ARIA with edema. Symptoms are headache, nausea, aphasia, weakness, or seizure	44 drugs interact with donanemab. Major interactions occur with aspirin, ticagrelor, warfarin, apixaban, clopidogrel, dabigatran
Aducanumab				
A humanized IgG1 monoclonal antibody directed against aggregated forms of amyloid beta	Treats early-stage AD by reducing amyloid beta plaque	Initial titration of 10 mg/kg. Medication must be diluted and administered as an IV infusion over 1 hour every 4 wk	ARIA with edema. Symptoms are headache, nausea, aphasia, weakness, or seizure	44 drugs interact with aducanumab. Major interactions occur with aspirin, ticagrelor, warfarin, apixaban, clopidogrel, dabigatran
Atypical Antipsychotic				
Brexpiprazole				
The efficiency of brexpiprazole may be mediated through a combination of partial agonist activity at serotonin 5-HT1A and dopamine D2 receptors, and antagonist activity at serotonin 5-HT2A receptors	Treats agitation resulting from AD	0.5–3 mg/day	Cold symptoms, dizziness, high blood sugar, and stroke	Amiodarone can decrease the effects of brexpiprazole. Amisulpride can increase the activity of the antipsychotic, and amitriptyline can increase orthostatic hypotensive activities

BID, twice a day; NMDA, *N*-methyl-D-aspartic acid; NSAIDs, nonsteroidal anti-inflammatory drugs.
Adapted from National Institute on Aging (NIA). (2023). How is Alzheimer's disease treated? https://www.nia.nih.gov/health/alzheimers-treatment/how-alzheimers-disease-treated#treatment

Anticholinergic medications should be avoided in patients with AD if possible. See Box 39.5 for examples of medications that are commonly prescribed in older adults that have anticholinergic properties.

Psychosocial Interventions

Psychosocial interventions support cognitive functioning and target symptoms. A variety of interventions can be implemented.

Memory Enhancement

The sooner patients begin taking AChEIs, the slower the cognitive decline will be. However, pharmacologic agents are only a small part of the intervention picture. The nursing goal is to maintain memory function as long as possible. When caring for a patient with AD, a concerted effort should be made to reinforce short- and long-term memory. For example, reminding patients what they had for breakfast, which activity was just completed, or who their visitors were a few hours ago will reinforce short-term memory. Encouraging patients to tell the stories of their earlier years will help bring long-term memories into focus. In the earlier stages of AD, there is considerable frustration when the patient realizes that they have short-term memory loss. In a matter-of-fact manner, help "fill in the blanks" and then redirect to another activity. Pictures of familiar people, places, and activities are also important tools in memory retrieval. Using scents (perfume, shaving lotions, spices, different foods) to stimulate memory retrieval and asking patients to relate their memories are also useful.

BOX 39.4

Medication Profile: Memantine and Donepezil

DRUG CLASS: *N*-methyl-D-aspartate (NMDA) receptor antagonist and cholinesterase inhibitor

RECEPTOR AFFINITY: Low to moderate affinity uncompetitive (open-channel) NMDA receptor antagonist, which binds preferentially to the NMDA receptor, a reversible inhibitor of the enzyme acetylcholinesterase.

INDICATIONS: For treatment of moderate to severe dementia of the Alzheimer type in patients stabilized on 10 mg of donepezil hydrochloride once daily

ROUTES AND DOSAGE: 7-, 14-, 21-, and 28-mg tablets

For patients stabilized on donepezil hydrochloride 10 mg and not currently on memantine hydrochloride, the recommended starting dose is 7/10 mg, taken once a day in the evening. The dose should be increased in 7-mg increments of the memantine hydrochloride component to the recommended maintenance dose of 28/10 mg once daily. The minimum recommended interval between dose increases is 1 week. The dose should only be increased if the previous dose has been well tolerated. The maximum dose is 28/10 mg once daily.

HALF-LIFE (PEAK EFFECT): Terminal half-life, 60 to 80 hours (peak effect, 3 to 7 hours). Excreted predominantly in the liver.

SPECIFIC PATIENT AND FAMILY EDUCATION: Caregivers should be instructed in the recommended administration (twice per day for doses above 5 mg) and dose escalation (minimum interval of 1 week between dose increases).

- This drug does not alter the Alzheimer disease process, and the efficacy of the medication may decrease over time.
- Continue using other medications for dementia as prescribed by the health care provider.
- Review the patient information.
- Instruct patients and caregivers to take memantine and donepezil only once daily in the evening, or as prescribed.
- If a patient misses a single dose of memantine and donepezil the patient should not double up on the next dose. The next dose should be taken as scheduled.
- Instruct patients and caregivers that memantine and donepezil capsules should be swallowed whole. Alternatively, memantine and donepezil capsules may be opened and sprinkled on applesauce and the entire contents consumed. The capsules should not be divided, chewed, or crushed. Warn patients and caregivers not to use any capsules of memantine and donepezil that are damaged or show signs of tampering.
- Advise patients and caregivers that memantine and donepezil may cause headache, diarrhea, dizziness, anorexia, vomiting, nausea, and ecchymosis.
- Do not discontinue the drug or change the dose unless advised by the health care provider.
- Do not increase the dose of memantine if Alzheimer disease symptoms do not appear to be improving or appear to be getting worse; notify the health care provider.
- Memantine and donepezil may cause drowsiness or dizziness. Use caution while driving and performing other activities requiring mental alertness and coordination until tolerance is determined.
- Do not use any prescription or over-the-counter medications, dietary supplements, or herbal preparations unless advised by the health care provider.
- Follow-up visits may be required to monitor therapy and to keep appointments.

BOX 39.5

Medications With Anticholinergic Effects

- Amitriptyline
- Captopril
- Codeine
- Cimetidine
- Citalopram
- Digoxin
- Diphenhydramine
- Dipyridamole
- Donepezil
- Escitalopram
- Furosemide
- Fluoxetine
- Isosorbide
- Mirtazapine
- Nifedipine
- Oxybutynin ER
- Paroxetine
- Phenytoin
- Prednisolone
- Ranitidine
- Theophylline
- Triamterene and hydrochlorothiazide
- Tolterodine
- Warfarin

Adapted from Healthline Media LLC (2025). Anticholinergics. https://www.healthline.com/health/anticholinergics

Formalized reminiscence groups also help patients relive their earlier experiences and support maintenance of long-term memories.

Orientation

To enhance cognitive functioning, attempts should be made to remind patients of the day, time, and location. However, if the patient begins to argue that they are really at home or falsely believes that it is 1992, the patient need not be confronted by facts. Any confrontation could easily escalate into an argument. Instead, either redirect the patient or focus on the topic at hand (Box 39.6).

Maintaining Language

Losing the ability to name an object (i.e., agnosia) is frustrating. For example, the patient may describe a flower in terms of color, size, and fragrance, but never be able to name the flower. When this happens while interacting with a patient, immediately say the name of the item. This reinforces cognitive functioning and prevents disruption in the interaction. Referral to speech therapists may also be useful if the language impairment impedes communication.

BOX 39.6

Therapeutic Dialogue: The Patient With Dementia of the Alzheimer Type

Lois's daughter has told the home health agency nurse that on several occasions Lois has been found cowering and fearful under the kitchen table, saying she was hiding from voices. The nurse also knows that Lois denies having any difficulty with her memory or her ability to care for herself.

INEFFECTIVE APPROACH

Nurse: I'm here to see you about your health issues.

Lois: I have no issues. Why are you here?

Nurse: I'm here to help you.

Lois: I do not need any help. I think there is a mistake.

Nurse: Oh, there is no mistake. Your name is Ms. W, isn't it?

Lois: Yes, but I don't know who you are or why you are here. I'm very tired; please excuse me.

Nurse: OK. I will return another day.

EFFECTIVE APPROACH

Nurse: Hello, my name is Susan Miller. I'm the home health nurse, and I will be spending some time with you.

Lois: Oh, alright. Come in. Sit here.

Nurse: Thank you.

Lois: There is nothing wrong with me, you know.

Nurse: Are you wondering why I am here? (Open-ended statement)

Lois: I know why you are here. My children think that I cannot take care of myself.

Nurse: Is that true? Can you take care of yourself? (Restatement)

Lois: Of course I can care for myself. When people get older, they slow down. I'm just a little slower now, and that upsets my children.

Nurse: You are a little slower? (Reflection)

Lois: I sometimes forget things.

Nurse: Such as … (open-ended statement)

Lois: Sometimes I cannot remember a telephone number or the name of a food.

Nurse: Does that cause issues?

Lois: According to my children, it does!

Nurse: What about you? What causes issues for you?

Lois: Sometimes the radio says terrible things to me.

Nurse: That must be frightening. (Acceptance)

Lois: It's terrifying. Then, my daughter looks at me as if I am crazy. Am I?

Nurse: It sounds like your mind is playing tricks on you. Let's see if we can figure out how to control the radio. (Validation)

Lois: Oh, OK. Will you tell my daughter that I am not crazy?

Nurse: Sure, I would be happy to meet with both you and your daughter if you would like. (Acceptance)

CRITICAL THINKING CHALLENGE

1. In the first scenario, how did the nurse's underlying assumption that the patient would welcome the nurse lead to rejection by the patient?
2. In the second scenario, what communication techniques did the nurse use to open communication and establish a sense of trust?

Supporting Visuospatial Functioning

The patient with visuospatial impairments loses the ability to sequence automatic behaviors, such as getting dressed or eating with silverware. For example, patients often put their clothes on backward, inside out, or with undergarments over outer garments. After they are dressed, they become confused as to how they arrived at their current state. If this happens, it may help to place clothes for dressing in a sequence for the patient so the patient can move from one article to the next in the correct sequence. This same technique can be used in other situations, such as eating, bathing, and toileting.

Suspiciousness, Illusions, and Delusions

Delusions often occur when patients are placed in a situation they cannot master cognitively. The principle of nonconfrontation is most important in dealing with the formation of suspiciousness and delusion. Efforts should be directed at determining the circumstances that trigger suspicion or delusion formation and creating a means of avoiding these situations.

Frequent causes of suspicion occur when changes in daily routine occur. The common accusations that "someone has entered my room" or "someone has changed my room" can be managed by asking, "Do you want to see if anything is missing?" Such accusations usually arise when a patient cannot remember what the room looked like or when the room was rearranged or cleaned.

Patients with AD often have delusions that a spouse, child, or other significant individual is an impostor. If this situation occurs, it is important to assert in a matter-of-fact manner, "This is your wife, Barbara" or "I am your daughter Jenny." More vigorous assertions, such as offering various types of proof, tend to increase puzzlement as to why an individual would go so far as to impersonate the spouse or child.

When patients experience illusions, find the source of the illusion and remove it from the environment if possible. For example, if a patient is watching a television program featuring animals and then verbalizes that the animal is in the room, switch the channel and redirect the conversation.

Some patients with AD may no longer recognize the reflections in the mirror as themselves and become agitated, thinking that a stranger is staring at them. Potentially misleading or disturbing stimuli, such as mirrors or artwork, can be easily covered or removed from the environment.

Hallucinations

Reassurance and distraction may be helpful for the hallucinating patient. For example, an 89-year-old patient with AD in a residential care facility would get up each night, walk to the nursing station, and whisper to the nurses, "There's a man in my bed who won't let me sleep. You should patrol this place better!" If the hallucination is not too disturbing for the patient, it can often be dismissed calmly with diversion or distraction. Because this patient did not seem too concerned by the "man" in her bed, the nurse may gently respond by saying, "I'm sorry you have to put up with so much. Just wait here (or come with me) and I'll make sure your room is ready for you." The nurse should then take the patient back to her room and help her into bed.

Frightening hallucinations and delusions usually require antipsychotic medications to dampen the patient's emotional reactions, but they can also be dealt with by optimizing perceptual cues (e.g., cover mirrors, turn off the television) and by encouraging patients to stay physically close to their caregivers. For example, one patient complained to their visiting nurse that they were being poisoned by deadly bugs that crawled up and down their arms and legs while they tried to sleep at night. Antipsychotic medication may help this patient sleep at night, and she would also likely benefit from reassurance and protection.

Mood Changes

Strategies for Depression

Psychotherapeutic nursing interventions for depression that accompanies AD are similar to interventions for any depression. It is important to spend time alone with patients and to personalize their care as a way of communicating the patient's value. Encouraging expression of negative emotions is helpful because patients can talk honestly to a nonjudgmental individual about their feelings. Although depressed patients with AD are likely to be too disorganized to attempt suicide, it is wise to remove potentially harmful objects from the environment.

Coping With Stress and Anxiety

Cognitively impaired patients are particularly vulnerable to anxiety. Patients with AD become unsure of their surroundings or of what is expected of them and then tend to react with fear and distress. They may feel lost, insecure, and left out. Failure to complete a task formerly regarded as simple creates anxiety and agitation. Often, they cannot explain the source of their anxiety. In many cases, lowering the demands, simplifying routines, and reducing the number of choices alleviate the anxiety.

Catastrophic Reactions

If a patient reacts catastrophically, remain calm, minimize environmental distractions (quiet the environment), get the patient's attention, and softly assure the patient that they are safe. Give information slowly, clearly, and simply, one step at a time. Let the patient know that you understand the fear or other emotional response, such as anger or anxiety.

As nursing skills are developed in identifying antecedents to the patient's catastrophic reactions, it becomes possible to avoid situations that provoke such reactions. Patients with AD respond well to structure but poorly to change. Attempts to argue or reason with them will only escalate their dysfunctional responses.

Apathy and Withdrawal

As the patient withdraws and becomes more apathetic, it becomes more challenging to engage the patient in meaningful activities and interactions. Providing this level of care requires knowing the premorbid functioning level of the patient. Close contact with family helps provide ideas about meaningful activities.

Behavioral Interventions

Restlessness and Wandering

Restlessness and wandering are major concerns for caregivers, especially in the community (home) or long-term care setting. The principal means of dealing with restless patients who wander into other patients' rooms or out the door is to have an adequate number of staff (or caregivers in the home setting) to provide supervision, as well as electronically controlled exits. Wandering behavior may be interrupted in more cognitively intact patients by distracting them verbally or visually. Patients who are beyond verbal distraction can be distracted by physically joining them on their walk and then interrupting their course of action and gently redirecting them back to the house or facility. Many times, wandering is a result of a patient's inability to find their own room or may represent other agenda-seeking behaviors such as trying to find a bathroom.

Agitated Behavior

Agitated behavior is likely to occur when patients are pressed to assist in their own care. A calm, unhurried, and undemanding approach is usually most effective. Attempts at reasoning may only aggravate the situation and increase the patient's resistance to care. If unable to determine the source of the patient's anxiety, the patient's restless energy can often be channeled into activities such as walking. Relaxation techniques also can be effective for reducing behavioral issues and anxiety in patients with AD. Under the guidance of an aromatherapist, essential oils are being used in some settings for reduction of agitation (Leach et al., 2021).

Aberrant Behavior

When patients are picking in the air or wringing hands, simple distraction may work. Hypervocalizations, which may have meaning to the patient, may mean the individual is in pain or discomfort. It is important to determine the underlying cause of the frequent vocalizations. If an underlying cause cannot be determined, the nurse can implement strategies to reduce the frequency of vocalizations and aberrant behavior. See Table 39.4.

Reducing Disinhibition

Anticipation of disinhibiting behavior is the key to nursing interventions for this issue. Disinhibition can take many forms, from undressing in a public setting to touching someone inappropriately to making cruel but factual statements. This behavior can usually be viewed as expected by itself, but unexpected within its social context. Keen behavioral assessment of the patient increases the ability to anticipate the likely socially inappropriate behavior and redirect the patient or change the context of the situation. If the patient starts undressing in the dining room, offering a robe and gently escorting them to another part of the room might be all that is needed. If a patient is trying to fondle a staff member, having the staff member leave the immediate area or redirecting the patient may alleviate the situation.

Complementary Therapies

Music therapy has been long recognized as an important therapy for people with AD because music abilities can be preserved even though language is lost. Evidence shows that music therapy improves memory, language, and orientation (Jiménez-Palomares et al., 2024). Anti-inflammatory effects of yoga have been suggested as the reason this intervention improves cognition in people with AD (Grzenda et al., 2024). Research supports the effectiveness of acupuncture in the treatment of AD. Acupuncture is thought to modulate the gut microbiota and reduce neuroinflammation, which in turn improves cognition (Yan et al., 2024).

Spiritual Interventions

Spiritual connections can provide emotional support for the patient, caregivers, and family throughout the disease progression. Encouraging patients and caregivers to reach out to local spiritual leaders can help reduce the social isolation that is often a part of AD (Padala et al., 2024).

Psychoeducation for Families

Especially in AD, the needs of family members should also be considered. Caring for a family member with dementia takes its toll. Over eighty percent of the home care is provided by family caregivers. Two-thirds of the caregivers are people assigned female at birth, and 30% are over the age of 65 years. Caregivers' health often declines and directly affects their ability to provide care (Alzheimer's Association, 2025f). Caregivers are faced with extreme pressures and often feel isolated, frustrated, and trapped. The potential for patient abuse is significant, especially if agitated and aggressive behaviors are present in the relative.

Caregivers should be encouraged to attend support groups and carve out personal time. Educational and training programs may help in understanding the

TABLE 39.4 MESSAGES, MEANINGS, AND MANAGEMENT STRATEGIES

Possible Underlying Meanings	Related Management Strategies
"I'm hurt!" (e.g., from arthritis, fractures, pressure ulcers, degenerative joint disease, cancer)	• Observe for pain behaviors (e.g., posture, facial expressions, and gait in conjunction with vocalizations). • Treat suspected pain judiciously with analgesics and nonpharmacologic measures (e.g., repositioning, careful manipulation of the patient during transfers and personal care, warm or cold packs, massage, relaxation).
"I'm ***tired***." (e.g., sleep disturbances possibly related to altered sleep–wake cycle with day–night reversal, difficulty falling asleep, frequent night awakenings)	• Increase daytime activity and exercise to minimize daytime napping and promote nighttime sleep. • Promote typical sleep patterns and biorhythms by strengthening natural environmental cues (e.g., provide light exposure during the day; avoid bright lights at night), provide large calendars and clocks. • Establish a bedtime routine. • Reduce night awakenings: avoid excess fluids, diuretics, caffeine at bedtime, minimize loud noises, consolidate nighttime care activities (e.g., changing, medications, treatments).
"I'm ***lonely.***"	• Encourage social interactions between patients and their family, caregivers, and others. • Increase time the patient spends in group settings to minimize time in isolation. • Provide opportunity to interact with pets.
"I need ..." (e.g., food, a drink, a blanket, to use the toilet, to be turned or repositioned)	• Anticipate needs (e.g., assist the patient to toilet soon after breakfast when the gastrocolic reflex is likely). • Keep patient comfort and safety in mind during care (e.g., minimize body exposure to prevent hypothermia).
"I'm ***stressed.***" (e.g., Inability to tolerate sensory overload)	• Promote rest and quiet time. • Minimize "white noise" (e.g., vacuum cleaner) and background noise (e.g., televisions and radios). • Avoid harsh lighting and busy, abstract designs. • Limit patient's contacts with other agitated people. • Reduce behavioral expectations of patient, minimize choices, and promote a stable routine.
"I'm ***bored.***" (e.g., lack of sensory stimulation)	• Maximize hearing and visual abilities (e.g., keep external auditory canals free from cerumen plugs, ensure that glasses and hearing aids are worn, provide reading material of large print, soften lighting to reduce glare). • Play soft classical music for auditory stimulation. • Offer structured diversions (e.g., outdoor activities).
"What are you doing to me?" (e.g., personal boundaries are invaded)	• Avoid startling patients by approaching them from the front. • Always speak before touching the patient. • Inform patients what you plan to do and why before you do it. • Allow for flexibility in patient care.
"I don't feel well." (e.g., a urinary or upper respiratory tract infection, metabolic anomaly, fecal impaction)	• Identify the etiology through patient history, examination, possible tests (e.g., urinalysis, blood work, chest radiography, neurologic testing). • Treat underlying causes.
"I'm ***frustrated—I have no control.***" (e.g., loss of autonomy)	• When possible, allow patient to make their own decisions. • Maximize patient involvement during personal care (e.g., offer the patient a washcloth to assist with bathing). • Treat patients with dignity and respect (e.g., dress or change patients in private).
"I'm ***lost.***" (e.g., memory impairment)	• Maintain familiar routines. • Label the patient's room, bathroom, drawers, and possessions with large name signs. • Promote a sense of belonging through displays of familiar personal items, such as old family pictures.
"I ***feel strange.***" (e.g., side effects from medications that may include psycho tropics, corticosteroids, beta-blockers, NSAIDs)	• Minimize the overall number of medications; consider nondrug interventions when possible. • Begin new medications one at a time; start with low doses and titrate slowly. Suspect a drug reaction if the patient's behavior (e.g., vocal) changes. • Educate caregivers about the patient's medications.
"I need to be loved!"	• Provide human contact and purposeful touch. • Acknowledge or verify the patient's feelings. • Encourage alternative, nonverbal ways to express feelings, such as through music, painting, or drawing. • Confirm a sense of purpose in life, acknowledge achievement, and reaffirm that the patient is still needed.

NSAID, nonsteroidal anti-inflammatory drug.

Reprinted from Clavel, D. S. (1999). Vocalizations among cognitively impaired elders: What is your patient trying to tell you? *Geriatric Nursing, 20*(2), 90–93.

BOX 39.7

Tips for Caregivers

When caring for the patient with dementia, be sure to include the caregivers, as appropriate, and address the following topic areas in the teaching plan:

- Psychopharmacologic agents, if used, including drug action, dosage, frequency, and possible adverse effects
- Rest and activity
- Consistency in routines
- Nutrition and hydration
- Sleep and comfort measures
- Protective environment
- Communication and social interaction
- Diversional measures
- Community resources

complex nature of the disorder (Boxes 39.7 and 39.8). Community resources, such as day care centers, home health agencies, and other community services, can be an important aspect of nursing care for the patient with dementia.

Promoting Safety

In the early stages of the illness, safety may not seem to be a prime issue because the individual is cognitively intact. However, early behaviors suggesting AD are often related to safety, such as the patient getting lost while driving or going the wrong way on the highway. Patients may be prevented from driving even though they can continue to live at home. Safety continues to be an issue in the home when patients engage in unsupervised cooking, cleaning, or household tasks. Day care centers provide a structured yet safe environment for these individuals. Family members should be encouraged to assess continually the abilities of members to live at home safely.

During hospitalizations or nursing home care, the safety issues are different. Most geropsychiatric units are kept locked and a dementia unit often has an electronic alarm system to alert staff about patients attempting to leave the secured floor. Staff and visitors need to be vigilant for perilous situations.

Implementing Milieu Therapy

Overstimulating activities (e.g., social outing, family visit) can result in an outburst of delusional accusations or agitation. The nurse should attempt to determine each patient's optimal level of stimulation at various times of the day. It may be that stimulating environments can be tolerated early in the morning but not in the afternoon, when the patient is tired.

Socialization Activities

Overlearned social skills are rarely lost in patients with AD. It is not unusual for patients with dementia to respond appropriately to a handshake or smile well into the disease process. Even patients who are no longer able to communicate coherently will carry on long discussions with people who are willing to listen and respond (to language that does not make sense). The risk for social isolation is strong in patients with AD because of communication difficulties. Reinforcing social remarks and gestures, such as eye contact, smiling, greetings, and farewells, can promote a sense of competency and self-esteem. Pet therapy and "stuffed animal" therapy can also enhance social interaction in cognitively impaired

BOX 39.8

Research for Evidenced-Based Practice: Caregiver Burden and Quality of Life

Possin, K. L., Dulaney, S., Sideman, A. B., Wood, A. J., Allen, I. E., Bonasera, S. J., Merrilees, J. J., Lee, K., Chiong, W., Braley, T. L., Hooper, S., Kanzawa, M., Gearhart, R., Medsger, H., Harrison, K. L., Hunt, L. J., Kiekhofer, R. E., Chow, C., Miller, B. L., & Guterman, E. L. (2024). Long-term effects of collaborative dementia care on quality of life and caregiver well-being. Alzheimer's & Dementia, *21(1), e14370. https://doi.org/10.1002/alz.14370*

THE QUESTION: Does a monthly telephone-based collaborative care model with care navigation for dementia (Care Ecosystem) reduce the burdens of caregiving?

METHODS: Dyads (an individual living with dementia and their caregiver) were recruited for this study because of high caregiver burden at baseline. Caregivers included either spouses or adult children. A total of 456 dyads were included in the study. Each dyad completed a telephone survey at baseline and every 6 months or until death of the individual with dementia. The intervention was delivered by an unlicensed care team navigator who provided resources under the supervision of a clinical team and guided by care protocols. The navigators responded to immediate needs first, and then screened for behavior, function, safety, medication changes, and unmet caregiver needs. Measurement included the cumulative 5-year treatment effects on the quality of life and health care utilization of the individual with dementia, and on the caregiver's depression, self-efficacy, and burden.

FINDINGS: Individuals living with dementia with a spouse caregiver experienced significant improvement in quality of life and fewer hospitalizations over the 5-year period than the individuals with dementia living with a child caregiver. Adult child caregivers experienced improvements in caregiver burden and depression. Both spouse and adult child caregivers experienced improvements in self-efficacy. The greatest benefit was during the first 2 years.

IMPLICATIONS FOR NURSING: Caregivers of individuals with dementia are at high risk for poorer quality of life than the general population. Nurses should encourage caregivers to seek help in navigating the health care system to support the changing needs of individuals living with dementia.

individuals. It is important to remember that patients with AD do not lose their ability to laugh and play, and the psychosocial benefits of humor are well known.

Activities that elicit pleasant memories from an earlier time in the patient's life (reminiscence) may produce a soothing effect. Eliciting pleasant memories may be enhanced by gentle stimulation of the patient's senses, for example, viewing and discussing photo albums, looking at personal memorabilia, providing a favorite food item, playing a musical instrument, or listening to music the individual preferred in younger years. It may be useful to incorporate movement or dance along with a singing exercise.

If the patient with AD resists structured exercise, it may be because of a fear of falling or injury or of demonstrating to others that their health is failing. Patients with AD often forget how to move or how to coordinate their movements in relation to objects. Therefore, exercise should be light and enjoyable. Encourage the patient to take rest periods at intervals throughout the activity to minimize stress.

Evaluation

The objectives of nursing interventions are to help the patient with AD remain as independent as possible and to function at the highest cognitive, physical, emotional, spiritual, and social levels. The maximum level of functional ability can be promoted when nursing care is related to and based on the remaining abilities of the patient.

Continuum of Care

The goal of in-home and community-based long-term care services is to maintain patients in a self-determining environment that provides the most home-like atmosphere possible, allows maximum personal choice for care recipients and caregiver, and encourages optimal family caregiving involvement without overwhelming the resources of the family network. All services for patients with AD and their families must be provided within a context of continuity of care, a concept that mandates access to various health and supportive services over an unpredictable and changing clinical course.

Nurses working with patients with AD are especially knowledgeable about all aspects of the illness and care. These nurses are often involved in local organizations, such as the Alzheimer's Association. Issues of care and safety and reimbursement for services often require professional expertise and influence.

Inpatient-Focused Care

Comprehensive admission assessment followed by the development of an individualized (and constantly updated) care plan that involves the patient, significant others, and diverse health care professionals is the foundation of an effective and efficient postdischarge plan. Attention to all aspects of this process is necessary to ensure that the goal of continuity of care is achieved. The hospital-based nurse may initiate family education and counseling as part of discharge planning.

Community Care

It is estimated that more than 60% to 70% of older adults with AD live at home, with 83% of home care provided by family and friends. In 2023, unpaid caregivers provided $350 billion of economic worth (Alzheimer's Association, 2025f). Use of community-based services (e.g., home health aides, home-delivered meals, adult day care centers, respite care, caregiver support groups) often extends the amount of time an individual with AD or a related disorder can safely remain in the home.

Nursing Home

As the AD progresses, many patients are placed in a nursing home for care. Nursing care in a nursing home is usually delivered by nurses' aides, who need support and direction. Interestingly, people with AD require complex nursing care, but the skill level of people caring for these individuals often is minimal. Education and support of the direct caregiver is the focus of most nursing homes.

Integration With Primary Care

People with AD usually have multiple physical health issues and are most likely to be treated by primary care providers. Dementia is often treated in the primary care health care settings until behavioral disturbances emerge. People with advancing dementia are then referred to mental health or specialized geriatric providers for treatment of these psychiatric symptoms. The other health care needs continue to be treated by primary care. The mental health specialist integrates care, with the medical health care being provided by the primary care nurse or providers. If patients are treated with medications, the primary care nurse must be monitoring the patient for changes in target symptoms, side effects, and drug–drug interactions.

OTHER DEMENTIAS

Dementia symptoms may occur as a result of a number of disorders and underlying etiologies. The subsequent sections provide a brief description of some of the dementias listed in the *DSM-5-TR*. In each case, the classic symptoms of dementia (e.g., memory impairment with a number of other cognitive deficits) must be present. Nursing interventions for all dementias are similar to those described for individuals with AD.

Vascular Neurocognitive Disorder

Vascular neurocognitive disorder (also known as *vascular dementia*) is a decline in thinking skill caused by conditions that block or reduce blood flow to the brain, and the second most common type of dementia. Slightly more in people assigned male at birth than those assigned female at birth. Vascular dementia results when a series of small strokes damage or destroy brain tissue. These are commonly referred to as "ministrokes" or TIAs; several TIAs may occur before the affected individual becomes aware of the symptoms of vascular dementia. Most often, a blood clot or plaques (fatty deposits) block the vessels that supply blood to the brain, causing a stroke. However, a stroke can also occur when a blood vessel bursts in the brain (Alzheimer's Association, 2025g).

Symptoms of vascular neurocognitive disorder usually begin more suddenly rather than in AD. Often, the neurologic symptoms associated with a TIA are minimal and may last only a few days, including slight weakness in a limb, dizziness, or slurred speech. Thus, the clinical progression is often described as intermittent and fluctuating or of step-like deterioration, with the patient's cognitive and functional status improving or plateauing for a period of time followed by a rapid decline in function after another series of TIAs. Treatment aims to reduce the primary risk factors for vascular dementia, including hypertension, diabetes mellitus, and additional strokes.

Dementia Caused by Parkinson Disease

In individuals with Parkinson disease, 80% will develop neurocognitive dementia (APA, 2022). Although investigators do not know why, pathologic overlap is considerable between Parkinson disease and AD. The evidence consistently suggests that low cerebrospinal fluid levels of amyloid-beta predict future cognitive decline and dementia in Parkinson disease. Cognitive-enhancing medications have some effect, but there is no convincing evidence that the progression of dementia can be delayed (Frost et al., 2024; Rose et al., 2024).

Dementia Caused by Huntington Disease

Huntington disease is a progressive, genetically transmitted, autosomal dominant disorder characterized by choreiform movements and mental anomalies. The onset is usually between the ages of 35 and 45 years, but onset occurs before 20 years of age in the juvenile form or as late as 70 years of age in the late-onset form. The disease affects people of all genders. An individual with Huntington disease usually lives for approximately 10 to 20 years after diagnosis (APA, 2022). The dementia syndrome of Huntington disease is characterized by insidious changes in behavior and personality. Typically, the dementia is frontal, which means that the individual demonstrates prominent behavioral issues and disruption of attention.

FRONTOTEMPORAL NEUROCOGNITIVE DISORDER

Progressive development of behavioral and personality change and/or language impairment characterizes frontotemporal neurocognitive disorder, which has distinct patterns of brain atrophy and distinctive neuropathology. Individuals with this disorder have varying degrees of apathy or disinhibition. They may lose interest in socialization, self-care, and personal responsibilities. Family members report socially inappropriate behaviors, but afflicted individuals show little insight. The cognitive deficits are typically in the area of planning, organization, and judgments. These individuals are easily distracted (APA, 2022).

NEUROCOGNITIVE DISORDER WITH LEWY BODIES

Progressive cognitive decline with visual hallucination, REM sleep disorder, and spontaneous parkinsonism characterizes dementia with Lewy bodies, a major neurocognitive disorder. Cognitive symptoms occur several months before motor symptoms. These symptoms fluctuate and may resemble delirium. These individuals are at high risk for falls because of periods of syncope and transient episodes of consciousness. Orthostatic hypotension and urinary incontinence may occur. The cause is unknown, but evidence implies genetic factors and neuroinflammation (Haider et al., 2023). The pathology involves Lewy bodies found in the cortical location in the brain, which are thought to be responsible for the disorder.

The estimated prevalence of this dementia ranges from 0% to 1.2% of the general older population, with people assigned male at birth slightly more affected (APA, 2022). This onset of disorder is typically in the sixth to ninth decades and is progressive with a 5- to 7-year survival rate. These individuals are more functionally impaired than those with other types of dementia (e.g., AD) and are very sensitive to psychotropic medication, especially antipsychotics.

NEUROCOGNITIVE DISORDER DUE TO PRION DISEASE

Neurocognitive disorder due to prion-related symptoms comprises a group of spongiform encephalopathies including Creutzfeldt–Jakob disease, a rare, rapidly fatal, brain disorder, and mad cow disease, which is a bovine disorder. A prion is a small infectious particle composed of unexpectedly folded protein that causes progressive neurodegeneration. Many of the symptoms seen in

Creutzfeldt–Jakob disease are similar to those found in AD and other dementias. However, changes in the brain tissue are different in Creutzfeldt–Jakob disease and are best differentiated with surgical biopsy or during autopsy (APA, 2022). Common symptoms include fluctuating fever, difficulty swallowing, incontinence, tremors, seizures, and sensitivity to touch and environmental noise.

At present, no effective treatment for the disease exists and nothing has been found to slow progression of the illness, although antiviral drug studies are ongoing. Person-to-person transmission of Creutzfeldt–Jakob disease is rare (but possible), and it can be transmitted from people to animals and between animals. Because of the transmissible nature of Creutzfeldt–Jakob disease and because the virus is not easily destroyed, strict criteria for the handling of infected tissues and other contaminated materials have been developed.

NEUROCOGNITIVE DISORDER DUE TO TRAUMATIC BRAIN INJURY

TBI affects about 2.87 million people in the United States each year, resulting in various symptoms including neurologic, cognitive, behavioral, and emotional impairments (APA, 2022). Repeated concussions can lead to brain injury with long-term TBI. Evidence suggests that even mild TBI is a significant risk factor for developing dementia (Pszczołowska et al., 2024).

SUBSTANCE- OR MEDICATION-INDUCED NEUROCOGNITIVE DISORDER

If dementia results from the persisting effects of a substance (e.g., drugs of misuse, a medication, exposure to toxins), substance-induced neurocognitive disorder can develop. Other causes of dementia (e.g., dementia caused by a general medical condition) must always be considered even in an individual with a dependence on or exposure to a substance. For example, head injuries often result from substance use and may be the underlying cause of the neurocognitive changes.

OTHER NEUROCOGNITIVE DISORDERS

MILD COGNITIVE IMPAIRMENT

Mild cognitive impairment (MCI) is diagnosed if a modest cognitive decline from a previous level of function is found in one or more of the cognitive domains, but the cognitive deficits do not interfere with independence in daily activities (Alzheimer's Association, 2025a). MCI is thought to be related to multiple causes and some, but not all, progress to AD. MCI is categorized according to type of memory loss. In **amnestic MCI,** an individual may start to forget important information such as appointments, conversations, or events. In **nonamnestic MCI**, impairment occurs in visual perception, the ability to make sound decisions, or the capacity to judge the time or sequence of steps needed to complete a complex task. (Alzheimer's Association, 2025a).

SUMMARY OF KEY POINTS

- Neurocognitive disorders are characterized clinically by significant deficits in cognition or memory that represent a clear-cut change from a previous level of functioning. In some disorders, the loss of cognitive function is progressive, such as in AD. It is important to recognize the differences because the interventions and expected outcomes of the two syndromes are different.
- Delirium is characterized by a disturbance in consciousness and a change in cognition that develops over a short period of time. It requires rapid detection and treatment.
- The primary goal of treatment of individuals with delirium is prevention or resolution of the acute confusion episode with return to previous cognitive status and interventions focusing on (1) elimination or correction of the underlying cause and (2) symptomatic and safety, and supportive measures.
- Dementia is characterized by the gradual onset of decline in cognitive function, especially memory, usually accompanied by changes in behavior and personality.
- AD is an example of a progressively degenerative dementia. Treatment efforts currently focus on the reduction of cognitive symptoms (e.g., memory loss; confusion; and issues with learning, speech, and reasoning) in attempts to improve the quality of life for both patients and their caregivers.
- Research efforts continue to focus on understanding the relationship among the development of the beta-amyloid plaques, neurofibrillary tangles, and cell death.
- Nursing care of an individual with dementia depends on the stage of the disease and the availability of family caregivers.
- Educating and supporting families and caregivers through the progressive cognitive decline and behavior changes is essential to ensuring proper care.
- Several mental health strategies (exercise, education, cognitive stimulation) support and protect an individual's cognitive reserve. A healthy cognitive reserve is thought to be protective against neuropathologic insults.
- Other neurocognitive dementias may be related to specific brain changes (Lewy bodies), infections (prion

disease), genetic diseases (Huntington disease), and substances/medications.

- Modest cognitive decline is referred to as MCI (mild cognitive impairment). MCI may not be a precursor to AD, but should be viewed as an unexpected occurrence, and underlying cause determined.

DEVELOPING CLINICAL JUDGMENT

1. What factors should be considered in differentiating AD from vascular neurocognitive disorder?
2. Suggest reasons that older adults are particularly vulnerable to the development of neurocognitive disorders.
3. Compare the nursing care of an individual with delirium versus one with dementia. What are the similarities and differences in the care?
4. The physical environment is particularly important to the patient with dementia. Visualize your last experience in a health care setting (e.g., hospital, nursing home, day care program, home care setting). Identify environmental factors that could be misleading or stress producing to an individual with impaired cognition (dementia) and identify ways to modify this environment to alleviate some of the stressors or misleading stimuli.
5. Mr. J. has been recently diagnosed with mild AD and is asking for advice about deciding on his care in the future. His wife and daughter believe that he does not have the ability to make these decisions and asks for the nurse's advice. How should the nurse respond?

MOVIES, TV, OR STREAMING PROGRAMS

***Three of Us*: 2022.** This Indian Hindi-language film, with English subtitles, is a simple story of Shailaja's (Shefali Shah) attempt to regain childhood memories that are being lost through dementia. Shailaja and her husband Depankar return to her childhood home and she reconnects with schoolmates and friends. The story centers around the reconnection of her memories with her childhood love Pradeep, whose wife encourages the relationship. It is not until the end of the movie that Shailaja's husband explains the progressive dementia that his wife is experiencing.

Viewing Points:

1. In the beginning of the movie, does Shailaja demonstrate any symptoms of dementia?
2. How can Shailaja have fairly clear memories of her childhood and have memory issues in everyday life?
3. How would you explain the difference in relationship between Shailaja and Depankar and Shailaja's relationship with Pradeep?

REFERENCES

2024 Alzheimer's disease facts and figures. (2024). *Alzheimer's & Dementia, 20*(5), 3708–3821. https://doi.org/10.1002/alz.13809

Alzheimer's Association. (2025a). *Mild cognitive impairment (MCI)*. https://www.alz.org/alzheimers-dementia/what-is-dementia/related_conditions/mild-cognitive-impairment

Alzheimer's Association. (2025b). *Women and Alzheimer's*. https://www.alz.org/alzheimers-dementia/what-is-alzheimers/women-and-alzheimer-s

Alzheimer's Association. (2025c). *Black Americans and Alzheimer's*. https://www.alz.org/help-support/resources/black-americans-and-alzheimers

Alzheimer's Association. (2025d). *What are the causes and risk factors of Alzheimer's and other dementias*? https://www.alz.org/alzheimers-dementia/what-is-alzheimers/causes-and-risk-factors

Alzheimer's Association. (2025e). *Differential diagnosis of Down Syndrome*. https://www.alz.org/professionals/health-systems-medical-professionals/dementia-diagnosis/differential-diagnosis/differential-diagnosis-of-down-syndrome

Alzheimer's Association. (2025f). *2025 Alzheimer's Disease facts and figures*. https://www.alz.org/alzheimers-dementia/facts-figures

Alzheimer's Association. (2025g). *Vascular dementia*. https://www.alz.org/alzheimers-dementia/what-is-dementia/types-of-dementia/vascular-dementia

Alzheimer's Society. (2021). *Hallucinations and dementia*. Retrieved January 14, 2025 from https://www.alzheimers.org.uk/about-dementia/symptoms-and-diagnosis/hallucinations#:~:text=What%20are%20hallucinations?,experienced%20by%20people%20with%20dementia

American Brain Foundation. (2024). *Alzheimer's Disease in Latino communities highlights disparities in brain health care*. Retrieved April 14, 2025 https://www.americanbrainfoundation.org/alzheimers-disease-in-latino-communities-highlights-disparities-in-brain-health-care/#:~:text=According%20to%20the%20Alzheimer's%20Association,or%20another%20form%20of%20dementia

American Psychiatric Association. (2022). *Diagnostic and statistical manual of mental disorders* (5th ed.) text revision. Author.

Azargoonjahromi, A. (2024). The duality of amyloid-β: Its role in normal and Alzheimer's disease states. *Molecular Brain, 17*(1), 44. https://doi.org/10.1186/s13041-024-01118-1

Azizan, Z., Zali, H., Mirmotalebisohi, S. A., Bazrgar, M., & Ahmadiani, A. (2024). Deciphering molecular bridges: Unveiling the interplay between metabolic syndrome and Alzheimer's disease through a systems biology approach and drug repurposing. *PloS One, 19*(5), e0304410. https://doi.org/10.1371/journal.pone.0304410

Biogen. (2023). *Aduhelm (aducanumab-avwa). Prescribing Information*. Retrieved January 12, 2025, from https://www.accessdata.fda.gov/drugsatfda_docs/label/2023/761178s011lbl.pdf

Borson, S., Scanlan, J. M., Chen, P., & Ganguli, M. (2003). The Mini-Cog as a screen for dementia: Validation in a population-based sample. *Journal of the American Geriatrics Society, 51*(10), 1451–1454.

Chen, J., Peng, G., & Sun, B. (2024a). Alzheimer's disease and sleep disorders: A bidirectional relationship. *Neuroscience, 557*, 12–23. https://doi.org/10.1016/j.neuroscience.2024.08.008

Chen, L., Li, D., Tang, K., Li, Z., & Huang, X. (2024b). Sleep duration and leisure activities are involved in regulating the association of depressive symptoms, muscle strength, physical function and mild cognitive impairment. *Heliyon, 10*(13), e33832. https://doi.org/10.1016/j.heliyon.2024.e33832

Cloak, N., Schoo, C., & Al Khalili, Y. (2024). Behavioral and psychological symptoms in dementia. In *StatPearls*. StatPearls Publishing. https://www.ncbi.nlm.nih.gov/books/NBK551552/?report=printable

Dalal, S., Ramirez-Gomez, J., Sharma, B., Devara, D., & Kumar, S. (2024). MicroRNAs and synapse turnover in Alzheimer's disease. *Ageing Research Reviews, 99*, 102377. https://doi.org/10.1016/j.arr.2024.102377

Devlin, J. W. (2024). Pharmacologic treatment strategies for delirium in hospitalized adults: past, present, and future. *Seminars in Neurology, 44*(6), 762–776. https://doi.org/10.1055/s-0044-1791246

Dominguez, L. J., Veronese, N., Parisi, A., Seminara, F., Vernuccio, L., Catanese, G., & Barbagallo, M. (2024). Mediterranean diet and lifestyle in persons with mild to moderate Alzheimer's disease. *Nutrients, 16*(19), 3421. https://doi.org/10.3390/nu16193421

Ekundayo, B. E., Obafemi, T. O., Adewale, O. B., Obafemi, B. A., Oyinloye, B. E., & Ekundayo, S. K. (2024). Oxidative stress, endoplasmic reticulum stress and apoptosis in the pathology of Alzheimer's disease. *Cell Biochemistry and Biophysics, 82*(2), 457–477. https://doi.org/10.1007/s12013-024-01248-2

Eli Lilly and Company. (2024). *Kisunla (donanemab-abt). Prescribing Information*. Retrieved January 12, 2025, from https://www.accessdata.fda.gov/drugsatfda_docs/label/2024/761248s000lbl.pdf

Eisai Inc. and Biogen. (2024). *Leqembi (lecanemab-irmb). Prescribing Information*. Retrieved January 12, 2025, from https://www.accessdata.fda.gov/drugsatfda_docs/label/2024/761269s008lbl.pdf

Frost, E. D., Shi, S. X., Byroju, V. V., Pitton Rissardo, J., Donlon, J., Vigilante, N., Murray, B. P., Walker, I. M., McGarry, A., Ferraro, T. N., Hanafy, K. A., Echeverria, V., Mitrev, L., Kling, M. A., Krishnaiah, B., Lovejoy, D. B., Rahman, S., Stone, T. W., & Koola, M. M. (2024). Galantamine-memantine combination in the treatment of Parkinson's disease dementia. *Brain sciences*, *14*(12), 1163. https://doi.org/10.3390/brainsci14121163

Galvin, J. E., Roe, C. M., Powlishta, K. K., Coats, M. A., Muich, S. J., Grant, E., Miller, J. P., Storandt, M., & Morris, J. C. (2005). The AD8: A brief informant interview to detect dementia. *Neurology*, *65*(4), 559–564.

Galvin, J. E., Roe, C. M., Xiong, C., & Morris, J. C. (2006). Validity and reliability of the AD8 informant interview in dementia. *Neurology*, *67*(11), 1942–1948.

Gogia, B., & Fang, X. (2023). Differentiating delirium versus dementia in the elderly. In *StatPearls*. StatPearls Publishing. https://www.ncbi.nlm.nih.gov/books/NBK570594

Gonzales, P. N. G., Villaraza, S. G., & Rosa, J. C. D. (2024). The association between sleep and Alzheimer's disease: A systematic review. *Dementia & Neuropsychologia*, *18*, e20230049. https://doi.org/10.1590/1980-5764-DN-2023-0049

Grzenda, A., Siddarth, P., Milillo, M. M., Aguilar-Faustino, Y., Khalsa, D. S., & Lavretsky, H. (2024). Cognitive and immunological effects of yoga compared to memory training in older women at risk for Alzheimer's disease. *Translational Psychiatry*, *14*(1), 96. https://doi.org/10.1038/s41398-024-02807-0

Haider, A., Spurling, B. C., & Sánchez-Manso, J. C. (2023). Lewy body dementia. In *StatPearls*. StatPearls Publishing. https://www.ncbi.nlm.nih.gov/books/NBK482441

He, M., Lian, T., Liu, Z., Li, J., Qi, J., Li, J., Guo, P., Zhang, Y., Luo, D., Guan, H., Zhang, W., Zheng, Z., Yue, H., Zhang, W., Wang, R., Zhang, F., & Zhang, W. (2024). An investigation into the potential association between nutrition and Alzheimer's disease. *Frontiers in Nutrition*, *11*, 1306226. https://doi.org/10.3389/fnut.2024.1306226

Huang, Y. Y., Gan, Y. H., Yang, L., Cheng, W., & Yu, J. T. (2024). Depression in Alzheimer's disease: Epidemiology, mechanisms, and treatment. *Biological Psychiatry*, *95*(11), 992–1005. https://doi.org/10.1016/j.biopsych.2023.10.008

Jack, C. R., Jr, Andrews, J. S., Beach, T. G., Buracchio, T., Dunn, B., Graf, A., Hansson, O., Ho, C., Jagust, W., McDade, E., Molinuevo, J. L., Okonkwo, O. C., Pani, L., Rafii, M. S., Scheltens, P., Siemers, E., Snyder, H. M., Sperling, R., Teunissen, C. E., & Carrillo, M. C. (2024). Revised criteria for diagnosis and staging of Alzheimer's disease: Alzheimer's Association Workgroup. *Alzheimer's & Dementia*, *20*(8), 5143–5169. https://doi.org/10.1002/alz.13859

Jackson, R. J., Hyman, B. T., & Serrano-Pozo, A. (2024). Multifaceted roles of APOE in Alzheimer disease. *Nature Reviews. Neurology*, *20*(8), 457–474. https://doi.org/10.1038/s41582-024-00988-2

Jiménez-Palomares, M., Garrido-Ardila, E. M., Chávez-Bravo, E., Torres-Piles, S. T., González-Sánchez, B., Rodríguez-Mansilla, M. J., De Toro-García, Á., & Rodríguez-Mansilla, J. (2024). Benefits of music therapy in the cognitive impairments of Alzheimer's-type dementia: A systematic review. *Journal of Clinical Medicine*, *13*(7), 2042. https://doi.org/10.3390/jcm13072042

Krishnamurthy, H. K., Jayaraman, V., Krishna, K., Wang, T., Bei, K., Changalath, C., & Rajasekaran, J. J. (2024). An overview of the genes and biomarkers in Alzheimer's disease. *Ageing Research Reviews*, *104*, 102599. https://doi.org/10.1016/j.arr.2024.102599

Leach, M. J., Sangalli, M., Breakspear, I., & Walsh, S. (2021). Essential oils for agitation in dementia [rELOAD]: A pragmatic, cluster-randomized, placebo-controlled, pilot feasibility trial. *Integrative Medicine Research*, *10*(4), 100747. https://doi.org/10.1016/j.imr.2021.100747

Liao, Y., Chen, H. W., Qiu, C., Shen, H., He, Z. Y., Song, Z. C., & Zhou, W. (2025). Detection of amyloid-β peptides in gingival crevicular fluid and its effect on oral pathogens. *Molecular Oral Microbiology*, *40*(2), 94–103. https://doi.org/10.1111/omi.12488

Lindroth, H., Liu, K., Szalacha, L., Ashkenazy, S., Bellelli, G., van den Boogaard, M., Caplan, G., Chung, C. R., Elhadi, M., Gurjar, M., Heras-La-Calle, G., Hoffman, M., Jeitziner, M. M., Krewulak, K., Mailhot, T., Morandi, A., Nawa, R. K., Oh, E. S., Collet, M. O.,…WDAD Study Team. (2024). World delirium awareness and quality survey in 2023-a worldwide point prevalence study. *Age and Ageing*, *53*(11), afae248. https://doi.org/10.1093/ageing/afae248

Liu, E., Zhang, Y., & Wang, J. Z. (2024). Updates in Alzheimer's disease: from basic research to diagnosis and therapies. *Translational Neurodegeneration*, *13*(1), 45. https://doi.org/10.1186/s40035-024-00432-x

Mather, M., & Scommegna, P. (2024). *Fact sheet: Aging in the United States*. Population Reference Bureau. https://www.prb.org/resources/fact-sheet-aging-in-the-united-states/

National Institute on Aging (NIA). (2024a). *What is dementia? Alzheimer's & Related Dementias*. Retrieved January 14, 2025, from https://www.alzheimers.gov/alzheimers-dementias/what-is-dementia

National Institute on Aging (NIA). (2024b). *Alzheimer's disease fact sheet*. Alzheimer's and Related Dementias Education and Referral Center. National Institute on Aging. NIH Publication No. 24-AG-6323. https://order.nia.nih.gov/sites/default/files/2024-07/nia-alzheimers-fact-sheet.pdf

National Institute on Aging (NIA). (2023). *Alzheimer's and related dementia resources for professionals*. National Institute on Aging. Retrieved January 12, 2025, from https://www.nia.nih.gov/health/alzheimers-dementia-resources-for-professionals

Ning, L., Shen, R., Xie, B., Jiang, Y., Geng, X., & Dong, W. (2024). AMPA receptors in Alzheimer disease: Pathological changes and potential therapeutic targets. *Journal of Neuropathology and Experimental Neurology*, *83*(11), 895–906. https://doi.org/10.1093/jnen/nlae093

Padala, A. P., Ramakrishnan, P., & Crawford, C. G. (2024). Spirituality for social isolation in a patient with cognitive impairment: A case report. *Journal of Alzheimer's Disease Reports*, *8*(1), 447–452. https://doi.org/10.3233/ADR-220028

Patti, L., & Gupta, M. (2023). Change in mental status. In *StatPearls*. StatPearls Publishing. https://www.ncbi.nlm.nih.gov/books/NBK441973

Perneczky, R., Dom, G., Chan, A., Falkai, P., & Bassetti, C. (2024). Anti-amyloid antibody treatments for Alzheimer's disease. *European Journal of Neurology*, *31*(2), e16049. https://doi.org/10.1111/ene.16049

Pszczołowska, M., Walczak, K., Miśków, W., Antosz, K., Batko, J., Kurpas, D., & Leszek, J. (2024). Chronic traumatic encephalopathy as the course of Alzheimer's disease. *International Journal of Molecular Sciences*, *25*(9), 4639. https://doi.org/10.3390/ijms25094639

Qu, L., Li, Y., Liu, F., Fang, Y., He, J., Ma, J., Xu, T., Wang, L., Lei, P., Dong, H., Jin, L., Yang, Q., Wu, W., & Sun, D. (2024). Microbiota-gut-brain axis dysregulation in Alzheimer's disease: Multi-pathway effects and therapeutic potential. *Aging and Disease*, *15*(3), 1108–1131. https://doi.org/10.14336/AD.2023.0823-2

Ramírez Echeverría, M. D. L., Schoo, C., Paul, M., & Doerr, C. (2022). Delirium (nursing). In *StatPearls*. StatPearls Publishing. https://www.ncbi.nlm.nih.gov/books/NBK568723

Rose, O., Huber, S., Trinka, E., Pachmayr, J., & Clemens, S. (2024). Treatment of Parkinson's disease psychosis-a systematic review and multi-methods approach. *Biomedicines*, *12*(10), 2317. https://doi.org/10.3390/biomedicines12102317

Ryan, S. L. (2024). Nonpharmacological prevention and management of delirium: Past, present, and future. *Seminars in Neurology*, *44*(6), 777–787. https://doi.org/10.1055/s-0044-1791696

Sakusic, A., & Rabinstein, A. A. (2025). ICU delirium. *Neurologic Clinics*, *43*(1), 1–13. https://doi.org/10.1016/j.ncl.2024.07.001

Samuelsson, J., Kern, S., Zetterberg, H., Blennow, K., Rothenberg, E., Wallengren, O., Skoog, I., & Zettergren, A. (2021). A Western-style dietary pattern is associated with cerebrospinal fluid biomarker levels for preclinical Alzheimer's disease—A population-based cross-sectional study among 70-year-olds. *Alzheimer's & Dementia (New York, N. Y.)*, 7(1), e12183. https://doi.org/10.1002/trc2.12183

Seddon, A. R., MacArthur, C. P., Hampton, M. B., & Stevens, A. J. (2024). Inflammation and DNA methylation in Alzheimer's disease: Mechanisms of epigenetic remodelling by immune cell oxidants in the ageing brain. *Redox*, *29*(1), 2428152. https://doi.org/10.1080/13510002.2024.2428152

Taylor, C., Peakman, G., Mackinnon, L., Mohamadzade, N., Han, W., Mackie, L., Gandhi, J., Mitchell, O., Bateman-Champain, C., Hetherington, J., Belarbi, F., & Alg, G. (2024). Improving delirium assessments in acute senior health: A quality improvement project for care of the older person. *BMC Geriatrics*, *24*(1), 781. https://doi.org/10.1186/s12877-024-05273-x

Torbic, H., Chen, A., Lumpkin, M., Yerke, J., Mehkri, O., Abraham, S., Wang, X., Duggal, A., & Scheraga, R. G. (2024). Antipsychotic use for ICU delirium and associated inflammatory markers. *Journal of Intensive Care Medicine*, *39*(4), 313–319. https://doi.org/10.1177/08850666231201567

Wang, J., Fourriere, L., & Gleeson, P. A. (2024). Advances in the cell biology of the trafficking and processing of amyloid precursor protein: impact of familial Alzheimer's disease mutations. *The Biochemical Journal*, *481*(19), 1297–1325. https://doi.org/10.1042/BCJ20240056

Yan, L., Li, H., Qian, Y., Liu, Q., Cong, S., Dou, B., Wang, Y., Wang, M., & Yu, T. (2024). Acupuncture modulates the gut microbiota in Alzheimer's disease: current evidence, challenges, and future opportunities. *Frontiers in Neuroscience*, *18*, 1334735. https://doi.org/10.3389/fnins.2024.1334735

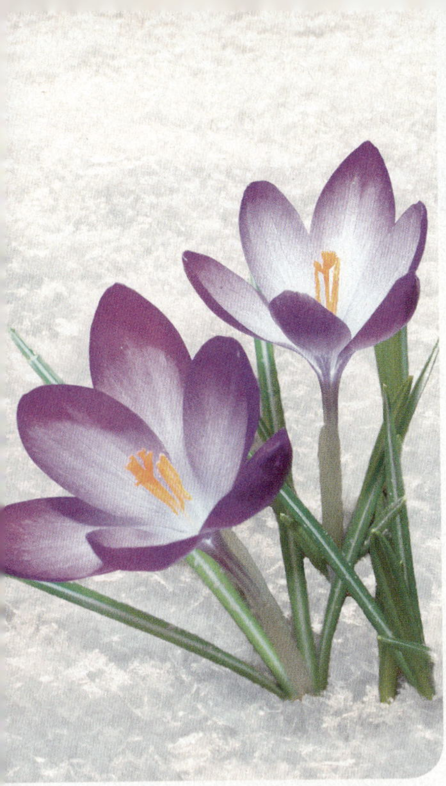

UNIT IX
Care of Special Populations

40
Care of Veterans With Mental Health Needs*

Mary Ann Boyd

KEYCONCEPTS

- military sexual trauma
- military veteran
- moral injury
- veteran identity

LEARNING OBJECTIVES

After studying this chapter, you will be able to:

1. Describe the military culture.
2. Trace the mental health needs of veterans during various military campaigns.
3. Describe the changing role of females in the military.
4. Discuss the inclusion of individuals who are members of underrepresented groups in the military.
5. Analyze mental health needs of veterans.
6. Using a clinical judgment model, formulate a person-centered, recovery-oriented nursing care approach for veterans with mental health needs.
7. Describe the mental health services available to veterans.

KEY TERMS

• active duty • active-duty (regular) service member • anxious-arousal • battle fatigue • betrayal • chronic pain • combat stress reaction (CSR) • combat-related trauma • housing instability • index trauma • microaggression • minority stress • musculoskeletal pain • National Guard members • non–combat-related trauma • nostalgia • numbing symptoms • perpetration • post-9/11 group • re-experiencing • reservist • service-connected disability • sexual assaults • sexual harassment • shell shock • soldier's disease • soldier's heart • traumatic brain injury (TBI) • war neurosis • witnessing

INTRODUCTION

The defense and protection of the United States (U.S.) depend upon the U.S. military armed forces. Wars and conflicts not only shape the history of the United States but also affect the long-term health and mental health of military service members and veterans. Different health and mental health issues are associated with various wars. Veterans' health and mental health issues reflect the time of service. The aim of this chapter is to discuss the mental health needs and recovery-oriented nursing care for veterans.

*In this chapter, "male" refers to a person assigned male at birth, and "female" refers to a person assigned female at birth.

U.S. MILITARY ORGANIZATIONS

The U.S. military is a complex institution consisting of three departments (Army, Navy, and Air Force) reporting to the Department of Defense (DOD). The Navy and Marines fall under the Department of the Navy and the Air Force and the Space Force under the Department of Air Force. The Coast Guard, which is a military service and a branch of the Armed Forces, is organizationally housed in the Department of Homeland Security (U.S. Department of Defense, 2025).

There are also seven reserve components that provide trained units and qualified people available for **active duty** in time of war or national emergency. The Army, Navy, Marine Corps, Air Force, and Coast Guard reserves are under federal control and are activated when they are needed. The Army National and Air National Guards are under the authority of their respective states with the exception of the District of Columbia National Guard, which is exclusively a federal organization. All national guard units can be ordered into federal service if needed (Congressional Research Service, 2024).

The operational names of the conflicts in Iraq and Afghanistan are used frequently to differentiate the time and focus of the military engagement (Box 40.1). The military gives names for different operational phases of a war or conflict. See Table 40.1 for an overview of the military wars and conflicts of the United States (Council on Foreign Relations, 2022; Torreon, 2024).

Active-duty (regular) service members are employed full time by the military; the **reservists** and **National Guard members** are not on full-time active duty but may live on a military base and can be deployed at any time. Enlistment time varies from 2 years to more than 20 years depending on the career goals of the service member. Once service members are discharged from the military, they become veterans and are entitled to varying privileges according to their time in service, rank, and situation.

In 1973, the United States ended conscription (compulsory enlistment of males) and transitioned to an all-volunteer force. The U.S. military consists of 2.86 million people worldwide and, in 2023, was the world's third largest active military by size. An estimated 1.29 million currently serve as active-duty personnel, and over 806,000 as national guard/reserves and members of the Coast Guard, which is less than one half of 1% of the U.S. population. In addition, there are another 779,000 civilian workers. The Army is the largest U.S. military service (USA Facts, 2024).

TABLE 40.1 U.S. MILITARY WARS/CONFLICTS

Wars/Conflicts	Periods of War[a]
Revolutionary War	1775–1783
War of 1812	1812–1815
Mexican American War	1846–1848
American Civil War	1861–1865
Spanish American War	1898–1902
World War I	1917–1918
World War II	1939–1946
Korean Conflict	1950–1955
Vietnam Era	1955–1975
Gulf War	1990–1991
Conflict in Afghanistan	2001–2021
Iraq Conflict	2003–2011
Islamic State-Operation Inherent Resolve (OIR)	2014–Ongoing

[a]Dates may vary depending on proclamations, declarations, laws, or treaties.

Source: Torreon, B. S. (2024). U.S. periods of war and dates of recent conflicts. Congressional Research Service. RS21405 and Council on Foreign Relations. (2022). *The U.S. War in Afghanistan 1999–2021*. Retrieved January 16, 2025, from https://www.cfr.org/timeline/us-war-afghanistan

BOX 40.1

Names of Operational Phases of Conflicts in Iraq and Afghanistan

Conflict	Operation Name	Period of Conflict[a]
Afghanistan (Global War on Terror—GWOT)	Operation Enduring Freedom (OEF)	2001–2014
	Operation Freedom's Sentinel (OFS)	2014–present
Iraq	Operation Iraqi Freedom (OIF)	2003–2011
	Operation New Dawn (OND)	2010–2014
Afghanistan	Operation Freedom's Sentinel (OFS)	2015–2021
	Islamic State-Operation Inherent Resolve (OIR)	2014–Present

[a]Dates may vary depending on proclamations, declarations, laws, or treaties.

Source: Torreon, B. S., & Miller, C. A. (2024). U.S. periods of war and dates of recent conflicts. Congressional Research Service. RS21405. Retrieved January 24, 2025, from https://sgp.fas.org/crs/natsec/RS21405.pdf

Military Culture

The military culture is structured to protect and defend the United States. The values, beliefs, and behaviors acquired in the military often last a lifetime. As a hierarchal organization, there is a chain of command with defined authority and responsibility. Leaders protect and maintain the health and well-being of their subordinates. Officers are expected to transmit values of honor, pride, discipline, and loyalty, instill warrior beliefs, and display self-sacrifice behaviors. There is a clear separation of officers and enlisted members with order and discipline being instilled in both groups. Officers and enlisted members are expected to maintain separate social networks. Within the military, there is little room for individuality. Symbols of military order include uniforms and rituals such as saluting officers and military march (Center for Deployment Psychology, 2021).

The Changing Role of Females in the Military Throughout History

Before World War II (WWII), females could only serve in the Women's Army Auxiliary Corps and the Army Nurse Corps which were temporary auxiliary components. They were activated only during times of national need such as during a war. These individuals were released from duty at the end of each war. Their work was often stigmatized and mocked. Sexual harassment was common (National WWII Museum, 2024).

The *Women's Armed Services Integration Act* signed into law on June 12, 1948, recognized females as full members of the armed forces. This meant that they could claim the same benefits as their male counterparts, and it allowed females to make a career in the armed forces. The law limited the number of females who could serve in the military to 2% of total forces in each branch. As a result of a regulation, females with dependent children were ineligible to serve in the military (Lopez, 2023).

During the Vietnam War, an estimated 10,000 females in the American military served in Southeast Asia, 90% of whom were nurses (Singleton, 2024). When the draft ended in 1973, females represented just 2% of enlisted forces and 8% of the officer corps (Council on Foreign Relations, 2020). Following the elimination of the draft, the need for service members became apparent, and females were actively recruited into the military. Females were finally admitted into America's service academies in 1976. Nearly 41,000 females were deployed to the Persian Gulf region during both gulf wars (Operation Desert Shield and Desert Storm). In 2020, females represented 16% of the enlisted forces and 19% of the officers. More than 300,000 females have served in Iraq and Afghanistan post-9/11 (DeSimone, 2023).

Inclusion of Individuals Who Are Members of Underrepresented Groups in the Military

Information related to individuals who are members of underrepresented groups in the military is very general because of federal racial and ethnic categorization. Federal agencies categorize race according to five groups—White, Black or African American, American Indian or Alaska Native, Asian, and Native Hawaiian or other Pacific Islander. Ethnicity is divided into two groups: (a) Hispanic or Latino and (b) not Hispanic or Latino. Based upon federal data, we know that a greater proportion of individuals who are members of underrepresented groups are found primarily in the lower rather than the higher military ranks. The majority of all service members are White, with the overwhelming majority of officers also White. In all the services, females are underrepresented when compared to male recruits (Statista Research Department, 2024).

For most of the U.S. military history, people who identified as lesbian, gay, bisexual, transgender, and queer or questioning (LGBTQ+) were excluded from military service. In 1993, a DOD *Directive 1304.26*, known as the "Don't Ask, Don't Tell policy," was issued that prohibited military personnel from asking or requiring recruits and service members to reveal their sexuality. People were no longer barred from military service based on sexual orientation. Even though LGBTQ+ individuals could serve in the military service if they concealed their sexual orientation, they could be excluded if they engaged in same-sex activities (or intended to do so), or if they attempted or accomplished same-sex marriage (DOD Directive, 1993, December 21). This directive remained in place until 2011 when the policy was repealed following a decision by a federal appeals court that barred further enforcement of the military's ban on openly gay members. In 2016, President Obama allowed transgender individuals to serve openly in the armed forces, but the policy was later reversed by President Trump. In 2021, President Biden lifted the ban and individuals who identified as LGBTQ+ could serve openly in the military. In 2025, re-elected President Trump again issued an executive order banning transgender individuals from serving in the military; this is currently being challenged in the court system as unconstitutional.

VETERANS OF THE U.S. MILITARY

KEYCONCEPT Military veteran refers to people who served in the armed services.

Every year, about 200,000 service members transition to civilian life (U.S. Department of Veterans Affairs, 2024a). In 2023, there were more than 18 million veterans in the United States or about 6% of the U.S. population. The veteran population has been declining for years and the decline is expected to continue. By 2048, it is projected that there will be about 12.1 million veterans living in the United States (Schaffer, 2023).

The veteran population served in several different departments, wars, and conflicts. The largest cohort of veterans served during the Vietnam Era (5.6 million) which lasted from 1964 to 1975. More than three quarters (78%) of veterans served during wartime and 22% during peacetime (Schaffer, 2023). The median age of veterans today is 65. The **post-9/11 group** (military service after September 2001) is the youngest with a median age of about 37 years. Vietnam Era veterans have a median age of about 71 years, and WWII veterans are the oldest with a median age of about 93 years (Vespa, 2020).

Veteran Identity

The veteran population consists of people of varying ages, ethnicities, races, and military experiences. The common element for all veterans is that their experience in the military helped to shape their adult life and form a veteran identity.

KEYCONCEPT A veteran identity is the prominence of past military service, beliefs, and norms on an individual's post-military sense of self (Dolan et al., 2022, pp. 231).

For veterans, this identity can be their primary view of themselves and defines their relationship with the world. Veterans have a distinct culture and social identity. A strong veteran identity can be compared to ethnicity, with cultural forces influencing the sense of self. For individuals with a strong veteran identity, it is important that others know them as veterans (Dolan et al., 2022).

The presence of a strong veteran identity is variable. Some people who are discharged from the military do not identify as veterans. Research shows that the strength of the veteran identity depends on several factors. For example, the extent of engagement with veteran service organizations and peers, identity reinforcement by civilian employment, and combat experience influence the strength of the veteran identity. Mental health issues as a result of the military experience, such as depression or posttraumatic stress disorder (PTSD), also play a role in forming a veteran identity (Dolan et al., 2022).

Post-military experiences can have a positive or negative impact on the strength of a veteran identity. For example, assimilation into a civilian world can pressure the individual to let go of the veteran identity. Contact with other veterans can support the veteran identity, which in turn can strengthen friendships, self-esteem, and reintegration into the civilian world (Guerrero et al., 2021; Miller & Saling, 2024).

Female Veterans

Females make up a growing share of veterans (U.S. Department of Veterans Affairs, 2022a). In 2023, about 11.3% of veterans or 2.1 million were females. By 2040, the number of female veterans is projected to increase to 18%. In 2023, the median age of female veterans was 52 years compared to 65 years for their male counterparts. The middle adulthood group (45 to 64 years old) represent the largest group of female patients in the Veterans Health Administration (VHA) (U.S. Department of Veterans Affairs, 2024b).

Females tend to be younger and more likely college graduates than their male counterparts (holding similar positions or functions). Females were more likely to serve during the Afghanistan/Iraq War, be deployed in National Guard/Reserve units, and less likely to experience high combat exposure. The female veteran population is more racially diverse than their male counterparts and is less likely to serve multiple tours. Female veterans are more likely to have low resilience and report poor health. female veterans are more likely to contemplate suicide and experience depression, but less likely to misuse alcohol than their male counterparts (Adams et al., 2021).

HEALTH CARE FOR VETERANS

The United States has an extensive system of integrated care for veterans. This health care system addresses the unique health and mental health needs of military veterans.

Health Issues of Veterans

Veterans have distinctive health issues related to the military service. They are more likely to suffer from trauma-related injuries, substance use, and mental health disorders than people who have never served in the armed forces. About one third (30%) of all veterans have a **service-connected disability**, an injury, disease, or disability that active duty either caused or aggravated. The post-9/11 veterans have the highest number of service-connected disabilities, with a 50% chance of reporting a high service-connected disability. The post-9/11 veterans have the highest proportion of disabilities for all groups (Vespa & Carter, 2024).

It is thought that the high rate of post-9/11 veterans service-connected disabilities is related to several factors such as extended tours of duty or difficult service conditions that were not experienced by the other cohorts. Another reason is that medical advances allow veterans to survive injuries that would have been fatal in past wars. Black, Hispanic, and veterans who are members of other underrepresented groups are more likely than White veterans to have a service-connected disability (Vespa, 2020). Although the type and severity of most injuries have remained constant across time, this is not true of PTSD. PTSD is more likely to be reported today than during previous periods (Vespa & Carter, 2024).

Transition to Civilian Life

Providing access and care immediately upon separation from the military is critical. The transition from the structured military life to civilian life can be difficult and

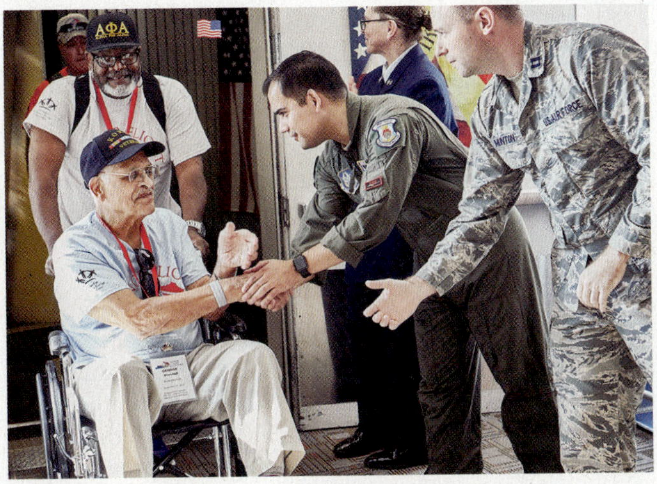

FIGURE 40.1 Active service members thanking veterans for their service.

stressful. The first year after discharge from the military is a high-risk period. Many newly separated veterans report chronic physical or mental health conditions and are less satisfied with their health than their work or social relations. Work satisfaction often deteriorates shortly after beginning a civilian job. Enlisted personnel consistently report poorer health, vocational, and social outcomes compared to their officer counterpart. War-zoned deployed service members report more health concerns; females have more mental health concerns when compared to their non-deployed female and male peers (Markowitz et al., 2023; Sachdev & Dixit, 2024).

The *Transition Assistance Program* supported by the departments of Defense, Veterans Affairs, and Homeland Security provides seamless access to mental health care and suicide prevention resources, particularly during the first year after separation or retirement. This program provides information on veteran benefits, mental health resources, training, and other resources to service members as they transition from military to civilian life. Psychosocial and peer support are also provided. Registration in the Veterans Administration Health Care System is facilitated to assure access to health care. Veterans can choose to seek health care in the private community systems or the VHA (Fig. 40.1).

Veterans Health Administration and U.S. Government Support of Veterans

The U.S. federal government has provided some care for veterans since the first Soldier's Home opened after the Civil War in 1865. By 1946, the Veterans Administration operated 87 hospitals. In 2024, the VHA is one of the two components of the Department of Veterans Affairs led by the Secretary of Veterans Affairs for Health and operates numerous medical and health care centers. The VHA has grown from 54 hospitals in 1930 to 1,600 health care facilities including 144 VA Medical Centers and 1,232 outpatient sites of care. The VHA operates one of the largest integrated health care systems in the world (U.S. Department of Veterans Affairs, 2024c).

In 2007, the Department of Veterans Affairs established the VA Nurse Academy which later became the VA Nursing Academic Partnerships. The goal is to enhance the care of the Veterans through developing relationships with nursing schools and providing educational opportunities for students (U.S. Department of Veterans Affairs, 2022b).

MENTAL HEALTH NEEDS OF VETERANS

Mental health needs are pervasive in the veteran population. Post-deployment depression, PTSD, and substance use disorders are disabling to the veterans and their families. Veterans are also at risk for suicide, traumatic brain injury (TBI), and housing instability.

Protective Factors

A strong veteran identity contributes to a positive self-esteem and self-definition and it can be protective of mental health issues such as suicidal ideation (Guerrero et al., 2021). Protective factors also include serving multiple tours, having a rank as an officer, and living in a rural area. Other protective factors include sense of duty toward others, employment, being able to meet basic needs, self-care, living stability, social support, spirituality, resilience, and self-determination (Moore et al., 2023).

Risks for Mental Health Issues

Veterans who are exposed to stressors and traumatic events during military deployments are at greater risk for mental disorders than the general population. Common risk factors for major depressive disorder and PTSD include having high combat exposure, history of concussion, high stressful life events within the past year, and low social support. Other predictors of PTSD include being female, high lifetime trauma, and low social capital (few connections with neighborhood and neighbors). Female veterans have a greater risk than their male counterparts for lifetime PTSD, depression, suicidal thoughts, and for lifetime use of psychological services (Fig. 40.2) (Boscarino et al., 2020).

Female veterans are less likely to experience combat and concussions than their male counterparts, but more likely to experience low unit support. Female veterans are more likely to meet criteria for lifetime PTSD, lifetime depression, and lifetime suicidal ideation than male veterans. Female veterans have an increased risk for PTSD, depression, likelihood of using psychiatric services (Adams, 2021).

National guard and reservists are at risk for post-deployment mental health issues which are more

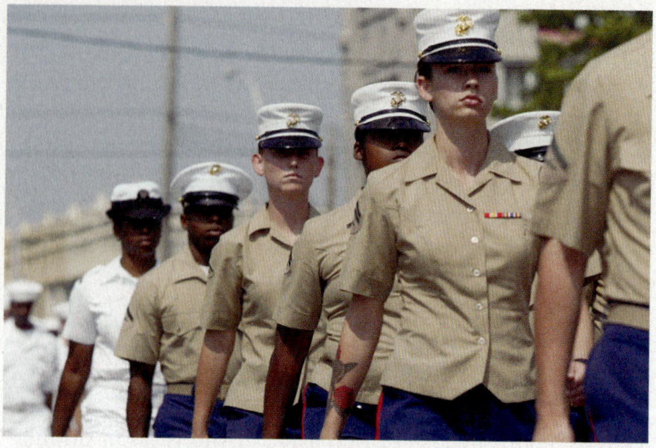

FIGURE 40.2 Female service members are integrated into military formation.

common in the national guard and reserve components than the active-duty component. It was initially thought that the national guard and reservists had higher rates of mental disorders because of being less prepared and having less support than the active component. But research shows that the mental health needs of national guard and reservists were related to combat exposure, lifetime traumatic stress exposures, current life stressors, and current social support (Boscarino et al., 2020).

POSTTRAUMATIC STRESS DISORDER

Trauma and stress during military combat are not new. During the 17th to 19th centuries, the term **nostalgia** described a condition where a longing to return home was experienced by young people in the military. In nostalgia, service members experienced sadness, insomnia, and anorexia which were sometimes linked to psychic trauma. Nostalgia could lead to death (Battesti, 2016). During the American Civil War (1861–1865), a disorder known as **soldier's heart** developed after combat and was expressed as fatigue, shortness of breath, sighing respirations, palpitations, rapid heart rate, and sweating, with no observable cardiologic anomaly (Da Costa, 1871; Ursano & Stein, 2022). During the First World War (WWI) (1914–1918), a condition known as **shell shock** or **war neurosis** was identified and shared similar, but not all, characteristics of modern-day posttraumatic disorder (Pedroso et al., 2017; Stein & Rothbaum, 2018). In WWII, the terms **combat stress reaction (CSR)** and **battle fatigue** described a psychological condition that soldiers developed. This syndrome was characterized by anxiety, intense autonomic arousal, reliving, and sensitivity to stimuli (Andreasen, 2010). Up to half of the military discharges during WWII were said to be related to combat exhaustion (Friedman, n.d.).

The Korean and Vietnam wars brought attention to the traumatic experiences of service members. When the *Diagnostic and Statistical Manual III* was published in 1980, a stress disorder category was included (American Psychiatric Association [APA], 1980). The PTSD diagnostic criteria have evolved into the current diagnosis published in the *DSM-5-TR*. See Chapter 29. PTSD is now understood to be a complex interplay of biologic and psychological symptoms that are experienced as a result of other traumatic experiences besides the trauma of war.

Epidemiology

The prevalence of PTSD in veterans is difficult to estimate because of the various diagnostic criteria that have been used over several decades. Reliable data on the prevalence of PTSD in veterans from WWII to Vietnam War are not available. Most experts believe the prevalence is much greater than reported. Estimated prevalence data of PTSD from OEF and OIF veterans is 29%. Experts agree that veterans who served Iraq and Afghanistan report higher rates of PTSD than nonveteran population. Co-occurring disorders, particularly alcohol use disorder (AUD), are common in veterans with PTSD (U.S. Department of Veterans Affairs, n.d.).

Trauma

To meet the criteria for a PTSD diagnosis, there must be exposure "to actual or threatened death, serious injury, or sexual violence" (APA, 2022, p. 306). The trauma can be experienced, witnessed, or learned about such as an accidental or violent event of a family or friend (APA, 2022). An **index trauma** is defined as either the worst single event or closely related multiple events (Nester et al., 2024). When there are multiple traumatic events, it may be difficult to identify one single event that precipitated the PTSD symptoms.

Service members deployed to areas of combat are at high risk for trauma, such as Iraq and Afghanistan. In the recent Iraq/Afghanistan Wars battlefield lines were not linear. There was no clearly defined front line or area in the rear where safe operations could be performed. Attacks occurred without warning and battle lines shifted. Witnessing and experiencing combat events in these high-risk locations have provoked traumatic responses and initiated PTSD.

Typical PTSD symptoms related to military trauma include startle reaction with hypervigilance, avoidance of memories with avoidance of external reminders, anhedonia with detachment, being upset when reminded of the event (physiologic reactivity), and dreams with sleep disturbance (Mojallal et al., 2024).

Combat- Versus Non–Combat-Related Trauma

Military trauma can be categorized as combat- or non–combat-related. **Combat-related trauma** occurs while engaging in warfare activities that involve injuries, loss of comrades on the battlefield, and improvised explosive devices. **Non–combat-related trauma** occurs outside of direct combat and includes trauma such as military sexual trauma (MST), witnessing violence, and serious accidents. Both types of traumas can result in PTSD. When combat-related traumas are compared with non–combat-related traumas, differences in PTSD symptom patterns emerge.

In a study of 944 veterans, 63.5% experienced combat-related trauma. They were more likely to be male, White or Hawaiian/Pacific Islander, married or widowed, serve in Vietnam, or OEF/OIF/Operation New Dawn (OND). This cohort experienced self-blame, intrusive memories with dreams, detachment, and reckless behavior with lack of positive emotion. The veteran group that experienced non–combat-related trauma were more likely to be female, Black and African American, divorced, separated, or never married and to have either not deployed to a war zone or served in wars other than Vietnam and OEF/OIF/OND. The PTSD symptoms of this group included exaggerated startle, self-blame with distorted beliefs, and concentration issues related to anhedonia (Macia et al., 2020).

Moral Injury

Moral injury has emerged as a significant construct in understanding the consequences of exposure to traumatic events (Phelps et al., 2024). Moral injury occurs when there is a betrayal of what is right by an individual in legitimate authority in a high-stakes situation (Shay, 2014). The concept was originally used to explain the experience of some Vietnam combat veterans with mental and behavioral health issues.

> **KEYCONCEPT Moral injury** is "the lasting psychological, biological, spiritual, behavioral, and social impact of perpetrating, failing to prevent, or bearing witness to acts that transgress deeply held moral beliefs and expectations" (Litz et al., 2009, p. 699).

Moral injurious experiences violate moral beliefs or cause one to question the justness of the world. Three types of moral injury have been identified. **Perpetration** is an act that transgresses or goes beyond personal moral values. **Witnessing** is observing transgression by others. **Betrayal** is being wronged by others' transgressions. For moral injury to occur, there must be an awareness of the discrepancy between personal morals and the injurious experience which results in dissonance and inner conflict. Consequences of moral injury may include self-harming behaviors and demoralization (Litz, 2025).

When exposure to potentially morally injurious events were examined in post-9/11 veterans ($N = 48{,}965$), 27.9% experienced witnessing events, 18.8% reported perpetration by commission or omission, and 41% reported being betrayed by leadership, fellow service members, or others outside the U.S. military. When separating the findings according to sex assigned at birth, females were more likely to experience psychological distress by witnessing and betrayal, whereas males experienced all three—perpetration, witnessing, and betrayal (Maguen et al., 2020).

The consequences of moral injury are apparent in the lives of the veterans. For example, for males who are parents/caregivers who experienced perpetrating events such as the killing of children in war, they may fear harm to their own children who serve as a reminder of those who were killed. For females, betrayal, such as MST, may be a strong driver of impaired functioning leading to demoralization and self-blame (Maguen et al., 2020).

Violent Combat and Caring for the Wounded

Violent combat is associated with a greater risk of developing **re-experiencing**, a cognitive–sensory experience with an emotional response to current stimuli that resembles the aspects of the index trauma. Violent combat also is associated with **numbing symptoms** (feeling flat physically and emotionally, unable to fully participate in life), that are likely a result of intrusive memories, nightmares, distress, and physiologic reactivity (Moore et al., 2023).

Being close to the wounded or dying is associated with re-experiencing and **anxious-arousal** symptoms (cognitive impairment with autonomic symptoms). For example, military personnel who gave aid to the wounded and seriously wounded or handled bodies of killed service members are more likely to re-experience the trauma and exhibit anxious-arousal symptoms (Spaegele et al., 2024).

Microaggressions and Stress in Individuals Who Are Members of Underrepresented Groups

Veterans who identify as LGBTQ+ are under stress because of social attitudes, stigma, and prevailing policies that may include exclusion from the service or reduction of benefits. They can have PTSD from experiencing the trauma of war, plus discrimination, **microaggressions** (brief verbal, behavioral, or environmental indignities, whether intentional or unintentional, that communicate hostile, derogatory, or negative slights and insult), and **minority stress** (high levels of stress experienced by individuals who are stigmatized because they are members of underrepresented groups). These individuals report experiencing paranoia, hypervigilance, drug use, sexual risk taking, and heightened anxiety and depression (Harper et al., 2024; Parker et al., 2024).

EVIDENCE-BASED NURSING CARE FOR VETERANS WITH PTSD

As with any patient, a comprehensive, patient-centered, and culturally informed assessment will guide veteran care. Veterans have unique needs which should be considered during the assessment process. Some veterans have a strong veteran identity, but others do not. It is important to determine the significance of the veteran experience and the relationship of the current PTSD symptoms to the military experience. Safety is always a concern. Is the patient having suicide thoughts or behaviors? For combat-related veterans, evidence of detachment, avoidance of people and places, and lack of social support are important indications that the veteran is experiencing PTSD symptoms.

The nurse should help the veteran identify the PTSD symptoms and refer patient to PTSD services. Encouragement from friends and family will increase the likelihood of engaging in therapy and the need for interpersonal therapy.

MILITARY SEXUAL TRAUMA

KEYCONCEPT Military sexual trauma (MST) refers to sexual assault and sexual harassment experienced during a veteran's military service (U.S. Department of Veterans Affairs, 2021b).

MST includes any sexual activity during military service where a veteran is involved against their will. MST can occur on or off the military base (see Box 40.2). People who conduct MST can be anyone—males or females, military personnel or civilians, commanding officers or subordinates, strangers, friends, or intimate partners.

MST is not a new phenomenon but has become more visible because people who have experienced MST are more likely to report the incident. In earlier wars, such as WWII and Vietnam, MST was underreported. If reported, the prevailing attitude was that the individual who experienced MST was responsible because something they did had caused the abuse. **Sexual harassment** (e.g., jokes, images involving sexual innuendos, and comments regarding sexual activity) is documented by female veterans from before 1973 through 1993. This harassment often occurred in public and work locations. **Sexual assaults** (i.e., intentional sexual touching without the individual's consent, groping, rape, and forcing an individual to engage in a sexual act) were more likely to occur when a female was alone and on duty. People who conduct MST were more likely to be ranked higher than the person who experienced the abuse (Wolff & Mills, 2016).

BOX 40.2

Military Sexual Trauma (MST)

MST BEHAVIORS

- Pressured into sexual activities—threats of negative consequences for not cooperating
- Unable to consent to sexual activities (i.e., when intoxicated)
- Physically forced into sexual activities
- Unwanted sexual touching or grabbing
- Threatening, offensive remarks about an individual's body, or sexual activities
- Threatening and unwelcome sexual advance

REACTIONS OF PEOPLE WHO HAVE EXPERIENCED MST

- Strong emotions (depressed, intense emotions, angry, and irritable)
- Feelings of numbness
- Trouble sleeping
- Difficulties with attention, concentration, and memory
- Misuse of alcohol or other drugs
- Difficulty with reminders of experience
- Difficulties in relationship
- Physical health issues

Adapted from U.S. Department of Veterans Affairs. (n.d.). Military sexual trauma. Mental Health. Retrieved January 22, 2025, from https://www.mentalhealth.va.gov/msthome/index.asp

Epidemiology

MST occurs primarily to females, but also to males. One in three females and 1 in 50 males have told their VA health care provider that they experienced sexual trauma in the military (U.S. Department of Veterans Affairs, 2021a). LGBTQ+ individuals are at an increased risk for sexual harassment. There is an increased risk of sexual harassment and assault for those who identify as transgender (Zelkowitz et al., 2024).

Mental Health Issues Related to MST

MST is a life-changing event. MST is highly associated with mental health disorders including PTSD, depression, anxiety disorders, eating disorders, suicide, lower satisfaction with interpersonal relationships, and substance use. There is evidence that many people who have experienced MST do not seek mental health care or disclose the trauma. MST represents a morally injurious experience that can profoundly affect an individual's view of the world (Nichter et al., 2024). There are several barriers that prevent people who have experienced MST from reporting abuse including self-stigma and fear of loss of relationships (Iverson et al., 2024). Females who experience MST are often hesitant to seek treatment at the male-dominated VA Medical Centers (Rose et al., 2024).

Depression, PTSD, substance use, suicidal ideation, and severe self-directed violence are associated with MST (Yancey et al., 2024). Self-directed violence such as suicide attempt or nonsuicidal self-injury following MST occurs in both males and females, but females have a greater risk of self-directed violence (Wiblin et al., 2021).

EVIDENCE-BASED NURSING CARE FOR VETERANS WITH MST

Screening for MST should be included in any nursing assessment of veterans. If the veteran screens positive for

BOX 40.3

Research for Evidence-Based Practice: Yoga and MST

Zaccari, B., Sherman, A. D. F., Higgins, M., & Ann Kelly, U. (2024). Trauma center trauma-sensitive yoga versus cognitive processing therapy for female veterans with PTSD who experienced military sexual trauma: A feasibility study. Journal of the American Psychiatric Nurses Association, 30*(2), 343–354. https://doi.org/10.1177/10783903221108765*

THE QUESTION: Is it feasible to implement Trauma Center Trauma-Sensitive Yoga (TCTSY) as a clinical intervention for female veterans with PTSD related to MST?

METHODS: In previous studies of the benefits of yoga to veterans, female veterans were underrepresented. For this study, 41 female veterans were recruited from a Veterans Care Health Care System in the southeastern United States. Participant ages ranged from 30 to 72 years (Md = 45; SD = 9.9) and the median highest education level obtained was 15 years. The majority were African American—non-Hispanic (80.5%), nearly one third (29.3%) had served in a war zone, and one quarter had been hospitalized for psychiatric or mental health treatment and/or had attempted suicide in their lifetime. TCTSY—a standardized Hatha yoga for use by females with treatment-resistant, complex PTSD–was implemented for 10 weekly sessions (n = 17). Cognitive processing therapy, a cognitively based, trauma-focused treatment and gold standard therapy for PTSD treatment, was implemented for 12 weekly sessions (n = 24). Feasibility was determined by demand, practicality, fidelity, and acceptability. Expressed interest, attendance, program completion, barriers to care, and satisfaction were measured.

FINDINGS: Feasibility was supported as a TCTSY intervention and the intervention protocol did not require changes or adaptations. Future studies would benefit from TCTSY-certified facilitators and video-recorded sessions.

IMPLICATIONS FOR NURSING: The results of this study indicate that implementation of yoga is feasible within a trauma center with females with PTSD following MST. Nurses should continue to investigate the use of this complementary therapy when caring for female veterans with PTSD.

MST, the impact of the MST should be discussed and considered for a referral to an experienced therapist or service for MST. In caring for people with MST, nurses should follow similar care strategies as anyone who has had been physically or sexually abused (see Chapter 23). The VHA has developed programs to address the needs of veterans who have experienced MST. See Box 40.3.

DEPRESSION

Depression is common in the U.S. population and is associated with high rates of mortality and morbidity (see Chapter 25). Depression is more common in the veteran population than in the general U.S. population. An increasing number of veterans are reporting depressive symptoms. Depression is highly comorbid with PTSD and suicidal ideation. Trauma exposure is associated with both depression and PTSD, which can ultimately result in suicidal ideation. There is limited research on depression among U.S. veterans (Moore et al., 2023).

Epidemiology

The estimated prevalence of depression among U.S. service members is 3% to 27%. Only a portion of those with depression use mental health services (Sharifian et al., 2025). The most recent published data indicate that the rate of depression in veterans had increased post 9/11, with the rate peaking in 2011 to 2013 at 12.3% of veterans experiencing depression. Studies indicate that rates of depression are low in the veterans cohort because veterans are not likely to seek treatment (Panaite et al., 2024).

Protective Factors

Involvement in community groups and activities, which fosters a sense of belonging and identity, has been shown to be a protective factor for depression and PTSD in veterans. An optimistic disposition appears to be protective of depression. Veterans who are optimistic are more likely to use adaptive and problem-focused coping strategies such as positive reframing of issues and seeking social support (Nichter et al., 2020).

Risk Factors

Black or Hispanic veterans are at high risk for depression and PTSD (Merians et al., 2023). The number of lifetime traumas increases the risk for PTSD and depression. They experience more psychosocial stressors (minority stress and microaggressions) than White veterans that, in turn, increase the risk for depression (Nichter et al., 2020).

EVIDENCE-BASED NURSING CARE FOR VETERANS WITH DEPRESSION

Nursing care for veterans with depression is similar to care for nonveterans. Cognitive therapy, cognitive processing therapy, medications, and transcranial magnetic stimulation are used. The care should be tailored to the needs of the veteran.

Depression and loneliness in female veterans have been associated with impaired quality of life (QOL), which leads to functional decline and behavioral issues. Accessing treatment for depression in female veterans can be complicated by discrimination and sexual harassment by male veterans when accessing VHA health care facilities. When inappropriate or unwanted comments or behavior from male veterans occur, the females are more likely to report feeling unwelcome and unsafe. Hence, the treatment is delayed or appointments are missed (Fitzke et al., 2024). Depression and poor QOL improve with treatment that is timely, comprehensive, and gender-specific (Schafer et al., 2024).

SUICIDE

Suicide occurs in the military and in the veteran population. The following sections differentiate the occurrence of suicide among service members and veterans.

Suicide in the Military

Active-duty military personnel dying by suicide is a relatively new phenomenon. For example, WWII (1939–1945) had a reported suicide rate of 5 per 100,000. Between 1945 and 1991, the rate generally stabilized in the low to mid-teens (10 to 15 per 100,000). Some experts suggest that rates of suicide in earlier wars are likely underreported. They suggest that wars provide other ways to end lives such as rushing from a trench into enemy fire. The military suicide rate began increasing in 2004, peaking in 2012 during the Afghanistan and Iraq Wars with 29.7 per 100,000 reported suicides (Jones, 2019). From 2008 to 2019, the annual rate remained within a range of 20.2 to 29.7 per 100,000 (Smith et al., 2019). In 2022 (latest data), there were 34.7 per 100,000 suicides, with 13.5 per 100,000 for female veterans and 37.3 per 100,000 for male veterans. The rate for nonveterans in 2022 was 17.1 per 100,000, with 7.2 per 100,000 for females and 28.7 per 100,000 for males (Office of Suicide Prevention, 2024).

Suicide in the Veteran Community

The most common suicide method is firearms with 73.5% of suicide deaths due to a self-inflicted firearm injury (74.8% of males; 45.4% of females). Poisoning and suffocation are the next most frequent methods (Office of Suicide Prevention, 2024). Veterans have higher rates of firearm ownership than the general population and are at substantially increased risk of firearm suicide compared to nonveterans. They use firearms mainly for personal protection and generally favor unsecured storage practices. Providers are often hesitant to screen and counsel for firearms because of the lack of familiarity with guns, little confidence in intervention effectiveness, or philosophical reasoning related to constitutional rights (Dempsey et al., 2025; Office of Suicide Prevention, 2024).

Epidemiology

In 2022, suicide rates were highest among multiracial veterans followed by American Indian or Alaska Native veterans and lowest among Black or African American veterans. Veterans aged 18 to 34 had the highest suicide rate with 47.6 per 100,000 (17.1 per 100,000 females and 54.8 per 100,000 males), and veterans aged 75 and older had the lowest suicide rate (33.8 per 100,000) (Office of Suicide Prevention, 2024). Veterans identifying as LGBTQ+ are more likely to report suicidal ideation and screen positive for PTSD, depression, and AUD than heterosexual veterans (Harper et al., 2024).

Protective Factors

The *National Health and Resilience in Veterans Study* (NHRVS), initiated in 2011, is an ongoing study characterizing the longitudinal trajectories of mental and physical health outcomes in U.S. veterans. This study focuses on genetic and environmental risk and protective factors that contribute to these trajectories. Findings from this study show that perceived social support, curiosity, resilience, and acceptance-based coping are protective of suicide. In veterans who had been diagnosed with PTSD and/or major depressive disorder, greater purpose in life, curiosity, and optimism were inversely related to suicidal ideation. For veterans who experience moral injury, having a greater global purpose and meaning in life were important in combating suicidal thoughts (Fischer et al., 2025).

Risk Factors for Veteran Suicide

Several risk factors are associated with veteran suicide including severe moral injury, extensive combat exposure, self-stigmatizing views toward their military identity, recency of discharge from the military, and low general and psychological wellness. Translating military-related skills to civilian jobs contributes to lower income and housing instability. Other risks include loneliness, disability in instrumental daily living (e.g., shopping, cooking), somatic symptoms, and use of denial-based coping (Edwards et al., 2024; Larson et al., 2024).

Suicide rates are higher in veterans with mental health or substance use disorder diagnoses. The risk of suicide is greater in veterans who have been diagnosed with PTSD and/or major depressive disorder (Saulnier et al., 2024).

Childhood abuse is associated with suicide behavior in adulthood. Combat-exposed veterans with a history of childhood sexual abuse are nearly three times more likely to contemplate suicide compared to those without a history of abuse. Childhood sexual abuse is a stronger predictor of suicide attempts than either childhood physical abuse or combat exposure. Childhood sexual abuse leads to long-term psychological consequences such as chronic depression, PTSD, and suicide-related outcomes. When a veteran with a history childhood sexual abuse also experiences MST, the risk for suicide is even greater than if the veteran had not experienced the childhood trauma (Holliday et al., 2023).

EVIDENCE-BASED NURSING CARE FOR VETERANS WITH SUICIDAL IDEATION

The results of the NHRVS studies indicate that a considerable proportion of U.S. veterans experience suicidal ideation, but that ideation may fluctuate over time (Fischer et al., 2025). That is, there may be long periods where suicidal thoughts are absent. Monitoring suicidal ideation by primary care nurses becomes important in identifying veterans' high risk for suicide.

The nursing care of a veteran with suicidal ideation begins with engagement in the therapeutic relationship and treatment. The aim of the care is to keep the veteran safe and to help the individual develop a safety plan (see Chapter 22). The nurse should recognize that veterans often internalize the stigma that seeking mental health care means weakness and are less likely to engage in care. It is estimated that as many as two thirds of veterans with suicidal ideation are not engaged in mental health treatment (Nichter et al., 2021).

Older male veterans with suicidal ideation are less likely to engage in treatment than their younger female counterparts. Concerns about masculinity and gender role expectations are often barriers for male veterans. Veterans are more likely to engage in treatment if they have a diagnosis of depression, a prior suicide attempt, multiple medical issues, or lifetime traumas (Short et al., 2024).

There are several nursing approaches for the care of veterans. The nurse should always screen for suicidal ideation by using a standardized screening tool such as the Columbia Suicide Severity Rating Scale (see Chapter 10). Every veteran should know about the Veterans Crisis Line (Fig. 40.3). If the veteran screens positive for suicidal ideation, the nurse should refer the patient to a mental health professional. If the veteran is currently thinking about hurting or killing themselves, looking for ways to kill themselves, talking about death, dying, or suicide, or carrying out self-destructive acts such as drug misuse or using weapons, the nurse should not leave the patient alone and seek available mental health help.

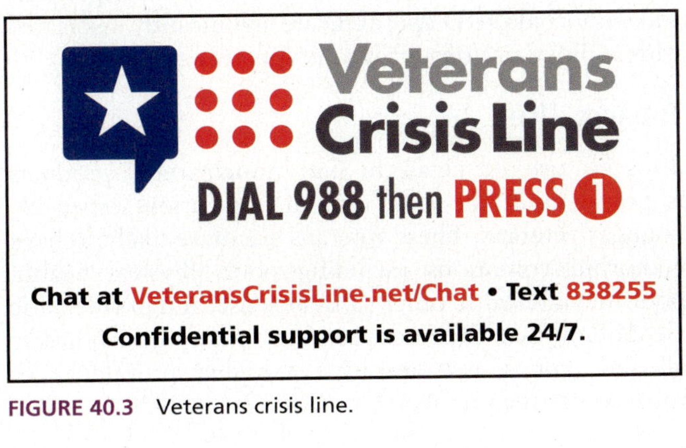

FIGURE 40.3 Veterans crisis line.

The VHA suicide prevention program is an important resource. Suicide prevention is a VHA clinical priority. Each VA Medical Center has a full-time suicide prevention coordinator who provides active preventive interventions and follows up with at-risk veterans. Suicide prevention teams provide community outreach, coordination of resources, and increase awareness of suicide risks. The VA provides medical screening and assessment of patients at risk for suicide. Patients with elevated suicide risk receive an enhanced level of care, including missed appointment follow-up, safety planning, follow-up visits, and care plans that directly address their risk factors for suicide (Office of Suicide Prevention, 2024).

SUBSTANCE USE

Service members and veterans use substances. Frequently, substance use begins in the military and continues following discharge.

Alcohol and Drug Use in the Military

Alcohol and drugs have long been associated with the military and war. Whiskey was used for wounded soldiers, but supplies would disappear and run consistently low. Drinking alcohol was a part of everyday life in the Civil War. Ulysses S. Grant had a well-documented alcohol issue (Chernow, 2017). Morphine was given as an anesthetic and a diarrhea cure, leaving many soldiers with a morphine dependency, or **soldier's disease**. During WWI, cocaine became the drug of misuse of the frontlines. Amphetamines were the most popular drugs used in WWII. Dextroamphetamine was a popular drug during the Vietnam War. During this war, antipsychotics were also given to soldiers (Tackett, 2024).

The misuse of alcohol and drugs in the military continues to be a problem in 2024. Deployment is associated with smoking initiation, unhealthy drinking, drug use, and risky behaviors. Many service members see drinking as part of the military culture. Military members are at higher risk of developing a drug or alcohol issue than civilians. Substance use is associated with combat, trauma, PTSD, and sexual and physical abuse (Moore et al., 2023).

Even though illicit drug use among active-duty personnel is relatively low, alcohol and rates of binge drinking are high compared to the general population. Cigarette smoking and misuse of prescription drugs have decreased in recent years (Moore et al., 2023).

Use of Substances

Substance use often continues long after military service ends. In the military, service members can face dishonorable discharge or criminal prosecution for a positive drug test. These consequences discourage illicit drug use. Once the service member transitions to civilian life, the protection of the service is gone and substance use becomes more likely. More than 1 in 10 veterans is diagnosed with a substance use disorder (Norman et al., 2023).

Alcohol Use

AUD is one of the most prevalent mental disorders in the United States (see Chapter 31). Veterans are more likely to use alcohol than other substances. They also are more likely to use alcohol than their nonveteran counterparts. In the U.S. veteran population, 42.2% met criteria for lifetime AUD (Panza et al., 2022).

Data from the NHRVS identified four veteran trajectories of alcohol consumption over 4 years ($N = 3{,}157$). *Rare drinkers* (65.3%) were abstinent or rarely drank alcohol; *moderate drinkers* (30.2%) consistently drank at a moderate level; *excessive drinkers* (2.6%) drank at elevated levels; and *recovering drinkers* (1.9%) drank excessively and decreased consumption over time. The researchers posited that the low percentage of excessive drinkers was related to the older age of the sample (Panza et al., 2022).

AUD is highly comorbid with PTSD, major depressive disorder, and suicide (Norman et al., 2023). Research shows that comorbidity varies among White, Black, and Hispanic veterans. Black and Hispanic veterans with AUD have greater psychiatric comorbidity relative to White veterans. Hispanic veterans with lifetime AUD have worse physical health, cognitive function, and QOL. Black and Hispanic veterans with lifetime AUD are more likely to screen positive for depressive disorder (Carr et al., 2021). These results suggest that individuals who are members of racial and ethnic underrepresented groups with AUD may have higher rates of mental disorders and poorer outcomes. There is a need for race/ethnicity-sensitive approaches to the care and treatment of AUD in veterans.

Risks and Protective Factors

Alcohol consumption and use of drugs are risks for the development of lifetime AUD. Other risk factors of AUD include trauma, exposure to military stress, and adjustment to civilian life. Due to the stigmatization of mental illness in the military culture, many veterans self-medicate with alcohol rather than access mental health services (Mathes et al., 2024).

Resilience, purpose in life, dispositional gratitude (believing that there is much in life to be thankful for), and religiosity/spirituality are protective factors for developing AUD. Social support and secure attachment style (feeling that it is easy to get close to others; feeling comfortable with others) are also protective.

Opioid Use

Opioid use disorder (OUD) is discussed in Chapter 31. The following discussion is specific to the unique challenges of veterans who use opioids.

Opioid Use in the Military

OUDs often begin with a prescription following an injury. Service members are at high risk for trauma and injury requiring the treatment of pain. Injured and sick military personnel are often prescribed pain medication. Because opioids can quickly become addictive, regular use of opioids can lead to dependency. The amount of pain medication prescribed to service members peaked in 2009 but began decreasing in 2011 in response to the prevention and appropriate prescribing initiatives of the DOD (Dowell et al., 2022).

Opioid Use by Veterans

An estimated 3% of veterans screen positively for OUD. These veterans use prescribed opioid pain relievers not as prescribed, or use opioids not prescribed for them. Characteristics of veterans with OUD include younger age, Black, non-Hispanic, lower income, and having more adverse childhood events compared to veterans who do not screen positively (Na et al., 2024).

Polysubstance Use, Comorbidity, and Overdose

Most veterans in the VHA diagnosed with OUD have at least one comorbid substance use disorder and many have multiple substance use disorders (Lin et al., 2021). OUD is strongly associated with psychiatric and substance use disorders. Opioid use is associated with suicide and unintentional overdose (Na et al., 2024).

Some veterans qualify to enroll in both the VA and Medicare Part D where they can receive opioid prescriptions from both systems. People who use both systems are at significantly higher odds of death from opioid overdose than those who receive opioids from the VA only (Ma et al., 2024). Veterans with an OUD have among the highest rates of suicide when compared to veterans with psychiatric disorders. Comorbid OUD and depression and comorbid OUD and AUD are significantly associated with additive risk of suicide attempts (Na et al., 2024).

Tobacco Use

Tobacco use of cigarette and noncigarette products is prevalent in the U.S. veteran population, especially younger veterans. These veterans are more likely to have comorbid conditions including poor physical health, poor mental health, other substance use, and problematic alcohol use than their nonveteran counterparts. In nearly all age groups, veterans have a higher prevalence of tobacco use than nonveterans (Ruiz et al., 2024).

EVIDENCE-BASED NURSING CARE FOR VETERANS WITH SUBSTANCE USE DISORDER

Nursing care for any veteran should include an assessment of substance use. Based on the research, veterans are at high risk for multiple substance use which significantly impacts their health and well-being. The U.S. veteran population has complex health needs that can be complicated by substance use.

The VHA health care system is prepared for treatment of substance use disorders, but not every veteran seeks care in the VHA system. Recognizing the relationship between the substance use and other health and mental health issues will guide the nurse in planning for the appropriate care. The approach to patients should always be nonjudgmental and foster a therapeutic partnership and help patients move toward recovery. The nurse should always conduct a medication assessment and determine where the prescriptions are filled. A medication assessment is especially important when the veteran is receiving care at the VA and non-VA facility to prevent overprescribing of medication, particularly opioids.

OTHER ISSUES IMPACTING VETERAN MENTAL HEALTH

The wellness and mental health of veterans are impacted by other conditions. These conditions are related to the mental health needs and recovery and are interrelated. It is important for nurses to stay informed about the issues and challenges that are unique to military veterans.

Pain

The prevalence of **chronic pain** (pain lasting longer than 3 to 6 months) occurs more frequently in veterans than nonveterans (Lakshman et al., 2024). General chronic pain prevalence estimate ranges from 25% to 72% of veterans. Pain type includes most parts of the body from head to neck, chest, and back (Reyes et al., 2021). Individuals with chronic pain experience high rates of disability, decreased QOL, and emotional distress (Benedict et al., 2024). Chronic back pain, jaw pain, severe headaches or migraine, and neck pain are frequently reported (Benedict et al., 2024).

Musculoskeletal pain (MSP) is caused by injuries or disorders of the joints, muscles, tendons, or ligaments to the bones, muscles, nerves, and/or connective tissue. Combat injuries (polytrauma, blast injuries) and noncombat injuries (muscle strain, overuse) can lead to chronic MSP. In an integrative review of the incidence, prevalence, and risk factors for MSP and headaches in active duty, inflammation and pain from overuse comprised the largest proportion of injury. The risk of MSP was highest among active duty, female, Army, and enlisted personnel, and those with greater time in a mother vehicle (a larger vehicle that transports smaller vehicles or equipment). For veterans who sustained a TBI, 92% reported headaches (Bader et al., 2018).

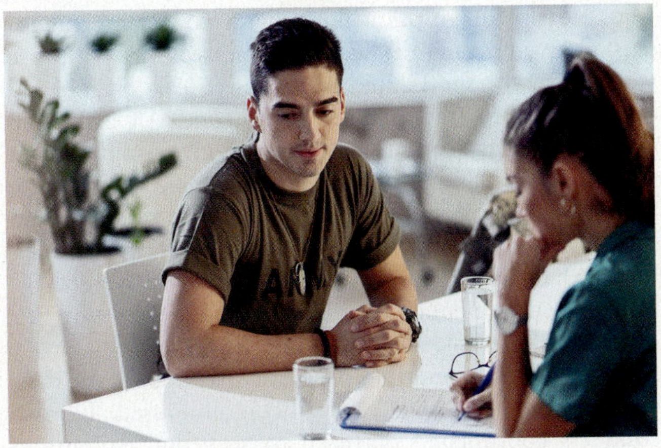

FIGURE 40.4 Veteran being assessed for health issues.

Considering the number of active-duty service members who transition each year to veteran status, chronic MSP is a major focus of treatment for this population (Santini et al., 2021). Pain is associated with an increase in allostatic load leading to physical manifestations of chronic stress including changes in endocrine dysfunction, sleep disturbance, orthopedic issues, substance use, depression, and suicide (Fig. 40.4) (Liang & Booker, 2024). Multifocal pain (i.e., multiple pain sites such as back, knees, hips, knees) is common and leads to poorer outcomes (Bushey et al., 2021).

Traumatic Brain Injury

Traumatic brain injury (TBI), disruption of expected brain function caused by a blow to the head or penetration of the skull, is often referred to as a "signature injury" of the post-9/11 conflict (OEF/OIF/OND). It is estimated that 49.5% to 78% of veterans with chronic pain use pain medication. It is estimated that more than 50% of veterans with general chronic pain have a history of TBI (Kumar et al., 2021). Hearing disturbance and headaches are the most frequently reported adverse outcomes of blast-related injuries. Frequent comorbidities associated with the blast-related injuries include PTSD, depression, anxiety, sleep disorders, attention disorders, and cognitive disorders (Mortimer, 2024).

Housing Instability

Housing instability (the challenge of paying rent for housing, living in overcrowded conditions, and moving frequently) is a problem for many veterans. U.S. veterans who are unhoused (no permanent housing) have served in wars from WWII to the recent wars in Afghanistan and

Iraq. Nearly half of the veterans with no living arrangements served during the Vietnam era; two thirds of those veterans served the United States for at least 3 years and one third were stationed in a war zone. An estimated 40,056 veterans are unhoused on any given night. Most are male, but a larger percentage of female veterans are unhoused when compared to males. Most veterans who are unhoused were enlisted and in the lower pay grades. Nearly half of veterans who were unhoused were diagnosed with a mental disorder (National Coalition for Homeless Veterans, n.d.).

The VHA has multiple programs to support veterans who are unhoused or at risk of being unhoused. The VA conducts coordinated outreach to seek out veterans in need of assistance. Veterans who are unhoused or at risk of being unhoused are connected with housing, health care, community employment services, and other required supports (U.S. Department of Veterans Affairs, 2025).

Multiple factors contribute to housing instability in the veteran population, including extreme shortages of affordable housing, inability to secure a livable income, and access to health care. Many displaced veterans live with the effects of PTSD and substance use, which are complicated by a lack of family and support networks. A higher proportion of veterans who are unhoused receive high-dose opioid therapy and have increased rates of fatal opioid overdoses (U.S. Department of Veterans Affairs, 2025).

Veterans who are unhoused often have multiple health and mental health issues. Although there are available services for veterans with housing instability, there are multiple barriers as well. Social stigma and perceived lack of support contribute to hesitancy to access services (Diaz, 2023). Veterans with children make up a considerable component of the female veterans who are unhoused. Veterans with families have additional stressors when compared to nonveteran unhoused families including military-related experiences, deployment, reintegration stress, and PTSD or MST (Ijadi-Maghsoodi et al., 2021).

SUMMARY OF KEY POINTS

- The U.S. military consists of three departments (Army, Navy, and Air Force). The Department of the Navy is responsible for the Navy and Marines and the Air Force is responsible for the Air Force and Space Force. There are seven reserve components that can be activated in time of war or national emergency. The Army is the largest U.S. military service with 35% of the active-duty members.
- The values, beliefs, and behaviors acquired in the military often last a lifetime.
- Historically, the number of females in the military was very small until the elimination of the draft when the need for service members became apparent. Females were admitted into the service academies in 1976.
- The majority of all service members are White, with the greater proportion of individuals who are members of underrepresented groups found primarily in lower ranks.
- Every year about 200,000 service members transition to civilian life. The transition year is a high-risk period for physical and mental health issues. The Transition Assistance Program provides support, resources, and training.
- A veteran identity is the degree to which the veteran role is essential or important to how they think about themselves.
- The VHA operates one of the largest integrated health care systems in the world. Nursing plays an important role in the care of the veterans through developing relationships with nursing schools and providing educational opportunities for students.
- Mental health needs are pervasive in the veteran population. Postdeployment depression, PTSD, and substance use disorders are disabling to the veterans and their families.
- Veterans are at risk for suicide, TBI, and housing instability. A strong veteran identity can support positive self-esteem and be protective of mental health issues.
- High combat exposure, history of concussions, stressful life events, and low social support are risk factors for depression and PTSD.
- PTSD is associated with both combat and noncombat trauma. PTSD symptoms from combat trauma include self-blame, intrusive memories with dreams, detachment, and reckless behavior. PTSD symptoms from noncombat trauma include exaggerated startle, self-blame with distorted beliefs, and concentration issues.
- Moral injury can be a consequence of exposure to traumatic events. Moral injury can be caused by perpetration, witnessing, and betrayal.
- Veterans who identify as LGBTQ+ experience the trauma of war plus microaggressions and minority stress.
- MST refers to sexual assault and sexual harassment. MST occurs primarily to females, but also to males. MST is a life-changing event and is highly associated with mental health disorders.
- Nursing care of veterans should always include a comprehensive assessment that screens for PTSD and MST. Veterans with these disorders should be referred to mental health specialists.
- Depression is more common in the veteran population than in the general U.S. population. Depression is highly comorbid with PTSD and suicidal ideation.

- Suicide is a major mental health issue in the veteran community. The most common method of suicide is firearms followed by poisoning and suffocation. Among veterans, childhood sexual abuse is a strong predictor of suicide. Experiences during deployment contribute to risks for suicidal ideation, especially morally injurious events.
- Veterans are more likely to use alcohol than other substances. Alcohol use often begins in the military service and continues after discharge. AUD is highly comorbid with PTSD, major depressive disorder, and suicide.
- Opioid use by veterans often begins with prescription pain medication putting them at risk of dependency and overdose. Veterans who have OUD are likely to have at least one comorbid substance use disorder. Opioid use is associated with suicide and unintentional overdose.
- Tobacco use is more prevalent by veterans than in the general population.
- Chronic pain, TBI, and housing instability contribute to health and mental health issues of veterans.

DEVELOPING CLINICAL JUDGMENT

1. Describe how the military culture influences the values, beliefs, and behaviors of a veteran.
2. Compare the mental health issues of World War I and II service members with those who served in Iraq and Afghanistan.
3. How did the Women's Armed Services Integration Act affect the military status of females?
4. Discuss the difficulties the LGBTQ+ community has experienced in the military and the impact of microaggression and minority stress on veterans.
5. M.J. was recently discharged from the U.S. Army. M.J. experienced combat in Afghanistan and was treated for PTSD but is reluctant to seek out care in the community. M.J. visits a clinic for an influenza injection and the nurse notices the Army insignia on the patient's wallet. Should the nurse ask about M.J.'s military service?
6. Differentiate combat-related trauma from non–combat-related trauma. Explain the different PTSD symptom patterns.
7. Define the types of a moral injury and explain their relationship to PTSD.
8. Discuss the nursing responsibility of screening for MST in veterans.
9. P.S., a Vietnam veteran, is attending a health screening at a local community clinic. The veteran is expressing worthlessness and sadness following the death of a life-long partner. Should the nurse conduct a suicide screening on the patient? Explain your answer.
10. During a health assessment, a 32-year-old veteran talks about consuming a six-pack of beer each night before going to bed to sleep. What additional assessment data are needed to determine the likelihood of an AUD?
11. Discuss the use of opioids and the treatment of pain in veterans. How should a nurse approach a veteran who is suspected of using excessive opioids for the treatment of pain?

MOVIES, TV, OR STREAMING PROGRAMS

Mending the Line: **2022.** John Colter (Siqua Walls) is a Marine Sargent who was wounded as he led his troops on their final day of deployment in Afghanistan. Several members of his command were wounded or killed, including his best friend. Colter was to serve as best man at his best friend's wedding. He develops severe PTSD and is sent to recover at a VA facility in Montana. Colter is hoping to be medically and psychiatrically cleared for another tour of duty.

Resisting any therapy attempts, Colter is referred to Ike Fletcher (Brian Cox), a Vietnam veteran who uses his passion for fly fishing to cope with his PTSD. Colter meets a local librarian, Lucy (Perry Mattfeld), as he pursues information about fly fishing. Lucy is still suffering from losing her fiancé from suicide 2 years previously. After a rocky start, Colter and Fletcher develop a relationship and a way to come to terms with their traumas. Lucy figures out a way to move on. The story revolves around their relationships, shared traumas, and healing through fly fishing.

Viewing Points:

1. How did Ike Fletcher's veteran identity differ from John Colter's veteran identity?
2. What symptoms characterized Colter's combat-related trauma?
3. How did Colter's alcohol use interfere with treatment?
4. If Colter, Ike, and Lucy were your patients, should a suicide screen be performed? What are their risk factors for suicide? Explain.

REFERENCES

Adams, R. E., Hu, Y., Figley, C. R., Urosevich, T. G., Hoffman, S. N., Kirchner, H. L., Dugan, R. J., Boscarino, J. J., Withey, C. A., & Boscarino, J. A. (2021). Risk and protective factors associated with mental health among female military veterans: Results from the veterans' health study. *BMC Women's Health*, *21*(1), 55. https://doi.org/10.1186/s12905-021-01181-z

American Psychiatric Association (APA) Committee on Nomenclature and Statistics. (1980). *Diagnostic and statistical manual of mental disorders* (3rd ed.). American Psychiatric Association.

American Psychiatric Association (APA). (2022). *Diagnostic and statistical manual of mental disorders* (5th ed., text rev.). Author.

Andreasen, N. C. (2010). Posttraumatic stress disorder: A history and a critique. *Annals of the New York Academy of Sciences, 1208*, 67–71. https://doi.org/10.1111/j.1749-6632.2010.05699.x

Bader, C. E., Giordano, N. A., McDonald, C. C., Meghani, S. H., & Polomano, R. C. (2018). Musculoskeletal pain and headache in the active duty military population: An integrative review. *Worldviews on Evidence-Based Nursing, 15*(4), 264–271. https://doi.org/10.1111/wvn.12301

Battesti, M. (2016). Nostalgia in the army (17th-19th centuries). *Frontiers of Neurology and Neuroscience, 38*, 132–142. https://doi.org/10.1159/000442652

Benedict, T. M., Nitz, A. J., Gambrel, M. K., & Louw, A. (2024). Pain neuroscience education improves post-traumatic stress disorder, disability, and pain self-efficacy in veterans and service members with chronic low back pain: Preliminary results from a randomized controlled trial with 12-month follow-up. *Military Psychology, 36*(4), 376–392. https://doi.org/10.1080/08995605.2023.2188046

Boscarino, J. A., Adams, R. E., Urosevich, T. G., Hoffman, S. N., Kirchner, H. L., Dugan, R. J., Boscarino, J. J., Withey, C. A., & Figley, C. R. (2020). Guard/Reserve service members and mental health outcomes following deployment: Results from the Veterans' Health Study. *General Hospital Psychiatry, 62*, 102–103. https://doi.org/10.1016/j.genhosppsych.2019.03.002

Bushey, M. A., Ang, D., Wu, J., Outcalt, S. D., Krebs, E. E., Yu, Z., & Bair, M. J. (2021). Multifocal pain as a predictor of pain outcomes in military veterans with chronic musculoskeletal pain: A secondary data analysis of a randomized controlled trial. *Pain Medicine, 22*(7), 1503–1510. https://doi.org/10.1093/pm/pnaa409

Carr, M. M., Potenza, M. N., Serowik, K. L., & Pietrzak, R. H. (2021). Race, ethnicity, and clinical features of alcohol use disorder among US military veterans: Results from the National Health and Resilience in Veterans Study. *The American Journal on Addictions, 30*(1), 26–33. https://doi.org/10.1111/ajad.13067

Center for Deployment Psychology. (2021). *Military culture: Enhancing clinical competence*. Uniformed Services University. Retrieved January 9, 2022, from https://deploymentpsych.org/Military-Culture-Enhancing-Competence-Course-Description

Chernow, R. (2017). *Grant*. Penguin Press.

Congressional Research Service. (2024). *Defense primer: Reserve forces*. Retrieved January 16, 2024, from https://fas.org/sgp/crs/natsec/IF10540.pdf

Council on Foreign Relations. (2020). *Demographics of the U. S. military*. Retrieved January 17, 2025, from https://www.cfr.org/backgrounder/demographics-us-military#:~:text=Now%2C%20there%20are%20about%201.3,percent%20of%20the%20U.S.%20population_

Council on Foreign Relations. (2022). *The U.S. War in Afghanistan 1999–2021*. Retrieved January 21, 2025, from https://www.cfr.org/timeline/us-war-afghanistan

Da Costa, J. M. (1871). On irritable heart: A clinical study of a form of functional cardiac disorder and its consequences. *American Journal of Psychiatry, 142*, 1341–1343.

Department of Defense (DOD). (1993, December 21). *Qualification standards for enlistment, appointment, and induction. Department of Defense*. Directive 1304.26. Retrieved January 23, 2025, from https://apps.dtic.mil/sti/tr/pdf/ADA275138.pdf

Dempsey, C. L., Benedek, D. M., Spangler, P. T., West, J. C., Bossarte, R. M., Nock, M. K., Zuromski, K. L., Georg, M. W., Ao, J., Haller, K., Probe, D. M., & Ursano, R. J. (2025). Gun ownership for safety/protection and unsecured firearm storage practices: Suicide risk and prevention among U.S. army servicemembers. *American Journal of Preventive Medicine, 68*(2), 311–319. https://doi.org/10.1016/j.amepre.2024.10.011

DeSimone, D. (2023). Over 200 years of service: The history of women in the U.S. military. Retrieved January 21, 2025, from https://www.uso.org/stories/3005-over-200-years-of-service-the-history-of-women-in-the-us-military#:~:text=In%20the%20Gulf%20War%2C%20from%20just%201990%2D1991%2C,serve%20in%20direct%20combat%20roles%20or%20assignments

Diaz, M. (2023). The negative health impacts of unsheltered homelessness. VA Homeless programs. Retrieved January 21, 2025, from https://www.va.gov/HOMELESS/featuredarticles/negative-health-impacts-of-unsheltered-homelessness.asp

Dolan, G., McCauley, M., & Murphy, D. (2022). Factors influencing the salience of military/veteran identity post discharge: A scoping review. *Journal of Veterans Studies, 8*(1), 231–246. https://doi.org/10.21061/jvs.v8i1.333

Dowell, D., Ragan, K. R., Jones, C. M., Baldwin, G. T., & Chou, R. (2022). CDC clinical practice guideline for prescribing opioids for pain–United States, 2022. *MMWR. Recommendations and reports, 71*(3), 1–95. https://doi.org/10.15585/mmwr.rr7103a1

Edwards, E., Osterberg, T., Coolidge, B., Greene, A. L., Epshteyn, G., Gorman, D., Ruiz, D., & El-Meouchy, P. (2024). Military experiences, connection to military identity, and time since military discharge as predictors of United States veteran suicide risk. *Military Psychology, 36*(5), 465–478. https://doi.org/10.1080/08995605.2023.2209006

Fischer, I. C., Nichter, B., Trachik, B., Bryan, C. J., & Pietrzak, R. H. (2025). Resilience and vulnerability: Suicide-specific cognitions in a nationally representative sample of US military veterans. *The Primary Care Companion for CNS Disorders*, 27(1), 24m03821. https://doi.org/10.4088/PCC.24m03821

Fitzke, R. E., Bouskill, K. E., Sedano, A., Tran, D. D., Saba, S. K., Buch, K., Hummer, J. F., Davis, J. P., & Pedersen, E. R. (2024). Barriers and facilitators to behavioral healthcare for women veterans: A mixed-methods analysis of the current landscape. *The Journal of Behavioral Health Services & Research, 51*(2), 164–184. https://doi.org/10.1007/s11414-023-09862-3

Friedman, M. (n.d.). *PTSD History and overview. PTSD: National Center for PTSD. U.S. Department of Veterans Affairs*. Retrieved January 24, 2025, from History of PTSD in Veterans: Civil War to DSM-5–PTSD: National Center for PTSD (va.gov). https://www.ptsd.va.gov/professional/treat/essentials/history_ptsd.asp

Guerrero, M., Wiedbusch, E. K., Abo, M. G., Nguyen, R. L., Soto-Nevarez, A., Principato, K., & Jason, L. A. (2021). "It's like a Brotherhood": Thematic analysis of veterans' identity processes in substance abuse recovery homes. *Journal of Community Psychology, 49*(6), 1531–1553. https://doi.org/10.1002/jcop.22623

Harper, K. L., Blosnich, J. R., Livingston, N., Vogt, D., Bernhard, P. A., Hoffmire, C. A., Maguen, S., & Schneiderman, A. (2024). Trauma exposure, mental health, and mental health treatment among LGBTQ+ veterans and nonveterans. *Psychological Trauma: Theory, Research, Practice and Policy*. https://doi.org/10.1037/tra0001735

Holliday, R., Nichter, B., Holder, N., Hill, M. L., Monteith, L. L., Norman, S. B., & Pietrzak, R. H. (2023). Childhood sexual abuse and military sexual trauma interact to increase suicide risk: Results from a nationally representative veteran sample. *Journal of Interpersonal Violence, 38*(5–6), 5354–5369. https://doi.org/10.1177/08862605221120909

Ijadi-Maghsoodi, R., Feller, S., Ryan, G. W., Altman, L., Washington, D. L., Kataoka, S., & Gelberg, L. (2021). A sector wheel approach to understanding the needs and barriers to services among homeless-experienced veteran families. *Journal of the American Board of Family Medicine, 34*(2), 309–319. https://doi.org/10.3122/jabfm.2021.02.200331

Iverson, K. M., Livingston, W. S., Vogt, D., Smith, B. N., Kehle-Forbes, S. M., & Mitchell, K. S. (2024). Prevalence of sexual violence and intimate partner violence among us military veterans: Findings from surveys with two national samples. *Journal of General Internal Medicine, 39*(3), 418–427. https://doi.org/10.1007/s11606-023-08486-9

Jones, D. S. (2019). In search of historical insight into the problem of military suicide. *JAMA Network Open, 2*(12), e1917498. https://doi.org/10.1001/jamanetworkopen.2019.17498

Kumar, R. G., Ornstein, K. A., Corrigan, J. D., Sayko Adams, R., & Dams-O'Connor, K. (2021). Association between lifetime history of traumatic brain injury, prescription opioid use, and persistent pain: A nationally representative study. *Journal of Neurotrauma, 38*(16), 2284–2290. https://doi.org/10.1089/neu.2020.7496

Lakshman, R., Tomlinson, E., & Bucknall, T. (2024). A systematic review of chronic pain management interventions among veterans of recent wars and armed conflicts. *Pain Management, 25*(3), 285–293. https://doi.org/10.1016/j.pmn.2024.03.008

Larson, R. M., Saxon, M., Phillips, M. A., Broussard, M. L., Straus, A. R., & Wright, W. A. (2024). The social determinants of suicide among female service members and veterans. *Journal of Community Health, 49*(5), 935–941. https://doi.org/10.1007/s10900-024-01359-0

Liang, Y., & Booker, C. (2024). Allostatic load and chronic pain: a prospective finding from the national survey of midlife development in the United States, 2004–2014. *BMC Public Health, 24*(1), 416. https://doi.org/10.1186/s12889-024-17888-1

Lin, L. A., Bohnert, A. S. B., Blow, F. C., Gordon, A. J., Ignacio, R. V., Kim, H. M., & Ilgen, M. A. (2021). Polysubstance use and association with opioid use disorder treatment in the US Veterans Health Administration. *Addiction, 116*(1), 96–104. https://doi.org/10.1111/add.15116

Litz, B. T. (2025). Moral injury: State of the Science. *Journal of Traumatic Stress, 38*(2), 187–199. https://doi.org/10.1002/jts.23125

Litz, B. T., Stein, N., Delaney, E., Lebowitz, L., Nash, W. P., Silva, C., & Maguen, S. (2009). Moral injury and moral repair in war veterans: A preliminary model and intervention strategy. *Clinical Psychology Review, 29*(8), 695–706. https://doi.org/10.1016/j.cpr.2009.07.003

Lopez, C. T. (2023). In 75 years since women's Armed Services Integration Act, female service members have excelled. Retrieved January 17, 2025, from https://www.defense.gov/News/News-Stories/Article/article/3425621/in-75-years-since-womens-armed-services-integration-act-female-service-members/

Ma, P., Cheng, Y., Goulet, J. L., Sandbrink, F., Brandt, C., Spevak, C., Kean, J. T., Becker, W., Libin, A., Shara, N., Sheriff, H. M., Houston, J. S., Butler, J., Workman, E. T., Agrawal, R. M., Kupersmith, J., & Zeng-Treitler, Q. (2024). Guideline concordant opioid therapy in Veterans receiving VA and community care. *BMC Health Services Research*, *24*(1), 1284. https://doi.org/10.1186/s12913-024-11742-1

Macia, K. S., Raines, A. M., Maieritsch, K. P., & Franklin, C. L. (2020). PTSD networks of veterans with combat versus non-combat types of index trauma. *Journal of Affective Disorders*, *277*, 559–567. https://doi.org/10.1016/j.jad.2020.08.027

Maguen, S., Griffin, B. J., Copeland, L. A., Perkins, D. F., Finley, E. P., & Vogt, D. (2020). Gender differences in prevalence and outcomes of exposure to potentially morally injurious events among post-9/11 veterans. *Journal of Psychiatric Research*, *130*, 97–103. https://doi.org/10.1016/j.jpsychires.2020.06.020

Markowitz, F. D., Dintzle, S., & Castro, C. A. (2023). Military-to-civilian transition strains and risky behavior among post-9/11 veterans. *Military Psychology*, *35*(1), 38–49.

Mathes Winnicki, B. M., Lee, D. J., Hawn, S. E., Livingston, N. A., Marx, B. P., & Keane, T. M. (2024). Alcohol consumption and dependence risk among male and female veterans: Trajectories and predictors. *Drug and Alcohol Dependence*, *257*, 111138. https://doi.org/10.1016/j.drugalcdep.2024.111138

Merians, A. N., Gross, G., Spoont, M. R., Bellamy, C. D., Harpaz-Rotem, I., & Pietrzak, R. H. (2023). Racial and ethnic mental health disparities in U.S. Military Veterans: Results from the National Health and Resilience in Veterans Study. *Journal of Psychiatric Research*, *161*, 71–76. https://doi.org/10.1016/j.jpsychires.2023.03.005

Miller, A., & Saling, L. L. (2024). Acculturative stress and identity challenges undermine the successful reintegration of Australian veterans. *Psychological Services*. https://doi.org/10.1037/ser0000888

Mojallal, M., Simons, R. M., Simons, J. S., & Swaminath, S. (2024). Daily exposure to combat-related cues and posttraumatic stress symptoms among veterans: Moderating effects of peri- and postdeployment experiences. *Journal of Traumatic Stress*, *37*(1), 57–68. https://doi.org/10.1002/jts.22991

Moore, M. J., Shawler, E., Jordan, C. H., & Jackson, C. A. (2023). Veteran and military mental health issues. In *StatPearls*. StatPearls Publishing. https://www.ncbi.nlm.nih.gov/books/NBK572092/

Mortimer, D. S. (2024). Military traumatic brain injury. *Physical Medicine and Rehabilitation Clinics of North America*, *35*(3), 559–571. https://doi.org/10.1016/j.pmr.2024.02.008

Na, P. J., Petrakis, I. L., Krystal, J. H., & Pietrzak, R. H. (2024). Problem opioid use among US Military Veterans: Prevalence, correlates, and psychiatric characteristics. *Journal of Addiction Medicine*, *18*(3), 313–318. https://doi.org/10.1097/ADM.0000000000001286

National Coalition for Homeless Veterans. (n.d.). *Background & statistics*. Retrieved January 21, 2025, from https://nchv.org/veteran-homelessness/

National WWII Museum. (2024). The women's army corps (WAC). Retrieved January 17, 2025, from https://www.nationalww2museum.org/war/articles/womens-army-corps-wac-world-war-ii#:~:text=Rogers%20introduced%20a%20bill%20on,personnel%2C%20and%20other%20noncombat%20roles.

Nester, M. S., Cook, M. H., Pugach, C. P., & Wisco, B. E. (2024). Exploring false negatives in self-reported trauma exposure status. *Psychological Trauma: Theory, Research, Practice and Policy*, *16*(8), 1409–1415. https://doi.org/10.1037/tra0001635

Nichter, B., Haller, M., Norman, S., & Pietrzak, R. H. (2020). Risk and protective factors associated with comorbid PTSD and depression in U.S. military veterans: Results from the National Health and Resilience in Veterans Study. *Journal of Psychiatric Research*, *121*, 56–61. https://doi.org/10.1016/j.jpsychires.2019.11.008

Nichter, B., Hill, M. L., Maguen, S., Norman, S. B., Fischer, I. C., & Pietrzak, R. H. (2024). Health and psychiatric impairment associated with moral injury, military sexual trauma, and their co-occurrence in U.S. combat veterans. *Journal of Psychosomatic Research*, *179*, 111617. https://doi.org/10.1016/j.jpsychores.2024.111617

Nichter, B., Stein, M. B., Norman, S. B., Hill, M. L., Straus, E., Haller, M., & Pietrzak, R. H. (2021). Prevalence, correlates, and treatment of suicidal behavior in US military veterans: Results from the 2019–2020 National Health and Resilience in Veterans Study. *The Journal of Clinical Psychiatry*, *82*(5), 20m13714. https://doi.org/10.4088/JCP.20m13714

Norman, S. Hicks, T., Klein, A., & Hamblen, J. (2023). Treatment of co-occurring PTSD and substance use disorder in VA. PTSD: National Center for PTSD. U. S. Department of Veterans Affairs. Retrieved January 20, 2025, from https://www.ptsd.va.gov/professional/treat/cooccurring/tx_sud_va.asp#backtotop

Office of Suicide Prevention. (2024). 2024 National Veteran Suicide Prevention Annual Report. U.S. Department of Veteran Affairs. Retrieved January 20, 2025, from https://www.mentalhealth.va.gov/docs/data-sheets/2024/2024-Annual-Report-Part-1-of-2_508.pdf

Panaite, V., Cohen, N. J., Luther, S. L., Finch, D. K., Alman, A., Schultz, S. K., Haun, J., Miles, S. R., Belanger, H. G., Kozel, F. A., Rottenberg, J., & Pfeiffer, P. N. (2024). Mental health treatment utilization patterns among 108,457 Afghanistan and Iraq veterans with depression. *Psychological Services*, *21*(3), 665–673. https://doi.org/10.1037/ser0000819

Panza, K. E., Kline, A. C., Na, P. J., Potenza, M. N., Norman, S. B., & Pietrzak, R. H. (2022). Epidemiology of DSM-5 alcohol use disorder in U.S. military veterans: results from the national health and resilience in veterans study. *Drug and Alcohol Dependence*, *231*, 109240. https://doi.org/10.1016/j.drugalcdep.2021.109240

Parker, V. L., Liechty, J. M., & Cantoni, N. P. (2024). Associations between trauma and health behaviors and outcomes among sexual minoritized adults: a scoping review. *Trauma, Violence & Abuse*, *25*(4), 2972–2985. https://doi.org/10.1177/15248380241233270

Pedroso, J. L., Linden, S. C., Barsottini, O. G., Filho, P. M., & Lees, A. J. (2017). The relationship between the First World War and neurology: 100 years of "Shell Shock." *Arquivos De Neuro-Psiquiatria*, *75*(5), 317–319. https://doi.org/10.1590/0004-282X20170046

Phelps, A. J., Adler, A. B., Belanger, S. A. H., Bennett, C., Cramm, H., Dell, L., Fikretoglu, D., Forbes, D., Heber, A., Hosseiny, F., Morganstein, J. C., Murphy, D., Nazarov, A., Pedlar, D., Richardson, J. D., Sadler, N., Williamson, V., Greenberg, N., Jetly, R., & Members of the Five Eyes Mental Health Research and Innovation Collaborative. (2024). Addressing moral injury in the military. *BMJ Military Health*, *170*(1), 51–55. https://doi.org/10.1136/bmjmilitary-2022-002128

Reyes, J., Shaw, L. E., Lund, H., Heber, A., & VanTil, L. (2021). Prevalence of chronic musculoskeletal pain among active and retired military personnel: A systematic review protocol. *JBI Evidence Synthesis*, *19*(2), 426–431. https://doi.org/10.11124/JBISRIR-D-19-00392

Rose, D. E., Farmer, M. M., Oishi, S. M., Klap, R. S., Bean-Mayberry, B. A., Canelo, I., Washington, D. L., & Yano, E. M. (2024). Does a welcoming environment influence women veterans' primary care experiences? *Women's Health Issues*, *34*(5), 540–548. https://doi.org/10.1016/j.whi.2024.07.002

Ruiz, R. A., Lehavot, K., Heffner, J. L., Kava, C. M., & Ornelas, I. J. (2024). Cigarette smoking motives and stages of change in smoking cessation among veterans: differences by gender and sexual orientation. *American Journal of Health Promotion*, *38*(3), 339–348. https://doi.org/10.1177/08901171231197147

Sachdev, S., & Dixit, S. (2024). Military to civilian cultural transition experiences of retired military personnel: A systematic meta-synthesis. *Military Psychology*, *36*(6), 579–592. https://doi.org/10.1080/08995605.2023.2237835

Santini, A., Petruzzo, A., Giannetta, N., Ruggiero, A., Di Muzio, M., & Latina, R. (2021). Management of chronic musculoskeletal pain in veterans: A systematic review. *Acta Bio-Medica*, *92*(S2), e2021011. https://doi.org/10.23750/abm.v92iS2.11352

Saulnier, K. G., Brabbs, S., Szymanski, B. R., Harpaz-Rotem, I., McCarthy, J. F., & Sripada, R. K. (2024). Suicide risk among veterans who receive evidence-based therapy for posttraumatic stress disorder. *JAMA Network Open*, *7*(12), e2452144. https://doi.org/10.1001/jamanetworkopen.2024.52144

Schaffer, K. (2023). The changing face of America's veteran population. Pew Research Center. Retrieved January 17, 2025, from https://www.pewresearch.org/short-reads/2023/11/08/the-changing-face-of-americas-veteran-population/

Schafer, K. M., Campione, M., & Joiner, T. (2024). Quality of life and loneliness among American military veterans. *The Journal of Nervous and Mental Disease*, *212*(7), 359–364. https://doi.org/10.1097/NMD.0000000000001776

Sharifian, N., LeardMann, C. A., Kolaja, C. A., Baccetti, A., Carey, F. R., Castañeda, S. F., Hoge, C. W., Rull, R. P., & Millennium Cohort Study Team. (2025). Factors associated with mental healthcare utilization among United States military personnel with posttraumatic stress disorder or depression symptoms. *American Journal of Preventive Medicine*, *68*(2), 289–299. https://doi.org/10.1016/j.amepre.2024.10.006

Shay, J. (2014). Moral injury. *Psychoanalytic Psychology*, *31*(2), 182–191.

Short, N. A., Allan, N. P., Ashrafioun, L., & Stecker, T. (2024). Beliefs about mental health treatment, treatment initiation, and suicidal behaviors among veterans and service members at-risk for suicide and not in treatment. *Suicide & Life-Threatening Behavior*, *54*(6), 1083–1091. https://doi.org/10.1111/sltb.13113

Singleton, M. (2024). Flashback Friday-After Vietnam, the ten-year battle to honor women veterans. University of Virginia School of Nursing. Retrieved January 17, 2025, from https://nursing.virginia.edu/news/flashback-vietnam-women-veterans/#:~:text=Today%2C%20it's%20generally%20estimated%20that,Medicine%20in%20San%20Antonio%2C%20Texas

Smith, J. A., Doidge, M., Hanoa, R., & Frueh, B. C. (2019). A historical examination of military records of US Army Suicide, 1819 to 2017. *JAMA Network Open*, *2*(12), e1917448. https://doi.org/10.1001/jamanetworkopen.2019.17448

Spaegele, N., Lewin, T., & Talmon, A. (2024). Trauma symptom patterns in a large sample of military personnel outpatients: Differential relations to trauma exposure, depression, and anxiety symptoms. *Psychological Trauma: Theory, Research, Practice and Policy*, *16*(8), 1290–1293. https://doi.org/10.1037/tra0001597

Statista Research Department. (2024). Distribution of active-duty enlisted women and men in the United States military in 2019, by race and ethnicity. Retrieved January 17, 2025, from https://www.statista.com/statistics/214869/share-of-active-duty-enlisted-women-and-men-in-the-us-military/

Stein, M. B., & Rothbaum, B. O. (2018). 175 years of progress in PTSD therapeutics: Learning from the past. *The American Journal of Psychiatry*, *175*(6), 508–516. https://doi.org/10.1176/appi.ajp.2017.17080955

Tackett, B. (2024). Drug use in wartime. American Addiction Centers. Retrieved January 19, 2025, from https://www.recovery.org/addiction/wartime/

Torreon, B. S. (2024). U.S. periods of war and dates of recent conflicts. Congressional Research Service. Retrieved January 16, 2025, from https://crsreports.congress.gov

Ursano, R. J., & Stein, M. B. (2022). From soldier's heart to shared genetic risk: PTSD and cardiovascular disease. *The American Journal of Psychiatry*, *179*(11), 785–787. https://doi.org/10.1176/appi.ajp.20220778

USA Facts. (2024). How many people are in the US military? A demographic overview. Retrieved January 16, 2025, from https://usafacts.org/articles/how-many-people-are-in-the-us-military-a-demographic-overview/

U.S. Department of Defense. (2025). Our forces. Retrieved January 21, 2025, from https://www.defense.gov/About/our-forces/

U.S. Department of Veterans Affairs. (n.d.) How common is PTSD in veterans? PTSD: National Center for PTSD. Retrieved January 18, 2025, from https://www.ptsd.va.gov/understand/common/common_veterans.asp

U.S. Department of Veterans Affairs. (2021a). *Top 10 things all healthcare and service professionals should know about VA services for veterans who experienced military sexual trauma (MST)*. Retrieved January 19, 2025, from https://www.mentalhealth.va.gov/docs/top_10_public.pdf 19

U.S. Department of Veterans Affairs. (2021b). Military sexual trauma fact sheet. Retrieved January 21, 2025, from https://www.mentalhealth.va.gov/docs/mst_general_factsheet.pdf

U.S. Department of Veterans Affairs. (2022a). Facts and statistics. Women Veterans Health Care. Retrieved January 18, 2025, from https://www.womenshealth.va.gov/materials-and-resources/facts-and-statistics.asp8

U.S. Department of Veterans Affairs. (2022b). Veterans Affairs nursing academic partnership. Retrieved January 18, 2025, from https://www.va.gov/charleston-health-care/work-with-us/internships-and-fellowships/veterans-affairs-nursing-academic-partnership-vanap/11

U.S. Department of Veterans Affairs. (2024a). Transition. Outreach, transition and economic development. Your VA Transition Assistance Program. Retrieved January 17, 2025, from https://benefits.va.gov/transition/index.asp

U.S. Department of Veterans Affairs. (2024b). Serving her country: Exploring the characteristics of women veterans. Retrieved January 18, 2025, from https://www.data.va.gov/stories/s/Women-Veterans-in-2023/wci3-yrsv/8

U.S. Department of Veterans Affairs. (2024c). VA History Summary. Retrieved January 18, 2025, from https://department.va.gov/history/history-overview/11

U.S. Department of Veterans Affairs. (2025). *VA Homeless Programs*. Retrieved January 21, 2025, from https://www.va.gov/homeless/

Vespa, J. E. (2020). Those who served: America's veterans from World War II to the War on Terror. *American Community Survey Report. U.S. Census Bureau*. Retrieved January 18, 2025, from https://www.census.gov/content/dam/Census/library/publications/2020/demo/acs-43.pdf

Vespa, J. E., & Carter, C. (2024). Trends in veteran disability status and service-connected disability: 2008–2022 *American Community Survey Report. U.S. Census Bureau*. Retrieved January 18, 2025, from https://www2.census.gov/library/publications/2024/demo/acs-58.pdf

Wiblin, J., Holder, N., Holliday, R., & Surís, A. (2021). Predictors of unbearability, unlovability, and unsolvability in veterans with military-sexual-trauma-related posttraumatic stress disorder. *Journal of Interpersonal Violence*, *36*(7–8), 3814–3830. https://doi.org/10.1177/0886260518777554

Wolff, K. B., & Mills, P. D. (2016). Reporting military sexual trauma: A mixed-methods study of women veterans' experiences who served from World War II to the war in Afghanistan. *Military Medicine*, *181*(8), 840–848. https://doi.org/10.7205/MILMED-D-15-00404

Yancey, J. R., Carson, C. N., McGlade, E. C., & Yurgelun-Todd, D. A. (2024). A literature review of mental health symptom outcomes in U.S. veterans and servicemembers following combat exposure and military sexual trauma. *Trauma, Violence & Abuse*, *25*(2), 1431–1447. https://doi.org/10.1177/15248380231178764

Zelkowitz, R. L., Livingston, W. S., Knutson, E. K., Kehle-Forbes, S., Vogt, D. S., Smith, B. N., & Mitchell, K. S. (2024). Associations of military sexual harassment and assault with nonsuicidal self-injury: Examining gender and sexual orientation as moderators. *Journal of Psychiatric Research*, *180*, 243–250. https://doi.org/10.1016/j.jpsychires.2024.10.015

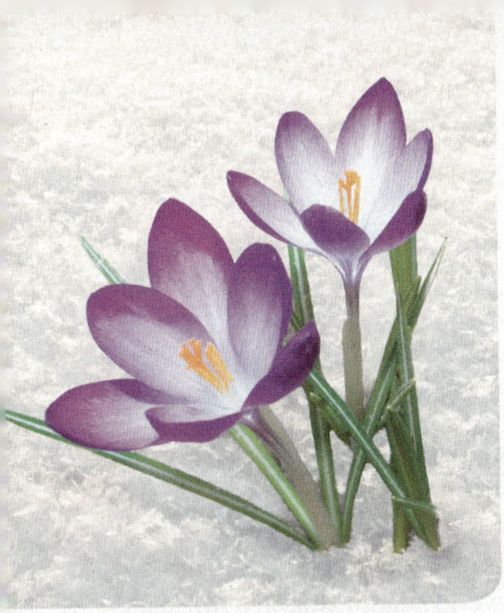

41 Care of People Experiencing Housing Instability and Mental Illness*

Rebecca Luebbert and Mary Ann Boyd

KEYCONCEPT

- housing instability

LEARNING OBJECTIVES

After studying this chapter, you will be able to:

1. Define sheltered and unsheltered housing instability.
2. Describe risk factors for housing instability.
3. Describe challenges of people who are experiencing housing instability and have a mental illness.
4. Discuss personal and societal attitudes and beliefs about housing instability.
5. Describe nursing care of people who are experiencing housing instability and have a mental illness.
6. Discuss the importance of advocacy for those who are experiencing housing instability and have a mental illness.

KEY TERMS

• assertive community treatment (ACT) • case management • continuum of care • day treatment • gentrification • housing first • safe havens • section 8 housing • shelter plus care program • sheltered housing instability • supportive housing • transitional housing • unsheltered housing instability

INTRODUCTION

Any person can find themselves without housing due to a variety of factors including lack of employment, crises, or a number of unanticipated events. Without a stable dwelling place, meeting basic needs is difficult. A person without stable housing may be carrying all of their possessions in a car, suitcase, bag, or shopping cart or storing necessities in a bus station locker or under the bed of a night shelter. They may have no place to store treasured objects, no closet for next season's clothing, no pantry with food to eat, no place to entertain friends or have solitude, and no place for a child to play.

People who experience housing instability tend to be ignored or not seen by the general population, who hurry on their own way. The community with housing instability is often treated poorly by society and may suffer from acts of violence. Many attacks go unreported. Hate crimes against the unhoused community are a vital issue in the United States. Perpetrators of these acts are most often males under the age of 40 (National Coalition for the Homeless, 2024).

This chapter explores issues relevant to individuals who are experiencing housing instability and who are also experiencing mental health issues. It presents nursing care measures and suggests ways to improve services for the population who is unhoused.

HOUSING INSTABILITY AND MENTAL ILLNESS

Children, adults, and families can experience housing instability from encountering a natural disaster, home fire, some situational crisis or unexpected overwhelming life situation, or economic hardship. Others find themselves without stable housing because of issues related to

In this chapter, "men," "women," "male," and "female" refer to people who identify as these genders.

BOX 41.1

Characteristics of People With Housing Instability and a Mentally Illness

People with a mental disorder:

- Are at greater risk for housing instability than the general population.

People with housing instability:

- Have an increase in mental health issues the longer the person is without stable housing.

People who are experiencing housing instability and have a mental illness:

- Have at least one psychiatric service encounter annually, usually in an ED rather than inpatient or outpatient units.
- Are without stable housing for longer periods, often years, than are those who are without housing and not mentally ill or substance dependent.
- Are more likely to be in poor physical health compared to other unhoused individuals.
- Have more contact with the legal system than those without mental illness.
- Are more likely to encounter employment barriers and are less likely to benefit from societal economic growth.
- Are less likely to have contact with family or friends, especially if they come from higher-income households.
- Are often eligible for, but have difficulty obtaining, income maintenance such as Social Security Disability Insurance, Veterans Affairs disability benefits, or other benefits.
- Are often willing to accept treatment after basic survival needs are met and a therapeutic relationship has been established.

Source: Substance Abuse and Mental Health Services Administration. (2021). *Behavioral health services for people who are homeless. Advisory. Treatment Improvement Protocol (TIP) Series* 55.

substance use or mental illness. Box 41.1 lists the characteristics of people who are experiencing housing instability and have a mental illness.

KEYCONCEPT Housing instability is characterized by a lack of a fixed, regular, and adequate nighttime residence, which includes places not designed for, or ordinarily used as, a regular sleeping accommodation (i.e., car, park, abandoned building, bus/train station), as well as publicly or privately operated shelters or **transitional housing**, including a hotel or motel paid for by government or charitable organization.

The following criteria define people experiencing housing instability in the United States (U.S. Department of Housing and Urban Development, 2025a):

- Individual or family who lacks a fixed, regular, and adequate nighttime residence
- Individual or family who will imminently lose their primary nighttime residence with no subsequent residence identified, and they lack resources or support networks to remain in housing
- Unaccompanied youth under 25 years of age, or families with children and youth who do not have permanent housing
- Any individual who is fleeing, or attempting to flee, domestic violence (includes dating violence, sexual assault, stalking, or other dangerous or life-threatening situations related to violence and lack resources or support networks to remain in housing.

Housing instability can be either sheltered or unsheltered. Individuals with **sheltered housing instability** obtain temporary or transitional housing operated by public and private agencies for individuals and families who do not have stable housing. Individuals with **unsheltered housing instability** live in places that are not used for housing, such as cars, parks, abandoned building, tents, or bus/train stations.

Since the COVID-19 pandemic, young adults have become particularly vulnerable to housing instability, highlighting health inequities, economic disparities, increased risk for mental health issues, and increased social isolation (Heerde et al., 2024).

Epidemiology

The unhoused population includes people of all ages, economic levels, racial and cultural backgrounds, and geographic areas. In January 2023, more than 653,000 people were without housing on a single night in the United States, more than a 12% increase over the previous year; nearly 30% of these are people living in families with children. Sixty percent of all people experiencing housing instability identify as men, and 20% of individuals are over the age of 55 (National Alliance to End Homelessness, 2024).

Among individuals experiencing housing instability, nearly two thirds are unsheltered. Black people, Indigenous people, and other People of Color are more likely to have housing instability due to systemic exclusion and discrimination, with Native Hawaiian people and Pacific Islander people being most likely (National Alliance to End Homelessness, 2024). Since 2015, rates of housing instability have increased most rapidly among Asian individuals (91% increase), Hispanic or Latino individuals (59% increase), American Indian or Alaskan Native individuals (53% increase), and Native Hawaiian or other Pacific Islander individuals (21% increase) (National Alliance to End Homelessness, 2024).

Approximately, two thirds of the unhoused population have a current mental health disorder. The most common disorders include substance use disorders, antisocial personality disorder, major depression, and psychotic disorders (Barry et al., 2024). Stigma and discrimination toward individuals with mental illness who are unhoused are pervasive across societies. Although people may consider members of this population to be a threat to public safety, these individuals are actually more likely to be targets of crimes than those who perpetrate them, with one study finding that approximately half of unhoused individuals reported being a target of violence. When people experiencing housing instability do perpetrate violence, it is often because of the need for self-protection (Xu et al., 2024).

Housing instability has been a major problem for veterans since the early 2000s. Since 2010, the number of veterans experiencing unstable housing has dropped by 55.6%; however, in 2024, still more than 32,000 veterans were without stable housing on a single night (U.S. Department of Veterans Affairs, 2024).

Risk Factors

There are a variety of factors that place individuals and families at risk for housing instability. Adolescents can become unhoused because of strained family relationships, family dissolution, transitional housing struggles, economic instabilities, and instability of residential placements (Armoon et al., 2024). The consequences of restrictions due to the COVID-19 pandemic, such as remote learning and stay-at-home orders increased the risk of housing instability for vulnerable youth. Unhoused youth are more likely to experience adverse outcomes, including physical health issues. They are more likely to participate in high-risk behaviors, including substance use and unsafe sexual behaviors (Farnish & Schoenfeld, 2024).

Immigrant and refugee populations are at increased risk for housing instability. Communication difficulties, lack of trust, concerns about confidentiality, and poor health literacy contribute to lack of resource utilization (Hynie et al., 2023). Migrant workers and their families lack residential stability as they move from one geographic region to another according to the growing and harvest season. These laborers and their families may be U.S. citizens or foreign born. According to Blackmore et al., 2020, they are economically disadvantaged and typically lack adequate living quarters and health care; in addition, physical health issues and depression are common in these families. After farm labor is completed, family members may be homeless until they can return to their place of origin or to a relative's home

Mental illness is significant risk factor for housing instability. Symptoms of mental illnesses often interfere with family relationships and impair judgments. Mental illness increases a person's vulnerability to exploitation or harm (see Box 41.2).

The Experience of Housing Instability

The person who is experiencing housing instability spends time hunting for shelter, food, and clothing and lacks consistent ways to meet basic needs. They are at higher risk for disease, infection, and exposure to the illness (Ogbonna et al., 2023). This lifestyle, plus grinding poverty and risk for exploitation, especially if the person has a mental illness, leaves little energy for change

BOX 41.2

Risk Factors for Housing Instability Among People With Mental Illness

INDIVIDUAL RISK FACTORS

- Symptoms of mental illness, including unpredictable behavior; an inability to manage everyday affairs; and an inability to communicate needs, which results in conflicts with family, employers, landlords, and neighbors
- Youth and adults with a concurrent mental disorder and substance use are at high risk for eviction, arrest, and incarceration or repeated admissions and short stays in psychiatric hospitals
- Coexisting demographic and societal factors of poverty, single-parent family (usually female-headed), dependent child; child in foster home; underrepresented groups; veteran status; unmarried adults, individuals who were previously incarcerated
- Coexisting physical illness or developmental disability
- Exposure to traumatic events repeatedly, resulting in posttraumatic stress disorder and deficits in independent living skills
- Exposure to physical and sexual abuse, especially if a family member was the person conducting the abuse
- Inability to cope with or manage the requirements of family, community, or group living home
- Lack of high school education or equivalence
- Is a war veteran

ENVIRONMENTAL RISK FACTORS

Mental Health System Factors

- Inadequate discharge planning with a lack of appropriate housing, treatment, and support services
- Lack of funding for community-based services
- Lack of integrated community-based treatment and support services for individual and group therapy, medication monitoring, and case management
- Lack of community-based crisis alternatives for housing, health care, and respite care for families with risk for rehospitalization and loss of residence
- Lack of attention to consumer preferences for autonomy, privacy, and integrated regular housing
- Changing environment, such as loss of home caused by natural or human-made disaster

SOCIETAL AND FAMILY FACTORS

- Lack of affordable housing; affluent economic times have caused housing prices to soar out of reach, to reduce construction of low-cost housing, and to create a tight rental market
- Insufficient disability benefits; Social Security income recipients are below the federal poverty level
- Lack of coordination between mental health and substance misuse systems
- Waiting lists to receive a subsidy that requires the person to pay only 30% of income for rent and utilities
- Lack of job opportunities for individuals with functional limitations
- Stigma and discrimination; resistance to community housing for people with mental illnesses is widespread
- Poor family relationships; willingness to help the ill person is exhausted as relatives cope with frightening or disturbing behavior and receive insufficient help from the community or medical profession

Source: Substance Abuse and Mental Health Services Administration. (2021). *Behavioral health services for people who are homeless. Advisory. Treatment Improvement Protocol (TIP) Series 55.*

or reentrance into mainstream society. Panhandling, scrambling for money, doing odd jobs, selling plasma, or getting money for aluminum cans are common sources of income, although some people who are without housing receive Social Security or veterans' pension benefits. The longer a person is without stable housing, the more likely the person is to experience mental illness or engage in substance use (Nishith et al., 2023).

The healthiest individuals dealing with housing instability seek support from others, maintain hope for the future, and strive to lead meaningful lives and embrace their sense of self. They believe they are resourceful, can handle uncertainty, and can maintain health. Women with children who are experiencing housing instability have described the need to keep going for the sake of, and to avoid losing, their children. However, women living in temporary or transitional shelters are confronted with insecurity, lack of privacy, isolation, stigma, and disempowerment. Some women have preexisting mental health issues that lead to housing instability, whereas others develop mental illness because of their lack of adequate housing. Domestic abuse is often an antecedent to housing instability (Rakus & Singleton-Jackson, 2024; Rempel et al., 2024; see Chapter 23).

Chronic Homelessness

A person is considered to be experiencing chronic housing instability when they spend more than a year without housing or have experienced a minimum of four episodes without housing over a 3-year period (U.S. Department of Housing and Urban Development, 2025b). The experience of experiencing housing instability for a long time results in a sense of depersonalization and fragmented identity; a loss of self-worth and self-efficacy. People who are without housing are often chronically ill, unemployed, or have recently lost all financial resources. Educational level varies greatly, from less than an eighth-grade education to doctoral degrees.

A person who is without housing for the first time or for a few months is more likely to have a more positive outlook than a person who has been experiencing unstable housing for a longer period of time because the chances of recovering economic and social status are greater. Biographies and research describe the tragedy and nightmare of being homeless (Mejia-Lancheros et al., 2020).

Housing Instability and Hope

Deprivation of needs, the sense of isolation and stigma, and the lack of accessible resources may be of short- or long-term duration. In turn, self-confidence and sense of competence can be eroded. People without housing who have mental illnesses have typically endured and coped with constraints or issues with extreme stressors or catastrophes and negative life events. Instilling a sense of hope and possibility of recovery from housing instability and mental illness is important. Many people who experience housing instability maintain hope and a positive attitude, which in turn helps them to reach out for help, take advantage of opportunities, and become part of the housed population (Moorkath et al., 2022).

Federal Assistance

There are several federal programs that provide assistance to people who are without housing. The McKinney–Vento Homeless Assistance Act (Public Law 100–77, first passed in 1987 as the McKinney Act), signed by President Ronald Reagan and confirmed by President Bill Clinton, provides federal money for housing shelter programs. This law established the U.S. Interagency Council on the Homeless that provided for the use of funds in a coordinated manner, and for programs to assist the unhoused, with special emphasis on older adults, people with disabilities, families with children, Native American individuals, and veterans. This program is funded through grants to the states.

Substance Abuse and Mental Health Services Administration (SAMHSA) recognizes that housing is critical to recovery from mental and substance use disorders and promotes safe, affordable, and permanent support housing in the community with access to benefits and services for individuals, families, and communities. SAMHSA has several initiatives to create safe places for people with mental illness and substance misuse. SAMHSA works closely with the U.S. Interagency Council on Homelessness to support and implement Opening Doors, the federal strategy to prevent and end housing instability. SAMHSA's programs emphasize the importance of employment and education as outcomes and core components of recovery (SAMHSA, 2023).

ETIOLOGY OF HOUSING INSTABILITY

Housing instability has no single cause. Generally, people want to have a home and be part of a family or social group. People do not choose or purposefully maintain housing instability. Many factors—unemployment, lack of skills, mental illness, substance use, domestic violence—typically combine, with time, to contribute to the person or family losing permanent housing. The series of events that result in having no home is the culmination of individual and environmental factors, including factors in the mental health system, society, and family or community (Box 41.3).

The reduction of psychiatric beds has had a huge impact on the increase in the number of people with mental illness who are without housing. The deinstitutionalization movement to move people with severe mental illness from state hospitals to receive less restrictive

BOX 41.3

Causes of Housing Instability

- Poverty, history of childhood family instability
- Lack of affordable housing, doubling up with relatives or friends until the situation is intolerable
- Mental illness or substance misuse and lack of needed services
- Low-paying jobs, unemployment
- Domestic violence, flight from a violent home or abandonment, youth aging out of services
- Eviction for not paying rent, multiple movers
- Limited life coping skills, disturbing behavior
- Changes or reductions in public assistance programs
- Veteran status
- Release from incarceration; having no money, job, or place to go

care in the community left many individuals falling through the cracks. Even today, people requiring emergent psychiatric care are often brought to hospitals and then released back to the community with an insufficient plan for follow-up (Silver, 2023). State hospitals that do exist dedicate most of their beds to those who have committed crimes and have court-ordered treatment. Even under these circumstances, there is often a 30-day to 6-month wait for a bed. Many "nonforensic" individuals are detained in emergency departments (EDs) until beds are available.

Gentrification, upgrading of inner-city property so that it is affordable to only people who have the resources of upper-middle or upper economic levels, is increasingly a factor in creating housing instability among urban residents. According to McIntosh et al., 2023, middle-class and upper-middle-class professionals, mostly White individuals, are relocating to the inner city; to appeal to this population, abandoned or substandard buildings in the inner city are demolished to build modern condominiums or "lofts," and people who formerly resided in these urban areas cannot afford the new housing in their regenerated neighborhood. They are often displaced and are at risk of becoming without housing (McIntosh et al., 2023).

FAMILY RESPONSE TO HOUSING INSTABILITY

Children who are unhoused have high rates of both acute and chronic health issues and are more likely than children who are not unhoused to be hospitalized, have delayed immunizations, and have elevated lead blood levels. In addition, they are at risk for developmental delays and emotional and behavioral difficulties. School attendance is disrupted frequently, and they are vulnerable to violence, either as targets or witnesses (Murran & Brady, 2023). Children who experience family housing instability, even for brief periods of time, are significantly more likely to demonstrate issues with behavior (Marçal, 2022).

Living in shelters is stressful for families for several reasons. Many shelters exclude men and adolescent males older than 12 years; thus, family members are separated. Overcrowding prevents privacy and promotes loss of personal control. Stressors of poverty and reduced social support compound the trauma of these experiences.

A history of abuse and assault is common among unhoused individuals. Women who are unhoused have increased mental health concerns, increased rates of diagnosed mental health issues, increased suicidal thoughts and attempts, and an increased rate of adverse childhood trauma. Unhoused women with children have often left abusive relationships and have difficulty accessing shelter and health care (Rakus & Singleton-Jackson, 2024).

RECOVERY-ORIENTED CARE FOR PEOPLE WITH MENTAL ILLNESS WHO HAVE HOUSING INSTABILITY

It is beyond the scope of most mental health services to meet many of the urgent needs of individuals with mental illness who are without stable housing. The mental health system is often the first contact for the person who is without housing or at risk for losing housing. The mental health team should have a working knowledge and relationships with community resources that provide housing, physical health care, financial support, and legal support.

Teamwork and Collaboration: Working Toward Recovery

SAMHSA (2021) recommends a five-stage process in housing rehabilitation for people with housing instability who have a mental illness:

1. *Outreach and engagement*, the first step in the process, involves facilitation of the individual into behavior changes. This stage involves recognizing the needs of people who are without housing for preventive and basic services and developing a trusting and supportive relationship with these individuals.
2. *Transition to intensive care* occurs when individuals agree to accept health and/or financial benefits, substance use/mental health treatment. During this phase, the clinician maintains a relationship with the individual and works to dispel any resistance or concerns the person has.
3. *Intensive care* phase emphasizes the person's participation in defining and managing their own goals. The primary focus of this phase is mental health treatment, accessing benefits, attending to medical issues, accessing housing, and seeking preventive services, such as skills training.

4. *Transition from intensive care to ongoing rehabilitation* is preparation for sustaining the process of recovery. Depending on the individual, some may move quickly into affordable housing and maintain an independent lifestyle. Others may need 1 or 2 more years of supportive recovery and housing.
5. *Ongoing rehabilitation* is an open-ended phase in which people gradually establish an identity as no longer being unhoused. This stage includes an active and continuing supportive counseling relationship, participation in mental health treatment as needed, and continued participation in prevention programs as appropriate (SAMHSA, 2021).

Safety Issues

Safety needs are always a priority. If an individual is a threat to others or self, safety interventions should be implemented. The person may be involuntarily hospitalized for stabilization of symptoms. Overdose of opioids or alcohol intoxication is also a priority care issue. People should be referred to emergency services. The nurse may be required to take immediate action to reverse the drug effects by administering naloxone. Other priority issues involve basic needs, including housing and food. Many people who are without stable housing are fearful of being incarcerated and resist any attempts to provide them with shelter.

Screening, Brief Interventions, and Referral to Treatment

Screening, brief interventions, and referral to treatment (SBIRT) integrates initial screening with brief interventions or referral to treatment for people who may have substance use disorders and co-occurring mental disorders (see Chapter 42). SBIRT is particularly useful for individuals who have housing instability. The screening requires little time—5 minutes to screen and 10 minutes to provide the interventions.

EVIDENCE-BASED NURSING CARE FOR A PERSON WITH A MENTAL ILLNESS WHO IS EXPERIENCING HOUSING INSTABILITY

A holistic perspective is essential for assessing any person or family unit who is experiencing housing instability. Assessing a person who has a mental disorder and does not have a home requires patience and skill. Generally, these individuals have not been following a recommended treatment regimen and are symptomatic.

The assessment begins at the point of the person's need; often, it is a physical need or health issue (Box 41.4). The person may be malnourished and most concerned about food and shelter. Because of negative past experiences with the health care system or providers or because of mental illness or substance use, the person may not allow a thorough physical examination or may refuse to answer questions about history at the first visit.

BOX 41.4
Assessment Tips for the Physical Assessment

- Use unobtrusive observation as a part of physical assessment. Some conditions will be immediately obvious. Other conditions may become apparent during the interview.
- Examine—look, touch, palpate, auscultate—the person to the extent that they allow. The person may resist anything more than a superficial conversation and observation. The nurse may need to perform initial palpation of the abdomen or auscultation of the lung through several layers of clothes. If the patient perceives the health care provider as too intrusive, the patient may leave the setting even though they are desperate for care.
- Listen carefully to what the patient does not say and pay attention to nonverbal as well as verbal expressions. Avoid unnecessary directness and probing. Give the person time to answer questions. The blood test or urine screen may have to wait; a patient, nonintrusive manner may ensure that the person returns for needed tests or screening.
- Determine whether the person has been prescribed medications in the past. Often, the person who is without stable housing is not taking medications, even if they are prescribed and essential. The person may have difficulty keeping pills dry and easily retrievable or paying for medications. A daily insulin injection, for example, may not seem practical. Or the person may have had their medication stolen.

Physical Health Assessment

The nurse should provide privacy for any assessment. They should be gentle, not be rushed, and explain the need for any physical examination. The person may feel very embarrassed about their physical appearance or body odor if there has been no opportunity for physical hygiene or clothing change. Observation of mucous membrane and skin integrity, including the face, torso, limbs, and feet, is essential. The nurse should explain their concern about the person's health status and the need to remove clothing, including shoes and socks, and to pull down underwear.

The nurse should realize that many people who are experiencing housing instability consider themselves well as long as they can get where they need to go. Be aware of the many health issues that may be present (Box 41.5). Children and adolescents who are experiencing housing instability may experience any of those listed, plus diseases that are specific to their age group. If a person is pregnant and experiencing housing instability, assess indications that the person is at high risk for maternal or fetal complications.

BOX 41.5

Common Physical Health Issues Experienced by People With Housing Instability

- Injuries, fractures, epistaxis, or edema from trauma, falls, burns, assault, gunshot wounds
- Influenza, colds, bronchitis, asthma, shortness of breath
- Hypothermia, hyperthermia
- Arthritis, musculoskeletal disorders, headaches, fatigue
- Diabetes mellitus
- Hypertension
- Cardiovascular and peripheral vascular diseases
- Malnutrition
- Pulmonary tuberculosis
- Infestations, such as lice or scabies
- Dermatitis, sunburn or frostbite, bruises
- Foot injury, blisters, calluses
- Sexually transmitted diseases
- Hypothyroidism or hyperthyroidism
- Kidney or liver disease
- Cancer
- Epilepsy
- Impaired vision, glaucoma, cataracts
- Impaired hearing
- Dental caries, periodontal disease

Psychosocial Assessment

Mental Status and Appearance

The mental status examination (see Box 41.6) may have to be completed over several sessions. Symptoms of schizophrenia may be difficult to differentiate from emotional responses to the stressors of experiencing a lifestyle without stable housing. Required hypervigilance may augment suspicion or paranoid beliefs. The need for constant awareness of possibilities for meeting basic needs can augment self-preoccupation. Blunted affect, lack of communication, loose associations, evidence of psychosis, ambivalence, isolation, and uncertainty may be the result of life on the streets and living in various places. Such symptoms or behaviors may be part of the experience of being without housing and reflect healthy coping mechanisms and creative survival techniques rather than pathology.

BOX 41.6

Assessment Tips for the Psychological Assessment

- Observe and listen to what the person defines as a problem and potential solution and what they consider to be a strength or coping strategy; validate and reinforce when applicable.
- View the person and their situation from the individual's perspective; be a patient, nonthreatening listener. Such an approach encourages the person to return regularly; the nurse can then observe the patterns of behavior.
- Determine the extent of stability or integration of the person's sense of self, cognitive appraisals, and overt behavior. Lack of integration or stability indicates the need for continued monitoring and therapy.
- Observe for behavior that suggests the person may be hallucinating, and try to validate.
- Listen for delusional thinking or denial over time; try to sense what purpose these serve.

Substance dependence should be considered because it is common among people with housing instability, including people with mental illnesses. Because people who are experiencing housing instability, especially those with psychiatric disorders, are often targets of crime and violence, the incidence of posttraumatic stress disorder among them may be higher than in the general population. Women without stable housing are especially in danger of being a target of physical and/or sexual assault (Greene et al., 2024).

When a child or adolescent is without stable housing, the nurse should ask about educational history, whether they are enrolled in school, and about perceived progress. Children without housing often have difficulty with school; the school district may change every time the parent/caregiver changes shelters or moves from a temporary residence. The nurse should determine whether the child has behavioral or emotional difficulties and whether they need special education services.

Behavioral Responses

The behavioral assessment should follow the one presented in Chapter 10. The nurse should recognize that the person who with housing instability has their own way of being in the world. The person may not have insight into their illness and deny that they have a mental health issue. Much of the behavioral assessment will be conducted through observation and listening to the person's explanation of events.

Stress and Coping Skills

Housing instability is stressful. It is important that the nurse understands how the person who is experiencing unstable housing copes on a day-to-day basis. The nurse should ask the person how basic needs are met: How does the client eat and sleep? How does the person cope with experiencing a lack of housing?

Cultural Assessment

Cultural value differences exist between people who are experiencing housing instability and people in the dominant American culture, to which most providers of health care subscribe. Thus, providers and the person who is without housing and needs health care may experience cultural conflict in their norms of health and illness, basic value systems and priorities, and perceptions about health care. Health care providers expect patients, including those who are without housing and have a mental illness or substance dependency, to problem solve, become more independent, and be future oriented. These values affect assessment, treatment, and interactions with the person

BOX 41.7

Assessment Tips for the Social Assessment

- Ask about support systems, people who could be helpful, and what services the person has used or could use.
- Determine whether the person is isolated from their biologic family, and if so, if it is by personal choice rather than by family choice.
- Respect that the person who feels isolated may avoid talking about their biologic family.
- Explore if the patient views a homeless peer, local pastor, counselor, or another health care provider as "family" or as a support system.
- Convey genuine interest in the person, and convey that others may also care.

and can interfere with the nursing process and patient response to the health care system. The nurse should consider how the person perceives their everyday life and vary the assessment and therapy approach accordingly.

Support Network and Support System Assessment

Housing instability is an expression of and response to certain family, societal, or environmental conditions, as well as to individual factors. See Box 41.7 for factors included in the social and family assessment. It is also important to consider that childhood abuse and prior trauma may be continuing to affect the person as a stressor or contribute to interpersonal crises.

Spiritual Assessment

The nurse should listen for expressions that convey a spiritual faith, a connection to a transcendent being, or a belief system that helps the person endure. Questions about the spiritual dimension may convey an invitation to talk about an aspect of life that is often ignored but that may be very important to the beliefs, and preferred practices will help determine relevant therapy approaches.

CLINICAL JUDGMENT

A person who is experiencing housing instability has several immediate needs. The first priority is safety from immediate harm to self or others. The next priority will depend upon the current housing situation—do they have safe shelter at night? Physical health needs should be a priority before addressing mental health needs.

THERAPEUTIC RELATIONSHIP

Self-awareness on the part of the nurse is important. Nurses, who are accustomed to caring for others and giving attention to people who ask for it, may find themselves considering various myths if a person who is without housing approaches them with requests for food, money, or interpersonal communication (Table 41.1). To respond appropriately, one must first examine these myths and one's own feelings about people who are without housing and have a mental illness. Relating to people who are unhoused requires a gentle and compassionate approach.

MENTAL HEALTH NURSING INTERVENTIONS

Interventions are directed at the social system as well as at the individual or family level. Interventions should take advantage of community resources and the inner resources and support systems of the individual or family. Box 41.8 describes interventions that focus on the individual and social system.

Establishing Recovery and Wellness Goals

Prioritizing the patient's goals will guide nursing care. The individual may only want to get a warm coat and a bus pass. The nurse should encourage the patient to identify meaningful goals, but it is important that their primary needs are met. Hospitalization may be needed to treat illness symptoms and to provide immediate shelter. The nurse should advocate for finding permanent housing, which is associated with mental health recovery (see Box 41.9).

BOX 41.8

Interventions for People Experiencing Housing Instability

- Stabilize physical health status.
- Provide a list with addresses and telephone numbers of shelters and restaurants that provide free food; discourage rooting through dumpsters and panhandling.
- Provide a list of facilities that are safe, including shelters that provide clothing, a safe place to sleep, and opportunities for basic hygiene and laundry.
- Give information on city ordinances that forbid sleeping on park benches, in building doorways, on sidewalk grates, at bus or train stations, in vacant buildings, or in viaducts.
- Explore sources of income, such as gathering and selling aluminum cans or engaging in temporary day labor. Discourage selling blood or plasma.
- Assist the person directly or by referral to pursue entitlements, such as Social Security, veterans, or other benefits.
- Explore how to stay safe. Even in a night shelter, the person who is without housing may not be safe from assault. It is difficult for the person without housing to know who is trustworthy; carrying a bag or case is usually considered a marker for being robbed on the streets.
- Explore how to secure privacy, which is difficult to achieve, and how to cope with loneliness, which can be overwhelming.
- Give a list of names, addresses, and telephone numbers of agencies that offer services and socialization, such as the local mental health agency, the local chapter of NAMI, or the local mental health support group.
- If the person is using substances, give information about meetings of Alcoholics Anonymous, Narcotics Anonymous, Cocaine Anonymous, or other support groups.

TABLE 41.1 MYTHS AND FACTS ABOUT PEOPLE WITH PSYCHIATRIC DISORDERS WHO ARE EXPERIENCING HOUSING INSTABILITY

Myth	Fact
People choose to be without stable housing.	Most people with housing instability want what most people want: to support themselves, have jobs, have attractive and safe housing, be healthy, and help their children do well in school.
Housing is a reward for abstinence and medication adherence, and society should not house people who have active substance use or mental disorders.	Housing may be the first step to becoming abstinent and/or entering treatment to address a variety of issues. From a public health perspective, adequate housing reduces risk for exploitation, hypothermia or hyperthermia, infectious diseases, and other risks to the population as a whole.
People who are without stable housing are unemployed.	Many people who are without housing are employed full or part-time.
Families without stable housing are rare.	About 30% of the unsheltered population is made up of families.
People who are without stable housing are not smart.	Being able to function while without housing takes ingenuity and experience. People who are homeless often have well-developed street skills, resourcefulness, and knowledge of the service system.
Those with substance use or mental disorders need to "bottom out," so housing instability is okay and provides a motivator to make behavioral changes.	People who have substance use and mental disorders are more responsive to interventions before they become without housing or when placed in housing.
Everyone stands an equal risk of housing instability.	Although anyone could find themselves without housing in their lifetime, some people are at higher risk than others. If people at special risk of housing instability can be identified, early intervention may prevent the devastating effects experienced by people who are without housing and have accompanying mental and/or substance use disorders.
All clients with substance use and mental disorders who are without housing require extensive, long-term care.	The process of recovery from substance use and mental illness is an ongoing and sometimes lifelong process, yet healing often begins with short-term, strategic interventions. Screening, brief intervention, and referral to treatment is a proven method for early intervention with substance use and mental disorders, and it can significantly reduce the impact and progression of illness.

Source: Substance Abuse and Mental Health Services Administration. (2021). *Behavioral health services for people who are homeless. Treatment Improvement Protocol (TIP) Series 55. HHS Publication No. (SMA) 13–4734.*

Overcoming Barriers to Care

Cost and lack of insurance are the biggest barriers to health and hospital care for people with housing instability. Another barrier is the inability of unhoused individuals to carry out treatment recommendations; survival is their first priority. Adherence to medication and treatment regimens is difficult because successful treatment requires collaboration, monitoring, time for medication and other measures to be effective, and a secure place to keep medication. People with mental disorders who are experiencing housing instability often cannot routinely

BOX 41.9

Research for Best Practice: Experiences With Supported Housing, Recovery, and Health Promotion

Hammervold, U. E., Gytri, S., Storm, M., Lid, T. G., & Sagvaag, H. (2024). What is known about persons with co-occurring problems' experiences with supported housing, recovery, and health promotion? A scoping review. BMC Health Services Research, 24*(1)*, 1366.

THE QUESTION: What are the experiences of individuals with co-occurring substance use and mental health issues with supported housing, including experiences of recovery and health promotion?

METHODS: A scoping review was conducted in the following databases: Ovide MEDLINE, Embase, PsycInfo, CINAHL, Social Services Abstracts, Web of Science, Scopus, and Oria.

FINDINGS: Forty publications were reviewed, 30 of which were peer-reviewed articles. Four main themes were identified related to individuals' experiences with supported housing: (1) the importance of safe and permanent housing; (2) the importance of housing for physical health; (3) the importance of relationships and support; and (4) the value of choice and independence.

IMPLICATIONS FOR NURSING: Safety and long-term housing are essential components in recovery in people with co-occurring substance use and mental health issues. Supported housing may contribute to health promotion, particularly when autonomy is valued and there is access to authentic relationships and support.

get prescriptions filled. Medicine may be stolen. It is necessary for the person or family unit to have a place to keep medications that can be reached at the necessary times and to have access to primary care services for regular check-ups, assessment for adverse drug responses, and necessary blood monitoring.

NCLEXNOTE The priority for people who are experiencing housing instability is meeting their basic needs—food, shelter, and so on. Treating the mental illness is secondary. The nurse should consider Maslow's hierarchy of needs as the guiding framework when planning interventions.

Improving Quality of Life

Interventions that improve quality of life include providing food, clothing, and assistance with housing; addressing physical health issues; promoting safety and self-esteem; and educating the person to decrease the risk of being targeted. A trusting relationship with the care provider and ongoing follow-up care is also necessary.

People who have been without stable housing for several years have greater difficulty readjusting to stability and need more time for healing, depending on illness severity, comorbidity, and available support systems. People who are experiencing housing instability, including those with psychiatric disorders, become creative at surviving on the streets. The nurse should explore available resources with the individual or family (see Box 41.8 for appropriate interventions).

Meeting Spiritual Needs

Depending on the person's beliefs, the nurse may explore ways to meet spiritual needs. Some ways a nurse may provide spiritual support include praying together, facilitating participation in religious services, discussing the meaning of life and the afterlife, and providing spiritual literature (Jensen et al., 2023).

NCLEXNOTE Providing physical resources, social services, and social and legislative advocacy counter the negative social and emotional effects of housing instability for the person and family.

Evaluation and Treatment Outcomes

Priority goals for people with housing instability who also have a mental illness include recovery from their mental disorder and living in a housing of choice. In some instances, after the mental disorder is treated and in remission, housing, a job, and positive interpersonal relationships follow. In other instances, finding housing sets the stage for strengthening coping skills to address the mental disorder.

COMMUNITY SERVICES

Diverse services and integrated systems are essential to address all aspects of the life situations of people who are without a home and experiencing psychiatric disorders. Essential components include **Safe Havens** or stable shelters or residences, accessible outreach, integrated case management, accessible and affordable housing options, treatment and rehabilitation services, general health care services, vocational training and assistance with employment, income support, and legal protection. The agencies that provide these services must develop a physical and emotional atmosphere that conveys a sense of caring and community. Often, community agencies are located at one site, much like a shopping mall, so that the person or family does not have to travel to numerous separately located agencies to have their needs met.

Emergency Services

Some agencies provide a street or mobile outreach program. As part of this program, a van travels to areas where unhoused people are located. Food, warm coffee, hygiene kits, and blankets are the first steps in building trust between staff and people with housing instability. The person who is without housing may accept an offer to be driven to a local shelter for the night. Following up the next day by van or bicycle provides a way to recontact the individual and invite them to the agency programs or take them to other social services or health care services. Luncheon sites for people with unstable housing are a basic step in emergency services. Some agencies have a health clinic on site for treatment of minor issues.

Integration With Primary Care

Integrating crisis intervention with physical and medical care is essential for individuals with psychosis who are seeking service in a hospital ED. The ED is likely to emphasize triage and rapid disposition while administering essential care. Physical care supersedes care for the emotional status of the person. Medication should be supplemented by crisis intervention techniques. The developmental level of the person, regardless of age, should also be considered. Emergency shelters typically provide refuge at night, along with an evening meal and morning coffee. Shelters for women and children without housing usually allow them to remain during daytime hours as well, although children leave the shelter for school and women may attend educational classes, counseling, **day treatment**, rehabilitation, or employment programs.

Housing Resources

Transitional housing may consist of a halfway house, a short-stay residence or group home, or a room at a hotel designated for people with housing instability. Some agencies have a transitional home and stabilization center where the atmosphere and staff are a model for residents, who work on specific goals and a treatment plan. Sharing housekeeping tasks; obtaining psychiatric stabilization; and attending residence group meetings, social skills and budgeting classes, day treatment programs, and vocational training are steps to independent housing and employment. A holistic program reduces readmission to the hospital and reentry to street dwelling.

Housing First is an approach that prioritizes permanent housing for people experiencing housing instability. This approach is adopted by communities by providing services to people who are homeless. It is guided by the belief that people need basic necessities like food and housing before they can attend to other issues such as recovery from a mental illness, secure a job, and develop meaningful relationships. Case management, living skills classes, and other services are provided as "wrap-around" interventions as needed. There is a direct relationship between the safety and security provided by the Housing First program and a decrease in psychiatric symptoms and chronic housing instability, with an increase in a sense of independence, choice, and mastery of living skills (O'Campo et al., 2022; Sullivan et al., 2023).

The HEARTH Act of 2009 consolidated the McKinney–Vento homeless assistance program, **Shelter Plus Care Program**, and Section 8 Moderate Rehabilitation single room occupancy (SRO) Program into one program known as the **Continuum of Care**. Shelter Plus Care provides long-term housing and supportive services for people who are homeless with disabilities, primarily those with serious mental illness, chronic issues with alcohol or drug use, or AIDS or related diseases (USDHUD, 2025c). **Section 8 housing** has been helpful to this population for many years. Section 8 federally subsidized housing units are supervised or operated by the state or city, for which tenants are responsible for paying one third of the monthly income (e.g., Supplemental Security Income or Social Security Disability Insurance) toward rent. The difference between the tenant payment and the maximum fair market rental price is calculated as the federal Section 8 housing contribution to the housing provider.

Safe Haven programs are found throughout the United States and provide 24-hour residence for an unspecified duration. Safe Havens serve hard-to-reach people with severe mental illness who are on the streets and have been unwilling or unable to participate in traditional supportive services. A Safe Haven provides private or semi-private accommodations and limits overnight occupancy to 25 people (Veterans Administration, 2025a).

Supportive housing, permanently subsidized housing with attendant social services, was previously considered too expensive. Today, communities are realizing that such programs for people who have mental illness and are without stable housing are a good investment. The person who is safely housed is less likely to use other acute care and publicly funded services, such as shelters, although case management services are needed. Use of acute psychiatric and medical services is reduced, and the person is less likely to be arrested or incarcerated.

U.S. Military Veterans Services

The Veterans Administration has a national service dedicated to the care of unhoused veterans with mental health issues. The Health Care for Homeless Veterans (HCHV) Program provides community-based residential treatment for veterans without housing. The HCHV serves as a hub for housing and other services that provide the Veterans Health Administration with a way to reach and assist Veterans with housing instability (Veterans Administration, 2025b; see Chapter 40).

Case Management

Case management is essential in addressing an individual's needs and preventing the person from becoming lost in the complexity of community services (SAMHSA, 2021). Case management involves systematic assessment, planning, goal setting, counseling and other interventions, coordination of services, referral as necessary, and monitoring of the person's or family's needs and progress. It enhances self-care capability and quality of care, decreases fragmentation, provides for cost containment, and reduces unnecessary duplication of services or hospitalization. The case manager is the gatekeeper and facilitator who may at first network with services on the person's or family's behalf and then encourage them to deal directly with other service providers to obtain bus passes and transportation, children's services and supplies, medical or obstetric care, or housing. The nurse is the ideal team member or case manager because of knowledge about both psychiatric and physical diseases and the ability to develop therapeutic relationships and stay connected with people or families who are unhoused and with the health care system.

Rehabilitation and Education

Day Treatment Programs

Day treatment provides a bridge between institutional and community care for people with mental illness or substance dependence. Participation in structured day treatment programs can provide emotional and practical support and strengthen ties to community services and potentially to family and friends. A day treatment program can provide legal assistance, help with finding employment and independent housing, and a mailing address for people who are homeless. It can provide case management, assistance with goal setting and problem solving, and psychiatric or medical care. The day treatment program may incorporate adult basic education classes to increase literacy and survival skills, and general education development (GED) classes for those who want a high school diploma, and computer skills to improve employment options. A Living Skills Program typically includes content in nutrition, budgeting, parenting, household and family management, tenant responsibilities and rights, and employment readiness. Such classes are especially useful to people who will no longer be receiving welfare benefits. The person can receive assistance applying for government benefits, if qualified, and obtaining identification, such as a birth certificate, if needed. The informal environment of day treatment programs promotes a feeling of camaraderie, self-confidence, trust in staff, and aspirations for independent living.

Alcohol and Substance Use Treatment

The structure of some day treatment programs included alcohol and substance use treatment. Sobriety or harm reduction is the goal; the person attends daily meetings, receives necessary psychiatric and medical treatment, and participates in all of the other activities and services available at the day treatment program. No one is terminated for relapse; the person is referred to more intensive services, including hospitalization, if necessary.

Employment Services

Job placement is most likely when an employment program teaches basic job-seeking skills (e.g., resume writing; interview skills; appropriate attire, hygiene, and behavior; and computer skills) and offers job training in settings that prepare the person for the real world and real jobs. Case management during employment training can increase self-confidence, teach budgeting skills and methods of coping with the stresses of regular employment, and link the person with community resources. It can also help to teach various skills for job retention and career development. The employment service should periodically follow up with both the employee and their employer to ensure a successful record and movement to independence.

Integrated Services

Assertive Community Treatment (ACT) programs, enacted by a transdisciplinary team of 10 to 12 specialists with a 1:10 staff–client ratio, focus on service delivery to individuals with housing instability and mental illness. A single, integrated, mobile staff team uses outreach, case management, practical assistance and support, and rehabilitation services to maximize the possibility that even consumers with significant functional limitations may live independently in the community and have a good quality of life. The team provides counseling and advocacy; monitors the person's management of housing, income, medication use, and leisure activities; and provides opportunities for employment if appropriate. Substance use management and physical health care are provided as needed.

Ongoing social support groups; membership in day treatment programs; attendance at substance use support meetings; or the local National Alliance on Mental Illness (NAMI) or Mental Health Association can help the person remain in the community and live independently or with family. Support groups foster peer socialization and problem solving, enhance self-esteem, and offer many activities (e.g., art and recreation therapy, legal assistance).

Advocacy

Nurses can share experiences and research findings with the local chapter or national headquarters of NAMI and with state legislators and members of Congress who are involved in developing legislation and policies related to people who are homeless, have a mental illness, or have substance dependence. Continued advocacy is essential to convey the perceptions and needs of this population and to influence allocations for needed programs and services.

SUMMARY OF KEY POINTS

- People experiencing housing instability are a heterogeneous, diverse group, some of whom have a mental disorder and/or a substance use disorder.
- There are many risk factors contributing to housing instability.
- People do not want to be without stable housing.
- Meeting the needs of people who have a mental illness and are experiencing housing instability requires more than mental health services. Housing services are critical.
- The nursing assessment must be holistic; the nurse must listen to the person's perceptions and observe carefully.
- People who have a mental illness or substance use disorder and are without a home may have various physical health issues.
- Intervention must be oriented to the person's or family's perceived needs, culturally sensitive, and compassionate.
- People who have mental disorders and are experiencing housing instability may avoid traditional health care services.
- Nurses must incorporate new trends in providing and improving services for health care and social integration.

DEVELOPING CLINICAL JUDGMENT

1. How do the effects of mental illness, substance use, and housing instability interact with one another?
2. What factors might interfere with the ability of a person who has a mental illness and without stable housing to participate in treatment?
3. What barriers to communication might the nurse experience when working with a person who has housing instability and a mental illness?

MOVIES, TV, OR STREAMING PROGRAMS

***Americans with No Address:* 2024.** The documentary "Americans with No Address" investigates the housing instability crisis in America, capturing the untold stories of individuals experiencing homelessness. It explores the systemic issues contributing to housing instability while also highlighting the hope that can be engendered in unhoused individuals by organizations that aim to help.

Viewing Points:

1. What health care challenges faced by individuals with housing instability does the documentary highlight?
2. What role does mental health play in the lives of unhoused individuals?
3. What social determinants of health are evident in the documentary?
4. How can nurses contribute to addressing the needs of people with housing instability?
5. How does the documentary challenge common stereotypes of housing instability?
6. What impact does being unhoused have on a person's overall well-being?

REFERENCES

Armoon, B., Mohammadi, R., & Griffiths, M. D. (2024). The global prevalence of non-suicidal self-injury, suicide behaviors, and associated risk factors among runaway and homeless youth: A meta-analysis. *Community Mental Health Journal, 60*(5), 919–944.

Barry, R., Anderson, J., Tran, L., Bahji, A., Dimitropoulos, G., Ghosh, S. M., Kirkham, J., Messier, G., Patten, S. B., Rittenbach, K., & Seitz, D. (2024). Prevalence of mental health disorders among individuals experiencing homelessness: A systematic review and meta-analysis. *JAMA Psychiatry, 81*(7), 691–699.

Blackmore, R., Boyle, J. A., Fazel, M., Ranasinha, S., Gray, K. M., Fitzgerald, G., Misso, M., & Gibson-Helm, M. (2020). The prevalence of mental illness in refugees and asylum seekers: A systematic review and meta-analysis. *PLoS Medicine, 17*(9), e1003337. https://doi.org/10.1371/journal.pmed.1003337

Farnish, K. A., & Schoenfeld, E. A. (2024). Implications of the COVID-19 pandemic for youth housing and homelessness services. *Child & Adolescent Social Work Journal, 41*(1), 75–94.

Greene, A., Korchmaros, J. D., & Frank, F. (2024). Trauma experience among women who have substance use disorders and are homeless or near homeless. *Community Mental Health Journal, 60*(2), 233–243.

Heerde, J. A., McMorris, B. J., Gewirtz, O'Brien, J. R., Bailey, J. A., & Toumbourou, J. W. (2024). Health and social vulnerabilities among unstably housed and homeless young adults during the COVID-19 pandemic. *Health Promotion Practice, 25*(5), 768–773.

Hynie, M., Oda, A., Calaresu, M., Kuo, B. C. H., Ives, N., Jaimes, A., Bokore, N., Beukeboom, C., Ahmad, F., Arya, N., Samuel, R., Farooqui, S., Palmer-Dyer, J.-L., & McKenzie, K. (2023). Access to virtual mental healthcare and support for refugee and immigrant groups: A scoping review. *Journal of Immigrant & Minority Health, 25*(5), 1171–1195.

Jensen, F. B., Supiano, K. P., Towsley, G. L., Ellington, L., & Cloyes, K. G. (2023). Experiences of homeless recipients of social model hospice care. *Journal of Hospice and Palliative Nursing, 25*(5), E71–E84.

Marçal, K. (2022). Pathways from food and housing insecurity to adolescent behavior problems: The mediating role of parenting stress. *Journal of Youth & Adolescence, 51*(4), 614–627.

McIntosh, A., Anguelovski, I., & Cole, H. (2023). "The trauma machine expands faster than our services": Health risks for unhoused people in an early-stage gentrifying area. *Health & Place, 83*, 103035.

Mejia-Lancheros, C., Lachaud, J., O'Campo, P., Wiens, K., Nisenbaum, R., Wang, R., Hwang, S. W., & Stergiopoulos, V. (2020). Trajectories and mental health-related predictors of perceived discrimination and stigma among homeless adults with mental illness. *PLoS One, 15*(2), e0229385. https://doi.org/10.1371/journal.pone.0229385

Moorkath, F., Vranda, M. N., & Naveen Kumar, C. (2022). Eventful past, stagnant present, and hopeful future: A time order analysis of experiences of homeless women with chronic mental illness residing in shelter care homes. *International Journal of Social Psychiatry, 68*(8), 1790–1794.

Murran, S., & Brady, E. (2023). How does family homelessness impact on children's development? A critical review of the literature. *Child & Family Social Work, 28*(2), 360–371.

National Alliance to End Homelessness. (2024). *State of homelessness: 2024 edition*. https://endhomelessness.org/homelessness-in-america/homelessness-statistics/state-of-homelessness/

National Coalition for the Homeless. (2024). *Violence and hate against unhoused Americans: 2020–2022*. https://nationalhomeless.org/wp-content/uploads/2024-Hate-Crimes-Report_for-web.pdf

Nishith, P., Huang, J., Tsai, J., Morse, G. A., Dell, N. A., Murphy, A., & Mueser, K. T. (2023). The relationship between serious mental illness and criminal offending in persons experiencing homelessness: The role of substance use disorder. *The Psychiatric Quarterly, 94*(4), 645–653.

O'Campo, P., Stergiopoulos, V., Davis, O., Lachaud, J., Nisenbaum, R., Dunn, J. R., Ahmed, N., & Tsemberis, S. (2022). Health and social outcomes in the Housing First model: Testing the theory of change. *EClinicalMedicine, 47*, 101387.

Ogbonna, O., Bull, F., Spinks, B., Williams, D., Lewis, R., & Edwards, A. (2023). The impact of being homeless on the clinical outcomes of COVID-19: Systematic review. *International Journal of Public Health, 68*, 1605893.

Rakus, M., & Singleton-Jackson, J. (2024). Homelessness and intimate partner violence: Women's experiences with accessing formal support services and the impact of their intersecting identities. *Affilia: Feminist Inquiry in Social Work, 39*(4), 628–643.

Rempel, E., Donelle, L., Hall, J., & Wathen, N. (2024). Examining second-stage shelters: insights into housing instability and tailored support for IPV survivors. *BMC Public Health, 24*(1), 397.

Silver, S. (2023). *Research weekly: Promoting a continuum of care for people with SMI who experience homelessness*. Treatment Advocacy Center. [Online]. https://www.tac.org/research-weekly-promoting-a-continuum-of-care-for-people-with-smi-who-experience-homelessness/

Substance Abuse and Mental Health Services Administration. (2021). *Advisory: Behavioral health services for people who are homeless. Treatment Improvement Protocol (TIP) Series 55*. https://library.samhsa.gov/product/tip-55-behavioral-health-services-people-who-are-homeless/sma15-4734

Substance Abuse and Mental Health Services Administration. (2023). *Homelessness programs and resources*. [Online]. https://www.samhsa.gov/communities/homelessness-programs-resources

Sullivan, C. M., Simmons, C., Guerrero, M., Farero, A., López-Zerón, G., Ayeni, O. O., Chiaramonte, D., Sprecher, M., & Fernandez, A. I. (2023). Domestic violence housing first model and association with survivors' housing stability, safety, and well-being over 2 years. *JAMA Network Open, 6*(6), e2320213.

U.S. Department of Housing and Urban Development. (2025a). *CoC and ESG homeless eligibility: Four categories in the homeless definition*. [Online]. https://www.hudexchange.info/homelessness-assistance/coc-esg-virtual-binders/coc-esg-homeless-eligibility/four-categories/

U.S. Department of Housing and Urban Development. (2025b). *Definition of chronic homelessness*. [Online]. https://www.hudexchange.info/homelessness-assistance/coc-esg-virtual-binders/coc-esg-homeless-eligibility/definition-of-chronic-homelessness/

U.S. Department of Housing and Urban Development. (2025c). "*Shelter Plus Care Program*" [Online]. https://www.hudexchange.info/programs/spc/

U.S. Department of Veterans Affairs. (2024). *The state of veteran homelessness: 2024*. [Online]. https://www.va.gov/HOMELESS/docs/The-State-of-Veteran-Homelessness-2024.pdf

Veterans Administration. (2025a). *Housing interventions and practices*. [Online]. https://www.va.gov/homeless/nchav/program-development-implementation/housing-interventions-practices/

Veterans Administration. (2025b). *VA programs for homeless veterans*. [Online]. https://www.va.gov/homeless/for_homeless_veterans.asp

Xu, K. Y., Gold, J. A., Szlyk, H. S., Rolin, S. A., & Shields, M. C. (2024). Mental illness and violence among people experiencing homelessness: An evidence-based review. *Missouri Medicine, 121*(1), 14–20.

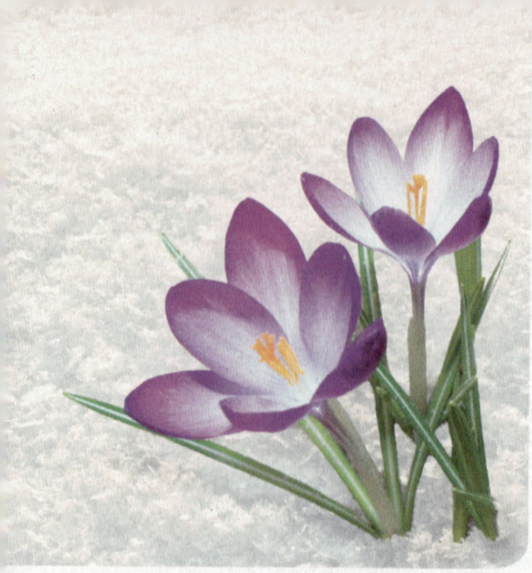

42 Care of People With Co-occurring Mental Disorders

Mary Ann Boyd

KEYCONCEPTS

- co-occurring disorder (COD)
- relapse cycle

LEARNING OBJECTIVES

After studying this chapter, you will be able to:

1. Examine the concept of co-occurring disorder (COD).
2. Relate the cycle of relapse to people with COD.
3. Analyze barriers to the treatment of patients with COD.
4. Using a clinical judgment model, formulate a person-centered, recovery-oriented nursing plan for people with COD.
5. Discuss the significance of a therapeutic relationship with people with COD.
6. Discuss the significance of integrated health care for people with COD.
7. Discuss patterns of substance use with co-occurring mental disorders.
8. Support the integration of health care and mental health care for people with COD.

KEY TERMS

• active treatment • assertive community treatment (ACT) • brief intervention • brief treatment • dual disorder • engagement • harm reduction • integrated treatment • level of care quadrants • personal motivation • referral to treatment • relapse prevention • recovery • SBIRT (screening, brief intervention, and referral to treatment) • screening • self-medicate

INTRODUCTION

When an individual experiences more than one mental disorder simultaneously, an array of symptoms occur that can be very confusing to both the individual and provider. If a mental disorder and a substance use disorder (SUD) co-occur in one individual, a diagnosis of co-occurring disorder (COD) is made. Each disorder is present in the same individual and they are independent from each other. The term **dual disorder** is sometimes used interchangeably with the term COD. In COD, the individual's experience, symptoms, and outcomes are influenced by the interaction of the two disorders.

> **KEYCONCEPT** The term **co-occurring disorder** (COD) refers to coexistence of a mental disorder and a substance use disorder (SUD) in the same individual.

The goal of treatment for patients with COD is a comprehensive recovery plan for the complex issues presented—one that offers the patient a way out of what can be a downward spiral of debilitation. Effective treatment of COD requires an integrated approach based on both an understanding of mental disorder and substance dependency. Integrated treatment, that is, coordinated substance use and mental health interventions, requires modifying traditional approaches to both the mental disorder and substance dependency (Office of Disease Prevention and Health Promotion, 2022).

This chapter presents the epidemiology and etiologic patterns of COD. It highlights methods of assessing COD and offers nursing care interventions to address this complex yet common presentation in psychiatric and substance use treatment settings. Specific mental disorders and substance use are discussed.

CO-OCCURRING DISORDERS OVERVIEW

The presence of COD was inadvertently magnified during the community mental health reform movement when there was a rational movement toward deinstitutionalization of people with mental disorders (see Chapter 1). Large numbers of people with mental disorders were left unhoused, lost to local and state mental health systems. Their long-standing mental disorders and protected life in a state hospital increased their vulnerability to exploitation by others, particularly the more astute and streetwise individuals with SUD. Along with being unhoused came the increased use of drugs and alcohol and discrimination (Singh & Agustines, 2024; see Chapter 41).

It is impossible to make any meaningful distinction between simple recreational use of a substance and actual substance use with this population because even small amounts of alcohol or other drugs can be damaging to people who have concurrent psychiatric issues. Substances of misuse exert profound effects on mental states, perception, psychomotor function, cognition, and behavior. The specific neurochemical and other biologic mechanisms that evoke these psychological features are discussed in Chapter 31. Table 42.1 lists the psychological effects of substances of misuse.

Clinical Course and Relapse

Although two types of disorders are diagnosed independently, people with COD cope with the interaction of two mental disorders. In many instances, the use of substances serves as a coping strategy for dealing with psychiatric symptoms. Without alternative, effective coping behaviors, the patient will continue to **self-medicate** (using substances, over-the-counter medications or medications without prescription or supervision to alleviate an illness or condition). People with COD have higher rates of infection with human immunodeficiency virus (HIV), relapse, rehospitalization, depression, and suicide risk than those with only one disorder (Brown et al., 2024).

A frequent issue of this group is relapse, which leads to repeated hospitalizations. When symptoms of the mental disorder are stabilized, the hospitalized patient is discharged. Once in the community, the patient does not follow the therapeutic regimen and resumes the use of alcohol or drugs. Reappearance of symptoms leads to another episode of hospitalization (Dion et al., 2024; Hyatt et al., 2024). The relapse cycle is characterized by a pattern of decompensation, hospitalization, stabilization, discharge, and then decompensation (Fig. 42.1).

TABLE 42.1 PSYCHOLOGICAL EFFECTS OF SUBSTANCES OF MISUSE

Substance	Psychological Effects
Alcohol	Alcohol amnestic syndrome, dementia Agitation, anxiety disorders, sleep disorders Ataxia, slurred speech Withdrawal symptoms, which may include hallucinations, confusion, illusions, delusions; protracted withdrawal delirium can occur Depression, increased rate of suicide, disinhibition
Cocaine	Anxiety, agitation, hyperactivity, sleep disorders, delusions, paranoia, euphoria, internal sense of interest, and excitement Rebound withdrawal symptoms, such as prolonged depression, somnolence, anhedonia
Amphetamines	Similar to cocaine but more prolonged hyperactivity, agitation, anxiety, increased energy
Hallucinogens (MDMA, or ecstasy) and phencyclidine	Hallucinations, delusions, paranoia, confusion Withdrawal can produce severe depression and somnolence Hallucinations, illusions, delusions, perceptual distortions, paranoia, rage, anxiety, agitation, confusion
Marijuana	Acute reactions: panic, anxiety, paranoia, sensory distortions, rare psychotic episodes; patients with schizophrenia use these reactions to distance themselves from painful symptoms and to gain control over symptoms Antimotivational syndrome: apathy, diminished interest in activities and goals, poor job or school performance, memory and cognitive deficits
Opiates	Confusion, somnolence Withdrawal can produce anxiety, irritability, and depression and can trigger suicidal ideation
Sedative–hypnotics	Confusion, slurred speech, ataxia, stupor, sleep disorders, withdrawal delirium, dementia, amnestic disorder, sleep disorders
Volatile solvents	Hallucinations, delusions, hyperactivity, sensory distortions, dementia

MDMA, 3,4-methylenedioxy-methamphetamine.

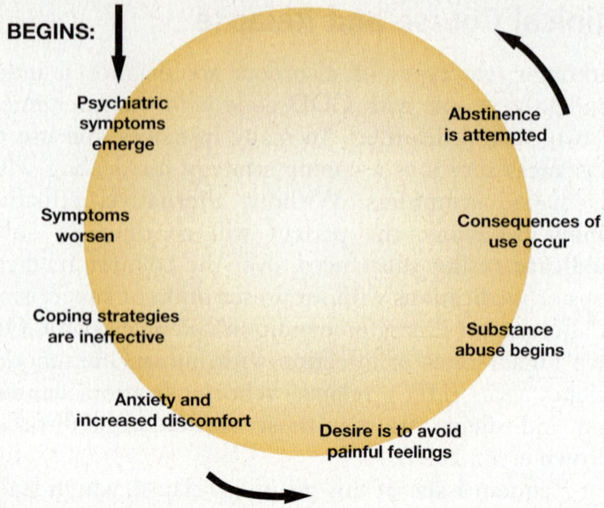

FIGURE 42.1 Relapse cycle.

> **KEYCONCEPT** In the **relapse cycle**, reemerging psychiatric symptoms lead to ineffective coping strategies, increased anxiety, substance use to avoid painful feelings, adverse consequences, and attempted abstinence until psychiatric symptoms reemerge and the cycle repeats itself.

Epidemiology

The pattern of alcohol and illicit drug use by those with a mental disorder varies, but it is estimated that as many as 21.5 million adults have both disorders. The most commonly used drug substance is alcohol, followed by marijuana and cocaine. Prescription drugs such as opioids and sleeping medicines may also be misused (SAMHSA, 2024a).

The risk for substance use varies among mental disorders. Anxiety, depression, posttraumatic stress disorder (PTSD), psychosis, and borderline and antisocial personality disorders are strongly associated with SUDs (NIMH, 2024). Having any SUD was associated with more lifetime suicide events when compared with those having no SUD (Diefenbach et al., 2024).

Etiology

There is no one model that explains why mental disorders and substance use occur together so frequently. In one pattern of occurrence, the mental disorder precedes substance use. The symptoms of the mental disorder appear first and then substances are used for self-medication. For example, as adolescents with emerging mental disorders are exposed to drug use, their disinhibition and impulsivity lead to drug experimentation. Substances are used to self-medicate the underlying mental disorders (SAMHSA, 2024a). Drugs that are misused (cocaine, alcohol, marijuana) temporarily potentiate neurotransmission in the brain's reward system, relieving the depression and anxiety for a short period of time. Self-administration of drugs can temporarily mask or suppress the aversive psychological effects of the dysregulated neuronal systems (see Chapter 31).

In the second pattern, the SUD appears first and leads to the mental disorder. Psychiatric symptoms have long been associated with dysregulation of the monoamines and neuropeptides. For example, lysergic acid diethylamide (LSD) or cocaine use may change the neurotransmission in the brain that results in panic attacks or psychosis. In the third pattern, there are common causes, either genetic or environmental, that lead to the onset or persistence of both disorders.

BARRIERS TO TREATMENT

High morbidity rates point to the need for effective treatment of individuals with COD (SAMHSA, 2024a). Although it was recognized that integrated treatment should be the standard of care, these patients often face major barriers in obtaining proper treatment. There are many well-documented barriers such as perceived shortcomings of substance use treatment systems, funding barriers, difficulty in communicating with substance use treatment providers, and difficulty reconciling different treatment approaches, and lack of staff (Mirzaian et al., 2024). The following discussion highlights some other barriers.

Nature of Co-occurring Disorders

Patients often deny an issue with substances and do not seek treatment because they do not view themselves as needing it. They do not fully understand their mental disorder or the effects of substance use on their mood or behavior. Even those who recognize their disorders are often reluctant to seek mental health treatment. It is confusing to be expected to abstain from alcohol and illicit drugs yet be prescribed medication that also affects their thoughts and feelings. If they take the substance of choice, they experience fleeting moments of joy and escape even though doing so will prompt a decline in overall function and worsen psychiatric symptoms. If they accept prescribed treatments, including medications, they will have higher levels of functioning and better treatment outcomes, but they lose their moments of joy and escape.

Staff Attitudes

Mental health professionals in psychiatric treatment programs are often frustrated in their efforts to assist patients with SUDs. Behavior often associated with substance dependency, such as denial of substance use and nonadherence with health-related protocols, is often regarded as a sign of treatment failure. This type of behavior can provoke hostility from the staff and can make planning for mental health recovery difficult.

Mental health professionals sometimes have difficulty understanding the compelling nature of drug or alcohol cravings, may not understand differences in drug use patterns and behaviors associated with particular drugs of misuse, and may not believe in some treatment approaches (Feder et al., 2025). In addition, patients or their therapists may recognize substance use because of the patients' psychiatric symptoms.

Stigma

Patients may be stigmatized and regarded as criminals because they purchase, use, or distribute illicit drugs. Strong public feelings about alcohol-related motor vehicle accidents, negative experiences with family members or friends with alcohol use disorder, and cultural biases against public intoxication can prejudice interactions with patients who drink alcohol (Magnan et al., 2024).

Health Issues

Numerous health hazards are associated with alcohol and drug use (see Chapter 31). The use of alcohol and illicit substances in addition to medications prescribed for mental disorders can lead to drug interactions and may exacerbate side effects of these medications. Housing instability can increase these patients' medical issues with inadequate nutrition, poor hygiene, and the adverse effects of exposure to the elements adding to their difficulties. Health care providers often become frustrated with patients' nonadherence and with what they see as behaviors that are difficult to manage. Their frustration may negatively affect the way they treat patients with COD. Because of the confusion about what is the primary and most immediate issue to treat, these patients are often underserved and only partially treated.

RECOVERY-ORIENTED CARE FOR PEOPLE WITH CO-OCCURRING DISORDERS

Recovery for individuals with COD can be conceptualized in two approaches. The first approach, known as SBIRT (described below), targets people who do not yet meet criteria for SUD and provides strategies for early intervention before the need develops for specialized treatment. The second approach targets people with SUDs.

Screening, Brief Intervention, and Referral to Treatment (SBIRT)

SBIRT (screening, brief intervention, and referral to treatment) is a comprehensive, integrated public health model which provides for services on a full continuum of care, not only the substance use specialty. This intervention model consists of universal screening, secondary prevention (detecting risky or hazardous substance use or dependence), timely referral, and treatment for people with SUD. This model has been implemented widely in the United States and other countries throughout the world (SAMHSA, 2024b; see Fig. 42.2).

Screening

The **screening** process identifies individuals who might be misusing substances but does not identify the exact kind of issue or its seriousness. Screening determines whether an issue exists or whether further screening is needed. Screening should be conducted using a validated instrument to classify the individual's pattern of alcohol or drug use. Screening should take 5 to 10 minutes and can be repeated at various intervals over time. The Alcohol Use Disorders Identification Test (AUDIT)

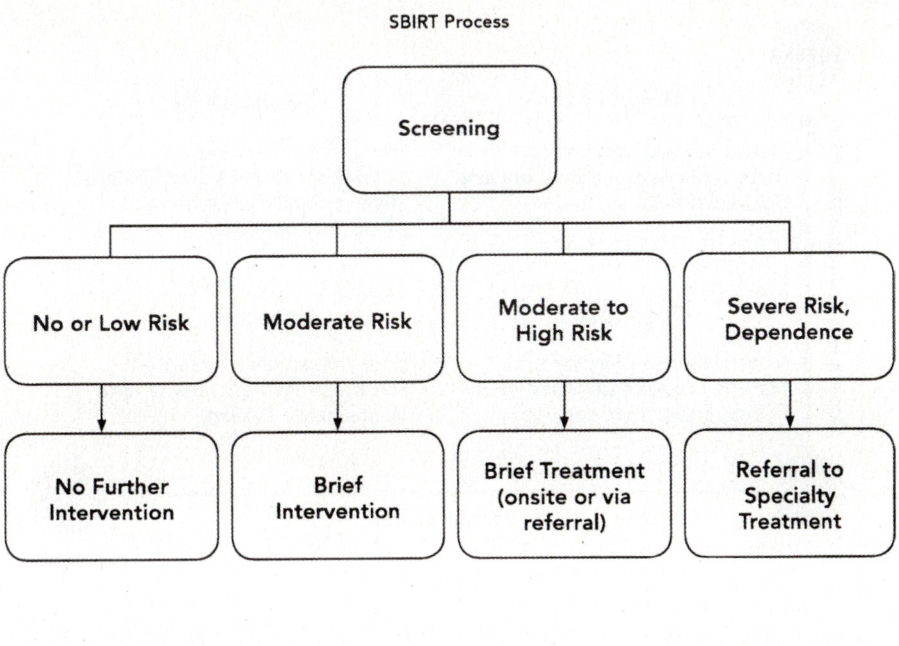

FIGURE 42.2 SBIRT process. (Reprinted from Substance Abuse and Mental Health Services Administration. [2013]. Systems-level implementation of screening, brief intervention, and referral to treatment. Technical Assistance Publication [TAP] Series 33. HHS Publication No. [SMA] 13–4741. Substance Abuse and Mental Health Services Administration.)

(Babor et al., 2001) and the National Institute on Drug Abuse (NIDA) offer examples of several instruments (NIDA, 2023). Screening can identify people across the whole spectrum of use—from risky to dependence.

Brief Intervention

A **brief intervention** is appropriate for people who are at moderate risk for SUD. This is a motivational intervention that typically consists of one to several sessions during which the patient becomes interested in seeking treatment. This intervention focuses on increasing an individual's insight into and awareness about substance use and behavior change. The primary goal of this stage is to educate the patient and increase their motivation to reduce risky behavior (Emery & Wimme, 2023).

Referral to Treatment

For patients who need additional services, a **referral to treatment** follows the assessment and brief intervention phases. The individual is referred to specialty programs focusing on recovery and is provided with the appropriate resources.

Level of Care Quadrants

Recovery programs for individuals with COD must address both the mental disorder and the SUD. The **level of care quadrants** model is a conceptual framework that classifies patients according to symptom severity, not diagnosis (Fig. 42.3). Developed in 2014, the level of care quadrants model continues to be used in 2025. The quadrants can guide an individual's treatment and site of delivery of care. In an integrated treatment model, treatment for both disorders is combined in a single session or interaction or series of interactions.

Stages of Recovery

Patients with COD enter treatment at various stages of recovery, which involves much more than avoiding alcohol and drugs. Flexible treatment programs that can meet each patient's needs are the most effective. Recovery is sought through commonly recognized stages of treatment, including **engagement, motivation, active treatment**, and **relapse prevention** (SAMHSA, 2024b).

Engagement

Engagement entails establishing a treatment relationship and enhancing motivation to make behavior changes and a commitment to treatment. Research has shown that engaged patients are more likely to stay in treatment and have positive outcomes (Zuccarini & Stiller, 2024). Patients who are misusing substances may experience repeated cycles of detoxification and relapse. They may have prolonged cycles of admissions and persistent medication nonadherence before acknowledging the need to engage in continuous treatment (Allaudeen et al., 2024). Each admission is a "window of opportunity."

Relapse does not mean that a treatment intervention, the health care provider, or the patient has failed (Sinha, 2024). Readmission and clear, realistic goals can further the patient's engagement in the treatment process. Effective programs emphasize a combination of empathic, long-term relationship building, and the use of leverage and possible confrontation by family, other caregivers, or the legal system.

Engagement in treatment is a process that may take many contacts with a patient and requires patience. Patients who struggle with authority and control issues must be convinced that the treatment team members

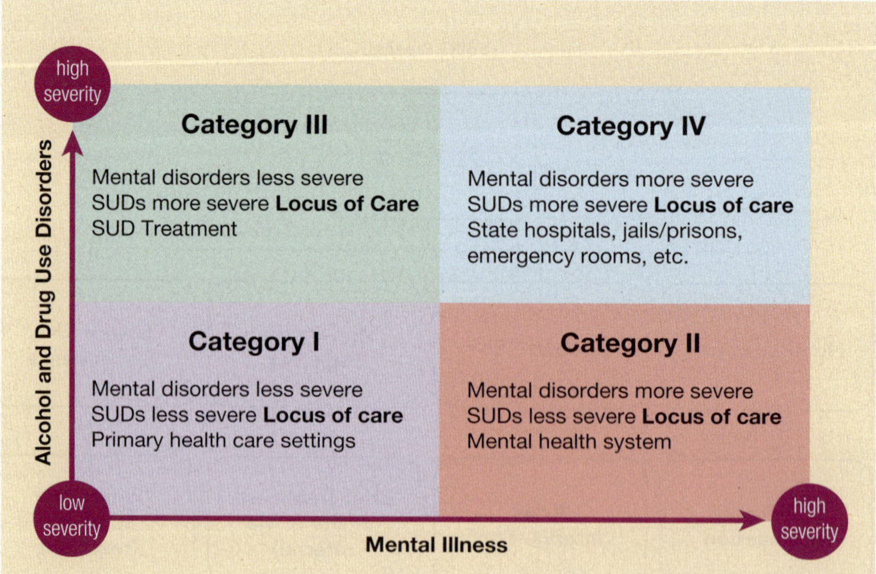

FIGURE 42.3 Level of care quadrants. (Reprinted from Substance Abuse and Mental Health Services Administration. [2020]. *Substance Use Disorder Treatment for People With Co-Occurring Disorders.* Treatment Improvement Protocol [TIP] Series, No. 42. SAMHSA Publication No. PEP20-02-01-004. Substance Abuse and Mental Health Services Administration. Retrieved February 5, 2025, from https://library.samhsa.gov/sites/default/files/pep20-02-01-004.pdf.)

have something to offer and are worth listening to before patients begin to trust them. The engagement process is enhanced if staff can deal with presenting crises concretely (e.g., provide help in avoiding legal penalties and obtaining food, housing, entitlements, relief from psychiatric symptoms, vocational opportunities, recreation, and socialization). **Harm reduction**, an evidence-based approach that equips individuals who use drugs with life-saving tools and the resources to create positive change in their lives, may be a first step toward a goal of abstinence (SAMHSA, 2024c).

The process of engagement is often characterized by approach–avoidance behavior by the patient. Lengthy intake and assessment procedures may discourage the patient from engagement or be intolerable if they are protracted and begin with asking the patient numerous pointed personal questions. These procedures may have to be adjusted to tailor treatment and accommodate the needs or reactions of the patient with COD.

Motivation

Once the individual is engaged in treatment, the next step is for the patient to identify **personal motivation** for seeking recovery such as personal values, aspirations, and desire for a better future. This is an important step and will help to remind the patient the reasons change is necessary.

Active Treatment

During **active treatment**, the individual is participating in treatment. There are several approaches to active treatment.

Brief Treatment

Brief treatment is a specialty outpatient treatment modality. It is a systematic, focused process that relies on patient engagement and implementation of change strategies. The treatment consists of 6 to 20 sessions of evidence-based, highly focused, and structured clinical sessions (e.g., solution-focused therapy, cognitive–behavioral therapy, motivation enhancement). The goals of brief treatment are to change the immediate behaviors or thoughts about a risky behavior, to address long-standing issues with harmful drinking and drug misuse, and to help patients with higher levels of disorder obtain more intensive care. One goal of this intervention is to increase engagement in treatment and help the patient identify their own goals (Jones et al., 2024).

Assertive Community Treatment

In **assertive community treatment (ACT)**, the delivery of services is in the community (rather than a clinic), with shared caseloads, 24-hour responsibilities for patients, and direct provision of most services. This model was developed for patients with severe mental disorders who do not use outpatient services, are prone to frequent relapses and rehospitalization, and have severe psychosocial impairment (Sudbeck et al., 2024).

Relapse Prevention

People with COD are highly prone to relapse even after they have achieved full remission. **Relapse prevention** focuses on identifying and preventing high-risk situations that could interfere with recovery. Although many relapse factors are the same for those with mental disorders as with the general population, such as interpersonal issues, negative emotions, social stresses, lack of involvement in more satisfying activities, and attempts to escape from painful experiences, there are additional factors that affect the population of individuals with COD. Symptoms of the mental disorders recur, and there are inadequate treatment resources in many settings. Many people with mental disorders live in extreme poverty, which forces them into high-crime, drug-infested neighborhoods, which makes them easy targets for crimes. Employment rates are low for this population even though many want to work (Tanarsuwongkul et al., 2025). Finally, the same neurobiologic dysfunctions may underlie both substance dependency and mental disorders (Lauretani et al., 2024).

Because people with mental disorders face more challenges, emerging evidence suggests that relapse prevention for this population should be different than for the general population. Relapse prevention needs to account for the pervasive cognitive and social dysfunctions that are inherent in many people with COD. Patients usually need assistance in finding and maintaining housing and employment. Learning new skills may be difficult because of cognitive impairments that reduce the effectiveness of learning new skills. Social deficits can lead to isolation and victimization. Relapse prevention for COD involves the following:

- A stable and safe place to live
- A specific, individualized plan for managing stressful times
- Making informed, healthy choices that support physical and emotional well-being
- Purposeful and meaningful daily activities such as a job, school, volunteering, family caretaking, or creative endeavors
- Relationships and social networks that provide support, friendship, love, and hope
- Support for meeting spiritual needs and finding a sense of meaning in life
- Independence, income, and resources to participate in society (SAMHSA, 2021)

EVIDENCED-BASED NURSING CARE FOR PEOPLE WITH CO-OCCURRING DISORDERS

It is crucial for patients with COD to be thoroughly assessed for responses to both psychiatric and SUDs. In some cultural groups, recognition of psychiatric and SUDs is difficult because of the lack of access and stigma associated with COD. Nurses in nonpsychiatric, community settings may be the only health care professional contact that some groups have. Assessment should include determination of the patient's willingness to change or level of motivation for treatment. Nursing care of specific co-occurring mental disorders and SUDs are discussed later in the chapter.

RECOGNIZING CUES: RELEVANT ASSESSMENT INFORMATION

It is important to delineate the relative contribution of each diagnosis to the severity of the current responses presented and to establish priorities accordingly. Because patients with COD often make unreliable historians or distort the reality of their mental health issues and the severity of their substance use, obtaining objective data is especially important. Ideally, one should obtain an objective history of the patient from family, significant others, board and care operators, other health care providers, or anyone familiar enough with the patient to provide an accurate history. Box 42.1 lists basic assessment tools and methods used for patients with COD. The following concepts are paramount when assessing people with COD:

- Psychiatric and SUDs can coexist.
- Responses (psychosis, agitation) to both disorders can be similar.
- Substance use can mask other symptoms and syndromes.
- Psychiatric behaviors can mimic alcohol and other drug use disorders.

NCLEXNOTE Patients with both mental disorders and SUDs have responses to both disorders. Prioritizing nursing care depends on the immediate issue, but responses to both disorders should be assessed.

Psychological testing and other methods of assessment determine the patient's level of cognitive functioning in order to select the appropriate treatment. It is also important to determine the extent of the mental disorder and the substance use. The nurse assesses the patient's abilities for self-care, independent living, impulse control, control of assaultive behavior, direction taking, and development of new responses to new situations and ideas. The nurse must also evaluate changes in mental status during the past 6 months and examine previous treatment outcomes.

BOX 42.1

Assessment of Co-occurring Disorders

Obtain a history and physical examination and laboratory tests (e.g., liver function tests, complete blood count) to confirm medical indicators related to substance use and to rule out medical disorders with psychiatric presentations.

- Obtain substance use history and severity of consequences and physical symptoms.
- Identify core cultural values; explore meaning of the symptoms.
- Assess mental status examination and severity of symptoms (e.g., suicidal, homicidal, florid psychosis).
- Explore social context—socioeconomic, environment, literacy, and support system.

Interview with and assess family members to verify or determine (1) the accuracy of the patient's self-reported substance use or mental health history; (2) the patient's history of past mental health issues during periods of abstinence; and, if possible, (3) the sequence of the diagnoses (i.e., what symptoms appeared first).

- Conduct interviews with the patient's partner, friends, social worker, and other significant people in the patient's life.
- Review court records, medical records, and previous psychiatric and substance use treatment.
- Perform urine and blood toxicity screens; use a breath analyzer to test the patient's blood–alcohol level.

Revise initial assessment by observation of the patient in the clinical setting; full assessment of the underlying psychiatric issue may not be possible until there is a long (up to 6 months) period of total abstinence.

- Observe the patient for reappearance of psychiatric symptoms after a period of sobriety.
- Assess the patient's motivation to seek treatment, desire to change behavior, and understanding of diagnoses.

ANALYZING CUES AND DEVELOPING HYPOTHESES

Many patients seeking treatment for CODs experience transitory cognitive impairment when they are detoxing from substances, which usually resolves within the first month of abstinence. Patients often experience difficulties with disorientation, clouding of consciousness, incoherent thoughts, memory loss, and delirium, which may hinder their ability to learn new concepts. These issues are a result of the neurobiologic insult on the brain by these substances and psychosocial factors such as fear of legal or relationship difficulties, depression, grief, and feelings of guilt and shame. However, if Wernicke syndrome, a reversible alcohol-induced amnestic disorder caused by a thiamine-deficient diet, or Korsakoff psychosis, characterized by a loss of recent memory and confabulation (or filling in the blanks in memory by making up facts to cover this deficit) is present, cognitive issues may last longer. Patients with this condition are highly suggestible, have poor judgment, and cannot reason critically. Korsakoff psychosis often follows Wernicke encephalopathy and is also associated with prior peripheral neuropathy (see Chapter 31).

PLANNING RECOVERY AND WELLNESS OUTCOMES: GENERATING SOLUTIONS

To move toward recovery, establishing a positive social network is critical. Isolation and alienation from prior sources of support is an issue that most people with co-occurring mental disorders and substance use share. Some patients relate poorly to their families, others are overly dependent on their families, and others have difficulty establishing and maintaining social relationships. Some patients' only "families" are peers within the drug subculture who reinforce substance-misusing behavior.

Following an agreed-on treatment plan is integral to recovery. Comprehensive planning within a multidisciplinary team approach is highly successful in the care of such patients. Part of a comprehensive relapse-prevention plan is to establish or reinforce the patient's social support network so that they can obtain (1) opportunities for substance-free socializing, (2) crisis counseling to prevent readmission to a hospital, and (3) support for sobriety. Community organizations are valuable sources of support as well.

Planning for housing is also essential for patients with COD. Supportive housing is especially crucial for patients who are being discharged from the hospital because the risk for relapse is greatest during the first few months after discharge. Halfway houses for people with SUD may deemphasize medication adherence, and housing designed for chronically mentally ill individuals may not emphasize abstinence enough. Thus, an important part of the multidisciplinary team approach to discharge planning for patients with COD is to help them find the best possible living situation.

Younger patients with a mental disorder may want and expect to find appropriate employment, but some of these patients may be unrealistic about potential professions. However, this desire can be a significant motivator and a useful tool in a treatment program. Referring patients to halfway houses or residential substance use treatment programs that stress vocational skill training can be beneficial. Use of community vocational rehabilitation services and educational opportunities can be an important part of a discharge plan.

THERAPEUTIC RELATIONSHIP

Patients with CODs are likely to seek mental health care more frequently than those individuals with one psychiatric disorder. Nurses in various care settings such as ICU, ED, and mental health are likely to have frequent contact with these patients. It is important for nurses to recognize the complexity and interaction of the disorders. Developing a positive, nonjudgmental relationship that is based on recovery principles is critical. Providing patients with hope for the future and assurance that there are a variety of ways to recover will support the patient during critical times.

TAKING ACTION: NURSING INTERVENTIONS

The nurse who provides care to patients with COD faces numerous challenges. Nurses implement interventions according to their level of practice and knowledge. Many of the interventions that are indicated for people with COD are discussed in previous chapters. Box 42.2 presents features of a COD outpatient program. Opportunities to socialize, access to positive recreational

BOX 42.2

Features of a Co-occurring Disorders Outpatient Program

- *Community meeting and goal setting:* Patients set small, realistic goals for themselves for the day, which aid them in their ultimate goal of better living in recovery.
- *Anger management and social communication:* Patients learn appropriate ways to express anger and how to socialize with others.
- *Group therapy:* Patients discuss interpersonal issues, get feedback from their peers, and learn problem-solving skills.
- *Dual recovery anonymous meetings:* Patient-run meetings (a modified AA meeting) address the specific needs of patients with COD.
- *Leisure planning:* Patients learn skills to enjoy leisure involving clean and sober fun.
- *Complementary therapies:* Art therapy, music therapy, yoga; these methods provide alternatives to the use of alcohol and other drugs.
- *Health education:* Patients learn about the effects of drugs and alcohol on the body and about other relevant medical topics.
- *Medication education:* Patients learn about psychiatric medications, their uses, their side effects, and interactions with drugs or alcohol.
- *Relapse-prevention planning:* Patients talk about their last relapse; triggers, feelings, and stresses that contributed to the relapse; and the consequences and formulate relapse-prevention plans.
- *Individual counseling:* Patients receive individual counseling to develop goals and work on problem-solving techniques.
- *Psychiatric consultation:* Patients are evaluated and followed up for medication and other psychiatric interventions.

Note: Patients are *not* discharged from the program if they are intoxicated or relapse. They are asked not to come to the program intoxicated but to return when they are sober to continue work on their recovery.

activities, and a supportive peer group are stabilizing influences on patients who may otherwise drop out of treatment altogether. The following discussion highlights interventions that are modified because of the special needs of this population.

Medication Management

One essential feature of COD treatment is medication management. Medication for a known mental disorder should never be discontinued on the grounds that the patient is using substances. Discontinuing prescribed medications is associated with increased behavior issues after discharge and is a direct cause of relapse and rehospitalization. Impulsive behavior in response to transient exacerbations of psychotic symptoms, depressed mood, or anxiety symptoms may lead to relapse.

Errors in medication management include treating temporary psychiatric symptoms resulting from withdrawal as if they were a permanent feature of the individual, withholding needed medication for a psychiatric disorder, or setting arbitrary limits on medication based on a belief that medication for all psychiatric symptoms should be suspended until the COD is treated. Overall, patients need ongoing help with adhering to a prescribed medication regimen.

Collaboration between the patient's prescriber and other treatment providers is important to minimize the possible misuse of prescription drugs such as forging prescriptions, acquiring drugs from nonmedical sources, frequent visits to EDs, or seeking multiple prescribers. In addition, caution is essential in prescribing medications that can increase the patient's potential for relapse into misusing the drug of choice.

Substance Use Counseling

With the patient with COD, substance use counseling is slower and less confrontational than in many traditional substance misuse programs. Content needs to be repeated frequently and motivation for treatment continually assessed.

Cognitive–Behavioral Interventions

Cognitive–behavioral interventions help patients to (1) analyze which situations are most likely to trigger relapses; (2) examine cognitive, emotional, and behavioral components of high-risk situations; and (3) develop cognitive, behavioral, and effective coping strategies and environmental supports. Role-playing ways out of high-risk situations is a technique that these groups often use. Homework assignments help patients create relapse-prevention plans that address new coping strategies for these high-risk situations (Tranberg et al., 2024).

Patient Education

Patient education is an essential element in treating COD. Patients need to learn about their specific mental disorder, substance use and misuse, and their effects. Relapse prevention and recovery should be highlighted. Education can be conducted in individual sessions, but group sessions encourage interaction among patients. Sharing their experiences with their peers, patients can enhance these presentations.

Topics should be clear; relevant to the group members; and illustrated with charts, handouts, or appropriate films. Each session should be relatively short and not contain too many new or difficult concepts. Reinforcing and reviewing previous discussions can be helpful to remind patients of particularly relevant concepts. Box 42.3 lists some suitable topics for nurse-led discussion groups. Individual patient education can focus on areas of knowledge deficits and reinforce topics discussed in group settings. Group sessions can also assist patients in learning interpersonal skills (e.g., assertiveness) and problem-solving skills and in relapse-prevention planning (Hesse et al., 2022).

For patients with cognitive or memory impairment, clear, direct, simple interventions that avoid extraneous

BOX 42.3

Topics for Education Groups for Patients With Co-occurring Disorders

- The effects of alcohol and drugs on the body
- Alcohol, drugs, and medication—what can go wrong?
- What is a healthy lifestyle?
- Triggers for relapse
- What is Alcoholics (or Narcotics) Anonymous?
- What is a sponsor in Alcoholics (or Narcotics) Anonymous?
- What is recovery from mental illness and substance use?
- What are the tools of recovery?
- The disease of substance dependency
- The relapse cycle
- How to cope with feelings without using alcohol or other drugs?
- Relapse prevention: what works?
- What are cognitive distortions?
- HIV prevention and education
- Leisure time management
- How to manage stress?
- Relaxation training
- Assertiveness and recovery
- Common slogans to live by
- Pitfalls in treatment
- The process of recovery
- Creating a relapse-prevention plan
- What are my goals? How does the use of alcohol and drugs affect them?
- Coping with thoughts about alcohol and drugs
- Problem-solving basics
- Coping with anger
- Negative thinking and how to manage it
- Enhancing social support networks

issues and theoretical discussion may be useful. Examples include:

- Reading material that is relevant to recovery and that can be referred to in short study sessions
- First-person accounts of substance dependency and recovery found in Alcoholics Anonymous (AA) and Narcotics Anonymous (NA) literature
- Basic concepts of recovery, such as those in AA slogans and on patients' need for continuing care after discharge
- Films with scenes illustrating relevant family issues or other issues related to substance use; movies can be more effective than lectures

Mutual Self-Help Groups

Several mutual self-help groups are appropriate for many patients with COD. Peer-led self-help approaches specifically for people with COD are being tried with some success. The most common groups are 12-step programs, such as AA and NA (see Chapter 31). The advisability of a patient enrolling in a 12-step program needs to be evaluated on an individual basis. A health care provider familiar with 12-step concepts can often facilitate patients' attempts to use these programs. The numerous advantages of self-help groups make them a potentially powerful support for continued recovery. Alternative mutual self-help programs similar to 12-step programs are available in some geographic areas. Rational Recovery and Secular Organization for Sobriety are groups that downplay the concept of powerlessness and the spiritual aspects associated with 12-step programs.

Family Support and Education

The families of patients with COD need education and support. Family psychoeducation interventions address mental disorders, substance use, and their interactions. The focus of family support groups, such as those under the auspices of the National Alliance on Mental Illness, has been both to educate and to help the family cope with a mentally ill relative. AA and NA take a similar approach to providing peer support to families of people with SUD. These self-help groups aid family members in balancing confrontation of the issue, detachment from forcing a solution to it, and support of the treatment process.

Continuum of Care

An integrated approach that combines mental health and substance use interventions at the clinical site has been shown to be the most effective. In an integrated system, the same team provides coordinated mental health and substance use interventions and guides the patient toward learning to manage these intertwined disorders. When the mental health and substance use systems are truly integrated, patient outcomes are positive (Archambault et al., 2024). Social interaction skills and coping skills learned in treatment can be reinforced in community settings to create or enhance a stable living situation and possible vocational opportunities.

When Hospitalization Is Necessary

Often, patients with COD can be treated effectively in community mental health settings if their symptoms are stable, they are following their treatment plan, they take medications as prescribed, and they remain alcohol and drug free. Patients are hospitalized when they have a need for detoxification, exacerbation of co-occurring psychiatric or medical disorders, suicidal or homicidal ideation, or a disorder that prevents abstinence or outpatient treatment. Interventions that support housing and employment are important, or deterioration may occur despite gains made during hospitalization.

Crisis Stabilization

Setting priorities is essential for hospitalized patients with COD. The first priorities are gathering data from a physical examination and nursing assessments, stabilizing psychiatric symptoms, and treating withdrawal symptoms (see Chapter 31). After these issues are addressed, the patient enters the rehabilitation phase of treatment for both diagnoses. Rehabilitative therapy is appropriate if the patient (1) can participate in a group process, (2) can focus attention on groups or reading material, (3) does not engage in behavior that is detrimental to the group process, (4) can listen to and receive feedback from others, and (5) can benefit from the group process.

Evaluation

Evaluation of the patient's ability to deal with both the substance use and mental disorder is an ongoing process. Because the goal of recovery is to have quality of life (QoL) in the community of choice, treatment outcomes should be evaluated for QoL as well as management of two disorders.

SPECIFIC CO-OCCURRING MENTAL AND SUBSTANCE USE DISORDERS

The following section describes key assessment and intervention areas for specific mental disorders and SUDs. A more complete discussion of the specific mental disorders and SUDs is found in Unit VI.

Schizophrenia and Substance Use Disorder

Research shows schizophrenia and SUD is a common dual disorder. There are several possible explanations for the frequency of substance use in individuals with schizophrenia. People with schizophrenia and SUD often experience poor physical health, poor social support, double stigma, and care access difficulties (Neyra et al., 2024).

Assessing the needs of people with schizophrenia, who also use substances, is complicated by the changing interaction among psychotic symptoms, the antipsychotic effects of medications, and the side effects of medications. People with a psychotic disorder may have an altered thought process or delusional thinking and may experience auditory hallucinations. They may also be cognitively impaired and have poor memory. These patients can have negative symptoms, such as poor motivation and poor hygiene. They often have low self-esteem and poor social skills and may have a general sense of not belonging to a community. Their sense of self in relation to the world may be altered.

As with all CODs, a multifaceted, integrated treatment approach is needed. Atypical antipsychotics continue to be the primary pharmacologic agent for the treatment of patients with co-occurring schizophrenia with substance use. Not only do these agents treat the symptoms of schizophrenia, but they also appear to reduce cue-trigger cravings of the substances and prevent relapse. Long-acting injectable (LAI) antipsychotics are promising treatments because the patient is no longer required to remember to take daily medication (Neyra et al., 2024). While monitoring side effects of antipsychotics, the nurse's attention needs to focus on liver functioning because drugs and alcohol are also metabolized by the liver. Relapse is frequently secondary to medication nonadherence, especially if patients experience side effects associated with the use of antipsychotics. Nursing interventions that focus on medication adherence may reduce the chance of relapse.

A confrontational interactive approach does not benefit this population and could even alienate patients. A supportive, collaborative approach is appropriate in which relapses are treated as an expected part of the recovery process. Addressing relapse risk is part of treatment planning. Focus on examining behavior, feelings, and the thinking process that led to the relapse. The nurse must avoid blame and guilt-inducing statements (Neyra et al., 2024).

Social skills training may be needed to help the patient learn ways of avoiding peer pressure and social situations that could lead to substance use. The goal is to successfully interact in a sober living situation, develop problem-solving skills, and refine behaviors (Barlati et al., 2024).

Mood Disorders and Substance Use

Substance use in patients with depression contributes to treatment nonadherence and less positive outcomes such as falls, orthostatic hypotension, sedation, and hyponatremia (Srifuengfung et al., 2024). Many who use substances self-medicate an underlying mood disorder. Because many of the symptoms of substance use are the same as those of mood disorders, it is difficult to differentiate between them. This is especially true in the case of stimulant use and bipolar disorder. It is often impossible to determine the presence of an underlying mood disorder until there has been a period of abstinence.

Screening for suicidal ideation is a priority during the assessment of these individuals. Both mood disorders and substance use are related to suicide (see Chapters 22, 25, and 31). Depression during withdrawal from alcohol, cocaine, opiates, and amphetamines also puts patients at severe risk for suicide. An individual's presenting behaviors may not have included depression, but depression may develop as the withdrawal syndrome unfolds. Hyperactivity often appears with stimulant use and at times with alcohol use. Patients may be treated for hypomania or bipolar disorder when they are actually hyperactive. Symptoms usually improve as the individual maintains abstinence.

Determining whether mood disorders are the cause or the effect of protracted substance use is difficult. An important nursing assessment is to determine how drug use relates to mood states. Patients may be attempting to alleviate uncomfortable symptoms, such as depression or agitation, or to enhance a mood state (e.g., hypomania). Symptoms that persist during periods of abstinence are a clue to the degree that the mood disorder contributes to the presenting symptoms.

There is little research regarding pharmacologic interventions for co-occurring mood disorders and substance use. Consequently, treatment is similar to that of mood disorders without substance use or misuse. When a pharmacologic agent is selected, attention is paid to its interaction with drugs and alcohol and its potential for dependence. The selective serotonin reuptake inhibitors (SSRIs) are frequently used for co-occurring depression. Higher doses may be required because of the possibility that alcohol use may induce hepatic microsomal activity. In the bipolar disorders, mood stabilizers are used.

Treatment for bipolar disorders and substance use should be individualized to accommodate the specific needs, personal goals, and cultural perspectives of these individuals in different stages of change. Using interventions centered on examining cognitive distortions (e.g., "I'll never get better; no one likes me; alcohol is my only friend") and cognitive therapy techniques can help improve mood. Use of positive self-talk can be helpful for both the depression and the SUDs.

Anxiety Disorders and Substance Use

Research is scant regarding the relationship of anxiety disorders to substance use. Because there are a variety of anxiety disorders with differing clinical symptoms and

BOX 42.4

Research for Evidence-Based Practice: Anxiety and Opioid Use Disorder

McHugh, R. K., Fitzmaurice, G. M., Votaw, V. R., Geyer, R. B., Ragnini, K., Greenfield, S. F., & Weiss, R. D. (2024). Cognitive behavioral therapy for anxiety and opioid use disorder: Development and pilot testing. Journal of Substance Use and Addiction Treatment, 160, *209296. https://doi.org/10.1016/j.josat.2024.209296*

THE QUESTION: What is the feasibility, acceptability, and clinical outcome of a pilot project that added cognitive-behavioral treatment for people with co-occurring opioid use disorder and anxiety disorder?

METHODS: Forty-two adults with dual diagnosis (anxiety and opioid use disorders) participated in an open pilot (*n* = 5) and RCT (*n* = 37 – 6 discontinued the study). Participants received 12 sessions of treatment within 14 weeks and completed baseline and posttreatment assessments. Session content was based on evidence-based principles for cognitive-behavioral treatment of substance use disorder and anxiety disorders. All participants received medication for the opioid use disorder.

FINDINGS: The results of the pilot program were positive. Participants experienced reduced anxiety symptoms, and most were abstinent in the prior month at the end of treatment. The results support of the use of a cognitive-behavioral approach. The benefit appears to be similar to the other psychosocial approaches that include medication treatment.

IMPLICATIONS FOR NURSING: Cognitive-behavioral approaches can be considered when caring for people with co-occurring opioid and anxiety disorders when their medication to promote abstinence is not adequate. Patients can be encouraged to engage in cognitive-behavioral approaches while taking medication for their disorder.

numerous substances of misuse, it is difficult to develop studies addressing all the anxiety disorders.

The symptoms of anxiety may result from an anxiety disorder, such as panic attack, or may be secondary to drug or alcohol use as part of a withdrawal syndrome. Symptoms are so subjectively disturbing that they can lead to drug or alcohol use as self-medication for the emotional pain; therefore, they require prompt evaluation and treatment. There are many unanswered questions regarding the relationship of the anxiety symptoms, stress, and changes in the hypothalamic–pituitary–adrenal axis response to substance use. More research is sorely needed in this area (Lin et al., 2024).

Pharmacologic treatment of patients with anxiety is difficult because the traditional medications used, the benzodiazepines, are subject to misuse. Long-term treatment of the anxiety disorders with the SSRIs maintains and improves QoL. Co-occurring anxiety disorders and substance use require psychosocial interventions along with pharmacologic treatment. See Box 42.4. Complementary therapies, such as yoga, are showing promise in the treatment of substance use and anxiety disorders (Krishnan, 2024).

Patients with anxiety disorders should also pay particular attention to their physical health. Regular, balanced meals; exercise; and sleep are ways to decrease and manage stress levels. Patients should avoid excessive consumption of caffeine and sugars. If the patient has a fear of crowds, they may benefit from gradual desensitization techniques (Nardi et al., 2024).

PTSD and Substance Use

PTSD is of particular concern because it has been shown to increase the risk of substance use relapse and is associated with poor treatment outcomes (Swannelll et al., 2025). For PTSD, other medications such as the atypical antipsychotics, non-SSRI antidepressants, and mood stabilizers also appear to result in improvements (see Chapter 29).

Personality Disorders and Substance Use

Personality disorders are frequently present in those who use alcohol and other substances. Antisocial personality and borderline disorders carry a high risk of having a co-occurring SUD (Chapman et al., 2024; Low et al., 2024). The assessment of people with co-occurring personality disorders and substance use focuses on the issues related to the particular personality disorder, as well as the substance use. Individuals with antisocial personality disorder are likely to have a family history of other psychiatric disorders and issues with hostility.

SUMMARY OF KEY POINTS

- In co-occurring mental disorder and SUD, each disorder is considered a primary disorder. Patients should be treated concurrently with an integrated approach.
- People with COD are at high risk for relapse. The relapse cycle repeats itself without treatment.
- There is not one model that explains why mental disorders and substance use occur together so frequently. The most common pattern is the onset of the mental disorder, followed by the issues with substance use, leading to misuse. It appears that the substance use is an attempt to self-medicate the psychiatric symptoms.
- Barriers for treatment include housing instability, unemployment, and lack of social support. Other

barriers include the complexity of the COD, staff attitudes, stigma, and health issues that interfere with treatment.

- Interdisciplinary treatment is through an integrated approach. Patients are moved toward recovery through engagement, motivation, assertive outreach and treatment, and relapse prevention.
- Recovery through commonly recognized stages of treatment—engagement, motivation, active treatment, and relapse prevention—involves much more than avoiding alcohol and drugs.
- Nursing assessment of COD often depends on objective data obtained from interviews with family members, reviews of court records, laboratory test results, and physical examination findings. Assessment should include a determination of the willingness to change and motivation for treatment.
- Interventions that are tailored to the special needs of the patient with a COD are medication management, substance use counseling, cognitive–behavioral interventions, patient education, and family support and education. Participation in peer-led self-help groups has had some success.
- An ideal continuum of care is an integrated approach with one team coordinating the mental health and substance use interventions. Patients should not have to negotiate treatment with two separate systems. Hospitalization may be required during periods of crises. Most treatment occurs in the community, where recovery is the goal.
- Treatment and nursing care need to be individualized within the context of the specific mental disorder and substances used.

DEVELOPING CLINICAL JUDGMENT

1. An 18-year-old patient, newly diagnosed with schizophrenia, is relatively adherent with their medication and treatment. This patient was recently at a social event where they were experimenting with alcohol and marijuana. What are key teaching points for this patient?
2. A nurse in an emergency department recommends AA for every patient who is admitted for detoxification. Is that an appropriate referral for an individual with co-occurring mental disorder and substance use?
3. A community health nurse wants to refer a young individual who lives in an underserved rural area to an integrated treatment program several miles away. However, the patient does not have reliable transportation and is unlikely to be able to access the services. Discuss alternative treatment options for this patient.
4. How would you respond to a patient with COD who states, "Once my medication is stable, I will be able to drink again"?
5. Compare traditional substance use approaches to an integrated treatment program.
6. A patient with a COD tells the nurse, "All chemicals are bad for you. I do not want to take my medication." Develop a response to this statement that reflects the use of engagement.
7. Discuss the differences in behavior of an individual with schizophrenia who uses cocaine and an individual with a mood disorder who uses marijuana.
8. Which COD concepts should be included in patient education?

MOVIES, TV, OR STREAMING PROGRAMS

***The Outrun:* 2024.** This film is about Rona (Saoirse Ronan), a 30-year-old single adult who has alcohol use disorder and is only happy when drinking. Rona grew up in the Orkney Islands in Scotland with a father who had bipolar disorder and a mother who used religion to cope with her husband's illness. The story begins in London where Rona is living with her boyfriend, who eventually leaves her because of her drinking. She makes several attempts at sobriety that result in relapses. Finally, she returns to the Orkney Islands where she hopes to heal. During the healing process, she visits memories of her traumatic childhood.

Viewing Points:

1. Would Rona be considered to have a co-occurring disorder? If so, what is the disorder?
2. There is no evidence that Rona used any medication to treat her alcohol use disorder or depression. What strategies did she use to treat both disorders?
3. Does Rona develop a positive attitude as she becomes sober?

REFERENCES

Allaudeen, N., Akwe, J., Arundel, C., Boggan, J. C., Caldwell, P., Cornia, P. B., Cyr, J., Ehlers, E., Elzweig, J., Godwin, P., Gordon, K. S., Guidry, M., Gutierrez, J., Heppe, D., Hoegh, M., Jagannath, A., Kaboli, P., Krug, M., Laudate, J. D.,…Gunderson, C. G. (2024). Medications for alcohol-use disorder and follow-up after hospitalization for alcohol withdrawal: A multicenter study. *Journal of Hospital Medicine*, *19*(12), 1122–1130. https://doi.org/10.1002/jhm.13458

Archambault, L., Bertrand, K., Martel, M. O., Bérubé, M., Belhouari, S., & Perreault, M. (2024). The current state of knowledge on care for co-occurring chronic pain and opioid use disorder: A scoping review. *Journal of Clinical Nursing*, *33*(8), 3056–3076. https://doi.org/10.1111/jocn.17139

Babor, T. F., Higgins-Biddle, J. C., Saunders, J. B., & Monteiro, M. G. (2001). *AUDIT: The alcohol use disorders identification test: Guidelines for use in primary health care* (2nd ed.). World Health Organization. https://apps.who.int/iris/handle/10665/67205

Barlati, S., Nibbio, G., & Vita, A. (2024). Evidence-based psychosocial interventions in schizophrenia: A critical review. *Current Opinion in Psychiatry*, *37*(3), 131–139. https://doi.org/10.1097/YCO.0000000000000925

Brown, J. L., Gause, N. K., Braun, R., Punches, B., Spatholt, D., Twitty, T. D., Sprunger, J. G., & Lyons, M. S. (2024). Substance use and mental health screening within an emergency department-based HIV screening program: Outcomes from 1 year of implementation. *Health Promotion Practice, 25*(6), 1049–1057. https://doi.org/10.1177/15248399231193005

Chapman, J., Jamil, R. T., Fleisher, C., & Torrico, T. J. (2024). Borderline personality disorder. In *StatPearls*. StatPearls Publishing. https://www.ncbi.nlm.nih.gov/books/NBK430883/

Diefenbach, G. J., Stubbing, J., Rice, T. B., Lord, K. A., Rudd, M. D., & Tolin, D. F. (2024). Uncovering the role of substance use in suicide attempts using a mixed-methods approach. *Suicide & Life-Threatening Behavior, 54*(1), 70–82. https://doi.org/10.1111/sltb.13019

Dion, K. M., Ferland, F., Farand, L., Gauvin, L., & Fleury, M. J. (2024). Reasons for high emergency department use among patients with common mental disorders or substance-related disorders. *Healthcare Policy, 19*(4), 55–69. https://doi.org/10.12927/hcpol.2024.27333

Emery, R. L., & Wimmer, M. (2023). Motivational interviewing. In *StatPearls*. StatPearls Publishing. https://www.ncbi.nlm.nih.gov/books/NBK589705/

Feder, K. A., Li, Y., Burke, K. N., Byrne, L., Desai, I. K., Saloner, B., & Krawczyk, N. (2025). Client and program-level factors associated with planned use of medications for opioid use disorder in specialty substance use treatment programs: Evidence from linked administrative data and survey data. *Journal of Substance Use and Addiction Treatment, 168*, 209545. https://doi.org/10.1016/j.josat.2024.209545

Hesse, M., Del Palacio-Gonzalez, A., & Thylstrup, B. (2022). Impulsive lifestyle counselling versus treatment as usual to reduce offending in people with co-occurring antisocial personality disorder and substance use disorder: a post hoc analysis. *BMC Psychiatry, 22*(1), 392. https://doi.org/10.1186/s12888-022-04025-8

Hyatt, A., Mullin, B., Hasler, V., Madore, D., Progovac, A. M., Cook, B. L., & DeLisi, L. E. (2024). Predictors of relapse and engagement in care one year after ending services in an urban safety net coordinated specialty care program for first episode psychosis. *Schizophrenia Research, 264*, 140–146. https://doi.org/10.1016/j.schres.2023.12.022

Jones, M., Seel, C. J., & Dymond, S. (2024). Electronic-screening, brief intervention and referral to treatment (e-SBIRT) for addictive disorders: Systematic review and meta-analysis. *Substance Use & Addiction Journal, 45*(4), 736–752. https://doi.org/10.1177/29767342241248926

Krishnan, A. (2024). Integrative treatment for substance use disorders: Improving outcomes through evidence-based practice of yoga-derived breathwork and meditation. *Journal of Addiction Medicine, 18*(2), 103–109. https://doi.org/10.1097/ADM.0000000000001263

Lauretani, F., Giallauria, F., Testa, C., Zinni, C., Lorenzi, B., Zucchini, I., Salvi, M., Napoli, R., & Maggio, M. G. (2024). Dopamine pharmacodynamics: New insights. *International Journal of Molecular Sciences, 25*(10), 5293. https://doi.org/10.3390/ijms25105293

Lin, E. R., Veenker, F. N., Manza, P., Yonga, M. V., Abey, S., Wang, G. J., & Volkow, N. D. (2024). The limbic system in co-occurring substance use and anxiety disorders: A narrative review using the RDoC framework. *Brain Sciences, 14*(12), 1285. https://doi.org/10.3390/brainsci14121285

Low, A., Stiltner, B., Nunez, Y. Z., Adhikari, K., Deak, J. D., Pietrzak, R. H., Kranzler, H. R., Gelernter, J., & Polimanti, R. (2024). Association patterns of antisocial personality disorder across substance use disorders. *Translational Psychiatry, 14*(1), 346. https://doi.org/10.1038/s41398-024-03054-z

Magnan, E., Weyrich, M., Miller, M., Melnikow, J., Moulin, A., Servis, M., Chadha, P., Spivack, S., & Henry, S. G. (2024). Stigma against patients with substance use disorders among health care professionals and trainees and stigma-reducing interventions: A systematic review. *Academic Medicine, 99*(2), 221–231. https://doi.org/10.1097/ACM.0000000000005467

Mirzaian, C. B., Deavenport-Saman, A., Hudson, S. M., & Betz, C. L. (2024). Barriers to mental health care transition for youth and young adults with intellectual and developmental disabilities and co-occurring mental health conditions: Stakeholders' perspectives. *Community Mental Health Journal, 60*(6), 1104–1116. https://doi.org/10.1007/s10597-024-01262-x

Nardi, W. R., Kelly, P., Roy, A., Becker, S., Brewer, J., & Sun, S. (2024). A systematic review and meta-analysis of psychosocial interventions for persons with comorbid anxiety and substance use disorders. *Journal of Substance Use and Addiction Treatment, 165*, 209442. https://doi.org/10.1016/j.josat.2024.209442

National Institute of Mental Health (NIMH). (2024). Substance use and co-occurring mental disorders. Retrieved January 26, 2025, from https://www.nimh.nih.gov/health/topics/substance-use-and-mental-health

National Institute on Drug Abuse (NIDA). (2023). Screening and assessment tools chart. Retrieved January 28, 2023, from https://nida.nih.gov/nidamed-medical-health-professionals/screening-tools-resources/chart-screening-tools

Neyra, A., Parro-Torres, C., Ros-Cucurull, E., Carrera, I., Echarri, E., & Torrens, M. (2024). Management of schizophrenia and comorbid substance use disorders: Expert review and guidance. *Annals of General Psychiatry, 23*(1), 40. https://doi.org/10.1186/s12991-024-00529-7

Office of Disease Prevention and Health Promotion. (2022). Increase the proportion of people with co-occurring substance use disorders and mental health disorders who receive treatment for both disorders. *Healthy People 2030*. Retrieved January 26, 2025, from https://odphp.health.gov/healthypeople/objectives-and-data/browse-objectives/mental-health-and-mental-disorders/increase-proportion-people-substance-use-and-mental-health-disorders-who-get-treatment-both-mhmd-07

Singh, M., & Agustines, D. (2024). Humanism and psychosis: Working with patients who have potential medical comorbidities along with mental illness. *Cureus, 16*(8), e66903. https://doi.org/10.7759/cureus.66903

Sinha, R. (2024). Stress and substance use disorders: risk, relapse, and treatment outcomes. *The Journal of Clinical Investigation, 134*(16), e172883. https://doi.org/10.1172/JCI172883

Srifuengfung, M., Lenze, E. J., Roose, S. P., Brown, P. J., Lavretsky, H., Karp, J. F., Reynolds, C. F., 3rd, Yingling, M., Sa-Nguanpanich, N., & Mulsant, B. H. (2024). Alcohol and substance use in older adults with treatment-resistant depression. *International Journal of Geriatric Psychiatry, 39*(6), e6105. https://doi.org/10.1002/gps.6105

Substance Abuse and Mental Health Services Administration (SAMHSA). (2021). *Employee assistance program prescription drug toolkit and fact sheets*. Publication No. PEP20-03-02-001.

Substance Abuse and Mental Health Services Administration (SAMHSA). (2024a). *Co-occurring disorders and other health conditions*. Retrieved January 26, 2025, from https://www.samhsa.gov/substance-use/treatment/co-occurring-disorders

Substance Abuse and Mental Health Services Administration (SAMHSA). (2024b). *Screening, brief intervention, and referral to treatment (SBIRT)*. Retrieved January 28, 2025, from https://www.samhsa.gov/substance-use/treatment/sbirt

Substance Abuse and Mental Health Services Administration (SAMHSA). (2024c). *Harm reduction*. Retrieved February 7, 2025, from https://www.samhsa.gov/substance-use/harm-reduction

Sudbeck, D., Jorgensen, S., & Dixon, L. B. (2024). Assertive community treatment. *Psychiatric Services, 75*(5), 508–509. https://doi.org/10.1176/appi.ps.24075007

Swannell, M., Bradlow, R. C. J., Pham, D., Gabriel, J., Manahan, Y., & Arunogiri, S. (2025). Pharmacological treatments for co-occurring PTSD and substance use disorders: A systematic review. *Journal of Substance Use and Addiction Treatment, 169*, 209601. https://doi.org/10.1016/j.josat.2024.209601

Tanarsuwongkul, S., Liu, J., Spaulding, M., Perea-Schmittle, K., Lohman, M., & Wang, Q. (2025). Associations between social determinants of health and mental health disorders among U.S. population: a cross-sectional study. *Epidemiology and Psychiatric Sciences, 34*, e4. https://doi.org/10.1017/S2045796024000866

Tranberg, K., Colnadar, B., Nielsen, M. H., Hjorthøj, C., & Møller, A. (2024). Interventions targeting patients with co-occurring severe mental illness and substance use (dual diagnosis) in general practice settings—A scoping review of the literature. *BMC Primary Care, 25*(1), 281. https://doi.org/10.1186/s12875-024-02504-3

Zuccarini, M. M., & Stiller, C. (2024). The effect of peer support on treatment engagement for opioid use disorder. *Journal of the American Psychiatric Nurses Association, 30*(3), 709–715. https://doi.org/10.1177/10783903221128062

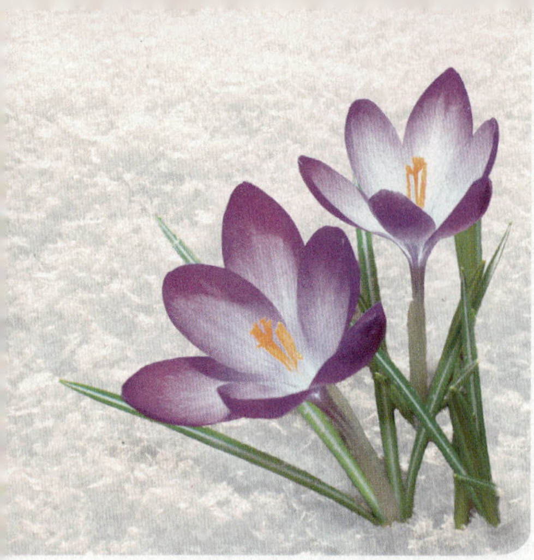

43 Care of People Who Are Medically Compromised*

Dorothy M. Corrigan

KEYCONCEPTS

- chronic medical illness
- comorbid condition
- implicit bias
- mortality gap
- multimorbid conditions
- secondary mental disorders

LEARNING OBJECTIVES

After studying this chapter, you will be able to:

1. Identify medically ill populations at risk for psychosocial issues.
2. Discuss the impact that both a mental disorder and a medical issue have on patients and their families.
3. Examine the relationship between social determinants of health and people who are medically compromised with mental health issues.
4. Discuss the multimodal approach to treatment of pain, especially for those experiencing chronic pain.
5. Using a clinical judgment model, formulate a nursing care plan for patients who are experiencing mental health issues associated with trauma or central nervous system (CNS) disorders.
6. Discuss the importance of integrating the medical aspects of care into psychiatric care for patients with mental health issues.

KEY TERMS

• acute pain • allodynia • Barthel index • Beck Depression Inventory • beta-endorphins • bidirectional illnesses • biopsychosocial–spiritual model of pain management • cancer • cardiovascular disease (CVD) • chronic pain • empathy gap • gate-control theory • Graded Chronic Pain Scale-Revised (GCPS-R) • health stereotyping • high-impact chronic pain (HICP) • hyperalgesia • hyperesthesia • hypothalamic–pituitary adrenal axis • ischemic cascade • Loeser model of pain • mechanism-based pain management • metabolic syndrome (MetS) • multimodal pain intervention • multimorbidity • nociceptive pain • nociceptors • pain behavior • pain chronification • pain resilience • pain vulnerability • Parkinson disease • persistent postconcussive syndrome (PPCS) • physiologic trauma • post stroke depression • prodrome • prostaglandins • psychological injury • sequela • social determinants of health • substance P • traumatic brain injury (TBI) • type 2 diabetes

INTRODUCTION

People with chronic mental disorders often have one comorbid condition that exists simultaneously with another disorder. In some cases, multimorbid conditions overlap each other and influence medical and psychiatric disease complexity and care.

KEYCONCEPTS A comorbid condition is the presence of one physical illness, injury, or disability that exists simultaneously with another disorder or illness. **Multimorbid conditions** exist when two or more disorders are present simultaneously.

It is estimated that one in four people with a severe mental disorder have physical **multimorbidity** (presence

**In this chapter, "male" refers to an individual assigned male at birth, and "female" refers to an individual assigned female at birth.*

of two or more long-term health conditions) (Halstead et al., 2024). When compared with the general population, people with serious mental disorders develop comorbid and multimorbid conditions at a much younger age. In addition, these conditions tend to cluster together, and males tend to have more multimorbidities (Launders, 2022).

Though medical and psychiatric disorders are often intertwined, mental health providers may not recognize a medical illness and medical providers may not screen and treat for mental health issues. Some medical providers believe that people with mental disorders are more dangerous than the general population and are then reluctant to treat them. Other providers may demonstrate implicit bias by attributing physical symptoms to the patient's mental disorder which can significantly compromise or endanger their health (Decker et al., 2022). Holistic and integrated approaches to care may not be a priority or even a possibility in some clinical settings.

KEYCONCEPT Implicit bias is the use of unconscious attitudes or stereotypes with respect to an individual or a group. These positive or negative attitudes can affect one's behaviors toward that individual or group. Health care may be compromised by implicit bias.

This chapter will discuss some common medical disorders that are experienced by people who also have mental disorders. It will also explore some mental disorders which are linked to primary medical illnesses. Three special populations will be also be presented: those with comorbid pain, those who have experienced physiologic trauma, and those with mental health issues related to CNS disorders.

Risk Factors Related to Comorbid Medical and Mental Disorders

Certain groups are at risk of developing comorbid medical and mental disorders. The following section discusses selected groups.

Sex Assigned at Birth Considerations

Although few discrete studies on sex assigned at birth exist on the relationship between mental disorders and multimorbid physical health issues, recent evidence suggests that a diagnosis of depression in females increases rates of CVD occurrence more than in males. Females who develop CVD also experience higher levels of depression than males after being diagnosed (Möller-Leimkühler, 2022). Females have a higher incidence of depressive symptoms after acute myocardial infarction (AMI) than do males who experience AMI (Liblik et al., 2022). Females with mental health issues are not adequately screened for cancer and other diseases, and they are more likely to begin initial treatment when the disease is already well advanced (O'Neill et al., 2023).

LGBTQ+ Considerations

LGBTQ+ individuals often experience social isolation, stigma, prejudice, and overt and covert discrimination. Mental health issues, expectations of rejection, feeling pressured to perform as a heterosexual/cisgender individual, internalized stigma, and compromised coping processes can contribute to gaps in health care (Alday-Mondaca & Lay-Lisboa, 2021). It is important that nurses are sensitive to the negative experiences common to LGBTQ+ individuals and use an empathic approach to patient care.

THE MORTALITY GAP AND SOCIAL DETERMINANTS OF HEALTH

Some medical illnesses experienced by individuals with mental disorders can result in death. Mental health issues and social determinants of health impact both morbidity and mortality.

The Mortality Gap

Although the principal causes of death (cancer and cardiovascular disease [CVD]) among the general population are the same as that of people with serious mental disorders, those with serious mental disorders die prematurely of these and other multimorbid disorders (Hancox et al., 2022). On average, in the United States, people with mental disorders may die 10 to 20 years earlier than those in the general population (Sud et al., 2021). With respect to COVID-19, for example, people with schizophrenia or bipolar disorder who were unvaccinated have a greater risk of mortality than the general unvaccinated population (Hassan et al., 2023). This chasm between the life expectancy of the general population and that of people with mental disorders has been referred to as the mental health mortality gap (Minhas et al., 2022; Ross et al., 2021; Solmi et al., 2021a; Sud et al., 2021b).

KEYCONCEPT The **mortality gap** is a widening of differences in life expectancy between two populations.

Impact of Social Determinants of Health on Medical Illnesses and Mental Disorders

Robust clinical research is ongoing as to why mental disorders remain an independent risk factor for many health issues, some of which will be noted throughout this chapter. However, **social determinants of health** such as poverty, lack of safe recreation space for exercise, food insecurity and limited access to full-service grocery stores, unemployment, undereducation, and housing insecurity also contribute to the presence of medical complexities as well as to the overall experience of decreased health and wellness among those with a mental disorder (Hancox et al., 2022).

Chronic stress from economic disadvantage, unstable neighborhoods, and other social factors has been shown to contribute to the destabilization of the neuroendocrine, immune, metabolic, and cardiovascular systems (Halling et al., 2022). In addition, some people may simply not have adequate access to health care, may not feel safe or respected at a health clinic, especially if they are LGBTQ+, or their clinic may not sufficiently integrate primary care with mental health care (Maria et al., 2024).

As a result, care for people who are medically compromised, especially care that exists in a complex medical–social–cultural–ecologic milieu, can become fragmented and difficult to negotiate. To avoid negative health outcomes, care for people who are medically compromised requires culturally sensitive engagement of patients and their families thorough screening and assessment, systematic monitoring, and comprehensive treatment planning among interdisciplinary team members.

COMMON COMORBID PHYSICAL ILLNESSES AMONG PEOPLE WITH MENTAL DISORDERS

CVD, metabolic syndrome (MetS), type 2 diabetes, chronic obstructive pulmonary disease (COPD), kidney disease, cancer, hepatitis B, hepatitis C, and human immunodeficiency virus (HIV) are among the many chronic illnesses that are more prevalent for people with serious mental disorders than for the rest of the population (Davies et al., 2021). This section will address MetS, CVD, cancer, and type 2 diabetes,

Metabolic Syndrome

Metabolic syndrome (MetS), also called cardiometabolic syndrome, is a combination of usually modifiable metabolic unexpected results which includes central obesity, elevated blood pressure (BP), elevated triglycerides (TGs), reduced high-density lipoprotein cholesterol (HDL-C), and elevated fasting plasma glucose (FPG). Any one of these unexpected results tends to introduce a disease cascade in which some or all of the other unexpected results subsequently occur.

People with psychotic disorders are especially vulnerable to the development MetS, and they seem to have a more severe disorder than does the general population (Perez et al., 2022). Females who have mental disorders and who are over 60 years of age appear to be the most vulnerable to the development of MetS (Tzeng et al., 2020). MetS has long been considered a major risk factor for both CVD and type 2 diabetes in all populations (Seyres et al., 2022).

NCLEXNOTE The metabolic unexpected results in MetS are modifiable. Weight loss, diet, increased physical activity, smoking cessation, and other lifestyle changes can reduce risks for CVD and type 2 diabetes while improving patient sense of well-being. It is important that the connection between risk of developing MetS and mental disorders be carefully explained and care plans to make needed lifestyle changes are reviewed with the patient.

Cardiovascular Disease

Cardiovascular disease (CVD) is a constellation of disorders that includes ischemic heart disease, coronary artery disease, stroke, heart failure, hypertension, hypertensive heart disease, congestive heart failure, and arrhythmias, to name a few. Among people with mental disorders, CVD is estimated to be two to three times higher than the general population and is the most common cause of death in people with severe mental disorders (Minhas et al., 2022). Disparity in both CVD screening and treatment has been shown to account for the severity and mortality of people with comorbid mental disorders and CVD (Solmi, 2021b). Although CVD has usually been linked to the use of antipsychotic medications and subsequent MetS development, new research has suggested that use of antipsychotic medication can *decrease* CVD-related mortality by 50%, especially for people with schizophrenia (Solmi et al., 2021b). Posttraumatic stress disorder (PTSD) has also been linked to the development of CVD as have MetS, autoimmune disorders, and gynecologic conditions such as endometriosis and polycystic ovary syndrome (Halling et al., 2022). Patients with traumatic brain syndrome (TBI) have increased risk of developing CVD and endocrine disorders (Izzy et al., 2022).

EMERGENCY CARE ALERT BPs equal to or higher than 180/120 may represent an urgent hypertensive crisis. Immediate medical advice should be sought by nurses if several subsequent BP readings remain this high during any patient encounter. When this reading is accompanied by anxiety, blurred vision, chest pain, confusion, nausea and vomiting, seizures, severe headache, fever, or shortness of breath emergent care is immediately required.

Cancer

Cancer is the second leading cause of mortality in all populations globally (Ahmad et al., 2023). However, mortality rates for people with mental disorders and cancer are significantly higher than the general population. The cancer mortality gap has been linked to failure by providers to screen people with mental disorders properly, thereby undermining the success of early detection for cure. For example, females who have mental disorders are screened for breast cancer at a rate of almost one third that of the general population (Ross et al., 2021). Nurses can be key partners in improving the screening process for various cancers and other disorders among those with mental disorders.

Type 2 Diabetes

Type 2 diabetes is an illness in which the beta cells in the pancreas fail to produce sufficient insulin to regulate the movement of glucose into cells. Cells then only partially respond to the decreased insulin when it does arrive, resulting in a buildup of glucose in the blood. Type 2 diabetes is often a **sequela** (related disorders or conditions that evolve directly from a preexisting illness or medical complication) of MetS. It occurs twice as often in people with mental disorders than in the general population, and such individuals are at a higher risk for complications (Busili et al., 2024).

Risk for type 2 diabetes among the general population typically escalates with age. However, younger people with mental disorders have been found to represent the highest number of people with type 2 diabetes (Lindekilde et al., 2022a). Among people with type 2 diabetes 40% have a sleep disorder, 21% have a binge-eating disorder, 16% have a substance use disorder, 16% have an anxiety disorder, 14% have a bipolar disorder, 11% have schizophrenia, 10% have mixed psychiatric disorders, 9% have depression, and 8% have an intellectual disability (Lindekilde et al., 2022b). Type 2 diabetes is among the most psychologically burdensome of chronic conditions for all populations, and proper daily self-management for people with mental disorders is crucial to prevent further mental and physical health deterioration (Busili et al., 2024).

CHRONIC MEDICAL ILLNESSES WITH SECONDARY MENTAL DISORDERS

A chronic medical illness is a stressful process that can alter an individual's perception of the physical, social, emotional, and spiritual self and increases the burden of suffering for patients and caregivers alike. Those with a chronic medical illness frequently fear a recurrence of their disease or an increase in the severity of symptoms (Türkel et al., 2025). During the COVID-19 pandemic, fear and anxiety about becoming ill were common features of daily life for many. However, those with chronic medical illnesses, who also had anxiety specifically about COVID-19, had increased risk of severe morbidity and mortality from their present chronic disorders *as well as* from COVID-19 (Alkouri et al., 2022).

> **KEYCONCEPT** A **chronic medical illness** is a health condition that lasts more than 1 year, requires ongoing medical care and treatment, and limits activities of daily living (ADLs; Centers for Disease Control and Prevention [CDC], 2022).

People with chronic medical illnesses are at risk for developing comorbid mental disorders such as anxiety disorders, substance use disorders, depressive episodes, and other mood disorders. Examples of chronic diseases that may increase an individual's risk for developing a mental disorder include autoimmune diseases (rheumatoid arthritis, inflammatory bowel disease, systematic lupus erythematosus), stroke, CVD, multiple sclerosis, COPD, cancer, diabetes, and HIV.

Mental health issues that newly accompany an acute or chronic medical condition are referred to as secondary mental disorders. Approximately 75% of patients in primary care settings will experience mental health issues related to their physical health (Schrager, 2021). Depression and anxiety often complicate the clinical picture in patients with hyperthyroidism and hypothyroidism, Cushing syndrome (hypercortisolism), and Addison disease (hypoadrenalism) (Yi Seah et al., 2024; Zhang et al., 2024). Malignancies have also been associated with anxiety and depression (Martinez-Calderon et al., 2024).

> **KEYCONCEPT Secondary mental disorders** are newly diagnosed mental issues that accompany an acute or chronic medical disorder or disability.

Depression

Depressed mood is a common affective prodrome of many medical disorders and its presence is associated with a higher risk of death (Herrera et al., 2021). A disease **prodrome** refers to the early signs and symptoms of an illness and typically occurs before major signs or symptoms of the illness emerge. Depression increases the risk for a cancer diagnosis (Mössinger & Kostev, 2023). Depressive symptoms are often prodromal to endocrine disorders, metabolic disturbances, malignancies, viral infections, inflammatory disorders, and cardiopulmonary conditions (Berk et al., 2023).

Chronic illness in adults, especially those with chronic pain, is a risk factor for depression and self-harm (Rogers et al., 2021). Children with a chronic illness are twice as likely to develop depression than their peers (Hards et al., 2023). Table 43.1 lists medical conditions associated with depression.

Psychosis

Psychosis can complicate a chronic medical illness by interfering with treatment and psychological well-being. Individuals with psychosis are more likely to be unable to follow treatment regimens. They may refuse to eat or take medication and may experience pronounced deterioration in their mental health and chronic health issues (Singh & Agustines, 2024). Delusions and hallucinations can lead to thoughts of self-harm. Patients with psychosis who are medically ill are at risk for suicide attempts (Chalker et al., 2024).

TABLE 43.1 MEDICAL ILLNESSES ASSOCIATED WITH SYMPTOMS OF DEPRESSION

Medical Illness	Symptoms of Depression
Endocrinopathies	Hypothyroidism and hyperthyroidism Hypoparathyroidism and hyperparathyroidism Cushing syndrome (steroid excess) Adrenal insufficiency (Addison disease) Hyperaldosteronism
Malignancies	Abdominal carcinomas—especially pancreatic Brain tumors (temporal lobe) Breast cancer Gastrointestinal cancer Lung cancer Prostate cancer Metastases
Neurologic disorders	Ischemic stroke Subarachnoid hemorrhage Parkinson disease Normal-pressure hydrocephalus Multiple sclerosis Closed head injury Epilepsy
Metabolic imbalance	Serum sodium and potassium reductions Vitamin B12, niacin, vitamin C deficiencies; irondeficiency (anemias) Metal intoxication (thallium and mercury) Uremia
Viral or bacterial infection	Infectious hepatitis Encephalitis Tuberculosis AIDS
Hormonal imbalance	Premenstrual, premenopausal, postpartum periods
Cardiopulmonary	Acute myocardial—infarction Postcardiac arrest Postcoronary artery bypass graft Post-heart transplantation Cardiomyopathy
Inflammatory disorders	Rheumatoid arthritis

Bidirectional Illnesses

CVD, type 2 diabetes, chronic pain, autoimmune disease, and irritable bowel syndrome (IBS), to name a few examples, are all independent risk factors for depression, and this relationship appears to be bidirectional. **Bidirectional illnesses** refer to a parallel biologic relationship between two separate disease processes, each of which is a risk factor for the other, such as heart disease influencing the development of depression and depression influencing the development of heart disease. Bidirectional illnesses evolve together and influence each other. Bidirectional markers involving existing depression and emerging CVD include alteration in platelet activity related to thrombus formation, increase in inflammatory cytokines, elevated cortisol, and heart rate variability. Some research has shown that people with major depression have a 56% higher risk of developing ischemic heart disease than the general population (Yu et al., 2022). This complex relationship between depression and CVD has been described in several studies (Zhang et al., 2022).

Psychosocial Aspects of Medical Illness

People typically respond to the loss of health with anxiety or depressed mood, particularly when the illness is debilitating, life threatening, and without a clear prognosis. People who have chronic illness are frequently distressed by loss of function and limitations imposed on their daily activities. The individual's usual social support systems may also be impacted as they withdraw from usual activities outside of the home as a consequence of functional loss or pain. Sometimes, relationships are also changed that can further affect healthy coping.

The Empathy Gap

There is a significant need for mental health care for LGBTQ+ individuals, who are 2.5 times more likely to experience depression than heterosexual people in the larger population (American Psychiatric Association [APA], 2025). Often, the hostility and implicit or overt bias from the local community are extended into the clinic or health care facility as well; LGBTQ+ individuals may be refused care or receive unequitable and/or lower-quality care (Sha & Aleshire, 2023).

One explanation for the hostility found in the health care community is the lack of empathy for LGBTQ+ individuals. An **empathy gap** (a tendency to underestimate the influence of an emotional state on decisions and behaviors and to overestimate intellectual decisions on decision-making) is a cognitive bias that makes it difficult to understand others (Mangione, 2024). The impact of this implicit bias with respect to care of LGBTQ+ individuals may be profound (Surace et al., 2024). Nurses and other health care providers can help bridge this gap by providing empathic, equitable, and informed care.

Health Stereotyping

One of the key issues encountered by LGBTQ+ people in health care settings is health stereotyping (Rice et al., 2021). **Health stereotyping** is a form of implicit bias in which a provider assumes that every member of a racial, ethnic, sexual/gender underrepresented group, or other demographic group will *always* present with illnesses, disorders, and disabilities that are common health issues in their specific population. An example of this would be a nurse assuming that a gay adult should be tested for HIV during the appointment even though he wants to discuss how his depressed mood has affected his diabetes

BOX 43.1

Reflection of a Nurse: LGBTQ+ Health Stereotypes

Incident

Karen—a married, 65-year-old lesbian patient with a history of hyperthyroidism, high BP, heart palpitations and generalized anxiety disorder—presents to her primary care clinic for a follow-up on side effects of her escitalopram PO 10 mg daily. The primary care nurse read somewhere that lesbians have a greater incidence of alcohol use disorder and wants to make sure that this topic is covered thoroughly in the appointment today. The nurse begins to ask intrusive questions about substance use. Karen quickly interrupts the nurse and states that she has never had any alcohol to drink whatsoever in her entire life, to the clear surprise of the nurse. The patient then says that she made the appointment to talk about how her anxiety medication is affecting her libido and her marriage, and she asks if there someone else she can talk to about this today.

Reflection

Upon reflection, the nurse realizes that though she was trying to be empathetic, her attempts at alliance with the patient were not successful.

1. What truth disputes the stereotype held by the nurse in this scenario?
2. What interventions would have been more effective to nurture a health care alliance with this patient?

Source: Kidd, J. D., Paschen-Wolff, M. M., Mercile, A. A., Caceres, B. A., Drabble, L. A., & Hughes, T. J. (2022). A scoping review of alcohol, tobacco, and other drug use treatment interventions for sexual and gender minority populations. *Journal of Substance Abuse Treatment*, *133*, 108539. https://doi.org/10.1016/j.jsat.2021.108539

self-care. Health stereotyping affects both assessment and treatment because pertinent health issues are ignored or missed and the patient's dignity, needs, and well-being are diminished (Saunders et al., 2024). See Box 43.1.

EVIDENCE-BASED NURSING CARE OF PEOPLE WITH CHRONIC MEDICAL ILLNESS AND SECONDARY MENTAL DISORDERS

Ideally, an interdisciplinary team of care providers that includes medical and mental health providers and nurses should work closely together to deliver optimal treatment of complex medical and mental disorders. In reality, the nurse on the medical team usually provides the mental health nursing care. The following discussion focuses on the mental health nursing care provided within a primary medical setting.

Recognizing Cues: Relevant Assessment Information

Mental health assessment should be part of every patient visit regardless of current health status. The mental status assessment (see Chapter 10) can be helpful to determine baseline functioning. Documenting mental health status at each appointment helps establish a baseline and provides for early intervention when there are changes.

For patients who have risk factors such as family history of mental health disorders, new psychosocial stressors, current primary mental disorders, or who have chronic medical illnesses, especially chronic pain, CVD, and diabetes, a thorough assessment at each visit should always be a priority so that issues can be identified and treated as early as possible. If possible, family and/or caregivers should be engaged as well so that clinical staff can monitor for changes in family dynamics or other new psychosocial issues that could impact the patient's progress and recovery.

It is important to discern the difference between a patient who has the capacity to exercise the right to refuse lifesaving treatment and a patient who is medically ill, has depression and delusions, and is expressing hopelessness and a desire to die. A clinical evaluation of the effect of depression on patients' capacity to make competent decisions regarding their care is imperative. Ethics consultations are often utilized to clarify the ethical issues and to provide a forum to discuss possible patient care interventions, including hospice. Patients with primary mental disorders and comorbid chronic medical illness may pose similar challenges when their medical condition deteriorates while admitted to a hospital. The use of advanced directives helps to address these complex and sensitive issues.

Analyzing Cues and Developing Hypotheses

The main challenge is to determine which signs and symptoms are part of a medical illness and its treatment and which symptoms signify the presence of a new or worsening mental health disorder. Factors to be considered in assessing mental health issues in patients with medical illnesses are outlined in Box 43.2. Sometimes, the presenting symptoms are a mix of a mental disorder(s) and chronic medical illness.

Some chronic medical illnesses have similar symptoms to mental disorders, such as decreased appetite, sleep

BOX 43.2

Factors to Consider in Assessing Mental Health Issues in Patients With Medical Illness

- One or more specific medical illnesses
- Past psychiatric history of the patient (before the medical illness)
- Family history of mental health issues
- Current mood, sense of hopelessness, suicidal ideation excessive worry, anxiety
- Current mental health issues, treatment, response to treatment
- Change in sleep or eating (not related to medical illness)
- Patient's sex assigned at birth
- LGBTQ+ status

disturbances, and loss of energy. However, when coupled with feelings of failure, low self-esteem, difficulty concentrating, feelings of hopelessness, and/or feelings of being punished, a mental health issue such should be considered. Side effects of medications for chronic medical illness may be causing the mood disturbance and should also be evaluated. Finally, it is important to recall that changes in mood may signal the beginning of another medical illness for the patient.

Planning Recovery and Wellness Outcomes: Generating Solutions

Current psychosocial stressors and patient coping mechanisms should be monitored and taken into consideration in developing all plans of care. Mutually agreed-upon goals and therapy should actively involve the patient. Ideally, planning should also include input of caregivers and family members whenever possible. Outcomes should be appropriate for the medical and mental disorder.

Therapeutic Relationship

Since the mental health care for people with medical illnesses typically occurs within the medical or primary care setting, the patient may be hesitant to discuss mental health issues with a nonmental health provider or nurse. It is important to spend time establishing rapport and trust with the patient as the mental health care is usually considered secondary concern to the medical disorder.

Taking Action: Nursing Interventions

Undiagnosed and untreated mental disorders in people who are medically ill are potentially life threatening because stable moods and adequate cognitive functioning are essential to adherence with the interdisciplinary treatment plan and recovery (Schenk et al., 2024). In addition, the underuse or overuse of analgesics and reluctance to perform self-care and rehabilitative activities hinder recovery and expose the individual to other potential complications (Golden et al., 2024). Subsequently, the diagnosis, treatment, and follow-up of comorbid mental disorders in patients with medical illnesses are crucial.

Medication

Medications for patients with comorbid or multimorbid disorders are usually prescribed at the minimal dose initially, with the dose advanced slowly; frequent blood-level monitoring is performed, if appropriate. The individual's weight should be carefully monitored at each appointment. Because of pathophysiologic changes associated with the medical illness and likely subsequent changes in pharmacokinetics of medications, doses required to achieve therapeutic blood levels may be less than the usual therapeutic dose and may take longer to titrate.

Medications used to treat medical disorders are known to be associated with agitation, anxiety, and depressed mood as side effects. See Table 43.2. When a drug is suspected of causing mood or mental status changes, it will most likely be withdrawn and an adequate alternative tried. When this is not possible, the dosage will be decreased to an effective level at which mood symptoms resolve.

Antidepressants, SSRIs (selective serotonin reuptake inhibitors) and SNRIs (serotonin–norepinephrine reuptake inhibitors) are frequently used in the treatment of depression and anxiety in patients with chronic medical illness. Both potential interactions and side effects of all medications should be monitored.

Psychosocial Interventions

Cognitive and behavioral strategies including individual therapy, group therapy, and family therapy are often implemented. Assisting the patient and family to understand the nature and relationship of the medical and psychiatric diagnoses may strengthen the support system, alter the perception of caregiver burden, and identify appropriate coping strategies. Cognitive intervention should address the areas of the patient's life that can be controlled, despite major lifestyle changes, so that feelings of competence and self-efficacy can be reinforced.

At some point, psychodynamic conflicts and maladaptive coping strategies may need to be explored. A referral to clergy or other spiritual support individual may also be of value for some patients and their family. In summary, secondary mental disorders can be approached using many of the same strategies that are effective for primary mental health disorders.

PAIN WITH MENTAL HEALTH DISORDERS

Pain is one of the most powerful and complex of human experiences and can affect all levels of an individual's biopsychosocial–spiritual functioning. Pain can negatively impact the mental health and well-being of anyone and can exacerbate existing medical conditions. It is one of the most common reasons adults seek medical care (Bifulco et al., 2021).

People with mental disorders can experience pain as a result of their medical condition and, in some cases, as a consequence of their mental disorder or related treatment. Pain is a frequent comorbidity in people diagnosed with PTSD, depressive disorders, anxiety disorders, alcohol use disorder, opioid use disorder, bipolar disorder, Alzheimer disease and related dementias, and sleep disorders (Bhatt et al., 2024; De Aquino et al., 2024; Rikard et al., 2023). Chronic pain in children is associated with a 1.34 times higher risk for the development of major depression later in life (Bergmans & Smith, 2022). The presence of pain is a prominent risk factor for self-harm (Balit et al., 2024).

TABLE 43.2 MEDICATIONS ASSOCIATED WITH SYMPTOMS OF MENTAL DISORDERS IN PATIENTS WITH MEDICAL ILLNESS

Drug Class	Medication
Analgesics and NSAIDs	Ibuprofen Indomethacin Opiates Pentazocine Phenacetin Phenylbutazone
Antihypertensives	Clonidine Hydralazine Methyldopa Propranolol Reserpine
Antimicrobials	Ampicillin (gram-negative agents) Clotrimazole Cycloserine Griseofulvin Metronidazole Nitrofurantoin Streptomycin Sulfamethoxazole (sulfonamides)
Neurologic agents	L-Dopa Levodopa
Antiparkinsonism drugs	Amantadine
Anticonvulsants	Carbamazepine Phenytoin
Antispasmodics	Baclofen Bromocriptine
Cardiac drugs	Digitalis Guanethidine Lidocaine Oxprenolol Procainamide
Psychotropic drugs	Benzodiazepines
Stimulants and sedatives	Amphetamines Barbiturates Chloral hydrate Chlorazepate Diethylpropion Ethanol Fenfluramine Haloperidol
Steroids and hormones	Adrenocorticotropic hormone Corticosteroids Estrogen Oral contraceptives Prednisone Progesterone Triamcinolone
Antineoplastic drugs	Bleomycin C-Asparaginase Trimethoprim Vincristine
Other miscellaneous drugs	Anticholinesterases Cimetidine Diuretics Metoclopramide

A comprehensive review of pain neuroscience and pain management is beyond the scope of this chapter. However, this section will briefly explore important areas of pain etiology, classification, assessment, and management that are essential for effective nursing care of people with mental health disorders.

Types of Pain

Knowledge of pain types is useful to determine prevention, assessment, treatment, and follow-up care. Pain is usually defined by how long the individual has been experiencing it. **Acute pain** is described as pain that lasts between 3 and 6 months, and **chronic pain** lasts over 6 months. **High-impact chronic pain (HICP)** refers to chronic pain that severely limits physical functioning and quality of life (QoL).

The *American Nurses Association* (ANA) and *the American Society for Pain Management Nursing* (ASPMN) encourage nursing professionals to reconceptualize pain type along four main classifications of pain: (1) *temporal pattern*—acute, chronic, and episodic; (2) *etiology*—cancer, postoperative, etc.; (3) *tissue injury*—nociceptive and neuropathic; and (4) *mixed*—different pain types and/or the simultaneous presence of both acute and chronic pain (ANA & ASPMN, 2016). See Box 43.3.

BOX 43.3

Classification of Pain

Acute pain: Lasts 3 to 6 months and has an identifiable cause, e.g., surgery, injury. Described by patients as sharp, throbbing, aching. Resolves when tissues heal and function returns.

Chronic or persistent pain: Occurs longer than 6 months or beyond usual healing time and may not have an identifiable cause. Alternation in the dorsal horn of the spinal cord and neuroplastic changes in the brain are thought to be the possible causes. Often associated with mental health comorbidities.

Nociceptive pain: Pain that elicits the typical response from the nociceptive pathway and is an expected response to noxious stimuli from tissue injury.

Neuropathic pain: In contrast to nociceptive pain, neuropathic pain originates in a primary lesion of the peripheral or CNS. Described by patients as tingling, burning, numbness, and/or shooting. Allodynia may also be described.

Cancer-related pain: Can be acute, chronic, or recurrent and is a caused by tumor or metastases, or cancer therapies such as chemotherapy and/or radiation. Often accompanied by malaise, fever, insomnia, and nausea.

Breakthrough pain: Pain that occurs over baseline pain in a more intense level.

Procedural pain: Pain associated with any medical intervention.

Adapted from American Nurses Association (ANA) and American Society for Pain Management Nursing (ASPMN). (2016). *Pain management nursing scope and standards* (2nd ed.). American Nurses Association.

Pain Vulnerability and Pain Resilience

Recent advances in neuroscience are decoding why the experience of pain is so individualized. One explanation is that early pain exposure in some neonates alters and then "primes" pain pathways in the brain. It is theorized that for some people these changes lead to later **pain vulnerability**, a hypersensitivity to nociceptive trauma (Denk et al., 2014). Ongoing research continues to examine this explanation (Selvanathan et al., 2024).

Genetics may also play a significant role in mediating the experience of pain. Some people may produce more or different **beta-endorphins** (neurotransmitters that exhibit opioid-like behavior). When activated, they diminish pain perception (Bonifácio de Assis et al., 2021). In doing so they may also improve **pain resilience**, which can be thought of as a diminished susceptibility to suffering from pain over time (Chen & Nakagawa, 2023). Many other genetic possibilities for pain vulnerability are being explored. Pain vulnerability and pain resilience can be conceptualized by nurses as a continuum in which patients may be in different pain toleration "locations" over time.

Epidemiology and Risk Factors

Age, ethnicity, marital status, military veteran status, sex assigned at birth, immune responsivity, socioeconomic status, comorbid medical and mental diagnoses, past psychological or physical trauma, and stress are also factors that contribute to pain vulnerability and pain resilience (Pak et al., 2024; Wilson et al., 2024). Military veterans who have been diagnosed with PTSD and comorbid pain experience worse pain than veterans who have chronic pain but not PTSD (Bair et al., 2020). Almost 54% of people with comorbid mental disorders who are unhoused have chronic pain (Vogel et al., 2021).

In the United States in 2021, 51.6 million adults experienced chronic pain, with 17.1 million adults over the age of 65 years accounting for most of the HICP (Rikard et al., 2023). Chronic pain is reported in 20% to 80% of patients who have experienced trauma (Gasperi et al., 2021).

Older adults who have experienced the biologic changes of aging such as systematic inflammation, altered autonomic function, and changes in neuronal structure suffer chronic pain, and they are routinely undertreated for this type of pain (Singh et al., 2023). Exposure to trauma with subsequent PTSD is linked to persistent pain in older adults (Maccarrone et al., 2021). Adults identifying as bisexual, non-Hispanic American Indian and Alaska Native adults, and adults who are divorced and separated experience a higher prevalence of both chronic pain and HICP than the general population (Rikard et al., 2023). For children in the United States, chronic pain has been reported to be as high as one in five children and adolescents (Chambers et al., 2024).

Many factors must be considered when caring for people in pain. The presence of mental health issues can certainly complicate pain management. Knowledge of the various biopsychosocial–spiritual risk factors and attentiveness to the uniqueness of each individual will ensure adequate pain assessment and appropriate pain interventions. Pain is a serious public health issue that contributes to high health care costs, lower worker productivity, and increased disability.

Biologic Explanations of Pain

Pain can be approached from several different perspectives. This section focuses on the common biologic explanations of pain.

Gate-Control Theory

Although current research has further refined the more than half-century-old pain model, gate-control theory continues to offer an adequate general framework for understanding the pain response, especially **nociceptive pain**, a protective response to noxious stimuli that serves as a warning of tissue injury, inflammation, and pathologic processes that lowers the threshold of sensitization. **Gate-control theory** postulates that there is not a single-pain mechanism but that the processing of pain occurs on at least three levels—peripheral, spinal, and supraspinal.

Gate-control theory holds that there are neurologic gates that can either inhibit or allow pain signals to be transmitted to the brain. At the site of the tissue injury, pain receptors **(nociceptors)** cause the release of **prostaglandins** (an unsaturated fatty acid that helps control smooth muscle contraction, BP, inflammation, and body temperature) and **substance P** (a peptide found in body tissues, especially nervous tissue, which is involved in the transmission of pain and in inflammation). Potassium, histamine, leukotrienes (short-range chemical messengers that help regulate the state of blood vessels and airways and influence the activities of some white blood cells), and bradykinin (chemical that dilates blood vessels) are also released. These substances function as transmitters of a relay signal sent to the dorsal horn of the spinal cord that in turn increases the flow of impulses relayed to the brain. See Box 43.4. The excitability of this pathway can be altered by inhibitory interneurons at the site of the dorsal horn, closing the gate and lesser or no pain may be experienced. If the cytokines or projection neurons are released, they sensitize and stimulate central pain receptors to spread the pain experience and activate areas of the brain responsible for memory, emotion, and personality. As these ascending pathways signal higher centers, descending noradrenergic and serotonergic pathways are activated and inhibit the release of substance P, which closes the gate and thereby reduces the pain

BOX 43.4

Neurotransmitters Active in Pain Sensation and Induced Plasticity

C-FIBER NEUROPEPTIDES (CYTOKINES) RELEASED BY PERIPHERAL NOXIOUS STIMULATION

- Bradykinin
- Calcitonin gene–related peptide (CGRP)
- Cholecystokinin
- Histamine
- Prostaglandins
- Somatostatin
- Substance P
- Vasoactive intestinal polypeptide (VIP)

EXCITATORY AMINO ACIDS WITH WIDESPREAD ACTIVITY IN THE CENTRAL NERVOUS SYSTEM (THALAMUS AND SOMATOSENSORY CORTICES)

- L-glutamate
- *N*-methyl-D-aspartate (NMDA)

NEUROTRANSMITTERS ACTIVE AS PAIN MODULATORS

- Endorphins
- Serotonin

Pain Chronification

For some people who have sustained an injury or trauma, the accompanying acute pain will resolve as the injury heals. For other people, acute pain does not resolve when the injury heals and instead acute pain transitions into chronic pain. This transition process is known as **pain chronification** and represents potentially permanent changes and modifications throughout the pain pathways and within the brain itself.

In pain chronification, neurobiologic alterations in dendrites, opioidergic and dopaminergic receptors, and cytokine production occur. These changes do not occur with acute pain (Kiriţoshi et al., 2024). People suffering from chronic pain report **hyperalgesia** (increased sensation of pain), **allodynia** (pain unrelated to noxious stimuli, lowered pain threshold), and/or **hyperesthesia** (increased nociceptor sensitivity). As with pain in general, vulnerability to the transition from acute pain to chronic pain is driven by a variety biopsychosocial and spiritual risk factors that are unique to the individual. Pain medication itself, including opioids, nonsteroidal antiinflammatory drugs (NSAIDs), and triptans, has also been linked to pain chronification in some people (Echeverria-Villalobos et al., 2023; Manhapra, 2022).

Psychosocial Aspects of Chronic Pain

The impact of chronic pain on QoL can be devastating. When pain persists for an extended period, mood, coping skills, interpersonal relations, and financial and social resources are affected. Pain becomes a preoccupying daily burden. Demoralization, sadness, isolation, loss of interest in life, feelings of worthlessness, self-reproach, excessive guilt, indecisiveness, and thoughts of self-harm are often associated with chronic pain. See Box 43.5.

Physiologic pain is uniquely personal. It involves a series of complex, neuropsychological events that culminate in a highly subjective and deeply individualized experience of discomfort and distress that can be modulated by a variety of factors, including various affective states and mental disorders. For some people with pain and mental disorders, pain perception unexpected results may occur, especially for those with schizophrenia and major depression (Kim et al., 2022).

This section discusses two biopsychosocial models that can be used as frameworks for understanding the pain experience.

BOX 43.5

Research for Evidence-Based Practice: Addressing Disparities in Pain Care in the LGBTQ+ Population

Zajacova, A., Grol-Prokopczyk, Liu, H., & Nahin, R. (2023). Chronic pain among U.S. sexual minority adults who identify as gay, lesbian, bisexual, or "something else." Pain, *164(9), 1942–1953. https://doi.org/10.1097/j.pain0000000000002891*

THE QUESTION: Do health care disparities exist between the LGBTQ+ population and the general population with respect to pain assessment and management?

METHODS: A quantitative design using Poisson regression and nonlinear covariates for analysis based on data from the National Health Interview Survey, 2013 to 2018, a leading cross sectional health survey of the United States was used. Chronic pain and pain from three or more body sites were the focus of the data analysis. Covariates: demographic, socioeconomic, health care, and psychological distress measures. Cohort age: 18 to 64 years old.

FINDINGS: The age-adjusted prevalence of both chronic pain and pain in three or more body sites was twice as high in adults who self-identified as bisexual or "something else" and 50% higher among gay males and lesbians when compared with the general population. Psychological distress was the most salient correlate of the disparities. The study's authors called for more research on distressing social factors of LGBTQ+ people's experiences, including discrimination, prejudice, and stigma as potential key upstream factors that drive pain disparities in the LGBTQ+ population.

IMPLICATIONS FOR NURSING: Significant health disparities appear to exist with respect to pain in LGBTQ+ individuals. Informed empathy by nurses regarding the unique kind of social challenges LGBTQ+ people experience can promote trusting health care alliances that empower good screening and assessment, especially for pain.

Biopsychosocial–Spiritual Model

A **biopsychosocial–spiritual model of pain management** for substance use, introduced to nursing in 2014, is organized according to intrinsic (spiritual, individual, and mental health) factors and extrinsic factors (previous pain experience, social and financial stressors, role modeling, encouragement, and social support) (Matteliano et al., 2014). In this model the experience of pain occurs within each individual's biopsychosocial–spiritual ecology where a unique, personal meaning to pain is created. The model proposes that prescription of an opioid for persistent pain in an individual who uses substances and has a mental disorder such as depression increases the risk of misuse. This model is used today as a framework for understanding the pain experience and implementing nonpharmacologic interventions for pain management (Umberger & Wilson, 2024). Nursing education programs incorporate components of this model in their comprehensive nursing education (International Association for the Study of Pain, 2021).

Loeser Model of Pain

The **Loeser model of pain** acknowledges the biopsychosocial experience of pain but importantly identifies pain behavior as the end outcome of the pain experience (Loeser & Ford, 1983). **Pain behavior** may be thought of as the actions and reactions an individual has in response to pain, including their behaviors with respect to anticipated pain. Given the Loeser model, it is easy to see how comorbid pain complicates care of all patients and especially those with mental health diagnoses. Behaviors such as anger, agitation, isolation, insomnia, change in appetite, lack of focus, and/or depressed mood may represent pain, a change in mental health status, or a combination of both and always require careful nursing assessment. The Loeser model of pain continues to be relevant in 2025 and is used as a model for understanding chronic pain (Volinn & Loeser, 2022).

EVIDENCE-BASED NURSING CARE OF PEOPLE WITH PAIN AND MENTAL DISORDERS

The treatment of pain, especially chronic pain, is complex and is always interdisciplinary. It requires careful assessment of the patient's pain and the systematic analysis of the likely mechanisms that are responsible for the experience of pain.

Recognizing Cues: Relevant Assessment Information

Appropriate diagnosis and treatment of pain begin with a comprehensive biopsychosocial–spiritual history as well as a physical examination. A functional assessment that investigates how the patient's pain affects their daily living should also be completed. Attentiveness to any recent falls due to pain, difficulty completing ADLs and instrumental activities of daily living (IADLs), and other diminishments of QoL is important. When discussing pain, a patient should be asked to describe the pain characteristics, including location and severity, and information about possible factors that may be influencing or producing pain. Patients should also be encouraged to express their feelings, beliefs, and values around pain and suffering. If the patient is a child, parents/caregivers should also be included in the discussion.

A direct relationship between the severity or extent of detectable disease and the intensity of the patient's pain may not be evident during the first interaction between nurse and patient. Pain assessment instruments can aid in evaluation. However, using an instrument designed to measure acute pain, such as asking the patient to rate pain on a scale of 1 to 10, is inadequate for assessing chronic pain because the pain may always be a 3 or 4, but the chronic nature of the pain is the issue (Robinson et al., 2024). The **Graded Chronic Pain Scale-Revised (GCPS-R)** may be a helpful tool to assess chronic pain (Von Korff et al., 2020).

All pain occurs in a time frame, so alertness as to whether pain episodically waxes and wanes, is worse at night, or improves with sleep, to name a few factors, is important. Among patients who are critically ill in an inpatient setting, failure to assess pain expeditiously and correctly can result in a variety of complications, including hyperglycemia and increased risk of infection, which among complications may unnecessarily lengthen a hospital stay. Attentiveness to the patient's pain, pain behaviors, levels of pain vulnerability and pain resilience, and acute and chronic medical and psychiatric comorbidities is crucial. Objective data and the patient's own subjective experience of pain must be carefully analyzed so that comprehensive pain management can occur. See Box 43.6.

Planning Recovery and Wellness Outcomes

Pain syndromes, especially chronic pain, are quite common in the primary care setting. See Box 43.7. The overall goal is to decrease or eliminate the pain. The nurse can help the patient identify circumstances when the pain was diminished and use this information to adjust existing strategies or develop new ones. Encouraging the patient to engage in all elements of the pain management plan is key. If the patient is taking medications, the nurse should closely monitor therapeutic and untoward effects. Education with the patient and family about approaches to pain mitigation and the patient's particular pain care helps to build positive outcomes.

BOX 43.6

Assessing Patients Who Report Pain

QUESTIONS TO ASSESS PAIN

The following questions can guide the nurse in reflecting on the significance of the chronic pain to the individual and family:

- What is the extent of the patient's disease or injury (physical impairment)?
- What is the magnitude of the illness? That is, to what extent is the patient suffering, experiencing disability, and unable to enjoy usual activities?
- Does the individual's behavior seem appropriate to the disease or injury, or is there evidence of amplification of symptoms for psychological or social reasons or purposes?
- How often and for how long does the patient perform specific behaviors, such as reclining, sitting, standing, and walking?
- How often does the patient seek health care and take analgesic medication (frequency and quantity)?

PAIN BEHAVIOR CHECKLIST

Pain behaviors have been characterized as interpersonal communications of pain, distress, or suffering. Pain behavior may be a more accurate indication of intensity and tolerance than verbal reports. Check the box of each behavior you observe or infer from the patient's comments.

- ☐ Facial grimacing, clenched teeth
- ☐ Holding or supporting of affected body area
- ☐ Asking questions such as, "Why did this happen to me?"
- ☐ Distorted gait, limping
- ☐ Frequent shifting of posture or position
- ☐ Requests to be excused from tasks or activities, avoidance of physical activity
- ☐ Taking medication as often as possible
- ☐ Moving extremely slowly
- ☐ Sitting with a rigid posture
- ☐ Moving in a guarded or protective fashion
- ☐ Moaning or sighing
- ☐ Using a cane, cervical collar, or other prosthetic device
- ☐ Requesting help in ambulation; frequent stopping while walking
- ☐ Lying down during the day
- ☐ Irritability

BOX 43.7

Pain Syndromes Seen in the Primary Care Setting

Cancer pain: Pain from malignant tumors that is caused by local infiltration or metastatic spread involving specific organs, bones, peripheral or cranial nerves, or the spinal cord. Pain therapy is aimed at providing sufficient relief to allow maximum possible daily functioning and a relatively pain-free death.

Chronic benign orofacial pain: Temporomandibular joint pain, trigeminal neuralgia.

Low back pain: Pain arising from the vertebral column or surrounding muscles, tendons, ligaments, or fascia. Causes range from simple muscle strain to arthritis, fracture, or nerve compression from a ruptured disk.

Migraine headache: A cerebrovasomotor disorder in which a focal reduction of cerebral blood flow initiates an ischemic headache. It may be preceded by a visual aura and followed by nausea, vomiting, and incapacitating head pain.

Myofascial pain: Pain in palpable bands (trigger points) of muscle; associated with stiffness, limitation of motion, and weakness

Neuropathic pain

- *Diabetic neuropathy:* neuropathy caused by diabetes mellitus; marked by diminished sensation secondary to vascular changes
- *Herpetic neuralgia:* pain associated with the dermatomal rash of acute herpes zoster
- *Inflammatory neuropathy:* neuropathy related to the presence of chemical or micro-organic pathogens
- *Peripheral or central neuralgia:* abrupt, intense, paroxysmal pain caused by intrinsic nerve injury or extrinsic nerve compression
- *Plexopathy:* neuropathy involving a peripheral nerve plexus
- *Polyneuropathy:* neuropathy involving multiple peripheral nerves
- *Radiculopathy:* pain radiating along a peripheral nerve tract, such as sciatica
- *Traumatic neuropathy:* neuropathy caused by avulsion or compression

Reflex sympathetic dystrophy: A painful burning syndrome that occurs after peripheral nerve injury. Associated with hyperesthesia, vasomotor disturbances, and dystrophic changes caused by sympathetic hyperactivity.

Rheumatoid arthritis: More than 100 different types of joint disease produce inflammation of the joints. Associated with varying degrees of pain and stiffness and eventual loss of use of the affected joints.

Vaso-occlusive pain: Thrombotic crisis of sickle cell anemia in joints and peripheral muscles that is caused by ischemia.

Therapeutic Relationship

The nurse–patient relationship is primary for healing, and nurses have an important role in helping the patient manage pain. The nurse's therapeutic use of self can help instill hope and improve the patient's self-efficacy and pain resilience. Listening and acknowledging the pain is important because others may ignore or invalidate the impact of the pain.

Taking Action: Nursing Interventions

The continuing opioid epidemic in the United States and elsewhere has initiated a long overdue scrutiny of the ways in which we conceptualize, assess, and manage pain. In this new era of pain management, the use of opioids alone, for example, is no longer considered the only first-line therapy for pain management, though there are exceptions especially for cancer patients (Meilhac et al., 2024; Paice et al., 2023). Innovative, person-centered approaches to pain have now become clinical necessities.

Multimodal Pain Management

One promising approach is **mechanism-based pain management**, which attempts to target the many unique pain-producing mechanisms along the subcellular and molecular pain pathways (Chen et al., 2024). Mechanism-based pain management uses simultaneous, multimodal interventions to elicit pain mitigation and relief. **Multimodal pain interventions** attempt to modulate the transduction, conduction, transmission, perception of and adaptation to pain (da Nobrega et al., 2023). Once the mechanisms of pain are identified or suspected within the pain pathway, lower-dose traditional analgesia may be used with lower-dose nontraditional analgesia along with nonpharmacologic/complementary interventions. See Figure 43.1.

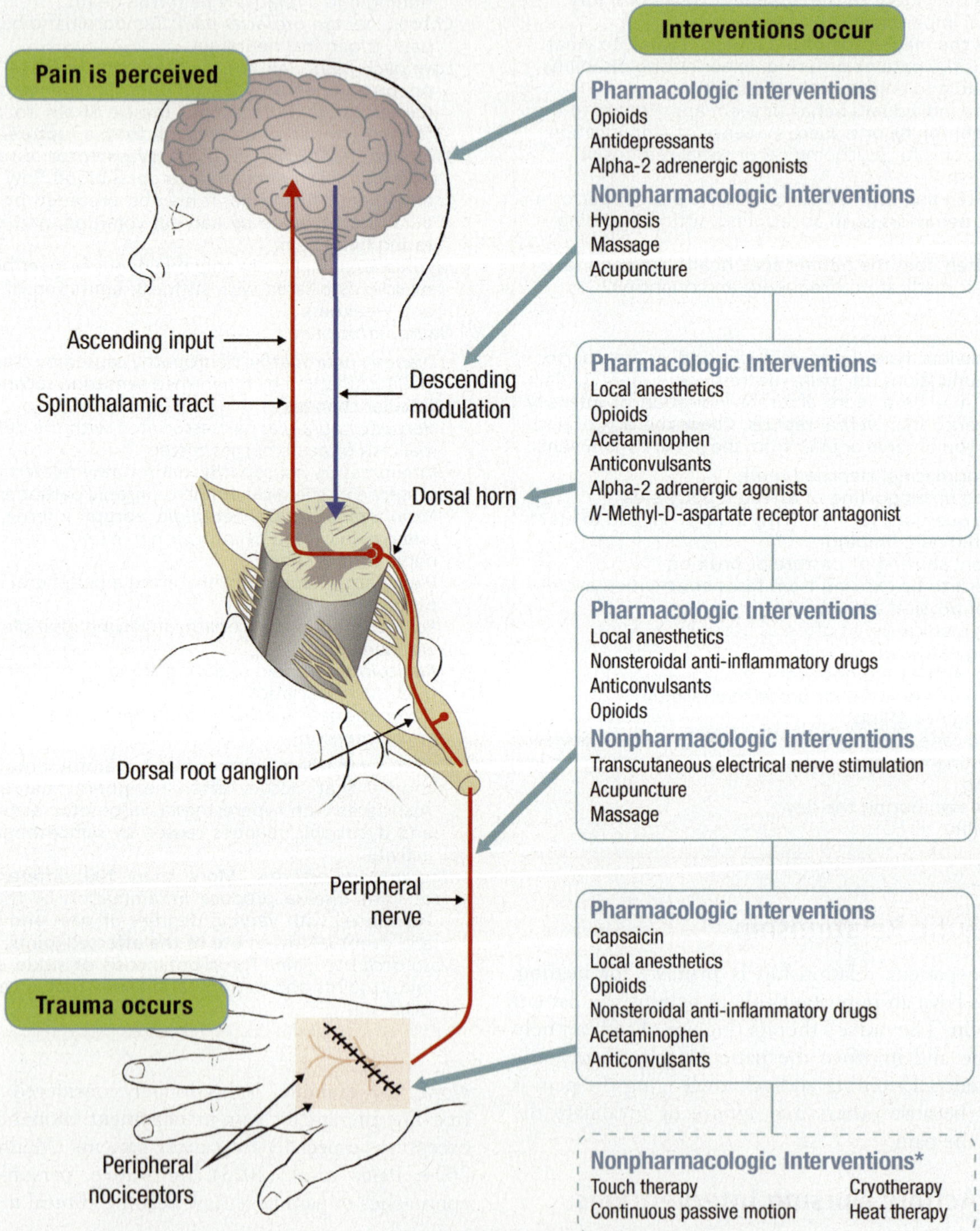

FIGURE 43.1 Mechanism-based pain: A multimodal approach identification of the pain pathway can guide selection of intervention. (Reprinted with permission from Manworren R. C. [2015]. Multimodal pain management and the future of a personalized medicine approach to pain. *AORN Journal, 101*(3), 308–318. https://doi.org/10.1016/j.aorn.2014.12.009)

Combinations of traditional analgesics such as local anesthetic agents to block nerve conduction, acetaminophen to inhibit prostaglandin synthesis, NSAIDs to block peripheral and central cyclooxygenase, and/or opioids that can address multiple sites of pain action may be used in combination with choices of nontraditional analgesics including anticonvulsants to inhibit neuronal firing, NMDA-receptor antagonists like ketamine to inhibit glutamate activation, antidepressants to activate ascending pain pathways, and alpha-2 adrenergic agonists like clonidine to inhibit substance P. Combinations of nonpharmacologic interventions such as transcutaneous electrical nerve stimulation, cognitive–behavioral therapies (CBTs), massage therapy, music therapy, and acupuncture, among many complementary options, complete the multimodal approach.

It is important to point out that in the mechanism-based pain management the many types of legitimate complementary treatments are no longer considered "alternative" or "adjunct." Instead, they are viewed as essential modalities of care to be integrated into the entire pain management plan. Emerging research has also demonstrated the importance of spiritual interventions for pain relief in patients for whom spirituality can helpful (Peng-Keller et al., 2021). Ritual, prayer, individual and group spiritual direction, and other interventions can be included as part of a care plan for some patients. See Box 43.8.

Interventions for People With Pain and Comorbid Substance Use Disorder

Patients diagnosed with acute or chronic pain who have comorbid alcohol or substance use disorders or a history of these disorders can present more complex treatment issues. Social stigma associated with various substance use disorders may prevent such patients from receiving timely and adequate pain management. However, having a current or past substance use disorder does not preclude patients from receiving adequate pain relief including the use of opioids, if necessary, as part of a mechanism-based, multimodal pain management plan.

Nurses are morally obligated to advocate for these patients so that adequate pain relief can occur. However, nurses must also be alert to the legitimate concerns of those same patients who may fear an exacerbation or relapse of substance use disorders. Patient preference regarding pain management options must always be taken into consideration. Multimodal pain management strategies are especially indispensable for these patients. Nurses are also ethically responsible for addressing behaviors with the patient that are not part of the pain management plan. Such behaviors may include lost prescriptions, asking for early refills of pain medications, and/or taking more medications than what was prescribed. When these behaviors occur, involvement of the interdisciplinary care team by the nurse is crucial to assure proper pain management as well as potential referrals for substance misuse assessment and treatment.

Wellness Challenges

There are many challenges to effective pain management. See Box 43.9. Providers may fail to acknowledge or accurately assess pain or may be fearful of providing enough pain relief, especially with pain medications. Patients may experience reluctance to acknowledge the pain and to communicate their distress or discomfort. Maladaptive coping by patients with respect to pain can lead to a fear of pain or a catastrophizing about how intense the pain will become or how long it will last. This can generate hopelessness, despair, and thoughts of self-harm for some. Improper pain management may also contribute to pain chronification.

Nonadherence with sequential prescription changes and combined treatments can be problematic as well. Strategies to assess adherence include awareness of the patient's pain mosaic and monitoring for new changes in it such as recent loss of housing, loss of employment, family stress, and new medical diagnoses, to name a few areas. Encouragement of regular self-report by the patient, biochemical assays that check for the presence of medications, and regular outcome assessments can also promote adherence to the treatment plan.

MENTAL HEALTH DISORDERS RELATED TO PHYSIOLOGIC TRAUMA

Physiologic trauma can be thought of as sudden onset, severe injury caused by blunt, penetrating, and/or burn mechanisms. Physiologic trauma activates the overall stress response of the autonomic nervous system. Massive catecholamine release causes certain cardiovascular, muscular, gastrointestinal, and respiratory symptoms that release energy stores and support survival. Tissue destruction, musculoskeletal pain, physical disability, and body image changes all contribute to the physiologic and psychological stress response, which continues long after the traumatic physical insult. Common behavioral responses are hypervigilance, fear, anxiety, and a sense of being overwhelmed. Psychological sequelae may include social isolation, agitation, PTSD, depression, and, in extreme cases, dissociative identity disorders. It may be difficult to distinguish trauma response from existing mental health issues in some people.

Biologic Basis of the Trauma Response

Changes in the brain result from any physiologic trauma. These changes set into motion the long-term psychological consequences of a physiologic trauma.

BOX 43.8

Treatment Approaches to Pain

PRINCIPLES OF PAIN TREATMENT

- Establish the correct diagnosis within the context of the individual's pain symptoms.
- Recognize that pain reduction, rather than complete pain control, is a reasonable goal.
- Utilize an interdisciplinary, multimodal approach. Opioids are not first-line or routine therapy for chronic pain alone.
- Control other symptoms besides pain. This includes addressing the symptoms that were present before treatment (e.g., depression and anxiety) and any adverse effects associated with the pain therapy. Monitor for signs and symptoms of opioid use disorder.
- Monitor for new mental health issues, including catastrophizing about pain, fear of pain, suicidal ideation, anxiety, depression, mania, psychosis, delirium.
- Treat physical conditions that may initiate or exacerbate the pain.
- Treat the adverse effects of all the agents used.

Examples of Traditional Analgesia Used in Mechanism-Based Pain Management

- Nonsteroidal antiinflammatory drugs (NSAIDs)
- Acetaminophen
- Acetylsalicylic acid
- Oral local anesthetics
- Topical agents
- Capsaicin
- EMLA (lidocaine and prilocaine mixture)
- Lidocaine gel
- Trigger point injection (TPI)
- Epidural steroid injection (ESI)
- Facet joint injection (FJI)
- Nerve root blocks
- Opioids

Examples of Non-Traditional Analgesia Used in Mechanism-Based Pain Management

- Baclofen
- Neuroleptics
- Pimozide
- Corticosteroids
- Pulsed glucocorticoids
- Calcitonin
- Benzodiazepines
- Clonazepam
- Valium
- Drugs for sympathetically maintained pain
- Nifedipine
- Phenoxybenzamine
- Prazosin
- Propranolol
- Tricyclic and tetracyclic antidepressants
- Amitriptyline
- Clomipramine
- Desipramine
- Doxepin
- Imipramine
- Maprotiline
- Nortriptyline
- Mirtazapine
- Selective and nonselective serotonin reuptake inhibitors (SSRIs)
- Bupropion
- Citalopram
- Escitalopram
- Fluoxetine
- Fluvoxamine
- Nefazodone
- Olanzapine
- Paroxetine
- Sertraline
- Trazodone
- Venlafaxine
- Serotonin–norepinephrine or dopamine reuptake inhibitors
- Desvenlafaxine
- Duloxetine
- Ziprasidone
- Anticonvulsants
- Carbamazepine
- Divalproex
- Neurontin
- Phenytoin

Examples of Non-Medication Treatments: Restorative Therapies, Interventional Procedures, Behavioral Interventions, and Complementary Health Options

- Transcutaneous electrical nerve stimulation (TENS)
- High-frequency spinal cord stimulation (10 kHz)
- Cryotherapy
- Heat therapy
- Massage therapy
- Physical therapy
- Recreational therapy
- Art therapy
- Music therapy
- Occupational therapy
- Cognitive–behavioral therapy
- Acceptance and commitment therapy
- Self-regulatory or psychophysiological therapies: Biofeedback
- Pain support groups
- Individual and group psychotherapy
- Hypnosis
- Tai-Chi
- Acupuncture
- Healing touch therapy
- Energy therapies
- Meditation/mindfulness
- Yoga
- Prayer
- Individual and group spiritual direction
- Ritual

Note: If the patient does not respond to all standard treatments, psychiatric evaluation for underlying issues should be emphasized.

BOX 43.9

Wellness Challenges

CHALLENGES OF HEALTH CARE PROFESSIONALS

- Inadequate knowledge and experience with pain management
- Poor assessment of pain especially in LGBTQ+ populations
- Concern about regulation of controlled substances
- Fear of patient tolerance and substance dependency
- Concern about side effects of analgesics

CHALLENGES OF PATIENTS

- Reluctance to report pain
- Concern about primary treatment of underlying disease
- Fear that pain means the disease is worse
- Concern about being a good patient and not a complainer
- Reluctance to take pain medications
- Fear of tolerance and substance dependency
- Fear of unmanageable side effects

CHALLENGES OF HEALTH CARE SYSTEM

- Cost or inadequate reimbursement
- Restrictive regulation of controlled substances
- Problems with availability of treatment or access to it

The Role of Neurotransmitters and the Hypothalamic–pituitary Adrenal (HPA) Axis

The neurotransmitters responsible for behavioral responses to fear and anxiety are usually held in balance to maintain a level of arousal appropriate for environmental threat. Information from the sensory processing areas in the thalamus and cortex alerts the amygdala (the lateral and central nucleus). Events that are appraised as threatening activate **hypothalamic–pituitary adrenal axis (HPA)**, which releases adrenal steroids initiating the generalized stress response (see Chapter 19). When the perceived threat is sustained, complex neurochemical processes involving norepinephrine, gamma-aminobutyric acid (GABA), dopamine, and serotonin are overwhelmed, leading to a general dysregulation of the HPA axis. As a result of this complex cascade, high levels of catecholamines are released and circulated until the perceived threat is diminished.

Trauma Memory Storage

Adaptation to trauma is related to such factors as the severity of the trauma, developmental status and age when the trauma occurs, available social support, and the individual's ability to mobilize coping strategies. During adaptation to prolonged stress, the patient's cognitive thought processes and coping behaviors cause dopamine and serotonin and other neurotransmitters to be released in the prefrontal cortex of the brain. Noradrenergic systems are presumed to play a major role in physiologic and emotional coping responses, storage of the trauma experience into memory in the hippocampus and amygdala, and possibly the development of PTSD. See Chapters 19 and 29.

Psychological Response to Trauma

An individual's psychological response to trauma depends on the extent of endocrine and autonomic activity that occurs during stress coupled with prior experience, developmental history, physical status, and existing social support. Psychological manifestation of sustained stress and trauma may be manifested as flashbacks, intrusive recurring thoughts, panic or anxiety attacks, paranoia, inappropriate startle reactions, social isolation, and nightmares (see Chapter 29). The patient may become so withdrawn and depressed that they stop participating in activities of daily living. Toward the other extreme, the patient may become agitated and combative, perceiving any treatment as a continued threat.

Recognizing Cues: Relevant Assessment Information

Complete physical assessment after physical traumatic injury is imperative in life-threatening circumstances. Multiple trauma and head injuries are the major causes of death and disability in young adults in society. Highly trained emergency and intensive care providers look for signs and symptoms of physiologic injury and intervene to stabilize primary and secondary trauma in the general medical setting.

Trauma assessment requires evaluation beyond physical injury. After physical stabilization, the patient should be examined for **psychological injury** through observation and interview to determine prevalent signs and symptoms of accompanying psychological disorders.

The nurse evaluates the patient's adjustment and coping skills, their personal way of dealing with the trauma, past traumatic events or accidents, as well as current social circumstances, and environmental and life stressors. The evaluation should include assessment of the patient's perception of experienced stress, feelings related to the stress, dominant mood, cognitive functioning, defense and coping mechanisms, and available support systems. In addition, assessment of the risk for self-harm should be ongoing.

Taking Action: Nursing Interventions

Psychiatric clinicians provide an important aspect of emergency care. Interventions that establish trust, reduce anxiety, promote positive adaptive coping, and cultivate a sense of control help the patient to begin recovery and maintain emotional health. Physical trauma involving children has been connected to serious, long-term psychological complications, making early intervention and support critical (Fuller-Thompson et al., 2021). Crisis intervention methods, stress management, CBTs, psychotherapy, and psychotropic medications, alone or in combination, may be useful in achieving the best possible outcome.

Traumatic death is often sudden and unexpected. When trauma causes the patient's death, the family must be informed of the death and allowed to grieve to prevent the development of a pathologic or prolonged grief response. Surviving family members may have a severe emotional reaction to the death. Unhealthy family dynamics, especially maladaptive coping, may become evident during this period. Ideally, the nurse can use family intervention strategies to enhance or improve relationships while the family's motivation to do all that is possible is high.

MENTAL HEALTH ISSUES RELATED TO CENTRAL NERVOUS SYSTEM DISORDERS

Several medical disorders are associated with changes in the CNS. This section presents an overview of generalized changes that can occur and a discussion of specific disorders.

Overview of Neurologic Events

Changes to the CNS occur after a physical insult to the brain. These changes can affect the total functioning of the CNS.

Neurologic Impairment

Neurologic impairment is most often related to brain cell (neuron) destruction. The primary causes of neuronal damage are traumatic injury, ischemia, infarction (cerebrovascular accident [CVA]), anomalous neuron growth (brain tumor), and metabolic poisoning associated with systemic disease. Brain cell loss may also be the result of degenerative processes, such as those that occur in Alzheimer or Parkinson disease. Psychiatric disorders are often complications of these neurologic diseases and may be difficult to distinguish from the neuropathology itself. Therefore, appropriate intervention depends on skilled assessment to discriminate and detect mental status changes related to organic brain injury as well as disorders of mood and thought.

The Ischemic Cascade

An injury to the brain can destroy brain cells directly or initiate a cascade of cell breakdown from ischemia. This **ischemic cascade** begins with hypoxia and is followed by paralysis of the ion exchange across the cell membrane, edema, calcium influx, free radical production, and lipid peroxidation (oxidative degradation of lipids). Complete ischemia results in brain cell death or infarction, commonly known as stroke. The resulting neurologic impairment is related to the size and location of the affected brain area. The severity of brain injury is related to the degree and duration of ischemia (Majumder, 2024).

Traumatic Brain Injury

Traumatic brain injury (TBI) is an intracranial injury that occurs when an outside mechanical force or acceleration-deceleration event injures the brain. Microstructural changes from the force of the trauma occur in the brain tissue, which can lead to disturbances in sleep, cognitive processes, body coordination, and behavior. Injury-related metabolites in the brain can take days to months to clear, depending on the scope of brain tissue damage. As the metabolites clear, symptoms usually improve over time. TBI is a major cause of disability for wounded US soldiers who served in Iraq and Afghanistan. Almost a half million military personnel suffered some form of TBI between 2000 and 2022 (Department of Defense [DOD], 2023).

An individual is described as having **persistent post-concussive syndrome (PPCS)** if symptoms including fatigue, sleep issues, difficulty concentrating, sensitivity to light and noise, issues with memory, sleep disturbances, and other mood-related symptoms occur for 4 weeks or longer following a TBI. Sleep issues are usually worse for females (Martens et al., 2023). See Box 43.10. TBI, depressive disorders, and PTSD often coexist as distinct, but related, phenomena among military veterans with TBI. Major depression has been reported to occur in up to 50% of those with TBI, and PTSD has been found to occur in 39% of veterans with TBI (Shi et al., 2023). Patients with TBI have a two-fold risk for suicide

BOX 43.10

Clinical Judgment Vignette: Traumatic Brain Injury (TBI) Complications in a Young Athlete

Debralee, a healthy 26-year-old female, plays on the local semi-pro soccer team. She is being seen in primary care today for a follow-up appointment to a concussion without loss of consciousness that she suffered 5 weeks ago. Aside from a headache the next day and the need for 7 sutures along her right eyebrow, she reports no continued headaches, blurred vision, difficulty concentrating, or dizziness. She has returned to work and her usual activities and is now asking to be cleared to play soccer again. The only two changes in her usual baseline are that she has had "terrible sleep" and "I am both really grumpy and really depressed probably because I can't sleep."

Building Clinical Judgment

1. What complication of TBI is Debralee likely experiencing?
2. How are Debralee's symptoms different that those of males?
3. What other key questions should be asked?

(Campbell-Sills et al., 2021). The triad of PPCS, PTSD, and depressive disorders may become evident in the acute recovery phase or during rehabilitation and often negatively affects survival and recovery. Early evaluation assists in the detection of these and other mental health complications after brain injury.

NCLEXNOTE Early identification of PPCS is critical to patient recovery and to preventing health complications during recovery. There is also increased risk for self-harm. Nurses should observe and assess for symptoms noted above, which may differ in kind and severity among females in comparison to males.

Ischemic Stroke

Depressive disorder and anxiety are frequent complications of ischemic stroke. **Post stroke depression** (PSD) occurs in about a third of people who have had a stroke (Guo et al., 2022). These mood changes are not only a result of the changes in the autonomic and endocrine systems but also a result of the breakdown of biogenic amines after ischemia and brain cell death. Other symptoms, such as sleep disturbances, cognitive dysfunction, poor concentration, difficulty making decisions, somatic discomfort, poor appetite, social withdrawal, and fatigue or agitation, often accompany the mood disturbance. Minor and moderate depression may go unrecognized and undiagnosed when patients with stroke describe somatic symptoms and demonstrate lack of motivation in ADLs.

Parkinson Disease

In **Parkinson disease (PD)** and other neurodegenerative diseases, the motor pathways in the brain degenerate due to a loss of dopamine secretion. This dysregulation affects still other neurotransmitters and results in movement dysfunction. Other non-motor symptoms, which are often prodromal and represent PD pathology in the cholinergic, glutamatergic, noradrenergic, and serotonergic systems, include sensory dysfunction, which is mostly olfactory, sleep disturbances, and neuropsychiatric issues (Bang et al., 2021). About 30% of patients with PD experience depression that contributes to impairment in daily functioning. However, only about 60% of these patients are diagnosed and receive treatment (Liu et al., 2022). Treatment of depression in patients with PD is critical to ensure QoL and because depression has been linked to cardiovascular dysautonomia in these patients, which can result in sudden death (Siddiqi & Fox, 2024).

Recognizing Cues: Relevant Assessment Information

A thorough neurologic examination of patients suffering from these and other neurologic disorders is key to determining the location and degree of impairment but is even more critical in establishing the locus of retained function. Cognitive functioning, mood, and functionality are key assessment areas. Many scales exist that accurately assess these areas, are easy to administer, and are generally accepted as reliable tools to detect the degree and limitations of disability.

Cognition can be measured using the mental status examination (see Chapter 39), and function ability for self-care can be measured using the **Barthel index** (Mahoney & Barthel, 1965). Evaluation of mood using the **Beck Depression Inventory** (Beck et al., 1961) or another instrument provides important information for designing intervention strategies for the at-risk neurologic patient. Findings of depressive symptoms indicate the need for a more definitive neuropsychological referral.

NCLEXNOTE Neurologic exams are incomplete unless cognitive functioning, mood, and general functionality are assessed. Nurses should be familiar with Barthel index, Beck Depression Inventory, and other instruments to accomplish a complete assessment,

Taking Action: Nursing Interventions for Central Nervous System Disorders

Isolation, lack of companionship, bereavement, and poverty are associated with depressive symptoms in the general population and compound the relative risk of depression developing after brain damage. Prevention strategies should be used as early and include (1) the assessment and provision of social support resources while the patient is hospitalized and as an important component of discharge planning to rehabilitation services; (2) early identification of potential mental health issues with a referral for complete evaluation; (3) education of patient and family about the mental health complications of CNS disorders so they will know when to seek medical attention and treatment to avert major issues; (4) encouragement to seek treatment for mental health issues, including pharmacologic strategies; and (5) enhancement of competence in performing ADLs, with a focus on the use of retained function rather than on adaptation to disabilities only.

SUMMARY OF KEY POINTS

- Over two thirds of adults with a mental disorder have at least one medical comorbidity and many other people with mental disorders have multimorbidities. These medical illnesses are developed at a much younger age, tend to cluster together, and males tend to have more multimorbidities than the general population. A mortality gap exists between the general population and people with mental disorders.
- Implicit bias may play a role in the disparity in care for people with both mental disorders and medical disorders. Some providers may not screen, assess, and treat people with mental disorders in the way they would the general population.

- People with a mental disorder often must negotiate care that exists in fragmented and complex social milieus in which they may not have equal access to health care, food, housing, transportation, other forms of social support. Some providers may be afraid of or otherwise not understand people with mental disorders. Negative health outcomes are common.
- MetS is a common comorbidity for people with mental disorders and it is most common to females over 60. The risk of developing CVD is higher among people with mental disorders than the general population and is the most common cause of their death. Type 2 diabetes occurs more frequently in people with mental disorders than in the general population. Cancer rates for people with mental disorders are significantly higher than the general population and females with mental disorders are at higher risk for breast cancer.
- A mortality gap exists between the general population and people with mental disorders due to a failure to screen early for these illnesses, among other reasons.
- Secondary mental disorders are common to many diseases, especially chronic disease and most patients in primary care clinics will experience mental health issues related to their health. Depression is one of the most frequent concerns of patients, especially those with chronic pain. Depression is a frequent prodrome of other health issues and it has been described as bidirectional to CVD, chronic pain syndromes, type 2 diabetes, IBS, and other illnesses. There are notable gender considerations, especially for females, who have increased levels of depression following AMI or CVD diagnosis.
- Pain is one of the most common reasons adults seek medical care. One in six children also experiences chronic pain. HIPC limits QoL.
- The BPSS Model for Pain Management and Delivery and the Loesser Model of Pain are two models for care of people experiencing pain, especially chronic pain. The pain vulnerability-pain resilience continuum is one way nurses may conceptualize a patient's pain coping over time. Pain is a complex of risk factors that is unique to each individual. People with chronic pain are at high risk for depression and self-harm.
- Gate-control theory is useful for understanding nociceptive pain. Mechanism-based pain management targets pain-producing mechanisms along the subcellular and molecular pain pathways and utilizes multimodal interventions to address pain. Nurse attentiveness to a patient's pain, pain behaviors, and pain vulnerability and resilience, is crucial to comprehensive pain management.
- Physical trauma often has behavioral responses including hypervigilance, fear, anxiety, social isolation, agitation, and pain. Noradrenergic systems are presumed to play a major role in coping responses, storage of the trauma experience in the hippocampus and amygdala for memory, and PTSD severity. Effective nursing interventions include those actions that establish trust, reduce anxiety, promote positive adaptive coping, and cultivate a sense of control.
- TBI is an intracranial injury that occurs when an outside mechanical force or acceleration–deceleration event injures the brain. Often patients develop PPCS following a TBI. Both TBI and PPCS carry a high risk for self-harm, so early evaluation is important.
- PSD occurs in about one third of people who have had a stroke but is frequently unrecognized by providers. Depression related to Parkinson disease is also commonly missed by health care staff. Multiple instruments exist to measure cognition, mood, and functional ability so that nurses can design intervention actions for at-risk neurologic patients.

DEVELOPING CLINICAL JUDGMENT

1. Discuss the relationship among mortality gaps, social determinants of health, and implicit bias. How do these factors affect the health of patients who are medically compromised? What nursing actions should be taken to ensure proper care of these patients?
2. An LGBTQ+ patient comes to a neighborhood primary care clinic for the first time for care of major depression and medical multimorbidities, including metabolic syndrome. What concerns and fears could the patient have about the visit? How can nursing staff build a trusting alliance with the patient so that they are able to be a partner in their health care?
3. Discuss the pain syndromes seen in the primary care setting.
4. A patient is being seen for chronic pain in your primary care clinic. What screenings and assessments will you do? What actions would you take to help the patient address the challenges of pain management?
5. You are a psychiatric–mental health nurse and have been asked to prepare a program for the medical–surgical nursing staff on psychiatric aspects of medical illnesses. What topics would you include?

MOVIES, TV, OR STREAMING PROGRAMS

Gaga: Five Foot Two: 2017. This is a contemporary documentary film in which the musical artist, Lady Gaga, navigates through preparations for a new album and a half-time performance and the Super Bowl. She does this while struggling with chronic hip pain from fracture and ligament repair surgery. There are several scenes where she is treated with ice, acupressure, and massage right before a performance. A subtheme in the film is her report of prodromal symptoms of fibromyalgia which present as depression, global pain, and exhaustion. She experiences these symptoms as well as ongoing chronic pain from her hip. In an emotional moment, Lady Gaga itemizes all the activities and projects she is expected to finish while battling through pain, irritability, low mood, and extreme fatigue. Six days after this film was released, Lady Gaga publicly disclosed her new diagnosis of fibromyalgia.

Viewing Points:

1. Discuss how chronic pain and chronic illness can affect a busy performance artist's personal life and professional responsibilities. What complicates care? What kind of support seemed to be helpful to Lady Gaga in the documentary?
2. Lady Gaga seems to have everything—success, talent, career, and family. How does her success interfere with mental well-being and pain management?
3. Describe financial challenges for those who are not famous and need specialized care.

REFERENCES

Ahmad, F. B., Cisewski, J. A., Xu, J., & Anderson, R. N. (2023). Provisional mortality data: United States, 2022. *Morbidity and Mortality Weekly Report*, *72*(18), 488–492. https://doi.org/10.15585/mmwr.mm7218a3

Alday-Mondaca, C., & Lay-Lisboa, S. (2021). The impact of internalized stigma on LGBT parenting and the importance of health care structures: A qualitative study. *International Journal of Environmental Research and Public Health*, *18*(10), 5373. https://doi.org/10.3390/ijerph18105373

Alkouri, O., Khader, Y., Hweidi, I. M., Gharaibeh, M. K., Jarrah, M., Hamdan, K. M., Marzouqi, A. A., & Khamaishe, K. (2022). COVID-19 fear and anxiety among patients with chronic heart failure: A cross sectional study. *Journal of Clinical Medicine*, *11*(21), 6586. https://doi.org/10.3390/jcm11216586

American Nurses Association (ANA), & American Society for Pain Management Nursing (ASPMN). (2016). (2nd ed.). *Pain management nursing scope and standards*. American Nurses Association.

American Psychiatric Association (APA). (2025). *Diversity & health equity education: Lesbian, gay, bisexual, transgender and queer/questioning*. Retrieved February 19, 2025, from https://www.psychiatry.org/psychiatrists/diversity/education/lgbtq-patients

Bair, M. J., Outcalt, S. D., Ang, D., Wu, J., & Yu, Z. (2020). Pain and psychological outcomes among Iraq and Afghanistan veterans with chronic pain and PTSD: ESCAPE trial longitudinal results. *Pain Medicine*, *21*(7), 1369–1376. https://doi.org/10.1093/pm/pnaa007

Balit, J., Erlangsen, A., Docherty, A., Turecki, G., & Orri, M. (2024). Association of chronic pain with suicide attempt and death by suicide: A two-sample Mendelian randomization. *Molecular Psychiatry*, *29*(7), 2043–2049. https://doi.org/10.1038/s41380-024-02465-0

Bang, Y., Lim, J., & Choi, H. J. (2021). Recent advances in the pathology of prodromal non-motor symptoms olfactory deficit and depression in Parkinson's disease: Clues to early diagnosis and effective treatment. *Archives of Pharmacal Research*, *44*, 588-604. https://doi.org/10.1007/s12272-021-01337-3

Beck, A. T., Ward, C. H., Mendelson, M., Mock, J., & Erbaugh, J. (1961). An inventory for measuring depression. *Archives of General Psychiatry*, *4*(6), 561–571. https://doi.org/10.1001/archpsyc.1961.01710120031004

Bergmans, R. S., & Smith, J. (2022). Associations of mental health and chronic physical illness during childhood with major depression in later life. *Aging & Mental Health*, *26*(9), 1813–1820. https://doi.org/10.1080/13607863.2021.1958143

Berk, M., Köhler-Forsberg, O., Turner, M., Penninx, B. W. J. H., Wrobel, A., Firth, J., Loughman, A., Reavley, N. J., McGrath, J. J., Momen, N. C., Plana-Ripoll, O., O'Neil, A., Siskind, D., Williams, L. J., Carvalho, A. F., Schmaal, L., Walker, A. J., Dean, O., Walder, K., … Marx, W. (2023). Comorbidity between major depressive disorder and physical diseases: A comprehensive review of epidemiology, mechanisms and management. *World Psychiatry*, *22*(3), 366–387. https://doi.org/10.1002/wps.21110

Bhatt, K., Palomares, A. C., Jutila, L., Rohde, I., Forget, P., & Societal Impact of Pain Platform (SIP). (2024). The pain and mental health comorbidity. *Epidemiology and Psychiatric Sciences*, *33*, e46. https://doi.org/10.1017/S204579602400057X

Bifulco, L., Anderson, D. R., Blankson, M. L., Channamsetty, V., Blaz, J. W., Nguyen-Louie, T. T., & Scholle, S. H. (2021). Evaluation of a chronic pain screening program implemented in primary care. *JAMA Network Open*, *4*(7), e2118495. https://doi.org/10.1001/jamanetworkopen.2021.18495

Bonifácio de Assis, E., Dias de Carvalho, C., Martins, C., & Andrade, S. (2021). Beta-endorphin as a biomarker in the treatment of chronic pain with non-invasive brain stimulation: A systematic scoping review. *Journal of Pain Research*, *14*, 2191–2200. https://doi.org/10.2147/JPR.S301447

Busili, A., Kumar, K., Kudrna, L., & Busaily, I. (2024). The risk factors for mental health disorders in patients with type 2 diabetes: An umbrella review of systematic reviews with and without meta-analysis. *Heliyon*, *10*(7), e28782. https://doi.org/10.1016/j.heliyon.2024.e28782

Campbell-Sills, L., Jain, S., Sun, X., Fisher, L. B., Agtarap, S. D., Dikmen, S., Nelson, L. D., Temkin, N., McCrea, M., Yuh, E., Giacino, J. T., Manley, G. T., & Stein, M. B. (2021). Risk factors for suicidal ideation following mild traumatic brain injury: A TRACK-TBI study. *The Journal of Head Trauma Rehabilitation*, *36*(1), E30–E39. https://doi.org/10.1097/HTR.0000000000000602

Centers for Disease Control and Prevention (CDC). (2022, July 21). *About chronic diseases*. https://www.cdc.gov/chronicdisease/about/index.htm

Chalker, S. A., Sicotte, R., Bornheimer, L. A., Parrish, E. M., Wastler, H., Ehret, B., DeVylder, J., & Depp, C. A. (2024). A call to action: informing research and practice in suicide prevention among individuals with psychosis. *Frontiers in Psychiatry*, *15*, 1378600. https://doi.org/10.3389/fpsyt.2024.1378600

Chambers, C. T., Dol, J., Tutelman, P. R., Langley, C. L., Parker, J. A., Cormier, B. T., Macfarlane, G. J., Jones, G. T., Chapman, D., Proudfoot, N., Grant, A., & Marianayagam, J. (2024). The prevalence of chronic pain in children and adolescents: A systematic review update and meta-analysis. *Pain*, *165*(10), 2215–2234. https://doi.org/10.1097/j.pain.0000000000003267

Chen, C., & Nakagawa, S. (2023). Recent advances in the study of the neurobiological mechanisms behind the effects of physical activity on mood, resilience and emotional disorders. *Advances in Clinical and Experimental Medicine*, *32*(9), 937–942. https://doi.org/10.17219/acem/171565

Chen, Y., Wang, E., Sites, B. D., & Cohen, S. P. (2024). Integrating mechanistic-based and classification-based concepts into perioperative pain management: An educational guide for acute pain physicians. *Regional Anesthesia and Pain Medicine*, *49*(8), 581–601. https://doi.org/10.1136/rapm-2022-104203

da Nobrega, R. Q., Ji, R. R., & Cheng, J. (2023). Mechanisms-based pain therapies. In R. R. Ji, J. Cheng, & J. Ji (Eds.), *Neuroimmune interactions in pain: Mechanisms and therapeutics* (pp. 321–334). Springer Nature. https://doi.org/10.1007/978-3-031-29231-6_14

Davies, S. J., Iwajomo, T., de Oliveira, C., Versloot, J., Reid, R. J., & Kurdyak, P. (2021). The impact of psychiatric and medical comorbidity on the risk of mortality: A population-based analysis. *Psychological Medicine*, *51*(2), 320–328. https://doi.org/10.1017/S003329171900326X

De Aquino, J. P., Sloan, M. E., Nunes, J. C., Costa, G. P. A., Katz, J. L., de Oliveira, D., Ra, J., Tang, V. M., & Petrakis, I. L. (2024). Alcohol use disorder and chronic pain: An overlooked epidemic. *The American Journal of Psychiatry*, *181*(5), 391–402. https://doi.org/10.1176/appi.ajp.20230886

Decker, V. B., Nelson, Z. E., Corveleyn, A., Gopalan, P. K., & Irwin, K. (2022). Caring for patients with serious mental illness: Guide for the oncology clinician. *Oncology*, *36*(7), 450–459. https://doi.org/10.46883/2022.25920966

Denk, F., McMahon, S. B., & Tracey, I. (2014). Pain vulnerability: A neurobiological perspective. *Nature Neuroscience*, *17*(2), 192–200. https://doi.org/10.1038/nn.3628

Department of Defense (DoD). (2023, June 12). *Numbers for traumatic brain injury worldwide*. https://www.health.mil/Military-Health-Topics/Centers-of-Excellence/Traumatic-Brain-Injury-Center-of-Excellence/DOD-TBI-Worldwide-Numbers

Echeverria-Villalobos, M., Tortorici, V., Brito, B. E., Ryskamp, D., Uribe, A., & Weaver, T. (2023). The role of neuroinflammation in the transition of acute to chronic pain and the opioid-induced hyperalgesia and tolerance. *Frontiers in Pharmacology*, *14*, 1297931. https://doi.org/10.3389/fphar.2023.1297931

Fuller-Thomson, E., Sawyer, J. L., & Agbeyaka, S. (2021). The toxic triad: Childhood exposure to parental domestic violence, parental addictions, and parental mental illness as factors associated with childhood physical abuse. *Journal of Interpersonal Violence*, *36*, 17–18. https://doi.org/10.1177/0886260519853407

Gasperi, M., Afari, N., Goldberg, J., Suri, P., & Panizzon, M. S. (2021). Pain and trauma: The role of criterion a trauma and stressful life events in the pain and PTSD relationship. *The Journal of Pain*, *22*(11), 1506–1517. https://doi.org/10.1016/j.jpain.2021.04.015

Golden, K., Borsi, L., Sterling, A., & Giacino, J. T. (2024). Recovery after moderate to severe TBI and factors influencing functional outcome: What you need to know. *The Journal of Trauma and Acute Care Surgery*, *97*(3), 343–355. https://doi.org/10.1097/TA.0000000000004305

Guo, J., Wang, J., Sun, W., & Liu, X. (2022). The advances of post-stroke depression: 2021 update. *Journal of Neurology*, *269*, 1236–1249. https://doi.org/10.1007/s00415-021-10597-4

Halling, M., Timmer-Murillo, S., Hunt, J. C., Geier, T., Beyer, K. M., Malecki, K. M., & deRoon-Cassini, T. A. (2022). Exposure to socioenvironmental stress as a predictor of physical and mental health. *Journal of Health Psychology*, *27*(9), 2091–2103. https://doi.org/10.1177/13591053211024712

Halstead, S., Cao, C., Høgnason Mohr, G., Ebdrup, B. H., Pillinger, T., McCutcheon, R. A., Firth, J., Siskind, D., & Warren, N. (2024). Prevalence of multimorbidity in people with and without severe mental illness: A systematic review and meta-analysis. *The Lancet Psychiatry*, *11*(6), 431–442. https://doi.org/10.1016/S2215-0366(24)00091-9

Hancox, L. E., Lee, P. S., Armaghanian, N., Hirani, V., & Wakefield, G. (2022). Nutrition risk screening methods for adults living with severe mental illness: A scoping review. *Nutrition & Dietetics*, *79*(3), 349–363. https://doi.org/10.1111/1747-0080.12652

Hards, E., Orchard, F., Khalid, S., D'souza, C., Cohen, F., Gowie, E., & Loades, M. (2023). Self-evaluation and depression in adolescents with a chronic illness: A systematic review. *Clinical Child Psychology and Psychiatry*, *28*(1), 382–397. https://doi.org/10.1177/13591045221115287

Hassan, L., Sawyer, C., Peek, N., Lovell, K., Carvalho, A. F., Solmi, M., Tilston, G., Sperrin, M., & Firth, J. (2023). Heightened COVID-19 mortality in people with severe mental illness persists after vaccination: A cohort study of greater Manchester residents. *Schizophrenia Bulletin*, *49*(2), 275–284. https://doi.org/10.1093/schbul/sbac118

Herrera, P. A., Campos-Romero, S., Szabo, W., Martínez, P., Guajardo, V., & Rojas, G. (2021). Understanding the relationship between depression and chronic diseases such as diabetes and hypertension: A grounded theory study. *International Journal of Environmental Research and Public Health*, *18*(22), 12130. https://doi.org/10.3390/ijerph182212130

International Association for the Study of Pain. (2021). *Incorporating pain competencies and IASP curriculum outlines into professional education*. Retrieved February 19, 2024, from https://www.iasp-pain.org/resources/fact-sheets/incorporating-pain-competencies-and-iasp-curriculum-outlines-into-professional-education/

Izzy, S., Chen, P. M., Tahir, Z., Grashow, R., Radmanesh, F., Cote, D. J., Yahya, T., Dhand, A., Taylor, H., Shih, S. L., & Albastaki, O. (2022). Association of traumatic brain injury with the risk of developing chronic cardiovascular, endocrine, neurological, and psychiatric disorders. *JAMA Network Open*, *5*(4), e229478. https://doi.org/10.1001/jamanetworkopen.2022.9478

Kim, D. J., Mirmina, J., Narine, S., Wachtel, J., Carbajal, J. M., Fox, H., & Cáceda, R. (2022). Altered physical pain processing in different psychiatric conditions. *Neuroscience & Biobehavioral Reviews*, *133*, 104510. https://doi.org/10.1016/j.neubiorev.2021.12.033

Kiritoshi, T., Yakhnitsa, V., Singh, S., Wilson, T. D., Chaudhry, S., Neugebauer, B., Torres-Rodriguez, J. M., Lin, J. L., Carrasquillo, Y., & Neugebauer, V. (2024). Cells and circuits for amygdala neuroplasticity in the transition to chronic pain. *Cell Reports*, *43*(9), 114669. https://doi.org/10.1016/j.celrep.2024.114669

Launders, N., Hayes, J. F., Price, G., & Osborn, D. P. (2022). Clustering of physical health multimorbidity in people with severe mental illness: An accumulated prevalence analysis of United Kingdom primary care data. *PLoS Medicine*, *19*(4), e1003976. https://doi.org/10.1371/journal.pmed.1003976

Liblik, K., Mulvagh, S. L., Hindmarch, C. C. T., Alavi, N., & Johri, A. M. (2022). Depression and anxiety following acute myocardial infarction in women. *Trends in Cardiovascular Medicine*, *32*(6), 341–347. https://doi.org/10.1016/j.tcm.2021.07.005

Lindekilde, N., Scheuer, S. H., Diaz, L. J., Rubin, K. H., Plana-Ripoll, O., Henriksen, J. E., Lasgaard, M., Andersen, G. S., & Pouwer, F. (2022a). Risk of developing type 2 diabetes in individuals with a psychiatric disorder: A nationwide register-based cohort study. *Diabetes Care*, *45*(3), 724–733. https://doi.org/10.2337/dc21-1864

Lindekilde, N., Scheuer, S. H., Rutters, F., Knudsen, L., Lasgaard, M., Rubin, K. H., Henriksen, J. E., Kivimäki, M., Andersen, G. S., & Pouwer, F. (2022b). Prevalence of type 2 diabetes in psychiatric disorders: An umbrella review with meta-analysis of 245 observational studies from 32 systematic reviews. *Diabetologia*, *65*, 440–456. https://doi.org/10.1007/s00125-021-05609-x

Liu, Y., Ding, L., Xianyu, Y., Nie, S., & Yang, J. (2022). Research on depression in Parkinson disease: A bibliometric and visual analysis of studies published during 2012–2021. *Medicine*, *101*(31), e29931. https://doi.org/10.1097/MD.0000000000029931

Loeser, J., & Ford, W. (1983). Chronic pain. In J. E. Carr & H. A. Dengerink (Eds.), *Behavioral science in the practice of medicine* (pp. 331–334). Elsevier Biomedical.

Maccarrone, J., Stripling, A., Iannucci, J., & Nierenberg, B. (2021). Exposure to trauma, PTSD and persistent pain in older adults: A systematic review. *Aggression and Violent Behavior*, *57*, 101488. https://doi.org/10.1016/j.avb.2020.101488

Mahoney, F. I., & Barthel, D. W. (1965). Functional evaluation: The Barthel Index: A simple index of independence useful in scoring improvement in the rehabilitation of the chronically ill. *Maryland State Medical Journal*, *14*, 61–65.

Majumder, D. (2024). Ischemic stroke: Pathophysiology and evolving treatment approaches. *Neuroscience Insights*, *19*, 26331055241292600. https://doi.org/10.1177/26331055241292600

Mangione, S. (2024). The empathy gap. *The American Journal of Medicine*, *137*(3), 290–291. https://doi.org/10.1016/j.amjmed.2023.12.008

Manhapra, A. (2022). Complex persistent opioid dependence: An opioid-induced chronic pain syndrome. *Current Treatment Options in Oncology*, *23*(7), 921–935. https://doi.org/10.1007/s11864-022-00985-x

Maria, S., Irwin, P., Gillan, P., Anderson, J., & Sengstock, B. (2024). Navigating mental health frontiers: A scoping review of accessibility for rural LGBTIQA+ communities. *Journal of Homosexuality*, 1–23. https://doi.org/10.1080/00918369.2024.2373798

Martens, G., Khosravi, M. H., Lejeune, N., Kaux, J. F., & Thibaut, A. (2023). Gender specificities in sleep disturbances following mild traumatic brain injury: A preliminary study. *Brain Sciences*, *13*(2), 323. https://doi.org/10.3390/brainsci13020323

Martinez-Calderon, J., García-Muñoz, C., Heredia-Rizo, A. M., & Cano-García, F. J. (2024). The prevalence of anxiety and depression in cancer around the world: An overview of systematic reviews evaluating 128 meta-analyses. *Journal of Affective Disorders*, *351*, 701–719. https://doi.org/10.1016/j.jad.2024.01.259

Matteliano, D., Marie, B. J. S., Oliver, J., & Coggins, C. (2014). Adherence monitoring with chronic opioid therapy for persistent pain: A biopsychosocial-spiritual approach to mitigate risk. *Pain Management Nursing*, *15*(1), 391–405. https://doi.org/10.1016/j.pmn.2012.08.008

Meilhac, M., Nesbit, S., Bowman, L. A., & Stewart, R. W. (2024). Know Your Guidelines Series: The CDC Clinical Practice Guideline for prescribing opioids for pain. *Southern Medical Journal*, *117*(7), 371–373. https://doi.org/10.14423/SMJ.0000000000001703

Minhas, S., Patel, J. R., Malik, M., Hana, D., Hassan, F., & Khouzam, R. N. (2022). Mind-body connection: Cardiovascular sequelae of psychiatric illness. *Current Problems in Cardiology*, *47*(10), 100959. https://doi.org/10.1016/j.cpcardiol.2021.100959

Möller-Leimkühler, A. M. (2022). Gender differences in cardiovascular disease and comorbid depression. *Dialogues in Clinical Neuroscience*, *9*(1), 71–83. https://doi.org/10.31887/DCNS.2007.9.1/ammoeller

Mössinger, H., & Kostev, K. (2023). Depression is associated with an increased risk of subsequent cancer diagnosis: A retrospective cohort study with 235,404 patients. *Brain Sciences*, *13*(2), 302. https://doi.org/10.3390/brainsci13020302

O'Neill, B., Yusuf, A., Lofters, A., Huang, A., Ekeleme, N., Kiran, T., Greiver, M., Sullivan, F., & Kurdyak, P. (2023). Breast cancer screening among females with and without schizophrenia. *JAMA Network Open*, *6*(11), e2345530. https://doi.org/10.1001/jamanetworkopen.2023.45530

Paice, J. A., Bohlke, K., Barton, D., Craig, D. S., El-Jawahri, A., Hershman, D. L., Kong, L. R., Kurita, G. P., LeBlanc, T. W., Mercadante, S., & Novick, K. L. (2023). Use of opioids for adults with pain from cancer or cancer treatment: ASCO guideline. *Journal of Clinical Oncology*, *41*(4), 914–930. https://doi.org/10.1200/JCO.22.02198

Pak, R., Mahmoud Alilou, M., Bakhshipour Roudsari, A., & Yousefpour, F. (2024). experiential avoidance as a factor in generalized psychological vulnerability: In the relationship between chronic pain and pain anxiety with pain disability. *Pain Management Nursing*, *25*(3), e256–e264. https://doi.org/10.1016/j.pmn.2024.01.007

Peng-Keller, S., Moergeli, H., Hasenfratz, K., Naef, R., Rettke, H., Hefti, R., Ljutow, A., Rittmeyer, I., Sprott, H., & Rufer, M. (2021). Including the spiritual dimension in multimodal pain therapy. Development and validation of the spiritual distress and resources questionnaire (SDRQ). *Journal of Pain and Symptom Management*, *62*(4), 747–756. https://doi.org/10.1016/j.jpainsymman.2021.02.021

Perez, C. S. H., Ciufolini, S., Sood, P. G., Krivoy, A., Young, A. H., Murray, R. M., Ismail, K., Atakan, Z., Greenwood, K., Smith, S., & Gaughran, F.

(2022). Predictive value of cardiometabolic biomarkers and depressive symptoms for symptom severity and quality of life in patients with psychotic disorders. *Journal of Affective Disorders*, *298*, 95–103. https://doi.org/10.1016/j.jad.2021.10.038
Rice, D. R., Hudson, S. K. T., & Noll, N. E. (2021). Gay= STIs? Exploring gay and lesbian sexual health stereotypes and their implications for prejudice and discrimination. *European Journal of Social Psychology*, *52*(2), 326–341. https://doi.org/10.1002/ejsp.2793
Rikard, S. M., Strahan, A. E., Schmit, K. M., & Guy Jr, G. P. (2023). Chronic pain among adults: United States, 2019–2021. *Morbidity and Mortality Weekly Report*, 72(15), 379. https://doi.org/10.15585/mmwr.mm7215a1
Robinson, C. L., Phung, A., Dominguez, M., Remotti, E., Ricciardelli, R., Momah, D. U., Wahab, S., Kim, R. S., Norman, M., Zhang, E., Hasoon, J., Orhurh, V., Viswanath, O., Yazdi, C., Chen, G. H., Simopoulos, T. T., & Gill, J. (2024). Pain scales: What are they and what do they mean. *Current Pain and Headache Reports*, *28*(1), 11–25. https://doi.org/10.1007/s11916-023-01195-2
Rogers, M. L., Joiner, T. E., & Shahar, G. (2021). Suicidality in chronic illness: An overview of cognitive–affective and interpersonal factors. *Journal of Clinical Psychology in Medical Settings*, *28*, 137–148. https://doi.org/10.1007/s10880-020-09749-x
Ross, E., Maguire, A., Mairs, A., Hall, C., Donnelly, M. J., & O'Reilly, D. P. (2021). Disparities in breast cancer screening uptake for women with mental illness in the United Kingdom. *American Journal of Preventive Medicine*, *60*(3), e123–e130. https://doi.org/10.1016/j.amepre.2020.09.010
Saunders, R. K., Carr, D. C., & Burdette, A. M. (2024). Health care stereotype threat and sexual and gender minority well-being. *Journal of Health and Social Behavior*, *65*(1), 20–37. https://doi.org/10.1177/00221465231205549
Schenk, A., Popa, C. O., Cojocaru, C. M., Marian, Ş., Maier, S., & Bălaşa, R. (2024). Neuroticism as a common factor in depression and anxiety associated with multiple sclerosis-A systematic review and meta-analysis. *International Journal of Environmental Research and Public Health*, *21*(10), 1264. https://doi.org/10.3390/ijerph21101264
Schrager, S. (2021). Integrating behavioral health into primary care. *Family Practice Management*, *28*(3), 3–4.
Selvanathan, T., Ufkes, S., Guo, T., Chau, V., Branson, H. M., Ibrahim, G. M., Ly, L. G., Kelly, E. N., Grunau, R. E., & Miller, S. P. (2024). Pain exposure and brain connectivity in preterm infants. *JAMA Network Open*, 7(3), e242551. https://doi.org/10.1001/jamanetworkopen.2024.2551
Seyres, D., Cabassi, A., Lambourne, J. J., Burden, F., Farrow, S., McKinney, H., Batista, J., Kempster, C., Pietzner, M., Slingsby, O., Cao, T. H., Quinn, P. A., Stefanucci, L., Sims, M. C., Rehnstrom, K., Adams, C. L., Frary, A., Ergüener, B., Kreuzhuber, R.,…Frontini, M. (2022). Transcriptional, epigenetic and metabolic signatures in cardiometabolic syndrome defined by extreme phenotypes. *Clinical Epigenetics*, *14*(1), 39. https://doi.org/10.1186/s13148-022-01257-z
Sha, S., & Aleshire, M. (2023). The impact of primary care providers' bias on depression screening for lesbian women. *Health Promotion Practice*, *24*(3), 536–545. https://doi.org/10.1177/15248399211066079
Shi, S., Almklov, E., Afari, N., & Pittman, J. O. (2023). Symptoms of major depressive disorder and post-traumatic stress disorder in veterans with mild traumatic brain injury: A network analysis. *PLoS One*, *18*(5), e0283101. https://doi.org/10.1371/journal.pone.0283101
Siddiqi, S. H., & Fox, M. D. (2024). Targeting symptom-specific networks with transcranial magnetic stimulation. *Biological Psychiatry*, *95*(6), 502–509. https://doi.org/10.1016/j.biopsych.2023.11.011
Singh, M., & Agustines, D. (2024). Humanism and psychosis: Working with patients who have potential medical comorbidities along with mental illness. *Cureus*, *16*(8), e66903. https://doi.org/10.7759/cureus.66903
Singh, S. P., Guindon, J., Mody, P. H., Ashworth, G., Kopel, J., Chilakapati, S., Adogwa, O., Neugebauer, V., & Burton, M. D. (2023). Pain and aging: A unique challenge in neuroinflammation and behavior. *Molecular Pain*, *19*, 17448069231203090. https://doi.org/10.1177/17448069231203090
Solmi, M., Fiedorowicz, J., Poddighe, L., Delogu, M., Miola, A., Høye, A., Heiberg, I. H., Stubbs, B., Smith, L., Larsson, H., Attar, R., Nielsen, R. E., Cortese, S., Shih, J. I., Fusar-Poli, P., Firth, J., Yathan, L. N., Carvalho, A. P., Castle, D. J.,…Correll, C. U. (2021a). Disparities in screening and treatment of cardiovascular diseases in patients with mental disorders across the world: Systematic review and meta-analysis of 47 observational studies. *American Journal of Psychiatry*, *178*(9), 793–803. https://doi.org/10.1176/appi.ajp.2021.21010031
Solmi, M., Tiihonen, J., Lähteenvuo, M., Tanskanen, A., Correll, C. U., & Taipale, H. (2021b). Antipsychotics use is associated with greater adherence to cardiometabolic medications in patients with schizophrenia: Results from a nationwide, within-subject design study. *Schizophrenia Bulletin*, *48*(1), 166–175. https://doi.org/10.1093/schbul/sbab087
Sud, D., Laughton, E., McAskill, R., Bradley, E., & Maidment, I. (2021a). The role of pharmacy in the management of cardiometabolic risk, metabolic syndrome and related diseases in severe mental illness: A mixed-methods systematic literature review. *Systematic Reviews*, *10*, 1–35. https://doi.org/10.1186/s13643-021-01586-9
Sud, D., Maidment, I., Bradley, E., & Tritter, J. (2021b). The experiences of the caring dyad: (Un)articulated realities of living with cardiometabolic risk, metabolic syndrome and related diseases in severe mental illness. *Health Expectations*, *24*(5), 1821–1832. https://doi.org/10.1111/hex.13322
Surace, A., Kang, A., Kahler, C. W., & Operario, D. (2024). "I'm gay with an asterisk": How intersecting identities influence LGBT strengths. *Journal of Homosexuality*, *71*(3), 841–861. https://doi.org/10.1080/00918369.2022.2132579
Türkel, A., Türkel, N. N., Kadıoğlu, A., Doğan, M., & Ertek, İ. E. (2025). The mediating effect of intrusive rumination on the relationship between illness uncertainty and fear of cancer recurrence in breast cancer survivors. *BMC Women's Health*, *25*(1), 41. https://doi.org/10.1186/s12905-025-03580-y
Tzeng, W. C., Chiang, Y. S., Feng, H. P., Chien, W. C., Tai, Y. M., & Chen, M. J. (2020). Gender differences in metabolic syndrome risk factors among patients with serious mental illness. *International Journal of Mental Health Nursing*, *29*(2), 254–265. https://doi.org/10.1111/inm.12670
Umberger, W., & Wilson, M. (2024). Translating the biopsychosocial-spiritual model into nursing practice. *Pain Management Nursing*, *25*(1), 1–3. https://doi.org/10.1016/j.pmn.2023.12.008
Vogel, M., Choi, F., Westenberg, J. N., Cabanis, M., Nikoo, N., Nikoo, M., Hwang, S. W., Somers, J., Schütz, C. G., & Krausz, M. (2021). Chronic pain among individuals experiencing homelessness and its interdependence with opioid and other substance use and mental illness. *International Journal of Environmental Research and Public Health*, *19*(1), 5. https://doi.org/10.3390/ijerph19010005
Volinn, E., & Loeser, J. D. (2022). What are the origins of chronic back pain of "obscure origins"? Turning toward family and workplace social contexts. *The Yale Journal of Biology and Medicine*, *95*(1), 153–163.
Von Korff, M., DeBar, L. L., Krebs, E. E., Kerns, R. D., Deyo, R. A., & Keefe, F. J. (2020). Graded chronic pain scale revised: Mild, bothersome, and high impact chronic pain. *Pain*, *161*(3), 651–661. https://doi.org/10.1097/j.pain.0000000000001758
Wilson, J. M., Steinhilber, K., Yamin, J. B., Edwards, R. R., & Meints, S. M. (2024). A dual-focus approach for evaluating contributors to chronic pain: The roles of psychosocial risk and resilience factors. *Current opinion in Psychology*, *62*, 101981. https://doi.org/10.1016/j.copsyc.2024.101981
Yi Seah, X., Tham, X. C., Aloweni, F., Kua, S. M. Y., Tham, W. Y., & Lim, S. H. (2024). Reducing anxiety and enhancing satisfaction in thyroid patients with DietLens application during radioactive iodine therapy: A quasi-experimental study. *Heliyon*, *10*(15), e35450. https://doi.org/10.1016/j.heliyon.2024.e35450
Yu, L., Chen, Y., Wang, N., Xu, K., Wu, C., Liu, T., & Fu, C. (2022). Association between depression and risk of incident cardiovascular diseases and its sex and age modifications: A prospective cohort study in Southwest China. *Frontiers in Public Health*, *10*, 765183. https://doi.org/10.3389/fpubh.2022.765183
Zhang, Y., Li, X., Chan, V. K., Luo, H., Chan, S. S., Wong, G. H., Wong, I. C., & Lum, T. Y. (2022). Depression duration and risk of incident cardiovascular disease: A population-based six-year cohort study. *Journal of Affective Disorders*, *305*, 188–195. https://doi.org/10.1016/j.jad.2022.03.005
Zhang, X., Lu, Q., Luo, Y., Wang, L., Tian, Y., & Luo, X. (2024). The causal relationship between major depression disorder and thyroid diseases: A Mendelian randomization study and mediation analysis. *Journal of Affective Disorders*, *359*, 287–299. https://doi.org/10.1016/j.jad.2024.05.097

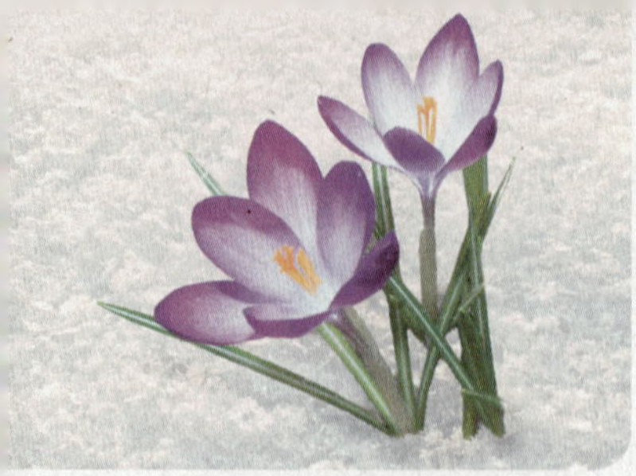

Appendix

Abnormal Involuntary Movement Scale (AIMS)

		None	Minimal	Mild	Moderate	Severe
Facial and Oral Movements	1: **Muscles of facial expression:** e.g., movements of forehead, eyebrows, periorbital area, cheeks; include frowning, blinking, smiling, grimacing	0	1	2	3	4
	2: **Lips and perioral area:** e.g., puckering, pouting, smacking	0	1	2	3	4
	3: **Jaw:** e.g., biting, clenching, chewing, mouth opening, lateral movement	0	1	2	3	4
	4: **Tongue:** Rate only increase in movement both in and out of mouth, *not* the inability to sustain movement	0	1	2	3	4
Extremity Movements	5: **Upper (arms, wrists, hands, fingers):** Include choreic movements (i.e., rapid, objectively purposeless, irregular, spontaneous), athetoid movements (i.e., slow, irregular, complex, serpentine); *do not* include tremor (i.e., repetitive, regular, rhythmic)	0	1	2	3	4
	6: **Lower (legs, knees, ankles, toes):** e.g., lateral knee movement, foot tapping, heel dropping, foot squirming, inversion and eversion of foot	0	1	2	3	4
Trunk Movements	7: **Neck, shoulders, hips:** e.g., rocking, twisting, squirming, pelvic gyrations	0	1	2	3	4
Global Judgment	8: **Severity of abnormal movements overall**	0	1	2	3	4
	9: **Incapacitation caused by abnormal movements**	0	1	2	3	4
	10: **Patient's awareness of abnormal movements:** Rate only patient's report					
		No awareness		0		
		Aware, no distress		1		
		Aware, mild distress		2		
		Aware, moderate distress		3		
		Aware, severe distress		4		
Dental Status	11: Current problems with teeth or dentures		No		0	
			Yes		1	
	12: Does patient usually wear dentures?		No		0	
			Yes		1	

Examination Procedure for AIMS

Either before or after completing the examination procedure, observe the patient unobtrusively, at rest (e.g., in the waiting room). The chair to be used in this examination should be a hard, firm one without arms.

1: Ask the patient whether there is anything in his or her mouth (e.g., gum, candy) and if there is, to remove it.

2: Ask the patient about the current condition of his or her teeth. Ask the patient if he or she wears dentures. Do teeth or dentures bother the patient now?

3: Ask the patient whether he or she notices any movements in the mouth, face, hands, or feet. If yes, ask to describe and to what extent they currently bother patient or interfere with his or her activities.

4: Have the patient sit in the chair with his or her hands on knees, legs slightly apart, and feet flat on floor. (Look at the entire body for movements while in this position.)

5: Ask the patient to sit with his or her hands hanging unsupported. If male, between legs, if female and wearing a dress, hanging over knees. (Observe hands and other body areas.)

6: Ask the patient to open his or her mouth. (Observe the tongue at rest within the mouth.) Do this twice.

7: Ask the patient to protrude his or her tongue. (Observe the tongue at rest within the mouth.) Do this twice.

*8: Ask the patient to tap his or her thumb, with each finger, as rapidly as possible for 10–15 seconds; separately with the right hand and then with the left hand. (Observe facial and leg movements.)

9: Flex and extend the patient's left and right arms (one at a time). (Note any rigidity and rate on NOTES.)

10: Ask the patient to stand up. (Observe in profile. Observe all body areas again, hips included.)

*11: Ask the patient to extend both arms outstretched in front with the palms down. (Observe trunk, legs, and mouth.)

*12: Have the patient walk a few paces, turn, and walk back to the chair. (Observe hand and gait.) Do this twice.

*Activated movements.

Reprinted from Guy, W. (1976). *ECDEU: Assessment manual for psychopharmacology* (DHEW Publ No 76–338). Washington, DC: Department of Health, Education, and Welfare, Psychopharmacology Research Branch.

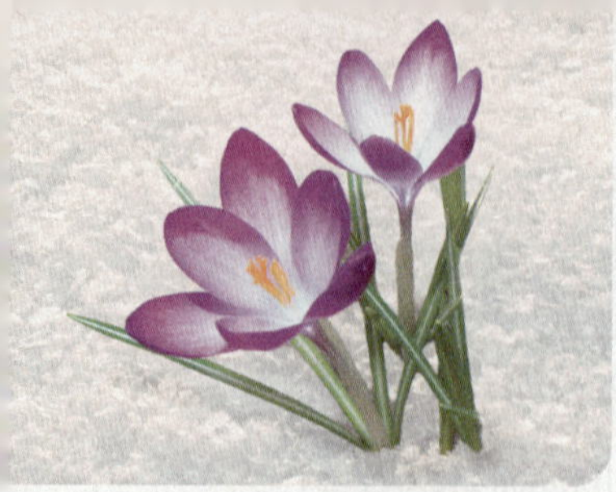

Index

Note: Page numbers followed by f, t, and b indicate figures, tables, and box respectively.

B

E

I

J

K

L

O

P

QUADM0925